The Kelalis–King–Belman

Textbook of

Clinical Pediatric Urology

The Kelalis–King–Belman Textbook of Clinical Pediatric Urology

Fifth edition

Editor-in-Chief

Steven G Docimo MD

Professor and Director Pediatric Urology
University of Pittsburgh School of Medicine
Children's Hospital of Pittsburgh
Pittsburgh, PA
USA

Associate Editors

Douglas A Canning MD

Director, Division of Urology
Children's Hospital of Pittsburgh
Pittsburgh, PA
USA

Antoine E Khoury MD FRCSC FAAP

Professor of Urology
Chief, Division of Urology
Hospital for Sick Children
University of Toronto
Toronto, Ontario
Canada

informa
healthcare

First published in the United Kingdom in 2007 by Informa UK Ltd,
4 Park Square, Milton Park, Abingdon, Oxon OX14 4RN
Informa Healthcare is a trading division of Informa UK Ltd,
Registered Office: 37/41 Mortimer Street, London W1T 3JH.
Registered in England and Wales Number 1072954.

Tel: +44 (0)20 7017 6000
Fax: +44 (0)20 7017 6336
Email: info.medicine@tandf.co.uk
Website: www.informahealthcare.com

A CIP record for this book is available from the British Library.
Library of Congress Cataloging-in-Publication Data

Data available on application

ISBN 10: 1 84184 504 3
ISBN 13: 978 1 84184 504 3

Distributed in North and South America by
Taylor & Francis
6000 Broken Sound Parkway, NW, (Suite 300)
Boca Raton, FL 33487, USA

Within Continental USA
Tel: 800 272 7737; Fax: 800 374 3401
Outside Continental USA
Tel: 561 994 0555; Fax: 561 361 6018
Email: orders@crcpress.com

Distributed in the rest of the world by
Thomson Publishing Services
Cheriton House
North Way
Andover, Hampshire SP10 5BE, UK
Tel: +44 (0)1264 332424
Email: tps.tandfsalesorder@thomson.com

Composition by Phoenix Photosetting, Chatham, Kent, UK
Printed and bound in India by Replika Press Pvt Ltd

Contents

Section IV: The Ureter

Section V: The Bladder and Prostate

Contributors

Mark C Adams MD FAAP
Professor of Urology and Pediatrics
Monroe Carell Jr Children's Hospital at Vanderbilt
Nashville, Tennessee
USA

Kourosh Afshar MD FRCSC
Assistant Professor of Surgery (Urology)
University of British Columbia
Pediatric Urologist, BC Children's Hospital
Vancouver, British Columbia
Canada

Cem Akbal MD
Department of Pediatric Urology
Indiana University School of Medicine
Indianapolis, Indiana
USA

Billy S Arant Jr MD
Professor of Pediatrics
University of Tennessee Health Science Center
Memphis, Tennessee
USA

Anthony Atala MD
Director
Department of Urology and Institute for Regenerative Medicine
Wake Forest University Baptist Medical Center
Winston Salem, North Carolina
USA

Paul F Austin MD FAAP
Assistant Professor of Surgery
St Louis Children's Hospital
Division of Urologic Surgery
Washington University School of Medicine
St Louis, Missouri
USA

Darius J Bägli MDCM FRCSC FAAP FACS
Associate Professor of Surgery
Associate Scientist, Research Institute
Hospital for Sick Children
Division of Urology
Institute of Medical Sciences
University of Toronto, Ontario
Canada

Linda Baker MD
Associate Professor of Urology
Director of Pediatric Urology Unit
University of Texas Southwestern
Children's Medical Center at Dallas
Dallas, Texas
USA

Laurence S Baskin MD
Chief Pediatric Urology
Professor of Urology and Pediatrics
UCSF Children's Hospital
San Francisco, California
USA

Stuart B Bauer MD FAAP
Professor of Surgery
Director Neuro-Urology
Surgery/Urology
Children's Hospital
Boston, Massachusetts
USA

Stephen Boorjian MD
Resident
Department of Urology
Hospital-Weill-Cornell Medical Center
New York, New York
USA

John W Brock III MD
Director of Pediatric Urology
Vanderbilt University
Nashville, Tennessee
USA

Stephen C Brown MD FRCPC
Director of Chronic Pain
Department of Anaesthesia
Hospital for Sick Children
Toronto, Ontario
Canada

Mark P Cain MD FAAP
Associate Professor
James Whitcomb Riley Hospital for Children
Indiana University School of Medicine
Indianapolis, Indiana
USA

Anthony A Caldamone MD
Chief, Pediatric Urology
Hasbro Children's Hospital
Professor of Surgery, Urology
Brown University School of Medicine
Providence, Rhode Island
USA

Douglas A Canning MD
Director
Division of Pediatric Urology
Children's Hospital of Philadelphia
Philadelphia, Pennsylvania
USA

Michael C Carr MD PhD
Assistant Professor of Surgery and Urology
Division of Pediatric Urology
Children's Hospital of Philadelphia
Philadelphia, Pennsylvania
USA

Lisa Cartwright MD
Pediatric Urology Fellow
Hospital for Sick Children
University of Toronto,
Toronto, Ontario
Canada

Patrick C Cartwright MD FAAP
Professor of Surgery and Pediatrics
University of Utah, HSC
Primary Children's Medical Center
Salt Lake City, Utah
USA

Anthony J Casale MD
Professor and Chairman
Department of Urology
University of Louisville School of Medicine
Louisville, Kentucky
USA

Pasquale Casale MD
Division of Pediatric Urology
Children's Hospital of Philadelphia
Philadelphia, Pennsylvania
USA

Marc Cendron MD
Associate Professor of Surgery (Urology)
Harvard School of Medicine
Department of Urology
Children's Hospital Boston
Boston, Massachusetts
USA

Martin Charron MD
Head of the Division of Nuclear Medicine
Head of Research for Diagnostic Imaging
Hospital for Sick Children
Professor of Radiology
University of Toronto
Toronto, Ontario
Canada

Earl Y Cheng MD FAAP FACS
Associate Professor of Urology
Children's Memorial Hospital
Chicago, Illinois
USA

Jeanne S Chow MD
Instructor in Radiology
Harvard Medical School
Childrens Hospital
Radiology
Boston, Massachusetts
USA

Christopher S Cooper MD
Associate Professor of Urology
Director, Pediatric Urology
University of Iowa and
Childrens Hospital of Iowa
Iowa City, Iowa
USA

Lawrence Copelovitch MD
Division of Pediatric Nephrology
Children's Hospital of Philadelphia
Philadelphia, Pennsylvania
USA

Douglas E Coplen MD
Director of Pediatric Urology
St Louis Children's Hospital
St. Louis, Missouri
USA

William DeFoor Jr MD
Assistant Professor
Division of Pediatric Urology
Cincinnati Children's Hospital Medical Center
Cincinnati, Ohio
USA

Romano T DeMarco MD FAAP
Assistant Professor of Urology and Pediatrics
Monroe Carell Jr Children's Hospital at Vanderbilt
Nashville, Tennessee
USA

Nafisa Dharamsi MD FRCSC
Fellow
Division of Pediatric Urology
Cincinnati Children's Hospital Medical Center
Cincinnati, Ohio
USA

David A Diamond MD
Associate Professor of Surgery
Harvard Medical School
Boston, Massachusetts
USA

Steven G Docimo MD
Professor and Director
Pediatric Urology
University of Pittsburgh School of Medicine
Children's Hospital of Pittsburgh
Pittsburgh, Pennsylvania
USA

Jack S Elder MD
Director of Pediatric Urology
Rainbow Babies and Children's Hospital
Cleveland, Ohio
USA

Alaa El-Ghoneimi MD PhD
Professor of Pediatric Surgery
Department of Pediatric Surgery and Urology
Hôpital Robert Debré,
Paris
France

James M Elmore MD
Clinical Assistant Professor of Urology
Emory University School of Medicine
Atlanta, Georgia
USA

Michael J Erhard MD
Chairman, Department of Surgery
Chief, Division of Pediatric Urology
Nemours Children's Clinic
Jacksonville, Florida
USA

Walid Farhat MD
Assistant Professor
Department of Surgery
University of Toronto
Division of Urology
Hospital for Sick Children
Toronto, Ontario
Canada

Fernando A Ferrer MD
Director
Connecticut Children's Medical Center
Hartford, Connecticut
USA

T Ernesto Figueroa MD
Chief, Division of Pediatric Urology
Alfred I duPont Hospital for Children
Wilmington, Delaware
USA

Julie Franc-Guimond MD
Pediatric Urology
CHU Sainte-Justine
Montréal, Québec
Canada

Israel Franco MD FACS FAAP
Associate Professor of Urology,
New York Medical College,
Valhalla, New York
USA

Leo Fung MD (deceased)
Associate Professor of Urologic Surgery and Pediatrics
University of Minnesota
Minneapolis, Minnesota
USA

Jens Goebel MD
Associate Professor of Pediatrics
Medical Director of Kidney Transplantation
Division of Nephrology and Hypertension
Cincinnati Children's Hospital Medical Center
Cincinnati, Ohio
USA

Richard W Grady MD
Associate Professor of Urology
Director, Clinical Research
University of Washington School of Medicine
Children's Hospital and Regional Medical Center
Seattle, Washington
USA

Larry Greenbaum MD PhD
Director
Division of Pediatric Nephrology
Emory University and Children's Healthcare of Atlanta
Atlanta, Georgia
USA

Mark Horowitz MD
Assistant Professor of Urology
Weill Medical College of Cornell University
Director, Pediatric Voiding Dysfunction Center
Weill Cornell Children's Hospital
New York, New York
USA

Anne-Marie Houle MD
CHU Sainte-Justine
Montréal, Québec
Canada

Hongying Huang MD
Department of Urology
New York University School of Medicine
New York, New York
USA

R Guy Hudson MD
Assistant Professor
Oregon Health and Science University
Pediatric Urology
Doembecher Children's Hospital
Portland, Oregon
USA

Douglas A Husmann MD
Professor of Urology
Mayo Clinic
Rochester, Minnesota
USA

Douglas H Jamieson MBChB FRCPC
Clinical Assistant Professor of Radiology
British Columbia Children's Hospital
Vancouver, British Columbia
Canada

Roman Jednak MD
Assistant Professor
Division of Urology
McGill University
Montréal, Québec
Canada

Susan John MD
Professor and Chairman
Department of Radiology
Houston Medical School
University of Texas
Houston, Texas
USA

David B Joseph MD FAAP FACS
Chief of Urology
Children's Hospital
Birmingham, Alabama
USA

Martin Kaefer MD
Associate Professor of Urology
Department of Pediatric Urology
Indiana University
Indianapolis, Indiana
USA

Bernard S Kaplan MB BCh
Director of Pediatric Nephrology
Children's Hospital of Philadelphia
Philadelphia, Pennsylvania
USA

George W Kaplan MD
Chief of Surgery
Children's Hospital and Health Center
San Diego, California
USA

William E Kaplan MD
Head of Urology and Director of Neuro-Urology
Children's Memorial Hospital
Chicago, Illinois
USA

Evan J Kass MD
Chief of Pediatric Urology
William Beaumont Hospital
Royal Oak, Michigan
USA

Michael A Keating MD
Medical Director, Spina Bifida Clinic
Department of Surgery
Division of Urology
Nemours Children's Clinic
Orlando, Florida
USA

William A Kennedy II MD
Assistant Professor
Department of Urology
Stanford University School of Medicine
Stanford, California
USA

Antoine E Khoury MD FRCSC FAAP
Professor of Urology
Chief, Division of Urology
Hospital for Sick Children
University of Toronto,
Toronto, Ontario
Canada

Christina Kim MD
Assistant Professor of Surgery
Connecticut Children's Medical Center
Hartford, Connecticut
USA

Andrew J Kirsch MD FAAP FACS
Professor of Urology
Emory University School of Medicine
Children's Healthcare of Atlanta
Atlanta, Georgia
USA

Thomas F Kolon MD
Assistant Professor of Urology
Children's Hospital of Philadelphia
Philadelphia, Pennsylvania
USA

Martin A Koyle MD FAAP FACS
Chairman, Department of Pediatric Urology
Children's Hospital
Denver, Colorado
USA

Bradley P Kropp MD FAAP FACS
Chief of Pediatric Urology
University of Oklahoma Health Sciences Center
Oklahoma City, Oklahoma
USA

Alberto Lais MD
Department of Urology
Children's Hospital
Boston, Massachusetts
USA

Yegappan Lakshmanan MD
Division of Pediatric Urology
Brady Urological Institute
Johns Hopkins Hospital
Baltimore, Maryland
USA

Steven E Lerman MD
Assistant Professor of Urology
UCLA Urology
Los Angeles, California
USA

Dennis B Liu MD
Fellow, Pediatric Urology
Children's Memorial Hospital
Chicago, Illinois
USA

Armando J Lorenzo MD
Senior Fellow, Pediatric Urology
Hospital For Sick Children
University of Toronto, Ontario
Canada

Irene M McAleer MD FAAP FACS
Department of Urology
Connecticut Children's Medical Center
Hartford, Connecticut
USA

Michael F MacDonald MD
Chief Resident
Wayne State University
Detroit, Michigan
USA

Patricia A McGrath PhD
Professor
Department of Anaesthesia
Hospital for Sick Children
Toronto, Ontario
Canada

Patrick H McKenna MD
Professor of Surgery
Division of Urology
Southern Illinois University School of Medicine
Springfield, Illinois
USA

Gordon A McLorie MD FAAP
Chief, Pediatric Urology
Department of Urology
Wake Forest University School of Medicine
Winston-Salem, North Carolina
USA

Andrew E MacNeily MD FRCSC FAAP
Associate Professor of Surgery (Urology)
University of British Columbia
Vancouver, British Columbia
Canada

Max Maizels MD
Director of Perinatal Urology
Feinberg School of Medicine at Northwestern University
Chicago, Illinois
USA

Padraig SJ Malone MCh FRCSI
Consultant Paediatric Urologist
Department of Paediatric Urology
Wessex Department of Paediatric Surgery
Southampton General Hospital
Southampton
UK

Timothy A Masterson, MD
Division of Urology
University of Utah Health Sciences Center
Salt Lake City, Utah
USA

Paul A Merguerian MD FRCSC FAAP
Professor of Surgery (Urology) and Pediatrics
Dartmouth-Hitchcock Medical Center
Dartmouth Medical School
Hanover, New Hampshire
USA

Peter D Metcalfe MD
Pediatric Urology Fellow
James Whitcomb Riley Hospital for Children
Indiana University School of Medicine
Indianapolis, Indiana
USA

Kevin EC Meyers MB BCH
Division of Pediatric Nephrology
Children's Hospital of Philadelphia
Philadelphia, Pennsylvania
USA

Eugene Minevich MD FACS FAAP
Associate Professor of Surgery
Cincinnati Children's Hospital Medical Center
Cincinnati, Ohio
USA

Rosalia Misseri
Assistant Professor of Pediatric Urology
Riley Children's Hospital
Indianapolis, Indiana
USA

Hiep T Nguyen MD FAAP
Assistant Professor in Surgery (Urology)
Harvard Medical School
Department of Urology
Children's Hospital
Urological Diseases Center
Boston, Massachusetts
USA

John M Park MD
Associate Professor of Urology
Director of Pediatric Urology
University of Michigan Medical School
Ann Arbor, Michigan
USA

Craig A Peters MD
Professor of Urology
University of Virginia Health System
Charlottesville, Virginia
USA

Joao Luiz Pippi Salle MD PhD
Associate Professor
Division of Urology
Hospital for Sick Children
University of Toronto, Toronto
Canada

Hans G Pohl MD FAAP
Assistant Professor of Urology and Pediatrics
Department of Pediatric Urology
Children's National Medical Center
George Washington University School of Medicine
Washington, DC
USA

John C Pope IV MD
Associate Professor Urologic Surgery
Vanderbilt Children's Hospital
Nashville, Tennessee
USA

Dix P Poppas MD
Chief Pediatric Urology
Children's Hospital of New York Presbyterian
Weill Medical College of Cornell University
New York, New York
USA

Pramod P Reddy MD
Program Director, Pediatric Urology Fellowship
Division of Pediatric Urology
Cincinnati Children's Hospital Medical Center
Cincinnati, Ohio
USA

Richard C Rink MD FAAP
Chief Pediatric Urology
James Whitcomb Riley Hospital for Children
Indiana University School of Medicine
Indianapolis, Indiana
USA

Michael L Ritchey MD
Professor of Urology
Mayo Clinic College of Medicine
Scottsdale, Arizona
USA

James M Robertson MD FRCPC
Assistant Professor
Department of Anesthesia
University of Toronto
Hospital for Sick Children
Toronto, Ontario
Canada

Jonathan H Ross MD
Head of Section of Pediatric Urology
Glickman Urological Institute
Cleveland Clinic Childrens Hospital
Cleveland, Ohio
USA

H Gil Rushton MD FAAP
Chairman, Department of Pediatric Urology
Children's National Medical Center
Washington, DC
USA

Michael Schwartz MD
Resident
Cornell University Weill Medical College
New York, New York
USA

Ellen Shapiro MD
Director Pediatric Urology
New York University School of Medicine
New York, New York
USA

Curtis A Sheldon MD
Professor of Surgery
Division of Pediatric Urology
Cincinnati Children's Hospital Medical Center
Cincinnati, Ohio
USA

Aseem R Shukla MD
Assistant Professor of Urologic Surgery
Nemours Children's Clinic
Jacksonville, Florida
USA

Steven J Skoog MD FACS FAAP
Professor and Director, Pediatric Urology
Oregon Health and Science University
Doembecher Children's Hospital
Portland, Oregon
USA

Warren T Snodgrass MD
Professor of Urology
University of Southwestern Medical Center at
Dallas,
Dallas, Texas
USA

Brent W Snow MD FAAP
Professor of Surgery and Pediatrics
University of Utah Health Sciences Center
Primary Children's Medical Center
Salt Lake City, Utah
USA

Howard M Snyder III MD
Associate Director, Pediatric Urology
Children's Hospital of Philadelphia
Philadelphia, Pennsylvania
USA

Julia Spencer Barthold MD
Associate Chief
Division of Urology
A.I. duPont Hospital for Children
Wilmington, Delaware,
USA

David FM Thomas MBBChir MA FRCP FRCS FRCPCH
Consultant Paediatric Urologist and Professor of Paediatric Surgery
Department of Paediatric Urology
St James's University Hospital
Leeds
UK

John C Thomas PhD
Adjunct Professor of Pharmacology
Vanderbilt University
Nashville, Tennessee
USA

Erica J Traxel MD
Resident
Division of Urologic Surgery
Washington University School of Medicine
St Louis, Missouri
USA

Julian Wan MD
Clinical Associate Professor of Urology
Pediatric Urology Division
University of Michigan Medical School
Ann Arbor
Michigan, Illinois
USA

Hsi-Yang Wu MD
Assistant Professor of Urology
Children's Hospital of Pittsburgh
Pittsburgh, Pennsylvania
USA

Stephen A Zderic MD
Professor of Surgery in Urology
University of Pennsylvania School of Medicine
Philadelphia, Pennsylvania
USA

J Michael Zerin MD
Chief, Department of Pediatric Imaging
Children's Hospital of Michigan
Detroit, Michigan
USA

Foreword

It is hard to believe that the time has come for a fifth edition of *Clinical Pediatric Urology*. It is even harder to realize that it has been over 30 years since our first edition was conceived and delivered. The history leading up to the first edition might be of some interest. Both Kelalis at the Mayo Clinic and King at Children's Memorial Hospital in Chicago had contracts to write or edit books. However, there was so much going on at that time in this new, young field of pediatric urology, clinically and academically, that there was little time for either to get the job done. It was a fertile, uncultivated field and a very exciting time. New discoveries and advances were being made daily. Kelalis and King ultimately joined forces, enlisting Belman, who was working with King in Chicago, as an author and associate editor, as well as most of the few other pediatric urologists in the field at the time to write chapters. The first edition was well received, with nearly 4000 of the two-volume text sold. The sales exceeded that of the edition of *Campbell's Urology* published about the same time.

The book was meant to continue in the tradition of Meridith Campbell, who had published a two-volume text entitled *Pediatric Urology* in 1937 and the original *Clinical Pediatric Urology* in 1951. The controversies of the day – such as the significance of vesicoureteral reflux, particularly in the absence of infection, the role of the urethra and bladder neck as causative factors of urinary tract infection and reflux, management of the child with neuropathology, and innovative surgical techniques – were all addressed in both Campbell texts as well as in our first edition of 1976. Most of these same questions are addressed in this current edition, although at a much more sophisticated and scientific level. Others have been resolved and the progress that has been made, particularly regarding the surgical treatment of hypospadias, bladder exstrophy and endoscopic treatment of reflux as well as other problems, as reported in this edition, is truly amazing.

Each of the editions that followed the first was meant to build on the previous one. Different authors were often chosen in following editions to keep the information 'fresh.' Of course, this became easier as the field grew and more experts became available. Often portions of previous chapters were incorporated to build upon by new authors and to offer historical perspective and depth. We continue to appreciate all the efforts by those who contributed to the first four editions.

This is the first edition in which none of the previous editors participated. This is a good thing, as it offers the opportunity to consider totally new perspectives of our growing field. We hope that the previous editions were of use to the current editors and authors and wish them well with their endeavor. We know from first-hand experience that 'doing a book' is a huge undertaking and often a frustrating experience. We wish them well. Our only regret is that Panos Kelalis is not here to see the fruits of his labors and take pride that his 'baby' has grown into this mature body.

Lowell R King
Professor Emeritus of Urology
Duke University School of Medicine
Professor of Urology
University of New Mexico School of Medicine
Albuquerque, New Mexico

A Barry Belman
Professor and Chairman Emeritus
Department of Urology
Children's National Medical Center
Washington, DC

Preface to the fifth edition

The textbook *Clinical Pediatric Urology*, known affectionately as 'Kelalis, King and Belman', has been the primary resource for pediatric urologists, residents and fellows for 30 years. We are honored to have the opportunity to edit the fifth edition. To commemorate the origins of this book, the title has been changed to *The Kelalis–King–Belman Textbook of Clinical Pediatric Urology*. We are fortunate to have the assistance of Barry Belman and Lowell King, who have supplied a Foreword to this text. Their contributions, along with Steven Kramer, who served as co-editor of the fourth edition, and of course the late Panayotis Kelalis cannot be overestimated. We are indebted to their vision, and the strong foundation they created, and upon which the current text is built.

The specialty of pediatric urology continues to grow and change rapidly. In the United States, pediatric urologists will soon have the opportunity to earn a Certificate of Added Qualification in pediatric urology, in addition to the Urology Boards. More pediatric urology is being done by full-time specialists, and less by general urologists. Areas of great controversy in the past, such as the utility of laparoscopy in pediatric urology, are now better defined, whereas areas for which we thought we had the answers, such as the management of vesicoureteral reflux, seem to be completely up in the air. We are on the verge of an era of translation of basic science discoveries to clinical therapies – most notably in pharmacotherapy and tissue engineering. We hope that this book will enlighten in all of these areas, and supply guidance where it is needed most.

We reorganized the textbook, starting with chapters of general interest, and then proceeding through each of the systems or anatomical areas of interest to urologists. Within each section, we have tried to incorporate a basic science chapter. Understanding that this is a clinical text, these authors have been tasked with enlightening the reader with those basic science efforts that are likely to impact clinical care now or in the future. The embryology and radiology chapters have been distributed throughout the book, according to system. Finally, minimally invasive surgery is no longer sequestered in a chapter of its own, but is incorporated in each section of the book. We are indebted to our returning authors, who graciously accepted and enhanced our new format, and to our many new authors who have infused the text with their energetic contributions.

As always, this is intended as a reference work, but not necessarily the last word. We have tried to present controversy where it exists, but in the end all recommendations are made based on the experience and best belief of the authors. The authors have been chosen in every case for their expertise, experience and rationality. Although we, as editors, may not have agreed with everything our authors have stated, we consider each of them a master in their area, and have tried to minimize our influence on their message.

We are especially indebted to our publisher, Alan Burgess of Informa Healthcare, without whose trust and guidance this work would not have begun; and his development editor Kelly Cornish, and to our production editor Cathy Hambly without whose hard work it would not have been finished.

Steven G Docimo
Douglas A Canning
Antoine E Khoury

Abbreviations

α_1-ANRB — α_1-adrenergic receptor-blocker
α-SMA — α-smooth muscle actin
AAP — American Academy of Pediatrics
ABL — allowable blood loss
ABU — asymptomatic bacteriuria
ACE — angiotensin-converting enzyme
ACEIs — angiotensin-converting enzyme inhibitors
ACKD — acquired cystic kidney disease
ACTH — adrenocorticotropic hormone
ADH — antidiuretic hormone
ADPKD — autosomal dominant polycystic kidney disease
AFP — alpha-fetoprotein
AGN — acute glomerulonephritis
AGT — alanine-glyoxylate aminotransferase
AIDS — acquired immunodeficiency syndrome
AIS — androgen insensitivity syndrome
ALPP — abdominal leak point pressure
ALT — alanine aminotransferase
AMD — dactinimycin
ANA — antinuclear antibodies
ANCA — antineutrophil cytoplasmic autoantibodies
ANGII — angiotensin II
AP — anteroposterior
APA — aldosterone-producing adenoma
APD — anteroposterior diameter
AR — androgen receptor
ARB — arterial blood gases
ARBs — angiotensin receptor blockers
ARF — acute renal failure
ARMS — alveolar rhabdomyosarcoma
ARMs — anorectal malformations
ARPKD — autosomal recessive polycystic kidney disease
ASO — antistreptolysin O (titer)
AST — aspartate aminotransferase
AT1, AT2 — angiotensin type 1 and 2 receptors
ATN — acute tubular necrosis
ATP — adenosine triphosphate
AUA — American Urological Association
AVM — arteriovenous malformation
BAH — bilateral adrenal hyperplasia
BAMA — bladder acellular matrix allografts
BAMG — bladder acellular matrix grafts
BAPS — British Association of Paediatric Surgeons
BC — bladder capacity
bFGF — basic fibroblast growth factor
BLE — bladder epithelium
BMP — bone morphogenetic protein
BNR — bladder neck reconstruction
BPH — benign prostatic hyperplasia
BRMS — botryoid rhabdomyosarcoma
bSMCs — bladder smooth muscle cells
BT — bleeding time
BUN — blood urea nitrogen
BWS — Beckwith–Wiedemann syndrome
BWT — bilateral Wilms' tumor
BXO — balanitis xerotica obliterans
C&S — culture and sensitivity
CA — cyproterone acetate
CAH — congenital adrenal hyperplasia
CAIS — complete androgen insensitivity (syndrome)
CAKUT — congenital abnormalities of the kidney and urinary tract
CAM — complementary/alternative therapies
CaMK — calcium–calmodulin dependent protein kinase
cAMP — cyclic adenosine monophosphate
CAN — chronic allograft nephropathy
CAPD — continuous ambulatory peritoneal dialysis
caspases — cysteinyl aspartate-specific proteinases
CBC — complete blood count
CCSK — clear cell carcinoma of the kidney
CDT — contralateral descended testes
CEC — central echogenic complex
CFU — colon-forming unit
cGMP — cyclic guanosine monophosphate
CGRP — calcitonin gene-related peptide
CI — calcineurin inhibitor
CIC — clean intermittent catheterization
CMC — corticomedullary crossover
CMN — congenital mesoblastic nephroma
CMs — cloacal malformations
CMV — cytomegalovirus
COX — cyclooxygenase
CPRE — complete primary repair for exstrophy
CPT — Current Procedural Terminology

CRF	chronic renal failure
CRH	corticotropin-releasing hormone
CRI	chronic renal insufficiency
CRP	C-reactive protein
CRRT	continuous renal replacement therapy
CSF	cerebrospinal fluid
CT	computed tomography
CURs	continent urinary reservoirs
CV	cardiovascular
CVA	costovertebral angle
CVP	central venous pressure
CWS	Cooperative Soft Tissue Sarcoma Study Group
DBP	dibutyl phthalate
DES	diethylstilbestrol
DES	dysfunctional elimination syndrome
DG	diacylglycerol
DGDH	D-glycerate dehydrogenase
DHEA	dehydroepiandrosterone
DHEAS	dehydroepiandrosterone sulfate
DHMEQ	dehydroxymethylepoxyquinomicin
DHT	dihydrotestosterone
DI	detrusor instability
DI	diabetes insipidus
DM	diabetes mellitus
DMSA	dimercaptosuccinic acid
DOC	deoxycorticosterone
DOX	doxorubicin
DRF	differential renal function
DRG	dorsal root ganglion
DRS	diuretic renal scintigraphy
DSD	detrusor–sphincter dyssynergia
DTPA	diethylenetriamine pentaacetic acid
DVSS	Dysfunctional Voiding Scoring System
DVSS	dysfunctional voiding system score questionnaire
Dx/HA	dextranomer/hyaluronic acid copolymer
EABV	effective arterial blood volume
EB	elementary body
EBV	Epstein–Barr virus
EBV	estimated blood volume
ECF	extracellular fluid
ECG	electrocardiogram
ECM	extracellular matrix
ECMO	extracorporeal membrane oxygenation
EDs	ejaculatory ducts
EFS	event-free survival
EGF	epidermal growth factor
EHL	electrohydraulic lithotripsy
ELISA	enzyme-linked immunosorbent assay
EM	ectomesenchymoma
EMG	electromyography (electromyogram)
EMT	epithelial–mesenchymal transition
EPO	erythropoietin
ER	estrogen receptor
ER	estrogen receptor
ERα	estrogen receptor α
ERβ	estrogen receptor β
ERK	extracellular signal-regulated kinase
ERKOα	estrogen receptor α knockout mouse
ERKOβ	estrogen receptor β knockout mouse
ERMS	embryonal rhabdomyosarcoma
ESR	erythrocyte sedimentation rate
ESRD	end-stage renal disease
ESWL	extracorporeal shock wave lithotripsy
EU	excretory urography
FDA	Food and Drug Administration
FDG	fluorodeoxyglucose
FENa	fractional excretion of sodium
FFP	fresh frozen plasma
FGF-2	fibroblast growth factor-2
FH	favorable histology
FISH	fluorescent in-situ hybridization
FJHN	familial juvenile hyperuricemic nephropathy
FKHR	fork head in rhabdomyosarcoma
Flk-1	fetal liver kinase-1
FNA	fine-needle aspiration
Fr	French
FSH	follicle-stimulating hormone
G6PD	glucose-6-phosphate dehydrogenase
GABA	γ-aminobutyric acid
GBM	glomerular basement membrane
GCKD	glomerulocystic kidney disease
GCSF	granulocyte colony-stimulating factor
GDNF	glial-cell-line-derived neurotrophic factor
GFN	genitofemoral nerve
GFR	glomerular filtration rate
GI	gastrointestinal
GnRH	gonadotropin-releasing hormone
GRA	glucocorticoid-remediable aldosteroniclm
GU	genitourinary
HBEGF	heparin-binding EGF-like growth factor
Hbf	minimal allowable hemoglobin
Hbi	initial hemoglobin
hCG	human chorionic gonadotropin
HDS	hematuria–dysuria syndrome
HIF	hypoxia inducible factor
HIV	human immunodeficiency virus

HLA	human leukocyte antigen
HNF-1β	hepatocyte nuclear factor –1β
HPA	hypothalamic–pituitary–adrenal (axis)
HPF	hepatocyte growth factor
HPF	high-power field
HPRT	hyperfractionated radiation therapy
HPRT	hypoxanthine–guanine phosphoribosyl transferase
HSK	horseshoe kidney
HUS	hemolytic uremic syndrome
ICAM-1	intercellular adhesion molecule 1
ICF	intracellular fluid
ICR	International Classification of Rhabdomyosarcoma
ICSI	intracytoplasmic sperm injection
ICU	intensive care unit
IE	ifosfamide + etoposide
IGF-1	insulin-like growth factor-1
IGF-1R	insulin-like growth factor-1 receptor
IGFBP-6	insulin-like growth factor binding protein-6
IL	interleukin (IL-2)
ILNR	intralobular nephrogenic rest
IMC	intermittent catheterization
iNOS	inducible nitric oxide synthase
INR	international normalized ratio
IOUS	in-office ultrasonography
IP_3	inositol 1,4,5-triphosphate
IRS IV	Intergroup Rhabdomyosarcoma Study IV
IRSG	Intergroup Rhabdomyosarcoma Group
IV	intravenous
IVC	inferior vena cava
IVP	intravenous pyelography (pyelogram)
IVU	intravenous urography
IZ	inner submucosal zone
JCAHO	Joint Commission on Accreditation of Health Care Organizations
JNK	c-Jun N-terminal kinase
KUB	kidney, ureter, and bladder (abdominal X-ray)
LBAA	laparoscopic bladder autoaugmentation
LDL	lactate dehydrogenase
LH	luteinizing hormone
LHRH	luteinizing hormone- releasing hormone
LIF	leukemia inhibitory factor
LOH	loss of heterozygosity
LPP	leak point pressure
LUTS	lower urinary tract symptoms
MACE	Malone antegrade continence enema
MAG3	mercaptoacetyltriglycine
MAPK	mitogen-activated protein kinase
MCDK	multicystic dysplastic kidney
MCKD	medullary cystic kidney disease
MCP-1	monocyte chemoattractant protein-1
MCU	mictating cystourethrogram
MDCT	multidetector computed tomography
MDK	multicystic dysplastic kidney
MDs	müllerian ducts
MEN 1	multiple endocrine neoplasia type I
MET	mesenchymal–epithelial transition
MIBG	metaiodobenzylguanidine
MIP	maximum intensity projection
MIS	müllerian inhibiting substance
MMC	myelomeningocele
MMK	Marshall–Marchetti–Krantz (procedure)
MMP	matrix metalloproteinase
MNE	monosymptomatic nocturnal enuresis
MNU	Mitrofanoff neourethra
MODY	maturity-onset diabetes of the young
MRA	magnetic resonance angiography
MRI	magnetic resonance imaging
MRU	magnetic resonance urography
MSK	medullary sponge kidney
MSRE	modern staged repair for exstrophy
MVA	motor vehicle accident
MVP	mitral valve prolapse
NAG	*N*-acetyl-β-D-glucosamidase
NE	nocturnal enuresis
NF-κB	nuclear factor-κB
NGF	nerve growth factor
NICU	neonatal intensive care unit
NO	nitric oxide
NPH	nephronophthisis
NSAIDs	non-steroidal anti-inflammatory drugs
NWTSG	National Wilms' Tumor Study Group
OS	overall survival
OTFC	oral transmucosal fentanyl citrate
PAH	para-aminohippurate
PAI-1	plasminogen activator-1
PAIS	partial androgen insensitivity
PBND	primary bladder neck dysfunction
PCA	patient-controlled analgesia
PCAP	pituitary adenylate cyclase-activating peptide
PDE	phosphodiesterase
PDGF-BB	platelet-derived growth factor-BB
PEC	percutaneous endoscopic colostomy
PEG	percutaneous endoscopic gastrostomy
PET	positron emission tomography

PFS	progression-free survival
PI3K	phosphatidylinositol 3-kinase
PIN	prostatic intraepithelial neoplasia
PLAP	placental alkaline phosphatase
PLNR	perilobular nephrogenic rest
PMC	pontine micturation center
PMTs	pseudosarcomatous myofibroblastic tumors
PNE	primary nocturnal enuresis
PNMC	Pediatric Nuclear Medicine Council
POG	Pediatric Oncology Group
POMC	pro-opiomelanocortin
PRA	plasma renin activity
PRBCs	packed red blood cells
PRE	prostatic epithelium
PSAP	posterior sagittal anoplasty
PSARP	posterior sagittal anorectoplasty
PSARUVP	posterior sagittal anorectal urethrovaginoplasty
PSPV	pressure-specific bladder volume
PT	prothrombin time
PTFE	polytetrafluoroethylene
PTH	parathyroid hormone
PTLD	post-transplant lymphoproliferative disorder
PTT	partial prothrombin time
PUJ	pelviureteral junction
PUV	posterior urethral valves
PV	processus vaginalis
PVR	postvoid residual urine
PZ	peripheral zone
QOLI	quality of life improvement
RAS	renin–angiotensin system
RB	reticulate body
RBCs	red blood cells
RBCs/HPF	red blood cells per high-power field
RBF	renal blood flow
RCC	renal cell carcinoma
RI	resistive index
RMS	rhabdomyosarcoma
RNC	radionuclide cystography
ROC	receiver operating characteristic
ROS	reactive oxygen species
RPGN	rapidly progressive glomerulonephritis
RR	relative risk
RTA	renal tubular acidosis
RTK	rhabdoid tumor of the kidney
RT-PCR	reverse transcription polymerase chain reaction
RTT	renal transit time
RUP	retrograde ureteropyelography
RVR	renal vascular resistance
RVT	renal venous thrombosis
SBE	subacute bacterial endocarditis
SERP	sonographically evident renal pyelectasis
SFU	Society for Fecal Urology
SG	specific gravity
SIADH	syndrome of inappropriate antidiuretic hormone
SIOP	International Society of Pediatric Oncology
SIS	small intestinal submucosa
SKM	skeletal muscle
SM	smooth muscle
SMN	second malignant neoplasm
SNARE	soluble N-methylmaleimide-sensitive factor attachment protein (SNAP) receptor
SNP	single nucleotide polymorphisms
SPA	suprapubic aspiration
SPECT	single-photon emission computed tomography
SPN	sacral parasympathetic nucleus
SQM	squamous metaplasia
SRC	steroid receptor coactivator
SRY	sex-determining region of the Y chromosome
SS	supersaturation
SSRIs	selective serotonin uptake inhibitors
StAR	steroid acute reaction protein
STING	subtrigonal injection
STS	Soft Tissue Sarcoma
SVM	seminal vesicle mesenchyme
TBW	total body water
TCC	transitional cell carcinoma
TF	transdermal fentanyl
Tfm	testicular feminization (syndrome)
TGF-β_1	transforming growth factor-β_1
TIMPs	tissue inhibitors of MMPs (matrix metalloproteinases)
TINU	tubulointerstitial nephritis and uveitis
TLR	toll-like receptor (TLR-2, TLR-4)
TLV	total lung volume
TNF-α	tumor necrosis factor-α
TS	tuberous sclerosis
TTP	thrombotic thrombocytic purpura
UA	urinalysis
UAH	unilateral adrenal hyperplasia
UDT	undescended testes
UGE	urogenital epithelium
UGM	urogenital mesenchyme
UGS	urogenital sinus

UKCCSG	United Kingdom Children's Cancer Study Group
UMC	undifferentiated mesenchyme
UPJ	ureteropelvic junction
UPJO	ureteropelvic junction obstruction
URA	unilateral renal agenesis
URGMs	urogenital sinus malformations
US	ultrasound, ultrasonography
UTI	urinary tract infection
UVJ	ureterovesical junction
UVJO	ureterovesical junction obstruction
VA	vincristine + dactinomycin
VAC	vincristine + dactinomycin + cyclophosphamide
VCH	Vanderbilt Children's Hospital
VCR	vincristine
VCUG	voiding cystourethrography (cystourethrogram)
VEGF	vascular endothelial growth factor
VHL	von Hippel–Lindau (disease)
VIP	vasoactive intestinal peptide
VLPP	Valsalva leak point pressure
VM	vincristine + melphalan
VP	ventriculoperitoneal (e.g. VP shunt)
VUDS	videourodynamics
VUJ	vesicoureteral junction
VUR	vesicoureteral reflux
vWF	von Willebrand factor
vWFRCo	vWF ristocetin cofactor activity
WAGR	Wilms' tumor, aniridia, genitourinary, retardation
WBCs	white blood cells
WD	wolffian duct
WT	wild-type
XRT	radiation therapy
YDL	Young–Dees–Leadbetter (procedure)

SECTION I

Evaluation of the Pediatric Urologic Patient

History and physical examination of the child

1

T Ernesto Figueroa

> Although the perfect history has never been taken by any physician, his careful, sympathetic and discerning questions frequently yield information from the sick person which enlarges the doctor's horizon of knowledge and experience as well as presenting him with unexpected examples of the dramatic or bizarre.
>
> David Seegal MD
> The Pharos of Alpha Omega Alpha
> 1963, 26: 7

The medical history

The path to caring for a patient and offering a solution to a medical condition commences with a well-taken and thorough medical history, and subsequent physical examination. These are the most basic of elements in medical care, and when properly conducted, allow for the understanding and appreciation of the medical condition, and the ability to initiate appropriate care for the patient. The extensive progress in medical technology has given the physician new tools for the diagnosis and treatment of most medical conditions; however, no technological advance can replace the sympathetic and discriminating ear of the physician, or the gentle and perceptive hand during the physical examination. In the diagnostic process, history accounts for 80% of the information, physical examination for 15%, and special investigations for 5%.[1] A thorough history is the clearly most enlightening component of the diagnostic process.[2]

The field of pediatrics presents a very different situation than the other branches of medicine in that the history is usually given by a second person instead of the patient, this being the mother, the father, other relatives, or a foster parent.[3] It is important to identify the person giving the history, and to clarify the relationship to the patient. As we first encounter the child and the parent, it is essential to introduce ourselves and offer our services to the patient and the family. The accompanying adult should be asked in a non-threatening way about his/her relationship to the patient. In an era of significant governmental regulatory oversight and the obligation to protect the patient's confidentiality and privacy, it is necessary to define the precise relationship to the patient early on in the interaction, and to determine who will be the recipient of the medical information related to the pediatric patient.[4] Current federal regulations establish limitations on the medical information that can be shared with individuals other than the patient, and there can be serious penalties for ignoring this federal directive. We should not assume that the accompanying adult has legal custody of the child.

Upon approaching an examination room, it is important to remember that small children will often move about the room, as the family waits for the physician. Prior to entering the room, the physician should first knock gently at the door to alert the parents to pick up the child who could be sitting behind the door, and then open the door cautiously. As we first encounter the child and accompanying adult, it is helpful to ask what the child likes to be called, and address the child in that manner. Also, it is beneficial to find an area of interest that will show patients that we care and are interested in them, such as asking what type of play they enjoy, offer a supportive commentary about their clothes, or inquire about their interests in sports or other activities. The child should feel that they are the primary interest of the interaction, and regardless of the age, the physician should look at the child and talk to him/her in words that the child can understand at various times during the encounter. A soft and courteous tone of voice and a sympathetic look are essential in developing a trusting relationship with the child, assuring the patient and the family that the physician is concerned about his/her condition. Abrupt, pressing and hurried interfaces often have a profoundly negative effect on the initial, and subsequent, patient–physician interactions. The physician should convey a willingness to listen, and demonstrate empathetic understanding for the information being gathered.[2] If a young child is not receptive to the interaction and is disruptive during the history taking, it is helpful to seek distraction techniques such as a toy box, coloring books, formula or snacks, or removal from the examination room, to allow adequate history gathering. A comfortable environment can enhance communication.[3] In essence, it is important to convey to the parent the interest in the child as well as the illness.[5]

The pediatric urologic history should be tailored to the condition of the patient, with some conditions being rather evident, such as the healthy newborn with hypospadias or undescended testis, and thus requiring a more focused and limited approach to the history. Other conditions, such as combined diurnal and nocturnal enuresis in an older patient, are likely to require a more detailed and comprehensive assessment of the medical history. Thus, not every patient seen by a pediatric urologist will require an extensive medical history with a need to cover all of the items traditionally listed in the medical history of a child. However, the role of the pediatric urologist is to determine what key questions are necessary to formulate the most accurate description of the patient's genitourinary condition. Once the pediatric urologist has established the main reason for the visit or interaction with the patient, additional information is necessary to complete the history. The family should be questioned about possible associated genitourinary symptoms including flank pain, abdominal pain, dysuria, hematuria, incontinence, frequency and urgency, difficulty with urination, previous urologic surgery, and scrotal pain and swelling. Other symptoms such as malaise, fever, weight loss, constipation, vomiting, or body posturing should be reviewed as part of the history of the present illness. The past medical history should include information about the prenatal history of the patient and pregnancy of the mother, including any fetal assessment, and illnesses or medication to which the mother was exposed. Any current or previous medications should be listed, as well as allergic reactions to medications. A comprehensive developmental history is not crucial to the pediatric urologic history, though a general awareness about the patient's ability to reach developmental milestones is important. Serious previous medical conditions and operations need to be documented. In assessing the review of systems, particular attention should be given to the overall state and growth of the patient, the presence or absence of reactive airway disease, and a history of congenital cardiac malformations.

Genitourinary surgery is one of the common indications for subacute bacterial endocarditis (SBE) prophylaxis in patients with some types of congenital heart disease, and the child's cardiologist should specify the need for antibiotic use for these patients. Other important elements of the review of systems include recurrent abdominal pain, constipation, diarrhea, or vomiting, and any nervous system abnormalities such as seizure disorders or attention deficit disorder. Recurrent abdominal pain and vomiting may be a presentation of intermittent hydronephrosis in a child. The assessment of the family history is important for many pediatric urologic conditions, including vesicoureteral reflux, urinary tract infections, genital malformations including hypospadias, and voiding disorders and enuresis. Finally, if not already obtained during the initial interaction, an assessment of the social history should be completed, including the marital status of the parents, who cares for the children when the mother is employed, number of siblings, progress at school, recent stressful experiences such as moving or loss of a family member, and the type of interactions with other children.[3,5,6] All of this information may elicit a diagnostic path possibly unrelated to the initial complaint of the patient.

The gathering of medical information occurs in many scenarios in the field of pediatric urology. The interaction with an expectant mother with a prenatally detected urologic malformation is very different from the interaction with an acutely ill boy with scrotal pain. Just as the types of questions and data gathering need to be adjusted according to a given medical scenario, so does the documentation of that encounter. In the 1990s, the 'Documentation Guidelines for Evaluation and Management Services' were developed by Health Care Financing Administration (HCFA) and the American Medical Association, and since then, many variations of these guidelines have evolved. The guidelines, commonly referred to as the E/M service guidelines, were developed with the premise that medical interactions should provide specific documentation of the history, physical examination, and decision-making process, in order to be processed and reimbursed by Medicare. Each interaction, be it with a new or an established patient, is coded according to the number of items (bullets) covered during the interaction. Three broad categories are used (office visits, hospital visits, and consultations), and each of these categories is further subdivided according to a new or established interaction with a patient.[7–9] In the context of this chapter, it is necessary to mention this newer component of the medical history and physical examination, though it is not the intent of this chapter to expand on these complex and controversial coding guidelines.

The physical examination

An important component of the physical examination occurs while obtaining the medical history, and that is the observation of the patient and the relationship with the family. While listening to the family, the physician can assess the level of comfort of the child and his/her overall physical health, and anticipate the approach to the physical examination. Perusing the vital signs, including the weight, blood pressure, temperature and pulse, prior to examining the child may point to the need to focus on specific areas of the examination. An elevated blood pressure is often seen in the agitated child, or when the blood pressure cuff is too small for the child, although it may also be the result of renal disease. Selecting the appropriate blood pressure cuff size for the child is vital to obtaining reliable blood pressure readings.[2]

When the time comes for the examination, the child should be informed in simple terms that are understandable to him/her that an examination is to take place. With younger children, having the parents stand or sit next to them during the examination can help reduce the fear of the experience. Young children, less than 1 year of age, can occasionally be examined while they recline in their mother's lap. Every effort should be taken to minimize separation anxiety in these children, common in children younger than 3 years of age. Preschoolers, ages 4–6 years, fear the possibility of bodily injury and mutilation, possibly castration, so the genital examination usually produces significant anxiety in this age group. In older children, and adolescents, privacy is very important, and respecting that privacy during the examination is vital, by asking the family members to look aside or to step out of the room. Examination of the adolescent should always be handled with sensitivity to avoid unnecessary embarrassment and preserve the dignity of the patient.[10]

Prior to placing the hands on the patient, the examining physician should wash his/her hands, and repeat this routine, though fundamental, exercise at the end of the examination. A cold pair of hands can tense the patient unexpectedly. The physician owes to the patient the courtesy of a warm pair of hands during the examination.[10] Upon placing the patient on the examining table, the pediatric urologist can determine if the child will cooperate with the examination. If the child is cooperative, the examination should include an assessment of the configuration of the chest and abdomen, appearance of the breast tissue in both boys and girls, presence of axillary hair, palpation of all four quadrants of the abdomen for abdominal wall tension, masses, rigidity, guarding or tenderness, and the presence of umbilical hernias. Auscultation of the chest for clear symmetric breath sounds and abdomen for normal bowel sounds can be performed while the child is held by a parent, or after placing the child on the examination table. In small children, the sigmoid colon can often be palpated when it contains a large amount of fecal material.

Detection of an abdominal mass may be the first manifestation of a pathologic or non-pathologic process, such as a distended bladder, a multicystic dysplastic kidney, a hydronephrotic kidney, or Wilms' tumor.[11] Palpation of the abdomen should be initially soft, gentle, and superficial, and progress to a more deliberate, deeper palpation. The inguinal and scrotal areas can be assessed simultaneously, looking for asymmetry, hernias, hydroceles, and undescended testes.

Hydroceles should be closely examined to ensure that the testes can be palpated. Transillumination is frequently performed to demonstrate a fluid-filled hydrocele sac (Figure 1.1). Failure to identify a testis in a patient with a tense hydrocele should prompt further evaluation with a scrotal ultrasound if surgical exploration is not planned. Placing a hand over the inguinal area at the pubic tubercle before touching the scrotum will often prevent a retractile testis from ascending into the inguinal area (Figures 1.2 and 1.3). The position of the testes in the scrotum should be observed prior to touching the patient.

The examination of the scrotal contents should be performed during each visit despite the findings of scrotal testes on an earlier visit, to exclude the possibility of testicular ascent.[12] When a testis is undescended, sliding the examining hand lubricated with soap over the inguinal area will often demonstrate the location of the testis. The consistency and approximate size of the testes should be noted, as well as the stage of sexual development. As the boy reaches adolescence, the first sign of puberty is the growth of the testes, which usually occurs around 11–12 years of age, corresponding to a Tanner stage 2.[13,14] Secondary sexual development follows over the ensuing 1.5–3 years.

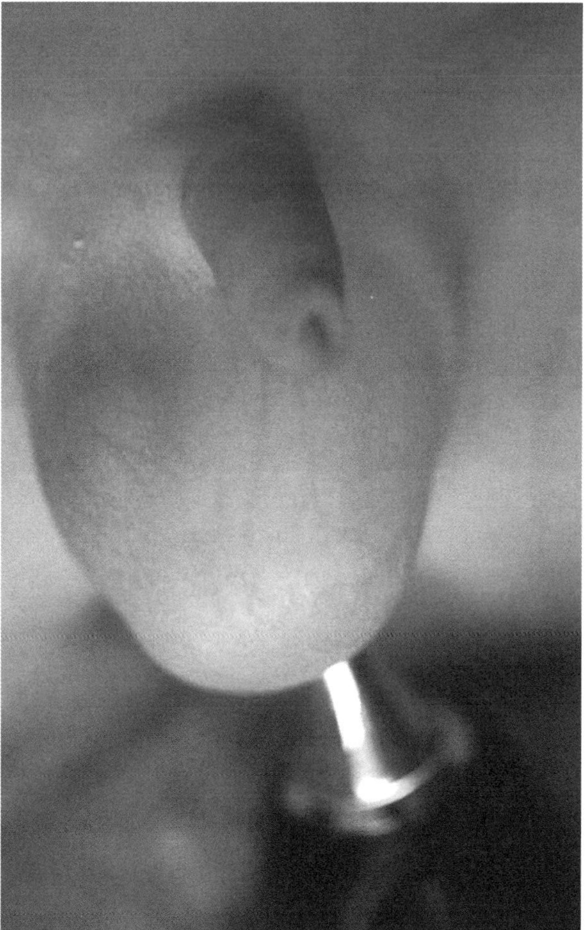

Figure 1.1 Transillumination of a hydrocele.

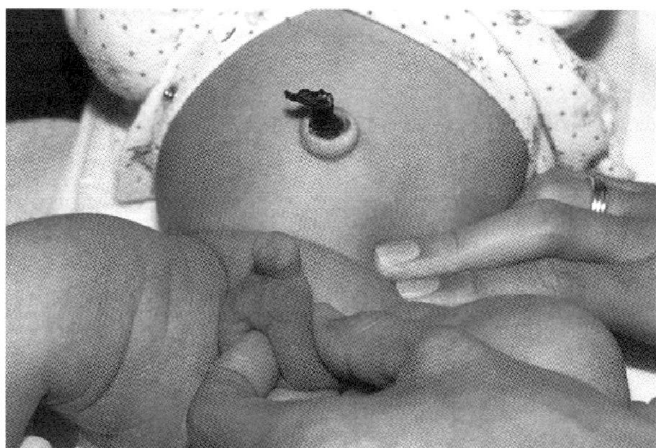

Figure 1.2 Physical examination of the groin and testis.

In girls, the first sign of puberty is usually breast development, followed by the appearance of pubic hair (Tanner stage 2). The onset of menses corresponds to a Tanner stage 4, and the corresponding external appearance for this stage of development is that of curly, coarse pubic hair, though less abundant

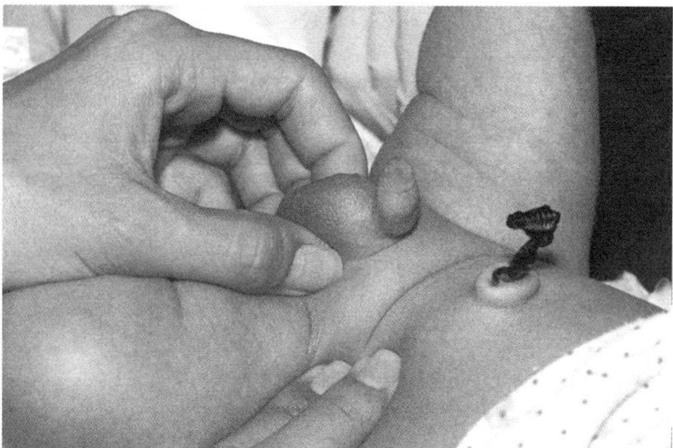

Figure 1.3 Physical examination of the testis.

than in adults, and the breast areola and papilla forming a secondary mound.[15]

In the male patient, the examination of the penis is conducted next. The child to this point should be comfortable with the examination, and the transition to the examination of the penis should be painless and well tolerated by the patient. The presence of a foreskin and appearance of the glans should be noted, as well as the presence of any penile abnormalities including hypospadias, penile torsion, and chordee. Occasionally, the urethral meatus may be in an ectopic location in boys with hypospadias (Figures 1.4 and 1.5). In circumcised boys, the glans should be assessed for the presence of mucosal adhesions (Figure 1.6) or skin bridging (Figure 1.7). A hidden penis should be differentiated from the rare but more serious micropenis (Figure 1.8). When a micropenis is suspected, measurement of the stretched penile length with a ruler is necessary, while pressing the prepubic fat away. If the child remains cooperative, the various abnormalities identified during the examination should be demonstrated to the parents as part of their education into the child's urologic condition. In the normally uncircumcised male, the foreskin should be retractile in 90% by 5 years of age, though some residual glanular preputial adhesions may remain. Gentle, atraumatic retraction of the prepuce should be attempted. The location and size of the meatus should be noted, remembering that a small meatus on examination is not always indicative of urethral meatal stenosis (Figure 1.9). The appearance of the deflected urinary stream during the assessment of the urinary flow in the toilet-trained patient will determine if urethral meatal stenosis is present.[16] After examining the penis, the child is asked to turn to his side, or helped to do the same, to assess the anus, which can be inspected while pulling the but-

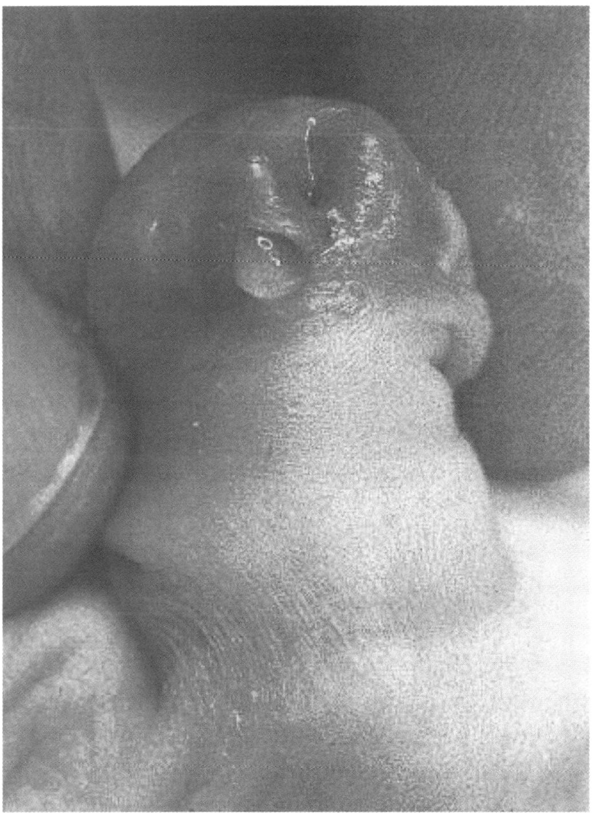

Figure 1.4 Ectopic meatus in hypospadias.

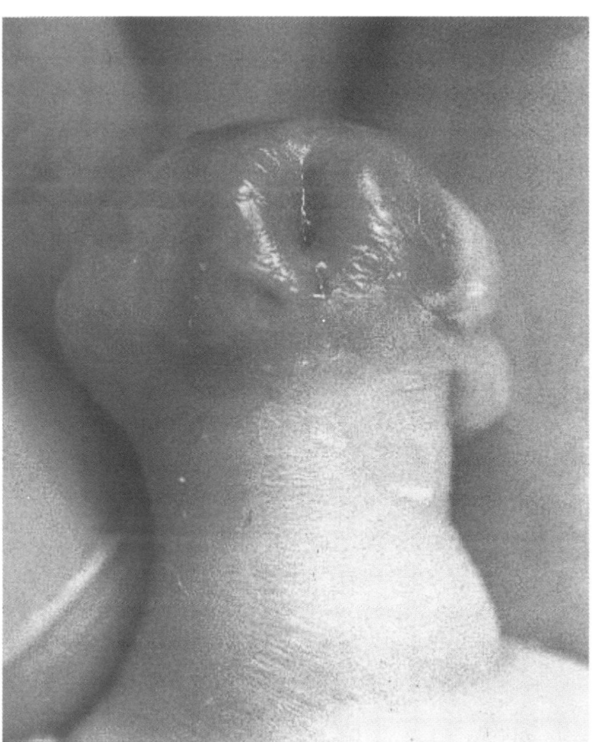

Figure 1.5 Ectopic meatus in hypospadias.

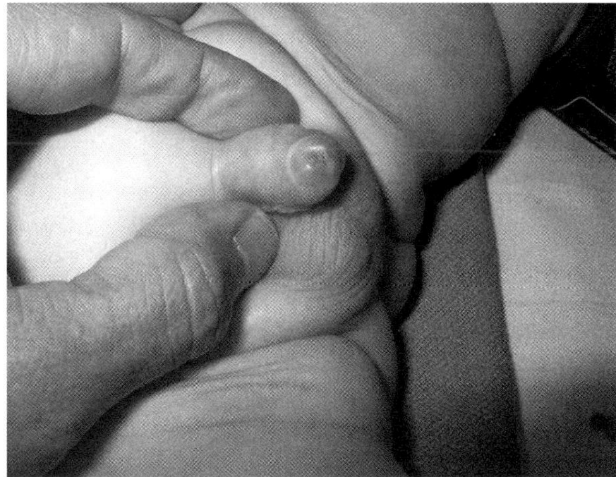

Figure 1.6 Foreskin adhesions.

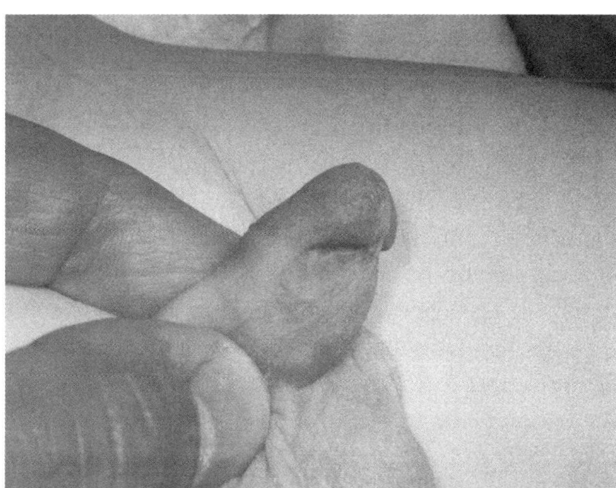

Figure 1.7 Penile skin bridge.

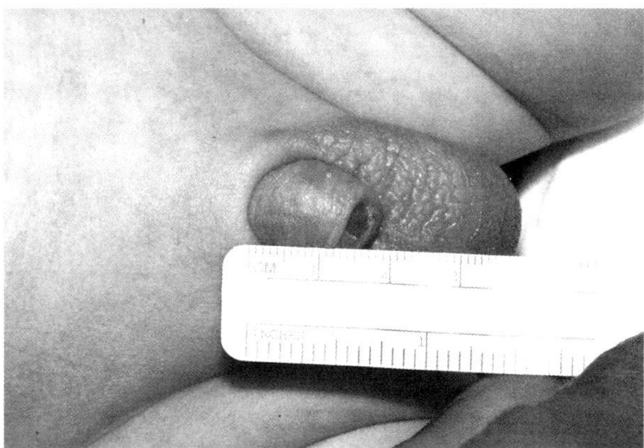

Figure 1.8 Micropenis.

tocks apart. Anal winking often occurs during this maneuver. With the exception of cases of congenital anorectal malformations such as imperforate or anteriorly placed anus, abnormalities of the anus are rare in this age group.[2] Inspection should reveal a sym-

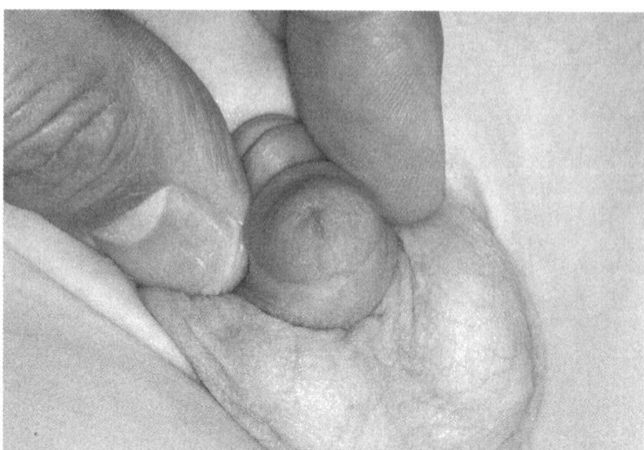

Figure 1.9 Meatal stenosis.

metrical pigmented perianal skin. A digital rectal examination should be reserved for special circumstances, such as a patient with urinary retention, assessment of the neurologically impaired child, or in cases of severe constipation, and it is best performed using a well-lubricated, gloved, small fifth finger. Examination of the lower backs and extremities completes the examination in the male child.

Examination of the genitalia in the preadolescent female is best conducted in the supine position with the legs in a frog-like position, with the soles of the feet touching each other. If this is not satisfactory, then a knee–chest position, asking the patient to perform Valsalva's maneuver, will allow satisfactory inspection of the introitus.[17] This should be the last part of the examination, and the girl may remain clothed until then. Practicing this part of the examination with a nurse prior to the physician conducting the genital examination may reduce the girl's apprehension related to the examination. To this effect, we often will tell the patient that a nurse is coming to help her undress, and to teach her a task. Talking to the girl and explaining what we are doing in a friendly, but professional, manner, is also helpful in comforting the patient. Depending on the age of the patient, the examination can be conducted while the girl remains in her mother's lap. If the child is placed on the examination table, the mother is encouraged to bend over to embrace the child and offer additional comfort. We ask the girl to try to touch the wall against the table with her knee, effectively encouraging her to flex and abduct her hips. After observing the external genital appearance, the labia majora are firmly, but not tightly, grasped between thumb and index finger, and pulled outwards and upwards, allowing full assessment of the open introitus, distal vaginal canal, and urethral meatus[18] (Figure 1.10). Any discharge or pooling of urine in the introitus should be further assessed with appropriate imaging studies. A pelvic examination, if necessary in the prepubertal female, should probably be conducted under general anesthesia, as manipulation and insertion of fingers or devices may have long-lasting psychologic consequences. Upon completion of the examination of the introitus, the girl is placed on her side to assess the appearance of the anus, as well as the cutaneous and bony aspects of the lower back. Attention should be given to the presence of dimples, scoliosis, discolored skin patches, or hairy nevi in this area. The examination of the lower extremities completes the examination, and particular attention should be given to symmetry, strength, and skin temperature.

When the child is uncooperative, the physician may rely on distraction techniques such as allowing him/her to play with a penlight, or toys, or hold an otoscope, to console the child. It is noteworthy that many patients who are uncooperative probably have had a negative experience with a healthcare provider in the past. If the child remains uncooperative, we should try to make the best of the situation, but never force an examination on the combative child. If an acute surgical condition is suspected, and the child is uncooperative, persevering with the examination with the use of assistants to gently restrain the combative child may be necessary. A useful technique to examine the abdomen and genitalia of anxious young boys is to have the mother embrace, and hold, the upper torso of the child against the examination table, while an assistant places the palms of their hands on the patient's thighs, close to the pelvis, to keep the body in place against the examination table. This allows the

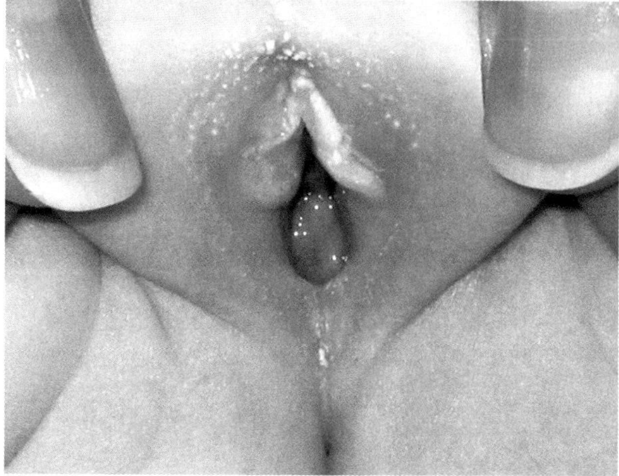

Figure 1.10 Examination of the female introitus in an infant.

examining physician to conduct a quick and effective examination while the child is reassured by the closeness to the mother.

In pre- and postpubertal males, the physical examination should always include examination of the scrotal contents while the patient is standing, specifically to determine if a varicocele is present.[19] Failure to include this step in the physical examination will result in missing this common condition.

Finally, an uncomplicated neurologic examination can be easily performed in most children, and, in the context of the urologic patient, this part of the examination is usually reserved for patients with voiding disorders. Normal-appearing patients with genital disorders will rarely have neurologic conditions that can be uncovered by the urologist, and neurologic examination of the infant and young child by the urologist is usually unnecessary. In the older child and adolescent, the neurologic exam includes assessment of mental status, muscle tone, deep tendon reflexes, cerebellar function, and sensory responses.[2]

Key points

History in pediatrics

- Identify caretaker
- Privacy and confidentiality issues
- Establish relationship with the child and the parent
- Present illness and past medical history:
  - Urologic symptoms
  - Prenatal and neonatal history
- ROS:
  - Growth and development
  - Pulmonary:
    - Reactive airway disease
  - Cardiac
  - Gastrointestinal:
    - Constipation
    - Diarrhea
  - Central nervous system:
    - Seizure disorder, ADD
- Family history
- Social history

Physical examination

- Vital signs
- The cooperative young child
- The uncooperative child
- Genital examination in the boy
- Techniques for examination of the female external genitalia

References

1. Robinson MJ. The clinical history and physical exam. In: Robinson MJ, Robertson DM, eds. Practical Pediatrics, 3rd edn. Philadelphia: Churchill-Livingstone, 1990: 67–74.
2. Drutz JE. The pediatric physical examination. In: Gonzales ET, Bauer SB, eds. Pediatric Urological Practice. Philadelphia: Lippincott, Williams & Wilkins, 1999: 1–33.
3. Boyle WE. The pediatric history. In: Hoekelman RA, ed. Primary Pediatric Care, 3rd edn. St Louis: Mosby, 1997: 45–54.
4. Health Insurance Portability And Accountability Act Of 1996 (HIPAA), Department of Labor, Health and Human Services, Public Law 104–191, 1996.
5. Barness LA. The pediatric history and physical examination. In: Oski FA, ed. Principles and Practice of Pediatrics, 2nd edn. Philadelphia: JB Lippincott, 1994: 29–45.
6. McCarthy PL, The well child. In: Behrman RE, Kliegman RM, Arvin AM, eds. Nelson Textbook of Pediatrics, 15th edn. Philadelphia: WB Saunders, 1996: 26–9.
7. American Urological Association. Coding tips for the urologist office. AUA 2003; 10:1–72.
8. Iglehart JK. The Centers for Medicare and Medicaid Services. N Engl J Med 2001; 345:1920–4.
9. American Medical Association, Evaluation and Service (E/M) Service Guidelines. In: Current Procedural Terminology (CPT) 2005 Professional Edition. Chicago: AMA Press, 2005: 1–7.
10. Seidell HM. Pediatric history and physical examination. In: Ziai M, ed. Pediatrics, 4th edn. Boston: Little Brown Company, 1990: 14–20.
11. Walker RD. Presentation of urogenital disorders in children. In: Kelalis PP, King LR, Belman AB, eds. Clinical Pediatric Urology, 2nd edn. Philadelphia: WB Saunders, 1985: 1–14.
12. Bloom DA, Wan J, Key D. Disorders of the male external genitalia and inguinal canal. In: Kelalis PP, King LR, Belman AB, eds. Clinical Pediatric Urology, 3rd edn. Philadelphia: WB Saunders, 1992: 1015–49.
13. Marshall WA, Tanner JM. Growth and physiological development during adolescence. Annu Rev Med 1968; 19:283–300.
14. Marshall WA, Tanner JM. Variations in the pattern of pubertal growth in boys. Arch Dis Child 1970; 45:13–23.
15. Marshall WA, Tanner JM. Variations in pattern of pubertal changes in girls. Arch Dis Child 1969; 44:291–303.
16. Kaplan GW, Scherz HC. Meatal stenosis. In: Kelalis PP, King LR, Belman AB, eds. Clinical Pediatric Urology, 3rd edn. Philadelphia: WB Saunders, 1992: 858.
17. Sanfilippo JS. Gynecologic problems of childhood. In: Behrman RE, Kliegman RM, Arvin AM, eds. Nelson Textbook of Pediatrics, 15th edn. Philadelphia: WB Saunders, 1996: 1554–5.
18. Redman JF. Techniques of genital examination and bladder catheterization in female children. Urol Clin North Am 1990; 17:1–4.
19. Belman AB. The adolescent varicocele. Pediatrics 2004; 114:1669–70.

Laboratory assessment of the pediatric urologic patient

2

Paul F Austin and Erica J Traxel

In general, laboratory assessment of the pediatric urologic patient is not as extensive as in the adult counterpart. Patients tend to be healthier and there are no recommended routine preoperative laboratory screening tests for pediatric urologic patients. However, there are certain instances when laboratory examination in pediatric urology is invaluable. This chapter will outline the most common laboratory tests used in pediatric urology, demonstrating the clinical scenarios in which each test should be employed.

Commonly ordered laboratory examinations

Urinalysis and urine culture and sensitivity

The most commonly utilized laboratory examinations in pediatric urology are urinalysis and urine culture and sensitivity. These urine tests are routinely ordered to identify a potential infection prior to invasive urologic procedures. A urinalysis with urine culture is also standard of care in investigating a fever of unknown origin in the infant. The prevalence of urinary tract infection (UTI) in pediatric patients with fever of unknown origin is 5%.[1] If a UTI is identified, the child requires more extensive testing to rule out further urologic pathology or anatomic abnormalities.

When children present with symptoms suggestive of a UTI such as dysuria, genital pain, diurnal enuresis, urgency, frequency, and urinary retention, it is important to understand that they may not have a UTI. These children may have a history of incomplete bladder emptying or a history of bladder and bowel holding termed 'dysfunctional elimination'.[2] A urinalysis and urine culture can help to discriminate between UTIs and the irritative voiding symptoms inherent to this group. Dysfunctional eliminators may have irritative voiding symptoms secondary to their behavior but they also have a higher risk of UTIs. When a UTI is identified, antibiotic treatment is essential acutely, but behavioral modification is the mainstay of treatment for children with dysfunctional elimination.[3]

It should be noted that there are certain instances in which the urinalysis should be interpreted with caution. In patients who perform clean intermittent catheterization, or who have undergone bladder reconstruction using intestinal segments, testing should be selective as a positive urinalysis in these patients may only represent colonization with bacteria. Antimicrobials are used when symptoms of infection, such as dysuria, pelvic pressure, and fever, accompany a positive urinalysis and urine culture. Overtreatment, however, may lead to the development of highly resistant organisms.[4–6]

Additionally, the method of collection can impact interpretation of laboratory urine tests. For example, a pediatric 'clean catch' urine specimen may yield growth not necessarily representative of an infectious process. In our practice we are careful to interpret urine collected from bagged specimens. Although a bagged specimen is a useful, non-invasive method for collecting urine from a non-toilet-trained child, this method can easily have a false-positive growth secondary to contamination from bacteria colonized on the genital and perineal skin. It is helpful when the bagged specimen results are negative or if there is a single isolate on the culture. It is also important to obtain both urinalysis and culture, as the absence of leukocytes in a specimen with positive culture should make one suspect contamination. If it is unclear whether there is truly infection, the urine specimen may need recollection via catheterization.

Serum blood urea nitrogen and creatinine

Serum blood urea nitrogen (BUN) and creatinine are frequently obtained as measures of renal function. When interpreting these tests, the clinician must be aware of the impact of the size of the child as well as their age. For example, the neonate's renal function is a reflection of maternal renal function at birth and the creatinine levels remains similar to the maternal serum creatinine for the first several days of life prior to decreasing to normal infant levels. Premature neonates in particular will have higher levels of creatinine and take longer to approach infant levels than full-term neonates.

Serum BUN and creatinine yield insight into renal function both as a baseline marker and as a method of longitudinal monitoring. With the diagnosis of prenatal and perinatal abnormalities, such as oligohydramnios (potentially secondary to bilateral renal agenesis, bilateral ureteropelvic junction (UPJ) obstruction, bilateral multicystic dysplastic kidney, or posterior urethral valves) or hydronephrosis (due to UPJ obstruction, congenital megaureter, posterior urethral valves, or vesicoureteral reflux), serum BUN and creatinine are important parameters that help determine the overall prognosis as well as monitoring therapeutic effectiveness. For example, a serum creatinine of more than 1.0 mg/dl at 1 year of age in a child with a history of posterior urethral valves is associated with poor renal outcome.[7] Other high-risk patients that require close monitoring of serum creatinine include patients with renal scarring that can be associated with vesicoureteral reflux[8] or with a neurogenic bladder.[9]

Complete blood cell count and coagulation studies

A complete blood cell count (CBC) and coagulation studies are not routinely obtained prior to most pediatric urology interventions. This is primarily due to the outpatient nature of pediatric urology procedures that are associated with low morbidity. There are certain patient populations, however, for whom these hematologic laboratory tests are indicated. These include children with chronic anemia or coagulopathic tendencies.

Important preoperative hematologic tests consist of a CBC, prothrombin time (PT), international normalized ratio (INR), and partial thromboplastin time (PTT). A lower than average hematocrit can be seen in children with sickle cell anemia and does not necessarily require intervention. If a value represents a significant change from baseline or if the patient is symptomatic or unstable, then hematologic intervention is recommended. Patients with von Willebrand disease will have poorly functioning platelets and possibly deficient levels of von Willebrand factor (vWF) VIII, with ensuing bleeding tendencies. In these patients it is advisable to obtain serum levels of vWF VIII, vWF ristocetin cofactor activity (vWFRCo), bleeding time (BT), as well as a CBC, PT, and PTT. Oncology patients are often pancytopenic, and procedures should be coordinated with chemotherapy cycles and administration of colony-stimulating factors, in order to maximize preoperative blood counts and minimize the chances for bleeding and infection. Clinical practice guidelines for platelet transfusion in patients with cancer have recently been published by the American Society of Clinical Oncology[10] and are essentially the same for children as for adults. With respect to surgery, or invasive procedures, these guidelines state the following: in the absence of associated coagulation abnormalities, a platelet count of 40 000/μl to 50 000/μl is sufficient to perform major invasive procedures with safety. For minor procedures, a lower threshold of 10 000/μl to 20 000/μl can be used.[10,11] If platelet transfusions are administered before a procedure, it is critical that a post-transfusion platelet count be obtained to prove that the desired platelet count has been reached. Platelets should also be available on short notice in case intraoperative or postoperative bleeding occurs. In summary, hematologic values must be considered within the context of careful clinical evaluation of each individual patient as well as the morbidity of the surgical procedure. Good communication with the pediatric hematologist will help steer the appropriate laboratory testing.

Common pediatric urologic clinical scenarios and requisite laboratory tests

Hematuria

When a child presents with hematuria, a number of tests are potentially indicated. Depending upon the degree of hematuria, and whether it is gross or microscopic, there are many potential etiologies (Table 2.1). Most hematuria originates in the renal parenchyma and is termed nephrologic hematuria. It is incumbent on the urologist to distinguish nephrologic bleeding from that caused by surgically significant sources.

Table 2.1 Differential diagnosis of hematuria in the pediatric population

Glomerular origin
IgA nephropathy
Alport's syndrome
Benign familial hematuria
Membranoproliferative glomerulonephritis
Acute post-streptococcal glomerulonephritis
Rapidly progressive glomerulonephritis
Systemic lupus erythematosus
Membranous nephropathy
Henoch–Schönlein purpura
Goodpasture's disease
Focal segmental glomerulosclerosis
Interstitial and tubular origin
Acute interstitial nephritis
Acute pyelonephritis
Tuberculosis
Hematologic disorders:
sickle cell disease, von Willebrand disease, renal vein thrombosis, thrombocytopenia
Urinary tract origin
Infection:
bacterial or viral, such as adenovirus
Nephrolithiasis
Structural/congenital anomalies:
UPJ obstruction, hydronephrosis, vascular malformation, polycystic kidney disease
Trauma
Tumors:
renal cell carcinoma, Wilms' tumor, transitional cell carcinoma
Exercise
Medications:
aminoglycosides, amitriptyline, anticonvulsants, aspirin, Coumadin (warfarin), cyclophosphamide, diuretics, penicillin, Thorazine (chlorpromazine)

Hematuria is often first noticed on a urine dipstick performed at the primary care office. A microscopic analysis of the urine should follow a positive dipstick. A freshly voided urine specimen should be used for this purpose. An approximately 10–15 ml aliquot of urine is spun in a centrifuge at 1500 rpm for about 5 minutes. The supernatant is decanted, and the sediment is resuspended in the remaining liquid and placed on a glass slide with a cover slip. Careful examination of the urine sample is then conducted under high-power magnification. All noncellular and cellular elements seen should be noted and recorded. The presence of more than 5 red blood cells (RBCs) per high-powered field (hpf) is generally considered abnormal. The detection of RBC casts is indicative of a glomerulotubular source of hematuria (Figure 2.1). The absence of RBCs and RBC casts despite a positive dipstick test is suggestive of hemoglobinuria or myoglobinuria. This is important because a positive urine dipstick for RBCs may have a completely negative microscopic examination and thus represent a false-positive result. Microscopic abnormal-shaped RBCs or dysmorphic RBCs are more commonly associated with nephrologic causes of hematuria, and normal-shaped or eumorphic RBCs are more commonly associated with urologic causes. The presence of proteinuria with dysmorphic RBCs further strengthens a nephrologic origin of the hematuria.[12]

Another practical test for microscopic hematuria in the outpatient clinic is a 'spot' urine calcium/creatinine ratio.[13–15] A ratio of >0.21 on two or three separate urine samples indicates hypercalciuria, although ratios can be significantly higher in infants. Hypercalciuria does not necessarily result in nephrolithiasis but is a reported risk factor.[16] A recent report indicates that the vast majority of children with hypercalciuria have a benign course and resolve with observation; therefore the rationale for doing this test routinely is less clear.[17,18]

It is important to note that the laboratory tests ordered for the evaluation of hematuria must be based on the clinical history and the physical examination. The physician should avoid automatically requesting tests that may be unnecessary. A panel of serum tests are selectively performed if renal and bladder sonog-

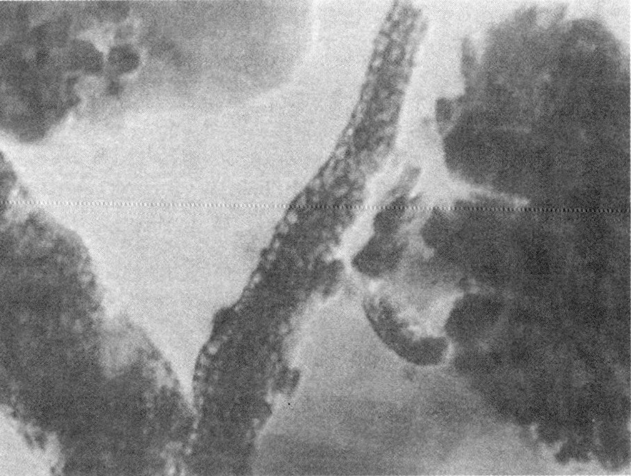

Figure 2.1 Red blood cell (RBC) casts. The RBCs are easily identified as biconcave disks embedded in the cast matrix. RBC casts are pathologic and their presence is usually indicative of severe injury to the glomerulus. Occasionally, RBC casts may be seen in an individual who has been playing contact sports. The urine will usually return to normal within 24–48 hours.

raphy are negative and the urine microscopy suggests a nephrologic origin. These tests, which include CBC, basic metabolic panel, serum complement levels, antistreptolysin O (ASO) titer, and antinuclear antibodies (Table 2.2), may subsequently indicate hematologic- or immunologic-mediated diseases affecting the kidney.

Testicular mass

A child presenting with a testicular mass should have testicular tumor markers obtained: these markers, including alpha-fetoprotein (AFP), human chorionic gonadotropin (HCG), lactate dehydrogenase (LDH), and placental alkaline phosphatase (PLAP), can be checked in the outpatient office setting or may be obtained in the operating room during the placement of the intravenous lines. These levels are important for staging as well as monitoring progress during treatment.

A serum AFP level will be elevated in tumors containing some component of yolk sac tumor, which is the most common nonseminomatous germ cell tumor in children. It will not be present in histologically pure choriocarcinoma or seminoma. Of note, serum AFP level at birth is relatively high and will remain so for the first several months of life, due to the yolk sac elements present during gestation (Table 2.3).[19] Additionally, AFP can be produced by the liver, pancreas, stomach, and lung; consequently, it may be elevated in diseases of these organs. In addition to ascertaining levels of tumor markers for testicular tumors, it is helpful to check liver function tests, as an elevation in these could indicate metastatic disease to the liver, which may or may not be visible on imaging.

Nephrolithiasis

The prevalence of nephrolithiasis in children is much smaller than in the adult population[20] and extensive laboratory assessment is recommended upon initial presentation. As opposed to the adult patient, nephrolithiasis in the pediatric population is more likely attributable to a metabolic abnormality. In the office, a urine dipstick can be performed to measure the urine specific gravity and pH. Microscopic examination of the spun urine can be performed to assess for RBCs and urinary crystals.[21,22] Calcium oxalate dihydrate crystals are seen as colorless squares with intersecting lines (resembling an envelope) (Figure 2.2). Calcium oxalate monohydrate crystals vary in size and may have a spindle, oval, or dumbbell shape. Most commonly, they appear as flat, elongated, hexagonal 'fence picket' crystals. Triple phosphate (struvite; magnesium ammonium phosphate) crystals usually appear as colorless, prism-like 'coffin lids' (Figure 2.3). Uric acid crystals may appear as yellow to brown rhombic plates, needles, or rosettes,

Table 2.2 Serum panel for nephrologic hematuria

CBC
Basic metabolic panel
C3 complement level
Antistreptolysin O (ASO) titer
Antinuclear antibodies (ANA)

Table 2.3 Average normal serum alpha-fetoprotein levels of infants

Age	Mean ± SD (ng/ml)
Premature	134,734 ± 41,444
Newborn	48,406 ± 34,718
Newborn to 2 weeks	33,113 ± 32,503
Newborn to 1 month	9,452 ± 12,610
2 weeks to 1 month	2,654 ± 3,080
2 months	323 ± 278
3 months	88 ± 87
4 months	74 ± 56
5 months	46.5 ± 19
6 months	12.5 ± 9.8
7 months	9.7 ± 7.1
8 months	8.5 ± 5.5

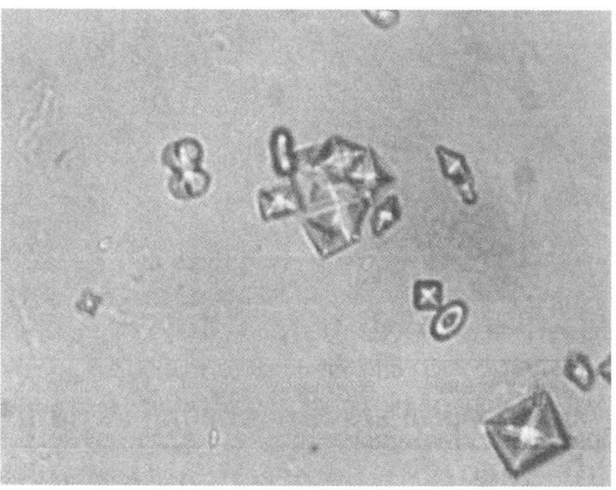

Figure 2.2 Calcium oxalate crystals. Calcium oxalate crystals most frequently have an 'envelope' shape and appear in acid, neutral, or slightly alkaline urine.

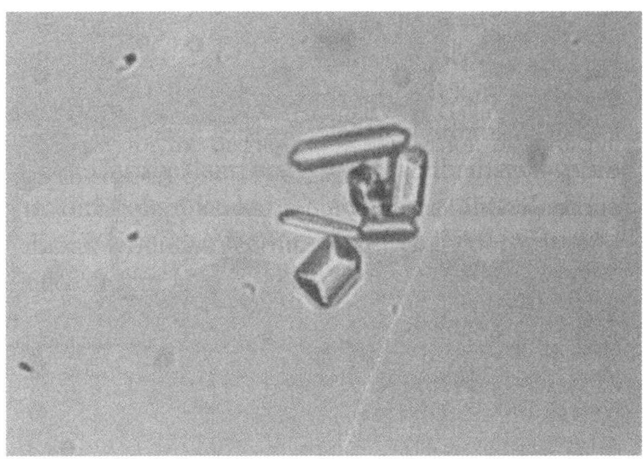

Figure 2.3 Triple phosphate crystals. These crystals are common in urine sediment. Triple phosphate crystals have a 'coffin-lid' shape, are colorless, and appear in alkaline urine. These crystals may be found with struvite or magnesium ammonium phosphate stones.

whereas cystine crystals have a characteristic hexagonal appearance (Figure 2.4).

Standard metabolic evaluation for pediatric nephrolithiasis includes serum tests and a 24-hour urine study (Table 2.4). A serum CBC, electrolytes, bicarbonate, calcium, phosphorus, BUN, creatinine, alkaline phosphatase, magnesium, and uric acid should be obtained. Elevated serum calcium suggests the possibility of hyperparathyroidism and a serum intact parathyroid hormone level should subsequently be checked. A 24-hour urine collection should be obtained on a regular diet, to check calcium, phosphorus, magnesium, oxalate, sodium, uric acid, citrate, cystine, creatinine, and volume.[23] The most common abnormalities seen on the 24-hour urine collection are

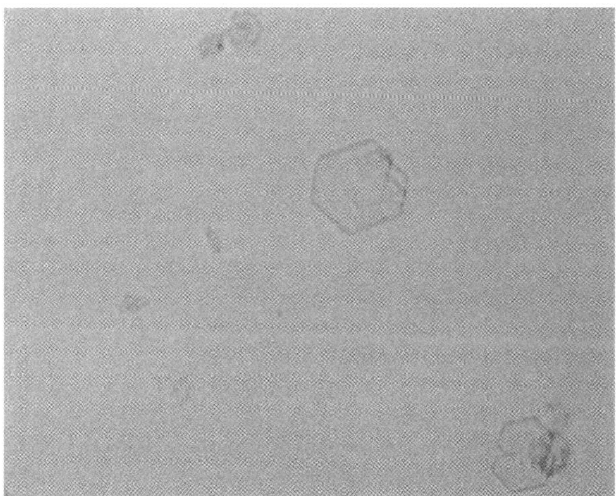

Figure 2.4 Cystine crystals. Cystine crystals are thin, hexagonal-shaped (6-sided) structures and appear in urine of children with cystinuria.

Table 2.4 Metabolic evaluation of pediatric nephrolithiasis

Serum	Urine – 24 hour
CBC	Volume
Basic metabolic panel	Calcium
Calcium	Oxalate
Uric acid	Citrate
Magnesium	Phosphorus
Phosphorus	Magnesium
Alkaline phosphatase	Sodium
	Uric acid
	Cysteine

diminished urinary volume indicative of poor hydration, hypocitraturia, and hypercalciuria.[24–27]

Intersex

The first laboratory tests ordered after a careful history and physical examination should be electrolyte assessment, a karyotype, and serum 17-hydroxyprogesterone (17-OH progesterone) levels. Obtaining electrolytes is important to identify any metabolic imbalances such as 'salt-wasting' seen in congenital adrenal hyperplasia (CAH) that would require prompt intervention. Serum 17-OH progesterone is obtained early because elevated levels identify CAH, which is the most common intersex condition. Formerly, the child's karyotype was obtained by a buccal smear but is now obtained by chromosome analysis of peripheral blood lymphocytes. A fluorescent in-situ hybridization (FISH) analysis may be done in conjunction with the chromosome analysis for rapid evaluation of sex chromosome presence. Although the FISH results will yield a karyotype within 24 hours, these results need verification from the formal chromosome analysis which takes 2–3 days. Further testing will then be directed accordingly (see Chapter 61).

Cryptorchidism

Nonpalpable testis in association with hypospadias requires an intersex work-up. Unilateral nonpalpable testis in the presence of normal external genitalia does not require additional laboratory investigation, although a newborn with bilateral nonpalpable testes and normal male genitalia must be evaluated for female pseudohermaphroditism due to CAH. Determination of the presence or absence of the unilateral undescended testicle is accomplished via surgical exploration or diagnostic laparoscopy. In the case of bilateral, non-palpable undescended testes in an older child, further laboratory assessment can be done to ascertain the presence of testicular tissue.

A karyotype should be performed as well as measurement of serum testosterone in cases of bilateral, nonpalpable cryptorchidism. Additionally, the serum gonadotropins, follicle-stimulating hormone (FSH) and luteinizing hormone (LH), can be measured and if these are elevated in the face of low testosterone, this is suggestive of anorchia.[28] It is important to note that serum testosterone is normally elevated during infancy in the neonate, at 2–3 months of age as well as at puberty. Subsequently, serum testosterone can be measured in the neonate or during this natural surge of infancy. If this window of opportunity is missed or if evaluation is being done in the newborn period, then either a human chorionic gonadotropin (HCG) stimulation test may be obtained or a measurement of serum Müllerian inhibiting substance (MIS).

The level of serum MIS produced by the Sertoli cell is the most sensitive indicator of testicular presence,[29,30] but unfortunately the enzyme-linked immunosorbent assays (ELISAs) are not readily available in many centers. Subsequently, an HCG stimulation test is more frequently obtained. Several methods of HCG stimulation have been described.[31,32] One method is to administer HCG intramuscularly (100 IU/kg or 5000 IU/1.7 m^2) one time and measure serum testosterone and dihydrotestosterone 72 and 96 hours later.[31] Another method involves three intramuscular injections of HCG on successive days at a daily dose dependent on the child's age (≤1 year old, 500 units; 1–10 years old, 1000 units; ≥10 years old, 1500 units).[32] The HCG should stimulate testicular Leydig cells, if present, to produce testosterone, resulting in a level >200 ng/dl. If there is an appropriate increase in testosterone, then some functioning testicular tissue is present. If there is no response to HCG, then presumably the child is anorchid. However, there is also the possibility of Leydig cell dysfunction, in that the Leydig cells do not respond appropriately to HCG. For this reason, many pediatric urologists still perform exploratory surgery, regardless of laboratory results.

Nocturnal enuresis

Screening tests for nocturnal enuresis are necessary to rule out any organic etiology.[33] These tests include a urinalysis or urine dipstick to assess the urine specific gravity and the presence of glucose. If the specific gravity on the urinalysis is low, correlating to dilute urine, the possibility of diabetes insipidus (DI) is suggested. If the urinalysis or urine dipstick demonstrates large amounts of glucose, diabetes mellitus (DM) may be present. Subsequent work-up and testing can then be tailored accordingly.

References

1. Practice parameter: the diagnosis, treatment, and evaluation of the initial urinary tract infection in febrile infants and young children. American Academy of Pediatrics. Committee on Quality Improvement. Subcommittee on Urinary Tract Infection. Pediatrics 1999; 103(4 Pt 1):843–52.
2. Koff SA, Wagner TT, Jayanthi VR. The relationship among dysfunctional elimination syndromes, primary vesicoureteral reflux and urinary tract infections in children. J Urol 1998; 160(3 Pt 2):1019–22.
3. Austin PF, Ritchey ML. Dysfunctional voiding. Pediatr Rev 2000; 21(10):336–41.
4. Lau SM, Peng MY, Chang FY. Resistance rates to commonly used antimicrobials among pathogens of both bacteremic and non-bacteremic community-acquired urinary tract infection. J Microbiol Immunol Infect 2004; 37(3):185–91.
5. Farrell DJ, Morrissey I, De Rubeis D, Robbins M, Felmingham D. A UK multicentre study of the antimicrobial susceptibility of bacterial pathogens causing urinary tract infection. J Infect 2003; 46(2):94–100.
6. Pape L, Gunzer F, Ziesing S et al. [Bacterial pathogens, resistance patterns and treatment options in community acquired pediatric urinary tract infection]. Klin Padiatr 2004; 216(2):83–6. [German]
7. Connor JP, Burbige KA. Long-term urinary continence and renal function in neonates with posterior urethral valves. J Urol 1990; 144(5):1209–11.
8. Kohler JR, Tencer J, Thysell H, Forsberg L, Hellstrom M. Long-term effects of reflux nephropathy on blood pressure and renal function in adults. Nephron Clin Pract 2003; 93(1):C35–46.
9. Kochakarn W, Ratana-Olarn K, Lertsithichai P, Roongreungsilp U. Follow-up of long-term treatment with clean intermittent catheterization for neurogenic bladder in children. Asian J Surg 2004; 27(2):134–6.
10. Schiffer CA, Anderson KC, Bennett CL et al. Platelet transfusion for patients with cancer: clinical practice guidelines of the American Society of Clinical Oncology. J Clin Oncol 2001; 19(5):1519–38.
11. Rebulla P. Platelet transfusion trigger in difficult patients. Transfus Clin Biol 2001; 8(3):249–54.
12. Ward JF, Kaplan GW, Mevorach R, Stock JA, Cilento BG Jr. Refined microscopic urinalysis for red blood cell morphology in the evaluation of asymptomatic microscopic hematuria in a pediatric population. J Urol 1998; 160(4):1492–5.
13. Lee MC, Lin LH. Ultrasound screening of neonatal adrenal hemorrhage. Acta Paediatr Taiwan 2000; 41(6):327–30.

14. Gokce C, Gokce O, Baydinc C, et al. Use of random urine samples to estimate total urinary calcium and phosphate excretion. Arch Intern Med 1991; 151(8):1587–8.
15. Ring E, Borkenstein M. [Use of the calcium-creatinine ratio in diagnosis and therapy]. Padiatr Padol 1987; 22(3):245–50. [German]
16. Stapleton FB. Idiopathic hypercalciuria: association with isolated hematuria and risk for urolithiasis in children. The Southwest Pediatric Nephrology Study Group. Kidney Int 1990; 37(2):807–11.
17. Parekh DJ, Pope JCt, Adams MC, Brock JW 3rd. The association of an increased urinary calcium-to-creatinine ratio, and asymptomatic gross and microscopic hematuria in children. J Urol 2002; 167(1):272–4.
18. Alon US, Berenbom A. Idiopathic hypercalciuria of childhood: 4- to 11-year outcome. Pediatr Nephrol 2000; 14(10–11):1011–15.
19. Wu JT, Book L, Sudar K. Serum alpha fetoprotein (AFP) levels in normal infants. Pediatr Res 1981; 15(1):50–2.
20. Stapleton FB. Nephrolithiasis in children. Pediatr Rev 1989; 11(1):21–30.
21. Simerville JA, Maxted WC, Pahira JJ. Urinalysis: a comprehensive review. Am Fam Physician 2005; 71:1153–62.
22. Fogazzi GB, Garigali G. The clinical art and science of urine microscopy. Curr Opin Nephrol Hypertens 2003; 12(6):625–32.
23. Bartosh SM. Medical management of pediatric stone disease. Urol Clin North Am 2004; 31(3):575–87, x–xi.
24. Lande MB, Varade W, Erkan E, Niederbracht Y, Schwartz GJ. Role of urinary supersaturation in the evaluation of children with urolithiasis. Pediatr Nephrol 2005; 20(4):491–4.
25. Battino BS, De FW, Coe F et al. Metabolic evaluation of children with urolithiasis: are adult references for supersaturation appropriate? J Urol 2002; 168(6):2568–71.
26. Miller LA, Stapleton FB. Urinary volume in children with urolithiasis. J Urol 1989; 141(4):918–20.
27. Erbagci A, Erbagci AB, Yilmaz M et al. Pediatric urolithiasis – evaluation of risk factors in 95 children. Scand J Urol Nephrol 2003; 37(2):129–33.
28. Jarow JP, Berkovitz GD, Migeon CJ, Gearhart JP, Walsh PC. Elevation of serum gonadotropins establishes the diagnosis of anorchism in prepubertal boys with bilateral cryptorchidism. J Urol 1986; 136(1 Pt 2):277–9.
29. Lee MM, Misra M, Donahoe PK, MacLaughlin DT. MIS/AMH in the assessment of cryptorchidism and intersex conditions. Mol Cell Endocrinol 2003; 211(1–2):91–8.
30. Yamanaka J, Baker M, Metcalfe S, Hutson JM. Serum levels of Müllerian inhibiting substance in boys with cryptorchidism. J Pediatr Surg 1991; 26(5):621–3.
31. Kolon TF, Miller OF. Comparison of single versus multiple dose regimens for the human chorionic gonadotropin stimulatory test. J Urol 2001; 166(4):1451–4.
32. Davenport M, Brain C, Vandenberg C et al. The use of the hCG stimulation test in the endocrine evaluation of cryptorchidism. Br J Urol 1995; 76(6):790–4.
33. Homsy YL, Austin PF. Dysfunctional voiding disorders and nocturnal enuresis. In: Belman AB, King LR, Kramer SA, eds. Clinical Pediatric Urology, 4th edn. London: Martin Dunitz, 2002: 345–69.

Fetal urology and prenatal diagnosis

3

David F M Thomas

Introduction

The era of prenatal diagnosis dates from the late 1970s when case reports of the prenatal detection of urologic malformations first began to appear in the literature. Since that time prenatal diagnosis has rapidly become an established and routine feature of clinical pediatric urology throughout the developed world. Many aspects of prenatal diagnosis and the natural history of urinary tract malformations have been clarified by studies published in the last two decades, but some important questions relating to long-term outcomes remain unresolved. A detailed consideration of the investigation and practical management of the various anomalies detected by prenatal ultrasonography is detailed in the relevant chapters elsewhere in this book. This chapter will therefore focus predominantly on the following areas of fetal and perinatal urology:

- pathophysiology of urinary tract malformations
- current status of fetal intervention
- value of prenatal ultrasound in screening
- a rational approach to early postnatal investigation
- significance of mild dilatation ('pyelectasis')

Functional development of the normal urinary tract

Detailed embryology is beyond the scope of this chapter, and is covered elsewhere. A pivotal event in functional development occurs at around 32 days of gestation when the ureteric bud fuses with the metanephric mesenchyme to initiate the formation of excretory nephrons. Nephrogenesis proceeds by a process of reciprocal induction until the 36th week of pregnancy, with the glomeruli, proximal tubules, and loops of Henle being derived from the metanephros, whereas the collecting ducts, calyces, and renal pelvis are derivatives of the ureteric bud. In man, nephrogenesis ceases at 36 weeks, and thereafter the number of nephrons remains fixed at between 0.7 and 1 million per kidney. Major developmental defects dating from the first trimester of gestation are characterized by agenesis or dysplasia (arrested differentiation that is characterized histologically by immature tubules and the presence of aberrant mesenchymal derivatives such as smooth muscle and cartilage).

Urine production and excretory function

The primitive nephrons begin to excrete urine at around the 9th week of gestation. Initially, its composition resembles an ultrafiltrate of plasma, but as gestation progresses and tubular function matures, fetal urine begins to acquire the low electrolyte, high creatinine composition that characterizes normal urine in postnatal life.[1] Fetal urinary output at different stages in gestation has been documented by ultrasonography of the fetal bladder in healthy fetuses. By the third trimester, the hourly fetal urine production is as high as 30–40 ml/h and it constitutes around 90% of the amniotic fluid[2] (Figure 3.1). In the fetus the role of the kidney lies principally in fluid excretion, since homeostatic regulation of extracellular fluid composition is undertaken by the placenta. For this reason, creatinine clearance does not provide a meaningful measure of fetal renal function. However, extrapolation of values derived from iothalamate studies in the fetal lamb suggest that the fetal glomerular filtration rate (GFR) at 36 weeks of gestation approximates to only 5% of the surface corrected adult value.[3]

The kidney lung loop

Amniotic fluid, of which fetal urine is the major constituent, has long been recognized as playing a critical

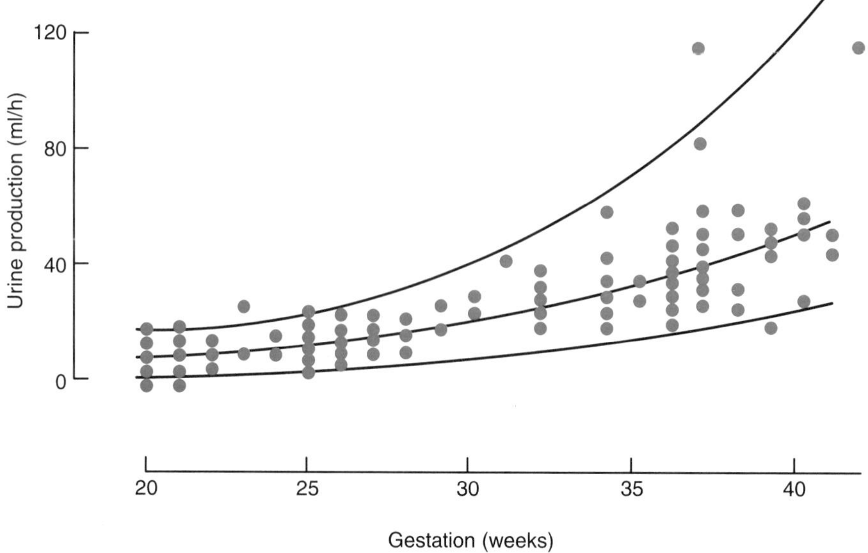

Figure 3.1 Fetal urine production at difference stages in normal pregnancy. (Adapted from Rabinowitz et al.[2])

role in lung development, and reduced amniotic fluid volume (oligohydramnios) is associated with varying degrees of pulmonary hypoplasia depending upon the timing and severity of the reduction in fetal urinary output. The role of amniotic fluid in promoting lung development probably extends beyond simple mechanical stenting of the airways, and renal-derived growth factors and other active agents are thought to be implicated in the regulation of early lung development.[4]

Changes at the time of birth

In the later stages of pregnancy, the fetus maintains a physiologic state of volume expansion. A high fluid intake of swallowed amniotic fluid is matched by a high obligatory urine output. If a comparable diuresis was maintained after birth, dehydration and volume depletion would rapidly supervene, but at the time of delivery, renal physiology rapidly switches to a fluid-restrictive mode, prompted in part by high circulating levels of aldosterone, vasopressin, and catecholamines. In addition, parenchymal perfusion and GFR increase dramatically in response to a fall in peripheral renovascular resistance and greatly increased renal perfusion. But, despite these adaptive changes, renal function remains marginal, with a corrected GFR at birth averaging only 30 ml/1.73 m^2. It is not until after 2 years of age that the GFR reaches the normal surface corrected adult value of approximately 125 ml/1.73 m^2.[5]

Pathophysiology of fetal uropathy

Defective nephrogenesis

Experimental ablation of the mesonephric duct (the origin of the ureteric bud) results in ipsilateral renal agenesis.

Renal dysplasia can be caused by a number of different mechanisms, including defective interaction between the ureteric bud and metanephric mesenchyme, intrinsic defects of differentiation, and a variety of extrinsic insults, notably obstruction. The classic observational studies of Mackie and Stephens[6] demonstrated the association between ureteral ectopia, faulty induction of nephrogenesis, and renal dysplasia in duplex systems. This 'ureteric bud hypothesis' can also be invoked to explain the association between renal dysplasia and high-grade reflux associated with ureteric ectopia.

More recently, studies using targeted gene ablation in 'knockout' mice have successfully reproduced a range of congenital abnormalities of the kidney and urinary tracts (CAKUT). Targeted mutations of the *AGTR2*,[7] *PAX2*,[8] and *UP3*[9] genes have been shown to give rise to congenital anomalies, including vesicoureteral reflux (VUR), with varying degrees of penetrance in experimental rodents. But while mutations of these and other genes have sometimes been implicated in the causation of urinary tract anomalies forming part of specific syndromes,[10] screening studies in children with isolated, non-syndromic urologic abnormalities have been almost entirely unrewarding.[11]

Fetal urinary tract obstruction

Upper tract

Experimentally, even brief periods of obstruction during nephrogenesis have been shown to induce apoptosis, aberrations of cell proliferation, and transdifferentiation of mesenchyme into the phenotypes that characterize renal dysplasia. Gene expression is also disrupted by obstruction.[12] However, the results of experimentally created obstruction in animal models must be interpreted with some caution in view of the difficulty in reproducing a model of chronic, partial upper tract obstruction – the pattern most commonly encountered in clinical practice.

Lower tract: bladder outlet obstruction

Experimentally induced infravesical obstruction was extensively studied by Harrison and his colleagues in San Francisco in the 1980s.[13] For example, these authors induced partial urethral obstruction in fetal lambs at 93–107 days of gestation. They then showed that the hydronephrosis, urinary ascites, and fatal pulmonary hypoplasia which ensued in untreated fetal lambs was reversed when the obstructed bladder was subsequently decompressed in utero. These and other studies underpinned the scientific rationale for introducing intrauterine bladder drainage in clinical practice. Unfortunately, subsequent experience with fetal intervention in the clinical setting suggests that some of the findings in the fetal lamb model may not translate to man. The current status of fetal intervention is considered in more detail below.

Fetal vesicoureteral reflux

The pattern of severe damage associated with grade V reflux can reasonably be ascribed to dysplasia resulting from a ureteric bud defect. By contrast, kidneys exposed to mild or moderate reflux in utero often appear normal or show global reduction in size with smooth outline (hypoplasia) on technetium 99m (^{99m}Tc) dimercaptosuccinic acid (DMSA) imaging. Focal scarring is predominantly a feature of postnatal infection.[14]

Very little is known of the mechanisms of renal damage seen in conjunction with sterile fetal reflux but in one fetal lamb model, experimentally induced VUR has been shown to exert significant changes on tubular function and on postnatal DMSA appearances of the kidneys.[15] In addition, clinical evidence is accumulating to indicate that even in the absence of infection high-grade bilateral primary reflux in males carries a greater risk of renal impairment than was previously recognized.[16] While the 'water hammer' effect of sterile urine has been largely discounted as a cause of ongoing postnatal renal damage, this mechanism may exert a more significant impact in the fetus.

Fetal intervention

In contrast to the evidence-based approach developed by Harrison's group in San Francisco, obstetricians in many other centers enthusiastically adopted fetal intervention on an uncritical and unreported basis in the 1980s. Where results were published, they were uniformly disappointing. The Fetal Surgery Register[17] reported an overall mortality rate of 59% in 73 fetuses – but this was probably an overoptimistic assessment, since an accurate urologic diagnosis was not established in many cases. By the end of the 1980s, enthusiasm for fetal intervention was waning. Mandell et al[18] identified 24 related publications between 1982 and 1985, but only 7 publications between 1985 and 1989, of which two were single-case reports. Although bladder decompression was initially achieved by open fetal surgery, this was soon abandoned in favor of vesicoamniotic shunting using an ultrasound-guided suprapubic pigtail catheter[19] (Figure 3.2). This remains the favored approach,

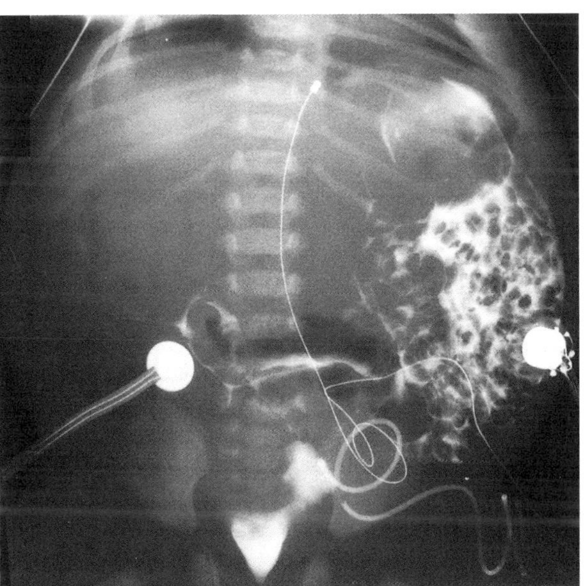

Figure 3.2 Complication of vesicoamniotic shunting. A postnatal contrast study reveals intraperitoneal placement of shunt with extravasation of contrast and urinary ascites. Despite shunting, this neonate succumbed to pulmonary hypoplasia.

although fetoscopy and intrauterine valve ablation have also been described.[20] Medium- to long-term outcome results have been reported by some centers which continue to undertake fetal intervention on a responsible and audited basis. In Detroit, Freedman and associates[21] documented the outcome of vesicoamniotic shunting in 34 fetuses treated during the period 1987–1996. Of these, only 17 survived to term, of whom 14 were assessed after 2 years minimum follow-up. Eight of these 14 children had already progressed into end-stage renal failure and 5 had been transplanted at the time of the study. Thus, of the original total of 34 shunted fetuses, only 6 were alive with normal renal function when assessed after 2 years of age. In another long-term study, the San Francisco group[22] analyzed the late outcome of 36 fetuses treated in the period 1981–1999. All had been selected for treatment on the basis of favorable urinary biochemistry. Of the 36 treated fetuses, 14 had a diagnosis of posterior urethral valves – of whom 6 did not survive to term. However, 8 infants with prenatally detected urethral valves treated in utero did survive and were evaluated at the mean of 11.6 years – when 5 were in renal failure. In all, only 3 (21%) of the 14 fetuses with posterior urethral valves survived with normal renal function. From a meta-analysis of published series totaling 342 fetuses, Clark et al[23] concluded that 'amongst controlled studies bladder drainage appeared to improve perinatal survival relative to no drainage.' Nevertheless, these authors cautioned that this positive conclusion might be influenced by a subgroup of fetuses with poor prognosis who had experienced a particular benefit in terms of early survival.

In summary, if survival is taken as the endpoint, there is reasonable evidence that intrauterine intervention ('fetal surgery') is effective, probably by facilitating lung development. Unfortunately, this does not appear to be true of renal development, since a high proportion of infants who have been treated in utero nevertheless progress rapidly into end-stage renal failure – with significant implications for their quality of survival in childhood and later life.

Prognostic indicators: selection for fetal intervention

Ultrasound

Bladder dilatation, regardless of the underlying cause, tends to carry a poor prognosis when detected before 24 weeks of gestation. A study in the author's unit demonstrated a marked difference in outcome between boys with prenatally detected posterior urethral valves identified before 24 weeks of gestation when compared with boys whose second trimester scans were normal and dilatation only became apparent on scans in later pregnancy. In the first group, 24% of boys died of pulmonary or renal failure following delivery and a further 29% progressed into early-onset renal failure. By contrast, when the second trimester scan was normal, none of the boys with posterior urethral valves succumbed in infancy and 93% had normal renal function at the time of follow-up.[24]

A high risk of poor prognosis and early-onset renal failure can be predicted from the following features:

1. Detection of dilatation before 24 weeks of gestation.
2. Male fetus.
3. Distended and/or thick-walled bladder.
4. Moderate or severe upper tract dilatation: corresponding to renal pelvic anteroposterior (AP) diameter of >10 mm before 24 weeks of gestation.
5. Abnormal renal parenchyma: microcystic or 'bright' parenchyma on ultrasound.
6. Oligohydramnios.

Biochemical markers

Since measures of renal function such as creatinine clearance are invalid in the fetus, the assessment of fetal renal function has relied mainly on analysis of biochemical markers in the fetal urine.

Urinary constituents that have been identified as predictors of poor functional outcome include a urinary sodium of >100 mEq/L after 20 weeks of gestation, elevated urinary calcium (>1.2 mmol/L), and elevated levels of urinary β_2 microglobulin.[25] Although serial sampling improves prognostic sensitivity, specificity is often poor, with considerable scatter and overlap of normal and abnormal values. Nicolini and Spelzini[26] have documented instances of fetuses with significant renal dysplasia where the initial urinary parameters were normal but then deteriorated progressively throughout the pregnancy. In the hope of improving sensitivity, attention has switched from markers of excretory renal function to molecules which are expressed during renal differentiation and which are regulated in renal dysplasia, such as transforming growth factor-β_1 (TGF-β_1).[27]

Summary: current status of fetal intervention

Long-term outcome studies and a growing body of anecdotal evidence indicate that fetal intervention does have the potential to increase survival by reducing the risk of pulmonary hyperplasia. By contrast, there is very little evidence that the prognosis for renal function is significantly improved by fetal intervention – probably because this is largely determined by dysplasia which predates diagnosis and treatment.

Indeed, it seems highly likely that some infants who might otherwise have succumbed to pulmonary hypoplasia have survived as a result of fetal intervention only to progress rapidly into end-stage renal failure in infancy or early childhood. Ransley[28] has consistently argued that our perception of fetal intervention has been colored by poor outcomes in bad prognosis cases and has suggested that the potential benefits of fetal intervention might be more apparent if it was extended to include all male fetuses with evidence of outflow obstruction in the second trimester. Unfortunately, it would require a prospective controlled study extending over many years to put Ransley's hypothesis to the test, since the full extent of renal insufficiency associated with congenital outflow obstruction is often not apparent until late childhood or adolescence. In addition, one might anticipate that parents who have been fully counseled on the implications of renal failure (dialysis, repeated hospitalization, transplantation including the likely requirement for a second transplant), would opt either for fetal intervention or termination of pregnancy rather than participate in the control arm of any study.

Screening for urologic anomalies

In countries with comprehensive healthcare systems the overwhelming majority of women are scanned by ultrasound at least once in pregnancy. Screening occurs at two levels: first, as part of formal screening for major fetal anomalies; and secondly, as an informal, ad-hoc screening process in which urinary tract anomalies are detected incidentally during the course of the third trimester scanning – usually for obstetric indications.

Nuchal pad transluscency is being used increasingly for screening at 10–12 weeks of gestation in high-risk pregnancies, particularly for Down syndrome. Although some structural abnormalities can be detected at this stage in gestation, the urinary tract is barely functional and the sensitivity of ultrasound for the detection of urinary tract anomalies in the general fetal population is unacceptably low.

Fetal anomaly screening

By contrast, the diagnositic sensitivity of ultrasonography is greatly increased by 17–20 weeks, the time when fetal anomaly scanning is routinely undertaken in the United Kingdom. In a 3½ year prospective study in the Yorkshire region, 2261 anomalies were identified on ultrasound, of which 369 (16%) prompted termination of pregnancy.[29] Autopsy and cytogenetic evaluation was performed in 97% of aborted fetuses. Central nervous system malformation accounted for almost 50% of terminations, whereas the genitourinary tract was the second most commonly affected system, accounting for 35 (9.5%) of the 369 terminations. Bilateral renal agenesis and multicystic renal dysplasia (Figure 3.3) were the most common lethal anomalies, followed by urethral obstruction and polycystic kidneys. No false-positive results were encountered, confirming a high level of

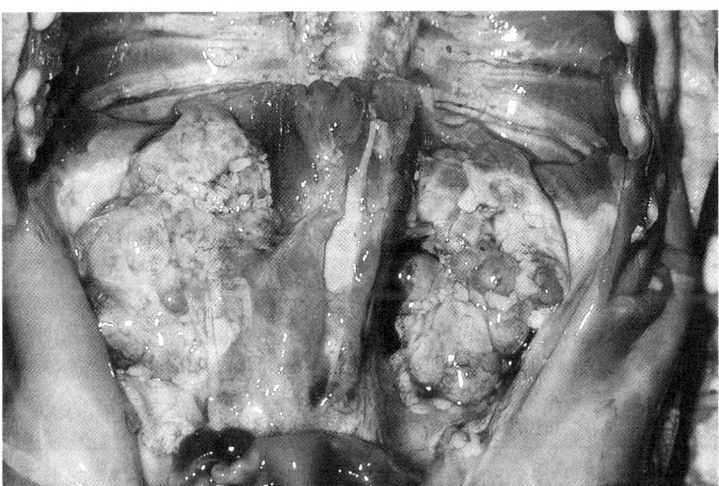

Figure 3.3 Bilateral multicystic renal dysplasia: autopsy findings following termination of pregnancy.

specificity for second trimester fetal anomaly screening for the detection of major urinary tract malformations.

Scott[30] analyzed 560 deaths in 2857 fetuses, neonates, and infants with urinary tract anomalies during a 6-year period in the Northern Region Congenital Abnormality Survey in the UK.

Of these 560 deaths, 68% occurred in utero (termination of pregnancy, intrauterine death, and stillbirth), whereas 32% occurred postnatally, most commonly from pulmonary hypoplasia.

Termination of pregnancy

Attitudes to termination of pregnancy ('therapeutic abortion') for severe congenital anomalies vary considerably between different countries. In most western European countries, including those that espouse Roman Catholicism, termination of pregnancy for fetal anomalies is legal (subject to gestational age and obstetric criteria), and is widely practiced. The situation is somewhat different in the United States where access to antenatal care (including second trimester ultrasonography), is more limited in certain socioeconomic groups and where abortion is a more divisive political issue.

Termination of pregnancy is already exerting a striking impact on pediatric urologic practice. Cromie et al[31] documented the outcome of 163 431 pregnancies recorded on the malformation surveillance program in Boston between 1974 and 1994. These authors found that elective termination of pregnancy had been undertaken in 65% of pregnancies following detection of myelomeningocele, 46% of pregnancies following prenatal diagnosis of posterior urethral valves, 31% for prune belly syndrome and 25% for bladder exstrophy. In the UK, termination of pregnancy is almost certainly being undertaken on a comparable or greater scale. The numbers of newborn infants being born with open spina bifida has declined dramatically over the last two decades and it is increasingly rare to encounter new cases of prune-belly syndrome (Figure 3.4). Similarly, the numbers of newborns with severe but nonlethal and potentially reconstructable anomalies such as 'classical' bladder exstrophy or cloacal exstrophy (Figure 3.5) are rapidly declining. As a consequence of the diminishing bladder exstrophy workload only two referral centers in England and Wales are now authorized to treat new cases.

Males with obstructive uropathy (predominantly posterior urethral valves) account for up to 90% of children aged 0–4 years old requiring renal replacement therapy (dialysis and/or transplantation).[32] These individuals can now be identified with considerable accuracy in the second trimester, and if parents were to opt increasingly for termination of pregnancy this would be reflected in declining numbers of children on end-stage renal failure programs in the first 5 years of life. In turn, this would have implications for pediatric nephrology workload.

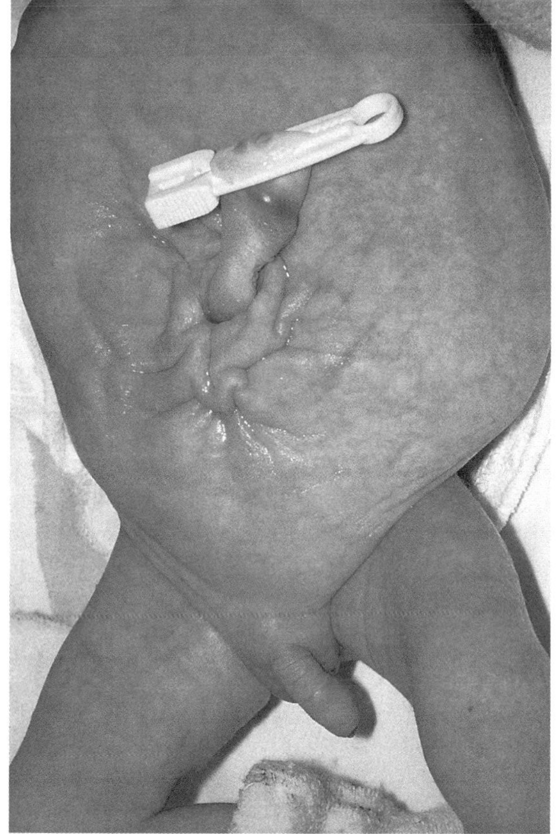

Figure 3.4 Newborn infant with characteristic features of prune belly syndrome, which is a disappearing disorder. Most major centers report a dramatic decline in incidence following the advent of prenatal diagnosis and termination of pregnancy.

Screening for nonlethal uropathies

The increasing use of ultrasound for a variety of obstetric indications in the third trimester constitutes a further, informal means of detecting urologic abnormalities.

But whereas ultrasonography detects severe, potentially lethal anomalies with a high degree of sensitivity it is far less reliable for detecting anomalies of mild to moderate severity. The diagnostic sensitivity

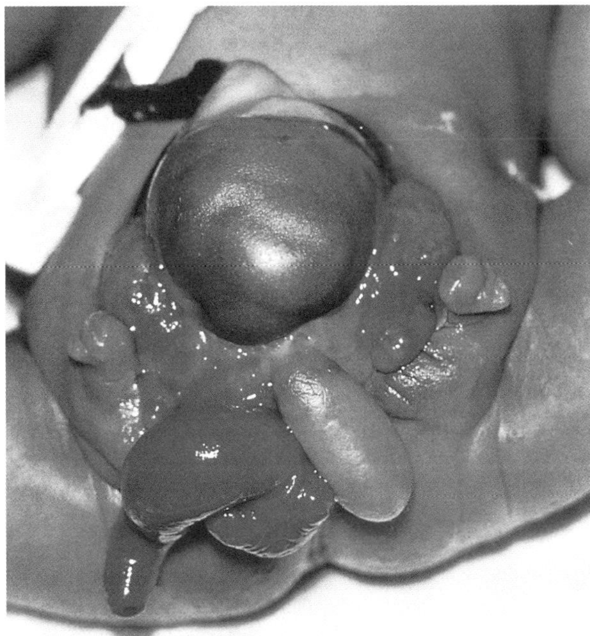

Figure 3.5 Cloacal exstrophy. Although cloacal and uncomplicated forms of bladder exstrophy are not generally associated with a significant risk of renal failure, prenatal diagnosis and possible termination of pregnancy raise serious ethical issues relating to quality of life.

of the ultrasound finding of isolated upper tract dilatation ('fetal hydronephrosis') is low, since these appearances may denote active obstruction, nonobstructive dilatation, a simple anatomic abnormality ('extrarenal pelvis'), or VUR. Ureteral dilatation may be due to reflux, obstructive or non-obstructive megaureter, or upper tract changes due to bladder dysfunction or infravesical obstruction. In the majority of instances, therefore, it is impossible to establish a definitive urologic diagnosis without the additional information provided by appropriate postnatal imaging. However, unilateral multicystic dysplastic kidney and duplex kidney are examples of anomalies which can be diagnosed with reasonable certainty – although confirmatory postnatal imaging is still required.

Defining 'pathologic' dilatation

Many studies have tried to establish a predictive 'cutoff' value for the AP diameter of the renal pelvis which is indicative of clinically significant pathology. Although 1 cm has been widely used, Livera et al[33] found that fewer than 50% of infants with this degree of dilatation detected at 28 weeks subsequently proved to have significant pathology.

Scott and Renwick[34] undertook a comprehensive analysis of 1301 fetal renal pelvic measurements at different gestational ages and correlated the values with postnatal outcomes. These authors concluded that 'a measurement of the fetal renal pelvis of 7 mm or greater at gestational age of 18 weeks is a strong indication that the urinary tract may be abnormal and should be carefully observed during the later stages of pregnancy.' In the author's unit, a study of 35 children with prenatally detected ureteropelvic junction (UPJ) obstruction demonstrated a broad correlation between the AP diameter of the renal pelvis in the second trimester and the severity of functional impairment on postnatal renography.[35] However, this only reached statistical significance in a small group of kidneys with an AP diameter >15 mm in the second trimester (in which postnatal mean differential function was reduced to 26.5%), whereas in the AP diameter range 6–15 mm (the range most commonly encountered in clinical practice) the predictive value was less consistent, with considerable scatter of values for postnatal function.

Dhillon et al[36] found that when the AP diameter was ≤15 mm, this measurement had a strong negative predictive value, since the risk of functional deterioration due to UPJ obstruction was only 2% (Table 3.1).

To summarize, severe dilatation confined to the renal collecting system, particularly when detected in the second trimester, is a reasonably sensitive predictor of significant obstruction. However, by the later stages of pregnancy the risk of obstruction causing functional impairment is largely confined to those kidneys with an AP diameter >15 mm.

Postnatal evaluation: general considerations

The most immediate threat faced by a newborn infant with a urologic abnormality is urinary infection – particularly when this is associated with outflow obstruction or high-grade reflux. Initial investigation should therefore be aimed at identifying infants at greatest risk, principally boys with posterior urethral valves or high-grade primary reflux. On the other hand, the importance of identifying the relatively small proportion of infants with serious pathology must be balanced by the need to avoid submitting large numbers of healthy asymptomatic infants to needless and often invasive investigations. A selective approach is

Table 3.1 Prenatally detected ureteropelvic junction obstruction: correlation between maximum recorded anteroposterior (AP) diameter of renal pelvis and likelihood of impaired differential function on initial postnatal evaluation or during follow-up

Maximal AP diameter of renal pelvis (mm)	Requirement for surgical intervention (based on functional criteria) (%)
<15	2
15–20	7
20–30	29
30–40	61
40–50	67
>50	100

Findings derived from prospective studies undertaken at the Hospital for Sick Children, Great Ormond Street, London.[36]

required, guided initially by the pre- and postnatal ultrasound findings.

Ultrasonography

Since the urinary output of newborn infants is reduced in the first 24 hours of life, it is generally recommended that ultrasonography is deferred for 24–48 hours until a more physiologic urinary output has been re-established. Although this remains the ideal, the risk of missing significant pathology as opposed to mild dilatational reflux has probably been overstated. Moreover, with the trend to earlier hospital discharge following delivery, this optimal timing may not be feasible. In the author's view, the principal indications for an early (24–48 hours) scan prior to discharge are as follows:

1 *Distended and/or thick-walled bladder, bilateral upper tract dilatation, ureteral dilatation.* These prenatal ultrasound findings suggest lower urinary tract obstruction. Relevant clinical findings may also be present, such as a palpable bladder or poor urinary stream.
2 *Bilateral renal dilatation without bladder or ureteral dilatation.* These findings are of greater significance in males, in whom they may denote posterior urethral valves or high-grade primary reflux. Nevertheless, ultrasound imaging can reasonably be deferred until 3–7 days of age if it is not feasible to proceed to imaging in the first 48 hours of life.

Where prenatal ultrasonography has demonstrated isolated unilateral renal dilatation, a duplex kidney, or a unilateral multicystic dysplastic kidney with a normal contralateral kidney, the initial postnatal scan can reasonably be deferred for up to 10–14 days, although a scan between 3 and 7 days remains preferable.

Formal measurement of the anteroposterior diameter of the renal pelvis is now routinely performed in most specialist centers. Although influenced by the state of hydration and other factors, measurement of the AP diameter is still preferable to subjective descriptions such as 'mild' or 'moderate' dilatation, 'full' or 'baggy' renal pelvis, etc. The grading system developed by the Society for Fetal Urology (SFU)[37] encompasses the appearances of the collecting system, 'central renal complex' and renal parenchymal thickness (Table 3.2), and these aspects of the ultrasonographic appearances should still be documented even if the formal SFU protocol is not followed. Evidence of ureteral dilatation should be sought and the bladder should be assessed for features such increased wall thickness and postvoid residual.

Voiding cystourethrography

Although opinion remains divided on the precise role of voiding cystourethrography (VCU) in postnatal evaluation, there is a growing consensus in many specialist units that a VCU is no longer mandatory in infants with isolated unilateral renal pelvic dilatation. A more selective approach has the benefit of reducing the numbers of healthy children subjected to an unnecessary and invasive investigation. In the author's practice the indications for an early VCU are as follows:

1 Abnormal appearances of the bladder – particularly thick-walled bladder or other evidence of outflow obstruction (e.g. 'keyhole' configuration indicative of posterior urethral valves).

Table 3.2 Classification of prenatal hydronephrosis (Society for Fetal Urology)

Renal image		
Grade of hydronephrosis	Central renal complex (intrarenal pelvis, calices)	Renal parenchymal thickness
0	Intact	Normal
1	Slight splitting	Normal
2	Evident splitting, complex confined within renal border	Normal
3[a]	Wide splitting, pelvis dilated outside renal border, *and* calices *uniformly* dilated	Normal
4	Further dilatation of pelvis and calices (calices may appear convex)	Thin

Grade of ureteral dilatation (UD Gr)	
UD Gr	Diameter of ureter (mm)
1	<7
2	7–10
3	>10

[a]An extrarenal pelvis extending outside the renal border which is not accompanied by caliceal dilatation corresponds to grade 2 hydronephrosis.
The grading system was devised as a guide to postnatal assessment but can also be used in the third trimester to counsel parents on the clinical significance, or otherwise, of prenatal sonogram findings.
From Maizels et al.[37]

2 Ureteral dilatation visualized on either pre- or postnatal ultrasound.
3 Duplex kidneys – in view of the high incidence of lower pole reflux.
4 Bilateral upper tract dilatation in a male fetus or infant.

Voiding cystourethrography should always be undertaken under antibiotic cover using a catheter or feeding tube – which should be left in the bladder when urethral obstruction is demonstrated. If there is already strong presumptive evidence of posterior urethral valves, it may be advantageous to perform the VCU via a percutaneously inserted neonatal suprapubic catheter.

Antibiotic prophylaxis

There is very little evidence on which to base reliable guidelines. As a rule, however, antibiotic prophylaxis is a prudent precaution for all newborn infants with prenatally detected uropathies, pending the outcome of postnatal investigations (particularly VCU). However, antibiotic prophylaxis may not be required for the following, although it is still generally prescribed:

- isolated renal dilatation with an AP diameter of 10 mm or less
- unilateral multicystic dysplastic kidney with a normal contralateral kidney and no evidence of contralateral or ipsilateral ureteric dilatation
- an ectopic but otherwise normal kidney.

Isotope imaging

By contrast to infection, obstruction per se rarely poses an urgent threat and thus the information provided by functional imaging does not usually influence immediate management. ^{99m}Tc DMSA is best suited for confirming total absence of function in a multicystic dysplastic kidney or for documenting differential function and patterns of parenchymal damage associated with VUR. Dynamic renography with ^{99m}Tc mercaptoacetyltriglycine (MAG3) is used primarily for the diagnosis of obstruction. Whereas furosemide washout is an essential element of the study, the interpretation of drainage curves is often problematic in young infants during the period of 'transitional' renal function.

Since the information derived from diuretic renography is rarely crucial in the first few weeks or months of life, this investigation can generally be deferred for 4–6 weeks, when the results can be interpreted more reliably.

Suggested protocols for postnatal imaging

Suggested protocols for postnatal imaging are illustrated in Figures 3.6–3.9. The investigative pathway is determined initially by pre- and postnatal ultrasound findings and it may occasionally be necessary to switch to a different plan of imaging if the original diagnosis is revised in the light of further information.

Commonly prenatally detected uropathies

A detailed consideration of the investigation and management of individual urinary tract malformations appears elsewhere in the relevant chapters of this book but some of the key points can be briefly summarized as follows.

Ureteropelvic junction obstruction

The management of prenatally detected UPJ obstruction has generated considerable controversy and the evolution of a more selective approach to surgery can be largely credited to Ransley's group[39] and Koff.[40] In addition to documenting the potential for the condition to resolve spontaneously, these and other authors have confirmed the relative safety of selective conservative management. Some of the more consistent themes to emerge from the literature are:

1 Significant loss of function which has occurred in utero does not usually recover despite relief of obstruction by pyeloplasty.
2 The probability of significant functional impairment at the time of birth or the subsequent risk of functional deterioration is linked to the severity of dilatation, with the risk of functional impairment being <10% where the AP diameter of the renal pelvis is <20 mm.
3 Conversely, an AP diameter of >35 mm denotes obstruction carrying a significant risk of functional impairment.
4 The risk of functional deterioration on conservative management is low, providing differential function in the obstructed kidney exceeds 40% and the maximum recorded AP diameter of the renal pelvis is <30 mm.

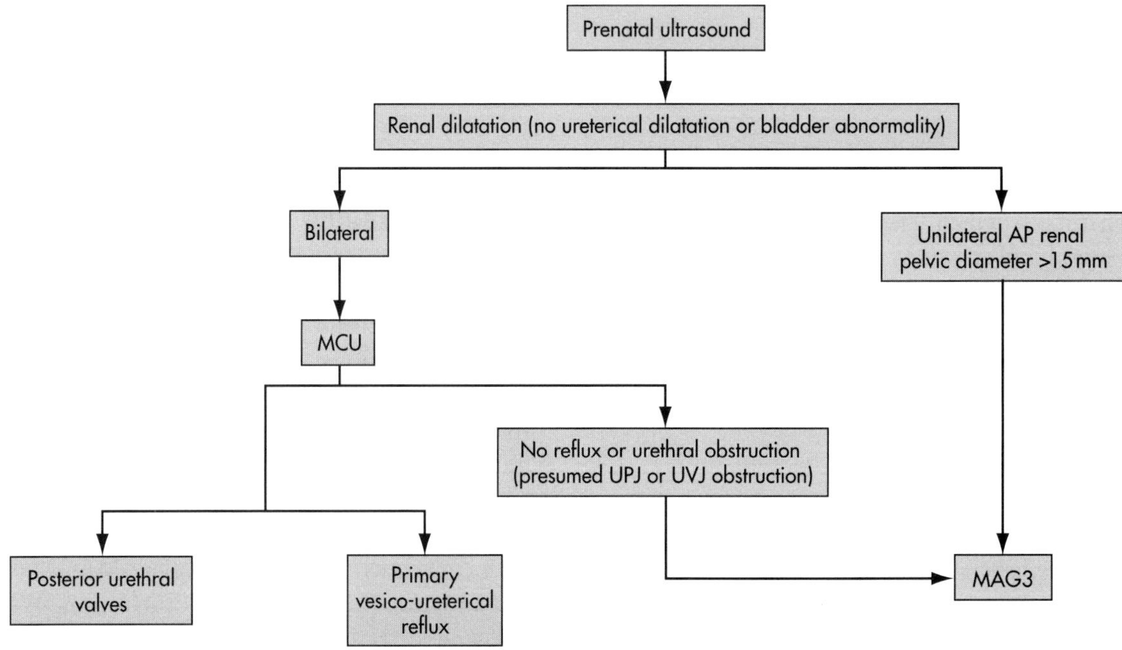

Figure 3.6 Postnatal diagnostic protocol for renal dilatation confined to the collecting system with no evidence of ureteral dilatation or bladder abnormality. MAG3, technetium 99m mercaptoacetyltriglycine; DMSA, technetium 99m dimercaptosuccinic acid. MCU = micurating cytourethrogram; UVJ = ureterovesical junction; UPJ = ureteropelvic junction; AP, anteroposterior. (Reproduced with permission from Dhillon.[38])

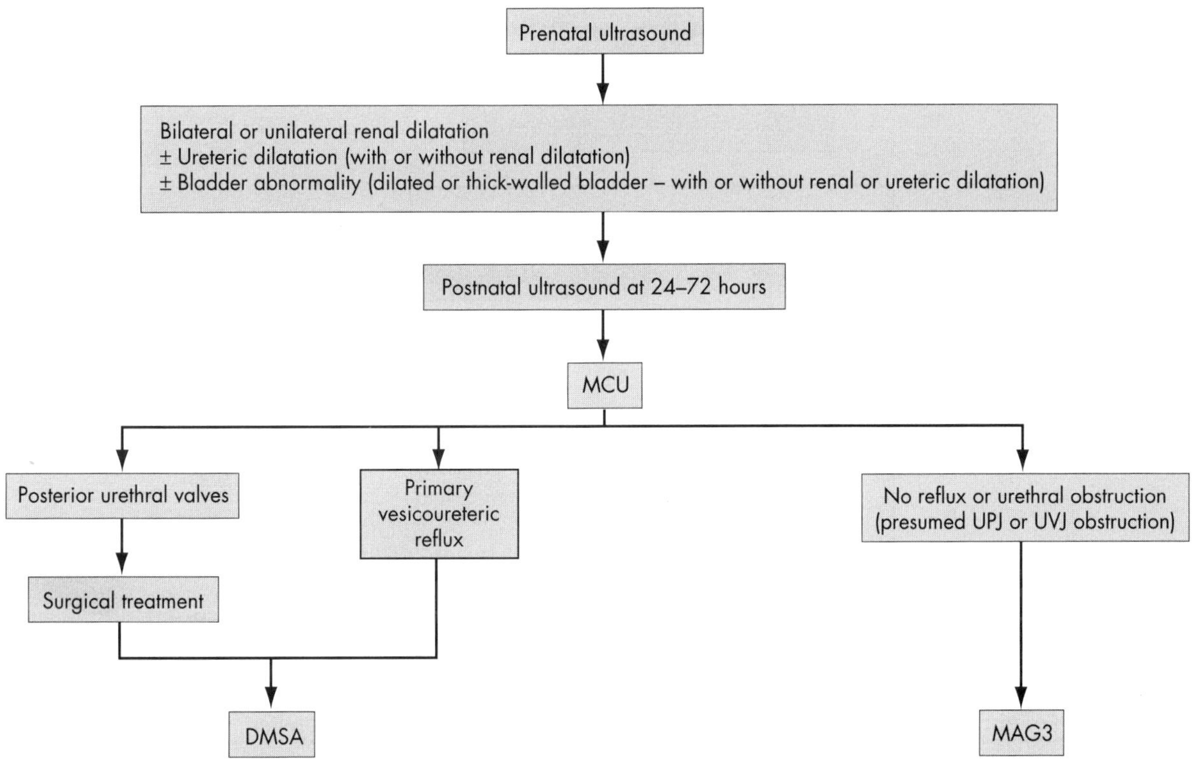

Figure 3.7 Postnatal diagnostic protocol for renal dilatation accompanied by abnormal appearances of the bladder and or ureteral dilatation. For abbreviations, see Figure 3.6. (Reproduced with permission from Dhillon.[38])

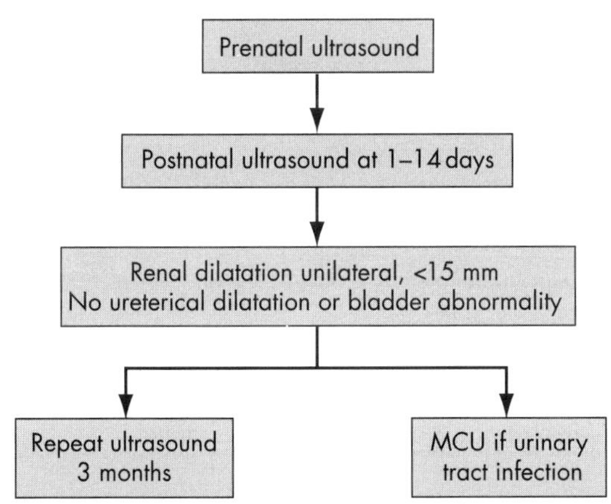

Figure 3.8 Postnatal diagnostic protocol for mild unilateral dilatation localized to the renal collecting system, with anteroposterior renal pelvic diameter <15 mm and without coexisting ureteral dilatation or bladder abnormality. MCU, micturating cystourethrogram. (Reproduced with permission from Dhillon.[38])

Posterior urethral valves

In many healthcare systems, between 50% and 80% of boys with this condition are now identified prenatally (Figures 3.10 and 3.11). Prenatal diagnosis has undoubtedly been a major factor in the dramatic reduction in early mortality since the 1980s, but the impact of prenatal diagnosis on the long-term burden of end-stage renal failure is less certain. It is becoming clear that even when prenatal diagnosis has resulted in prompt and optimal management, a sizeable proportion of individuals with this condition are nevertheless continuing to progress into end-stage renal failure in late childhood or adolescence. Whether the greater use of fetal intervention would reduce this burden of long-term morbidity remains an unanswered question.

Vesicoureteral reflux

Primary VUR accounts for 15–20% of prenatally detected uropathies. In addition, low-grade non-dilating VUR may be identified as an incidental finding on a VCU performed as part of the routine evaluation of a coexisting prenatally detected uropathy. Prenatally detected VUR is predominantly a disorder of male infant, with males outnumbering females by a ratio of up to 5 to 1.[41] Urodynamic studies in male infants with high-grade VUR have revealed marked bladder dysfunction,[42–44] which has been attributed by some authors to the legacy of transient urethral obstruction in utero – for example, by Cowper's duct cysts.

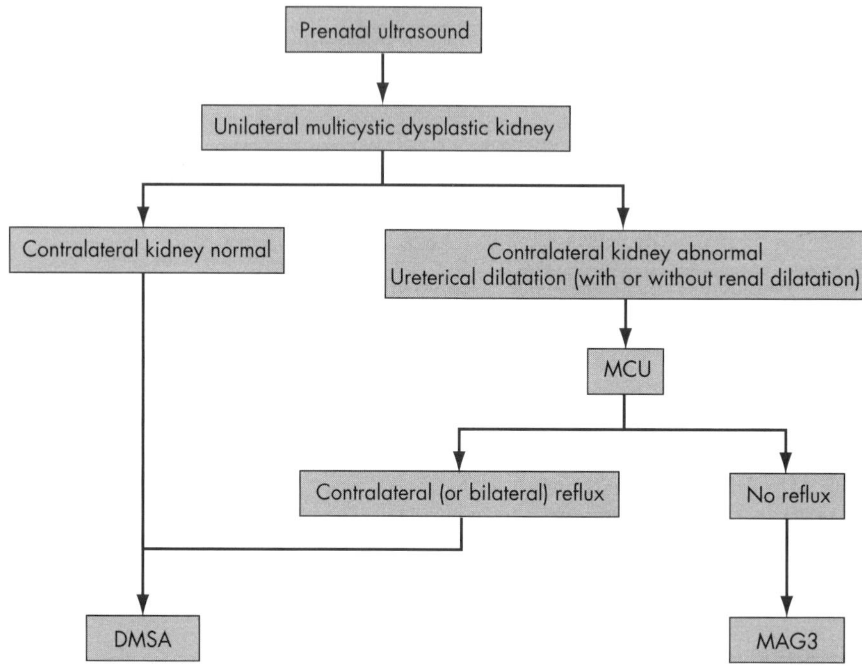

Figure 3.9 Postnatal diagnostic protocol for investigation of prenatal ultrasound findings suggesting multicystic dysplastc kidney. For abbreviations see Figure 3.6. (Reproduced with permission from Dhillon.[38])

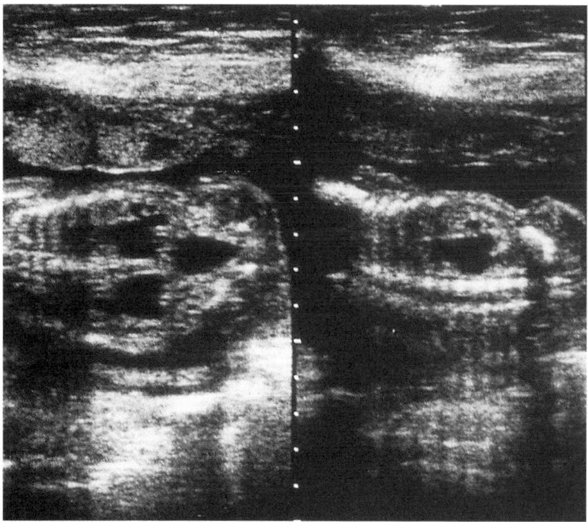

Figure 3.10 Posterior urethral valves: the fetal spine and thoracic cage are clearly visualized. Bilateral hydronephrosis and bladder distention can be seen.

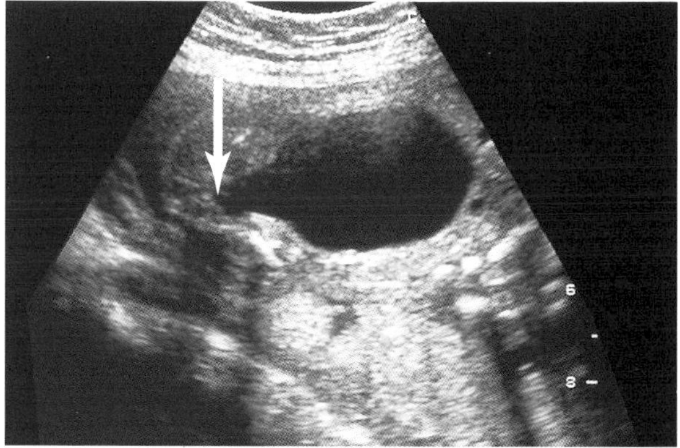

Figure 3.11 'Keyhole' sign. Dilatation of fetal bladder accompanied by distinctive dilatation of posterior urethra (arrow) and posterior urethral valves.

Regardless of any underlying cause, prenatally detected VUR seems to have a greater potential to resolve spontaneously than clinically presenting reflux. Reviewing the outcome of 413 prenatally detected refluxing units reported in 7 published series, Elder[45] noted an overall figure for spontaneous resolution of 78% for grades I–III VUR and 36% for grades IV and V. Conservative management was effective in the majority, with only 13% of children developing urinary infections during the course of follow-up.

Where breakthrough urinary infection necessitates surgical intervention in the early months of life, the author's preference is for cutaneous vesicostomy, but thereafter ureteral reimplantation is performed.

Multicystic dysplastic kidney

The introduction of prenatal ultrasonography revealed that the true prevalence of multicystic dysplastic kidney (MDK) is far higher than was previously recognized.[46,47] The natural history of prenatally detected MDKs is characterized by shrinkage or complete involution – which can also occur in utero, mimicking renal agenesis.[48]

Although there are reports of MDK occurring on a familial basis, it more commonly behaves as a sporadic anomaly. A study undertaken in the author's unit documented three affected families, one of whom demonstrated a pattern consistent with autosomal dominant inheritance with variable expressivity.[49] Ultrasound screening of 94 first-degree relatives of 29 children with prenatally detected MDK did not identify any significant renal anomaly. For this reason, we do not advocate formal screening on the families of children with MDK. The management of prenatally detected MDKs is considered elsewhere.

Mild dilatation (pelviectasis)

Mild collecting system dilatation, typically a renal pelvic diameter in the range 5–10 mm (Figure 3.12), is a feature of approximately 1 : 100 pregnancies. However, this is often a transient phenomenon. For example, Sairam[50] reported an 80% resolution rate for dilatation in the range 4–6 mm. Likewise, Chitty et al[51] followed 475 fetuses with mild dilatation detected between 16 and 26 weeks' gestation, and documented complete resolution or improvement in 66% on re-evaluation in the third trimester.

Pelviectasis is sometimes cited as a possible marker

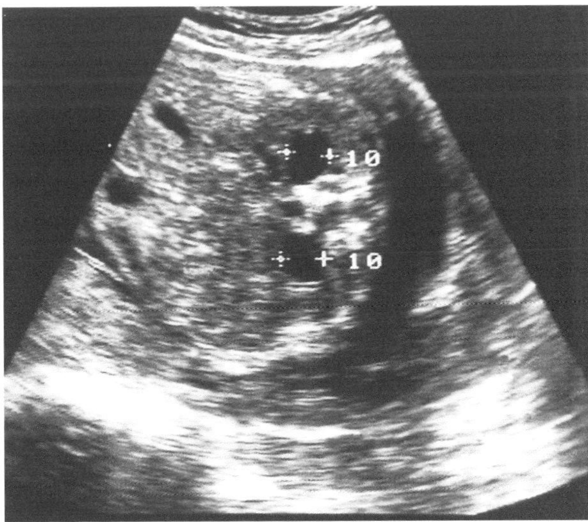

Figure 3.12 Bilateral renal pelvic dilatation. Anteroposterior diameter = 1.0 cm at 26 weeks' gestation. No underlying pathology was identified on postnatal investigation.

for aneuploidy. However, in a study of 25 586 unselected low-risk pregnancies, Havutcu et al[52] documented a 1.25% incidence of mild dilatation (mean AP diameter 6.4 mm, range 5–15 mm) but found no cases of aneuploidy. These authors concluded that the 'risk (of aneuploidy) in isolated fetal pyelectasis in low-risk populations is so small that it should not be an indication for invasive prenatal karyotyping.' Although the weight of reliable evidence indicates that isolated dilatation is not a marker of aneuploidy, when this finding occurs in conjunction with other anomalies it is more strongly indicative of an underlying genetically determined anomaly or syndrome.

Mild dilatation and vesicoureteral reflux

Although isolated mild dilatation (pelviectasis) can be largely discounted as an indicator of aneuploidy or significant upper tract obstructions, it can denote underlying VUR. In a prospective study of 5643 fetuses undertaken by Ismali et al,[53] mild dilatation or 'pyelectasis' (defined as AP diameter of >4 mm in the second trimester and an AP diameter in the range 7–15 mm in the third trimester) was found in 258 fetuses. Subsequent voiding cystourethrography in these individuals identified an overall incidence of VUR of 10.7%.

In a smaller study, Gloor et al[54] documented an incidence of VUR of 15% in 22 infants with dilatation in the range AP diameter 4–10 mm detected before 24 weeks' gestation. In practice, however, the morbidity generated by mild dilatation is minimal. In the author's unit, a follow-up study totaling 122 child-years of follow-up identified only two incidences of morbidity related to the urinary tract, neither of which were due to reflux.[55] DeJong et al[56] undertook a questionnaire case control study in children aged 4–9 years old to compare the incidence of urinary tract symptoms in children with a history of prenatally detected mild dilatation with normal controls. No difference was found in the incidence of either urinary tract infection or incontinence between the two groups.

Thus, there appears to be increasingly little justification for routinely submitting infants with prenatally detected isolated pelviectasis to voiding cystourethrography, an invasive and potentially distressing procedure which will yield negative results in 85–90% of cases. Some instances of predominantly low-grade, self-limiting VUR (mainly in boys) will be missed by this selective approach, but this risk is outweighed by the benefit of reducing the burden of unnecessary investigation in large numbers of healthy infants.

Nevertheless parents should be involved in the decision-making process, whenever possible, since there is a very small risk of VUR that might be destined to give rise to infection and scarring. If parents decide against a VCU, both they and their primary care physicians should be alerted to the need for the urine to be checked promptly for possible infection if the child develops an unexplained febrile illness or urinary symptoms.

Conclusion

Ultrasonography is now so firmly rooted in obstetric practice that it would be unthinkable for pediatric urology to return to the preultrasonography era. In general, prenatal diagnosis must be considered to have been beneficial, but it must also be acknowledged that the detection of mild dilatation and some asymptomatic anomalies has generated needless parental anxiety and unnecessary investigation. In many countries the impact of termination of pregnancy is already evident in a substantial decline in new cases of prune belly syndrome (see Figure 3.4), cloacal and 'classic' bladder exstrophy and neuropathic bladder associated with open meningomyelocele. As termination of pregnancy extends to include other severe, nonlethal fetal uropathies the number of infants and young children requiring renal replacement therapy and transplantation (predominantly males with urethral obstruction and renal dysplasia) may also diminish.

Prenatal ultrasonography has undoubtedly advanced our understanding of the functional development of the urinary tract and the pathophysiology of many urinary tract malformations. In the future, this will be complemented by important discoveries within the rapidly advancing science of developmental biology to provide pediatric urologists with a much greater understanding of the scientific foundations of the specialty.

References

1. Glick PL, Harrison MR, Golbus MS et al. Management of the fetus with congenital hydronephrosis II. Prognostic criteria and selection for treatment. J Pediatr Surg 1985; 20:376–87.
2. Rabinowitz R, Peters MT, Vyas S et al. Measurement of fetal urine production in normal pregnancy by real-time ultrasonography. Am J Obstet Gynecol 1989; 161:1264–6.
3. Haycock GB. Development of glomerular filtration and tubular sodium reabsorption in the human fetus and newborn. Br J Urol 1998; 81:33–8.
4. De Mello D, Reid LM. The kidney/lung loop. In: Thomas DFM, ed. Urological Disease in the Fetus and Infant. Oxford: Butterworth-Heinemann, 1997: 62–77.
5. Brocklebank JT. Renal function in the infant and management of renal failure. In: Thomas DFM, ed. Urological Disease in the Fetus and Infant. Oxford: Butterworth-Heinemann, 1997: 124–49.
6. Mackie GG, Stephens FD. Duplex kidneys: a correlation of renal dysplasia with position of the urethral orifice. In: Stephens FD, Smith ED, Hutson JM, eds. Congenital Anomalies of the Urinary and Genital Tract. Oxford: Isis, 1996: 307–16.
7. Oshima K, Miyazaki Y, Brock JW 3rd et al. Angiotension type II receptor expression and ureteral budding. J Urol 2001; 166:1848–52.
8. Keller SA, Jones JM, Boyle A et al. Kidney and retinal defects (Krd), a transgene-induced mutation with a deletion of mouse chromosome 19 that includes the Pax2 locus. Genomics 1994; 23:309–20.
9. Hu P, Deng FM, Liang FX et al. Ablation of uroplakin III gene results in small urothelial plaques, urothelial leakage, and vesicoureteral reflux. J Cell Biol 2000; 151:961–72.
10. Sanyansin P, Schimmenti LA, McNoe LA et al. Mutation of the PAX2 gene in a family with optic nerve colobomas, renal anomalies and vesicoureteral reflux. Nat Genet 1995; 9:358–64.
11. Jiang S, Gritlin J, Deng FM et al. Lack of major involvement of human uroplakin genes in vesicoureteral reflux: implications for disease heterogeneity. Kidney Int 2004; 66:10–19.
12. Gobet R, Cisek LR, Chang B et al. Experimental fetal vesicoureteral reflux induces renal tubular and glomerular damage, and is associated with persistent bladder instability. J Urol 1999; 162:1090–5.
13. Harrison MR, Nakayama DK, Noall R, de Lorimier AA. Correction of congenital hydronephrosis in utero II. Decompression reverses the effects of obstruction on the fetal lung and urinary tract. J Pediatr Surg 1982; 17:965–74.
14. Crabbe DCG, Thomas DFM, Gordon AC et al. Use of ^{99m}technetium-dimercaptosuccinic acid to study patterns of renal damage associated with prenatally detected vesicoureteral reflux. J Urol 1992; 148:1229–31.
15. Gobet R, Park B, Chang H et al. Dysregulation of the renal renin/angiotensin system caused by partial bladder outlet obstruction in foetal sheep. Br J Urol 1999; 83(3):79.
16. Caoine P, Villa M, Capozza N, De Gennaro M, Rizzoni G. Predictive risk factors for chronic renal failure in primary high-grade vesicoureteric reflux. BJU Int 2004; 93:1309–12.
17. Manning FA, Harrison MR, Rodeck C et al. Catheter shunts for fetal hydronephrosis and hydrocephalus. N Engl J Med 1986; 315:336.
18. Mandell J, Peters CA, Retik AB. Current concepts in the perinatal diagnosis and management of hydronephrosis. Urol Clin North Am 1990; 17:247–61.

tions on the renal drainage system. Normally the time to empty one-half of the collecting system activity ($T_{1/2}$) is less than 8–10 minutes. This value may be higher (up to 20 minutes) in grossly dilated pelves or after surgery. In cases where the $T_{1/2}$ is >10 minutes, retention at 20 minutes is calculated (counts at time '0' minus counts at 20 minutes divided by the counts at time '0') (Figure 5.2). If the patient has a $T_{1/2}$ of 20 minutes, the retention value at 20 minutes should be 50%; thus the two converge at this point. The Lasix washout study appears to reflect the state of urinary flow better than the Whitaker test in the postoperative period.

In children who have had repair of a UPJ junction obstruction or have had reimplantation of the ureters as an antireflux surgical procedure, there will be a significant delay in drainage that can persist for up to 6 months. When evaluated after that time, they usually drain normally.

Several important points have to be made regarding assessing diuretic washout curves. First, the $T_{1/2}$ is invalid when performed on normal kidneys that have already emptied their pelves. Secondly, when there is poor renal function, the kidneys cannot be evaluated as there may be poor, if any, response to the Lasix stimulation. Finally, in large hydronephrotic kidneys (pelvic volume greater than 75 ml) there will be a significant delay in emptying due to dilution, even though there may be no mechanical obstruction.

Renal transplant assessment

In children with a renal transplant, the renal scan has been used during the first 2 weeks to evaluate the effectiveness of the transplant surgery. As the art of renal transplantation has improved significantly, the need for an immediate renal evaluation is not so important. We now generally do one study in the first 48–72 hours if the urine output is normal and blood pressure and creatinine are as expected. At 2 weeks after the transplantation, we do the first GFR estimate and then on a regular basis until the child has only yearly re-evaluations. Most important observations are the glomerular filtration estimate and whether or not there is any evidence of renal infarct (Figure 5.3).

Urinary tract infection

In children with upper urinary tract infection (UTI), radionuclide techniques are the primary modalities. The direct radionuclide cystogram is the most sensitive method for detecting reflux, which is present in approximately one-third of children with upper UTI. Radionuclide cystography is a well-documented technique, with acceptable sensitivity and specificity.[3] Recently, computer-analyzed antegrade voiding cystograms have been tried and appear to be almost as accurate as the retrograde version according to some reports. This could be a preferred technique, as it is more physiologic due to the absence of bladder overfilling. However, the generally preferred method is still the catheter voiding cystogram (Figure 5.4). The monitoring of the bladder and ureters is constant throughout both filling and emptying, which is not feasible using fluoroscopy.

If the child has an upper UTI, an evaluation may be needed to determine whether or not acute pyelonephritis is present[4] with a DMSA planar or single-photon

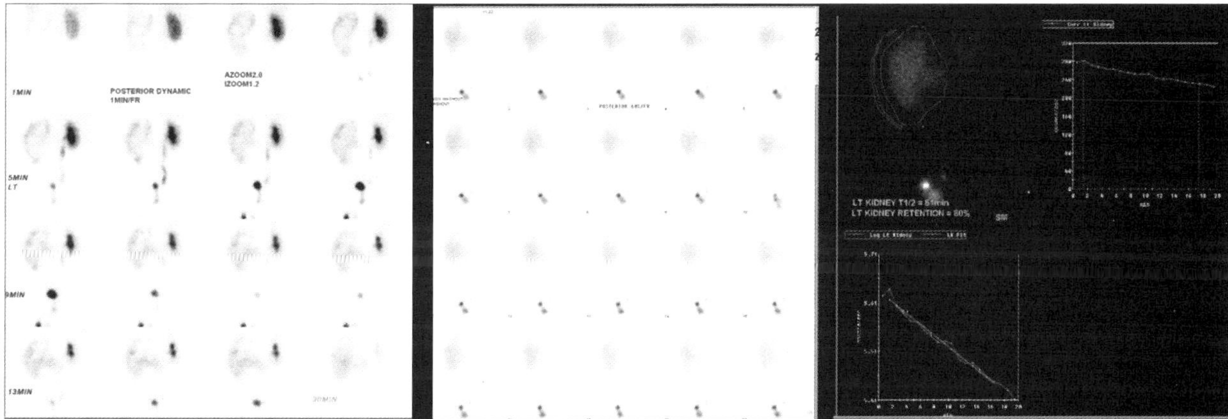

Figure 5.2 Ureteropelvic junction obstruction. The renogram images demonstrate the gross dilatation of the left renal collecting system. After Lasix (furosemide) injection there was markedly delayed drainage with a $T_{1/2}$ of 61 minutes and a 20-minute retention of 80%.

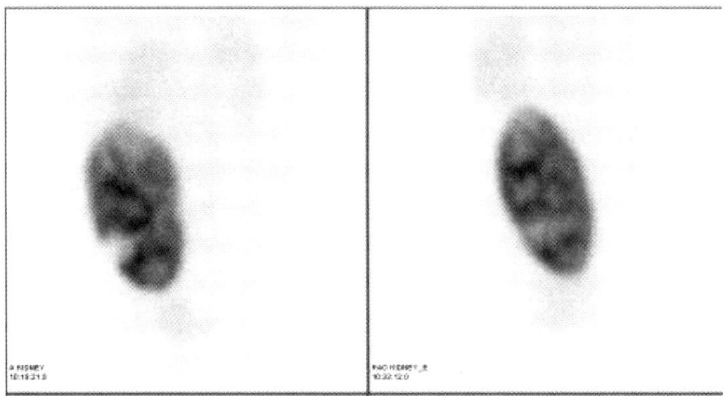

Figure 5.3 Postrenal transplant infarct. The wedged-shaped cortical defect is typical of a post-transplantation infarct.

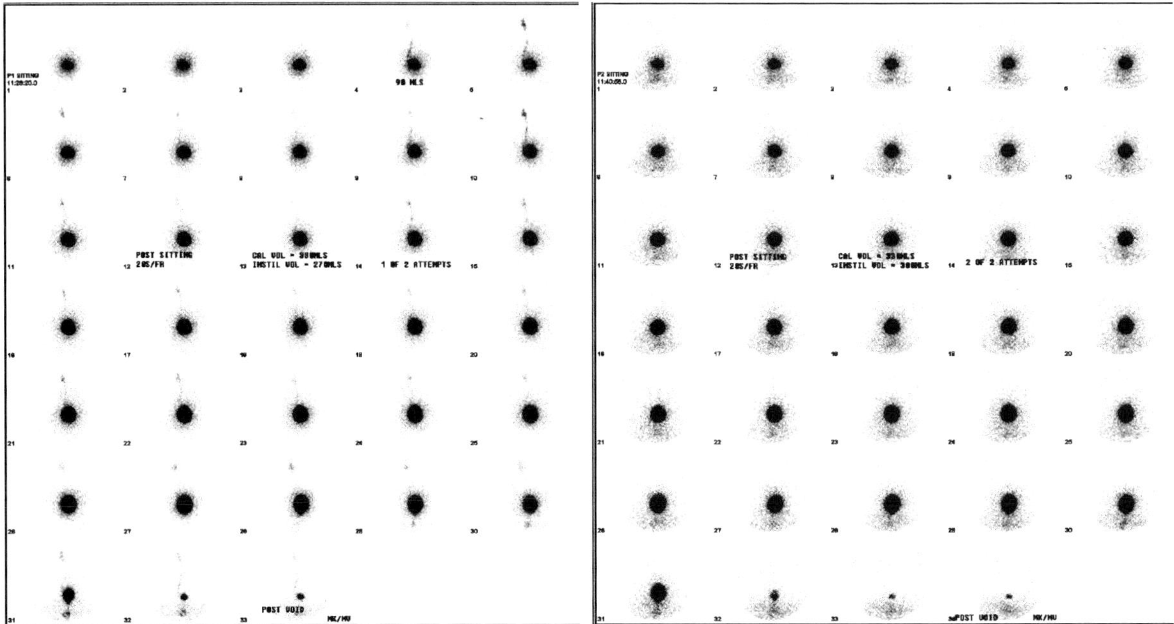

Figure 5.4 Left vesicoureteropelvic reflux. The reflux is seen to occur during filling and persist through voiding in the first attempt to fill the bladder to target capacity. In the second, no reflux occurred.

emission computed tomography (SPECT) study[4] (Figure 5.5). Recent data suggest that ultrasound should also be performed only if this a second or third UTI,[5] though most urologists have a low threshold to do a risk- and radiation-free study that can yield valuable information. Finally, a cystogram should be performed to see whether reflux is present.

Acute pyelonephritis appears as a non-segmental single or multifocal reduction in cortical accumulation of the ^{99m}Tc DMSA. In the acute phase, it is sometimes difficult to do SPECT imaging. Although it is better in defining the location of the lesions, it has only a marginal increase in sensitivity. Planar with oblique images is a satisfactory substitute. Subsequent ^{99m}Tc DMSA scans to monitor the progress of acute pyelonephritis should probably be done using SPECT imaging. In our hands and others, it has been shown that SPECT may have no increase in sensitivity in diagnosing disease, but is useful in diagnosing size and multiplicity of lesions.

A major concern after an episode of acute pyelonephritis is the development of scars. In this case, SPECT imaging appears to be the method of choice.[6] Not only is it easier to define whether scars are present or not but also location and definition are enhanced. In addition, it is much easier to determine whether splenic impression of the upper pole of the left kidney is present vs a true scar (Figure 5.6). Cortical mantle thickness is also much more readily defined.

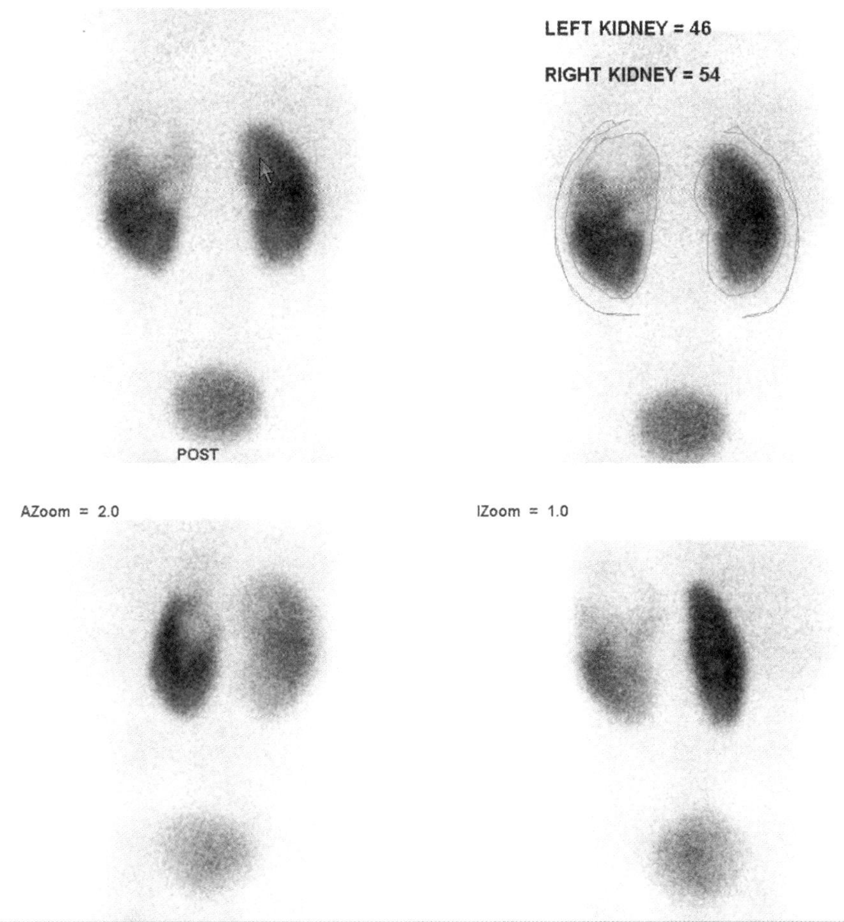

Figure 5.5 Acute pyelonephritis. A large photopenic area is seen in the upper pole of the left kidney. It is not associated with loss of cortical volume. This is the typical appearance of acute pyelonephritis.

Radionuclide cystography

Since a large number of children are seen because of UTI and VUR, isotope cystography is the preferred method for follow-up studies because of its accuracy and low radiation dose compared with conventional radiographic techniques. ^{99m}Tc pertechnetate or sulfur colloid may be instilled into the bladder via a catheter in conjunction with a saline infusion. In contrast to radiographic cystography, continuous recordings can be done during the bladder filling and voiding phases with no extra patient irradiation. Thus, chances of documenting reflux are theoretically enhanced. Conway has found good correlation with micturition cystography.[3] After the child voids, the residual counts can be used to quantify reflux and voiding volumes, since the concentration of isotope in the solution used to fill the bladder is known.

Antegrade cystography following a DTPA kidney study is an alternative method to detect VUR that avoids the problems of bladder catheterization.[7] However, it can only be carried out once the radioisotope has completely cleared from the upper tract and accumulated in the bladder. The child is then asked to void while reflux is assessed. This method compares favorably with micturating cystography and cystoscopy in some hands.

Kidney trauma

Traumatic lesions of the kidney can also be easily defined by DMSA SPECT imaging. Although ultrasound, CT, and IVPs are the common methods for evaluating trauma, sometimes the degree of functional impairment is important to know. In some institutions, SPECT imaging may be more easily and less expensively obtained. Sensitivity of SPECT ^{99m}Tc DMSA imaging for renal trauma is extremely high and is favorably compared with CT and superior to ultrasound and IVP. In fact, combined SPECT liver and spleen imaging as well as renal imaging is

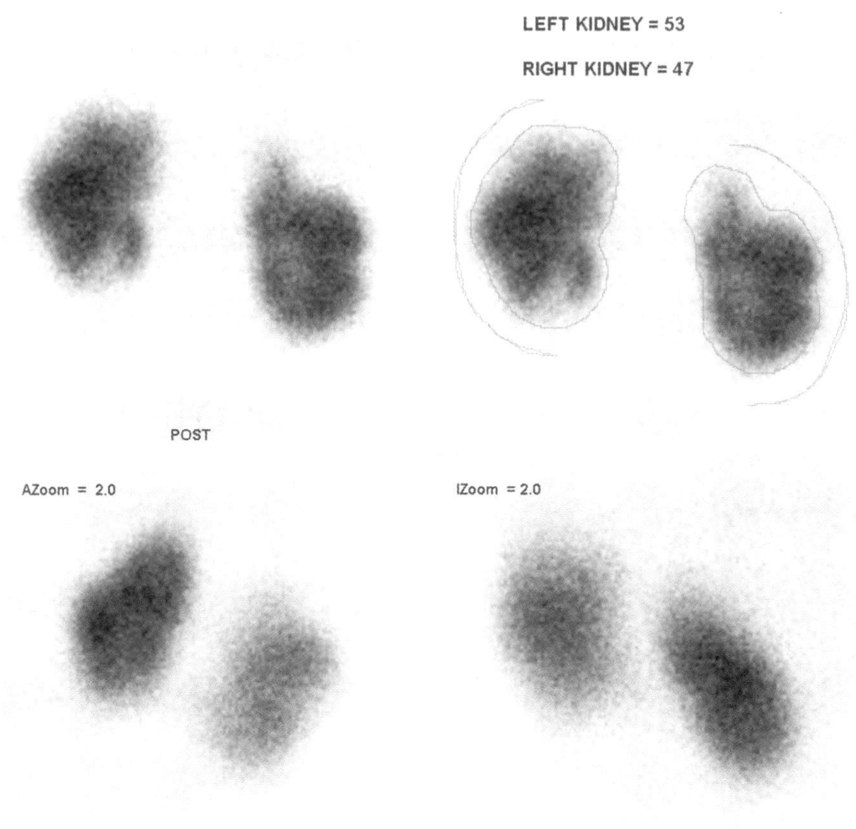

Figure 5.6 Pyelonephritic scars. Both kidneys demonstrate multiple defects with loss of cortical volume.

extremely sensitive to the overall detection of trauma of these organs. Usually, the abnormality is that of a band or section of the kidney which has depressed renal function due to fracture. Sometimes, the abnormality may be iatrogenic after interventional angiography and embolization.

Renal artery stenosis

Subsegmental or segmental renal artery stenosis is difficult to detect by the traditional nuclear medical techniques, even ^{99m}Tc DTPA imaging with captopril. In this case, we see a subsegmental or segmental reduction in ^{99m}Tc DMSA accumulation within the kidney. This is much more easily seen with SPECT than planar imaging.

Acute kidney lesions

Most of these lesions are related to hypovolemia with reduced renal perfusion. The net result in the kidney depends on the severity of the underlying clinical problem. The renal scan with its early angiogram phase has been shown to be useful in various pathologic states such as tubular necrosis, cortical necrosis, and renal vein thrombosis. The interpretation of the scan, however, must be made in light of the clinical circumstances, since other entities such as acute glomerulonephritis can look somewhat similar.

Children with acute tubular necrosis generally show good perfusion to the involved kidney. However, there is delayed excretion because radioactivity is retained within the renal parenchyma and often no activity is seen in the bladder by 30 minutes. There is no dilatation of the collecting systems to suggest hydronephrosis. In neonates the asphyxiated bladder syndrome may coexist and consists of gross bladder distention with urinary retention. Urate nephropathy of the newborn will look similar because it also causes intratubular obstruction. However, an episode of circulatory compromise is usually present to distinguish acute tubular necrosis.

Renal vein thrombosis

In renal vein thrombosis, there is poor perfusion to an enlarged kidney with poor excretion. The radiopharmaceutical injection should be into a suitable vein in the foot in order for the bolus to be visualized flowing up the inferior vena cava. Lack of flow implies caval thrombosis, with possible renal vein involvement. One must be wary in interpreting this, since crying, particularly in the neonate, may cause preferential flow up the paravertebral veins even with patent inferior vena cava and result in a false-positive test. It is often difficult to distinguish renal vein thrombosis from an arterial problem or intrarenal vascular problem, and this diagnosis should usually be confirmed by contrast angiography or Doppler ultrasound.

References

1. Pieretti R, Gilday D, Jeffs R. Differential kidney scan in pediatric urology. Urology 1974; 4:665–8.
2. Ash J, Gilday D. Renal nuclear imaging and analysis in pediatric patients. Urol Clin North Am 1980; 7:201–14.
3. Conway J, Kruglik GD. Effectiveness of direct and indrect radionuclide cystography in detecting vesicoureteral reflux. J Nucl Med 1976; 17:81–3.
4. Jantausch BA, Wiedermann BL, Hull SI et al. Escherichia coli virulence factors and 99mTc-dimercaptosuccinic acid renal scan in children with febrile urinary tract infection. Pediatr Infect Dis J 1992; 11:343–9.
5. Hoberman A, Charron M, Hickey RW et al. Imaging studies after a first febrile urinary tract infection in young children. N Engl J Med 2003; 348(3): 195–202.
6. Mouratidis B, Gilday DL, Ash JM. Comparison of bone and 67-gallium scintigraphy in the initial diagnosis of bone involvement in children with malignant lymphoma. Nuc Med Comm 1994; 15:144–7.
7. Pollet JE, Sharp PF, Smith FW. Radionuclide imaging for vesico-renal reflux using intravenous 99mTc-DTPA. Pediatr Radiol 1979; 8:165–7.

Prenatal and postnatal urologic emergencies

6

Patrick H McKenna and Fernando A Ferrer

Introduction

There are few true urologic emergencies. The object of this chapter is to cover the practical management of urgent consultations from the antenatal period through childhood. This includes a discussion of abdominal masses and intraoperative consultations. Several factors have impacted the identification and management of fetuses and children with urologically related anomalies. One of the most important factors has been the ability to identify urologic problems during fetal development. This has occurred because of increasingly accurate imaging, genetic screening, and the active participation of pediatric urologists in a multidisciplinary approach to urologic problems. As technology and genetic understanding continue to advance, the frequency with which diseases are identified in the prenatal period will continue to increase.

Antenatal period

Intervention during the antenatal period takes many forms, including medical treatment, termination of pregnancy, early induction of delivery, and surgical intervention. The incidence of prenatal surgical intervention is gradually increasing but remains rare. There are ethical, technical, and medical issues surrounding fetal surgery.[1]

Pertinent ethical issues also surround the decision to terminate a pregnancy. Discussion of the ethics of termination is beyond the scope of this chapter and is societal in nature. The pertinent ethical issues facing maternal fetal specialists and pediatric urologists that are germane to this discussion are the accuracy of the antenatal diagnosis and correct explanation of the long-term outcome of antenatally detected problems to the expecting parents. These issues are especially important in countries such as the USA where there is a time limit on the developmental date when elective termination can be performed.

Most initial screening antenatal sonograms are performed in an obstetric office. When significant abnormalities are identified, patients should be referred to centers with experience with these abnormalities to confirm the diagnosis and provide an accurate explanation of the consequences and long-term outcomes. The difficult task is providing an accurate assessment of the quality of life for patients with severe congenital abnormalities so that they can make an educated decision about intervention or pregnancy termination. Currently, severe urinary tract obstruction and congenital abnormalities, complications of intervention, and intersex disorders are the most commonly encountered antenatal problems that may involve an urgent antenatal consultation.

Urinary tract obstruction with oligohydramnios

It is estimated that only one in 30 000 pregnancies may be a candidate for antenatal intervention because of an obstructive lesion.[2–4] The most common form of intervention is the induction of early delivery after lung maturity is established. Treating the mother with corticosteroids may accelerate lung maturity in the fetus.[5] Since this is such a rare event, much of the effort of pediatric urologists has been spent in preventing unnecessary antenatal intervention. There are scant scientific data to support the efficacy of early intervention.[6–12] Published reports concerning results of intervention are mostly retrospective in nature and none has long-term follow-up.[13] In addition, the natural history of these lesions differs in the timing of presentation and their severity, even during the antenatal period, making case comparisons difficult.[14] Early severe obstruction impacts on lung development, leading to pulmonary hypoplasia.[15–17]

Urethral atresia is the most common cause of early severe hydroureteronephrosis. Posterior urethral valves (PUVs) (Figure 6.1) may present either early or late in the pregnancy with varying degrees of renal

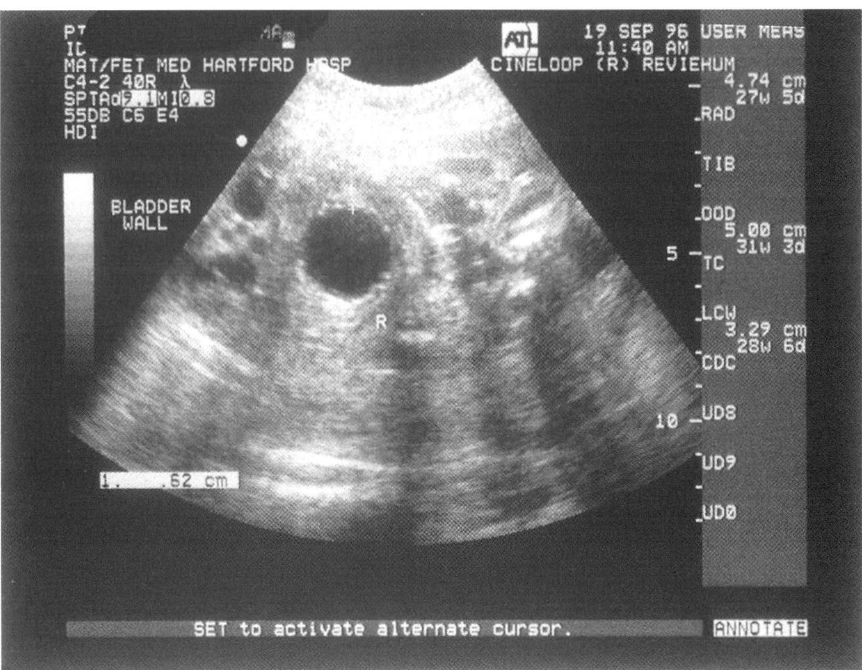

Figure 6.1 Prenatal posterior urethral valves: prenatal sonogram showing bilateral dilated renal pelvises and bladder with oligohydramnios.

injury. A ureterocele obstructing the bladder neck due to a ball-valve mechanism is another rare form of bladder neck obstruction more common in females.[18] These issues may be approached by working with maternal–fetal specialists to educate the general obstetricians on the differential diagnosis of antenatal urologic abnormalities. The flow diagram in Figure 6.2 is designed to focus the obstetrician on the importance of oligohydramnios when considering intervention. Education of obstetricians is important because ultimately they make the decisions and determine the timing of intervention. If the flow diagram is followed, only patients with oligohydramnios are even considered intervention candidates. Good prenatal sonography is accurate in making the diagnosis of PUV.[19] The correct management of these problems should involve a multidisciplinary approach since the bulk of the care resulting from the early intervention will fall to the pediatrician, nephrologist, and pediatric urologist.

In the rare instance where intervention is considered, oligohydramnios should be present, other severe congenital abnormalities should be ruled out, and evidence of recoverable renal function should be established (Figure 6.3).[20] Infusion of fluid into the amniotic space may be required to conduct an accurate sonographic survey for other severe congenital abnormalities incompatible with survival. In addition, chromosomal analysis should be obtained. Assessment of viable renal function is more difficult. It has been suggested that serial urine samples from the fetus be obtained to confirm renal function. Normal values (Table 6.1) may predict a better prognosis, as does the rate with which the bladder refills after tapping off the urine.[8,9,21–23] The reliability of these tests needs to be further documented.[24,25] In these studies, no assessment of quality of life issues in these patients was done. In cases of significant obstruction, the picture of increasing dilatation of the renal pelvis correlates with a greater likelihood of obstruction.[26] The in-utero progression of mild hydronephrosis is usually less than 15%.[27] No prospective studies have been performed comparing intervention to observation. Since these severe abnormalities are so rare,

Table 6.1 Fetal urine electrolytes suggesting good renal function (bladder aspirates)

	Value
Sodium	<100 mEq/L
Chloride	<90 mEq/L
Osmolarity	<210 mOsm/L
Urine output	>2 ml/h
β_2-Microglobulin	<6 mg/L

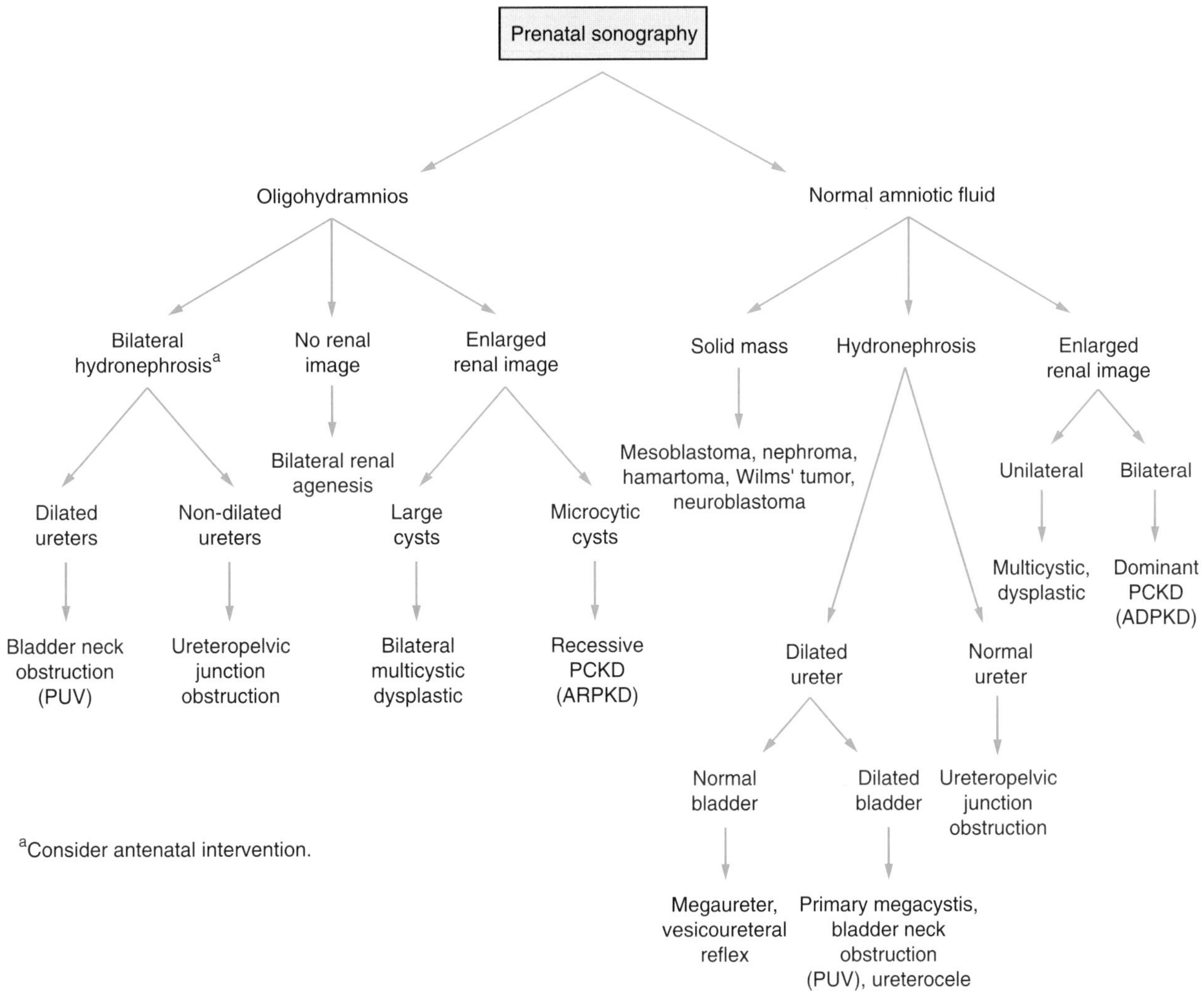

- Prenatal sonography
  - Oligohydramnios
    - Bilateral hydronephrosis[a]
      - Dilated ureters
        - Bladder neck obstruction (PUV)
      - Non-dilated ureters
        - Ureteropelvic junction obstruction
    - No renal image
      - Bilateral renal agenesis
    - Enlarged renal image
      - Large cysts
        - Bilateral multicystic dysplastic
      - Microcytic cysts
        - Recessive PCKD (ARPKD)
  - Normal amniotic fluid
    - Solid mass
      - Mesoblastoma, nephroma, hamartoma, Wilms' tumor, neuroblastoma
    - Hydronephrosis
      - Dilated ureter
        - Normal bladder
          - Megaureter, vesicoureteral reflex
        - Dilated bladder
          - Primary megacystis, bladder neck obstruction (PUV), ureterocele
      - Normal ureter
        - Ureteropelvic junction obstruction
    - Enlarged renal image
      - Unilateral
        - Multicystic, dysplastic
      - Bilateral
        - Dominant PCKD (ADPKD)

[a]Consider antenatal intervention.

Figure 6.2 Prenatal flow diagram. (PUV = posterior urethral value; PCKD = polycystic kidney disease.)

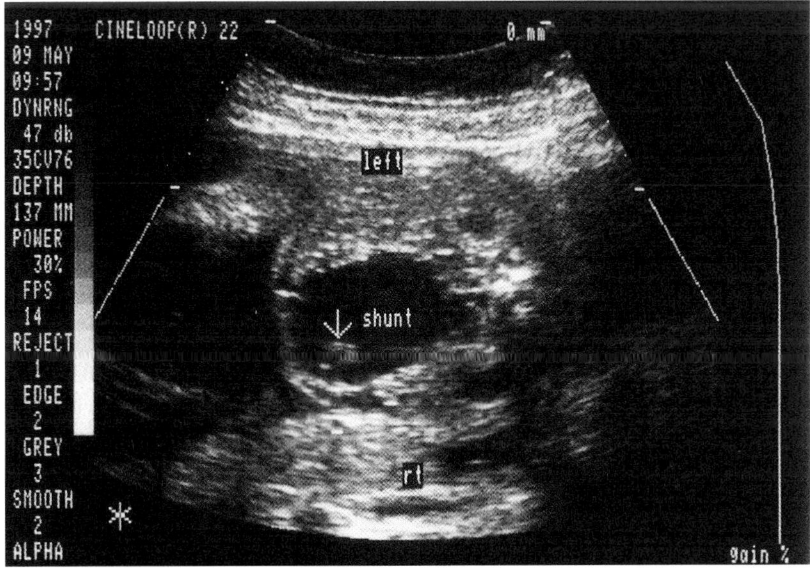

Figure 6.3 Antenatally detected posterior urethral valves with percutaneously placed vesicoamniotic shunt.

single-center experiences are always few. A multicenter registry was attempted in the past but only a small number of patients was entered and long-term follow-up was not obtained.[28] The single-center review of 14 patients with follow-up greater than 2 years revealed that five patients required renal transplantation, three had renal insufficiency, and six had normal renal function.[11] Ultimately, multicenter studies will be required to answer many of the questions concerning appropriateness of intervention. A survey of practicing pediatric urologists confirmed that few recommend antenatal intervention. When it is considered, the strict criteria outlined above should be followed.[29] Ideally, intervention should take place before any renal injury occurs. This approach can only take place if future studies can accurately identify obstruction very early in the antenatal period, which is currently rarely accomplished.

Complications of antenatal intervention

Intervention in the antenatal period can take various forms, from medical treatment to surgical intervention. The consequences of antenatal medical treatment for congenital adrenal hyperplasia (CAH) exemplify some of the ethical and practical problems with prenatal treatment of the fetus with medication. The risks to the fetus escalate the more invasive the form of antenatal intervention. Amniocentesis during the second trimester has become almost a routine procedure. When it is done with ultrasound guidance there is a 1% incidence of spontaneous abortion.[30,31] Fetal hemorrhage, cord laceration, direct fetal injury, uterine injury, and chorioamnionitis have been reported after amniocentesis. But, when amniocentesis is performed using specific guidelines by experienced teams, these risks are minimized.[32,33] Chorionic villus sampling historically had a fetal loss rate of approximately 3.5% and infection rates of 0.25–0.5%.[34,35] Recent data suggest that chorionic villus sampling may be safer than early amniocentesis.[36]

More invasive intervention, including percutaneous procedures and open surgery, are associated with more significant problems. The main abnormalities currently considered for intervention include fetal urinary tract obstruction, myelomeningocele, fetal diaphragmatic hernia, fetal cystic adenomatoid malformation, and fetal sacrococcygeal teratoma.[37,38] Even the most invasive procedures have minimal maternal risks or effect on future maternal fertility.[39]

The most common complication of hysterotomy for fetal intervention is subsequent uterine contractions with premature delivery.[40,41] Development of better tocolytic agents and other methods to prevent uterine contraction is crucial to successful prenatal surgery. The increased use of percutaneous laparoscopic surgery may decrease the problems of uncontrolled uterine contractions. However, laparoscopy is associated with an increased risk of percutaneous access wounds. Risks include injury to other fetal organs and to the abdominal wall.[42–49] Once intervention is anticipated, the pediatric team, including the maternal–fetal obstetrician, pediatric urologist, and neonatologist, should be available because complications such as uncontrolled uterine contraction or serious fetal injury may require immediate delivery, infant resuscitation, or surgical intervention.[4]

Classic bladder exstrophy

The antenatal identification of exstrophy is relatively straightforward. A combination of characteristics can be identified on a screening sonogram. The five most commonly identified findings are (1) no visualization of the bladder; (2) a lower abdominal bulge; (3) small penis and anteriorly placed scrotum; (4) a low-set umbilicus; and (5) abnormal widening of the iliac crests.[50] Omphaloceles are usually associated with a midline defect at the umbilical insertion, gastroschisis most frequently consists of a small, right-sided paraumbilical defect, and large lateral defects usually occur in the limb–body wall complex. In addition, specific organ evisceration and other associated abnormalities assist in the differential diagnosis.[51,52] More recently, the use of fetal MRI in the antenatal diagnosis and accurate determination of fetal gender has been reported by Hsieh[53] (Figure 6.4).

The challenge in the antenatal identification of these abnormalities is to provide counseling to the parents at the time when the abnormalities are identified.[54] The best approach is to involve a physician familiar with the long-term outcome of patients with these complex reconstructive problems. Initial work on the psychosocial and physical outcome of patients treated with various surgical approaches has begun but the outcome is known in a small number of patients.[55–57] Although some broad generalizations can be made, more outcomes data will be required to confirm early results. In the initial reviews, concerns centered primarily on worries about sexual function and sexual disfigurement, whereas education, family life, and employment appear to be essentially normal. The males were concerned about the appearance of

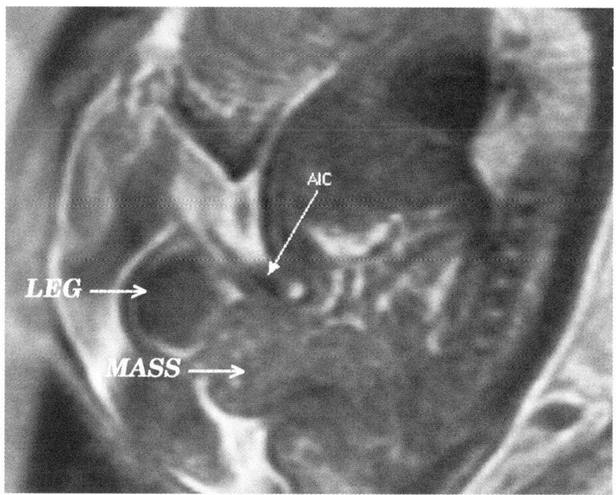

Figure 6.4 Determination of fetal gender using MRI.

their external genitalia, even though their sexual function was preserved. The female patients were less concerned about disfigurement and had normal sexual function, sexuality, and fertility. A complete understanding of the underlying anatomical abnormalities and the approach in the surgical reconstruction are requirements for the appropriate counseling of these patients.

Neural tube defects

Although not primarily a urologic abnormality, neural tube defects result in significant urinary tract morbidity. The accurate diagnosis of neural tube defects during the antenatal period can result from a combination of routine screening of maternal serum α-fetoprotein and targeted sonography.[58] Neuropathic bladder effects have been detected before birth.[59] The decreasing incidence of neural tube defects in the newborn period is due to the increased use of folic acid by childbearing women[60,61] and the increase in termination of affected fetuses during pregnancy.[62] The Public Health Service of the USA currently recommends that all women capable of childbearing consume 0.4 mg folic acid per day to decrease the risk of neural tube defects and anencephaly. Recently, it has been determined that the neurologic abnormalities associated with neural tube defects may result primarily from prolonged exposure of the neural tube to amniotic fluid. Intrauterine repair of spina bifida in fetuses with a ventricular size of <14 mm, fetuses who had surgery at or before 25 weeks, and fetuses with defects that were located at or below L4 were less likely to require postnatal ventriculoperitoneal shunting.[38] The fetal intervention may not improve the ultimate bladder function and these patients should be managed urologically similar to spina bifida patients that did not undergo fetal surgery.[63] The level of the defect, timing of repair, and type of repair all affect the outcome. Long-term follow-up of antenatally treated patients is not available and urologic participation in the postnatal evaluation and follow-up will be crucial to determine the possible benefits of the antenatal surgical approach.

Solid masses

The antenatal identification of a solid mass seldom requires early intervention but often generates an urgent consultation. The commonly detected antenatal masses include:

- adrenal hemorrhage
- neuroblastoma
- congenital mesoblastic nephroma
- Wilms' tumor
- pulmonary sequestration
- teratoma
- sacrococcygeal teratoma
- hepatic lesions
- rhabdomyosarcoma.

Since hydronephrotic and cystic lesions are easily distinguished by sonography the list is predominantly made up of rare but reported lesions. The recommendation should be to evaluate these patients thoroughly after delivery.

Intersex disorders

The identification of intersex disorders in the antenatal period is the result of better screening techniques and advances in the understanding of the inheritance of these diseases. Unlike the postnatal period, where the discovery of ambiguous genitalia is the initiating factor, amniocentesis, chorionic villus sampling, and better sonographic techniques allow early identification of many intersex disorders in the antenatal period.[64–68] The prenatal identification of these problems results in the need to provide adequate prenatal counseling.[69] Identifying CAH before birth provides the opportunity to treat the fetus in the hope of preventing androgen effects on fetal development, though presumptive early therapy is most effective in those known to have a familial risk.[70–76]

Most intersex disorders other than CAH are identified inadvertently.[77] In some cases this is the result of an amniocentesis because of a simple parental request to know the sex of the fetus. In other cases, there can be an issue of other known inheritable diseases such as determining the likelihood of an X-linked disorder (e.g. hemophilia). Knowing the sex may be helpful in confirming the cause of a structural disorder (e.g. PUV) that does not occur in girls. In cases with a family history of CAH genetic sampling can identify the inherited genetic disorder. The identification of an intersex disorder may also result from routine screening of an older mother. In situations where the genetic sex is known, but the genital screening by ultrasound does not appear to match the genotype, clinicians should consider the possibility of an intersex disorder. In the case of a 46,XY karyotype with female-appearing genitalia, the differential diagnosis should include gonadal dysgenesis or androgen insensitivity. In severely androgenized females with CAH, a 46,XX karyotype may be associated with ultrasound findings suggesting male genitalia. Table 6.2 lists the chromosomal analyses and possible intersex disorders.

The ability to identify and medically treat a disease in the antenatal period will probably become the norm in the future; however, the consequences of prenatal treatment need to be completely understood before it is openly embraced. Accuracy of the antenatal diagnosis and the effect of the medical treatment on other aspects of the fetus' development must be understood before treatment becomes routine. There is no better example of this controversy than the current debate over prenatal treatment of CAH.[78–80] Prenatal treatment of CAH needs to start before 6 weeks' gestation to completely prevent androgenic effects. Chorionic villus sampling to obtain fetal DNA cannot be done until 10–12 weeks' gestation.

The most common cause of CAH is 21-hydroxylase deficiency. This deficiency results in the inability to synthesize cortisol. The pituitary and hypothalamus overstimulate the adrenal gland, causing the overproduction of androstenedione. The androstenedione is further metabolized, predominantly to testosterone and dihydrotestosterone, resulting in the prenatal virilization of the female fetus. Early treatment with dexamethasone can prevent or minimize severe genital abnormalities in some patients.[73,81–83] The risk of having an infant with CAH for a mother with classic 21-hydroxylase deficiency is 1 in 8. The complications of prenatal treatment to the fetus, maternal risks, and long-term effects to the child are incompletely understood. Since antenatal treatment with dexamethasone needs to begin at 6 weeks' gestation, seven fetuses are treated unnecessarily to affect the external genital development of one fetus. This has significant ethical implications. The fetal metabolism of dexamethasone is not understood, and the doses recommended for treatment are greater than required to suppress the adrenal in the adult.[78] The effect on unaffected fetuses is not completely known. Despite these concerns, the possibility of preventing androgen imprinting of the brain in the affected female fetuses justifies a controlled long-term study.

Postnatal period

In the past, urologic problems identified at birth were primarily obvious congenital abnormalities such as

Table 6.2 Chromosomal analyses and possible intersex disorder

46,XX	Female pseudohermaphrodite (usually CAH) Male pseudohermaphrodite (i.e. SRY positive) True hermaphrodite Gonadal dysgenesis
46,XY	Male pseudohermaphrodite True hermaphrodite
46,XX/XY	True hermaphrodite
45,X, 45,X/46,XX, 45,X/46,XY, others	Gonadal dysgenesis Mixed gonadal dysgenesis Male pseudohermaphrodite True hermaphrodite

exstrophy. Now, the majority of urologic problems seen by urologists in the immediate postnatal period are identified by prenatal sonography and magnetic resonance imaging (MRI). In the evaluation and treatment of these problems physicians need to consider the unique aspects of bonding between the infant and the parents.[84,85] Bonding can be affected by separation of the infant from the parents and by severely disfiguring congenital anomalies.[86,87] These considerations should impact the treatment of infants with and without obvious congenital abnormalities. The support needs go beyond helping the family to come to grips with the congenital anomaly, and should include dealing with parental fears concerning job loss, financial difficulties, and effects on other family members.[86] One should encourage early discharge of infants who can be adequately managed as outpatients. When prolonged hospitalization is required, parental rooming-in with the infant is encouraged. A psychiatrist and staff educated on bonding issues should be actively involved in patient and parental management.[88–90]

Congenital anomalies noted at birth

Anorectal malformations

Anorectal malformations (imperforate anus) are congenital lesions of the cloaca (Figure 6.5). It is important for urologists to be familiar with these malformations because they are often associated with urologic abnormalities. There is also a high incidence of other congenital abnormalities associated with such malformations. There are multiple classification systems but none has gained wide acceptance. From a urologic perspective the simple distinction of 'high', 'intermediate', or 'low' anorectal lesions is probably sufficient: low lesions are those that occur inferior to the levator muscles, high lesions occur above the levator muscles, and intermediate ones in between (Figure 6.6).[91] From a clinical point of view most intermediate lesions are treated as high lesions. The surgical correction of these malformations is most often by a technique popularized by de Vries and Pena[92] using the posterior sagittal approach. Associated urologic abnormalities occur in up to 20% of patients with low lesions and up to 60% of those with high lesions.[93,94] The most common findings are vesicoureteral reflux (VUR), neuropathic bladder, renal agenesis, renal dysplasia, and cryptorchidism. It is not surprising that there is a high incidence of neuropathic bladder because of the likely

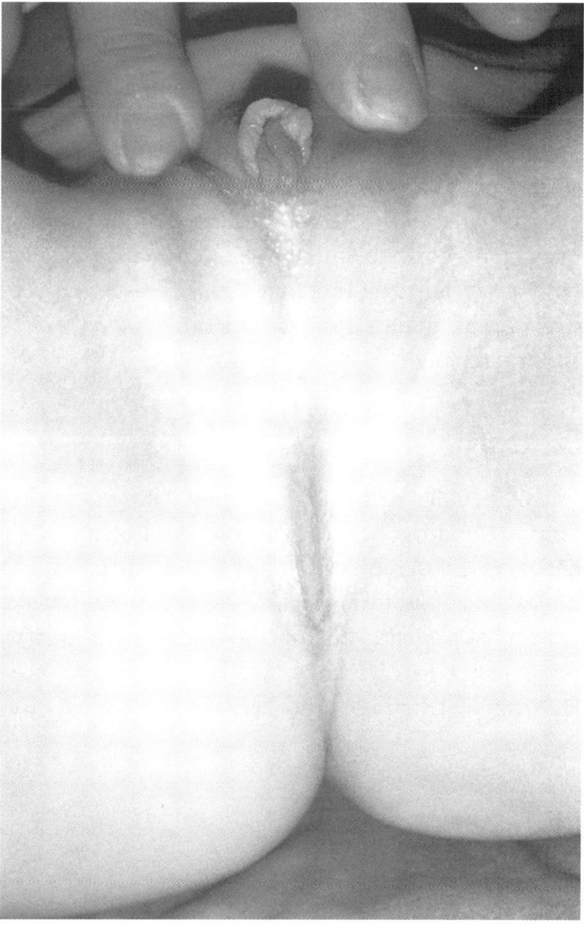

Figure 6.5 Patient with imperforate anus. (From Dr Donald W Hight, Connecticut Children's Medical Center, with permission.)

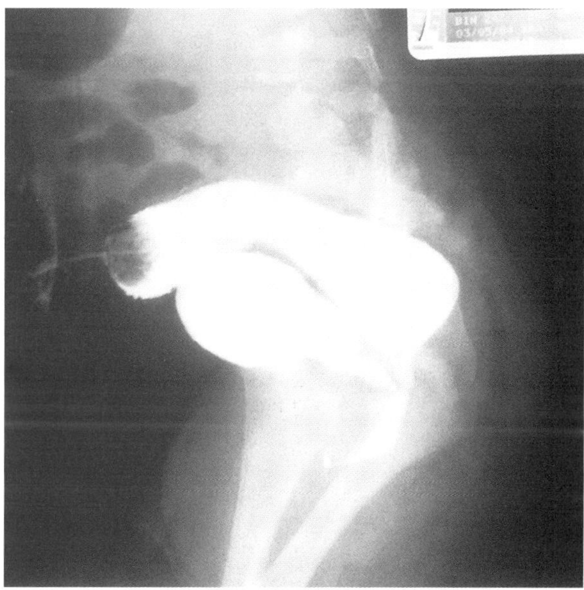

Figure 6.6 Radiographic picture of high bowel–urethral fistula. (From Dr Donald W Hight, Connecticut Children's Medical Center, with permission.)

association of vertebral abnormalities with anorectal malformations, especially with high lesions. Neuropathic bladder may occur in as many as 50% of patients.[93] The most common anatomic abnormality in patients with vertebral abnormalities is a tethered cord. Only recently has this association been identified and linked to the high incidence of neuropathic bladders and dysfunctional pelvic floors.[95] Patients with anorectal malformations should be studied urodynamically if they have high lesions and/or spinal abnormalities.

Exstrophy

Classic bladder exstrophy still most commonly presents at the time of birth despite the known specific antenatal sonographic findings[50] (Figure 6.7). The typical infant is male and is otherwise healthy. An exstrophic bladder, abdominal wall defect, epispadias, pelvic diastasis, VUR after bladder closure, and bilateral inguinal hernias characterize the anomaly. Initially, much time is spent with the family explaining the disease and planning the bladder closure. Patients should be managed by a urologist with exstrophy closure experience. The initial treatment is to protect the exposed bladder mucosa. If a plastic umbilical clamp was placed in the delivery suite it should be removed and replaced with a suture. If possible, nothing should come into contact with the bladder mucosa. A modified humidifier tent can be placed over the bladder, but for transport a cellophane non-adherent dressing may be utilized.[96]

The traditional methods of reconstruction used a staged strategy,[97,98] the first stage involving bladder and abdominal wall closure with pelvic osteotomy in most cases (Figure 6.8).[97,98] The epispadias is reconstructed in the next stage, and finally the incontinence and reflux. Several centers have advocated combining the first stages into one operation soon after birth (see Chapter 55). Initial reports are encouraging, but few patients have been treated in this way and there is little long-term follow-up.[96,99] Combined closure and

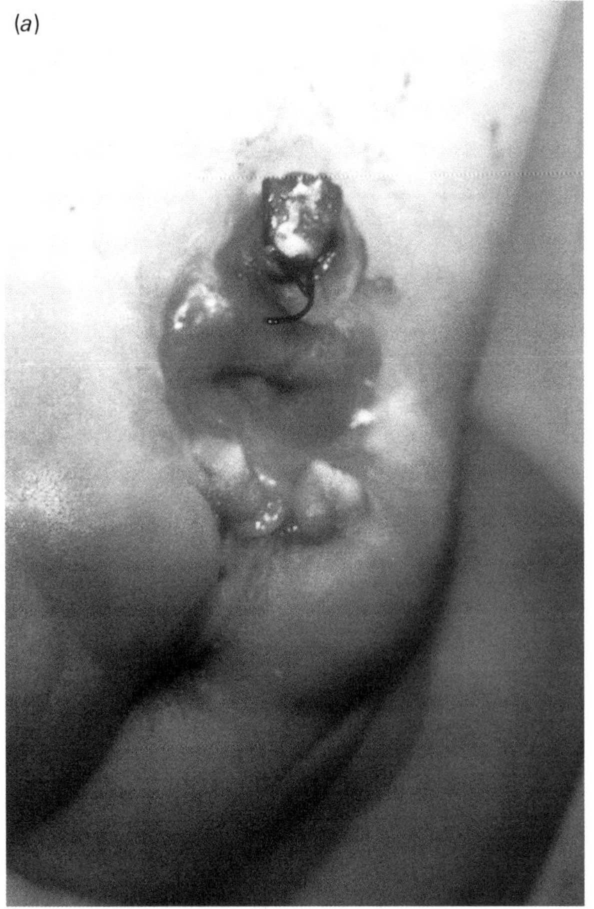

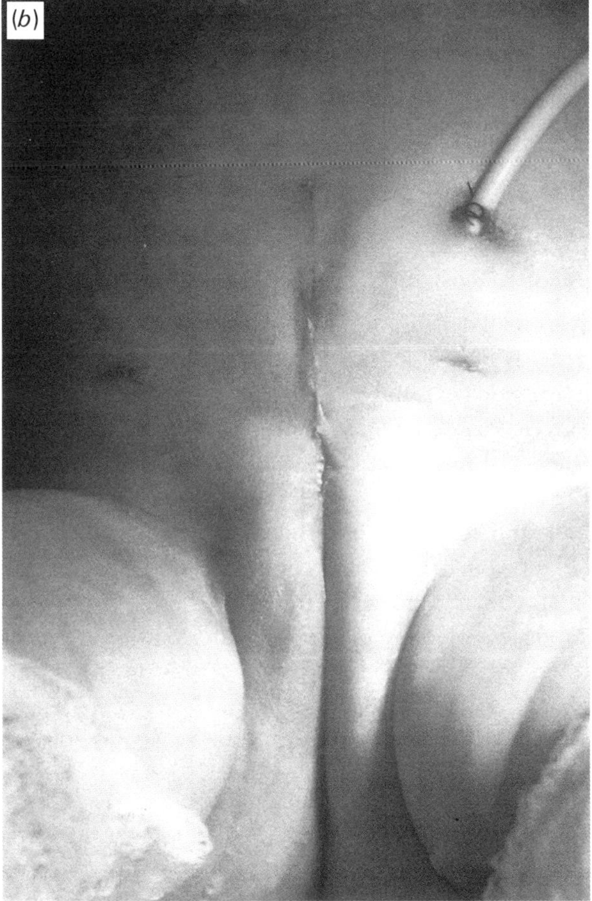

Figure 6.7 (*a*) Newborn female exstrophy patient; (*b*) 4 weeks after initial closure.

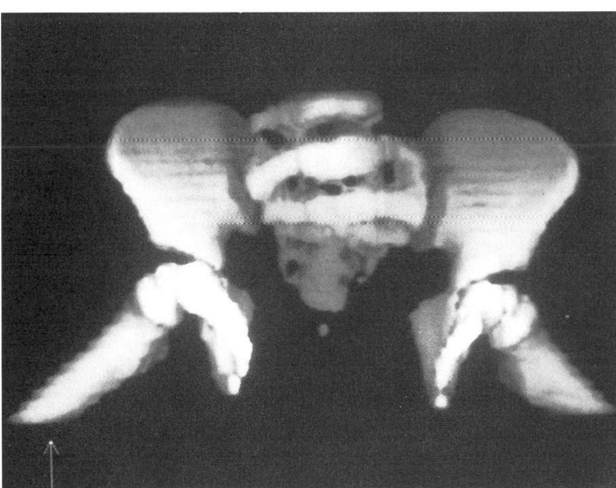

Figure 6.8 Three-dimensional CT reconstruction of a 5-year-old male with uncorrected classic bladder exstrophy showing a wide separation of the pubic bones and flattening of the ilial bones.

epispadias repair can lead to its own unique set of complications, including loss of the hemi-glans or glans, and hypospadias,[100] although either of these complications can potentially be seen after more traditional reconstruction.

Exstrophy reconstruction has led to a greater understanding of sphincter and pelvic floor anatomy and function. Patients have improved pelvic floor reconstruction and better continence rates after osteotomy.[101–104] This is likely to be due to better approximation of the pelvic floor muscle. In addition, there is a close relationship between bladder size and continence. In situations where capacity is inadequate, bladder augmentation, bladder neck closure, and a catheterizable stoma may provide the best alternative.[98]

Prune belly syndrome

Deficient abdominal wall musculature, cryptorchism, and urinary tract dilatation characterize this syndrome. Other names include triad syndrome, Eagle–Barrett syndrome, and abdominal muscular deficiency syndrome. The spectrum of this disease is wide. It ranges from in-utero demise, renal dysplasia and subsequent renal failure, to normal renal function. The pathogenesis is not completely understood.[105] The presumptive prenatal diagnosis has been made as early as 12 weeks' gestation.[106] In the most severe forms, identified antenatally, there is complete urethral obstruction. In the antenatal period these patients are often confused with patients who have severe PUV and may be inadvertently combined in retrospective reviews.[8] One terminated fetus had urethral atresia with histologically normal kidneys, which may mean that there is a role for intervention in cases identified very early.[107] The postnatal evaluation should include sonography, voiding cystourethrography (VCUG), and renal scan when indicated, though VCUG can be avoided to reduce the risk of early urinary tract infection. Although predominantly affecting males, a female variety has been described.[108] Initially, medical treatment (i.e. antibacterial prophylaxis and perhaps circumcision in babies with reflux) and close surveillance are indicated in all but the most severe cases where vesicostomy or upper tract diversion may be needed.[109–111] In the long term, a combination of continuous antibacterial prophylaxis, well-planned surgery, and close surveillance is the best means to ensure an optimal outcome.[110,112–115] Severity of the congenital renal dysplasia, nadir creatinine >0.7 mg/dl, recurrent pyelonephritis, and renal obstruction all correlate with eventual development of renal failure.[113,115] Treatment of the undescended testes should be similar to that recommended for other patients with abdominal testes. Early orchidopexy should be accomplished and may be facilitated by laparoscopy.[116] No prune belly patient has been known to father a child; however, early testis biopsy has identified spermatogonia, so fertility is possible using in-vitro fertilization.[117,118] The histologic findings of significantly reduced spermatogonia and marked Leydig cell hyperplasia suggest that the pathology of the testis in prune belly syndrome is secondary to more than just its abdominal location. Testis tumors have developed in these patients.[119–121]

Myelodysplasia

In the past myelodysplasia was the most common cause of neurogenic bladder dysfunction in children. Its incidence has been steadily decreasing because of early detection in the antenatal period resulting in termination of the pregnancy, and maternal folic acid treatment which markedly decreases the likelihood of developing spinal defects.[47,122–124] There is a slight increase in the incidence of myelodysplasia if other family members also have the condition.[125]

Open myelomeningoceles (Figure 6.9) are readily identifiable at birth. The level of the lesion does not correlate with the neurologic defect because some nerve roots may be left intact. An Arnold–Chiari

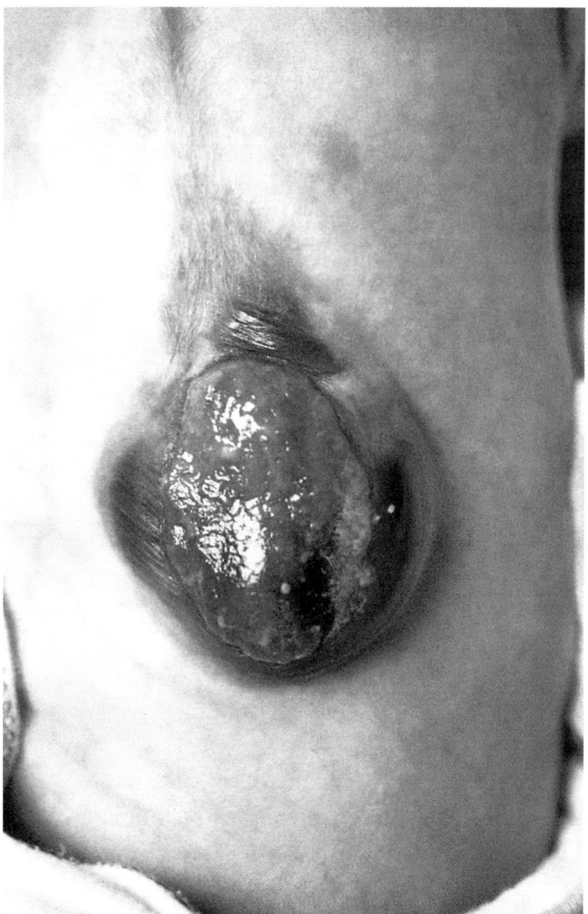

Figure 6.9 Newborn with myelomeningocele.

malformation can affect the brainstem and pontine micturition center. It is this malformation that is most likely to be prevented by fetal surgery. Tethering of the spinal cord and different growth rates in the distorted vertebral bodies can affect the final neurologic deficit.[126] Likewise, immediately after birth and during infancy and early childhood, a changing pattern is often seen in the urodynamics of these patients.[127–129] It is impossible to make broad generalizations, but in children with high thoracic lesions, patients may have an intact sacral reflex arc. Those with lesions at S1 and below can have normal bladder function but upper or lower motor lesions involving the bladder and/or pelvic floor are also seen. Complete urologic evaluation after closure of the defects including renal sonography, VCUG, and full urodynamic assessment is advisable because sphincter dyssynergia and uninhibited bladder contractions may be predictive of future upper tract deterioration.[127,130–133] Clear evidence exists that starting prophylactic treatment in situations where there is high risk for deterioration (uninhibited bladder contraction and elevated storage pressure in association with sphincter dyssynergy) is beneficial in decreasing the likelihood of upper tract and bladder deterioration.[134–136] Management usually involves initiation of clean intermittent catheterization (CIC) and anticholinergic medication. The dynamic nature of this disease requires routine surveillance throughout the patient's life, but particularly during periods of rapid linear growth, when spinal cord tethering may occur.[136,137]

Lipomeningocele

This abnormality is difficult to identify on physical examination. It is important to have a high level of suspicion and to examine the lower spine carefully because the vast majority of children with lipomeningocele have an identifiable superficial or cutaneous lesion. The neurologic changes occur because of an intradural lipoma. This lesion results in a broad spectrum of disease and presentation.[138] Typically, during early childhood, there are few outward physical abnormalities and only with complete urodynamic assessment is the effect on the bladder identified.[139] The most common urodynamic findings are consistent with an upper motor neuron lesion. Sphincter dyssynergy is less often identified in this group. In older children where the diagnosis has been delayed there are often neurologic changes in the lower extremities.[140] The bladder changes in the older group are mixed between detrusor hyperreflexia and detrusor areflexia. The best methods to identify and characterize these lesions are MRI and complete urodynamic assessment.[141]

Sacral agenesis

This lesion is even more difficult to identify on physical examination, and often the patient presents at an older age with failure to become continent.[142,143] Loss of the lower vertebral bodies can be easily seen on a lateral lower plain film of the spine or on an MRI study. White and Klauber[144] suggested that palpation of the coccyx could identify absent vertebral bodies, but radiographic confirmation is the best method. These patients have a stable neurologic lesion that does not progress with growth. However, the results of urodynamic studies are variable.[145] Patients may have no sign of denervation or hyperreflexia, areflexia, intact sphincter function, or sphincter dyssynergy, and some have absent control over the sphincter.[146] A high level of suspicion and complete urodynamics help to guide treatment.[142] Specific intervention is based on the identified findings.[143]

Scrotal masses

Palpation of a scrotal mass commonly results in an urgent consultation. When it is of an acute nature with pain, testicular torsion is the most important diagnosis to consider. This represents a true surgical emergency. It is best managed by early exploration, detorsion, and, when the testis is salvageable, fixation. If the testis is not salvageable it should be removed. In either instance, the contralateral testis should also be sutured to the scrotal wall.

The history should focus on the age of the patient, whether there is associated pain, and whether there is a history of trauma. The onset and severity of pain may be helpful in the differential diagnosis of torsion versus epididymitis. The physical examination should focus on identifying the location of the mass in relation to the testis. The orientation of the testis should be evaluated. Normally, the epididymis is posterior and lateral to the testis. Careful palpation will identify torsion of appendices such as the appendix testis, both anterior and superior appendices of the epididymis, and the hydatid of Morgagni that is located in the posterior inferior epididymal testicular ridge.[147] In non-acute masses, sonography is important to confirm the location and architecture of the mass. Possible scrotal masses are:

- hydrocele
- incarcerated hernia
- torsion of the testis
- appendage torsion
- testis tumor
- epididymitis
- epididymal cyst
- epididymal tumor
- paratesticular tumor
- varicocele
- Henoch–Schönlein purpura
- idiopathic edema
- cavernous hemangioma
- funiculitis
- lesions that result from a patent process vaginalis.

Neonatal scrotal masses

History plays very little role in the diagnosis in neonates.[148] The specific differential diagnosis of such masses includes:

- hydrocele
- incarcerated hernia
- torsion
- lesion secondary to patent processus vaginalis
- meconium
- testis tumors
- trauma.

The initial evaluation of these infants involves a complete physical examination. Perinatally, firm enlarged scrotal masses may be hydroceles but the diagnosis of bilateral torsion should be considered.[149] Positive transillumination can often aid the differential diagnosis. Occasionally a plain abdominal film may be helpful in identifying bowel gas in the scrotal mass that would indicate an inguinal hernia with bowel in the scrotum, or calcification suggesting old meconium. If the mass is associated with thickened cord structures or if it can be reduced, a hernia is also likely. Ultrasound examination can differentiate solid and cystic masses. Doppler ultrasound can often confirm blood flow, but can be misleading in the small child.

Prenatal testis torsion is also referred to as neonatal torsion, extravaginal, intrauterine torsion, antenatal torsion, perinatal torsion, and newborn torsion. There is controversy over the mechanism of the torsion, risk of bilaterality, and need for and timing of contralateral fixation.[150–152] When torsion occurs before delivery it has been thought to occur extravaginally, involving the entire spermatic cord and its tunics. Some physicians believe that this process can occur very early in the pregnancy and that it is responsible for most instances of testicular agenesis.[153–155] It is impossible to determine whether all cases are extravaginal and at least some probably represent intravaginal torsion, as seen in older boys. When torsion occurs prior to delivery the presentation is one of a non-tender, discolored, solid scrotal mass. Doppler ultrasound is generally accurate in confirming the diagnosis.[156–160] The torsion is most often unilateral but over 30 bilateral cases have been reported.[158,161,162] A strong case has been made for early exploration, with orchiectomy when the testis is necrotic, and contralateral fixation, as many examples of subsequent contralateral torsion have now been reported.[163–165] The arguments in favor of early exploration include: relative safety of anesthesia in the neonatal period; possibility of testicular salvage (10%), particularly the hormonal function; ability to fix the contralateral testis to prevent asynchronous torsion in the future; and to confirm the diagnosis.

Lesions that result from a patent processus vaginalis include meconium mass, hemoscrotum from intra-abdominal hemorrhage, and tumor seeding from renal or adrenal tumors.[166–170] Spontaneous rupture of the bowel can occur during fetal development, resulting in meconium peritonitis. If the processus vaginalis is still open at that time the meconium can fall into the scrotum and present as a solid mass at birth. Stippled calcification is usually present. Likewise, other anomalies such as adrenal hematomas, neuroblastoma, and Wilms' tumor can also seed the scrotum through a patent canal and should be considered in the differential diagnosis of neonatal scrotal masses. All of these suggest the utility of abdominal ultrasonography at discovery of the scrotal mass.

Testis tumors are also seen in the neonatal period but are rare (Table 6.3).[171] Yolk sac tumors, teratomas, gonadal stromal tumors and juvenile granulosa cell tumors are the most common. Early radical surgical removal is the recommended treatment for those with malignant potential, with chemotherapy in selected cases.

Pediatric scrotal masses

In older patients history plays a greater role in the differential diagnosis. Torsion has a bimodal distribution: in the perinatal period and at or before puberty.[172] When there is sudden onset of severe pain associated with nausea and scrotal swelling, torsion should be suspected and represents a true surgical emergency. On examination of the scrotum there is no spermatic cord swelling in acute torsion. The cremasteric reflex is generally absent, though this can be an inconsistent finding, and the testis is tense to palpation and rides high in the scrotum.[173] The epididymis will either not be palpable or is palpable in an abnormal location. Urinalysis is usually normal. Torsion is usually confirmed by surgical exploration; however, in centers with rapid access to color Doppler ultrasound the diagnosis can be confirmed before intervention.[174–176] In most cases history and physical examination are sufficient for diagnosis, and radiologic evaluation is only performed in those in whom the diagnosis is unlikely. Detorsion can take place prior to exploration by manually untwisting the involved testis. The most common direction of torsion is from lateral to medial (when viewing the scrotum from the patient's feet), so detorsion manually should be from medial to lateral (again viewing the scrotum from the patient's feet). If detorsion is unsuccessful, attempts in the other direction can be tried. Once the direction is determined, the testis will spin rapidly and complete resolution of pain confirms detorsion. The testis should still be fixed in place by suture to prevent recurrent torsion. Torsion in the pediatric period is usually intravaginal and secondary to a bell-clapper deformity. Torsion should be relieved within 4 hours to be certain of testis viability, but detorsion after 12 hours has resulted in viable testis tissue in some cases; by 24 hours there is almost uniform eventual atrophy if the testis is left in place.[177–179] Cases where there has been testicular salvage after longer periods probably represent intermittent or incomplete torsion. Spermatogonia appear to be more sensitive to ischemia then the Sertoli and Leydig cells.[180] Since the bell-clapper deformity can affect both testes, the contralateral testis should be fixed at the time that the involved testis is explored. In a typical pediatric emergency room, 16% of the patients who present with an acute scrotum will have testis torsion, 46% will have torsion of an appendix of the testis, 35% will be identified as epididymitis, and the remainder are other lesions.[181] It appears that treatment with human chorionic gonadotropin (hCG) may occasionally induce torsion in the undescended testes[182] (Figure 6.10).

Epididymitis should also be considered in boys with acute scrotal pain. It usually presents as scrotal swelling with gradually increasing pain. Physical examination isolates pain to the epididymis. The cremasteric reflex is often intact.[183] Elevation of the testis may improve the pain (Prehn's sign). When pyuria is present, this supports the diagnosis, but in children it is often not present. Sonography shows a hyperemic swollen epididymis.[184] The causes of epididymitis include trauma, infection, or reflux of sterile urine. Since the cause may not be identified at diagnosis, treatment should include scrotal elevation, bed rest, antibiotics if the urinalysis is positive, and an anti-inflammatory medication. In sexually active teenagers possible *Chlamydia trachomatis* infection should be treated, and in non-sexually active children treatment

Table 6.3 Neonatal testicular tumors

Tumor	Frequency (%)
Yolk sac	27
Gonadal stromal tumors	27
Juvenile granulosa cell tumors	27
Gonadal blastoma	9
Teratoma	5
Harmartoma	5

Adapted from Levy et al.[171]

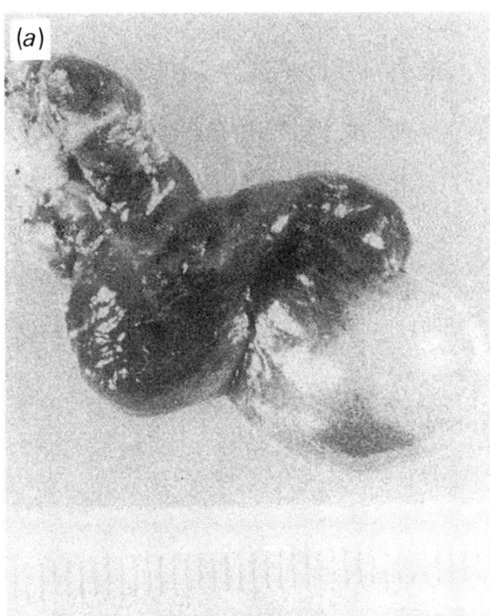
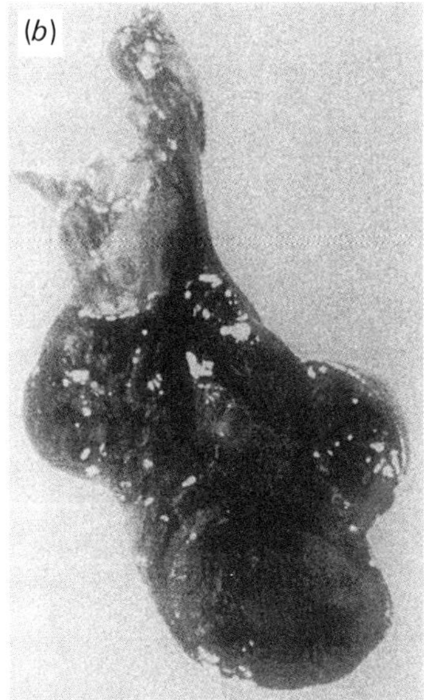

Figure 6.10 Infarcted testes and spermatic cord after treatment with hCG: (*a*) external appearance; (*b*) longitudinal sections. (From Sawchuk et al,[182] with permission.)

should be directed toward *Escherichia coli*. In boys with proven bacterial epididymitis there is a high probability of an anatomic abnormality. After treatment, full examination of the upper and lower urinary tract should be accomplished with ultrasound and a VCUG.[181]

Pediatric scrotal tumors are rare and include primary testis lesions, paratesticular tumors, and metastatic or lymphatic tumors:[185]

- mature teratoma
- teratocarcinoma
- yolk sac tumor
- paratesticular rhabdomyosarcoma
- gonadal stromal tumors
- granulosa cell tumors
- cavernous hemangioma
- gonadoblastoma
- metastatic tumors.

Ultrasound is helpful in locating the origin of these lesions but the diagnosis is made by surgical exploration through a groin incision. It is inadvisable to explore tumors through a scrotal incision because such intervention can theoretically change the direction of lymphatic spread of the tumor, though there is little evidence that this actually happens. Once the tumor is removed, pathologic evaluation determines the diagnosis. A combination of surgery, chemotherapy, and radiation has resulted in a high cure rate.[107,171] Benign testis lesions in prepubertal children can be removed by partial orchiectomy, avoiding loss of the entire testis.

Another scrotal lesion that may present as a scrotal mass is a varicocele. It is usually left sided and disappears when the patient lies flat. Intervention is indicated if it is associated with ipsilateral testicular growth failure. Other intrascrotal lesions are extremely rare, usually benign, and identified by history, physical examination, ultrasound, and biopsy[185–187] (Figure 6.11). The more common superficial lesions such as funiculitis and idiopathic edema should be considered when the scrotal contents are normal (Figure 6.12).

Intersex disorders

A consultation for ambiguous genitalia is one of the urgent problems that a urologist must face. The initial approach to managing intersex patients is to identify and treat possible life-threatening abnormalities.[188–190] In most instances sexual assignment is straightforward, and, where it is not, consideration should be given to delaying the decision to intervene surgically until the infant is older[189,191] (see Chapter 58).

CAH is the most common cause of ambiguous genitalia at birth. It is the only form of intersex that can be life threatening. The possible enzyme deficiencies include 21-hydroxylase, 11β-hydroxylase, 20,22-desmolase, and 3β-hydroxysteroid dehydrogenase. In 21-hydroxylase deficiency, lack of mineralocorticoid and glucocorticoid cause an electrolyte imbalance resulting in elevated serum potassium and low sodium that lead to dehydration or potentially lethal cardiac arrhythmias. The excess androstenedione that

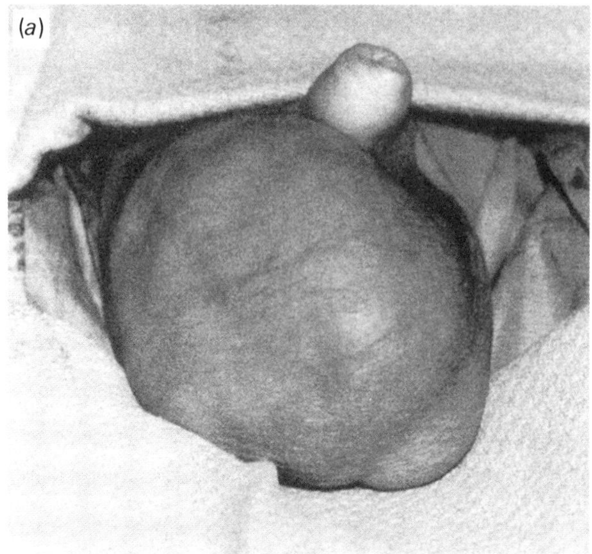

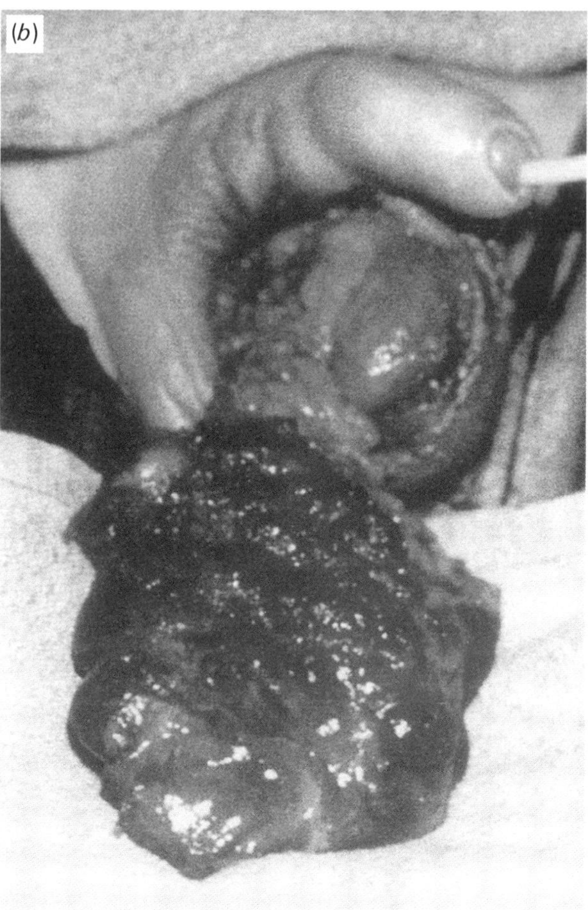

Figure 6.11 (*a*) Preoperative picture of scrotal cavernous hemangioma; (*b*) intraoperative picture of a cavernous hemangioma.

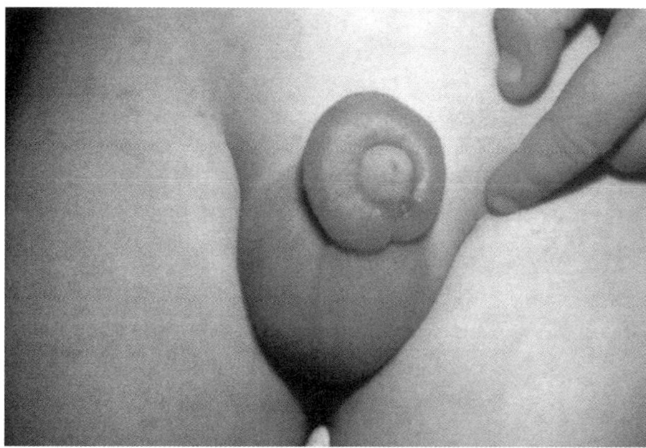

Figure 6.12 Idiopathic edema.

builds up behind the enzymatic block metabolizes to testosterone and dihydrotestosterone, causing virilization of the female infant (Figure 6.13). Physical examination and screening laboratory studies facilitate the differential diagnosis relatively rapidly. The infant will have varying degrees of masculinization, from hypertrophy of the clitoris and mild labioscrotal development to a normal-appearing male phallus and scrotum. The gonads are symmetrical and typically non-palpable. The Barr body is positive, and pelvic sonography identifies a uterus and ovaries. Müllerian inhibiting substance is undetectable, and the chromosome evaluation is 46,XX. Serum studies should include electrolytes, glucose, gonadotropin, dihydrotestosterone, testosterone, and adrenal steroid levels. Initial treatment involves glucocorticoid and mineralocorticoid replacement. It is strongly recommended that these patients be reared as female because of the chromosomal sex and potential fertility, but in the most virilized form questions have arisen as to the best sex of rearing.[192,193]

Although CAH is the most common intersex disorder, it is important to have a diagnostic plan for evaluating all intersex patients. The differential diagnosis method used by the authors is based on history, chromosome determination, serum tests, screening radiological studies, and pathology (Figure 6.14).

The initial history should focus on pedigree and

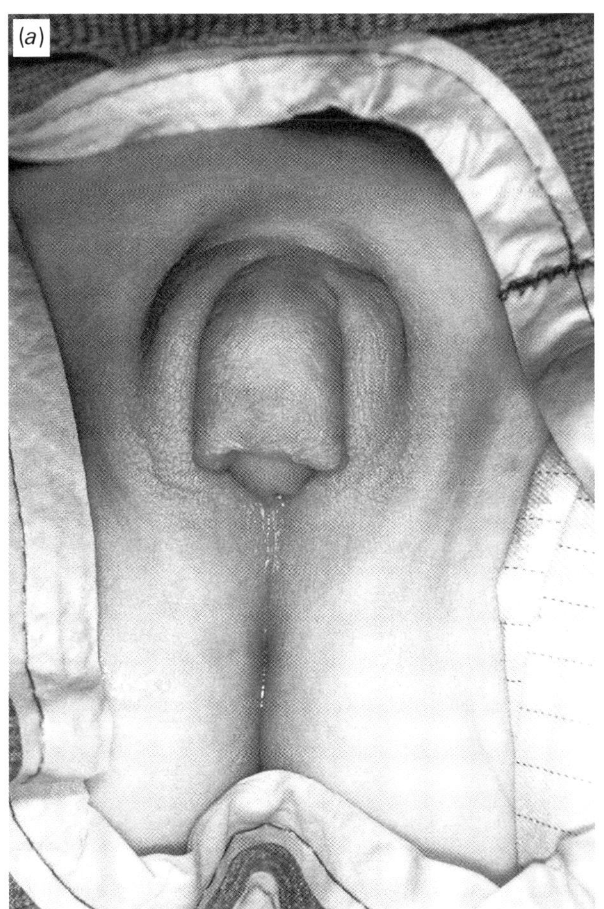

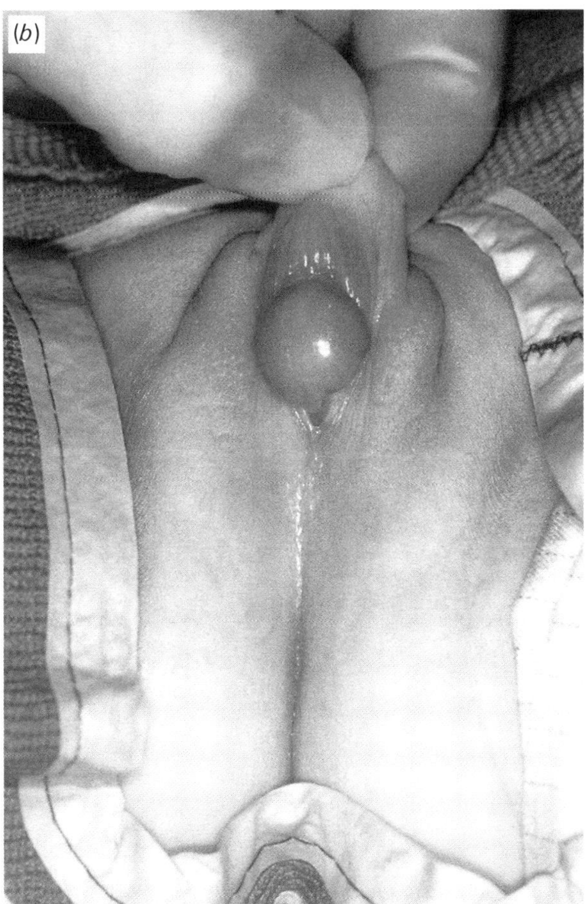

Figure 6.13 Severely androgenized patient with congenital adrenal hyperplasia.

drug ingestion history. Physical examination should concentrate on palpating the gonads. If no gonads can be palpated in the masculinized baby, one should consider female pseudohermaphroditism (FPH), gonadal dysgenesis (GD), male pseudohermaphroditism (MPH), and true hermaphroditism (TH). When only one gonad is palpable one should consider mixed gonadal dysgenesis (MGD), TH and MPH. When both gonads are palpated one should consider MPH and rarely TH. The next step involves targeted laboratory and radiologic screening. Initial evaluation should include measuring serum electrolytes, 17-hydroxyprogesterone, testosterone and dihydrotestosterone (DHT) levels, and determining karyotype. Screening sonography and genitography in appropriate situations are helpful in the evaluation.

When 17-hydroxyprogesterone is elevated, the karyotype is 46,XX, and a uterus is identified by ultrasound, one is dealing with CAH. Checking the 11-deoxycortisol levels can differentiate between 21α-hydroxylase and 11β-hydroxylase deficiency. If the 17-hydroxyprogesterone levels are normal and a uterus and ovaries are identified in a child with a 46,XX karyotype, a maternal virilizing syndrome should be considered.

In the remainder of cases, 17-hydroxyprogesterone will not be elevated. A combination of ultrasound findings and laparoscopy with or without biopsy is often required to make a definitive diagnosis. If two testes are identified, an hCG stimulation test should be performed. Serum testosterone, DHT, dehydroepiandrosterone (DHEA) and androstenedione should be measured before and after stimulation. This will identify MPH (46,XY, 46,XX, 45,X/46,XY). There are a number of causes of MPH, including testicular failure, dysgenetic testes, steroid deficiency secondary to male CAH, complete androgen insensitivity syndrome, and 5α-reductase deficiency.

When laparoscopy and biopsy identify a streak gonad, one should consider gonadal dysgenesis, which is pure gonadal dysgenesis with both gonads represented as streaks (45,X, 45,X/46,XX, 45,X/46,XY), or mixed gonadal dysgenesis with a streak gonad and testis (45,X/46,XY, 46,XY). In cases with both a testis and ovary or ovotestes, one should consider true hermaphroditism (46,XX, 46,XX/XY, 46,XY).

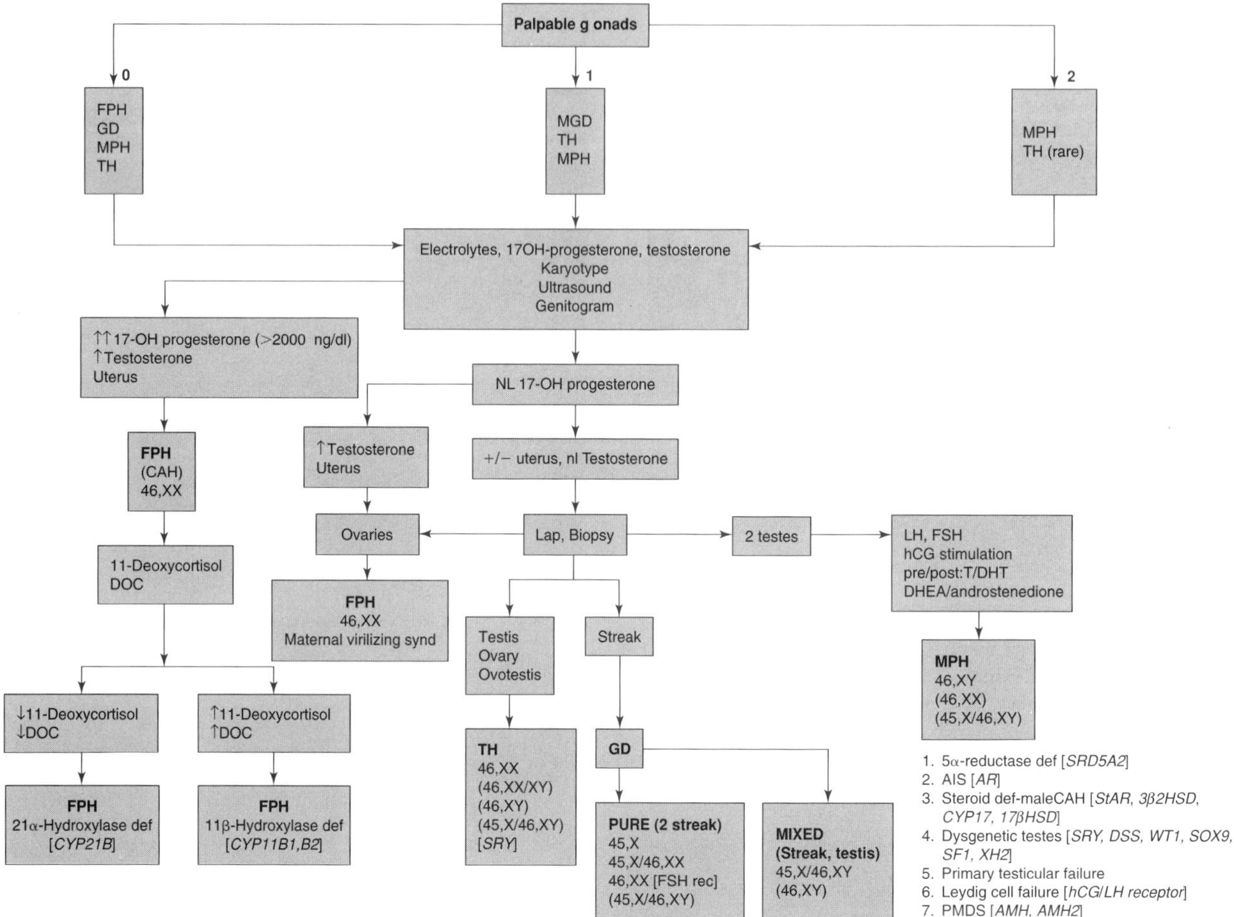

Figure 6.14 Differential diagnosis of intersex disorders. (Adapted from flow diagram presented to the Society for Fetal Urology in 1999 by Thomas Kolon MD.) (FPH = female pseudohermaphroditism; GD = gonadal dysgenesis; MPH = male pseudohermaphroditism; TH = true hermaphroditism; MGD = mixed gonadal dysgenesis; CAH = congenital adrenal hyperplasia; AIS = androgen insensitivity syndrome; PMDS = persistent Müllerian duct syndrome; genes are in italics (uncommon karyotypes in square brackets).

Posterior urethral valves and lower urinary tract abnormalities

This cause of lower urinary tract obstruction is now commonly diagnosed presumptively in the antenatal period. Previously, infants presented with failure to thrive, an abdominal mass, or urosepsis.[194] Common antenatal ultrasound findings include a distended thick-walled bladder, bilateral hydronephrosis, and oligohydramnios in some cases.[19,194,195] Although the outcomes of patients diagnosed antenatally may be worse than those diagnosed postnatally, this is indicative of a greater severity of disease and should not be taken to mean that antenatal diagnoses will not improve outcome in these patients.[196]

There is significant variability in the treatment of infants with PUV. Appropriate treatment is usually determined based on the overall medical condition of the infant, including renal function, hydrational status, presence of infection and lung maturity, as well as caliber of the urethra. In general, some basic tenets are applicable to most cases. Catheter drainage of the bladder will allow decompression of the urinary tract and prophylactic antibiotics should be initiated at birth. Initial measures of renal function are reflective of the mother's kidney function; therefore, catheter drainage should be maintained until the nadir creatinine is reached.[197–200] If the creatinine falls below 1 mg/dl, valve ablation with pediatric endoscopic equipment should be performed, after which careful monitoring of renal function, bladder function, and reflux should be continued while the child remains on antibiotic prophylaxis.[201,202]

Infants whose renal function does not substantially improve pose a much more difficult management problem. In these patients minimizing intrarenal pressure may have a positive effect on renal function. These patients may have either low or high urinary diversion.[197,198,203,204] Whereas upper tract diversion was commonly used in the past, vesicostomy is usually the initial step to decompress these kidneys. Upper tract diversion does not appear to have an adverse effect on bladder function.[205] Consideration to upper tract diversion may be given in severe cases in order to minimize intrapelvic pressures and in those with urinary infection, as this optimizes renal drainage. However, little evidence exists that upper tract diversion really helps, unless infection has been present, and it complicates subsequent reconstruction. Long-term outcome in these patients depends essentially on the degree of renal damage and on bladder function.[196,206] Older children may require anticholinergics and/or bladder augmentation for the 'valve bladder' with high storage pressures. Reimplantation to correct reflux may be necessary: The worst cases come to dialysis and eventual transplantation.

An ectopic ureterocele can present as an obstructing lesion at the bladder neck. This condition occurs with a female prevalence of approximately 3–4:1.[207–209] Cases in which the ureterocele creates a ball-valve obstructive mechanism have been reported and these have been detected antenatally.[209] Bilateral ureteroceles have also been diagnosed by ultrasound prior to birth. In general, these patients are managed initially by transurethral incision[210–214] (Figure 6.15). Once stabilized, they undergo final management, which may include treatment of reflux, excision of the ureterocele, and in some cases upper pole nephrectomy and ureterectomy.[207] As in all cases of lower urinary tract obstruction, treatment of long-term bladder dysfunction may be required. Infection is another indication for ureterocele incision.

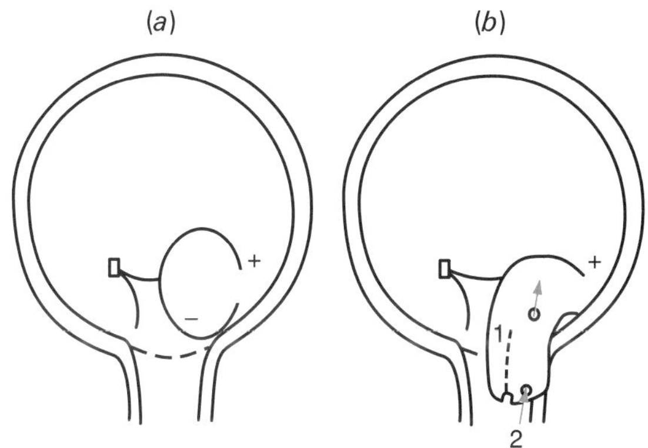

Figure 6.15 Technique for incision of ureteroceles: (*a*) incision for an intravesical ureterocele; (*b*) techniques for an ectopic ureterocele: (1) incising proximally, (2) puncturing urethal and intravesical segments separately. (From Blyth et al,[210] with permission.)

VUR can be the cause of the upper tract dilatation in as many as 35% of children with antenatal hydronephrosis.[67] Recent reviews suggest that this is less likely in African–Americans and more common in males than females[215,216] but all should be screened. Children with dilated upper tracts should have a VCUG to rule out reflux prior to treatment for other urinary tract abnormalities.[217]

Circumcision injuries

Circumcision is the most common surgical procedure performed in the USA, with approximately 600 000 to 700 000 operations performed annually.[218] A recent report suggests that circumcision rates are actually increasing in the USA. It was estimated in the period 1988–1991 ~48% of newborns underwent neonatal circumcision versus ~61% in the period 1997–2000.[219] Absolute indications for neonatal circumcisions are few.[220,221] In neonates with prenatally detected hydronephrosis, especially when reflux is identified, circumcision may be recommended because it decreases the likelihood of an early urinary tract infection (UTI).[67,222,223] Reports demonstrating a marked change in the periurethral and glanular bacterial flora in boys after circumcision support this practice.[224] Indications for circumcision in older children include persistent phimosis, paraphimosis, and recurrent balanitis. A viable alternative to circumcision in infants and older children is the use of steroid cream.[225,226] This is typically accomplished by applying 0.05% betamethasone cream to the prepuce twice daily for 4 weeks. Success rates of roughly 70–90% have been reported. Paraphimosis is best treated by pressure on the edemetous preputial skin and reduction of the paraphimotic skin. If the glans cannot be replaced, a dorsal slit incision in the phimotic skin allows reduction. Circumcision in infants with known bleeding disorders, hypospadias, and congenital anomalies of the penis, buried penis, or prematurity should be delayed to a later date.[227]

Complications of circumcisions are infrequent, occurring in 0.2–3%.[228]

1 Early acute complications:
   - bleeding
   - infection
   - laceration
   - amputation, usually partial
   - urinary retention

- skin loss
- necrosis, sometimes due to overuse of cautery.

2 Non-acute complications:
- skin excess
- skin asymmetry
- skin bridges
- skin chordee
- epidermal inclusion cysts
- concealed (buried) penis
- phimosis
- meatal stenosis
- urethrocutaneous fistula
- circumcision despite hypospadias, removing skin needed for repair
- plastibell specific
- lymphedema.

The majority of circumcision complications are minor.[229–236] The incidence of complications is probably higher than reported in the urologic literature since many are treated without referral and some do not present until the patient is much older. Complications are best prevented by strict attention to the details of the procedure, which include sterile technique, hemostasis, protection of the glans, and removing the appropriate amount of inner and outer preputial skin.[237–239] Certain anatomic variations may predispose to complications during neonatal circumcision. Caruso et al suggested that a prominent fat pad, penoscrotal webbing, or prematurity are associated with a higher incidence of circumcision complications.[240] When complications occur, immediate attention and treatment is the best management.[241–245] Bleeding is best managed by pressure, placing an absorbable stitch, or with electrocautery, though electrocautery should never be used with a metallic clamp device in place because of the risk of penile necrosis. Most of the cases that require immediate repair involve laceration or amputation of a portion of the glans (Figure 6.16). Commonly, these result from a circumcision done using a Mogen clamp placed at an angle incorporating the frenulum which draws up the glans into the clamp.[243] If the amputated portion of the glans can be retrieved it can be reapproximated with absorbable sutures. When amputation occurs, the amputated portion of the glans should be wrapped sterilely and kept cool on ice, but not submerged in saline. In most instances it can be reattached utilizing long-lasting absorbable sutures (i.e. PDS).[242,243,245,246] Amputation of a portion of the penis involving the urethra should also be repaired by immediate reconstruction. Results are best if reapproximation occurs within hours of the injury; however, successful reapproximation after delays of up to 18 hours have been reported.[247] Most urethral injuries should have a staged reconstruction, although fistulae can be closed immediately if recognized.[244]

Penile skin loss as a result of circumcision can usually be managed conservatively by application of antibiotic impregnated gauze. Ingrowth of skin usually results in a good cosmetic appearance. Skin grafting is rarely necessary. Sometimes an apparently normal penis with a complete circumferential prepuce is found to have a hypospadiac meatus when the skin

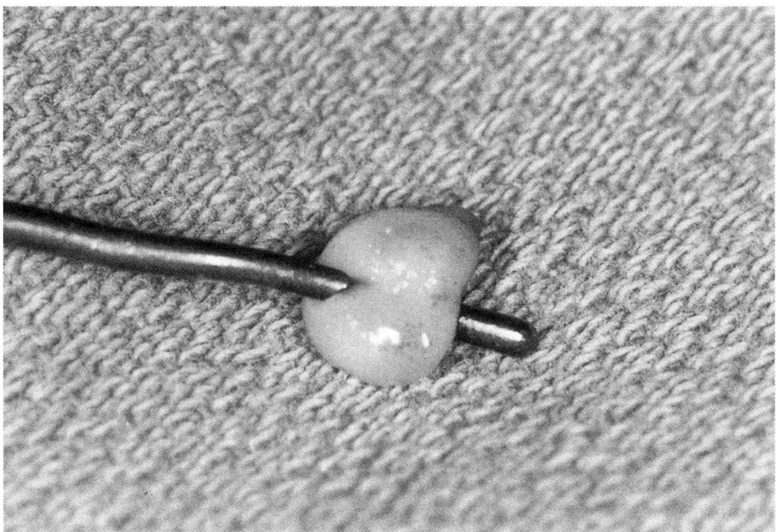

Figure 6.16 Amputation of the distal portion of the glans shown with urethra intubated. This was successfully reattached.

is incised or retracted. This rare form of hypospadias is called megameatus with intact prepuce. The circumcision should be discontinued and any remaining skin left attached for possible later use in hypospadias repair. Plastibell circumcisions have their own specific complications, including a higher incidence of delayed wound infections and retained plastic cuff. Concealed or buried penis can result when the glans penis recedes below the circumcision scar and the scar then contracts[248] due to insufficient removal of inner prepuce.

Recently, much emphasis has been placed on the appropriate form of analgesia for circumcision. The best method of providing a penile block is with a ring block using lidocaine.[249–253] Single injection on the dorsum is the next best approach. EMLA cream requires a prolonged exposure to provide deep superficial analgesia[254] and often results in moderate preputial edema; consequently, it has not been the authors' method of choice.[255] A recent double-blinded study has suggested that EMLA cream can provide equivalent analgesia to a bupivacaine dorsal penile block without complications, suggesting that this is a reasonable alternative.[256]

Abdominal masses in the infant

The neonate presenting with an abdominal mass is of particular importance to the pediatric urologist because the majority of such lesions arise in the retroperitoneum in general and the kidney specifically.[257,258] Traditionally, they presented with a palpable mass. Although some still present this way, masses are far more likely to be detected by prenatal sonography. At the time of presentation to the urologist most have already been categorized as solid, cystic, or hydronephrotic. The urologist must be familiar with the masses that originate from the genitourinary tract as well as the following broad spectrum of other potential etiologies:

1. Hydronephrotic and cystic lesions:
   - hydronephrosis
   - multicystic dysplastic kidney
   - cystic nephroma
   - autosomal recessive polycystic kidney disease
   - autosomal dominant polycystic kidney disease.
2. Midline-pelvic cystic lesions:
   - hydrometrocolpos
   - ovarian cyst
   - distended bladder
   - urinary ascites.
3. Solid lesions:
   - neuroblastoma
   - congenital mesoblastic nephroma
   - Wilms' tumor
   - rhabdoid tumor
   - clear cell sarcoma
   - angiomyolipoma
   - ossifying tumor of the kidney
   - renal vein thrombosis
   - renal artery thrombosis
   - adrenal hemorrhage.
4. Non-genitourinary lesions:
   - pulmonary sequestration
   - hepatic lesions
   - gastrointestinal lesions
   - germ cell tumors
   - sarcoma
   - sacrococcygeal teratoma.

Figure 6.17 provides a flow diagram that outlines the general framework used to evaluate the lesions identified antenatally. The evaluation of an infant with a mass often becomes a continuation of the evaluation that began prenatally. It is important to note that neonates with masses represent a diagnostic emergency for both parent and referring physician, but rarely do they require emergency surgery and prenatal intervention is almost never indicated.

Hydronephrotic lesions

Ureteropelvic junction (UPJ) obstruction causing hydronephrosis remains one of the most common causes of an abdominal mass in the neonate.[259] The diagnosis is almost always made by prenatal ultrasound.[260] Significant hydronephrosis has an incidence of approximately 1:600 infants; however, hydronephrosis causing an abdominal mass is much less common.[261] Barring the development of oligohydramnios or anhydramnios, most fetuses are observed until term delivery. UPJ obstruction is usually unilateral but can be bilateral in up to 20–40% of cases.[262]

Postnatal management includes prophylactic antibiotics and postnatal sonography. The authors typically wait 48 hours after birth to perform sonography to minimize the incidence of false-negative studies, although the data suggest that this traditional delay is unnecessary.[263] Clearly in the face of a neonate with a mass no delay is warranted. If hydronephrosis is detected and no ureter is visualized, the presumed diagnosis of UPJ is made. A VCUG will exclude the possibility of ipsilateral or contralateral reflux. This test should be performed before any intervention is considered. To establish the diagnosis,

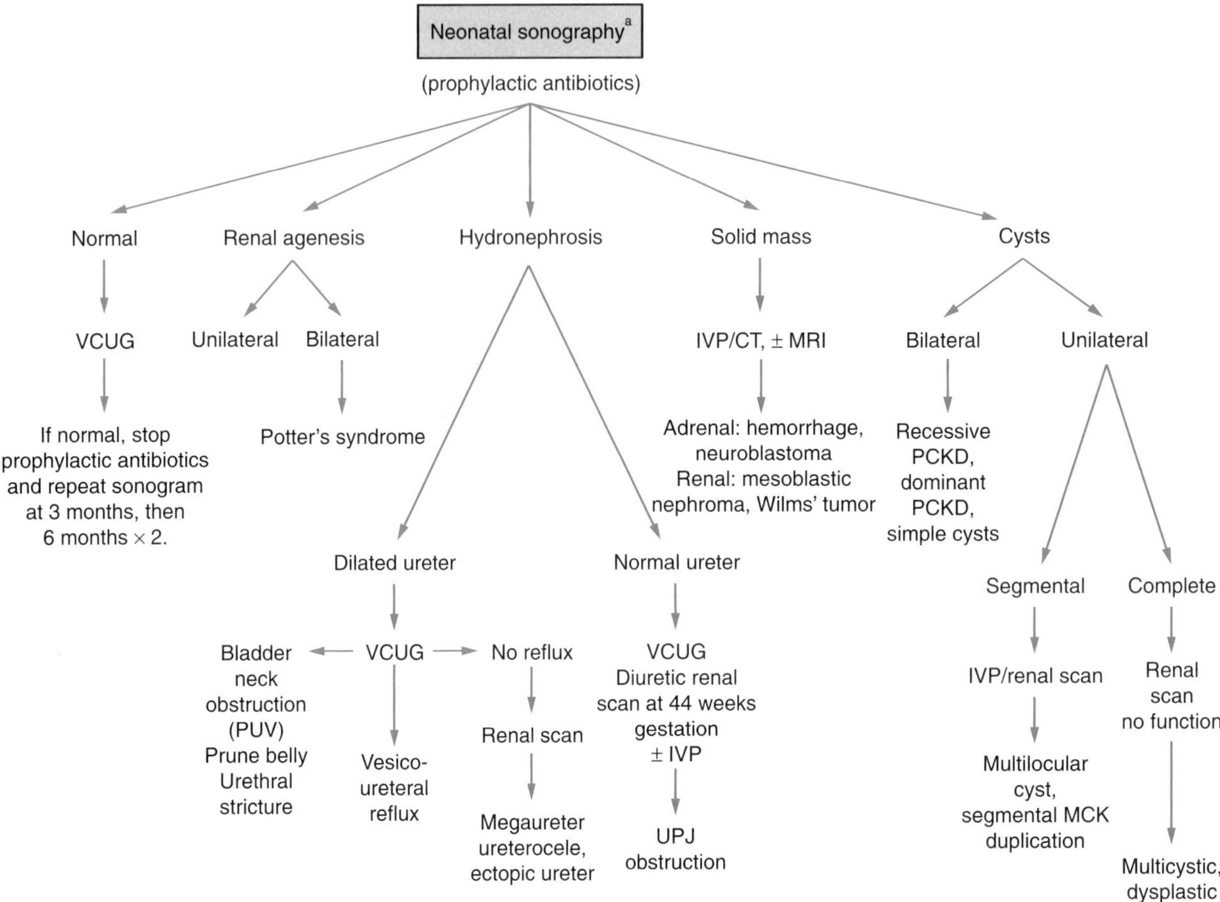

[a](1) Unilateral hydronephrotic and cystic lesions can be evaluated as an outpatient.
(2) Bilateral lesions should be evaluated prior to discharge.
(3) Masses should be evaluated prior to discharge.

Figure 6.17 Postnatal flow diagram. (VCUG = voiding cystourethrography; IVP = intravenous pyelogram; CT = computed tomography; MRI = magnetic resonance imaging; PCKD = polycystic kidney disease; PUV = posterior urethal valves; UPJ = ureteropelvic obstruction.)

a well-tempered renogram is performed. When performing Lasix (furosemide) renograms it is important to optimize the study by following an accepted protocol and ensuring that the infant is well hydrated.[264,265] Prophylactic antibiotics are discontinued when reflux and obstruction are excluded.

In cases where it is believed that the obstructed kidney may have minimal function, proceeding with evaluation and treatment earlier is often indicated because the neonatal kidney has significant ability to regain function. When presentation involves an abdominal mass from massive hydronephrosis, evaluation of viable renal parenchyma is difficult. In these cases a period of percutaneous drainage followed by nuclear scintigraphy to evaluate function may reveal a salvageable renal unit. A biopsy at the time of surgical correction has the best predictive value with regard to future renal function (Figure 6.18).[266] If no function is present on the renal scan the diagnosis of multicystic dysplastic kidney (MCDK) must be considered.

Treatment of the UPJ depends on the degree of obstruction and whether the lesion is unilateral or bilateral.[267] Clearly, children with significant bilateral obstruction require early intervention. Since surgical repair of UPJ in infants does not have a higher complication rate than in larger children, age does not affect the decision to intervene surgically.[268]

Renal cystic lesions

Increasingly, cystic mass lesions in the neonatal period are detected antenatally by sonography. In evaluating these lesions it is useful to divide them into

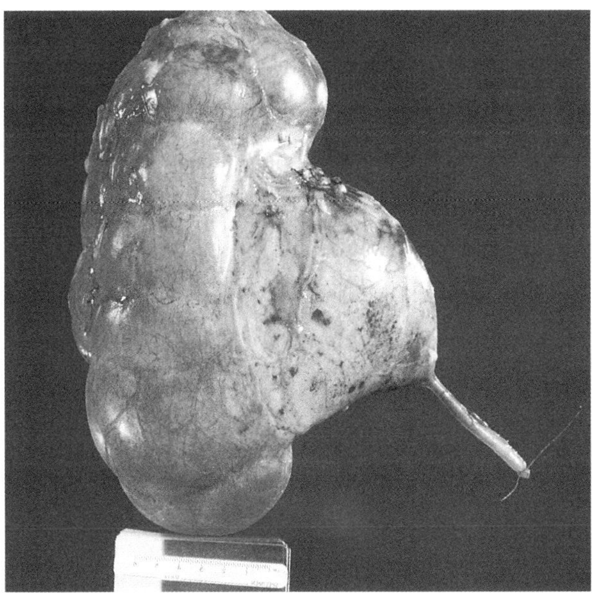

Figure 6.18 End-stage ureteropelvic junction obstruction showing how the dilated calices can mimic cystic structures.

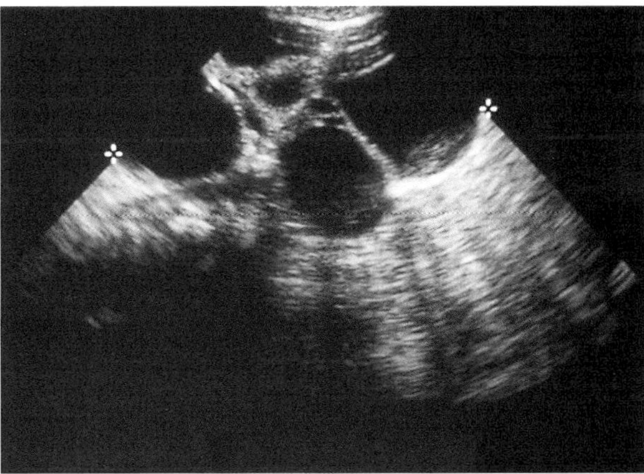

Figure 6.19 Sonogram of multicystic dysplastic kidney. (From Anthony Balcom, Milwaukee, WI, with permission.)

unilateral and bilateral categories. This allows a natural division of diagnostic possibilities.[269] Most lesions are detected antenatally but do not require intervention or further evaluation until after birth.

Unilateral lesions

MCDK is the second most common cause of an abdominal mass in infants.[270] Usually the mass is unilateral and may be palpable as a multilobular 'cluster of grapes' that transilluminates. These lesions may be quite large and can impede normal feeding because of compression of the stomach; alternatively, they may impinge on the diaphragm and affect respiration. Importantly, this lesion has a high incidence of associated contralateral renal abnormalities. Contralateral lesions are seen in upwards of 25% of these children.[271,272] The two most common kidney lesions are UPJ obstruction and contralateral VUR. Miller et al[273] recently reported an incidence of contralateral VUR of 26.4%. The majority (89%) of the VUR was low grade (I or II). The majority of the cases underwent spontaneous resolution. While US evaluation of the contralateral kidney should be performed, the need for a VCUG in cases where the contralateral kidney is normal by sonography is controversial.

Diagnosis of MCDK is usually made postnatally with a sonogram, which shows a multiloculated mass with little parenchyma (Figure 6.19). The cysts are generally non-connected. When the cysts appear to be connected, the diagnosis of severe UPJ obstruction should be entertained. Although there are reports of familial lesion, most are sporadic and familial screening in the absence of a significant familial history is not warranted.[274] The diagnosis is confirmed with a dimercaptosuccinic acid (DMSA) scan that demonstrates no function of the affected side. Contralateral imaging with sonography to rule out obstruction or bilateral MCDK is mandatory. Ureteral atresia is associated with a higher incidence of contralateral abnormalities than is renal pelvic atresia.[275]

Whereas previously nephrectomy was commonly performed, today serial sonography is the standard. Multicystic kidneys typically regress.[276,277] To date no reliable predictive features of regression have been identified, with the possible exception of initial size <62 mm.[278] Rare reports of malignancy have led some to suggest that these lesions should be removed if they persist, and only lesions that involute be managed non-operatively.[279,280] More recently, it is recognized that the likelihood of malignancy is extremely rare.[281] Rarely, lesions that compromise respiration or feeding, or are associated with hypertension, should also be excised.[282]

Bilateral cystic lesions

Autosomal recessive polycystic kidney disease (ARPKD) is an inherited nephropathy with an overall incidence of approximately 1:20 000 and presents with varying degrees of severity.[283] Children present with massively enlarged kidneys that are typically seen on antenatal or postnatal sonograms as homogeneously hyperechogenic. In severe cases oligohydramnios and Potter's facies may be present. The sonographic pattern is sufficiently different from that of MCDK and autosomal dominant polycystic kidney disease (ADPKD) to distinguish reliably between these. Pathologically the kidneys of these children exhibit ectasia and cystic dilatation of the collecting tubules. Associated conditions include pulmonary hypoplasia and hepatic fibrosis, which both contribute significantly to morbidity. Abnormalities of the the ARPKD gene, *PKHD1*, are responsible for this disease. Prognosis for these children depends on the spectrum of their disease, but is generally poor, with those surviving the neonatal period requiring hemodialysis and transplantation.[284] Up to 30% of children die as neonates, with 20–45% progressing to end-stage renal disease by age 15.[285]

ADPKD has an incidence of 1 in 500 to 1 in 1000 births, and two gene sequences on chromosome 16 (*PKD1*) and chromosome 4 (*PKD2*) have been associated with this disorder.[286,287] Approximately, 85% of cases are related to an abnormality of *PKD1*.[288] A third locus, *PKD3*, has been proposed but remains unidentified.[288] Although formerly called 'adult' polycystic kidney disease, this name is inaccurate as the condition has been identified in children. Patients with this disease may be diagnosed by prenatal sonogram. Sonography is also the primary modality used to screen potentially affected siblings.[289] Infants born with this disorder often have massive renomegaly and severely affected infants have poor survival. It is important to remember that in children the disease may initially present unilaterally or with asymmetry. A meta-analysis of the cases identified in utero revealed that 43% of cases died before the first year of life and a significant proportion (67%) developed hypertension by age 3.[290] Children who do not present in the neonatal period often come to attention later in life with hypertension, impaired renal function, proteinuria, or hematuria. Associated conditions include hepatic and pancreatic cysts as well as cerebral aneurysms. Although the outlook for these patients is improving, a significant number eventually develop renal failure.[291]

Midline cystic abdominal lesions

As with UPJ and MCDK, modern ultrasonography has greatly facilitated the diagnosis of other less common cystic abdominal masses in infants. Previously, children would often undergo laparotomy to establish such a diagnosis.

Hydrometrocolpos refers to the distention of the vagina with mucus and blood derived from uterine and cervical glands. Produced in response to maternal estrogens, it results from vaginal obstruction secondary to imperforate hymen or other obstructive vaginal anomalies such as transverse vaginal septum, or vaginal atresia.[292] In patients with a mid or high transverse septum or vaginal agenesis, a thorough search for associated genitourinary and gastrointestinal abnormalies should be performed.[293] It most commonly presents as a midline abdominal mass and/or an interlabial mass in the perineum, which is the bulging imperforate hymen. The diagnosis has also been made on antenatal sonography.[294,295] Careful physical examination will show that the mass is anterior to the rectum. Sonography will indicate that the lesion is behind the bladder. A common finding in these patients is lower urinary tract obstruction and hydronephrosis.[296] Once the diagnosis is made, incision of the hymen and drainage result in resolution of the mass. Hydronephrosis then usually resolves with time. Care must be taken because simple percutaneous drainage may result in reaccumulation of secretions within the vagina. Serial ultrasonography should be performed to ensure that the hydronephrosis resolves. Other causes of an interlabial mass in a newborn infant include hydro(metro)colpos, prolapsed urethra, prolapsed ureterocele, and paraurethral cyst.

Ovarian cysts are the third most common cause of an intra-abdominal mass in an infant, after renal and gastrointestinal causes. They may exist in up to 30% of neonates.[297] This diagnosis has been made prenatally by ultrasound as well as postnatally.[298] The classic prenatal sonographic appearance is that of an anechoic, unilocular mass in the fetal pelvis. Any internal echogenicity suggests cyst torsion or hemorrhage.[297] The majority of cysts regress and only require observation. Large cysts may compromise bowel or respiratory function. Adnexal torsion in females followed by cystic degeneration of the ovary may occur. This situation is typically managed by excision of the cystic mass (Figure 6.20). This can be accomplished by open surgery or may be achieved laparoscopically, even in infants[299] (Figure 6.21) .

Dilation of the urinary bladder or megacystis can also result in an abdominal mass. It is most typically associated with posterior urethral valves in male infants. The classic US findings include a dilated, thickened bladder and a dilated posterior urethra ('keyhole sign'). Other potential causes include urethral atresia, megacystis-microcolon syndrome, prune belly syndrome, and ureterocele obstructing the bladder outlet. Neonatal urinary ascites previously

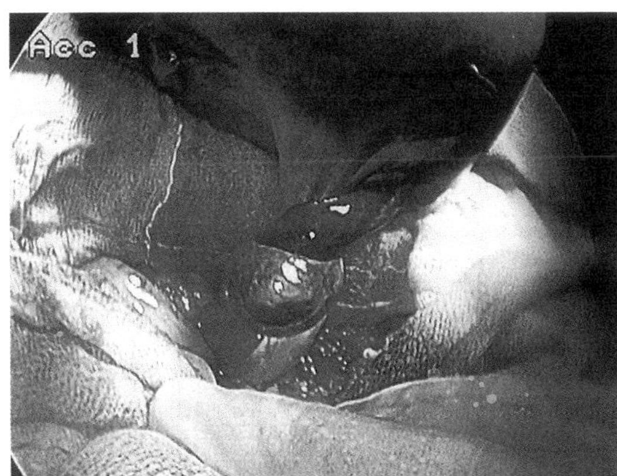

Figure 6.20 Torsion of the ovary presenting as a complex cyst.

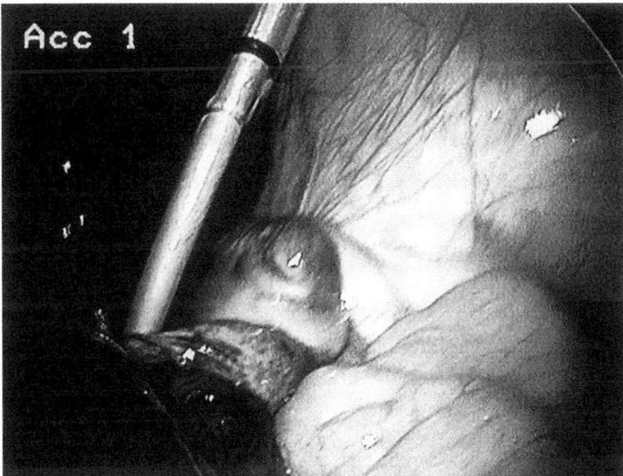

Figure 6.21 Laparoscopic identification of ovarian torsion.

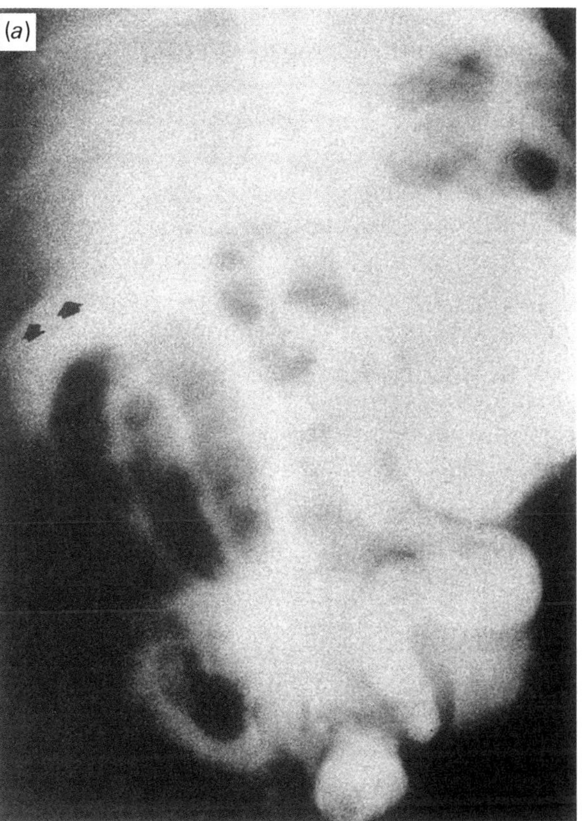

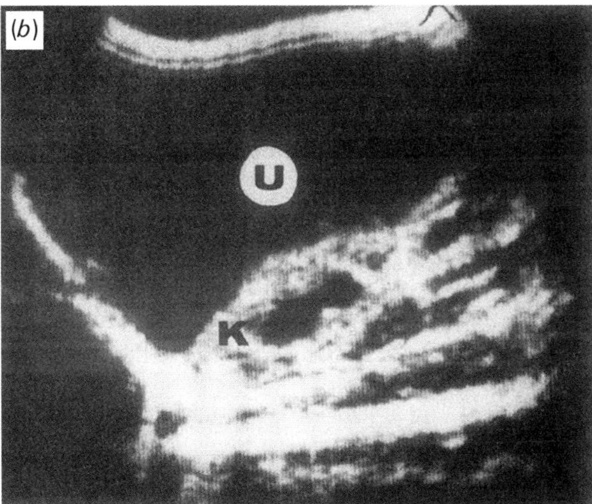

Figure 6.22 (*a*) Voiding cystourethrogram of urinary ascites: the black arrows point to the liver edge. (*b*) Ultrasound study showing a retroperitoneal urinoma. K, kidney; U, urine collection. (From Rittenberg et al,[308] with permission.)

presented as an enlarged abdomen in newborns; however, today the diagnosis is frequently made in utero by antenatal sonography.[300,301] Ascites in the fetus or newborn can be from urologic and non-urologic causes. *Urinary ascites accounts for about 30% of all cases of neonatal ascites.*[302] Among urologic causes, lower urinary tract obstruction and trauma are most common. Specifically, PUV, urethral stenosis, distal ureteral stenosis, and obstructing ureteroceles have all been associated with neonatal urinary ascites[302–307] (Figure 6.22). Less frequently, obstructed and hydronephrotic kidneys may also be the cause. In these cases, extravasation of urine occurs either from the bladder or, more commonly, from a forniceal rupture in the kidney.[309] Ascites from unilateral obstructive lesions has been reported, although far less commonly than in cases of bilateral obstruction.[310] Alternatively, perinatal trauma to the urinary tract may also cause neonatal ascites.[311] In particular, umbilical artery catheterization with inadvertent bladder perforation is an important cause of neonatal urinary ascites.[312,313]

Sonography and VCUG can usually determine the urologic abnormality and site of extravasation in those with neonatal urinary ascites. Historically, plain film X-ray findings of a ground-glass appearance of the abdomen with floating loops of bowel have been described in patients with ascites. Neonatal urinoma, which may or may not be associated with ascites, can be identified by a 'c' sign, a rim of opacified contrast around the kidney on intravenous pyelography (IVP).[314] Clinically, these patients can be quite ill. The characteristic laboratory findings include hyponatremia, hyperkalemia, and elevated serum creatinine.[315] Treatment is individualized, but urinary drainage with a urethral catheter allowing the intraperitoneal urine to be reabsorbed, along with urinary antibiotic prophylaxis, is often sufficient. Open drainage may be required in instances where infection of the urine occurs or when respiratory embarrassment is due to the mass effect. Previous reports of 70% mortality have improved to less than 15% in more recent series.[307,316,317] Recently, De Vries et al[318] reported long-term follow-up of a series of patients with severe obstruction that had good lower tract and renal function. Like others, the authors postulate that the development of ascites serves as a protective mechanism, allowing the kidney to decompress and minimizing damage from obstruction.[319–321] Non-urologic causes of neonatal ascites include erythroblastosis fetalis, cardiac or hepatic abnormalities, sepsis, and gastrointestinal perforation.[259]

Solid lesions

Solid lesions in children are being detected prenatally with increasing frequency. One of the best examples is neuroblastoma.[322,323] Whereas early detection of neuroblastoma does not necessarily change initial management, it results in the child receiving treatment sooner. In addition, patients with neuroblastomas detected early in life have a better outlook. Thus, early diagnosis probably improves the prognosis.[322] As a rule, solid lesions detected antenatally are followed before delivery, and then after birth are imaged by computed tomography (CT) scan or MRI. Occasionally, a postcontrast kidney, ureter, and bladder (KUB) film may clarify the diagnosis. No indications for antenatal intervention exist for solid lesions.

Sacrococcygeal teratoma represents the most common fetal neoplasm, with an estimated incidence of 1 in 40 000 births.[324] The majority occur in females. Intrapelvic lesions may be difficult to diagnose. The presumptive in-utero diagnosis has been made by ultrasound. When this lesion is suspected in the postnatal period it is best evaluated by CT or MRI.[325] The tumor may cause obstruction of the urinary tract with resultant hydronephrosis. Treatment typically consists of surgical excision

Neuroblastoma is the most common solid malignant tumor in neonates and is characterized by its variability in presentation.[326] This tumor effects 1:7000 children, with 40% of cases diagnosed in children <1 year of age.[327] The tumor is often identified prenatally.[328–331] In addition to prenatal ultrasound, fetal MRI can contribute to the prenatal evaluation.[332] Many factors, including age at detection and location, affect overall outcome. Early diagnosis and treatment may be critical in some cases.[333] However, information derived from countries with mandatory postnatal screening for neuroblastoma suggests that many tumors detected in the perinatal period regress. Therefore, some infants diagnosed very early may have unnecessary interventions.[334–336] More recently, well-designed studies have demonstrated that neonatal screening is unlikely to effect mortality in neonates.[327] The Children's Oncology Group currently is conducting an observation pilot study for children presenting with perinatal neuroblastoma. Specific inclusion criteria are: age <3 months; sonographically identified adrenal mass, which is <16 ml in volume, if solid, or <65 ml if at least 25% cystic, and which does not cross the midline.

On physical examination, neuroblastoma has been classically described as a firm, fixed lesion that may cross the midline. Children may also present with bulky metastatic disease that includes a palpable liver and subcutaneous nodules that characterize stage IV-S disease. This form usually undergoes spontaneous regression.[337] Imaging by ultrasound can usually suggest the diagnosis. Confirmation is made by CT scan or MRI. These studies show a lesion that displaces the kidney but does not arise from the kidney (Figure 6.23). The appearance of a tumor arising from the kidney will cause a beaking effect of the renal tissue (Figure 6.24). Despite modern imaging techniques the diagnosis of neuroblastoma may be confused with other less common conditions, such as pulmonary sequestration.[338] Cystic neuroblastomas detected prenatally have also been reported, so the diagnosis should not be excluded on the basis of a cystic component.[339–343] Most neuroblastomas cause elevations of urinary catecholamines, which should be checked in all such patients.

Treatment varies from observation to surgery for those patients with early-stage localized disease. Multimodal therapy, including chemotherapy and radiotherapy, is indicated in patients with advanced

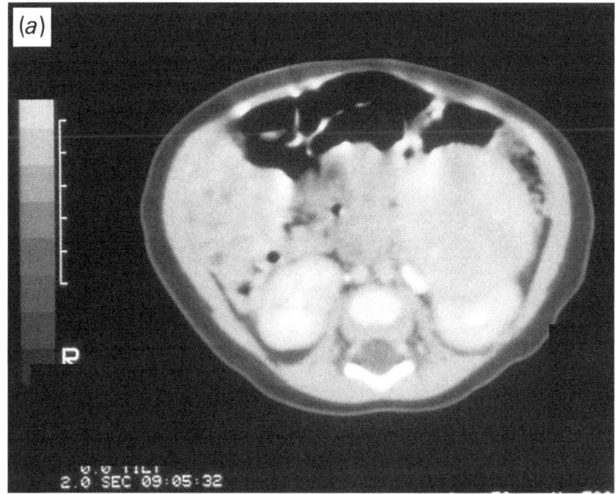

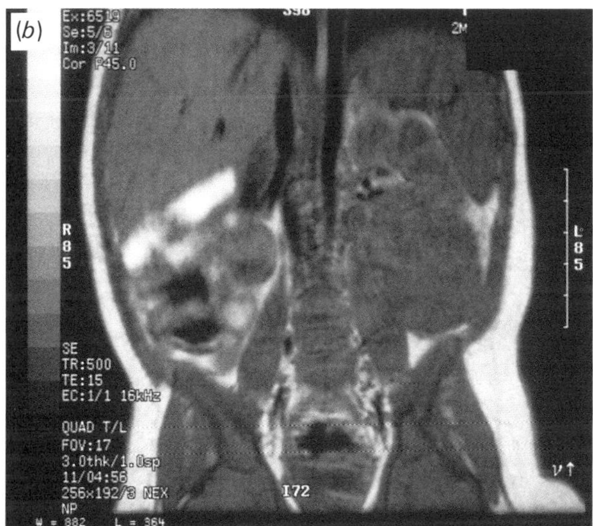

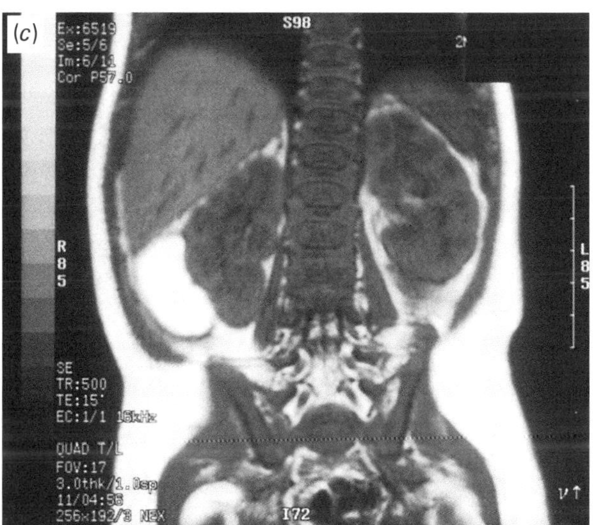

Figure 6.23 (*a*) CT scan showing displacement of the kidney by neuroblastoma (note no beaking of the renal tissue). (*b*) MRI showing neuroblastoma in relation to the kidney. (*c*) MRI showing normal renal contour confirming that the tumor is separate from the kidney.

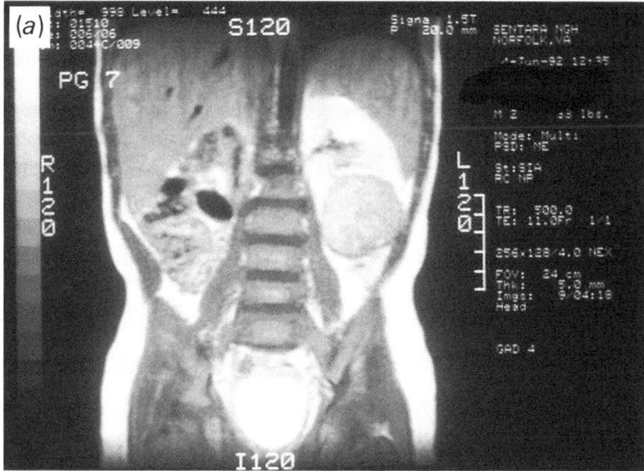

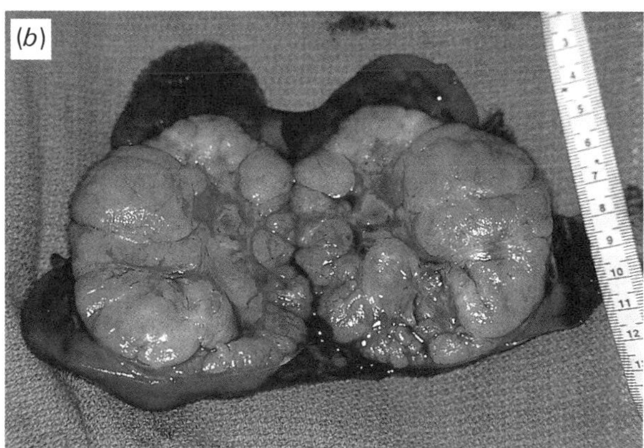

Figure 6.24 (*a*) Wilms' tumor showing beaking of the renal tissue, confirming its intrarenal location. (*b*) Bivalved tumor showing the beaking effect of the normal renal tissue around the mass.

disease. There are several clinical trials of experimental drugs in the high-risk group. Treatment protocols are available through the Children's Oncology Group.[333,334]

Although Wilms' tumor is the most common renal tumor in children, it occurs infrequently in the neonatal period.[345] In children <6 months of age, congenital mesoblastic nephroma is a more common cause of a solid renal lesion; however, Wilms' tumor, rhabdoid tumors, clear cell tumors, renal cell carcinoma, angiomyolipoma, and ossifyng tumors are known to occur.[346,347] Most of these present as a neonatal abdominal mass, less frequently as hematuria, paraneoplastic syndromes, or hypertension.[348] Wilms' tumor has also been detected by prenatal US evaluation.[349–351] Associated findings in the prenatal period include fetal hydrops and polyhydramnios.[348] Postnatally these children may have a palpable mass and in some cases hypertension. Children born with known associated syndromes such as aniridia, WAGR syndrome, Denys-Drash symdrome, or Beckwith–

Wiedemann syndrome develop tumors at a younger age and are more likely to have bilateral lesions; therefore surveillance US should be performed.[345] Bilateral nephroblastomatosis, aniridia, and 11p13 deletion result in the development of Wilms' tumor in close to 100% of affected individuals (Figure 6.25). These patients may develop bilateral Wilms' tumor, requiring nephron-sparing surgical techniques. Evaluation of the vascular anatomy is best performed with MR angiography[352] (Figure 6.26). The treatment is based on stage of the tumor and involves surgery, chemotherapy, and sometimes radiation therapy. The common chemotherapy agents utilized include vincristine, doxorubicin, and dactinomycin. Readers are referred to the Children's Oncology Group protocols for specific therapy recommendation.

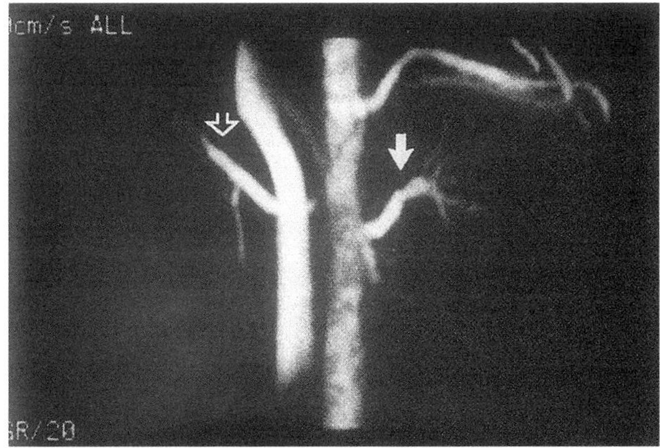

Figure 6.26 Phase-contrast magnetic resonance angiography. The open arrow indicates the superiorly displaced right renal artery from a Wilms' tumor. The solid arrow indicates the single left renal artery. (From Ferrer et al,[352] with permission.)

Congenital mesoblastic nephroma is a rare renal tumor that is the most common solid renal mass in children <6 months of age (50%). Eighty percent of these lesions are discovered in the first month of life.[353] Congenital mesoblastic nephroma may frequently be detected prenatally, where it is associated with polyhydramnios in approximately 70% of cases.[354] Typically, the lesion is noted as a solid intrarenal mass on sonogram that appears fibroid when removed[355] (Figure 6.27). A cystic form can also occur[353] (Figure 6.28). Pathologically, the tumor can be divided into two groups: classic and cellular. The classic lesion represents one-third of cases and is microscopically similar to a leiomyoma and does not metastasize.[356,357] The cellular variant has the potential for local recurrence and metastasis.[348,357] In-utero treatment usually consists of observation and management of polyhydramnios with its attendant complications. Postnatally, nephrectomy is recommended. In cases where metastases have occurred, chemotherapy may be warranted.[348,358] Hypercalcemia requiring treatment has been documented but usually resolves after nephrectomy.[348] Cases requiring urgent surgery following tumor rupture and hemorrhage have been reported.[359,360]

Renal vein thrombosis (RVT) may be the cause of a mass in a neonate. The characteristic clinical presen-

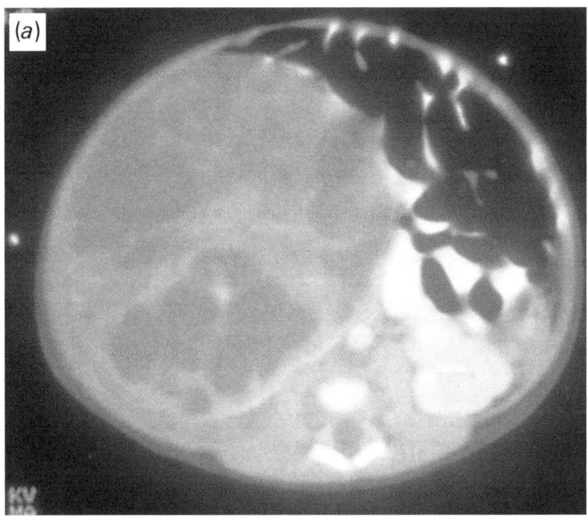

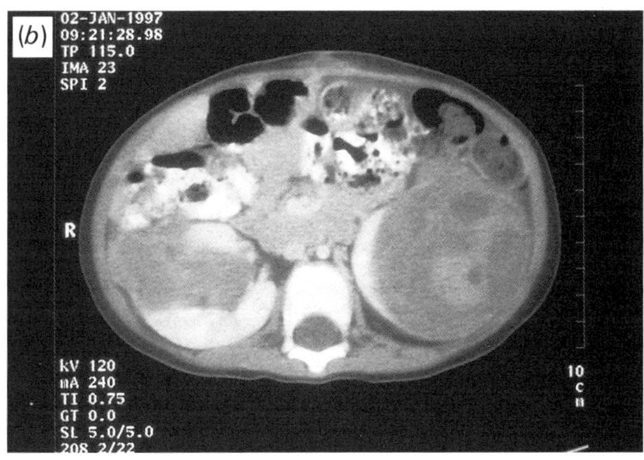

Figure 6.25 (*a*) CT scan of cystic mesoblastic nephroma. (*b*) Bilateral Wilms' tumor in a patient with aniridia.

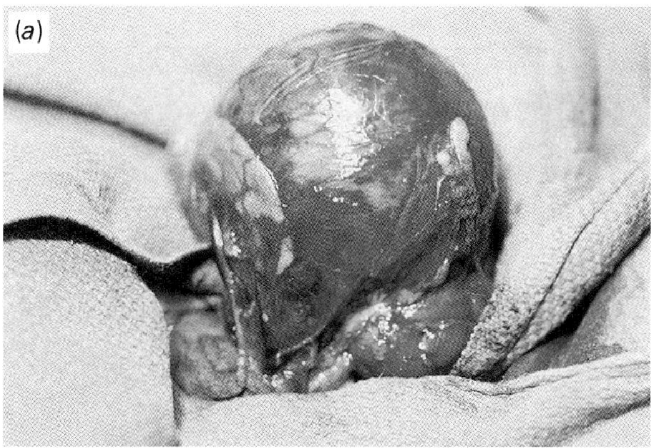

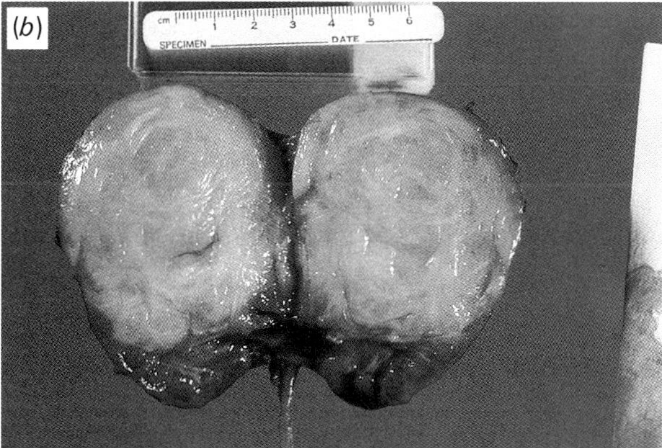

Figure 6.27 Solid mesoblastic nephroma in a 3-day-old patient: (*a*) surgical picture; (*b*) bivalved lesion showing a typical fibroid appearance.

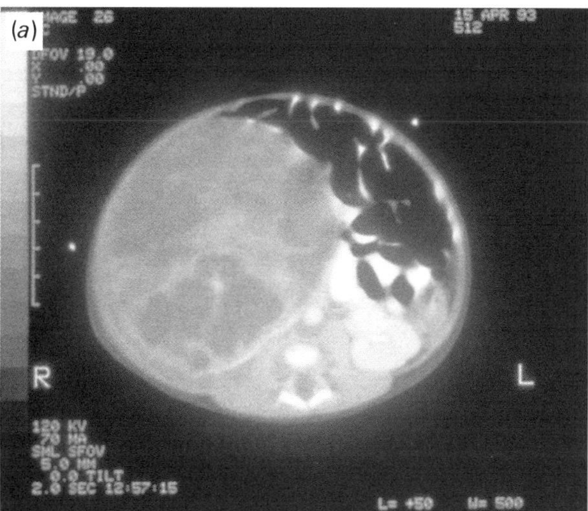

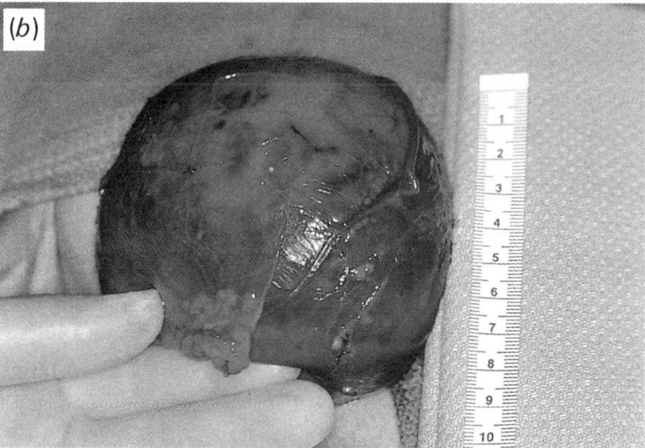

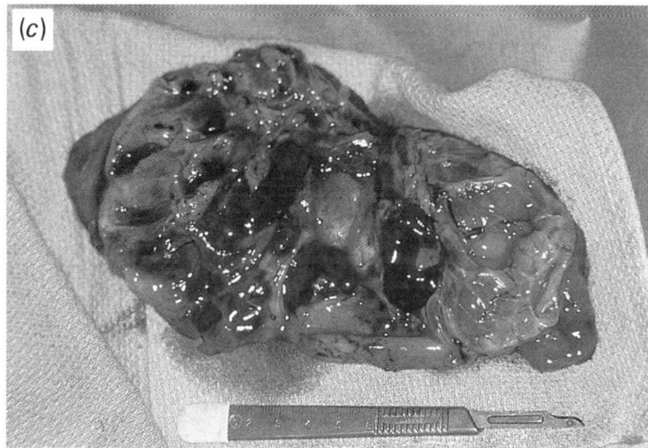

Figure 6.28 (*a*) CT scan of cystic mesoblastic nephroma. (*b*) Cystic mesoblastic nephroma after excision. (*c*) Bivalved cystic mesoblastic nephroma.

tation of RVT – an enlarged kidney, hematuria and proteinuria in an ill infant – is only present in a small percentage of patients (Figure 6.29). Low platelet counts due to consumption by the developing thrombus may be seen. Infants appear to be predisposed to this condition, because of lower renal arterial and venous flow rates, than older children and adults. Reports of prenatal diagnoses of RVT are now commonplace.[362,363] RVT is most commonly associated with risk factors that include dehydration, sepsis, birth asphyxia, maternal diabetes, polycythemia, cardiac disease, protein C deficiency, twin-twin transfusion, and presence of an umbilical catheter.[363] In addition, the significance of prothrombotic risk factors, such as factor V, are increasingly being recognized.[364,365] The thrombosis starts in the venules within the kidney and progressively extends to the major renal vein or veins. The diagnosis is most commonly made by ultrasound (Figure 6.30). Initially, the lesion appears as highly echogenic streaks within the kidney. Subsequently, the kidney becomes enlarged and echogenic, with loss of corticomedullary differentiation.[361] Treatment of unilateral RVT is supportive, with hydration and correction of any predisposing abnormalities.[366] Bilateral thrombosis requires more aggressive treatment and has a worse prognosis, but thrombus removal has not proven helpful. These patients warrant treatment with either heparin or systemic thrombolytic therapy in order

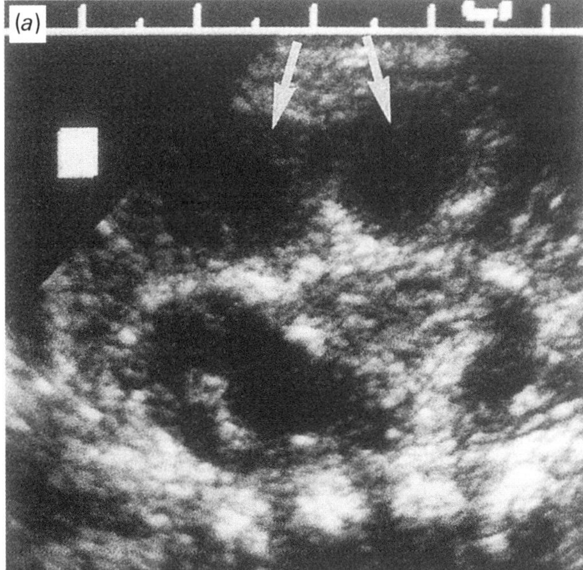

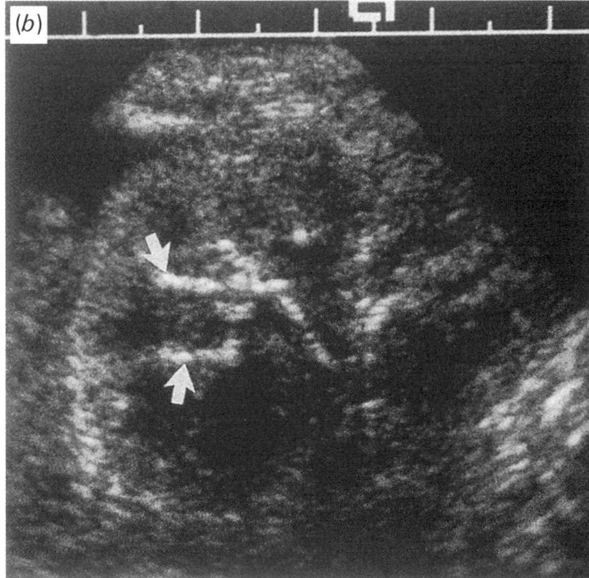

Figure 6.29 Renal vein thrombosis. (*a*) Enlarged left kidney with echogenic intermedullary streaks and echopoor medullary pyramids (arrows). (*b*) Same patient's right kidney showing swelling of the upper pole and focal echogenic intermedullary streaks. (From Hibbert et al,[361] with permission.)

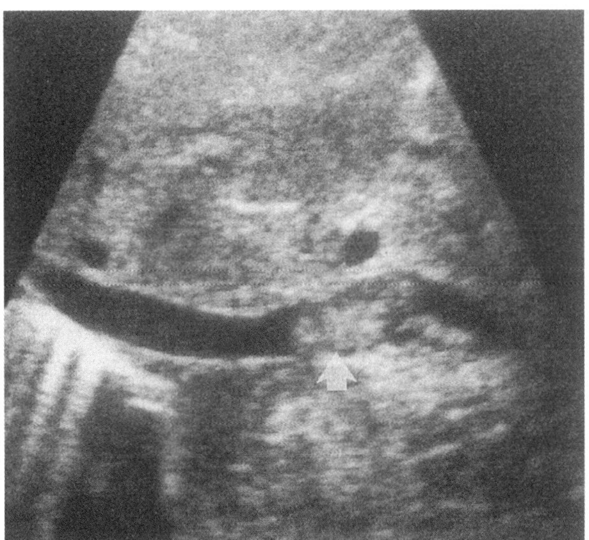

Figure 6.30 Renal vein thrombosis. Ultrasound through the IVC showing thrombus within the IVC at the level of the renal vein. (From Hibbert et al,[361] with permission.)

to minimize morbidity.[367,368] Recent reports suggest that those who receive aggressive therapy with anticoagulants fare better than those who do not.[363] Patients with unilateral thrombosis usually do well, whereas those with bilateral thrombosis have a higher rate of complications such as renal failure.[369] All patients must have long-term monitoring of renal function and evaluation for hypertension, which is common.[370,371]

Renal artery thrombosis does not commonly present as a neonatal mass.[372] The occurrence of this disorder has increased significantly in relation to the increased use of umbilical artery catheters, despite the fact that a causal relationship was identified some time ago.[373] The diagnosis is commonly made with Doppler ultrasound, which demonstrates the absence of flow in the renal artery. Treatment options include supportive measures, thrombolytics, and surgery, depending on the extent of thrombosis and whether or not aortic involvement exists.[374–377]

Neonatal adrenal hemorrhage is associated with traumatic or difficult labor, neonatal hypoxia, septicemia, or coagulopathy. Traditionally, it is believed that the relatively large size and vascularity of the newborn gland predisposes it to bleeding. A study using ultrasound to screen newborns for adrenal hemorrhage in 8374 pregnancies reported an incidence of 1.9 per 1000 births.[378] In this report, 13 cases were on the right, two on the left, and one was bilateral. These findings corroborate previous reports indicating a right-sided predominance and 10% bilaterality. Diagnosis is made by ultrasound, and antenatal diagnosis has been made in the second and third trimesters (Figure 6.31). Identification by ultrasound is usually reliable, but in some cases it is difficult to differentiate from an adrenal neuroblastoma[379–381] (Figure 6.32). In difficult cases, CT and MRI may be helpful in the diagnosis.[382,383] Negative urine catecholamines also support the diagnosis of adrenal hemorrhage.

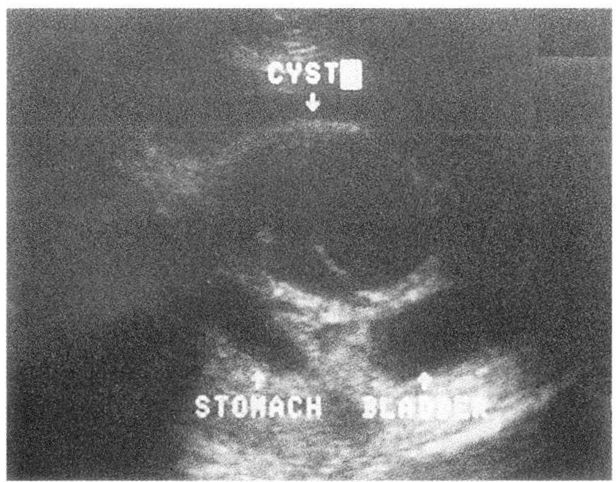

Figure 6.31 Prenatal adrenal hemorrhage identified as a complex cyst on sonogram. (From Burbige,[379] with permission.)

Experience has confirmed the initial belief that the majority of infants with adrenal hemorrhage require no treatment except for occasional phototherapy and, rarely, transfusion.[384,385] Resultant adrenal insufficiency is uncommon. Observation for resolution and monitoring of hematocrit and bilirubin should be routine. Occasionally, steroid replacement for temporary adrenal insufficiency is required.

Cystic nephroma is a rare benign renal neoplasm. Lesions may be unilateral or bilateral, and bilateral metachronous lesions have been reported.[386] Partial nephrectomy is appropriate when possible to preserve renal parenchyma (Figure 6.33).

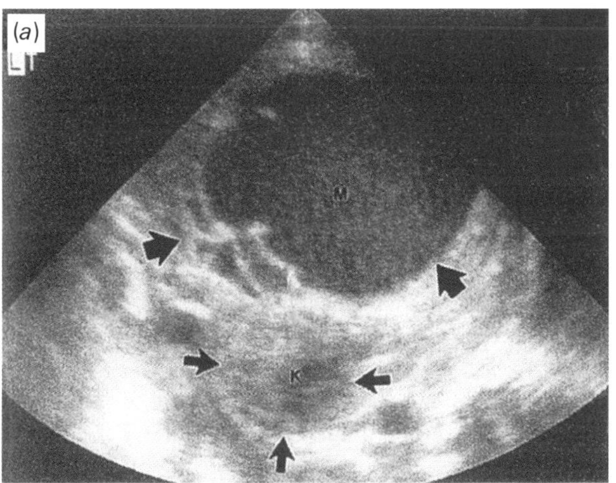

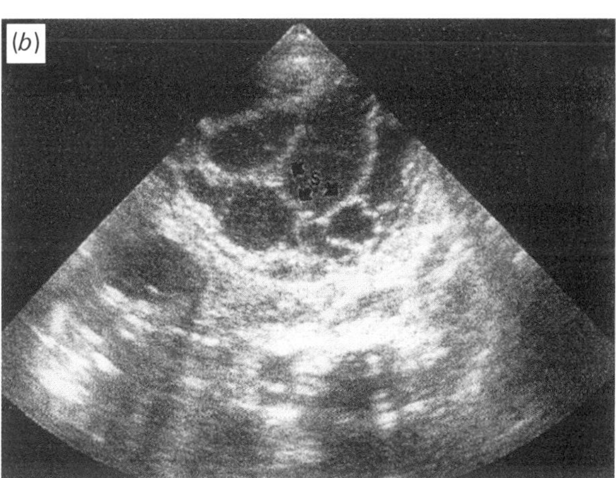

Figure 6.32 Postnatal confirmation of a complex cystic lesion superior to the kidney. Surgical exploration later confirms adrenal hemorrhage. (From Burbige,[379] with permission.)

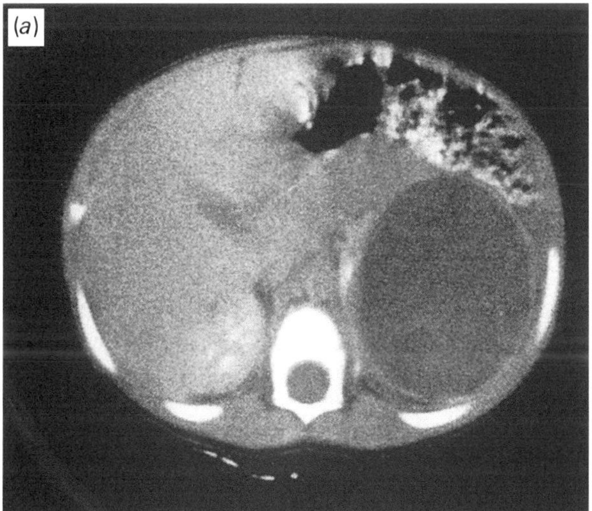

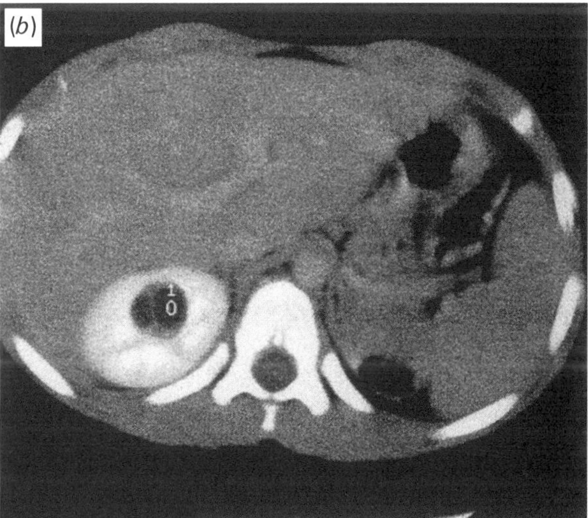

Figure 6.33 Multilocular cyst of the kidney (cystic nephroma). (*a*) CT scan of cystic nephroma in the left kidney with a normal right kidney. (*b*) CT scan of the same patient 2 years later with a solitary right kidney and metachronous cystic nephroma. (From Ferrer and McKenna,[386] with permission.)

Rhabdomyosarcoma is an uncommon neoplasm of the lower urinary tract in children. Lesions may occur in the bladder, prostate, vagina, or uterus (Figure 6.34). Presentation in infancy depends on the organ of origin and may include hematuria, vaginal bleeding, or obstruction of the urinary tract. Treatment is multimodal, including chemotherapy, radiation therapy, and exenteration followed by reconstructive surgery.[387,388] As a result of collaborative efforts by the Intergroup Rhabdomyosarcoma Study, treatment results for these patients are improving. Current efforts are focused on bladder preservation.[389] Dysfunctional bladders may result, however, from high doses of chemotherapy and radiation.

Germ cell tumors are rare in children and their presentation as a lower abdominal mass is extremely uncommon. They may occur as an ovarian mass or as a mass in an undescended testis.[390,391] Treatment for these tumors is dependent on stage at diagnosis but is usually multimodal including surgery and platinum-based chemotherapy, depending on histology.

Enterocystoplasty and the acute abdomen

Bladder augmentation with bowel segments is commonly performed in children with neuropathic bladders, bladder tumors, and exstrophy. Most of these patients require clean intermittent catheterization after bladder augmentation and have poor bladder sensation. A combination of poor sensation and overdistention can lead to a spontaneous augmentation rupture, an acute abdomen, and life-threatening sepsis. The presentation can be confusing because most patients have altered abdominal sensation, so identifying the source of sepsis can be difficult. A cystogram may not reveal extravasation and the best rapid screening study may be a sonogram that shows floating loops of bowel. Early surgical exploration is indicated. The rupture is usually located at the posterior suture line between the bladder and augmented bowel. Whenever a patient with a bladder augmentation presents with sepsis, this diagnosis should be considered.

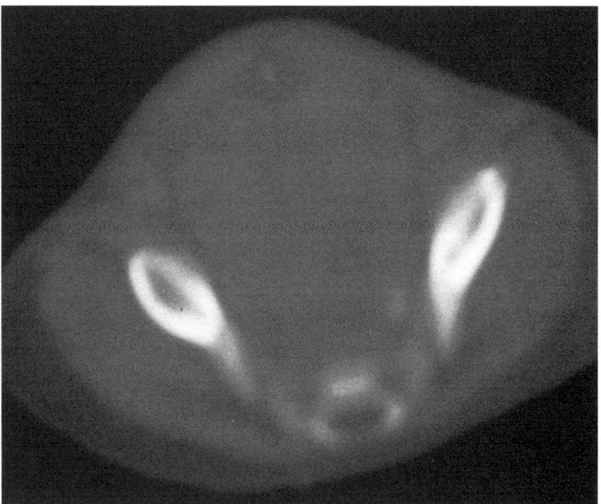

Figure 6.34 Pelvic sarcoma with displacement of the bladder superiorly. Note Foley balloon in the bladder.

Intraoperative consultations

The best approach to intraoperative consultations is to take the time to obtain a complete history. This is usually chart based but may include talking to the parents prior to making a quick decision about a complex question. This is also the case when one is asked about a surgical finding or called to address a surgical complication. After the chart review and appropriate history, it is best to scrub into the case and review the exact location of the lesion from the skin to the region of question. One must take a fresh look at the situation and not rely totally on the primary physician. When any questions arise that deal with surgical excision of a mass, multiple radiologic modalities can be used intraoperatively, and frozen section sampling is available. There is little to be lost in closing the patient who needs further evaluation, which cannot be undertaken in the operating room, and reoperating when the problem is better understood.

Many unusual structures may be found during a pediatric hernia repair. Among these is the finding of reproductive organs appropriate to the opposite sex. Although rare, this will usually generate an intraoperative consultation. In males, the finding of female organs, such as a fallopian tube or uterus, is termed persistent Müllerian duct syndrome[392] or hernia uterine inguinale. The cause of this anomaly is a failure of Sertoli cell production of Müllerian inhibiting substance (MIS), leading to feminization of pelvic structures. The testis should be undescended, but otherwise the patient is phenotypically male. Intraoperative biopsy confirms the presence of a normal testis. Excision of the female structures should be performed with care, avoiding injury to the adjacent functioning Wolffian duct structures. Excision is important because of the risk of future malignancy arising in these tissues.[393] Others have recommended that they be left in place to avoid potential injury.[394] In phenotypic females, the finding of male reproductive structures during hernia repair suggests testicular feminization. Here, the timing of excision of the male gonads is controversial: if removed early, exogenous estrogens must be administered to induce normal maturation at puberty; if left in situ until puberty, the testis must then be removed because of the high possibility of developing gonadoblastoma.[395] Laparoscopic removal of the testis allows for a minimally invasive approach yet permits direct molecular analysis of the specimen.[396] Over 40 other tissues have been identified in and around the hernia sac. They include normal structures drawn into the sac, organ duplications as 'rests', inflammatory lesions, tumors, and drainage from the abdomen into a patent processus vaginalis.[397]

1 Organs drawn into the hernia sac:
   - appendix
   - bladder
   - gonad
   - Meckel's diverticulum
   - omentum
   - bowel
   - pelvic kidney
   - ureter
   - uterus.
2 Aberrant rests:
   - adrenal
   - ectopic renal tissue
   - accessory spleen.
3 Inflammatory lesions:
   - abscess
   - funiculitis
   - granulomas
   - sarcoidosis
   - meconium granuloma
   - parasitic disease
   - peritonitis
   - polyarteritis nodosa
   - vasitis nodosa
   - xanthogranuloma.
4 Tumors and benign lesions:
   - adrenal tumor
   - dermoid cyst
   - epidermoid cyst
   - epididymal cysts and nodules
   - calculi
   - hemangioma
   - lymphangioma
   - mesenchymoma
   - neuroblastoma
   - paratesticular cyst/rhabdomyosarcoma
   - spermatic cord tumors
   - spermatocele
   - tunica albuginea cyst
   - tunica vaginalis cyst
   - venous thrombosis
   - Wilms' tumor.
5 Lesions that appear because of patent processus vaginalis:
   - adrenal hemorrhage
   - endometriosis
   - meconium
   - blood.

Unusual findings in the spermatic cord of which the urologist should be aware include those listed above, particularly ectopic adrenal tissue and accessory spleens.[398,399] In cases of ectopic adrenal tissue the yellow color and an appearance similar to the normal gland usually aid identification. Neuroblastoma has also been reported to present as a mass in the spermatic cord.[400] In addition to the more common scrotal masses, heterotopic Wilms' tumor and neuroblastoma have been reported.[401] Both adrenal and splenic tissue have also been found in the scrotum, and splenogonadal fusion is not uncommon with an undescended left testis. Excision of these masses is usually best, with careful pathologic evaluation to confirm the diagnosis.

Although vasal injuries are most commonly diagnosed later in life during the work-up of infertility, vasal injury during pediatric hernia repair mandates intraoperative pediatric urologic consultation. Previous studies have documented the ease with which vasal trauma may occur secondary to intraoperative manipulation.[402] In cases of transection, immediate microvascular repair is indicated. Crush injuries may result in future obstruction. In these situations the decision regarding treatment must be individualized. In most instances observation is indicated. However, when a severe crush injury has occurred, as when a clamp is applied and closed with obvious injury, excision and primary reanastomosis is indicated.

Intraoperative consultations relating to the bladder are usually a result of trauma or iatrogenic injury during surgery. Intraoperative injury to the bladder is rare but may occur secondary to percutaneous laparoscopic procedures or during inguinal hernia repair. When it happens it is best managed by primary closure, and bladder drainage in the postoperative period via a urethral catheter and/or suprapubic tube. Perivesical drainage is also appropriate in the immediate postoperative period. A cystogram to confirm the absence of extravasation should be performed prior to removal of drainage catheters. Rarely, during umbilical hernia repair, a urachal abnormality is discovered. In these cases the urachus should be traced to the dome of the bladder and excised with primary closure of the bladder.[401] If the diagnosis is uncertain, an intraoperative cystogram may clarify the picture.

Most consultations related to the kidney and ureter are in patients with renal trauma. *The basic recommendation is not to explore the flank even when an expanding mass is present until normal function of the contralateral kidney has been assured.* When an expanding retroperitoneal mass is explored after trauma, early renal vascular control should be the main objective. Traumatic separation of the ureter and pelvis occasionally occurs in children. Unlike many injuries where drainage and observation is indicated, complete avulsion of the ureter should be surgically repaired as quickly as possible. It is a more complex procedure than a standard UPJ repair because the pelvis is almost always intrarenal and mobilization of the kidney and ureter to prevent tension on the anastomosis can be difficult. The procedure is much more difficult if the correction is delayed because of edema with subsequent scar formation.

As a result of advances in imaging and thorough preoperative evaluations, consultations because of a previously undiagnosed renal mass, formerly common, are now unusual. Despite this, the urologic surgeon should bear in mind that occasionally an ectopic or a pelvic kidney may be confused with a pelvic mass and indicate intraoperative consultation. Reports of inadvertent nephrectomy in patients with solitary ectopic kidneys are found in the literature.[401] When it is unclear whether the mass in question is a solitary kidney, intraoperative imaging may be necessary to clarify the situation. This is critical, as reports indicate that up to 10% of all pelvic kidneys are solitary.[403] Intraoperatively, it is important to remember that ectopic kidneys may not be reniform in shape and tend to have an anomalous blood supply derived from the aorta and iliac vessels, or the superior mesenteric artery.[403] Simple needle aspiration to confirm the presence of urine may also be useful in identifying a kidney. Fusion anomalies and horseshoe kidneys may also be a source of confusion and prompt urologic consultation.

Occasionally, the urologist will be called to evaluate an infant for difficulty in placing a urethral catheter. Initially, properly lubricating the urethra by injecting 2% lidocaine jelly facilitates catheter insertion. Most commonly, these will be male neonates who have had multiple attempts at catheterization before urologic consultation. In these cases a good option may be to use a curved-tip 'coude' catheter, which has recently become available in pediatric sizes. When these catheters are not available, or will not pass, a small catheter guide may be placed within a pediatric feeding tube and manipulated into the bladder. If no guides are available, bending a heavy wire suture for use as a catheter guide may be successful.[404,405] Lubricating jelly must be placed on the guide to facilitate its removal. In cases where this fails, proceeding directly to cystoscopy to evaluate the possibility of a false passage is warranted. Use of a guidewire placed under direct vision followed by catheter placement over the wire ensures proper catheter placement. When the bladder is palpable, a percutaneous cystotomy may be performed under local anesthesia or in the operating room. Alternatively, a large-gauge needle placed into the distended bladder will permit insertion of a guidewire, dilation of the tract, and placement of a suprapubic catheter.

References

1. Boyle RJ, Salter R, Arnander MW et al. Ethics of refusing parental requests to withhold or withdraw treatment from their premature baby. J Med Ethics 2004; 30:402–5; discussion 406–9.
2. Housley HT, Harrison MR. Fetal urinary tract abnormalities. Natural history, pathophysiology, and treatment. Urol Clin North Am 1998; 25:63–73.
3. Freedman AL, Johnson MP, Smith CA, Gonzalez R, Evans MI. Long-term outcome in children after antenatal intervention for obstructive uropathies. Lancet 2000; 354:374–7.
4. Herndon CDA, Ferrer FA, Freedman AL, McKenna PH. Consensus on the prenatal management of antenatally detected urological abnormalities. J Urol 2000; 164:1052–6.
5. Leviton LC, Goldenberg RL, Baker CS et al. Methods to encourage the use of antenatal corticosteroid therapy for fetal maturation: a randomized controlled trial. JAMA 1999; 281:46–52.
6. Elder JS, Duckett JW Jr, Snyder HM. Intervention for fetal obstructive uropathy: has it been effective? Lancet 1987; 2:1007–10.
7. Crombleholme TM, Harrison MR, Golbus MS et al. Fetal intervention in obstructive uropathy: prognostic indicators and efficacy of intervention. Am J Obstet Gynecol 1990; 162:1239–44.
8. Johnson MP, Bukowski TP, Reitleman C et al. *In utero* surgical treatment of fetal obstructive uropathy: a new comprehensive approach to identify appropriate candidates for vesicoamniotic shunt therapy. Am J Obstet Gynecol 1994; 170:1770–6.
9. Johnson MP, Corsi P, Bradfield W et al. Sequential fetal urine analysis provides greater precision in the evaluation

of fetal obstructive uropathy. Am J Obstet Gynecol 1995; 173:59–65.

10. Freedman AL, Bukowski TP, Smith CA et al. Fetal therapy for obstructive uropathy: specific outcomes diagnosis. J Urol 1996; 156:720–4.
11. Freedman AL, Johnson MP, Smith CA et al. Long-term outcome in children after antenatal intervention for obstructive uropathies. Lancet 1999; 354:374–7.
12. Chevalier RL. Perinatal obstructive nephropathy. Semin Perinatol 2004; 28:124–31.
13. McCurdy CM Jr, Seeds JW. Oligohydramnios: problems and treatment. Semin Perinatol 1993; 17:183–96.
14. Hutton KAR, Thomas DFM, Arthur RJ et al. Prenatally detected posterior urethral valves: is gestational age at detection a predictor of outcome? J Urol 1994; 152:698–701.
15. Harrison MR, Nakayama DK, Noall R, deLorimier AA. Correction of congenital hydronephrosis in utero II: decompression reverses the effects of obstruction on the fetal lung and urinary tract. J Pediatr Surg 1982; 17:965–74.

16a. Peters CA, Docimo SG, Luetic T et al. Effect of in utero vesicostomy on pulmonary hypoplasia in the fetal lamb with bladder outlet obstruction and oligohydramnios: a morphometric analysis. J Urol 1991; 146:1178–83.

16b. Peters CA, Reid LM, Docimo S et al. The role of the kidney in lung growth and maturation in the setting obstructive uropathy and oligohydramnios. J Urol 1991; 146:597–600.

17. Chevalier RL, Klahr S. Therapeutic approaches in obstructive uropathy. Semin Nephrol 1998; 18:652–8.
18. Ashmead GG, Mercer B, Herbst M, Moodley J, Bota A, Elder JS. Fetal bladder outlet obstruction due to ureterocele: in utero 'colander' therapy. J Ultrasound Med 2004; 23:565–8.
19. Cohen HL, Zinn HL, Patel A et al. Prenatal sonographic diagnosis of posterior urethral valves: identification of valves and thickening of the posterior urethral wall. J Clin Ultrasound 1998; 26:366–70.
20. Golan A, Lin G, Evron S et al. Oligohydramnios: maternal complications and fetal outcome in 145 cases. Gynecol Obstet Invest 1994; 37:91–5.
21. Glick PL, Harrison MR, Globus MS et al. Management of the fetus with congenital hydronephrosis II: prognostic criteria and selection for treatment. J Pediatr Surg 1985; 20:376–87.
22. Evans MI, Sacks AJ, Johnson MP et al. Sequential invasive assessment of fetal renal function and the intrauterine treatment of fetal obstructive uropathies. Obstet Gynecol 1991; 77:545–50.
23. Lipitz S, Ryan G, Samuell C et al. Fetal urine analysis for the assessment of renal function in obstructive uropathy. Am J Obstet Gynecol 1993; 168:174–9.
24. Wilkins IA, Chitkara U, Lynch L et al. The nonpredictive value of fetal urinary electrolytes: preliminary report of outcomes and correlations with pathologic diagnosis. Am J Obstet Gynecol 1987; 157:694–8.
25. Guez S, Assael BM, Melzi ML et al. Shortcomings in predicting postnatal renal function using prenatal urine biochemistry in fetuses with congenital hydronephrosis. J Pediatr Surg 1996; 31:1401–4.
26. Anderson N, Clautice-Engle T, Allan R et al. Detection of obstructive uropathy in the fetus. AJR Am J Roentgenol 1995; 164:719–23.
27. Bobrowski RA, Levin RB, Lauria MR et al. *In utero* progression of isolated renal pelvis dilation. Am J Perinatol 1997; 14:423–6.
28. Manning FA, Harrison MR, Rodeck C. Catheter shunts for fetal hydronephrosis and hydrocephalus. Report of the International Fetal Surgery Registry. N Engl J Med 1986; 315:336–40.
29. Herndon CDA, McKenna PH. Survival after vascular injury with prenatal intervention: review of the complications. Soc Fetal Urol 1998; 5(2):4.
30. Tabor A, Philip J, Madsen M et al. Randomised controlled trial of genetic amniocentesis in 4606 low-risk women. Lancet 1986; i:1287–93.
31. Hsieh TT, Lee JD, Kuo DM et al. Perinatal outcome of chorionic villus sampling versus amniocentesis. Taiwan I Hsueh Hui Tsa Chih 1989; 88:894–9.
32. Bahado-Singh R, Schmitt R, Hobbins JC. New technique for genetic amniocentesis in twins. Obstet Gynecol 1992; 79:304–7.
33. Cederholm M, Haglund B, Axelsson O. Infant mortality following amniocentesis and chorionic villus sampling for prenatal karyotyping. BJOG 2005; 112:394–402.
34. Rhoads GG, Jackson LG, Schlesselman SE et al. The safety and efficacy of chorionic villus sampling for early prenatal diagnosis of cytogenetic abnormalities. N Engl J Med 1989; 320:609–17.
35. Kuliev A, Jackson L, Froster U et al. Chorionic villus sampling safety. Report of World Health Organization/EURO meeting in association with the Seventh International Conference on Early Prenatal Diagnosis of Genetic Diseases, Tel-Aviv, Israel, May 21, 1994. Am J Obstet Gynecol 1996; 174:807–11.
36. Brambati B, Tului L. Chorionic villus sampling and amniocentesis. Curr Opin Obstet Gynecol 2005; 17:197–201.
37. Farmer DL. Fetal surgery: a brief review. Pediatr Radiol 1998; 28:409–13.
38. Bruner JP, Tulipan N, Reed G et al. Intrauterine repair of spine bifida: preoperative predictors of shunt-dependent hydrocephalus. Am J Obstet Gynecol 2004; 190:1305–12.
39. Farrell JA, Albanese CT, Jennings RW et al. Maternal fertility is not affected by fetal surgery. Fetal Diagn Ther 1999; 14:190–2.
40. Longaker MT, Golbus MS, Filly RA et al. Maternal outcome after open fetal surgery. A review of the first 17 human cases. JAMA 1991; 265:737–41.
41. Harrison MR. Fetal surgery. Am J Obstet Gynecol 1996; 174:1255–64.
42. Robichaux AG III, Greene MJ, Greene MF et al. Fetal abdominal wall defect: a new complication of vesicoamniotic shunting. Fetal Diagn Ther 1991; 6:11–13.
43. Estes JM, MacGillivray TE, Hedrick MH et al. Fetoscopic surgery for the treatment of congenital anomalies. J Pediatr Surg 1992; 27:950–4.
44. Quintera RA, Johnson MP, Romero R et al. In-utero percutaneous cystoscopy in the management of fetal lower obstructive uropathy. Lancet 1995; 346:537–40.

45. Coplen DE, Hare JY, Zderic SA et al. 10-year experience with prenatal intervention for hydronephrosis. J Urol 1996; 156:1142–5.
46. Coplen DE. Prenatal intervention of hydronephrosis. J Urol 1997; 157:2270–7.
47. Lewis DP, Van Dyke DC, Stumbo PJ, Berg MJ. Drug and environmental factors associated with adverse pregnancy outcomes. Part II: improvement with folic acid. Ann Pharmacother 1998; 32:947–61.
48. Lewis KM, Pinckert TL, Cain MP, Ghidini A. Complications of intrauterine placement of a vesicoamniotic shunt. Obstet Gynecol 1998; 91:825–7.
49. Oberg KC, Robles AE, Ducsay CA et al. Endoscopic intrauterine surgery in primates: overcoming technical obstacles. Surg Endosc 1999; 13:420–6.
50. Gearhart JP, Ben-Chaim J, Jeffs RD, Sanders RC. Criteria for the prenatal diagnosis of classic bladder exstrophy. Obstet Gynecol 1995; 85:961–4.
51. Emanuel PG, Garcia GI, Angtuaco TL. Prenatal detection of anterior abdominal wall defects with US. Radiographics 1995; 15:517–30.
52. Dykes EH. Prenatal diagnosis and management of abdominal wall defects. Semin Pediatr Surg 1996; 5:90–4.
53. Hsieh K, O'Loughlin MT, Ferrer FA. Bladder exstrophy and phenotypic gender determination on fetal magnetic resonance imaging. Urol 2005; 65:998–9.
54. Cacciari A, Pilu GL, Mordenti M et al. Prenatal diagnosis of bladder exstrophy: what counseling? J Urol 1999; 161:259–61.
55. Woodhouse CRJ, Ransley PC, Williams DI. The exstrophy patient in adult life. Br J Urol 1983; 55:632–42.
56. Feitz WF, Van Gruns-Venn EJ, Froeling FM, de Vries JD. Outcome analysis of psychosexual and socioeconomic development of adult patients born with bladder exstrophy. J Urol 1994; 152:1417–19.
57. Ben-Chaim J, Jeffs RD, Reiner WG, Gearhart JP. The outcome of patients with classic bladder exstrophy in adult life. J Urol 1996; 155:1251–2.
58. Vintzileos AM, Ananth CV, Fisher AJ et al. Cost–benefit analysis of targeted ultrasonography for prenatal detection of spina bifida in patients with an elevated concentration of second-trimester maternal serum alpha-fetoprotein. Am J Obstet Gynecol 1999; 180:1227–33.
59. Kopp C, Greenfield SP. Effects of neurogenic bladder dysfunction in utero seen in neonates with myleodysplasia. Br J Urol 1993; 71:739–42.
60. Christensen B, Rosenblatt DS. Effects of folate deficiency on embryonic development. Baillieres Clin Haematol 1995; 8:617–37.
61. Neuhouser ML, Beresford SA, Hickok DE, Monsen ER. Absorption of dietary and supplemental folate in women with prior pregnancies with neural tube defects and controls. J Am Coll Nutr 1998; 17:625–30.
62. Cromie WJ, Lee K, Houde K, Holmes L. Implications of the decrease in major genitourinary malformations in the United States, 1972–1974. American Academy of Pediatrics, Annual Meeting, San Francisco, CA; 1998: Abstract 106.
63. Holzbeierlein J, Pope JC IV, Adams MC, Bruner J, Tulipan N, Brock JW 3rd. The urodynamic profile of myelodysplasia in childhood with spinal closure during gestation. J Urol 2000; 164:1336–9.
64. Elejalde BR, de Elejalde MM, Heitman T. Visualization of the fetal genitalia by ultrasonography: a review of the literature and analysis of its accuracy and ethical implications. J Ultrasound Med 1985; 4:633–9.
65. Doran TA. Chorionic villus sampling as the primary diagnostic tool in prenatal diagnosis. Should it replace genetic amniocentesis? J Reprod Med 1990; 35:935–40.
66. Mandell J, Bromley B, Peters CA, Benacerraf BR. Prenatal sonographic detection of genital malformations. J Urol 1995; 153:242–6.
67. Herndon CDA, McKenna PH, Kolon TF et al. A multicenter outcomes analysis of patients with neonatal reflux presenting with prenatal hydronephrosis. J Urol 1999; 162:1203–8.
68. Shapiro E. The sonographic appearance of normal and abnormal fetal genitalia. J Urol 1999; 162:530–3.
69. Kemp J, Davenport M, Pernet A. Antenatally diagnosed surgical anomalies: the psychological effect of parental antenatal counseling. J Pediatr Surg 1998; 33:1376–9.
70. David M, Forest MG. Prenatal treatment of congenital adrenal hyperplasia resulting from 21-hydroxylase deficiency. J Pediatr 1984; 105:799–803.
71. Evans MI, Chrousos GP, Mann DW et al. Pharmacologic suppression of the fetal adrenal gland in utero. Attempted prevention of abnormal external genital masculinization in suspected congenital adrenal hyperplasia. JAMA 1985; 253:1015–20.
72. Speiser PW, Laforgia N, Kato K et al. First trimester prenatal treatment and molecular genetic diagnosis of congenital adrenal hyperplasia (21-hydroxylase deficiency). J Clin Endocrinol Metab 1990; 70:838–48.
73. Forest MG, David M, Morel Y. Prenatal diagnosis and treatment of 21-hydroxylase deficiency. J Steroid Biochem Mol Biol 1993; 45:75–82.
74. Mercado AB, Wilson RC, Cheng KC et al. Prenatal treatment and diagnosis of congenital adrenal hyperplasia owing to steroid 21-hydroxylase deficiency. J Clin Endocrinol Metab 1995; 80:2014.
75. Lajic S, Wedell A, Bui T-H et al. Long-term somatic follow-up of prenatally treated children with congenital adrenal hyperplasia. J Clin Endocrinol Metab 1998; 83:3872–80.
76. New MI, Carlson A, Obeid J et al. Prenatal diagnosis for congenital adrenal hyperplasia in 532 pregnancies. J Clin Endocrinol Metab 2001; 86:5651–7.
77. Ross HL, Elias S. Maternal serum screening for fetal genetic disorders. Obstet Gynecol Clin North Am 1997; 24:33–47.
78. Miller WL. Dexamethasone treatment of congenital adrenal hyperplasia in utero: an experimental therapy of unproven safety. J Urol 1999; 162:537–40.
79. Speiser PW. Prenatal treatment of congenital adrenal hyperplasia. J Urol 1999; 162:534–6.
80. Lajic S, Nordenstrom A, Ritzen EM, Wedell A. Prenatal treatment of congenital adrenal hyperplasia. Eur J Endocrinol 2004; 151(Supp 3):1163–9.
81. Pang SY, Pollack MS, Marshall RN, Immken L. Prenatal treatment of congenital adrenal hyperplasia due to 21-hydroxylase deficiency. N Engl J Med 1990; 322:111–15.

82. Speiser PW, New MI. Prenatal diagnosis and management of congenital adrenal hyperplasia. Clin Perinatol 1994; 21:631–8.
83. New M, White P. Genetic disorders of steroid hormone synthesis and metabolism. Baillieres Clin Endocrinol Metab 1995; 9:525–54.
84. Klaus M, Kennell J. Interventions in the premature nursery: impact on development. Pediatr Clin North Am 1982; 29:1263–73.
85. Crouch M, Manderson L. The social life of bonding theory. Soc Sci Med 1995; 41:837–44.
86. Riski JE. Parents of children with cleft lip and plate. Clin Commun Disord 1991; 1(3):42–7.
87. Bradbury ET, Hewison J. Early parental adjustment to visible congenital disfigurement. Child Care Health Dev 1994; 20:251–66.
88. Drotar D, Baskiewicz A, Irvin N et al. The adaptation of parents to the birth of an infant with a congenital malformation: a hypothetical model. Pediatrics 1975; 56:710–17.
89. Quine L, Pahl J. First diagnosis of severe handicap: a study of parental reactions. Dev Med Child Neurol 1987; 29:232–42.
90. Varni JW, Setoguchi Y. Effects of parental adjustment on the adaptation of children with congenital or acquired limb deficiencies. J Dev Behav Pediatr 1993; 14:13–20.
91. Belman AB, King LR. Urinary tract abnormalities associated with imperforate anus. J Urol 1972; 108:823–4.
92. deVries PA, Pena A. Posterior sagittal anorectoplasty. J Pediatr Surg 1982; 17:638–43.
93. McLorie GA, Sheldon CA, Fleisher M, Churchill BM. The genitourinary system in patients with imperforate anus. J Pediatr Surg 1987; 22:1100–4.
94. Levitt MA, Rodriguez G, Gaylin DS, Pena A. The tethered spinal cord in patients with anorectal malformations. J Pediatr Surg 1997; 32:462–8.
95. Boemers TM. Neurogenic bladder in infants born with anorectal malformations: comparison with spinal and urologic status. J Pediatr Surg 1999; 34:1889–90.
96. Surer I, Baker LA, Jeffs RD, Gearhart JP. Combined bladder neck reconstruction and epispadias repair for exstrophy-epispadias complex. J Urol 2001; 165:2425–7.
97. Jeffs RD, Guice SL, Oesch I. The factors in successful exstrophy closure. J Urol 1982; 127:974–7.
98. Gearhart JP, Jeffs RD. Augmentation cystoplasty in the failed exstrophy reconstruction. J Urol 1988; 139:790–3.
99. Grady RW, Mitchell ME. Complete primary repair of exstrophy. J Urol 1999; 162:1415–20.
100. Gearhart JP. Complete repair of bladder exstrophy in the newborn: complications and management. J Urol 2001; 165:2431–3.
101. McKenna PH. A functional classification of ectopic ureteroceles based on renal unit jeopardy. Dialog Pediatr Urol 1993; 16:9.
102. McKenna PH, Khoury AE, McLorie GA et al. Anterior diagonal mid-innominate osteotomy. Dialog Pediatr Urol 1993; 16:1.
103. McKenna PH, Khoury AE, McLorie GA et al. Iliac osteotomy: model to compare options in bladder and cloacal exstrophy reconstruction. J Urol 1994; 151:182–6, discussion 186–7.
104. Sponseller PD, Jani MM, Jeffs RD, Gearhart JP. Anterior innominate osteotomy in repair of bladder exstrophy. J Bone Joint Surg Am 2001; 83-A:184–93.
105. Wheatley JM, Stephens FD, Hutson JM. Prune belly syndrome: ongoing controversies regarding pathogenesis and management. Semin Pediatr Surg 1996; 5:95–106.
106. Hoshino T, Ihara Y, Shirane H, Ota T. Prenatal diagnosis of prune belly syndrome at 12 weeks of pregnancy: case report and review of the literature. Ultrasound Obstet Gynecol 1998; 12:362–6.
107. Shigeta M, Nagata M, Shimoyamada H et al. Prune belly syndrome diagnosed at 14 weeks' gestation with severe urethral obstruction but normal kidneys. Pediatr Nephrol 1999; 13:135–7.
108. Hirose R, Suita S, Taguchi T et al. Prune belly syndrome in a female, complicated by intestinal malrotation after successful antenatal treatment of hydrops fetalis. J Pediatr Surg 1995; 30:1373–5.
109. Burbige KA, Amodio J, Berdon WE et al. Prune belly syndrome: 35 years of experience. J Urol 1987; 137:86–90.
110. Woodard JR, Zucker I. Current management of the dilated urinary tract in prune belly syndrome. Urol Clin North Am 1990; 17:407–18.
111. Druschel CM. A descriptive study of prune belly in New York state, 1983 to 1989. Arch Pediatr Adolesc Med 1995; 149:70–6.
112. Reinberg Y, Manivel JC, Fryd D et al. The outcome of renal transplantation in children with the prune belly syndrome. J Urol 1989; 142:1541–2.
113. Reinberg Y, Manivel JC, Pettinato G, Gonzalez R. Development of renal failure in children with the prune belly syndrome. J Urol 1991; 145:1017–19.
114. Bukowski TP, Perlmutter AD. Reduction cystoplasty in the prune belly syndrome: a long-term followup. J Urol 1994; 152:2113–16.
115. Noh PH, Cooper CS, Winkler AC et al. Prognostic factors for long-term renal function in boys with the prune belly syndrome. J Urol 1999; 162:1399–401.
116. Docimo SG, Moore RG, Kavoussi LR. Laparoscopic orchidopexy in the prune belly syndrome: a case report and review of the literature. Urology 1995; 45:679–81.
117. Woodhouse CR, Snyder HM III. Testicular and sexual function in adults with prune belly syndrome. J Urol 1985; 133:607–9.
118. Orvis BR, Bottles K, Kogan BA. Testicular histology in fetuses with the prune belly syndrome and posterior urethral valves. J Urol 1988; 139:335–7.
119. Woodhouse CR, Ransley PG. Teratoma of the testis in the prune belly syndrome. Br J Urol 1983; 55:580–1.
120. Massad CA, Cohen MB, Kogan BA, Beckstead JH. Morphology and histochemistry of infant testes in the prune belly syndrome. J Urol 1991; 146:1598–600.
121. Parra RO, Cummings JM, Palmer DC. Testicular seminoma in a long-term survivor of the prune belly syndrome. Eur Urol 1991; 19:79–80.
122. Stein SC, Feldman JG, Freidlander M, et al. Is myelomeningocele a disappearing disease? Pediatrics 1982; 69:511–13.

123. Anon. Use of folic acid for prevention of spina bifida and other neural tube defects. Morb Mort Weekly Rep 1991; 40:513–16.
124. Cromie WJ. Implications of antenatal ultrasound screening in the incidence of major genitourinary malformations. Semin Pediatr Surg 2001; 10:204–11.
125. Scarff TB, Fronczak S. Myelomeningocele: a review and update. Rehabil Lit 1981; 42:143–6.
126. Lais A, Kasabian NG, Dyro FM et al. The neurosurgical implications of continuous neurourological surveillance of children with myelodysplasia. J Urol 1993; 150:1879–83.
127. Bauer SB. Management of neurogenic bladder dysfunction in children. J Urol 1984; 132:544–5.
128. Roach MB, Switters DM, Stone AR. The changing urodynamic pattern in infants with myelomeningocele. J Urol 1993; 150:944–7.
129. Sillén U, Hansson E, Hermansson G et al. Development of the urodynamic pattern in infants with myelomeningocele. Br J Urol 1996; 78:596–601.
130. van Gool JD, Kuijten RH, Donckerwolcke RA, Kramer PP. Detrusor-sphincter dyssynergia in children with myelomeningocele: a prospective study. Z Kinderchir 1982; 37:148–54.
131. McGuire EJ, Woodside JR, Borden TA et al. Prognostic value of urodynamic testing in myelodysplasia patients. J Urol 1981; 126:205–9.
132. Dator DP, Hatchett L, Dyro FM et al. Urodynamic dysfunction in walking myelodysplastic children. J Urol 1992; 148:362–5.
133. Andros GJ, Hatch DA, Walter JS et al. Home bladder pressure monitoring in children with myelomeningocele. J Urol 1998; 160:518–21.
134. Perez LM, Khoury J, Webster GD. The value of urodynamic studies in infants less than 1 year old with congenital spinal dysraphism. J Urol 1992; 148:584–7.
135. Wu HY, Baskin LS, Kogan BA. Neurogenic bladder dysfunction due to myelomeningocele: neonatal versus childhood treatment. J Urol 1997; 157:2295–7.
136. Bauer SB. Editorial: the challenge of the expanding role of urodynamic studies in the treatment of children with neurological and functional disabilities. J Urol 1998; 160:527–8.
137. Bauer SB, Lais A, Scott RM. Continuous urodynamic surveillance of babies with myelodysplasia: implications for further neurosurgery. Eur J Pediatr Surg 1992; 1(Suppl 2):35–6.
138. Foster LS, Kogan BA, Cogan PH, Edwards MSB. Bladder function in patients with lipomyelomeningocele. J Urol 1990; 143:984–6.
139. Atala A, Bauer SB, Dyro FM et al. Bladder functional changes resulting from lipomeningocele repair. J Urol 1992; 148:592–4.
140. Bruce DA, Schut L. Spinal lipomas in infancy and childhood. Brain 1979; 5:192–203.
141. Colak A, Pollack IF, Albright AL. Recurrent tethering: a common long-term problem after lipomyelomeningocele repair. Pediatr Neurosurg 1998; 29:184–90.
142. Guzman L, Bauer SB, Hallet M et al. The evaluation and management of children with sacral agenesis. Urology 1983; 23:506–9.
143. Gotoh T, Shinno Y, Kobayashi S et al. Diagnosis and management of sacral agenesis. Eur Urol 1991; 20:287–92.
144. White RI, Klauber GT. Sacral agenesis. Analysis of 22 cases. Urology 1976; 8:521–5.
145. Koff SA, DeRidder PA. Patterns of neurogenic bladder dysfunction in sacral agenesis. J Urol 1977; 118:87–9.
146. Borrelli M, Bruschini H, Nahas WC et al. Sacral agenesis: why is it so frequently misdiagnosed? Urology 1985; 26:351–5.
147. Noske HD, Kraus SW, Altinkilic BM, Weidner W. Historical milestones regarding torsion of the scrotal organs. J Urol 1998; 159:13–16.
148. Herman TE, Siegel MJ. Special imaging casebook. Neonatal spermatic cord torsion and testicular infarction. J Perinatol 1994; 14:431–2.
149. Gross BR, Cohen HL, Schlessel JS. Perinatal diagnosis of bilateral testicular torsion: beware of torsions simulating hydroceles. J Ultrasound Med 1993; 12:479–81.
150. Baptist EC, Amin PV. Perinatal testicular torsion and hard testicle. J Perinatol 1996; 16:67–8.
151. Pinto KJ, Noe HN, Jerkins GR. Management of neonatal testicular torsion. J Urol 1997; 158:1196–7.
152. Driver CP, Losty PD. Neonatal testicular torsion. Br J Urol 1998; 82:855–8.
153. Huff DS, Wu H, Snyder HM III et al. Evidence in favor of the mechanical (intrauterine torsion) theory over the endocrinopathy (cryptorchidism) theory in the pathogenesis of testicular agenesis. J Urol 1991; 146:630–1.
154. Cilento BG, Najjar SS, Atala A. Cryptorchidism and testicular torsion. Pediatr Clin North Am 1993; 40:1133–49.
155. Gong M, Geary ES, Shortliffe LMD. Testicular torsion with contralateral vanishing testis. Urology 1996; 48:306–7.
156. Cartwright PC, Snow BW, Reid BS, Shultz PK. Color Doppler ultrasound in newborn testis torsion. Urology 1995; 45:667–70.
157. Stone KT, Kass EJ, Cacciarelli AA, Gibson DP. Management of suspected antenatal torsion: what is the best strategy? J Urol 1995; 153:782–4.
158. Groisman GM, Nassrallah M, Bar-maor JA. Bilateral intra-uterine testicular torsion in a newborn. Br J Urol 1996; 78:800–1.
159. Hernanz-Schulman M, Yenicesu F, Heller RM, Brock JW III. Sonographic identification of perinatal testicular torsion. J Ultrasound Med 1997; 16:65–7.
160. Zinn HL, Cohen HL, Horowitz M. Testicular torsion in neonates: importance of power Doppler imaging. J Ultrasound Med 1998; 17:385–8.
161. Tripp BM, Homsy YL. Prenatal diagnosis of bilateral neonatal torsion: a case report. J Urol 1995; 153:1990–1.
162. Cooper CS, Snyder OB, Hawtrey CE. Bilateral neonatal testicular torsion. Clin Pediatr 1997; 36:653–6.
163. LaQuaglia MP, Bauer SB, Eraklis A et al. Bilateral neonatal torsion. J Urol 1987; 138:1051–4.
164. Das S, Singer A. Controversies of perinatal torsion of the spermatic cord: a review, survey and recommendations. J Urol 1990; 143:231–3.
165. Calleja R, Archer TJ. Bilateral testicular torsion in a neonate. Br J Urol 1996; 78:793–804.
166. Putnam MH. Neonatal adrenal hemorrhage presenting as a right scrotal mass. JAMA 1989; 261:2958.

167. Ring KS, Axelrod SL, Burbige KA, Hensle TW. Meconium hydrocele: an unusual etiology of a scrotal mass in the newborn. J Urol 1989; 141:1172–3.
168. McAlister WH, Sisler CL. Scrotal sonography in infants and children. Curr Probl Diagn Radiol 1990; 19: 201–42.
169. Stokes S III, Flom S. Meconium filled hydrocele sacs as a cause of acute scrotum in a newborn. J Urol 1997; 158:1960–1.
170. Han K, Mata J, Zaontz MR. Meconium masquerading as a scrotal mass. Br J Urol 1998; 82:765–7.
171. Levy DA, Kay R, Elder JS. Neonatal testis tumors: a review of the Prepubertal Testis Tumor Registry. J Urol 1994; 151:715–17.
172. Melekos MD. Re: Testicular torsion in a 62-year-old man. J Urol 1988; 140:387–9.
173. Caldamone AA, Valvo JR, Altebarmakian VK, Rabinowitz R. Acute scrotal swelling in children. J Pediatr Surg 1984; 19:581–4.
174. Kass EJ, Stone KT, Cacciarelli AA, Mitchell B. Do all children with an acute scrotum require exploration? J Urol 1993; 150:667–9.
175. Patriquin HB, Yazbeck S, Trinh B et al. Testicular torsion in infants and children: diagnosis with Doppler sonography. Radiology 1993; 188:781–5.
176. Yazbeck S, Patriquin HB. Accuracy of Doppler sonography in the evaluation of acute conditions of the scrotum in children. J Pediatr Surg 1994; 29:1270–2.
177. Brandell RA, Brock JW III. Common problems in pediatric urology. Compr Ther 1993; 19:11–16.
178. Tryfonas G, Violaki A, Tsikopoulos G et al. Late postoperative results in males treated for testicular torsion during childhood. J Pediatr Surg 1994; 29:553–6.
179. Rampaul MS, Hosking SW. Testicular torsion: most delay occurs outside hospital. Ann R Coll Surg Engl 1998; 80:169–72.
180. Mikuz G. Testicular torsion: simple grading for histological evaluation of tissue damage. Appl Pathol 1985; 3:134–9.
181. Lewis AG, Bukowski TP, Jarvis PD et al. Evaluation of acute scrotum in the emergency department. J Pediatr Surg 1995; 30:277–82.
182. Sawchuk T, Costabile RA, Howards SS, Rodgers BM. Spermatic cord torsion in an infant receiving human chorionic gonadotropin. J Urol 1993; 150:1212–13.
183. Kadish HA, Bolte RG. A retrospective review of pediatric patients with epididymitis, testicular torsion, and torsion of testicular appendages. Pediatrics 1998; 102:73–6.
184. Hamm B. Differential diagnosis of scrotal masses by ultrasound. Eur Radiol 1997; 7:668–9.
185. Sugita Y, Clarnette TD, Cooke-Yarborough C et al. Testicular and paratesticular tumours in children: 30 years' experience. Aust NZ J Surg 1999; 69:505–8.
186. Ferrer FA, McKenna PH. Cavernous hemangioma of the scrotum: a rare benign genital tumor of childhood. J Urol 1995; 153:1262–4.
187. Aragona F, Pescatori E, Talenti E et al. Painless scrotal masses in the pediatric population: prevalence and age distribution of different pathological conditions – a 10 year retrospective multicenter study. J Urol 1996; 155:1424–26.
188. Donahoe PK, Powell DM, Lee MM. Clinical management of intersex abnormalities. Curr Probl Surg 1991; 28:513–79.
189. Donahoe PK, Schnitzer JJ. Evaluation of the infant who has ambiguous genitalia, and principles of operative management. Semin Pediatr Surg 1996; 5:30–40.
190. Lee MM, Donahoe PK. The infant with ambiguous genitalia. Curr Ther Endocrinol Metab 1997; 6:216–23.
191. Meyer-Bahlburg HF. Gender assignment and reassignment in 46,XY pseudohermaphroditism and related conditions. J Clin Endocrinol Metab 1999; 84:3455–8.
192. Meyer-Bahlburg HF, Heino FL. New York State Psychiatric Institute, Dept of Psychiatry, Columbia University, New York, NY. Gender assignment and reassignment in intersexuality: controversies, data, and guidelines for research. In: Zderic SA, Canning DA, Snyder HM III, Carr MC, eds. Pediatric Gender Reassignment: A Critical Reappraisal. New York: Plenum, 1999: 12–24.
193. Colapinto J. The true story of John/Joan. Rolling Stone 1997; Feb:55–96.
194. Dinneen MD, Dhillon HK, Ward HC et al. Antenatal diagnosis of posterior urethral valves. Br J Urol 1993; 72:364–9.
195. Dewan PA, Goh DG. Variable expression of the congenital obstructive posterior urethral membrane. Urology 1995; 45:507–9.
196. Reinberg Y, De Castano I, Gonzalez R. Prognosis for patients with prenatally diagnosed posterior urethral valves. J Urol 1992; 148:125–6.
197. Churchill BM, McLorie GA, Khoury AE et al. Emergency treatment and long-term followup of posterior urethral valves. Urol Clin North Am 1990; 17:343–60.
198. Gonzales ET. Alternatives in the management of posterior urethral valves. Urol Clin North Am 1990; 17:335–42.
199. Merguerian PA, McLorie GA, Churchill BM et al. Radiographic and serologic correlates of azotemia in patients with posterior urethral valves. J Urol 1992; 148:1499–503.
200. Tietjen DN, Gloor JM, Husmann DA. Proximal urinary diversion in the management of posterior urethral valves: is it necessary? J Urol 1997; 158:1008–10.
201. Smith GHH, Canning DA, Schulman SL et al. The long-term outcome of posterior urethral valves treated with primary valve ablation and observation. J Urol 1996; 155:1730–4.
202. Close CE, Carr MC, Burns MW, Mitchell ME. Lower urinary tract changes after early valve ablation in neonates and infants: is early diversion warranted? J Urol 1997; 157:984–8.
203. Walker RD, Padron M. The management of posterior urethral valves by initial vesicostomy and delayed valve ablation. J Urol 1990; 144:1212–14.
204. Farhat W, McLorie G, Capolicchio G, Choury A, Bagli D, Merguerian PA. Outcomes of primary valve ablation versus urinary tract diversion in patients with posterior urethral valves. Urology 2000; 56:653–7.
205. Ghanem MA, Nijman RJ. Long-term follow up of bilateral high (sober) urinary diversion in patients with posterior urethral valves and its effect on bladder function. J Urol 2005; 173:1721–4.

206. Parkhouse HF, Woodhouse CRJ. Long-term status of patients with posterior urethral valves. Urol Clin North Am 1990; 17:373–8.
207. Mor Y, Ramon J, Raviv G et al. A 20-year experience with treatment of ectopic ureteroceles. J Urol 1992; 147:1592–4.
208. Sherer DM, Hulbert WC. Prenatal sonographic diagnosis and subsequent conservative surgical management of bilateral ureteroceles. Am J Perinatol 1995; 12:174–7.
209. Gloor JM, Ogburn P, Matsumoto J. Prenatally diagnosed ureterocele presenting as fetal bladder outlet obstruction. J Perinatol 1996; 16:285–7.
210. Blyth B, Passerini-Glazel G, Camuffo C et al. Endoscopic incision of ureteroceles: intravesical versus ectopic. J Urol 1993; 149:556–60.
211. Smith C, Gosalbez R, Parrott TS et al. Transurethral puncture of ectopic ureteroceles in neonates and infants. J Urol 1994; 152:2110–12.
212. Di Benedetto V, Morrison-Lacombe G, Bagnara V, Monfort G. Transurethral puncture of ureterocele associated with single collecting system in neonates. J Pediatr Surg 1997; 32:1325–7.
213. Coplen DE. Editorial: neonatal ureterocele incision. J Urol 1998; 159:1010.
214. Pfister C, Ravasse P, Barret E et al. The value of endoscopic treatment for ureteroceles during the neonatal period. J Urol 1998; 159:1006–9.
215. Avni EF, Schulman CC. The origin of vesico-ureteric reflux in male newborns: further evidence in favour of a transient fetal urethral obstruction. Br J Urol 1996; 78:454–9.
216. Yeung CK, Godley ML, Dhillon HK et al. The characteristics of primary vesico-ureteric reflux in male and female infants with pre-natal hydronephrosis. Br J Urol 1997; 80:319–27.
217. Tibballs JM, De Bruyn R. Primary vesicoureteral reflux – how useful is postnatal ultrasound? Arch Dis Child 1996; 75:444–7.
218. Poland RL. The question of routine neonatal circumcision. N Engl J Med 1990; 322:1312–15.
219. Nelson CP, Dunn R, Wan J, Wei JF. The increasing incidence of newborn circumcision: data from the nationwide inpatient sample. J Urol 2005; 173:978–81.
220. Gordon A, Collin J. Save the normal foreskin: widespread confusion over what the medical indications for circumcision are. BMJ 1993; 306:1–2.
221. Wiswell TE, Tencer HL, Welch CA, Chamberlain JL. Circumcision in children beyond the neonatal period. Pediatrics 1993; 92:791–4.
222. Barnhouse DH, Chin DL, Lewis DD et al. Circumcision and urinary tract infection. JAMA 1992; 268:54–5.
223. Spach DH, Stapleton AE, Stamm WE. Lack of circumcision increases the risk of urinary tract infection in young men. JAMA 1992; 267:679–82.
224. Gunsar C, Kurutepe S, Alparslan O. The effect of circumcision status on periurethral and glanular bacterial flora. Urol Int 2004; 72:212–15.
225. Elmore JM, Baker LA, Snodgrass WT. Topical steroid therapy as an alternative to circumcision for phimosis in boys younger than 3 years. J Urol 2002;168(4 Pt 2):1746–7; discussion 1747.
226. Ashfield JE, Nickel Kr, Siemens DR, MacNeily AE, Nickel JC. Treatment of phimosis with topical steroids in 194 children. J Urol 2003 Mar;169(3):1106–8.
227. Alter GJ, Horton CE Jr, Horton CE Jr. Buried penis as a contraindication for circumcision. J Am Coll Surg 1994; 178:487–9.
228. Christakis DA, Harvey E, Zerr DM, Feudtner C, Wright JA, Connell FA. A trade-off analysis of routine newborn circumcision. Pediatrics 2000; 105(1 Pt 3):246–9.
229. Williams N, Kapila L. Complications of circumcision. Br J Surg 1993; 80:1231–6.
230. Eason JD, McDonnell M, Clark G. Male ritual circumcision resulting in acute renal failure. BMJ 1994; 309:660–1.
231. Smith DJ, Hamdy FC, Chapple CR. An uncommon complication of circumcision. Br J Urol 1994; 73:459–60.
232. Persad R, Sharma S, McTavish J et al. Clinical presentation and pathophysiology of meatal stenosis following circumcision. Br J Urol 1995; 75:91–3.
233. Neulander E, Walfisch S, Kaneti J. Amputation of distal penile glans during neonatal ritual circumcision – a rare complication. Br J Urol 1996; 77:924–5.
234. Strimling BS. Partial amputation of glans penis during Mogen clamp circumcision. Pediatrics 1996; 97:906–8.
235. Bliss DP Jr, Healey PJ, Waldhausen JHT. Necrotizing fasciitis after Plastibell circumcision. J Pediatr 1997; 131:459–62.
236. Ozdemir E. Significantly increased complication risks with mass circumcisions. Br J Urol 1997; 80:136–9.
237. Kaplan GW. Complications of circumcision. Urol Clin North Am 1983; 10:543–9.
238. Niku SD, Stock JA, Kaplan GW. Neonatal circumcision. Urol Clin North Am 1995; 22:57–65.
239. Davenport M. Problems with the penis and prepuce. (ABC of general surgery in children) BMJ 1996; 312:299–301.
240. Mayer E, Caruso DJ, Ankem M, Fisher MC, Cummings KB, Barone JG. Anatomic variants associated with newborn circumcision complications. Can J Urol 2003; 10:2013–16.
241. Gearhart JP, Rock JA. Total ablation of the penis after circumcision with electrocautery: a method of management and long-term followup. J Urol 1989; 142:799–801.
242. Gluckman GR, Stoller ML, Jacobs MM, Kogan BA. Newborn penile glans amputation during circumcision and successful reattachment. J Urol 1995; 153:778–9.
243. Sherman J, Borer JG, Horowitz M, Glassberg KI. Circumcision: successful glanular reconstruction and survival following traumatic amputation. J Urol 1996; 156:842–4.
244. Baskin LS, Canning DA, Snyder HM III, Duckett JW Jr. Surgical repair of urethral circumcision injuries. J Urol 1997; 158:2269–71.
245. Ozkan S, Gurpinar T. A serious circumcision complication: penile shaft amputation and a new reattachment technique with a successful outcome. J Urol 1997; 158:1946–7.
246. Sotolongo JR Jr, Hoffman S, Gribetz ME. Penile denudation injuries after circumcision. J Urol 1985; 133:102–3.

247. Hashem FK, Ahmen S, al-Malaq AA, AbuDaia JM. Successful replantation of penile amputation (post-circumcision) complicated by prolonged ischaemia. Br J Plast Surg 1999; 52:308–10.
248. Kon M. A rare complication following circumcision: the concealed penis. J Urol 1983; 130:573–4.
249. Stang HJ, Gunnar MR, Snellman L et al. Local anesthesia for neonatal circumcision: effects on distress and cortisol response. JAMA 1988; 259:1507–9.
250. Snellman LW, Stand HJ. Prospective evaluation of complications of dorsal penile nerve block for neonatal circumcision. Pediatrics 1995; 95:705–9.
251. Hardwick-Smith S, Mastrobattista JM, Wallace PA, Ritchey ML. Ring block for neonatal circumcision. Obstet Gynecol 1998; 91:930–4.
252. Horger EO III, Arnett RM, Jones JS et al. Local anesthesia for infants undergoing circumcision. (Letter to the Editor). JAMA 1998; 279:1169.
253. Howard CR, Howard FM, Garfunkel LC et al. Neonatal circumcision and pain relief: current training practices. Pediatrics 1998; 101:423–8.
254. Benini F, Johnston CC, Faucher D, Aranda JV. Topical anesthesia during circumcision in newborn infants. JAMA 1993; 270:850–3.
255. Lander J, Brady-Fryer B, Metcalfe JB et al. Comparison of ring block, dorsal penile nerve block, and topical anesthesia for neonatal circumcision: a randomized controlled trial. JAMA 1997; 278:2157.
256. Choi WY, Irwin MG, Hui TW, Lim HH, Chan KL. EMLA cream versus dorsal penile nerve block for postcircumcision analgesia in children. Anesth Analg 2003; 96:396–9, table of contents.
257. Caty MG, Shamberger RC. Abdominal tumors in infancy and childhood. Pediatr Clin North Am 1993; 40:1253–71.
258. Xue H, Horwitz JR, Smith MB et al. Malignant solid tumors in neonates: a 40-year review. J Pediatr Surg 1995; 30:543–5.
259. Griscom NT, Colodny AH, Rosenberg HK et al. Diagnostic aspects of neonatal ascites: report of 27 cases. AJR Am J Roentgenol 1977; 128:961–70.
260. Dhillon HK. Prenatally diagnosed hydronephrosis: the great Ormond Street experience. Br J Urol 1998; 81:39–44.
261. Dudley JA, Haworth JM, McGraw ME, Frank JD, Tizard EJ. Clinical relevance and implications of antenatal hydronephrosis. Arch Dis Child Fetal Neonatal Ed 1997; 76:F31–4.
262. Murphy JP, Holder TM, Ashcraft KW et al. Ureteropelvic junction obstruction in the newborn. Pediatr Surg 1984; 19:642–8.
263. Docimo SG, Silver RI. Renal ultrasonography in newborns with prenatally detected hydronephrosis: why wait? J Urol 1997; 157:1387–9.
264. Conway JJ, Maizels MJ. The 'well tempered' diuretic renogram: a standard method to examine the asymptomatic neonate with hydronephrosis or hydroureteronephrosis. A report from combined meetings of The Society for Fetal Urology and members of The Pediatric Nuclear Medicine Council–The Society of Nuclear Medicine. Nucl Med 1992; 33:2047–51.
265. O'Reilly P, Aurell M, Britton K et al. Consensus on diuresis renography for investigating the dilated upper urinary tract. J Nucl Med 1996; 37:1872–76.
266. Erbagci A, Yagi F, Sarica K, Bakir K. Predictive value of renal histological changes for postoperative renal function improvement in children with congenital ureteropelvic junction stenosis. Int J Urol 2002; 9:279–84.
267. Palmer LS, Maizels M, Cartwright PC et al. Surgery versus observation for managing obstructive grade 3 to 4 unilateral hydronephrosis: a report from the Society for Fetal Urology. J Urol 1998; 159:222–8.
268. King LR, Coughlin PW, Bloch EC et al. The case for immediate pyeloplasty in the neonate with ureteropelvic junction obstruction. J Urol 1984; 132:725–8.
269. McVicar M, Margouleff D, Chandra M. Diagnosis and imaging of the fetal and neonatal abdominal mass: an integrated approach. Adv Pediatr 1991; 38:135–49.
270. Pathak IG, Williams DI. Multicystic and cystic dysplastic kidneys. Br J Urol 1964; 36:318–31.
271. Glassberg KI, Stephens FD, Lebowitz RL et al. Renal dysgenesis and cystic disease of the kidney: a report of the Committee on Terminology, Nomenclature and Classification, Section on Urology. American Academy of Pediatrics. J Urol 1997; 138:1085–92.
272. Al-Khaldi N, Watson AR, Zuccollo J et al. Outcome of antenatally detected cystic dysplastic kidney disease. Arch Dis Child 1994; 70:520–2.
273. Miller DC, Rumohr JA, Dunn RL, Bloom DA, Park JM. What is the fate of the refluxing contralateral kidney in children with multicystic dysplastic kidney? J Urol 2004; 172(4 Pt 2):1630–4.
274. Belk RA, Thomas DF, Mueller RF, Godbole P, Markham AF, Weston MJ. A family study and the natural history of prenatally detected unilateral multicystic dysplastic kidney. J Urol 2002; 167(2 Pt 1):666–9.
275. De Klerk DP, Marshall FF, Jeffs RD. Multicystic dysplastic kidney. J Urol 1977; 118:306–8.
276. Kessler OJ, Ziv N, Livne PM et al. Involution rate of multicystic renal dysplasia. Pediatrics 1998; 102:E73.
277. Perez LM, Naidu SI, Joseph DB. Outcome and cost analysis of operative versus nonoperative management of neonatal multicystic dysplastic kidneys. J Urol 1998; 160:1207–11.
278. Rabelo EA, Oliveira EA, Silva JM et al. Conservative management of multicystic dysplastic kidney: clinical course and ultrasound outcome. J Pediatr (Rio J) 2005; 81:400–4.
279. Birken G, King D, Vane D, Lloyd T. Renal cell carcinoma arising in a multicystic dysplastic kidney. Pediatr Surg 1985; 20:619–21.
280. Dimmick JE, Johnson HW, Coleman GU, Carter M. Wilms tumorlet, nodular renal blastema and multicystic renal dysplasia. Urology 1989; 142:484–5; discussion 489.
281. Narchi H. Risk of Wilms' tumour with multicystic kidney disease: a systematic review. Arch Dis Child 2005; 90:147–9.
282. Susskind MR, Kim KS, King LR. Hypertension and multicystic kidney. Urology 1989; 34:362–6.
283. Zerres K, Rudnik-Schoneborn S, Steinkamm C et al. Autosomal recessive polycystic kidney disease. J Mol Med 1998; 76:303–9.

284. Cole BR, Conley SB, Stapleton FB. Polycystic kidney disease in the first year of life. Pediatrics 1987; III:693–9.
285. Harris PC, Rossetti S. Molecular genetics of autosomal recessive polycystic kidney disease. Mol Genet Metab 2004; 81:75–85.
286. Reeders ST, Germino GG. The molecular genetics of autosomal dominant polycystic kidney disease. Semin Nephrol 1989; 9:122–34.
287. Peters DJ, Spruit L, Saris JJ et al. Chromosome 4 localization of a second gene for autosomal dominant polycystic kidney disease. Nat Genet 1993; 5:359–62.
288. Paterson AD, Pei Y. Is there a third gene for autosomal dominant polycystic kidney disease? Kidney Int 1998; 54:1759–61.
289. Papadopoulou D, Tsakiris D, Papadimitriou M. The use of ultrasonography and linkage studies for early diagnosis of autosomal dominant polycystic kidney disease (ADPKD). Ren Fail 1999; 21:67–84.
290. MacDermot KD, Saggar-Malik AK, Economides DL, Jeffery S. Prenatal diagnosis of autosomal dominant polycystic kidney disease (PKD1) presenting in utero and prognosis for very early onset disease. J Med Genet 1998; 35:13–16.
291. Glassberg KI. Unilateral renal cystic disease. Urology 1999; 53:1227–8.
292. Hahn-Pedersen J, Kvist N, Nielsen OH. Hydrometrocolpos: current views on pathogenesis and management. J Urol 1984; 132:537–40.
293. Tran AT, Arensman RM, Falterman KW. Diagnosis and management of hydrohematometrocolpos syndromes. Am J Dis Child 1987; 141:632–4.
294. Hill SJ, Hirsch JHA. Sonographic detection of fetal hydrometrocolpos. Ultrasound Med 1985; 4:323–5.
295. Banerjee AR, Clarke O, MacDonald LM. Sonographic detection of neonatal hydrometrocolpos. Br J Radiol 1992; 65:268–71.
296. Turner JH, Leonard JC. Renal scintigraphic findings in a patient with hydrometrocolpos. Clin Nucl Med 1997; 22:394–6.
297. Meizner I, Levy A, Katz M, Maresh AJ, Glezerman M. Fetal ovarian cysts: prenatal ultrasonographic detection and postnatal evaluation and treatment. Am J Obstet Gynecol 1991; 164:874–8.
298. Armentano G, Dodero P, Natta A et al. Fetal ovarian cysts: prenatal diagnosis and management. Report of two cases and review of literature. Clin Exp Obstet Gynecol 1998; 25:88–91.
299. Decker PA, Chammas J, Sato TT. Laparoscopic diagnosis and management of ovarian torsion in the newborn. JSLS 1999; 3:141–3.
300. Blessed WB, Sepulveda W, Romero R et al. Prenatal diagnosis of spontaneous rupture of the fetal bladder with color Doppler ultrasonography. Am J Obstet Gynecol 1993; 169:1629–31.
301. Adams MC, Ludlow J, Brock JW III, Rink RC. Prenatal urinary ascites and persistent cloaca: risk factors for poor drainage of urine or meconium. J Urol 1998; 160:2179–81.
302. Machin GA. Diseases causing fetal and neonatal ascites. Pediatri Pathol 1985; 4:195–211.
303. Mann CM, Leape LL, Holder TM. Neonatal urinary ascites: a report of 2 cases of unusual etiology and a review of the literature. J Urol 1974; 111:124–8.
304. Forrest JR, Buschi AJ, Howards SS. Neonatal urinary ascites secondary to distal ureteral stenosis. J Urol 1980; 124:919–20.
305. Kay R, Brereton RJ, Johnson JH. Urinary ascites in the newborn. Br J Urol 1980; 52:451–4.
306. Cass AS, Khan AU, Smith S, Godec C. Neonatal perirenal urinary extravasation with posterior urethral valves. Urology 1981; 18:258–61.
307. Greenfield SP, Hensle TW, Berdon WE, Geringer AM. Urinary extravasation in the newborn male with posterior urethral valves. Pediatr Surg 1982; 17:751–6.
308. Rittenberg M, Hulbert WC, Snyder HM 3rd et al. Protective factors in posterior urethal valves. J Urol 1988; 140:993–6.
309. Sahdev S, Jhaveri RC, Vohra K, Khan AJ. Congenital bladder perforation and urinary ascites caused by posterior urethral valves: a case report. J Perinatol 1997; 17:164–5.
310. Chun KE, Ferguson RS. Neonatal urinary ascites due to unilateral vesicoureteric junction obstruction. Pediatr Surg Int 1997; 12:455–7.
311. Smith DP. Can perinatal events cause neonatal urinary ascites? Urology 1998; 159:1652–3.
312. Mata JA, Livne PM, Gibbons MD. Urinary ascites: complication of umbilical artery catheterization. Urology 1987; 30:375–7.
313. Diamond DA, Ford C. Neonatal bladder rupture: a complication of umbilical artery catheterization. J Urol 1989; 142:1543–4.
314. Barry JM, Anderson JM, Hodges CV. The subcapsular C sign: a rare radiographic finding associated with neonatal urinary ascites. J Urol 1994; 112:836–9.
315. Clarke HS Jr, Mills ME, Parres JA, Kropp KA. The hyponatremia of neonatal urinary ascites: clinical observations, experimental confirmation and proposed mechanism. Urology 1993; 150:778–81.
316. Scott TW. Urinary ascites secondary to posterior urethral valves. Urology 1976; 116:87–91.
317. Tank ES, Carey TC, Seifert AL. Management of neonatal urinary ascites. Urology 1980; XVI:270–3.
318. De Vries SH, Klijn AJ, Lilien MR, De Jong TP. Development of renal function after neonatal urinary ascites due to obstructive uropathy. J Urol 2002; 168:675–8.
319. Parker RM. Neonatal urinary ascites. A potentially favorable sign in bladder outlet obstruction. Urology 1974; III:589–94.
320. Wasnick RJ. Neonatal urinary ascites secondary to ureteropelvic junction obstruction. Urology 1987; 30:470–1.
321. Reha WC, Gibbons MD. Neonatal ascites and ureteral valves. Urology 1989; 33:468–71.
322. Fowlie F, Giacomantonio M, McKenzie E et al. Antenatal sonographic diagnosis of adrenal neuroblastoma. Can Assoc Radiol J 1986; 37:50–1.
323. Giulian BB, Chang CCN, Yoss BS. Prenatal ultrasonographic diagnosis of fetal adrenal neuroblastoma. J Clin Ultrasound 1986; 14:225–7.
324. Flake AW. Fetal sacrococcygeal teratoma. Semin Pediatr Surg 1993; 2:113–20.

325. Chisholm CA, Heider AL, Kuller JA et al. Prenatal diagnosis and perinatal management of fetal sacrococcygeal teratoma. Am J Perinatol 1999; 16:47–50.
326. Lukens JN. Neuroblastoma in the neonate. Semin Perinatol 1999; 23:263–73.
327. Woods WG, Gao RN, Shuster JJ. Screening of infants and mortality due to neuroblastoma. N Engl J Med 2002; 346:1041–6.
328. Liyanage IS, Katoch D. Ultrasonic prenatal diagnosis of liver metastases from adrenal neuroblastoma. J Clin Ultrasound 1992; 20:401–3.
329. Ho PTC, Estroff JA, Kozakewich H et al. Prenatal detection of neuroblastoma: a ten-year experience from the Dana-Farber Cancer Institute and Children's Hospital. Pediatrics 1993; 92:358–64.
330. Jennings RW, LaQuaglia MP, Leong K et al. Fetal neuroblastoma: prenatal diagnosis and natural history. J Pediatr Surg 1993; 28:1168–74.
331. Toma P, Lucigrai G, Marzoli, Lituania M. Prenatal diagnosis of metastatic adrenal neuroblastoma with sonography and MR imaging. AJR Am J Roentgenol 1994; 162: 1183–14.
332. Houlihan C, Jampolsky M, Shilad A, Principe D. Prenatal diagnosis of neuroblastoma with sonography and magnetic resonance imaging. J Ultrasound Med 2004; 23:547–50.
333. Haase GM, Perez C, Atkinson JB. Current aspects of biology, risk assessment, and treatment of neuroblastoma. Semin Surg Oncol 1999; 16:91–104.
334. McWilliams NB. Screening infants for neuroblastoma in North America. Pediatrics 1987; 79:1048–9.
335. Woods WG, Tuchman M. Neuroblastoma: the case for screening infants in North America J Natl Cancer Int 1997; 89:373–80.
336. Erttman R, Tafese T, Berthold F et al. 10 years' neuroblastoma screening in Europe: preliminary results of a clinical and biological review from the Study Group for Evaluation of Neuroblastoma Screening in Europe (SENSE). Eur J Cancer 1998; 34:1391–7.
337. van Noesel MM, Hahlen K, Hakvoort-Cammel FG, Egeler RM. Neuroblastoma 4S: a heterogeneous disease with variable risk factors and treatment strategies. Cancer 1997; 80:834–43.
338. Matzinger MA, Matzinger FR, Matzinger KE, Black MD. Antenatal and postnatal findings in intra-abdominal pulmonary sequestration. Can Assoc Radiol J 1992; 43:212–14.
339. Eklof O, Mortensson W, Sandstedt B. Suprarenal haematoma versus neuroblastoma complicated by haemorrhage. Acta Radiol Diag 1986; 27:3–10.
340. Croitoru DP, Sinsky AB, Laberge J. Cystic neuroblastoma. J Pediatr Surg 1992; 27:1320–1.
341. Richard ML, Gundersen AE, Williams MS. Cystic neuroblastoma of infancy. J Pediatr Surg 1995; 30:1354–7.
342. Acharya S, Jayabose S, Kogan SJ et al. Prenatally diagnosed neuroblastoma. Cancer 1997; 80:304–10.
343. Hamada Y, Ikebukuro K, Sato M et al. Prenatally diagnosed cystic neuroblastoma. Pediatr Surg Int 1999; 15:71–4.
344. Hosoda Y, Miyano T, Kimura K et al. Characteristics and management of patients with neuroblastoma. J Pediatr Surg 1992; 27:623–5.
345. Bove KE. Wilms' tumor and related abnormalities in the fetus and newborn. Semin Perinatol 1999; 23:310–18.
346. Pinto E, Guignard JP. Renal masses in the neonate. Biol Neonate 1995; 68:175–84.
347. Lowe LH, Isuani BH, Heller RM et al. Pediatric renal masses: Wilms' tumor and beyond. Radiographics 2000; 20:1585–603.
348. Glick RD, Hicks MJ, Nuchtern JG, Wesson DE, Olutoye OO, Cass DL. Renal tumors in infants less than 6 months of age. J Pediatr Surg 2004; 39:522–5.
349. Applegate KE, Ghei M, Perez-Atayde AR. Prenatal detection of a Wilms' tumor. Pediatr Radiol 1999; 29:65–7.
350. Beckwith JB. Pernatal detection of a Wilms' tumor. Pediatr Radiol 1999; 29:64–5.
351. Vadeyar S, Ramsay M, James D, O'Neill D. Prenatal diagnosis of congenital Wilms' tumor (nephroblastoma) presenting as fetal hydrops. Ultrasound Obstet Gynecol 2000; 16:80–3.
352. Ferrer FA, McKenna PH, Donnal JF. Noninvasive angiography in preoperative evaluation of complicated pediatric renal masses using phase contrast magnetic resonance angiography. Urology 1994; 44:254–9.
353. Campagnola S, Fasoli L, Flessati P et al. Congenital cystic mesoblastic nephroma. Urol Int 1998; 61:254–6.
354. Haddad B, Haziza J, Touboul C et al. The congenital mesoblastic nephroma: a case report of prenatal diagnosis. Fetal Diagn Ther 1996; 11:61–6.
355. Chan HSL, Cheng M, Mancer K et al. Congenital mesoblastic nephroma: a clinicoradiologic study of 17 cases representing the pathologic spectrum of the disease. J Pediatr 1987; III:64–70.
356. Charles AK, Vujanic GM, Berry PJ. Renal tumours of childhood. Histopathology 1998; 32:293–309.
357. Leob DM, Hill DA, Dome JS. Complete response of recurrent cellular congenital mesoblastic nephroma to chemotherapy. J Pediatr Hematol Oncol 2002 Aug; 24:478–81.
358. Heidelberger KP, Ritchey ML, Dauser RC et al. Congenital mesoblastic nephroma metastatic to the brain. Cancer 1993; 72:2499–502.
359. Arensman RM, Belman AB. Ruptured congenital mesoblastic nephroma: chemotherapy and irradiation as adjuvants to nephrectomy. Urology 1980; XV:394–6.
360. Matsumura M, Nishi T, Sasaki Y et al. Prenatal diagnosis and treatment strategy for congenital mesoblastic nephroma. J Pediatr Surg 1993; 28:1607–9.
361. Hibbert J, Howlett DC, Greenwood KL et al. The ultrasound appearances of neonatal renal vein thrombosis. Br J Radiol 1997; 70:1191–4.
362. Cozzolino DJ, Cendron M. Bilateral renal vein thrombosis in a newborn: a case of prenatal renal vein thrombosis. Urology 1997; 50:128–31.
363. Zigman A, Yazbeck S, Emil S, Nguyen L. Renal vein thrombosis: a 10-year review. J Pediatr Surg 2000; 35:1540–2.
364. Heller C, Schobess R, Kurnik K et al. Abdominal venous thrombosis in neonates and infants: role of prothrombotic risk factors – a multicentre case-control study. For the Childhood Thrombophilia Study Group. Br J Haematol 2000; 111:534–9.

365. Kosch A, Kuwertz-Broking E, Heller C et al. Renal venous thrombosis in neonates: prothrombotic risk factors and long-term follow-up. Blood 2004; 104:1356–60.
366. Belman AB, King LR. The pathology and treatment of renal vein thrombosis in the newborn. J Urol 1972; 107:852–5.
367. Duncan BW, Adzick NS, Longaker MT et al. In utero arterial embolism from renal vein thrombosis with successful postnatal thrombolytic therapy. Pediatr Surg 1991; 26:741–3.
368. Nuss R, Hays T, Manco-Johnson M. Efficacy and safety of heparin anticoagulation for neonatal renal vein thrombosis. Am J Pediatr Hematol Oncol 1994; 16:127–31.
369. Keidan I, Lotan D, Gazit G et al. Early neonatal renal venous thrombosis: long-term outcome. Acta Paediatr 1994; 83:1225–7.
370. Jobin J, O'Regan S, Demay G et al. Neonatal renal vein thrombosis – long-term follow-up after conservative management. Clin Nephrol 1982; 17:36–40.
371. Laplante S, Patriquin HB, Robitaille P et al. Renal vein thrombosis in children: evidence of early flow recovery with Doppler US. Radiology 1993; 189:37–42.
372. Durante D, Jones D, Spitzer R. Neonatal renal arterial embolism syndrome. Pediatrics 1976; 89:978–81.
373. Bauer SB, Feldman SM, Gellis SS, Retik AB. Neonatal hypertension. A complication of umbilical-artery catheterization. N Engl J Med 1975; 293:1032–3.
374. Kavaler E, Hensle TW. Renal artery thrombosis in the newborn infant. Urology 1997; 50:282–4.
375. Griscom NT, Colodny AH, Rosenberg HK. Diagnostic aspects of neonatal ascites: report of 27 cases. AJR Am J Roentgenol 1977; 128:961–9.
376. Greenberg R, Waldman D, Brooks C et al. Endovascular treatment of renal artery thrombosis can be caused by umbilical artery catheterization. J Vasc Surg 1998; 28:949–53.
377. Gunnarsson B, Heard CM, Martin DJ, Brecher ML, Steinhorn RH. Successful lysis of an obstructive aortic and renal artery thrombus in a neonate on extracorporeal membrane oxygenation. J Perinatol 2000; 20(8 Pt 1):555–7.
378. Felc A. Ultrasound in screening for neonatal adrenal hemorrhage. Am J Perinatol 1995; 12:363–6.
379. Burbige KA. Prenatal adrenal hemorrhage confirmed by postnatal surgery. J Urol 1993; 150:1867–9.
380. Chen C, Shih S, Chuang C et al. In utero adrenal hemorrhage: clinical and imaging findings. Acta Obstet Gynecol Scand 1998; 77:239–41.
381. Fang SB, Lee HC, Sheu JC et al. Prenatal sonographic detection of adrenal hemorrhage confirmed by postnatal surgery. J Clin Ultrasound 1999; 27:206–9.
382. Willemse AP, Coppes MJ, Feldberg MA et al. Magnetic resonance appearance of adrenal hemorrhage in a neonate. Pediatr Radiol 1989; 19:210–1.
383. Hoeffel C, Legmann P, Luton JP et al. Spontaneous unilateral adrenal hemorrhage: computerized tomography and magnetic resonance imaging findings in 8 cases. J Urol 1995; 154:1647–51.
384. Khuri FJ, Alton DJ, Hardy BE et al. Adrenal hemorrhage in neonates: report of 5 cases and review of the literature. J Urol 1980; 124:684–7.
385. Sherer DM, Kendig JW, Sickel JZ et al. In utero adrenal hemorrhage associated with fetal distress, subsequent transient neonatal hypertension, and a nonfunctioning ipsilateral kidney. Am J Perinatol 1994; 11:302–4.
386. Ferrer FA, McKenna PH. Partial nephrectomy in a metachronous multilocular cyst of the kidney (cystic nephroma). J Urol 1994; 151:1358–60.
387. Duel BP, Hendren WH, Bauer SB et al. Reconstructive options in genitourinary rhabdomyosarcoma. J Urol 1996; 156:1798–804.
388. Merguerian PA, Agarwal S, Greenberg M et al. Outcome analysis of rhabdomyosarcoma of the lower urinary tract. J Urol 1998; 160: 1191–14, discussion 1216.
389. Hays DM, Raney RB, Wharam MD et al. Children with vesical rhabdomyosarcoma (RMS) treated by partial cystectomy with neoadjuvant or adjuvant chemotherapy, with or without radiotherapy. A report from the Intergroup Rhabdomyosarcoma Study (IRS) Committee. J Pediatr Hematol Oncol 1995; 17:46–52.
390. Lazar EL, Stolar CJ. Evaluation and management of pediatric solid ovarian tumors. Semin Pediatr Surg 1998; 7:29–34.
391. Mukai M, Takamatsu H, Noguchi H, Tahara H. Intra-abdominal testis with mature teratoma. Pediatr Surg Int 1998; 13:204–5.
392. Sloan WR, Walsh PC. Familial persistent Mullerian duct syndrome. J Urol 1976; 115:459–61.
393. Allen TD. Disorders of sexual differentiation. Urology 1976; 7(Suppl 4):1–32.
394. Rajfer J, Walsh PC. Testicular descent. Normal and abnormal. Urol Clin North Am 1978; 5:223–35.
395. Verp MS, Simpson JL. Abnormal sexual differentiation and neoplasia. Cancer Genet Cytogenet 1987; 25:191–218.
396. Kanayama H, Naroda T, Inoue Y et al. A case of complete testicular feminization: laparoscopic orchietomy and analysis of androgen receptor gene mutation. Int J Urol 1999; 6:327–30.
397. Bloom DA, Wan J, Key D. Disorders of the male external genitalia and inguinal canal. Clin Pediatr Urol 1992; 2:1015–49.
398. Mares AJ, Shkolnik A, Sacks M, Feuchtwanger MM. Aberrant (ectopic) adrenocortical tissue along the spermatic cord. Pediatr Surg 1980; 15:289–92.
399. Paul R, Bielmeier J, Breul J et al. Accessory spleen of the spermatic cord. Urologe A 1997; 36:262–4.
400. Knoedler CJ, Kay R, Knoedler JP Sr, Wiig Th. Pelvic neuroblastoma. J Urol 1989; 141:905–7.
401. Kay R. Pediatric urologic intraoperative consultation. Urol Clin North Am 1985; 12:461–8.
402. Shandling B, Jank JJ. The vunerability of the vas deferens. J Pediatr Surg 1981; 16:461–4.
403. Zabbo A, Montie JE. Intraoperative consultation for the kidney. Urol Clin North Am 1985; 12:405–10.
404. Gerber WL. Catheter guide for neonates. Urology 1982; 20:87.
405. Redman JF. A catheter guide to obviate difficult urethral catheterization in male infants and boys. J Urol 1994; 151:1051–2.

Urinary tract infections in children

7

Hans G Pohl and H Gil Rushton

Introduction

In prior editions, this chapter was introduced with the concept that recently discovered bacterial virulence factors, such as those promoting adherence to uroepithelial cells, were assuming a greater importance in the pathophysiology of urinary tract infections (UTIs) in children. However important these genetically encoded bacterial factors might be in enhancing the potential of uropathogenic bacteria to cause symptomatic disease, mounting evidence suggests that deficient host defense factors and tissue repair mechanisms may contribute more significantly to an individual's susceptibility to urinary infection.

Epidemiology

Urinary tract infections in children may be symptomatic or asymptomatic. Symptomatic infections may be confined to the bladder (cystitis), or they may involve the upper collecting system (ureteritis, pyelitis), or extend into the renal parenchyma (pyelonephritis). Age, gender, race, circumcision status, the method of detection, and presentation all influence the prevalence of symptomatic versus asymptomatic urinary infection.

Overall, the incidence of neonatal bacteriuria has been reported as 1–1.4%.[1–3] The male-to-female ratio in infants is reversed from that seen in older children. From a compilation of screening studies of healthy newborns reviewed by Stamey, 1.5% of boys versus only 0.13% of girls had bacteriuria.[4] However, the actual incidence of UTI during infancy has probably been underestimated in the past, partly because of the difficulty in diagnosing UTI in this age group. In a 3-year prospective study of 3581 infants (aged 0–1 year) in Goteborg, Sweden, asymptomatic bacteriuria was confirmed by suprapubic aspiration of urine in 2.5% of boys and 0.9% of girls.[5] Symptomatic urinary infection occurred equally often in both sexes (1.2% of boys and 1.1% of girls). Overall, 3.7% of boys and 2% of girls had positive urine cultures during the first year of life. The male predominance noted in the Goteborg study during the first few months of life has also been reported by others.[6–9] Uncircumcised infant boys are eight to ten times more likely to have symptomatic urinary infection as compared to their circumcised counterparts.[10]

During preschool and school age, the male-to-female ratio observed in neonates is reversed, making screening bacteriuria more prevalent in girls[8,9] (Table 7.1). In several large studies of school-age children the aggregate risk of screening bacteriuria has been reported to be 0.7–1.95% of girls and 0.04–0.2% of boys.[12–16] However, in as many as one-third of these children a prior history of UTI or voiding symptoms could be elicited (Table 7.2). Based on an average annual incidence figure of 0.4%, Kunin (1964) estimated that bacteriuria will develop in approximately 5% of girls prior to graduation from high school. Additional data collected by Kunin[12] revealed that infection will recur in up to 80% of all white girls and 60% of black girls within 5 years of initial infection.[12]

In a prospective population-based study of symptomatic UTIs in children living in Goteborg, Sweden, Winberg et al estimated that the aggregate risk for symptomatic UTI up to age 11 was at least 3% for girls and 1.1% for boys.[11] In an update of a previous study, the incidence of culture-documented UTIs was

Table 7.1 Gender ratio of urinary tract infections

Age range	Females	Males
Neonate	0.4	1
1–6 months	1.5	1
6–12 months	4.0	1
1–3 years	10.0	1
3–11 years	9.0	1
11–16 years	2.0	1

From Belman and Kaplan, 1981, modified from Winberg et al.[11]

Table 7.2 The clinical history and symptoms of 109 children with 'screening' bacteriuria

History/symptoms	Prevalence (%)
All symptoms (excluding nocturnal enuresis)	70
Urgency	54
Frequency	53
Nocturnal enuresis	51
Diurnal enuresis	47
Previous urinary tract infection	20
Dysuria	13
Unexplained fever	7
Flank pain	4
Nocturia	4

Modified from Savage et al.[17]

twice as high as previously estimated, affecting 7.8% of girls and 1.6% of boys during the first 6 years of life.[18] To confirm these findings, Marild and Jodal recently performed a retrospective population-based study of 41 000 children of Goteborg, Sweden.[19] The cumulative incidence rate of symptomatic UTIs was 6.6% for girls and 1.8% for boys. These data probably do not reflect an increasing incidence of UTIs since the publication of the earliest report, but instead a greater detection rate. In these epidemiologic studies, the incidence of febrile UTIs was greatest in infant boys and girls as compared to children over 2 years of age. Gender differences in the incidence rates of first-time febrile and non-febrile UTIs were most evident in children >2 years old. Girls >2 years old were much more likely to present with first-time UTI, both with and without fever, as compared to their age-matched male counterparts (Figure 7.1a and b).

Once treated, infants with symptomatic urinary infections are at risk for recurrent infection (26%), usually in the first 3 months of follow-up. In older girls the risk for recurrence following symptomatic

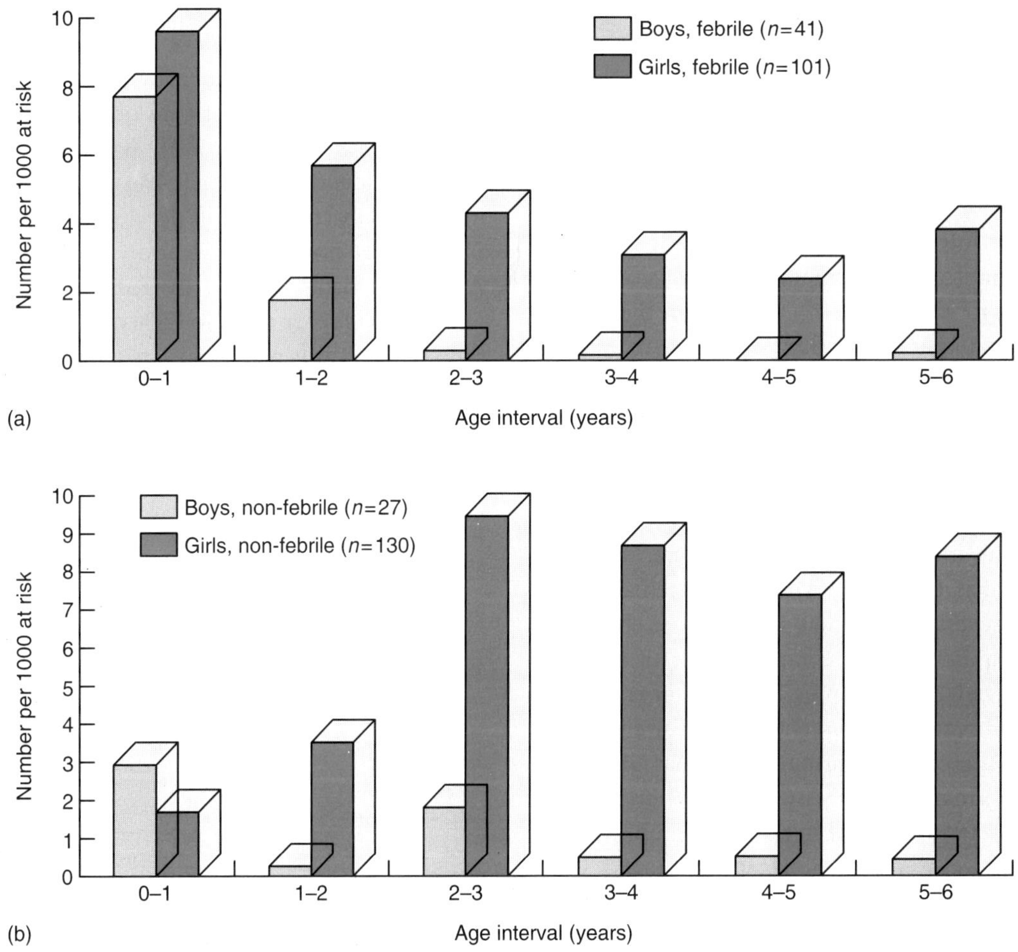

Figure 7.1 Annual incidence rate in 1 year intervals of febrile urinary tract infection in children studied during a 20-month period between 1979 and 1981. (*a*) Incidence of febrile infections in boys compared with girls. (*b*) Incidence of non-febrile infections in boys compared with girls. (Adapted from Marild and Jodal.[19])

urinary infection is as high as 40–60% within 18 months. This risk persists into adulthood.[8] In one study, 60 girls with childhood bacteriuria followed into adulthood (9–18-year follow-up) were compared with 38 non-bacteriuric controls.[20] During pregnancy, a significantly greater incidence of bacteriuria was diagnosed in the group with the history of positive urine cultures in childhood (63.8%) when compared with the controls (26.7%). Interestingly, the propensity for urinary infection persisted in the children born to bacilluric women, whereas none of the children born to healthy controls demonstrated urinary infection.

Further evidence supporting a lifelong risk for symptomatic urinary infection in individuals presenting during childhood is reported by the Goteborg Childhood UTI Research Group. These authors followed 111 women with renal scarring or recurrent UTIs. Febrile UTIs were more prevalent than nonfebrile UTIs during the first 10 years of life but continued to occur into the third decade. Although the prevalence of febrile UTIs diminished in adulthood, women with renal scarring during childhood were significantly more likely to have subsequent febrile UTIs. Overall, the median incidence of symptomatic UTIs was 7 per individual.[21,22]

Bacteriology

The organisms that colonize the urinary tract are specifically adapted towards this purpose. Research has identified specific virulence factors that determine an organism's pathogenic potential, thus differentiating strains commonly associated with asymptomatic bacteriuria, cystitis, or acute pyelonephritis. However, uropathogenic strains do not rigorously conform to predicted behavior. Rather, a few general principles are applicable, such as the presence of surface molecules important for adhesion and toxins that assist tissue invasion.

A large family of Gram-negative, aerobic bacilli known as Enterobacteriaciae cause the majority of uncomplicated UTIs. Included in this family are the genera *Escherichia*, *Klebsiella*, *Enterobacter*, *Citrobacter*, *Proteus*, *Providencia*, *Morganella*, *Serratia*, and *Salmonella*. Of these, *E. coli* is by far the most frequently isolated organism, being responsible for approximately 80% of UTIs. This family of bacteria is generally characterized by a negative reaction to the oxidase test and the capacity to ferment glucose and reduce nitrates to nitrite. *Pseudomonas* is also a Gram-negative, aerobic bacillus but is distinct and unrelated to Enterobacteriaciae. Most *Pseudomonas* recovered from the urine are of relatively low virulence and do not tend to invade tissue unless host defense mechanisms are compromised.

The most common Gram-positive organisms found in UTIs are *Staphylococcus* and *Enterococcus*. Anaerobic fecal flora rarely produce UTIs despite being 100 to 1000 times more abundant than *E. coli* in stool.[23] Occasionally, unusual or fastidious organisms may produce infections that are difficult to detect because they do not grow well in commonly used culture media. For example, *Haemophilus influenzae* has been reported to cause urinary infections,[24] as well as epididymo-orchitis in infant males.[25] Other unusual organisms include *Salmonella* sp. and *Shigella*. Although lactobacilli, corynebacteria, and alpha streptococcus may rarely cause UTI, they probably should be considered contaminants unless they are found in culture of specimens obtained by suprapubic aspiration or by catheterization.

The bacteriologic findings in the Goteburg study suggest that 'the [predisposing] environmental conditions in the periurethral region and the host defense mechanisms vary with age and sex'.[11] This study identified four characteristic bacteriologic trends in childhood urinary tract infections:

1. A high frequency of *Proteus* sp. infections in older boys (most of whom were uncircumcised), and greater variability in infecting organisms in boys than in girls.
2. A greater likelihood of staphylococcal infection in adolescence, especially in girls.
3. A greater frequency of *E. coli* urinary infection in neonatal boys than in girls of that age.
4. A decreased frequency of *Klebsiella* urinary infection in older children (Table 7.3)

Other general rules include the fact that the majority of uncomplicated infections are caused by a single organism. Patients with complicated infections, particularly those children who have been managed with long-term catheterization, may have multiple organisms. Sometimes the strain of bacterium is suggestive of underlying urinary pathology, such as the relationship of *Proteus* sp. and struvite stones.

Serology

E. coli, the most common species of uropathogens, can be typed serologically by three major groups of antigenic structures capable of producing specific antibodies. There are more than 150 O (cell wall)

Table 7.3 Infecting bacteria (%) isolated from 'first-time' urinary infection in children categorized by age and gender

	Females (%)			Males[a] (%)	
Infecting organism	All neonates (*n* = 73)	1 month to 10 years[b] (*n* = 30)	10–16 years (*n* = 30)	1 month to 10 years (*n* = 62)	10–16 years (*n* = 42)
E. coli	**57% (females) 83% (males)**	**83%**	**60%**	**85%**	**33%**
Klebsiella	11	4	0	2	2
Proteus sp.	0	3	0	5	33
Enterococcus	3	2	0	0	2
Staphylococcus	1	4	30	0	12
Other, mixed or unknown	9	11	10	8	17

Modified from Winburg et al.[11]
[a] Males not routinely circumcised in Scandinavia.
[b] No difference between girls 1 month to 1 year old and 1 to 10 years old.

antigens, more than 50 H (flagellar) antigens, and approximately 100 K (capsular) antigens. Not all strains are typable. Serologic classification in UTI is restricted mainly to O antigens. Early studies have attempted to correlate serologic markers with increased virulence or tissue invasiveness. Most of these were epidemiologic studies that were conducted prior to discovery of the special role of specific virulence factors, such as adhesins (attachment structures). In contrast to patients with cystitis or asymptomatic bacteriuria, patients with pyelonephritis have been found to be more frequently infected with certain O typable strains and strains having certain K antigens. Eight O antigen types (O1, O2, O4, O6, O7, O18, O25, O75) were the cause of 80% of cases of pyelonephritis in one report.[26] Another study reported that *E. coli* possessing five K antigens (K1, K2, K3, K12, K13) accounted for 70% of isolates from patients with pyelonephritis.[27] These serologic studies have been extended to identify more specific O:K:H combination serotypes characteristic of pyelonephritogenic strains.

Virulence factors

The term virulence simply refers to the ability of microorganisms to cause disease. The concept of uropathogenic bacteria refers to certain strains that are selected from the fecal flora, not by chance or prevalence, but because of the presence of specific virulence factors that enhance colonization of the uroepithelium. Other virulence factors aid in persistence of bacteria in the urinary tract and provide these organisms with the capacity to induce inflammation of the urethra, bladder, or renal parenchyma. Recognized *E. coli* virulence factors include but are not limited to (1) adherence to uroepithelial cells, (2) elaboration of endotoxin, (3) ability to evade phagocytosis, (4) ability to damage host cells and other bacteria, (5) ability to acquire iron, and (6) resistance to serum bactericidal activity. Studies of pyelonephritogenic strains of *E. coli* reveal the presence of a limited number of bacterial clones that possess specific virulence factors that are expressed only in certain O groups.[28] In a mouse model of acute pyelonephritis, it was determined that each virulence factor has a role causing UTI. Although the presence of P-fimbriae and hemolysin was significantly associated with mortality, additional factors functioned synergistically to augment a strain's pathogenicity.[29]

Adherence

Bacterial adherence or attachment is an essential initiating step in all infections. Perineal colonization by uropathogenic bacteria has been found to precede clinical UTI in women and children at risk for UTI.[6,30–33] Tissue invasion, inflammation, and cell damage are secondary events. Uropathogenic bacteria, especially *E. coli*, can attach to specific receptor sites (bacterial tropism) by means of specialized proteins (adhesins) on the ends of attachment structures (fimbria). Non-specific adherence also occurs by electrostatic and hydrophobic forces. In addition to recognizing constituents of uroepithelial cell surface, fimbriae also attach to constituents of the basement membrane. By virtue of such attachment, virulent strains of bacteria can ascend into the upper urinary

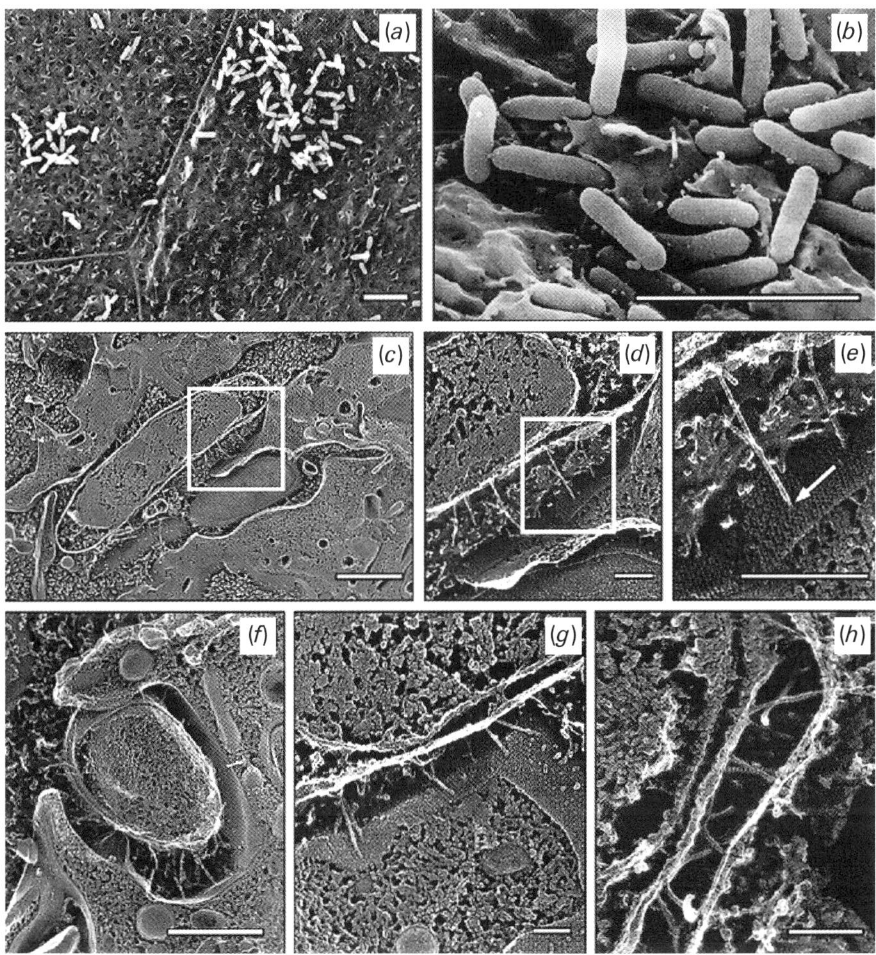

Figure 7.2 Type 1 pilus-mediated bacterial adherence to the bladder epithelium. Mouse bladders were processed for (*a, b*) scanning electron microscopy (SEM) and high-resolution EM at 2 h after infection with *E. coli* NU14. The boxed areas in (*c*) and (*d*) are shown magnified in (*d*) and (*e*), respectively. The arrow in (*e*) indicates the FimH-containing tip. In (*h*), type 1 pili span from the host cell membrane on the right to the bacterium on the left. Scale bars = 5 μm (*a, b*), 0.5 μm (*c, f*), and 0.1 μm (*d–h*). (From Malvey et al.[34])

tract even in the absence of structural abnormalities such as vesicoureteral reflux (VUR).

Several different types of fimbriae have been identified. Type 1 fimbriae mediate agglutination between bacteria and cells in culture. Type 1 fimbriae bind specifically to mannose-terminated glycoproteins on uroepithelial cell surfaces. Since this agglutination can be competitively inhibited by a mannose-rich solution, type 1 fimbriae are often termed mannose-sensitive. Alternatively, P-fimbriae recognize a glycolipid commonly found on uroepithelial cells of the upper urinary tract through a mannose-resistant interaction (Figure 7.2). Uropathogenic bacteria rely on both mannose-sensitive type 1 fimbriae and mannose-resistant P-fimbriae to colonize the urinary tract. The expression of type 1 and P-fimbriae varies between 'on' and 'off' states, and is likely regulated by environmental conditions.[35] In addition to type 1 and P-fimbriae, uropathogenic bacteria employ several other adhesins, both fimbrial and non-fimbrial. Unfortunately, little epidemiologic evidence exists that clarifies the role of these additional adhesins on *E. coli* (S-fimbriae, FIC-fimbriae, S/FIC-related fimbriae), *Klebsiella* (MR/K HA), and *Proteus* sp. (MR/P HA, PMF, ATF, NAF, UCA) in the pathogenesis of UTI.

In addition to promoting attachment, type 1 fimbriae mediate bacterial invasion into the uroepithelial cells themselves, thus protecting bacteria from antibiotics that do not penetrate the cell's membrane, such as aminoglycosides.[34] In fact, viable internalized bacteria can be isolated from uroepithelial cells 48 hours after infection, and may account for recurrent infection by the same bacterial strain (Figure 7.3). Once type 1 fimbriated *E. coli* attach, the uroepithelial cells

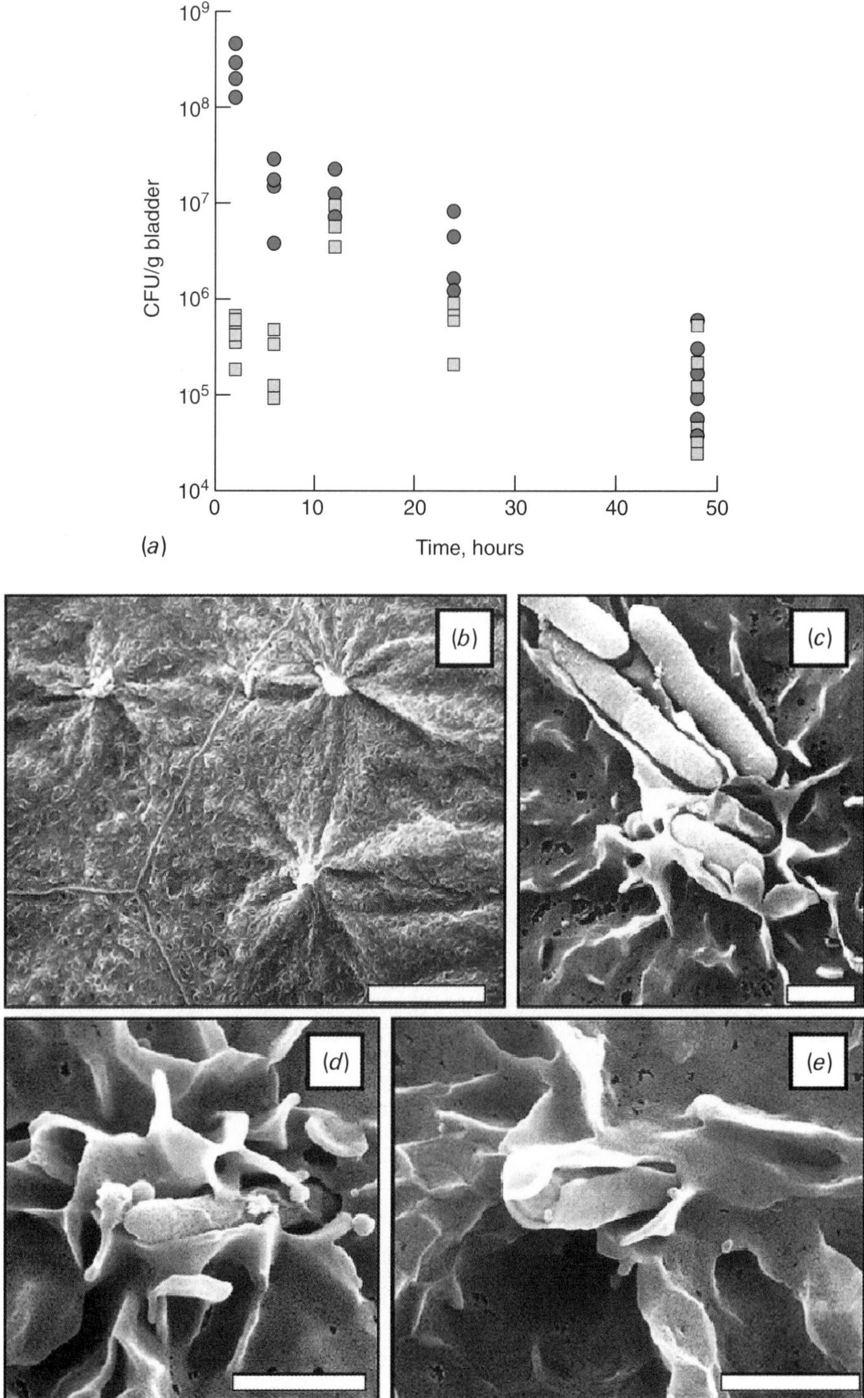

Figure 7.3 Kinetics of bacterial reduction in *E. coli* NU14-infected bladders and the persistence of intracellular bacteria. (*a*) The total numbers of bacteria per gram of mouse bladder (circles) and the numbers of gentamicin-protected bacteria (boxes) were examined per time point. (*b–e*) Bacteria in various stages of internalization into superficial cells at 2 h after infection with *E. coli* NU14 were detected by scanning electron microscopy (SEM). Scale bars = 10 μm (*b*) and 1 μm (*c–e*). (From Malvey et al.[34])

undergo apoptosis (programmed cell death) that results in bladder mucosal ulceration.

Although the entire urothelial surface, including the upper urinary tract, contains glycoprotein receptors for type 1 fimbriae, no evidence exists that implicates type 1 fimbriae directly in the pathogenesis of pyelonephritis. However, it has been demonstrated in experimental models and clinical studies that once pyelonephritis occurs, the presence of type 1 fimbriae significantly increases a strain's ability to persist in the urinary tract and to stimulate inflammation.[36–39]

Clinical and experimental studies have shown that pyelonephritic *E. coli* frequently possess fimbriae that can recognize and agglutinate erythrocytes of the P-1 blood group. Hence, this type of pili have been termed P-fimbriae. The P-fimbriae attach to the carbohydrate portion (α-D-galactopyranosyl-(1–4)-β-D-galactopyranoside) of the glycolipid antigen in the P blood group series, which is also expressed by human uroepithelial cells.[40,41] The components of P-fimbriae are encoded by 11 genes in the pyelonephritis-associated pilus (pap) gene cluster, of which pap E, F, and G, encode for the adhesin subunits.

Further research has identified that not all P-fimbriae are alike. Proteins located at the tip (G-tip proteins or tip adhesins) determine the fimbria's specific attachment properties. Three classes have been identified, of which only class II and class III P-fimbriae have uropathogenic potential. In-vitro studies have found that the class III P-fimbriae bind receptors found in higher density on bladder uroepithelium. In contrast, class II tip adhesins may be more important in the evolution of acute pyelonephritis by virtue of an increased density of class II specific receptors located on the uroepithelium of the upper urinary tract.[42] James-Ellison et al have described a statistically significant greater likelihood of clinical and histologic indicators of acute pyelonephritis in primates inoculated with class II fimbriated *E. coli* than when primates are inoculated with class III fimbriated *E. coli*.[43]

Epidemiologic studies in children have provided considerable evidence that the presence of P-fimbriae on *E. coli* is a significant virulence factor, particularly in upper urinary tract infections. These studies have shown that 76–94% of pyelonephritogenic strains of *E. coli* are P-fimbriated compared with 19–23% of cystitis strains, 14–18% of strains isolated from patients with asymptomatic bacteriuria, and 7–16% of fecal isolate strains.[28,44] Other evidence supporting the importance of P-fimbriae in causing upper urinary tract infections comes from animal model studies. Inoculation of the bladders of non-refluxing primates with P-fimbriated *E. coli* resulted in pyelonephritis in 66% of animals. In contrast, pyelonephritis was not seen in any of the monkeys inoculated with non-P-fimbriated *E. coli*.[45]

In addition to their role in the pathogenesis of pyelonephritis through attachment to renal epithelial cells, P-fimbriae also function to promote intestinal carriage by the host, as well as enhancing perineal colonization (see host factors) and persistence in the urinary tract. Although the data regarding intestinal carriage and perineal colonization (see host factors) by P-fimbriated *E. coli* strongly implicate the P-fimbriae in the pathogenesis of infection, the data regarding bacterial persistence are less clear.

Although fimbriae appear to be the primary method by which bacteria colonize the urinary tract, there is also attachment to non-exposed 'receptors' located in the interstitium. Secondary binding to fibronectin occurs by means of fimbriae encoded by pap, papG, sfa, afa and prsG DNA sequences; a feature also more common in pyelonephritogenic strains than in strains causing cystitis or asymptomatic bacteriuria.[46,47] Other adhesins may actually play a protective role by preventing UTI through competitive binding. For example, S-fimbriae and type 1 fimbriae bind to Tamm–Horsfall protein and low molecular weight substances, respectively. Once bound, clearance of bacteria by periodic shedding of these soluble bacteria–protein complexes in the urine offers a theoretical advantage by reducing the number of infecting organisms.

Some data suggest that an organism's phenotype is variable, first facilitating colonization of the uroepithelium, then undergoing specific changes (phase variation) to evade eradication by the host's immune response, as well as promote ascent within the urinary tract.[48] *E. coli* alternately express type 1 then P-fimbriae as UTI progresses from colonization to cystitis, then to pyelonephritis. Some type 1 bacteria do reach the renal parenchyma (as in the case of VUR). These bacteria, however, must then escape type 1 fimbria-specific neutrophil receptors. In-vitro studies have demonstrated that neutrophils elicit a more severe inflammatory response in the presence of type 1 fimbriated strains than when in the presence of a mutant strain lacking the type 1 fimbria.[37] Phase variation to non-type 1 fimbriated strains is known to occur, thereby conferring a potentially protective advantage. Despite this apparently unified view of bacterial virulence, several studies also exist to challenge any attempt to simplify the complex interaction between bacteria and host.[49,50] In fact, the appearance of P-fimbriated strains in the periurethral region of girls at risk for cystitis does not inevitably result in urinary infection.[51] Thus, bacterial virulence properties should not be the sole focus of blame in the development of UTI. Host risk factors probably are of equal, if not greater, significance.

Despite its significance, bacterial adherence is only one of several factors believed to have a role in infection. Other bacterial virulence factors and host defense factors may play an even greater role in tissue invasion and inflammation. In an experimental study in mice, the presence of P-fimbriae was necessary for colonization of the upper urinary tract but did not produce tissue invasion unless combined with other virulence factors.[52] Similarly, in a clinical study that employed dimercaptosuccinic acid (DMSA) renal scans to document acute parenchymal inflammation in children with febrile UTI, no difference in the prevalence of P-fimbriated *E. coli* was found in children with an abnormal scan compared with those who had a normal scan.[53] Likewise, renal scarring has been reported to be more common following pyelonephritis caused by non-*E. coli* organisms when compared to those caused by P-fimbriated *E. coli*.[42,54]

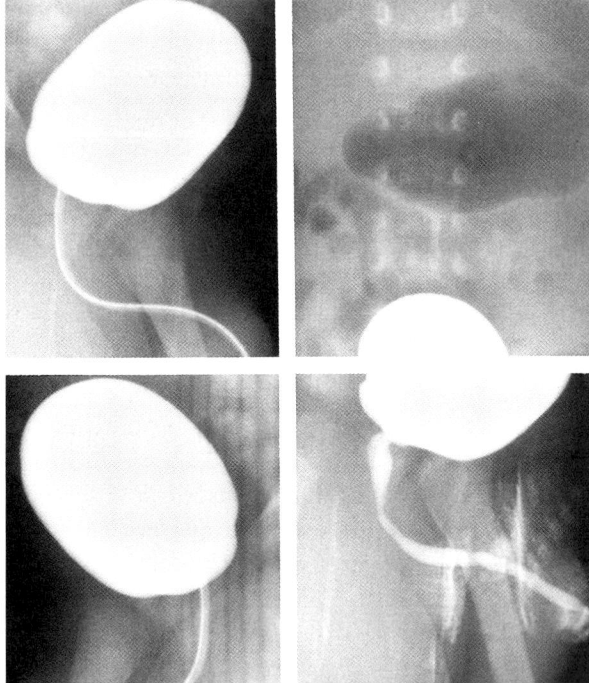

Figure 7.4 Voiding cystourethrogram demonstrating the absence of vesicoureteral reflux and obstructive pathology (posterior urethral valves, ureterocele) in an uncircumcised infant boy with acute pyelonephritis confirmed by ^{99m}Tc DMSA renal scan.

Other virulence factors

1 Endotoxin. A lipopolysaccharide present in the bacterium's cell wall, endotoxin, is responsible for initiating the acute inflammatory response common to Gram-negative infections.
2 K antigen. Capsular polysaccharides afford K antigen specificity to *E. coli.* K antigen has been shown to shield bacteria from complement lysis and phagocytosis and to enhance persistence of bacteria in the kidneys of experimental mice.[55–59] It is more commonly isolated from children with clinical pyelonephritis than in those from children with cystitis or healthy controls.[57–60]
3 Hemolysins. Cytotoxic proteins, such as hemolysins, are another recognized virulence property capable of damaging renal tubular cells, in vitro. Hemolytic strains of *E. coli* produce more severe experimental pyelonephritis in mice.[61]
4 Colicin: Another protein elaborated by pyelonephritogenic *E. coli,* colicin kills other bacteria in the vicinity of the *E. coli* producing it. The colicin V plasmid is also thought to encode for an iron uptake system that further promotes the survival and pathogenicity of colicin-producing organisms.[62]
5 Iron-binding capacity: Most bacteria require iron for optimal growth and metabolism and have developed mechanisms to acquire iron when there is limited supply. Mediated by such proteins as aerobactin, iron-binding capacity has also been shown to be associated with increased virulence in epidemiologic studies.[63,64]
6 Serum resistance: In the presence of fresh human serum, many strains of *E. coli* are killed following activation of complement. Serum resistance to such killing action is another property that has been related to virulence of Gram-negative bacteria both in UTIs and Gram-negative bacteria.[65,66]

Although these virulence factors have been considered separately, their effect appears to be additive. In contrast to those with cystitis or asymptomatic bacteriuria, the majority of bacterial isolates in patients with non-reflux acute pyelonephritis express three or four virulence properties.[42] Interestingly, the frequency of P-fimbriae and other virulence factors is significantly lower in patients who have VUR (Figures 7.4 and 7.5). This would appear logical since, in the presence of reflux, virulence properties such as adherence are not necessary for bacteria to reach the upper urinary tract. It has been suggested that efforts aimed at interfering with 'virulent' bacteria, such as by vaccination, may be of less value in patients with recurrent pyelonephritis and reflux, the group in whom renal scars are more likely to develop. However, others have not demonstrated a significant difference in virulence traits among pyelonephritogenic strains in patients with and without reflux.[67]

Role of bacterial virulence in renal scarring

Regardless of their role in the etiology of urinary tract infection, some studies suggest that there may be a

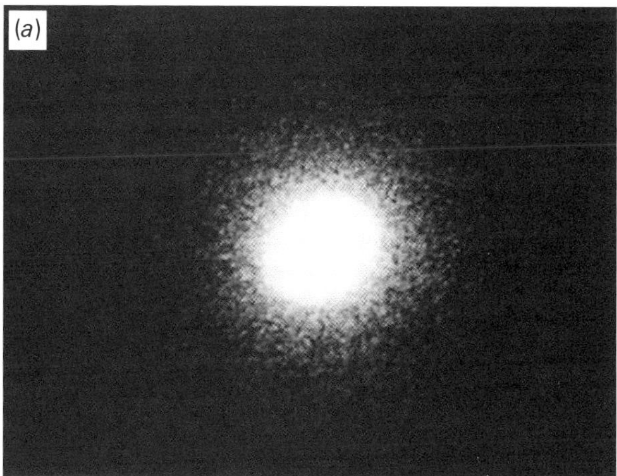

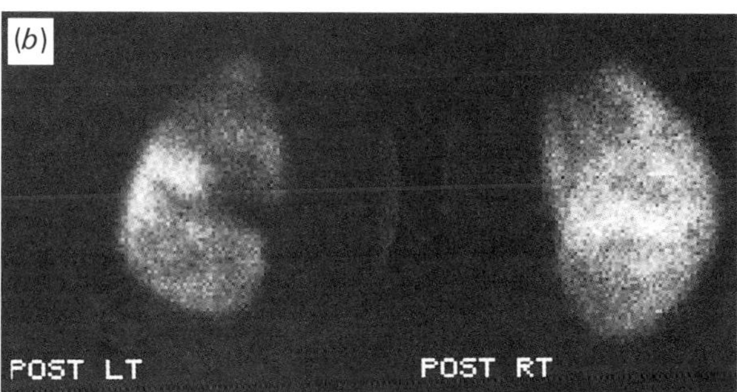

Figure 7.5 (*a*) Isocystogram demonstrating the absence of vesicoureteral reflux in a child with (*b*) ^{99m}Tc DMSA renal scan documented acute pyelonephritis (upper and lower poles are affected).

paradoxical relationship between bacterial virulence, defined by P-fimbriated binding, and renal scarring. In one study of patients with recurrent pyelonephritis, virulent clones expressing P-fimbriae occurred significantly less often in those who developed scarring (22%) than in those who did not develop renal scars (62%).[42] Although the frequency of scarring among girls with VUR was 57% in contrast to 8% of those without reflux, this alone did not explain the selection of bacteria of low virulence in those patients with scar development. Lomberg et al[42] concluded that reduced host resistance was essential for the tendency to renal scarring after acute pyelonephritis (APN).

In rodent models of APN, type 1 fimbrae have been implicated in the pathogenesis of renal scarring by virtue of stimulating neutrophil chemotaxis, the oxidative burst necessary to generate reactive oxygen species, and the release of lysosomal proteins from neutrophils.[68–70] Other evidence suggests that more virulent bacteria, as measured by the presence of adhesins, may elicit a more rigorous inflammatory response than less virulent clones and are thus cleared more rapidly. An alternative explanation would be that children infected with more virulent bacteria present earlier with symptoms such as fever, resulting in more prompt diagnosis and treatment. Observations in patients with bladder dysfunction and asymptomatic bacteriuria have demonstrated a low prevalence of P-fimbriated *E. coli* (less than 20%), suggesting that the presence of specific attachment structures may not be necessary for bacterial persistence in the urinary tract.[56,71,72] Moreover, coincident with an inflammatory response, P- and type-1 fimbriated *E. coli* were demonstrated to be more rapidly cleared than non-fimbriated strains from individuals with bladder abnormalities.[73]

Host defense factors

Interacting with bacterial virulence properties are an equally important and complex number of mechanical, hydrodynamic, anti-adherence, receptor-dependent, and immunologic host factors that affect an individual's susceptibility to UTI. By necessity, these factors are closely interrelated to the pathogenesis of UTIs, beginning with the route of entry of bacteria into the urinary tract.

Perineum

Hematogenous seeding of the urinary tract is an uncommon source of urinary infection in children. When this is the cause of a renal infection, a cortical abscess rather than classic pyelonephritis is more likely to occur. Considerable clinical and experimental evidence has clearly established an ascending or retrograde urethral route of entry of bacteria in the majority of UTIs. The same bacterial strains causing urinary infections can be found on perineal cultures prior to bladder invasion. This is in contrast to negative perineal cultures in healthy controls.[74–77] The usual organisms originate from fecal flora that colonizes the perineum.[78]

An infant's initial exposure to uropathogenic bacteria occurs at the time of birth, subjecting infants born to bacilluric mothers to a fourfold greater risk of urinary tract infections.[79,80] It has been postulated that other host defense factors mature during the first year of life, resulting in a decrease of both periurethral colonization and frequency of UTI. Overall, the quantities and species of colonizing bacteria in the periurethral area diminish during the first year of life until few remain at age 5 years. Meanwhile, normal periurethral flora may even be protective against urinary infection by competitive interference with attachment of uropathogenic bacteria.[81,82] This potential protective effect can be altered by the administration of antimicrobial agents, given for any reason. In a study of children with first-time acute pyelonephritis, significantly more children had been recently treated with antibiotics, usually for non-UTIs, compared with controls.[83] In general, the genitalia of infant boys are more heavily colonized than are those of infant girls, and, when colonized, boys carry *E. coli* more frequently than do girls. These data concur with Winburg's epidemiologic findings that UTI occurs less frequently with advancing age and more frequently in boys younger than 6 months than in their female counterparts.

Ultimately, an infant's own intestinal tract may become colonized by bacteria with uropathogenic potential. Wold et al[84] reported on 13 girls with asymptomatic bacteriuria who underwent characterization of fecal flora. Resident strains isolated from affected girls more commonly expressed P-fimbria, were adherent to colonic epithelium in a mannose-resistant fashion, and were one of several uropathogenic serotypes present when compared with transient strains of *E. coli*. Plos et al[85] confirmed these findings in a prospective review of fecal isolates from children with UTIs. Affected children demonstrated intestinal colonization with P-fimbriated *E. coli* more frequently than healthy controls both during infection (86% versus 29%) and during infection-free intervals (40% versus 29%).

Since Bollgren and Winburg's original work in 1976 in school-age girls with a history of recurrent UTIs,[86] three additional studies have reported on the natural history of periurethral colonization. Despite the widely accepted concept of an ascending route of infection, the mere presence of uropathogenic bacteria on the perineum did not portend symptomatic UTI. Schlager et al[51] studied the association between periurethral colonization and recurrent UTI in a cohort of seven toilet-trained girls (3–6 years of age). Each girl underwent weekly periurethral and urinary cultures during a 6-month period immediately following her first UTI. Almost half (43%, 53/122) of the periurethral cultures were positive; however a positive perineal culture was obtained equally as often in the absence of urinary infection as it was prior to a symptomatic recurrence. Moreover, in only one of the four recurrences was the causative organism isolated from a perineal culture. Similarly, although heavy periurethral colonization has been reported in 75–80% of healthy infants and toddlers of both sexes,[86] only 1–3% become infected.[11] In a study similar to Schlager's, Brumfitt et al[87] found that perineal colonization by the responsible organism did not precede the symptomatic recurrent UTI in up to 34% of the adult women studied. These data may reflect the transient nature of bacterial species colonizing the perineum. Alternatively, these findings may reflect the short time course between initiation of perineal colonization and symptomatic UTI by uropathogenic bacteria in certain individuals.

Although it is not unreasonable to suspect that an abrupt change in the expression of certain key virulence factors might precipitate ascent from the perineum to the bladder, some data exist to refute this hypothesis. Schlager et al[51] characterized the expression of six virulence factors among *E. coli* colonizing the bladder in the absence of symptoms and those causing symptomatic UTI in seven girls. Although P-fimbriae were commonly identified in infecting species of *E. coli*, none of the six virulence factors, including P-fimbriae, accurately predicted which colonizing species would ultimately cause symptomatic infection. Thus, although sufficient evidence exists to support bacterial ascent into the bladder from the perineum as the mode of entry, the facilitating events in that mechanism remain poorly understood.

Prepuce

A hematogenous route of infection, rather than ascent into the urinary tract from the perineum, has been suggested in the newborn. This proposal was based on the more frequent finding of bacteremia associated with UTI in this age group.[6] However, others have not substantiated a higher incidence of bacteremia in neonates compared with other infants and children with febrile UTIs.[3,18] Furthermore, the increased risk for UTI (including pyelonephritis) in uncircumcised boys compared with both girls and circumcised boys provides additional convincing support for an ascending route of infection even during the first several months of life. In fact, over 90% of boys with febrile UTIs during the first year of life are uncircumcised.[6,88] In 1985, Wiswell et al[10] initially found a 20-fold higher rate of UTI among infant boys who were not circumcised than among those who were (4.12% vs 0.21%). Subsequently, two larger cohort studies by the same investigator, encompassing 637 097 infants, found the rate of UTI among uncircumcised boys to be less than that originally described, but still significantly greater (10-fold) than the incidence of UTI among those circumcised[88,89] (Table 7.4). Rushton and Majd[88] prospectively found that 92% of boys under 6 months of age hospitalized with febrile UTIs were uncircumcised compared with 49% of a control

Table 7.4 Incidence of urinary tract infection (UTI) in female and circumcised and uncircumcised male infants (0–1 year old) born in US army hospitals (1974–83)

	Total No.	No. with UTI	Rate per 1000
All males	217 116	661	3.0
Circumcised	175 317	193	1.1
Uncircumcised	41 799	468	11.2
Females	205 212	1164	5.7

Modified from Wiswell and Roscelli.[91]

group of infant boys hospitalized with febrile respiratory infections.

Evidence exists to implicate the prepuce as a reservoir for uropathogenic bacteria. Wijesina et al prospectively cultured the periurethral flora before and after circumcision in 25 boys. Prior to circumcision 52% (13/25) of the boys were colonized by potentially uropathogenic organisms as opposed to none of the boys after circumcision. Other studies have demonstrated that uropathogenic P-fimbriated *E. coli* adhere well to the mucosal surface of the prepuce, whereas non-pathogenic *E. coli* do not.[30,88,90]

One must wonder what differs in neonatal boys recognizing that the incidence of pyelonephritis declines throughout childhood despite the persistence of foreskin and periurethral colonization. In a retrospective study, Kim suggested that the increased risk of UTI in neonates might be related to the inability to retract the foreskin.[92] However, many boys cannot retract their prepuces until adolescence. Despite this conflicting evidence, the periurethral area of the uncircumcised infant is a closed space, harboring bacteria with the potential to cause serious urinary infection in some boys.[30,93] Consequently, circumcision may help to prevent UTI in male infants by removal of the mucosal surface necessary for bacterial adherence to occur. However, since even in uncircumcised boys the incidence of UTI is low, the debate regarding routine circumcision as a preventive health measure will likely continue. Justification for circumcision in boys who have other risk factors for UTI such as antenatally detected hydronephrosis associated with posterior urethral valves, megaureters, or high-grade VUR, is more easily argued.

Urethra

The short urethra in girls appears to be the most obvious explanation for the increased relative incidence of UTIs in girls as compared with boys after the first 6–12 months of life. Narrowed urethral caliber, historically blamed as the pre-eminent factor influencing susceptibility to lower UTIs in girls, does not play a role. It has long been established that the intrinsic urethral luminal size is not significantly narrower in those girls who are bacteriuric compared with those who never have been infected.[94,95] In fact, both of these studies demonstrated that the urethral diameter was slightly larger in infected groups than in those never infected. Consequently, there is no role for urethral dilation or other cystoscopic procedures in the routine management of childhood UTIs.

Other commonly held misconceptions related to the etiology of UTIs are that improper wiping techniques and bubble baths predispose to urinary infections. There is no evidence to support these myths. The strongest evidence against improper wiping techniques being a cause of UTIs is that over 95% of non-toilet-trained infants never develop urinary infection despite daily exposure to soiled diapers. Although bubble baths may occasionally cause dysuria from local meatal or vaginal irritation, there is no association with bacterial cystitis. More important for urethral ascent into the bladder is the ability of uropathogenic bacteria to attach to uroepithelial cells. Similar to the findings with periurethral cells,[96] increased adherence of bacteria to uroepithelial cells has been demonstrated in children prone to urinary infections.[97] This implies a difference in host receptor density or affinity that influences an individual's susceptibility to infection.

Dysfunctional elimination

One of the most important host risk factors for recurrent UTIs is voiding dysfunction. Common voiding disorders in children prone to UTI range from the small-capacity, unstable bladder characterized by frequency, urgency, posturing, and wetting to the infrequent voider ('lazy bladder syndrome') characterized by very infrequent voiding, a large-capacity bladder, paradoxical incontinence (wet despite a large bladder capacity), and constipation. The prevalence of some of these is listed in Table 7.5.[98] Numerous reports have linked dysfunctional voiding and recurrent UTIs in children.[99–105] Attention has also been focused on the association between dysfunctional voiding and the presence of VUR in infants and children with recurrent UTIs.[103,106,107] Chen and coworkers performed a multivariate logistic analysis to identify the association between VUR, UTI, and dysfunctional elimination in 2759 girls and boys. Dysfunctional

Table 7.5 Prevalence of symptoms characteristic of dysfunctional elimination in 7–8 year-old schoolchildren: results of Danish Epidemiological Questionnaire Survey

	Girls (%)	Boys (%)
Urge symptoms	20	21
Day wetting	13	9
Night wetting	13	22
Nocturia	7	6
Encopresis	5	8
Emptying difficulties	8	7

From Hansen et al.[98]

elimination was present in 36% of the girls and 20% of the boys with VUR. UTI was not associated with dysfunctional elimination in children without VUR; however, those with VUR and UTI had a twofold greater risk of dysfunctional elimination.[107] The predisposition to recurrent UTIs and VUR in children with dysfunctional voiding is related to the presence of residual volume resulting from inadequate emptying of the bladder, increased intravesical pressure created by uninhibited bladder contractions, and bladder overdistention from infrequent voiding habits.[108] The elimination of bacteria from the bladder by frequent and complete emptying plays a significant role in preventing infection.[109] In a group of girls followed with asymptomatic bacteriuria (ABU), the incidence of recurrent bacteriuria correlated directly to bladder emptying. The average postvoid residual urine volume in those with ABU was 23.7 ml, whereas in normal controls it was 1.1 ml. On follow-up, recurrent bacteriuria was present in 75% of those with more than 5 ml of postvoid residual urine as compared with only 17% of those with less than 5 ml of residual urine.[26] The establishment of normal voiding habits in these children has been shown to reduce the incidence of recurrent UTIs.[110–112]

Paramount to identifying the dysfunctional voider is a thorough voiding history. Squatting, delayed or infrequent micturition, urgency, constipation and/or encopresis are significant symptoms which frequently can be elicited in 50–90% of children with urinary tract infection.[102,104,113–118] Hellstrom et al[18] reported an abnormal voiding history in up to 49% of girls presenting between 3 and 5 years of age with their first urinary tract infection. Specifically, the presence of daytime urinary symptoms strongly correlated with the risk for subsequent infection. In a related study of the same children, Hansson[100] found that a majority of girls with 'covert' bacteriuria had urodynamic evidence of dysfunctional bladders when compared with controls. Wan et al[119] evaluated the relationship between toileting habits and anatomic abnormalities that predispose to infection in 101 children with UTI (77 girls and 24 boys). Ninety percent of the children without structural abnormalities demonstrated dysfunctional elimination as a contributing factor to their urinary infections, compared with 40% of those patients found to have a structural abnormality such as VUR.

Similarly, there is a definite correlation between constipation and urinary incontinence, VUR, and recurrent UTIs in children.[120,121] Constipation classically is characterized by infrequent bowel movements that are large caliber and firm. This may be associated with perineal and/or abdominal pain from colonic distention. Paradoxically, children with constipation may be referred for encopresis (fecal soiling), a manifestation of the elimination of loose stool around feces impacted within the rectal vault. Unfortunately, physical examination of the constipated child is unreliable and often a soft abdomen or empty rectal vault is encountered even when significant constipation is present radiographically. Likewise, the diagnosis of constipation can be difficult in children under 5 years who are unable to provide an accurate history.

A growing body of evidence suggests that constipation is an important facet of disordered elimination that, if appropriately managed, can help reduce the number of recurrent UTIs and promote resolution of VUR. Although this theoretically may be the result of mechanical factors related to compression of the bladder and bladder neck by a hard mass of stool, it is more likely due to the frequent coexistence of constipation with dysfunctional voiding and incomplete bladder emptying. In an epidemiologic questionnaire surveying 1597 Danish children 7–8 years old (863 girls, 728 boys, 6 gender unknown) the overall prevalence of encopresis was 13.9% (5.6% girls, 8.3% boys)[98] (Table 7.6). Among the girl respondents, 75 had a history of UTI and 13% of these suffered from encopresis vs only 6% of the girls without UTIs. Moreover, in a prospective study of 234 chronically constipated children, approximately one-third of the children demonstrated associated daytime incontinence (24%) and nighttime incontinence (34%), which reflects the degree to which bowel and bladder elimination disorders are interrelated.[111] The resolution of constipation resulted in disappearance of day- and nighttime incontinence in a majority of children (89% and 63%, respectively). Most significant was

Table 7.6 Difference in micturition symptoms in girls with and without prior urinary tract infection (UTI)

Symptoms	Prior UTI (n = 75) (%)	No history of UTI (n = 723) (%)	p-Value
Day wetting	29.3	12.9	<0.0002
Bed wetting	25.3	12.4	<0.002
Prolonged voiding	33.3	17.8	<0.002
Incomplete emptying	32.0	17.3	<0.002
Poor stream	29.3	15.8	<0.003
Manual compression of abdomen	17.3	7.3	<0.003
Staccato voiding	30.6	17.4	<0.006
Straining	17.3	8.6	<0.02
Does not reach the toilet	40.0	27.9	<0.03
Encopresis	13.3	6.0	<0.03

Modified from Hansen et al.[98]

Table 7.7 Prevalence of elimination symptoms among 143 children with primary vesicoureteral reflux (VUR)

Symptom	Prevalence (%)
Constipation	23
Bladder instability	19
Infrequent voiding	16

From Koff et al.[122]

the impact on the frequency of UTIs (approximately 10% of total), that completely disappeared in children without structural abnormalities.

Chronic constipation also plays a role in the etiology of recurrent UTIs in children with primary VUR. Recently, Koff et al[122] have demonstrated that up to 50% of the children with VUR who might otherwise be considered 'normal' have significant disorders of elimination (Table 7.7). Of the dysfunctional elimination symptoms, chronic constipation was the most prevalent in the presence of recurrent UTIs.[122] Many children without a history of UTI had detrusor instability in the absence of infection. Of those studied who had VUR, dysfunctional elimination significantly increased the risk of breakthrough UTIs, resulting in more frequent reimplantation surgery in these children. Additionally, it took 1.5 years longer for primary VUR to resolve in children with dysfunctional elimination (constipation included) compared with those without any elimination symptoms, despite a lower mean grade of reflux in those with dysfunctional elimination.

Immunologic factors

Heredity

Evidence that heredity plays a role in determining individual susceptibility to UTI is accumulating. The daughters of mothers who had been bacteriuric in childhood show a higher incidence of UTI, and female siblings tend also to show a higher incidence of bacteriuria.[20,123] Children with first-time pyelonephritis significantly more often have relatives with a history of UTI than do controls.[83] Racially dependent differences in the prevalence of UTIs and in the rate of bacteriuria have also been reported. Kunin[12] reported a 1.2% bacteriuria prevalence rate in white girls vs a rate of 0.5% in black girls in the same age group. In a retrospective review, the number of black girls evaluated following UTI who were found to have VUR was one-third that of white girls at an institution where equal numbers of black and white girls were hospitalized.[124] This observation was subsequently confirmed by a prospective study of patients admitted to this same institution with febrile UTIs.[7] Experimental urinary tract infection in mice is also significantly influenced by heredity, as evidenced by a slower response to treatment in certain strains of inbred mice as compared to others in which the UTI resolves more rapidly.[125] These same studies have also demonstrated that the acute inflammation and acquired immune response (antibody production) that follows urinary infection differs among genetically different strains of mice. As stated, '[this] result strongly suggests that the presence or absence of specific host genes will determine how effectively an *E. coli* UTI will be resolved.'

Table 7.8 Distribution of antigens in secretions and on epithelial cells and erythrocytes in the secretor and non-secretor phenotype

	Secretor	Non-secretor
Secretions (saliva, mucus)	ABH antigens	No ABH antigens
Epithelial cell	Le^{b+}, Le^{y+}	Le^{a+}, Le^{x+}
Erythrocytes	Le^{a-}, Le^{b+}	Le^{a+}, Le^{b-}
	Le^{a-}, Le^{b-}	Le^{a-}, Le^{b-}

Subsequent work has determined that innate immunity is the critical effector of inflammation and reparative processes that influence the resolution of UTI. Most of the research in this field has focused on genetic determinants within this cascade that influence the risk of acquired renal cortical scarring. Specifically, polymorphisms within the angiotensin-converting enzyme gene (ACE I/D) and tumor necrosis factor-alpha (TNF-α G308A) gene have been strongly associated with acquired renal scarring, whereas genetic abnormalities of cytokines and transforming growth factor-beta (TGF-β) have been less strongly correlated.[126–130]

Antiadherence

Epidemiologic and in-vitro data support the hypothesis that some blood group antigens behave as bacterial receptors in addition to their long-recognized role in determining red cell phenotypes. Of the many carbohydrate antigens, the role of ABH, Lewis antigens (Le^a, Le^b, Le^x, and Le^h), P, Kell, Duffy, MNS, and Kidd systems in host susceptibility to urinary infection is becoming better understood. Blood group antigens can be found on the surfaces of many epithelial cells in the body, including vaginal and uroepithelial cells, and as secreted antigens in mucus in addition to on erythrocytes.[131] Presumably, bacterial colonization of epithelial surfaces is facilitated by cell-surface-bound antigens, whereas secreted antigens mitigate against colonization by virtue of competitive inhibition.

Individuals belong to one of two distinct phenotypes based on the expression of ABH and Lewis antigens on cell surfaces and in secretions (Table 7.8). The secretor phenotype is characterized by ABH antigens in saliva, Le^b and Le^y antigens on epithelial cell surfaces, and $Le(a^- b^+)$ erythrocytes. Non-secretors have mucus devoid of ABH antigens, express Le^a and Le^x antigens on epithelial cells, and have $Le(a^+ b^-)$ erythrocytes. Those with $Le(a^- b^-)$ erythrocytes can be secretors or non-secretors, depending on the presence of ABH antigens in secretions.

Since bacterial attachment to glycoprotein (type 1 fimbriae) or glycolipid (P-fimbriae) receptors are critical steps in colonization and tissue invasion, respectively, an individual's risk for UTI may be influenced by the composition of surface receptors available for bacterial attachment. Observations by Schaeffer and coworkers in healthy women found that the profile of antigen expression on vaginal cells and in vaginal mucus correlated with the ABO phenotype and secretor status.[132] They also noted that individuals within the same blood group phenotype expressed different amounts of ABH and Lewis antigens. Moreover, longitudinal analysis demonstrated that the level of expression of these antigens fluctuated over time.[133] However, utilizing quantitative immunohistochemical techniques, Schaeffer's group did not identify an association between a particular phenotype and a positive history of UTI when controlling for secretor status.[134] Thus, despite the appealing hypothesis that some individuals may be more susceptible to bacterial colonization by virtue of genetically determined cell-surface antigens, these data do not support this notion in adult women.

In children, similar associations between blood group phenotypes and the risk of UTI have been sought. Sheinfeld et al[135] studied the expression pattern of blood group antigens in 72 tissue specimens from children who underwent urologic surgery for anatomic abnormalities of the urinary tract. Sixty-six percent (48/72) had a history of UTI and the remainder served as controls. Although an increased susceptibility to UTI was noted among non-secretors as compared with secretors, the high risk of UTI was most likely a consequence of the prevalence of structural abnormalities in this study population.[135] Jantausch et al[136] performed a more extensive analysis of blood group antigens in seven different systems and found that only the $Le(a^-b^-)$ phenotype correlated with a positive history of febrile UTIs in children, yielding a threefold relative risk. Recently, Albarus et al[137] sought to confirm the association between blood group phenotypes and the susceptibility to childhood febrile UTIs. In a well-matched case–control study of children with a febrile UTI during the first year of life, no such association existed. If blood group phenotypes and secretor status do not influence the risk of UTI, as some data might suggest, then perhaps the susceptibility to UTI is mediated by urinary or epithelial factors that are as yet unidentified.

Urinary inhibitors

Although urine commonly provides the appropriate environmental conditions for successful bacterial growth, several constituents within urine have been identified that inhibit bacterial growth. Normally, the pH of urine fluctuates between 4.6 and 7.2 in accordance with physiologic needs. Since the optimal pH range for bacterial growth is between 6 and 7, increases in urine acidity can limit bacterial growth. Extremes of urine osmolarity can also inhibit bacterial growth by virtue of the limited nutrients available to support replication in dilute urine (hypo-osmolarity) or of the dehydration that ensues in concentrated urine (hyperosmolarity). Tamm–Horsfall protein, a glycoprotein secreted by luminal cells of the ascending loop of Henle, may also be protective. This glycoprotein has been shown to contain abundant mannose residues and is identical to uromucoid. In-vitro studies have shown adherence of large numbers of *E. coli* with type 1 fimbria to uroepithelial cells coated with uromucoid in contrast to poor adherence to uroepithelial cells devoid of uromucoid.[138] It has been postulated that free Tamm–Horsfall protein in the urine may trap *E. coli* possessing type 1 fimbriae, thereby inhibiting attachment to uroepithelium. In fact, two studies have demonstrated such binding between type 1 and S-fimbriae and Tamm–Horsfall protein.[139,140] Tamm–Horsfall protein has also been demonstrated to bind to neutrophils, and it is believed that this interaction mediates recognition of bacterial invasion by neutrophils.[141] A study of UTIs in infants revealed a significantly lower mean concentration of Tamm–Horsfall protein in those with documented *E. coli* infections compared with healthy controls.[142]

Receptors

Bacterial adherence, particularly by P-fimbriae on certain strains of *E. coli*, appears to be particularly significant in the pathogenesis of upper urinary tract infections. As discussed earlier, a special class of glycosphingolipids, possessing Gal 1–4 Gal oligosaccharide, act as receptors for P-fimbriated *E. coli*.[40,41] These receptors are antigens in the P blood group system. It is felt that host susceptibility to bacterial adherence is conferred by the P1 blood group phenotype, since this group is over-represented in children with recurrent pyelonephritis in contrast to normal controls.[143,144] However, this over-representation of the P1 blood group phenotype is seen only in patients with pyelonephritis who do not have associated VUR.[143] Despite the tenuous association between non-secretor status and an increased susceptibility to UTI, apparently as a result of diminished secretion of antiadherence factors, a recent study has identified the presence of specific attachment structures for *E. coli* in non-secretors. Stapleton et al[145] have identified glycosphingolipids on vaginal and renal epithelial cells that bind each of the three major classes of *E. coli* adhesins. Of the glycosphingolipids studies, sialosyl galactosyl globoside was determined to be the preferred binding receptor for uropathogenic *E. coli.* Bergsten et al[146] have shown that bacterial attachment through P-fimbriae is sufficient to activate the innate host response. Thus, an individual's risk for UTI may be more strongly influenced by the presence of receptors for bacterial attachment, rather than the absence of blocking antigens.

Immunity

The immunologic response to UTI has been studied at both the kidney and bladder level. Understanding the immune response to infection is particularly important because immunization is currently being explored as a possible means of preventing recurrent UTIs. The antibody response to infection has also been used diagnostically to localize the level of urinary infection to the upper or lower urinary tract.[147,148]

Antibody response

The focus of most of the clinical and experimental immunologic studies of UTI has been the immune response to pyelonephritis. During acute pyelonephritis a systemic antibody response occurs with antibody production primarily against the O antigen of the infecting bacteria. A diminshed response is seen toward the K antigen.[61,149] Counteracting bacterial adherence to host epithelial cells are protective antibodies that may be passively acquired (from mother to fetus) or actively acquired through previous exposure to infection. Conversely, in the absence of protective antibodies some individuals are at greater risk for UTI.[150] Antibodies of the immunoglobulin M (IgM), IgG, IgA, and secretory IgA (sIgA) type have all been demonstrated in the serum and urine of children and experimental animals with acute pyelonephritis.[151,152] High IgG, IgA, and secretory IgA antibody levels have also been found in the urine of girls with pyelonephritis.[152] The presence of antibodies within the renal parenchyma enhances bacterial opsonization, the process by which bacteria are coated by proteins, which leads to further phagocytosis.

Antibody response to pili has also been found following pyelonephritis.[153] Secretory IgA directed against pili has been recovered from the urine of patients with acute pyelonephritis and has been shown to prevent in-vitro adherence of *E. coli* to human uroepithelial cells.[154]

Mannose-specific interactions between *E. coli* and the carbohydrate moiety of secretory IgA have been reported.[155] Secretory IgA, when bound to the uroepithelium, may thus offer a receptor site for bacteria. When excreted, it may result in competitive inhibition of binding.

With regard to the immune response of the bladder to urinary infection, a systemic circulating antibody response to cystitis is not seen.[152,156] However, an elevation of secretory IgA antibody in the urine has been observed in children with UTI, suggesting local antibody production.[152,157] A more recent study reported a decreased excretion rate of secretory IgA in uninfected children with a history of symptomatic infections compared with healthy controls. However, when these girls were subsequently studied at the time of symptomatic UTI, secretory IgA excretion rates were significantly higher than in controls.[158] Other evidence supporting a role for secretory IgA as a host defense factor comes from animal studies. Attempts at local immunization of the urinary tract have shown that intravesical immunization is effective against experimentally induced ascending UTI in rats.[159] The presence of secretory IgA in the urine following local bladder or vaginal immunization has been shown to decrease adherence to uroepithelial cells in this experimental model.[160,161]

The urine of newborns has nearly undetectable levels of sIgA that increase during the first year of life, particularly in breastfed as compared with non-breastfed infants. Case-control studies have identified a diminished incidence of UTI in breastfed infants, presumably related to soluble substances that are absorbed enterically and excreted into the urine. Using high-performance liquid chromatography to purify oligosaccharides in breast milk, Coppa et al[162] identified small molecular weight, neutral oligosaccharides that significantly decreased adhesion between human uroepithelial cells and *E. coli* isolated from an infant with UTI. Additionally, breast milk contains T and B lymphocytes, cytokines, growth factors and, most importantly, antibodies that may act synergistically to decrease the breastfed infant's risk of UTI.

No differences have been noted in the levels of urinary sIgA among boys and girls, and thus impaired immunity does not explain the higher incidence of UTI in infant boys as compared to girls. Instead, the predominance of UTI in infant boys likely reflects local periurethral factors (especially among uncircumcised boys).[43]

Cell-mediated immunity

The protective role, if any, of cell-mediated immunity in UTI is controversial.[163] T and B lymphocytic response is seen in the kidney during experimental pyelonephritis.[164] However, others have shown a depressed cell-mediated response during the early phase of renal infection when bacterial replication is maximal.[165] Although such studies have documented cell-mediated host responsiveness to bacterial infection, they have not defined the role of this process in the pathogenesis of UTI. There is no strong clinical evidence to support abnormality of cell-mediated immunity in patients prone to UTI. Experimental UTI in mice has demonstrated no increased susceptibility to *E. coli* in athymic animals (with dysfunctional cellular immune systems) and normal controls.[166] Similarly, in patients with compromised immune systems, an increased susceptibility to UTIs has not been reported. Studies to better define the role of cell-mediated immunity in UTI are obviously needed.

Innate immunity

Normally, uroepithelial cells have the capacity to produce cytokines when exposed to bacteria in vivo and in cell culture systems. Whereas these molecules serve as chemoattractants for inflammatory cells, they also participate in the uroepithelial cells' own response to invasion by pathogenic bacteria (see Table 7.3). The specific stimulus for uroepithelial cell cytokine production and release appears to be components of P- and type-1 fimbriae, since urinary levels of interleukin-6 (IL-6) are significantly greater in the presence of adhering bacteria and adhesin positive P-fimbriae.[161–169] Further in-vitro studies have determined that in response to direct contact between bacterial fimbriae and receptors located on the uroepithelial cell membrane, the uroepithelial cell is able to suppress bacterial growth.[170] These receptors have subsequently been identified as the 'toll-like receptor', an evolutionarily old system of pathogen recognition that is homologous to the interleukin-1 receptor. Moreover, utilizing human uroepithelial cells in culture, Mannhardt and coworkers[170] have demonstrated that, in individuals with a history of recurrent UTIs, a transmembrane defect impedes signal transduction within the urothelial cell, thus rendering the cell incapable of responding to bacterial attachment. Among the 10 identified toll-like receptors, TLR-2 and -4 are the most relevant to the investigation of APN since these recognize antigens present on the surface of uropathogenic bacteria: peptidoglycans and lipoproteins (TLR-2) and lipopolysaccharide (TLR-4). TLR-2 and -4 participate with other membrane-bound proteins to stimulate transcription of cytokine genes, including TGF-β, which has been implicated in tissue fibrosis.[171] In mice, disruption of the downstream effects of TLR-2 and -4 stimulation results in delayed bacterial clearance and renal cortical scarring.[172] These data lend support to the concept that the most important arm of cellular immunity in the urinary tract may not be T and B cells, as classically described, but instead the inherent ability of the uroepithelium to respond to bacterial invasion.

Vaccines

Much of the significance of clarifying the immune response to UTI relates to the possibility of developing an effective vaccine to prevent urinary infections. Experimental evidence has accumulated to suggest that this may be possible in the near future. Protection against experimental ascending pyelonephritis in rats has been demonstrated using isolated capsular antigen to stimulate antibody production directed at K antigen.[159] Similarly, immunization with *E. coli* P-fimbriae in both mice and primates confers protection against ascending pyelonephritis, presumably by interfering with adherence of the organism to the uroepithelium.[173–175] Immunization of rats with purified type-1 fimbriae also affords substantial protection against experimental ascending pyelonephritis.[176] Thankavel et al have identified the specific subunit region within the FimH determinant of type-1 fimbriae that is responsible for attachment to uroepithelial cells. Antibodies directed specifically against this region of only 25 amino acids, and not other regions on FimH or FimA subunits of type 1 fimbriae, reduced experimental pyelonephritis in mice.[177] Some evidence suggests a potential role for immunization with hemolysins as well.[52]

Recent clinical investigations have demonstrated the efficacy of acquired immunity as prophylaxis against recurrent UTIs in women and children. Both vaginal and intramuscular immunization with inactivated uropathogenic bacteria has resulted in significantly increased levels of sIgA.[178] In a small trial involving only 10 girls with recurrent UTIs and an equal number of healthy controls, intramuscular immunization also resulted in significantly fewer recurrences in the girls vaccinated.[179] Although these results are promising, the full value of such vaccines to prevent pyelonephritis will be critically assessed only by appropriately controlled, large clinical trials.

Anatomical abnormalitites of the upper urinary tract

Vesicoureteral reflux

Numerous reports have documented that vesicoureteral reflux is present in 25–50% (average 35%) of children with culture documented UTIs.[180] In contrast, in a survey of the literature Bailey reported an incidence of VUR in children without UTI of only 0.4–1.8%.[181] Similar findings were reported by Ransley, who compiled voiding cystograms in 535 children without a history of UTI and found VUR in only 7 children (1.3%).[182] Vesicoureteral reflux, when present, continues to be the most significant host risk factor in the etiology of childhood pyelonephritis. The risk for both acute pyelonephritis and subsequent renal scarring is directly related to the severity of VUR. In one prospective study of children with febrile UTIs, approximately 80% of patients with VUR demonstrated changes consistent with acute pyelonephritis on technetium-99m (^{99m}Tc) DMSA renal scans, including 100% of patients with moderate to severe reflux (grades III–V/V).[53] In contrast, only 60% of patients without demonstrable reflux had evidence of acute pyelonephritis on the DMSA scan. Kidneys associated with moderate or severe reflux were twice as likely to demonstrate abnormalities on DMSA scans (67%) when compared with kidneys with mild (32%) or no reflux (34%). In a compilation of 10 published clinical studies of children with febrile UTIs, DMSA renal scan abnormalities have been reported in 50–80% of children.[183] When VUR was present, approximately 80–90% of patients had abnormal studies, including almost all with moderate or severe VUR.

The presence of VUR appears to compensate for decreased virulence of *E. coli* in patients with recurrent pyelonephritis.[42] When there is reflux of infected urine from the bladder into the upper urinary tract, bacteria do not require special virulence properties, such as cellular attaching ability, to ascend from the bladder to the kidney. In one study of girls with recurrent pyelonephritis, infections were caused by P-fimbriated *E. coli* in only 36% of those with VUR compared with 71% of those without VUR.[42] Despite the important role that VUR plays when it is present, studies of children with febrile UTIs have reported that the majority of patients (60–68%) with abnormal DMSA renal scans demonstrating acute pyelonephritic changes do not have demonstrable VUR at the time of investigation.[183]

In children with dysfunctional voiding, the presence of residual urine and elevated voiding pressures during urinary tract infection is more likely to result in significant post-pyelonephritic renal scarring than anticipated for the grade of VUR present. Perhaps because of more frequent breakthrough infections while on antibacterial prophylaxis, these children have been found to be at greater risk for progressive renal scarring (up to 44%).[184]

Obstruction

Urinary obstruction may occur at the ureteropelvic junction, the ureterovesical junction, or the posterior urethra in boys with valves. Patients with obstruction may present with severe infection. Ectopic ureters, with or without associated ureteroceles, also represent obstructed pathology. However, such anomalies are present in only a minority of children with UTIs. In fact, recent prospective studies of children presenting with first-time febrile UTIs have reported significant obstructive uropathy in fewer than 1%.[185] Perhaps this lower incidence is due in part to the increased detection of hydronephrosis on prenatal ultrasonography prior to the development of clinical infection. The increased predisposition to infection presumably results from impairment of urinary flow with resultant stasis that compromises bladder and renal defense mechanisms. Both obstruction and high-grade reflux result in an increase in the residual volume of urine in the bladder or dilated urinary tract, permitting the multiplication of bacteria in the urine.[109] Obstruction also inhibits the mechanical washout or flushing effect associated with ureteral peristalsis and effective micturition and may alter other local defense factors as well. All of these factors result in increased susceptibility of the parenchyma to infection and damage.

Diagnosis of urinary tract infection

Urinary tract infection can be reliably diagnosed only by urine culture. Symptoms of dysuria, urgency, frequency, and enuresis are non-specific and may be the result of vulvitis, urethritis, dysfunctional voiding, or non-specific causes, such as dehydration associated with febrile illness. In 34 children with lower urinary symptoms alone, urine culture demonstrated significant bacteriuria in only 18%; 40% of those with sterile urine had upper respiratory tract infection.[186] Similarly, Heale et al[187] found that of 378 children with specific urinary complaints, only 14.3% had urinary infection. Thirty-three percent with flank pain, frequency, and/or dysuria and 31.5% with the recent onset of wetting had UTI, whereas only 4.2% with chronic nocturnal enuresis were infected. Of those without specific complaints, 4.4% had UTI (there was little difference from those who were wet only at night).

Urinalysis

Although routine urinalysis can be helpful in calling attention to those who might be infected, the association of inflammatory cells in the urine by itself is at best only about 70% reliable.[6,188,189] The finding of significant pyuria on routine urinalysis varies with the volume of urine centrifuged and examined, the force and duration of centrifugation, the volume in which cells are resuspended, and observer error.[190] Urine microscopy for bacteria significantly improves the reliability of urinalysis for the detection of urinary infection, particularly when one combines this with examination of urinary sediment for pyuria.[191] Jenkins et al reviewed approximately 40 publications reporting urine microscopy for bacteria and found a wide variation in methodology and diagnostic criteria. They concluded that the least reliable method was examination of unstained, uncentrifuged urine. When stained, centrifuged urine was examined, the sensitivity using the criteria of one or more organisms per oil immersion field was greater than 95% when compared with urine culture growing ($\geq 10^5$ colony-forming units (CFUs) per ml. The specificity was at least 95% when more than 5 organisms per oil immersion field were viewed. Hoberman et al have compared quantitative urine cultures with an 'enhanced' urinalysis for the detection of pyuria and bacteriuria in urine specimens obtained by catheterization in children presenting with fever. The data obtained demonstrated that UTI is best defined by more than 10 leukocytes/mm^3 on urinalysis combined with urine cultures yielding more than 50 000 CFU/ml.[192] In contrast, dipstick determination for the presence of leukocyte esterase and nitrite yielded sensitivities of only 52.9% and 31.4%, respectively, in detecting clinically significant bacteriuria (greater than 50 000 CFU/ml). In both this and another study of febrile infants, the findings of urinalysis were compared with the results of ^{99m}Tc (DMSA) renal scans. Both studies concluded that acute pyelonephritis in febrile infants is almost always associated with the finding of pyuria on urinalysis.[192,193]

Partly as a result of the technique and operator-dependent variability with urine microscopy, a number of enzymatic methods for detection of bacteriuria or pyuria have been developed. The two most popular are the leukocyte esterase and the nitrite reductase tests. These studies are inexpensive, rapid, and easy to perform.

Leukocyte esterase test

The leukocyte esterase dipstick test demonstrates the presence of pyuria by histochemical methods that specifically detect esterases in the neutrophils. When compared with chamber count methods, studies have reported sensitivity as high as 88–95% for the detection of pyuria using a cutoff of 10 or more leukocytes/mm^2.[32,194] However, in a study which evaluated 110 children with fever and positive urine cultures, the leukocyte esterase test had sensitivities of only 52.9% and 66.7% in detecting ≥10 and ≥20 leukocytes/mm^3, respectively.[189] Furthermore, one would not anticipate this test to be any more sensitive than the finding of pyuria alone for the identification of children with positive urine cultures.

Nitrite test

Bacteria convert urine nitrate to nitrite. The nitrite method employs reagent paper impregnated with sulfanilic acid and α-naphthylamine that form a red azo dye when in contact with nitrite. Thus, a positive colorimetric assay implies the presence of bacteria in the bladder. However, a relatively long incubation period (4 hours) is required for conversion of nitrate to nitrite. For this reason, first morning urine sample in a toilet-trained child is the best specimen to test. A single test on a randomly collected urine specimen was reported to have a sensitivity of only 29.2–44% on 790 urine specimens using dipsticks from two manufacturers. However, the specificity was 98% when the test was positive.[194,195] This test is not a reliable office screening method when used alone.[194]

Combining the leukocyte test and the nitrite test on a single dipstick has improved the accuracy to detect or exclude UTI. In a review of rapid methods to detect UTIs, Pezzlo reported a sensitivity of 78–92% and a specificity of 60–98% when using the combination test.[196] However, the accuracy is affected by the probability of the patient being infected based on clinical findings.[196,197] Accordingly, urine culture may be omitted when the dipstick test is negative only when there is limited suspicion for UTI based on clinical symptoms. Conversely, urine culture should be obtained in any patient suspected of having a UTI or in whom the dipstick test is positive.

Others have evaluated the role of urinary *N*-acetyl-β-glucosaminidase (NAG) (a renal tubular enzyme thought to be a marker of tubular damage), β_2-microglobulin (β_2M) (a low molecular weight circulating protein with increased fractional excretion in children with tubulointerstitial disease) and IL-8 in the diagnosis of pyelonephritis in febrile children. Unfortunately, NAG and β_2M have been found in both children with febrile UTIs and in children with sterile urine who had severe renal scarring associated with high-grade VUR. Elevated IL-8 urinary levels are also non-specific, as they have been seen in inflammatory disorders other than acute pyelonephritis. Thus, these markers are currently unreliable for the diagnosis of acute pyelonephritis.[135,198–200]

Urine culture

In the pre-toilet-trained group, the urine specimen is often obtained by applying a collection bag. The results of a bag urine specimen are reliable *only* when the specimen is negative. Contamination is directly related to the length of time the bag is in place. If a specimen has not been obtained within 30 minutes of application, reliability begins to decrease. Removing the appliance and plating or refrigerating the urine immediately after the child voids is paramount. Having the parent apply the bag before leaving for the physician's office in an effort to shorten the wait is acceptable only when the cultured specimen is negative. When confirmation of voided urine or immediate treatment is necessary, bladder catheterization or suprapubic aspiration (SPA) should be employed. A feeding tube (8–10 Fr) inserted only a few centimeters into the bladder is ideal for catheterization. In girls and boys who can void on command, midstream specimens are more reliable than bag-collected specimens.

SPA has achieved popularity in some centers. Young children are particularly favorable candidates for SPA because of the abdominal location of their urinary bladders. However, the procedure cannot be expected to be successful when the bladder is empty. This is the major drawback of SPA. If urine is not obtained initially, time should not be wasted in a sick child who requires antibiotic treatment. Urethral catheterization should be done. SPA is performed after first cleaning the suprapubic area with an antiseptic solution. A 21–25 gauge needle is inserted perpendicular to the patient in the midline, one finger-breadth above the symphysis. Although a local anesthetic can first be infiltrated, this appears unnecessary and may actually cause more pain than a quick in-and-out aspiration. It is practical to apply a U-bag to the perineum prior to cleansing the abdomen. Many times the child voids during preparation for aspiration, obviating the necessity for the procedure if the voided urine is immediately plated or refrigerated.

It has often been stated that 'any number of bacteria' obtained by SPA are significant. Since the bladder is a reservoir and this method of collection depicts the number of bacteria in that reservoir, one should not anticipate colony counts significantly different from those properly collected by other means. Ginsburg and McCraken found ≥100 000 CFU/ml in 96% and 40 000–80 000 in the remaining 4% of 100 febrile infants with bacteriuria demonstrated on SPA.[6] None showed fewer than 40 000 colonies. Nelson and Peters had previously reported similar results in a study of premature and term infants.[201] Hoberman et al recently reported the results of positive urine cultures on specimens obtained by catheterization in 110 febrile infants <2 years old.[192] Of 110 urine cultures with ≥10 000 CFU/ml, 92 (84%) had ≥100 000 CFU/ml, 10 (9%) had 50 000–99 000 CFU/ml, and only 8 (7%) had 10 000–49 000 CFU/ml. Furthermore, urine specimens with 10 000–49 000 were much more likely to yield Gram-positive or mixed organisms than specimens with >50 000 CFU/ml. These authors concluded that UTI is best defined by ≥10 leukocytes/mm^3 and colony counts of ≥50 000 on catheterized specimens. Thus, colony counts from the bladder <50 000 CFU/ml are suspect regardless of the manner in which the urine was collected.

Clinical presentation and localization

As one would anticipate, the classic signs and symptoms for UTI are usually lacking in the very young.

Table 7.9 Prominent symptoms in neonatal non-obstructive urinary tract infection: combined results of four studies (n = 255)

Symptom	Prevalence (%)
Failure to thrive or weight loss	51
Fever	41
Jaundice	12
Cyanosis/pallor	30
Vomiting	35
Diarrhea	29
Convulsions/CNS symptoms	20

Instead, non-specific symptoms – such as irritability, poor feeding, failure to gain weight, vomiting, and diarrhea – may be the only signs suggestive of an underlying problem (Table 7.9). In one study of children with symptomatic urinary infections, only 9% of 78 infants were initially referred with a suspected diagnosis of UTI.[202] Often absent in neonates, fever is present in most infants between 1 and 12 months old who present with symptomatic UTIs.[5,11,19] In fact, urinary tract infections have recently been described as one of the most common serious bacterial illnesses among febrile infants and young children, with a reported prevalence ranging from 4.1% to 7.5%.[192] In one study of 945 infants who presented to a pediatric ER with fever, the overall prevalence of UTI was 5.3%.[203] The prevalence was highest in Caucasian girls, 17% of whom had a positive urine culture. In contrast, the prevalence of UTI among African-American girls was only 3.5% and among boys it was 2.5%. Another prospective study reported UTI in 7.5% of 442 infants (less than 8 weeks of age) presenting to the emergency room with fever ≥100.6 °F (38.1 °C), only half of whom had abnormal urinalyses suggestive of UTI (>5 white blood cells per high-power field or any bacteria present).[204] Thus, a urine specimen for culture, preferably collected by catheterization, should be obtained routinely whenever a non-verbal, non-toilet-trained child presents with unexplained fever.

As the child becomes verbal and is toilet-trained, urinary tract symptomatology is more easily detected. Fever continues to be relatively common in toddlers with first-time symptomatic infection. However, fever is not as frequently associated with recurrent and/or long-standing infection. In older children urgency, frequency, enuresis, and dysuria are common presenting symptoms. Failure to become toilet-trained at the proper age may occasionally

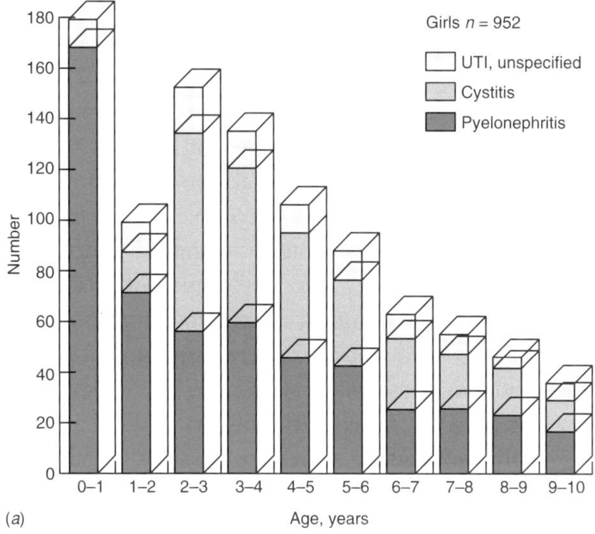

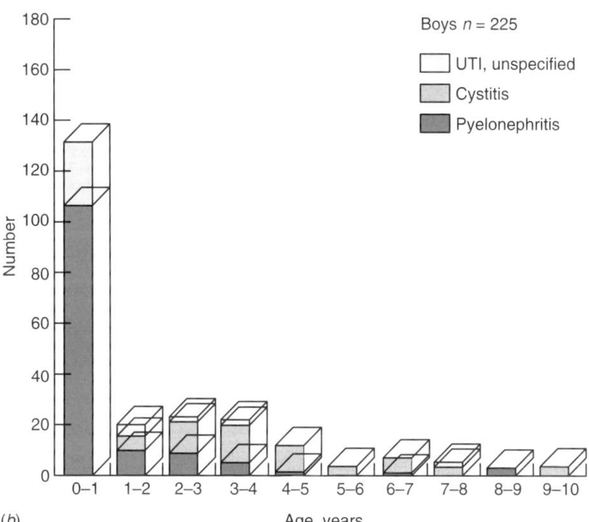

Figure 7.6 Children with first-time diagnosis of urinary tract infection at the Children's Hospital in Goteborg, Sweden, according to age and clinical diagnosis. (Reprinted from Jodal[206], with permission.)

herald underlying chronic lower urinary infection. Although urinary tract symptoms such as vaginal pain, urinary frequency, dysuria, and enuresis are common following childhood sexual abuse, actual urinary infection is not.[205]

There are few population-based studies of symptomatic UTIs in childhood. The classic epidemiologic study by Winberg et al[11] was carried out between 1960 and 1966 in Goteborg, Sweden. The special organizational structure of that city's pediatric medical care has afforded unique opportunities to perform ongoing epidemiologic studies of UTIs in children. Jodal[5] reported a follow-up prospective epidemiologic study conducted in Goteborg from 1970 to 1979. There were 952 females and 225 males (4.2:1) below age 10 years of age who were treated for a first-time symptomatic urinary infection (Figure 7.6).[206] Of the 225 boys, 59% presented during the first year of life. The number of boys diagnosed in the higher age groups was low, especially over age 5. The number of first infections in girls was also highest in the first year of life (19%). A gradual decrease in number of girls with first-time infections was associated with increasing age. In both girls and boys, febrile infections, presumed to be pyelonephritis, predominated during the first year of life. Acute cystitis was most commonly seen between 2 and 5 years of age in both sexes, with a marked peak frequency in girls during the third year of life. As expected, infections during infancy were the most difficult to characterize as pyelonephritis or cystitis.

Asymptomatic bacteriuria

The natural history and uroradiographic findings in patients with asymptomatic or covert bacteriuria vary according to the age of the patient and prior episodes of symptomatic infections. Screening bacteriuria does not necessarily represent asymptomatic bacteriuria, as approximately one-third of school-aged girls with screening bacteriuria have a prior history of symptoms related to the urinary tract and some have had previous symptomatic UTIs. It is unclear whether the prognosis is any different for children who have primary asymptomatic bacteriuria compared with those in whom asymptomatic bacteriuria develops following treatment of a symptomatic infection.

A study of asymptomatic and symptomatic bacteriuria in infants under 1 year of age reveals interesting differences in the two populations.[5] In 2 of 50 patients with asymptomatic bacteriuria, clinical acute pyelonephritis developed within 2 weeks of detection. The others remained free of symptoms. 46 (92%) of the patients with asymptomatic bacteriuria were evaluated with voiding cystourethrography (VCUG) and mild reflux (grades I to II) was found in only 5 (11%). Of 45 left untreated, 36 spontaneously cleared the bacteriuria and 8 others became abacteriuric following antibiotic treatment for other reasons. Although asymptomatic recurrences developed in 6 (12%), no pyelonephritic recurrences occurred in this group during follow-up of at least 1 year. Follow-up urography, done in 36, did not reveal any evidence of renal scarring. In contrast, among 40 infants with symptomatic infections, 1 patient had a significant ureteropelvic junction obstruction and 14 of 39 (36%) had VUR, including 3 with grade III or greater. Fourteen of 40 (35%) experienced recurrences, including 6 with acute pyelonephritis and 3 with cystitis, whereas asymptomatic bacteriuria was noted in 5 patients. It was concluded that infants with asymptomatic bacteriuria represent a low-risk group with a tendency to spontaneously become abacteriuric, usually within a few months.

Considerable variation in uroradiographic findings has been reported in school-aged children found to have bacteriuria on screening. These studies have reported VUR in 19–35% and renal scarring in 10–26%.[12,15,16,207] However, many of these children had a prior history of symptomatic UTIs and others undoubtedly had infections during infancy that were overlooked or misdiagnosed. Although, recurrent infections following treatment occur in up to 80%, the risk for development of acute pyelonephritis in a girl older than 4 years of age with untreated asymptomatic bacteriuria is small and seems to be associated with a change in bacterial strain, perhaps as a result of antibiotic treatment.[12,208] Follow-up by the Cardiff–Oxford Bacteriuria Study Group revealed that those schoolchildren who presented initially with a radiographically normal urinary tract remained normal in spite of persistent asymptomatic bacteriuria.[209] Only in those children who had previous renal scarring did new scars or progression of scarring develop, and all of these children had VUR. Other studies have shown that asymptomatic bacteriuria is associated with low-virulence bacterial strains lacking the ability to adhere and cause symptoms.[44,154,210] Furthermore, there is considerable evidence that these organisms may be commensal with the host and may even protect against infection by more virulent strains.[211]

Cystitis

Acute cystitis in children is rarely associated with significant long-term morbidity. Typical symptoms that accompany acute cystitis in toilet-trained children include dysuria, frequency, urgency, and/or secondary-onset enuresis. Fever and systemic complaints are generally not a feature of the clinical picture. As previously mentioned, however, these same irritative lower tract symptoms are often seen in the absence of bacterial cystitis, mandating that a specimen for urine culture be obtained prior to institution of therapy.

Although the recurrence rate of lower UTIs is high, most cases can be considered little more than a nuisance and recurrences tend to decrease or disappear by adolescence. However, it is worth noting that many children prone to recurrent lower UTIs have voiding dysfunction, particularly infrequent voiding. Typically, these children do not void for 1 or 2 hours after awakening in the morning and then may void only two or three times throughout the day. Consequently, bladder capacity is abnormally large and bladder emptying is often incomplete. Often these children also have chronic constipation, including encopresis in some. Other children with recurrent cystitis have underlying bladder instability associated with urinary frequency, urgency, urge incontinence, and posturing associated with a reduced functional bladder capacity. Girls with a history of UTI are significantly more likely to report a variety of chronic voiding disturbances as compared to girls without a history of UTI[18,201] (see Table 7.6). In some cases, recurrent UTIs may be a precipitating factor to the child's voiding disturbance. Conversely, primary bladder instability may itself contribute to an increased susceptibility to UTIs. In contrast to daytime voiding disorders, isolated bedwetting is rarely associated with a history of previous UTI.[18]

Approximately 10% of susceptible girls will have a recurrent infection shortly after completion of a course of antibiotic therapy. These children have chronic symptoms of bladder instability. Squatting or posturing in response to unstable bladder contractions is common in this group. Many have voiding dyssynergia associated with high voiding pressures and incomplete bladder emptying. Some also have chronic inflammatory changes of the bladder. Historically, endoscopic evaluation of these children often revealed multiple raised 'cysts' in the area of the bladder neck and trigone. Histologically, submucosal lymphoid follicles were present. Clinically, this entity has been termed cystitis cystica, although the histologic appearance suggests it would be more accurately referred to as cystitis follicularis. The presence of these follicles suggests an immunologic response to chronic infection.[212] It should be noted that treatment of these children is no longer predicated on the basis of these endoscopic findings: rather, treatment is determined by the recurrence rate of infection and the type of underlying voiding and bowel disorder.

Pyelonephritis

Pathophysiology of acute pyelonephritis

Acute pyelonephritis represents the most serious type of UTI in children. It is not only responsible for greater acute morbidity but it also has the potential for causing irreversible damage. Acute pyelonephritis in older children typically presents with fever and flank pain or tenderness associated with pyuria and positive urine culture. In the majority of cases, laboratory evaluation reveals an elevated serum white blood cell (WBC) count, erythrocyte sedimentation rate (ESR), and/or C-reactive protein (CRP). However, when compared directly with localization studies such as DMSA renal scans, these clinical and laboratory parameters are associated with high false-positive and/or false-negative rates.[183] This is particularly true in neonates and young infants, an age group at greatest risk for renal scarring following pyelonephritis. Neonates in particular present with non-specific symptoms such as irritability, poor feeding, failure to thrive, vomiting, and diarrhea (Table 7.9). When one considers that approximately half of all children with febrile UTIs present during the first year of life, the importance of early and accurate diagnosis becomes obvious.

Experimental studies by Roberts and others have found that bacterial adherence to uroepithelium elicits an inflammatory cascade proportional to the virulence of the infecting organism. The same acute inflammatory response that is responsible for the eradication of bacteria is also responsible for the damage to renal tissue and subsequent renal scarring.[213] Through a series of experimental studies using the primate model, Roberts has developed a unified theory of the chain of events involved in the process that ultimately leads to renal scarring (Figure 7.7).[214] The initiating event is bacterial inoculation of the renal parenchyma that elicits both immune and inflammatory responses. Whereas the immune response can be stimulated by live or heat-killed bacteria, the acute inflammatory response occurs only following inoculation by live bacteria.[213] Since heat-killed bacteria do not cause renal scarring, it appears that it is the acute inflammatory response that is more important as a cause for the subsequent development of permanent renal damage. Potent cytokines induce chemotaxis of granulocytes and cellular- and humoral-mediated bacterial killing.

Studies have also reported that focal ischemia may be a consequence of acute pyelonephritis. Kaack et al have shown that granulocyte aggregation within capillaries leads to vascular occlusion. Renal ischemia is then evidenced by a transient rise in circulating renin levels.[215] Hill and Clark found evidence of marked cortical vasoconstriction in areas of acute inflammation in rabbits with acute renal infection, with inflammatory cells obstructing the peritubular capillaries.[216] Androulakakis et al found microvascular changes in acute pyelonephritis in pigs using microradiologic and stereomicroscopic techniques. Focal ischemia in areas involved by the acute inflammatory response was evidenced by compression of glomeruli, small peritubular capillaries, and vasa rectae, presumably from interstitial edema.[217] Using the microsphere technique, Majd and Rushton evaluated renal blood flow changes associated with acute pyelonephritis in the refluxing piglet model. Focal renal blood flow was decreased in sites of acute pyelonephritis identified by diminished uptake of DMSA and subsequently confirmed by histopathology. Uninvolved areas of the affected kidneys demonstrated normal blood flow comparable to that of the contralateral normal kidney.[218]

Since host-derived cytotoxins are central in the genesis of tissue suppuration, investigators have tried to understand and modify the inflammatory response. Granulocytes kill bacteria, releasing toxic enzymes (lysozymes) both within the granulocyte and into the lumen of renal tubules, which causes renal cell damage. The respiratory burst, a phenomenon universal to acute inflammatory responses, generates oxygen radicals (superoxides) that have classically been felt to mediate bacterial killing, as well as that of granulocytes and surrounding tubular cells.[219]

The role of reactive oxidants, inducible nitric oxide (iNOS), and tissue-destructive proteinases in the acute inflammatory response has only recently been elucidated. In an extensive review of the literature spanning 70 years, Weiss proposes that neutrophil-derived superoxide and oxygen radicals are merely highly reactive intermediates in the production of toxic chlorinated oxidants (e.g. hypochlorous acid and chloramines). If these chlorinated oxidants are the true mediators of tissue destruction, then inhibiting their generation should lessen tissue injury. In fact, in-vitro models have demonstrated that cellular destruction could be prevented in the presence of specific inhibitors of the H_2O_2–halide–myeloperoxidase system, effectively preventing HOCl (hypochlorous acid) generation.[220] Despite this compelling evidence, Weiss' 'enthusiasm' for HOCl as the sole agent in inflammation-mediated tissue destruction is tempered by the fact that living tissue perfused with HOCl solutions remains viable.[221] However, evidence suggests that the primary role for HOCl and chloramines is to neutralize circulating enzyme inhibitors that prevent the untimely digestion of host tissues by neutrophils. These oxidants do have mild direct cytotoxic effects. Thus, in the absence of significant inflammation, any enzymes released from neutrophilic lysosomes are

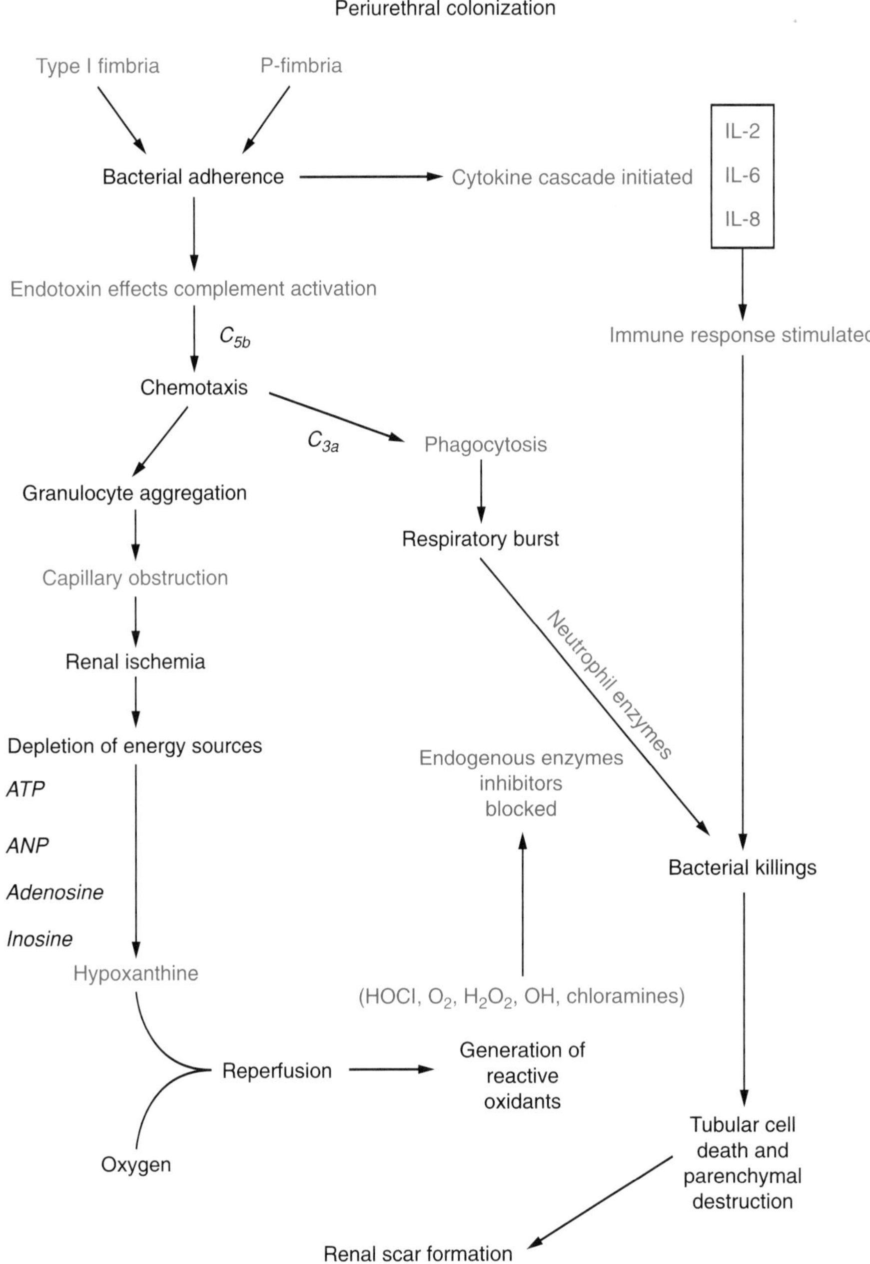

Figure 7.7 Diagram of the pathophysiologic events (from bacterial adherence to renal scar formation) that are characteristic of acute pyelonephritis. (Modified from Roberts.[214])

immediately inactivated. However, once stimulated, the neutrophil can release the aforementioned oxidants into its immediate surroundings and can create a microenvironment capable of inactivating enzyme inhibitors, activating latent neutrophil-derived enzymes, and rapidly degrading microbes, host cells, and connective substratum.[222] Tubular cell death releases the toxic inflammatory agents into the interstitium, causing further damage.

Oxygen radicals are also produced by cell reaction during reperfusion of ischemic tissue. Focal parenchymal ischemia, resulting from intravascular granulocyte aggregation and edema, occurs with bacterial infection of the renal parenchyma.[215,219,223] In ischemic tissue, hypoxanthine is produced during anaerobic metabolism of adenosine monophosphate. During reperfusion, hypoxanthine in the presence of xanthine oxidase and oxygen yields superoxides and hydrogen peroxide.[223] Treatment with allopurinol, an inhibitor of xanthine oxidase, protects against tissue damage from reperfusion injury and from that associated with bacteria in the renal parenchyma.[223]

It appears that the interstitial damage associated with the acute inflammatory response of pyelonephritis results from ischemia-related injury and from toxic enzymes. Additionally, bacterial virulence factors, such as hemolysins and lipopolysaccharides, work in concert with neutrophil-derived mediators to disrupt cellular membranes and degrade the extracellular matrix. The inflammatory process extends through the renal interstitium, thus contributing to the damage that ultimately results in irreversible renal scarring.

Recently, the impact of adjunctive corticosteroids on post-inflammatory renal scarring was evaluated in the treatment of experimental pyelonephritis in the refluxing piglet model. Following induction of acute pyelonephritis as confirmed by DMSA scintigraphy, animals were randomized to receive either standard antibiotic therapy or antibiotics and prednisolone (2 mg/kg daily). Two months later, DMSA scintigraphy was repeated and kidneys were harvested for gross and microscopic examination. The risk of focal scarring corresponded to the severity of the initial acute pyelonephritic lesion, based on the percentage of renal parenchyma involved. In kidneys with mild and moderate acute pyelonephritic lesions, antibiotics alone were equally effective in preventing scarring when compared to treatment with antibiotics and steroids. However, severe pyelonephritic lesions were three times as likely to heal without scarring in animals treated with antibiotics in conjunction with steroids as compared to antibiotics alone.[224]

Detection of acute pyelonephritis

Dimercaptosuccinic acid (DMSA) renal scan

The diagnosis of acute pyelonephritis traditionally has been made on the basis of the classic signs and symptoms of fever and flank pain or tenderness asssociated with pyuria and positive urine culture. However, accurate diagnosis based solely on these parameters is often difficult, particularly in neonates and infants.[53,225] Despite the fact that the majority of patients (50–80%) with fever and systemic clinical findings consistent with acute pyelonephritis have abnormal DMSA scan findings, there is still a high false-positive and/or -negative rate based on routine clinical and laboratory parameters, including fever, elevated WBC, elevated CRP, elevated ESR, and the presence of VUR.[183]

Direct techniques have been used to localize the level of UTI to the upper or lower urinary tract. These include split-urine cultures collected by ureteral catheterization, bladder washout, and thin-needle aspiration of renal pelvic urine under ultrasonic guidance.[226,227] Although these efforts may accurately localize infection to the upper or lower urinary tract, they are obviously invasive and do not assess the extent of renal parenchymal involvement.

Renal cortical scintigraphy with ^{99m}Tc DMSA has emerged as the imaging agent of choice for the detection and evaluation of acute pyelonephritis and renal scarring in children. Early clinical reports showed that renal cortical scintigraphy using ^{99m}Tc DMSA or glucoheptonate was significantly more sensitive than IVU and renal sonography in the detection of acute pyelonephritis.[228–230] Subsequently, to evaluate the true sensitivity and specificity of renal cortical scintigraphy, experimental studies in an animal model were conducted using strict histopathologic criteria as the standard of reference.[231,232] In these two investigations, pyelonephritis was created in young piglets by surgically inducing unilateral VUR of infected urine. Typical DMSA renal scan findings of acute pyelonephritis included focal areas of diminished uptake of DMSA with preservation of the renal contour (Figure 7.8).[233] The DMSA scan was determined to be highly sensitive and reliable for the

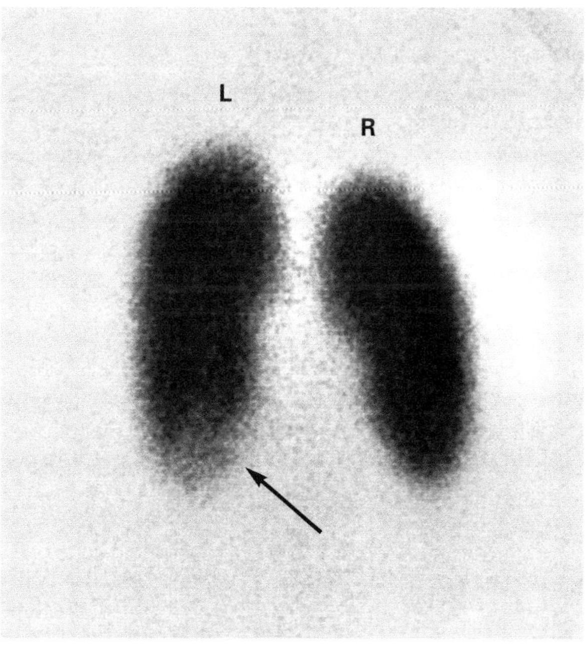

Figure 7.8 ^{99m}Tc DMSA renal scan obtained 1 week after introduction of infection in young pig with experimentally produced left vesicoureteral reflux. Focal decrease in uptake with preservation of renal contour is noted in left lower pole (arrow). Pathologic examination confirmed left lower pole pyelonephritis. (Reprinted from Rushton and Majd,[233] with permission.)

detection and localization of experimental acute pyelonephritis, with a sensitivity of 87–89% and specificity of 100% in both. When individual pyelonephritic lesions were analyzed, DMSA scan findings correlated with histopathologic changes with an overall agreement rate of 89–94%. Those lesions not detected were microscopic foci of inflammation not evident on gross examination and not associated with significant parenchymal damage.

Not only is DMSA scintigraphy highly sensitive and specific for the diagnosis of acute pyelonephritis but it also provides important information regarding renal function and the extent of renal parenchymal inflammation. Documentation of renal parenchymal damage associated with acute pyelonephritis is fundamental to understanding the roles of infection and VUR in the etiology of pyelonephritis and renal scarring.

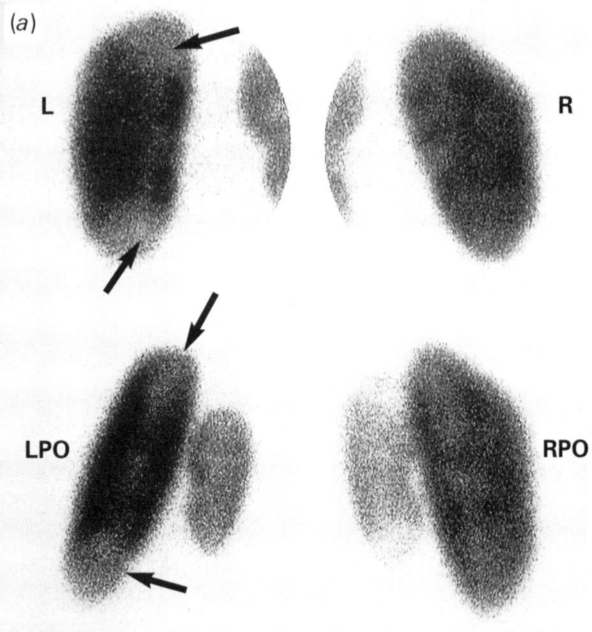

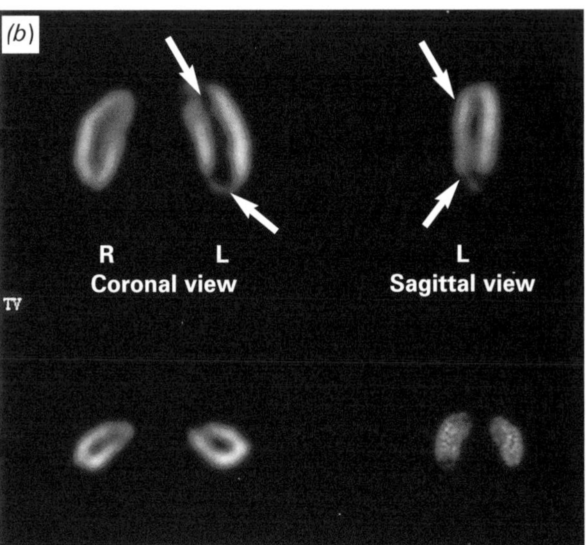

Figure 7.9 (*a*) Posterior and posterior oblique pinhole and (*b*) coronal and sagittal SPECT images of ^{99m}Tc DMSA renal scan in a young pig with bilateral vesicoureteral reflux and acute left pyelonephritis 48 h after introduction of *E. coli* broth into the bladder. Photopenic lesions in the left upper and lower poles are demonstrated by both modalities (arrows).

Single-photon emmision computed tomography (SPECT)

The application of SPECT to DMSA scintigraphy reportedly further enhances the sensitivity of DMSA in the detection of acute pyelonephritis.[234–236] In clinical studies, a greater number of defects have been detected by SPECT compared with standard pinhole imaging. Obviously, in these clinical trials, histopathologic confirmation of the abnormal findings demonstrated by renal scintigraphy was not possible. To further evaluate the accuracy of SPECT imaging in the detection of acute pyelonephritis, SPECT was compared with pinhole imaging of DMSA renal scans for the detection and localization of acute pyelonephritis in 16 piglets (32 kidneys) with bilateral reflux of infected urine.[237] Animals were evaluated with both imaging modalities immediately prior to sacrifice at 1, 2, 3, and 10 days following the introduction of infection into their bladders. The overall sensitivity for detection of affected renal zones with histologic evidence of pyelonephritis was 86% for pinhole imaging and 91% for SPECT. The specificity was 95% for pinhole imaging and 82% for SPECT. Overall accuracy for the presence or absence of kidney involvement was 88% for both (Figure 7.9). Thus, SPECT imaging appears to be slightly more sensitive than standard pinhole imaging, but its application may result in more false-positive findings. Furthermore, it is easier to differentiate acute inflammatory changes from chronic renal scarring with pinhole imaging. Whether pinhole or SPECT imaging is utilized is to some extent dependent on the availability and experience of the imaging unit.

Sonography and intravenous pyelography (IVP)

Several clinical studies have clearly demonstrated that renal sonography is not as reliable as DMSA scintigraphy for the detection of acute pyelonephritis.[238–244]

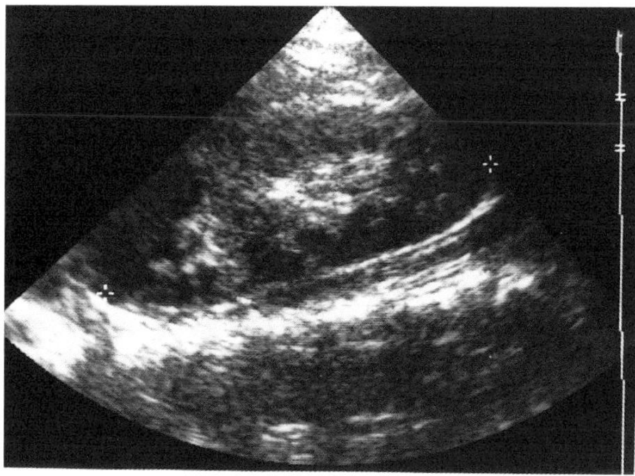

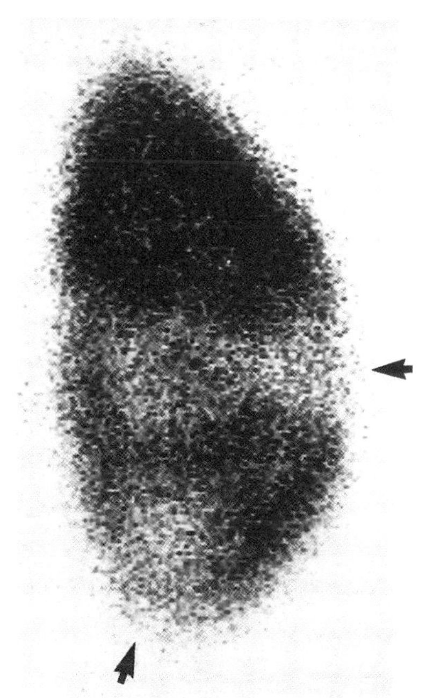

Figure 7.10 Normal sonogram and grossly abnormal ^{99m}Tc DMSA renal scan of right kidney showing large mid-zone and moderate lower pole photopenic lesions characteristic of acute pyelonephritis in a 4-year-old girl who presented with her first documented febrile UTI (arrows). VCUG was negative for vesicoureteral reflux.

In one prospective study of 91 children with culture-documented febrile UTIs, DMSA renal scans showed changes consistent with acute pyelonephritis in 63% of the patients.[238] In contrast, sonography revealed changes consistent with acute pyelonephritis in only 39% of the same patients. More recently, MacKenzie et al prospectively compared the results of renal ultrasound with DMSA renal scans in 112 children with their first documented symptomatic UTI.[239] Although ultrasound was particuarly effective in detecting dilatation of the collecting system and renal swelling, it failed to detect over half of those patients with abnormal DMSA scans demonstrating photon-deficient areas consistent with acute inflammatory changes of pyelonephritis (Figure 7.10). Intravenous pyelography has been shown to be very insensitive for the detection of acute pyelonephritis.[245]

Other renal isotopes

The usefulness of an early ^{99m}Tc mercaptoacetyl-triglycine(MAG3) renal scan in predicting renal alterations seen on DMSA renal scans has been evaluated by Piepz et al.[244] These investigators concluded that the accuracy of the MAG3 renal scan was population dependent. When the DMSA scan was normal or very abnormal, the MAG3 image correctly reflected the findings of the DMSA renal scan. However, when the DMSA abnormalities were less pronounced, the early MAG3 scan failed to detect about half of the cases.

^{99m}Tc glucoheptonate has also been used in the detection of acute inflammatory changes associated with acute pyelonephritis.[229,230,247] Although the sensitivity and specificity of ^{99m}Tc-labeled glucoheptonate and DMSA have not been directly compared, certain observations can be made. Approximately 60% of the administered dose of ^{99m}Tc DMSA is tightly bound to the proximal tubular cells, and only a small amount is excreted slowly in the urine. Consequently, DMSA allows for excellent visualization of the renal parenchyma without interference from retained tracer in the collecting systems. In contrast, only about 20% of the administered dose of ^{99m}Tc glucoheptonate is firmly bound to the tubular cells. Most of the administered dose is excreted in the urine, which allows for moderately good visualization of the renal collecting systems on the early images. This additional information makes glucoheptonate the preferred agent of some clinicians.[247] However, the quality of the delayed renal cortical images is clearly better with DMSA.

MRI, CT scans, power Doppler sonography

The use of magnetic resonance imaging (MRI) with UTIs has also been reported. In a clinical study for detection of acute pyelonephritic damage in children, the sensitivity and specificity of gadolinium-enhanced MRI was equal to that of ^{99m}Tc DMSA scanning.[246] In a more recent animal study, SPECT imaging using DMSA was compared with spiral computed tomography (CT) scanning (pre- and postcontrast), gadolinium-enhanced MRI, and power Doppler sonography in 35 infected piglets with 70 refluxing

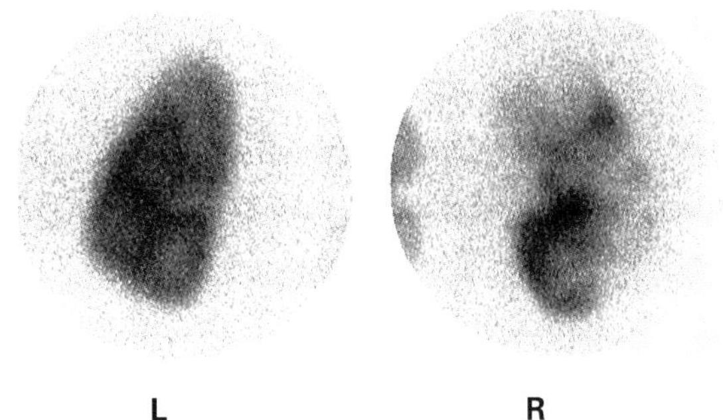

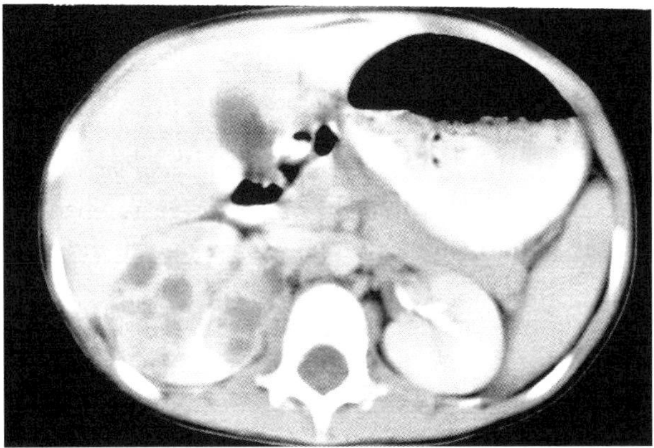

Figure 7.11 Severe multifocal acute pyelonephritis in the right kidney is well demonstrated on both a ^{99m}Tc DMSA renal scan and CAT scan in a 3-year-old girl with her first febrile UTI. Photopenic areas on DMSA scan correspond to attenuated hypodense lesions on CAT scan. Note diffuse right renal swelling on CAT scan.

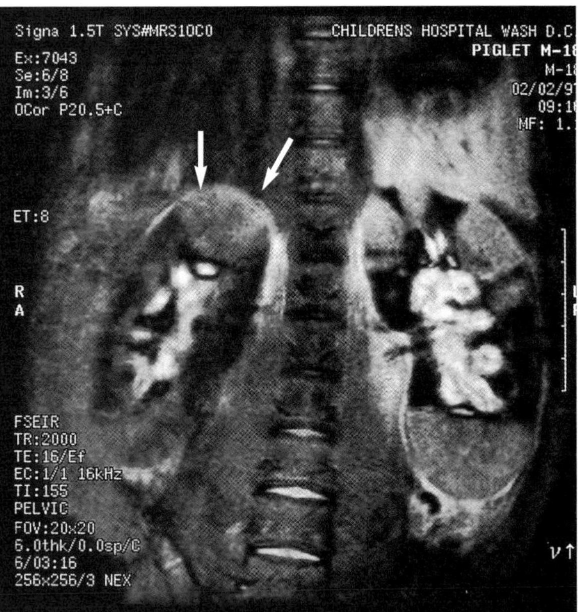

Figure 7.12 Gadolinium-enhanced MRI in a young pig with bilateral vesicoureteral reflux (VUR) demonstrates multiple acute pyelonephritic lesions in both kidneys as evidenced by bright parenchymal lesions (arrows).

kidneys.[249] The imaging modalities were interpreted independently and compared in a blinded fashion with histopathologic findings. SPECT DMSA, spiral CT, and MRI were equally sensitive and reliable for the detection and localization of acute pyelonephritis (Figures 7.11 and 7.12). Power Doppler sonography was significantly less accurate in this porcine model. However, a recent clinical study comparing Doppler sonography to DMSA scanning in 62 children, found favorable positive- and negative-predictive values (93.1% and 85.7%, respectively) for Doppler studies.[250] Nevertheless, with increased experience and enhanced applications, clinical use of spiral CT and MRI is likely to gain popularity in the evaluation of the pediatric urinary tract.

Evaluation of the child with urinary tract infection

Controversy continues to exist regarding when and how a child with documented UTI should be evaluated. A recent systematic overview of the literature to assess the evidence on which current recommendations for routine diagnostic imaging are based found that there were no controlled trials or analytic studies which evaluated the need for routine diagnostic imaging.[251] All reports were descriptive and the majority were retrospective. Furthermore, none provided evidence of the impact of routine imaging on the development of renal scars and clinical outcomes in children with their first UTI.

Most pediatric urologists would agree that all children under 5 years of age, boys of any age, and all with febrile UTI or documented acute pyelonephritis should be evaluated when infection is first recognized. The key to this recommendation is adequate documentation of UTI.

The arguments in favor of early evaluation of young children following their first documented UTI are based on both experimental and clinical data. Clinical and experimental studies have proved that significant renal scarring can occur after a single UTI.[252,253] A higher incidence of renal scarring has been reported in children with VUR and recurrent UTIs than in those with reflux who have had only a single infection.[254,255] Similarly, Jodal reported a strong association between the number of pyelonephritic episodes and the incidence of renal scarring.[5] Recurrence of UTI within 1 year of a preceding infection occurs in approximately 30% of girls with one, 60% with two, and 75% with three prior infections.[11] Furthermore, the non-specificity of signs and symptoms that typically accompany urinary infection in infants and toddlers often makes it impossible to determine whether an infection actually represents the first episode.[11] Additional justification for early evaluation is based on the high yield of uropathology obtained from the evaluation of children with culture-documented UTIs. Cystography in Caucasian girls with symptomatic UTIs consistently demonstrates the presence of VUR in approximately 30–50% of cases, regardless of whether the study is requested by pediatric subspecialists (urology/nephrology) or other clinicians (pediatricians, family practitioners, adult urologists).[5,256,257] The exception is found in African-American girls with UTI in whom the relative incidence of VUR is about one-third that of Caucasian girls.[7,124] Unfortunately, other clinical parameters have proven unreliable in distinguishing those children with UTI who also have VUR.[118] All of the aforementioned factors offer a convincing argument to pursue early evaluation of young children following their first documented UTI. Waiting until a child has had two or more UTIs before proceeding with evaluation clearly increases the risk that permanent scarring, which might have otherwise been prevented, may occur.

History

Evaluation of the child with a UTI should always begin with a careful history. Because bladder emptying plays an important role in the etiology and prevention of UTI, a careful voiding history is an essential component of the work-up of toilet-trained children with UTIs.[258] Many of these children also have associated constipation that may only be detected when specific questions are directed toward the patient and parents. Family history should also be obtained, since heredity appears to play a role in an individual's predisposition toward infection, as evidenced by familial studies showing an increased incidence of bacteriuria in female siblings.[123] Similarly, a significant familial risk for VUR has been demonstrated when a sibling or parent has a history of having reflux.[259]

Physical examination

Physical examination of the child presenting with UTI should include palpation of the abdomen for flank masses, bladder distention, and/or abdominal masses caused by fecal impaction. Although genital examination in boys should exclude significant meatal stenosis, this is an extremely rare cause of UTI. Considering the epidemiologic evidence demonstrating an increased risk for UTI in uncircumcised boys, the circumcision status is of particular importance in male infants. Abnormal genital findings in girls include vulvovaginitis or the presence of labial adhesions that might predispose the child to perineal colonization by bacteria. More often labial adhesions increase the risk for contamination of 'clean-catch' urine specimens for culture. In children with a significant history of voiding dysfunction associated with constipation and/or encopresis, a brief neurologic examination should include evaluation of perineal sensation, of peripheral reflexes in the lower extremities, and of the the lower back for sacral dimpling or cutaneous abnormalities that suggest an underlying spinal abnormality (occult spinal dysraphism). Rectal examination for fecal impaction may be indicated if the history suggests severe constipation or encopresis.

Imaging

Recommended imaging studies for a child with a history of a culture-documented UTI are based, to some extent, on the experience of the radiologist and the availability of imaging modalities. Age, gender, race, and the type and frequency of UTIs must also be taken into consideration. For many years, the emphasis on the investigation of the child with UTI has centered on diagnosis of VUR. Some authors have suggested that the emphasis should be on whether the child has renal scarring or is at risk for renal scarring.[260–265] They argue that if there is no evidence of renal damage at the time of the infection, then it is not necessary to evaluate for VUR as the risk for future renal scarring is minimal. Consequently, these authors have recommended that the initial evaluation in children older than 1–2 years should be of the kidney, including sonography to exclude surgical conditions which predispose to infection and DMSA scintigraphy to detect acute pyelonephritic inflammation. With this approach, cystography is reserved for infants under 1–2 years and older children with abnormal DMSA scan findings or recurrent UTIs. One critical review found that such an approach might miss approximately 8% (7/80) of children with grade III VUR who have normal DMSA scans. However, VUR resolved or significantly improved in 86% (6/7) and no child had recurrent UTI.[266] This algorithm is further supported by the observations that while clinically significant acute lesions may be present in the presence or absence of VUR, significant renal scarring is most likely to occur in those with grade III and IV VUR.[267] In contrast, most American urologists, pediatricians, and radiologists still recommend that the evaluation of infants and toddlers should always include a cystogram to detect the presence of VUR, ureteroceles, posterior urethral valves in boys, or bladder wall thickening and a sonogram to look for obstruction, hydronephrosis, or other congenital malformations.[268,269] Whether one accepts the recommendation that DMSA scintigraphy should precede voiding cystourethrography in the evaluation of children with UTIs is determined in part by the goal of management of these patients. For those whose ultimate goal of treatment is the cessation of VUR, when present, then VCUG will continue to be the initial study of choice. For others, whose primary goal is the detection and future prevention of pyelonephritis and new renal damage, DMSA scintigraphy may well replace VCUG as the initial investigation of children with symptomatic UTIs. It should be recognized that, to date, no studies have analyzed the relative advantages of any specific imaging approach with regard to documentation of their impact on the development of renal scars or other clinical outcomes.[251]

Timing of evaluation

The timing of evaluation is often a concern of the urologist, radiologist, and pediatrician. Many recommend that children requiring hospitalization should at least be screened for obstruction with an ultrasound scan prior to discharge. For patients evaluated with cystography, it has been suggested that this be delayed 4–6 weeks following the acute infection to avoid demonstrating transient mild reflux secondary to inflammatory changes of the ureterovesical junction. However, it is rare for reflux to be detected during infection and then disappear after treatment.[270,271] Furthermore, since the significance of reflux is greatest at the time of bacterial infection, demonstration of even transient reflux may be very meaningful. One potential disadvantage of obtaining a cystogram early in the course of a febrile infection is that ureteral dilatation secondary to the effect of endotoxins may result in overestimation of the grade of reflux.[272,273] Nevertheless, a prolonged 'waiting period' is not necessary. The cystogram can usually be performed whenever the patient is no longer symptomatic and when the urine is sterile.[274] Regardless of when studies are performed, antibiotic prophylaxis should be maintained until that time, particularly in infants or in children with a previous febrile UTI, in order to prevent reinfection.[253,274]

For patients evaluated with DMSA renal scintigraphy, the timing of the study is in part determined by the reason for the study. If one is attempting to document acute pyelonephritic inflammatory changes, the DMSA renal scan is best obtained early within the first several days of the acute episode.[275] However, if the primary goal is to document irreversible renal scarring following an episode of infection, then the study should be delayed for 6 months following the acute infection since transient acute changes on DMSA scans can persist for up to 5 months prior to resolving.[276]

Cystography

Both direct and indirect cystography techniques are used. Direct cystography involves filling the bladder by urethral catheterization or percutaneous suprapubic infusion. Both standard contrast medium and radiolabeled nuclides are satisfactory. In boys, contrast cystography is preferred because it provides for visualization of the urethra and for grading reflux (Figure 7.13).[277] It is also more reliable for detecting duplication, ureteral ectopia with or without ureteroceles, posterior urethral valves, bladder trabeculation, bladder diverticula, and foreign bodies. Many also prefer its use for the initial examination in girls because the grade of reflux can be determined. Several methods for grading are used. The International Reflux Study method is most widely accepted.[277] A disadvantage of standard contrast cystography is the high gonadal radiation dose it entails, particularly with multiple studies or fluoroscopic monitoring. The addition of digital fluoroscopy reduces gonadal radiation exposure.[278] Using a low-dose fluoroscopic system with a computer-based video frame grabber, the ovarian radiation dose has been reported to compare favorably to radionuclide cystography.[279]

Direct radionuclide cystography allows continuous monitoring for reflux throughout the study without additional radiation exposure. It is reported to be more sensitive than contrast cystography for the diagnosis of reflux.[280–282] Whereas precise grading of VUR is limited, it can usually be categorized as mild, moderate, or severe (Figure 7.14). Although radionuclide cystography has been criticized for being unable to detect grade I/V VUR, a recent study found that direct radionuclide cystography demonstrated VUR

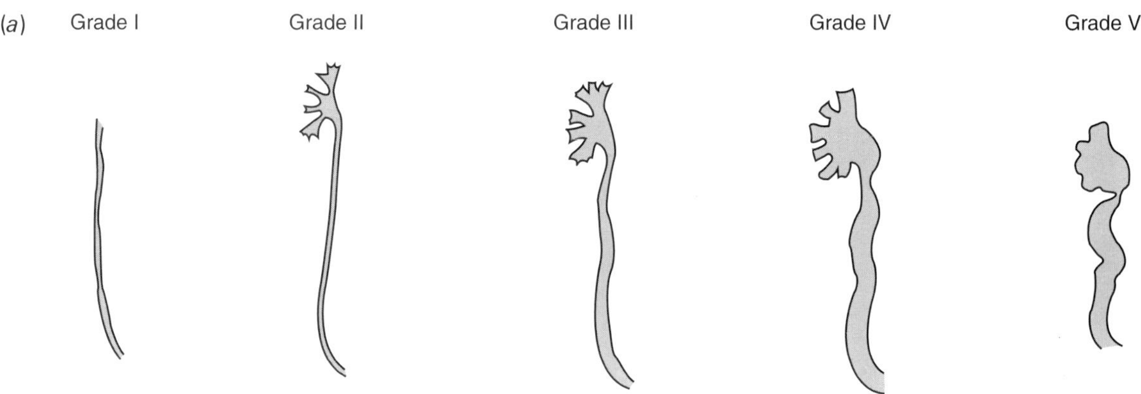

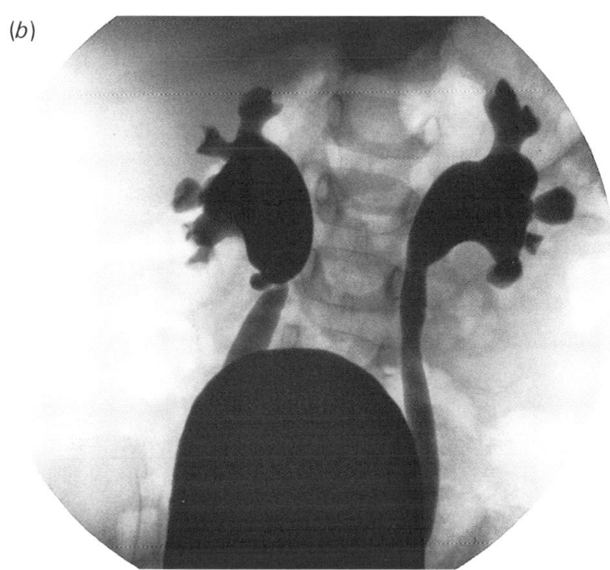

Figure 7.13 (*a*) International classification of vesicoureteral reflux: grade I, ureter only; grade II, ureter, pelvis, calices, no dilatation, normal caliceal fornices; grade III, mild or moderate dilatation and/or tortuosity of ureter, and mild or moderate dilatation of the pelvis, but no or slight blunting of the fornices; grade IV, moderate dilatation and/or tortuosity, of ureter and mild dilatation of renal pelvis and calices, complete obliteration of sharp angle of fornices but maintenance of papillary impressions in majority of calices, grade V, gross dilatation and tortuosity of ureter, gross dilatation of renal pelvis and calices, papillary impressions are no longer visible in majority of calices. (Modified from International Reflux Committee[277].) (*b*) Voiding cystogram shows grade III VUR on the right with moderate dilatation and tortuosity of ureter, moderate dilatation of the pelvis, but slight blunting of the fornices. Grade IV reflux is seen on the left with similar dilatation of the ureter and pelvis but with obliteration of sharp angle of fornices. Papillary impressions are maintained in the majority of the calices.

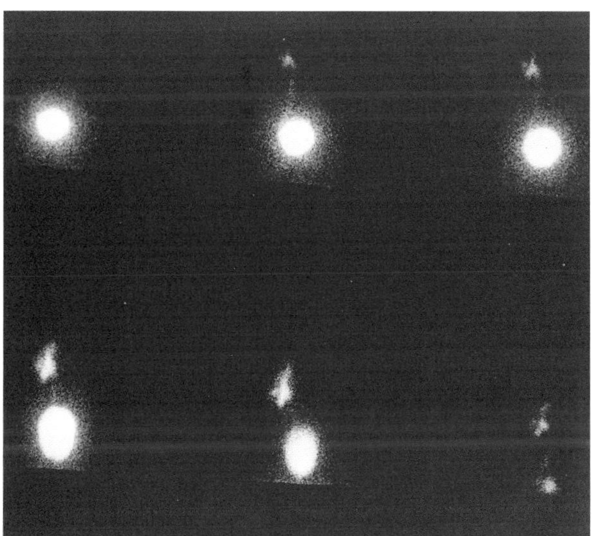

Figure 7.14 Isotope cystogram demonstrates mild left vesicoureteral reflux during filling (*top row*), which becomes moderate reflux when the bladder is full and during voiding (*bottom row*).

to the renal pelvis in all 17 kidneys with grade I/V VUR on contrast cystography.[283] The radiation dose from radionuclide cystography reportedly is 50–200 times less than that with standard techniques using contrast cystography, making it ideal for the follow-up of children with VUR and for following results of antireflux surgery.[284]

Indirect radionuclide cystography uses ^{99m}Tc DTPA (technetium-99m-labeled diethylenetriamine pentaacetic acid), which is excreted by glomerular filtration. The presence of reflux can be assumed when radioisotope counts increase in the renal areas after voiding. Indirect cystography is less reliable for the detection of VUR than direct radionuclide cystography, with false-negative rates ranging from 22 to 51%.[285,286] More recently indirect radionuclide cystography using ^{99m}Tc MAG3 was reported to also be unreliable for the detection of VUR, missing approximately two-thirds of refluxing kidneys[286] (Figure 7.15).[287]

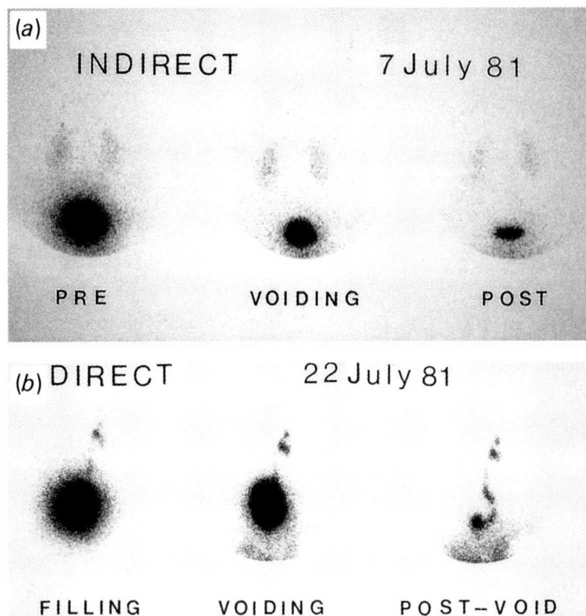

Figure 7.15 (*a*) False-negative indirect radionuclide cystogram in a 6-year-old girl. Images before and after voiding demonstrate no evidence of vesicoureteral reflux. (*b*) Selected images from a direct radionuclide cystogram in the same patient obtained 2 weeks after the indirect study show moderate reflux on the right during filling and voiding, and after voiding. (Reprinted from Majd et al,[287] with permission.)

Upper tract imaging

Recommendations for evaluating the upper urinary tract in children presenting with UTI also vary from institution to institution. The ideal study should be painless, safe, cost-effective, and associated with minimal or no radiation and yet should be capable of detecting clinically significant structural malformations as well as renal scarring. Unfortunately, such an all-encompassing study does not exist.

One approach is initial screening of all patients being evaluated for a history of UTI with a renal–bladder sonogram.[288] In children, sonography has been found to be as sensitive as IVP for the detection of any significant renal abnormality, except for uncomplicated duplication anomalies and focal renal scarring.[288–291] Sonography is painless, non-invasive, simple to perform, radiation-free, and independent of renal function. It is critical that appropriate images of the ureters, bladder, and true pelvis be routinely obtained in order to detect the presence of ureteroceles or dilated ureters secondary to ureteral ectopia, ureterovesical junction obstruction, or severe VUR. To do so, the bladder should be full during the examination. A postvoiding residual also can be demonstrated at the completion of the study. In the absence of reflux, hydronephrosis revealed by sonography is best evaluated with diuretic renography using ^{99m}Tc DTPA or ^{99m}Tc MAG3.[292] When combined with the findings of the renal bladder sonogram, the site of obstruction can be reliably determined in almost all cases.[136] When needed, further evaluation is best accomplished with percutaneous antegrade pyelography and pressure–perfusion studies (Whitaker test).

Considering the very low incidence of surgically significant hydronephrosis presenting as UTI, some authors have questioned the role of sonography in the investigation of UTIs in children, recommending instead a cortical renal scan as the initial upper tract study of choice.[239,247,293,294] Still other authors have suggested a tailored approach to the evaluation of children with UTI, beginning with a voiding cystogram.[295,296] If no reflux is present, a renal ultrasound scan is done to exclude hydronephrosis or other upper tract malformations. Otherwise, if reflux is demonstrated, the next study would be a renal cortical scan to detect renal scarring (Figure 7.16).[297] This approach seems reasonable for the majority of cases.

In clinical practice, the use of DMSA scintigraphy is best reserved for those occasions when it will influence management. DMSA scintigraphy can be helpful in the initial evaluation and follow-up of patients with VUR. For example, not all patients with VUR and breakthrough UTIs require immediate surgical intervention, particularly those with asymptomatic bacteriuria[298] (Figure 7.17). In contrast, when new renal damage associated with a breakthrough UTI is objectively demonstrated by DMSA scintigraphy, anti-

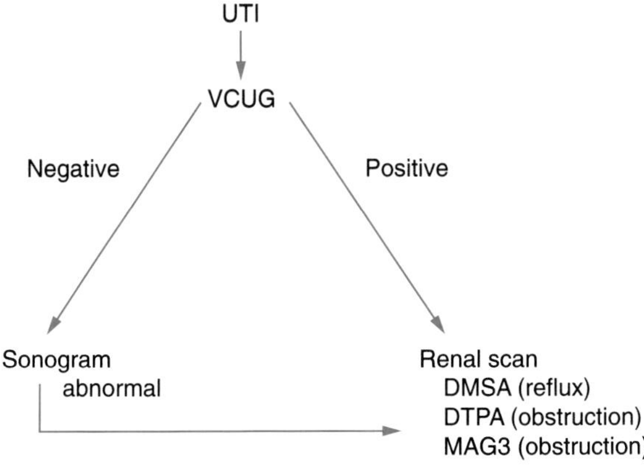

Figure 7.16 Algorithm for evaluation of children with urinary tract infection. (Adapted from Rushton[297], with permission.)

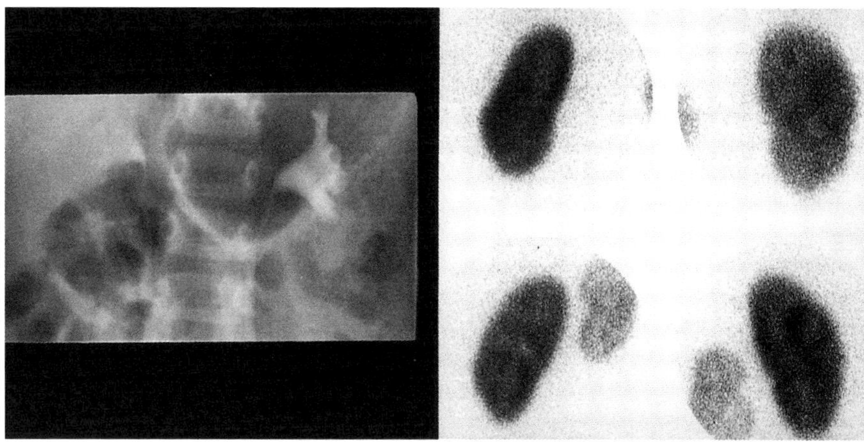

Figure 7.17 A 3-year-old girl with bilateral grade II vesicoureteral reflux (*left*) developed a breakthrough febrile UTI while on antibiotic prophylaxis. A ^{99m}Tc DMSA renal scan (*right*) at the time of the infections did not demonstrate any evidence of pyelonephritis or scarring. Her prophylaxis was changed and repeat isotope cystogram 1 year later revealed complete resolution of her reflux.

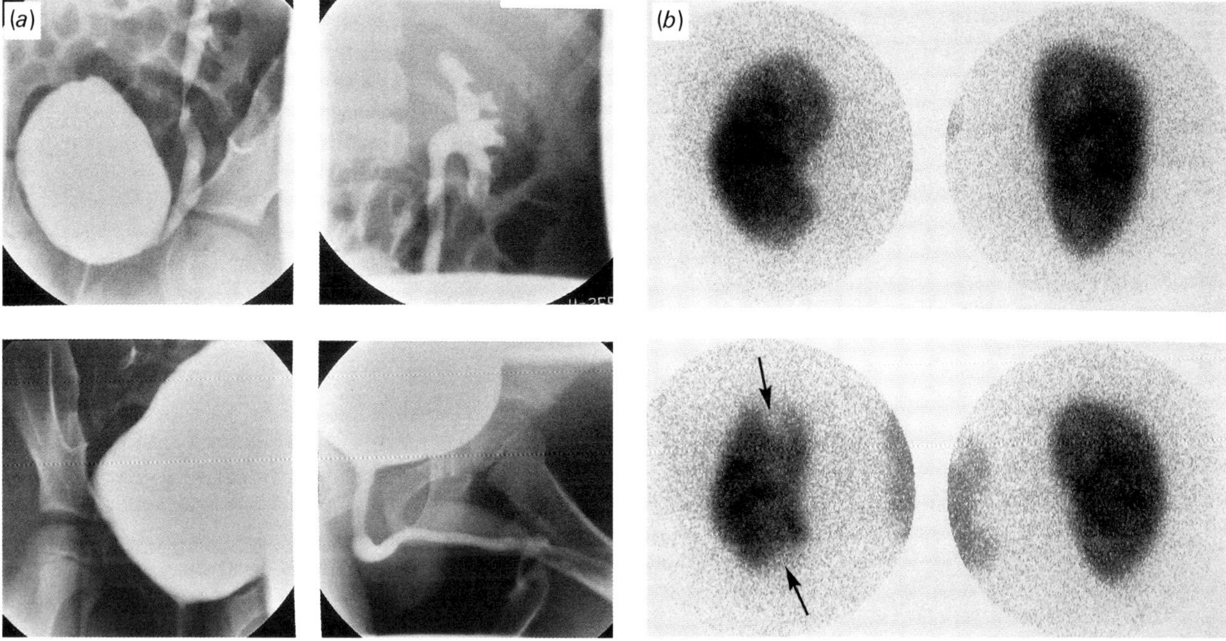

Figure 7.18 A 2-year-old girl presented with her first culture- documented UTI. (*a*) Voiding cystogram demonstrates left grade III vesicoureteral reflux. (*b*) (*Top*) Initial ^{99m}Tc DMSA renal scan was normal. (*Bottom*) Repeat ^{99m}Tc DMSA renal scan following a breakthrough febrile UTI reveals acute pyelonephritic changes in the left upper and lower poles (arrows). Left ureteral reimplantation was performed.

reflux surgery becomes imperative (Figure 7.18). It has been suggested that DMSA scan abnormalities are predictors of breakthrough UTIs (odds ratio 6.0) in children with VUR.[299] Likewise, DMSA scintigraphy is important in the initial evaluation of infants with prenatally detected VUR, as many of these patients will have significant congenital reflux nephropathy.

DMSA scintigraphy is also particularly helpful for establishing the correct diagnosis of pyelonephritis in situations when the diagnosis is unclear based on clinical and laboratory findings, such as in neonates and young infants. Not infrequently, the diagnosis in these young children is obscured by improper urine collection techniques or the institution of antibiotics before

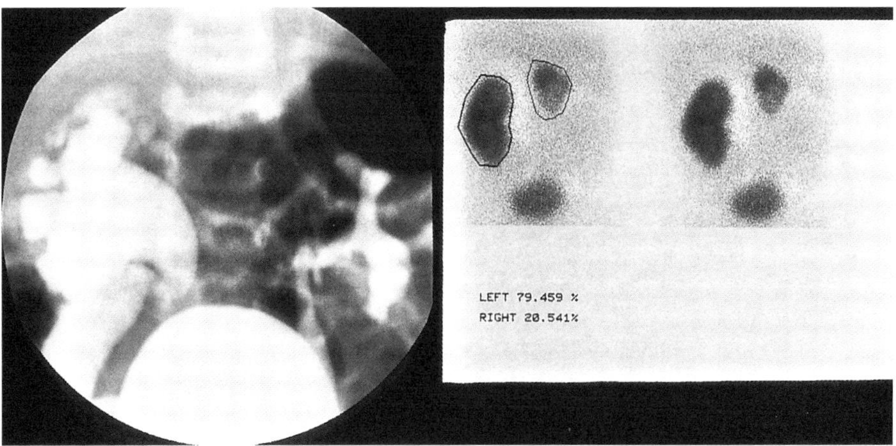

Figure 7.19 One-month-old boy with prenatally detected hydronephrosis. (*Left*) Voiding cystogram shows right grade V (note intrarenal reflux) and left grade III vesicoureteral reflux. (*Right*) ^{99m}Tc DMSA scan reveals a hypoplastic right kidney with markedly reduced differential renal function. He had been on antibiotic prophylaxis since birth and urine cultures were negative.

a urine culture is obtained. Other difficult diagnostic situations include children with neuropathic bladders managed by clean intermittent catheterization.[300,301] These children are usually chronically bacteriuric; therefore, the diagnostic significance of a positive urine culture at the time of a febrile episode is lost.

Renal scarring

Partly because most renal scars that are detected in children with prior urinary tract infection(s) have become established by the time of initial evaluation, the pathogenesis of renal scarring remains controversial.[15,207,254] Furthermore, it has become increasingly clear that the term renal scarring has been applied to the end result of more than one type of pathophysiologic process, including both abnormalities that are congenital and those that are acquired postnatally. The correlation between the severity of VUR and renal scarring is also well established.[5,302–304] Although the vast majority of cases of renal scarring associated with VUR are detected during the evaluation of children with UTI, recent studies of prenatally detected hydronephrosis secondary to high-grade VUR have also confirmed cases of congenital functional abnormalities documented by DMSA renal scintigraphy even in the absence of infection[305–10] (Figure 7.19). Furthermore, a higher prevalence of renal scarring has been reported in children with secondary VUR associated with functional or anatomic bladder outlet obstruction, including posterior urethral valves and neuropathic bladders,

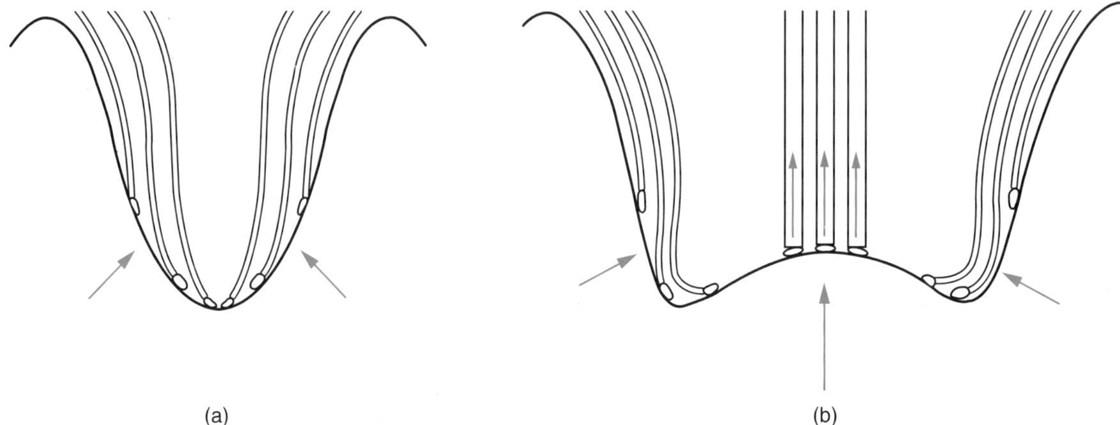

Figure 7.20 Papillary configuration in intrarenal reflux. (*a*) Convex papilla (non-refluxing): crescentric or slit-like orifices of collecting ducts opening obliquely onto the papilla. (*b*) Concave or flat papilla (refluxing papilla): round, gaping orifices of collecting ducts opening at right angles onto flat papilla. (Reprinted Ransley,[312] with permission.)

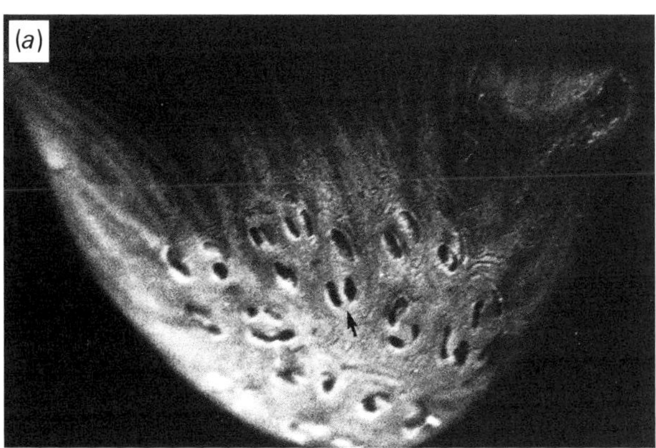

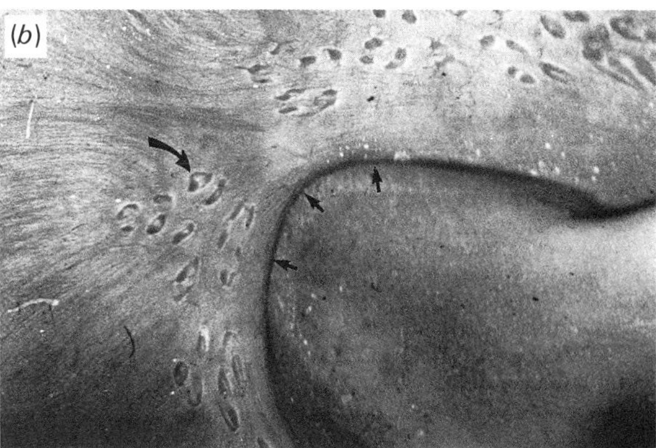

Figure 7.21 (*a*) Non-refluxing simple papilla with convex conical configuration and slit-like orifices of collecting ducts (arrow). (*b*) Refluxing compound papilla with concave configuration (arrows) and gaping oval to round orifices of collecting ducts (curved arrow). (Reprinted from Rushton et al,[231] with permission.)

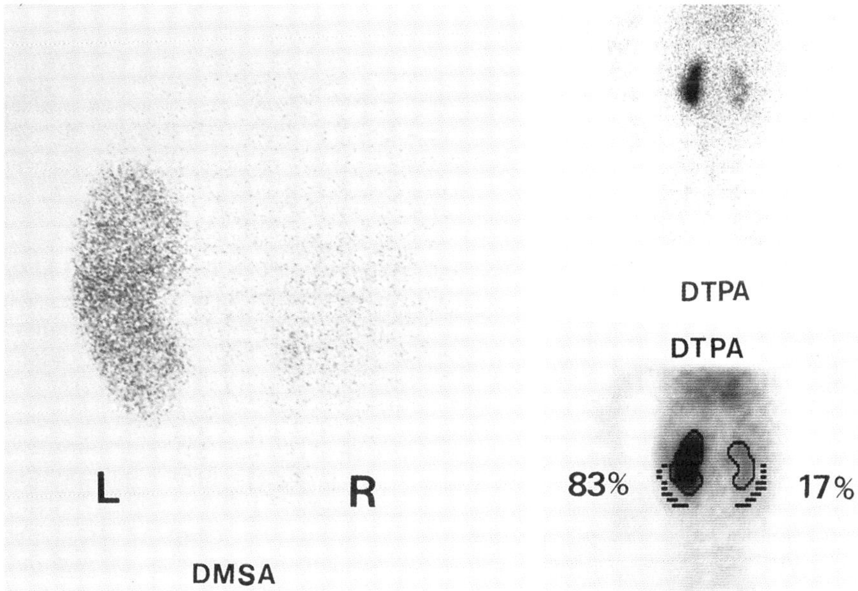

Figure 7.22 A 9-month-old girl hospitalized with her first febrile UTI. VCUG demonstrated right grade IV vesicoureteral reflux. Sonography showed moderate right hydronephrosis. (*a*) Initial ^{99m}Tc DMSA renal scan at the time of hospitalization demonstrates marked diffuse decreased uptake (function) in the right kidney, consistent with acute pan-pyelonephritis. (*b*) Follow-up ^{99m}Tc DTPA renal scan 1 month later shows partial recovery of function, but the kidney is contracted and scarred with a differential function of only 17%. (Reprinted from Rushton,[297] with permission.)

than in children with primary VUR.[54] Lumping renal sequelae from all of these pathophysiologic entities under the terms 'renal scarring' or 'reflux nephropathy' has hampered attempts at understanding the pathogenic mechanisms involved.

The critical role that infection plays in the pathogenesis of renal scarring associated with reflux was clarified in Ransley and Risdon's classic experimental studies of VUR in piglets.[311] They demonstrated that, in the face of VUR and normal voiding pressures, renal scarring occurs only when urinary infection is present. Reflux in the absence of infection caused renal changes only when bladder outlet resistance was increased, so that obstruction, not reflux, was the pathophysiologic explanation for renal damage. It was suggested that the portions of the kidney at risk for scarring are those susceptible to pyelotubular backflow (intrarenal reflux), based on papillary morphology and configuration (Figures 7.20 and 7.21).[312]

Clinically, new or progressive scarring is almost always associated with a history of UTI. Experimental studies and clinical experience have shown that a single episode of pyelonephritis can lead to significant renal damage (Figure 7.22).[252,313] Furthermore, a

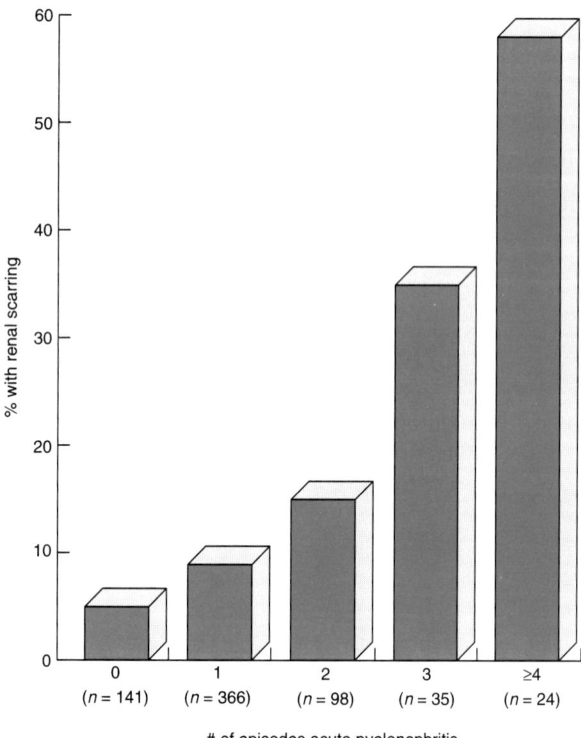

Figure 7.23 Relationship of renal scarring to number of episodes of acute pyelonephritis. (Adapted from Jodal.[5])

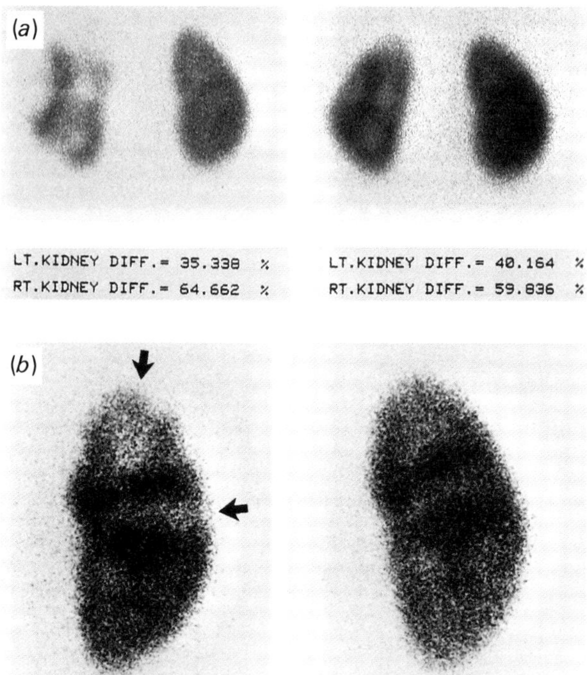

Figure 7.24 (*a*) ^{99m}Tc DTPA renal scan in a 3.5-year-old girl with left grade IV vesicoureteral reflux and multiple recurrent UTIs. (*Left*) Multifocal acute pyelonephritis is demonstrated in the upper and lower poles and mid-zone of the left kidney. (*Right*) Follow-up ^{99m}Tc DMSA renal scan 1 year later reveals significant improvement in function of the left kidney. (Reprinted with permission from Rushton.[314]) (*b*) (*Left*) ^{99m}Tc DMSA renal scan in 4.5-year-old girl with acute pyelonephritis evidenced by typical changes of photopenia with preservation of the renal contour in the upper pole and mid-zone of the right kidney (arrows). (*Right*) Repeat DMSA renal scan 15 months later demonstrates complete resolution of acute inflammatory changes without residual scarring or loss of cortex. (Reprinted from Rushton and Majd,[233] with permission.)

clear association between the number of pyelonephritic attacks and incidence of renal scarring has been reported (Figure 7.23).[5,22,254] Both experimental and clinical studies have also shown that some renal scarring can be prevented or diminished by early antibiotic treatment of acute pyelonephritis (Figures 7.24 and 7.25).[31,252,315–316] Furthermore, when reflux is present, progressive renal scarring can be successfully prevented by keeping the patient free of infection.[303,304,317] Based on all of the above, it is clear that infection, not reflux alone, is a prerequisite for acquired renal scarring.

Congenital renal scarring associated with reflux

Severe reflux may be associated with significant renal dysplasia thought to result from abnormal induction of the nephrogenic cord during embryogenesis.[318, 319] Several reports have described DMSA scan renal functional abnormalities in patients with primary VUR detected prenatally.[305–309] The reported incidence of renographic abnormalities in these studies has varied widely, ranging from 17% to 60%.[306–308] Many of these infants were evaluated by renal scintigraphy

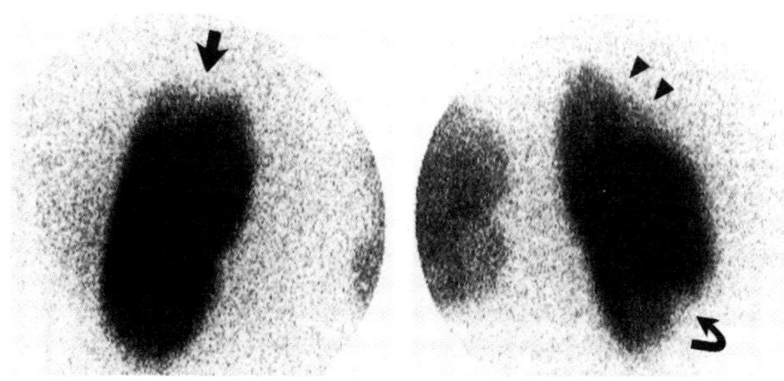

Figure 7.25 ^{99m}Tc DMSA renal scan in a 7-year-old girl 7 months after her first documented febrile UTI. A VCUG revealed bilateral grade II vesicoureteral reflux. Renal scarring is present in both kidneys. The left upper pole is flattened (arrow). There is a wedge-shaped defect in the right lower pole (curved arrow) and thinning of the right upper pole (arrowheads). (Reprinted from Rushton,[314] with permission.)

prior to any known episodes of infection, confirming that the functional abnormalities present at birth represent a congenital fetal nephropathy rather than a secondary acquired abnormality. In one study, nephrectomy specimens in a few of these severely 'scarred' kidneys with minimal function demonstrated severe dysplasia and growth arrest.[308] This would suggest that both congenital and acquired scarring may occur in the same kidney.

Imaging of renal scarring

In the past, the primary imaging modality for the detection of renal scarring was the intravenous pyelogram. However, limitations of the IVP have actually hindered our understanding of the pathogenesis of renal scarring. Although relatively sensitive for the detection of renal scarring, the IVP is very insensitive in the detection of acute pyelonephritis.[245] Furthermore, pyelographic evidence of new renal scarring may take 2 or more years to develop after a documented UTI.[253,320] Consequently, this has forced investigators to speculate retrospectively about the etiology of renal scarring.

In contrast, DMSA renal cortical scintigraphy is capable of detecting both the acute inflammatory changes of pyelonephritis and renal scarring. Several studies comparing the DMSA renal scan to the IVP in the detection of renal scarring have demonstrated a greater sensitivity with isotope imaging, especially in younger children.[242,321–325] Merrick et al compared the findings of IVP to DMSA scans in 79 children who had proven UTI and had been followed for a period of 1–4 years.[321] The sensitivity of IVP for the detection of renal scars was 80% and the specificity was 92%, whereas cortical scintigraphy had a sensitivity of 92% and a specificity of 98%. When both IVP and DMSA scintigraphy demonstrate scars, an excellent correlation on a site-by-site basis has been reported.[321–323,325,326] When compared with histology in an animal model, the sensitivity and specificity of the DMSA scan for the detection of renal scarring in 60 piglets with reflux and infected urine was 85% and the specificity was 97%.[327] Thus, DMSA renal cortical scintigraphy offers a superior opportunity to study the progression of renal damage or functional loss from the time of the initial insult until either complete healing or irreversible scarring develops.

Studies that have compared ultrasonography with DMSA scintigraphy for the detection of renal scarring have consistently reported greater sensitivity with DMSA renal scans.[239,242,243] In one study, Yen and associates compared ultrasound, IVP, and both planar

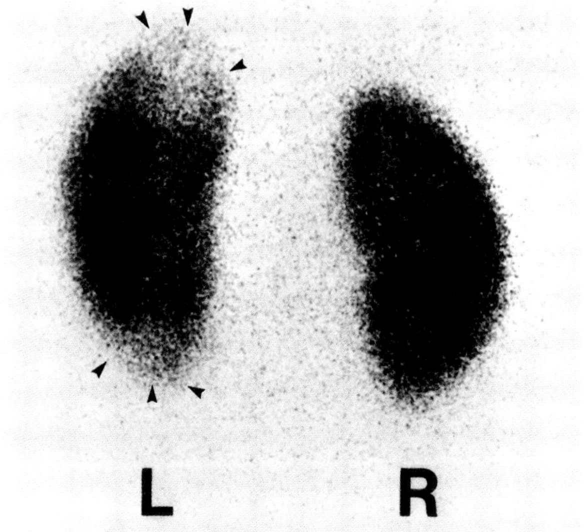

Figure 7.26 ^{99m}Tc DMSA renal scan demonstrates typical changes of acute pyelonephritis in the upper and lower poles of the left kidney. Diminished uptake of isotope is seen with an intact renal cortical outline without volume loss or contraction (arrowheads). (Reprinted from Cohen et al,[300] with permission.)

and SPECT DMSA renal scintigraphy in the evaluation of 130 children with UTI (42 patients), VUR (37 patients), and unilateral or bilateral small kidneys (51 patients).[244] SPECT imaging of DMSA scans detected the highest number of defects, followed by planar imaging.

Renal scars detected by DMSA scintigraphy appear as focal or generalized areas of diminished uptake of radioisotope associated with loss or contraction of functioning renal cortex. This may appear as thinning or flattening of the cortex in some kidneys, while in others renal scars appear as classic discrete wedge-shaped parenchymal defects (see Figure 7.25). In more severe cases, generalized damage may be associated with multifocal or diffusely scarred kidneys and reduced differential renal function. In contrast, defects associated with acute pyelonephritis are more typically characterized by focal areas of diminished uptake but with preservation of the normal renal contour (Figure 7.26). Although it is often possible for an experienced observer to distinguish acute versus chronic lesions, it should be recognized that this differentiation may be less apparent in those kidneys with acute pyelonephritis superimposed on pre-existent renal scarring.

New or acquired scarring

Until recently a common assumption was that VUR was an absolute prerequisite for new or acquired renal

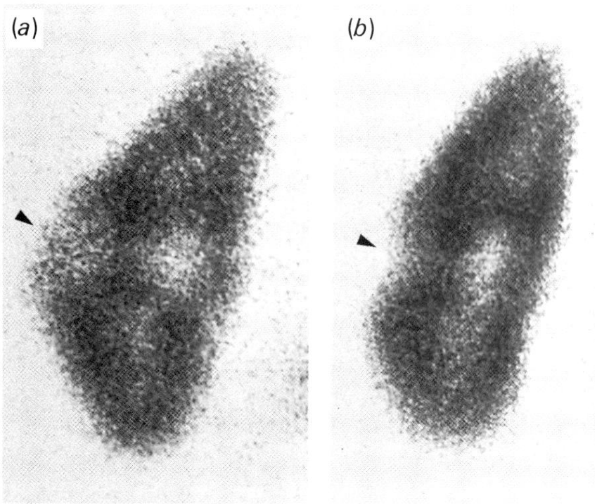

Figure 7.27 ^{99m}Tc DMSA renal scan in a 13-month-old girl with an acute febrile UTI. (*a*) Left posterior oblique view on the initial DMSA scan demonstrates acute pyelonephritis of the mid-zone of the left kidney evidenced by a photopenic lesion with preservation of the renal contour (arrowhead). (*b*) Follow-up DMSA renal scan reveals progression to renal scar in the exact same site characterized by contraction and loss of functioning renal cortex (arrowhead). (Reprinted from Rushton et al,[54] with permission.)

scarring. This mindset was further perpetuated by earlier investigations of new or acquired renal scarring, most of which focused retrospectively on patients with known VUR. However, in one earlier study which selected patients on the basis of infection alone, only half of the 37 children who formed new renal scars had VUR.[316]

Several investigators have now evaluated the evolution of the acute inflammatory changes associated with pyelonephritis using serial DMSA renal scans.[233,276,328–330] The interval from the initial DMSA scan obtained at the time of acute infection until the repeat scan ranged from 3 months to 2 years. Acute DMSA renal scan defects persisted as renal scarring in 36–52% of kidneys. The sites of new renal scarring corresponded exactly to those sites of acute pyelonephritis seen on the initial DMSA renal scans, confirming the primary role of the acute inflammatory response to infection in the etiology of acquired renal scarring (Figure 7.27). Contralateral normal kidneys and initially uninvolved areas of abnormal kidneys have almost always remained normal on follow-up DMSA renal scans. Surprisingly, reflux has been present in only 25–50% of kidneys that developed new renal scarring. This is attributable in part to the fact that the majority of patients (63–75%) with acute inflammatory changes on the initial DMSA renal scans did not have VUR. Nevertheless, in one prospective study of 38 kidneys with initially abnormal DMSA scans, scarring developed in 6 of 15 (40%) kidneys with associated VUR and in 10 of 23 (42%) kidneys without demonstrable reflux.[54] Similar findings have been observed by others.[331] These observations provide convincing clinical evidence that renal parenchymal infection, rather than VUR, is the prerequisite for acquired (postnatal) renal scarring. Once bacteria have invaded the renal parenchyma, the inflammatory response appears similar and the propensity for renal scarring is equally as great whether or not reflux is present.

Despite these findings, the importance of VUR (particularly grades III or higher) as a risk factor for renal scarring should not be discounted. Clearly, patients with moderate and severe reflux are much more likely to develop acute pyelonephritic damage than children with mild or no reflux.[53,332] Furthermore, although 62% of the kidneys with postpyelonephritic renal scarring in one study were drained by non-refluxing ureters, renal scarring was still significantly more common in those kidneys with grade III or higher VUR compared with kidneys with mild or no reflux.[331] Thus, the increased propensity for scarring in patients with higher grades of VUR is attributable in part to the increased risk of these kidneys for acute inflammatory damage at the time of the initial infection.[53,240,331] Coupled with this, reflux (pyelotubular backflow of urine from the pelvis into the collecting ducts) of infected urine or scarring of adjacent papillae may transform marginally competent, non-refluxing papillae into papillae that do reflux, thereby predisposing the kidney to greater pyelonephritic damage.[53,311] Indeed, in one study which attempted to quantitate the area of acute pyelonephritic parenchymal damage, the presence of grade ≥3 reflux was associated with a significantly greater frequency of kidneys demonstrating large defects (defined as >10% of the kidney demonstrating DMSA uptake <2 SD of the control kidney) when compared with kidneys with no vesicoureteral reflux (p <0.02).[332] Thus, when present, moderate or severe reflux (grade ≥3) remains the most significant host risk factor for acute pyelonephritis and renal scarring.

Other risk factors for the development of renal scarring include associated bladder pathology, regardless of whether reflux is present. In one study, the frequency of new renal scarring was significantly higher in kidneys associated with overt bladder pathology compared with those with normal bladders (86% vs 32%; $p = 0.028$).[233] Marked bladder thickening and trabeculation, suggesting either functional or anatomic bladder outlet obstruction, was present in 67% of the patients with bladder pathology who developed new scarring. Urodynamic evaluation of children with neuropathic bladders associated with spina bifida has demonstrated that increased intravesical pressure may lead to upper tract deterioration, with or without VUR.[333] Animal studies have also shown an increased propensity for renal scarring when infection and reflux occur in the presence of bladder outlet obstruction.[311]

Two studies have also analyzed the association of various clinical and bacteriologic parameters with the development of new renal scarring.[233,331] In both, children who developed new renal scars were actually older at the time of acute pyelonephritis, although the difference was statistically significant in only one.[330] An elevated WBC count at the time of the initial infection was not associated with renal scarring. When comparing those patients with and without new scarring, no significant differences were noted in race, gender, duration of fever, maximum temperature, or acute inflammatory signs (CRP, ESR) at the time of the acute pyelonephritic episode. *E. coli* was cultured from the urine of 88–95% of the patients in both studies. Interestingly, new scarring occurred in 33–41% of patients infected with *E. coli* compared with 100% of patients in both studies who were infected with other bacteria. In one study no significant association was found between bacterial virulence factors (hemolysin, colicin, P-fimbriae) and renal scarring, although colicin production was found almost twice as often in the bacteria isolated from patients with new renal scarring.[54] In a more recent report of 157 children evaluated with a DMSA renal scan 1 year following their first-time symptomatic UTI, children with high levels of CRP, high fever, and dilating VUR were 10 times more likely to have scarring than children with normal or slightly elevated CRP levels, no or mild fever, and no reflux.[275]

Sequelae of renal scarring

Hypertension

Renal scarring is reported to be a common cause of hypertension in children and young adults.[334–337] The risk of hypertension in patients with renal scarring varies, based on length of follow-up and severity of scarring. In follow-up studies of children with renal scarring, approximately 6–13% of children with scarring will develop hypertension.[22,187,337,338] In some cases, it may be associated with progressive renal insufficiency.[339] A recent report of an older cohort of 294 patients (mean age at presentation, 17.3 years) with reflux nephropathy noted that the risk of hypertension increased with age and length of follow-up.[340] Whereas 8.5% of these patients had hypertension at presentation, 38% became hypertensive later on (mean age 34.2 years). Hypertension was significantly more common in those with severe bilateral parenchymal scarring. Similarly, in another series 13% (11/83) of children with renal scarring were hypertensive at initial evaluation and another 17% (14/83) developed hypertension over the subsequent 4–20 years.[341]

The development of hypertension is clearly related to the severity of renal scarring and is more often observed in patients with a history of recurrent episodes of pyelonephritis associated with moderate or severe VUR.[187,339] The actual risk for hypertension in children with milder degrees of scarring is unknown, but is undoubtedly less. The etiology of hypertension associated with renal scarring is controversial. Some investigators report no evidence that the renin–angiotensin–aldosterone (RAS) system contributes;[342,343] others report that it does.[344–347] Despite these controversies, most would agree that the risk for hypertension in patients with severe renal scarring is significant, and long-term follow-up is mandatory, since hypertension may take 10–20 years to develop.

Renal insufficiency

The actual risk of renal insufficiency secondary to postpyelonephritic renal scarring is unknown. The annual incidence of new patients presenting with end-stage renal disease (ESRD) associated with 'reflux nephropathy' in Australia and New Zealand between 1985 and 1989 was 3.9 and 4.89 per million of the population, respectively.[348] Overall, this represented 7% of all new cases of ESRD commencing treatment during this time period, including 24% in the teenage group. In a more recent study of 102 patients with ESRD seen at a pediatric hospital over a 10-year period, only 3 had reflux nephropathy, including 1 patient with no history of UTI and 1 patient with a single, afebrile UTI.[349] Only 1 child with grade II–III bilateral reflux had a history of recurrent UTIs.

Studies have shown that the incidence of renal insufficiency in patients with postpyelonephritic renal scarring increases with age. The incidence of renal insufficiency in a report by Martinell et al of 30 adults who were diagnosed with severe renal scarring as children was 10%.[22] Another study of an older cohort of 294 patients (mean age at presentation 17.2 years) with reflux nephropathy found a 2% incidence of renal insufficiency glomerular filtration rate (GFR) – defined as <40–69 ml/min – at presentation, that increased to 24% at last follow-up (mean age 34.2 years). The more extensive the renal scarring, the higher proportion with renal insufficiency.[339] Most patients (90–100%) with reflux nephropathy and ESRD have focal segmental glomerulosclerosis, almost always associated with proteinuria.[350–353]

Treatment

The obvious goals of treatment of UTI are symptomatic relief and prevention of new or progressive renal damage, especially in infants and young children who are at greatest risk for renal scarring. Initial treatment, ideally, should be based on in-vitro sensitivity studies. Frequently, such testing is not done or treatment is instituted before the results are available. Fortunately, because the common uropathogens are susceptible to multiple antibiotics and the response to antibiotics correlates best with urine levels that are usually more highly concentrated than serum level, high cure rates have been reported in most therapeutic trials.[354]

Asymptomatic bacteriuria

Treatment of true asymptomatic bacteriuria does not appear to be necessary if the urinary tract is otherwise normal.[355–357] The risk for pyelonephritis in infants and young girls with untreated asymptomatic bacteriuria is small, and many demonstrate spontaneous remission.[5,11] In a prospective follow-up of 50 infants with initial screening bacteriuria, 37 were followed for a minimum of 6 years.[358] Of the original 50, 2 infants developed pyelonephritis within 2 weeks after bacteriuria was diagnosed. In 45, bacteriuria was left untreated. Spontaneous clearance was observed in 36, while in 8 clearance followed treatment with antibiotics for respiratory infections. Recurrences of bacteriuria were observed in 10 of 50 children, of whom one had pyelonephritis. No child had more than one recurrence. Follow-up urography in 36 of 50 children after a median of 32 months showed no evidence of renal damage in any of them.

In contrast to infants with screening bacteriuria, treatment of school-age girls with asymptomatic bacteriuria is followed by high recurrence rates of up to 80%.[12] Most are caused by new strains, which may carry the risk of being more virulent.[359,360] In contrast, when left untreated, spontaneous changes of strain are uncommon.[361]

Several studies in the 1970s reported that non-treatment of asymptomatic bacteriuria was associated with normal growth of kidneys without the development of new scars provided the urinary tract initially appeared normal radiographically.[208,209,362,363] In a 4-year follow-up by the Cardiff–Oxford Bacteriuria Study Group in children 5–12 years of age with untreated covert bacteriuria, new or progressive renal scarring did not occur unless VUR was present.[209] Similarly, the presence of asymptomatic bacteriuria in the absence of VUR is not a risk factor for renal scarring in children with neuropathic bladders who perform clean intermittent catheterization.[301]

Hansson et al compared, retrospectively, treatment vs non-treatment of asymptomatic bacteriuria in older girls (median age 8 years) with pre-existent renal scarring.[361] Many also had mild grade I–II/V VUR. Of 21 girls who were given a short course of antibiotics, 17 acquired a new infection within a year including 7 with pyelonephritic recurrences. Of 23 girls treated with antibiotic prophylaxis for 2–3 years, one-half developed breakthrough infections, and recurrences after completion of long-term prophylaxis were as common as after short-term treatment. Overall, in girls who received short- or long-term antibiotic treatment, 14 patients developed 21 episodes of acute pyelonephritis during a total of 140 patient-years of observation. In contrast, ABU was left untreated in 29 girls for a total of 74 patient years of observation. Only one patient developed acute pyelonephritis.

Based on this information it is reasonable that true asymptomatic bacteriuria, particularly in older girls, be left untreated.[154,211] However, in the presence of VUR, the risks of non-treatment of asymptomatic bacteriuria have not been clearly established, particularly in infants and younger children. It should also be recognized that bladder dysfunction is commonly found in girls with so-called asymptomatic bacteriuria, including detrusor instability and incomplete emptying.[101] This explains in part the marked tendency for recurrent infection after treatment of asymptomatic bacteriuria with antibiotics alone. Treatment of the underlying voiding dysfunction is key to the successful long-term management of these patients.

Uncomplicated lower urinary tract infection

Agents that have been used successfully for acute, uncomplicated lower urinary infections include sulfonamides, trimethoprim–sulfamethoxazole (TMP-SMX), nitrofurantoin, trimethoprim, and oral cephalosporins (see Appendix). Unfortunately, ampicillin and amoxicillin are used commonly by primary healthcare physicians. High intestinal levels of these two antibiotics often result in rapid development of resistant enteric organisms, which then become the reinfecting bacteria. The emergence of resistant strains to ampicillin or amoxicillin has limited its initial efficacy in treating urinary infections compared with other antibiotics.[364] Resistance rates to ampicillin–amoxicillin have been recently reported to be as high as 54% in children with their first documented symptomatic UTI.[365] This drawback of the synthetic penicillins has been diminished by the relatively recent combination of clavulanic acid with amoxicillin (Augmentin). Clavulanic acid inhibits the bacterial β-lactamase enzymes, which render the β-lactamic antibiotics ineffective. This combination has proved effective in eradication of UTIs in children, even when in-vitro susceptibility testing demonstrated resistance to amoxicillin alone.[366,367] However, ampicillin–clavulanic acid is associated with a high incidence of side effects, is expensive, and is no more effective than the usual drugs.

The fluoroquinolones have been shown to have a wide spectrum of activity that includes most Gram-positive and Gram-negative organisms, including *Pseudomonas aeruginosa* and *Proteus*.[368] These are bactericidal agents and are believed to work by inhibiting the essential bacterial enzyme deoxyribonucleic acid (DNA) gyrase, which is essential for DNA replication in bacterial cells.[369] Concern regarding adverse arthropathic effects, based on animal studies showing cartilage toxicity, has prevented its approval for use in children.[370] However, the same experimental toxic effects have been reported with all quinolones, including nalidixic acid, which is licensed for use and has been used in children for decades.[371] A retrospective match-controlled study of nalidixic acid in 11 children treated for 10–600 days with follow-up examination 3–12 years later did not reveal any differences in arthropathic adverse effects compared with controls.[372] Furthermore, clinical evidence of cartilage toxicity has not been reported in more than 100 children with cystic fibrosis treated with varying courses of high-dose ciprofloxacin.[373] Despite the lack of clinical evidence demonstrating cartilage toxicity in children, the use of fluoroquinolones in growing children generally should be avoided until definitive studies have been performed.

Duration of treatment

The optimal duration of treatment of acute uncomplicated lower UTIs in children is controversial. Recently, several randomized, controlled studies have been published reporting the efficacy of single-dose or short-course antimicrobial therapy in children. The potential advantages of short-course therapy include decreased costs, improved compliance, decreased antibiotic-related side effects, and decreased effect on the fecal flora.

In 1988, Moffatt and associates reported a methodologic analysis by four independent reviewers of 14 randomized, controlled trials of short-course antimicrobial therapy for uncomplicated lower UTIs in children. Short-course therapy varied in these 14 studies. Conventional therapy ranged from 7 to 10 days. In two trials, short-course therapy was less effective.[374] One study compared single-dose vs 10-day amoxicillin therapy, and one compared 1-day vs 10-day cefadroxil therapy.[375,376] The other 12 studies showed no difference in outcome. The authors concluded that there was insufficient evidence to recommend short-course therapy for UTIs in children.

In a more recent review article by Khan, the findings in 12 of these reports were re-evaluated by pooling the data on 320 infants and children.[377] He reported that single-dose therapy achieved an overall cure rate of 89% (63–100%), defined as a negative follow-up culture at 1 week and the lack of a subsequent recurrence with the same organism. However, the response varied with the antimicrobial agents. Intramuscular aminoglycosides, used in 178 (56%), achieved the highest cure rate (96%), followed by TMP–SMX or a sulfa drug (90%). The cure rate of amoxicillin was significantly less (75%; $p < 0.01$). Another large clinical study investigated single-dose vs multidose antibiotic therapy in 132 children with a culture-documented 'first-time' acute UTI. There was no difference in the bacteriologic cure rate for single-dose (93%) vs multidose regimens (96%), but recurrence rates at 10–12 days or 28–37 days after treatment were significantly higher in the single-dose group (20.5%) compared with the 3-day (5.6%) and 7-day (8%) groups.[378]

Two other studies have compared relatively short 3-day vs conventional 10-day courses of antibiotics for treatment of uncomplicated UTIs in children. In one prospective, randomized, open multicenter study of 264 girls 1–15 years old, similar results were observed when short-course treatment with either 3 days of sulfamethizole or pivmecillinam was compared with 10 days of sulfamethizole.[379] Specifically, there was no difference in the number of girls with no or insignificant growth on urine cultures after treatment, or in the recurrence-free interval after treatment among the three groups. In another study of 110 children, no difference in initial cure or subsequent relapse rates was found in children treated with 3-day therapy vs 10 days using either co-trimoxazole or nitrofurantoin.[380]

Based on the available data, it appears reasonable to treat acute lower uncomplicated infections in children with a 'relatively' short 3-day course of antibiotics. However, young children with their first-time infection or those with febrile infections should then continue to receive low-dose antimicrobial prophylaxis until radiographic evaluation is completed.

Pyelonephritis

The child with suspected pyelonephritis requires a greater degree of assurance of immediate therapeutic success, since the degree of scarring and renal damage resulting from an infection may be influenced by the rapidity of effective therapy.[31,252,315,316,381] Oral medication can be initiated in older children who are not septic or vomiting, as long as good compliance is ensured. TMP–SMX can be anticipated to be effective in most cases. Cephalosporins are also a good choice for initial therapy in the febrile child who does not require parenteral therapy. New third-generation cephalosporins such as cefixime offer the advantage of once-daily dosing and have been shown to be as effective as twice-daily TMP–SMX.[382,383] Treatment can be changed to include less expensive agents when the antibiotic sensitivities become available.

Although most would concur with a 10–14 day course of antibiotic therapy for pyelonephritis, there is considerable controversy over the need for hospitalization and treatment with parenteral antibiotics vs outpatient therapy with oral drugs. In a recent survey of 445 general practitioners, 143 pediatricians, and 45 pediatric nephrologists, there were significant differences in the recommendation for initial hospitalization by the general practitioners and pediatricians (17%) compared with the pediatric nephrologists (69%).[384] The pediatric nephrologists were evenly split between single and combined antibiotic therapy, whereas general practitioners and pediatricians preferred monotherapy. Intravenous antibiotics were preferred by 78% of the pediatric nephrologists compared with only 23–27% of pediatricians and general practitioners. This may suggest a greater concern and/or awareness on the part of the nephrologists regarding the potential for renal damage associated with pyelonephritis in children. However, in a recent prospective randomized clinical trial of 306 children 1–24 months old with febrile UTIs, outpatient treatment with oral third-generation cephalosporins was equally effective when compared with initial treatment with intravenous antibiotics. There was no significant difference in treatment success, duration of fever, or subsequent renal scarring on DMSA scans.[383]

Clearly, there is a need for controlled therapeutic trials for UTI in children with old and new drugs in different dosages and for varying lengths of treatment. These trials should categorize patients into different age groups such as: (1) neonates aged 0–28 days; (2) infants aged 1 month to <2 years; (3) older children ≥2 years; and (4) adolescents.[385] Meanwhile, until such clinical trials are conducted, non-toxic children and infants >3 months of age can be treated as outpatients as long as compliance is not an issue. It is reasonable to initiate therapy with 1–2 days of a long-acting, third-generation cephalosporin, such as ceftriaxone, administered intramuscularly, followed by 10–14 days of oral antibiotics and prophylaxis until evaluated. Ceftriaxone is active against most Gram-negative uropathogens and it achieves very high levels in both the urine and renal parenchyma following single daily doses. This approach virtually assures compliance and adequate antimicrobial coverage until the urine culture and sensitivity results are known. Alternatively, if compliance does not seem to be a problem, initial therapy with appropriate, broad-spectrum oral antibiotics may be as effective in the treatment of acute pyelonephritis and in the prevention of irreversible renal damage.[383]

In contrast, the toxic child and infants <3 months of age with suspected acute pyelonephritis should be considered candidates for immediate hospitalization and parenteral therapy. In these patients combination therapy, including an aminoglycoside and ampicillin, are appropriate choices until the urine culture results are known. Alternatively, one of the newer third-generation cephalosporins may be used, but these are more expensive and do not provide comprehensive coverage of Gram-positive organisms, including *Enterococcus*. Parenteral antibiotic therapy should be continued for 7–10 days in neonates, although oral outpatient therapy to complete a full 10–14 day course can be substituted in patients >2 months when afebrile for 24–48 hours. Follow-up specimens for urine culture should be obtained at the completion of therapy, and prophylaxis should be instituted until evaluation of the urinary tract is completed.

Prophylaxis

Long-term, continuous antibiotic prophylaxis is recommended in children with VUR (particularly under

8 years of age) and those with frequent symptomatic recurrences. Antibiotic prophylaxis should also be considered in young children (under age 1) with non-reflux acute pyelonephritis when acute or chronic renal damage is documented by cortical scintigraphy. These children, in particular, appear to have bacterial virulence–host defense factors that appear to place them at significant risk for pyelonephritic damage.

In children with VUR, prophylaxis is usually continued until the reflux spontaneously resolves or is surgically corrected. Some advocate stopping prophylaxis in children older than 7 or 8 years of age who have mild or even moderate (grades I–III) VUR, particularly when there is no evidence of prior renal scarring.[386] If infection recurs during that time and reflux persists, correction shoud be considered for those with clinical or DMSA scan-documented pyelonephritis. Regardless of whether reflux is present, girls with a history of recurrent UTIs should be advised of the importance of surveillance urine cultures during pregnancy because they are at increased risk for pyelonephritis. In one review, a group of 41 women who had UTIs in childhood were followed through 65 pregnancies.[21] They were compared with age-matched controls. Of those with a history of childhood UTIs, 19 had renal scarring and 22 did not. The incidence of bacteriuria was higher in those with renal scarring (47%) than in those without renal scarring (27%), but both were significantly greater ($p < 0.001$ and $p < 0.01$, respectively) than in controls without a history of UTI (2%). This is true regardless of whether or not reflux is present.[20] Even those who underwent successful surgical correction of reflux during childhood continue to be at increased risk for pyelonephritis during pregnancy.[387–389]

Children with recurrent pyelonephritis and those with frequent recurrent symptomatic lower UTIs (three in 6 months, four in a year) should also be considered for prophylaxis for a minimum of 6–12 months, even in the absence of VUR. Periodic urine specimens for culture should be obtained every 3–6 months to monitor the success of prophylaxis. Medication should then be reinstituted for an additional 12 months if infection recurs within 3 months of discontinuation. It is not necessary to discontinue treatment to obtain urine specimens for culture. When breakthrough infection occurs, the offending organism will be resistant to the current agent. Therefore, the culture media will not be sterilized by the excreted drugs.

Although prophylaxis effectively prevents infection, it cannot be expected to reduce the recurrence rate of urinary infection after therapy has been discontinued. In one trial using TMP–SMX, all the children were treated for 2 weeks and then were randomized to receive no treatment or 6 months of prophylaxis.[390] Although prophylaxis was highly effective in preventing infection, the rate of recurrent infection after stopping prophylaxis was virtually identical to that observed after 2 weeks of treatment. Similarly, Smellie et al reported a high recurrence rate (42%) in children with a history of recurrent urinary infections following discontinuation of long-term antimicrobial prophylaxis.[180] In those with cystitis cystica (cystitis follicularis), 80% experience recurrences within 1 year after 6–12 months of continuous prophylaxis.[391] Nevertheless, it is helpful to achieve an infection-free period in those children with a history of multiple, symptomatic urinary infections. During this period of time, aggressive efforts should be made to improve the voiding and bowel habit patterns in those children who have clinical and/or urodynamic evidence of dysfunctional voiding, a common finding in this difficult group of patients.

Antimicrobials with proven efficacy in the prevention of recurrent urinary infections include nitrofurantoin, TMP–SMX or TMP–sulfadiazine, and TMP alone.[180,357,392–394] In one study that compared prophylaxis with nitrofurantoin vs trimethoprim alone in a double-blind study in 130 children, nitrofurantoin demonstrated superior efficacy in those chldren with abnormal urography and/or reflux.[395] However, no differences were seen in children without urinary tract abnormalities. Nitrofurantoin did not alter the pattern of resistance of intestinal bacterial flora, whereas trimethoprim significantly increased the percentage of trimethoprim-resistant bacteria during prophylaxis. Side effects, primarily gastrointesinal, were more frequent in the nitrofurantoin group (37%) compared with the trimethoprim group (21%) ($p = 0.05$). The authors recommended nitrofurantoin as the first choice for prophylaxis in children with recurrent UTI and urinary tract abnormalities. Pure SMX is less effective, and synthetic penicillins are particularly poor prophylactic agents because of the frequent emergence of resistant organisms.

Prophylactic doses are generally less than those used to treat acute infection. Smellie et al effectively used SMX 10 mg + TMP 2 mg/kg/day, or nitrofurantoin 1–2 mg/kg/day in one to two doses.[391,392] Our practice is to administer one-third to one-half of the therapeutic dose once daily. Alternatively, intermittent prophylaxis with low-dose TMP–SMX every other day has also been reported to be effective both in children with VUR and preadolescent girls with recurrent infection.[396,397] In difficult cases of children who develop breakthrough UTIs on single-drug antimicrobial prophylaxis, double prophylaxis with nitrofurantoin and TMP–SMX has been shown to be effective in reducing recurrences. In one study of 31 girls with recurrent breakthrough infections on single-drug therapy, 68% had VUR, 49% had voiding dysfunction, and 26% had both.[398] When treated with double drug prophylaxis, the rate of infection was reduced from 17.4 UTIs/100 patient-months to 3.6 UTIs/100 patient-months (p <0.001). These patients were also treated with anticholinergics and frequent timed voiding.

Renal abscess

In the past the majority of renal abscesses, a rare form of renal infection, were not caused by ascending infection. Historically, *Staphylococcus aureus* has been the offending agent as a result of hematogenous seeding from a peripheral cutaneous site of origin, or seeding of the contused renal parenchyma after blunt abdominal trauma.[399,400] Diagnosis is often delayed in these patients because urine cultures are negative in most. With the advent of early recognition and effective therapy, the frequency of staphylococcal bacteremia and renal abscesses has decreased. More cases of Gram-negative infections in the presence of VUR or other anatomic abnormalities of the urinary tract are now being seen.[401]

Most patients with a renal abscess present with high fever, leukocytosis, and an elevated ESR, often accompanied by flank pain. A variety of imaging techniques have been used to diagnose renal abscesses, including IVP and angiography, gallium-67 scintigraphy, sonography and CT[402–405] (Figure 7.28). The classic treatment of renal abscess has been surgical drainage in addition to appropriate antibiotic therapy. However, improved antibiotics and diagnostic techniques, together with the ability to obtain culture by percutaneous aspiration or drainage under ultrasonic control, have often obviated the necessity for surgical intervention. In 7 patients reported by Schiff et al, 10

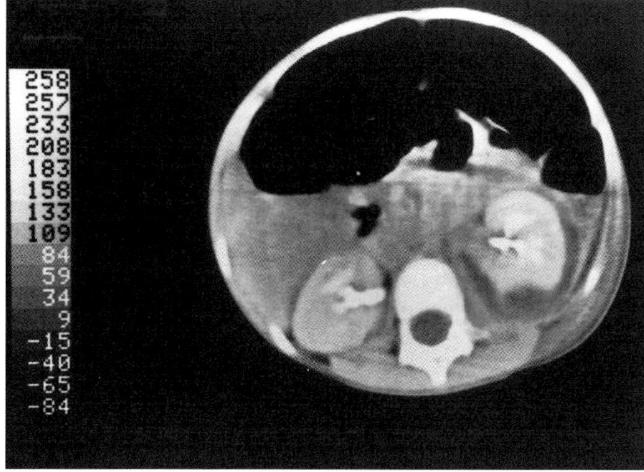

Figure 7.28 CT scan reveals a filling defect in upper pole of left kidney consistent with a renal abscess in a child with flank pain and fever. (Reprinted from Rushton,[297] with permission.)

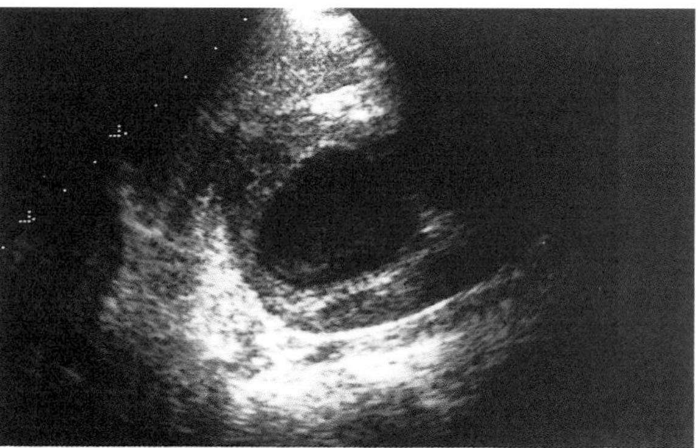

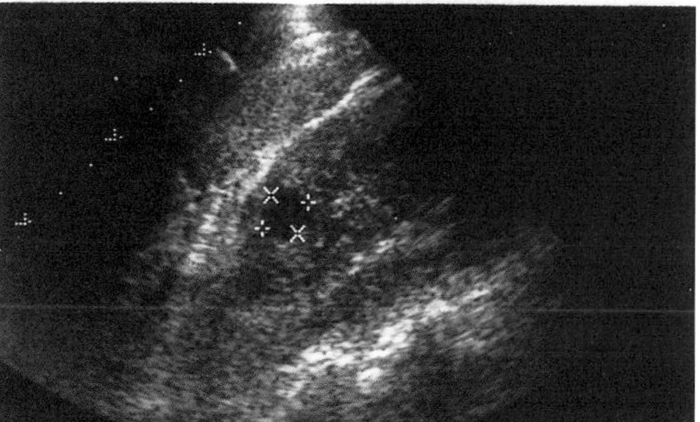

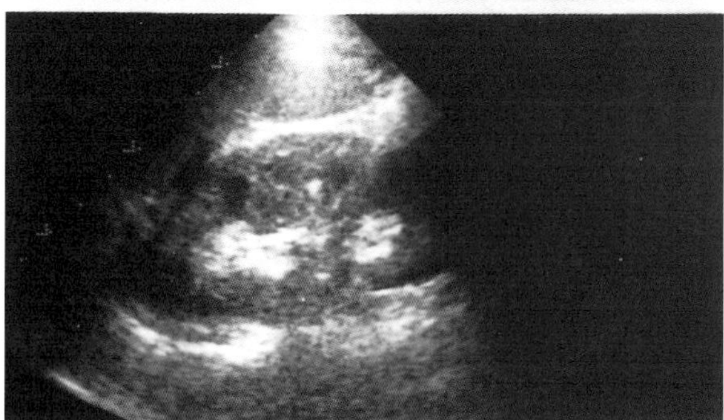

Figure 7.29 Sonogram in a 16-year-old girl who presented with fever and flank pain. (*Top*) Sonolucent mass in the left upper pole consistent with a renal abscess. Needle aspiration under sonographic guidance yielded purulent material that grew *E. coli.* Following 2 weeks of parenteral and 4 weeks of oral antibiotic therapy, sonograms 7 weeks later (*middle*) and 17 weeks later (*bottom*) show progressive resolution of abscess cavity. (Reprinted from Rushton,[297] with permission.)

days of parenteral antibiotic treatment alone followed by an additional 2 weeks of appropriate oral therapy was successful.[406] However, in a review of the literature performed by Steele et al, 62% (16/26) of the children with renal abscesses ultimately required surgical intervention.[407] Unfortunately, no controlled data exist that rigorously compare the resolution rate between children treated with antibiotics alone vs those treated with antibiotics and drainage. Currently, most cases of renal abscess initially can be managed without intervention, percutaneous drainage being reserved for persistent infection (Figure 7.29). Children who are immunocompromised by virtue of malnutrition or infection with the human immunodeficiency virus (HIV) are at particular risk for developing recurrent renal abscesses and abscesses containing unusual organisms (*Listeria monocytogenes*).[408,409] In these circumstances, more aggressive surgical or percutaneous intervention is often necessary early to eradicate the infection.

Treatment in renal failure

The dynamics of antibiotic detoxification and excretion are usually deranged in the child with renal failure. Antibacterial doses need to be adjusted in such patients to avoid adverse reactions. Certain drugs – those that are dependent on renal function for efficacy – are useless in these patients. The frequency of administration of those drugs that are effective in the face of renal failure – rather than their dosages – should be modified based on the degree of renal insufficiency.

Dysfunctional elimination

In addition to appropriate antimicrobial therapy, other factors must be taken into consideration in patient management. Voiding frequency and control of constipation are the two most common variables that are readily changeable and may be the most important in effecting changes in susceptibility to infection, particularly for children who are infrequent voiders. Establishing a voiding schedule in children may be extremely difficult and may provoke conflict in the parent–child relationship. The physician can interject his influence by explaining the treatment goal to the child and requesting that a regular voiding pattern be instituted and maintained. Children should be told that they will be reminded by their parents to void regularly and that they should follow this request even if they do not feel the urge to void at that time. Multialarm wrist watches can be a useful and inexpensive reminder for older school-age children.

The mainstay of treatment of children with recurrent UTIs and underlying bladder instability involves the long-term use of anticholinergic medicine, primarily oxybutynin (Ditropan). Other anticholinergic and antispasmodic agents include hyoscyamine (Levsinex) and tolterodine (Detrol). Koff et al reported that after initial clearing of urinary infection, 31 of 58 (58%) children with recurrent UTIs and uninhibited bladder contractions who were treated with anticholinergics alone maintained sterile urine. The necessity for long-term antibiotic prophylaxis in these patients is then determined by the frequency of subsequent recurrences and/or the presence of VUR.[103] For children older than 6 years, the usual dosage of oxybutynin is 2.5–5 mg, given two to three times daily. A new long-acting formulation, Ditropan XL, is now available which only requires once-daily dosing. The usual dose for hyoscyamine in this age group is one 0.375 mg cap twice daily. Although not yet approved for children, tolterodine has been used successfully with doses of 1–2 mg twice daily. Reportedly, tolterodine has a more specific action on the bladder and is associated with fewer side effects. Comparative efficacy among these medications has not been established in children. Timed voidings should always be used in conjunction with anticholinergic therapy.

In more difficult cases of voiding dysfunction with detrusor–sphincter dyssynergia, pelvic floor relaxation biofeedback therapy has been used successfully in the treatment of recurrent UTIs.[410] In a recent report, 42 girls with recurrent UTIs and urodynamically confirmed dysfunctional voiding were treated with a multimodal approach involving pelvic floor relaxation biofeedback, a voiding and drinking schedule, anticholinergics in those with bladder instability, and antibiotic prophylaxis.[112] This combined therapeutic approach was effective in preventing recurrent UTIs in 35 (83%).

For constipation, an intensive therapeutic approach is often required. Initially, in severe cases, enemas given for several days may be necessary to disrupt a high fecal impaction and relax an overstretched colon. Increased intake of fiber and fluid and regular toilet habits must then be instituted. In refractory cases, regular use of a fiber-based laxative may be necessary. In most cases, these are long-term requirements, and failure to continue this regimen generally results in recurrence of both constipation and UTI.[411] A recent study of 234 constipated and encopretic children found that urinary infection was present in 11%, daytime urinary incontinence in 29%, and nocturnal incontinence in 34%.[111] During follow-up of at least 12 months after initiation of treatment for constipation, recurrent UTIs were effectively prevented in all patients who had no anatomic abnormality of the urinary tract. Daytime urinary incontinence resolved in 89% and nocturnal incontinence resolved in 63% of patients.

Urinary stasis for any other reason needs to be addressed if infection cannot be otherwise controlled with antibiotic prophylaxis. Causes may include severe reflux with secondary poor bladder emptying (megacystis–megaureter syndrome), dilatation in the absence of obstruction, bladder diverticula, or residual ureteral stumps. Since otherwise unexplained urinary infection is so common, it is incumbent upon the physician to document the influence of any of these entities on infection prior to recommending surgical correction. For example, a specimen for culture may be obtained by needle aspiration of a dilated, non-obstructed upper collecting system to ascertain its involvement prior to surgical revision.

Tuberculosis

The advent of effective antituberculous agents has made genitourinary tuberculosis an uncommon occurrence in the Western world. In 1984, 21 197 cases were reported in the United States and nearly 2000 people died of the disease.[412] The infection rate in children living in the United States whose parents were born there ranges between one and two cases per 10 000 per year. Genitourinary tuberculosis accounts for approximately one-fifth of the cases of extrapulmonary tuberculosis.[412]

Tuberculosis in children occurs most often in lower socioeconomic groups. Case rates are higher in black children and other minorities than in white children. Transmission of tuberculous infection from mother to infant via the placenta or amniotic fluid has been reported in 130–200 patients.[413]

Pathogenesis

Mycobacterium tuberculosis, the tubercle bacillus, is a slow-growing, acid-fast organism that is usually acquired through inhalation of respiratory droplets from an infected person. Renal tuberculosis is always preceded by a focus of infection in some other organ system, usually pulmonary.[414] The tubercle bacilli gain access to the kidneys by means of hematogenous dissemination, and therefore renal infection must be considered bilateral in nature.

Pathology

Genitourinary tuberculosis occurs in 4–15% of patients with tuberculosis;[415,416] it accounts for 73% of the cases of extrapulmonary tuberculosis.[417] Renal tuberculosis is a late and uncommon complication of pulmonary disease, and occurs less than 4–5 years after primary infection. Predisposing conditions, such as malnutrition, diabetes mellitus, and chronic corticosteroid administration play a significant role in the development of genitourinary tuberculosis. Like all blood-borne renal infections, the tuberculosis bacillary emboli are deposited initially in the glomerular and cortical arterioles and cause small tubercles to develop. These tubercles undergo necrosis, with eventual caseation and cavitation of sloughed material into the caliceal walls at the papillary tips. The lesions may extend throughout the renal parenchyma and cause total destruction of the renal pyramids. Rupture of the bacilli into the calyx and collecting system results in extension of disease to other calices, renal pelvis, ureter, and bladder.

Local progression results in fibrosis causing stenosis of the caliceal neck, infundibulum, ureteropelvic junction, mid-ureter, and ureterovesical junction. Ureteral fibrosis results in straightening and shortening of the ureter and ultimately produces the classic gaping ureteral orifice with vesicoureteral reflux. Alternatively, ureteral stricture may produce hydroureteronephrosis and ultimately non-functioning 'autonephrectomized' kidney.[418] Involvement of the bladder by tubercle bacilli causes ulceration and bleeding with destruction of the vesical mucosa.

Tuberculosis of the genital tract is uncommon in both sexes before puberty. In males, involvement of the genital tract usually occurs either hematogenously or through retrograde passage of infected urine through the posterior urethra in the prostatic ducts. Tuberculous epididymitis or epididymo-orchitis can occur in early childhood and may be the initial method of presentation. The fallopian tubes are involved in approximately 90%, the endometrium in 50%, the ovaries in 20–30% and the cervix in 2–4% of females with genital tuberculosis.[413]

Symptoms

The majority of children with genitourinary tuberculosis have no symptoms during the initial infection.[419] Due to the lagtime between pulmonary infection and the clinical onset of renal tuberculosis, symptoms of frequency, dysuria, hematuria, and pyuria occur late in the course of disease, when the lesions ulcerate through the calices and renal pelvis, and tubercle bacilli are disseminated to the bladder. Genitourinary tuberculosis must be suspected in children with sterile pyuria, draining sinuses, and those with a history of tuberculosis elsewhere in the body. One child with a tuberculous vesicovaginal fistula and total urinary incontinence has been reported.[420] With treatment of the tuberculosis, the fistula closed and the incontinence was corrected.

Diagnosis

Microscopic hematuria and pyuria are usually present. Routine urine specimens for culture are often negative; however, 15–20% of patients with tuberculous bacilluria may have coexistent bacterial infection. The diagnosis of genitourinary tuberculosis is suggested by the demonstration of acid-fast bacilli in the stained urinary sediment and is confirmed by culture, usually guinea pig inoculation. Collection of fresh morning urine specimens appears to be just as accurate as 24-hour urinary concentrates in providing the diagnosis.[421] The acid-fast tubercle bacilli are discharged intermittently, and therefore at least three separate specimens should be collected for study. Tetracycline and sulfa medications exert mild bacteriostatic effects on tuberculosis cultures, and these drugs should be discontinued before urine collection.[422] Skin tests for tuberculosis (PPD) are usually positive except in cases of overwhelming infection, or with human immunodeficiency virus (HIV) infection. The erythrocyte sedimentation rate (ESR) may be increased, and anemia may be seen in advanced disease.

Plain films of the abdomen may reveal punctate calcification overlying the renal parenchyma.[423] In approximately 10% of patients with renal tuberculosis, calculi are present. The earliest radiographic findings on the excretory urogram are minimal caliceal dilatation or erosion of the papillary tip. As the infection proceeds, there is increased destruction of the calices. With advanced disease, there may be cavitation and cicatricial deformity of the collecting system, progressing to pyonephrosis and non-function. Conversely, a normal excretory urogram does not rule out active genitourinary tuberculosis. In patients with hydroureteronephrosis or non-functioning renal units, ureteral catheterization may be helpful for selective urinary collection and retrograde pyelography may be necessary to provide accurate delineation of pyelocaliceal architecture.

Cystoscopic examination reveals only minimal inflammatory changes in the early stages of disease. With coalescence of the tubercles, there may be areas of white or yellow raised nodules with a halo of hyperemia. With advanced localized disease, bladder capacity may become markedly diminished, with fixed and incompetent ureteral orifices, mucosal ulceration and diffuse cystitis.

Treatment

The advent of short-course chemotherapy has changed the surgical management of genitourinary tuberculosis.[424] The current recommendation is for surgery to restore function or to remove irreparable disease. Surgery can be performed 6 weeks after the start of chemotherapy.

Antituberculosis drugs inhibit multiplication of tubercle bacilli and arrest the course of disease progression. Various antituberculosis agents are currently available.[413,425,426] The efficacy of combination chemotherapy compared with single-drug administration has been well documented and treatment with orally administered agents is as effective as parenteral drug administration.

Isoniazid

The dosage of isoniazid (INH) is 10–20 mg/kg of body weight per day, up to 300 mg daily, given in one dose. The drug is the most effective of the antituberculosis agents available and remains the keystone of all therapeutic regimens. Isoniazid is metabolized in the liver and is excreted primarily through the kidney. It is available in liquid form (50 mg/5 ml) and in tablets, which may be dissolved in fruit juice or water; this makes drug administration easier in infants and young children. Peripheral neuritis is the most common side effect and is probably caused by inhibition of pyridoxine metabolism. Neurotoxic side effects have not been reported in children younger than 11 years of age, and thus pyridoxine supplementation is not recommended unless nutrition is inadequate. Hepatotoxicity, which is seen often in older patients, rarely occurs in children.

Rifampin

The dosage of rifampin is 10–20 mg/kg/day, up to 600 mg daily. Rifampin is extremely effective and virtually non-toxic for administration in children. Rare cases of minor hepatic and renal dysfunction and thrombocytopenia have been reported. This drug is indicated for the initial treatment of genitourinary tuberculosis and for cases requiring re-treatment.

Rifampin is excreted in the bile and urine and may cause orange discoloration of urine, tears and sweat. In older females taking rifampin, contraceptive drugs should be avoided because rifampin changes the kinetics of the estrogen component.

Ethambutol

The dosage of ethambutol is 15–20 mg/kg/day, up to 2500 mg daily, divided into two to three doses. This is an extremely effective antituberculosis drug, which has replaced *p*-aminosalicylic acid for use in most adults. It is rapidly absorbed and excreted in the urine. Optic neuritis is a major toxic effect of ethambutol, and monthly visual examinations are required. This drug is not recommended for use in small children who are not able to cooperate in examination of visual acuity and color vision.

Streptomycin

The dosage of streptomycin is 20–40 mg/kg/day given intramuscularly, up to 1000 mg daily. Although streptomycin is still a useful drug for the treatment of genitourinary tuberculosis, the risk of eighth nerve damage prohibits use of this medication for longer than 12 weeks.

p-Aminosalicylic acid (PAS)

The dosage of PAAS is 200 mg/kg/day, up to 10 g daily. PAS is an effective bactericidal drug for the treatment of renal tuberculosis when used in combination with other antituberculosis medications. However, PAS is not effective when used alone. Major side effects are gastrointestinal problems, including nausea, vomiting, diarrhea, and anorexia. It is best to give PAS after meals and in the form of sodium and potassium PAS to decrease gastrointestinal irritability.

Pyrazinamide

The dosage of pyrazinamide is 30 mg/kg/day, up to 2 g/day. The drug is bactericidal, seldom hepatotoxic and well tolerated by children.

Ethionamide

The dosage of ethionamide is 15–20 mg/kg/day, up to a maximum of 1 g/day. The drug is well tolerated by children, is bacteriostatic, and occasionally is useful for drug-resistant cases. A physician experienced with this drug should be consulted prior to its use.

Other drugs

Cycloserine, kanamycin, and capreomycin may be useful in treating drug-resistant cases of genitourinary tuberculosis.

Specific therapy for genitourinary tuberculosis

The accepted treatment for genitourinary tuberculosis is triple-drug chemotherapy administered daily for 2 years.[427] Short-course chemotherapy (6 month treatment regimen) has been advocated in an attempt to (1) increase patient compliance, (2) decrease the cost of medication, (3) lower drug toxicity, and (4) produce an equally successful regimen comparable with the standard therapy.[424,428] Short-course chemotherapy must include rifampin as one of the drugs.[412]

The recommendation of the American Academy of Pediatrics for treatment of genitourinary tuberculosis is 9 months of INH and rifampin. In the first 2 months of therapy, a third drug should be added. This may include pyrazinamide, streptomycin, or ethambutol in children older than 5 years of age. If the infection is associated with HIV infection, treatment should include three drugs and may need to be longer than 9 months.[425]

The majority of relapses occur within the first 2 years. Females in the childbearing years should avoid pregnancy until therapy is completed.[429] Women who are delivered of a baby while they have genitourinary tuberculosis may infect the infant with tuberculosis.[430]

With the rapid bactericidal activity of drugs like rifampin, recent recommendations call for 1-year follow-up unless calcification is seen on abdominal radiographs.[412] If calcification is present, long-term follow-up is required to be sure that the disease does not progress. During the follow-up period, urinalysis is performed every 2 months. The upper urinary tracts should be monitored prior to, during, and after treatment to assess for obstruction because strictures are common.

Surgical therapy in patients with genitourinary tuberculosis is essentially of historical significance.[431,432] The result of chemotherapy are so impressive that surgical intervention is limited to exceptional cases such as ureteral stricture,[418] ureterovesical junction reconstruction, or augmentation cystoplasty in children with small contracted bladders.[433]

Xanthogranulomatous pyelonephritis

Xanthogranulomatous pyelonephritis is an atypical form of severe chronic renal parenchymal infection characterized by unilateral destruction of parenchyma and accumulation of lipid-laden macrophages (xanthoma cells) either surrounding abscess cavities or as discrete yellow nodules. More than 50 cases of xanthogranulomatous pyelonephritis have been reported in children.[434–436] The age of presentation has ranged from infancy to 16 years. Most patients present with non-specific symptoms of chronic infection, including weight loss, recurrent fever, failure to thrive, pallor, and lethargy, although those with the focal form often appear healthy.[434,435] A palpable abdominal mass is present in approximately one-third of cases. Bacterial specimens for culture can be obtained from the urine or renal abscess in the majority of cases, with *Proteus* being the most common organism isolated.

Both diffuse and focal forms of the disease have been reported, with the focal form being more common in children than in adults.[435,437] The pathologic and radiologic differences between focal and diffuse xanthogranulomatous pyelonephritis have been described.[438] Radiologic evaluation in the diffuse form of the disease often reveals non-function of the entire kidney. Calcification or stones may be present, although this is less common in the focal form of the disease. Characteristic sonographic or CT appearances of xanthogranulomatous pyelonephritis have also been reported.[439] However, these features are non-specific and often mimic neoplasia or other forms of chronic inflammatory renal parenchymal disease. Consequently, the correct diagnosis is seldom made preoperatively. Nephrectomy is curative, although partial nephrectomy may be adequate in focal disease, assuming that the diagnosis can be established. No incidence of recurrence in the contralateral kidney has been reported.

Appendix: antibacterial agents

Sulfonamides

Sulfonamides act by competitively blocking the conversion of para-aminobenzoic acid to folic acid.[422] About 75% of the oral dose is absorbed. Free sulfonamide is excreted into urine by filtration and tubular secretion. Although high tissue levels are not achieved, excellent urine levels result. Sulfonamides are most effective against *E. coli* but also may be effective against other Gram-negative and Gram-positive organisms.

Sulfonamides are well tolerated by children, are inexpensive, and produce few side effects. They affect the gastrointestinal flora when used for long-term prophylaxis but are effective agents for short-term acute therapy of uncomplicated infections. They displace protein-bound bilirubin and hence in the neonate have the potential to interfere with bilirubin excretion and cause jaundice. Once the infant has passed through the period of 'physiologic jaundice,' these agents can be utilized safely. Some patients are allergic to sulfa drugs, but fortunately most reactions are of a minor cutaneous nature, such as urticaria. There have been some problems with major hypersensitivity reactions, such as the Stevens–Johnson syndrome, but these are rare. The most widely used agent is sulfisoxazole, employed in a dose of 120–150 mg/kg of body weight per day, given acutely in four to six divided doses orally.[441,442]

Trimethoprim–sulfamethoxazole

The TMP–SMX combination is useful both in the management of simple cystitis and for long-term antibacterial prophylaxis. This combination has a diminished effect on bowel flora and offers the advantage of trimethoprim entering vaginal secretions in the adult female.[443] This latter characteristic appears to be of particular utility in its effectiveness as a prophylactic agent. In addition, trimethoprim has also been shown in vitro to induce phase variation of fimbriated *E. coli* to a non-fimbriated state.[444] This and the high concentration in vaginal secretions work to prevent vaginal and periurethral colonization with organisms that could potentially cause urinary tract infection. Trimethoprim interferes with dihydrofolic acid reductase, and sulfa methoxazole blocks the conversion of para-aminobenzoic acid to dihydrofolic acid. The combination is effective against many Gram-negative as well as Gram-positive organisms. It is well absorbed, attains high levels in both serum and urine, and is well tolerated by children. Neutropenia and thrombocytopenia are not uncommon with its use. However, the significance of these changes is unknown.[445]

The combination is available as a suspension containing 40 mg of trimethoprim and 200 mg of sulfamethoxazole per 5 ml. The dose employed in children over 2 months of age is TMP 6–12 mg and SMX 30–60 mg/kg/day, in two divided doses.[441]

Nitrofurantoin

Nitrofurantoin is quite useful in the treatment of simple cystitis and is also a very effective agent for long-term, low-dose prophylaxis. It is thought to interfere with early stages of the bacterial Krebs cycle.[442] It is well absorbed from the gastrointestinal tract and has minimal effect on bowel flora. Tissue levels are low because it is excreted almost entirely in the urine by glomerular filtration. Urinary levels tend to be quite high. Urinary alkalinization increases urine levels, whereas acidification increases tissue levels. It works well against most *E. coli* and enterococci but is not particularly effective against *Klebsiella, Proteus,* or *Pseudomonas*.

Nausea and vomiting are frequent troublesome side effects in children; however, these can be minimized by administering the agent immediately following a meal or by utilizing nitrofurantoin macrocrystals supplied in capsule form. For the small child, the contents of the capsule can be emptied and administered in potatoes or apple sauce.

In neonates, nitrofurantoin has the potential to cause a hemolytic anemia because of glutathione instability. Consequently, it should not be used in this age group. Additionally, the drug is ineffective in patients with significant renal impairment. Other side effects are rare but do include peripheral neuropathy and pulmonary infiltrates. The usual dose in children older than 3 months of age is 5–7 mg/kg/day given orally in three to four divided doses.[441]

Penicillin

The penicillins as a class are probably the most widely used antibiotics. All act by blocking mucopeptide synthesis in the cell walls so that the bacterium is unprotected from its high internal osmotic pressure. This effect occurs only in growing cells.

Penicillin G

Extremely high urine levels can be achieved with penicillin G in patients with normal renal function, and under these circumstances this drug may be very effective against both *E. coli* and *Proteus*. Its major toxic effect is allergy manifested by rash or anaphylaxis.

Ampicillin

Ampicillin is the most widely used penicillin in the treatment of UTIs. It is not well absorbed from the gastrointestinal tract; therefore, high fecal levels do occur and diarrhea is common. High serum and urine concentrations are achievable. This agent should not be administered to patients with a known history of penicillin allergy. The usual dose is 50–100 mg/kg/day given every 6 hours. It can be administered either orally or intravenously.[442]

Amoxicillin

Amoxicillin is a derivative of ampicillin that is absorbed more readily and therefore produces less diarrhea. It is administered orally in a dose of 20–40 mg/kg/day every 6–8 hours.[442]

Carbenicillin

Carbenicillin is an agent that may be useful in the treatment of *Pseudomonas* and indole-positive *Proteus*; however, its usefulness is often diminished by the emergence of resistant strains. It is available as tablets and as a parenteral solution. When it is used parenterally for UTI in children, the usual dose is 50–200 mg/kg/day given every 4 hours; for severe infections, the dose can be increased to 400–500 mg/kg/day.[446] The oral form is not predictably effective in children.

Ticarcillin

Ticarcillin is available for parenteral therapy only. Like carbenicillin, it is active against *Pseudomonas* and indole-positive *Proteus*, which may be resistant to other drugs. It is often used with an aminoglycoside for a synergistic effect. This combination may also delay the emergence of resistant strains. Sodium overload is less likely to occur with ticarcillin compared with carbenicillin. The usual dose in children for treatment of UTI is 50–100 mg/kg/day given every 4–6 hours. In life-threatening infections, the dose can be increased to 200–300 mg/kg/day.[446]

Piperacillin

Piperacillin has essentially the same antimicrobial spectrum as carbenicillin and ticarcillin, but is more effective on a weight basis. Piperacillin may have some advantage in allowing lower doses and therefore less sodium load compared with carbenicillin and ticarcillin. The dosage in children is 50 mg/kg/day given every 4–6 hours.[426]

Cephalosporins

Cephalosporins are usually effective against most of the Gram-negative and many of the Gram-positive pathogens. Excretion is by both glomerular filtration and tubular secretion. Although there can be some cross-reactivity in patients who are allergic to penicillin, in general these agents can be cautiously administered to patients with penicillin allergy.

Oral drugs

Oral cephalexin, a 'first-generation' cephalosporin, is well absorbed from the gastrointestinal tract, and can be given in a dose of 25–50 mg/kg/day every 6 hours.[441]

Cefaclor, a 'second-generation' oral cephalosporin, is somewhat more active against Gram-negative bacteria but is more expensive than cephalexin. The dosage is 20–40 mg/kg/day given every 8 hours.[441] Other oral cephalosporins include cephradine (first generation) and cefadroxil (second generation). A new 'third-generation' cephalosporin for oral administration, cefixime, is now available. In addition to broader coverage of Gram-negative organisms, an advantage of cefixime is a prolonged half-life, allowing for once- or twice-daily dosage. The recommended dose for children is 8 mg/kg/day in one or two divided doses.[447]

Parenteral drugs

Numerous cephalosporins are available for parenteral use. The first-generation cephalosporins (cephalothin, cefazolin, cepharadine, cephapirin) are useful agents for urinary infections caused by most strains of *E. coli*, *Klebsiella*, and *Proteus*, but not *Pseudomonas*. As with all cephalosporins, they are inactive against enterococci. The second-generation parenteral cephalosporins (cefamandole, cefoxitin) are more active than the first-generation agents against many enteric Gram-negative bacteria, but not *Pseudomonas*. Cefoxitin is the most active cephalosporin against anaerobes, including *Bacteroides fragilis*. There are a number of new third-generation cephalosporins (cefoperazone, cefotaxime, ceftazidime, ceftriaxone). These drugs have been developed because of their relatively greater activity against Gram-negative bacteria. Although most retain some activity against Gram-positive bacteria, they are much less active than first-generation cephalosporins for staphylococci or other Gram-positive bacteria. Ceftriaxone has a longer half-life, allowing for once- or twice-daily dosage. It is also more active than cefoperazone against most Gram-negative bacteria.

Other cephalosporins

There are so many new cephalosporins that it is difficult to choose among them. It is recommended that the physician become familiar with the use of one oral and one parenteral drug in each generation. Dosage in children varies with each cephalosporin.

Aminoglycosides

The aminoglycosides are well tolerated by children and are of special utility in the treatment of complicated gram-negative UTI. They interfere with protein synthesis by binding proteins of the bacterial ribosomes.

Gentamicin

Gentamicin is probably the most widely used of the aminoglycosides in children and is especially effective against *Pseudomonas*. The usual pediatric dose is 5–7.5 mg/kg/day parenterally in two divided doses, depending upon age.[441] It achieves high tissue concentration and can be ototoxic, particularly to the vestibular cells. Nephrotoxicity also occurs in a small percentage of patients and should be watched for by checking serum creatinine periodically during the course of therapy. Nephrotoxicity occurs particularly frequently when gentamicin is given in combination with cephalosporins. Both ototoxicity and nephrotoxicity are usually transient.

Tobramycin

Tobramycin has the advantage of particular efficacy against *Pseudomonas*. It is said to be less nephrotoxic than gentamicin.[448] The dosage is 4–7.5 mg/kg/day given every 8–12 hours, depending upon age.[441]

Amikacin

A newer aminoglycoside, amikacin, was developed to improve activity against emerging resistant strains of *Pseudomonas*. As with other aminoglycosides, it is potentially both nephrotoxic and ototoxic. The dosage is 15–22.5 mg/kg/day given every 8–12 hours, depending upon age.[441]

Nalidixic acid

Nalidixic acid is an antibacterial agent that produces good urinary levels and is effective against Gram-negative organisms. It is especially effective against *Proteus*. Previous negative reports regarding the effectiveness of this agent can probably be accounted for by inadequate dosage.[449] Nalidixic acid is readily absorbed from the gastrointestinal tract and is well tolerated by children. It is rapidly inactivated by the liver. It is thought to interfere with DNA synthesis. The development of pseudotumor cerebri has been reported as a complication of its use in children. Nalidixic acid is available in both tablet and suspension form. The recommended dose is 55 mg/kg/day in four divided doses.[441]

Methenamine mandelate and methenamine hippurate

These agents are readily absorbed from the intestinal tract and remain inactive until they are excreted by the kidney and concentrated in the urine. Methenamine is converted to the bactericidal agent formaldehyde in acidic urine; however, this conversion takes a minimum of 2 hours to achieve adequate bactericidal levels. Mandelic and hippuric acids are urinary acidifiers that have some additional inherent but weak antibacterial agent. Efficacy of methenamine may be enhanced further by supplementary urinary acidification, such as with ascorbic acid. Both can cause dysuria when administered in high doses, and methenamine mandelate has, on rare occasions, produced hemorrhagic cystitis.[450] The recommended dose for these agents initially is 100 mg/kg/day given orally in four divided doses, followed by 50 mg/kg/day in four divided doses.[441]

Tetracyclines

Tetracyclines should not be used in children under 8 years of age because they stain the permanent teeth. The need for tetracycline is extremely unusual in modern-day pediatrics.

References

1. Abbott GD. Neonatal bacteriuria: a prospective study in 1,460 infants. BMJ 1972; 1(795):267–9.
2. O'Dougherty NJ. Urinary tract infection in the neonatal period and later in infancy. In: Urinary Tract Infection. London: Oxford University Press, 1968.
3. Littlewood JM, Kite P, Kite BA. Incidence of neonatal urinary tract infection. Arch Dis Child 1969; 44:617.
4. Stamey TA. Urinary infections in infancy and childhood. In: Pathogenesis and Treatment of Urinary Tract Infections. Baltimore: Williams and Wilkins, 1980.
5. Jodal U. The natural history of bacteriuria in childhood. Infect Dis Clin North Am 1987; 1:713–29.
6. Ginsburg CM, McCracken GH Jr. Urinary tract infections in young infants. Pediatrics 1982; 69(4):409–12.
7. Majd M, Rushton HG, Jantausch B et al. Acute febrile urinary infection in children: a prospective clinical, laboratory, and imaging study. J Pediatr 1991; 119:578.
8. Bergstrom T, Larson H, Lincoln K et al. Studies of urinary tract infections in infancy and childhood. XII. Eighty consecutive patients with neonatal infection. J Pediatr 1972; 80(5):858–66.
9. Drew JH, Acton CM. Radiological findings in newborn infants with urinary infection. Arch Dis Child 1976; 51:628–30.
10. Wiswell TE, Smith FR, Bass JW. Decreased incidence of urinary tract infections in circumcised male infants. Pediatrics 1985; 75(5):901–3.
11. Winberg J, Andersen HJ, Bergstrom T et al. Epidemiology of symptomatic urinary tract infection in childhood. Acta Paediatr Scand 1974; 252(Suppl):1.
12. Kunin CM. The natural history of recurrent bacteriuria in schoolgirls. N Engl J Med 1970; 282(26):1443–8.
13. Savage JP. The deleterious effect of constipation upon the reimplanted ureter. J Urol 1973; 109(3):501–3.
14. Saxena SR, Collis A, Laurence BM. Bacteriuria in preschool children. Lancet 1974; 2:517.
15. Newcastle Asymptomatic Bacteriuria Research Group. Asymptomatic bacteriuria in school children in Newcastle-upon-Tyne. Arch Dis Child 1975; 50:90.
16. Lindberg U, Claesson I, Hanson LA et al. Asymptomatic bacteriuria in school girls: I. Clinical and laboratory findings. Acta Paediatr Scand 1975; 64:425.
17. Savage DCL, Wilson MI, McHardy M et al. Covert bacteriuria of childhood: a clinical and epidemiological study. Arch Dis Child 1973; 48:8.
18. Hellstrom A, Hanson E, Hansson S, Hjalmas K, Jodal U. Association between urinary symptoms at 7 years old and previous urinary tract infection. Arch Dis Child 1991; 66(2):232–4.
19. Marild S, Jodal U. Incidence rate of first-time symptomatic urinary tract infection in children under 6 years of age. Acta Paediatr 1998; 87:549–52.
20. Gillenwater JY, Harrison RB, Kunin CM. Natural history of bacteriuria in schoolgirls. A long-term case-control study. N Engl J Med 1979; 301(8):396–9.
21. Martinell J, Jodal U, Lidin-Janson G. Pregnancies in women with and without renal scarring after urinary infections in childhood. BMJ 1990; 300(6728):840–4.
22. Martinell J, Lidin-Janson G, Jagenburg R et al. Girls prone to urinary infections followed into adulthood. Indices of renal disease. Pediatr Nephrol 1996; 10(2):139–42.
23. Brook I. Anaerobes as a cause of urinary tract infection in children [Letter]. Lancet 1981; 1(8224):835.
24. Granoff DM, Roskes S. Urinary tract infection due to Haemophilus influenzae, type b. J Pediatr 1974; 84(3):414–16.
25. Rytand DA, Spreiter S. Prognosis in postural (orthostatic) proteinuria: forty to fifty-year follow-up of six patients after diagnosis by Thomas Addis. N Engl J Med 1981; 305(11):618–21.
26. Lindberg U, Hanson LA, Lidin-Janson G et al. Asymptomatic bacteriuria in school girls: II. Differences in E. coli causing asymptomatic and symptomatic bacteriuria. Acta Paediatr Scand 1975; 64:432.
27. Kaijser B. Immunology of Escherichia coli K antigen and its relation to urinary tract infections in children. Lancet 1977; 1:633.
28. Vaisanen-rhen V, Elo J, Vaisanen E et al. P-fimbriated clones among uropathogenic Escherichia coli strains. Infect Immun 1984; 43:149–55.
29. Yamamoto S, Nakata K, Yuri K et al. Assessment of the significance of virulence factors of uropathogenic Escherichia coli in experimental urinary tract infection in mice. Microbiol Immunol 1996; 40(9):607–10.
30. Fussell EN, Kaack MB, Cherry R, Roberts JA. Adherence of bacteria to human foreskins. J Urol 1988; 140(5):997–1001.
31. Glauser MP, Lyons JM, Brande AI. Prevention of chronic experimental pyelonephritis by suppression of acute suppuration. J Clin Invest 1978; 61:403.

32. Gillenwater JYJ. Detection of urinary leukocytes by chemstrip-1. J Urol 1981; 125:383.
33. Fussell EN, Kaack MB, Cherry R et al. Bacteriuria in families of girls with recurrent bacteriuria. Clin Pediatr 1977; 16:1132.
34. Malvey MA, Lopez-Bondo Y, Wilson C et al. Induction and evasion of host defenses by type-1 piliated uropathogenic Escherichia coli. Science 1998; 282:1494–7.
35. Blomfield IC. The regulation of pap and type 1 fimbriation in Escherichia coli. Adv Microb Physiol 2001; 45:1–49.
36. Hagberg L, Hull R, Hull S et al. Contribution of adhesion to bacterial persistence in mouse urinary tract. Infect Immun 1983; 40:265–72.
37. Connell I, Agace W, Klemm P et al. Type-1 fimbrial expression enhances Escherichia coli virulence for the urinary tract. Proc Natl Acad Sci USA 1996; 93(18): 9827–32.
38. Marild S, Jodal U, Orskov I et al. Special virulence of Escherichia coli O1:K1:H7 clone in acute pyelonephritis. J Pediatr 1989; 115:40–5.
39. Gunther NW 4th, Lockatell V, Johnson DE, Mobley HL. In vivo dynamics of type 1 fimbria regulation in uropathogenic Escherichia coli during experimental urinary tract infection. Infect Immun 2001; 69:2838–46.
40. Kallenius G, Mollby R, Svensson SB et al. The pK antigen as receptor for the hemagglutination of pyelonephritogenic Escherichia coli. FEMS Microbiol Lett 1980; 7:297.
41. Leffler H, Svanborg-Eden C. Chemical identification of a glycosphingolipid receptor for Escherichia coli attaching to human urinary tract epithelial cells and agglutinating human erythrocytes. FEMS Microbiol Lett 1980; 8:127.
42. Lomberg H. Properties of Escherichia coli in patients with renal scarring. J Infect Dis 1989; 159:579–82.
43. James-Ellison MY, Roberts R, Verrier-Jones K, Williams JD, Topley N. Mucosal immunity in the urinary tract: changes in sIgA, FSC, and total IgA with age and in urinary tract infection. Clin Nephrol 1997; 48(2):69–78.
44. Kallenius G, Mollby R, Svenson SB et al. Occurrence of P-fimbriated Escherichia coli in urinary tract infections. Lancet 1981; 2(8260–61):1369–72.
45. Roberts JA, Suarez GM, Kaack B et al. Experimental pyelonephritis in the monkey VII: ascending pyelonephritis in the absence of vesicoureteral reflux. J Urol 1985; 133:1068.
46. Daigle F, Harel J, Fairbrother JM et al. Expression and detection of pap-, sfa-, and afa-encoded fimbrial adhesin systems among uropathogenic Escherichia coli. Can J Microbiol 1994; 40(4):286.
47. Johanson M, Plos K, Machlund BI, Svanborg C. Pap, papG, and prsG DNA sequences in Escherichia coli from the fecal flora and the urinary tract. Microb Pathog 1993; 15(2):121–9.
48. Roberts JA. Factors predisposing to urinary tract infections in children. Pediatr Nephrol 1996; 10(4):517.
49. Perugini MK, Vidotto MC. Frequency of pap and pil operons in Escherichia coli strains associated with urinary infections. Braz J Med Biol Res 1996; 29(3):351–7.
50. Bartkova G, Ciznar I, Lehotska V et al. Characterization of adhesion associated surface properties of uropathogenic Escherichia coli. Folia Microbiol 1994; 39(5):373.
51. Schlager TA, Whittam TS, Hendley JO et al. Comparison of expression of virulence factors by Escherichia coli causing cystitis and E. coli colonizing the periurethra of healthy girls. J Infect Dis 1995; 172(3):772–7.
52. O'Hanley P, Lark D, Falkow S, Schoolnik G. Molecular basis of Escherichia coli colonization of the upper urinary tract in BALB/C mice. Clin Invest 1985; 75:347.
53. Majd M, Rushton HG, Jantausch B, Wiedermann BL. Relationship among vesicoureteral reflux, P-fimbriated Escherichia coli, and acute pyelonephritis in children with febrile urinary tract infection. J Pediatr 1991; 119(4): 578–85.
54. Rushton HG, Majd M, Jauntausch B et al. Renal scarring following reflux and non-reflux pyelonephritis in children: evaluation with 99m-technetium dimercaptosuccinic acid distribution patterns in acute pyelonephritis. J Urol 1992; 147(5):1327–32.
55. Horowitz MA, Silverstein SC. Influence of Escherichia coli capsule on complement fixation and on phagocytosis and killing by human phagocytes. J Clin Invest 1980; 65:82.
56. Svanborg-Eden C, Hagberg L, Hull R et al. Bacterial virulence versus host resistance in the urinary tracts of mice. Infect Immun 1987; 55:124.
57. Siegfried L, Kmetkova M, Pazova H, Molokacova M, Filka J. Virulence-associated factors in Escherichia coli strains isolated from cultures of blood specimens from urosepsis and non-urosepsis patients. Microbiologia 1994; 10(3):249.
58. Blanco M, Blanco JE, Alonso MP, Blanco J. Virulence factors and O groups of Escherichia coli strains isolated from cultures of blood specimens from urosepsis and non urosepsis patients. Microbiologia 1994; 10(3):249.
59. Blanco M, Blanco JE, Alonso MP, Blanco J. Virulence factors and O groups of Escherichia coli isolates from patients with acute pyelonephritis, cystitis, and asymptomatic bacteriuria. Eur J Epidemiol 1996; 12(2):191.
60. Kaijser B. Immunology of Escherichia coli: K antigen and its relation to urinary-tract infection. J Infect Dis 1973; 127(6):670–7.
61. Waalwijk C, MacLaren DM, de Graaff J. In vivo function of hemolysin in the nephropathogenicity of Escherichia coli. Infect Immun 1983; 42:245–9.
62. Williams PH. Novel iron uptake system specified by Col V plasmids: an important component in the virulence of invasive strains of Escherichia coli. Infect Immun 1979; 26:295.
63. Carbonetti NH, Boonchai S, Paary SH et al. Aerobactin-mediated iron uptake by Escherichia coli isolates from human extraintestinal infections. Infect Immun 1986; 51:966.
64. Jacobson SN, Hammarlind M, Lidelfeldt K. Incidence of aerobactin-positive Escherichia coli strains in patients with symptomatic urinary tract infection. Eur J Clin Microbiol Infect Dis 1988; 7:630.
65. McCabe WR, Kaijser B, Olling S et al. Escherichia coli in bacteremia: K and O antigens and serum sensitivity of strains from adults and neonates. J Infect Dis 1978; 138:33–41.

66. Olling S, Hansson LA, Holmgren JU et al. The bactericidal effect of normal human serum on E. coli strains from normals and from patients with urinary tract infections. Infect Immun 1973; 1:24.
67. Arthur M, Johnson CE, Rubin RH. Molecular epidemiology of adhesin and hemolysin virulence factors among uropathogenic Escherichia coli. Infect Immun 1989; 57:303–13.
68. Topley N, Steadman R, Mackenzie R. Type 1 fimbriate strains of Escherichia coli initiate renal parenchymal scarring. Kidney Int 1998; 4:609–16.
69. Mizunoe Y, Matsumoto T, Sakumoto M et al. Renal scarring by mannose-sensitive adhesin of Escherichia coli type 1 pili. Nephron 1997; 77(4):412–16.
70. Mundi H, Bjorksten B, Svanborg C et al. Extracellular release of reactive oxygen species from human neutrophils upon interaction with Escherichia coli strains causing renal scarring. Infect Immun 1991; 59(11):4168
71. Hagberg L, Jodal U, Korkonen T et al. Adhesion, hemagglutination, and virulence of Escherichia coli causing urinary tract infections. Infect Immun 1981; 31:564–70.
72. Svanborg-Eden C, Eriksson B, Hanson LA. Adhesion of Escherichia coli to human uroepithelial cells in vitro. Infect Immun 1977; 21:767–74.
73. Anderson P, Engberg I, Lidin-Janson G. Persistence of Escherichia coli bacteriuria is not determined by bacterial adherence. Infect Immun 1991; 59:2915–21.
74. Bollgren I, Winburg J. The periurethral aerobic bacterial flora in girls highly susceptible to urinary infections. Acta Paediatr Scand 1976; 65:81.
75. Stamey TA, Timothy M, Millar M et al. Recurrent urinary infections in adult women. The role of introital enterobacteria. Calif Med 1971; 115:1.
76. Leadbetter G Jr, Slavins S. Pediatric urinary tract infections: significance of vaginal bacteria. Urology 1974; 3:581.
77. Stamey TA. The role of introital bacteria in recurrent urinary infections. J Urol 1973; 109:467.
78. Gruneberg RN. The relationship of infecting organisms to fecal flora in patients with symptomatic urinary infection. Lancet 1969; 2:766.
79. Patrick MJ. The influence of maternal renal infection on the foetus and infant. Arch Dis Child 1967; 42:208.
80. Gareau FE, Mackel DC, Boring JR et al. The acquisition of fecal flora by infants from their mothers during birth. J Pediatr 1959; 54:313.
81. Chan RCY, Bruce AW, Reid G. Adherence of cervical, vaginal and distal urethral normal microbial flora to human uroepithelial cells and inhibition of adherence of gram-negative uropathogens by competitive exclusion. J Urol 1984; 131:596.
82. Chan RCY, Reid G, Irvin RT et al. Competitive exclusion of uropathogens from human uroepithelial cells by lactobacillus whole cells and cell wall fragments. Infect Immun 1985; 47:84.
83. Marild S, Jodal U, Mangelus L. Medical histories of children with acute pyelonephritis compared with controls. J Pediatr Infect Dis 1989; 8:511.
84. Wold AE, Caugant DA, Lidin-Janson G et al. Resident E. coli strains frequently display uropathogenic characteristics. J Infect Dis 1992; 165(1):46.
85. Plos K, Connell H, Jodal U et al. Intestinal carriage of P fimbriated Escherichia coli and the susceptibility to urinary tract infection in young children. J Infect Dis 1995; 171(3):625–31.
86. Bollgren I, Winburg J. The periurethral aerobic bacterial flora in healthy boys and girls. Acta Paediatr Scand 1976; 65:74.
87. Brumfitt W, Gargan RA, Hamilton-Miller JM. Periurethral enterobacterial carriage preceding urinary infection. Lancet 1987; 1(8537):824–6.
88. Rushton HG, Majd M. Pyelonephritis in male infants: how important is the foreskin? J Urol 1992; 148:733.
89. Wiswell TE, Enzenauer RW, Holton ME, Cornish JD, Hankins CT. Declining frequency of circumcision: implications for changes in the absolute incidence and male to female sex ratio of urinary tract infections in early infancy. Pediatrics 1987; 79(3):338–42.
90. Wiswell TE, Hachey WE. Urinary tract infections and the uncircumcised state: an update. Clin Pediatr 1993; 32(3):130–4.
91. Wiswell TE, Roscelli JD. Corroborative evidence for the decreased incidence of urinary tract infection in circumcised male infants. Pediatrics 1986; 78:66.
92. Kim KK. Preputial condition and urinary tract infections. J Korean Med Sci 1996; 11(4):332.
93. Roberts JA. Neonatal circumcision: an end to the controversy? South Med J 1996; 89(2):167–71.
94. Graham JB, King LR, Kropp KA et al. The significance of distal urethral narrowing in young girls. J Urol 1967; 97:1045.
95. Immergut MA, Wahman GE. The urethral caliber of female children with urinary tract infection. J Urol 1968; 99:189.
96. Kallenius G, Winberg J. Bacterial adherence to periurethral epithelial cells in girls prone to urinary-tract infections. Lancet 1978; 2(8089):540–3.
97. Svanborg-Eden C, Jodal U. Attachment of Escherichia coli to sediment epithelial cells from UTI prone and healthy children. Infect Immun 1979; 26:837.
98. Hansen A, Hansen B, Dahm TL. Urinary tract infection, day wetting and other voiding symptoms in seven- to eight-year-old Danish children. Acta Pediatr 1997; 86:1135–9.
99. Allen TD. The non-neurogenic bladder. J Urol 1977; 117:232.
100. Hansson S. Urinary incontinence in children and associated problems. Scand J Urol Nephrol Suppl 1992; 141:47–55.
101. Hansson S, Hjalmas K, Jodal U, Sixt R. Lower urinary tract dysfunction in girls with untreated asymptomatic or covert bacteriuria. J Urol 1990; 143:333–5.
102. Hinman F. Urinary tract damage in children who wet. Pediatrics 1974; 54(2):143–50.
103. Koff SA, Murtagh DS. The uninhibited bladder in children: effect of treatment on recurrence of urinary infection and on vesicoureteral reflux resolution. J Urol 1983; 130(6):1138–41.
104. Snodgrass W. Relationship of voiding dysfunction to urinary tract infection and vesicoureteral reflux in children. Urology 1991; 38:341.
105. Van Gool J, Tanagho E. External sphincter activity and urinary tract infections in girls. Urology 1977; 10:348.

106. Mayo ME, Burns MW. Urodynamic studies in enuresis and the non-neurogenic bladder. Br J Urol 1990; 65:641.
107. Chen JJ, Mao W, Homayoon K, Steinhardt GF. A multivariate analysis of dysfunctional elimination syndrome, and its relationships with gender, urinary tract infection and vesicoureteral reflux in children. J Urol 2004; 171(5):1907.
108. van Gool JD. Dysfunctional voiding: a complex of bladder/sphincter dysfunction, urinary tract infections and vesicoureteral reflux. Acta Urolog Belg 1995; 63:27–33.
109. Cox CE, Hinman F. Experiments with induced bacteriuria, vesical emptying, and bacterial growth on the mechanisms of bladder defense to infection. J Urol 1961; 86:739.
110. Schulman SL, Quinn CK, Plachter N, Kodman-Jones C. Comprehensive management of dysfunctional voiding. Pediatrics 1999; 103(3):e31.
111. Loening-Baucke V. Urinary incontinence and urinary tract infection and their resolution with treatment of chronic constipation of childhood. Pediatrics 1997; 100(2 Pt 1):228–32.
112. De Paepe H, Hoebeke P, Renson C et al. Pelvic-floor therapy in girls with recurrent urinary tract infections and dysfunctional voiding. Br J Urol 1998; 81(Suppl 3):109–13.
113. Koff SA, Lapides J, Piazza DH. Association of urinary tract infection and reflux with uninhibited bladder contractions and voluntary sphincteric obstruction. J Urol 1979; 122(3):373–6.
114. Seruca H. Vesicoureteral reflux and voiding dysfunction: prospective study. J Urol 1989; 142:494.
115. Williams MA, Noe HN, Smith RA. The importance of urinary tract infection in the evaluation of the incontinent child. J Urol 1994; 151(1):188–90.
116. Van Gool JD, Kuijten RH, Donekerwolcke RA et al. Bladder-sphincter dysfunction, urinary infection and vesicoureteral reflux with special reference to cognitive bladder training. Contrib Nephrol 1984; 39:190.
117. Hjalmas K. Functional daytime incontinence: definitions and epidemiology. Scand J Urol Nephrol 1992; 141 (Suppl):39.
118. Van Gool JD, Vijverberg MA, de Jong TP. Functional daytime incontinence: clinical and urodynamic assessment. Scand J Urol Nephrol 1992; 141:58.
119. Wan J, Kaplinsky R, Greenfield S. Toilet habits of children evaluated for urinary tract infection. J Urol 1995; 154(2 Pt 2):797–9.
120. Neumann PZ, DeDomenico IJ, Nogrady MB. Constipation and urinary tract infection. Pediatrics 1973; 52(2):241–5.
121. O'Regan S, Yazbeck S, Schick E. Constipation, bladder instability, urinary tract infection syndrome. Clin Nephrol 1985; 23:152.
122. Koff SA, Wagner TT, Jayanthi VR. The relationship among dysfunction elimination syndromes, primary vesicoureteral reflux and urinary tract infections in children. J Urol 1998; 160:1019–22.
123. Fennell RS, Wilson SG, Garin EH et al. Bacteriuria in families of girls with recurrent bacteriuria. Clin Pediatr 1977; 16:1132.
124. Askari A, Belman AB. Vesicoureteral reflux in black girls. J Urol 1982; 127(4):747–8.
125. Hopkins WJ, Gendron-Fitzpatrick A, Balish E, Uehling DT. Time course and host response to Escherichi coli urinary tract infection in genetically distinct mouse strains. Infect Immun 1998; 66(6):2798–802.
126. Cotton SA, Gbadegesin RA, Williams S et al. Role of TGF-β1 in renal parenchymal scarring following childhood urinary tract infection. Kid Int 2002; 61:61–7.
127. Solari V, Ennis S, Cascio S, Puri P. Tumor necrosis factor-alpha gene polymorphism in reflux nephrapathy. J Urol 2004; 172(4 Pt2): 1604–6; discussion 1606.
128. Ozen S, Alikasifoglu M,Tuncbilek E et al. Polymorphisms in angiotensin converting enzyme gene and reflux nephropathy: a genetic predisposition to scar formation? Nephrol Dial Transplant 1997; 12(9):2031.
129. Erdogan H, Mir S, Serdaroglu E et al. Is ACE gene polymorphism a risk factor for renal scaring with low-grade reflux? Pediatr Nephrol 2004; 19:734–7.
130. Hohenfellner K, Wingen AM, Nauroth O et al. Impact of ACE I/D gene polymorphism on congenital renal malformations. Pediatr Nephrol 2001; 16(4):356
131. Marcus DM. The ABO and Lewis blood-group system. Immunocytochemistry, genetics and relation to human disease. N Engl J Med 1969; 280:994–1006.
132. Navas EL, Venegas MF, Duncan JL et al. Blood group antigen expression on vaginal and buccal epithelial cells and mucus in secretor and nonsecretor women. J Urol 1993; 149:1492.
133. Schaeffer AJ, Navas EL, Venegas MF et al. Variation of blood group antigen expression on vaginal cells and mucus in secretor and nonsecretor women. J Urol 1994; 152(3):859–64.
134. Navas EL, Venegas MF, Duncan JL et al. Blood group antigen expression on vaginal cells and mucus in women with and without a history of urinary tract infections. J Urol 1994; 152(2 Pt 1):345–9.
135. Sheinfeld J, Cordon-Cardo C, Fair WR, Wartinger DD, Rabinowitz R. Association of type 1 blood group antigens with urinary tract infections in children with genitourinary structural abnormalities. J Urol 1990; 144(2 Pt 2):469–73; discussion 474.
136. Jantausch BA, Criss VR, O'Donnell R et al. Association of Lewis blood group phenotypes with urinary tract infection in children. J Pediatr 1994; 124(6):863–8.
137. Albarus MH, Salzano FM, Goldraich NP. Genetic markers and acute febrile urinary tract infection in the first year of life. Pediatr Nephrol 1997; 11(6):691–4.
138. Chick S, Harver MJ, MacKenzie R et al. Modified method for studying bacterial adhesion to isolated uroepithelial cells and uromucoid. Infect and Immun 1981; 34:256.
139. Orskov I, Ferencz A, Orskov F. Tamm–Horsfall protein or uromucoid is the normal urinary slime that traps Type-1 fimbriated Escherichia coli. Lancet 1980; 2:887.
140. Parkkinen J, Virkola R, Korhonen TK. Escherichia coli strains binding neuraminyl α2-3 galactosides. Biochem Biophys Res Commun 1983; 11:456–61.
141. Toma G, Bates J, Kumar S. Uromodulin (Tamm–Horsfall protein) is a leukocyte adhesion molecule. Biochem Biophys Res Commun 1994; 200:275–82.
142. Israele V, Darabi A, McCracken GH Jr. The role of bacterial virulence factors and Tamm–Horsfall protein in the

pathogenesis of Escherichia coli urinary tract infection in infants. Am J Dis Child 1987; 141(11):1230–4.
143. Lomberg H, Hanson LA, Jacobsson B et al. Correlation of P blood group, vesicoureteral reflux, and bacterial attachment in patients with recurrent pyelonephritis. N Engl J Med 1983; 308(20):1189–92.
144. Tomisawa S, Kogure T, Kuroume T et al. P blood group and proneness to urinary tract infections in Japanese children. Scand J Infect Dis 1989; 21:403.
145. Stapleton AE, Stroud MR, Hakomori SI, Stamm WE. The globoseries glycosphingolipid sialosyl galactosyl globoside is found in urinary tract tissues and is a preferred binding receptor in vitro for uropathogenic Escherichia coli expressing pap-encoded adhesins. Infect and Immun 1998; 66(8):3856–61.
146. Bergsten, G, Samuelsson M, Wullt B et al. PapG-dependent adherence breaks mucosal inertia and triggers the innate host response. J Infect Dis 2004; 189(9):1734–42.
147. Hellerstein S, Kennedy E, Nussbaum L, Rice K. Localization of the site of urinary tract infections by means of antibody-coated bacteria in the urinary sediments. J Pediatr 1978; 92(2):188–93.
148. Thomas V, Shelokov A, Forland M. Antibody-coated bacteria in the urine and the site of urinary-tract infection. N Engl J Med 1974; 290:588–90.
149. Hanson LA, Ahlstedt S, Fasth A et al. Antigens of Escherichia coli, human immune response, and the pathogenesis of urinary tract infections. J Infect Dis 1977; 136(Suppl):S144–9.
150. Hopkins WJ, Xing Y, Dahmer LA, Balish E, Uehling DT. Western blot analysis of anti-Escherichia coli serum immunoglobulins in women susceptible to recurrent urinary tract infections. J Infect Dis 1995; 172(6):1612–6.
151. Mattsby-Baltzer I, Claesson I, Hanson LA et al. Antibodies to lipid A during urinary tract infection. J Infect Dis 1981; 144(4):319–28.
152. Sohl-Akerlund A, Ahlstedt S, Hanson LA et al. Antibody responses in urine and serum against Escherichia coli in childhood urinary tract infections. Acta Pathol Microbiol 1979; 87:29.
153. Rene P, Silverblatt FJ. Serological response to Escherichia coli in pyelonephritis. Infect Immun 1982; 37:749.
154. Svanborg-Eden C, Svennerholm AM. Secretory immunoglobulin A and G antibodies prevent adhesion of Escherichia coli to human urinary tract epithelial cells. Infect Immun 1978; 22:790.
155. Wold AE, Mestecky J, Svanborg-Eden C. Agglutination of E. coli by secretory IgA – a result of interaction between bacterial mannose-specific adhesins and immunoglobulin carbohydrate? Monogr Allergy 1988; 24:307–9.
156. Clark H, Ronal AR, Turck M. Serum antibody response in renal versus bladder bacteria. J Infect Dis 1971; 123:539.
157. Uehling DT, Steihm ER. Elevated urinary secretory IgA in children with urinary tract infection. Pediatrics 1971; 47(1):40–6.
158. Fleidner M, Mehls O, Rauterberg EW et al. Urinary SIgA in children with urinary tract infection. J Pediatr 1986; 109:416.
159. Kaijser B, Larsson P, Olling S. Protection against ascending Escherichia coli pyelonephritis in rats and significance of local immunity. Infect Immun 1983; 20:78–81.
160. Uehling DT, Jensen J, Balish E. Vaginal immunization against urinary tract infection. J Urol 1982; 128:1382.
161. Uehling DT, Mizutani K, Balish E. Effect of immunization on bacterial adherence to urothelium. Invest Urol 1978; 16:145.
162. Coppa GV, Gabrielli O, Giorgi P et al. Preliminary study of breastfeeding and bacterial adhesion to uroepithelial cells. Lancet 1990; 335(8689):569–71.
163. Hahn H, Kaufmann SHE. The role of cell-mediated immunity in bacterial infections. Rev Infect Dis 1981; 3:1221.
164. Hjelm EM. Local cellular immune response in ascending urinary tract infection: occurrence of T-cells, immunoglobulin-producing cells, and Ia-expressing cells in rat urinary tract tissue. Infect Immun 1984; 44:627.
165. Miller TE, Scott L, Stewart E et al. Modification by suppressor cells and serum factors of the cell-mediated immune response in experimental pyelonephritis. J Clin Invest 1978; 61:864.
166. Svanborg-Eden C, Briles D, Hagberg L, McGhee J, Michael S. Genetic factors in host resistance to urinary tract infection. Infection 1984; 12:118–23.
167. Svensson M, Lindstedt R, Radin N et al. Epithelial glycosphingolipid expression as a determinant of bacterial adherence and cytokine production. Infect Immun 1994; 62:4404–10.
168. Hedges S, Svensson M, Svanborg C. Interleukin–6 response of epithelial cell lines to bacterial stimulation in vitro. Infect Immun 1992; 60:1295–301.
169. Agace W, Hedges S, Ceska M et al. IL–8 and the neutrophil response to mucosal Gram negative infection. J Clin Invest 1993; 92:780–5.
170. Mannhardt W, Becker A, Putzer M et al. Host defense within the urinary tract. I. Bacterial adhesion initiates an uroepithelilal defense mechanism. Pediatr Nephrol 1996; 10(5):568–72.
171. Takeda K, Akira S. Toll receptors and pathogen resistance. Cell Microbiol 2003; 5(3):143–53.
172. Hang L, Frendeus B, Godaly G et al. Interleukin-8 receptor knockout mice have subepithelial neutrophil entrapment and renal scarring following acute pyelonephritis. J Infect Dis 2000; 182(6):1738–48.
173. Pecha B, Low D, O'Hanley P. Gal-Gal pili vaccines prevent pyelonephritis by piliated E. coli in a murine model. J Clin Invest 1989; 83:2102.
174. Roberts JA, Hardaway K, Kaack B et al. Prevention of pyelonephritis by immunization with p-fimbria. J Urol 1984; 131:602.
175. Roberts JA, Kaack MB, Baskin G et al. Antibody responses and protection from pyelonephritis following vaccination with purified Escherichia coli PapDG protein. J Urol 2004; 171(4):1682.
176. Silverblatt FJ, Weinstein R, Rene P. Protection against experimental pyelonephritis by antibodies to pili. Scand J Infect Dis 1982; 33:79.
177. Thankavel K, Madison B, Ikeda T et al. Localization of a domain in the FimH adhesin of Escherichia coli type 1 fimbriae capable of receptor recognition and use of a domain-

specific antibody to confer protection against experimental urinary tract infection. J Clin Invest 1997; 100(5):1123–36.
178. Uehling DT, Hopkins WJ, Balish E, Xing Y, Heisey DM. Vaginal mucosal immunization for recurrent urinary tract infection: phase II clinical trial. J Urol 1997; 157(6):2049–52.
179. Nayir A, Evare S, Sinin A et al. The effects of vaccination with inactivated uropathogenic bacteria in recurrent urinary tract infections in children. Vaccine 1995; 13(11):987–90.
180. Smellie JM, Gruneberg RN, Leakey A, Atkin WS. Long-term low-dose co-trimoxazole in prophylaxis of childhood urinary tract infection: clinical aspects. BMJ 1976; 2(6029):203–6.
181. Bailey RR. The relationship of vesico-ureteric reflux to urinary tract infection and chronic pyelonephritis-reflux nephropathy. Clin Nephrol 1973; 1:132.
182. Ransley PG. Vesicureteral reflux: continuing surgical dilemma. Urology 1978; 12:246.
183. Rushton HG. The evaluation of acute pyelonephritis and renal scarring with technetium 99m-dimercaptosuccinic acid renal scintigraphy: evolving concepts and future directions. Pediatr Nephrol 1997; 11:108–20.
184. Naseer SR, Steinhardt GF. New renal scars in children with urinary tract infections, vesicoureteral reflux and voiding dysfunction: a prospective evaluation. J Urol 1997; 158(2):566–8.
185. Hobermann A, Wald ER. Urinary tract infections in young febrile children. Pediatr Infect Dis 1997; 16(1):11–17.
186. Dickinson JA. Incidence and outcome of symptomatic urinary tract infection in children. BMJ 1979; 1:1330–2.
187. Heale WF, Weldone DP, Hewstone AS. Reflux nephropathy: presentation or urinary infection in children. Med J Aust 1977; 1:1138.
188. Corman LI, Forsage WS, Kotchmar GS. Simplified urinary microscopy to detect significant bacteriuria. Pediatrics 1982; 70:133.
189. Pryles CV, Eliot CR. Pyuria and bacteriuria in infants and children: the value of pyuria as a diagnostic criterion of urinary tract infections. Am J Dis Chil 1965; 110:628.
190. Stamm WE. Measurement of pyuria and its relationship to bacteriuria. Am J Med 1983; 75(Suppl):53.
191. Robins DG, Rogers KB, White RHR. Urine microscopy as an aid to detection of bacteriuria. Lancet 1975; 1:476.
192. Hoberman A, Wald ER, Reynolds EA, Penchansky L, Charron M. Pyuria and bacteriuria in urine specimens obtained by catheter from young children with fever. J Pediatr 1994; 124(4):513–19.
193. Landau D, Turner ME, Brennan J, Majd M. The value of urinalysis in differentiating acute pyelonephritis from lower urinary tract infection in febrile infants. Pediatr Infect Dis 1994; 13:777.
194. Kusumi RK, Glover PJ, Kunin CM. Rapid detection of pyuria by leukocyte esterase activity. JAMA 1981; 254:1653.
195. James GP, Paul KL, Fuller JB. Urinary nitrate in urinary tract infection. Am J Clin Pathol 1978; 70:671.
196. Pezzlo M. Detection of urinary tract infection by rapid methods. Clin Microbiol Rev 1988; 1:268.
197. Bolann BJ, Sandberg S, Digranes A. Implications of probability analysis for interpreting results of leukocyte esterase and nitrite test strips. Clin Chem 1989; 35:1663.
198. Tomlinson PA, Smellie JM, Prescod N et al. Differential excretion of urinary proteins in children with vesicoureteric reflux and reflux nephropathy. Pediatr Nephrol 1994; 8:21.
199. Miyakita H, Puri P. Urinary levels of N-acetyl-beta-D-glucosaminidase – a simple marker for predicting tubular damage in higher grades of vesicoureteric reflux. Eur Urol 1994; 25:135.
200. Taha AS, Grant V, Kelly RW. Urinalysis for interleukin-8 in the non-invasive diagnosis of acute and chronic inflammatory diseases. Postgrad Med J 2003; 79(929):159–63.
201. Nelson JD, Peters PC. Suprapubic aspiration of urine in preterm and term infants. Pediatrics 1965; 36:132.
202. Smellie JM, Hodson CJ, Edwards D et al. Clinical and radiological features of urinary infection in childhood. BMJ 1964; 2:1222.
203. Hoberman A, Chao HP, Keller DM et al. Prevalence of urinary tract infection in febrile infants. J Pediatr 1993; 123(1):17–23.
204. Crain EF, Gershel JC. Urinary tract infections in febrile infants younger than 8 weeks of age. Padiatrics 1990; 86(3):363–7.
205. Klevan JL, De Jong AR. Urinary tract symptoms and urinary tract infection following sexual abuse. Am J Dis Child 1990; 144(2):242–4.
206. Jodal U. Urinary tract infection in children. In: Holliday M, Barratt TM, Avner Ed, eds. Pediatric Nephrology, 3rd edn. Baltimore, MD: Williams and Wilkins, 1994.
207. McLachlan M, Mellor S, Verrier-Jones E et al. Urinary tract infection in school girls with covert bacteriuria. Arch Dis Child 1975; 50:253.
208. Lindberg U, Claesson I, Hanson LA et al. Asymptomatic bacteriuria in schoolgirls: VIII. Clinical course during a three-year follow-up. J Pediatr 1978; 92:194.
209. Cardiff–Oxford Bacteriuria Study Group. Sequelae of covert bacteriuria in school children. Lancet 1978; 1:889.
210. Svanborg-Eden C, Hanson CA, Jodal U, Lindberg U, Sohl-Akerlund A. Variable adherence to normal human urinary tract epithelial cells of Escherichia coli strains associated with various forms of urinary infection. Lancet 1976; 11:490.
211. Linshaw M. Asymptomatic bacteriuria and vesicoureteral reflux in children. Kidney Int 1996; 50:312.
212. Uehling DT, King LR. Secretory immunoglobulin A excretion in cystitis cystica. Urology 1973; 1:305.
213. Roberts JA. Etiology and pathophysiology of pyelonephritis. Am J Kidney Dis 1991; 17:1.
214. Roberts JA. Mechanisms of renal damage in chronic pyelonephritis (reflux neuropathy). In: Current Topics in Pathology. Heidelberg: Springer, 1995.
215. Kaack MB, Dowling KJ, Patterson GM, Roberts JA. Immunology of pyelonephritis: E. coli causes granulocytic aggregation and renal ischemia. J Urol 1986; 136:1117–22.
216. Hill GS, Clarck RL. A comparative angiographic, microangiographic, and histologic study of experimental pyelonephritis. Invest Radiol 1972; 7:33.

217. Androulakakis PA, Ransley PG, Risdon RA. Microvascular changes in the early stage of reflux pyelonephritis: an experimental study in the pig kidney. Eur Urol 1987; 13:219–23.
218. Majd M, Rushton HG. Renal cortical scintigraphy in the diagnosis of acute pyelonephritis. Semin Nucl Med 1992; 22:98–111.
219. Roberts KB, Charney E, Sweren RJ et al. Urinary tract infection in infants with unexplained fever: a collaborative study. J Pediatr 1983; 103(6):864–7.
220. Weiss SJ. Tissue destruction by neutrophils. N Engl J Med 1989; 320(6):365–75.
221. Dakin HD. On the use of certain antiseptic substances in the treatment of infected wounds. BMJ 1915; 2:318–20.
222. Ginsburg I, Kohen R. Cell damage in inflammatory and infectious sites might involve a coordinated 'cross-talk' among oxidants, microbial haemolysins and ampiphiles, cationic proteins, phospholipases, fatty acids, proteinases, and cytokines (an overview). Free Rad Res 1995; 22(6):489–517.
223. Roberts JA, Ruth JK, Dominique GL et al. Immunology of pyelonephritis in the primate model: effect of superoxide dismutase. J Urol 1982; 128:1394.
224. Pohl HG, Rushton HG, Park JS et al. Adjunctive oral corticosteroids reduce renal scarring: the piglet model of reflux and acute experimental pyelonephritis. J Urol 1999; 162(3 Pt 1):815–20.
225. Busch R, Huland H. Correlation of symptoms and results of direct bacterial localization in patients with urinary tract infections. J Urol 1984; 132(2):282–5.
226. Stamey TA, Govan DE, Palmer JM. The localization and treatment of urinary tract infections: the role of bactericidal levels as opposed to serum levels. Medicine 1965; 44:1.
227. Fairley KF, Carson NE, Gutch RC et al. Site of infection in acute urinary-tract infection in general practice. Lancet 1971; 2(7725):615–18.
228. Handmaker H. Nuclear renal imaging in acute pyelonephritis. Semin Nucl Med 1982; 12:246.
229. Traisman ES, Conway JJ, Traisman HS. The localization of urinary tract infection with 99m Tc glucoheptonate scintigraphy. Pediatr Radiol 1986; 16:403.
230. Sty JR, Wells RG, Starshak RJ, Schroeder BA. Imaging in acute renal infection in children. AJR Am J Roentgenol 1987; 148(3):471–7.
231. Rushton HG, Majd M, Chandra R, Yim D. Evaluation of 99m-technetium-dimercaptosuccinic acid renal scans and experimental acute pyelonephritis in piglets. J Urol 1988; 140:1169–74.
232. Parkhouse HF, Godley ML, Cooper J, Risdon RA, Ransley PG. Renal imaging with 99m-Tc-labelled DMSA in the detection of acute pyelonephritis: an experimental study in the pig. Nucl Med Commun 1989; 30:1219.
233. Rushton HG, Majd M. Dimercaptosuccinic acid renal scintigraphy for the evaluation of pyelonephritis and scarring: a review of experimental and clinical studies. J Urol 1992; 148(2 Pt 2):1726–32.
234. Tarkington MA, Fildes RD, Levin K et al. High resolution single photon emission computerized tomography (SPECT) 99m-technetium-dimercaptosuccinic acid renal imaging: a state of the art technique. J Urol 1990; 144:598–600.
235. Itoh K, Asano Y, Tsukamoto E et al. Single photon emission computed tomography with Tc-99m-dimercaptosuccinic acid in patients with upper urinary tract infection and/or vesicoureteral reflux. Ann Nucl Med 1991; 5(1):29–34.
236. Itoh K, Yamashita T, Tsukamoto E et al. Qualitative and quantitative evaluation of renal parenchymal damage by 99mTc-DMSA planar and SPECT scintigraphy. Ann Nucl Med 1995; 9:23–8.
237. Majd M, Rushton HG, Chandra R et al. ^{99m}Tc-DMSA renal cortical scintigraphy for the detection of experimental acute pyelonephritis in piglets: comparison of planar (pinhole) and SPECT imaging. J Nucl Med 1996; 37:1731–4.
238. Bjorgvinsson E, Majd M, Eggli DK. Diagnosis of acute pyelonephritis in children: comparison of sonography and 99m-Tc DMSA scintigraphy. AJR Am J Roentgenol 1991; 157:539.
239. MacKenzie JR, Fowler K, Hollman AS et al. The value of ultrasound in acute urinary tract infection. Br J Urol 1994; 74(2):240.
240. Melis K, Vandevivere J, Hoskens C et al. Early 99m Tc-dimercaptosuccinic acid scintigraphy in symptomatic first time urinary tract infection. Acta Pediatr 1992; 85(4):430.
241. Benador D, Benador N, Slosman DO et al. Cortical scintigraphy in the evaluation of renal parenchymal changes in children with pyelonephritis. J Pediatr 1994; 124(1):17–20.
242. Shanon A, Feldman W, McDonald P et al. Evaluation of renal scars by technetium-labeled dimercaptosuccinic acid scan, intravenous urography, and ultrasonography: a comparative study. J Pediatr 1992; 120:399–403.
243. Tasker AD, Lindsell DR, Moncrieff M. Can ultrasound reliably detect renal scarring in children with urinary tract infection? Clin Radiol 1993 47(3):177–9.
244. Yen TC, Chen WP, Chang SL et al. A comparative study of evaluating renal scars by 99m-Tc-DMSA planar and SPECT renal scans, intravenous urography, and ultrasonography. Ann Nucl Med 1994; 8:147–52.
245. Silver TM, Kass EJ, Thornbury JR et al The radiological spectrum of acute pyelonephritis in adults and adolescents. Radiology 1976; 118:65.
246. Piepsz A, Pintelon H, Verboven M, Keuppens F, Jacobs A. Replacing 99mTcm-DMSA for renal imaging? Nucl Med Commun 1992; 13:494–6.
247. Sreenarasimhaiah V, Alon US. Uroradiologic evaluation of children with urinary tract infection: are both ultrasonography and renal cortical scintigraphy necessary? J Pediatr 1995; 127(3):373–7.
248. Lonergan GJ, Pennington DJ, Morrisson JC et al. Childhood pyelonephritis: comparison of gadolinium-enhanced MR imaging and renal vortical scintigraphy for diagnosis. Radiology 1998; 207:377–85.
249. Majd M, Nussbaum-Blask AR, Markle BM et al. Acute pyelonephritis: comparison of diagnosis with 99mTc-DMSA, SPECT, spiral CT, MR imaging, and power Doppler US in an experimental pig model. Radiology 2001; 218(1):101–8.
250. Halevy R, Smolkin V, Bykov S et al. Power Doppler ultrasonography in the diagnosis of acute childhood pyelonephritis. Pediatr Nephrol 2004; 19(9):987–91.

251. Dick PT, Feldman W. Routine diagnostic imaging for childhood urinary tract infections: a systematic overview. J Pediatr 1996; 128(1):15–22.
252. Ransley PG, Risdon RA. Reflux nephropathy: effects of antimicrobial therapy on the evolution of the early pyelonephritic scar. Kidney Int 1981; 20:733–42.
253. Smellie JM, Ransley PG, Normand IC, Prescod N, Edwards D. Development of new renal scars: a collaborative study. BMJ Clin Res Ed 1985; 290(6486):1957–60.
254. Smellie JM, Normand ICS, Katz G. Children with urinary infection: a comparison of those with and without vesicoureteric reflux. Kidney Int 1981; 20:717.
255. Winberg J, Bergstrom T, Jacobsson B. Morbidity, age, and sex distribution, recurrences and renal scarring in symptomatic urinary tract infection in childhood. Kidney Int 1975; 8:S101.
256. Smellie J, Edwards D, Hunter N et al. Vesicoureteral reflux and renal scarring. Kidney Int 1975; 8(Suppl):65.
257. Sargent MA, Stringer DA. Voiding cystourethrography in children with urinary tract infection: the frequency of vesicoureteric reflux is independent of the specialty of the physician requesting the study. AJR Am J Roentgenol 1995; 164(5):1237–41.
258. Koff SA. A practical approach to evaluating urinary tract infections in children. Pediatr Nephrol 1991; 5:398–400.
259. Jerkins GR, Noe HN. Familial vesicoureteral reflux: a prospective study. J Urol 1982; 128:7743.
260. MacKenzie JR. A review of renal scarring in children. Nucl Med Commun 1996; 17:176–90.
261. Ditchfield MR, De Campo JF, Cook DJ et al. Vesicoureteral reflux: an accurate predictor of acute pyelonephritis in childhood urinary tract infection? Radiology 1994; 190(2):413–15.
262. Haycock GB. A practical approach to evaluating urinary tract infection in children. Pediatr Nephrol 1991; 5:401–2.
263. Gleeson FV, Gordon I. Imaging in urinary tract infection. Arch Dis Child 1991; 66(11):1282–3.
264. Verboven M, Ingels M, Delree M, Piepsz A. 99m Tc-DMSA scintigraphy in acute urinary tract infection in children. Pediatr Radiol 1990; 20:540–2.
265. Verber IG, Strudley MR, Meller ST. 99mTc dimercaptosuccinic acid (DMSA) scan as first investigation of urinary tract infection. Arch Dis Child 1988; 63(11):1320–5.
266. Hansson S, Dhamey M, Sigstrom O et al. Dimercaptosuccinic acid scintigraphy instead of voiding cystourethrography for infants with urinary tract infection. J Urol 2004; 172(3):1071–3; discussion 1073–4.
267. Gonzalez E, Papazyan JP, Girardin E. Impact of vesicoureteral reflux on the size of renal lesions after an episode of acute pyelonephritis. J Urol 2005; 173(2):571–4.
268. Nash MA, Siegele RL. Urinary tract infections in infants and children. Adv Pediatr Infect Dis 1996; 11:403–8.
269. AAP Committee on Quality Improvement. Practice parameter: the diagnosis, treatment and evaluation of the initial urinary tract infection in febrile infants and children. Pediatrics 1999; 103:843–52.
270. Gross GW, Lebowitz RL. Infection does not cause reflux. AJR Am J Roentgenol 1981; 137(5):929–32.
271. Craig JC, Knight JF, Sureshkumar P et al. Vesicoureteric reflux and timing of micturating cystourethrography after urinary tract infection. Arch Dis Child 1997; 76(3):275–7.
272. Hellstrom M, Jodal U, Marild S, Wettergren B. Ureteral dilatation in children with febrile urinary tract infection or bacteriuria. AJR Am J Roentgenol 1987, 148(3):483–6.
273. Roberts JA. Experimental pyelonephritis in the monkey. III. Pathophysiology of ureteral malfunction induced by bacteria. Invest Urol 1975; 13:117–20.
274. Lebowitz RL, Mandell J. Urinary tract infection in children: putting radiology in its place. Radiology 1987; 165(1):1–9.
275. Stokland E, Hellstrom M, Jacobsson B, Jodal U, Sixt R. Renal damage one year after first urinary tract infection: role of dimercaptosuccinic acid scintigraphy. J Pediatr 1996; 129(6):815–20.
276. Jakobsson B, Svensson L. Transient pyelonephritic changes on 99m-technetium-dimercaptosuccinic acid scan for at least five months after infection. Acta Paediatr 1997; 86(8):803–7.
277. International Reflux Committee. Medical versus surgical treatment of primary, vesicoureteral reflux. Pediatrics 1981; 67:392.
278. Cleveland RH, Constantinou C, Blickman J et al. Voiding cysoturethrography in children: value of digital fluoroscopy in reducing radiation dose. Am J Radiol 1991; 158:137.
279. Diamond DA, Kleinman PK, Spevak M et al. The tailored low-dose fluoroscopic voiding cystogram for fmilial reflux screening. J Urol 1996; 155:681–2.
280. Conway JJ, King LR, Belman AB. Detection of vesicoureteral reflux with radionuclide: a comparison study with roentgenographic cystography. AJR Am J Roentgenol 1972; 115:720.
281. Nasrallah PF, Sreeramulu N, Crawford J. Clinical applications of nuclear cystography. J Urol 1982; 128:550.
282. Jaya G, Bal CS, Padhy AK. Radionuclide studies in the evaluation of urinary tract infections in children. Indian Pediatr 1996; 33:635–40.
283. Saraga M, Stanicic A, Markovic V. The role of direct radionuclide cystography in the evaluation of vesicoureteral reflux. Scand J Urol Nephrol 1996; 30: 367–71.
284. Willi UV, Treves ST. Radionuclide Voiding Cystography. New York: Springer-Verlag, 1985: 105–20.
285. Majd M, Kass EJ, Belman AB. The accuracy of the indirect (intravenous) radionuclide cystogram in children. J Nucl Med 1983; 24:23.
286. De Sadeleer C, De Boe V, Keuppens F et al. How good is technetium-99m mercaptoacetyltriglycine indirect cystography? Eur J Nucl Med 1994; 21:223–7.
287. Majd M, Kass EJ, Belman AB. Radionuclide cystography in children: comparison of direct (retrograde) and indirect (intravenous) techniques. Am Radiol 1985; 28:322–8.
288. Kangarloo H, Gold RH, Fine RN, Diament MJ, Boechat MI. Urinary tract infection in infants and children evaluated by ultrasound. Radiology 1985; 154(2):367–73.
289. Horgan JG, Rosenfeld NS, Weiss RM et al. Is renal ultrasound a reliable indicator of nonobstructed duplication anomaly? Pediatr Radiol 1984; 14:388.

290. Jequier S, Forbes PA, Negrady MB. The value of ultrasound as a screening procedure in first documented urinary tract infections in children. J Ultrasound Med 1985; 4:393.
291. Leonidas JC, McCauley RG, Klauber GC, Fretzayas AM. Sonography as a substitute for excretory urography in children with urinary tract infection. AJR Am J Roentgenol 1985; 144(4):815–19.
292. Majd M. Nuclear medicine in pediatric urology. In: Clinical Pediatric Urology, 3rd edn. Philadelphia: WB Saunders, 1992.
293. Mucci B, Macguire B. Does routine ultrasound have a role in the investigation of children with urinary tract infection? Clin Radiol 1994; 49:324–5.
294. Alon US, Ganapathy S. Should renal ultrasonography be done routinely in children with first urinary tract infection? Clin Pediatr 1999; 38:21–5.
295. Ben-Ami T, Rozin M, Hertz M. Imaging of children with urinary tract infection: a tailored approach. Clin Radiol 1989; 40:64.
296. Blickman JG, Taylor GA, Lebowitz RL. Voiding cystourethrography: the initial radiologic study in children with urinary tract infection. Radiology 1985; 156(3): 659–62.
297. Rushton HG. Genitourinary infections: nonspecific infections. In: Kelalis PP, King LR, Belman AB, eds. Clinical Pediatric Urology, 3rd edn. Philadelphia: WB Saunders, 1992.
298. Hansson S, Jodal U, Noren L, Bjure J. Untreated bacteriuria in asymptomatic girls with renal scarring. Pediatr 1989; 84:964–8.
299. Mingin GC, Hinds A, Nguyen HT, Baskin LS. Children with a febrile urinary tract infection and a negative radiologic workup: factors predictive of recurrence. Urology 2004; 63(3):562–5.
300. Cohen RA, Rushton HG, Belman AB et al. Renal scarring and vesicoureteral reflux in children with myelodysplasia. J Urol 1990; 144:541–54.
301. Ottolini MAC, Schaer CM, Rushton HG et al. Relationship of asymptomatic bacilluria and renal scarring in children with neuropathic bladders who are practicing intermittent catheterization. J Pediatr 1995; 127:368.
302. Bisset GS III, Strife JL, Dunbar JS. Urography and voiding cystourethrography: findings in girls with urinary tract infection. AJR Am J Roentgenol 1987; 148(3):479–82.
303. Skoog SJ, Belman AB. A nonsurgical approach to the management of primary vesicoureteral reflux. J Urol 1987; 138(4 pt 2):941–6.
304. Bellinger MF, Duckett JW. Vesicoureteral reflux: a comparison of non-surgical and surgical management. In: Contributions to Nephrology. Reflux Nephropathy Update 1983, Vol. 39; 1984.
305. Burge DM, Griffiths MD, Malone PS, Atwell JD. Fetal vesicoureteral reflux: outcome following conservative postnatal management. J Urol 1992; 148(5 Pt 2):1743–5.
306. Crabbe DC, Thomas DF, Gordon AC et al. Use of ^{99m}technetium-dimercaptosuccinic acid to study patterns of renal damage associated with prenatally detected vesicoureteral reflux. J Urol 1992; 148(4):1229–31.
307. Sheridan M, Jewkes F, Gough DCS. Reflux nephropathy in the 1st year of life – the role of infection. Pediatr Surg Int 1991; 6:214.
308. Anderson PAM, Rickwood AMK. Features of primary vesicoureteric reflux detected by prenatal sonography. Br J Urol 1991; 67:267.
309. Najmaldin A, Burge DM, Atwell TD. Reflux nephropathy secondary to intrauterine vesicoureteric reflux. J Pediatr Surg 1990; 25:387–90.
310. Gordon I. Urinary tract infection in paediatrics: the role of diagnostic imaging. Br J Radiol 1990; 63(751):507–11.
311. Ransley PG, Risdon RA. Reflux in renal scarring. Br J Radiol 1978; 51 (Suppl 14):1.
312. Ransley PG. Intrarenal reflux: anatomical, dynamic and radiological studies. Part I. Urol Res 1977; 5:61.
313. Smellie JM, Preece MA, Paton AM. Somatic growth in girls receiving low dose prophylactic co-trimoxazole. BMJ Clin Res Ed 1983; 287(6396):875.
314. Rushton HG. Reflux versus nonreflux pyelonephritis. In: Gonzales ET, Paulson DF, eds. Problems in Urology. Advances in Pediatric Urology, Vol. 8, Philadelphia: WB Saunders, 1994.
315. Winberg J, Bollgren I, Kallenius G, Mollby R, Svenson SB. Clinical pyelonephritis and focal renal scarring. A selected review of pathogenesis, prevention, and prognosis. Pediatr Clin North Am 1982; 29(4):801–14.
316. Winter AL, Hardy BE, Alton DJ, Arbus GS, Churchill BM. Acquired renal scars in children. J Urol 1983; 129(6):1190–4.
317. Edwards D, Normand IC, Prescod N, Smellie JM. Disappearance of vesicoureteric reflux during long-term prophylaxis of urinary tract infection in children. BMJ 1977; 2(6082):285–8.
318. Mackie GG, Stephens FD. Duplex kidneys: a correlation of renal dysplasia with position of the ureteral orifice. J Urol 1975; 114:2743.
319. Sommer JT, Stephens FD. Morphogenesis of nephropathy with partial ureteral obstruction and vesicoureteric reflux. J Urol 1981; 125:67.
320. Filly R, Friedland GW, Govan DE, Fair WR. Development and progression of clubbing and scarring in children with recurrent urinary tract infections. Radiology 1974; 113(1):145–53.
321. Merrick MV, Uttley WS, Wild SR. The detection of pyelonephritic scarring in children by radioisotope imaging. Br J Radiol 1980; 53(630):544–56.
322. Goldraich NP, Ramos DL, Goldraich JH et al. Urography versus DMSA scan in children with vesicoureteral reflux. Pediatr Nephrol 1987; 3:1.
323. Monsour M, Azmy AF, MacKenzie JR. Renal scarring secondary to vesicoureteric reflux. Critical assessment and new grading. Br J Urol 1987; 32(5):375–8.
324. Elison BS, Taylor D, Van der Wall H et al. Comparison of DMSA scintigraphy with intravenous urography for the detection of renal scarring and its correlation with vesicoureteral reflux. J Urol 1992; 69:294–302.
325. Farnsworth RH, Rossleigh MA, Leighton DM, Bass SJ, Rosenberg AR. The detection of reflux nephropathy in infants by ^{99m}technetium dimercaptosuccinic acid studies. J Urol 1991; 145(3):542–6.

326. Stokland E, Hellstrom M, Jacobsson B, Jodal U, Sixt R. Evaluation of DMSA scintigraphy and urography in assessing both acute and permanent renal damage in children. Acta Radiol 1998; 4:447–52.
327. Arnold AJ, Brownless SM, Carty HM, Rickwood AM. Detection of renal scarring by DMSA scanning – an experimental study. J Pediatr Surg 1990; 25(4):391–3.
328. Rosenberg AR, Rossleigh MA, Brydon MP et al. Evaluation of acute urinary tract infection in children by dimercaptosuccinic acid scintigraphy: a prospective study. J Urol 1992; 148(5 Pt 2):1746–9.
329. Wallin L, Bajc M. Typical technetium dimercaptosuccinic acid distribution patterns in acute pyelonephritis. Acta Paediatr 1993; 82(12):1061–5.
330. Stokland E, Hellstrom M, Hansson SA et al. Reliability of ultrasonography in identification of reflux nephropathy in children. BMJ 1994; 309(6949):235–9.
331. Jakobsson B, Berg U, Svensson L. Renal scarring after acute pyelonephritis. Arch Dis Child 1994; 70:111.
332. Jakobsson B, Nolstedt L, Svensson L, Soderlundh S, Berg U. ^{99m}Tc-dimercaptosuccinic acid (DMSA) in the diagnosis of acute pyelonephritis in children: relation to clinical and radiological findings. Pediat Nephrol 1992; 6:328–34.
333. McGuire EJ, Woodside JR. Diagnostic advantages of fluoroscopic monitoring during urodynamic evaluation. J Urol 1981; 125(6):830–4.
334. Londe S. Cause of hypertension in the young. Pediatr Clin North Am 1978; 25:55–65.
335. Still JL, Cottom D. Severe hypertension in childhood. Arch Dis Child 1967; 42:34.
336. Gill DG, Mendes da Costa B, Cameron JS et al. Analysis of 100 children with severe and persistent hypertension. Arch Dis Child 1976; 51:951.
337. Wanner C, Lusher T, Groth H et al. Unilateral parenchymatous kidney disease and hypertension: results of nephrectomy and medical treatment. Nephron 1985; 41:250–7.
338. Goonasekera CD, Shah V, Wade AM, Barratt TM, Dillon MJ. 15-year follow-up of renin and blood pressure in reflux nephropathy. Lancet 1996; 347(9002):640–3.
339. Jacobson SH, Eklof O, Eriksson CG et al. Development of hypertension and uraemia after pyelonephritis in childhood: twenty-seven year follow-up. BMJ 1989; 299:703.
340. Zhang Y, Bailey RR. A long term follow up of adults with reflux nephropathy. N Z Med J 1995; 108:142–4.
341. Smellie JM, Normand ICS. Reflux nephropathy in childhood. In: Reflux Nephropathy. New York: Masson, 1979:14–20.
342. Bailey RR, McRae CU, Maling TMJ et al. Renal vein renin concentration in the hypertension of unilateral reflux nephropathy. J Urol 1978; 120:21.
343. Bailey RR, Lynn KL, McRae CU. Unilateral reflux nephropathy and hypertension. Contrib Nephrol 1984; 39:116.
344. Savage JM, Koh CT, Shah V, Barrett TM, Dillon MJ. Five-year prospective study of plasma renin activity and blood pressure in patients with longstanding reflux nephropathy. Arch Dis Child 1987; 62:678.
345. Jacobson SH, Kjellstrend CM, Lins LE. Role of hypervolaemia and renin in the blood pressure control of patients with pyelonephritic renal scarring. Acta Med Scand 1988; 224:47.
346. Holland NH, Kotchen T, Bhathena D. Hypertension in children with chronic pyelonephritis. Kidney Int 1975; 8:S243.
347. Luscher TF, Wanner C, Hauri D, Siegenthaler W, Vetter W. Curable renal parenchymatous hypertension: current diagnosis and management. Cardiology 1985; 72 (Suppl):33–45.
348. Disney APS. Reflux nephropathy in Australia and New Zealand: prevalence, incidence and management – 1975–1989. Second CJ Hodson Symposium on Reflux Nephropathy. Christ Church, New Zealand: Design Printing Services, 1991:53–9.
349. Sreenarasimhaiah S, Hellerstein S. Urinary tract infections per se do not cause end-stage kidney disease. Pediatr Nephrol 1998; 12:210–113.
350. Zimmerman SW, Uehling DT, Burkholder PM. Vesicoureteral reflux nephropathy. Evidence for immunologically mediated glomerular injury. Urology 1973; 2:534–8.
351. Torres VE, Velosa JA, Holley KE Progression of vesicoureteral reflux nephropathy. Ann Intern Med 1980; 92:776–84.
352. Bhathena DB, Weiss JH, Holland NH et al. Focal and segmental glomerulosclerosis in reflux nephropathy (chronic pyelonephritis). Am J Med 1980; 68:886.
353. Kincaid-Smith P. Glomerular lesions and atrophic pyelonephritis in reflux nephropathy. Kidney Int 1975; 8:S–81.
354. Stamey TA, Fair WR, Timothy MM et al. Serum versus urinary antimicrobial concentrations in cure of urinary-tract infections. N Engl J Med 1974; 291(22):1159–63.
355. Eichenwald HF. Some aspects of the diagnosis and management of urinary tract infection in children and adolecents. Pediatr Infect Dis J 1986; 5:760.
356. Hansson S, Caugant D, Jodal U, Svanborg-Eden C. Untreated asymptomatic bacteriuria in girls: I. – Stability of urinary isolates. BMJ 1989; 298:853–5.
357. White RHR. Management of urinary tract infection. Arch Dis Child 1987; 62:421.
358. Wettergren B, Hellstrom M, Stokland E, Jodal U. Six year follow up of infants with bacteriuria on screening. BMJ 1990; 301:845–8.
359. Bergstrom T, Lincoln K, Orskov F et al. Studies of urinary tract infections in infancy and children. VIII Reinfection vs relapse in recurrent urinary tract infections: evaluation by means of identification of infecting organisms. J Pediatr 1967; 72:13.
360. McGeachie J. Recurrent infection of the urinary tract: reinfection or recrudescence? BMJ 1966; 1:952.
361. Hansson S, Jodal U, Noren L. Treatment vs. nontreatment of asymptomatic bacteriuria in girls with renal scarring. Host–Parasite Interactions in Urinary Tract Infections. Chicago: University of Chicago Press, 1989:289–91.
362. Savage DCL, Howie G, Adler K, Wilson MI. Controlled trial of therapy in covert bacteriuria in childhood. Lancet 1975; 1:358–61.
363. Newcastle Asymptomatic Bacteriuria Research Group. Asymptomatic bacteriuria in school children in Newcas-

tle-upon-Tyne: a 5-year followup. Arch Dis Child 1981; 56:585–92.

364. Russo RM, Gururaj VJ, Laude TA, Rajkumar SV, Allen JE. The comparative efficacy of cephalexin and sulfisoxazole in acute urinary tract infection in children. Clin Pediatr 1991; 16(1):83–4.
365. Craig JC, Irwig LM, Knight JF, Sureshkumar P, Roy LP. Symptomatic urinary tract infection in preschool Australian children. J Paediatr Child Health 1998; 34:154–9.
366. Al Roomi LG, Sutton AM, Cockburn F et al. Amoxycillin and clavulanic acid in the treatment of urinary infection. Arch Dis Child 1984; 59(3):256–9.
367. Ruberto U, D'Eufemia P, Martino F, Giardini O. Amoxycillin and clavulanic acid in the treatment of urinary tract infections in children. J Int Med Res 1989; 17:168–71.
368. Barry HC, Ebell MH, Hickner J. Evaluation of suspected urinary tract infection in ambulatory women: a cost–utility analysis of office-based strategies. J Family Pract 1997; 44(1):49–60.
369. Hooper DC, Wolfson TS, Ng EY et al. Mechanism of action and resistance to ciprofloxacin. Am J Med 1987; 82(Suppl 4A):12.
370. Schluter G. Toxicology of ciprofloxacin. First International Ciprofloxacin Workshop, Proceedings 1986; 61.
371. Bouissou H, Caujolle D, Caujolle F, Milhand G. [Cartilaginous tissue and nalidixic acid]. C R Acad Sci Hebd Seances Acad Sci D 1978; 286(23):1743–6. [French]
372. Schaad UB, Wedgwood-Krucko J. Nalidixic acid in children: a retrospective matched controlled study for cartilage toxicity. Infection 1978; 15:165.
373. Ball P. Ciprofloxacin: an overview of adverse experiences. J Antimicrob Chemother 1986; 18(Suppl D):187.
374. Moffatt M, Embree J, Grimm P, Law B. Short-course antibiotic therapy for urinary tract infections in children. A methodological review of the literature. Am J Dis Child 1988; 142(1):57–61.
375. Avner ED, Ingelfinger JR, Herrin JT et al. Single-dose amoxicillin therapy of uncomplicated pediatric urinary tract infections. J Pediatr 1983; 102(4):623–7.
376. McCracken GH Jr, Ginsburg CM, Namasonthi V, Petruska M. Evaluation of short-term antibiotic therapy in children with uncomplicated urinary tract infections. Pediatrics 1981; 67(6):796–801.
377. Khan AJ. Efficacy of single-dose therapy of urinary tract infection in infants and children: a review. J Nat Med Assoc 1994; 86:690–6.
378. Madrigal G, Odio CM, Mohs E et al. Single dose antibiotic therapy is not as effective as conventional regimens for management of acute urinary tract infections in children. Pediatr Infect Dis J 1988; 7:316.
379. Petersen KE. Short term treatment of acute urinary tract infections in girls. Copenhagen Study Group of Urinary Tract Infections in Children. Scand J Infect Dis 1991; 23:213–20.
380. Ruberto U, D'Eufemia P, Ferretti L, Giardini O. Effect of 3- vs 10-day treatment of urinary tract infections. J Pediatr 1984; 104(3):483–4.
381. Smellie JM, Poulton A, Prescod NP. Retrospective study of children with renal scarring associated with reflux and urinary infection. BMJ 1994; 308(6938):1193–6.
382. Dagan R, Einhorn M, Lang R et al. Once daily cefixime compared with twice daily trimethoprim/sulfamethoxazole for urinary tract infection in infants and children. Pediatr Infect Dis J 1992; 11:198–203.
383. Hoberman A, Wald ER, Hickey RW et al. Oral versus initial intravenous therapy for urinary tract infections in young febrile children. Pediatrics 1999; 104:74–86.
384. Cornu C, Cochat P, Collet JP et al. Survey of the attitudes to management of acute pyelonephritis in children. Pediatr Nephrol 1994; 8:275–7.
385. Helwig H. Therapeutic strategies for urinary tract infections in children. Infection 1994; 22(S):12.
386. Belman AB. A perspective on vesicoureteral reflux. Urol Clin North Am 1995; 22(1):139–50.
387. Austenfeld MS, Snow BW. Complications of pregnancy after reimplantation for vesicoureteral reflux. J Urol 1988; 140:1103.
388. Mansfield JT, Snow BW, Cartwright PC, Wadsworth K. Complications of pregnancy in women after childhood reimplantation for vesicoureteral reflux: an update with 25 years of followup. J Urol 1995; 154(2 Pt 2):787–90.
389. Bukowski TP, Betrus GG, Aquilina JW, Perlmutter AD. Urinary tract infections and pregnancy in women who underwent antireflux surgery in childhood. J Urol 1998; 159(4):1286–9.
390. Stansfeld JM. Duration of treatment for urinary tract infections in children. BMJ 1975; 3(5975):65–6.
391. Belman AB. Clinical significance of cystitis cystica in girls: results of a retrospective study. J Urol 1978; 127:7474.
392. Smellie JM, Katz G, Gruneberg RN. Controlled trial of prophylactic treatment in childhood urinary-tract infection. Lancet 1978; 2(8082):175–8.
393. Lidin-Janson G, Jodal U, Lincoln K. Trimethoprim-och nitrofurantoin for profylax mot UVI hos barn. Recip Reflex 1980; Suppl VI:38.
394. Smellie JM, Bantock HM, Thompson BD. Co-trimoxazole and the thyroid [Letter]. Lancet 1982; 2(8289):96.
395. Brendstrup L, Hjelt K, Petersen KE et al. Nitrofurantoin versus trimethoprim prophylaxis in recurrent urinary tract infection in childhood. A randomized, double-blind study. Acta Paediatr Scand 1990; 79:1225–34.
396. Harding GK, Ronald AR, Boutros P, Lank B. A comparison of trimethoprim–sulfamethoxazole with sulfamethoxazole alone in infections localized to the kidneys. Can Med Assoc J 1975; 112(13 Spec No):9–12.
397. Hori C, Hiraoka M, Tsukahara H et al. Intermittent trimethoprim–sulfamethoxazole in children with vesicoureteral reflux. Pediatr Nephrol 1997; 11:328–30.
398. Smith EM, Elder JS. Double antimicrobial prophylaxis in girls with breakthrough urinary tract infections. Urology 1994; 43:708–12.
399. Rote AR, Bauer SB, Retik AB. Renal abscess in children. J Urol 1978; 119:254.
400. Vachvanichsanong P, Dissaneewate P, Patrapinyokul S, Pripatananont C, Sujijantararat P. Renal abscess in healthy children: report of three cases. Pediatr Nephrol 1992; 6(3):273–5.
401. Timmons JW, Perlmutter AD. Renal abscess: a changing concept. J Urol 1976; 115:299.

402. Koehler PR. The roentgen diagnosis of renal inflammatory masses – special emphasis on angiographic changes. Radiology 1974; 112:257–66.
403. Hopkins GB, Hall RL, Mende CW. Gallium–67 scintigraphy for the diagnosis and localization of perinephric abscesses. J Urol 1976; 115:126.
404. Kumar B, Coleman RE, Anderson PO. Gallium citrate Ga-67 imaging in patients with suspected inflammatory processes. Arch Surg 1975; 110:1237.
405. Wippermann CF, Schofer O, Beetz R et al. Renal abscesses in childhood: diagnostic and therapeutic progress. Pediatr Infect Dis J 1991; 10(6):446–50.
406. Schiff M Jr, Glickman M, Weiss RM et al. Antibiotic treatment of renal carbuncle. Ann Intern Med 1977; 8:305.
407. Steele BT, Petrou C, de Maria J. Renal abscesses in children. Urology 1990; 36(4):325–8.
408. Brandeis JM, Baskin LS, Kogan BA, Wara D, Corenbaum A. Recurrent Staphylococcus aureus renal abscess in a child positive for the human immunodeficiency virus. Urology 1995; 46(2):246–8.
409. Gomber S, Revathi G, Krishna A, Gupta A. Perinephric abscess (presenting as abdominal pain) due to Listeria monocytogenes. Ann Trop Paediatr 1998; 18(1):61–2.
410. Sugar EC, Firlit CF. Urodynamic biofeedback: a new therapeutic approach for childhood incontinence/infection (vesical voluntary sphincter dyssynergia). J Urol 1982; 128(6):1253–8.
411. Yazbeck S, Schick E, O'Regan S. Relevance of constipation to enuresis, urinary tract infection and reflux. A review. Eur Urol 1987; 13(5):318–21.
412. Weinberg AC, Boyd SD. Short-course chemotherapy and role of surgery in adult and pediatric genitourinary tuberculosis. Urol 1988; 31:95.
413. Smith MHD, Marquis IR. Tuberculosis and other mycobacterial infections. In: Feigin RD, Cherry ID (eds) Textbook of Pediatric Infectious Diseases, Vol 1. Philadelphia: WB Saunders, 1981.
414. Cotran RS, Kumar V, Robbins SL. Robbins Pathologic Basis of Disease, 4th ed. Philadelphia: WB Saunders, 1989. pp 374–80.
415. Cinman AC. Genitourinary tuberculosis. Urol 1982; 20:353.
416. Cos LR, Cockett ATK. Genitourinary tuberculosis revisited. Urol 1982; 20:111.
417. García-Rodriguez IA, García Sanchez IE, Gómez-García AC et al. Extrapulmonary tuberculosis in a university hospital in Spain. Eur J Epidemiol 1989; 5:154.
418. Murphy DM, Fallon B, Lane V et al. Tuberculosis stricture of the ureter. Urol 1982; 20:382.
419. Ehrlich RM, Lattimer JK. Urogenital tuberculosis in children. Urol 1971; 105:461.
420. Singh A, Fazal AR, Sinha SK et al. Tuberculosis vesicovaginal fistula in a child. Br J Urol 1988; 62:615.
421. Kenney M, Loechel AB, Lovelock FJ. Urine cultures in tuberculosis. Am Rev Respir Dis 1960; 82:564.
422. Lattimer JK, Vasquez G, Wechler H. New drugs for treatment of genitourinary tuberculosis: a comparison of efficacy. J Urol 1960; 83:493.
423. Hartmann GW, Segura JW, Hattery RR. Infectious diseases of the genitourinary tract. In: Witten DM, Myers GH Jr, Utz DC (eds) Emmett's Clinical Urography: An Atlas and Textbook of Roentgenologic Diagnosis, Vol 2, 4th ed. Philadelphia: WB Saunders 1977, 898–918.
424. Gow JG. Genitourinary tuberculosis. In: Walsh PC, Critter RF, Perlmutter AD et al (eds) Campbell's Urology, Vol 1, 5th ed. Philadelphia: WB Saunders 1986, 1037–69.
425. American Academy of Pediatrics. Report of the Committee on Infectious Diseases, 21st ed. EIK Grove Village, IL: American Academy of Pediatrics, 1988.
426. Glassroth I, Robins AG, Snider DE Jr. Letter to the editor. N Engl J Med 1980; 303:940.
427. Weschler H, Lattimer JK. An evaluation of the current therapeutic regimen for renal tuberculosis. J Urol 1975; 113:760.
428. Fox W. The chemotherapy of pulmonary tuberculosis: a review. Chest 1979; 76:785.
429. Gow JG, Barbosa S. Genitourinary tuberculosis: a study of 1117 cases over a period of 34 years. Br J Urol 1984; 56:449.
430. Shaaf HS, Smith I, Donald PR et al. Tuberculosis presenting in the neonatal period. Clin Pediatri (Phila) 1989; 28:474.
431. Flechner SM, Gow JG. Role of Rephrectomy in the treatment of non-functioning or very poorly functioning unilateral tuberculous kidney. J Urol 1980; 123:822.
432. Wong SH, Lau WY. The surgical management of nonfunctioning tuberculous kidneys. J Urol 1980; 124:187.
433. Zinman L, Libertino IA. Antirefluxing ileocecal conduit. Urol Clin North Am 1980; 7:503.
434. Yazaki T, Ishikawa S, Ogawa Y et al. Xanthogranulomatous pyelonephritis in childhood: case report and review of English and Japanese literature. J Urol 1982; 127(1):80–3.
435. Watson AR, Marsden HB, Cendron M et al. Renal pseudotumors caused by xanthogranulomatous pyelonephritis. Arch Dis Child 1982; 57:635.
436. Goodman TR, McHugh K, Lindsell DR. Paediatric xanthogranulomatous pyelonephritis. Int J Clin Pract 1998; 52(1):43–5.
437. Schulman CC, Denis R. Xanthogranulomatous pyelonephritis in childhood [Letter]. J Urol 1977; 117:398.
438. Bagley FH, Stewart AM, Jones PF. Diffuse xanthogranulomatous pyelonephritis in children: an unrecognized variant. J Urol 1977; 118:434.
439. Subramanyam BR, Megibow AJ, Raghavendra BN et al. Diffuse xanthogranulomatous pyelonephritis: analysis by computed tomography and sonography. Urol Radiol 1982; 4:5.
440. Feingold DS. Antimicrobial chemotherapeutic agents: the nature of their action in selected toxicity. N Engl J Med 1963; 269:900.
441. Behrman RF, Vaughan VCI. Nelson Textbook of Padiatrics, 13th edn. Philadelphia: WB Saunders, 1987.
442. American Medical Association. AMA Drug Evaluations. Chicago: AMA, 1971.
443. Stamey TA, Condy M, Mihara G. Prophylactic efficacy of nitrofurantoin macrocrystals and trimethoprim–sulfamethoxazole in urinary infections: biologic effects on the vaginal and rectal flora. N Eng J Med 1977; 296:780.

444. Vaisanen V, Lounatmaa R, Korhonen TK. Effects of sublethal concentrations of antimicrobial agents on the hemagglutination, adhesion, and ultrastructure of pyelonephritogenic Escherichia coli strains. Antimicrob Agents Chemother 1982; 22:120–7.
445. Asmar BI, Maqbool S, Dajani AS. Hematologic abnormalities after oral trimethoprim–sulfamethoxazole therapy in children. Am J Dis Child 1981; 135(12): 1100–3.
446. Kunin CM. Detection, Prevention and Management of Urinary Tract Infections, 4th edn. Philadelphia: Lea and Febiger, 1987.
447. Drug Newsletter. Facts and Comparisons Div. 8:56 edition. St Louis: JB Lippincott, 1989.
448. Kurnin GD. Clinical nephrotoxicity of tobramycin and gentamicin: a prospective study. JAMA 1980; 244:1808.
449. Stamey TA, Bragonje J. Resistance to nalidixic acid. A misconception due to underdosage. JAMA 1976; 236:1857–60.
450. Ross R Jr, Conway GF. Hemorrhagic cystitis following an accidental overdosage of methenamine mandelate. Am J Dis Child 1970; 119:86.

Fungal, parasitic, and other inflammatory diseases of the genitourinary tract

8

William A Kennedy II

Fungal infections of the urinary tract

Candidiasis

Pediatric fungal inflammations of the genitourinary tract are becoming more common with both the increasing number of preterm infants surviving aggressive intensive care unit (ICU) management and the increasing number of immunocompromised children living with either malignancies, human immunodeficiency virus (HIV), or solid organ and bone marrow transplantation. Preterm neonates are often intubated for weeks, receive long-term hyperalimentation, and receive broad-spectrum antibiotics. Baley et al[1] report that systemic candidiasis will develop in as many as 4% of those weighing 1500 g and 10% of those weighing 1000 g. Prolonged survival of profoundly immunocompromised pediatric patients has likewise led to the emergence of fungal infections as the major cause of mortality and morbidity in advanced disease states. *Candida* is the leading bloodstream isolate from children hospitalized with opportunistic infections.[2]

Candida albicans is a yeast that belongs to the commensal flora of the mouth, intestinal tract, vagina, and skin. *Candida* is the most common of the opportunistic mycoses. Systemic disease occurs almost exclusively in patients with impaired host resistance. Conditions that predispose to candidemia include contamination of intravenous catheters, long-term antibiotic therapy, steroid administration, immunosuppressive agents, cytotoxic drug therapy, burns, and open surgical wounds.[3] Mokaddas et al[4] have also identified ICU stay, prior broad-spectrum antibiotic therapy, and surgery on the gastrointestinal tract as being additional risk factors for candidemia in the pediatric surgery patient.

The diagnosis of candiduria is made by urine culture. In the neonate, urine is obtained by suprapubic bladder tap or by percutaneous renal aspirate if renal candidiasis is suspected. Colony counts of greater than 10 000 *Candida* per 1 ml of urine signify infection.[5] Colony counts of 15 000/ml in midstream voided urine in males or straight catheterized specimens in females are evidence of renal *Candida* infection.[6] Urine specimens taken from indwelling catheters may have colony counts as high as 100 000/ml with no relationship to upper tract candidal infection.

Pediatric patients with renal candidiasis present with symptoms of urosepsis. Ureteral obstruction due to fungus ball infestation has been reported.[7] Anuria in infants can result from bilateral pelvic fungus balls.[8] Radiologic evaluation of these patients with ultrasound may demonstrate unilateral or bilateral hydronephrosis with an intrapelvic mass. Renal scan generally demonstrates that the involved kidney exhibits poor function. In patients with localized candidal cystitis, symptoms often consist of urinary urgency, frequency, and dysuria, or may be asymptomatic.

The treatment of candiduria is dependent on the extent of the infection. Candiduria that occurs in otherwise healthy children after long-term broad-spectrum antibiotic therapy should clear after the use of the antibiotic has stopped and usually requires no treatment except for local care when secondary skin irritation occurs. Infections limited to the bladder may be controlled and eradicated by urinary alkalinization and/or intermittent instillation or irrigation with a solution of amphotericin B (5% in sterile water, shielded from light) via a three-way bladder catheter or intermittent catheterization.[9] Candidiuria confined to the upper collecting system may require treatment with oral 5-flucytosine (5-FC) or nephrostomy irrigation with amphotericin solution; however, 5-FC should not be used in children with azotemia or bone marrow depression. Infants with obstructing renal fungus balls may at times require surgical removal via pyelotomy or percutaneous aspiration, followed by nephrostomy tube irrigation. Alkalay et al[10] also report the therapeutic use of forced diuresis with furosemide to clear fungus balls from the renal pelvis. Fluid intake and furosemide therapy were adjusted to keep a urine output at a level of 4 ml/kg/h to wash out the fungal bezoar.

The treatment of choice for systemic candidiasis is intravenous amphotericin B with or without the addition of 5-FC. Amphotericin B is nephrotoxic and must be carefully titrated to obtain appropriate serum levels. Peak serum levels should be twice the mean inhibitory concentration for the infectious organism and trough levels should be equal to the mean inhibitory concentration. The duration of therapy is dependent upon the extent of the disease; however, administration is often required for several weeks to eradicate systemic infections. Toxic side effects include fever, nausea and vomiting, generalized malaise, and renal failure. Monitoring of serum creatinine on an every other day schedule is necessary.

Other antifungal medications exist for the treatment of candidiasis. These include fluconazole, which has less associated nephrotoxicity and is therefore preferred by some physicians. Its use has steadily increased in such closed populations as the neonatal nursery. The gold standard of treatment still remains amphotericin B in the management of neonatal candidiasis, as the incidence of fluconazole resistance will probably increase given its recent widespread use in the neonatal nursery.[11,12]

Aspergillosis

Aspergillosis refers to a group of diseases caused by mycelial fungus of the genus *Aspergillus*. Aspergillosis is the second most common fungal infection in immunocompromised children.[13] Aspergilli are distributed worldwide, and spores are readily isolated from soil and decaying plants. Outbreaks of invasive disease usually occur among groups of immunocompromised children as a result of exposure to aerosolized spores at large construction sites near hospitals. Once the infection is acquired from inhalation of airborne spores, it is widely disseminated through hematogenous spread. The organisms may also be introduced through operative wounds, or indwelling foreign bodies such as intravenous or urinary catheters.

Microscopic hematuria and pyuria are often present in patients with aspergillosis. The fungi may be identified as branched septate hyphae on potassium hydroxide preparations of infected urine. Results of urine cultures are often inconclusive and multiple cultures may be required to make a diagnosis. Obstructive uropathy resulting from an aspergilloma in the renal pelvis may be the initial mode of presentation.[14] Invasive aspergillosis of the renal parenchyma is characterized by focal microabscess formation and occasional papillary necrosis.

Treatment of invasive aspergillosis remains high-dose intravenous amphotericin B. In patients with fungus balls in the renal pelvis, upper tract irrigation through a nephrostomy tube is indicated. Percutaneous or open surgical removal of obstructing aspergillomas is sometimes indicated.

Coccidioidomycosis

Coccidioidomycosis is an infection caused by a dimorphic fungus, *Coccidioides immitis*, that is found in the soil of the Western Hemisphere. Endemic areas in the United States are confined to the southwestern states, including Texas, New Mexico, Arizona, and California.

Genitourinary involvement occurs with disseminated disease. Autopsy studies[15] of patients with disseminated coccidioidomycosis indicate that renal involvement occurs in approximately 60% of the cases. Fungal involvement of the kidney is confined to the cortex as small miliary granulomas or microabscesses. Large, obstructive lesions within the renal pelvis do not occur as with other fungal infections. The radiographic findings of advanced renal coccidioidomycosis are similar to those of renal tuberculosis. They include infundibular stenosis, blunted or sloughed calices, and calcified granulomas.

Antifungal chemotheraphy is indicated for those at high risk for severe coccidioidomycosis and those with recognized disseminated disease. Currently available antifungal agents for use in treatment of coccidioidomycosis include amphotericin B, fluconazole, and ketoconazole. In the pediatric patient with rapidly progressing coccidioidomycosis, it is generally agreed that amphotericin B should be administered.

Parasitic infections of the urinary tract

Schistosomiasis

Schistosomiasis is a parasitic disease that infects more than 200 million individuals, primarily children and young adults. Urinary schistosomiasis, or bilharziasis, is a vascular parasitic infection caused by the blood fluke *Schistosoma haematobium*. The disease is endemic in Egypt and has spread to areas of Africa, Asia, South America, and the Caribbean. Prevalence is increasing in many areas, as population density increases and new irrigation projects provide broader habitats for vector snails. Rare cases are seen in the United States and always originate from an endemic area.

Humans are infected through contact with water contaminated with crecariae, the free-living infective stage of the parasite. These organisms emerge from infected snails and penetrate the intact human skin. The crecariae change into schistosomula in the subcutaneous tissues and then migrate to the portal circulation where they reach sexual maturity. Adult worms then migrate to the perivesical and periureteral venous plexus. Upon fertilization, female worms deposit eggs in the small venules which eventually reach the lumen of the urinary tract. Eggs are passed into freshwater, where they hatch, infect freshwater snails, and begin the cycle anew (Figure 8.1).

Humans become infected with *Schistosoma* after coming in contact with contaminated water. Children of any age are most at risk due to activities such as swimming, bathing, and drinking this water. Acute schistosomiasis occurs between 3 and 9 weeks after infection and coincides with deposition of eggs in the bladder wall. The classic findings are terminal hematuria and dysuria. Bleeding can be so severe as to result in anemia. During the inactive phase of the infection, fibrosis and contracture of the bladder and distal ureter occur. The disease process is insidious and gross hydroureteronephrosis with renal insufficiency may occur before clinical symptoms appear.

Vester et al[16] recently defined the prevalence of schistosomiasis infection in an endemic region of Mali by screening 824 villagers. Infection ranged from 77% in adolescents to 51% in adults older than 40 years of age. Intensity of infection was generally low, with 91% excreting less than 100 ova per 10 ml

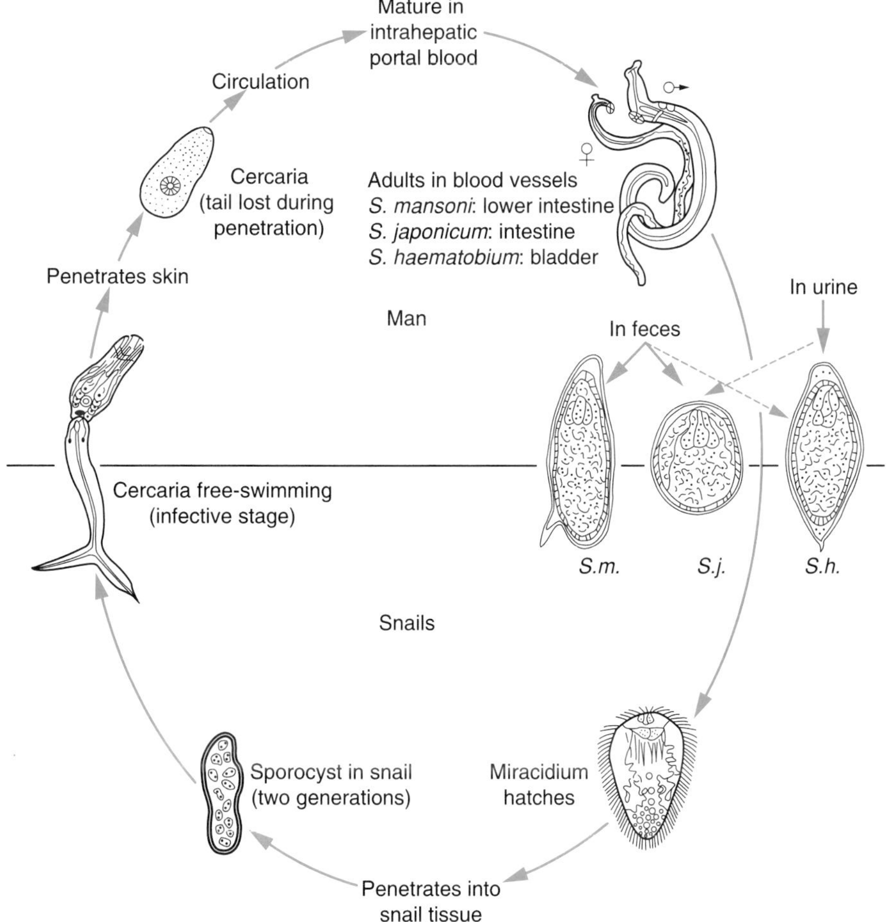

Figure 8.1 The life cycle of the schistosome. (Used with permission of the US Department of Health & Human Services, Public Health Services Publications, US Government Printing Office, Washington, DC, 1964.)

urine. Bladder wall enlargement and irregularities, bladder masses, and dilatation of the upper tracts were found ultrasonographically in approximately one-third of the individuals. Bladder lesions were more frequent in children than adults and correlated well with the intensity of the infection in younger age groups. The prevalence of urinary tract pathology dropped significantly with age, suggesting that either spontaneous resolution of urinary tract pathology occurs or the incidence in the population is increasing.

Schistosoma eggs produce a pronounced eosinophilic infiltrate within the bladder wall. As the disease progresses, collagen infiltration of the bladder occurs. There is deposition of calcareous material and ultimately sclerosis of the bladder due to calcification. Mucosal hyperplasia, squamous metaplasia, and epithelial dysplasia of the urothelium may occur at any stage of the disease process. Involvement of the trigone and bladder neck is most pronounced. Eventual bladder neck fibrosis may lead to outlet obstruction. Stasis of urine and urinary infections can predispose these patients to vesical calculi, whereas chronic bladder irritation predisposes these patients to squamous cell carcinoma. Vesicoureteral reflux is commonly reported in up to 50% of these patients as a result of fibrosis and lateral displacement of the intramural ureter.[17]

The diagnosis of schistosomiasis is established by the presence of terminal-spined eggs in the urine. A 24-hour urine collection with microscopic examination of the sediment is recommended. If infection is suspected and evaluation of the urine is negative, then cystoscopy and bladder biopsy may be performed. Peripheral blood examination will usually show eosinophilia. Anemia may be present with chronic infection due to destruction of erythrocytes by the blood fluke.

Calcification of the bladder wall presenting an eggshell appearance on plain film of the lower abdomen is classic for chronic urinary schistosomiasis. Hydronephrosis secondary to ureteral stricture may be found on imaging studies of the urinary tract. On cystoscopic evaluation of the bladder, bilharzial tubercles predominate over the trigone and posterior bladder wall.[17] Overdistention of the bladder results in bleeding. In patients with chronic disease, fibrosis and calcification of the tubercles in the submucosa form dull, granular 'sandy patches' that resemble grains of sand under water.

Various drugs are available for the treatment of urinary schistosomiasis. Most carry with them significant side effects. Management of children with schistosomiasis should be based on an appreciation of the intensity of the infection and the extent of the disease. The current drug of choice is praziquantel, which is effective against all species of *Schistosoma*. It is administered orally as a single or divided dose to a total of 40–60 mg/kg.[18]

Surgical intervention in schistosomiasis should be reserved until the effects of medical management can be assessed. Fibrosis and contracture of the bladder may require autoaugmentation, intestinal augmentation, or bladder replacement. Bilharzial strictures of the lower ureter can produce obstructive uropathy. Extensive fibrosis of the ureteral wall and the bladder mucosa usually precludes ureteroneocystostomy by traditional submucosal tunneling. Bazeed et al[19] suggest a method of partial flap ureteroneocystostomy to alleviate the obstruction. They report it to be effective in improving or stabilizing the upper tracts in 83% of individuals. Vesicoureteral reflux may develop in as many as 30% of these individuals after surgery.

Echinococcosis

Echinococcosis is the most prevalent human cestode infection in the world. It is commonly called hydatid cyst disease. There is virtually no part of the human anatomy that is immune from hydatid cyst disease. It is caused by the dog tapeworm *Echinococcus granulosus*. Although uncommon in the USA, it is endemic in the sheep-raising areas of the world such as Argentina, Australia, Spain, and Greece.

Humans are an intermediate host for the larval eggs of the adult tapeworm. The adult tapeworm lives in the intestinal tracts of dogs and sheds larval eggs which are excreted in the dog feces. Humans, as well as sheep, cattle, and pigs, may accidentally ingest these larval eggs through orofecal contamination. Dogs initially acquire the disease by swallowing the parasite scolices, which have become encysted in the liver or lungs of sheep, thus completing the life cycle of this parasitic worm.

In humans, the larval eggs pass through the intestinal wall and are widely disseminated throughout the body. Dissemination may occur by direct, vascular, or lymphatic invasion.[20] The primary organ affected in humans is the liver. Genitourinary involvement has been documented in the kidney, ureter, bladder, prostate, and epididymis.[21] The most common location for hydatid cyst disease in humans is the kidney. It is estimated that approximately 3% of all echinococcal infection involves the kidney.[22]

The largest series of pediatric echinococcosis was reported by Auldist and Myers,[23] who document 114 cases of hydatid cyst disease. Children of all ages were infected; however, manifestations of the disease are infrequently evident in children under 5 years of age. This is probably a result of the slow growth pattern of the hydatid cyst. The growth rate of hydatid cysts is estimated at 1 cm/year.[24] The cyst is typically very large at the time of initial presentation. The most common site of genitourinary infestation in the pediatric population is also the kidney. Hydatid cysts of the kidney usually present as a painful flank mass. Microscopic hematuria is present in the majority of the cases. Acute flank pain may be caused by rupture of the hydatid cyst into the collecting system. The passage of scolices (daughter cysts) may be associated with gross hematuria and urinary obstruction.[25]

Sonography has proved to be the most valuable tool in the diagnosis of hydatid disease. Hydatid cysts are easily uncovered on ultrasonographic evaluation of the abdomen in children. The coexistence of hydatid disease in other organs assists in the diagnosis. Plain films or computed tomography (CT) of the abdomen and pelvis may also reveal calcification within the walls of these cysts. The diagnosis of echinococcosis is usually suspected when there is a history of contact with sheep dogs in an endemic area of the world.

As humans are infected with only an intermediate stage of *Echinococcus*, the actual parasite cannot be routinely recovered from any easily accessible body fluid. If the hydatid cyst has ruptured into the collecting system, the recovery of scolices from the urine is pathognomonic for genitourinary echinococcosis. Serologic studies can also be useful in confirming the diagnosis of echinococcosis. Apt and Knierim[26] report that eosinophilia is present in one-third of the children affected with echinococcosis. Indirect hemagglutination and enzyme-linked immunosorbent assay (ELISA) testing are the most sensitive immunologic methods to diagnose human hydatidosis; however, false-positive reactions with other parasitic infections are possible.[20] Immunoelectrophoresis to detect specific antibodies against antigens isolated from hydatid cyst fluid is currently the most specific method of diagnosis of echinococcosis.[27]

Albendazole is the preferred drug for medical management of cystic hydatidosis. This drug therapy (15 mg/kg/day divided in three doses for 28 days) may be repeated for as many as four courses with 15 day drug-free intervals. A positive response may be seen in 40–60% of pediatric patients treated.[24] Ultrasonographic indications of successful therapy include flattening of the cyst, increase in echogenicity, and detachment of membranes from the cyst capsule. The factors predictive of success with chemotherapy are age of the cyst (>2 years old), low internal complexity of the cyst, and small size.[28]

Although previously thought to be contraindicated because of risk of anaphylaxis, percutaneous drainage of cysts under ultrasound guidance during albendazole therapy has become increasingly more successful for complete resolution of cystic disease. Spillage of cyst fluid is uncommon during aspiration. Nevertheless, systemic anaphylactic reactions are always possible with spillage of cyst fluid.

Surgical therapy is also an option for solitary lesions or failed medical management. Considerable care must be taken at the time of surgical resection to assure that there is no rupture of the cyst or spillage of cyst fluid during removal, as viable protoscolices may contaminate the surgical field, each capable of forming a secondary cyst wherever it lodges. There is also a risk of developing anaphylaxis as a result of spillage of cyst fluid at the time of surgical resection.

Enterobiasis

Pinworm infestation (enterobiasis) is caused by the nematode *Enterobius vermicularis*. Humans are infected by ingesting the eggs, which are usually carried on fingernails, clothing, or bedding. The adult worm lives in the large intestines of humans. The gravid adult female worm migrates at night to the rectum and deposits her eggs in the perianal and perineal skin. Perianal irritation during oviposition by female worms induces scratching. Eggs carried underneath the fingernails promotes reinfection and dissemination of the disease to others. The peak age of infection is between 5 and 14 years of age.

Enterobiasis has been implicated as a factor in acute and chronic urinary tract infections (UTIs). In a study of female children, Kropp et al[29] demonstrated that 22% of girls with documented UTIs had pinworm infestations compared with only 5% of an age-matched control population. They also report that the recovery of pinworms from the perianal region is higher in girls with enteric organisms present on a swab of their introitus.

Definitive diagnosis is established by either finding the parasitic eggs or recovering worms. Eggs can be easily detected by pressing adhesive tape against the perianal region early in the morning. The tape is then applied to a glass slide and it is examined under low-power magnification. Repeated examinations, usually totaling three, are necessary to make a negative diagnosis.

Drug therapy should be given to all infected individuals. Pyrantel pamoate (11 mg/kg or maximum dose of 1 g) with a repeat dose at 2 weeks is the drug treatment of choice. Mebendazole (100 mg dose) with a repeat dose at 2 weeks is an alternative treatment. Neither is recommended in children under 2 years of age. Kropp et al[29] report a greater than 50% success rate in eradicating multiple recurrent UTIs in girls with concomitant pinworm infestation when the infestation is definitively treated.

Other inflammatory diseases of the urinary tract

Chlamydial infection

Chlamydia are obligate intracellular bacteria that are distinguished by a unique developmental cycle. Although they possess their own DNA and RNA, contain ribosomes, and have a cell wall, they lack the ability to generate adenosine triphosphate (ATP) and are therefore considered an energy parasite. *Chlamydia* alternate between an infectious metabolically inactive extracellular form, the elementary body (EB), and a non-infectious, metabolically active form, the reticulate body (RB). It is the EB that binds to specific receptor proteins on the cell membrane and enters the cell by endocytosis. Within 12 hours of ingestion, the EB then differentiates into the RB form and undergoes binary fission. This results in the typical intracytoplasmic inclusion bodies characteristic of a chlamydial infection. After approximately 36 hours, the RB differentiates back into an EB and is then released from the cell by a process of exocytosis.

Chlamydia trachomatis is the only one of the four chlamydial species that commonly infects the human genitourinary tract and causes human oculogenital diseases. *Chlamydia trachomatis* is thought to be responsible for the majority of non-gonococcal urethritis and pelvic inflammatory diseases in adolescents. Rettig and Nelson[30] also documented the coexistence of *Chlamydia* in boys with anogenital gonorrhea.

Chlamydial infections in children should be divided into two categories: perinatally transmitted infections and sexually transmitted infections in older children. Cervical chlamydial infections are reported in approximately 25% of pregnant women. Active chlamydial infections at the time of pregnancy may be transmitted to the infant at the time of vaginal delivery. The risk of transmission from mother to child is about 50%.[31] Conjunctivitis and pneumonia are the most common perinatally transmitted chlamydial infections. Genitourinary sites of perinatal transmission include the vagina and urethra. Perinatally transmitted vaginal, urethral, or rectal infections may persist for 3 years with minimal or no symptoms; therefore, the presence of *Chlamydia* is not necessarily an indication of child abuse.

The most common chlamydial infections in older infants and children include vaginitis in girls and urethritis and epididymitis in boys. In boys, the most common symptom of chlamydial urethritis is a clear mucoid urethral discharge. It may be associated with or without urinary urgency and frequency. In girls, acute inflammatory changes in the vagina or cervix may lead to mucopurulent discharge.

The definitive diagnosis of chlamydial infection includes isolation by culture of the organism from the urethra in boys and endocervical region in girls. Several non-culture methods have also been approved by the US Food and Drug Administration (FDA) and include a direct fluorescent antibody test or an enzyme immunoassay. Newer tests for the diagnosis of chlamydial infections include a DNA probe and a polymerase chain reaction assay. These two assays have not yet been approved for testing in children.

Antibiotics are the mainstay of therapy for chlamydial infections in children. These antimicrobials, usually sulfonamides, erythromycin, and tetracyclines, are typically given for 10–14 days; tetracyclines should not be administered to children under the age of 8 years because of the resulting dental discoloration that may occur.

Viral cystitis

Viral cystitis causes irritative voiding symptoms and hematuria in infants and children. In the toilet-trained and older child, it is characterized by severe urinary frequency, urgency, incontinence, and gross hematuria with a negative urine culture for bacteria. Severe hemorrhagic viral cystitis is seen more frequently in pediatric patients undergoing bone marrow transplantation.[32] Viral cystitis also commonly occurs in the child infected with HIV. Viral infections can often be life threatening in these immunocompromised patients.

The usual causative viruses are adenovirus types 11 and 21, influenza A, and cytomegalovirus.[33] Studies of acute hemorrhagic cystitis in Japanese and US children revealed adenovirus type 11 as the most common cause. It was noted that 51% of the Japanese children and 23% of the US children had adenoviruria during their episode of hemorrhagic cystitis. In both populations male outnumbered female patients by a ratio of nearly 2–3:1.[33] Viral shedding may continue throughout the duration of the illness and may last from 4 days to 2 weeks. Herpes zoster involving the bladder may also cause bladder irritative symptoms.

The diagnosis of adenoviral cystitis can be made by the immunofluorescence of adenoviral antigen in exfoliated bladder epithelial cells in the urine of these patients, although this is not commonly done.[34] Since viral cystitis is not an ascending infection, routine voiding cystourethrography (VCUG) as part of the evaluation is not necessary if the diagnosis is confirmed. Radiographic changes within the bladder are remarkable and often resemble that of a bladder sarcoma, and ultrasonography may show a diffusely thickened bladder wall (Figure 8.2). These changes usually resolve within 2–3 weeks. If complete resolution of sonographic bladder wall thickening occurs, then cystoscopy is unnecessary. These infections are self-limited and supportive care with hydration is often all that is necessary.

Polyoma BK virus is frequently identified in the urine of bone marrow transplant patients with hemorrhagic cystitis.[35] The diagnosis of BK viruria is made by identification of epithelial cells within the urine containing intranuclear inclusion bodies suggestive of BK virus and a positive polymerase chain reaction test for BK virus in the urine. Arthur et al[36] report that the viruria occurred exclusively in patients who were seropositive at transplantation, indicating a reactivation of the virus. Many immunocompromised patients do not respond to traditional therapies for hemorrhagic cystitis and may progress to acute renal failure (Figure 8.3), which may be fatal.[37]

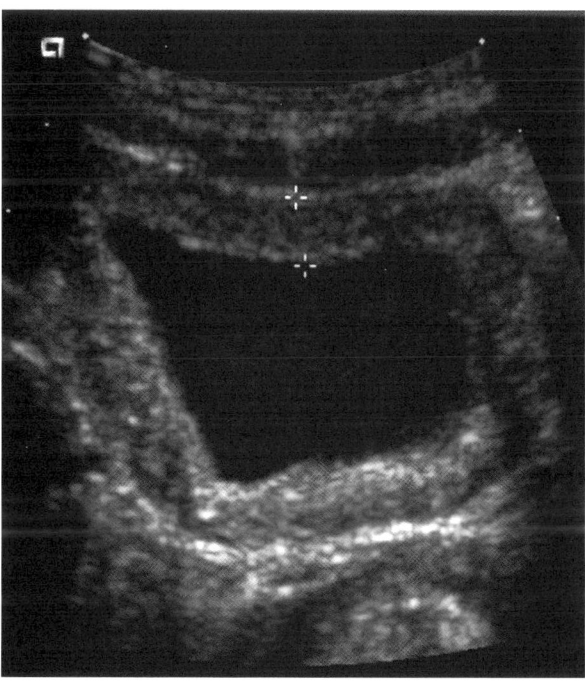

Figure 8.2 Diffusely thickened bladder wall of a 6-year-old boy with adenovirus cystitis.

The immunocompromised pediatric patient may require additional management. The use of ribavirin, an intravenous antiviral agent, has been suggested for treatment of acute adenovirus hemorrhagic cystitis.[38] If treatment with aggressive fluid hydration and forced diuresis with furosemide has failed to control symptoms of hemorrhagic cystitis, some clinicians have advocated the instillation of prostaglandin E_1 into the bladder for up to 7 days[39] before resorting to chemical fulguration with alum or formalin for those with intractable bleeding. Laszlo et al[40] have recommended direct instillations of prostaglandin E_2 into the bladder of patients infected with BK virus presenting with hemorrhagic cystitis. They report resolution of hematuria in all cases within 5 days of initial treatment. Novel therapies such as hyperbaric oxygen treatment have also been reported in cases that are refractory to all conventional treatments.[41]

Eosinophilic cystitis

Eosinophilic cystitis is a rare inflammatory disorder of the urinary bladder, also characterized by irritative voiding symptoms. Symptoms are non-specific, with the most common being dysuria, frequency, lower abdominal discomfort, and hematuria.[42] Children may present with a palpable suprapubic mass on physical examination. Occasionally, this may be mistaken for a pelvic sarcoma.[43] Often the child will have a history of allergies. Eosinophils in the urine or peripheral blood eosinophilia, although diagnostically helpful, are frequently not found.[44]

Imaging studies of the bladder usually begin with sonography. Focal thickening of the bladder wall may be evident as well as hydronephrosis and hydroureter if the lesion affects the region of the ureteral orifice. These findings are similar to those of bladder sarcoma.[45] The definitive diagnosis is established by cystoscopy and bladder biopsy. Cystoscopic findings include erythematous, velvety, raised plaques. The

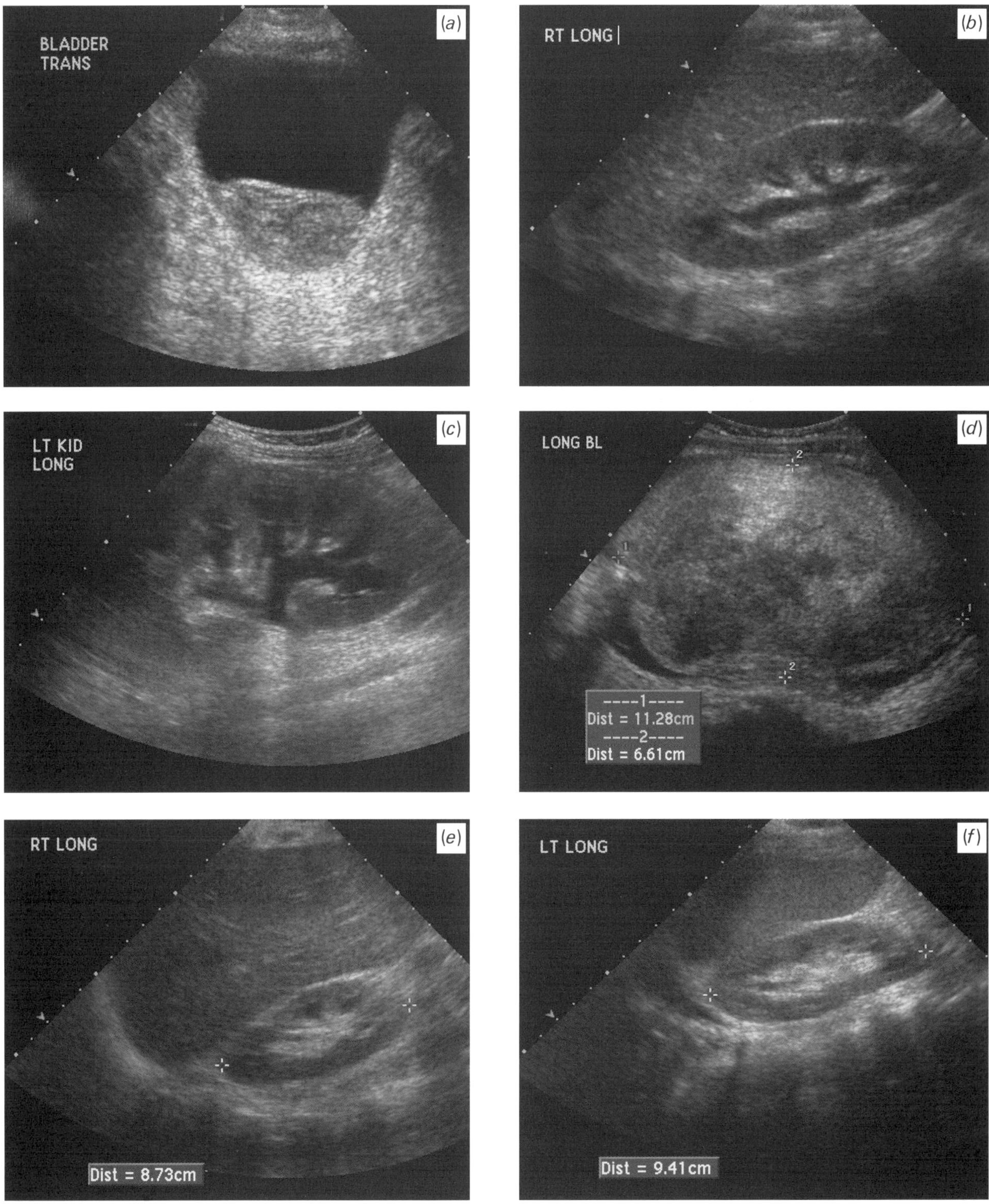

Figure 8.3 Urinary sonography of a 4-year-old boy s/p status post bone marrow transplant with hemorrhagic cystitis due to BK viruria. (*a–c*) Bladder, right kidney, and left kidney at time of initial presentation; (*d–f*) bladder, right kidney, and left kidney at time of death due to renal failure.

mucosa is often edematous with areas of ulceration.[46] Eosinophilic cystitis in children affects all parts of the bladder. Urethral involvement has been seen in only one case.[47]

Biopsy shows a classic eosinophilic infiltration in the lamina propria and muscle layers of the bladder. There may be muscle necrosis or significant muscle fibrosis. Giemsa stain for eosinophils and trichrome stain for muscle fibrosis are helpful in making the diagnosis.[48] Electron microscopy is also a useful diagnostic aid. If eosinophils are degenerating, ultrastructural examination may be the only way of documenting their presence.

The true etiology of eosinophilic cystitis remains unknown. An immunoglobulin E (IgE)-mediated allergic cause has been suggested given the strong allergic histories of the patients. Food allergens, drugs, and other substances have been implicated.[49] It has been postulated that various inciting agents such as bacteria and foreign protein act as antigenic stimuli in the bladder to produce an eosinophilic infiltration. The antigens form immune complexes, resulting in the release of lysosomes that break down bladder tissue and result in inflammation.

The treatment of eosinophilic cystitis involves removing the antigenic stimulus if present and identifiable. Identification of the antigenic stimulus may be difficult in a pediatric population. In a cohort of 8 pediatric patients who presented with eosinophilic cystitis, an identifiable cause (i.e. parasitic infection) could be found in only one case. The role of antihistamines and steroids is unclear. Sutphin and Middleton[50] reported that of these 8 patients with biopsy-proven eosinophilic cystitis, only 2 received antihistamines and steroids. These individuals showed resolution of their symptoms and radiographic findings within 2 weeks. The other untreated pediatric patients also resolved their symptoms; however, the mean interval to resolution was greater than 7 weeks. The prognosis for children with eosinophilic cystitis is generally very good. Almost all reported cases in the literature resolved within 12 weeks.

Despite the apparent self-limited course of eosinophilic cystitis, it should be kept in mind that recurrence of this disease is possible. Documented recurrences have been reported several years after the initial event.[51] It has been hypothesized that local surgical trauma to the bladder or an anesthetic agent may be the cause for recurrence. A recommendation for pretreatment with steroids and antihistamines prior to bladder surgery has been made for patients with a previous history of eosinophilic cystitis.[51]

Malacoplakia

Malacoplakia is an unusual benign granulomatous condition that was first recognized by Michaelis and Gutmann in 1902.[52] It has been postulated that the cause is the defective digestion of phagocytosed bacteria due to an intracellular abnormality of macrophage function.[53] Microscopically, malacoplakia consists of large macrophages mixed with lymphocytes and plasma cells. Michaelis–Gutmann bodies are evident on histologic evaluation. They are rounded intracytoplasmic inclusions with a concentric 'owl-eye' appearance (Figure 8.4). The Michaelis–Gutmann bodies contain incompletely digested bacterial components mineralized with iron and calcium phosphate salts.

In an adult population, malacoplakia affects the bladder in about 40% of cases.[55] Conversely, in a pediatric population, a wide variety of organs such as the tongue, gastrointestinal tract, lungs, brain, adrenals, and retroperitoneum may be involved, but the most common genitourinary site appears to be the kidney as opposed to the bladder. Although Witherington et al[54] describe a case of bladder malacoplakia in a child with recurrent UTIs, vesicoureteral reflux, and a selective IgA deficiency, in general renal malacoplakia is reported more frequently and may involve one or both kidneys.

Pediatric genitourinary malacoplakia occurs in the setting of recurrent UTIs, usually with *Escherichia coli*.[55] Renal malacoplakia is suspected in the pediatric patient when response to traditional antimicrobial therapy does not occur. These patients often have persistent nephromegaly without abscesses demonstrated by either ultrasonography or CT. Diagnosis is usually confirmed by renal biopsy (either open or percutaneous), showing chronic parenchymal inflammation with Michaelis–Gutmann bodies. Recent reports[56]

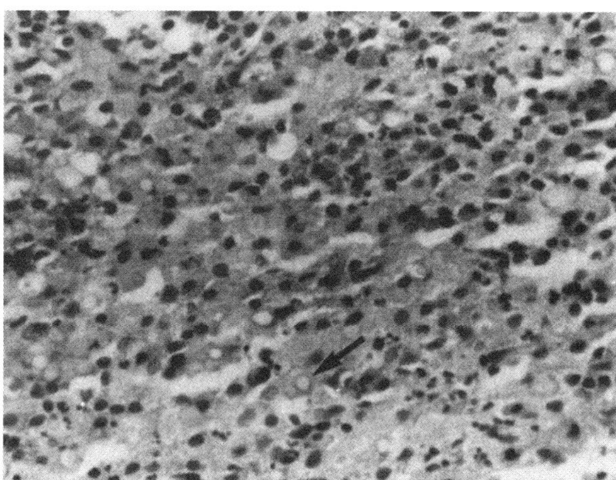

Figure 8.4 Bladder biopsy from a 2.5-year-old boy with *E. coli* urinary tract infection and hematuria. Inflammatory reaction with Michaelis–Gutmann body (arrow) seen in the lamina propria. (Reproduced with permission of Witherington et al.[54])

have confirmed the diagnosis by cytologic evaluation of a renal fine-needle aspirate.

Previously, bilateral renal malacoplakia in the pediatric population was considered a fatal disease. Unilateral disease was frequently treated with nephrectomy. Honjo et al[57] suggest a conservative treatment plan consisting of an immunomodulating regimen. Patients should receive antimicrobial therapy using an antimicrobial agent with intracellular activity (i.e. trimethoprim–sulfamethoxasole), with immunomodulating pulse therapy with methylprednisolone and intravenous G-CSF (granulocyte colony-stimulating factor). If a patient is on immunosuppressive therapy, they recommend appropriate reductions. With the advent of such treatment, nephrectomy may no longer be mandatory in renal malacoplakia and the disease is no longer fatal in the pediatric population.

Other inflammatory diseases of the genitourinary tract

Epididymitis

Epididymitis has been traditionally thought of as a rare occurrence in a pediatric population. It results from an inflammatory reaction of the epididymis to an infectious agent, a chemical irritant, or a non-specific cause. Although infection with bacteria or viral organisms is thought to be the cause of epididymitis, the majority of documented cases are not associated with culture-proven UTIs.[58] Sterile urine in the epididymis may also be sufficient to incite an inflammatory reaction. Epididymal infection may therefore occur as a result of retrograde passage of urine through the ejaculatory ducts,[59] hematogenous spread from a systemic infection, or direct extension from a pre-existing orchitis.

Boys with epididymitis usually present with scrotal pain and edema. They are exquisitely tender to palpation in the region of the epididymis and the vas deferens. A reactive hydrocele may also be present. The differential diagnosis of epididymitis in a child must always include testicular torsion, torsion of an appendix testis, and idiopathic scrotal edema. The onset of pain in boys with epididymitis is often more insidious than in boys with torsion of the testis or appendix testis. Careful physical examination and radiologic imaging studies with either Doppler ultrasound or radionuclide testicular scanning will often aid in making the correct diagnosis. If a definitive diagnosis of epididymitis cannot be arrived at, then surgical exploration may be required to exclude testicular torsion.

The use of a urinalysis in making the diagnosis of epididymitis would seem to be a valuable discriminator; however, it is often inconclusive. Gislason et al[60] showed that only 24% of patients with epididymitis had greater than 10 white blood cells per high power field on urinalysis at the time of presentation. Urinalyses have also been abnormal in 10% of boys that present with testicular torsion.[61] Urine cultures are also unrewarding in making the diagnosis of epididymitis, as only 12.5% were positive in the cohort of boys with epididymitis that were retrospectively studied by Gislason et al.[60]

The evaluation of a boy with epididymitis should not end once the diagnosis has been confirmed. This relatively rare problem in boys is often enigmatic in its etiology. In prepubertal boys, infection in the epididymis may result from an anatomic defect such as a urethral obstruction (urethral valves or meatal stenosis) or an ectopic ureter draining into the seminal vesicle or vas deferens.[62] Urologic investigational procedures after resolution of the inflammation should be performed. Urologists vary widely in their recommendations for radiologic examinations. Most agree that at a minimum an upper tract evaluation with an ultrasound should be performed for culture-proven bacterial epididymitis. Excretory urography would be the imaging study of choice for an ectopic ureter draining to the seminal vesicles, while VCUG would demonstrate urethral anomalies and reflux of urine into the ejaculatory ducts. If the epididymitis was associated with a documented bacterial UTI, VCUG should be performed.

Dysfunctional voiding in older boys has been proposed as an etiology for epididymitis.[63] External sphincter spasm is thought to facilitate retrograde urine flow through the vas deferens. A report of 56 boys with epididymitis revealed that nearly 25% had dysfunctional voiding tendencies associated with epididymitis. Therefore, the addition of a detailed voiding history and use of non-invasive urodynamic testing with uroflow, patch electromyography, and ultrasonographic residual urine assessment has been advocated for boys over the age of 5 years that present with epididymitis. Congenital urologic anomalies are a less frequent cause of epididymitis in the absence of documented bacterial infection.

The treatment of acute epididymitis includes scrotal support and elevation, and analgesic and anti-inflammatory medications. If a bacterial infection is likely, an antibiotic may be started after obtaining a urine culture. Once the acute infection is treated, age-appropriate studies to determine the etiology of the epididymitis should be undertaken.

Vulvovaginitis

Vulvovaginal inflammation is the most common gynecologic complaint of the prepubertal girl. Most cases are initially treated by the primary care physician, with referral to the pediatric urologic specialist only when symptoms persist.

The majority of girls have a profuse, thick vaginal discharge during the newborn period that is primarily a response to the perinatal stimulation of circulating maternal hormones. This should not be mistaken for a pathologic process. At puberty, both the vulvar and vaginal tissues are once again stimulated by circulating estrogens and therefore swelling and discharge may be expected.

Vulvovaginitis is most commonly seen in prepubertal females between the ages of 2 and 7 years. The child is typically brought to the physician with complaints of discharge, discomfort, pruritus, and often urinary symptoms such as burning with voiding. The parents frequently note a discharge present in the child's diaper or undergarments. An abnormal odor and/or redness of the vulva may also be described.

There are several reasons to explain why young girls are particularly susceptible to vulvovaginitis. Anatomically, the vulva of the young girl is relatively unprotected, lacking the labial fat pads and pubic hair of the postpubertal girl. Vulvar skin is also thin, sensitive, and easily irritated by minor trauma. In addition, the vaginal mucosa is also thin in this age group. The vaginal cavity in these prepubertal girls is also an excellent culture medium for bacteria with its neutral pH and warm, moist environment. These obvious structural and biologic differences make the vulvovaginal environment of prepubertal girls particularly sensitive to inflammation. In addition, children tend to have poor hygiene habits when compared with adolescents. They do not practice good handwashing and often play in areas that expose them to dirt and sand, creating chronic irritation of the vulva. The presence of a foreign body or suspected sexual abuse must also be considered in the list of risk factors for vulvovaginitis in the prepubertal girl.[64]

In evaluating the young child with vulvovaginitis, the preceding risk factors should be kept in mind. A complete history and detailed perineal examination must be performed. The history should include information concerning the onset of the condition and any therapies previously instituted for treatment. A history of potential chemical irritants should be elicited (i.e. bubble baths, soaps, powders). A previous surgical history and family history of diabetes, eczema, or contact sensitivities should be addressed. The child's social setting should also be reviewed for information regarding potential child abuse (i.e. primary care giver, day care, contact with older children). The physical examination should look for evidence chronic illness, dermatologic problems, or traumatic injury. Most girls can be comfortably examined in the frog-leg position without the aid of sedation. Some sexual abuse experts recommend a knee–chest position for a complete examination. Cultures may be obtained by a sterile saline-moistened swab or a saline flush of the vaginal introitus. If bleeding or malodorous discharge raises the issue of a foreign body, then formal vaginoscopy may need to be undertaken under anesthesia. If a persistent and continuous flow from the vaginal introitus is present, then an ectopic ureter may enter the differential diagnosis. In this situation, ultrasonography or excretory urography will assist in confirming the diagnosis.

The treatment of vulvovaginitis depends entirely on the etiology of the inflammation. Non-specific vaginitis accounts for the majority of these prepubertal cases. It is thought to involve alterations in the normal flora of the vagina, resulting in vulvar and distal vaginal inflammation. The vagina of a prepubertal girl is typically colonized with the same variety of bacteria as observed in older women. It may be appropriate to request colony counts on all organisms recovered from culture, as overgrowth by one particular organism may warrant antimicrobial therapy directed at that organism. Routine treatment of non-specific vaginitis is usually directed toward improved hygiene, avoidance of irritating stimuli, and techniques to promote drying of the vulva, such as wearing loose-fitting clothing at night.

Specific vaginitis in prepubertal girls may be the result of infections with *Candida albicans* and *Enterobius vermicularis*. Treatments of these infections have been previously outlined. Other causes of specific vaginitis include sexually transmitted organisms, resulting in gonorrhea, chlamydia, and herpes. The treatment of these infections is outlined in Table 8.1. These organisms may be acquired during passage of the newborn through the birth canal or may result from sexual abuse. The age at presentation, along with social history and physical examination, will suggest the etiology.

Table 8.1 Treatment of specific vulvovaginitis

Specific infection	Treatment
Gonorrhea	Ceftriaxone sodium 50–75 mg/kg IM *not to exceed* adult dose of 250 mg IM (one-time IM dose only) If allergic: tetracycline[a] 40 mg/kg for 7 days
Chlamydia	Tetracycline[a] 40 mg/kg PO for 7 days
Gardnerella vaginalis	Metronidazole 15 mg/kg PO
Herpes	Acyclovir 1200 mg/day PO for 7–10 days

[a] Not to be used in children under 8 years old.

Malodorous discharge with associated vaginal bleeding should alert the clinician to the possibility of the presence of a foreign body within the vagina. Eighty percent of all foreign bodies present within the vagina are wads of toilet tissue lodged in the vaginal vault.[65] This may result in both an infectious and inflammatory response. Various other foreign bodies have been recovered, including coins, safety pins, pen tops, fruit pips, and small toys.[66] The probability of foreign bodies being recovered from the vagina of prepubertal girls presenting with vulvovaginitis is 4%.[67] The inflammatory response associated with the presence of the foreign body resolves with the removal of the object.

Idiopathic scrotal and penile edema

It is well known that acute scrotal swelling in children may be primarily due to conditions such as testicular torsion, torsion of the appendix testis, epididymo-orchitis, acute hydrocele, or incarcerated inguinal hernia. There is, however, a lesser-known clinical entity called idiopathic scrotal edema which is characterized by painful scrotal swelling. This is a distinct diagnosis that may be responsible for up to 20% of cases of acute scrotal inflammation.[58] It will typically present in boys between the ages of 1 and 14 years.[68]

The largest single series of idiopathic scrotal edema was reported by Evans and Snyder,[69] in which they retrospectively reviewed 30 cases in 26 patients over an 8-year study period. These boys usually exhibited a sudden 1 day onset of unilateral or bilateral scrotal erythema, which was minimally tender. The edema may frequently extend onto the anterior abdominal wall or the perineum. The child is frequently afebrile, with a normal urinalysis and normal peripheral white blood cell count. Occasionally, eosinophilia is present. When examined early in the process of scrotal swelling, the spermatic cord and testes should feel normal. Characteristically, the clinical findings resolve in 1–2 days. Kaplan[68] reported that in his series of 6 patients, the examiner had the distinct impression that the edema was confined to the superficial layers of the scrotum and that it rarely extended to the penis. Lau and Ong[70] reported that a similar benign and self-limiting condition of the penis exists which is suspected to be a variant of idiopathic scrotal edema.

If the diagnosis is uncertain, then imaging studies may be necessary. Radionuclide testicular scanning or Doppler ultrasonography may be necessary to exclude testicular pathology. On physical examination, this can often be assessed by manipulation of the testis into the superficial inguinal pouch where it can be noted to be palpably normal and non-tender. In rare instances when diagnostic uncertainty still exists, surgical exploration to rule out testicular pathology will reveal a normal testis and epididymis with inflammation confined to the scrotal wall.

There has been much speculation on the etiology of acute idiopathic scrotal edema. Infection with cellulitis was thought to be the etiology until multiple studies revealed negative intraoperative cultures, no elevation of peripheral white blood cell count, and normal urinalysis and culture.[69] The process is also self-limiting and resolves without the use of antibiotics. Insect bites were also entertained as an etiology; however, the lack of a lesion characteristic of a bite has made this less likely. Allergy has also been suggested as an etiology, especially given the presence of eosinophilia in selected cases. In no case, however, has a particular allergen been identified, and the majority of these patients are not characterized as having an allergic diathesis.[68]

Evans and Snyder[69] suggest that idiopathic scrotal edema bears a strong resemblance to angioedema, which is characterized by a localized painless swelling of the subcutaneous tissue of various body parts. The overlying skin is usually normal in color and temperature, but slightly reddened. The chief sensation is one of distention. The individual lesion may persist from 1 to 3 days. Angioedema results from a dilation of small blood vessels, with a transudation of fluid through the capillaries. These vascular changes are believed to be mediated by a local derangement of histamine release. Recommended therapy should consist of reassurance and perhaps a short course of antihistamines.

Interstitial cystitis

Interstitial cystitis is a chronic, debilitating bladder disease of unknown etiology that is seldom reported to occur in children. The first report of the disease was made by Skene in 1878.[71] Since that initial report, there are only a handful of manuscripts that document this disease process in the pediatric population.[72–74]

Patients with interstitial cystitis typically have severe sensory urgency with urinary frequency and bladder pain that may be alleviated with voiding. Cystoscopy after hydrodistention in these patients will show changes varying from petechial hemorrhage in regions with no ulcers to other regions with classic Hunners's ulcers.[75] Middle-aged women constitute the majority of patients with interstitial cystitis. It is less frequently reported in men and rarely documented in children.

Chenoweth and Clawater[72] were the first to report interstitial cystitis in children. In their series of seven cases, they describe the presenting signs and symptoms as:

- day and night frequency of urination
- abdominal pain
- decreased bladder capacity
- negative urinalysis and culture.

In addition, these children were described as being extremely nervous and tense, resting poorly, crying frequently, and having poor appetites. Farkas et al[73] report that the pediatric cases of interstitial cystitis are more common in adolescent girls.

Close et al[74] reported the first large retrospective analysis of interstitial cystitis in the pediatric population, distinguishing this group of patients from the hundreds of individuals that present with voiding dysfunction. They characterized a group of 16 individuals who presented over a 12-year period. Unlike previous pediatric and adult reports, there is less of a female preponderance, with 70% girls and 30% boys in the study population. The most common presenting symptom was urinary frequency and urgency (88%), followed by abdominal pain relieved by voiding (81%). All patients had negative urinalysis and urine culture.

Diagnostic evaluation of pediatric patients suspected of having interstitial cystitis consists of cystoscopy with hydrodistention. Close et al[74] report that all patients had diffuse glomerulations and terminal hematuria after hydrodistention (60–70 cmH_2O for 1–2 minutes). Bladder biopsies, obtained in select cases, revealed chronic inflammation with lymphocytic infiltrate. No mast cells or eosinophils were noted. Urodynamic evaluation demonstrated early bladder filling sensation with no evidence of involuntary bladder contractions. Bladder capacity is also significantly reduced in these individuals. Poor bladder compliance was only documented in approximately 40% of patients.[74]

Treatment of interstitial cystitis in children is met with the same disappointing results as in adults. Bladder distention may temporarily alleviate symptoms.[72–74] Repeated hydrodistentions were required by 50% of the patients reported by Close et al.[74] In rare circumstances chlorpactin instillations have been utilized with temporary and incomplete relief of symptoms.[72] Although bladder augmentation with intestine has been reported as a treatment option,[73] inflammatory changes consistent with interstitial cystitis have been found in the bowel segment on follow-up. Surgical management of this disease in children should be considered only when all other treatment options have failed and the diagnosis has been absolutely confirmed.

References

1. Baley JE, Annable WL, Kliegman RM. Candida endophthalmitis in the premature infant. J Pediatr 1981; 98:458–61.
2. Muller FMC, Groll AH, Walsh TJ. Current approaches to diagnosis and treatment of fungal infections in children infected with HIV. Eur J Pediatr 1999; 158:187–99.
3. Stone HH, Kolb LD, Currie CA et al. Candida sepsis: pathogenesis and principles of treatment. Ann Surg 1974; 179:697–711.
4. Mokaddas EM, Ramadan SA, Abo el Maaty SH et al. Candidemia in pediatric surgery patients. J Chemother 2000; 12:332–8.
5. Kozinn PJ, Taschdjian CL, Goldberg PK et al. Advances in the diagnosis of renal candidiasis. J Urol 1978; 119:184–7.
6. Wise GJ, Goldberg P, Kozinn PJ. Genitourinary candidiasis: diagnosis and treatment. J Urol 1976; 116:778–80.

7. Schonebeck J, Andersson L, Lingardh G, Winblad B. Ureteric obstruction caused by yeast-like fungi. Scand J Urol Nephrol 1970; 4:171–5.
8. Eckstein C, Koss EJ, Koff SA. Anuria in a newborn secondary to bilateral ureteropelvic fungus balls. J Urol 1982; 127:109–10.
9. Wise GJ, Kozinn PJ, Goldberg P. Amphotericin B as a urological irrigant in the management of noninvasive candiduria. J Urol 1982; 128:82–4.
10. Alkalay AL, Srugo I, Blifeld C et al. Noninvasive medical management of fungus ball uropathy in a premature infant. Am J Perinatol 1991; 8:1330–2.
11. Rowen JL, Tate JM. Management of neonatal candidiasis. Pediatr Infect Dis J 1988; 17:1007–11.
12. Pappas PG, Rex JH, Lee J et al. A prospective observational study of candidemia: epidemiology, therapy, and influences on mortality in hospitalized adult and pediatric patients. Clin Infect Dis 2003; 37:634–43.
13. Walmsley S, Devi S, King S et al. Invasive Aspergillus infections in a pediatric hospital: a ten-year review. Pediatr Infect Dis J 1993; 12:673–82.
14. Eisenberg RL, Hedgcock MW, Shanser JD. Aspergillus mycetoma of the renal pelvis associated with UPJ obstruction. J Urol 1977; 118:466–7.
15. Conner WT, Drach GW, Bucher WC. Genitourinary aspects of disseminated coccidioidomycosis. J Urol 1975; 113:82–8.
16. Vester U, Kardorff R, Traore M et al. Urinary tract morbidity due to Schistosoma haematobium infection in Mali. Kidney Int 1997; 52:478–81.
17. Hanash KA, Bissada NK. Genitourinary schistosomiasis, Part I. King Faisal Specialist Hosp Med J 1982; 1:59–64.
18. King CH, Mahmoud AA. Drugs five years later: praziquantel. Ann Intern Med 1989; 110:290–6.
19. Bazeed MA, Ashamalla A, Abd-Alrzek AA et al. Partial flap ureteroneocystostomy for bilharzial strictures of the lower ureter. Urology 1982; 20:237–41.
20. Angulo JC, Escribano J, Diego A et al. Isolated retrovesical and extrarenal retroperitoneal hydatidosis: clinical study of 10 cases and literature review. J Urol 1998; 159:76–82.
21. Halim A, Vaezzadeh K. Hydatid disease of the genitourinary tract. Br J Urol 1980; 52:75–8.
22. Silber SJ, Moyad RA. Renal echinococcus. J Urol 1972; 108:669–72.
23. Auldist AW, Myers NA. Hydatid disease in children. Aust NZ J Surg 1974; 44:402–7.
24. Blanton R. Echinococcosis. In: Behrman RE, Kliegman RM, Arvin AM, eds. Nelson Textbook of Pediatrics. Philadelphia: WB Saunders, 1996: 995–7.
25. Gilsanz V, Lozano F, Jimenez J. Renal hydatid cysts: communicating with collecting system. AJR Am J Roentgenol 1980; 135:357–61.
26. Apt W, Knierim F. An evaluation of the diagnostic tests for hydatid disease. Am J Trop Med Hyg 1970; 19:943–6.
27. Babba H, Messedi A, Masmoudi S et al. Diagnosis of human hydatidosis: comparison between imagery and six serologic techniques. Am J Trop Med Hyg 1994; 50:64–8.
28. Todorov T, Mechkov G, Vutova K et al. Factors influencing the response to chemotherapy for human cystic echinococcosis. Bull WHO 1992; 70:347–58.
29. Kropp KA, Cichocki GA, Bansal NK. Enterobius vermicularis, introital bacteriology and recurrent UTIs in children. J Urol 1978; 120:480–2.
30. Rettig PJ, Nelson JD. Genital tract infection with Chlamydia trachomatis in prepubertal children. J Pediatr 1981; 99:206–10.
31. Hammerschlag MR. Chlamydia. In: Behrman RE, Kliegman RM, Arvin AM, eds. Nelson Textbook of Pediatrics, Philadelphia: WB Saunders, 1996: 827–32.
32. Shields AF, Hackman RC, Fife KH, Corey L, Meyers JD. Adenovirus infections in patients undergoing bone marrow transplantation. N Engl J Med 1985; 312:529–33.
33. Mufson MA, Belshe RB. A review of adenovirus in the etiology of acute hemorrhagic cystitis. J Urol 1976; 115:191–4.
34. Belshe RB, Mufson MA. Identification by immunofluorescence of adinoviral antigen in exfoliated bladder epithelial cells from patients with acute hemorrhagic cystitis. Proc Soc Exp Biol Med 1974; 146:754–8.
35. Leung AY, Suen CK, Lie AK et al. Quantification of polyoma BK viruria in hemorrhagic cystitis complicating bone marrow transplant. Blood 2001; 98:1971–8.
36. Arthur PR, Shah KV, Charache P et al. BK and JC virus infections in recipients of bone marrow transplants. J Infect Dis 1988; 158:536–9.
37. Iwamoto S, Azuma E, Hori H et al. BK virus-associated fatal renal failure following late-onset hemorrhagic cystitis in an unrelated bone marrow transplant. Pediatr Hematol Oncol 2002; 19:255–61.
38. Jurado M, Navarro JM, Hernandez J et al. Adenovirus-associated haemorrhagic cystitis after bone marrow transplantation successfully treated with intravenous ribavirin. Bone Marrow Transplant 1995; 15:651–2.
39. Trigg ME, O'Reilly J, Morgan D et al. Prostaglandin E_1 bladder instillations to control severe hemorrhagic cystitis. J Urol 1990; 143:92–4.
40. Laszlo D, Bosi A, Guidi S et al. Prostaglandin E_2 bladder instillation for the treatment of hemorrhagic cystitis after allogeneic bone marrow transplantation. Haematologica 1995; 80:421–5.
41. Hughes AJ, Schwarer AP, Millar IL. Hyperbaric oxygen in the treatment of refractory haemorrhagic cystitis. Bone Marrow Transplant 1998; 22:585–6.
42. Okafo BA, Jones HW, Dow D et al. Eosinophilic cystitis: pleomorphic manifestations. Can J Surg 1985; 28:17–18.
43. Thijssen A, Gerridzen RG. Eosinophilic cystitis presenting as invasive bladder cancer: comments on pathogenesis and management. J Urol 1990; 144:977–9.
44. Thauscher JW, Shaw DC. Eosinophilic cystitis. Clin Pediatr 1981; 20:741–3.
45. Champion RH, Ackles RC. Eosinophilic cystitis. J Urol 1966; 96:729–32.
46. Littleton RH, Farah RN, Cerny JC. Eosinophilic cystitis: an uncommon form of cystitis. J Urol 1982; 127:132–3.
47. Sujka SK, Fisher JE, Greenfield SP. Eosinophilic cystitis in children. Urology 1992; 40:262–4.
48. Hellstrom HR, Davis BK, Shonnard JW. Eosinophilic cystitis: a study of 16 cases. Am J Clin Pathol 1979; 72:777–84.

49. Wenzl JE, Greene LF, Harris LE. Eosinophilic cystitis. J Pediatr 1994; 64:746–9.
50. Sutphin MS, Middleton AW. Eosinophilic cystitis in children: a self limited process. J Urol 1984; 132:117–19.
51. Axelrod SL, Ring KS, Collins MH et al. Eosinophilic cystitis in children. Urology 1991; 37:549–52.
52. Michaelis L, Gutmann C. Uber einschlusse in blasentumoren. Clin Med 1902; 47:208–16.
53. Curran FT. Malakoplakia of the bladder. Br J Urol 1987; 59:559–63.
54. Witherington R, Branan WJ, Wray BB et al. Malakoplakia associated with vesicoureteral reflux and selective immunoglobin A deficiency. J Urol 1984; 132:975–7.
55. Long JP, Althausen AF. Malakoplakia: a 25 year experience with a review of the literature. J Urol 1989; 141:1328–31.
56. Kapasi H, Robertson S, Futter N. Diagnosis of renal malakoplakia by fine needle aspiration cytology. Acta Cytol 1998; 42:1419–23.
57. Honjo K, Sato T, Matsuo M et al. Renal malakoplakia in a four week old infant. Clin Nephrol 1997; 47:341–4.
58. Qvist O. Swelling of the scrotum in infants and children, and non-specific epididymitis; a study of 158 cases. Acta Chir Scand 1956; 110:417–21.
59. Megalli M, Gursel E, Lattimer JK. Reflux of urine into ejaculatory ducts as a cause of recurring epididymitis in children. J Urol 1972; 108:978–9.
60. Gislason T, Noronha RF, Gregory JG. Acute epididymitis in boys: a 5-year retrospective study. J Urol 1980; 124:533–4.
61. Ransler CW, Allen TD. Torsion of the spermatic cord. Urol Clin North Am 1982; 9:245–50.
62. Siegal A, Snyder HM, Duckett JW. Epididymitis in infants and boys: underlying urogenital anomalies and efficacy of imaging modalities. J Urol 1987; 138:1100–3.
63. Bukowski TP, Lewis AG, Reeves D et al. Epididymitis in older boys: dysfunctional voiding as an etiology. J Urol 1995; 154:762–5.
64. Farrington PF. Pediatric vulvovaginitis. Clin Obstet Gynecol 1997; 40:135–40.
65. Henderson P, Scott R. Foreign body vaginitis caused by toilet tissue. Am J Dis Child 1966; 111:529–32.
66. Hepp J, Everhart W. Foreign body in the immature vagina. Am J Surg 1950; 79:589–91.
67. Paradise J, Willis E. Probability of vaginal foreign body in girls with genital complaints. Am J Dis Child 1985; 139:472–6.
68. Kaplan GW. Acute ideopathic scrotal edema. J Pediatr Surg 1977; 12:647–9.
69. Evans JP, Snyder HM. Idiopathic scrotal edema. Urology 1977; 9:549–51.
70. Lau JTK, Ong GB. Acute idiopathic penile edema: a separate clinical entity. J Urol 1981; 126:704–5.
71. Skene AJC. Cystitis. In: Diseases of the Bladder and Urethra in Women. New York: William Wood and Co., 1878; 167–72.
72. Chenoweth CV, Clawater EW Jr. Interstitial cystitis in children. J Urol 1960; 83:150–2.
73. Farkas A, Waisman J, Goodwin WE. Interstitial cystitis in adolescent girls. J Urol 1976; 118:837 9.
74. Close CE, Carr ME, Burns MW et al. Interstitial cystitis in children. J Urol 1996; 156:860–2.
75. Hunner GL. Elusive ulcer of the bladder: further notes on a rare type of bladder ulcer with a report of 25 cases. Am J Obstet 1918; 78:374–95.

Pain management for the pediatric urologic patient

9

Stephen C Brown and Patricia A McGrath

Introduction

When we were asked to contribute a chapter in a major textbook in urology, I was keen on the idea for several reasons. If you look at many surgical textbooks from 10 years ago, pain was often not even mentioned. In the last few years, pain has made it to the radar screen, but only in a cursory fashion. In this chapter we wish to expand on the surgeon's ability to assess, treat, and more fully understand the complex entity of pain, with the result being to further decrease pain in children. Should a psychological theme in treating pain be explored in a surgical textbook of urology? I feel it is not only important but also essential.

Pain control is an integral component for the pediatric patient undergoing procedures and ongoing care by the urologist. Children may experience many different types of pain from invasive procedures or operations, the cumulative effects of toxic therapies, progressive disease, or psychological factors. While acute postoperative pain is often straightforward to treat, some cases can be complex, with pain resulting from multiple nociceptive and neuropathic components. In addition, several situational factors usually contribute to children's pain, distress, and disability. Thus, to adequately treat pain in children receiving care by the urologist, we must evaluate the primary pain sources. Some cases may require us to ascertain which situational factors are relevant for which children and families, where treatment emphasis would shift accordingly from an exclusive disease-centered framework to a more child-centered focus.

In this chapter, we describe a child-centered framework for understanding and controlling pain for children undergoing procedures and ongoing care by the urologist. Pain control should include regular pain assessments, appropriate analgesics administered at regular dosing intervals, adjunctive drug therapy for symptom and side-effects control, and non-drug interventions to modify the situational factors that can exacerbate pain and suffering. This chapter describes the unique nature of children's pain, including the primary factors that affect their pain and quality of life, presenting guidelines for selecting and administering drug therapy in accordance with the nociceptive and neuropathic components, and recommending practical non-drug therapies for integration within a hospital or home setting.

Guidelines for assessment, analgesic selection and administration, and non-pharmacologic interventions

The principles of analgesic therapy, the guidelines for drug administration, and the guidelines for a supportive cognitive-behavioral approach are those that should be followed in all pediatric care.

Pain assessment

Pain assessment is an integral component of diagnosis and treatment for children. A thorough medical history, physical examination, and assessment of pain characteristics and contributing factors are necessary to establish a correct clinical diagnosis. Subsequent assessments of pain intensity enable us to determine when treatments are effective and to identify those children for whom they are most effective. Healthcare providers need pain measures that are convenient to administer and whose resulting pain scores provide meaningful information about children's pain experiences. An extensive array of pain measures have been developed and validated for use with infants, children, and adolescents.[1–3]

Like adult pain measures, children's pain measures

are classified as physiologic, behavioral, and psychological, depending on what is monitored – physical parameters (e.g. heart rate, sweat index, blood pressure, cortisol level), distress behaviors (e.g. grimaces, cries, protective guarding gestures), or children's own descriptions of what they are experiencing (e.g. words, drawings, numerical ratings). Physiologic and behavioral measures provide indirect estimates of pain because healthcare providers must infer the location and strength of a child's pain solely from his or her responses. In contrast, psychological measures can provide direct information about the location, strength, quality, affect, and duration of the pain.

The criteria for an accurate pain measure are similar to those required for any measuring instrument. A pain measure must be valid, in that it measures a specific aspect of pain, so that changes in pain ratings reflect meaningful differences in a child's pain experience. The measure must be reliable, in that it provides consistent and trustworthy pain ratings, regardless of the time of testing, the clinical setting, or who is administering the measure. The measure must be relatively free from bias, in that children should be able to use it similarly, regardless of differences in how they may wish to please adults. The pain measure should be practical and versatile for assessing different types of pain (e.g. disease-related, procedural pain) in many different children (according to age, cognitive level, cultural background) and for use in diverse clinical and home settings.

Physiologic and behavioral pain scales

Although physiologic parameters can provide valuable information about a child's distress state, more research is required to develop a sensitive system for interpreting how these parameters reflect pain strength. At present, there are no valid physiologic pain scales for children.

Most behavioral pain scales are checklists of the different distress behaviors that children exhibit when they experience a certain type of pain.[1,4,5] To develop these scales, trained healthcare providers carefully observe children when they are in pain (e.g. after surgery) and document any behaviors that seem caused by the pain. They then list these 'presumed pain' behaviors (e.g. crying, facial expression, limb rigidity) on an itemized checklist. Parents complete the pain scale by checking which of the listed behaviors they see when children are ill. On many scales, parents also rate the intensity of the behaviors. The intensity scores for each of the observed behaviors are summed to produce a composite pain score. Although most behavioral scales measure acute pain, recent attention is focused on the need to develop sensitive measures for children who are cognitively or physically impaired.[6]

Psychological pain scales

Psychological or self-report pain scales directly capture a child's subjective experience of pain. Interviews, questionnaires, adjective checklists, and numerous pain intensity scales are available for children, each with some evidence of validity and reliability.[1,7] Clinical interviews are ideally suited for learning about the sensory characteristics of pain, the aversive component, and contributing cognitive, behavioral, and emotional factors. Interviews should also include a simple rating scale to document pain strength. Children choose a level on the scale that best matches the strength of their own pain (i.e. a level on a number or thermometer scale, a number of objects, a mark on a visual analogue scale, a face from a series of faces varying in emotional expression, or a particular word from adjective lists). Pain intensity scales are easy to administer, requiring only a few seconds once children understand how to use them. Many of these scales yield pain scores on a 0–10 scale. Visual and colored analogue scales are versatile for use with acute, recurrent, and chronic pain and provide a convenient and flexible pain measure for use in hospital and at home.

Healthcare providers must consider the age and cognitive ability of a child when selecting a pain scale. Most toddlers (approximately 2 years of age) can communicate the presence of pain, using words learned from their parents to describe the sensations they feel when they hurt themselves. They use concrete analogies to describe their perceptions. Gradually children learn to differentiate and describe three levels of pain intensity: 'a little,' 'some or medium,' and 'a lot'. By the age of 5, most children can differentiate a wider range of pain intensities and many can use simple pain intensity scales.

Children's understanding and descriptions of pain naturally depend on their age, cognitive level, and previous pain experience. Children begin to understand pain through their own hurting experiences; they learn to describe the different characteristics of their pains (intensity, quality, duration, and location) in the same way that they learn specific words to describe different sounds, tastes, smells, and colors. Most children can communicate meaningful information about their pain. Gradually they develop an increasing ability to describe specific pain features – the quality (aching, burning, pounding, sharp), intensity (mild to severe), duration and frequency (a few seconds to years), location (from a diffuse location on their skin to more precise internal localization), and unpleasantness (mild annoyance to an intolerable discomfort). Children's understanding of pain and the language that they use to describe pain comes from the words and expressions used by their families and peers and from characters depicted in books, videos, and movies. (For a more extensive review of developmental factors in children's pain, see References 8–14.)

Physicians should always ask children directly about their pain. Pain onset, location, frequency (if recurring), quality, intensity, accompanying physical symptoms, and pain-related disability should be assessed as part of children's clinical examination. Healthcare providers should also assess relevant situational factors in order to modify their pain-exacerbating impact, especially the factors listed in Table 9.1.

Table 9.1 Situational factors that increase children's acute pain

Cognitive factors
Lack of age-appropriate information about pain source
Inaccurate expectation of uncontrolled pain
Lack of knowledge about practical non-drug therapies
Lack of choice and little perceived control during treatments
Inaccurate information about child's prognosis
Behavioral factors
Overt physical distress
Inconsistent or inappropriate responses from staff or parents during treatments
Altered parenteral and sibling behaviors toward child within the family
Emotional factors
Anticipatory anxiety toward treatments
Heightened distress during treatments
Fear about continuing pain, increasing disability, or death
Frustration about disruption to activities
Depression about condition or treatments

Reprinted with permission from McGrath and Hillier.[15]

Pain management

Oral analgesics

Pain control should include regular pain assessments, appropriate analgesics and adjuvant analgesics administered at regular dosing intervals, adjunctive drug therapy for symptom and side-effects control, and non-drug therapies to modify the situational factors that can exacerbate pain and suffering. Analgesics include acetaminophen, non-steroidal anti-inflammatory drugs (NSAIDs), and opioids. Adjuvant analgesics include a variety of drugs with analgesic properties that were initially developed to treat other health problems, such as anticonvulsants and antidepressants. The use of adjuvant analgesics has become a cornerstone of pain control in pediatric chronic pain. They are especially crucial when pain has a neuropathic component.

The guiding principles of analgesic administration are 'by the ladder', 'by the clock', 'by the child', and 'by the mouth'. 'By the ladder' refers to a three-step approach for selecting drugs according to their analgesic potency based on the child's pain level – acetaminophen to control mild pain, codeine to control moderate pain, and morphine for strong pain.[16] The ladder approach was based on our scientific understanding of how analgesics affect pain of nociceptive origin. If pain persists despite starting with the appropriate drug, recommended doses, and dosing schedule, move up the ladder and administer the next more potent analgesic. Even when children require opioid analgesics, they should continue to receive acetaminophen (and NSAIDs if appropriate) as supplemental analgesics. The analgesic ladder approach is based on the premise that acetaminophen, codeine, and morphine should be available in all countries and that doctors and healthcare providers can relieve pain in the majority of children with a few drugs.

However, increasing attention is focusing on 'thinking beyond the ladder' in accordance with our improved understanding of pain of neuropathic origins.[17,18] Children should receive adjuvant analgesics to more specifically target neuropathic mechanisms. Regrettably, two of the main classes of adjuvant analgesics, antidepressants and anticonvulsants, have unfortunate names. Proper education of healthcare providers, parents, and children should lead to a wider acceptance and use of these medications for pain management. For example, amitriptyline may require 4–6 weeks to affect depression, but often requires only 1–2 weeks to affect pain. The newer classes of antidepressants, the selective serotonin reuptake inhibitors (SSRIs), may be beneficial to treat depression for a child with pain but have not been shown to be beneficial for pain management. The other main class of adjuvant analgesics are the anticonvulsants. The two principal medications used for this purpose in pediatrics are carbamazepine and gabapentin. With gabapentin, the main dose-limiting side effect is sedation, so that a slow titration to maximal dose is required. Because of its greater number of significant side effects, the use of carbamazepine has decreased recently and the use of gabapentin has increased. We still await published studies to support the wide use of gabapentin.

NSAIDs are similar in potency to aspirin. They are used primarily to treat inflammatory disorders and to lessen mild to moderate acute pain. They should be used with caution in patients with hepatic or renal impairment, compromised cardiac function, hypertension (since they may cause fluid retention, edema), and a history of gastrointestinal (GI) bleeding or ulcers. NSAIDs may also inhibit platelet aggregation, and thus must be monitored closely in patients with prolonged bleeding times. NSAIDs have been used for many years in pediatrics and with their minimal side effects, and many advantages (no effect on ventilation, no physical dependence, morphine-sparing effect, etc.), their use should be encouraged.

The specific drugs and doses are determined by the needs of each child. The drugs listed in this chapter are based on guidelines from our institution.[19] Recommended starting doses for analgesic medications to control children's disease-related pain are listed in Table 9.2 and Table 9.3; starting doses for adjuvant analgesic medications to control pain, drug-related side effects, and other symptoms are listed in Table 9.4. (For further review of analgesics and adjuvant analgesics in children, see References 18, 20–23.)

Children should receive analgesics at regular times, 'by the clock', to provide consistent pain relief and prevent breakthrough pain. The specific drug schedule (e.g. every 4 or 6 h) is based on the drug's dura-

Table 9.2 Non-opioid drugs to control pain in children

Drug	Dosage	Comments
Acetaminophen	10–15 mg/kg PO, every 4–6 h	Lacks GI and hematologic side effects; lacks anti-inflammatory effects (may mask infection-associated fever) Dose limit of 65 mg/kg/day or 4 g/day, whichever is less
Ibuprofen	5–10 mg/kg PO, every 6–8 h	Anti-inflammatory activity Use with caution in patients with hepatic or renal impairment, compromised cardiac function or hypertension (may cause fluid retention, edema), history of GI bleeding or ulcers, may inhibit platelet aggregation Dose limit of 40 mg/kg/day; max dose of 2400 mg/day
Naproxen	10–20 mg/kg/day PO, divided every 12 h	Anti-inflammatory activity. Use with caution and monitor closely in patients with impaired renal function. Avoid in patients with severe renal impairment Dose limit of 1 g/day
Diclofenac	1 mg/kg PO, every 8–12 h	Anti-inflammatory activity. Similar GI, renal, and hepatic precautions as noted above for ibuprofen and naproxen Dose limit of 50 mg/dose

Note: Increasing the dose of non-opioids beyond the recommended therapeutic level produces a 'ceiling effect', in that there is no additional analgesia but there are major increases in toxicity and side effects.
IM, intramuscular; PO, by mouth; GI, gastrointestinal.
Reprinted with permission from McGrath and Brown.[20]

Table 9.3 Opioid analgesics: usual starting doses for children

Drug	Equianalgesic dose (parenteral)	Starting dose IV	IV:PO ratio	Starting dose PO/ transdermal	Duration of action
Morphine	10 mg	Bolus dose = 0.05 mg/kg–0.1 mg/kg every 2–4 h Continuous infusion = 0.01–0.04 mg/kg/h	1:3	0.15–0.3 mg/kg/dose every 4 h	3–4 h
Hydromorphone	1.5 mg	0.015–0.02 mg/kg every 4 h	1:5	0.06 mg/kg every 3–4 h	2–4 h
Codeine	120 mg	Not recommended		1.0 mg/kg every 4 h (dose limit 1.5 mg/kg/dose)	3–4 h
Oxycodone	5–10 mg	Not recommended		0.1–0.2 mg/kg every 3–4 h	3–4 h
Meperidine[a]	75 mg	0.5–1.0 mg/kg every 3–4 h	1:4	1.0–2.0 mg/kg every 3–4 h (dose limit 150 mg)	1–3 h
Fentanyl[b]	100 µg	1–2 µg/kg/h as continuous infusion		25 µg patch	72 h (patch)

Note: Doses are for opioid-naive patients. For infants under 6 months, start at one-quarter to one-third the suggested dose and titrate to effect.

Principles of opioid administration:

1. If inadequate pain relief and no toxicity at peak onset of opioid action, increase dose in 50% increments.
2. Avoid IM administration.
3. Whenever using continuous infusion, plan for hourly rescue doses with short-onset opioids if needed. Rescue dose is usually 50–200% of continuous hourly dose. If greater than 6 rescues are necessary in 24-h period, increase daily infusion total by the total amount of rescues for previous 24 h/24. An alternative is to increase infusion by 50%.
4. To change opioids – because of incomplete cross-tolerance: if changing between opioids with short duration of action, start new opioid at 50% of equianalgesic dose. Titrate to effect.
5. To taper opioids – anyone on opioids over 1 week must be tapered to avoid withdrawal: taper by 50% for 2 days, and then decrease by 25% every 2 days. When dose is equianalgesic to an oral morphine dose of 0.6 mg/kg/day, it may be stopped. Some patients on opioids for prolonged periods, may require much slower weaning.

[a]Avoid use in renal impairment. Metabolite may cause seizures.
[b]Potentially highly toxic. Not for use in acute pain control.
PO, by mouth; IV, intravenous; IM, intramuscular.
Modified from McGrath and Brown.[20]

tion of action and the child's pain severity. Although breakthrough pain episodes have been recognized as a problem in adult pain control, they may represent an even more serious problem for children. Unlike adults, who generally realize that they can demand more potent analgesic medications or demand more frequent dosing intervals, children have little control, little awareness of alternatives, and fear that their pain cannot be controlled. They may become progressively frightened, upset, and preoccupied with their symptoms. Thus, it is essential to establish and maintain a therapeutic window of pain relief for children.

Analgesic doses should be adjusted 'by the child'. There is no one dose that will be appropriate for all children with pain. The goal is to select a dose that prevents children from experiencing pain before they receive the next dose. It is essential to monitor the child's pain regularly and adjust analgesic doses as necessary to control the pain. The effective opioid dose to relieve pain varies widely among different children or in the same child at different times. Some children require large opioid doses at frequent intervals to control their pain. If such doses are necessary for effective pain control, and the side effects can be managed by adjunctive medication so that children are comfortable, then the doses are appropriate. Children receiving opioids may develop altered sleep patterns so that they are awake at night, fearful and complaining about pain, and they sleep intermittently throughout the day. They should receive adequate

Table 9.4 Adjuvant analgesics: doses for children

Drug category	Drug, dosage	Indications	Comments
Antidepressants	Amitriptyline, 0.2–0.5 mg/kg PO Titrate upward by 0.25 mg/kg every 2–3 days. Maintenance: 0.2–3.0 mg/kg Alternatives: nortriptyline, doxepin, imipramine	Neuropathic pain (i.e. vincristine-induced, radiation plexopathy, tumor invasion, CRPS-1) Insomnia	Usually improved sleep and pain relief within 3–5 days Anticholinergic side effects are dose-limiting. Use with caution for children with increased risk for cardiac dysfunction
Anticonvulsants	Gabapentin, 5 mg/kg/day PO Titrate upward over 3–7 days. Maintenance: up to 15–50 mg/kg/day PO divided tid. Carbamazepine, Initial dosing: 10 mg/kg/day PO divided od or bid. Maintenance: up to 20–30 mg/kg/day PO divided every 8 h. Increase dose gradually over 2–4 weeks Alternatives: phenytoin, clonazepam	Neuropathic pain, especially shooting, stabbing pain	Side effects: gastro-intestinal upset, ataxia, dizziness, disorientation, somnolence Monitor for hematologic, hepatic, and allergic reactions with carbamazepine
Sedatives, hypnotics, anxiolytics	Diazepam, 0.025–0.2 mg/kg PO every 6 h Lorazepam, 0.05 mg/kg/dose SL Midazolam, 0.5 mg/kg/dose PO administered 15–30 min prior to procedure; 0.05 mg/kg/dose IV for sedation	Acute anxiety, muscle spasm Premedication for painful procedures	Sedative effect may limit opioid use. Other side effects include: depression and dependence with prolonged use
Antihistamines	Hydroxyzine, 0.5 mg/kg PO every 6 h Diphenhydramine, 0.5–1.0 mg/kg PO/IV every 6 h	Opioid-induced pruritus, anxiety, nausea	Sedative side effects may be helpful
Psychostimulants	Dextroamphetamine, methylphenidate, 0.1–0.2 mg/kg bid Escalate to 0.3–0.5 mg/kg as needed	Opioid-induced somnolence Potentiation of opioid analgesia	Side effects include agitation, sleep disturbance, and anorexia Administer second dose in afternoon to avoid sleep disturbances
Corticosteroids	Prednisone, prednisolone, and dexamethasone dosage depends on clinical situation (i.e. dexamethasone initial dosing: 0.2 mg/kg IV. Dose limit 10 mg. Subsequent dose 0.3 mg/kg/day IV divided every 6 h)	Headache from increased intracranial pressure, spinal or nerve compression; widespread metastases	Side effects include edema, dyspeptic symptoms, and occasional gastro-intestinal bleeding

CRPS-1 = complex regional pain syndrome, type 1; PO, by mouth; IV, intravenous; SL, sublingual; tid, three times daily; bid, twice day; od, once daily.
Modified from McGrath and Brown.[20]

analgesics at night with antidepressants or hypnotics as necessary to enable them to sleep throughout the night. To relieve ongoing pain, opioid doses should be increased steadily until comfort is achieved, unless the child experiences unacceptable side effects such as somnolence or respiratory depression (Table 9.5).

'By the mouth' refers to the oral route of drug administration. Medication should be administered to children by the simplest and most effective route, usually by mouth. Since children are afraid of painful injections they may deny that they have pain or they may not request medication. When possible, children should receive medications through routes that do not cause additional pain. Although optimal analgesic administration for children requires flexibility in selecting routes according to children's needs, parenteral administration is often the most efficient route for providing direct and rapid pain relief. Since intravenous, intramuscular, and subcutaneous routes cause additional pain for children, serious efforts have been expended on developing more pain-free modes of administration that still provide relatively direct and rapid analgesia. Attention has focused on improving the effectiveness of oral routes. As an example, oral transmucosal fentanyl citrate (OTFC) provides rapid-onset analgesia via a pleasant route for children receiving painful medical procedures. OTFC produces significant serum concentrations after 15–20 minutes.[24] Children aged 2–14 years have shown good cooperation and sedation when given OTFC as a premedication.[25,26] OTFC produced safe and effective analgesia for outpatient wound care in

Table 9.5 Opioid side effects

Side effect	Management
Respiratory depression	Reduction in opioid dose by 50%, titrate to maintain pain relief without respiratory depression
Respiratory arrest	Naloxone, titrate to effect with 0.01 mg/kg/dose IV/ETT increments or 0.1 mg/kg/dose IV/ETT, repeat prn. Small frequent doses of diluted naloxone or naloxone drip preferable for patients on chronic opioid therapy to avoid severe, painful withdrawal syndrome. Repeated doses often required until opioid side effect subsides
Drowsiness/sedation	Frequently subsides after a few days without dosage reduction; methylphenidate or dextroamphetamine (0.1 mg/kg administered twice daily, in the morning and mid-day so as not to interfere with night-time sleep). The dose can be escalated in increments of 0.05–0.1 mg/kg to a maximum of 10 mg/dose for dextroamphetamine and 20 mg/dose for methylphenidate
Constipation	Increased fluids and bulk, prophylactic laxatives as indicated
Nausea/vomiting	Administer an antiemetic (e.g. ondansetron, 0.1 mg/kg IV/PO every 8 h) Antihistamines (e.g. dimenhydrinate 0.5 mg/kg/dose every 4–6 h IV/PO) may be used. Prechemotherapy, nabilone 0.5–1.0 mg PO and then every 12 h may also be used
Confusion, nightmares, hallucinations	Reassurance only, if symptoms mild. A reduced dosage of opioid or a change to a different opioid or add neuroleptic (e.g. haloperidol 0.1 mg/kg PO/IV every 8 h to a maximum of 30 mg/day)
Multifocal myoclonus; seizures	Generally occur only during extremely high-dose therapy; reduction in opioid dose indicated if possible. Add a benzodiazepine (e.g. clonazepam 0.05 mg/kg/day divided bid or tid increasing by 0.05 mg/kg/day every 3 days prn up to 0.2 mg/kg/day. Dose limit of 20 mg/day)
Urinary retention	Rule out bladder outlet obstruction, neurogenic bladder, and other precipitating drug (e.g. tricyclic antidepressant). Particularly common with epidural opioids. Change of opioid, route of administration, and dose may relieve symptom. Bethanechol or catheter may be required

IV, intravenous; PO, by mouth; ETT, endotracheal tube; prn, as needed; bid, twice a day; tid, three times a day.
Reprinted with permission from McGrath and Brown.[20]

children and the taste was preferred to oral oxycodone.[27]

Many hospitals have restricted the use of intramuscular injections because they are painful and drug absorption is not reliable; they advocate the use of intravenous lines into which drugs can be administered directly without causing further pain. Topical anesthetic creams should also be applied prior to the insertion of intravenous lines in children. The use of portacatheters has become the gold standard in pediatrics, particularly for children with cancer under the care of the urologist, who require administration of multiple drugs at weekly intervals.

Continuous infusion has several advantages over intermittent subcutaneous, intramuscular, or intravenous routes. This method circumvents repetitive injections, prevents delays in analgesic drug administration, and provides continuous levels of pain control without children experiencing increased side effects at peak level and pain breakthroughs at trough level. Continuous infusion should be considered when children have pain for which oral and intermittent parenteral opioids do not provide satisfactory pain control, when intractable vomiting prevents the use of oral medications, and when intravenous lines are not desirable. Children receiving a continuous infusion should continue to receive 'rescue doses' to control breakthrough pain, as necessary. As outlined in Table 9.3, the rescue doses should be 50–200% of the continuous infusion hourly dose. If children experience repeated breakthrough pain, the basal rate can be increased by 50% or by the total amount of morphine administered through the rescue doses over a 24-h period (divided by 24 h).

Patient-controlled analgesia

Patient-controlled analgesia (PCA) enables children to administer analgesic doses according to their pain level. PCA provides children with a continuum of analgesia that is prompt, economical, not nurse dependent, and a lower overall narcotic use.[28–31] It has a high degree of safety, allows for wide variability between patients, and there is no delay in analgesic administration. (For review, see Reference 32.) It can now be regarded as a standard for the delivery of analgesia in children aged >5 years old.[33] However, there are opposing views about the use of background infusions with PCA. Although they may improve efficacy, they may increase the occurrence of adverse effects such as nausea and respiratory depression. In a comparison of PCA with and without a background infusion for children having lower extremity surgery, the total morphine requirements were reduced in the PCA-only group and the background infusion offered no advantage.[34] In another study comparing background infusion and PCA, children between 9 and 15 years old achieved better pain relief with PCA, whereas children between 5 and 8 years old showed no difference.[35] Our current standard is to add a background infusion to the PCA if the pain is not controlled adequately with PCA alone. The selection of opioid used in PCA is perhaps less critical than the appropriate selection of parameters such as bolus dose, lockout, and background infusion rate. The opioid choice may be based on an adverse-effect profile rather than on efficacy. Clearly, patient-controlled analgesia offers special advantages to children who have little control and who are extremely frightened about uncontrolled pain. PCA is, as it states, patient-controlled analgesia: when special circumstances require that other people administer the medication, we do allow both nurse- and parent-controlled analgesia. Under these circumstances, parents require our nurse educators to fully educate them on the use of PCA. A recent alert by the Joint Commission on Accreditation of Health Care Organizations (JCAHO) advised that serious adverse events can result when family members, caregivers, or clinicians who are not authorized become involved in administering the analgesia for the patient 'by proxy'.[36,37]

Transdermal fentanyl

Fentanyl is a potent synthetic opioid, which like morphine binds to mu (μ) receptors. However, fentanyl is 75–100 times more potent than morphine. The intravenous preparation of fentanyl has been used extensively in children. A transdermal preparation of fentanyl was introduced in 1991 for use with chronic pain. This route provides a non-invasive but continuously controlled delivery system. Although limited data are available on transdermal fentanyl (TF) in children, its use is increasing for children with pain. In a 2001 study, TF was well tolerated with effective pain relief in 11 of 13 children and provided an ideal approach for children where compliance with oral analgesics was problematic.[38] In another study, when children were converted from oral morphine doses to TF; the investigators noted diminished side effects and improved convenience with TF.[39] The majority of parents and investigators considered TF to be better than previous treatment. No serious adverse events were attributed to fentanyl, suggesting that TF was both effective and acceptable for children and their families. Similarly, no adverse effects were noted in a study of TF for children with pain due to sickle cell crisis.[40] This study showed a significant relationship between TF dose and fentanyl concentration; pain control with the use of TF was improved in 7 of 10 patients in comparison to PCA alone. In a multicenter crossover study in adults, TF caused significantly less constipation and less daytime drowsiness in comparison to morphine, but greater sleep disturbance and shorter sleep duration.[41] Of those patients able to express a preference, significantly more preferred fentanyl patches. As with all opioids, fatal adult complications have been noted with the use of multiple transdermal patches.[42]

Regional anesthesia

Topical

Topical anesthetics have proved invaluable in assisting with not only decreasing pain for minor procedures such as intravenous insertion but also for some procedures that are more invasive. At the Hospital for Sick Children, a number of these topical anesthetics are employed and include EMLA (lidocaine/prilocaine cream), Ametop (tetracaine hydrochloride), or Maxilene 4 (lidocaine cream). Each of these agents has advantages and disadvantages – EMLA requires approximately 1 hour to onset and causes vasoconstriction compared with Ametop, which is quicker in onset at approximately 30 minutes. Maxilene 4 has the advantage of being effective in approximately 10 minutes and does not require an occlusive barrier with application.

EMLA has been shown to be an effective and simple method to produce postcircumcision analgesia,[43] is simple to use, and avoids the rare but serious complications of a dorsal penile nerve block. A meta-analysis of three randomized controlled trials using EMLA prior to circumcision demonstrated a statistically significant reduction in pain.[44]

Local infiltration

The surgeon or the anesthesiologist should not underestimate the importance of postoperative pain relief. One of the simplest methods of postoperative analgesia is local infiltration of the wound with a long-acting local anesthetic such as bupivacaine. The adult literature is confusing at times, with various reports showing either a benefit or showing no demonstrative positive results. On the other hand, the pediatric literature is quite clear on the benefits of local infiltration. Beginning in the 1980s, two different studies were reported in the journal *Anaesthesia*: the first report compared wound infiltration to the use of the ilioinguinal nerve block[45] and the second report compared wound infiltration to the caudal block.[46] Wound infiltration provided comparable results to both the ilioinguinal and caudal block. In the 1990s, two more studies compared wound infiltration again to the caudal block[47] and to an ilioinguinal/iliohypogastric block.[48] The results were similar as to before, with wound infiltration providing satisfactory analgesia. Bupivacaine is our standard local anesthetic for this type of procedure at the Hospital for Sick Children, but this is not the important point. Doing the block is!

Peripheral nerve blockade

Two of the most commonly used blocks performed by the urologist are the penile block and the ilioinguinal and iliohypogastric nerve block. Both blocks are safe, easy to learn and perform, and provide good analgesia.

The penile block provides excellent analgesia, and is especially useful for the commonly performed circumcision. The penile block is easily learned by residents,[49] with over a 90% success rate possible in the first 10 blocks performed. The subpubic approach is preferred: a short-bevel needle is inserted 0.5–1 cm lateral to the midline, bilaterally into the subpubic space (deep to Scarpa's fascia), where the nerves run before entering the base of the penis, and a small volume of local anesthetic (0.1 ml/kg of body weight – usually 1–2 ml per side) is injected. Dalens et al[50] achieved a 100% success rate on 100 patients employing this technique. Our preferred local anesthetic is 0.5% bupivacaine, without epinephrine. For a full description of the technique see Reference 51. An alternative approach is the subcutaneous ring block of the penis. In a prospective study[52] it was shown that the penile block provided significantly better analgesia than the subcutaneous block.

The other commonly performed block is the ilioinguinal/iliohypogastric nerve block. This block is especially useful for procedures such as inguinal herniorrhaphy, hydrocele, and orchiopexy. The goal of this block is to anesthetize the ilioinguinal, iliohypogastric, and the genital branch of the genitofemoral nerve. A short-bevel needle is employed and is inserted 1 cm medial and 1 cm inferior to the anterior superior iliac spine. The needle is inserted through skin, external oblique, and the internal oblique muscles. The local anesthetic is then inserted in a fan-shaped motion as well as a subcutaneous wheal. I personally use 0.2–0.4 ml/kg of 0.25% bupivacaine with 1:200 000 epinephrine (to a maximum dose of 10 ml). These volumes have to be adhered to strictly because of the possibility of increased bupivacaine concentrations after ilioinguinal block in pediatric patients.[53] For an excellent description of this procedure see Reference 51. The ilioinguinal/iliohypogastric block compares favorably with the caudal block, as confirmed by a prospective comparative study from 1986 which demonstrated that both blocks provide excellent postoperative analgesia.[54]

Caudal epidural blocks

The caudal approach to the epidural space is one of the most frequently used approaches to provide anesthesia and postoperative analgesia for the pediatric urology patient. Easy access to the caudal space can be made at the level of the sacrococcygeal ligament, thus reducing the risk of neurologic injury. There are well-known variations to the sacral hiatus though,[55] and thus if after several attempts at placing a caudal block you are unsuccessful, alternative methods of analgesia must be found. The procedure is performed frequently on our patients at the Hospital for Sick Children for cases such as herniorrhaphy and orchiopexy and for most hypospadias repairs. With the ease of procedure, good safety profile, and the excellent results it provides, it seems logical that it remains one of our gold standards. In a 1989 retrospective study of caudal analgesia in 750 pediatric patients, Dalens and Hasnaoui found no major complications or neurologic sequelae, and good patient and parent acceptance of caudal anesthesia. Their overall success rate was 96%, with most failures occurring in children >7 years old.[56] Although the addition of preoperative or postoperative acetaminophen showed no increased effect on the duration and intensity of postoperative analgesia obtained by caudal bupivacaine,[57] we continue to recommend its use perioperatively in a dosage of 30–40 mg/kg given as a rectal suppository. In some cases that may have a prolonged surgical time or that may require admission of the patient to hospital, a catheter may be left in place that can be 'topped up' by the anesthesiologist at the end of the case. Alternatively, this catheter may be employed to run an infusion in a manner similar to a formal epidural. In a recent study, both caudal and epidural analgesia combined with intravenous rescue analgesics provided adequate pain control following intravesical ureteroneocystostomy.[58]

Epidural and spinal analgesia

The use of regional techniques (epidural and spinal) for the administration of local anesthetics and analgesics for children continues to be an integral part of pain control in children.[59] Experience from many centers suggests that these techniques can be extremely useful for children undergoing extensive surgery with resulting pain that may be difficult to control by more conventional means.

When one undertakes the administration of potent analgesics and anesthetics, whether by intravenous or a regional anesthetic technique such as an epidural or spinal approach, appropriate monitoring is paramount for the safety of the patient. This involves:

- the education and training of staff
- the immediate availability of resuscitative drugs and equipment
- an accurate and timely pain record, consisting of vitals signs, pain, and sedation scores.

A complete set of intravenous and epidural monitoring guidelines is shown in Table 9.6.

Complementary/alternative therapies

An extensive array of non-drug therapies are available to treat children's pain, including counseling, guided imagery, hypnosis, biofeedback, behavioral management, acupuncture, massage, homeopathic remedies, naturopathic approaches, and herbal medicines. In a 2002 self-report questionnaire of 1013 pediatric patients seeking primary care, the most common types of complementary/alternative therapies (CAM) were herbs (41%), prayer healing (37%), folk/home remedies (28%), massage therapy (19%), and chiropractic (18%).[60] Non-drug therapies are generally regarded as safe, with few contraindications for their use in otherwise healthy children. However, little is known about the safety and effectiveness of certain therapies for children. The problem of major adverse events and the high degree of uncertainty regarding a causal relationship of these events and the therapy is frequently noted. The size of the problem and its importance relative to the well-documented risks of conventional treatments is presently unknown.[61] Although Sampson et al[62] reported 908 randomized controlled trials (RCTs) in the field of CAM and Moher et al[63] have assessed the quality of 47 CAM systematic reviews, where they found the overall qual-

Table 9.6 Analgesia monitoring guidelines

Baseline assessment
Obtain RR, HR, BP, O_2 saturation, sedation score, and pain score before administering a single or intermittent dose or initiating continuous infusion
Intermittent intravenous administration
RR, HR, BP, and sedation score every 5 min × 4, then every 30 min × 2, and then as per child's condition/pre-existing orders
Pain score every 20–30 min
Continuously monitor O_2 saturation only for children whose underlying condition predisposes them to respiratory depression
Intravenous additive (to run over 15–20 min)
RR, HR, BP, and sedation score every 10 min × 2, then every 30 min × 2, and then as per child's condition
Pain score at completion of the flush, then every 30 min × 2, and then as per child's condition/pre-existing orders
Continuously monitor O_2 saturation only for children whose underlying condition predisposes them to respiratory depression
Continuous IV infusion/PCA
RR, HR, BP, pain score, and sedation score every 1 h × 4, then RR and sedation score every 1 h, and then HR, BP, and pain score every 4 h
Continuously monitor O_2 saturation and document reading every 1 h
Intermittent epidural administration
RR, HR, and BP every 5 min for the first 20 min following a bolus dose, and then RR and sedation score every 1 h
HR, BP, pain score, and motor block score every 4 h
Continuously monitor only for children whose underlying condition predisposes them to respiratory depression
Continuous epidural infusion[a,b]
RR, HR, BP, sedation score, pain score and motor block score every 1 h × 4 h, then RR and sedation score every 1 h, and HR, BP, pain score, and motor block score every 4 h
Continuously monitor O_2 saturation and document reading every 1 h

[a] Opioids used with bupivacaine.

[b] **Note:** After any change in drug dose, infusion rate, or if transferred between patient care areas, return to assessments every 1 h for 4 h.

Continuous respiratory rate/apnea monitoring may provide additional benefits for certain children who are receiving continuous opioid infusions by alerting the nurse to a decreasing respiratory rate. Respiratory rate monitoring is not, however, a substitute for frequent patient observation and vital sign monitoring.

ECG monitoring is not routinely required, but may be ordered if the child's underlying condition predisposes them to ECG abnormalities.

RR, respiratory rate; HR, heart rate; BP, blood pressure; ECG, electrocardiogram.

Adapted from 2001–2002 Drug Formulary, the Hospital for Sick Children, Toronto, Ontario, Canada.

Reprinted with permission from McGrath and Brown.[20]

ity of reporting similar to conventional therapy, researchers continue to call for more studies in this area.[64] Thus, the efficacy of complementary therapies for treating children's pain is unclear, even though children are increasingly using complementary therapies.[65] Madsen et al[66] reported in 2003 that 53% of pediatric patients had tried CAM as a supplement to conventional medicine, which compares with an Australian study of 33% of parents having used CAM for their inpatient child.[67] The percentages were even higher for children with cancer using CAM (65%) compared with a control group (51%).[68]

Cognitive and behavioral methods of pain management

Cognitive and behavioral therapies can mitigate some of the factors that intensify pain, distress, and disability for children. In contrast to complementary therapies, the evidence base supporting the efficacy of cognitive and behavioral approaches is strong.[15,28,69–81] Cognitive therapies are directed at a child's beliefs, expectations, and coping abilities. They encompass a wide range of approaches from basic patient education to formal psychotherapy. Most children and families benefit from supportive counseling. Accurate information about what will happen and what children may feel should improve children's understanding, increase their control, lessen their distress, and reduce their pain. In addition, healthcare providers can teach children how to use a few pain control methods to lessen pain and guide families to recognize the particular circumstances that exacerbate pain and distress. These methods provide children with some independent strategies – either to relieve mild pain or to complement the medication needed to relieve strong pain. Children seem more adept than adults at using non-drug therapies, presumably because they are usually less biased than adults about their potential efficacy.

Distraction is a simple and effective pain control method. When children intently attend to something other than their pain, they can lessen its intensity and unpleasantness. Distraction is often incorrectly perceived as a simple diversionary tactic; the implication is that the pain is still there but the child is momentarily focused elsewhere. However, when children's attention is fully absorbed in some engaging topic or activity, distraction is a very active process that can reduce the neuronal responses to a noxious stimulus. Children do not simply ignore their pain, but are actually reducing it. The essential feature for achieving pain relief is a child's ability to attend fully to and concentrate on something else besides the pain. Therefore, the choice of a distraction is crucial and varies according to children's ages and interests. Young children usually need to be actively involved with their parents or peers, whereas older children and adolescents can distract themselves more independently. Children should work with their parents or a therapist to choose distracting activities that they can practically incorporate into their lives.

There is considerable overlap among the interventions of attention/distraction, guided imagery, and hypnosis. Hypnosis usually begins with an induction procedure in which a child's full attention is focused gradually on the therapist and his/her suggestions. The therapist guides the child into a very relaxed physical and mental state, an altered level of consciousness – distinct from an alert or sleep state. The induction procedure typically includes guided imagery for the child and progressive muscle relaxation for the adolescent. The induction can be very simple for young children. They can be guided into an hypnotic state as they vividly imagine their favorite television shows, movies, books, or cartoon characters.[82–84] As they imagine an activity, scene, or character, they gradually receive suggestions for relaxation, reduced anxiety, increased control, and pain reduction. The therapist provides consistent positive suggestions, rather than authoritative commands. The emphasis is on the child's own natural abilities, as in, 'Notice that your back, legs (painful body areas) feel lighter, the heaviness and pain are starting to lessen. It seems as if your back doesn't hurt as much as before. You are doing well at turning down the pain switch.'

During an hypnotic state, individuals become extremely susceptible to suggestions, including suggestions for pain relief. Children become so involved in thoughts or ideas that they dissociate from a 'reality orientation'.[83] Hypnosis enables children to redirect attention from the painful sensation or to reinterpret the sensation as something more pleasant/less aversive and/or less bothersome.[84] Like adults, children differ in their ability to be hypnotized. Children's ability to use their imagination is the key component in determining their hypnotic susceptibility.

Behavior therapy is often used in combination with cognitive therapy. The goals are to lessen the specific behaviors (i.e. child, family, and staff) that may increase pain, distress, or disability, while concomitantly increasing healthy behaviors that engage children in living as fully as possible. Relaxation training is a common method used for children who require painful procedures or who experience chronic pain. Therapists train children how to achieve a state of mental and physical relaxation, so that those children can eventually relax independently when they experience pain or feel stressed and fearful about their condition. Therapists may use guided imagery, hypnosis, deep breathing, or progressive relaxation exercises to train children.

Conclusion

In this chapter we have briefly reviewed the management of pain for the pediatric patient as it applies to the urologist. In surveys carried out at the Hospital for Sick Children in Toronto and elsewhere, the assessment and management of pain in our patients was inadequate in the past and continues to this day. A full multidisciplinary 'pain team' that involves all the techniques and skills of the anesthesiologist perioperatively and the pain team postoperatively is essential. The day when intramuscular Demerol (meperidine) could end pain and suffering is surely over. The pharmacologic and non-pharmacologic tools that we now have in our pain armamentarium must be used to end pain in our patients.

References

1. McGrath PA, Gillespie J. Pain assessment in children and adolescents. In: Turk D, Melzack R, eds. Handbook of Pain Assessment, 2nd edn. New York: Guilford Press, 2001:97–118.
2. Finley GA, McGrath PJ. Measurement of Pain in Infants and Children. Seattle: IASP Press, 1998.
3. Royal College of Nursing Institute. Clinical Guideline for the Recognition and Assessment of Acute Pain in Children: Recommendations. London: Royal College of Nursing Institute, 1999.
4. McGrath PJ. Behavioral measures of pain. In: Finley GA, McGrath PJ, eds. Measurement of Pain in Infants and Children. Seattle: IASP Press, 1998:83–102.
5. Sweet SD, McGrath PJ. Physiological measures of pain. In: Finley GA, McGrath PJ, eds. Measurement of Pain in Infants and Children. Seattle: IASP Press, 1998:59–81.
6. Hunt AM, Goldman A, Mastroyannopoulou K, Seers K. Identification of pain cues of children with severe neurological impairment. In: Proceedings of the 9th World Congress on Pain. Seattle: IASP Press, 1999: Abstract 84.
7. Champion GD, Goodenough B, von Bayer CL, Thomas W. Measurement of pain by self-report. In: Finley GA, McGrath PJ, eds. Measurement of Pain in Infants and Children. Seattle: IASP Press, 1998:123–60.
8. McGrath PA. Pain in Children: Nature, Assessment and Treatment. New York: Guilford Publications, 1990.
9. Ross DM, Ross SA. Childhood Pain: Current Issues, Research, and Management. Baltimore: Urban & Schwarzenberg, 1988.
10. Bush JP, Harkins SW, eds. Children in Pain: Clinical and Research Issues from a Developmental Perspective. New York: Springer-Verlag, 1991.
11. Gaffney A, McGrath PJ, Dick B. Measuring pain in children: developmental and instrumental issues. In: Schechter NL, Berde CB, Yaster M, eds. Pain in Infants, Children, and Adolescents, 2nd edn. Philadelphia: Lippincott Williams and Wilkins, 2003:128–42.
12. McGrath PJ, Unruh AM. Pain in Children and Adolescents. Amsterdam: Elsevier, 1987.
13. Peterson L, Harbeck C, Farmer J, Zink M. Developmental contributions to the assessment of children's pain: conceptual and methodological implications. In: Bush JP, Harkins SW, eds. Children in Pain: Clinical and Research Issues from a Developmental Perspective. New York: Springer-Verlag, 1991:33–58.
14. Pichard-Leandri E, Gauvain-Piquard A, eds. La Douleur Chez l'Enfant. Paris: Medsi/McGraw-Hill, 1989.
15. McGrath PA, Hillier LM. Modifying the psychological factors that intensify children's pain and prolong disability. In: Schechter NL, Berde CB, Yaster M, eds. Pain in Infants, Children, and Adolescents, 2nd edn. Philadelphia: Lippincott Williams and Wilkins; 2003:85–104.
16. World Health Organization. Cancer Pain Relief and Palliative Care. Geneva: World Health Organization, 1990.
17. Staats PS. Cancer pain: beyond the ladder. J Back Musculoskeletal Rehab 1998; 10:69–80.
18. Krane EJ, Leong MS, Golianu B, Leong YY. Treatment of pediatric pain with nonconventional analgesics. In: Schechter NL, Berde CB, Yaster M, eds. Pain in Infants, Children, and Adolescents, 2nd edn. Philadelphia: Lippincott Williams and Wilkins, 2003:225–41.
19. The Hospital for Sick Children. The 2004–2005 Formulary, 23rd edn. Toronto: the Hospital for Sick Children, 2004–2005.
20. McGrath PA, Brown SC. Paediatric palliative medicine – pain control. In: Doyle D, Hanks G, Cherny N, Calman K, eds. Oxford Textbook of Palliative Medicine, 3rd edn. Oxford: Oxford University Press, 2004:775–89.
21. Maunuksela EL, Olkkola KT. Nonsteroidal anti-inflammatory drugs in pediatric pain management. In: Schechter NL, Berde CB, Yaster M, eds. Pain in Infants, Children, and Adolescents, 2nd edn. Philadelphia: Lippincott Williams and Wilkins, 2003:171–81.
22. Yaster M, Kost-Byerly S, Maxwell LG. Opioid agonists and antagonists. In: Schechter NL, Berde CB, Yaster M, eds. Pain in Infants, Children, and Adolescents, 2nd edn. Philadelphia: Lippincott Williams and Wilkins, 2003:181–225.
23. Yaster M, Tobin JR, Kost-Byerly S. Local anesthetics. In: Schechter NL, Berde CB, Yaster M, eds. Pain in Infants, Children, and Adolescents, 2nd edn. Philadelphia: Lippincott Williams and Wilkins, 2003:241–65.
24. Schutzman SA, Liebelt E, Wisk M, Burg J. Comparison of oral transmucosal fentanyl citrate and intramuscular meperidine, promethazine, and chlorpromazine for conscious sedation of children undergoing laceration repair. Ann Emerg Med 1996; 28(4):385–90.
25. Dsida RM, Wheeler M, Birmingham PK et al. Premedication of pediatric tonsillectomy patients with oral transmucosal fentanyl citrate. Anesth Analg 1998; 86(1):66–70.
26. Malviya S, Voepel-Lewis T, Huntington J, Siewert M, Green W. Effects of anesthetic technique on side effects associated with fentanyl Oralet premedication. J Clin Anesth 1997; 9(5):374–8.
27. Sharar SR, Carrougher GJ, Selzer K et al. A comparison of oral transmucosal fentanyl citrate and oral oxycodone for pediatric outpatient wound care. J Burn Care Rehabil 2002; 23(1):27–31.
28. Schechter NL, Berde CB, Yaster M, eds. Pain in Infants, Children, and Adolescents, 2nd edn. Philadelphia: Lippincott Williams and Wilkins, 2003.
29. Hill HF, Chapman CR, Kornell JA et al. Self-administration of morphine in bone marrow transplant patients reduces drug requirement. Pain 1990; 40(2):121–9.
30. Rodgers BM, Webb CJ, Stergios D, Newman BM. Patient-controlled analgesia in pediatric surgery. J Pediatr Surg 1988; 23(3):259–62.

31. Shapiro BS, Cohen DE, Howe CJ. Patient-controlled analgesia for sickle-cell-related pain. J Pain Symptom Manage 1993; 8(1):22–8.
32. Berde CB, Solodiuk J. Multidisciplinary programs for management of acute and chronic pain in children. In: Schechter NL, Berde CB, Yaster M, eds. Pain in Infants, Children, and Adolescents, 2nd edn. Philadelphia: Lippincott Williams and Wilkins, 2003:471–86.
33. McDonald AJ, Cooper MG. Patient-controlled analgesia: an appropriate method of pain control in children. Paediatr Drugs 2001; 3(4):273–84.
34. McNeely JK, Trentadue NC. Comparison of patient-controlled analgesia with and without nighttime morphine infusion following lower extremity surgery in children. J Pain Symptom Manage 1997; 13(5):268–73.
35. Bray RJ, Woodhams AM, Vallis CJ, Kelly PJ, Ward-Platt MP. A double-blind comparison of morphine infusion and patient controlled analgesia in children. Paediatr Anaesth 1996; 6(2):121–7.
36. Patient controlled analgesia by proxy. Joint Commission of Healthcare Organizations. Sentinel Event Alert 2004; 33:1–2.
37. Maddox RR, Williams CK, Fields M. Respiratory monitoring in patient-controlled analgesia. Am J Health Syst Pharm 2004; 61(24):2628–9.
38. Noyes M, Irving H. The use of transdermal fentanyl in pediatric oncology palliative care. Am J Hosp Palliat Care 2001; 18(6):411–16.
39. Hunt A, Goldman A, Devine T, Phillips M. Transdermal fentanyl for pain relief in a paediatric palliative care population. Palliat Med 2001; 15(5):405–12.
40. Christensen ML, Wang WC, Harris S, Eades SK, Wilimas JA. Transdermal fentanyl administration in children and adolescents with sickle cell pain crisis. J Pediatr Hematol Oncol 1996; 18(4):372–6.
41. Ahmedzai S, Brooks D. Transdermal fentanyl versus sustained-release oral morphine in cancer pain: preference, efficacy, and quality of life. The TTS-Fentanyl Comparative Trial Group. J Pain Symptom Manage 1997; 13(5):254–61.
42. Edinboro LE, Poklis A, Trautman D et al. Fatal fentanyl intoxication following excessive transdermal application. J Forensic Sci 1997; 42(4):741–3.
43. Choi WY, Irwin MG, Hui TW, Lim HH, Chan KL. EMLA cream versus dorsal penile nerve block for postcircumcision analgesia in children. Anesth Analg 2003; 96(2):396–9.
44. Taddio A. Pain management for neonatal circumcision. Paediatr Drugs 2001; 3(2):101–11.
45. Reid MF, Harris R, Phillips PD et al. Day-case herniotomy in children. A comparison of ilio-inguinal nerve block and wound infiltration for postoperative analgesia. Anaesthesia 1987; 42(6):658–61.
46. Fell D, Derrington MC, Taylor E, Wandless JG. Paediatric postoperative analgesia. A comparison between caudal block and wound infiltration of local anaesthetic. Anaesthesia 1988; 43(2):107–10.
47. Schindler M, Swann M, Crawford M. A comparison of postoperative analgesia provided by wound infiltration or caudal analgesia. Anaesth Intensive Care 1991; 19(1):46–9.
48. Anatol TI, Pitt-Miller P, Holder Y. Trial of three methods of intraoperative bupivacaine analgesia for pain after paediatric groin surgery. Can J Anaesth 1997; 44(10):1053–9.
49. Schuepfer G, Johr M. Generating a learning curve for penile block in neonates, infants and children: an empirical evaluation of technical skills in novice and experienced anaesthetists. Paediatr Anaesth 2004; 14(7):574–8.
50. Dalens B, Vanneuville G, Dechelotte P. Penile block via the subpubic space in 100 children. Anesth Analg 1989; 69(1):41–5.
51. Dalens B. Regional anesthetic techniques. In: Bissonnette B, Dalens BJ, eds. Pediatric Anesthesia. New York: McGraw-Hill, 2002:528–75.
52. Holder KJ, Peutrell JM, Weir PM. Regional anaesthesia for circumcision. Subcutaneous ring block of the penis and subpubic penile block compared. Eur J Anaesthesiol 1997; 14(5):495–8.
53. Smith T, Moratin P, Wulf H. Smaller children have greater bupivacaine plasma concentrations after ilioinguinal block. Br J Anaesth 1996; 76(3):452–5.
54. Markham SJ, Tomlinson J, Hain WR. Ilioinguinal nerve block in children. A comparison with caudal block for intra and postoperative analgesia. Anaesthesia 1986; 41(11):1098–103.
55. Sekiguchi M, Yabuki S, Satoh K, Kikuchi S. An anatomic study of the sacral hiatus: a basis for successful caudal epidural block. Clin J Pain 2004; 20(1):51–4.
56. Dalens B, Hasnaoui A. Caudal anesthesia in pediatric surgery: success rate and adverse effects in 750 consecutive patients. Anesth Analg 1989; 68(2):83–9.
57. Ozyuvaci E, Altan A, Yucel M, Yenmez K. Evaluation of adding preoperative or postoperative rectal paracetamol to caudal bupivacaine for postoperative analgesia in children. Paediatr Anaesth 2004; 14(8):661–5.
58. Merguerian PA, Sutters KA, Tang E, Kaji D, Chang B. Efficacy of continuous epidural analgesia versus single dose caudal analgesia in children after intravesical ureteroneocystostomy. J Urol 2004; 172(4 Pt 2):1621–5; discussion 1625.
59. Wilder RT. Regional anesthetic techniques for chronic pain management in children. In: Schechter NL, Berde CB, Yaster M, eds. Pain in Infants, Children, and Adolescents, 2nd edn. Philadelphia: Lippincott Williams and Wilkins, 2003:396–416.
60. Sawni-Sikand A, Schubiner H, Thomas RL. Use of complementary/alternative therapies among children in primary care pediatrics. Ambul Pediatr 2002; 2(2):99–103.
61. Ernst E. Serious adverse effects of unconventional therapies for children and adolescents: a systematic review of recent evidence. Eur J Pediatr 2003; 162(2):72–80.
62. Sampson M, Campbell K, Ajiferuke I, Moher D. Randomized controlled trials in pediatric complementary and alternative medicine: where can they be found? BMC Pediatr 2003; 3(1):1.
63. Moher D, Soeken K, Sampson M, Ben-Porat L, Berman B. Assessing the quality of reports of randomized trials in pediatric complementary and alternative medicine. BMC Pediatr 2002; 2(1):2.
64. Scrace J. Complementary therapies in palliative care of

children with cancer: a literature review. Paediatr Nurs 2003; 15(3):36–9.
65. Spigelblatt L, Laine-Ammara G, Pless IB, Guyver A. The use of alternative medicine by children. Pediatrics 1994; 94(6 Pt 1):811–14.
66. Madsen H, Andersen S, Nielsen RG et al. Use of complementary/alternative medicine among paediatric patients. Eur J Pediatr 2003; 162(5):334–41.
67. Fong DP, Fong LK. Usage of complementary medicine among children. Aust Fam Physician 2002; 31(4):388–91.
68. Friedman T, Slayton WB, Allen LS et al. Use of alternative therapies for children with cancer. Pediatrics 1997; 100(6):E1.
69. World Health Organization. Cancer Pain Relief and Palliative Care in Children. Geneva: World Health Organization, 1998.
70. Dahlquist LM, Gil KM, Armstrong FD, Ginsberg A, Jones B. Behavioral management of children's distress during chemotherapy. J Behav Ther Exp Psychiatry 1985; 16(4):325–9.
71. Dash J. Hypnosis for symptom amelioration. In: Kellerman J, ed. Psychologic Aspects of Childhood Cancer. Springfield, Illinois: CC Thomas, 1980:215–30.
72. Hartman GA. Hypnosis as an adjuvant in the treatment of childhood cancer. In: Deasy-Spinetta P, ed. Living with Childhood Cancer. St Louis: Mosby, 1981:143–52.
73. Hilgard JR, LeBaron S. Relief of anxiety and pain in children and adolescents with cancer: quantitative measures and clinical observations. Int J Clin Exp Hypn 1982; 30(4):417–42.
74. Hilgard JR, LeBaron S. Hypnotherapy of pain in children with cancer. Los Altos, California: Kaufmann, 1984.
75. Jay SM, Elliott CH, Ozolins M, Olson RA, Pruitt SD. Behavioral management of children's distress during painful medical procedures. Behav Res Ther 1985; 23(5):513–20.
76. Katz ER, Kellerman J, Ellenberg L. Hypnosis in the reduction of acute pain and distress in children with cancer. J Pediatr Psychol 1987; 12(3):379–94.
77. LaBaw W, Holton C, Tewell K, Eccles D. The use of self-hypnosis by children with cancer. Am J Clin Hypn 1975; 17(4):233–8.
78. McGrath PA, Hillier LM. A practical cognitive-behavioral approach for treating children's pain. In: Gatchel R, Turk DC, eds. Psychological Approaches to Pain Management. New York: Guilford Press, 2002:534–52.
79. Olness K. Imagery (self-hypnosis) as adjunct therapy in childhood cancer: clinical experience with 25 patients. Am J Pediatr Hematol Oncol 1981; 3(3):313–21.
80. Olness K. Hypnosis in pediatric practice. Curr Probl Pediatr 1981; 12(2):1–47.
81. Zeltzer L, LeBaron S. Hypnosis and nonhypnotic techniques for reduction of pain and anxiety during painful procedures in children and adolescents with cancer. J Pediatr 1982; 101(6):1032–5.
82. Hall H. Hypnosis and pediatrics. In: Tennes R, ed. Medical Hypnosis: An Introduction and Clinical Guide. New York: Churchill Livingstone, 1999:79–93.
83. LeBaron S, Zeltzer L. Children in pain. In: Barber J, ed. Hypnosis and Suggestion in the Treatment of Pain: A Clinical Guide. New York: WW Norton, 1996:305–40.
84. Olness K, Kohen DP. Hypnosis and Hypnotherapy with Children, 3rd edn. New York: Guilford Press, 1996.

Office pediatric urology 10

Patrick C Cartwright, Timothy A Masterson, and Brent W Snow

Introduction

The environment of a medical office can play a pivotal role in making pediatric patients and their families comfortable. Engaging decorations, bright colors, toys, and play areas often help calm nervous children. A bulletin board with patient photos and cards may soften the feel of the office. Every effort should be made to allow parents to be with their child at all times to provide reassurance. Each physician's style and personality is different, but often those who deal with children forego the formality of a white coat so that the encounter might be more familiar to the patient. It is important upon entering the examination room first to engage the patient in gentle conversation, when possible, to develop rapport and place the child at ease. If the child is old enough, history taking generally begins with the child and is supplemented by parental input.

The physical examination is generally performed on the examining table with a parent standing beside the physician at the head of the bed. It is important to let the child know that he will not be poked or hurt but gently checked. As children approach puberty, they may be relieved to have one or both of their parents leave for the examination when given this opportunity by the physician. After the examination is completed, it is important to let patients know that they are finished so they will no longer be ill at ease. Upon leaving the office, children are often rewarded for their good behavior so that they will look forward to return visits.

Most physicians find that dealing with children in an honest, straightforward manner is best. It is appropriate to tell the child before any uncomfortable procedures are undertaken to develop trust in the provider. Surprising a child with an unpleasant examination or injection results in a loss of trust and faith in the physician, which is difficult to regain. Parents are encouraged to tell their children honestly about diagnostic X-ray examinations and office visits so that the children can be appropriately prepared. Under these circumstances, the examination and history may be completed accurately with little threat to the child.

The penis

Foreskin and phimosis

The appropriate management of penile problems in childhood is based upon an understanding of genital embryology and postnatal penile development. Genital differentiation takes place between the 9th and 13th weeks of gestation. The glans penis forms from the genital tubercle and is covered with a prepuce which is adherent to its surface. The preputial attachments persist throughout gestation and the epithelial layer of the inner prepuce and the glans penis are fused at birth. The newborn foreskin cannot be retracted without disrupting this natural adherence. Subsequently, glandular secretions and desquamated epithelial debris, collectively called smegma, collect between the inner prepuce and the glans penis, gradually separating these two layers. The build up of this material can be impressive and patients may present with a mass that can be seen through the thin foreskin. This has been referred to as a foreskin pearl. Treatment is not required as the smegma eventually erupts at the foreskin meatus, disrupting the adherence and resulting in partial separation of the foreskin.[1] This sequence is often misdiagnosed as a penile infection, with the smegma presumed to be 'pus'. Reassurance usually quiets parental concerns.

The physiologic adherence (physiologic phimosis) resolves spontaneously, but may remain present for several years. Texts suggest that most physiologic phimosis resolves by the age of 3–5 years, such that the glans penis can be fully exposed.[2] In the authors' experience, limited adherence of little significance may remain for years longer. In a longitudinal study, Oster[3] reported that physiologic phimosis in school-aged boys resolved over time (Table 10.1).

Physiologic phimosis should be distinguished from

Table 10.1 Incidence of phimosis in children

Age (years)	Phimosis (%)	Tight prepuce (%)
6–7	8	1
8–9	6	2
10–11	6	2
12–13	3	3
14–15	1	1
16–17	1	1

pathologic or true phimosis. Physiologic phimosis exists when the adherence between the inner prepuce and glans penis persists as filmy attachments. True phimosis occurs when the foreskin cannot be retracted after it has been previously retractable, if there is a densely thickened prepuce that will not retract, or one that remains non-retractile after a patient has completed pubertal development.

The easiest way to differentiate physiologic phimosis from pathologic phimosis is careful examination. Forceful separation of foreskin adhesions is not recommended because of pain and trauma to the patient, but gentle proximal traction of the foreskin may enable one to differentiate between normal and abnormal. If the foreskin retracts part way and then lays flat against the glans penis and effaces or thins, the remaining attachments are probably physiologic and more time is required for natural separation to occur. If, when the foreskin is retracted to the point of attachment there is a thickened, rolled edge, this is likely pathologic phimosis due to scarring and inflammation (Figure 10.1). This is unlikely to resolve spontaneously and may require circumcision. Ballooning of the foreskin during voiding is often associated with true phimosis as well. There have been recent studies suggesting that steroids applied to the prepuce and glans penis will help separate physiologic adhesions, aiding in the resolution of this diagnostic dilemma.[4]

Questions often arise about care of the uncircumcised penis. The genital area should be cleaned as any other skin area and the foreskin may be gently retracted to the extent allowable without discomfort for cleaning. Forcible retraction may result in tearing of the foreskin meatus, inflammation, and secondary scarring leading to true phimosis.

Postcircumcision phimosis (entrapped penis)

Following routine neonatal circumcision with any standard circumcision clamp, an unusual type of secondary phimosis can develop. Since the circumcision scar is circumferential, and the process of wound healing involves contracture, this may cause narrowing of the shaft skin at the circumcision site. If the circumcision site is mobile and sufficient inner foreskin remains, the circumcision site can migrate distally over the glans and begin to contract in this position (Figure 10.2). This contraction and scarring may be tight enough that the glans penis can no longer be seen and occasionally urinary flow may be restricted. This type of phimosis (penile entrapment, secondary phimosis) can be avoided by firmly seating the bell of the newborn clamp at the coronal margin so that there is no redundant inner prepuce remaining which might let the circumcision scar ride distally over the coronal margin. This seems to be a more common problem in young boys with an abundant pubic fat pad who may not be candidates for circumcision in the first place (Figure 10.3). If secondary phimosis is discovered early after circumcision, aggressive fore-

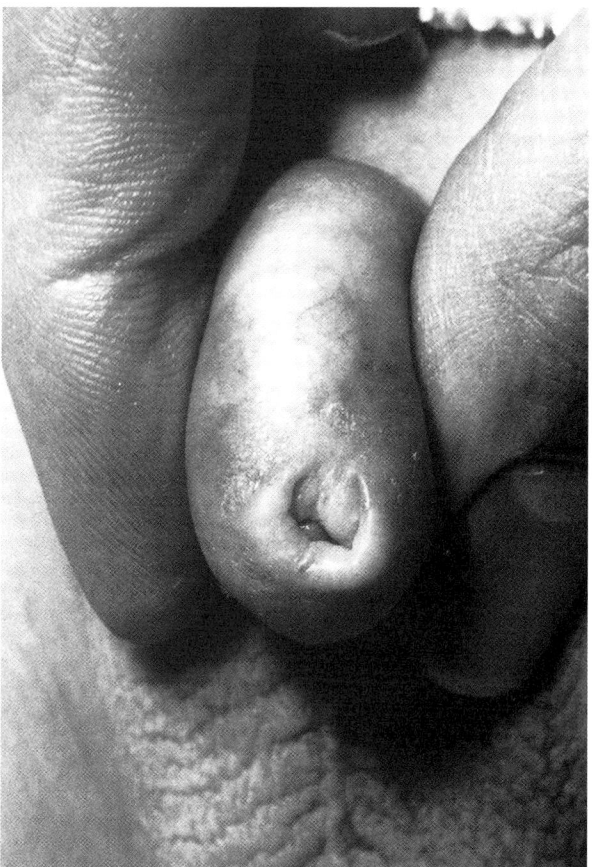

Figure 10.1 This prepuce displays a true 'phimotic ring' laterally and inferiorly with thickened skin, whereas superiorly the skin shows a more normal, effaced (thin) appearance when the foreskin is pushed gently toward the base of the penis.

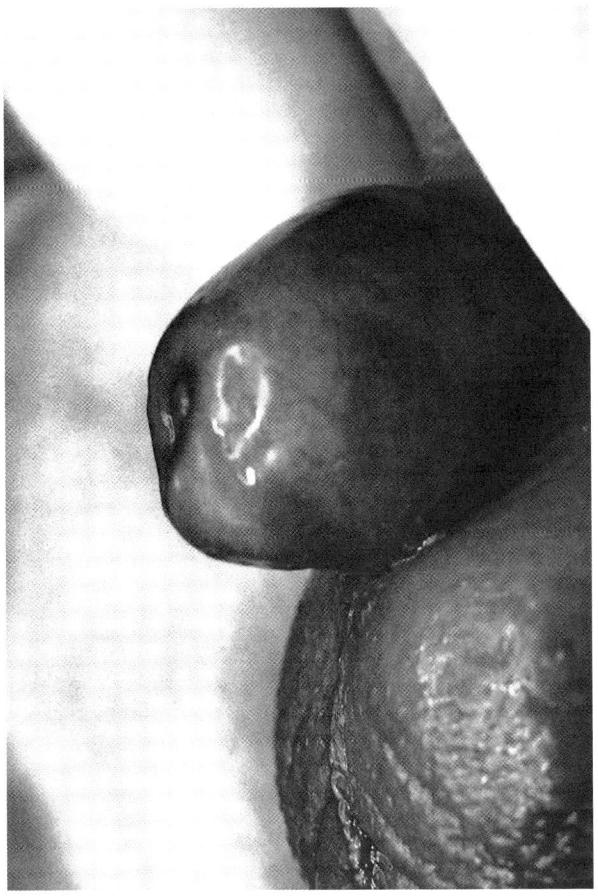

Figure 10.2 Entrapped penis following circumcision (secondary phimosis).

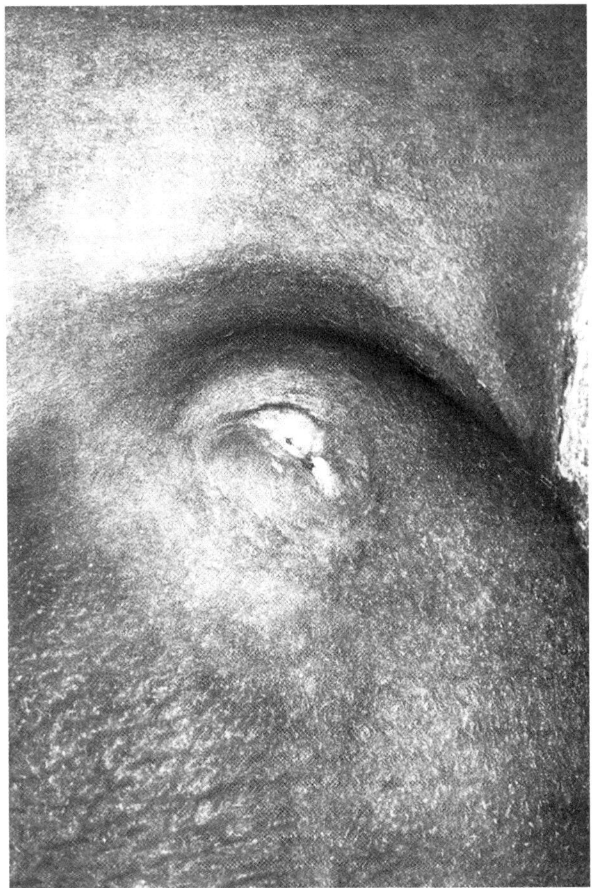

Figure 10.3 Severe penile entrapment. This required incision of the phimotic ring in two locations followed by horizontal closure of the vertical incision lines.

skin retraction by stretching the ring with a hemostat dilates the scar and the need for later revision of the circumcision is avoided. In other cases, the phimotic ring may be anesthetized and snipped in the office, incising vertically and closing horizontally to create a wider circumference. This may not resolve the problem in all patients and formal circumcision revision may be necessary in some, reducing the inner foreskin length so that the circumcision scar cannot migrate past the coronal margin; occasionally, removal of more shaft skin becomes necessary.

Penile glanular adhesions (skin bridges)

After newborn circumcision, the glans epithelium is denuded owing to separation of the physiologic adhesions with the foreskin. The circumcision site is also a raw surface and if the glans epithelium and the circumcision site rest together for a prolonged period, a postsurgical adhesion may form (Figure 10.4). These are dense adhesions that cannot be teased apart in the office. These adhesions usually occur as skin bridges so that an instrument tip can be passed underneath them, and their blood supply comes from both the shaft skin and the glans. Surgical division of such skin bridges is required.

This technique usually requires some sort of analgesic agent, which may be EMLA® cream, or local injection in the office, or if more extensive, general anesthesia. After appropriate analgesia, a hemostat is used to crush the bridge near the glans and the adhesion is divided with scissors, rotating the blade and cutting the skin bridge nearly flush with the glans epithelium. Sometimes a second cut flush with the shaft skin will be necessary for good cosmesis. It is important not to cut the skin bridge in the middle because this often leaves a skin tag of shaft skin on the glans penis, which is a noticeable cosmetic problem. Suturing may be necessary for bleeding or wound approximation. Ointment is then placed on the penis twice daily for 7–10 days; gently retracting the shaft skin prevents the two edges from coming into contact to reform the adhesion.

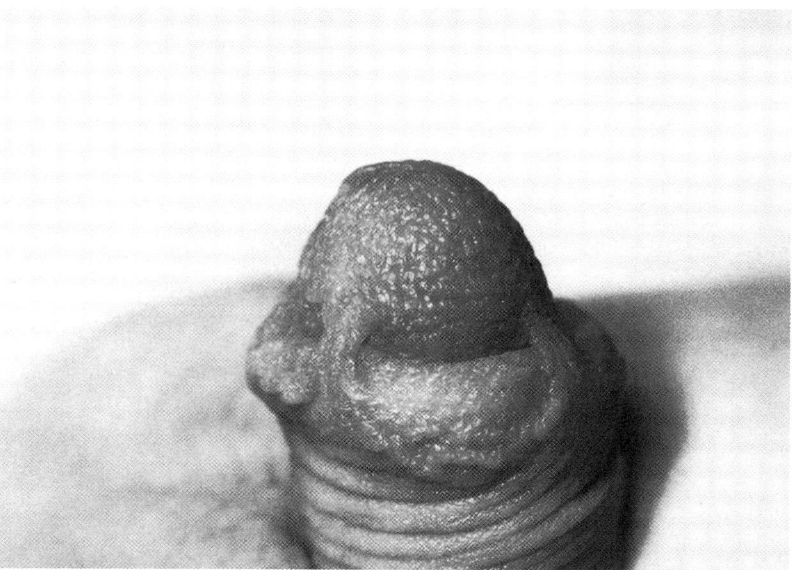

Figure 10.4 Postcircumcision skin bridges.

Paraphimosis

Paraphimosis is the term applied when the foreskin has been retracted and cannot then be brought back over the glans penis (Figure 10.5). This can happen after the foreskin has been forcefully separated for the first time, disrupting the preputial adherence to the glans. In the hospital this often occurs when the foreskin has been retracted for the placement of an indwelling catheter. Once the catheter has been secured, medical personnel neglect to replace the foreskin over the glans penis. With the tight foreskin proximal to the glans penis, venous congestion leads to progressive swelling. When paraphimosis is recognized, it is imperative that the foreskin be immediately placed back over the glans to allow the blood flow to return to the prepuce and glans. If there is significant edema, this can be difficult. The best technique is to hold a gauze sponge with the index and third fingers of each hand proximal to the foreskin, with the gauze covering the fingers for traction. The thumbs push the glans penis back through the paraphimotic ring between the other four fingers that are supporting it. A minute or two of steady pressure may be required to decompress the glans and force the foreskin edema proximally and allow for the glans to suddenly slip through to the paraphimotic ring. Placing ice on the penis before this procedure has been advocated and a penile anesthetic block may be administered before the manual reduction. Additionally, infiltration of the edematous foreskin with hyaluronidase has been reported to facilitate decompression.[5] If manual reduction is unsuccessful, immediate dorsal slit of the tight preputial ring will restore venous drainage from the distal tissue. A formal circumcision can be completed at a later date if necessary.

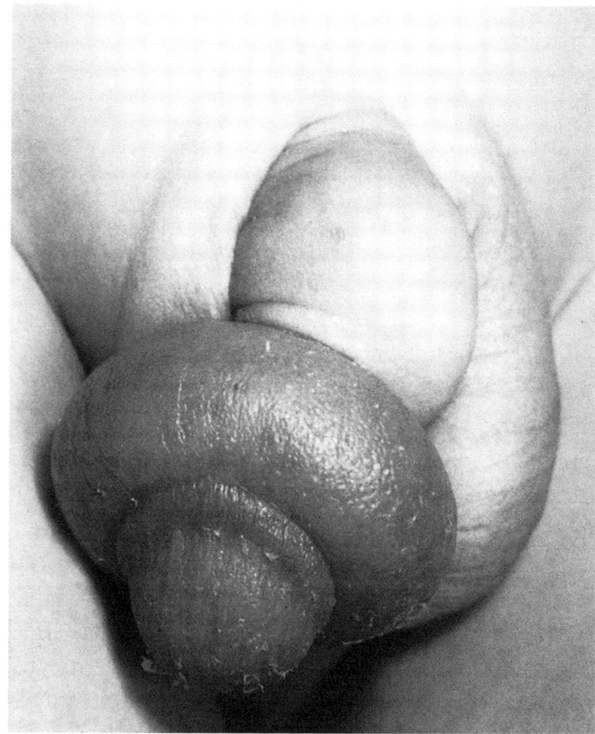

Figure 10.5 Paraphimosis with edematous, discolored prepuce trapped proximal to glans penis.

Meatal stenosis

Stenosis of the urethral meatus seems to be largely an acquired problem of circumcised boys. Recurrent meatitis or meatal inflammation secondary to prolonged exposure of the meatus to the moist and irritating environment of the diaper (ammoniacal dermatitis) or other inflammatory skin diseases can induce this problem. The delicate meatal skin edges lose their superficial epithelial lining when inflamed, and as a result become adherent in a side-to-side fashion. This almost always occurs ventrally and progresses dorsally, and boys are left with a small or even pinpoint meatus at the apex of the glans. Some authors have suggested that the advent of disposable diapers has led to increasing prevalence of this problem since the 1980s. The occurrence of meatal stenosis is distinctly unusual in an uncircumcised boy and therefore is best considered a potential side-effect of circumcision.

Causes beyond simple irritation which can induce strictures of the meatus include prior hypospadias repair or other penile surgery, prolonged urethral catheterization, trauma, or balanitis xerotica obliterans (BXO). These diagnoses are often apparent on examination or when reviewing the child's history. BXO induces a characteristic whitish circumferential discoloration of much of the glans and may induce a narrowing of the urethra extending more proximal than simple irritative meatal stenosis. BXO is more difficult to treat.

Normal meatal caliber based on age has been reported in boys. In general, a boy under the age of 1 year should have a meatus that easily accepts a 5 Fr feeding tube. Between the ages of 1 and 6 years this increases to at least an 8 Fr size. It can be difficult to estimate meatal size accurately when inspecting this visually. However, gentle lateral traction on the meatal edges to open the meatus side to side reveals the typical fused appearance of the ventral edges, confirming some degree of stenosis. On the other hand, if normal urethral mucosa can be everted, meatal size is probably adequate. Final confirmation is obtained by observing voiding. There is a characteristic dorsal deflection of the stream due to a ventral lip of scar tissue as a result of fusion of the meatal edges. The patient also demonstrates a very fine-caliber, forceful stream with a long voiding distance. This is due to the acute decrease in the size of the lumen of the urethra distally and the secondary accelerated velocity of the urine. Some patients will learn to direct their penis towards their feet during voiding so that the stream will enter the toilet bowl, whereas others seem not to catch on and miss the bowl entirely.

Meatal stenosis is uncommonly diagnosed prior to a boy becoming toilet trained. There may be intermittent dysuria with discomfort at the tip of the glans and occasional blood spotting in the underwear due to recurrent inflammation at the meatus. Patients with meatal stenosis demonstrate a prolonged voiding time and some boys decide that it is simpler to sit during voiding rather than try to direct their streams while standing. It should be noted that meatal stenosis is an unlikely cause of recurring urinary tract infection (UTI) or true obstruction to the lower urinary tract. When the history, examination, and observation of the urinary stream suggest meatal stenosis, no other diagnostic evaluation is required.

When any of the above symptoms are present, and voiding is characteristic, treatment of meatal stenosis is generally warranted. Simple dilatation of the urethral meatus will often result in tearing of the skin edges and a high rate of recurrent stenosis. Urethral meatotomy is, therefore, the preferred method of treatment. Meatotomy is a very simple procedure in which one prong of a hemostat is inserted within the urethral meatus and directed toward the ventrum in the midline of the glans a few millimeters proximal to the stenotic pinpoint meatus. The skin edges are crushed together for 1–2 minutes. Once the clamp is removed, fine scissors are used to incise the ventral midline, thus reopening the meatus (Figure 10.6). The crushed skin remains together, generating appropriate hemostasis.

Options exist in terms of anesthetic techniques for meatotomy. The procedure may be performed under a general anesthetic in the operating room as a quick and simple outpatient procedure; however, this is generally not necessary. Some urologists have performed this procedure in an office setting by injecting a small amount of lidocaine with epinephrine directly into the ventral meatal skin using a small-caliber needle. This provides analgesia and hemostasis. However, most boys will not tolerate this since the injection is distinctly uncomfortable.

More recently, the authors have reported using topical EMLA cream (eutectic mixture of local anesthetics) applied over the entire glans to anesthetize the meatus and perimeatal skin for urethral meatotomy.[6,7] Others have recently reported a similar use for EMLA cream.[8] The EMLA cream is applied liberally over the entire glans, especially on the ventrum. It is secured in place with an occlusive dressing and left in contact with the glans skin for 1–1.5 hours before the procedure (Figure 10.7). The cream is removed and the meatotomy is completed. The vast majority of patients experience no discomfort when EMLA cream

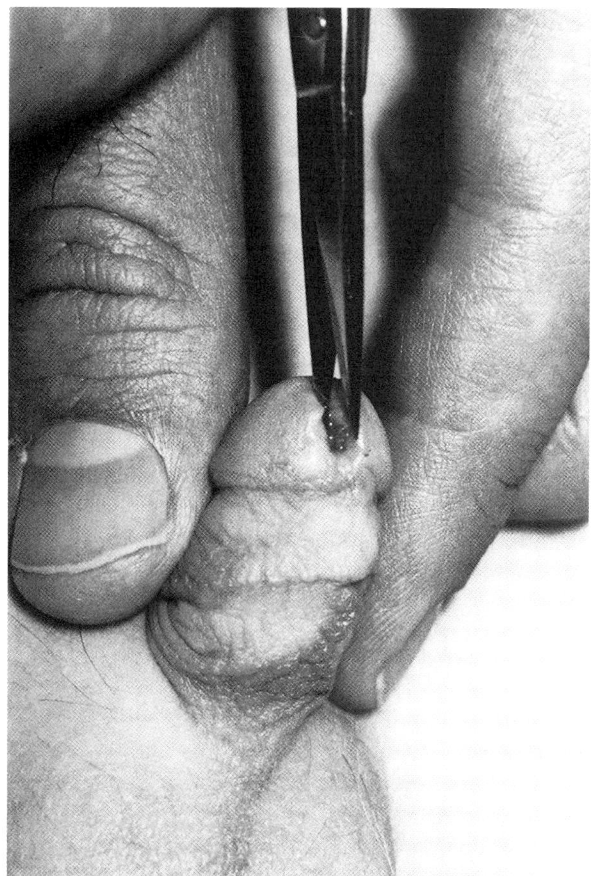

Figure 10.6 Vertical incision for meatotomy following 60 seconds of clamping with a hemostat.

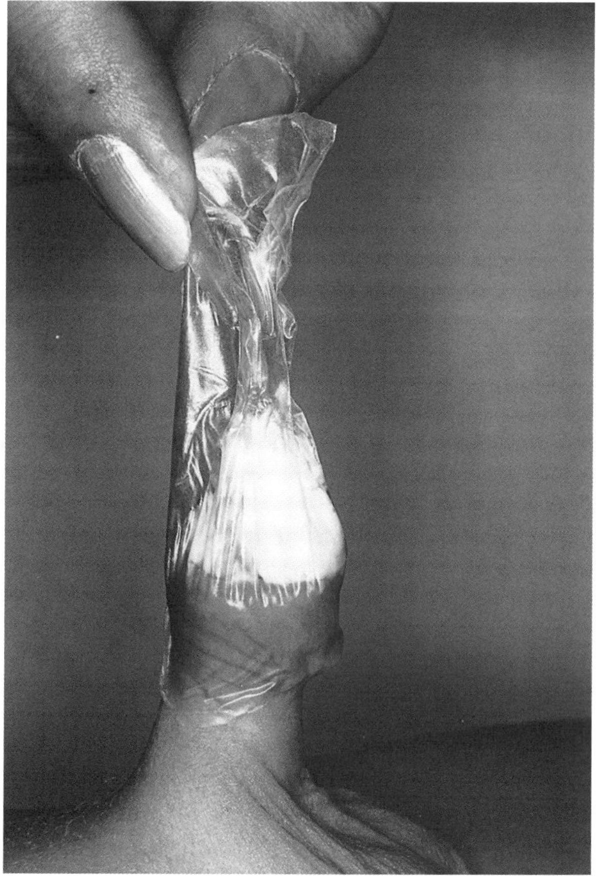

Figure 10.7 EMLA cream is applied over entire glans prior to meatotomy. This remains for at least 60 minutes before the procedure.

is used with this technique. Occasionally, there will be a sensation of pressure when the hemostat is clamped. This is almost always at the most proximal point of clamping. In an occasional patient the EMLA cream may be supplemented with a small amount of injected lidocaine with epinephrine, which seems to be minimally uncomfortable when given following EMLA. Uncommonly, a patient may require a suture on each side of the meatotomy for oozing from the meatal edges following the procedure.

Patient tolerance of the procedure overall is quite good as long as a caring and patient approach is taken to reassure boys before and during the procedure. The room is quiet with minimal lighting and parents bring some of the child's books and hand-held toys for the waiting period after the EMLA is applied. Parents stay in the room during the procedure and this further reassures the child. The authors have chosen, based on parental preference and patient personality, to use midazolam hydrochloride as an anxiolytic with good results in some patients. However, the general observation has been that midazolam is unnecessary for the majority of patients.

Following meatotomy, it is crucial to keep the edges of the meatus separated so that restenosis does not occur. Immediately following meatotomy, while still in the office, the parent is shown how to apply antibiotic ointment within the meatus. The parent then continues this at home, using one hand to separate the meatus while the other index finger is used to place a small amount of ointment directly into the meatus. This is continued twice daily for the first 2 weeks and then once daily for another 4 weeks. Alternatively, a small tube of ophthalmic ointment (Lacri-Lube) may be used as a meatal dilator. A small amount of the ointment is extruded from the metal tip for lubrication and the tip is then passed within the meatus. It is of appropriate size to serve as a dilator for most boys undergoing meatotomy. The use of meatal dilation may be helpful in certain cases if readherence of meatal edges is problematic, but the authors do not feel that it is routinely required.

Patients may be expected to experience mild dysuria for the first 1–2 days postoperatively. It has generally been helpful to have them take ibuprofen or acetaminophen 2 hours preoperatively to decrease discomfort. Boys at the age of 3 or 4 years may respond to meatotomy by holding the urine for prolonged periods of time. Placing them in a warm tub often stimulates voiding in this circumstance. One value of keeping ointment over the meatal edges is that it functions as a barrier to shield the surface from the passage of urine and the resulting discomfort. It should also be noted that increasing the fluid intake for the first day or two following the procedure dilutes the urine and leads to less dysuria. Minor blood spotting in the underwear following meatotomy is common for 1–2 days. Printed handouts are given to parents with these recommendations and they are warned of the risk for restenosis when the instructions are not followed. In addition, boys who remain wet following meatotomy, from either still being in a diaper or having problems with persistent incontinence, are at risk for redeveloping stenosis based upon recurrent inflammation of the meatus. This group may not be candidates for treatment until dryness is achieved. Two out of 226 patients seen by the authors required a second meatotomy. Over the same period that they have used EMLA cream for analgesia, the authors have chosen to perform meatotomy in the operating room in three boys due to patient behavioral issues, including extreme attention deficient disorder. As experience has been gained, it has become apparent that midazolam works well in the moderately overactive, anxious, or difficult young boy, and meatotomy in the operating room should be reserved for the patient with BXO or posthypospadias meatal stenosis.

Non-neonatal circumcision

The pros and cons of newborn circumcision have been and will continue to be debated. Less discussion surrounds circumcision after the newborn period, when it is estimated that 1 in 100 uncircumcised boys will require circumcision.[9] During childhood the most common indication for circumcision is phimosis. This develops because of preputial irritation leading to inflammation, scarring, and thickening of the preputial opening so that the foreskin cannot retract. Hygiene then becomes a problem and, occasionally, this process is so severe that urine flow is affected and the preputial sac dilates with urine dribbling out after voiding. In some patients with chronic skin irritation and inflammation, fissures of the prepuce develop. This makes spontaneous erections and retraction of the foreskin painful, and discomfort occasionally awakens the patient during sleep. Steroid ointments may reduce inflammation, but circumcision is indicated if fissures persist.

Balanoposthitis is an infection of the glans and preputial sac. This infection occurs uncommonly, but can be painful. Skin flora are usually the predominant organisms found on culture. If the balanoposthitis is mild, sitz baths and topical antibiotic ointment (bacitracin) may be sufficient. If cellulitis and fever are present, then a systemic antibiotic is added. The first episode of balanoposthitis is not a mandatory indication for circumcision. Recurrent episodes strengthen the argument for circumcision. Penile hygiene should be reviewed with the parents and patient.

UTIs are more common in uncircumcised boys, especially during the first 6 months of life. Some consider a UTI in a boy an indication for circumcision. After 1 year of age the increased risk for UTI in the uncircumcised male diminishes.

Penile cancer is known to be prevented by newborn circumcision. It is thought that the development of penile cancer closely correlates with penile hygiene, and in developed countries where hygiene is good, the rate of penile cancer is very low regardless of circumcision status. Since penile cancer is very uncommon, the likelihood of a serious circumcision complication may be higher than the eventual possibility of penile cancer.

Occasionally, trauma to the prepuce leads to circumcision. Zipper trauma is the most common occurrence. Usually, with local anesthesia, the zipper can be dislodged by simple advancement or at times by cutting the median bar of the zipper, thereby allowing the teeth to separate. Occasionally, circumcision may be warranted acutely.

After the newborn period the indications for circumcision are relatively few. Circumcision is generally performed under general anesthesia after the newborn period, although a recent report documents the use of local blocks and circumcision in boys beyond this period.[10] Depending upon the age of the patient and the size of the penis, surgical excision and suturing or newborn clamps may be used. The procedure is usually successful, with low complication rates, and is performed on an outpatient basis. Recovery is generally prompt, with the older patients experiencing more discomfort and having a longer recovery period.

Genital holding

Children who hold or clutch their genitalia are often of concern to their parents. This behavior begins shortly after toilet training and may last through the prepubertal years. It is more common in boys than girls. In boys, some degree of genital holding is almost universal. This behavior is thought to have no significant sexual or psychological implications;[1] is thought to be normal and does not warrant any diagnostic studies. Seldom is there any underlying physical cause and evaluation beyond physical examination and urinalysis is not warranted. The best advice for parents is to have them redirect the child's attention without placing great emphasis on this behavior. Generally, over time, children learn more acceptable public behavior without the apparent preoccupation for genital holding. Occasionally, very persistent holders may be told that the behavior may make others uncomfortable, and that for this reason, if they must hold themselves, they should do this in private. Parental education and reassurance is the best course of management.

Female-specific problems

Urethral prolapse

The circumferential eversion of urethral mucosa through the urethral meatus may be seen in girls and is termed urethral prolapse. It is associated with vascular congestion and possible strangulation of the prolapsed tissue. It is possible to have a partial or incomplete prolapse, but complete urethral prolapse is more common.[11] The etiology of urethral prolapse is unclear. Suggested causes include: poor attachment between the inner longitudinal and outer circular and oblique smooth muscle layers of the urethra associated with antecedent episodes of increased abdominal pressure, mucosal redundancy and vaginal mucosal atrophy, estrogen deficiency leading to lax periurethral fascia, neuromuscular disorders, urethral malposition, increased width of the urethra, poor bladder support, and deficient elastic tissues.[12] Predisposing Valsalva maneuvers such as chronic coughing, asthma, and constipation, as well as UTI and trauma, have been reported.[13–16]

Urethral prolapse is often misdiagnosed as the cause of urogenital bleeding in girls. The correct diagnosis at presentation has been reported at only 21%.[17] It is important to recognize that the prolapse appears as a doughnut-shaped mass protruding at the vulva (Figure 10.8). The mucosa is edematous, friable, bright red, or blue-black. As time goes on it may become infected, ulcerated, necrotic, or gangrenous.[11] The differential diagnosis of urethral prolapse includes a prolapsing ectopic ureterocele, prolapsed urethral polyp, ectopic ureter, prolapsed bladder, urethral cyst, hydrometrocolpos, condyloma acuminatum, sarcoma botryoides, and periurethral abscess. The diagnosis of urethral prolapse is visual and based on the typical circumferential appearance of the lesion around the meatus. None of the other stated conditions has a similar appearance. At times, diagnostic confirmation is made by placing a catheter or an instrument tip demonstrating that the urethra is actually in the center of the edematous tissue. Imaging studies are not necessary, but a voiding cystourethrogram (VCUG) can show a narrow, distal urethra.[18] The age range at diagnosis in pediatric series is from 5 days to 11 years, with a mean of 4.5–6 years.[14,16,17,19,20] Urethral prolapse has been reported in identical twins.[21] Also, ≥90% of girls with urethral prolapse are of African descent in most reports.[14,17,22]

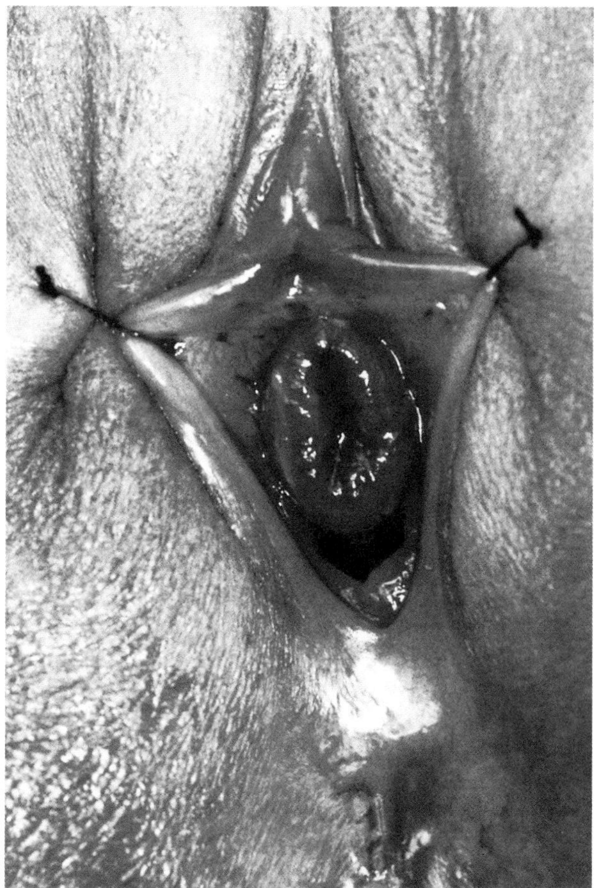

Figure 10.8 Urethral prolapse: note the doughnut appearance with urethral meatus centrally.

In addition to bleeding, symptoms include dysuria or frequency in 25% of girls;[14,16,17,19] 9% of the patients are asymptomatic, with the urethral mucosa showing no tenderness.[11,16] Urogenital bleeding from a urethral prolapse may be mistaken as being from a vaginal source.[14,16,17,19,23]

Treatment options vary for urethral prolapse. Simple treatments should be tried first, including observation alone, topical antibiotic ointment, topical estrogen cream, and sitz baths. Surgical treatments include primary excision, reduction and catheterization, suture ligation of the prolapsed tissue over a catheter, and in adult women cryoablation has been reported.[24] Most published series recommend conservative therapy.[14,17,19,23,25,26] Surgical treatment should be reserved for those rare instances of recurrence or persistent, symptomatic prolapse.[12,14,17,19,23]

Labial adherence

Labial adherence, midline fusion of the labia minora, is a common acquired lesion in young girls. Before puberty the labia minora are covered with a thin hypoestrogenized epithelium.[22,27] An irritating event, such as infection, trauma, or inflammation, causes the area to become denuded and inflamed, and the medial labial surfaces adhere with a fibrinous exudate over their surfaces.[22] Perhaps the most common inciting event is ammoniacal irritation. Adherence generally begins posteriorly and progresses anteriorly, leaving a small opening for the urine just inferior to the glans clitoris[28] (Figure 10.9). Occasionally the process begins near the clitoris, forming a 'preputial fusion'.[22] Labial adherence is also known as labial adhesions, labial agglutination, gynatresia, vulvar fusion, coalescence of the labia minora, vulvar synechiae, labial fusion, and occlusion of the vaginal vestibule. Differential diagnosis includes scarring of the labia minora, imperforate hymen, vaginal agenesis, clitoral hypertrophy, and intersex disorders.[27]

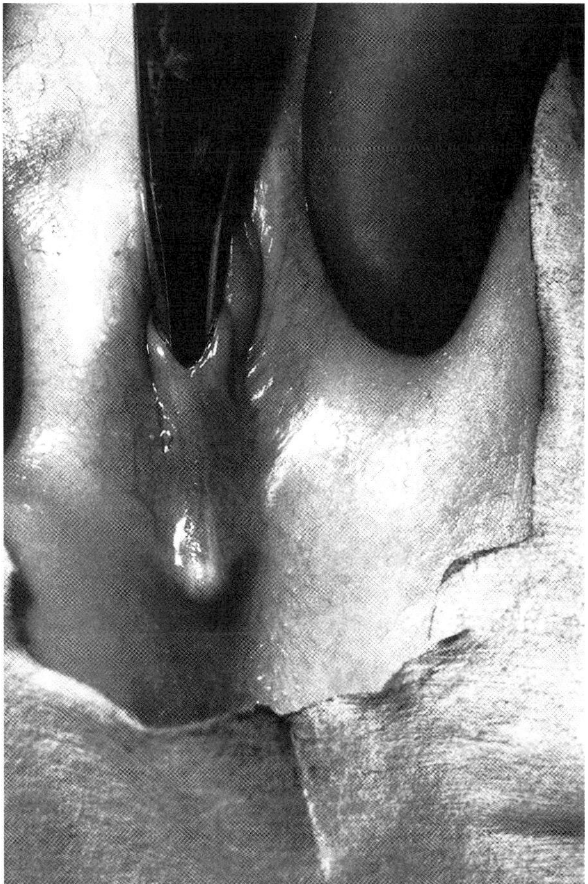

Figure 10.9 Labial adhesions characterized by fusion of the labia minora. There is generally a small opening anteriorly.

Labial adherence is fairly common and accounts for a large number of the genital abnormalities seen in girls. The peak incidence is between birth and 2 years old and again around the age of 6–7 years, although fusion can be seen until puberty.[28,29] Most girls with fused labia are asymptomatic but some have a deflected urinary stream or vaginal pooling of urine. Dysuria, generally secondary to the underlying inflammatory process, may be a persistent complaint. Patients may present with the diagnosis of UTI;[28] however, the suspected infection may simply be a contaminated specimen, as urine pools beneath the fused labia before exiting. True adhesion of the labia can occur in sexually abused girls with an incidence of approximately 3%.[27,30] This scarring is often thick and irregular in texture, and involves deeper layers.[31]

Treatment of adherent labia minora is not routinely required. Parents and referring primary care physicians should be reassured that they will lyse spontaneously given time. If treatment is thought to be necessary, estrogen cream can be applied daily, with success reported to be as high as 90% at 8 weeks.[27] The side effects of the estrogen cream will include vulvar pigmentation in all of the patients and breast tenderness in 6%, which resolves after the estrogen therapy is discontinued.[28] However, the long-term effects of estrogen given to prepubertal girls are unknown and treatment beyond a few weeks is probably unwarranted. Persisting adherence can be separated in the office using topical anesthetic (EMLA) and gentle, blunt separation.[22,27,28] An oral anxiolytic may be considered in such girls for this procedure.

Following separation, daily separation of the labia with application of an ointment should be continued for a time to prevent recurrence.[27,28] Forceful separation without analgesia is not recommended.

Vaginal cysts

Incidental vaginal cysts are uncommon and are often found in the newborn period, possibly as a consequence of stimulation by maternal estrogens. They are usually single and between 1 and 3 cm in diameter. When recognized in newborns, evaluation should include passage of a catheter or instrument into the vaginal introitus to assure patency. Rarely, ultrasonography may be necessary to ensure that the vagina is normal and not obstructed. These cysts almost always rupture spontaneously or resolve over a few weeks and need no further treatment. Introital cysts are of several types, including Gartner's duct cyst, Müllerian duct cyst, and epithelial inclusion cyst.

Gartner's duct is the distal rudimentary portion of the wolffian (mesonephric) duct in girls. These ducts in girls usually regress and almost completely disappear. If remnants persist, they are usually found along the anterolateral walls of the vagina. Flat, cuboidal cells line the cyst.[32] Gartner's duct cysts present as a perivaginal mass and usually appear in infants.[33] These cysts can be large enough to protrude from the vaginal introitus or fill the vagina and block its opening.[30,33,34]

Müllerian duct cysts are remnants of non-fused portions of the Müllerian ducts. They are generally asymptomatic and do not usually cause problems until menarche.

Most epithelial inclusion cysts are remnants of the urogenital sinus. Following trauma or surgery, buried vulvar or vaginal epithelium may also cause epithelial inclusion cysts. These are rare in children, although not uncommon in older women.[32] They usually occur posteriorly and in the midline of the vagina.[35] The cysts contain thick caseous material with a squamous epithelium lining their inner surface.[32] Surgical excision is the treatment of choice.[34]

Hydrocolpos

Distention of the vagina with fluid or mucus secretions is called hydrocolpos. If the uterus is involved, the term is hydrometrocolpos. The vagina can be obstructed from an imperforate hymen, transverse vaginal septum, or atretic vaginal introitus.[36] This produces a bulging, shiny, pearly gray protuberance observed over the vaginal introitus.[33,36] The urethral meatus can be noted anterior to the mass (Figure 10.10). Large abdominal masses can be palpable or identified on ultrasonography (U/S). Occasionally, urinary retention can be due to a mass effect. Ultrasonography shows a retrovesical oval cystic mass occasionally causing hydroureteronephrosis.[37] Treatment consists of drainage of the obstructed vagina perineally, but occasionally temporary abdominal vaginostomy may be necessary.

Other interlabial masses

Paraurethral cysts are known to occur along the distal one-third of the urethrovaginal wall.[32] The urethral meatus can be displaced, causing compression and a deflected urinary stream or dysuria. These cysts usually rupture spontaneously.[36,38]

Vaginitis

Vulvovaginitis is the most common cause of vaginal bleeding in the pediatric age group.[39] Vulvitis is vulvar irritation secondary to trauma, topical allergens,

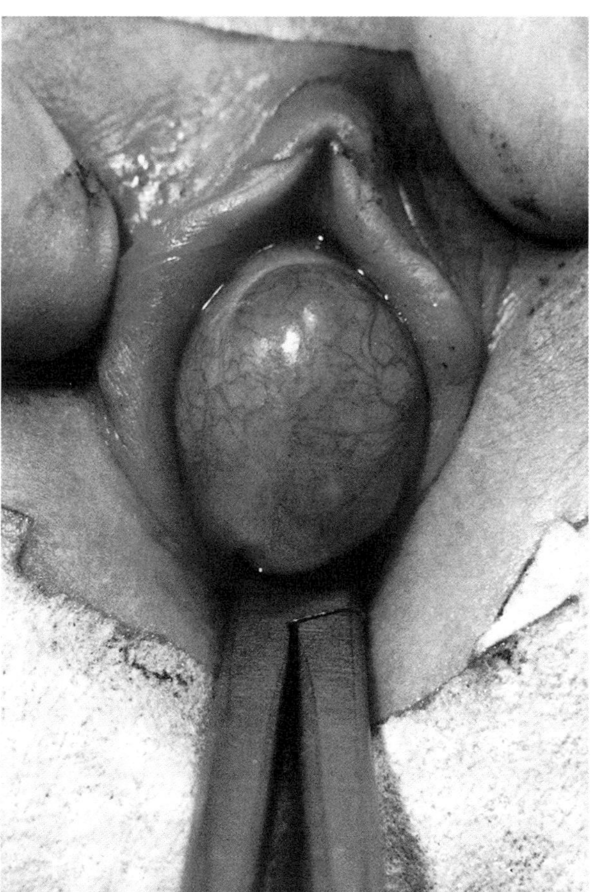

Figure 10.10 Hydrocolpos with duplicated vagina. The urethral meatus is seen splayed above the bulging mass while the hemostat is placed in the patent (second) vaginal opening.

mechanical irritation, chemical irritation, or poor hygiene.[40] Vaginitis is erythema and inflammation of the vaginal mucosa generally associated with discharge. Vulvovaginitis is very often a self-limiting problem and immediate work-up is not necessary. As the symptoms persist or become more annoying, work-up should include sampling of the vaginal pool for pH, wet mount, potassium hydroxide swab, and examination for chlamydia and gonorrhea. A urinalysis with culture may be diagnostic. If specific treatment is desired, a definitive diagnosis must be made.[39] Non-infectious causes in infants and children should be investigated, including ruling out the presence of a foreign body. Foreign body vaginitis symptoms are similar to other types of vaginitis. Toilet paper remnants are the most common objects found in the vagina.

Non-specific vulvovaginitis

Non-specific vulvovaginitis refers to a non-purulent, non-odorous discharge with a neutral pH and normal flora on wet mount. It accounts for 25–75% of all vulvovaginitis seen in premenarchal girls.[38] The etiology includes poor hygiene, urinary soiling, tight clothing, or chemical irritants such as harsh soaps. When testing is normal, treatment consists of reassurance and encouragement of good hygiene and appropriate clothing.

Newborn physiologic leukorrhea

It is normal for newborn girls under maternal estrogen stimulation to have a vaginal discharge. It is usually clear with white–gray mucus not associated with odor or irritation. Wet mount shows numerous epithelial cells without pathogenic bacteria or leukocytes. The discharge diminishes once maternal estrogen stimulation subsides. The tendency towards treatment with vaginal creams and antibiotics should be discouraged.

Genital infections of the young

Sexually transmitted diseases

A common sexually transmitted disease is chlamydial infection caused by *Chlamydia trachomatis*, which is an obligate intracellular Gram-negative organism capable of infecting the atrophic cuboidal epithelium of the prepubertal non-estrogenized vagina.[40] Young children may acquire chlamydia by passing through an infected birth canal or by sexual abuse. In newborns, chlamydia may infect the conjunctiva, pharynx, vagina, or anus. It is estimated that 50–75% of newborns become infected if their mothers were infected with chlamydia.[41]

Gonorrhea is the most common sexually transmitted disease found in abused children and is not likely to occur in children who are not sexually abused.[40,42] It is important to recognize gonorrhea to prevent sequelae and to recognize the child who is sexually abused. Infants can be contaminated through vaginal secretions in the birth canal colonizing the oropharynx, vagina, and rectum. The infection may remain asymptomatic. However, a white, yellow, or greenish, thick vaginal discharge with odor may be present. Labial erythema, urethral irritation, proctitis, or dysuria may be present.

Yeast infections

Other than the cutaneous variety associated with diaper rash, yeast infections are more common in adult females than in prepubertal girls. The alkaline vaginal pH of childhood is hostile to yeast.[40] Most yeast vaginitis is caused by *Candida albicans*. Most often yeast infections are secondary to such predisposing host factors as broad-spectrum antibiotic use or depressed cellular immunity.

Bacterial vaginosis

Less commonly, vaginal infections can be due to bacteria and are often listed as non-specific or *Gardnerella* vaginitis. This is now recognized to be caused by a mixed flora that includes anaerobic bacteria.

Pediatric hematuria

The presence of blood in the urine is a common clinical entity resulting in referral to pediatric urologists. It is a manifestation of abnormalities localized to the urinary tract from the kidneys to the urethra. Hematuria may be visible grossly or seen only on microscopic examination. Urine dipstick measures the presence of hemoglobin in urine and can be falsely positive for hematuria when hemoglobinuria and myoglobinuria are present. Verification of a positive urine dipstick for blood using microscopy can be performed to identify red blood cells (RBCs) within the specimen. To be considered significant for hematuria, urinalysis (UA) requires 5 RBCs per high-power field of a spun urinary specimen. RBC casts, dysmorphic or fragmented RBCs, and RBC blebs on UA signify a glomerular source for hematuria. Gross hematuria accounted for an estimated 1–2 patient visits per 1000 in pediatric emergency clinics.[43,44] The incidence of microscopic hematuria in asymptomatic children ranged from 14 to 41 per 1000 individuals when a minimum of 4 urine specimens were collected.[45,46]

The evaluation of a child with hematuria should be guided in a systematic fashion as determined by history, physical examination, and laboratory tests. Questions regarding the timing of hematuria relative to gastrointestinal, cutaneous, and respiratory infections are important. The presence of UTI symptoms including dysuria, flank pain, fevers, chills, frequency, and urgency, and a history of recent trauma, prolonged or vigorous exercise add direction to the initial assessment. The character of blood in urine (terminal versus throughout voiding), passage of clots, signs of stone passage including flank pain, nausea, vomiting, and radiating pain associated with hematuria, should be recorded. Documentation of any family history of renal failure, deafness, sickle cell trait or disease, and recurrent hematuria should clue the clinician to a hereditary source of hematuria. Medications, such as non-steroidal anti-inflammatory drugs (NSAIDs), and certain chemotherapeutic drugs, can be causative in the development of hematuria.

Physical examination should identify the presence or absence of flank or abdominal tenderness, extremity edema, pharyngitis, cutaneous rashes, deafness, fever, and hypertension. Urinalyses demonstrating proteinuria and/or abnormalities of RBC morphology are present in diseases involving the glomerulus or its basement membrane. Nitrites, leukocyte esterase, white blood cells (WBCs), and bacteria should prompt urine culture to tailor antibiotic treatment. Further laboratory and radiographic testing should be based upon clinical suspicion.

Asymptomatic microscopic hematuria is often identified when routine screening urine dipsticks are obtained in children. The absence of an inciting event (i.e. trauma), proteinuria, infection, hypertension, lower extremity edema, and renal insufficiency is reassuring and most of these patients can be observed with follow-up UA in 3–6 month-intervals until they normalize. When attributable to vigorous exercise or medications (i.e. NSAIDs), repeat UA can be performed every 1–2 weeks after discontinuation of the offending source to confirm resolution of the hematuria. Diagnostic tests such as radiographic examinations (U/S or VCUG) or invasive procedures, including renal biopsy or cystoscopy, are not warranted in these patients.[47] If asymptomatic gross hematuria or persistent microscopic hematuria occurs, diagnostics testing can be tailored, based upon history and physical examination.

When persistent microscopic hematuria develops without a contributory history or physical examination, obtaining calcium/creatinine (Ca/Cr) ratio, parental urinalysis, and hemoglobin electrophoresis (if the patient is of African–American descent), is helpful in assessing for hypercalciuria, benign familial hematuria, and sickle cell disease/trait, respectively. The spot calcium/creatinine ratio is considered abnormal when >0.21 in children >6 years of age.[48] Alternatively, a 24-hour urine collection demonstrating a urine calcium level >4 mg/kg/day is diagnostic for hypercalciuria.[49] In a small retrospective study of children referred for microscopic hematuria,[47] evaluation of serum electrolytes, creatinine, cystoscopy, VCUGs and U/S of the kidneys and bladder failed to show abnormalities. However, serum creatinine and renal U/S are often utilized to assist in the initial evaluation despite their apparent low yield. When normal, parents can be reassured that their child's prognosis is excellent. Nonetheless, these patients should be followed yearly to assess for the development of proteinuria, hypertension, new symptoms, or resolution of hematuria that would alter current management.

When microscopic hematuria is associated with symptoms, patient evaluation should be tailored based on clinical presentation. The concomitant presence of proteinuria, hypertension, and peripheral edema should prompt an assessment to distinguish between glomerular etiologies of hematuria. Laboratory tests including chemistry panel, complete blood count (CBC), C3, C4, albumin, antistreptolysin-O (ASO) and anti-DNAase-B antibodies will facilitate discriminating between the different immune and basement membrane abnormalities. Prompt referral to a pediatric nephrologist should occur in the presence of an acutely ill child, rapidly progressing or chronic glomerulonephritis, patients exhibiting symptoms of nephritic syndrome, uncertainty of a correct diagnosis, or the need of assistance in management and therapy.[50] However, when microscopic hematuria is associated with a small amount of proteinuria, a conservative course with close follow-up can be instituted with further investigation utilizing the above algorithm if evidence of persistence or clinical progression occurs.

If a history of recent trauma is present, computed tomography (CT) and retrograde urethrography are warranted based upon the clinical scenario and judgment. When signs or symptoms worrisome for a UTI occur, protocols should include obtaining urine cultures, instituting antibiotic therapy based on culture sensitivities, and repeating a formal UA and culture after the infection has been treated to assess for resolution of the hematuria. Non-contrast CT and urine calcium analysis are helpful if urolithiasis is suspected; abdominal imaging (U/S or CT) if an abdominal mass is palpated.

The presence of gross hematuria can be differentiated based upon its appearance. Tea- or cola-colored urine suggests a glomerular source. Bright red urine with normal morphology on microscopic examination suggests a urinary tract etiology for the hematuria.[51] The absence of RBCs on microscopic examination in light of a positive dipstick may be indicative of hemoglobinuria or myoglobinuria. Subsequent work-up for gross hematuria is driven primarily by clinical presentation. Signs and symptoms suggestive of stones, infection, recent trauma, or glomerulonephropathies can follow similar protocols as described for symptomatic microscopic hematuria.

Idiopathic urethrorrhagia is seen in prepubertal boys who present with blood spotting in the underwear between voiding. In a review at our institution, dysuria was reported in ~30% of patients and mean age at presentation was 10.1 years old.[52] Laboratory and radiographic studies – intravenous pyelography (IVP), U/S, and VCUG – are routinely normal, although RBCs can be seen in up to 57% of patients.[52,53] Symptoms can persist, ranging from a few weeks to 3 or 4 years. Etiology is unknown, although anterior and posterior urethritis have been documented.[52,54] Cystoscopy is generally considered unnecessary unless symptoms persist >24 months as urethral stricture may be identified. This process is self-limited and resolves by puberty without treatment.

For a review of the diagnostic algorithms presented for pediatric hematuria, please refer to Figure 10.11.

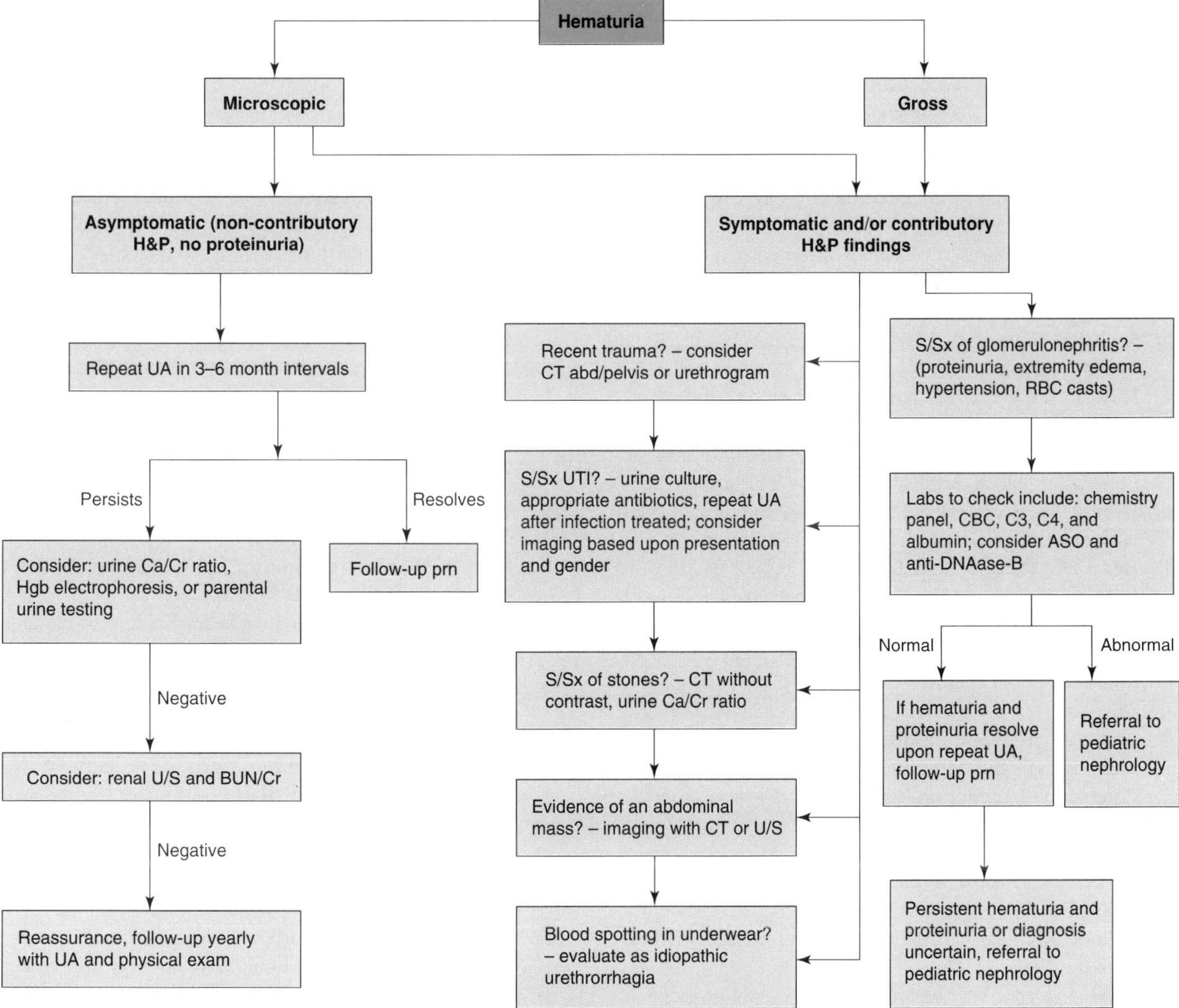

Figure 10.11 Diagnostics algorithm for pediatric hematuria. For abbreviations see text. In addition: BUN, blood urea nitrogen; S/Sx, signs and symptoms; prn, as required; H&P, history and physical examination; Hgb, hemoglobin.

References

1. Caldamone AA, Schulman S, Rabinowitz R. Outpatient pediatric urology. In: Gillenwater JY, Grayhack JT, Howards SS, Duckett J, eds. Adult and Pediatric Urology. St Louis: Mosby, 1996: 2730–1.
2. Walker RD. Presentation of genitourinary disease and abdominal masses. In: Kelalis PP, King LR, Belman AB, eds. Clinical Pediatric Urology. Philadelphia: WB Saunders, 1992: 218–43.
3. Oster J. Further fate of the foreskin: incidence of preputial adhesions, phimosis and smegma among Danish schoolboys. Arch Dis Child 1968; 43:200–3.
4. Chu C, Chen K, Diau G. Topical steriod treatment of phimosis in boys. J Urol 1999; 162:861–3.
5. DeVries CR, Miller AK, Packer MG. Reduction of paraphimosis with hyaluronidase. Urology 1996; 48(3):464–5.
6. Cartwright P, Snow B, McNees D. Urethral meatotomy in the office utilizing topical EMLA cream for anesthesia. J Urol 1996; 156:857–9.
7. Brown MR, Cartwright PC, Snow BW. Common office problems in pediatric urology and gynecology. Pediatr Clin North Am 1997; 44:1091–115.
8. Hoebeke P, Dupawn P, Van Laecke E et al. The use of EMLA cream as anaesthetic for minor urological surgery in children. Acta Urol Belg 1997; 65:25–8.
9. Bloom DA, Wan J, Key D. Disorders of the male external genitalia and inguinal canal. In: Kelalis PP, King LR, Belman AB, eds. Clinical Pediatric Urology. Philadelphia: WB Saunders, 1992: 1015–18.
10. Jayanthi VR, Burns JE, Koff SA. Postneonatal circumcision with local anesthesia: a cost-effective alternative. J Urol 1999; 161:1301–3.
11. Shah BR, Tunnessen WW. Picture of the month. Arch Pediatr Adolesc Med 1995; 149:462–3.
12. Kleinjan JH, Vos P. Strangulated urethral prolapse. Urology 1996; 47:599–601.
13. Kamat MH, DelGaizo A, Seebode JJ. Urethral prolapse in female children. Am J Dis Child 1969; 118:691–3.
14. Jerkins GR, Verheeck K, Noe HN. Treatment of girls with urethral prolapse. J Urol 1984; 132:732–3.
15. Lowe FC, Hill GS, Jeffs RD et al. Urethral prolapse in children: insights into etiology and management. J Urol 1986; 135:100–3.
16. Fernandes ET, Dekermacher S, Sabadin MA et al. Urethral prolapse in children. Urology 1993; 41:240–2.
17. Anveden-Hertzberg L, Gauderer WL, Elder JS. Urethral prolapse: an often misdiagnosed cause of urogenital bleeding in girls. Pediatr Emerg Care 1995; 11:212–14.
18. Potter BM. Urethral prolapse in girls. Radiology 1971; 98:287–9.
19. Richardson DA, Hajj SN, Herbst AL. Medial treatment of urethral prolapse in children. Obstet Gynecol 1982; 59:69–74.
20. Bullock KN. Strangulated prolapse of female urethra. Urology 1983; 21:46–8.
21. Mitre A, Nahas W, Gilbert A et al. Urethral prolapse in girls: familial case. J Urol 1987; 137:115.
22. Rock JA, Azziz R. Genital anomalies in childhood. Clin Obstet Gynecol 1987; 30:682–96.
23. Trotman MD, Brewster EM. Prolapse of the urethral mucosa in prepubertal West Indian girls. Br J Urol 1993; 72:503–5.
24. Friedrich EG. Cryosurgery for urethral prolapse. Obstet Gynecol 1977; 50:359–61.
25. Redman JF. Conservative management of urethral prolapse in female children. Urology 1982; 19:505–6.
26. Carlson NJ, Mercer LJ, Hajj SN. Urethral prolapse in the premenarcheal female. Int J Gynaecol Obstet 1987; 25:69–71.
27. Starr NB. Labial adhesions in childhood. J Pediatr Health Care 1996; 10:26–7.
28. Clair DL, Caldamone AA. Pediatric office procedures. Urol Clin North Am 1988; 15:715–23.
29. Starr A. Ureteral plication. A new concept in ureteral tapering for megaureter. Invest Urol 1979; 17:153–8.
30. Muram D. Labial adhesions in sexually abused children. JAMA 1988; 259:352–3.
31. McCann J, Voris J, Simon M. Labial adhesions and posterior fourchette injuries in childhood sexual abuse. Am J Dis Child 1988; 142:659–63.
32. Klein FA, Vick CW, Broecker BH. Neonatal vaginal cysts: diagnosis and management. J Urol 1986; 135:371–2.
33. Muram D, Jerkins GR. Urinary retention secondary to a Gartner's duct cyst. Obstet Gynecol 1988; 72:510–11.
34. Gallup DG, Talledo OE. Benign and malignant tumors. Clin Obstet Gynecol 1987; 30:662–70.
35. Beazley JM. Congenital anomalies of the female genital tract excluding intersex. Clin Obstet Gynecol 1977; 20:533–44.
36. Nussbaum AR, Lebowitz RL. Interlabial masses in little girls: review and imaging recommendations. AJR Am J Roentgenol 1983; 141:65–71.
37. Patel VH, Merchant SA, Kedar RP et al. Isolated hydrocolpos: ultrasound findings and the importance of confident preoperative diagnosis. J Clin Ultrasound 1992; 20:85–6.
38. Emans SJ, Goldstein DP. Pediatric and Adolescent Gynecology, 3rd edn. Boston: Little, Brown and Co., 1990.
39. Fishman A, Paldi E. Vaginal bleeding in premenarchal girls: a review. Obstet Gynecol Surv 1991; 46:457–60.
40. Jenny C. Sexually transmitted diseases and child abuse. Pediatr Ann 1992; 21:497–503.
41. Hammerschlag MR. Chlamydia trachomatis in children. Pediatr Ann 1994; 23:349–53.
42. Judson FN, Ehret J. Laboratory diagnosis of sexually transmitted infections. Pediatr Ann 1994; 23:361–9.
43. Ingelfinger JR, Davis AE, Grupe WE. Frequency and etiology of gross hematuria in a general pediatric setting. Pediatrics 1977; 59:557–61.
44. Anand SK. Hematuria and glomerular disorders. In: Osborn LM, DeWitt TG, First LR, Zenel JA, eds. Pediatrics, 1st edn. Philadelphia: Elsevier Mosby, 2005: 713–19.
45. Vehaskari VM, Rapola J, Koskimies O et al. Microscopic hematuria in school children: epidemiology and clinicopathologic evaluation. J Pediatr 1979; 95:676–84.
46. Dodge WF, West EF, Smith EH, Bruce H 3rd. Proteinuria and hematuria in schoolchildren: epidemiology and early natural history. J Pediatr 1976; 88:327–47.

47. Feld LG, Meyers KE, Kaplan BS, Stapleton FB. Limited evaluation of microscopic hematuria in pediatrics. Pediatrics 1998; 102:E42.
48. Sargent JD, Stukel TA, Kresel J, Klein RZ. Normal values for random urinary calcium to creatinine ratios in infancy. J Pediatr 1993; 123:393–7.
49. Parks JH, Coe FL. A urinary calcium–citrate index for the evaluation of nephrolithiasis. Kidney Int 1986; 30:85–90.
50. Patel HP, Bissler JJ. Hematuria in children. Pediatr Clin North Am 2001; 48:1519–37.
51. Tomita M, Kitamoto Y, Nakayama M, Sato T. A new morphological classification of urinary erythrocytes for differential diagnosis of glomerular hematuria. Clin Nephrol 1992; 37:84–9.
52. Walker BR, Ellison ED, Snow BW, Cartwright PC. The natural history of idiopathic urethrorrhagia in boys. J Urol 2001; 166:231–2.
53. Kaplan GW, Brock WA. Idiopathic urethrorrhagia in boys. J Urol 1982; 128:1001–3.
54. Renouard C, Gauthier F, Valayer J. [Urethrorrhagia in boys]. Chir Pediatr 1984; 25:106–9.

Principles of minimally invasive surgery

11

Walid A Farhat and Pasquale Casale

Introduction

Laparoscopy is becoming increasingly popular in pediatric urology, reducing the invasiveness of treatment and shortening the period of convalescence.[1] With the development of new instruments, better designed for pediatrics, laparoscopy in all ages may be now a safe and effective way to treat many urologic disorders. Nearly any procedure performed in a body cavity can be accomplished using the instrumentation available to us today and the variety of laparoscopic procedures that can be performed in pediatric patients is virtually unlimited.[2] To master this technique, the novice must perform a large number of cases and understand that the learning curve is steep so as not to get discouraged.

Anesthesia

Induction and maintenance of anesthesia may be with either inhalational or intravenous agents or a combination of both. Nitrous gas increases bowel distention, potentially bringing the peritoneum closer to the area of dissection for retroperitoneal procedures and decreasing working space in transperitoneal procedures. Intraoperative monitoring should include a routine electrocardiogram (ECG), non-invasive blood pressure, SpO_2, temperature, and inspired oxygen concentration.[3] Although end-tidal CO_2 may not accurately reflect arterial CO_2 tension, its use is helpful in planning appropriate ventilation strategies. In infants and children with respiratory illness, capillary or arterial blood gas analysis might be needed to accurately monitor CO_2 tension. Maintenance intravenous fluid is usually sufficient unless there is unanticipated bleeding. Finally, it is preferable to insert the intravenous line in the arm on the side of the surgery for a patient in the flank position for easy access.

Anesthesia and physiology

Patient positioning during laparoscopic surgery may potentiate the impact of gas insufflation. For instance, the Trendelenburg position during laparoscopy will increase heart rate and vascular resistance while decreasing mean arterial pressure and cardiac output, whereas the opposite effect is seen in the reverse Trendelenburg position.[4] Furthermore, flank positioning, especially with the kidney rest up and patient flexed, will accentuate impaired venous return and increase cardiac strain. In fact, the left lateral decibitus position produces more significant hemodynamic and respiratory changes than the right flank position.

Pressure effects

As gas is placed in a closed space, it moves depending on the partial pressure gradients. Once the pressure rises, a plethora of cardiovascular, pulmonary, and renal effects may be seen. The heart rate and mean arterial pressure increase while the venous return and cardiac output decrease. These parameters are seen even when pressure is set at a standard working level of 10–15 mmHg. Above this level more profound hemodynamic alterations are anticipated to occur, with further decrease in cardiac output. Furthermore, limitation of diaphragmatic mobility may cause respiratory restriction, manifested by increased airway pressure, requiring an increase in the peak end-inspiratory pressure to maintain a set tidal volume. Finally, renal effects occur secondary to gas insufflation, manifested by decreased glomerular filtration rate (GFR) and urine output. Animal studies have shown that gas insufflation causes renal vein compression, inducing decreased renal blood flow, decreased urine output, and diminished creatinine clearance.[5,6] These effects do not appear to cause renal damage in humans, however.

Absorption effects

Insufflated CO_2 is absorbed into the blood by diffusion, which is limited and determined by many variables; most important are the pressure differential and the cross-sectional area of the absorbing surface. The effects of gas absorption are either pulmonary or hemodynamic. The pulmonary effects are increased CO_2 retention and increased end-tidal CO_2, exacerbated by decreased functional residual capacity and decreased diaphragmatic excursion. The hemodynamic effects of hypercarbia are increased heart rate, vasodilation, and increased cardiac contractility. Although in healthy children there is little if any added cardiorespiratory risk from laparoscopic procedures, children with cardiopulmonary compromise require close and careful monitoring.[3]

Instrumentation

Rapid progress in video technology and the miniaturization of instruments to <2 mm in diameter have made the performance of a variety of pediatric laparoscopic procedures possible.[4] Instruments of this size and larger come in nearly every variety (scissors, needle holders, dissectors, graspers, clamps, suction devices, energy delivery devices, etc.) and facilitate the performance of the most complex cases. The surgical procedure, in combination with the size of the patient, will determine the surgeon's selection of instruments and telescope size. Laparoscopic trocars are available in 3 mm, 5 mm, and 10–12 mm sizes, with corresponding instruments and reducers. Telescopes are available in 3.3 mm, 5 mm, and 10 mm sizes, with varying degrees for optimal visualization. For most ablative or reconstructive urologic procedures, 3 mm or 5 mm trocars are sufficient. However, sometimes 10–12 mm trocars may be necessary if a stapling device needs to be utilized, or when specimen extraction is anticipated.

Access

For all laparoscopic procedures, whether transperitoneal or retroperitoneal, there are two techniques to gain access into the peritoneum: blind access and access through visualization. The blind closed approach is facilitated through the use of a Veress insufflation needle. A stab wound is made with either a #15 or a #11 blade, the Veress needle is inserted through the 1 mm opening, passed through all layers of tissue, and verification of placement is confirmed by opening the stopcock and infusing a small amount of saline into the channel to verify placement typically in the retroperitoneal approach. For transperitoneal procedures, it is more accurate to attach the insufflation needle to the insufflator and monitor pressures. Low pressures (<10 mmHg) are a reliable indication of being intraperitoneal. The second technique is the open (Hasson) approach and is facilitated through the use of direct and telescopic visualization of all tissue during insertion of the trocar with a blunt obturator to gain access into the working space. This technique is generally preferred in children and is especially ideal for obese patients. All proposed trocar sites are injected with bupivacaine 0.5%, with 1:100 000 epinephrine after insufflation and prior to accessory trocar placement.[3] Placement of accessory ports should be carried out using direct vision from within. The location of the accessory trocars depends on the operation to be performed, and specifics of all trocar placements are described below in the transperitoneal and retroperitoneal laparoscopy subsections of this chapter.

Trocar fixation

For all laparoscopic procedures a short (~1 cm) section of rubber, plastic tubing, or cone can be placed around the trocar shaft, about one-third the way from the tip to the hub of the trocar. This prevents the trocar from being pushed into the surgical cavity as instruments are advanced. Prior to CO_2 insufflation, a 2-0 Vicryl (UR-6 needle) suture may be placed around the trocar and in the fascia as a purse-string suture. Once the depth of the trocar is well delineated, this suture is tied to the side of the port and serves several purposes: it prevents the trocar from moving in or out during instrument manipulation; it decreases the possibility of subcutaneous emphysema or leakage of CO_2 from around the trocar site; and it can be used to lift the abdominal wall to enlarge the retroperitoneal space.

Insufflation

Newer insufflators can deliver a great volume of gas rapidly; this may be dangerous in an infant weighing less than 2 kg. In addition to pressure fluctuation, CO_2 insufflation with unwarmed high-flow gas may cool a tiny infant quickly.[3–5] Whereas the rule is to insufflate with just enough pressure to have unobstructed visualization, pressures of 15 mmHg appear to be well tolerated in any size patient with the only issue being ventilatory compromise in infants with marginal lung function. For all laparoscopic procedures, CO_2 insufflation should be started at a pressure of 12–15 mmHg for children >2 years old and 8–10 mmHg for children <2 years old.

Both the peritoneal and retroperitoneal spaces are closed yet expansible. The physiologic consequences of CO_2 insufflation may be related to the compressive effects of the gas or the metabolic consequences of the gas absorption. With insufflation, the gas will attempt to reach equilibrium with the surrounding environment; such equilibrium is monitored with the use of insufflators that not only control the flow of gas but also monitor the feedback pressure generated from the insufflation.

Operative approaches

Indications for retroperitoneal or transperitoneal laparoscopy

- Total nephrectomy.
- Partial nephrectomy for duplicated renal system.
- Distal ureterectomy for duplication anomaly.
- Pyeloplasty.
- Pyelolithotomy and ureterolithotomy. Extracorporeal lithotripsy and endourologic procedures have almost eliminated the need for open surgery to remove urinary stones. On the other hand, in patients who have unusual anatomy such as ectopic kidneys, a laparoscopic approach may be used either to perform pyelolithotomy or to help in getting direct percutaneous access to the kidney.
- Adrenalectomy for cortical adenoma associated with congenital adrenal hyperplasia.

Contraindications to laparoscopy

Contraindications to laparoscopy in infants, children, and adolescents are the same as for any other surgical procedure, except for evidence of limited lung reserve function, which may be considered as a relative contraindication. If the patient is septic, in shock, or exhibits a coagulopathy, these should be corrected before surgery is contemplated. If surgery is deemed essential under these circumstances, then it probably should be performed open.[4]

Strong contraindications

- Cardiopulmonary morbidity.
- Uncorrected coagulopathy.
- Sepsis.
- Malignant tumors. Although laparoscopy may play a role in the staging of malignant pediatric abdominal tumors such as Wilms' tumor or neuroblastoma, its role in the management of these tumors has yet to be defined. Morcellation of specimens for extraction has raised concerns about accurate pathologic staging; hence, large-sized tumors mandate an incision to retrieve them. In addition, the fragile consistency of the tumor makes it more prone to rupture, and hence may obviate the use of this technique.[5]

Retroperitoneal laparoscopic approach

Relative contraindications

- Prior retroperitoneal scar (kidney surgery, kidney biopsy, or pyeloplasty).
- Previous infectious or inflammatory retroperitoneal process (xanthogranulomatous pyelonephritis), except for experienced surgeons in this approach.

Advantages

- The technique mimics the open urologic surgical procedure through the retroperitoneal approach.
- This direct approach to the organs of the genitourinary tract requires less dissection to the colon or the spleen to expose the kidneys and adrenals.
- Previous transperitoneal surgery does not preclude retroperitoneoscopy.
- Trocar sites have less postoperative hernias than an open incision.
- It facilitates the view of the posterior surface of the kidney hence rapid access to the renal hilum.

Disadvantages

- Manipulation of instruments may be initially difficult due to a restricted working space: e.g. in reconstructive surgery such as a pyeloplasty, suturing and knot tying may be difficult, as well as in ablative surgery, the degree of technical difficulty increases in the presence of large-sized specimens.
- Achieving anatomic orientation may initially be a challenge for the inexperienced laparoscopist.[6]

Anatomic considerations for retroperitoneal laparoscopy

An understanding of the retroperitoneal surgical anatomy is mandatory before embarking on retroperitoneoscopic surgery. The boundaries of the retroperitoneal space are:

- posteriorly and laterally – the paraspinous, psoas, and quadratus lumborum muscles, which are anatomically fixed structures
- anteriorly – the mobile posterior parietal peritoneum and its contents
- superiorly – the diaphragm
- inferiorly – contiguous with the extraperitoneal portions of the pelvis.

The retroperitoneum contains the great vessels, kidneys, adrenals, and ureters, in addition to the perirenal adipose and aerolar tissues. Since there is no preformed space, pneumoretroperitoneum is only accomplished after breaking up the adipose aerolar tissue in the retroperitoneum.

Patient preparation and positioning

Bowel preparation for retroperitoneoscopic renal surgery may be recommended in adults; however, this has not been our practice in children.

Although a retroperitoneoscopic approach may be accomplished with the patient prone, we prefer the flank position as it increases the anteroposterior dimensions of the retroperitoneal space and displaces the peritoneal reflection anteriorly, decreasing the chance of inadvertently opening it. The patient is positioned in the full 90° flank position as close to the posterior edge of the table as possible. To further increase the retroperitoneal space, the table is flexed and the kidney rest elevated. Pressure points are meticulously padded and an axillary roll is placed to prevent postoperative complications such as brachial plexus palsy. The patient should be taped to the table using 3-inch adhesive tape placed across the shoulder and the hips so that the patient will remain secured while the table is moved during the surgery.

We prefer to have the surgeon and assistant standing on the same side of the table and we use only one monitor. We believe that having both surgeon and assistant in the same line of vision facilitates eye–hand coordination, particularly that of the assistant surgeon.

Laparoscopic technique

Access to the retroperitoneum is preferably achieved by the open (Hasson) technique, which provides visual guidance. As children have a small retroperitoneal space, and close proximity between the abdominal wall and the major vessels, the closed technique is not recommended. In addition, since there is no actual pre-existing retroperitoneal space, the placement of a Veress needle is not precise and may cause either injury to the great vessels or pneumoperitoneum.

In the midaxillary line, a 1 cm long incision is made 1–2 cm below the tip of the 12th rib. The muscles are split in the direction of their fibers and then the lumbodorsal fascia is incised to enter the retroperitoneum. The method for the development of the retroperitoneal space using a blunt instrument or the balloon dissector is up to the surgeon. Although commercial balloon dissectors are readily available, an inexpensive balloon can be made using the finger of a surgeon's glove tied around a catheter. The balloon is inserted anterior to the psoas muscle and outside Gerota's fascia, and approximately 400–500 ml of air is used to inflate the balloon, creating the space. Instead of using a balloon we introduce a wet gauze close to the posterior muscular wall to create the retroperitoneal space.

Insertion of the primary trocar in the correct space is of paramount importance because inserting the trocar too far medially may result in peritoneal entry or colon injury, whereas entering posteriorly in the quadratus or psoas muscles may cause bleeding. If Gerota's fascia is easily visible, it is incised and opened for direct CO_2 insufflation, although this technique may be associated with inadvertent peritoneotomy. For this reason, it is preferable to create the retroperitoneal space outside Gerota's fascia, dissect the peritoneum medially, and then insert the posterior secondary 5 mm trocar, open Gerota's fascia under vision, and proceed with the creation of the retroperitoneal space by medially dissecting the peritoneal reflection for the third trocar insertion.

We exclusively create the retroperitoneal space using blunt dissection. Through the incision and with the psoas muscle as a reference point, a 10 mm trocar with the laparoscope (0°) is inserted to confirm correct placement. Initially, the posterior–inferior aspect of Gerota's fascia and the lower pole are visualized. Identification of the psoas muscle posteriorly is crucial; on the other hand anteriorly, the edge of the peritoneum is identified and swept medially to expose the underside of the transversalis fascia. To avoid tearing the peritoneum, it is dissected medially by manipulating the laparoscope in a lateral to medial fashion close to the abdominal wall to expose the internal surface of the transversalis muscle. Having created the working space, two 5 mm secondary trocars are inserted. The posterior secondary port is first inserted approximately midway between the 12th rib and the iliac bone, and lateral to the border of the paraspinous muscles. Using a grasper through this trocar, the peritoneum is further mobilized medially to create the pelvic extraperitoneal space. The anterior secondary trocar is inserted at the anterior axillary line 2 cm superior to the iliac crest. The two secondary ports should be inserted as far apart as possible to improve ergonomics.

In order to place the secondary trocars under vision, a 30° laparoscope may be used. However, we use the 0° telescope, and we insert the trocars in the following fashion for both the retroperitoneal and the transperitoneal approach. A small skin stab is made using a #11 blade; then, using sharp-tipped obturators, the trocars are advanced through the muscles and fascia. Once in the retroperitoneal space, a blunt-tipped obturator is exchanged for a sharp one and the trocars are advanced into the retroperitoneum. This safety tip prevents injury to the peritoneum or the major vessels. In addition, while inserting the trocar, it should be directed toward the area of dissection because if the trocar is advanced away from the site of dissection, this might result in constant tension on the skin during surgery or a greater chance of gas leakage at the trocar site.

Although the sites of the telescope and other trocars are the same for all retroperitoneal renal and adrenal laparoscopic procedures, the sequence of operative strategy and the need for accessory trocars depend on the surgical procedure. In event that more than three ports are required, laparoscopic guidance and bimanual palpation are recommended for accurate placement. For instance, during retroperitoneoscopic pyeloplasty, an additional port may be required to maintain traction on the ureteropelvic junction for better exposure; in this case, a fourth trocar (3 or 5 mm) is placed along the anterior axillary line at the tip of the 11th rib. In order to avoid inadvertent peritoneotomy, adequate dissection of the peritoneal reflection medially at the trocar insertion point is mandatory.

The following laparoscopic landmarks are useful for orientation in any retroperitoneoscopic renal procedure: the psoas muscle and posterior aspect of the kidney are identified first. This approach allows rapid visualization of the 'vertically' oriented main artery and vein. To further facilitate exposure of the renal pedicle, save dissection of the anterior surface of the kidney to the last step. This will maintain retraction on the renal pedicle in case a nephrectomy or a partial nephrectomy is contemplated. In addition, this approach will suspend the kidney anteriorly, exposing the ureteropelvic junction in case a pyeloplasty is performed.

For identifying the renal hilum, locate the psoas muscle, then find the great vessels medially and these will lead to the renal pedicle. In addition, identifying the distal ureter and following it proximally, with the pulsations of the renal artery, aorta, or vena cava, may help to locate the renal hilum. On the right side, initial identification of the inferior vena cava on the medial aspect of the psoas muscle facilitates identification of the gonadal, renal, and possibly the suprarenal veins, which are all located in the same plane. On the left side, the pulsations of the aorta are often visualized and help guide the surgeon to the renal artery.

Transperitoneal laparoscopic approach

Transperitoneal procedures provide exceptional exposure since the intraperitoneal space is large.

Patient preparation and positioning

For upper transperitoneal procedures, positioning the patient in a flank or modified flank position at the edge of the table is crucial. This positioning allows the surgeon to full access of the abdominal cavity without limitations caused by the edge of the table. For the modified flank, a roll should be placed under the torso to provide a 60° patient angulation from the table. The patient should be secured, so that the table may be repositioned as necessary during the procedure. The main monitor should be placed on the lesion side of the operative table, with a slave monitor behind the surgeon. All cables, lines, and wires for the instruments should preferably go off the opposite side to the surgeon. This positioning and port placement is used for the majority of renal interventions such as nephrectomy, heminephrectomy, pyeloplasty, and other renal extirpative and reconstructive procedures. The transabdominal approach also allows access to the pelvis by altering the port use via placing the camera through the subcostal port and instruments through the umbilical and lateral ports.

For lower transperitoneal procedures in infants, it is most convenient to position the patient at the foot of the bed, across the bottom, and to stand at the side of the bed (at the patient's head) to operate.[4] This is a good approach to the bladder. For older patients a mid-table, supine position with a sacral roll to thrust the pelvis up is preferable. Usually the side opposite the lesion is chosen, and the telescope placed centrally in or near the umbilicus. The instrument trocars are placed lateral to the rectus muscle after insufflation, sufficiently superior and inferior to the telescope cannula so that the instruments can be introduced at a 45° angle relative to the operative field. The monitor should be located towards the foot end of the operative table. Only one monitor is necessary in this scenario. All cables, lines, and wires should be off the foot of the bed for optimal ergonomics.

This approach is extremely helpful for gynecologic and urologic procedures in the pelvis, including transvesical approaches. The new transvesical procedures such as ureteral reimplantation require cannula fixation so that the bladder mucosa does not strip and dissect away from the detrusor muscle. One way to achieve this is to perform a cystostomy at the skin incision to help hold the bladder wall and mucosa to the anterior abdominal wall. A balloon-tipped cannula may also be helpful here, but the size of the balloon tip may impair instrument manipulation in a small child.

Laparoscopic technique

Transabdominal access is best achieved through the umbilicus using the open technique previously discussed, whereby the umbilical scar is lifted using an Allis clamp; then, using a #11 blade, the skin and subcutaneous tissue is incised and peritoneum is entered.

Instruments can be placed directly through a stab wound without the need for a trocar if the surgeon does not anticipate repeatedly withdrawing and reinserting instruments through this site.[6–9]

In infants and thin children, the laxity of the abdominal wall might allow large trocars or heavy instruments to compress the abdominal wall, obscuring vision and limiting CO_2 distention. Once access is attained, sometimes bowel, bladder, or other structures can obstruct the view. It can be helpful to pass one or more sutures through the abdominal wall, through the structure, and back out through the abdominal wall for retraction. These can be tied to a self-retaining retractor or can simply be tied at the distended abdominal wall if that is sufficient.[4]

Technical laparoscopic tips

Suturing

Intracorporeal suturing requires two needle holders or a needle holder and a grasping device. Several sutures can be placed with one length of suture material. A 6 or 7 cm length of suture with its curved needle may be directly passed through 5 mm trocars, but not through 3.5 mm trocars unless the curved needle is first straightened. The suture may also be passed through the abdominal wall to avoid the need for a 5 mm trocar if ≤3 mm trocars are being utilized.

Laparoscopic extracorporeal-assisted tying is possible, but requires a large cannula at one of the port sites. There are a variety of automatic suturing devices and suture assistants; however, it is important for the endoscopic surgeon to become proficient with non-assisted suturing techniques. This is because suture assist devices require larger trocars and are more costly than non-assisted intracorporeal suturing. Furthermore, the majority of devices have a limited choice of suture material and size, and most are not acceptable for complex delicate reconstruction.[10]

An innovative technique for intracorporeal suturing is to tie together the ends of two 5 cm segments of 6-0 Vicryl, one dyed and one undyed, both on a small taper needle, prior to insertion into the peritoneal cavity. The knot tied initially secures the first suture into the renal pelvis and both decreases trauma to the tissue and expedites the anastomosis. The color differentiation facilitates suturing and decreases any confusion and need for repetitive suturing.

Hemostasis

Vessels may be ligated with laparoscopic clip-applying devices that are available in 5 and 10 mm. Laparoscopic tie assisting devices are also available if clips are not preferable. They typically require a ≥5 mm cannula and either have an cinch knot technology or allow extracorporeal tying and knot placement with a pusher device. Freehand laparoscopic tying can also be performed, but is time consuming and does not seem to be beneficial with the current hemostatic devices available.

Laparoscopic stapling devices are available for hemostasis. They are an excellent alternative for large vessels and for transecting thick tissue such as bowel mesentery. The laparoscopic stapling devices require a ≥10 mm trocar for access and come in different lengths, deployment widths, and angulation capabilities. The tissue or vessel is transected as the staples are deployed. One must ensure the device completely traverses the target before deployment, otherwise hemorrhage can occur, especially with large vessels or thick vascular tissue. Stapling devices have been routinely utilized for main organ vessels as well as mesentery with reproducible success. If dividing vascular structures, one must be certain that the device contains vascular and not gastrointestinal staples.

Care should be taken when dividing tissue or establishing hemostasis with high-energy devices, as injury to adjacent structures is possible. A 3–5 mm right-angled hook cautery is a useful device for dividing tissue and preventing hemorrhage. It is important to make contact with the tissue prior to activation of the monopolar electrocautery in order to avoid arcing of current, which may cause a delayed thermal injury to internal structures. Another form of electrocautery that is available is the 3 mm bipolar cautery forceps, which allows for greater control of the current than with standard monopolar cautery.

Tissue extraction

The benign nature of most pediatric renal diseases allows specimen removal with little concern for spillage. In transperitoneal laparoscopic approaches, most structures can be extracted from the umbilical trocar site, whereas in retroperitoneal approaches the site for the specimen extraction depends on its size. This includes segments of bowel, cysts, adrenal gland, biopsies, and nearly anything else compressible. In an infant, these tissues are brought directly through the trocar wound since there are few bags small enough to be of much use. In older children, if a 10 mm trocar is utilized, then endoscopic retrieval bags may be utilized. Larger structures such as intact solid kidneys or heminephroureterectomy specimens may require enlarging a trocar incision to facilitate removal. The umbilical trocar site is typically utilized or a small Pfannenstiel incision can be performed if it is convenient and remains inconspicuous.

Closure

The same technique is used for all laparoscopic procedures. For wounds <3 mm, application of a tissue adhesive or adhesive paper strips is sufficient. Closing the fascia for all wounds >3 mm in diameter is recommended. Fascial closure devices facilitate closure, especially in the obese patient.

Possible pitfalls and solutions

Malfunction of the equipment

Well-trained nurses capable of quickly recognizing and correcting equipment malfunction are mandatory. Since the success of the laparoscopic procedures depends heavily on the proper functioning of the equipment, these cases are best performed when skilled staff are available.

Fogging of the lens

Initially warming the laparoscope in warm saline/povidone-iodine solution or using commercial defogging fluid may avoid fogging of the lens. Inadequate vision, on the other hand, may result from a gas leak around the primary trocar. This usually leads to complete collapse of the retroperitoneal space, and an extra purse-string suture around the trocar may help to decrease the leak. Another possible reason for inadequate vision during retroperitoneoscopy is a peritoneal tear causing intraperitoneal insufflation. It is then necessary either to convert to a transperitoneal laparoscopic approach or attempt venting the peritoneum using the technique described below. Whether a patient has undergone retroperitoneal surgery before or not, dissection of a previously inflamed retroperitoneum may be suboptimal and frustrating and also dangerous; hence, conversion to open surgery may be considered at any time and should not be considered a failure. Families must be aware of this possibility.

Bleeding

Bleeding may occur while bluntly dissecting, especially the retroperitoneal space: in this case, posterior secondary trocars should be placed and the small vessels must be handled carefully using electrosurgical scissors or the bipolar cautery forceps to secure hemostasis.

Subcutaneous emphysema

Subcutaneous emphysema may occur due to leakage of CO_2 into the skin around the area of the ports, as that area is larger than the size of the trocar. Signs of this problem include readily palpable crepitus over the flank and abdomen. Treatment for this complication includes either placement of a purse-string suture around the leaking port, changing the trocar to a larger size, or reduction of the insufflation pressure.

Intraperitoneal CO_2 insufflation during retroperitoneal laparoscopic surgery

If this insufflation occurs prior to the insertion of the two 5 mm accessory trocars, consider transperitoneal or open conversion.

If this insufflation occurs while inserting the secondary trocars (mainly the medial one, superior to the iliac spine), then consider insertion of a Veress needle or an angiocath at the level of the umbilicus intraperitoneally to deflate the peritoneum and change the site

Radiologic assessment of the adrenal

15

Kourosh Afshar, Douglas H Jamieson, and Andrew E MacNeily

Diagnostic imaging is an essential part of the investigation of adrenal disorders. Modalities such as ultrasound, magnetic resonance imaging (MRI), and computed tomography (CT) have replaced older techniques such as intravenous urography and angiography. In this chapter we discuss the imaging characteristics of the more common childhood adrenal abnormalities (Table 15.1).

Table 15.1 Differential diagnosis of antenatally detected adrenal masses

Adrenal hemorrhage
Neuroblastoma
Renal duplication anomaly
Pulmonary sequestration
Enteric duplication

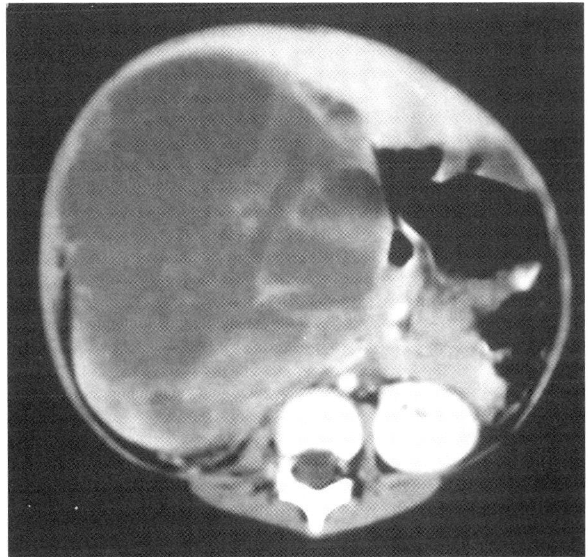

Figure 15.1 Contrast-enhanced CT demonstrates a large heterogeneous mass with areas of non-enhancing low density. It is difficult to separate a mass arising from the upper pole of the right kidney from an adrenal mass. The tumour renal interface is indistinct.

Solid masses of the adrenal

Neuroblastoma

If a solid adrenal mass is encountered when a child is imaged, neuroblastoma must always be considered. These are malignant tumors originating from neural crest cells with a peak age incidence of 2.5 years. They arise from the adrenal medulla in 40% of cases, the remainder being extra-adrenal in origin. Although they can be detected incidentally at the time of imaging for other indications, neuroblastoma usually presents as a large abdominal mass and is metastatic in 70% of cases at the time of presentation.[1]

Calcification, which is amorphous and speckled, is seen on up to 50% of plain abdominal radiographs and 80% of CT scans.[2] On ultrasound, tumors are solid, heterogeneously echogenic with occasional hypoechoic areas.[3]

Cross-sectional imaging (CT or MRI) depicts a large irregular mass and punctuate calcification with or without enlarged lymph nodes or visceral metastases.[4] Neuroblastoma tends to cross the midline and encase vascular structures. It displaces the kidney laterally and inferiorly (Figures 15.1 and 15.2). These features are helpful to differentiate neuroblastoma from a large Wilms' tumor.[5] On CT, areas of low attenuation often represent areas of cystic necrosis or hemorrhage (Figure 15.3, 15.4a–b).[5] On MRI, the mass has low or intermediate signal intensity on T1- and high intensity on T2-weighted images.[6] CT- or MRI-based myelograms are useful in selected cases to assess the extent of intraspinal extension, which presents as a dumbbell-shaped tumor (Figure 15.5a–b,

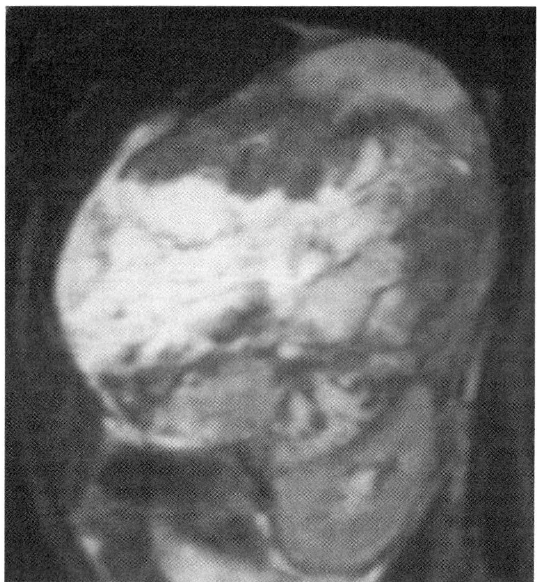

Figure 15.2 Sagittal T2-weighted MRI image clearly demonstrates tumor mass displacing the right kidney inferiorly confirming adrenal mass. The tumor mass has large areas of increased T2 signal intensity corresponding to the low density areas on CT (Fig. 15.1). Areas of tumor necrosis or old areas of hemorrhage are suspected.

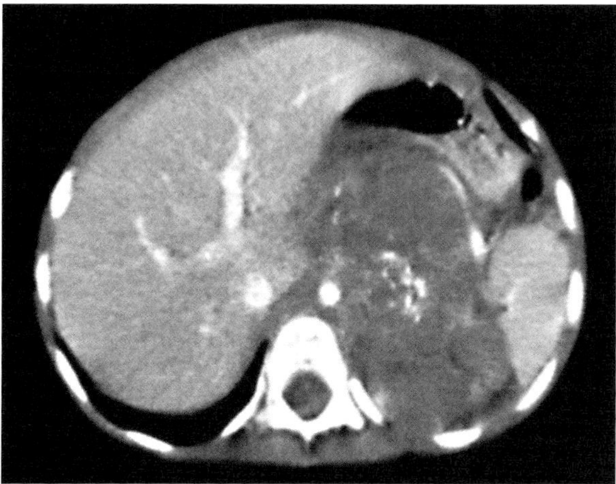

Figure 15.3 Contrast-enhanced CT in a 4-year-old child presenting ill, with weight loss and a hard abdominal mass. There is a large mass in the left adrenal/retroperitoneal location. Dense areas of opacity indicate calcification. The mass enhances poorly and inhomogeneously. Lymphadenopathy surrounds the aorta, displacing it away from the vertebral body. Histology confirmed neuroblastoma.

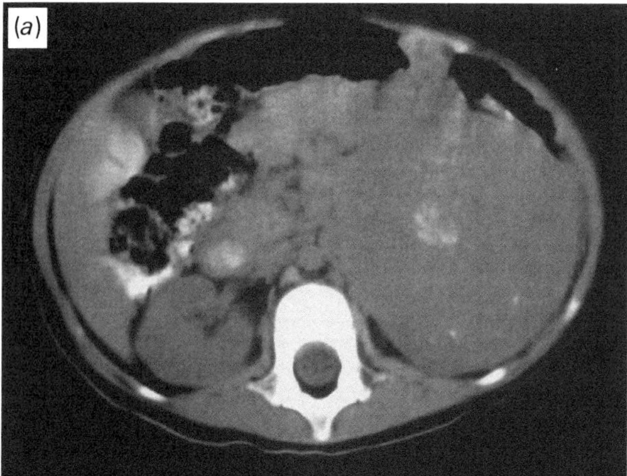

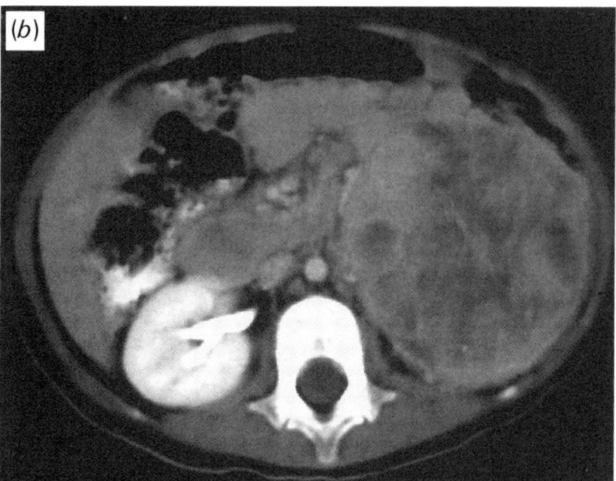

Figure 15.4 (*a*) Non-enhanced CT demonstrates a large left neuroblastoma mass with calcification. Note the nodal spread to right renal hilar region also has calcification. (*b*) Contrast-enhanced CT slightly inferior to *a* shows marked inhomogeneity of enhancement.

and 15.6a–c).[7] Iodine^{132} or I^{131} or I^{123} metaiodobenzylguanidine (MIBG) scintigraphy demonstrates uptake by the primary tumor and any metastatic sites, such as bone.[8,9] However, MIBG has up to 30% false-negative results in diagnosing primary tumors and is less sensitive than 99m technetium methylene diphosphonate (^{99m}Tc MDP) at diagnosing bony metastases. In practice, the two tests are used to compliment each other.[5,10] A recent study concluded that both CT and MRI have poor accuracy for estimating local extension, but when either modality is combined with ^{99m}Tc MDP scintigraphy they are equally useful in diagnosing stage 4, with an accuracy of 90%.[11]

Ganglioneuroma and ganglioneuroblastoma

These benign tumors arise from sympathetic ganglions and represent a more differentiated form of neuroblastoma. On CT they manifest as an oval, discrete mass with variable enhancement. Calcification that is usually not as extensive as in neuroblastoma is seen in 20% of cases. On MRI, the mass has a low-

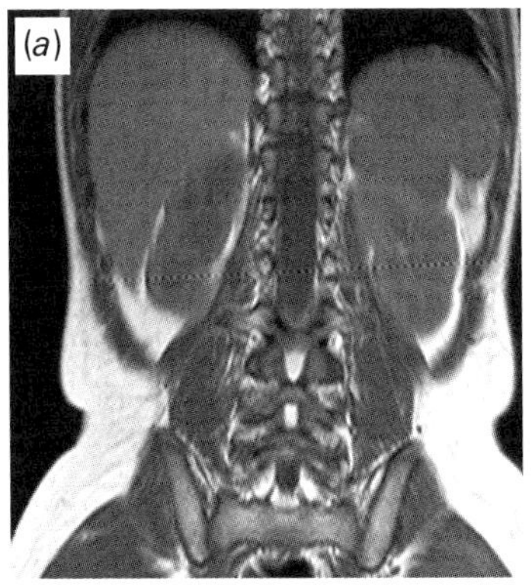
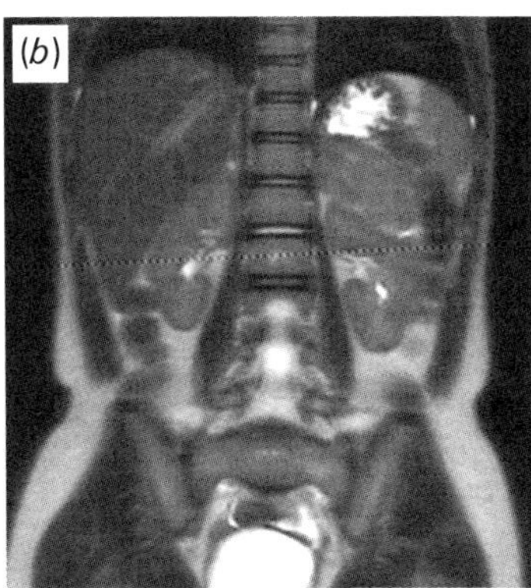

Figure 15.5 Coronal T1 MRI (*a*) and coronal T2 MRI (*b*) demonstrate a left adrenal mass that is homogenous and has soft tissue signal characteristics. This is usual for smaller neuroblastoma where tumor necrosis and hemorrhage are less encountered. Note MRI can easily miss calcification, although this has little impact on diagnosis.

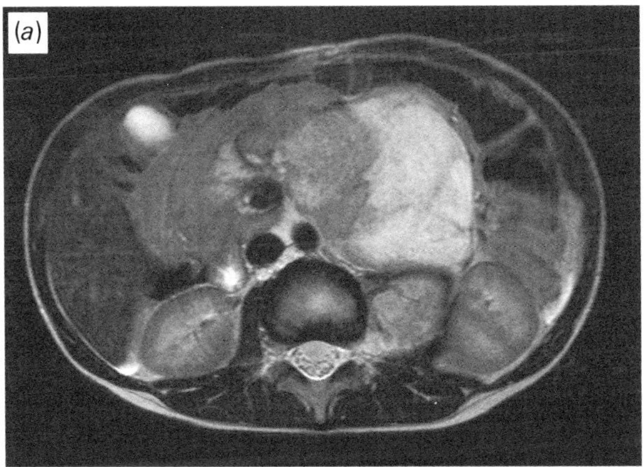
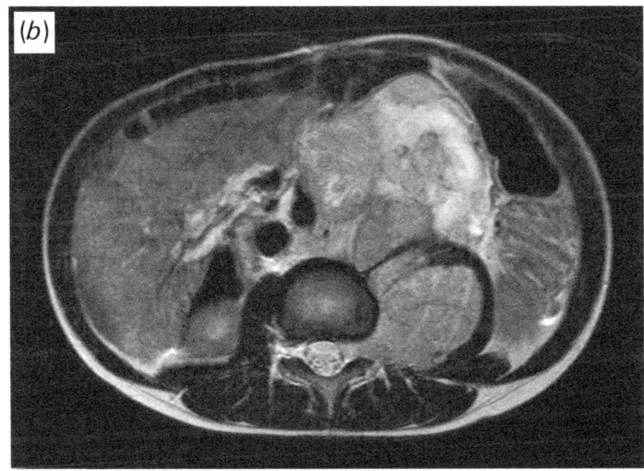
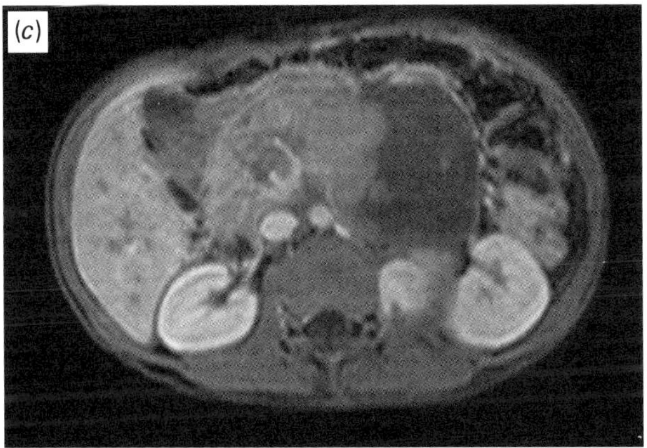

Figure 15.6 Axial T2 MRI (*a*, *b*) and gadolinium-enhanced fat-saturated T1-weighted MRI (*c*). A large heterogeneous tumor mass crossing the midline is well delineated. The extensive left-sided area of increased T2 signal intensity shows no contrast enhancement and suggests tumor necrosis. It would be important to direct biopsy away from this area to obtain appropriate diagnostic information. Note also the tumor encroachment on the left-sided neural foramen (*b*). Evaluation of tumor extent into the spinal canal is superbly imaged by MRI.

intensity signal on T1 and high intensity on T2 images with a characteristic whorled appearance.[12] Ganglioneuroblastoma is an intermediary tumor of sympathetic tissue containing both benign and malignant elements. It has variable imaging features, depending on the composition of the tumor.[12]

Pheochromocytoma

Also a tumor of neural crest cells, pheochromocytoma tends to occur in older children compared to neuroblastoma. The main presentation is headache due to hypertension.[13] On ultrasound, the tumor is seen as a hypoechoic mass, occasionally containing small cysts. Generally, CT and MRI are both highly (>90%) sensitive and specific in diagnosing and staging pheochromocytomas; but because of the possibility of a hypertensive crisis, induced by the iodinated contrast material, some authors prefer MRI as the first choice for cross-sectional imaging. However, at least one study has demonstrated that non-ionic contrast agents are safe in the setting of a confirmed pheochromocytoma.[14] On non-enhanced scans, tumors are isodense to the surrounding soft tissue but enhance intensely following intravenous (IV) contrast.[15] MRI generally characterizes these tumors as possessing low signal intensity on T1-weighted images and a characteristic marked increased signal intensity on T2 images secondary to their high vascularity.[16] MIBG scans have a sensitivity and specificity of 90% in detecting functioning tumors but without the anatomic resolution provided by cross-sectional imaging.[4,17]

Cortical neoplasms

These are rare tumors of childhood mostly associated with endocrine syndromes.[18] In the absence of metastasis the distinction between adenoma and carcinoma is very difficult, even with histologic study of the removed tumor.

On ultrasound, these tumors present as round or ovoid masses, commonly lobulated. They may be hypo- or hyperechoic and the larger tumors are inhomogeneous.[19,20] On CT, they manifest as circumscribed and heterogeneous masses. The criteria used in adults to differentiate between adenoma and carcinoma, such as non-enhanced densiometry and size, have not been studied adequately in children. On MRI, cortical neoplasms have intermediate-intensity T1 and high-intensity T2 signals.[21]

Myelolipoma

This rare benign tumor is composed of adipose and bone marrow elements. The diagnosis is made based on demonstration of fat on CT or MRI.[22]

Adrenal metastasis

Metastatic lesions presenting as an adrenal mass are rare in children. The imaging criteria to differentiate primary adrenal adenomas from secondary tumors as described in adults, such as attenuation values more than 10 Hounsfield units (HU) or signal loss less than 20% in chemical shift MRI,[23] have not been studied in children.

Renal lesions

Lesions in the upper pole of the kidney should be included in the differential diagnosis of an adrenal mass. Wilms' tumor, renal cell carcinoma, and a

Table 15.2 Imaging characteristics of pediatric adrenal masses

Adrenal mass	Ultrasound	CT scan	MRI	Nuclear scan
Neuroblastoma	Solid mass, heterogeneous echotexture	Heterogeneous, low attenuation areas of hemorrhage or necrosis, calcification up to 80%	Heterogeneous signal on T1 and high signal on T2	MIBG avid in 70% 99 Tc MDP more accurate for bone metastasis
Ganglioneuroma	Solid oval or lobulated mass	Homogeneous attenuation lower than muscle, varying degree of enhancement	Homogeneous low signal on T1 and whorled appearance on T2 with varying degree of enhancement	MIBG may be positive
Pheochromocytoma	Solid tumor, possible cystic area	Intense enhancement with contrast, low attenuation areas of necrosis/ hemorrhage	Low intensity T1, extremely high intensity T2 signal	90% MIBG avid
Adrenal cortical neoplasm	Lobulated solid mass	Heterogeneous attenuation	Low T1 and high T2 signal intensity	
Metastasis		Attenuation <10 HU	Signal drop <20% in chemical shift MRI	
Adrenal hemorrhage	Initially hyperechoic with gradual liquefaction	Initial high attenuation (50–60 HU) with no enhancement	Initially: Low signal T1 Intermediate (1–5 weeks): High signal T1 and T2 Late (weeks to months): Low signal T1 and T2	

HU = Hounsfield unit.

hydronephrotic upper pole moiety of a duplicated system can all masquerade as a primary adrenal mass.

Cystic masses of the adrenal

Cystic adrenal masses are rare in childhood. They are usually unilateral and asymptomatic. These lesions may be classified as pseudocysts, endothelial, epithelial, and parasitic cysts. Pseudocysts are formed following hemorrhage into normal or abnormal adrenal tissue. Examples include bleeding into or necrosis of a neuroblastoma or adrenal carcinoma. Calcification is common. Endothelial cysts are the most common category in some series.[24] They may have a vascular or lymphatic origin, and are lined by the corresponding endothelium.[25] Epithelial cysts may be true glandular cysts, embryonal or cystic adenoma.[26] Hydatid cysts constitute the majority of parasitic cysts described in the literature.[27] Typically, cysts are hypoechoic on ultrasound. They possess low intensity on T1-weighted MRI and high intensity on T2. Treatment of adrenal cysts depends on the underlying pathology and ranges from percutaneous aspiration of cysts containing water density fluid, to laparoscopic or open adrenalectomy for more complex lesions.[28]

Antenatally detected adrenal masses

With the advent of routine maternal fetal ultrasound the detection of fetal adrenal masses is becoming increasingly common. Most of these lesions are detected in the third trimester, with the majority being cystic or cystic/solid in nature.. Ultrasound is the modality of choice for initial and follow-up evaluation of these findings. In neonates the normally large adrenal glands are clearly visualized and consist of a hypoechoic cortex and a thin echogenic medulla. The differential diagnosis for antenatally detected adrenal masses is shown in Table 15.2. The intensity of imaging and clinical management of these incidental findings must strike a balance between aggressive surgical intervention for a presumed malignancy and watchful waiting for a benign condition, or one which has a natural history of spontaneous involution.

In a retrospective study of 30 prenatally diagnosed adrenal masses reported from Paris, 13 (43%) were ultimately found to be neuroblastoma, the remainder representing mainly adrenal hemorrhage with the rare pulmonary sequestration (Figure 15.7).[29] Antenatally detected neuroblastoma can be either cystic or solid.

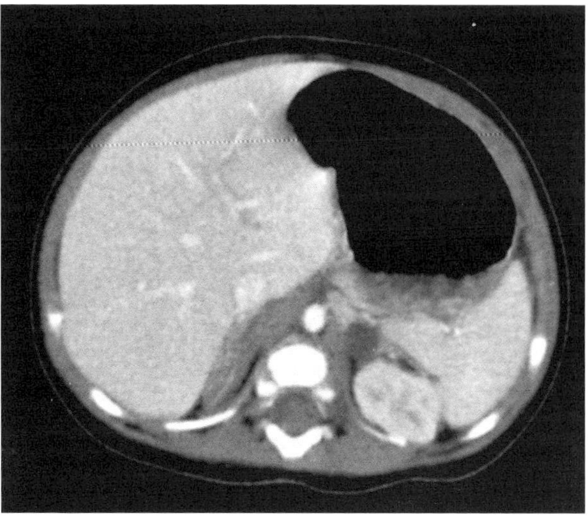

Figure 15.7 Contrast-enhanced CT scan confirmed the antenatal and postnatal detection of a left adrenal cystic lesion. Surgical removal confirmed the diagnosis of a pulmonary sequestration.

Of importance is the fact that MIBG scanning only provided a 70% sensitivity and a 55% negative predictive value for neuroblastoma in this population. Similarly, urinary catecholamines provided only 36% sensitivity and 72% negative predictive value. Postnatal features suggestive of neuroblastoma include large size (>3 cm), homogenous solid nature, and growth on serial follow-up. Conversely, development of calcification in follow-up, shrinkage in size, or development of internal echoes suggests a resolving adrenal hemorrhage (Figure 15.8a–b).[30]

Although adrenal hemorrhage classically occurs in the first few days of life in association with neonatal sepsis or other stressors, it may be observed in the second or third trimester of pregnancy and therefore clinical features alone are inadequate to determine a diagnosis.[31] It is the most common neonatal adrenal mass, and occurs on the right side in 70% of cases. This latter characteristic is thought to be secondary to adrenal compression between the liver and kidney anteriorly and the spine posteriorly.[32]

Early ultrasound of an adrenal hemorrhage depicts a hyperechoic mass. Over the initial few days, the hematoma gradually liquefies (Figure 15.9, 15.10). Complete resolution takes up to 6 weeks with occasional calcification or pseudocyst formation.[33] CT and MR scanning are necessary only in selected cases to determine whether blood is the sole component of a mass, a finding that most likely indicates a benign cause. Acutely, CT of an adrenal hemorrhage is manifested as a well or poorly defined mass with increased

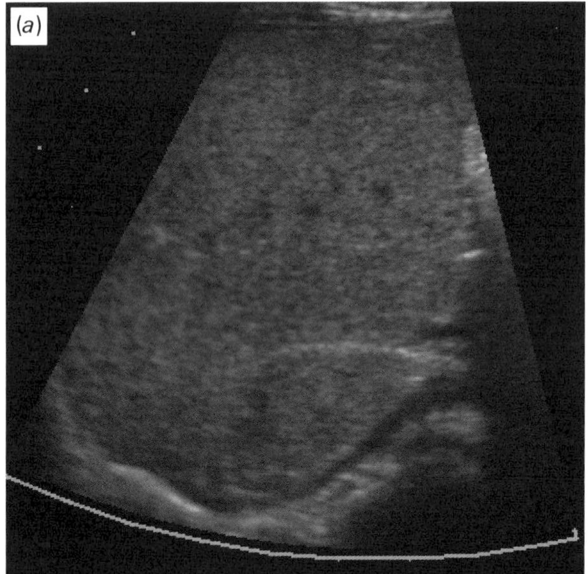

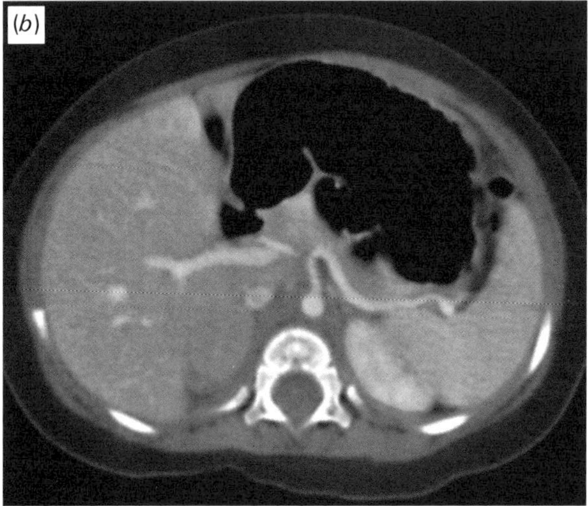

Figure 15.8 (*a*) Neonatal ultrasound performed in follow-up of an antenatally detected right supra-renal mass demonstrates a solid, fairly homogeneous right adrenal mass lesion. Serial images failed to demonstrate involution over the course of several weeks. (*b*) Subsequent contrast-enhanced CT shows a solid homogeneous right adrenal mass, confirmed to be neuroblastoma upon excision.

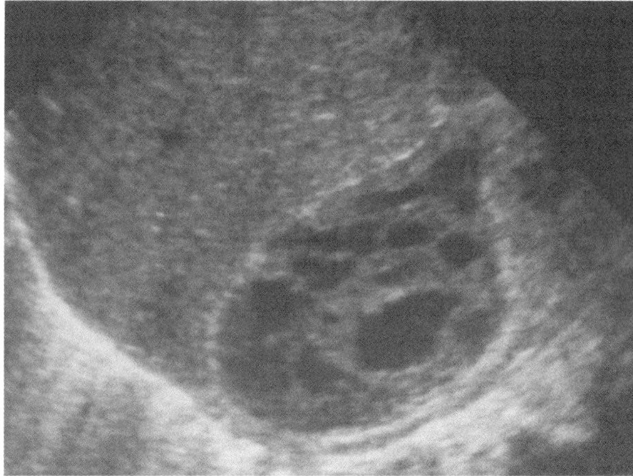

Figure 15.9 Ultrasound obtained in a 5-day-old neonate following traumatic delivery demonstrates a multiseptated right adrenal mass typical of an organizing hematoma.

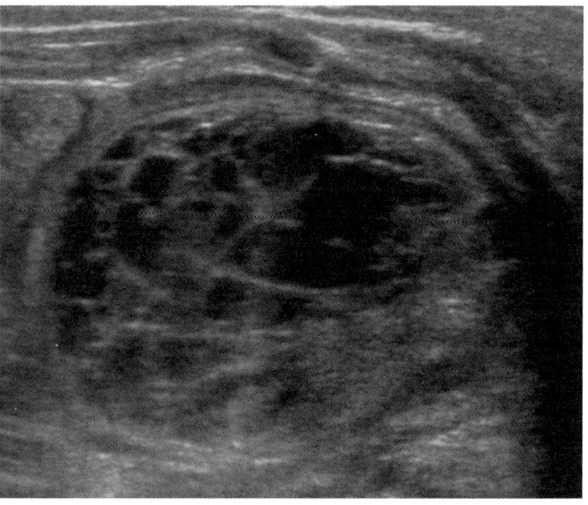

Figure 15.10 Sonogram on day 3 of life, requested to exclude renal anomalies in a patient with transposition of the great vessels. Unexpected but typical findings of a septated left adrenal hematoma. The incident causing the hematoma probably occurred in utero.

attenuation (50–60 HU) that does not enhance with IV contrast (Figure 15.11; Table 15.2). In the acute phase, MRI of hematomas demonstrates a reduced signal on T1-weighted images. Methemoglobin in the subacute phase (1–5 weeks) causes a high signal on both T1- and T2-weighted images. Chronic hemorrhage (5 weeks to 10 months) demonstrates the gradual formation of low-signal hemosiderin.[32,33]

For small antenatally detected lesions, an initial postnatal ultrasound, MIBG scan, and urinary catecholamines should be routine. If initial investigations are suggestive of a benign process, then monthly ultrasounds for the first 6 months suffice. Surgical removal is recommended for an increase in size, elevated urinary catecholamines, or failure of involution with observation.[34]

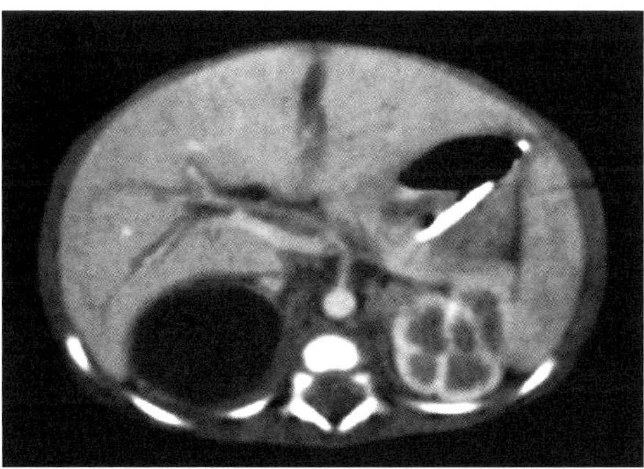

Figure 15.11 Contrast-enhanced CT on the same day as ultrasound Fig 15.9. In the right adrenal location, a non-enhancing low-density mass typical of an adrenal hematoma is apparent. Note that the septations are not apparent on the CT.

Calcified adrenal lesions

Adrenal calcification detected on abdominal imaging of a child has a broad differential diagnosis (Table 15.3) but it usually prompts investigations for a tumor, most commonly neuroblastoma.[33] The aforementioned affinity of neuroblastoma for skeletal tracer is independent of the presence of calcification, and its mechanism is unknown.[35] Ganglioneuromas and ganglioneuroblastomas can also calcify, and they are radiographically indistinguishable from neuroblastomas.

Granulomatous diseases often result in childhood adrenal calcification either unilaterally or bilaterally.[36–38] Distinguishing from the various granulomatous infections is impossible by imaging alone.

Table 15.3 Differential diagnosis of pediatric calcified adrenal masses

Neural crest tumors:
Neuroblastoma[a]
Ganglioneuroblastoma[a]
Ganglioneuroma
Resolving hemorrhage[a]
Adrenal cortical carcinoma
Pheochromocytoma
Adrenal cortical adenoma
Granulomatous infection
Storage disorders:
Wolman's disease
Niemann–Pick disease
Myelolipoma

[a] Denotes most common findings.

Wolman's disease is an uncommon autosomal recessive inborn error of metabolism leading to the accumulation of lipid in the abdominal organs. The condition is usually fatal by 6 months of age. On plain film the adrenal glands are enlarged and densely calcified. Ultrasound demonstrates concomitant hepatosplenomegaly. CT confirms the adrenal origin of the calcifications. MRI demonstrates the adrenal high signal intensity on T1 sequences due to lipid deposition.[39,40]

As mentioned above, perinatal adrenal hemorrhage can subsequently calcify. Imaging characteristics can vary from a peripheral rim of calcification to complete replacement of the gland. Incomplete resolution of hematoma can result in a peripherally calcified rim around a non-enhancing pseudocyst.[40]

References

1. Ritchey M. Pediatric urologic oncology. In: Walsh PC, Retik AB, Stamey TA, Vaughan ED Jr, eds. Campbell's Textbook of Urology, 6th edn. Philadelphia: WB Saunders, 2002: 2470.
2. Brodeur GM, Pritchard J, Berthold F et al. Revisions of the international criteria for neuroblastoma diagnosis, staging, and response to treatment. J Clin Oncol 1993; 11(8):1466–77.
3. Bousvaros A, Kirks DR, Grossman H. Imaging of neuroblastoma: an overview. Pediatr Radiol 1986; 16(2):89–106.
4. Agrons GA, Lonergan GJ, Dickey GE, Perez-Monte JE. Adrenocortical neoplasms in children: radiologic–pathologic correlation. Radiographics 1999; 19(4):989–1008.
5. Chaaya S. Neuroblastoma. In: Grainger MB, Adam A, Dixon AK, eds. Grainger & Allison's Diagnostic Radiology: A Textbook of Medical Imaging. Edinburgh: Churchill Livingstone, 2001: 1486.
6. Meyer JS, Harty MP, Khademian Z. Imaging of neuroblastoma and Wilms' tumor. Magn Reson Imaging Clin N Am 2002; 10(2):275–302.
7. Azizkhan RG, Haase GM. Current biologic and therapeutic implications in the surgery of neuroblastoma. Semin Surg Oncol 1993; 9(6):493–501.
8. Geatti O, Shapiro B, Sisson JC et al. Iodine-131 metaiodobenzylguanidine scintigraphy for the location of neuroblastoma: preliminary experience in ten cases. J Nucl Med 1985; 26(7):736–42.
9. Parisi MT, Greene MK, Dykes TM et al. Efficacy of metaiodobenzylguanidine as a scintigraphic agent for the detection of neuroblastoma. Invest Radiol 1992; 27(10):768–73.
10. Gordon I, Peters AM, Gutman A et al. Skeletal assessment in neuroblastoma – the pitfalls of iodine-123-MIBG scans. J Nucl Med 1990; 31(2):129–34.

11. Siegel MJ, Ishwaran H, Fletcher BD et al. Staging of neuroblastoma at imaging: report of the radiology diagnostic oncology group. Radiology 2002; 223(1):168–75.
12. Rha SE, Byun JY, Jung SE et al. Neurogenic tumors in the abdomen: tumor types and imaging characteristics. Radiographics 2003; 23(1):29–43.
13. Abramson SJ. Adrenal neoplasms in children. Radiol Clin North Am 1997; 35(6):1415–53.
14. Mukherjee JJ, Peppercorn PD, Reznek RH et al. Pheochromocytoma: effect of nonionic contrast medium in CT on circulating catecholamine levels. Radiology 1997; 202(1):227–31.
15. Quint LE, Glazer GM, Francis IR, Shapiro B, Chenevert TL. Pheochromocytoma and paraganglioma: comparison of MR imaging with CT and I-131 MIBG scintigraphy. Radiology 1987; 165(1):89–93.
16. Weishaupt D, Debatin JF. Magnetic resonance: evaluation of adrenal lesions. Curr Opin Urol 1999; 9(2):153–63.
17. Francis IR, Gross MD, Shapiro B, Korobkin M, Quint LE. Integrated imaging of adrenal disease. Radiology 1992; 184(1):1–13.
18. Neblett WW, Frexes-Steed M, Scott HW Jr. Experience with adrenocortical neoplasms in childhood. Am Surg 1987; 53(3):117–25.
19. Hamper UM, Fishman EK, Hartman DS, Roberts JL, Sanders RC. Primary adrenocortical carcinoma: sonographic evaluation with clinical and pathologic correlation in 26 patients. AJR Am J Roentgenol 1987; 148(5):915–19.
20. Prando A, Wallace S, Marins JL, Pereira RM, de Oliveira ER. Sonographic findings of adrenal cortical carcinomas in children. Pediatr Radiol 1990; 20(3):163–5; discussion 169.
21. Hanson JA, Weber A, Reznek RH et al. Magnetic resonance imaging of adrenocortical adenomas in childhood: correlation with computed tomography and ultrasound. Pediatr Radiol 1996; 26(11):794–9.
22. Kenney PJ, Wagner BJ, Rao P, Heffess CS. Myelolipoma: CT and pathologic features. Radiology 1998; 208(1):87–95.
23. Sahdev A, Reznek RH. Imaging evaluation of the nonfunctioning indeterminate adrenal mass. Trends Endocrinol Metab 2004; 15(6):271–6.
24. Tung GA, Pfister RC, Papanicolaou N, Yoder IC. Adrenal cysts: imaging and percutaneous aspiration. Radiology 1989; 173(1):107–10.
25. Tanuma Y, Kimura M, Sakai S. Adrenal cyst: a review of the Japanese literature and report of a case. Int J Urol 2001; 8(9):500–3.
26. Foster D. Adrenal cysts. Review of literature and report of case. Arch Surg 1966; 92:131–43.
27. Krebs TL, Wagner BJ. The adrenal gland: radiologic–pathologic correlation. Magn Reson Imaging Clin N Am 1997; 5(1):127–46.
28. Sroujieh AS, Farah GR, Haddad MJ, Abu-Khalaf MM. Adrenal cysts: diagnosis and management. Br J Urol 1990; 65(6):570–5.
29. Sauvat F, Sarnacki S, Brisse H et al. Outcome of suprarenal localized masses diagnosed during the perinatal period: a retrospective multicenter study. Cancer 2002; 94(9):2474–80.
30. Lin JN, Lin GJ, Hung JJ, Hsueh C. Prenatally detected tumor mass in the adrenal gland. J Pediatr Surg 1999; 34(11):1620–3.
31. Fang SB, Lee HC, Sheu JC, Lo ZJ, Wu BL. Prenatal sonographic detection of adrenal hemorrhage confirmed by postnatal surgery. J Clin Ultrasound 1999; 27(4):206–9.
32. Kawashima A, Sandler CM, Ernst RD et al. Imaging of nontraumatic hemorrhage of the adrenal gland. Radiographics 1999; 19(4):949–63.
33. Paterson A. Adrenal pathology in childhood: a spectrum of disease. Eur Radiol 2002; 12(10):2491–508.
34. Granata C, Fagnani AM, Ganbini C et al. Features and outcome of neuroblastoma detected before birth. J Pediatr Surg 2000; 35(1):88–91.
35. Podrasky AE, Stark DD, Hattner RS, Gooding CA, Moss AA. Radionuclide bone scanning in neuroblastoma: skeletal metastases and primary tumor localization of 99mTc-MDP. AJR Am J Roentgenol 1983; 141(3):469–72.
36. Wang YX, Chen CR, He GX, Tang AR. CT findings of adrenal glands in patients with tuberculous Addison's disease. J Belge Radiol 1998; 81(5):226–8.
37. Kawashima A, Sandler CM, Fishman EK et al. Spectrum of CT findings in nonmalignant disease of the adrenal gland. Radiographics 1998; 18(2):393–412.
38. Buxi TB, Vohra RB, Sujatha et al. CT in adrenal enlargement due to tuberculosis: a review of literature with five new cases. Clin Imaging 1992; 16(2):102–8.
39. Fulcher AS, Das Narla L, Hingsbergen EA. Pediatric case of the day. Wolman disease (primary familial xanthomatosis with involvement and calcification of the adrenal glands). Radiographics 1998; 18(2):533–5.
40. Hindman N, Israel GM. Adrenal gland and adrenal mass calcification. Eur Radiol 2005; 15(6):1163–7.

Adrenal tumors and functional consequences

16

Julie Franc-Guimond and Anne-Marie Houle

Introduction

The pathogenesis, diagnosis, and management of adrenal tumors have recently evolved[1,2] mainly because of easier discovery of clinically silent, incidentally detected adrenal tumors using more sensitive imaging procedures such as computed tomography (CT) and magnetic resonance imaging (MRI).[3] Even if these tumors are rarely seen in children, it is important that the physician recognizes the clinical manifestations of these tumors as soon as possible, leading to an earlier diagnosis, prompt intervention, and improved survival.

Adrenal neoplasms

Although adrenal neoplasms in pediatrics are fortunately rare, representing less than 1% of all solid tumors, they may be potentially fatal. Tumors can arise from the medullary or the cortical portions of the adrenals and can be benign or malignant. Malignant cancers are rare, accounting for 0.05–0.2% of all cancers in the overall population, with an incidence of less than 2 new cases per million yearly.[4,5] Occurring at all ages,[6–11] adrenocortical carcinomas tend to present according to a bimodal age distribution, with the first peak occurring before age 5 years, and the second in the fourth to fifth decade.[12] Females clearly predominate in all series, accounting for 65–90% of the cases reported in the literature.[2] Even though some authors have reported a left-sided prevalence, others have not: bilaterality has been observed in 2–10% of cases.[2,9] Most adrenal masses found in children are functional, which renders the establishment of the diagnosis, as well as the medical and the surgical treatment, even more challenging.

Diseases of the adrenal cortex

Cortical tumors may be benign (adenoma, cyst, myolipoma) or malignant (adrenocortical carcinoma): all are rarely seen in children.[13–15] Furthermore, it may be very difficult to distinguish between them and the ultimate confirmation of the diagnosis is by histopathology; however, at times, the clinical outcome may not even correlate well with the histologic features.[16] The incidence of adrenocortical carcinomas is approximately 1 in 1.7 million in the general population.[17] They are seen in older patients compared with adenomas[18] and are more frequently encountered in females.[6] Moreover, they tend to be functional and may be part of hereditary syndromes. A retrospective review revealed that 92% of patients found to have a carcinoma presented with a mixed endocrine syndrome vs 32% of adenoma patients.[19] The latter commonly presented with a virilization syndrome only (92%).

Hormone-producing syndromes in patients with adrenal cortical neoplasms

Associated endocrine syndromes resulting from secretion of cortisol and/or adrenal androgens and their precursors, or, rarely, estrogen or mineralocorticoids, may be seen in patients with hormone-secreting adrenocortical neoplasms.

A more gradual onset of signs of hormone hypersecretion is generally observed in patients with adenomas, unlike those with adrenocortical carcinoma who tend to have a more acute and progressive course.

Cushing's syndrome

Cushing's syndrome in children is most commonly caused by an adrenocortical carcinoma and is seen in one-third to one-half of these patients.[20] The classic Cushing's syndrome is a clinical disorder seen in cases of overproduction of cortisol, which leads to protein catabolism, subsequent increased glucogeneogenesis, and the typical symptoms associated with cortisol excess. Cushing's syndrome refers to patients presenting with the syndrome regardless of the cause; it differs from Cushing's disease which is caused by pituitary hypersecretion of adrenocorticotropic hormone (ACTH). One-fourth of the cases of endogenous Cushing's syndrome are caused by primary adrenal disease.

Aside from functional adrenocortical tumors and other usual causes, Cushing's syndrome can be particularly seen in children with primary pigmented nodular adrenocortical disease, which occurs as a component of Carney's complex. Also, infants found to have the McCune–Albright syndrome can present with ACTH-independent Cushing's syndrome with nodular hyperplasia or adenoma formation. Finally, islet cell carcinoma of the pancreas, neuroblastoma or ganglioneuroblastoma, hemangiopericytoma, Wilms' tumor, and thymic carcinoid can lead to ectopic production of ACTH in the pediatric population.

Pathophysiology

ACTH is secreted in response to corticotropin-releasing hormone (CRH) and vasopressin. It stimulates glucocorticoid cortisol secretion from the zona fasciculata and zona reticularis of the adrenal gland. Cortisol creates a negative feedback control on CRH, vasopressin, and ACTH. Cortisol is usually secreted in a circadian rhythm. Cushing's syndrome occurs when there is a loss of that rhythm, accompanied with a loss of the feedback mechanism of the hypothalamic–pituitary–adrenal axis, resulting in chronic exposure to excessive circulating cortisol levels.[21]

Clinical findings

Signs and symptoms associated with hypercortisolemia are variable; however, moon facies, truncal obesity, and typical evidence of Cushing's syndrome are generally obvious in children. More specifically, weight gain associated with growth retardation in the pediatric group should highlight the possibility of the diagnosis.[6] Other findings may include hirsutism, muscle weakness, bruising, vertebral fractures, hypertension, and diabetes mellitus, but these are rarely seen these days. Lethargy, depression, acne, and menstrual irregularity[22,23] could also be observed. Patients' photographs may help in showing the clinical progression to a Cushingoid state. In general, the findings are more obvious in infants than in older children.

Laboratory findings

The goal is to determine whether a patient has Cushing's syndrome rather than to identify the cause.[24] More specifically, Cushing's syndrome due to functioning adrenocortical tumors will exhibit elevated levels of several plasma and urinary steroids. These include cortisol following dexamethasone suppression test, dehydroepiandrosterone (DHEA) and its sulfate derivative (DHEAS), Δ^5-androstenediol, Δ^4-androstenedione, pregnenolone, 17-hydroxypregnenolone, and 11-deoxycortisol in the plasma, and free cortisol, 17-hydroxysteroids, 17-ketosteroids, and the tetrahydro metabolite of 11-deoxycortisol in the urine.[21] Measurements of other steroidogenic precursors, such as 17-hydroxyprogesterone and 11-deoxycortisol, may help if the presence of an adrenal malignancy in patients with Cushing's syndrome is suspected.[22] Autonomous activity of the adrenal glands will lead to a low plasma ACTH level, associated with elevated plasma cortisol concentration.

Tumor localization

Abdominal CT and/or MRI can document the existence of an adrenal lesion or bilateral nodular hyperplasia in cases of ACTH-dependent Cushing's syndrome. In patients with adrenal tumors, the contralateral adrenal should appear normal but could be atrophic since there is suppression of ACTH by the unilateral cortisol-secreting tumor.[25] Determining between adenomas and carcinomas is usually not feasible, but tumors >5 cm should be considered malignant until proven otherwise. Nevertheless, the ultimate confirmation of the diagnosis is histopathologic.[26,27]

Treatment

The treatment of Cushing's syndrome secondary to adrenal tumors is surgical. Adrenalectomy will either be performed unilaterally if there is a mass or bilaterally in patients with ACTH-dependent Cushing's syndrome not cured by other modalities. Preoperative preparation requires measures to correct the hypercortisolemia and its metabolic sequelae. Moreover, cortisol administration perioperatively should take place to prevent a state of hypoadrenalism. This would occur in cases of total bilateral adrenalectomy but also in cases of unilateral adrenalectomy, because the removal of the source of excessive cortisol in the presence of an invariably atrophied contralateral gland will inevitably lead to temporary or permanent adrenal insufficiency.

Medical treatment is indicated in patients who cannot undergo surgery or in those who have had unsuccessful resection of their tumor (pituitary, ectopic, or adrenal) with or without metastatic spread. Metyrapone, ketoconazole, aminoglutethimide, mitotane, and etomidate have been used as inhibitors of steroid biosynthesis, and thus can be utilized in all cases of hypercortisolemia, regardless of cause, often with rapid improvement in the clinical features.

Prognosis

Removal of an adenoma offers an excellent prognosis, whereas the outlook for patients with malignant tumors is poor. Children tend to have a better prognosis, however.[28,29]

Virilizing adrenal tumors

Abnormal virilization is seen in cases of adrenocortical carcinomas in two-thirds of the adult patients,[30] whereas it is the most common hormonal syndrome in children with adrenocortical tumors.[2,8,10,31] Virilization is due to hypersecretion of adrenal androgens, including DHEA and its sulfate derivative DHEAS, Δ^5-androstenediol, and Δ^4-androstenedione, all of which may be converted to testosterone and 5α-dihydrotestosterone.

In adult females, the signs and symptoms include oligoamenorrhea, hirsutism, acne, excessive muscle mass, temporal balding, increased libido, and clitoromegaly. In young girls, precocious puberty occurs. Cushing's syndrome, combined with signs of virilization, is seen in 10–30% of all patients.[2,3,32]

Measurement of plasma adrenal androgens, testosterone, and 24-h urinary excretion of 17-ketosteroids may confirm the clinical diagnosis of adrenally induced virilization.

Feminizing adrenal tumors

Feminization seen as a single manifestation is quite rare. More commonly seen in males, feminization comes to one's attention because of newly observed gynecomastia and can be confirmed by measurements of elevated plasma estradiol and/or estrone.[33]

Aldosteronism

Aldosterone is the principal mineralocorticoid secreted by the adrenal gland. Increased secretion may be secondary to a primary defect (primary hyperaldosteronism) or result from factors that activate the renin–angiotensin system (secondary). Patients with primary hyperaldosteronism present with hypertension and/or hypokalemia; those with secondary do not. Primary aldosteronism will lead to a state of mineralocorticoid excess with low plasma renin activity (PRA). It may be caused by the following pathologies: an aldosterone-producing adenoma (APA), idiopathic bilateral (BAH) or unilateral (UAH) adrenal hyperplasia, glucocorticoid-remediable aldosteronism (GRA), or an aldosterone-producing adrenocortical carcinoma.

Although rare, unilateral APA has been described in children as young as 3.5 years and usually affects girls. Hypertension, hypokalemia, and metabolic alkalosis resulting from autonomous production of aldosterone by an adenoma was first reported by Conn in 1954. Since then, numerous studies have looked at the prevalence of primary aldosteronism and reported rates of between 0.05 and 14.4% among hypertensive individuals.[34–37] BAH tends to occur in older children and affects males more frequently. Primary aldosteronism due to UAH has been reported infrequently in the pediatric population.[38–41] Adrenal carcinomas, an exceedingly rare cause of primary aldosteronism, are usually large (>5 cm) at the time of diagnosis.

Other states of mineralocorticoid excess with low PRA may include cases of congenital adrenal hyperplasia or Liddle's syndrome.[42] In these two syndromes, non-aldosterone-mediated renal sodium reabsorption results in volume expansion and suppression of both PRA and plasma aldosterone (PA).

At the other end of the spectrum, other patients may present with a state of mineralocorticoid excess with high PRA. They may be hypertensive (renovascular disorders, coarctation of the aorta, renin-secreting tumors), normo- or hypotensive with reduced circulating blood volume (Gitelman's syndrome, Bartter syndrome, pseudohypoaldosteronism type I, diuretic use), or have reduced 'effective' circulating blood volume (congestive heart failure, hepatic cirrhosis, nephrotic syndrome).

Physiology of aldosterone regulation and action

Aldosterone synthesis is orchestrated by the renin–angiotensin system. Renin, produced in the juxtaglomerular apparatus, catalyzes the conversion of angiotensinogen to angiotensin I. Angiotensin I undergoes further enzymatic conversion by angiotensin-converting enzyme (ACE) to produce angiotensin II, which acts to stimulate the production of aldosterone from the zona glomerulosa. The renin–angiotensin II system is also expressed locally and regulates aldosterone production in a paracrine fashion. Aldosterone's release is positively and directly modified by potassium balance. It can also be modulated by other factors such as ACTH, dopamine, and atrial natriuretic peptide.

Clinical findings

Signs and symptoms of hyperaldosteronism are nonspecific, often resulting in or associated with hypertension with headache, dizziness, and visual disturbances. However, some individuals have minimal blood pressure elevations and, as a result, hypertension is not a sine qua non for this disorder.[12] In fact, the most common finding remains hypokalemia. Chronic hypokalemia may lead to 'clear cell nephrosis', polyuria, nocturia, enuresis, and polydipsia. Muscle weakness and discomfort, tetany, intermittent paralysis, fatigue, and growth failure may also be observed in these children. Classic features of moderate-to-severe hypertension, hypokalemia, and metabolic alkalosis are highly suggestive of mineralocorticoid excess. However, only subtle clues of hyperaldosteronism exist in the majority of cases such as the recent onset of refractory hypertension.

Laboratory findings

Hyperaldosteronism can generally be proven by measurements of aldosterone and PRA, 11-deoxycorticosterone and/or corticosterone, respectively. Plasma and urine levels of aldosterone are increased, and plasma levels of renin are persistently low.[43–45] In addition, the serum pH, carbon dioxide content, and sodium concentrations may be increased and the serum chloride and magnesium levels decreased. Serum levels of calcium are normal, even in children who manifest tetany. The urine is neutral or alkaline, and kaliuresis is present. Aldosterone does not decrease with sodium chloride administration and renin does not respond to salt and fluid restriction.

Differential diagnosis and tumor localization

All cases with a history of hypertension associated with 'spontaneous' or severe hypokalemia precipitated by diuretic therapy should suggest the diagnosis of primary aldosteronism. Suspicion is also warranted in all incidentally discovered adrenal masses, especially in a hypertensive individual.[46] Once the diagnosis is established, it is necessary to identify the underlying cause (APA, BAH, UAH, GRA, or an aldosterone-producing adrenocortical carcinoma).

All children should have a therapeutic trial with daily administration of dexamethasone before invasive studies are carried out, since this test is easy to perform. A marked suppression of aldosterone and disappearance of hypertension is observed in patients with the glucocorticoid-suppressible variant of hyperaldosteronism or GRA.

If there is no response, CT scanning or MRI may reveal a mass within the adrenal. In cases of inconclusive data or equivocal radiographic features, however, adrenal vein sampling of aldosterone and cortisol is recommended to differentiate between an adenoma and hyperplasia.[47–50]

Treatment

GRA is managed by daily administration of glucocorticoid. The treatment of an APA is surgical. Resection cures or ameliorates hypertension and invariably treats the hypokalemia. In one recent analysis, however, only one-third of patients became normotensive postoperatively.[51] In patients known to have an APA, suppression of aldosterone secretion in the contralateral adrenal gland is expected, thus resulting in a transient hyporeninemic hypoaldosterone state.[52] Therefore, sodium restriction could increase the risk of dehydration. Pharmacologic treatment of BAH with spironolactone or amiloride usually results in normalization of the blood pressure and serum potassium levels. Management of secondary hyperaldosteronism is directed toward the specific causative disorder.

Hereditary syndromes associated with adrenocortical tumor formation

Adrenocortical tumors have been associated with several genetic syndromes, which explains the origin of the familial adrenocortical tumors and the unusual associations with other tumors and/or conditions.[2] Among many, the multiple endocrine neoplasia type 1 (MEN 1) and the Beckwith–Wiedemann syndrome are the ones most commonly mentioned. The clinical features associated with MEN 1 are hyperparathyroidism and pancreatic–duodenal and pituitary tumors. The chromosomal anomalies are mutations at locus 11q13,[53,54] whereas the chromosomal defect found in the Beckwith–Wiedemann syndrome (neonatal macrosomia, macroglossia, and omphalocele) is an allelic loss of 11q15. Other syndromes associated with benign and/or malignant adrenocortical neoplasms include Carney's complex, congenital adrenal hyperplasia, Li-Fraumeni syndrome and McCune–Albright syndrome.

Diseases of the adrenal medulla

Pheochromocytoma

Pheochromocytomas are catecholamine-secreting tumors. Ninety percent arise from the medullary portion of the adrenals, whereas 10% occur in extra-adrenal chromaffin tissues (paragangliomas). About 10% are familial, multicentric, and bilateral, whereas the remainder are sporadic. The incidence in the hypertensive population varies between 0.05 and 0.1%.

Pheochromocytomas are uncommonly observed in children and the true incidence is unknown. Indeed, it appears that this tumor of neuroectodermal origin is more common in adults, and most data on its behavior and management have been obtained from the adult population. In comparison with the findings observed in adults, known facts regarding pheochromocytomas in children include an age at presentation of around 10 years, a male propensity in most series, an increased incidence of bilaterality (20%) and multifocality, a lower incidence of malignancy (2.4–3.5%), and a greater tendency for familial occurrence.[55]

Familial pheochromocytomas can occur with or without an association to known familial cancer syndromes (MEN 2, von Hippel–Lindau disease, neurofibromatosis type 1, Sturge–Weber syndrome, and familial carotid body tumors).[56] It appears that hereditary forms can evolve differently in terms of tumor growth rate and malignancy potential. Thus, individuals with familial pheochromocytomas are diagnosed at a younger age and tend to have bilateral or multifocal lesions that are usually benign.

Signs and symptoms

Signs and symptoms are related to excessive secretion of catecholamines produced in large amounts by pheochromocytes. Hypertension is the most common sign and it is more frequently sustained in young subjects rather than paroxysmal. Other signs and symptoms could include postural hypotension, headaches, increased sweating, pallor, flushing, tachycardia, weight loss, constipation, weakness, and visual complaints. Headaches, nausea, vomiting, constipation, weight loss, and visual complaints are frequently observed in children.[57,58] A palpable mass could also be present and in combination with sustained hypertension should strongly suggest the diagnosis. Nonetheless, a palpable mass could be the sole finding.

Diagnosis

The biochemical diagnosis is achieved from measurements of catecholamines and catecholamine metabolites in plasma or urine.[59–63] Norepinephrine and epinephrine are ubiquitously produced by the sympathoneuronal and sympathomedullary systems and, therefore, are not specific to pheochromocytomas. Other limitations relate to the fact that increased plasma catecholamine levels may be produced by a variety of conditions (e.g. emotional stress, physical activity, eating, fever), that in some patients pheochromocytomas may not secrete catecholamines, or that many pheochromocytomas secrete episodically. Glucagon stimulation and clonidine suppression tests are useful in some patients to further confirm the diagnosis of pheochromocytoma.[57,64,65]

Tumor localization

Pheochromocytomas can be imaged with CT, MRI, and/or scintigraphy after administration of ^{131}I- or ^{123}I-labeled metaiodobenzylguanidine (MIBG).[66–69] If an initial abdominal CT or MRI is positive, whole-body MIBG should be performed to confirm the diagnosis. If abdominal studies are negative, then whole-body evaluation by CT or MRI is indicated. If an initial MIBG scan is positive, then CT or MRI follows to precisely localize a mass. However, a negative MIBG scan does not exclude a pheochromocytoma. More recently, positron emission tomography (PET) has been used in particular cases.

Treatment

The definitive treatment is surgical excision of the tumor. Of particular interest, patients with pheochromocytomas should undergo pharmacologic blockade (α and β) of catecholamine effects and synthesis prior to surgery as well as aggressive correction of the hypovolemia perioperatively to avoid hypotension. Intra-adrenal pheochromocytomas can be removed successfully by laparoscopy, which minimizes catecholamine-induced hemodynamic changes during operation.[70]

The neuroblastic tumors

Neuroblastic tumors include ganglioneuroma, ganglioneuroblastoma, and neuroblastoma, which are tumors of the sympathetic nervous system.[71] They arise wherever sympathetic tissue exists and are found in the neck, posterior mediastinum, adrenal gland, retroperitoneum, and pelvis. The adrenal gland is the most common site; hence the need to discuss these pathologies.

The most benign tumor is the ganglioneuroma, which is composed of gangliocytes and mature stroma.[72,73] It arises from the medulla in less than half of the cases found to have an abdominal ganglioneuroma.[74–77] Patients of all ages are affected, predominantly children and young adults (42–60% of cases)[78–81] and they are often asymptomatic. Otherwise, abdominal pain or an abdominal mass is the most common finding.[79] Hormonally active tumors have been reported, and the secretion of catecholamines, vasoactive intestinal polypeptides, or androgenic hormones explains such symptoms as hypertension, diarrhea, and virilization.[78–80,82–84] The prognosis is excellent, and recurrence is rare after surgical removal.[79,85]

Ganglioneuroblastomas are transitional tumors of sympathetic cell origin that contain elements of both malignant neuroblastoma and benign ganglioneuroma. The most common tumor location is the abdomen. This tumor is most often seen in patients 2–4 years old and is rarely seen after 10 years.[86] The prognosis and response to therapy are significantly more favorable than with neuroblastomas.[87]

Neuroblastoma is the most immature, undifferentiated, and malignant tumor of the three that consist of primitive neuroblasts.[88] Neuroblastoma, however, may have a relatively benign evolution, even when metastatic. It is the third most frequent neoplasm in children after leukemia and central nervous system tumors.

These tumors are predominantly found in boys <10 years of age. Furthermore, approximately 80% of these neoplasms are found in children under the age of 5 years, with a median age of 22 months.[88] Two-thirds of neuroblastomas are located in the abdomen, and approximately two-thirds of these arise in the adrenal gland. The remaining ones originate in the paravertebral sympathetic chain or presacral area or organ of Zuckerkandl.[89] Neuroblastomas metastasize to bone, bone marrow, liver, lymph nodes, and skin and 35–70% of the cases have systemic disease when diagnosed.[88,90–96]

These tumors can also be observed in newborns or fetuses, as prenatal sonography may allow antenatal diagnosis.[86] In fact, neuroblastoma is the most common malignancy in the first month of life, accounting for 30–50% of all malignant tumors at this age. Both fetal and neonatal neuroblastomas have very good prognoses but differ somewhat in their patterns of metastatic spread and organ of origin.[97,98] Neonatal neuroblastoma has an adrenal origin in 45% of patients and 60% have metastases at the time of diagnosis, mostly to the liver, bone cortex, marrow, and skin. Tumor biologic behavior is usually favorable, and the survival rate is greater than 90%. However, mortality may occur, and is often caused by respiratory insufficiency from massive hepatic metastases.[97] Fetal neuroblastoma has been discovered as early as 19 weeks, although the mean age at discovery is 36 weeks.[98] It is almost always (90% of cases) of adrenal origin. It presents with hepatic and, less commonly, marrow metastases. An almost universally good outcome is expected and a conservative approach is advocated.[98] Because approximately 90% of neuroblastomas and ganglioneuroblastomas secrete vanillylmandelic acid (VMA) and homovanillic acid (HVA), screening of urinary catecholamines via urine assay grew in popularity in an attempt to improve outcome. Screening began in Japan in 1973 in 6-month-old infants. Unfortunately, epidemiologic analysis showed that the incidence in older children did not change, and that the tumors discovered at screening were of low stage and favorable histologic characteristics, suggesting that the tumors discovered via urinary screening were those likely to remain occult, regress, or mature. Other studies done in Quebec have shown similar data.[99] Therefore, it appears that screening in infancy does not reduce the incidence of advanced-stage disease in older children, nor does it increase survival in younger patients with more aggressive tumors. The value of screening after 1 year of age or later is unknown.[100,101]

The most frequent clinical finding observed in the presence of a neuroblastoma is abdominal pain followed by abdominal distention. Other symptoms include malaise, irritability, weight loss, shortness of breath, and peripheral neurologic deficit.[90] Of interest, neuroblastic tumors may rarely occur in combination with von Recklinghausen's disease, Beckwith–Wiedemann syndrome, Hirschsprung's disease, central failure of ventilation, or DiGeorge syndrome.[87,88,102]

Two classification systems are commonly used in North America to differentiate neuroblastic tumors into risk groups: the Shimada classification and the Pediatric Oncology Group (POG) classification. Both systems assess histologic features, such as cellular differentiation, to determine prognosis. The POG system is based solely on the degree of differentiation of the different histologic elements.[103,104] The Shimada classification combines histologic features and patient age at diagnosis.[105] The degree of cellular and extracellular maturation between the three tumors varies tremendously; immature tumors tend to be aggressive and occur in youngsters (median age under 2 years), whereas mature tumors occur in older patients (median age approximately 7 years) and tend to have a more benign behavior.[71] Also, prognosis varies according to additional features such as DNA content, tumor proto-oncogenes, and catecholamine synthesis. Also, another stratification tool, based on clinical, radiologic, and surgical features, was developed in 1986 by an international consensus group, the International Neuroblastoma Staging System (INSS).[106,107]

Treatment consists of surgery and, usually, chemotherapy. Radiation therapy may also be used. Children with low- or intermediate-risk tumors have a relatively good prognosis but, despite recent advances in treatment, including bone marrow transplantation, neuroblastoma remains a lethal tumor, accounting for 15% of cancer deaths in children.[108,109] More specifically, even with aggressive treatment of the high-risk tumors, the 3-year event-free survival rate for these patients is less than 15%[108] but improved 2-year survival after bone marrow transplantation has been documented in some studies; prolonged survival is currently being assessed.[109]

References

1. Vassilopoulou-Sellin R, Schultz PN. Adrenocortical carcinoma. Clinical outcome at the end of the 20th century. Cancer 2001; 92(5):1113–21.
2. Latronico AC, Chrousos GP. Extensive personal experience: adrenocortical tumors. J Clin Endocrinol Metab 1997; 82(5):1317–24.
3. Ross NS, Aron DC. Hormonal evaluation of the patient with an incidentally discovered adrenal mass. N Engl J Med 1990; 323(20):1401–5.
4. Third national cancer survey: incidence data. Natl Cancer Inst Monogr 1975; (41):i–x, 1–454.
5. Young JL Jr, Miller RW. Incidence of malignant tumors in U. S. children. J Pediatr 1975; 86(2):254–8.
6. Nader S, Hickey RC, Sellin RV, Samaan NA. Adrenal cortical carcinoma. A study of 77 cases. Cancer 1983; 52(4):707–11.
7. Henley DJ, van Heerden JA, Grant CS, Carney JA, Carpenter PC. Adrenal cortical carcinoma – a continuing challenge. Surgery 1983; 94(6):926–31.
8. Chudler RM, Kay R. Adrenocortical carcinoma in children. Urol Clin North Am 1989; 16(3):469–79.
9. Barzilay JI, Pazianos AG. Adrenocortical carcinoma. Urol Clin North Am 1989; 16(3):457–68.
10. Ribeiro RC, Sandrini Neto RS, Schell MJ et al. Adrenocortical carcinoma in children: a study of 40 cases. J Clin Oncol 1990; 8(1):67–74.
11. Pommier RF, Brennan MF. An eleven-year experience with adrenocortical carcinoma. Surgery 1992; 112(6): 963–70.
12. Kono T, Ikeda F, Oseko F, Imura H, Tanimura H. Normotensive primary aldosteronism: report of a case. J Clin Endocrinol Metab 1981; 52(5):1009–13.
13. Patil KK, Ransley PG, McCullagh M, Malone M, Spitz L. Functioning adrenocortical neoplasms in children. BJU Int 2002; 89(6):562–5.
14. Teinturier C, Brugieres L, Lemerle J, Chaussain JL, Bougneres PF. Adrenocortical carcinoma in children: retrospective study of 54 cases Arch Pediatr 1996; 3(3):235–40.
15. Stewart JN, Flageole H, Kavan P. A surgical approach to adrenocortical tumors in children: the mainstay of treatment. J Pediatr Surg 2004; 39(5):759–63.
16. Bergada I, Venara M, Maglio S et al. Functional adrenal cortical tumors in pediatric patients: a clinicopathologic and immunohistochemical study of a long term follow-up series. Cancer 1996; 77(4):771–7.
17. Hofmockel G, Dammrich J, Manzanilla Garcia H, Frohmuller H. Myelolipoma of the adrenal gland associated with contralateral renal cell carcinoma: case report and review of the literature. J Urol 1995; 153(1):129–32.
18. Kiely EM. Radical surgery for abdominal neuroblastoma. Semin Surg Oncol 1993; 9(6):489–92.
19. Daitch JA, Goldfarb DA, Novick AC. Cleveland Clinic experience with adrenal Cushing's syndrome. J Urol 1997; 158(6):2051–5.
20. McLorie GA, Bagli DJ. Adrenal tumors in children. In: Gearhart JP, Rink RR, Mouriquand P, eds. Pediatric Urology. Philadelphia: WB Saunders, 1999: 908–16.
21. Newell-Price J, Trainer P, Besser M, Grossman A. The diagnosis and differential diagnosis of Cushing's syndrome and pseudo-Cushing's states. Endocr Rev 1998; 19(5):647–72.
22. Orth DN. Cushing's syndrome. N Engl J Med 1995; 332(12):791–803. Erratum in: N Engl J Med 1995; 332(22):1527.
23. Ross EJ, Linch DC. Cushing's syndrome – killing disease: discriminatory value of signs and symptoms aiding early diagnosis. Lancet 1982; 2(8299):646–9.
24. Raff H, Findling JW. A physiologic approach to diagnosis of the Cushing syndrome. Ann Intern Med 2003; 138(12):980–91.
25. Doppman JL, Miller DL, Dwyer AJ et al. Macronodular adrenal hyperplasia in Cushing disease. Radiology 1988; 166(2):347–52.
26. Trainer PJ, Grossman A. The diagnosis and differential diagnosis of Cushing's syndrome. Clin Endocrinol (Oxf) 1991; 34(4):317–30.
27. Galifer RB, Couture A, Dyon JF et al. [Solid tumors of the adrenal gland in children (excluding neuroblastomas). A study of a series of 18 cases]. Chir Pediatr 1989; 30(5):209–14. [French]
28. Michalkiewicz EL, Sandrini R, Bugg MF et al. Clinical characteristics of small functioning adrenocortical tumors in children. Med Pediatr Oncol 1997; 28(3):175–8.

29. Mayer SK, Oligny LL, Deal C et al. Childhood adrenocortical tumors: case series and reevaluation of prognosis – a 24-year experience. J Pediatr Surg 1997; 32(6): 911–15.
30. Hayles AB, Hahn HB Jr, Sprague RG, Bahn RC, Priestley JT. Hormone-secreting tumors of the adrenal cortex in children. Pediatrics 1966; 37(1):19–25.
31. Danilowicz K, Albiger N, Vanegas M et al. Androgen-secreting adrenal adenomas. Obstet Gynecol 2002; 100(5 Pt 2):1099–102.
32. Phornphutkul C, Okubo T, Wu K et al. Aromatase p450 expression in a feminizing adrenal adenoma presenting as isosexual precocious puberty. J Clin Endocrinol Metab 2001; 86(2):649–52.
33. Sandrini R, Ribeiro RC, DeLacerda L. Childhood adrenocortical tumors. J Clin Endocrinol Metab 1997; 82(7):2027–31.
34. Gordon RD. Mineralocorticoid hypertension. Lancet 1994; 344(8917):240–3.
35. Hiramatsu K, Yamada T, Yukimura Y et al. A screening test to identify aldosterone-producing adenoma by measuring plasma renin activity. Results in hypertensive patients. Arch Intern Med 1981; 141(12):1589–93.
36. Young WF Jr, Hogan MJ, Klee GG, Grant CS, van Heerden JA. Primary aldosteronism: diagnosis and treatment. Mayo Clin Proc 1990; 65(1):96–110.
37. Lim PO, Rodgers P, Cardale K, Watson AD, MacDonald TM. Potentially high prevalence of primary aldosteronism in a primary-care population. Lancet 1999; 353(9146): 40.
38. Abasiyanik A, Oran B, Kaymakci A et al. Conn syndrome in a child, caused by adrenal adenoma. J Pediatr Surg 1996; 31(3):430–2.
39. Bryer-Ash M, Wilson DM, Tune BM et al. Hypertension caused by an aldosterone-secreting adenoma. Occurrence in a 7-year-old child. Am J Dis Child 1984; 138(7): 673–6.
40. Fallo F, Kuhnle U, Boscaro M, Sonino N. Abnormality of aldosterone and cortisol late pathways in glucocorticoid-remediable aldosteronism. J Clin Endocrinol Metab 1994; 79(3):772–4.
41. Gordon RD. Primary aldosteronism. J Endocrinol Invest 1995; 18(7):495–511.
42. Findling JW, Raff H, Hansson JH, Lifton RP. Liddle's syndrome: prospective genetic screening and suppressed aldosterone secretion in an extended kindred. J Clin Endocrinol Metab 1997; 82(4):1071–4.
43. Weinberger MH, Fineberg NS. The diagnosis of primary aldosteronism and separation of two major subtypes. Arch Intern Med 1993; 153(18):2125–9.
44. Blumenfeld JD, Sealey JE, Schlussel Y et al. Diagnosis and treatment of primary hyperaldosteronism. Ann Intern Med 1994; 121(11):877–85.
45. Montori VM, Young WF Jr. Use of plasma aldosterone concentration-to-plasma renin activity ratio as a screening test for primary aldosteronism. A systematic review of the literature. Endocrinol Metab Clin North Am 2002; 31(3):619–32, xi.
46. Thompson GB, Young WF Jr. Adrenal incidentaloma. Curr Opin Oncol 2003; 15(1):84–90.
47. Mulatero P, Stowasser M, Loh KC et al. Increased diagnosis of primary aldosteronism, including surgically correctable forms, in centers from five continents. J Clin Endocrinol Metab 2004; 89(3):1045–50.
48. Young WF Jr, Stanson AW, Grant CS, Thompson GB, van Heerden JA. Primary aldosteronism: adrenal venous sampling. Surgery 1996; 120(6):913–19; discussion 919–20.
49. Magill SB, Raff H, Shaker JL et al. Comparison of adrenal vein sampling and computed tomography in the differentiation of primary aldosteronism. J Clin Endocrinol Metab 2001; 86(3):1066–71.
50. Young WF Jr. Minireview: primary aldosteronism – changing concepts in diagnosis and treatment. Endocrinology 2003; 144(6):2208–13.
51. Sawka AM, Young WF, Thompson GB et al. Primary aldosteronism: factors associated with normalization of blood pressure after surgery. Ann Intern Med 2001; 135(4):258–61.
52. Kendrick ML, Curlee K, Lloyd R et al. Aldosterone-secreting adrenocortical carcinomas are associated with unique operative risks and outcomes. Surgery 2002; 132(6):1008–11; discussion 1012.
53. Stratakis CA, Ball DW. A concise genetic and clinical guide to multiple endocrine neoplasias and related syndromes. J Pediatr Endocrinol Metab 2000; 13(5): 457–65.
54. Langer P, Cupisti K, Bartsch DK et al. Adrenal involvement in multiple endocrine neoplasia type 1. World J Surg 2002; 26(8):891–6.
55. Reddy VS, O'Neill JA Jr, Holcomb GW 3rd et al. Twenty-five-year surgical experience with pheochromocytoma in children. Am Surg 2000; 66(12):1085–91.
56. Riccardi VM. Neurofibromatosis: past, present, and future. N Engl J Med 1991; 324(18):1283–5.
57. Bravo EL, Gifford RW Jr. Pheochromocytoma. Endocrinol Metab Clin North Am 1993; 22(2):329–41.
58. Ram CV, Fierro-Carrion GA. Pheochromocytoma. Semin Nephrol 1995; 15(2):126–37.
59. Bravo EL, Tarazi RC, Gifford RW, Stewart BH. Circulating and urinary catecholamines in pheochromocytoma. Diagnostic and pathophysiologic implications. N Engl J Med 1979; 301(13):682–6.
60. Chen F, Slife L, Kishida T et al. Genotype–phenotype correlation in von Hippel–Lindau disease: identification of a mutation associated with VHL type 2A. J Med Genet 1996; 33(8):716–17.
61. Duncan MW, Compton P, Lazarus L, Smythe GA. Measurement of norepinephrine and 3,4-dihydroxyphenylglycol in urine and plasma for the diagnosis of pheochromocytoma. N Engl J Med 1988; 319(3): 136–42.
62. Heron E, Chatellier G, Billaud E, Foos E, Plouin PF. The urinary metanephrine-to-creatinine ratio for the diagnosis of pheochromocytoma. Ann Intern Med 1996; 125(4):300–3.
63. Manu P, Runge LA. Biochemical screening for pheochromocytoma. Superiority of urinary metanephrines measurements. Am J Epidemiol 1984; 120(5):788–90.
64. Bravo EL. Evolving concepts in the pathophysiology, diagnosis, and treatment of pheochromocytoma. Endocr Rev 1994; 15(3):356–68.

65. Bravo EL, Tarazi RC, Fouad FM, Vidt DG, Gifford RW Jr. Clonidine-suppression test: a useful aid in the diagnosis of pheochromocytoma. N Engl J Med 1981; 305(11):623–6.
66. Eisenhofer G, Pacak K, Goldstein DS, Chen C, Shulkin B. ^{123}I-MIBG scintigraphy of catecholamine systems: impediments to applications in clinical medicine. Eur J Nucl Med 2000; 27(5):611–12.
67. Lynn MD, Shapiro B, Sisson JC et al. Pheochromocytoma and the normal adrenal medulla: improved visualization with I–123 MIBG scintigraphy. Radiology 1985; 155(3):789–92.
68. Shulkin BL, Shapiro B, Francis IR et al. Primary extra-adrenal pheochromocytoma: positive I–123 MIBG imaging with negative I–131 MIBG imaging. Clin Nucl Med 1986; 11(12):851–4.
69. Tsuchimochi S, Nakajo M, Nakabeppu Y, Tani A. Metastatic pulmonary pheochromocytomas: positive I–123 MIBG SPECT with negative I–131 MIBG and equivocal I–123 MIBG planar imaging. Clin Nucl Med 1997; 22(10):687–90.
70. Vargas HI, Kavoussi LR, Bartlett DL et al. Laparoscopic adrenalectomy: a new standard of care. Urology 1997; 49(5):673–8.
71. Shimada H, Ambros IM, Dehner LP et al. Terminology and morphologic criteria of neuroblastic tumors: recommendations by the International Neuroblastoma Pathology Committee. Cancer 1999; 86(2):349–63.
72. Joshi VV. Peripheral neuroblastic tumors: pathologic classification based on recommendations of international neuroblastoma pathology committee (Modification of shimada classification). Pediatr Dev Pathol 2000; 3(2):184–99.
73. Joshi VV, Cantor AB, Altshuler G et al. Conventional versus modified morphologic criteria for ganglioneuroblastoma. A review of cases from the Pediatric Oncology Group. Arch Pathol Lab Med 1996; 120(9):859–65.
74. Jain M, Shubha BS, Sethi S, Banga V, Bagga D. Retroperitoneal ganglioneuroma: report of a case diagnosed by fine-needle aspiration cytology, with review of the literature. Diagn Cytopathol 1999; 21(3):194–6.
75. Freeman BD, Zuckerman GR, Callery MP. Duodenal ganglioneuroma: a rare cause of upper GI hemorrhage. Am J Gastroenterol 1996; 91(12):2626–7.
76. Dellinger GW, Lynch CA, Mihas AA. Colonic ganglioneuroma presenting as filiform polyposis. J Clin Gastroenterol 1996; 22(1):66–70.
77. Mithofer K, Grabowski EF, Rosenberg AE, Ryan DP, Mankin HJ. Symptomatic ganglioneuroma of bone. A case report. J Bone Joint Surg Am 1999; 81(11):1589–95.
78. Moriwaki Y, Miyake M, Yamamoto T et al. Retroperitoneal ganglioneuroma: a case report and review of the Japanese literature. Intern Med 1992; 31(1):82–5.
79. Geoerger B, Hero B, Harms D et al. Metabolic activity and clinical features of primary ganglioneuromas. Cancer 2001; 91(10):1905–13.
80. Lucas K, Gula MJ, Knisely AS et al. Catecholamine metabolites in ganglioneuroma. Med Pediatr Oncol 1994; 22(4):240–3.
81. Bove KE, McAdams AJ. Composite ganglioneuroblastoma. An assessment of the significance of histological maturation in neuroblastoma diagnosed beyond infancy. Arch Pathol Lab Med 1981; 105(6):325–30.
82. Andrich MP, Shalaby-Rana E, Movassaghi N, Majd M. The role of 131 iodine-metaiodobenzylguanidine scanning in the correlative imaging of patients with neuroblastoma. Pediatrics 1996; 97(2):246–50.
83. Clerico A, Jenkner A, Castello MA et al. Functionally active ganglioneuroma with increased plasma and urinary catecholamines and positive iodine 131-meta-iodobenzylguanidine scintigraphy. Med Pediatr Oncol 1991; 19(4):329–33.
84. Yoshizawa K, Fukumoto T, Hori T, Miura K, Morita J. Mediastinal ganglioneuroma with the secretive activity of catecholamines, visualized by 131-I-MIBG scintigraphy Nippon Kyobu Geka Gakkai Zasshi 1991; 39(2):204–8.
85. Goldman RL, Winterling AN, Winterling CC. Maturation of tumors of the sympathetic nervous system. Report of long-term survival in 2 patients, one with disseminated osseous metastases, and review of cases from the literature. Cancer 1965; 18(11):1510–16.
86. Wilson LM, Draper GJ. Neuroblastoma, its natural history and prognosis: a study of 487 cases. Br Med J 1974; 3(5926):301–7.
87. Kilton LJ, Aschenbrener C, Burns CP. Ganglioneuroblastoma in adults. Cancer 1976; 37(2):974–83.
88. Bousvaros A, Kirks DR, Grossman H. Imaging of neuroblastoma: an overview. Pediatr Radiol 1986; 16(2): 89–106.
89. Morris JA, Shcochat SJ, Smith EI et al. Biological variables in thoracic neuroblastoma: a Pediatric Oncology Group study. J Pediatr Surg 1995; 30(2):296–302.
90. Matthay KK. Neuroblastoma: a clinical challenge and biologic puzzle. CA Cancer J Clin 1995; 45(3):179–92.
91. Dresler S, Harvey DG, Levisohn PM. Retroperitoneal neuroblastoma widely metastatic to the central nervous system. Ann Neurol 1979; 5(2):196–8.
92. Aronson MR, Smoker WR, Oetting GM. Hemorrhagic intracranial parenchymal metastases from primary retroperitoneal neuroblastoma. Pediatr Radiol 1995; 25(4):284–5.
93. Sener RN. CT of diffuse leptomeningeal metastasis from primary extracerebral neuroblastoma. Pediatr Radiol 1993; 23(5):402–3.
94. Tanabe M, Ohnuma N, Iwai J et al. Bone marrow metastasis of neuroblastoma analyzed by MRI and its influence on prognosis. Med Pediatr Oncol 1995; 24(5):292–9.
95. Panuel M, Bourliere-Najean B, Gentet JC et al. Aggressive neuroblastoma with initial pulmonary metastases and kidney involvement simulating Wilms' tumor. Eur J Radiol 1992; 14(3):201–3.
96. Rosenfield NS, Leonidas JC, Barwick KW. Aggressive neuroblastoma simulating Wilms tumor. Radiology 1988; 166(1 Pt 1):165–7.
97. Toma P, Lucigrai G, Marzoli A, Lituania M. Prenatal diagnosis of metastatic adrenal neuroblastoma with sonography and MR imaging. AJR Am J Roentgenol 1994; 162(5):1183–4.
98. Lukens JN. Neuroblastoma in the neonate. Semin Perinatol 1999; 23(4):263–73.
99. Acharya S, Jayabose S, Kogan SJ et al. Prenatally diagnosed neuroblastoma. Cancer 1997; 80(2):304–10.

100. Brodeur GM, Look AT, Shimada H et al. Biological aspects of neuroblastomas identified by mass screening in Quebec. Med Pediatr Oncol 2001; 36(1):157–9.
101. Report of the 1998 Consensus Conference on Neuroblastoma Screening. Med Pediatr Oncol 1999; 33(4):357–9.
102. Joshi VV, Cantor AB, Altshuler G et al. Age-linked prognostic categorization based on a new histologic grading system of neuroblastomas. A clinicopathologic study of 211 cases from the Pediatric Oncology Group. Cancer 1992; 69(8):2197–211.
103. Michna BA, McWilliams NB, Krummel TM, Hartenberg MA, Salzberg AM. Multifocal ganglioneuroblastoma coexistent with total colonic aganglionosis. J Pediatr Surg 1988; 23(1 Pt 2):57–9.
104. Askin FB, Perlman EJ. Neuroblastoma and peripheral neuroectodermal tumors. Am J Clin Pathol 1998; 109(4 Suppl 1):S23–30.
105. Brodeur GM, Pritchard J, Berthold F et al. Revisions of the international criteria for neuroblastoma diagnosis, staging, and response to treatment. J Clin Oncol 1993; 11(8):1466–77.
106. Shimada H, Ambros IM, Dehner LP et al. The International Neuroblastoma Pathology Classification (the Shimada system). Cancer 1999; 86(2):364–72.
107. Coldman AJ, Fryer CJ, Elwood JM, Sonley MJ. Neuroblastoma: influence of age at diagnosis, stage, tumor site, and sex on prognosis. Cancer 1980; 46(8): 1896–901.
108. Castleberry RP. Biology and treatment of neuroblastoma. Pediatr Clin North Am 1997; 44(4):919–37.
109. Pritchard J, McElwain TJ, Graham-Pole J. High-dose melphalan with autologous marrow for treatment of advanced neuroblastoma. Br J Cancer 1982; 45(1): 86–94.

Surgery of the adrenal

17

Stephen Boorjian, Michael Schwartz, and Dix P Poppas

Background

In 1936, Hugh Hampton Young described bilateral subtotal adrenalectomy for children with congenital adrenal hyperplasia (CAH).[1] Since that time, the physiology and pathophysiology of the adrenal gland has become increasingly understood, while imaging of the adrenal to localize disease processes has improved. These advancements have helped to define the role of surgery in the management of adrenal disorders. The spectrum of pediatric adrenal disease, as well as the pathophysiology of these processes, has been covered in the preceding chapters. Here, we focus primarily on the surgical management of adrenal disease. Specific pathologic conditions are addressed with regard to their influence on surgical approach.

Laparoscopic adrenalectomy

Since the first description of laparoscopic adrenalectomy by Gagner et al in 1992, the advantages of the laparoscopic approach have been well documented in the adult population, including shorter hospital stay, decreased postoperative pain, quicker return to preoperative activity level, and improved cosmesis.[2–6] However, there has been a relative delay in the application of laparoscopic adrenalectomy to the pediatric population. This delay has resulted in part from the higher incidence of malignant adrenal tumors among children compared with adults.[7–9] In addition, neuroblastoma, which represents the most common adrenal tumor in children, is characterized by an infiltrative growth pattern that has traditionally been seen as a contraindication to laparoscopic excision. Nevertheless, the growing experience with laparoscopy and the continued improvements in surgical instrumentation have fostered a trend toward increased use of minimally invasive techniques in pediatric adrenal surgery. To date, laparoscopic adrenalectomy has been reported for a variety of adrenal pathologies in children, including adrenal adenoma, carcinoma, hyperplasia, pheochromocytoma, and, more recently, select cases of neuroblastoma as well.[9–12]

The approach to laparoscopic adrenalectomy may be either transperitoneal or retroperitoneal. In both of these techniques, the central tenet of the procedure is to dissect the adrenal gland from the surrounding tissue with minimal manipulation of the gland itself; in essence, to remove the patient from the adrenal gland.[13]

Transperitoneal laparoscopic adrenalectomy

Patients are placed on a clear liquid diet on the day before surgery, and are given a mechanical bowel preparation. After general anesthesia is established, a Foley catheter is inserted into the bladder, and the stomach is decompressed with an oral gastric tube. We place the patient in the semilateral decubitus position, with the side of the lesion elevated approximately 45°, and flex the operating table. The patient is draped from the nipple line to the lower abdomen and across the midline, allowing for possible open conversion. The patient is rolled to a near-supine position, and pneumoperitoneum is established. We prefer the Hasson open cutdown technique for establishing pneumoperitoneum in the pediatric population. The first trocar, an 11–12 mm trocar, is placed in the midline just above the umbilicus. The peritoneal space is insufflated to 12–15 mmHg using CO_2, and the abdominal cavity is explored with a 10 mm, 30° laparoscope. The table is then rolled to a full flank position for additional trocar placement.

For left adrenalectomy, two accessory trocars are inserted: a 5 mm port 3–4 cm cephalad to the supraumbilical trocar, and a 5 mm port in the midclavicular line, below the costal margin (Figure 17.1). Port placement may vary slightly with the age and size of the child. Adhesions of the left upper quadrant to the anterior abdominal wall are first identified and

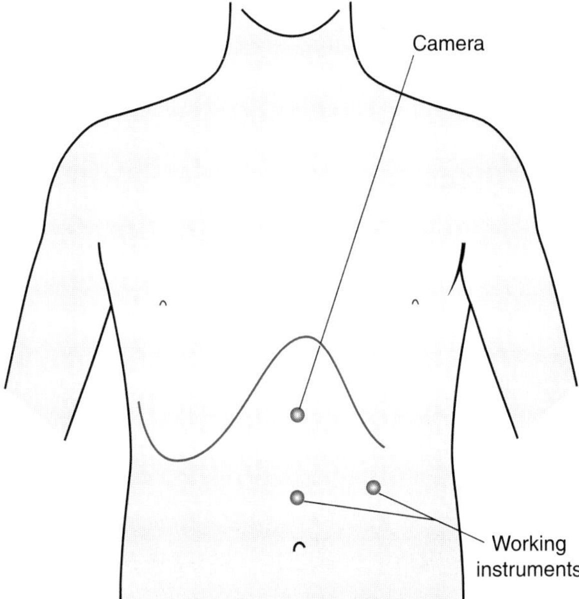

Figure 17.1 Port placement for transperitoneal laparoscopic left adrenalectomy. The supraumbilical working instrument trocar is 11–12 mm, to facilitate insertion of a clip applier.

incised using the harmonic scalpel. The splenic flexure of the left colon is then mobilized by incising the peritoneum along the line of Toldt. The spleen is mobilized by incising its attachments to Gerota's fascia, abdominal side wall, and diaphragm with the harmonic scalpel or electrocautery shears. Dissection of the lateral splenic attachments is carried out until the gastric fundus is visualized. At the conclusion of this dissection, the spleen should fall medially without the need for retraction.

Once the splenic flexure and spleen are mobilized, the plane between the tail of the pancreas and Gerota's fascia is developed to release the pancreas medially. The superior border of the adrenal gland is then dissected from lateral to medial. The inferior phrenic vessels are identified, clipped, and divided as they are encountered along the upper aspect of the adrenal. The lateral-most attachments of the gland are left intact to hold the gland in place, and thereby facilitate the remainder of the dissection. Dissection is carried medially along the gland, where the arterial supply to the adrenal from the aorta is encountered, clipped, and divided. Inferiorly, the left adrenal vein is identified entering the left renal vein, clipped, and divided.

Division of the left adrenal vein often reveals an inferior adrenal artery arising from the left renal artery; if encountered, this artery should be clipped and divided. Finally, the lateral attachments of the adrenal are divided, releasing the gland. The adrenal is placed in a retrieval bag inserted through the umbilical port. Visualization for the remainder of the procedure is accomplished with a 5 mm, 30° scope placed through the port in the midclavicular line. The bag containing the specimen is temporarily placed on the kidney, and the operative bed irrigated and inspected for bleeding. Once hemostasis is ensured, the specimen is then removed from the patient; the trocar site may be enlarged if necessary to facilitate the removal of larger glands. The remaining ports are then removed and closed.

Laparoscopic right adrenalectomy is performed using three accessory trocars, because of the need to retract the liver. After insufflation, a 5 mm port is placed 3–4 cm cephalad to the supraumbilical trocar (as for left adrenalectomy above), while two 5 mm ports are placed laterally, below the costal margin in the anterior axillary and midclavicular lines (Figure 17.2). After adhesions of the right upper quadrant to the anterior abdominal wall are incised, the liver is mobilized from the abdominal side wall and diaphragm by incising the triangular and coronary ligaments. The extent of mobilization of the liver necessary for exposure increases with age in children, as the distance between structures increases and the flexibility of tissues decreases. A liver retractor is then introduced through the anterior axillary line trocar to reflect the liver away from the adrenal (see Figure 17.2).

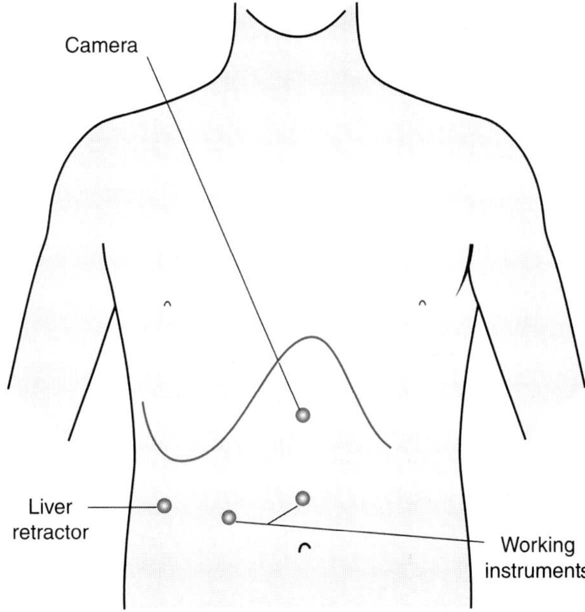

Figure 17.2 Port placement for transperitoneal laparoscopic right adrenalectomy. Note additional trocar in anterior axillary line for liver retractor.

With the liver mobilized, the anterior wall of the vena cava is identified, and the medial attachments of the adrenal gland are released. The duodenum is mobilized medially, exposing the renal hilum. As the dissection is carried cephalad on the anterior wall of the cava, the right adrenal vein is identified. We secure the vein by doubly clipping both the patient and specimen sides of the vein and then sharply dividing the vein between the clips (Figure 17.3).

Once the adrenal vein has been controlled, the superior and inferior aspects of the adrenal are sequentially dissected as for a left adrenalectomy, dividing the inferior phrenic vessels on the cephalad border and the inferior vascularized pedicle, which arises from the right renal hilum, on the caudal border of the gland. The adrenal gland is then mobilized off the upper pole of the kidney by incising Gerota's fascia at the junction of the upper pole and the adrenal using the harmonic scalpel. The lateral attachments, left intact to maintain the gland in position for dissection, are released last, and the adrenal removed.

Postoperatively, patients are started on clear liquids on the night of surgery, and their diet is advanced as tolerated. The Foley catheter is removed on the first postoperative day, and patients are typically discharged after passing a trial of voiding.

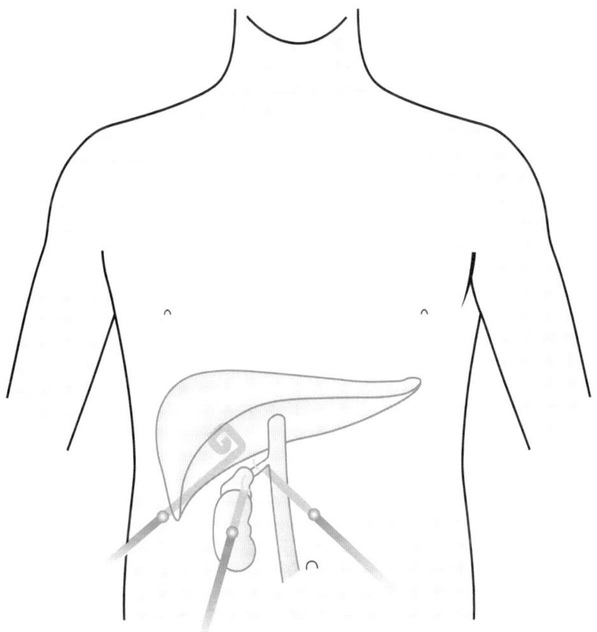

Figure 17.3 Transperitoneal laparoscopic exposure and ligation of the right adrenal vein. The camera port is not shown.

Retroperitoneal laparoscopic adrenalectomy

Since its description by Gaur in 1992, retroperitoneal laparoscopy has been well described for a variety of procedures, including adrenalectomy, in adults.[14] Proponents of the retroperitoneal laparoscopic approach argue that this technique offers a more direct access to the adrenals, without the need for dissection and retraction of intra-abdominal organs. This approach may be particularly suited for patients with a history of abdominal trauma or surgery, in whom dense intra-abdominal adhesions may be anticipated. In addition, by not opening the peritoneum, postoperative intestinal complications are potentially avoided.[15] Disadvantages of retroperitoneal laparoscopy include a limited working space, which is a particular challenge in the pediatric patient population.[16] To date, the application of retroperitoneal laparoscopic adrenalectomy in children has been limited. One study reported on 3 cases of retroperitoneal laparoscopic adrenalectomy in children, with one open conversion, while a second study reported on 10 cases without an open conversion.[17,18] As the experience with pediatric retroperitoneal laparoscopic nephrectomy becomes more widespread, however, and its efficacy and safety confirmed, the application of retroperitoneal adrenalectomy will probably increase as well.[16,19–22]

We position the patient in flank position, and gain initial access through an incision below the tip of the 12th rib, just superior to the anterior iliac spine. Dissection is carried bluntly through the external and internal oblique muscles and the transversus abdominus muscle into the retroperitoneum. The peritoneum is swept medially, and a working space in the retroperitoneum is established using balloon distention. We prefer fashioning a balloon for distention by securing the finger of a surgeon's glove to a 16 Fr red rubber catheter. Once the balloon is introduced into the retroperitoneal space, the glove tip is filled with 100–500 ml of saline and left inflated for 5 minutes to develop the retroperitoneal space. The balloon is then removed, a 10 mm Hasson trocar is introduced into the space, and pneumoretroperitoneum established to a pressure of 12 mmHg. Two additional 5 mm trocars are placed in the posterior and anterior axillary lines, superior to the Hasson trocar.

For right adrenalectomy, the vena cava is identified medial to the psoas muscle, and dissection is carried superiorly along the vena cava to identify first the renal hilum and then the right adrenal vein, which is ligated using hemoclips. The medial and inferior margins of the adrenal are dissected, dividing the adrenal arteries with the harmonic scalpel or clips as they are encountered. The superior aspect of the gland is mobilized as well, and the adrenal is then dissected free from the upper pole of the kidney. As with the transperitoneal laparoscopic adrenalectomy, the lateral attachments of the gland are released last, and the adrenal is removed.

The initial dissection for a retroperitoneal laparoscopic left adrenalectomy identifies the renal hilum. The left renal artery is retracted inferiorly, revealing the adrenal vein as it enters the left renal vein. The adrenal vein is ligated with hemoclips and divided. The adrenal gland is then dissected along its perimeter, using the harmonic scalpel and hemoclips as needed. For a left-sided retroperitoneal laparoscopic adrenalectomy, the medial attachments of the gland are left intact to facilitate dissection, while the superior, lateral, and inferior mobilization of the adrenal is completed. The medial attachments are released last, and the specimen extracted.

Results of laparoscopic adrenalectomy

There are no prospective studies in the pediatric population comparing laparoscopic versus open adrenalectomy. A recent retrospective analysis of adrenalectomy in children found a shorter hospitalization, decreased postoperative pain, more rapid return to preoperative activity level, and improved cosmesis in the laparoscopic cohort.[23] Moreover, a number of studies have confirmed the safety and efficacy of laparoscopic adrenalectomy in children (Table 17.1).[9–11]

Although no absolute upper limit has been set on the size of adrenal tumors that can be removed laparoscopically, larger tumors, especially of the right adrenal gland where lesions may grow behind the vena cava, present a greater technical challenge and increased operative risk. These lesions should be assessed on an individual basis, taking into account the likely tumor pathology as well as the surgeon's experience. In particular, tumors with clear evidence of local extension, requiring en bloc resection of adjacent organs, should be managed with open resection.

Open adrenalectomy

Given that the role of laparoscopic adrenalectomy in the pediatric population is still evolving, as well as the predominance of neuroblastomas (many of which may not be amenable to the laparoscopic resection) among adrenal lesions in children, pediatric urologists should be familiar with the various open approaches to adrenalectomy as well. As with laparoscopy, the central principle of open adrenal surgery is to dissect the patient from the tumor, with minimal manipulation of the gland.

Flank approach

The standard extrapleural, extraperitoneal flank approach to the adrenal gland may be performed for either left or right adrenalectomy. This technique offers the advantage of utilizing the positioning and initial exposure (Figure 17.4) familiar to urologists from radical nephrectomies. For right adrenalectomy, the retroperitoneal space is first identified by medial reflection of the colon and duodenum. The liver is dissected off the anterior surface of the adrenal, allowing ligation of the superior vasculature to the gland. This dissection is facilitated by inferior traction on the kidney, and the mobilization is continued along the posterior abdominal wall and diaphragm from lateral to medial. The small arterial branches to the adrenal should be divided with hemoclips as they are encountered. The inferior vena cava is then exposed, and the adrenal vein identified, dissected free, and divided with clips or ties. The inferior attachments of the adrenal to the kidney are released last, allowing removal of the gland.

Mobilization for left adrenalectomy begins with

Table 17.1 Published series of laparoscopic adrenalectomy in children

Study	No. of patients	Age (mean)	Lesion size (mean)	Hospital stay (mean)	Operative time (mean)	Rate of open conversion
Miller et al[10]	17	9.8 years	4.8 cm	1.5 days	120 min	5.8%
Castilho et al[11]	13	6.3 years	4.1 cm	5.5 days	107 min	15.4%
Kadamba et al[9]	10	4 years	5.3 cm	3 days	143 min	20%

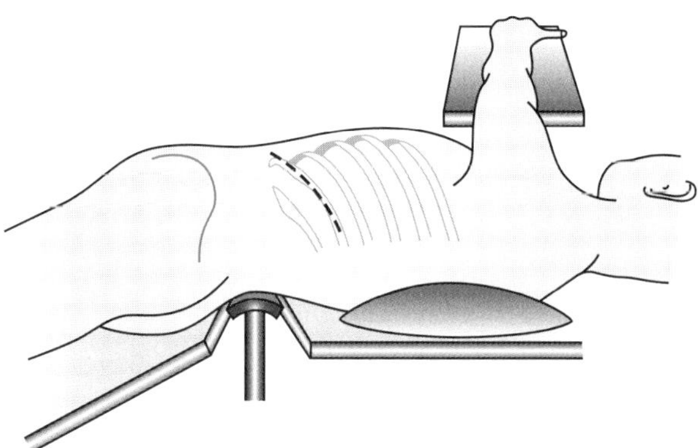

Figure 17.4 Positioning for flank approach to left adrenalectomy. Dotted line marks 11th rib incision.

division of the splenorenal ligament. Gerota's fascia can be swept medially, and the pancreas retracted superiorly and medially, exposing the adrenal. The superior attachments of the adrenal are released from lateral to medial, leading to the renal hilum. The adrenal vein is isolated at its entry to the renal vein, where it is divided. The inferior aspect of the gland is dissected off the upper pole of the left kidney, and the gland is then removed.

Thoracoabdominal adrenalectomy

The main indication for a thoracoabdominal approach to the adrenal gland is to provide maximum exposure for large tumors, particularly on the right side where the liver and vena cava can impede exposure. However, this technique may increase pulmonary complications, as the diaphragm is divided and the thoracic cavity entered.[24] The patient is positioned in approximately 45° flank, and the incision is made through either the 8th or 9th intercostal space (Figure 17.5). The intercostal muscles are encountered and divided, revealing the muscle fibers of the diaphragm, which are circumferentially divided. Adrenalectomy is then performed as described above for the flank approach. At the conclusion of the procedure, a thoracostomy tube is placed in the ipsilateral hemithorax, and the diaphragm is closed using interrupted silk sutures.

Posterior adrenalectomy

Currently, we use the open posterior approach to adrenalectomy primarily for simultaneous bilateral adrenalectomy: for example, in patients with Cushing's disease.[24] Patients are placed in the prone position, and an oblique incision is made overlying the 11th or 12th ribs (Figure 17.6). After subperiosteal

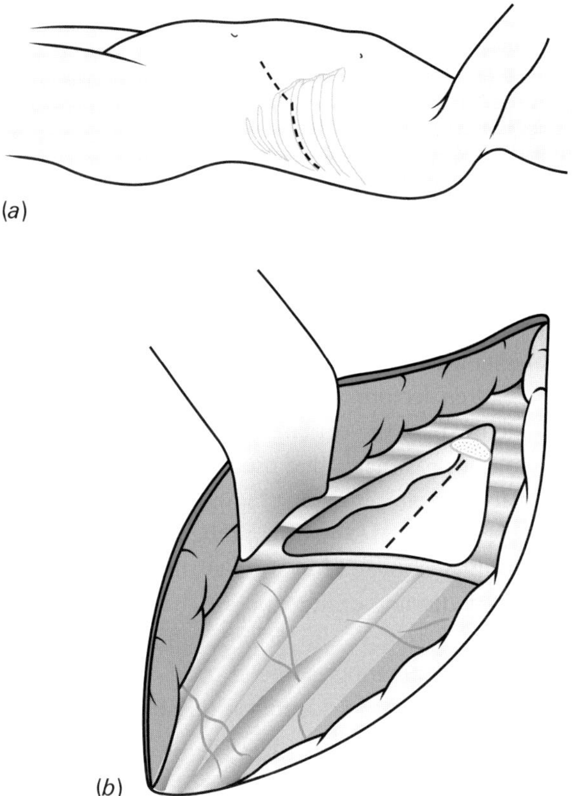

Figure 17.5 (*a*) Incision overlying 9th rib for thoracoabdominal left adrenalectomy. (*b*) Exposure after resection of rib (seen cut at top of figure). Dotted line marks incision in diaphragm muscle.

rib resection, the diaphragm and pleura are mobilized superiorly to expose the retroperitoneal space. For left adrenalectomy, the splenorenal ligament is first released laterally, and dissection then proceeds on the superior aspect of the gland from lateral to medial. This dissection may be facilitated by downward manual traction on the kidney. Medially, the left adrenal vein is identified and divided with clips or ties at its insertion to the left renal vein. Dissection is completed along the inferior aspect of the gland, and the adrenal is removed.

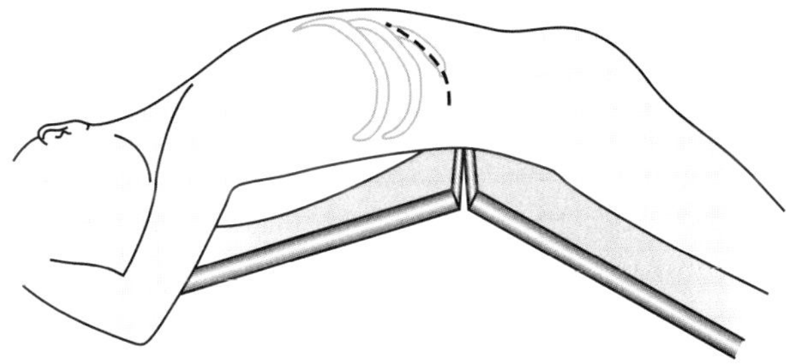

Figure 17.6 Positioning for (standard) posterior approach to adrenalectomy. Dotted line marks incision.

For a posterior right adrenalectomy, the liver is initially dissected off the adrenal and retracted cephalad. The superior vascular attachments of the gland are then divided from lateral to medial, until the vena cava is exposed. The lateral wall of the vena cava is dissected to the origin of the right adrenal vein, which can be clipped or tied and divided. After division of the vein, the inferior attachments of the gland are released, and the adrenal is removed. Given the often difficult exposure of the right adrenal vein through this (standard) posterior approach, we perform open right adrenalectomy via a modified posterior approach, where the patient's position on the operating table approximates that used during a Gil–Vernet dorsal lombotomy incision (Figure 17.7).[25] An 11th or 12th rib incision is made, and the liver is mobilized as described above. However, as the vena cava is exposed by division of the superior attachments of the gland, the adrenal vein is encountered coursing toward the operating surgeon (see Figure 17.7), thereby facilitating its identification and division. In the (standard) posterior approach, the vein lies in a posterior position and is thus at risk of avulsion during exposure.[15] The remainder of the dissection proceeds as for the standard posterior approach.

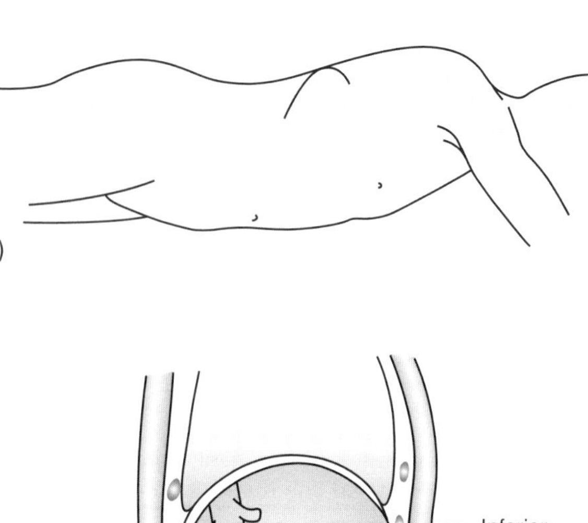

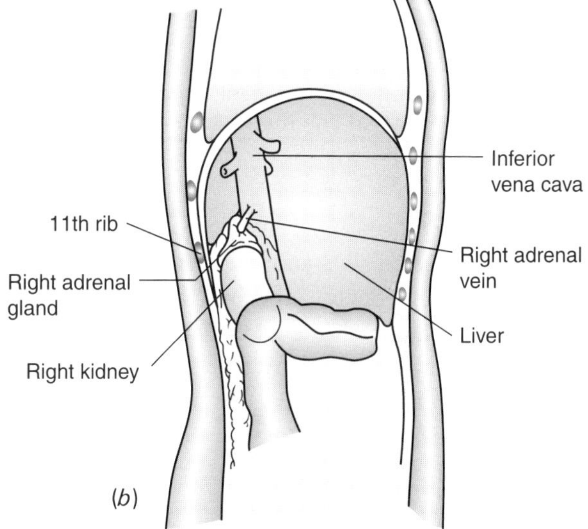

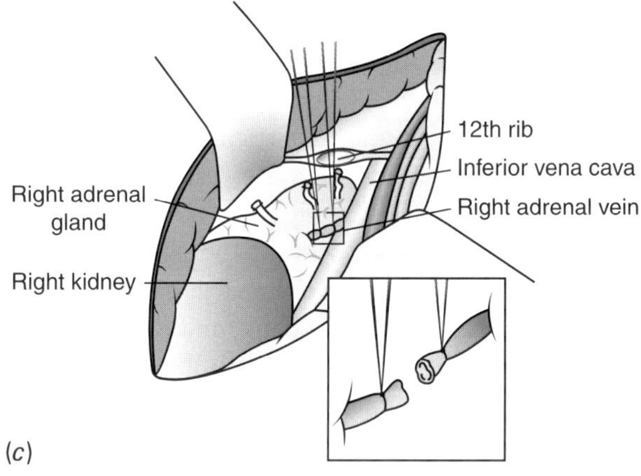

Figure 17.7 Modified posterior right adrenalectomy. (*a*) Positioning and incision. (*b*) View of adrenal bed, with right adrenal vein visible, seen during this approach. (*c*) Exposure and division of right adrenal vein.

Transabdominal adrenalectomy

Transabdominal adrenalectomy is indicated primarily to facilitate complete abdominal exploration, as in the case of multiple pheochromocytomas, patients with large adrenal carcinomas, and for adrenal lesions with involvement of the inferior vena cava. A chevron incision is used to gain access to the peritoneum (Figure 17.8), which is then systematically explored for lesions and/or metastases. Once this has been accomplished, right adrenalectomy may be performed by reflection of the hepatic flexure of the colon inferiorly and incision in the posterior peritoneum lateral to the kidney. This allows reflection of the liver superiorly and exposes the anterior vena cava, approximately at the level of the renal hilum. Cephalad dissection along the anterolateral wall of the vena cava leads to the right adrenal vein, which is then divided. The superior vasculature of the adrenal is released next, proceeding from medial to lateral and facilitated by downward manual traction on the kidney. Lastly, the inferior attachments of the adrenal to the right kidney are mobilized.

For left adrenalectomy, the colon is first reflected medially, and the renal hilum identified and dissected. The left adrenal vein is divided as it enters the left renal vein. The anterior adrenal surface is then exposed by mobilization of the pancreas and spleen. The remainder of the dissection proceeds from medial to lateral along the superior and inferior borders of the gland.

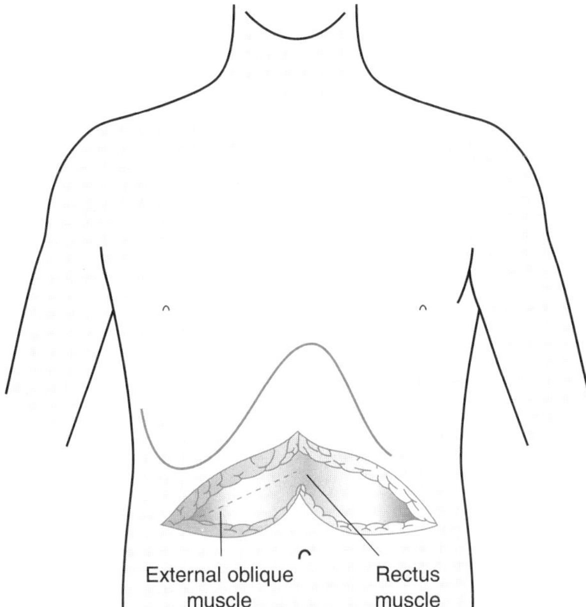

Figure 17.8 Chevron incision for transabdominal adrenalectomy. While such an incision facilitates exposure of both adrenal glands and abdominal exploration for metastases, improved imaging has increased the capacity for precise preoperative localization of lesions. In such cases, the incision can be limited on the contralateral side.

Complications of adrenal surgery

Bleeding may be encountered during either open or laparoscopic adrenalectomy. When operating on the left adrenal, particular care should be taken to avoid injury to Belsey's artery, a communicating branch between the left gastric and the inferior phrenic arteries. This vessel lies close to the esophageal hiatus, and is often accompanied by a phrenic vein.[26] When encountered, Belsey's artery, as well as any associated phrenic vessels, should be ligated to prevent avulsion.

Injury to adjacent organs may also occur during adrenalectomy, most commonly to the diaphragm and pleura. If recognized intraoperatively, the injury may be repaired without the need for thoracostomy tube placement. If such an injury occurs during open adrenalectomy, a red rubber catheter is placed through the defect, with the other end draining into a container of water. The defect is closed with a pursestring chromic suture during hyperinflation of the lung once no bubbles are seen exiting the water end of the catheter. The catheter is removed immediately prior to tightening the purse-string suture. Laparoscopic identification and suture repair of diaphragmatic injuries have also been reported.[27] In any case of diaphragmatic injury, a chest radiograph should be obtained postoperatively to evaluate for pneumothorax, and a thoracostomy tube may be placed at that time if necessary. Other adjacent organ injuries which may occur during adrenalectomy include capsular tears of the liver or spleen, which usually can be managed with a combination of manual tamponade, argon beam coagulation, and hemostatic gel packing.

Complications specific to the laparoscopic approach include trocar injury during placement and port-site hernia. Passage of trocars should be done under direct vision; if inadvertent organ injury is suspected, close inspection and repair should be performed. Moreover, when exchanging instruments during the case, they should be passed under direct visual guidance. With regard to postoperative port-site herniation, there is no consensus on the minimum port-site size that necessitates closure; however, the need for closure of smaller port sites depends on both the size of the child and the type of trocar used.

Special considerations

Neuroblastoma

Neuroblastoma, the most common extracranial solid tumor of childhood, can occur anywhere within the sympathetic nervous system. Most often, however, these tumors originate within the adrenal medulla. The growth pattern of neuroblastoma is variable, ranging from sharply demarcated tumors to highly infiltrative lesions. The often infiltrative growth pattern of neuroblastoma has led most surgeons to excise these tumors via open resection, with the choice of a transabdominal vs retroperitoneal approach guided by tumor location and adjacent organ involvement. More recently, however, laparoscopy has been employed for the biopsy and resection of neuroblastomas.[12,28] Patients with tumors of limited size with clearly defined margins on preoperative imaging have undergone resection, whereas patients with advanced tumors have undergone laparoscopic biopsy prior to chemotherapy.[12,28] Laparoscopic adrenalectomy may be particularly suited for neuroblastomas identified by mass screening programs, which have been associated with a more favorable biology and clinical outcome than clinically diagnosed tumors.[29–33] Currently, the place for laparoscopy in the treatment of neuroblastoma continues to evolve, and the decision regarding treatment approach should be individualized.

Pheochromocytoma

Pheochromocytoma is a rare tumor of chromaffin cell origin that usually arises in the adrenal medulla. Approximately 10% of cases of pheochromocytoma occur in children, and the presentation of these tumors in the pediatric age group may be similar to that in adults.[34] Pheochromocytomas are characterized by catecholamine production; as such, the clinical manifestations of these tumors result from the physiologic effects of catecholamine excess.

Close cooperation of the pediatric urology, medicine, and anesthesiology teams is required in the management of patients with a pheochromocytoma. Patients are typically treated preoperatively with alpha-blockade (phenoxybenzamine) to control their blood pressure. Beta-blockers may be added to alpha-blockers to prevent arrhythmias, but beta-blockade administered without prior alpha-blockade may cause a significant increase in peripheral vascular resistance due to unopposed alpha activity.[15] In addition, many patients have decreased intravascular volume, and therefore intravenous fluids are aggressively administered in the perioperative period to expand plasma volume and minimize intraoperative and postoperative hypotension.[34]

The central tenet of adrenal surgery – removing the patient from the adrenal without manipulation of the gland – is essential during pheochromocytoma excision. Severe intraoperative hemodynamic instability from catecholamine release may occur if the adrenal is manipulated. An additional key principle of adrenalectomy for pheochromocytoma is early control and division of the main adrenal vein, in order to prevent the systemic release of catecholamines during dissection of the gland. Given the potential for blood pressure fluctuation which may occur after ligation of the adrenal vein, the anesthesiologist should be notified at the time of the vein's division, and should be prepared with intravenous fluids and vasopressors if needed.

As for the choice of surgical approach to pheochromocytomas, laparoscopic adrenalectomy has been reported as a safe and effective option in select patients.[35] The presence of multiple sites of disease and the suspicion of lymph node involvement are indications for open removal, which in such cases should be performed through a transabdominal approach.[15] For patients with bilateral adrenal lesions, partial adrenalectomy has been reported in an effort to preserve steroid synthesis and thereby avoid the need for lifetime glucocorticoid replacement therapy.[36,37] However, recurrence has been reported in up to 20–33% of patients undergoing partial adrenalectomy, and therefore close follow-up of these patients is recommended.[38]

Congenital adrenal hyperplasia

Hugh Hampton Young first reported adrenalectomy as a treatment for CAH in the 1930s.[1] With the development of synthetic adrenal steroids, however, the management of these patients has become almost exclusively medical (apart from genital reconstructive surgery). For most patients, the dosage of exogenous steroids needed to retard adrenal androgen production does not result in severe hypercortisolism with its associated sequela. However, in some patients, suppression of adrenocorticotropic hormone (ACTH) is difficult, requiring large doses of exogenous steroids, which may cause obesity, hirsutism, acne, and other cushingoid features. In women, hypercortisolism may in addition result in menstrual irregularities, significant bone loss, and infertility.[39]

Van Wyk et al revisited the concept of adrenalectomy as a treatment for CAH patients who were difficult to manage on medical therapy.[40] In a study of 18 patients who underwent bilateral adrenalectomy for treatment of CAH and were followed an average of 59 months, virtually all patients had a significant decrease in androgen excess.[41] A separate investigation reported two women with CAH who had been infertile and oligomenorrheic who then experienced successful pregnancies following bilateral adrenalectomy.[42] In addition, although the majority of studies on adrenalectomy as a treatment for CAH have involved patients with 21-hydroxylase deficiency, patients with 11β-hydroxylase deficiency, who are prone to develop hypertension as part of their disease process, have been treated with bilateral adrenalectomy as well, with a subsequent improvement in blood pressure.[40,43–46]

Lastly, whereas the aforementioned studies employed adrenalectomy as a treatment for CAH patients, the role of prophylactic adrenalectomy has been explored for patients with CAH as well.[39] Until longer-term data are available, however, prophylactic adrenalectomy is still considered experimental.

Key points

1. Adrenalectomy may be performed in the pediatric patient population using any of a variety of laparoscopic and open techniques; the optimal approach for a particular patient should be individualized

based on the size of the tumor, the pathology of the adrenal, the age and body habitus of the patient, and the experience of the surgeon.
2. Adrenalectomy should be performed with minimal manipulation of the gland itself; essentially, the patient should be removed from the adrenal.
3. During transperitoneal laparoscopic adrenalectomy, the lateral attachments of the gland are released last; these attachments are left intact to hold the adrenal in place for the remainder of the dissection.
4. Preoperative blood pressure control with alpha-blockade, perioperative intravenous hydration, and early ligation of the adrenal vein during surgical excision are keys to the management of adrenal pheochromocytoma.
5. Adrenalectomy may be a treatment alternative for patients with severe congenital adrenal hyperplasia who experience the sequela of iatrogenic hypercortisolism.

References

1. Young HH. A technique for simultaneous exposure and operation on the adrenals. Surg Gynecol Obstet 1936; 63:179–88.
2. Gagner M, Lacroix A, Bolte E. Laparoscopic adrenalectomy in Cushing's syndrome and pheochromocytoma. N Engl J Med 1992; 327:1033.
3. Prinz RA. A comparison of laparoscopic and open adrenalectomies. Arch Surg 1995; 130:489–92.
4. Brunt LM, Doherty GM, Norton JA et al. Laparoscopic adrenalectomy compared to open adrenalectomy for benign adrenal neoplasms. J Am Coll Surg 1996; 183:1–10.
5. Gill IS, Schweizer D, Nelson D. Laparoscopic versus open adrenalectomy in 210 patients: Cleveland Clinic experience. J Urol 1999; 161(Suppl):21.
6. Imai T, Kikumori T, Ohiwa M, Mase T, Funahashi H. A case-controlled study of laparoscopic compared with open lateral adrenalectomy. Am J Surg 1999; 178:50–3.
7. Cagle PT, Hough AJ, Pysher TJ et al. Comparison of adrenal cortical tumors in children and adults. Cancer 1986; 57:2235–7.
8. Mayer SK, Oligny LL, Deal C et al. Childhood adrenocortical tumors: case series and reevaluation of prognosis – a 24-year experience. J Pediatr Surg 1997; 32:911–15.
9. Kadamba P, Habib Z, Rossi L. Experience with laparoscopic adrenalectomy in children. J Pediatr Surg 2004; 39:764–7.
10. Miller KA, Albanese C, Harrison M et al. Experience with laparoscopic adrenalectomy in pediatric patients. J Pediatr Surg 2002; 37:979–82.
11. Castilho LN, Castillo OA, Denes FT, Mitre AI, Arap S. Laparoscopic adrenal surgery in children. J Urol 2002; 168:221–4.
12. De Lagausie P, Berrebi D, Michon J et al. Laparoscopic adrenal surgery for neuroblastomas in children. J Urol 2003; 170:932–5.
13. Del Pizzo JJ. Transabdominal laparoscopic adrenalectomy. Curr Urol Rep 2003; 4:81–6.
14. Gaur DD. Laparoscopic operative retroperitoneoscopy: use of a new device. J Urol 1992; 148:1137–9.
15. Vaughan ED Jr, Blumenfeld JD, Del Pizzo JJ, Schichman SJ, Sosa RE. The adrenals. In: Walsh PC, Retik AB, Vaughan ED Jr, Wein AJ, eds. Campbell's Urology, 8th edn. Philadelphia: WB Saunders, 2002: 3507–69.
16. El-Ghoneimi A, Valla JS, Steyaert H, Aigrain Y. Laparoscopic renal surgery via a retroperitoneal approach in children. J Urol 1998; 160:1138–41.
17. Shanberg AM, Sanderson K, Rajpoot D, Duel B. Laparoscopic retroperitoneal renal and adrenal surgery in children. BJU Int 2001; 87:521–4.
18. Steyaert H, Juricic M, Hendrice C et al. Retroperitoneoscopic approach to the adrenal glands and retroperitoneal tumors in children: where do we stand? Eur J Pediatr Surg 2003; 13:112–15.
19. Valla JS, Guilloneau B, Montupet P et al. Retroperitoneal laparoscopic nephrectomy in children. Preliminary report of 18 cases. Eur Urol 1996; 30:490–3.
20. Kobashi KC, Chamberlin DA, Rajpoot D, Shanberg AM. Retroperitoneal laparoscopic nephrectomy in children. J Urol 1998; 160:1142–4.
21. Borer JG, Cisek LJ, Atala A et al. Pediatric retroperitoneoscopic nephrectomy using 2 mm instrumentation. J Urol 1999; 162:1725–9.
22. El-Ghoneimi A. Pediatric laparoscopic surgery. Curr Opin Urol 2003; 13:329–35.
23. Stanford A, Upperman JS, Nguyen N, Barksdale E Jr, Wiener ES. Surgical management of open versus laparoscopic adrenalectomy: outcome analysis. J Pediatr Surg 2002; 37:1027–9.
24. Novick AC, Howards SS. The adrenals. In: Gillenwater JY, Grayhack JT, Howards SS, Mitchell ME, eds. Adult and Pediatric Urology, 4th edn. Philadelphia: Lippincott Williams and Wilkins, 2002: 531–62.
25. Vaughan ED Jr, Phillips H. Modified posterior approach for right adrenalectomy. Surg Gynecol Obstet 1987; 165:453–5.
26. Vaughan ED Jr. Complications of adrenal surgery. In: Taneja SS, Smith RB, Ehrlich RM, eds. Complications of Urologic Surgery: Prevention and Management, 3rd edn. Philadelphia: WB Saunders, 2001: 362–9.
27. Del Pizzo JJ, Jacobs SC, Bishoff JT, Kavoussi LR, Jarrett TW. Pleural injury during laparoscopic renal surgery: early recognition and management. J Urol 2003; 169:41–4.
28. Iwanaka T, Arai M, Ito M et al. Surgical treatment for abdominal neuroblastoma in the laparoscopic era. Surg Endosc 2001; 15:751–4.
29. Matthay KK, Sather HN, Seeger RC, Haase GM, Hammond GD. Excellent outcome of stage II neuroblastoma is independent of residual disease and radiation therapy. J Clin Oncol 1989; 7:236–44.
30. Bessho F, Hashizume K, Nakajo T, Kamoshita S. Mass screening in Japan increased the detection of infants with neuroblastoma without a decrease in cases in older children. J Pediatr 1991; 119:237–41.

Renal anomalies

20

Michael L Ritchey and Susan John

Embryology

Renal anomalies may be the result of an arrest in development or a malformation. A complete understanding of the embryologic development of the genitourinary tract is a prerequisite for the evaluation of a child with a suspected anomaly. Anomalies of the urogenital tract are among the most common of all organ systems. Using real-time ultrasonography as a screening test in healthy infants, Steinhart et al found that 3.2% of infants had an abnormality of the genitourinary tract and half of these required surgical intervention.[1] Shieh et al noted a 0.5% incidence of renal abnormalities using portable ultrasound screening of school-age children.[2]

The development of the urinary tract can be divided into two segments, the nephric system and the vesicourethral system.[3] There are three stages in the formation of the nephric system. The two intermediate stages are the pronephros, which completely disappears, and the mesonephros. Although the mesonephros undergoes degeneration, its duct persists and extends caudally to communicate with the anterior cloaca. Vestigial remnants of the mesonephric tubules occur in both sexes and are associated with the reproductive tract. Early in the 4th–5th weeks, the ureteral bud begins to develop from the distal end of the mesonephric duct near its junction with the cloaca. The cranial end of the ureter then ascends to meet the nephrogenic cord of the intermediate mesoderm. This begins to develop into the metanephros and continues its cephalad migration. The cranial end of the ureteral bud begins a series of branchings to form the renal pelvis, the calices, and a portion of the collecting ducts.[4] This branching is associated with the simultaneous differentiation of the metanephrogenic cap, which becomes arranged around the branching collecting ducts, and ascends. The ascent of the kidneys occurs in part due to true migration and also secondary to differential somatic growth of the lumbar portion of the body. They reach their final level by the end of the 8th week of fetal life (Figure 20.1). The kidney also undergoes axial rotation medially of 90° during the 7th and 8th weeks before it assumes its final position. During ascent, each kidney receives its blood supply from the neighboring vessels. Initially, this is from the middle sacral artery, then the common iliac and inferior mesenteric arteries, and finally the aorta.

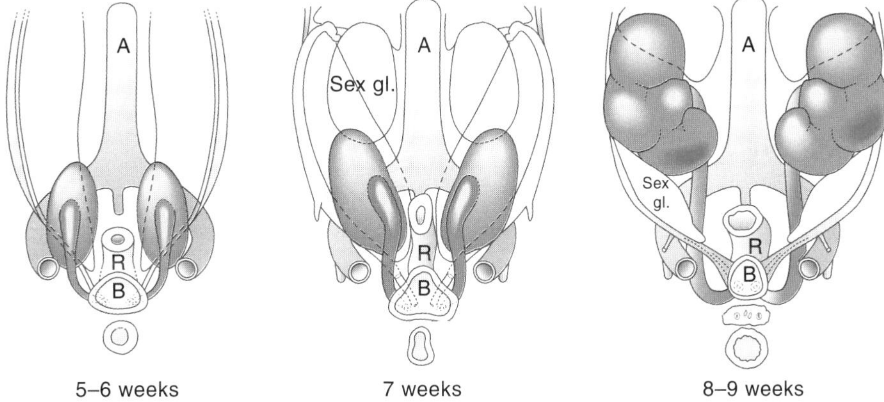

Figure 20.1 Ascent and rotation of kidneys during fetal life. The normal rotation of the kidney from facing forward to facing medially is shown. A, aorta; R, rectum; B, bladder; Sex gl, sex gland. (From Campbell.[5])

Anomalies in number

Supernumerary kidney

A supernumerary kidney is an uncommon anomaly, with no more than 100 cases reported in the literature.[6–9] The embryologic basis shares some similarities with that found in ureteral duplication. There are either two ureteral buds arising from the mesonephric duct, leading to double ureters, or a branching of the ureteral bud, that results in a bifid collecting system. The two ureteral buds then either join two separate metanephroi or a splitting of the nephrogenic blastema occurs. This later develops into twin metanephroi after induction by the two ureteral buds. It is not necessary for the two ureteral buds to be widely divergent.[8]

The supernumerary kidney is caudal to the ipsilateral kidney in 60% of cases. A supernumerary kidney associated with complete ureteral duplication is more likely to be in a cranial location. There is generally one extra kidney, but as many as five separate renal masses have been reported. This anomaly occurs more frequently on the left side. The ureter of the anomalous kidney joins the ipsilateral ureter about as commonly as it enters the bladder separately, but only rarely is the ureter ectopic. The extra kidney has its own renal capsule and blood supply. The supernumerary kidney is often smaller and one-third exhibit other pathologic changes (e.g. hydronephrosis, pyelonephritis). Renal function is frequently decreased in the smaller hypoplastic unit.

Most cases are diagnosed after the third decade of life. Presenting complaints are usually related to urinary obstruction or infection and include pain, fever, or an abdominal mass.[10] However, many patients remain asymptomatic throughout life and 20% of reported cases were discovered at autopsy.[11] The diagnosis can be readily established with current imaging modalities; nuclear renal scintigraphy will confirm the presence of functioning renal tissue.[12]

Unilateral renal agenesis

Renal agenesis results from a failure of induction of the metanephric blastema by the ureteral bud. This could result from agenesis of the ureteral bud or Wolffian duct, failure of the bud to reach the blastema, absence or abnormality of the metanephric blastema, or failure of the ureteral bud to invade the metanephric blastema.[13] It is unclear whether there is a genetic predisposition or if it is related to other prenatal factors. Parikh et al found diabetes and black maternal race were associated with an increased incidence of renal agenesis, but it is probably multifactorial, with both environmental and genetic factors playing a role.[14] A familial tendency has been reported, supporting the latter.[15] The reported incidence of this condition varies between series of patients collected from either clinical or autopsy data. Doroshow and Abeshouse estimated that unilateral renal agenesis (URA) is found in 1 of every 1100 autopsies.[16] A similar incidence has been noted in school-age children undergoing ultrasound screening.[2] The clinical incidence on imaging studies is 1 in 1500, suggesting that most cases are diagnosed during life.[17] Currently, most renal anomalies seen by pediatric urologists are detected prenatally and URA is no exception, but fetal ultrasound studies have detected renal agenesis with a much lower frequency.[18,19] Many patients previously reported with URA probably had prior involution of multicystic or dysplastic kidneys. This has been documented to occur prenatally,[20] and rapid involution of multicystic and dysplastic renal units has also been shown to occur early in postnatal life.[21,22] Hiraoaka et al have suggested that aplasia is the predominant cause of congenital solitary kidneys.[23] There is a slight male predominance, and the condition occurs more frequently on the left side. This male predominance may reflect the earlier differentiation of the Wolffian duct that takes place close to the time of ureteral bud formation. The ureteral bud is more likely to be influenced by abnormalities of the Wolffian duct than that of the Müllerian duct, which occurs later.

Associated anomalies

The ipsilateral ureter is absent in 50–87% of cases and only partially developed in the remainder.[24] On cystoscopy, a hemitrigone will be present in patients with complete ureteral agenesis. Anomalies of the contralateral kidney are common, with reflux the most frequent finding, followed by ureterovesical and ureteropelvic junction obstruction.[25–27] Limakeng and Retik reported an increased incidence of contralateral abnormality if a hypoplastic ureter was associated with the absent kidney.[28] The ipsilateral adrenal was found to be absent on autopsy in 8% of patients with URA.[24] One report noted ipsilateral adrenal agenesis in two of seven patients with URA examined with abdominal ultrasonography.[29]

The most commonly associated abnormalities are those of the female genitalia. The incidence ranges from 20 to 60%.[16,30] Likewise, patients with known genital anomalies have an increased incidence of renal anomalies.[31] Complete absence or hypoplasia of the vagina, the Mayer–Rokitansky–Küster–Hauser syndrome, is frequently associated with agenesis of the kidney.[32–34] Most of the genital anomalies in female patients with URA are asymptomatic, but such anomalies often assume greater clinical importance, leading to earlier evaluation and diagnosis of the absent kidney. The most common problems involve the uterus and vagina. There is often a unicornuate or bicornuate uterus (Figure 20.2), and the ipsilateral horn and fallopian tube may be rudimentary or absent.[35] A duplex uterus is attributable to a developmental anomaly of the urogenital septum, resulting in incomplete midline fusion of the Müllerian ducts and a longitudinal vaginal septum. The development of the Müllerian duct appears to be inhibited by the defective Wolffian duct if the defect occurs early in development.[36] Defects of the ureteral bud that occur after Müllerian duct fusion will affect only ureteral and renal development.[37] Obstruction of the lower genital tract can occur, leading to hydrocolpos or hematocolpos. Patients present with a pelvic mass or pain and fail to menstruate at puberty.[38] Patients with complete Müllerian arrest will require vaginal construction to achieve adequate sexual function but will be infertile.

The vas deferens, seminal vesicle, and ejaculatory duct are absent in 50% of males with URA.[39] Conversely, in those patients presenting with an absent vas, the reported incidence of renal agenesis varies greatly. Donahue and Fauver found an absent kidney in 22/26 (85%) patients with an absent vas deferens.[40] Goldstein and Schlossberg used computed tomography (CT) to evaluate 26 men with absence of the vas deferens.[41] Unilateral renal agenesis was noted in only four men, in all of whom the seminal vesicle was absent. Schlegel et al found an 11% incidence of renal agenesis in infertile men with unilateral agenesis of the vas.[42] Of interest, men with both agenesis of the vas and renal anomalies rarely had *CFTR* gene defects. Cysts of the seminal vesicle associated with URA or dysgenesis and an ectopic ureter have also been reported.[43] The ipsilateral testis is usually present.[24] Cystic dysplasia of the rete testis is associated with a high incidence of URA.[44]

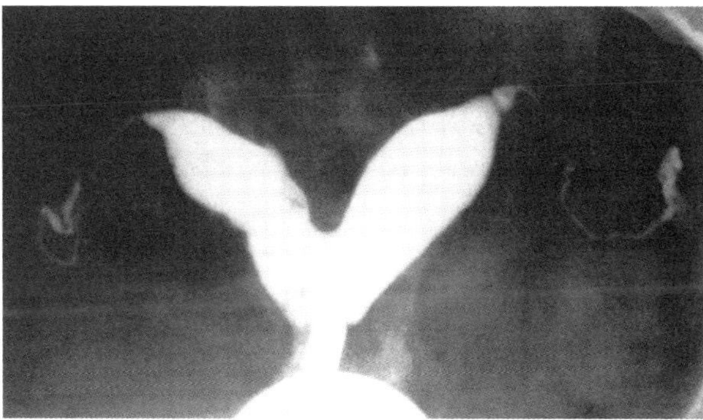

Figure 20.2 Bicornuate uterus seen on hysterosalpingogram with filling of both fallopian tubes. The vagina was normal in this patient with an absent right kidney.

Approximately 25–40% of patients with URA have anomalies of other organ systems. Most frequently affected are cardiovascular (30%), gastrointestinal (25%), and musculoskeletal (14%).[45] Unilateral renal agenesis is associated with several syndromes, including Turner's, Poland's,[46] Goldenhar's,[47] VACTERL association,[48] and Klippel–Feil syndromes.[49]

Diagnosis

Absence of the kidney may be suspected on a plain film of the abdomen if the gas pattern of the splenic or hepatic flexure of the colon is displaced into the renal fossa.[50] This non-specific finding is also found after the kidney has been surgically removed. The diagnosis is confirmed by an absent kidney and contralateral compensatory hypertrophy on excretory urography. Sonography will also reveal an empty renal fossa, but the hypertrophied adrenal gland can be mistaken for a small kidney.[51] In these cases, the adrenal gland loses its 'Y' and 'V' configuration and becomes flatter and more elliptical in shape. This flattened adrenal gland has been described as the 'lying down' sign and can also be noted in renal ectopy.[52] Radionuclide imaging should be performed in all children with the diagnosis of a solitary kidney, as it can identify small, poorly functioning kidneys missed by other imaging studies. Renography will also reveal kidneys that are ectopically located.[53] As noted above, cystography is recommended in all children with URA due to the increased risk of vesicoureteral reflux (VUR). Ultrasound and magnetic resonance imaging (MRI) are useful for examining the internal genital structures in females with a diagnosis of renal agenesis. In general, the uterus and cervix can be visualized in both infants and older girls. Renal sonography has been recommended for screening of parents and siblings of children born with renal agenesis. Roodhooft et al reported a 9% incidence of asymptomatic renal malformations in family members, with URA the most common finding.[54]

Prognosis

Hypertrophy of the solitary kidney occurs as an adaptive compensatory response. This hypertrophy has been shown to occur in utero.[55] There are both experimental and clinical studies suggesting that hyperfiltration of remnant nephrons may have an adverse effect on renal function, depending on the number of nephrons remaining.[56] There are reports of focal glomerulosclerosis, the renal lesion that develops in hyperfiltration, occurring in humans with URA.[57–59] Some studies have noted an increased rate of hypertension, proteinuria, and mild renal insufficiency.[60,61] However, others have noted normal renal reserve in patients with URA.[62] Although the risk of significant renal disease is low, we advise our patients to have annual measurement of blood pressure and urinalysis to assess for proteinuria.

Bilateral renal agenesis

The incidence of bilateral renal agenesis (Potter's syndrome) is 1 in 4000 births, with a slight male predominance (male : female ratio of 2.5 : 1).[63] A familial tendency has been reported, and the risk of recurrence in subsequent pregnancies is 2–5%.[64] These infants have a characteristic facies (Figure 20.3) that is found in conditions in which there is an absence of intrauterine renal function. The most constant finding is a prominent epicanthal fold that extends onto the cheek. The skin of these infants is very loose, particularly over the hands. Oligohydramnios during pregnancy is profound, except in rare instances. This causes intrauterine compression of the fetus, which results in other characteristic external features, including bowed legs and clubbed feet. The most significant sequelae of oligohydramnios is pulmonary hypoplasia. This is the result of compression of the thoracic cage, preventing lung expansion, lack of pulmonary fluid stenting the airways, or absence of renal factors, such as proline production.[65]

Approximately 40% of such infants are stillborn, and the remainder rapidly succumb to respiratory failure associated with the pulmonary hypoplasia unless aggressively treated. This poor prognosis has led to the recommendation of termination of the pregnancy if the diagnosis is made early in gestation.

The ultrasound criteria for diagnosis of a fetus with bilateral renal agenesis are the presence of severe oligohydramnios or anhydramnios occurring after 14–16 weeks' gestation, failure to visualize both kidneys, and non-visualization of the bladder. Prior to 16 weeks gestation, relatively little of the amniotic volume is due to fetal urine. Because fetal imaging is very difficult in severe oligohydramnios, non-visualization of the urinary bladder is a more reliable indication of fetal renal non-function than the inability to identify the fetal kidneys.[66] Caution must be used in accepting the antenatal diagnosis of bilateral renal agenesis, because false-positive diagnoses have been made. Color Doppler sonography is recommended to establish the presence or absence of renal arteries.[67] MRI may facilitate assessment of the fetus with possible bilateral renal agenesis.[68]

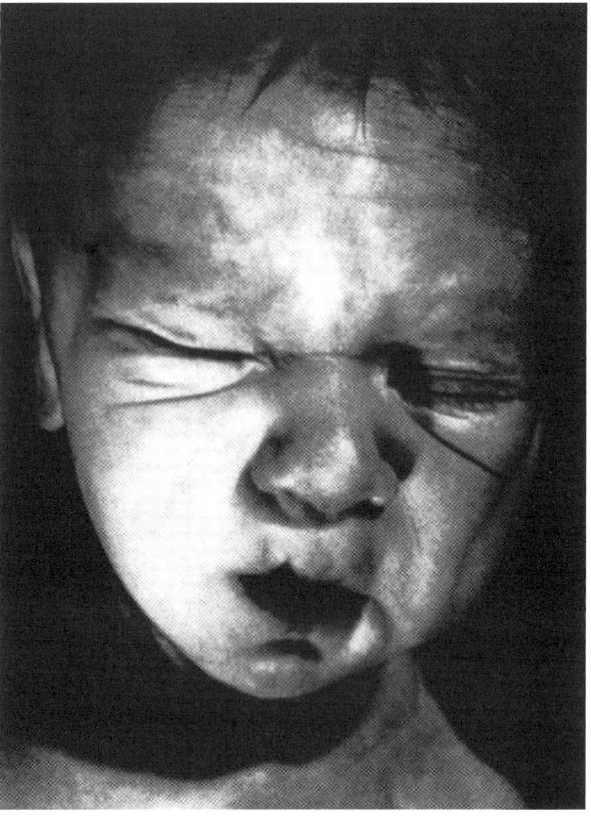

Figure 20.3 Potter's facies. (Courtesy of Dr Catherine Poole, University of Miami, Florida.)

The ureter is absent in the majority of cases and only partially developed in the remaining individuals.[24] The bladder is either absent or severely hypoplastic as a result of the absence of urine flow. The adrenal glands are rarely absent or malpositioned, but are flat.[52] External genital development is usually normal except when bilateral renal agenesis occurs in a sirenomelic monster. Testicular absence has been reported in up to 10%, but the vasa are usually present.[52] The presence of the vasa suggests that this anomaly is not due to failure of the Wolffian duct to develop. The organs most often abnormal in the female are derived from the Müllerian structures. In both sexes, there is an increased incidence of spina bifida and gastrointestinal malformations, imperforate anus in particular. A regional disturbance affecting the posterior portion of the cloaca and the adjacent mesonephros and Müllerian ducts is probably responsible for these associations.[63]

Anomalies of rotation

Abnormal rotation, or malrotation, is most commonly associated with an ectopic or fused kidney, but may also occur in kidneys that undergo complete ascent. In the normal adult kidney, the renal pelvis is oriented medially and the calices point laterally. The fetal kidneys undergo a 90° rotation during the 6th–8th weeks of embryonic development to achieve normal orientation (see Figure 20.1). The rotation of the fetal kidney has been proposed to be the result of differential growth, with more tubules being formed on the ventrolateral side than on the dorsomedial side.[69] This theory does not explain all of the abnormalities of rotation. Weyrauch suggested that the ureteral bud makes more lateral contact with the renal blastema. This may explain an anomalous initial position of the kidney, but does not explain normal renal rotation. Campbell reported only 17 cases of renal malrotation among 32 834 autopsies on adults.[70] Smith and Orkin found an incidence of 1 in 390 and stated that malrotation accounts for 10% of upper urinary tract anomalies.[71] The true incidence of this type of anomaly is probably understated because in many patients there are no clinical manifestations.

The different types of malrotation are depicted in Figure 20.4. The most common is an incomplete rotation, or non-rotation (Figure 20.5). The renal pelvis is anterior or between the fetal anterior and normal medial position in the adult. Other major types of anomalous rotation are reverse rotation and hyper-rotation (excessive rotation) in which the kidney faces laterally, but these are rare (Figure 20.6).[72] In reverse rotation, the renal pelvis rotates laterally and the renal vessels cross the kidney anteriorly to reach the hilum (Figure 20.7). In excessive rotation, the kidney rotates more than 180° but less than 360°. The pelvis faces laterally, but the renal vessels are carried posteriorly to the kidney. Less severe hyper-rotation may leave the renal pelvis in a dorsal position.[3]

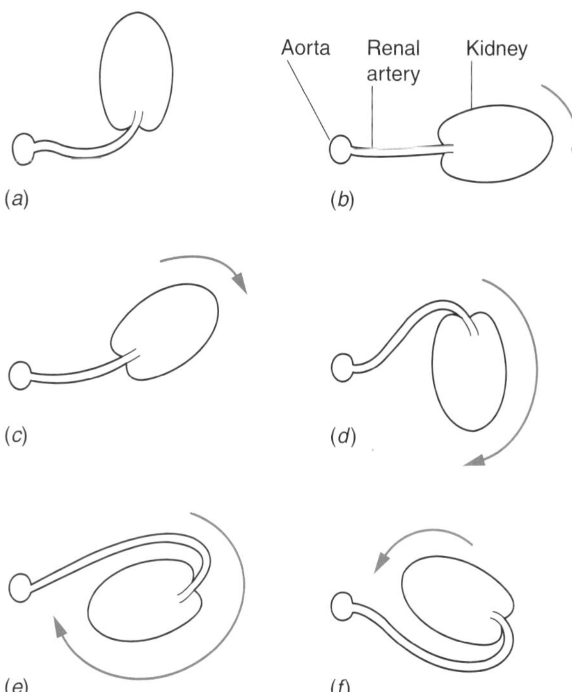

Figure 20.4 Rotation of the kidney during its ascent from the pelvis. The left kidney (with its renal artery) and the aorta are viewed in transverse section to show normal and abnormal rotation during its ascent to the adult site. (*a*) Primitive embryonic position, hilus faces ventrad (anterior). (*b*) Normal adult position, hilus faces mediad. (*c*) Incomplete rotation. (*d*) Hyper-rotation, hilus faces dorsad (posterior). (*e*) Hyper-rotation, hilus faces laterad. (*f*) Reverse rotation, hilus faces laterad. (From Parrott et al.[3])

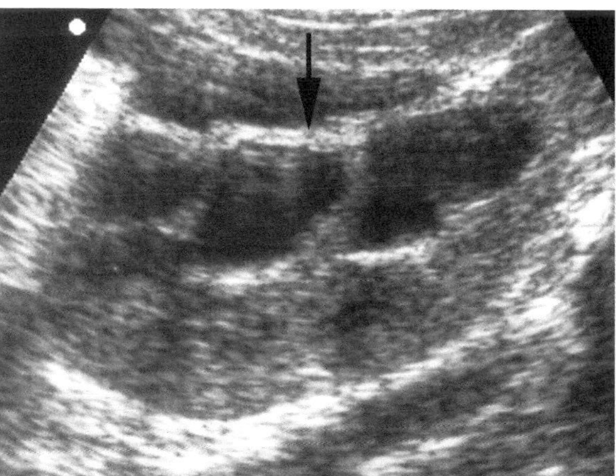

Figure 20.5 Ultrasound demonstrating malrotation of the right kidney. This results in an anterior location of the renal collecting structures (arrow) on ultrasound, rather than the usual posteromedial orientation.

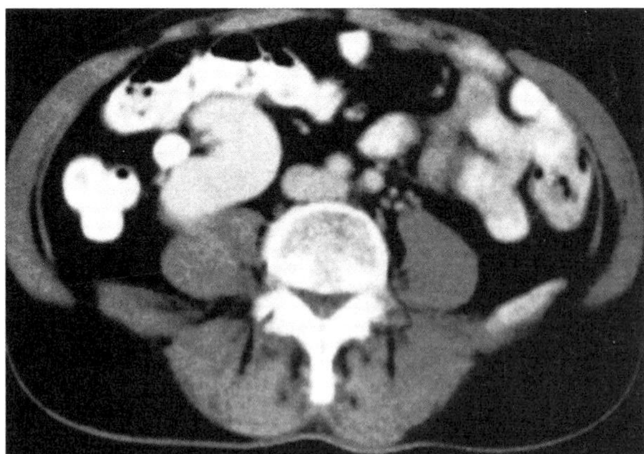

Figure 20.6 CT demonstrating excessive rotation of the right kidney.

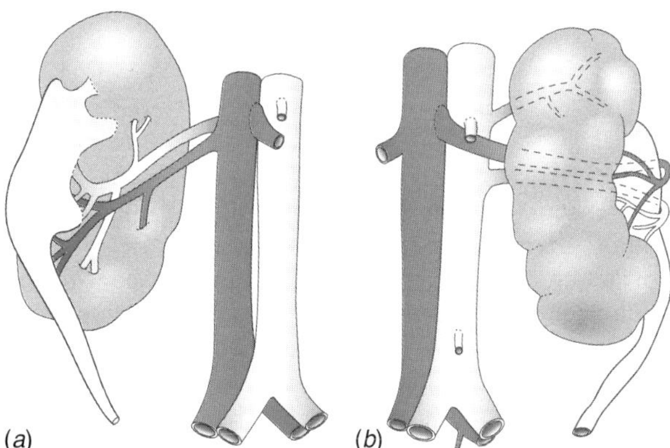

Figure 20.7 Abnormal renal rotation: (*a*) reverse rotation; (*b*) hyper-rotation. (Adapted from Weyrauch.[72])

Malrotation is usually discovered incidentally during imaging of the kidney. When symptoms occur, they are most often related to intermittent hydronephrosis and consist of abdominal pain often associated with vomiting. It is important to establish the correct diagnosis and to exclude other pathologic conditions that can produce similar distortion of the kidney. The upper third of the ureter may be displaced laterally and the renal pelvis may appear elongated, suggesting obstruction or effacement by an extrinsic mass. Obstruction may be secondary to compression of the ureter from an anomalous accessory vessel or other obstructive lesions that also occur in normally rotated kidneys. The calices are often distorted even without any associated obstruction. Helical CT can be very informative.[73] Treatment of malrotation is reserved for alleviation of associated obstruction, calculi, or infection secondary to poor drainage.

Anomalies of ascent

Renal ectopy

Renal ectopy is the term used to describe a kidney that lies outside the renal fossa. The kidney migrates cephalad early in gestation to reach its normal position. Failure of ascent can be due to a number of factors: abnormality of the ureteral bud or metanephric blastema, genetic abnormalities, teratogenic causes, or anomalous vasculature acting as a barrier to ascent.[74] During ascent, the kidney receives its blood supply from the middle sacral artery, iliac artery, and finally the aorta. The anomalous blood supply that is invariably present is dependent on the final position of the kidney and is probably not the cause of the malposition. However, the blood vessels are frequently short, rendering surgical mobilization very difficult.

The incidence of renal ectopy in postmortem studies varies from 1 in 500 to 1 in 1290.[75,76] The incidence of ectopic kidney is higher in autopsy series than in clinical studies, suggesting that many cases remain unrecognized throughout life.[74,76] There is a slight predilection for the left side, and 10% of cases are bilateral. Simple renal ectopy refers to a kidney that remains in the ipsilateral retroperitoneal space. The most common position is in the pelvis (sacral or pelvic kidney) opposite the sacrum or below the aortic bifurcation.[76] The lumbar or iliac ectopic kidney is one that is fixed above the crest of the ileum but below the level of L-2 and L-3. Crossed renal ectopy refers to a kidney that crosses the midline (see discussion on anomalies of fusion later in this chapter). Lastly, malrotation often accompanies renal ectopy (Figure 20.8).

The differentiation between a ptotic kidney and renal ectopia can be difficult, but there are several discerning features. The length of the ureter may be helpful. In renal ectopy ureteral length corresponds to the location of the kidney; in a ptotic kidney, the ureter appears redundant. The ptotic kidney is mobile and usually can be manipulated into its normal position.

Diagnosis

Most cases of renal ectopy diagnosed in childhood present with symptoms attributed to the genitourinary or gastrointestinal system, such as vague abdominal pain or renal colic secondary to ureteropelvic junction (UPJ) obstruction or urolithiasis. Urinary tract infection (UTI) is the presentation in 30% of children. The ectopic kidney may also be noted inci-

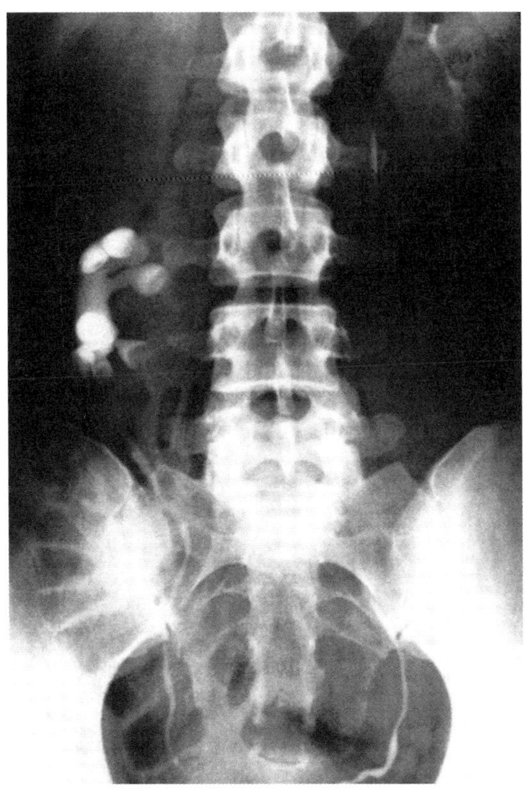

Figure 20.8 Malrotated ectopic kidney opposite lower lumbar vertebrae.

dentally, most frequently on prenatal ultrasound. A pelvic kidney is the most common finding in a fetus with an empty renal fossa and normal amniotic fluid volume.[77] They can also be detected during the evaluation of the other associated anomalies. Less often, the ectopic kidney can be detected as an abdominal mass on physical examination.

In past years, pelvic kidneys were often difficult to recognize on excretory urography because they overlie the bony structures (Figure 20.9). However, most can be now be identified by ultrasonography or radionuclide imaging.[53] Whenever a kidney is absent on ultrasound, radionuclide imaging is indicated to exclude an ectopic kidney. Voiding cystourethrography (VCUG) is recommended in all children with a diagnosis of pelvic kidney to exclude VUR, which is frequently associated with an ectopic kidney.[78] Hydronephrosis is frequently noted in ectopic kidneys.[79] Gleason et al found that half of the dilation could be attributed to ureteropelvic or ureterovesical obstruction. Obstruction in the ectopic kidney is frequently due to a high insertion of the ureter on the renal pelvis (Figure 20.10). High-grade reflux was

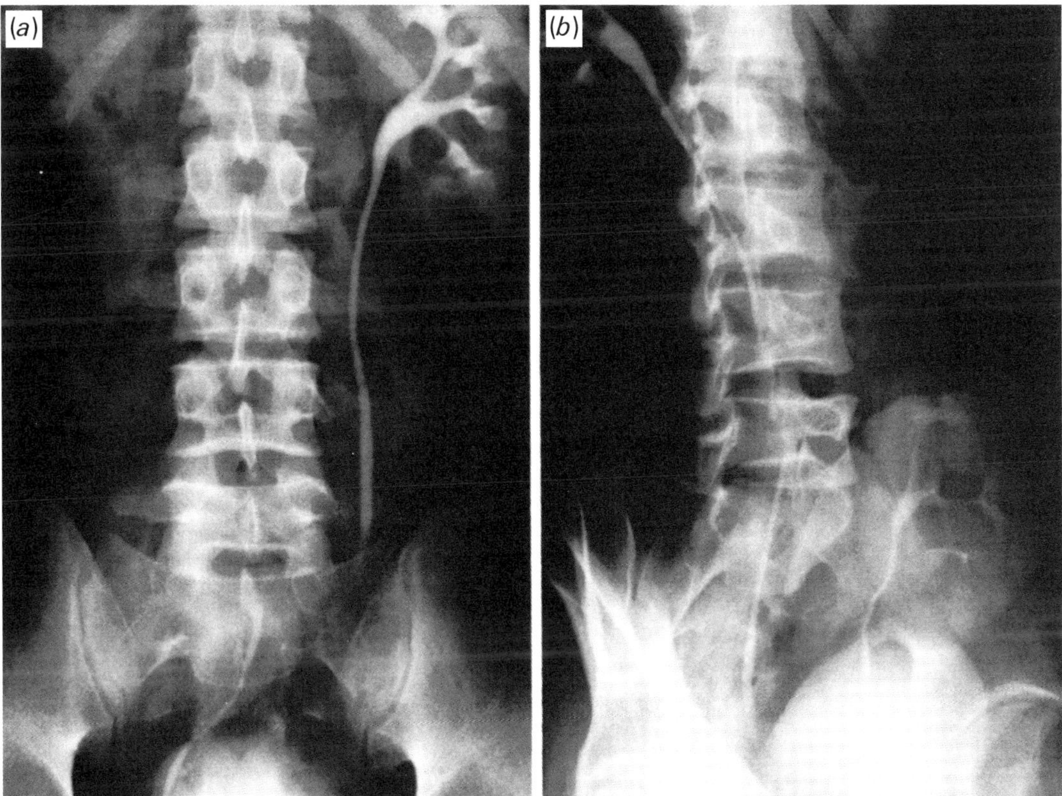

Figure 20.9 Excretory urogram in patient with a right pelvic kidney. (*a*) The short right ureter is seen overlying the bony structures. (*b*) Oblique film allows much better visualization of the collecting system and renal outline.

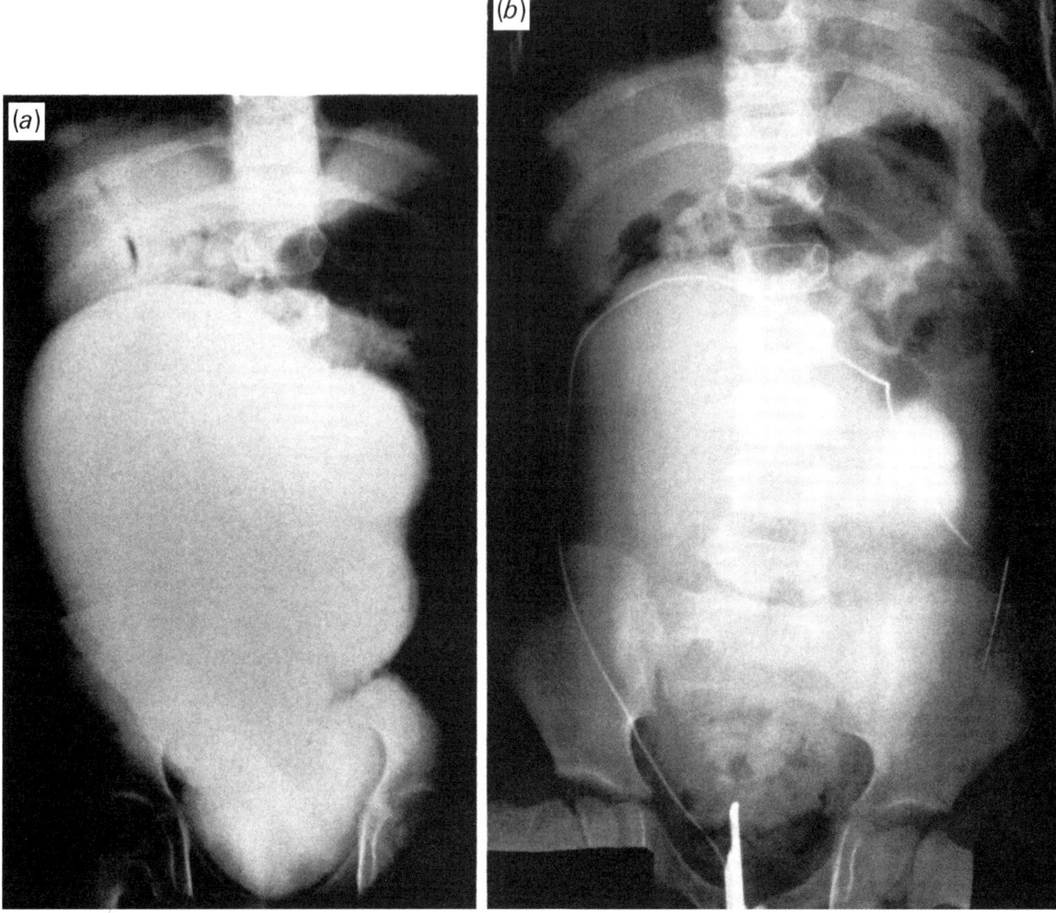

Figure 20.10 Ectopic solitary pelvic kidney in a 6-year-old boy with gross hematuria. (*a*) Excretory urogram showing giant hydronephrosis. (*b*) Retrograde pyelogram showing a catheter in the ureter with high insertion into pelvis.

responsible for 26% of hydronephrotic kidneys, and extrarenal collecting system with malrotation accounted for the remainder. Diuretic renography may be needed to distinguish these abnormal pyelocaliceal patterns from UPJ obstruction. The ectopic kidney can be clearly shown on the renal scan, but the gamma camera should be place anteriorly to obtain better images (Figure 20.11). However, if the kidney is totally non-functional, an ultrasound or CT scan may be the best method of localization. MR urography is a newer modality that shows promise for detection of small poorly functioning renal units.[80] Retrograde pyelography can be used to delineate the collecting system anatomy in selected cases (Figure 20.12). Renal arteriography is now seldom performed in the patient with an ectopic kidney. Most often the kidney is supplied by multiple vessels that arise from the distal aorta, aortic bifurcation, or the iliac artery. These can be identified at the time of surgery.

Associated anomalies

The contralateral kidney is abnormal in up to 50% of patients.[74] There is a 10% incidence of contralateral renal agenesis. Associated VUR is found in 70–85% of children with an ectopic kidney.[78,81] The adrenal gland is normally positioned in most cases of renal ectopy. Genital anomalies are common, with an incidence ranging from 10% in males to 75% in females.[32,76] In males, the most common abnormalities are hypospadias and undescended testes.[74,81] Anomalies of the reproductive organs in the female include duplication of the vagina, bicornuate uterus, and hypoplasia or agenesis of the uterus or vagina.[33] These may become clinically important during pregnancy, and may require cesarean section.[32]

Anomalies of other organ systems also occur with increased frequency. Skeletal anomalies are present in up to 50% of children. The most common include asymmetry of the skull, rib abnormalities, dysplastic

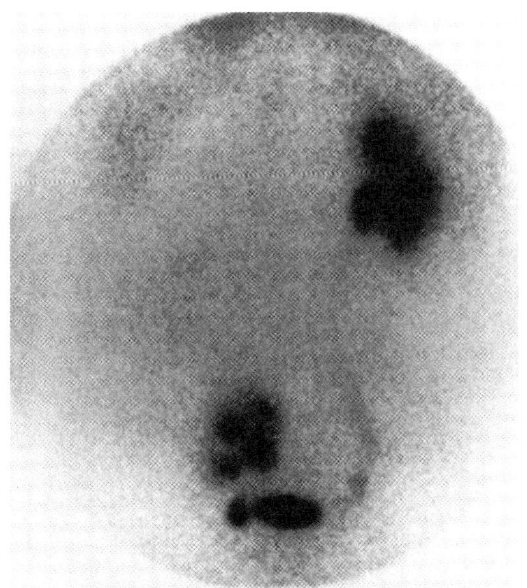

Figure 20.11 Renal scintigram of a right pelvic kidney. The camera was placed anteriorly in this patient with bilateral pyelocaliectasis.

vertebrae, and absent bones. Cardiovascular lesions were noted in 9 of the 21 children studied by Malek et al, and gastrointestinal abnormalities are found in one-third of patients.[74] Downs et al, however, reported a lower incidence of associated extragenitourinary anomalies.[32]

Management

Renal ectopy remains undiagnosed in many patients throughout life. Overall, renal disease will develop in 40% of patients with a solitary pelvic kidney.[32] The most common problem is UPJ obstruction.[79] This may be due to the malrotation and high ureteral insertion, or an anomalous vessel that partially obstructs the collecting system. Treatment should be individualized. Most cases have been managed via a transabdominal approach for pyeloplasty. The goal of surgery is to achieve dependent drainage, and in some cases ureterocalicostomy may be best. Endopyelotomy has been used in a small number of patients with some success.[82] Renal stones may develop in these kidneys (Figure 20.13). In the past, these were managed with open removal but now are amenable to extracorporeal shock wave lithotripsy (ESWL) or endourologic techniques, particularly if the ureter is dependent. An important consideration in management is that the contralateral kidney is frequently abnormal, so that every effort should be made to salvage renal tissue.

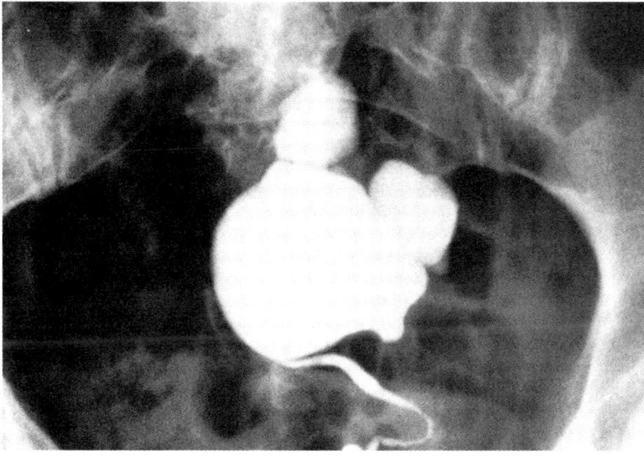

Figure 20.12 Retrograde pyelogram in a patient with a symptomatic ureteropelvic junction obstruction in a left pelvic kidney.

Thoracic kidney

Excessive cranial migration of the kidney results in a thoracic kidney. N'Guessan et al prefer to call this a 'superior ectopic kidney' because most high kidneys actually lie below the diaphragm.[83] A kidney is intrathoracic when either a portion or all extends

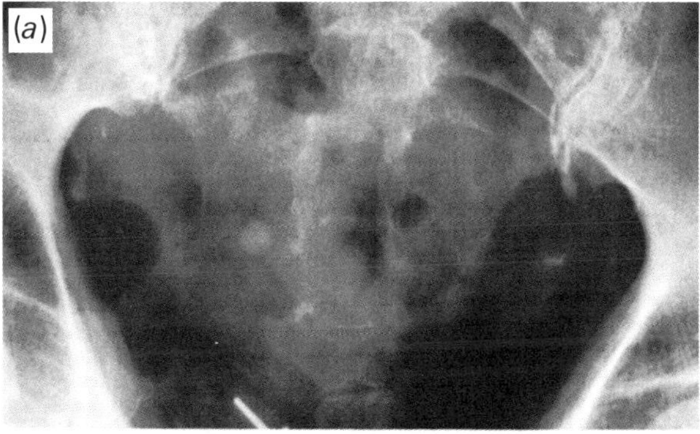

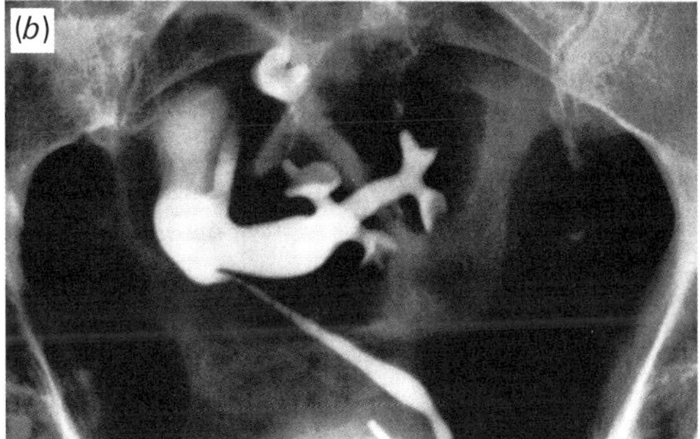

Figure 20.13 Left pelvic kidney. (*a*) Kidney–ureter–bladder (KUB) study revealed opaque calculus in the true pelvis. (*b*) Retrograde pyelogram confirmed the stone to be within the renal pelvis of the pelvic kidney.

above the diaphragm. This accounts for less than 5% of renal ectopy, with an incidence of 1 in 13 000 autopsies[75] with more than 140 cases reported.[84] The left side is more commonly involved and there is a male predominance. The condition is rarely bilateral.[83]

Renal ascent is normally complete by the 8th week of gestation. An intrathoracic kidney may be the result of accelerated ascent prior to diaphragmatic closure or delayed closure of the diaphragmatic anlage allowing continued ascent.[83,85] The renal vascular supply often arises from the normal site of origin on the aorta,[86] but may arise more superiorly. The kidney otherwise appears normal and has generally completed rotation.

In most cases, the kidney is actually subdiaphragmatic in location. A thin membranous portion of the diaphragm overlying the kidney has been described in patients examined at thoracotomy or necropsy. In the supradiaphragmatic kidney, the ureter and hilar vessels enter through the foramen of Bochdalek. The adrenal gland frequently remains caudal to the kidney in its normal location.[83] A superior ectopic kidney in association with a Bochdalek's hernia is uncommon. In this circumstance, there is herniation of other viscera through the diaphragm, and the kidney is mobile and can be easily withdrawn from the thorax.

In general, the thoracic kidneys function normally and most patients are asymptomatic. As with most renal anomalies, prenatal diagnosis is possible.[87] UPJ obstruction has been noted.[84] The condition is most often detected on routine chest radiographs as a suspected mediastinal mass. Excretory urography or CT scans confirm the diagnosis.

Anomalies of fusion

The congenital renal anomaly that produces some of the most bizarre-looking urograms is the result of fusion of two or more kidney masses. There are several proposed mechanisms. The kidneys cross the umbilical arteries as they ascend out of the pelvis. Malposition of the umbilical arteries may cause the developing nephrogenic blastemas to fuse in the midline, resulting in a horseshoe kidney. If during ascent, one kidney advances slightly ahead of the other, the inferior pole may come in contact with the superior pole of the trailing kidney. This would result in crossed ectopia with fusion. A single nephrogenic mass induced by ureteral buds from both sides could also produce crossed fused renal ectopia.[88] This latter theory, with the ureters crossing the midline, explains a solitary or bilaterally crossed ectopic kidney. Fusion of the two masses occurs early in embryogenesis, and malrotation is present in all cases.

Horseshoe kidney

The horseshoe kidney (HSK) is the most common renal fusion anomaly, with the two renal masses joined at the lower poles in more than 90% of cases (Figure 20.14). It is postulated that fusion of the lower poles occurs very early in gestation when they are in close proximity and is the result of abnormal migration of nephrogenic cells.[89] The isthmus crossing the midline joining the two kidneys consists of either renal parenchyma or fibrous tissue. The horseshoe kidney is usually positioned low in the abdomen, with the isthmus lying just below the junction of the inferior mesenteric artery and aorta. It is postulated

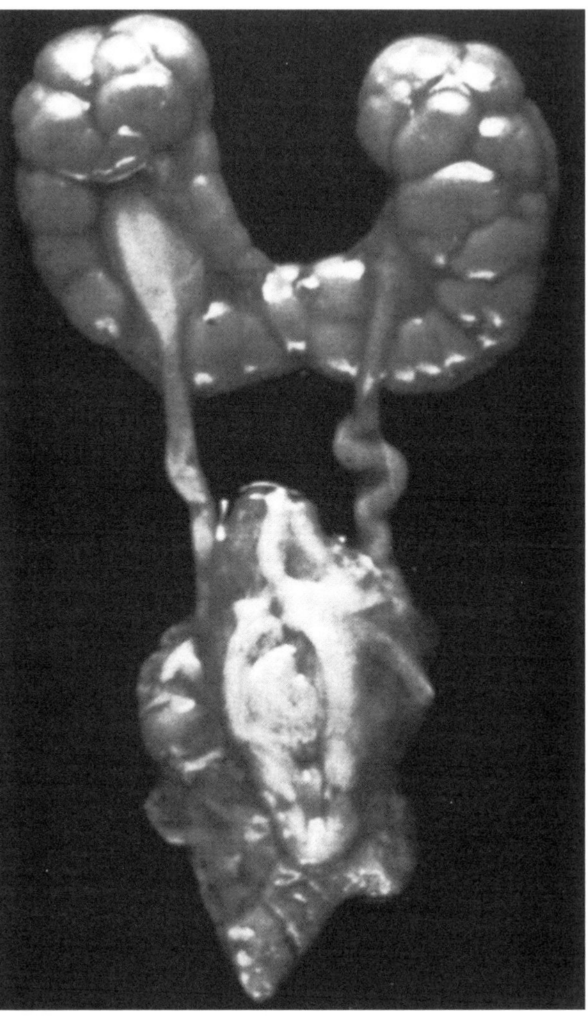

Figure 20.14 Horseshoe kidney, postmortem specimen.

that the inferior mesenteric artery obstructs the isthmus and prevents further ascent. Although usually situated anterior to the great vessels, the isthmus may cross posterior to the aorta and/or inferior vena cava.[90]

The reported incidence of horseshoe kidney varies from 1 in 400 to 1 in 1800.[70,91] The abnormality is more common in males. In autopsy series, this anomaly is found more commonly in children, which is attributed to the high incidence of associated congenital anomalies causing the demise of such children. This is in comparison to the 3.5% incidence of associated congenital malformation in adults discovered to have horseshoe kidneys. Horseshoe kidneys have been reported in identical twins and in several siblings within the same family.[92]

Diagnosis

Many horseshoe kidneys are now diagnosed on prenatal ultrasound.[77] Strauss et al reported that sonographic features are low-lying kidney, curved configuration of the kidney, tapering and elongation of the lower pole, and a poorly defined inferior border.[93] The diagnosis of the horseshoe kidney may be suspected from a plain radiograph of the abdomen if the renal outlines are visible. The classic features of HSK have been noted on excretory urography, but this is now seldom performed in children (Figure 20.15). Malrotation of the kidney is always present and is attributed to very early fusion of the kidneys before rotation is complete. The renal pelves remain anterior, with the ureters crossing the isthmus. The orientation of the calices is generally anteroposterior, but the lowermost calices invariably point towards the midline, medial to the ureter. These lower calices often overlie the vertebral column. The renal axis appears to be vertical or shifted outward, with the lower poles lying closer together than the upper poles. The course of the ureters is variable, but they often lie anterior to the pelvis. The upper ureter appears to be laterally displaced by a midline mass. Other pertinent urographic findings are low-lying kidneys, and the lower outer border of the kidney appears to continue across the midline. The radiographic appearance of a horseshoe kidney is frequently altered by associated abnormalities such as hydronephrosis and/or diminished renal function.

The diagnosis of a horseshoe kidney can be confirmed by a variety of imaging techniques, including ultrasound, CT, or MRI (Figure 20.16). In general, the fusion of the kidneys can be clearly visualized with either of these studies (Figure 20.17). Radionuclide imaging (Figure 20.18) can also be helpful in making the diagnosis when other imaging modalities are

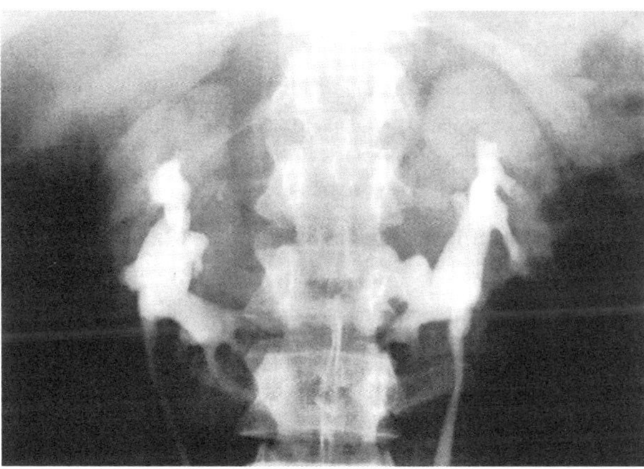

Figure 20.15 Typical appearance of horseshoe kidney on an excretory urogram.

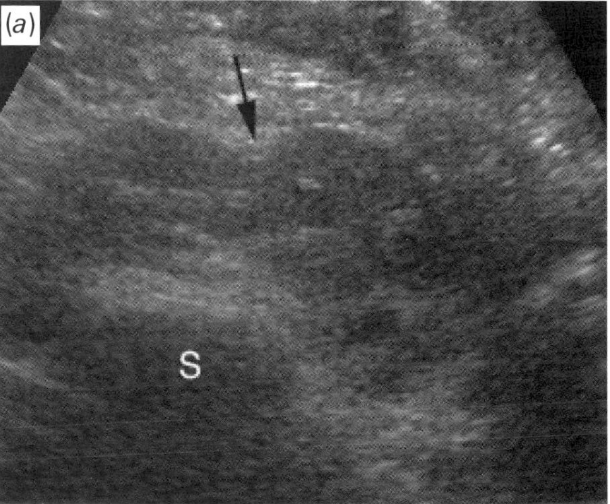

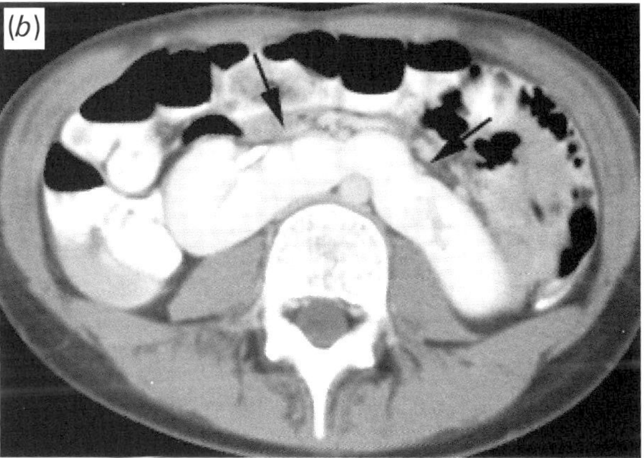

Figure 20.16 Horseshoe kidney. (*a*) Ultrasound demonstrates the isthmus (arrow), which is only partially visible anterior to the spine (S). (*b*) CT of the same patient better demonstrates the fused lower poles (arrows).

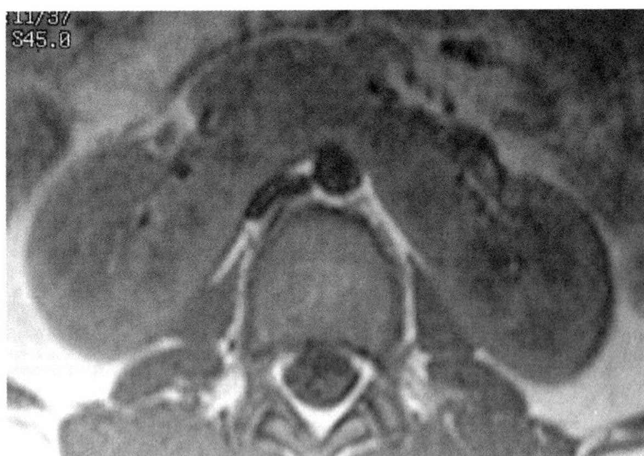

Figure 20.17 MRI of a patient with horseshoe kidney.

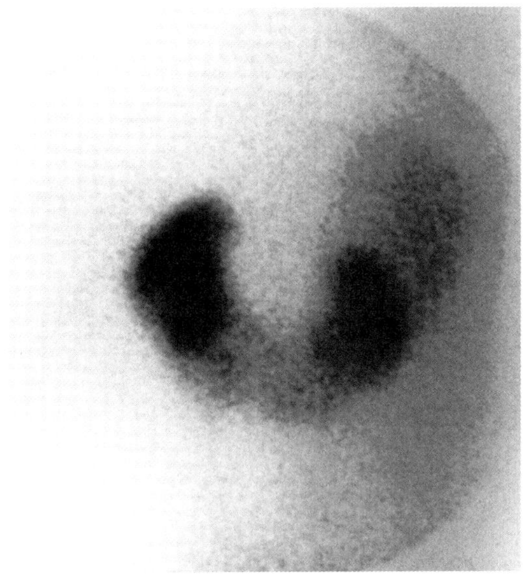

Figure 20.18 Renal scan in a patient with horseshoe kidney showing minimal function of the isthmus.

inconclusive.[94] Kao et al found that a DMSA (dimercaptosuccinic acid) renal scan identified the isthmus in 100% of children with HSK. In the past, renal arteriography was often performed before surgery to delineate the vascular blood supply. In the majority of cases, there are multiple renal vessels. The blood supply to the isthmus is particularly variable, often supplied by a separate vessel. This may arise from the aorta, common iliac, or inferior mesenteric arteries.

Associated anomalies

There is a frequent association of other anomalies in children with horseshoe kidney, especially when the horseshoe kidney is discovered in the newborn period. Zondek and Zondek examined the postmortem records of 99 individuals with horseshoe kidneys.[95] Infants who were stillborn or who died within the first year of life had a 78% incidence of other malformations. The most commonly affected organ systems were the gastrointestinal, skeletal, cardiovascular, and central nervous systems. Boatman et al reported that one-third of patients with horseshoe kidney had at least one other abnormality.[96]

Several well-known syndromes have a predisposition for HSK. Trisomy 18 is associated with a 21% incidence of renal fusion.[96,97] More than 60% of patients with Turner's syndrome have renal abnormalities, including HSK, ureteral duplication, or other minor abnormalities.[98] One study noted a 7% incidence of HSK in patients with Turner's syndrome who were evaluated with renal ultrasound scanning.[99] There is also an increased incidence of HSK in patients with neural tube defects.[100]

Other genitourinary abnormalities are also encountered with increased frequency in patients with HSK. Ten percent of patients have ureteral duplication, and VUR has been found in 10%[101] to 80% of children who undergo evaluation.[102] A more recent report by Cascio et al found VUR in 13/40 patients with HSK undergoing cystography.[103] Multicystic dysplasia[104] and autosomal dominant polycystic kidney disease have also been reported.[101] Hypospadias and undescended testes occur in 4% of the males, bicornuate uterus or septate vagina in 7% of females.[96] Retrocaval ureter has been found in association with a horseshoe kidney in six patients.[105]

Prognosis

A horseshoe kidney does not usually affect life expectancy. Nearly one-third of patients with a horseshoe kidney remain undiagnosed throughout life.[101] Most women are able to go through pregnancy and delivery without adverse effects.[106] In those patients with problems, symptoms are most often secondary to hydronephrosis, UTI, or urolithiasis. These patients generally present with vague abdominal pain. Patients can develop abdominal pain and nausea with hyperextension of the spine (Rovsing syndrome), presumably resulting from stretching of the isthmus. Operations to divide the isthmus were once performed to relieve pain, but this procedure has little merit.[101]

UPJ obstruction is the most common cause of hydronephrosis, occurring in 30% of patients diagnosed during life. Kao et al performed diuretic renography in 22 children with HSK detected on routine screening.[94] Only 1/44 renal units, 2.3%, was found to have obstructive hydronephrosis. This suggests that most cases of obstruction are acquired over time. The obstruction may be caused by a high ureteral insertion or an anomalous renal vessel. It must be recognized that the calices may have an abnormal appearance as a result of the malrotation alone and that not all of these kidneys are obstructed. Kao et al[94] showed that 25% of renal units had some stasis prior to administration of diuretic. In some children, the upper urinary tract dilatation may be secondary to VUR (Figure 20.19).

Urolithiasis develops in 20% of patients with a horseshoe kidney. The increased risk of stones is attributed to stasis secondary to hydronephrosis, but metabolic factors should not be overlooked.[107] A recent multicenter study showed that all patients with HSK and calculi had some metabolic abnormality.[108] Hypercalcuria, hypocitraturia, and low urine volumes were the most common defects.

Over 100 cases of renal malignancy have been reported in patients with horseshoe kidney,[109] with a number of tumors arising from the isthmus.[110] There appears to be an increased incidence of renal pelvic tumors and nephroblastoma in patients with HSK compared with the general population.[110,111] Wilms' tumor is the second most common tumor found in horseshoe kidneys. In a review of National Wilms' Tumor Study Group (NWTSG) patients, Mesrobian et al found that there was a sevenfold increased risk of a Wilms' tumor developing in patients with a horseshoe kidney.[112] Neville et al updated the NWTSG experience and identified 41 children with Wilms' tumor arising in a HSK.[113] The diagnosis of horseshoe kidney was missed preoperatively in 13 patients, even though CT was performed in the majority.

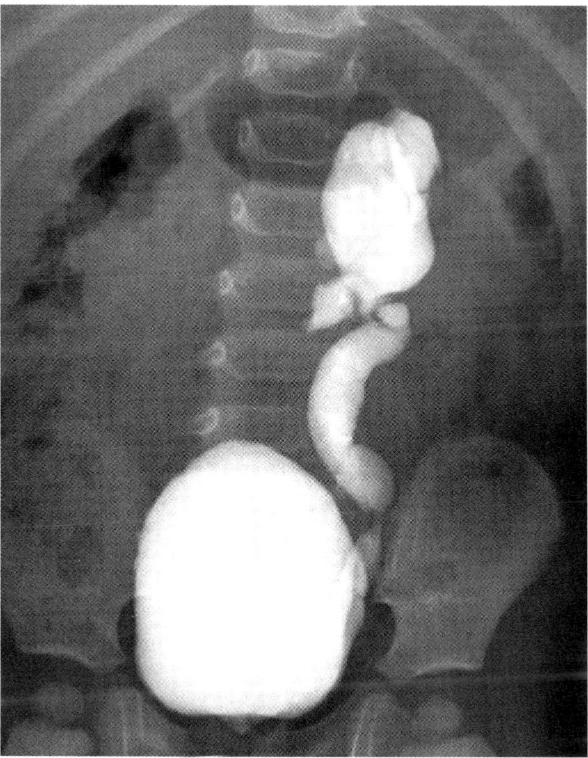

Figure 20.19 Horseshoe kidney. Voiding cystourethrogram demonstrating high-grade vesicoureteral reflux into the left renal moiety. Note the medial pointing calyx in the lower pole extending into the isthmus.

Management

Correction of UPJ obstruction is the most frequent indication for surgical intervention in a patient with a horseshoe kidney. The goal of dependent drainage following pyeloplasty may be difficult to achieve in these patients. Routine division of the isthmus was once recommended to avoid having the ureter cross the isthmus. However, it has become clear that the isthmus does not contribute to the obstruction and should not be routinely divided.[114] Donahoe and Hendren report that the kidneys remain in their original position following symphysiotomy because of fixation by the abnormal vasculature.[115] An extraperitoneal flank approach is utilized for unilateral operations. In those patients requiring bilateral procedures, a transperitoneal approach may be preferable in order to allow operation on both sides at once. Endourologic management, percutaneous endopyelotomy, or laparoscopic pyeloplasty are other options for these patients, but experience is limited.[82,116]

Treatment of renal calculi will be dependent on stone burden. Most patients with small renal stones can be managed with ESWL.[117] Calculi >2 cm are best managed percutaneously. Upper pole access and flexible nephroscopy are frequently required.[118]

Crossed renal ectopia

Crossed renal ectopia is the second most common fusion anomaly. The etiology of crossed ectopia is uncertain, although several theories have been expressed.[24] The ectopic kidney crosses the midline to lie on the opposite side from its ureteral insertion into the bladder (Figure 20.20). The four varieties of crossed renal ectopia are illustrated in Figure 20.21. The incidence of crossed ectopia has been placed at 1 in 7000 autopsies.[120] Crossed renal ectopia with fusion is the most common type and accounts for

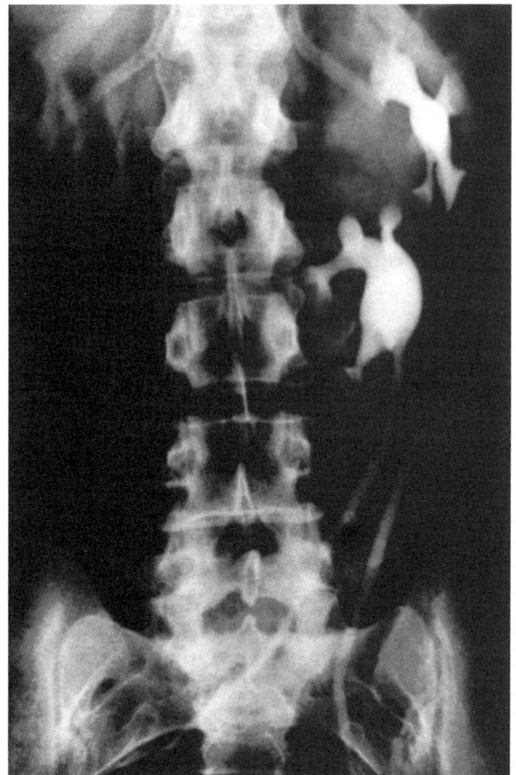

Figure 20.20 Crossed ectopia, with the right kidney crossing midline and fused to the lower pole of the left kidney.

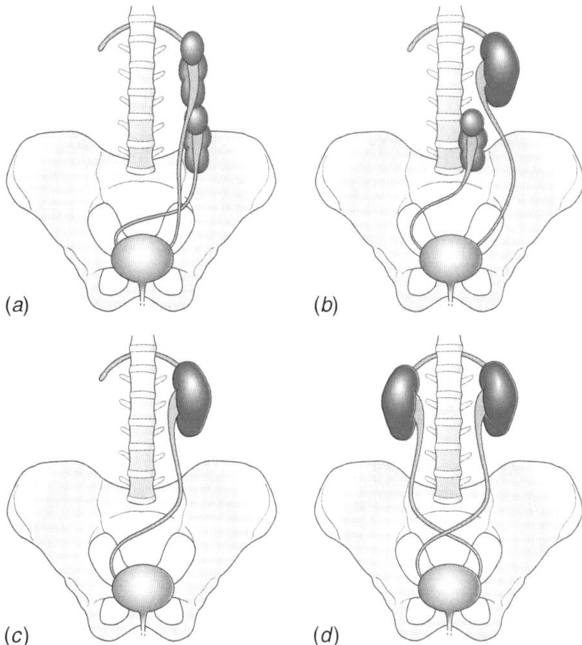

Figure 20.21 Four varieties of crossed renal ectopia: (*a*) with fusion; (*b*) without fusion; (*c*) solitary; and (*d*) bilateral. (Redrawn from McDonald and McClellan,[119] as reproduced by Abeshouse and Bhisitkul.[120])

85% of the cases. Crossed ectopia without fusion represents fewer than 10% of all cases, and solitary crossed ectopia and bilateral crossed ectopia are exceedingly rare.[119,121] With all of these abnormalities, there is a slight male predominance and crossing from left to right occurs more frequently than right to left.

The many variations of fusion can produce bizarre radiographic pictures, and determination of the exact type of crossed ectopia can be difficult. McDonald and McClellan described six different varieties of crossed ectopia with fusion (Figure 20.22).[119] The most common form is unilateral fused type with inferior ectopia, in which the upper pole of the crossed kidney is fused to the lower pole of the normally positioned kidney. The renal pelves remain in their anterior position, representing failure to complete rotation. The second most common type is the sigmoid, or S-shaped, kidney. The crossed kidney is inferior, but both kidneys have completed their rotation so that the two renal pelves face in opposite directions. The fusion of the two kidneys probably occurs later, after axial rotation is completed.

The other four types of fusion are much less common. The lump, or 'cake', kidney and the 'disk' kidney both involve extensive fusion of the two renal masses. In an L-shaped kidney, the crossed kidney assumes a transverse position. The least common type is the superior ectopic kidney, in which the crossed ectopic kidney lies superior to the normal kidney. The two kidneys may also fuse side to side and ascend together to the renal fossa (Figure 20.23).

Diagnosis

The classification described above was devised to stratify the patients in some logical fashion. There is a spectrum of abnormalities, and it is often difficult to categorize patients based on urographic findings. It also can be difficult to distinguish between crossed ectopia with fusion from crossed renal ectopy without fusion. This distinction may be possible on ultrasound or excretory urography if the two renal masses are widely separated. CT and MRI are more likely to establish the correct diagnosis. Radionuclide imaging is also useful.

The vascular supply to these kidneys is quite variable. Renal arteriography often demonstrates multiple anomalous branches to both kidneys arising from the aorta, or common iliac artery. Rarely will the renal artery cross the midline to supply the crossed kidney.[122]

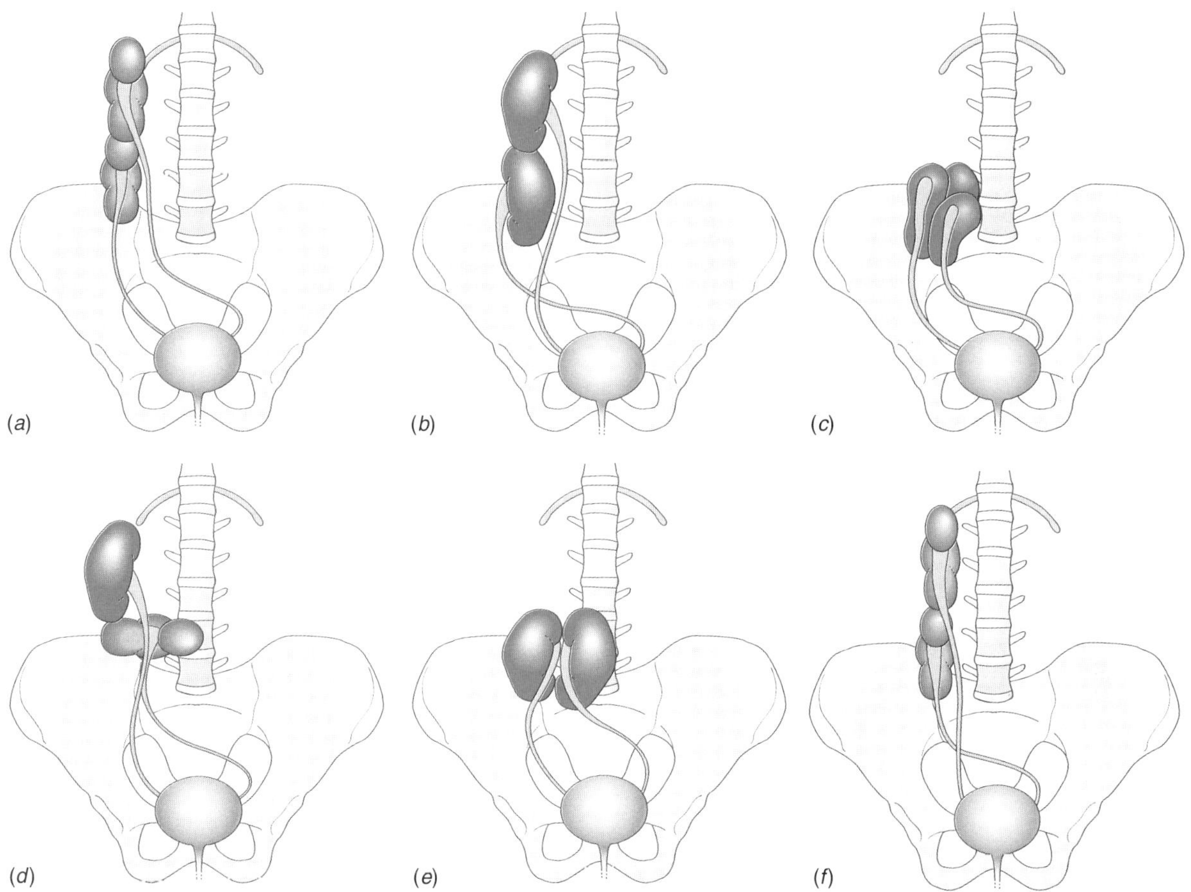

Figure 20.22 Six varieties of crossed renal ectopia with fusion: (*a*) unilateral fused kidney, superior ectopia; (*b*) sigmoid or S-shaped kidney; (*c*) 'lump' kidney; (*d*) L-shaped kidney; (*e*) 'disk' kidney; and (*f*) unilateral fused kidney, inferior ectopia. (Redrawn from McDonald and McClellan,[119] as reproduced by Abeshouse and Bhisitkul.[120])

Associated anomalies

There is an increased incidence of other malformations, including orthopedic or skeletal anomalies, imperforate anus, and cardiovascular anomalies.[120] A higher incidence of genital abnormalities is found in patients with solitary crossed ectopia similar to that found in unilateral renal agenesis.[78]

The ureter in the crossed ectopic kidney usually enters the bladder and its orifice is only rarely ectopic.[120] The most commonly associated abnormality is VUR, which is frequently noted in the ectopic kidney.[78,81] VCUG should be performed in all of these patients. Less common problems include UPJ obstruction, renal dysplasia,[123] and renal tumors.[124]

Prognosis

Most patients with crossed renal ectopia are discovered incidentally, often by antenatal sonography when two kidneys are not identified.[77] When symptoms do occur, they are often related to infection and obstruction. Abeshouse and Bhisitkul reported that one-third of patients had pyelonephritis and one-quarter had hydronephrosis (Figure 20.24).[120] The caliceal dilatation and distortion may be secondary to the malrotation or the presence of VUR. Urolithiasis has been found in up to one-third of patients.[97] Mininberg et al reported one infant who presented with hypertension secondary to a vascular lesion.[125] Other patients may be found to have an abdominal mass on physical examination or during surgical exploration. It is particularly pertinent in the patient with a fused pelvic kidney to recognize that this is the total functioning renal parenchyma.

Fetal lobulation

Fetal lobulation is commonly found in children and represents a persistence of normal fetal development (Figure 20.25). Another term used to describe this is

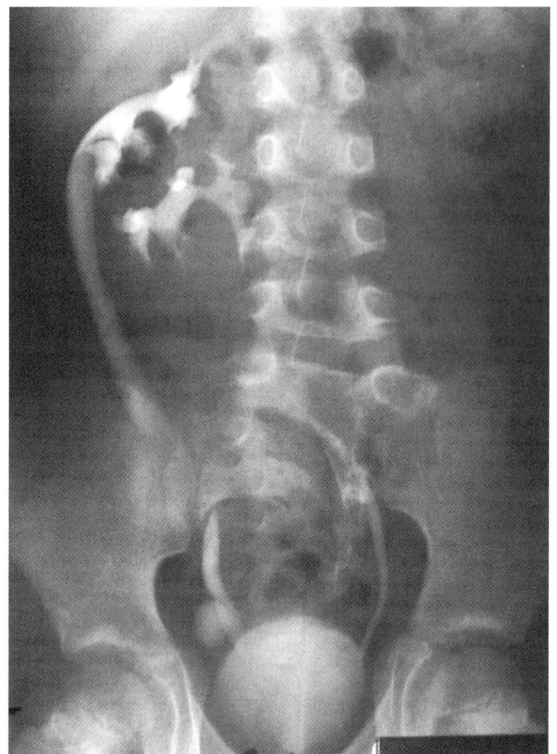

Figure 20.23 Crossed fused ectopia. Intravenous pyelogram of a child with crossed ectopia, without obstruction.

'renal' lobation, because it designates the larger renal lobe (pyramid plus surrounding cortex) rather than the lobule (medullary ray and surrounding glomeruli).[70] Fetal lobulation is found at autopsy in 17.6% of children and in 3.9% of adults. This condition is of no clinical importance, and should be recognized as a normal variant. Radiographically, it may appear as small notches in the renal margin that are placed midway between the calices.

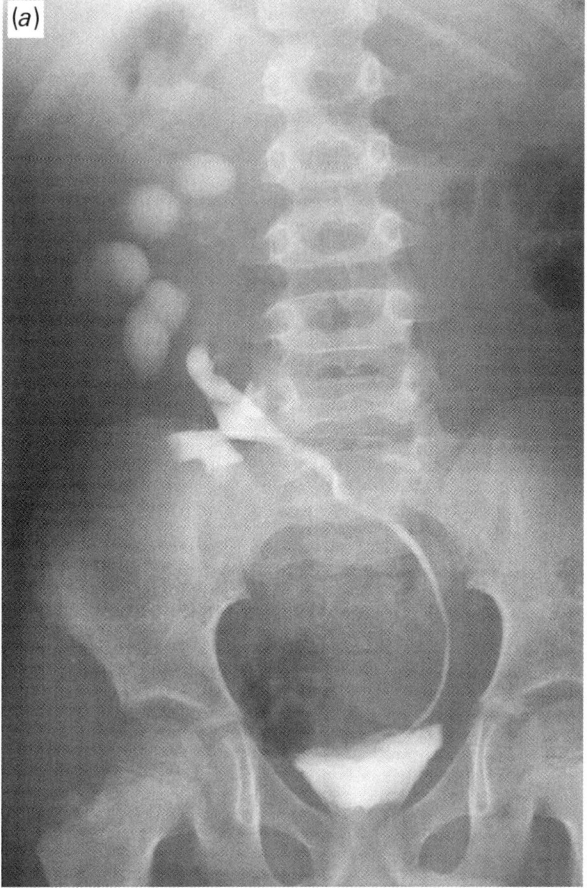

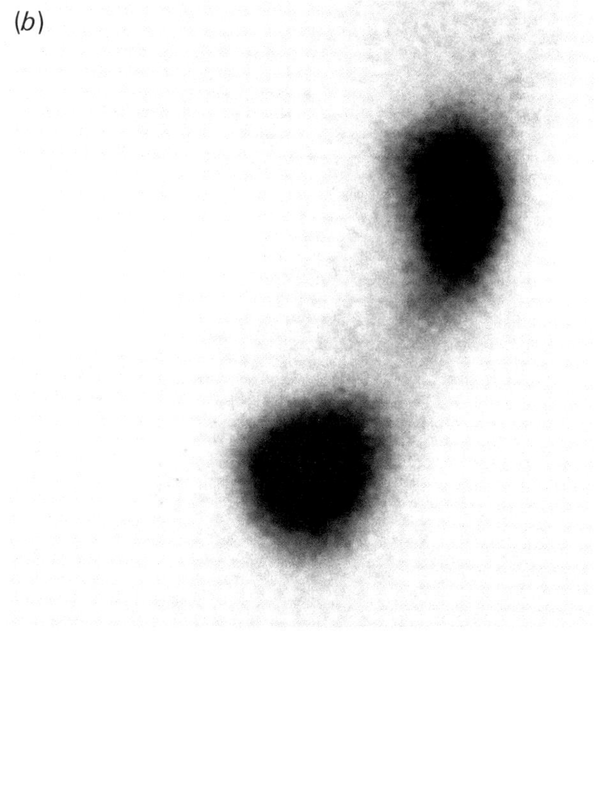

Figure 20.24 Crossed fused ectopia. (*a*) The left kidney crosses the midline. The presence of fusion is difficult to ascertain with confidence on this intravenous pyelogram. Obstruction is noted in the normally positioned right kidney. (*b*) ^{99m}Tc MAG3 radioisotope scan shows increased tracer activity in the right abdomen only.

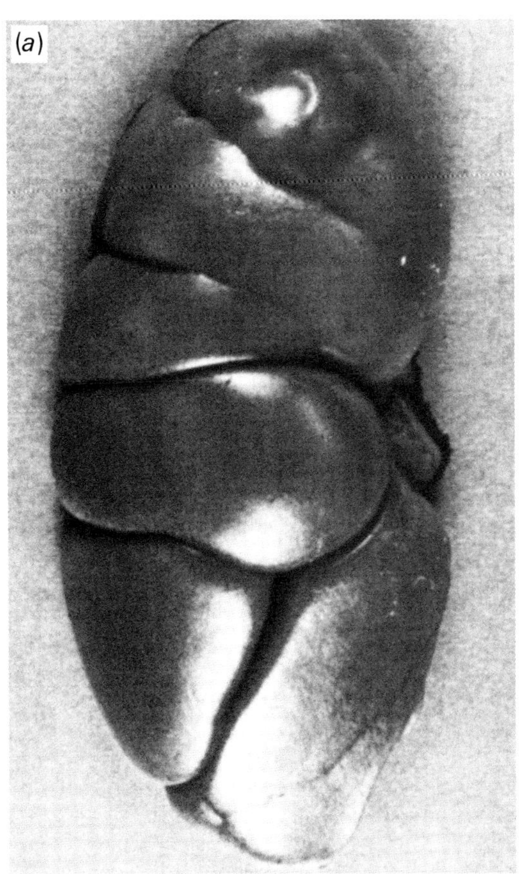

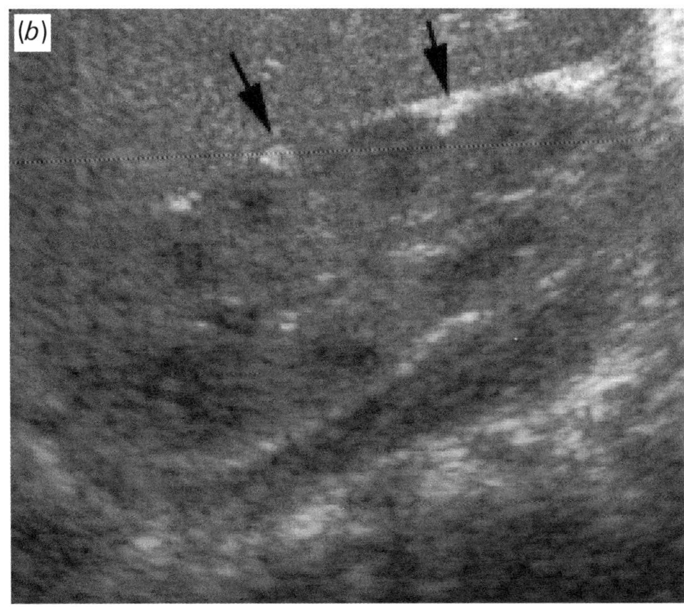

Figure 20.25 Fetal lobulation of the kidney. (*a*) Gross image. (*b*) Ultrasound: note the regularly spaced indentations along the margin of the kidney (arrows) in this normal child.

References

1. Steinhart JM, Kuhn JP, Eisenberg B et al. Ultrasound screening of healthy infants for urinary tract abnormalities. Pediatrics 1988; 82:609–14.
2. Shieh CP, Liu MB, Hung CS et al. Renal abnormalities in school children. Pediatrics 1989; 86:323.
3. Parrott TS, Shandalakis JE, Gray SW. The kidney and ureter. In: Shandalakis JE, Gray SW, eds. Embryology for Surgeons. The Embryological Basis for the Treatment of Congenital Anomalies, 2nd edn. Baltimore: Williams and Wilkins, 1994: 594–670.
4. Osathanondh V, Potter EL. Development of human kidney as shown in microdissection – 3 parts. Arch Pathol 1963; 76:271–302.
5. Campbell MF. Clinical Pediatric Urology. Philadelphia: WB Saunders, 1951.
6. Oto A, Kerimoglu U, Eskicorapci S, Hazirolan T, Tekgul S. Bilateral supernumerary kidney: imaging findings. JBR-BTR 2002; 85:300–3.
7. Wulfekuhler WV, Dube VE. Free supernumerary kidney: report of a case. J Urol 1971; 106:802–4.
8. Antony J. Complete duplication of female urethra with vaginal atresia and supernumerary kidney. J Urol 1977; 118:877–8.
9. N'Guessan G, Stephens FD. Supernumerary kidney. J Urol 1983; 130:649–53.
10. Bernik TR, Ravnic DJ, Bernik SF, Wallack MK. Ectopic supernumerary kidney, a cause of para-aortic mass: case report and review. Am Surg 2001; 67:657–9.
11. Carlson HE. Supernumerary kidney: a summary of 51 reported cases. J Urol 1950; 64:224–9.
12. Sy WM, Seo IS, Sze PC et al. A patient with three kidneys: a correlative imaging case report. Clin Nucl Med 1999 24:264–6.
13. Kamba T, Higashi S, Kamoto T et al. Failure of ureteric bud invasion: a new model of renal agenesis in mice. Am J Pathol 2001; 159:2347–53.
14. Parikh CR, McCall D, Engelman C, Schrier RW. Congenital renal agenesis: case-control analysis of birth characteristics. Am J Kidney Dis 2002; 39:689–94.
15. Arfeen S, Rosborough D, Luger AM, Nolph KD. Familial unilateral renal agenesis and focal and segmental glomerulosclerosis. Am J Kidney Dis 1993; 21:663–8.
16. Doroshow LW, Abeshouse BS. Congenital unilateral solitary kidney: report of 37 cases and a review of the literature. Urol Surv 1961; 11:219–29.
17. Longo VJ, Thompson GJ. Congenital solitary kidney. J Urol 1952; 68:63–8.
18. Helin I, Persson PH. Prenatal diagnosis of urinary tract abnormalities by ultrasound. Pediatrics 1986; 78:879–83.
19. Rosendahl H. Ultrasound screening for fetal urinary tract malformations: a prospective study in general population. Eur J Obstet Gynecol Reprod Biol 1990; 36:27–33.

20. Mesrobian HG, Rushton HG, Bulas D. Unilateral renal agenesis may result from in utero regression of multicystic renal dysplasia. J Urol 1993; 150:793–4.
21. Pedicelli G, Jequier S, Bowen A, Boisvert J. Multicystic dysplastic kidneys: spontaneous regression demonstrated with ultrasound. Radiology 1986; 161:23–6.
22. Avni EF, Thoua Y, Lalmand B et al. Multicystic dysplastic kidney: natural history from in utero diagnosis and postnatal follow-up. J Urol 1987; 138:1420–4.
23. Hiraoka M, Tsukahara J, Ohshima Y et al. Renal aplasia is the predominant cause of congenital solitary kidneys. Kidney Int 2002; 61:1840–4.
24. Ashley DJB, Mostofi FK. Renal agenesis and dysgenesis. J Urol 1960; 83:211–30.
25. Song JT, Ritchey ML, Zerin JM, Bloom DA. Incidence of vesicoureteral reflux in children with unilateral renal agenesis. J Urol 1995; 153:1249–51.
26. Cascio S, Paran S, Puri P. Associated urological anomalies in children with unilateral renal agenesis. J Urol 1999; 162:1081–3.
27. Kaneyama K, Yamataka A, Satake S et al. Associated urologic anomalies in children with solitary kidney. J Pediatr Surg 2004; 39:85–7.
28. Limakeng ND, Retik AB. Unilateral renal agenesis with hypoplastic ureter: observations on the contralateral urinary tract and report of 4 cases. J Urol 1972; 108:149–52.
29. Nakada T, Furuta H, Kazama T, Katayama T. Unilateral renal agenesis with or without ipsilateral adrenal agenesis. J Urol 1988; 140:933–7.
30. Thompson DP, Lynn HB. Genital anomalies associated with solitary kidney. Mayo Clin Proc 1966; 41:538–48.
31. Li S, Qayyum A, Coakley FV, Hricak H. Association of renal agenesis and Müllerian duct anomalies. J Comput Assist Tomogr 2000; 24:829–34.
32. Downs RA, Lane JW, Burns E. Solitary pelvic kidney: its clinical implications. Urology 1973; 1:51–6.
33. Griffin JE, Edwards C, Madden JD, Harrod MJ, Wilson JD. Congenital absence of the vagina: the Mayer–Rokitansky–Küster–Hauser syndrome. Ann Intern Med 1976; 85:224–36.
34. Basile C, De Michele V. Renal abnormalities in Mayer–Rokitansky–Küster–Hauser syndrome. J Nephrol 2001; 14:316–18.
35. Candiani GB, Fedele L, Candiani M. Double uterus, blind hemivagina, and ipsilateral renal agenesis: 36 cases and long-term follow-up. Obstet Gynecol 1997; 90:26–32.
36. Acien P, Acien M, Sanchez-Ferrer. Complex malformations of the female genital tract. New types and revision of classification. Hum Reprod 2004; 19:2377–84.
37. Magee MC, Lucey DT, Fried FA. A new embryologic classification for uro-gynecologic malformations: the syndromes of mesonephric duct induced müllerian deformities. J Urol 1979; 121:265–7.
38. Yoder IC, Pfister RC. Unilateral hematocolpos and ipsilateral renal agenesis: report of two cases and review of the literature. AJR Am J Roentgenol 1976; 127:303–8.
39. Charney CW, Gillenwater JY. Congenital absence of the vas deferens. J Urol 1965; 93:399–401.
40. Donahue RE, Fauver HE. Unilateral absence of the vas deferens. A useful clinical sign. JAMA 1989; 261:1180–2.
41. Goldstein M, Schlossberg S. Men with congenital absence of the vas deferens often have seminal vesicles. J Urol 1988; 140:85–6.
42. Schlegel PN, Shin D, Goldstein M. Urogenital anomalies in men with congenital absence of the vas deferens. J Urol 1996; 155:1644–8.
43. Shieh CP, Hung CS, Wei CF, Lin CY. Cystic dilatations within the pelvis in patients with ipsilateral renal agenesis or dysplasia. J Urol 1990; 144:324–7.
44. Burns JA, Cooper CS, Austin JC. Cystic dysplasia of the testis associated with ipsilateral renal agenesis and contralateral crossed ectopia. Urology 2002; 60:344.
45. Emanuel B, Nachman R, Aronson N, Weiss H. Congenital solitary kidney: a review of 74 cases. Am J Dis Child 1974; 127:17–19.
46. Mace JM, Kaplan JM, Schanberger JE et al. Poland's syndrome: report of seven cases and review of the literature. Clin Pediatr 1972; 11:98–102.
47. Ritchey ML, Norbeck J, Huang C, Keating MA, Bloom DA. Urologic manifestations of Goldenhar syndrome. Urology 1994; 43:88–91.
48. Kolon TF, Gray CL, Sutherland RW, Roth DR, Gonzales ET. Upper urinary tract manifestations of the VACTERL association. J Urol 2000; 163:1949–51.
49. Moore WB, Matthews TJ, Rabinowitz R. Genitourinary anomalies associated with Klippel–Feil syndrome. J Bone Joint Surg (Am) 1975; 57:355–7.
50. Mascatello V, Lebowitz RL. Malposition of the colon in left renal agenesis and ectopia. Radiology 1976; 120:371–6.
51. McGahan JP, Myracle MR. Adrenal hypertrophy: possible pitfall in the sonographic diagnosis of renal agenesis. J Ultrasound Med 1986; 5:265–8.
52. Hoffman CK, Filly RA, Cullen PW. The 'lying down' adrenal sign: a sonographic indicator of renal agenesis or ectopia in fetuses and neonates. J Ultrasound Med 1992; 11:533–6.
53. Pattaras JG, Rushton HG, Majd M. The role of ^{99m}technetium dimercapto-succinic acid renal scan in the evaluation of occult ectopic ureters in girls with paradoxical incontinence. J Urol 1999; 162:821–5.
54. Roodhooft AM, Birnhalz JC, Holmes LB. Familial nature of congenital absence and severe dysgenesis of both kidneys. N Engl J Med 1984; 310:1341–5.
55. Hill LM, Nowak A, Hartle R, Tush B. Fetal compensatory renal hypertrophy with a unilateral functioning kidney. Ultrasound Obstet Gynecol 2000; 15:191–3.
56. Hostetter TH, Olson JL, Rennke HG. Hyperfiltration in remnant nephrons: a potentially adverse response to renal ablation. Am J Physiol 1981; 241:F85–93.
57. Kiprov DD, Colvin RB, McClusky RT. Focal and segmental glomerulosclerosis and proteinuria associated with unilateral renal agenesis. Lab Invest 1981; 46:275–81.
58. Gutierrez-Millet R, Nieto J, Praga M et al. Focal glomerulosclerosis and proteinuria in patients with solitary kidneys. Arch Intern Med 1986; 146:705–9.
59. Nomura S, Osawa G. Focal glomerular sclerotic lesions in a patient with urinary oligomeganephronia and agenesis

of the contralateral kidney: a case report. Clin Nephrol 1990; 33:7–11.

60. Argueso L, Ritchey ML, Boyle ET Jr et al. Prognosis of patients with unilateral renal agenesis. Pediatr Nephrol 1992; 6:412–16.
61. Mei-Zahav M, Korzets Z, Cohen I et al. Ambulatory blood pressure monitoring in children with a solitary kidney – a comparison between unilateral renal agenesis and uninephrectomy. Blood Press Monit 2001; 6:263–7.
62. DeSanto NG, Anastasio P, Spitali P et al. Renal reserve is normal in adults born with unilateral renal agenesis and is not related to hyperfiltration or renal failure. Miner Electrolyte Metab 1997; 23:283–6.
63. Potter EL. Bilateral absence of ureters and kidneys: a report of 50 cases. Obstet Gynecol 1965; 25:3–12.
64. Rizza JM, Downing SE. Bilateral renal agenesis in two female siblings. Am J Dis Child 1971; 121:60–3.
65. Adzick N, Harrison MR, Glick PL, Villa RL. Finkbeiner W. Experimental pulmonary hypoplasia and oligohydramnios: relative contributions of lung fluid and fetal breathing movements. J Pediatr Surg 1984; 19:658–65.
66. Romero R, Cullen M, Grannum P et al. Antenatal diagnosis of renal anomalies with ultrasound. III. Bilateral renal agenesis. Am J Obstet Gynecol 1985; 151:38–43.
67. Sepulveda W, Stagiannis KD, Flack NJ, Fisk NM. Accuracy of prenatal diagnosis of renal agenesis with color flow imaging in severe second-trimester oligohydramnios. Am J Obstet Gynecol 1995; 173:1788–92.
68. Cassart M, Massez A, Metens T et al. Complementary role of MRI after sonography in assessing bilateral urinary tract anomalies in the fetus. AJR Am J Roentgenol 2004; 182:689–95.
69. Priman J. A consideration of normal and abnormal positions of the hilum of the kidney. Anat Rec 1929; 42:355–63.
70. Campbell MF. Anomalies of the kidney. In: Campbell MF, Harrison JH, eds. Urology, Vol 2, 3rd edn. Philadelphia: WB Saunders, 1970: 1416–86.
71. Smith EC, Orkin LA. A clinical and statistical study of 471 congenital anomalies of the kidney and ureter. J Urol 1945; 53:11.
72. Weyrauch HM Jr. Anomalies of renal rotation. Surg Gynecol Obstet 1939; 69:183–99.
73. Cocheteux B, Mounier-Vehier C, Gaxotte V et al. Rare variations in renal anatomy and blood supply: CT appearances and embryological background. Eur Radiol 2001; 11:779–86.
74. Malek RS, Kelalis PP, Burke EC. Ectopic kidney in children and frequency of association with other malformations. Mayo Clin Proc 1971; 46:461–7.
75. Campbell MF. Renal ectopy. J Urol 1930; 24:187–98.
76. Thompson GJ, Pace JM. Ectopic kidney: a review of 97 cases. Surg Gynecol Obstet 1937; 64:935–43.
77. Yuksel A, Batukan C. Sonographic findings of fetuses with an empty renal fossa and normal amniotic fluid volume. Fetal Diagn Ther 2004; 19:525-32.
78. Kramer SA, Kelalis PP. Ureteropelvic junction obstruction in children with renal ectopy. J Urol (Paris) 1984; 5:331–6.
79. Gleason PE, Kelalis PP, Husmann DA, Kramer SA. Hydronephrosis in renal ectopia: incidence, etiology and significance. J Urol 1994; 151:1660–1.
80. Perez-Brayfield MR, Kirsch AJ, Jones RA, Grattan-Smith JD. A prospective study comparing ultrasound, nuclear scintigraphy and dynamic contrast enhanced magnetic resonance imaging in the evaluation of hydronephrosis. J Urol 2003; 170:1330–4.
81. Guarino N, Tadini B, Camardi P et al. The incidence of associated urological abnormalities in 57 children with renal ectopia. J Urol 2004; 172:1757–9.
82. Jabbour ME, Goldfischer ER, Stravodimos KG, Klima WJ, Smith AD. Endopyelotomy for horseshoe and ectopic kidneys. J Urol 1998; 160:694–7.
83. N'Guessan G, Stephens FD, Pick J. Congenital superior ectopic (thoracic) kidney. Urology 1984; 24:219–28.
84. Hampton LJ, Borden TA. Ureteropelvic junction in a thoracic kidney treated by dismembered pyeloplasty. Urology 2002; 60:164.
85. Burke EC, Wenzl JE, Utz DC. The intrathoracic kidney: report of a case. Am J Dis Child 1967; 113:487–90.
86. Lundius B. Intrathoracic kidney. AJR Am J Roentgenol 1975; 125:678–81.
87. Masturzo B, Kalache KD, Cockell A, Pierro A, Rodeck CH. Prenatal diagnosis of an ectopic intrathoracic kidney in right-sided congenital diaphragmatic hernia using color Doppler ultrasonography. Ultrasound Obstet Gynecol 2001; 18:173–4.
88. Cook WA, Stephens FD. Fused kidneys: morphologic study and theory of embryogenesis. Birth Defects 1977; 13:327–40.
89. Domenech-Mateu JM, Gonzalez-Compta X. Horseshoe kidney: a new theory on its embryogenesis based on the study of a 16-mm human embryo. Anat Rec 1988; 222:408–17.
90. Dajani AM. Horseshoe kidney: a review of twenty-nine cases. Br J Urol 1966; 38:388–402.
91. Weizer AZ, Silverstein AD, Auge BK et al. Determining the incidence of horseshoe kidney from radiograph data at a single institution. J Urol 2003; 170:1722–6.
92. David RA. Horseshoe kidney: a report of one family. BMJ 1974; 4:571–2.
93. Strauss S, Dushnitsky T, Peer A et al. Sonographic features of horseshoe kidney: review of 34 patients. J Ultrasound Med 2000; 19:27–31.
94. Kao PF, Sheih CP, Tsui KH, Tsai MF, Tzen KY. The 99mTc-DMSA renal scan and 99mTc-DTPA diuretic renogram in children and adolescents with incidental diagnosis of horseshoe kidney. Nucl Med Commun 2003; 24:525–30.
95. Zondek LH, Zondek T. Horseshoe kidney in associated congenital malformations. Urol Int 1964; 18:347–56.
96. Boatman DL, Kolln CP, Flocks RH. Congenital anomalies associated with horseshoe kidney. J Urol 1972; 107:205–7.
97. Warkany J, Passarge E, Smith LB. Congenital malformations in autosomal trisomy syndromes. Am J Dis Child 1966; 112:502–17.
98. Smith DW. Turner syndrome. In: Smith DW, ed. Recognizable Patterns of Human Malformation. Genetic,

Embryologic and Clinical Aspects, 3rd edn. Philadelphia: WB Saunders, 1982: 72.

99. Lippe BL, Geffner ME, Dietrich RB, Boechat MI, Kangarloo H. Renal malformation in patients with Turner's syndrome: imaging in 141 patients. Pediatrics 1988; 83:852–6.
100. Whitaker RH, Hunt GM. Incidence and distribution of renal anomalies in patients with neural tube defects. Eur Urol 1987; 13:322–3.
101. Pitts WR Jr, Muecke EC. Horseshoe kidneys: a 40-year experience. J Urol 1975; 113:743–6.
102. Segura JW, Kelalis PP, Burke EC. Horseshoe kidney in children. J Urol 1972; 108:333–6.
103. Cascio S, Sweeney B, Granata C et al. Vesicoureteral reflux and ureteropelvic junction obstruction in children with horseshoe kidney: treatment and outcome. J Urol 2002; 167:2566–8.
104. Novak ME, Baum NH, Gonzales ET Jr. Horseshoe kidney with multicystic dysplasia associated with ureterocele. Urology 1977; 10:456–8.
105. Fernandes M, Scheuch J, Seebode JJ. Horseshoe kidney with retrocaval ureter: a case report. J Urol 1988; 140:362–4.
106. Bell R. Horseshoe kidney in pregnancy. J Urol 1946; 56:159–61.
107. Evans WP, Resnick MI. Horseshoe kidney and urolithiasis. J Urol 1981; 125:620–1.
108. Raj GV, Auge BK, Assimos D, Preminger GM. Metabolic abnormalities associated with renal calculi in patients with horseshoe kidneys. J Endourol 2004; 18:157–61.
109. Buntley D. Malignancy associated with horseshoe kidney. Urology 1976; 8:146–8.
110. Blackard CE, Mellinger GT. Cancer in a horseshoe kidney: a report of two cases. Arch Surg 1968; 97:616–27.
111. Dische MR, Johnston R. Teratoma in horseshoe kidneys. Urology 1979; 13:435–8.
112. Mesrobian HG, Kelalis PP, Hrabovsky E et al. Wilms' tumor in horseshoe kidneys: a report from the National Wilms' Tumor Study. J Urol 1985; 133:1002–3.
113. Neville H, Ritchey ML, Shamberger RC et al. The occurrence of Wilms tumor in horseshoe kidneys: a report from the National Wilms Tumor Study Group (NWTSG). J Pediatr Surg 2002; 37:1134–7.
114. Schuster T, Dietz HG, Schutz S. Anderson–Hynes pyeloplasty in horseshoe kidney in children: is it effective without symphysiotomy? Pediatr Surg Int 1999; 15:230–3.
115. Donahoe PK, Hendren WH. Pelvic kidney in infants and children: experience with 16 cases. J Pediatr Surg 1980; 15:486–95.
116. Bove P, Ong AM, Rha KH et al. Laparoscopic management of ureteropelvic junction obstruction in patients with upper urinary tract anomalies. J Urol 2004; 171:77–9.
117. Yohannes P, Smith AD. The endourological management of complications associated with horseshoe kidney. J Urol 2002; 168:5–8.
118. Raj GV, Auge BK, Weizer AZ et al. Percutaneous management of calculi within horseshoe kidneys. J Urol 2003; 170:48–51.
119. McDonald JH, McClellan DS. Crossed renal ectopia. Am J Surg 1957; 93:995–1002.
120. Abeshouse BS, Bhisitkul I. Crossed renal ectopia with and without fusion. Urol Int 1959; 9:63–91.
121. Kakei H, Kondo H, Ogisu BI, Mitsuya H. Crossed ectopia of solitary kidney: a report of two cases and a review of the literature. Urol Int 1976; 31:470–5.
122. Rubinstein ZJ, Heitz M, Shahin N, Deutsch V. Crossed renal ectopia: angiographic findings in six cases. AJR Am J Roentgenol 1976; 126:1035–8.
123. Nussbaum AR, Hartman DS, Whitley N, McCauley RG, Sanders RC. Multicystic dysplasia and crossed renal ectopia. AJR Am J Roentgenol 1987; 149:407–10.
124. Gerber WL, Culp DA, Brown RC, Chow KC, Platz CE. Renal mass in crossed-fused ectopia. J Urol 1980; 123:239–44.
125. Mininberg DT, Roze S, Pearl M. Hypertension associated with crossed renal ectopia in an infant. Pediatrics 1971; 48:454–7.

Fetal and neonatal renal function 21

Billy S Arant Jr

Introduction

The developing mammalian kidney is a remarkably complex organ. Although it has been characterized as small, immature, limited, and imbalanced and, as such, an impediment to the medical management of sick infants, this view is unwarranted. When it was first recognized that glomerular filtration rate (GFR) corrected for the body size of newborn infants was less than values measured in the adult,[1] the notion of limited renal function was introduced. Although the bulk of published studies on the various functions of the neonatal kidney seem to support limitation, many of these studies were misinterpreted and seemed to have conformed to the bias prevalent at the time.

It is somewhat difficult to imagine how the species survived the stress of fetal adaptation to the functional integrity of postnatal life if the neonatal kidney were indeed limited in its functional capacity. Many premature infants weighing <1000 g at birth survived even in the 1930s to become healthy infants long before the availability of supportive measures now referred to as neonatal intensive care.[2] Recent human and experimental animal studies provide some enlightenment and confirm the essential and unique role of the kidney at any stage of viability once the umbilical blood flow is interrupted at birth.

The kidney of the human neonate functions qualitatively like the adult kidney and is more than adequate to support functional development and growth of the infant following birth, at least within limits. These limits, however, are often exceeded by the demands imposed during the treatment of sick infants when most clinical decisions are made without concern for kidney function. Too often, perhaps, it is easier to fault the kidney because it is small rather than to understand the essence of its supporting role in health and disease. Failing to appreciate the unique responses of the neonatal kidney will, on occasion, compromise clinical decision making, especially when prescribing fluid therapy[2] and drugs eliminated primarily by renal excretion.[3,4]

Morphologic development

The human metanephros is formed about the 5th week after conception, when the sequential branching ureteric bud contacts the caudal mesenchyma and induces glomerulogenesis. All glomeruli are contained within the cortex. The first ones formed occupy a juxtamedullary position and have the longest loops of Henle. The ureteric bud forms the collecting duct for each nephron and continues to branch in a centrifugal pattern until 20 weeks of gestation. New glomeruli are formed until 34–36 weeks after conception when each kidney will contain approximately one million nephrons (Figure 21.1). When birth occurs prematurely, glomerulogenesis continues. But there is speculation that the total number of glomeruli at maturity may be deficient and contribute to morbidity, mainly hypertension and renal insufficiency in later life due to glomerular hyperfiltration.[6] Glomerular filtration is evident after 8 weeks' gestation, but the ureter may not be entirely patent until the 11th week. Ureteral obstruction is thought to provoke dilation of the proximal collecting system, the renal pelvis, and calices. The layers of smooth muscle and elastic fibers in the ureter are laid down after 36 weeks' gestation and continue to form for 8 weeks after birth at term. If there is an essential role of the fetal kidney, it must be to contribute the majority of amniotic fluid after the first trimester of pregnancy.

Physiologic adaptation at birth

Body composition

From the moment of conception, when the composition of the fertilized ovum is 99% salt and water,

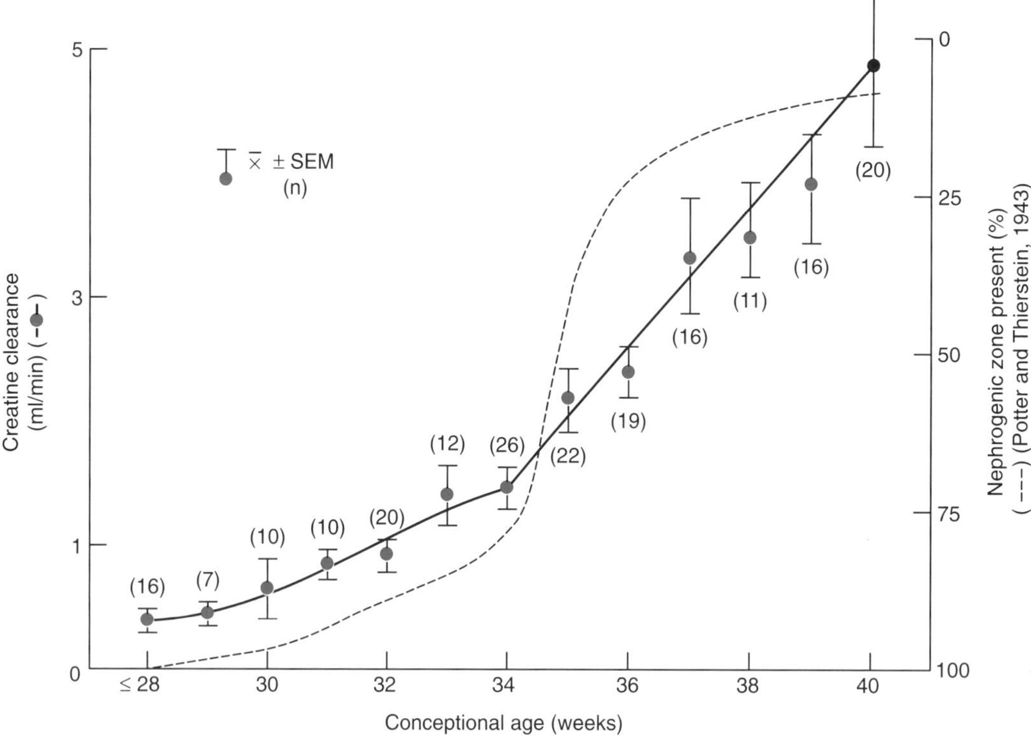

Figure 21.1 Developmental pattern of changes in creatinine clearance [glomerular filtration rate (GFR)] and the disappearance of the nephrogenic zone of the renal cortex compared with the conceptional age of human infants. (From Arant,[5] with permission.)

there is a gradual reduction in the relative body content of water and minerals with age. While the total amounts of minerals and water provided by the placenta increase as the fetus grows, organs are formed and tissue growth occurs which incorporate these elements into cytoplasm and extracellular matrix. The higher salt and water content of the fetus assures a relative abundance of extracellular fluid, which decreases from 60% of body weight at the beginning of the last trimester to 40% at birth; extracellular fluid represents only 20% of body weight in the adult.[7] Therefore, whether birth occurs before or at term, essentially all neonates have an expanded extracellular fluid volume that allows them to survive naturally without intake for a few days postnatally as the volume of the mother's breast milk increases. Extracellular fluid volume expansion in the neonate influences renal function just as it does in the adult. When birth occurs at term, the total body water content has been reduced to 75% and the sodium content has decreased from 120 mmol/kg body weight at 8 weeks after conception to 85 mmol/kg.[8] During the first week of life, there is an additional reduction in the relative body water and sodium content, mainly through urinary losses and, thus, extracellular fluid volume is reduced further. In premature infants, this abrupt reduction in total body water and sodium following birth is more pronounced and represents losses of up to 25% of body weight as water and 14 mmol/kg of sodium with no change in plasma sodium concentration or blood pressure.[9–11]

Cardiovascular hemodynamics

During fetal life, systemic vascular resistance is kept very low except in the pulmonary and renal circulations, where vascular resistance is high since neither organ contributes directly to the viability of the fetus.[5] The explanation for the regulation of the differences in these specialized circulations may be the local formation of vasoactive substances that cause vascular smooth muscle to contract (angiotensin) or relax (prostaglandins and nitric oxide). Cardiac output in the fetus is high and varies only with heart rate since stroke volume is always at a maximum.[12] Moreover, blood volume in the fetus and very preterm infant may be as high as 120 ml/kg body weight compared with 75 ml/kg in the adult.[13] With both cardiac output and blood volume high, how can blood pressure be so low? Normal mean arterial pres-

patients, there are protean extrarenal manifestations, including the potentially life-threatening possibility of a ruptured intracranial aneurysm. Severity varies greatly between patients and symptoms tend to develop over time. Fortunately, most children are asymptomatic; even middle-age adults may be unaware of their diagnosis. There are, however, children with severe and occasionally fatal disease. This underscores the importance of avoiding the term 'adult' PKD.

An increasing percentage of children with ADPKD are diagnosed from a positive family history or because of an incidental finding during an imaging study. This has caused a marked shift in the pediatric patient population, with many patients having no symptoms and requiring very limited intervention.

Genetics

ADPKD is a genetically heterogeneous condition; disease occurs owing to mutations in one of at least two separate genetic loci (Table 22.3). Patients with a mutation of the *PKD1* gene,[66] which is located on chromosome 16, account for approximately 85% of cases. Most remaining cases are due to a mutation in the *PKD2* gene on chromosome 4.[67] The presence of a third locus (*PKD3*) is inferred based on studies showing an absence of genetic linkage to either *PKD1* or *PKD2* in some families with ADPKD,[68–70] although the evidence for a third locus has been questioned.[71]

Table 22.3 Multiple gene defects that cause ADPKD

Gene	Chromosome location	Protein
PKD1	16p	Polycystin
PKD2	4q	Polycystin-2
PKD3	Unknown	Unknown

PKD1 encodes for a protein called polycystin, which is a transmembrane protein with multiple extracellular domains.[72] The *PKD2* gene product, polycystin-2, is also a transmembrane protein and has moderate homology to polycystin.[67] Polycystin and polycystin-2 interact with each other, and are localized within primary cilia.[73–75]

The variable development of cyst formation in ADPKD appears to be related to the need for a second inactivating mutation. The kidney cells of patients with the *PKD1* mutation initially have one normal gene for polycystin and one defective gene. Cyst formation occurs when there is a second somatic mutation that inactivates the good gene. This produces a cell that does not produce any normal polycystin. Additional cysts are due to a second mutation in other cells.[76,77] A similar mechanism takes place in patients with *PKD2*.[78,79] This helps to explain why cysts appear fairly randomly and increase in number over time.

There is a great deal of variability in the severity of ADPKD, some of which is based on the specific gene affected. Patients with PKD2 have less severe symptoms, including later mean age for the development of ESRD and a decreased incidence of hypertension, urinary tract infections (UTIs), and hematuria.[80] In one study, the median age of death or onset of ESRD was 53 and 69 years in patients with PKD1 and PKD2, respectively.[80] There is also evidence that the disease severity is influenced by the specific mutation (allelic heterogeneity) in the *PKD1* or *PKD2* genes.[81–83] Additional sources of variability may involve environmental factors and genetic differences at other loci.[84–86] For example, polymorphisms in the angiotensin-converting enzyme (ACE) gene modify renal disease severity in patients with PKD1.[87]

In cases of neonatal ADPKD, the affected parents have not had early-onset disease.[20,88,89] However, there appears to be an increased likelihood of early disease in affected siblings[20,88,90,91] and other members of the same kindred.[89] Early-onset disease may be more likely in families with mutations in *PKD1*.[92]

Pathology

The kidneys are typically enlarged and have random cysts, which can originate from any portion of the nephron (Figure 22.6). Except for cysts, the renal architecture is initially normal, although as the disease progresses fibrosis and glomerulosclerosis gradually increase.

Clinical features

Most children with ADPKD are asymptomatic, and increasing numbers of these patients are diagnosed based on a positive family history followed by a screening computed tomography (CT) scan or ultrasound. Others are diagnosed after kidney cysts are incidentally noted on an imaging study, including prenatal ultrasound.

Although children are often asymptomatic, there are reports of severe disease, including neonatally lethal

(a)

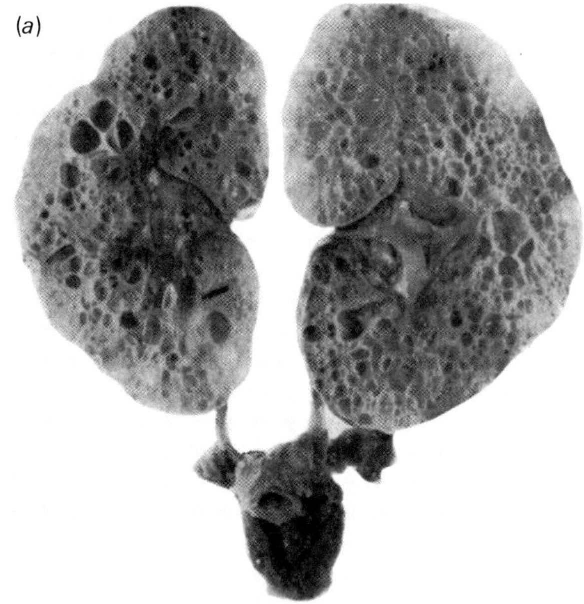

(b)

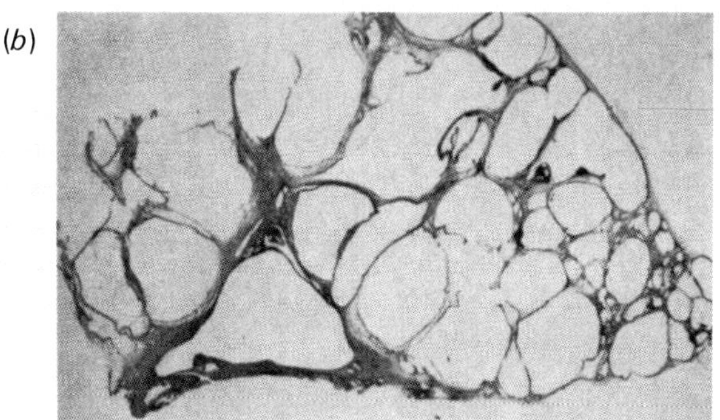

Figure 22.6 (*a*) Example of 'adult' polycystic kidney disease in a 3-month-old infant. Note the rounded cysts of varying size. (*b*) Low-power view of the same kidney. Foci of normal renal tissue are seen between the grossly dilated tubules. (Reproduced with permission from Blyth and Ockenden.[34])

Table 22.4 Presenting complaints in symptomatic children with ADPKD[a]

Symptom	Gagnadoux et al[22]	Fick et al[99]	Kääriäinen et al[91]
Hematuria	3	2	2
Abdominal pain	3	1	1
Hypertension	3	1	0
Renal mass	1	1	0
Frequency	0	2	0
UTI	0	1	1
Proteinuria	0	0	1

[a] This table excludes patients with severe neonatal disease.

disease.[20,88,93] Neonatal mortality is usually a result of respiratory failure and is associated with massively enlarged kidneys.[20,90,93] Most neonates diagnosed on the basis of on an abnormal prenatal ultrasound are asymptomatic. The majority of these children maintain normal renal function, but some will reach ESRD during childhood.[22,92–94] Maternal inheritance may be a risk factor for neonatal presentation.[95]

Most children with symptomatic ADPKD have a more subtle presenting complaint, typically in late childhood or adolescence.[20,22] Hematuria is quite common in adults with ADPKD[96] and can manifest in childhood.[20,22,97,98] Other presenting symptoms include hypertension, frequency, abdominal or flank pain, abdominal mass, UTI, and proteinuria (Table 22.4).[20,22,98,99] The majority of patients who are symptomatic during childhood do not have renal insufficiency as young adults,[22] but they may be at a higher risk for early kidney failure.[98]

The presence of symptoms in children correlates with the number of cysts. Children with more than 10 cysts have an increased incidence of flank or back pain, palpable kidneys, and hypertension.[99] Such children also have more complaints of palpitations and urinary frequency than their unaffected siblings.[99]

Hypertension and resultant end-organ damage occurs in children with ADPKD. When a group of mostly asymptomatic children were screened, 13% had hypertension (vs 0% of controls) and the hypertensive patients had left ventricular hypertrophy.[100] A smaller study using ambulatory blood pressure monitoring found no evidence of hypertension in patients <15 years, but there was an increase in left ventricular mass.[101] In addition, patients between 15 and 25 years had significant increases in blood pressure and ventricular mass.[101] Another study found hypertension at clinical presentation in 22% of children.[95] Not surprisingly, hypertension is more common in children who are symptomatic in the neonatal period.[20] The renin–angiotensin system is implicated in hypertensive adults with ADPKD and normal renal function,[102] although this mechanism has not been studied in children.

Some children with mild ADPKD have a subtle defect in urinary concentrating ability,[22] and this is more common in children with more than 10 cysts.[99] Children with more than 10 cysts also have an increased incidence of proteinuria.[103] Kidney stones, often presenting as acute flank pain, are increased in adults,[104] but are infrequent in children.

Kidney infections are more common in patients with ADPKD, and complications may include

Table 22.5 Extrarenal symptoms in ADPKD

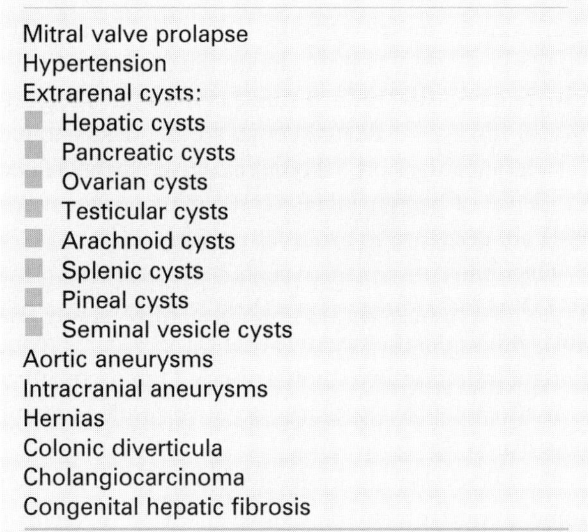

- Mitral valve prolapse
- Hypertension
- Extrarenal cysts:
  - Hepatic cysts
  - Pancreatic cysts
  - Ovarian cysts
  - Testicular cysts
  - Arachnoid cysts
  - Splenic cysts
  - Pineal cysts
  - Seminal vesicle cysts
- Aortic aneurysms
- Intracranial aneurysms
- Hernias
- Colonic diverticula
- Cholangiocarcinoma
- Congenital hepatic fibrosis

perinephric abscess, septicemia, and death;[105] there may be an increased risk of VUR.[106] Cyst infection is especially troublesome, since the urine culture may be negative and not all antibiotics achieve therapeutic levels in the cyst fluid.[105]

There are a large number of possible extrarenal manifestations in adults with ADPKD (Table 22.5). Extrarenal involvement is less common in childhood. Mitral valve prolapse (MVP) is found in 26% of adults with ADPKD.[107] Among a group of children, 12% had MVP (vs 3% of controls) and the incidence increased with age.[100] Inguinal hernias are substantially increased in both children[98,99] and adults.[108,109]

Liver cysts are the most common extrarenal manifestation in adults with ADPKD, with the prevalence increasing with age.[110,111] Women tend to have more and larger cysts[112] and pregnancy is an additional risk factor.[111] Some adults experience abdominal fullness and pain, but cysts almost never impair liver function or cause portal hypertension,[110,112] except in extreme cases.[113] Infected liver cysts present with pain, fever, and leukocytosis.[114] Liver cysts are rare in children.[99,115] Liver enlargement[20] has occasionally been described in children. A few patients with ADPKD have congenital hepatic fibrosis;[43,44,116] but this liver involvement is usually restricted to one member of the family and thus does not appear to be related to a unique ADPKD gene defect.

Pancreatic cysts are present in only 9% of patients over 30 years of age,[117] and almost never cause complications;[118] they are extremely unusual in children.[115] The claim that ovarian cysts are increased in ADPKD has been questioned.[119] The remaining cystic complications are quite rare.[120]

Ruptured intracranial aneurysms are a significant cause of mortality in adults with ADPKD.[121] In one study, the mean age of bleeding was 39.5 years, but 10% of patients were <20 years.[122] There are reports of young children with a subarachnoid hemorrhage,[20] a bleeding arteriovenous malformation (AVM),[123] and ruptured intracranial aneurysms.[124,125] Aneurysms cluster in families,[126–128] and thus a positive family history for intracranial hemorrhage or aneurysm is an important risk factor.

Gender differences in ADPKD include the predisposition to liver cysts in women. The rate of progression to kidney failure is faster in adult males with either PKD1[129] or PKD2.[80] No gender differences among children have been reported.[99]

Radiologic features

Ultrasound (Figure 22.7) and CT scan (Figure 22.8) are useful for detecting the macroscopic cysts of

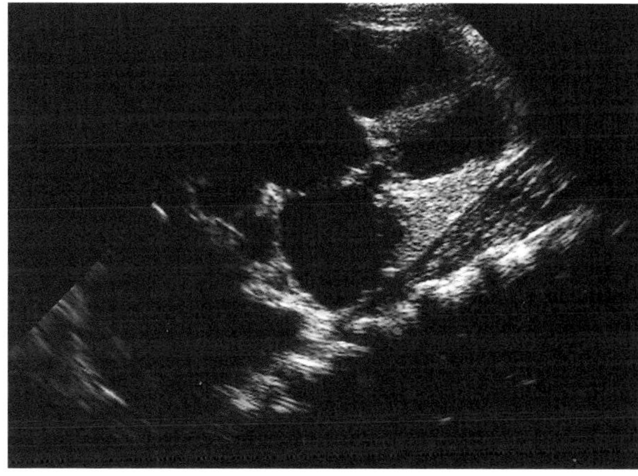

Figure 22.7 Ultrasound of an infant with severe ADPKD. The kidneys are enlarged owing to multiple cysts. (Courtesy of Dr J Sty, Children's Hospital of Wisconsin.)

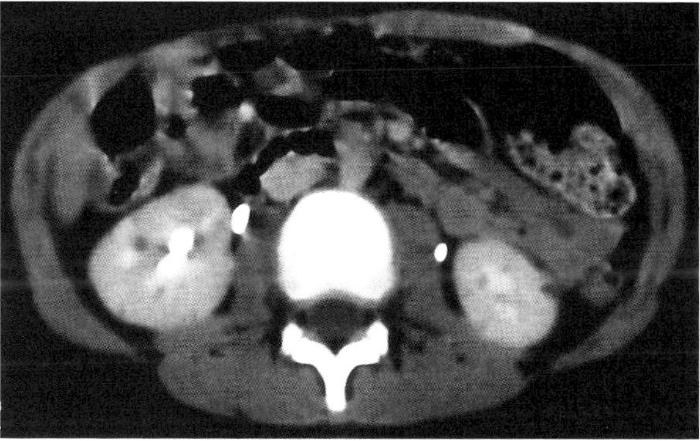

Figure 22.8 CT scan of a child with ADPKD. Macroscopic cysts are readily visible. (Courtesy of Dr J Sty, Children's Hospital of Wisconsin.)

ADPKD. The number and size of cysts in children increase with age, and those children with more cysts have increased kidney size.[99] Increased renal echogenicity may be seen in some children.[40] Occasionally, children can have marked disease asymmetry, which can create diagnostic confusion.[130] Liver cysts are quite unusual in children.[99]

Diagnosis

Rare, early-onset ADPKD can sometimes be diagnosed by prenatal ultrasound,[88,89,116,131] although most cases are identified in the last 10 weeks of gestation. The kidneys are large, with increased echogenicity, and cannot easily be distinguished from the kidneys of children with ARPKD. Occasionally, macrocysts are identified.[116] Early diagnosis in a fetus with an affected parent is possible using DNA analysis.[132,133]

Even after birth it is often difficult to distinguish early-onset ADPKD from ARPKD. Radiologic studies of the kidneys are often inconclusive. Liver imaging or biopsy is useful because hepatic fibrosis is always present in ARPKD and extremely rare in ADPKD. Kidney pathology is also helpful, given the absence of glomerular cysts in ARPKD. The presence of a parent with ADPKD is the most useful diagnostic clue. Yet, many parents are unaware of their own disease,[22,92] and thus screening imaging studies of 'normal' parents are mandatory. Because of the possibility of a false-negative radiologic study, screening of the grandparents is sometimes useful, especially if the parents are <30 years old.

Diagnosis in asymptomatic or mildly symptomatic children is usually accomplished by renal ultrasound. The sensitivity and specificity of this approach increases with the child's age (Table 22.6). CT scan, although perhaps more sensitive than ultrasound,[135] is usually not a front-line approach because of the greater ease of ultrasound. Unilateral cysts may be the only initial finding in children with ADPKD,[22,99,124,130,136,137] and in the context of a positive family history even a single cyst is highly suggestive of disease.[134] Bilateral cysts are frequently found on later investigation.[99] For adults, given the increased incidence of benign solitary cysts, more stringent criteria are necessary to avoid false positives.[138]

Table 22.6 Sensitivity and specificity of ultrasound for detecting ADPKD in children

Age	Specificity (%)	Sensitivity (%)
3 months–5 years	89	62
5 years–10 years	100	82
10 years–15 years	100	86
15 years–17.5 years	100	67

This table summarizes the results of ultrasound screening in a group of children with PKD1 by linkage analysis. The presence of a single cyst was interpreted as a positive ultrasound. Table adapted from Gabow et al.[134]

The ability to screen patients for mutations in the *PKD1* or *PKD2* genes is currently commercially available, although false-negative results can occur. Identifying a mutation in a known affected family member is useful for proving that a negative result is a true negative.

The increasing ability to diagnose ADPKD raises some important issues. Unlike many other genetic diseases, the morbidity and mortality in ADPKD typically occurs in older adults and problems are fairly modest in many patients. Nevertheless, among a group of adults at risk for the disease, 97% would like to receive genetic testing.[139] There is also enthusiasm for genetic testing of offspring, with 89% selecting this option.[139] However, knowledge of the presence of this disease has little impact on reproductive decisions. Only 11% of patients do not have children because of the risk of passing the disease to offspring and even fewer (4%) would terminate a pregnancy for ADPKD.[139]

Screening and monitoring

Many children have a parent with ADPKD and therefore have a 50% risk of carrying the defective gene. Undiagnosed, asymptomatic patients may have significant abnormalities such as hypertension, proteinuria, bacteriuria, and an increased creatinine.[140] Certainly, at-risk children need periodic screening, with special attention to the blood pressure. A possible algorithm is presented in Figure 22.9. Screening ultrasounds are not recommended because of concerns regarding obtaining health insurance.[141] A more aggressive approach will be necessary if an effective early treatment for ADPKD becomes available.[142] Figure 22.9 also presents a basic approach to monitoring the child with a diagnosis of ADPKD, with the caveat that monitoring needs to be customized for the individual patient.

Treatment

Children with severe disease receive standard therapy for chronic renal insufficiency. This should include

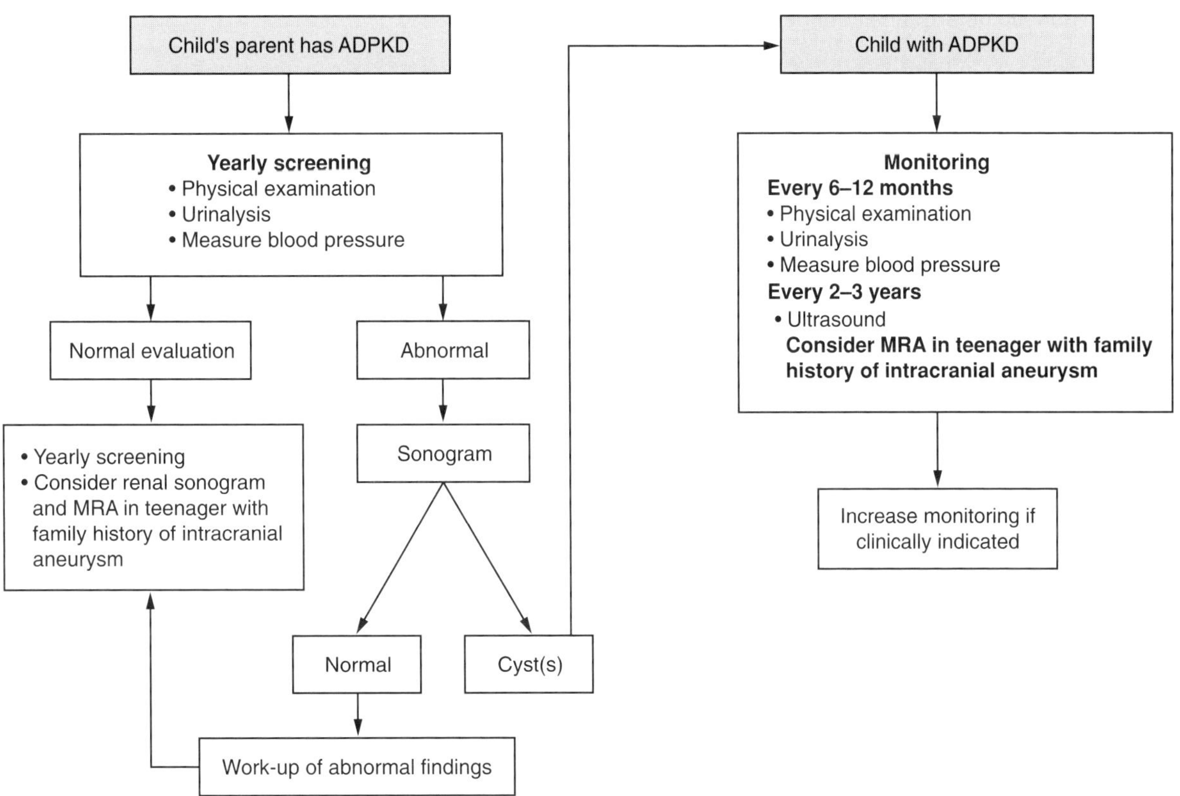

Figure 22.9 ADPKD: screening and monitoring of children. MRA, magnetic resonance angiography.

careful monitoring of nutrition and growth. In adults with moderate renal insufficiency, there was no benefit to protein restriction, although there was a marginal slowing in the rate of decline of the glomerular filtration rate (GFR) in patients with severe renal insufficiency.[143] Such an approach is not recommended in children because the benefits are minimal and there is potential for adverse effects on growth and development. A variety of other interventions to slow the progression of ADPKD have been tested in animal models, and a clinical trial of a vasopressin 2 receptor antagonist is currently underway in adults.[142]

Hypertension is fairly common in older children with ADPKD and should be treated. In adults with ADPKD, rigorous control of blood pressure was superior to standard control in reversing left ventricular hypertrophy.[144] There is not a consensus on the ideal class of antihypertensive agent to select for these patients. Despite the pathogenic role of the renin–angiotensin system[102] and the evidence that ACE inhibitors slow the progression of renal insufficiency in a variety of kidney diseases,[145,146] ACE inhibitors, when rigorously tested, do not slow the progression of chronic renal insufficiency in ADPKD.[146] ACE inhibitors do reverse left ventricular hypertrophy in hypertensive adults with ADPKD,[147] but there is a small risk of precipitating acute renal failure in patients with ADPKD, and thus they must be used cautiously.[148] Other agents, such as calcium channel blockers, have also been advocated.[149]

The goal of therapy is normalization of blood pressure using standard guidelines.[150] In adults with ADPKD, low targets for blood pressure may have a deleterious effect on renal function.[143]

Urinary tract infections should be treated promptly, with awareness for the increased risk of abscesses and septicemia. Cyst infection requires selection of an antibiotic that penetrates the cyst, such as trimethoprim–sulfamethoxazole[151] or ciprofloxacin;[152] occasionally, cyst aspiration may be necessary.[153] Patients with intractable pain from renal cysts can benefit from either cyst aspiration, surgical reduction, or thoracoscopic denervation.[154,155]

The possibility of a ruptured intracranial aneurysm is a frightening, albeit rare complication in pediatric patients. The advisability of screening patients is currently being debated. Magnetic resonance angiography (MRA) is a safe and sensitive approach for detecting an asymptomatic aneurysm.[126] However,

Table 22.7 Genetic heterogeneity of nephronophthisis (NPH)

Type	Chromosome locations	Gene mutated	Encoded protein	Clinical form
NPH type 1	2q13	*NPHP1*	Nephrocystin	Juvenile
NPH type 2	9q22	*NPHP2*	Inversin	Infantile
NPH type 3	3q22	*NPHP3*	Nephrocystin-3	Adolescent
NPH type 4	1p36	*NPHP4*	Nephrocystin-4	Juvenile

there is a need to balance the safety and efficacy of surgical intervention with the risk of aneurysm rupture. One decision analysis supported screening a 20-year-old patient with ADPKD,[156] although others have suggested a less aggressive approach.[157,158] Because of the familial predilection to aneurysm formation,[126,127] screening of older teenagers with a positive family history is a reasonable approach.[159] However, patient selection, timing, and frequency of screening continue to evolve.[160,161]

Prognosis

Most children with ADPKD will have minimal symptoms throughout childhood. The adult course of the disease is extremely variable.

There are currently limited data on the ultimate prognosis for patients diagnosed during childhood. This is especially true for patients with asymptomatic cysts; the impact of increased numbers of cysts on the risk of chronic renal failure is unknown. Children who are diagnosed after the neonatal period do not have a decrease in GFR, even in the subgroup with more cysts and symptoms.[99] In adults, the presence of the *PKD1* gene, younger age at diagnosis, male gender, hypertension, increased left ventricular mass, hepatic cysts in women, three or more pregnancies, gross hematuria, UTI in men, proteinuria, and renal volume are all independently associated with poor renal function.[129,162] In children, increased renal volume in early life or hypertension is associated with subsequent faster renal growth, a potential marker of a worse prognosis.[163] There seems to be a higher risk of early chronic renal failure when patients have more severe disease as children.[98]

Interestingly, many children diagnosed antenatally have normal renal function,[22] although follow-up is relatively limited. The cases diagnosed neonatally frequently have severe, often fatal, disease. These children are at risk for early chronic renal insufficiency and ESRD. However, others maintain normal renal function throughout childhood.[92]

Nephronophthisis

Nephronophthisis (NPH), also called 'juvenile nephronophthisis,' is one of the most common causes of chronic renal insufficiency in children.[164] NPH, which is recessively inherited, is often grouped with dominantly inherited medullary cystic disease because of an overlapping radiologic and histologic appearance. However, medullary cystic disease is genetically distinct, lacks extrarenal involvement, and usually presents in adulthood. We will therefore consider it separately later in this chapter.

Genetics

Mutations at four different loci may cause NPH (Table 22.7), and additional genetic heterogeneity is likely.[165] The majority of cases of NPH are due to mutations in the *NPHP1* gene.[166,167] Most patients with nephronophthisis type 1 are homozygous for a large deletion that affects the *NPHP1* gene.[166,168]

Pathology

Grossly the kidneys are often small and have a pale finely granular surface.[169,170] On light microscopy, there is diffuse interstitial fibrosis with a mononuclear cell infiltration.[169,171,172] Along with tubular atrophy, there is extreme thickening and lamination of the tubular basement membranes.[169,171] Electron microscopy confirms this thickening, and also shows splitting of the basement membrane.[169] In a child with a biopsy early in the course of the disease, tubular basement membrane thickening was the only histologic abnormality.[172] Cysts appear to originate from the distal convoluted tubules and collecting ducts.[171] The glomeruli may be normal or have periglomerular fibrosis with thickening of Bowman's capsule; glomerular obsolescence eventually develops.[169]

Clinical features

Polyuria and polydipsia are due to poor urinary concentrating ability, and this can lead to problems such as dehydration, nocturia, and primary or secondary nocturnal enuresis.[169,173,174] Renal sodium wasting[169] leads to salt craving in some children.[173] The urinalysis is notable for the absence of abnormalities,[169,170,173] although low levels of proteinuria, usually tubular in origin,[174] are sometimes present. Glucosuria is also occasionally present.[174,175] Probably due to the polyuria and salt wasting, hypertension is unusual,[170,176] except in patients with NPH type 2. Symptoms of chronic renal failure, such as fatigue, anorexia, and growth retardation, are frequently present.[170,173,174,177] Symptoms of renal osteodystrophy may be the initial complaint.[177] Children with NPH have an anemia that is out of proportion to their degree of renal failure, and thus often have very low hematocrits and notable pallor.[170,173,174,177,178] The anemia appears to be due to decreased erythropoietin production.[179]

The majority of patients with NPH type 1 develop ESRD at a mean age of about 10–13 years.[169,180] The defect in urine concentrating ability can lead to severe dehydration and acute renal failure, which may accelerate the development of chronic renal failure.[180]

NPH type 2 is distinct from the other forms of NPH. Renal failure occurs in infancy, and the kidneys are large with widespread cysts.[181,182] Hypertension is more common than in the other forms of NPH. *NPHP2* gene defects may also lead to situs inversus in a minority of children.[182] The timing of ESRD is fairly similar in NPH type 1 and NPH type 4, whereas ESRD develops at about a mean age of 19 years in NPH type 3.[180,183]

Senior–Løken syndrome is the combination of NPH with tapetoretinal degeneration.[184,185] In the early-onset form, called congenital amaurosis of Leber, nystagmus is usually present, and there is an absent pupillary response to light. The retina is markedly abnormal on funduscopic examination; findings include arteriolar narrowing, pale optic disks, and granular pigmentation of the fundus.[186] Most patients are blind or severely visually impaired, and have a flat electroretinogram.[174] There is a late-onset form of Senior–Løken syndrome in which visual impairment develops during childhood. Moreover, patients with a defect in the *NPHP1* gene may have ocular findings, including areas of retinal atrophy with flat or low-voltage electroretinograms. However, these patients are usually asymptomatic, and probably should not be considered to have Senior–Løken syndrome.[176,187,188] Senior–Løken syndrome has been described in children with mutations in the *NPHP3* and *NPHP4* genes.[165,189,190] The majority of children with NPH types 3 and 4 do not have Senior–Løken syndrome; there is no explanation for this variable expression.

Table 22.8 Extrarenal manifestations of nephronophthisis

Tapetoretinal degeneration
Liver fibrosis
Skeletal abnormalities
Mental retardation
Cerebellar ataxia

Some children with NPH have other extrarenal manifestations, including mental retardation,[169,178,191] hepatic fibrosis,[169,191–194] Dandy–Walker syndrome,[178] cerebellar ataxia,[193,195] coloboma,[169] and skeletal anomalies.[169,193,195–197] However, there is some question about the rigor of the renal diagnosis in some of these cases.[198]

Mutations in the *NPHP1* gene have been associated with extrarenal manifestations, including Joubert's syndrome,[199] Cogan's oculomotor apraxia,[200] and the combination of cerebellar ataxia and nystagmus.[201] Mutations in the *NPHP3* gene can cause hepatic fibrosis or tapetoretinal degeneration.[190] Mutations in the *NPHP4* gene can cause Cogan's oculomotor apraxia or tapetoretinal degeneration.[165,202]

The more common possible extrarenal manifestations of NPH are shown in Table 22.8. Many patients with extrarenal manifestations also have tapetoretinal degeneration, and thus are part of the Senior–Løken syndrome.

Radiologic features

By ultrasound, the kidneys are hyperechoic with loss of corticomedullary differentiation; they are of normal or slightly decreased size.[203–205] Medullary cysts are a hallmark of the disease, but they are not always detected by ultrasound.[173,203,204] CT is a more sensitive method for identifying medullary cysts[206] and thin-section CT is recommended.[173]

Diagnosis

The diagnosis of NPH can be challenging, especially in patients without extrarenal manifestations. A history of polyuria and polydipsia, salt craving, disproportionate anemia, a benign urinalysis, and the age of presentation are important clues. The detection of medullary cysts in the setting of chronic renal failure in a child and smallish, echogenic kidneys is virtually diagnostic. The presence of consanguinity or an affected sibling suggests an autosomal recessive disease and thus strongly supports the diagnosis. Renal histology is potentially helpful in uncertain cases. Genetic diagnosis is now possible because screening for the large chromosomal deletion in the *NPHP1* gene is relatively easy,[207] and this will identify approximately 60% of patients with NPH.[208] Moreover, sequencing of the entire *NPHP1* gene for mutations is commercially available for the small percentage of patients with NPH type 1 who do not have the large deletions. Genetic testing for the other forms of NPH is only available on a research basis. All patients should have an ocular examination to screen for Senior–Løken syndrome and a liver ultrasound to screen for hepatic fibrosis.

Treatment

There is no specific therapy for NPH. Families should be counseled regarding the risk of dehydration due to polyuria. The anemia responds to erythropoietin therapy. Children receive standard therapy for chronic renal insufficiency and ultimately require dialysis and transplantation. The disease does not recur in the kidney transplant and thus transplant is usually quite successful.[186,209] Appropriate specialist care is necessary in children with extrarenal manifestations.

Multicystic dysplastic kidney

Multicystic dysplastic kidney (MCDK) is the most common cystic disease diagnosed during childhood. Most cases are unilateral and asymptomatic; rare bilateral disease is usually fatal at birth as a result of Potter's syndrome.[210] The widespread use of prenatal ultrasound has led to more frequent diagnosis of MCDK, and the approach to the management of these patients is evolving.

The incidence of MCDK is estimated at 1 in 2500 newborns;[211] it is one of the most common fetal anomalies detected by prenatal ultrasound. It occurs slightly more commonly in the left kidney,[212] and the affected child is more likely to be male.[213,214] Given the low incidence of unilateral renal agenesis in neonates, and the much higher incidence of single kidneys in adults, the majority of adults with a single kidney had an MCDK that involuted over time.

MCDK is typically composed of cysts of varying size that do not appear to communicate, and a small amount of abnormal-appearing renal parenchyma. The ureter from the affected kidney is atretic. On microscopic examination, the tissue between the cysts is dysplastic, with undifferentiated mesenchymal cells, often with cartilage, and immature glomeruli and tubules. Occasionally, a few normal-appearing nephrons may be present, explaining the minimal renal function that is infrequently demonstrated on nuclear scan.

Most cases of MCDK are sporadic,[215] although families with putative autosomal dominant inheritance have been described.[215,216] The incidence of MCDK is increased in a variety of syndromes.[217] The pathogenesis of MCDK has been attributed to either early ureteral obstruction[218] or disruption of the normal mechanism of induction of the metanephric blastema by the ureteric bud.[219]

Currently, most cases of MCDK are diagnosed by prenatal ultrasound, with palpable abdominal mass, typically in the neonate, as the second most common presentation.[220–222] Rare cases of diagnosis result from symptoms such as emesis or respiratory compromise as a result of compressive effects.[223] In older children, MCDK is uncommonly diagnosed during the evaluation for abdominal pain or mass, hematuria, or hypertension. In all ages, MCDK may be discovered during the evaluation for UTI or as an incidental finding during abdominal imaging.[224,225]

The diagnosis of MCDK is typically made by ultrasound. In infants with a prenatal diagnosis, a postnatal ultrasound should be performed to confirm the presence of MCDK. The major diagnostic dilemma is differentiation from hydronephrosis.[226] In MCDK, there is typically no communication between cysts, and the larger cysts are not medial. In hydronephrosis, the calices extend outward from the dilated renal pelvis, and there is renal parenchyma surrounding the central cystic structure. The normal reniform shape is usually present with hydronephrosis, but usually absent in MCDK.[227] If the diagnosis is unclear, a radionuclide scan shows uptake of tracer if hydronephrosis is present, but usually no uptake with MCDK. Occasionally, MCDK demonstrates a small amount of uptake,[228,229] and other studies may then be useful in confirming the diagnosis.[226]

Children with MCDK are more likely to have abnormalities of the contralateral kidney.[213,230,231] VUR has been reported in from 4% to 31% of contralateral kidneys.[212,213,230–232] Other reported anomalies include ureteropelvic junction (UPJ) obstruction, ureteral ectopia, uterovesical junction obstruction, ureteroceles, and renal dysplasia.[213,230,231]

The natural history of MCDK is usually gradual involution. In one study, 18% were undetectable by ultrasound at 1 year of age, and 58% were undetectable by 6 years of age.[220] Some MCDK do increase in size during the first few years of life, and complete involution may take more than 20 years.

Hypertension, which is postulated to be renin mediated,[233] has been reported as a potential complication of MCDK.[212,234] There are reports of hypertension being cured following surgical removal of the MCDK.[233] Yet, others have questioned the validity of these reports. For example, in a series of 260 cases, there were only 4 patients with hypertension, which was described as minimal and probably unrelated to the MCDK.[235]

Malignancy is another possible complication of MCDK. There are cases of Wilms' tumor in younger children[236] and renal cell carcinoma in older teenagers and adults,[237] but some question the validity of these reports.[238] The true increase in risk is unclear. Less than 0.1% of the 7500 children enrolled in the National Wilms' Tumor Study Group had an MCDK.[238] A recent systematic review concluded that the risk of malignancy is extremely low.[239]

The management of MCDK is controversial.[234,240,241] There has been a shift from routine surgical removal to non-operative management, consisting of surveillance ultrasounds to screen for Wilms' tumor.[235] There is not a consensus on the frequency of these ultrasound evaluations, especially given the low risk of Wilms' tumor. Ultrasounds are usually done more frequently during the first year of life (e.g. every 3 months), and then less frequently (e.g. every 6–12 months) until approximately age 5 years.[220] Surgical removal (discussed in Chapter 29) is indicated if there is any change that is suspicious for a Wilms' tumor. Other indications for nephrectomy include mass effect, pain, hypertension, and parental preference.

Follow-up, and surgical repair when indicated,[213] of the contralateral kidney is also critical. The follow-up ultrasounds of the MCDK should evaluate the size and echogenicity of the contralateral kidney; there should be compensatory hypertrophy.[212,231] Given the high rate of VUR, a routine voiding cystourethrogram is frequently recommended,[242] although this has been questioned in the child with a normal-appearing contralateral kidney.[213,243]

Medullary cystic kidney disease

Medullary cystic kidney disease (MCKD) is frequently grouped with NPH as the juvenile nephronophthisis/medullary cystic disease complex.[244] However, MCKD is clearly a distinct entity, based on its autosomal dominant inheritance and later onset.[245] Renal failure typically develops during adulthood, although renal insufficiency may be apparent in some children.[202,245,246] In some families, the disease is not apparent until a mean age of over 60 years.[247] Hyperuricemia and gouty arthritis, occasionally diagnosed in childhood,[246] may be the presenting manifestation.[248,249] Other clinical features include polyuria, anemia, and hypertension.[250,251] The kidneys are usually of normal size or small, and renal imaging may show a few medullary cysts, but the absence of visible cysts is relatively common.[246] The urinalysis is typically benign, except for low-grade proteinuria in a minority of patients.[250] Histologic examination demonstrates interstitial nephritis; thickening and splitting of the basement membrane is the most notable feature.[246,252]

Mutations in *UMOD*, the gene encoding uromodulin (also called Tamm–Horsfall protein), cause MCKD type 2.[253] Mutations in *UMOD* also cause the autosomal dominant disorder, familial juvenile hyperuricemic nephropathy (FJHN).[253,254] It is now clear that MCKD type 2 and FJHN are the same disease, since they are genetically allelic and clinically indistinguishable.[246,253,255] The dominant features are chronic renal failure and gout.[252] Genetic diagnosis, by sequencing of exons 3 and 4, the site of most mutations in this disorder, is commercially available. The locus for MCKD type 1 has been identified on chromosome 1.[247] These patients tend to have fewer manifestations of hyperuricemia than patients with MCKD type 2 and a later onset of renal insufficiency.[250] There is evidence for additional genetic heterogeneity.[250,256]

Medullary sponge kidney

Medullary sponge kidney (MSK) is predominantly a disease of adults, but occasionally presents in childhood.[257–259] The intrapapillary collecting ducts are dilated and multiple small cysts may be present. Not all renal pyramids are always affected, providing an explanation for the often asymmetric and focal appearance. This does not appear to be an inherited disease, although a few family clusters are described.[260,261]

The diagnosis of MSK is based on the characteristic changes on IVP, which shows stagnation of contrast in one or more renal papillae due to dilation of

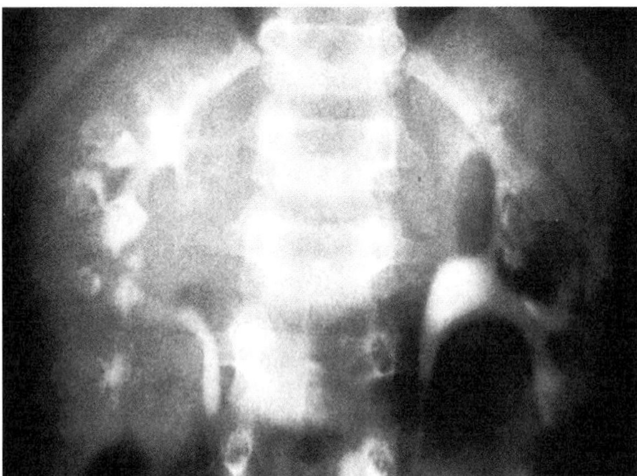

Figure 22.10 IVP demonstrating bilateral medullary sponge kidneys in a 9-year-old girl who presented with hematuria. Note the characteristic radial stretching and puddling that represent the contrast-filled dilated collecting tubules in this disease. (From Glassberg et al.[262])

the collecting ducts (Figure 22.10). The resultant image has been described as a 'pyramidal blush'.[263] These changes are sometimes misdiagnosed as papillary necrosis.[260] A CT scan is not as sensitive for making the diagnosis of MSK, but it has a superior ability to detect the papillary calcifications that frequently complicate MSK.[258,264,265] Ultrasound also frequently detects this nephrocalcinosis, which may not be visible on a plain film.[258]

Clinically, patients are at increased risk for hematuria, UTI, and nephrolithiasis. There may be impairment of urinary concentrating ability[258] or urinary acidification (renal tubular acidosis [RTA]), but the GFR is normal.[266,267] The urinary concentrating defect can lead to complaints of polyuria in a child.[258] The increased risk of nephrolithiasis and nephrocalcinosis[268–270] is probably secondary to stagnation in the dilated collecting tubules and an increased incidence of hypercalciuria,[271] hypocitraturia, and hypomagnesuria.[272,273] Patients with RTA are more likely to have hypercalciuria or hypocitraturia, and the acidification defect may be the primary problem.[271,272,274] Nevertheless, even patients without a defect in urinary ion excretion have an increased risk of nephrolithiasis,[270] arguing for a role of the dilated tubules.[275]

The RTA in MSK, when present in a child, can lead to growth retardation.[259] RTA is sometimes associated with severe potassium wasting and this can lead to symptomatic hypokalemia.[276]

Hematuria is usually mild, but massive bleeding is occasionally seen.[277] More commonly, MSK is the explanation for asymptomatic microscopic or gross hematuria, and these are frequent complaints in pediatric cases.[257,258]

The increased risk of UTI may be related to stasis in the dilated tubules and the presence of stones, which may cause obstruction or act as a nidus of infection. UTI in MSK is occasionally complicated by abscess formation.[278]

Associated anomalies reported with MSK include hemihypertrophy,[259,279–283] Caroli's disease,[284,285] hyperparathyroidism[286,287] and a variety of miscellaneous disorders.[261,288,289]

Most patients require limited treatment. Nephrolithiasis is successfully treated by the usual approaches, including extracorporeal shock wave lithotripsy (ESWL).[290] Patients with MSK and RTA have a good response to alkali therapy, with decreased hypercalciuria and stone formation.[271,291] UTIs are treated conventionally, with the caveat that an abscess should be suspected if the patient does not respond.[278]

Glomerulocystic kidney disease

Glomerular cysts are present in a variety of diseases (Table 22.9); the diagnosis is made by kidney biopsy. The term 'glomerulocystic kidney disease' is reserved for patients who do not have an underlying disease such as ADPKD. As detailed below, glomerulocystic kidney disease (GCKD) is not a uniform, well-defined entity; rather it describes a heterogeneous group of patients who have been grouped into categories based on apparent inheritance and kidney size.

Glomerular cysts may be seen in children with a variety of severe, usually inherited, malformation syndromes (see Table 22.9).[292–299] Many of these

Table 22.9 Diseases with glomerular cysts

Syndromes with glomerular cysts:

- Brachymesomelia–renal syndrome
- Oral–facial–digital syndrome
- Glutaric acidemia type II
- Trisomy 18
- Renal retinal dysplasia
- Short-rib polydactyly syndrome type II
- Tuberous sclerosis
- Zellweger syndrome
- Autosomal dominant polycystic kidney disease
- Sporadic glomerulocystic kidney disease
- Familial hypoplastic glomerulocystic kidney disease
- Autosomal dominant glomerulocystic kidney disease

patients have accompanying renal dysplasia. Again, these patients have glomerular cysts, but do not have GCKD.

Glomerular cysts are seen in ADPKD, but most patients also have cysts involving other segments of the nephron.[123,300,301] However, there are cases of GCKD in children with a strong family history of ADPKD.[90,302] This suggests that, in these patients, GCKD is a variant of ADPKD, with predominance of glomerular cysts. In fact, one child had GCKD on initial biopsy, but subsequently had pathologic findings consistent with ADPKD.[302] It has also been hypothesized that some patients with 'sporadic' GCKD may, in fact, have ADPKD, either due to a new mutation or because of incomplete family studies.

Children with sporadic GCKD have a variable presentation. The kidneys are frequently enlarged at birth, with a loss of corticomedullary differentiation.[303,304] Kidney size may normalize,[304] and occasionally the medulla is of normal echogenicity despite an echogenic cortex.[303] Ultrasound and MRI can identify cortical cysts.[41,305] Renal function may be normal[303,304] or decreased.[306,307] Other cases of sporadic GCKD present in adults; these patients may have mild[57,308] or severe[309–311] renal failure, typically with enlarged kidneys.

There is an autosomal dominant form of GCKD that is associated with small (hypoplastic) kidneys and malformed or absent calices.[312,313] These children have a decreased GFR at birth, but then renal function remains fairly stable. Some of these patients have been growth retarded,[313] and a few have a noticeable prognathism.[312,313] In some families, hypoplastic GCKD is secondary to mutations in hepatocyte nuclear factor (HNF)-1β.[314–316] Heterozygous mutations in HNF-1β may also cause maturity-onset diabetes of the young (MODY), and thus affected patients may have renal disease and diabetes.[314–316]

The remaining families with GCKD have normal or increased kidney size. In one family with apparent autosomal dominant inheritance, kidney size and kidney function were normal, but those affected had an abnormal ultrasound.[317] In another family, a 10-year-old girl with an affected father had a mildly depressed GFR.[318] Melnick et al[319] describe three siblings and their father; all had normal kidney size but a decreased GFR. Finally, a large family with GCKD was extensively studied by Sharp and colleagues.[320] These patients had hypertension, and renal function ranged from normal to ESRD. The kidneys were large and echogenic; pelvocaliectasis and a hypoechoic cortical rim were additional sonographic features. Inheritance was autosomal dominant and linkage analysis indicated that neither the *PKD1* gene nor the *PKD2* gene was responsible for this family's disease.[320]

Simple renal cysts

The increased use of radiologic testing has led to the identification of more children with simple cysts, which may be solitary or multiple. The incidence of simple cysts increases with age.[321–324] Fewer than 0.3% of children have simple renal cysts, and they are usually not associated with subsequent problems.[325] Cysts in children usually do not increase in size, and single cysts are commonly located in the right upper pole.[325] However, the presence of even a single cyst in the context of an appropriate family history supports a diagnosis of ADPKD.[134] The incidence of simple renal cysts is increased in children with acquired immunodeficiency syndrome (AIDS).[326] Simple renal cysts are rarely detected by fetal ultrasonography, and the majority resolve before delivery.[327]

Simple renal cysts do not impair renal function,[325,328] except in rare instances.[329] They may play a role in causing infection[330] or hypertension[322,329,331,332] in some patients. Cysts in children occasionally cause pain.[333,334] Symptomatic cysts can be treated by percutaneous drainage, although they usually recur unless a sclerosing agent is injected. Injection of the cyst with either alcohol[335,336] or tetracycline[333] prevents recurrence. Surgical marsupialization is rarely necessary. Because cysts frequently occur in the upper pole, it is sometimes difficult to differentiate a cyst from upper pole hydronephrosis due to an obstructed ureterocele or an ectopic ureter. Such a diagnostic dilemma can be resolved by cyst aspiration.[333,337] Cyst fluid has the same blood urea nitrogen (BUN) and creatinine concentration as the patient.[337] Most children with simple renal cysts only need routine ultrasound follow-up, unless the cysts are atypical and therefore suggestive of a malignancy.

Multilocular cysts

A multilocular cyst is a unilateral, benign tumor of the kidney. Approximately half the cases occur in children, with the remainder in middle-aged adults.[338] The children are more likely to be male, whereas the adults are more likely to be female. Children are usually <2 years of age, and the most common presenting complaint is an abdominal mass.[338,339]

Pathologically, the multilocular cyst is well encapsulated and non-infiltrating. The multiple cysts, which do not communicate, are typically separated by fibrous tissue, although embryonic tissue is sometimes present, especially in pediatric cases. The cysts are well visualized by a CT scan or ultrasound. The differential diagnosis includes Wilms' tumor, ADPKD, or a multicystic dysplastic kidney. Occasionally, a second multilocular cyst appears months later in the contralateral kidney.[340]

Because of the possibility of a cystic Wilms' tumor, surgical resection is recommended.[338] Nephrectomy is sometimes the only option, but increasing numbers of cases are managed with renal preserving surgery.[338,340]

Acquired cystic kidney disease

Kidney failure is sometimes associated with cyst formation in a previously non-cystic kidney. Acquired cystic kidney disease (ACKD) occurs in patients with renal failure, including dialysis patients, transplant patients, and chronic renal failure patients. ACKD occurs in children and the number of cysts increases over time.[341–345] Children with ACKD are at a low risk for gross hematuria and retroperitoneal hemorrhage.[342] More ominously, a small percentage of children develop renal cell carcinoma.[343,345] Because of this possibility, periodic ultrasound screening of dialysis patients is necessary and children with suspicious lesions should have a nephrectomy.

Syndromes with cystic kidneys

A large number of syndromes are associated with cystic kidneys. These are mostly rare diseases and many are neonatally fatal. We will briefly review the major features of a few prominent entities, emphasizing those with a defined genetic etiology.

Tuberous sclerosis

Although classified as one of the neurocutaneous syndromes, renal involvement is an important cause of morbidity and mortality in tuberous sclerosis (TS).[346,347] Patients with TS develop hamartomas in a variety of organs, including angiomyolipomas of the kidneys. The major extrarenal manifestations of TS are summarized in Table 22.10. Most of the features of TS become more prominent over time, except for cardiac rhabdomyomas, which tend to regress during childhood.[348] The hypopigmented macules (ash-leaf spots) are especially helpful diagnostically, since they are often visible at birth and are eventually present in over 97% of children;[349] use of a woods lamp, especially in light-skinned individuals, may aid in their identification. Facial angiofibromas, which may be confused with acne, and shagreen patches are also extremely common. Neurologic lesions include multiple calcified tubers, disorders of neuron migration, and giant cell astrocytomas. The neurologic manifestations, with both seizures and developmental delay, are often the dominant clinical feature. Tumors of the kidney are the most common cause of malignancy in TS, but a variety of extrarenal cancers are also seen in adults and children.[350,351]

TS is an autosomal dominant condition, but two-thirds of the cases are due to new mutations, so most patients will not have a positive family history. There is variable penetrance and thus affected parents usually have mild disease and may be undiagnosed. TS is caused by mutations in either the *TSC1* gene on chromosome 9[352] or the *TSC2* gene on chromosome 16.[353] Both of these genes encode tumor suppressors and the hamartomas arise because of mutations in the normal wild-type gene.[354,355] Intellectual disability is more common in patients with mutations in the

Table 22.10 Extrarenal manifestations of tuberous sclerosis

Neurologic:
- Cortical tubers
- Seizures
- Mental retardation
- Intracranial aneurysms
- Retinal hamartoma

Cutaneous:
- Hypopigmented macules
- Facial angiofibromas
- Shagreen patch
- Café-au-lait macules
- Molluscum fibrosum pendulum
- Forehead fibrous plaque
- Periungual fibromas
- Confetti-like macules

Cardiac:
- Rhabdomyomas
- Wolff–Parkinson–White syndrome

Bone:
- Sclerosis
- Cystic changes

Pulmonary lymphangiomyomatosis

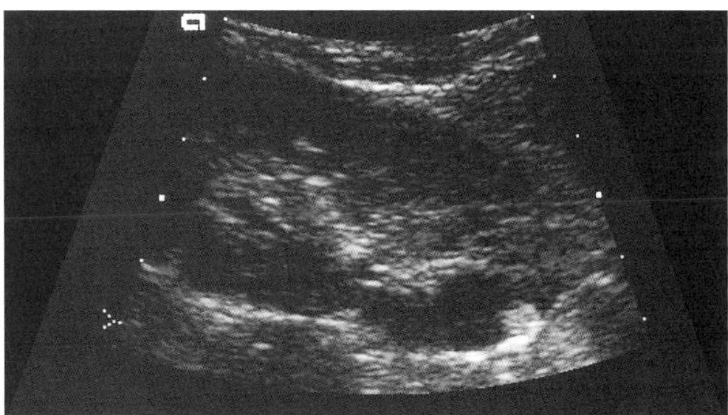

Figure 22.11 Ultrasound of a child with angiomyolipomas due to tuberous sclerosis. This case shows the hyperechoic fat (without shadowing) of an angiomyolipoma. (Courtesy of Dr J Sty, Children's Hospital of Wisconsin.)

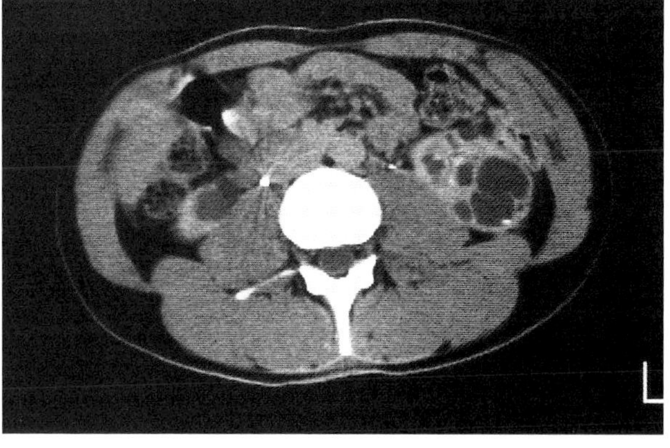

Figure 22.12 Renal CT of a child with cysts due to tuberous sclerosis. Multiple cysts are visible. (Courtesy of Dr J Sty, Children's Hospital of Wisconsin.)

TSC2 gene.[356,357] The *TSC2* gene is located adjacent to the *PKD1* gene on chromosome 16.[72] Some children have large chromosomal deletions that affect both the *TSC2* gene and the *PKD1* gene and these children tend to have severe polycystic kidney disease.[72,358] This contiguous gene syndrome is present in the majority of children with early, severe polycystic kidney disease and TS.[359]

Angiomyolipomas are the most common renal lesion in TS and are readily seen by CT or ultrasound (Figure 22.11). Angiomyolipomas are usually not detected in the first few years of life but they are ultimately found in most children with TS and they tend to increase in size during childhood.[360,361] Larger angiomyolipomas are sometimes associated with pain.[347] Hematuria is uncommon.[362] However, retroperitoneal bleeding from angiomyolipomas can be life threatening[346] and presents with sudden flank pain, a palpable abdominal mass, and symptoms of anemia. Clinical manifestations of angiomyolipomas are relatively uncommon in children.[363,364]

Renal cysts (Figure 22.12) are less common than angiomyolipomas and sometimes disappear on subsequent evaluation.[360] Renal malignancies, including renal cell carcinoma and malignant angiomyolipomas, are a serious concern in TS and both are seen in children, sometimes in early childhood.[350,360]

Both renal cysts and angiomyolipomas cause destruction of normal renal tissue, and this can lead to renal failure in adults[365] and children.[359] The risk of renal failure and hypertension is greater in patients with cystic disease.[366–368] Children with disruption of the contiguous *PKD1* and *TSC2* genes usually have severe cystic disease and are at high risk for hypertension and early kidney failure.[359]

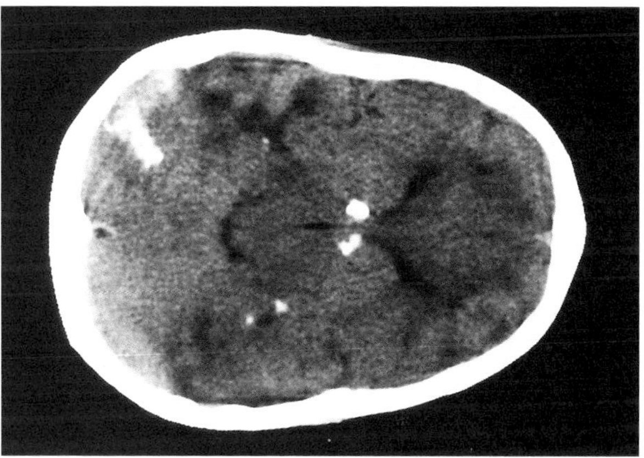

Figure 22.13 Head CT of the same child shown in Figure 22.12. Subendymal calcific densities are present in the region of the foramen magnum. (Courtesy of Dr J Sty, Children's Hospital of Wisconsin.)

The diagnosis of TS is based on the classic clinical features, although genetic testing is commercially available. The possibility of TS should be suspected in a young child with large renal cysts suggestive of early-onset ADPKD. These children may have the contiguous gene syndrome with a deletion affecting both the *PKD1* and *TSC2* genes. A family history of TS is often not present due to variable penetrance and a high rate of new mutations. A search for skin manifestations is usually helpful, although cutaneous manifestations are less prominent or sometimes absent in infants.[349] Young children have fewer cortical tubers than older patients but MRI is quite sensitive for detecting other subtle findings in infancy.[369] Although MRI is more sensitive, most children have the mineralized subendymal nodules that are visible by CT (Figure 22.13).

Children with TS require the input of multiple specialists. All children with TS should have a renal ultrasound at diagnosis and follow-up renal ultrasounds every 1–3 years, with frequency dictated by the specific clinical situation.[370] Patients with extensive or rapidly changing lesions require more frequent follow-up. Those with more severe kidney disease may require CT or MRI to screen for malignant changes. Differentiating angiomyolipomas from malignancy requires careful comparison of sequential images. Patients with kidney failure are treated with dialysis[365] and transplantation.[371] Because of the risk for renal hemorrhage and malignancy, there is an argument for bilateral nephrectomies in children who progress to ESRD, especially those with large angiomyolipomas.

Meckel's syndrome

Meckel's syndrome, sometimes called Meckel–Gruber syndrome, is a lethal autosomal recessive disorder. The most common extrarenal manifestations are posterior encephalocele, polydactyly, and hepatic fibrosis and cysts; however, a variety of other findings may also be present.[372,373] Cystic dysplasia of the kidneys is present in all cases.[372,373] Multiple genetic loci for Meckel's syndrome have been identified.[374–376]

Von Hippel–Lindau disease

Von Hippel–Lindau (VHL) disease is a rare autosomal dominant disorder with variable penetrance. The most prevalent manifestations are cerebellar hemangioblastoma, retinal angioma, pancreatic cysts, renal cell carcinoma, spinal hemangioblastoma, and pheochromocytoma.[377,378] Renal cysts are also common but, like renal cell carcinoma, they are rarely seen in childhood.[377,378] A mutation in a tumor-suppressor gene, located on chromosome 3, causes VHL disease;[379] genetic testing is commercially available.

References

1. Pazour GJ. Intraflagellar transport and cilia-dependent renal disease: the ciliary hypothesis of polycystic kidney disease. J Am Soc Nephrol 2004; 15:2528–36.
2. Menezes LF, Cai Y, Nagasawa Y et al. Polyductin, the PKHD1 gene product, comprises isoforms expressed in plasma membrane, primary cilium, and cytoplasm. Kidney Int 2004; 66:1345–55.
3. Praetorius HA, Spring KR. Bending the MDCK cell primary cilium increases intracellular calcium. J Membr Biol 2001; 184:71–9.
4. Nauli SM, Alenghat FJ, Luo Y et al. Polycystins 1 and 2 mediate mechanosensation in the primary cilium of kidney cells. Nat Genet 2003; 33:129–37.
5. Cole BR. Autosomal recessive polycystic kidney disease. In: Gardner KD Jr, Bernstein J, eds. The Cystic Kidney. Boston: Kluwer Academic, 1990: 327–50.
6. Zerres K. Autosomal recessive polycystic kidney disease. Clin Invest 1992; 70:794–801.
7. Ward CJ, Hogan MC, Rossetti S et al. The gene mutated in autosomal recessive polycystic kidney disease encodes a large, receptor-like protein. Nat Genet 2002; 30:259–69.
8. Onuchic LF, Furu L, Nagasawa Y et al. PKHD1, the polycystic kidney and hepatic disease 1 gene, encodes a novel large protein containing multiple immunoglobulin-like plexin-transcription-factor domains and parallel beta-helix 1 repeats. Am J Hum Genet 2002; 70:1305–17.
9. Furu L, Onuchic LF, Gharavi A et al. Milder presentation of recessive polycystic kidney disease requires presence of amino acid substitution mutations. J Am Soc Nephrol 2003; 14:2004–14.
10. Bergmann C, Senderek J, Sedlacek B et al. Spectrum of mutations in the gene for autosomal recessive polycystic kidney disease (ARPKD/PKHD1). J Am Soc Nephrol 2003; 14:76–89.
11. Deget F, Rudnik-Schoneborn S, Zerres K. Course of autosomal recessive polycystic kidney disease (ARPKD) in siblings: a clinical comparison of 20 sibships. Clin Genet 1995; 47:248–53.
12. Gang DL, Herrin JT. Infantile polycystic disease of the liver and kidneys. Clin Nephrol 1986; 25:28–36.
13. Barth RA, Guillot AP, Capeless EL, Clemmons JJ. Prenatal diagnosis of autosomal recessive polycystic kidney disease: variable outcome within one family. Am J Obstet Gynecol 1992; 166:560–1.
14. Osathanondh V, Potter EL. Pathogenesis of polycystic kidneys. Arch Pathol 1964; 77:466–73.
15. Lieberman E, Salinas-Madrigal L, Gwinn JL et al. Infantile polycystic disease of the kidneys and liver: clinical, pathological and radiological correlations and comparison with congenital hepatic fibrosis. Medicine (Baltimore) 1971; 50:277–318.
16. Landing BH, Wells TR, Claireaux AE. Morphometric analysis of liver lesions in cystic diseases of childhood. Hum Pathol 1980; 11:549–60.
17. Bernstein J. Hepatic involvement in hereditary renal syndromes. Birth Defects Orig Artic Ser 1987; 23:115–30.
18. Kaplan BS, Fay J, Shah V, Dillon MJ, Barratt TM. Autosomal recessive polycystic kidney disease. Pediatr Nephrol 1989; 3:43–9.
19. Isdale JM, Thomson PD, Katz S. Infantile polycystic disease of the kidneys. S Afr Med J 1973; 47:1892–6.
20. Kääriäinen H, Koskimies O, Norio R. Dominant and recessive polycystic kidney disease in children: evaluation of clinical features and laboratory data. Pediatr Nephrol 1988; 2:296–302.
21. Bean SA, Bednarek FJ, Primack WA. Aggressive respiratory support and unilateral nephrectomy for infants with severe perinatal autosomal recessive polycystic kidney disease. J Pediatr 1995; 127:311–13.
22. Gagnadoux MF, Habib R, Levy M, Brunelle F, Broyer M. Cystic renal diseases in children. Adv Nephrol Necker Hosp 1989; 18:33–57.

23. Hoyer PF. A young adult with so-called infantile cystic kidney disease. Nephrol Dial Transplant 1996; 11:377–8.
24. Cole BR, Conley SB, Stapleton FB. Polycystic kidney disease in the first year of life. J Pediatr 1987; 111:693–9.
25. Mattoo TK, Khatani Y, Ashraf B. Autosomal recessive polycystic kidney disease in 15 Arab children. Pediatr Nephrol 1994; 8:85–7.
26. Zerres K, Rudnik-Schoneborn S, Deget F et al. Autosomal recessive polycystic kidney disease in 115 children: clinical presentation, course and influence of gender. Arbeitsgemeinschaft fur Padiatrische, Nephrologie. Acta Paediatr 1996; 85:437–45.
27. Rahill WJ, Rubin MI. Hypertension in infantile polycystic renal disease. The importance of early recognition and treatment of severe hypertension in polycystic renal disease. Clin Pediatr (Phila) 1972; 11:232–5.
28. Guay-Woodford LM, Desmond RA. Autosomal recessive polycystic kidney disease: the clinical experience in North America. Pediatrics 2003; 111:1072–80.
29. Roy S, Dillon MJ, Trompeter RS, Barratt TM. Autosomal recessive polycystic kidney disease: long-term outcome of neonatal survivors. Pediatr Nephrol 1997; 11:302–6.
30. Anand SK, Chan JC, Lieberman E. Polycystic disease and hepatic fibrosis in children. Renal function studies. Am J Dis Child 1975; 129:810–13.
31. Alvarez F, Bernard O, Brunelle F et al. Congenital hepatic fibrosis in children. J Pediatr 1981; 99:370–5.
32. Jamil B, McMahon LP, Savige JA, Wang YY, Walker RG. A study of long-term morbidity associated with autosomal recessive polycystic kidney disease. Nephrol Dial Transplant 1999; 14:205–9.
33. Rossetti S, Torra R, Coto E et al. A complete mutation screen of PKHD1 in autosomal-recessive polycystic kidney disease (ARPKD) pedigrees. Kidney Int 2003; 64:391–403.
34. Blyth H, Ockenden BG. Polycystic disease of kidney and liver presenting in childhood. J Med Genet 1971; 8:257–84.
35. Neumann HP, Krumme B, van Velthoven V, Orszagh M, Zerres K. Multiple intracranial aneurysms in a patient with autosomal recessive polycystic kidney disease. Nephrol Dial Transplant 1999; 14:936–9.
36. Chapman AB, Rubinstein D, Hughes R et al. Intracranial aneurysms in autosomal dominant polycystic kidney disease. N Engl J Med 1992; 327:916–20.
37. Kääriäinen H, Jääskeläinen J, Kivisaari L, Koskimies O, Norio R. Dominant and recessive polycystic kidney disease in children: classification by intravenous pyelography, ultrasound, and computed tomography. Pediatr Radiol 1988; 18:45–50.
38. Chilton SJ, Cremin BJ. The spectrum of polycystic disease in children. Pediatr Radiol 1981; 11:9–15.
39. Metreweli C, Garel L. The echographic diagnosis of infantile renal polycystic disease. Ann Radiol (Paris) 1980; 23:103–7.
40. Avni FE, Guissard G, Hall M et al. Hereditary polycystic kidney diseases in children: changing sonographic patterns through childhood. Pediatr Radiol 2002; 32:169–74.
41. Mercado-Deane MG, Beeson JE, John SD. US of renal insufficiency in neonates. Radiographics 2002; 22: 1429–38.
42. Boal DK, Teele RL. Sonography of infantile polycystic kidney disease. AJR Am J Roentgenol 1980; 135: 575–80.
43. Cobben JM, Breuning MH, Schoots C, ten Kate LP, Zerres K. Congenital hepatic fibrosis in autosomal-dominant polycystic kidney disease. Kidney Int 1990; 38:880–5.
44. Lipschitz B, Berdon WE, Defelice AR, Levy J. Association of congenital hepatic fibrosis with autosomal dominant polycystic kidney disease. Report of a family with review of literature. Pediatr Radiol 1993; 23:131–3.
45. Consugar MB, Anderson SA, Rossetti S et al. Haplotype analysis improves molecular diagnostics of autosomal recessive polycystic kidney disease. Am J Kidney Dis 2005; 45:77–87.
46. Stapleton FB, Hilton S, Wilcox J, Leopold GR. Transient nephromegaly simulating infantile polycystic disease of the kidneys. Pediatrics 1981; 67:554–9.
47. Blankenberg TA, Ruebner BH, Ellis WG, Bernstein J, Dimmick JE. Pathology of renal and hepatic anomalies in Meckel syndrome. Am J Med Genet 1987; 3(Suppl): 395–410.
48. Boichis H, Passwell J, David R, Miller H. Congenital hepatic fibrosis and nephronophthisis. A family study. Q J Med 1973; 42:221–33.
49. Larson RS, Rudloff MA, Liapis H et al. The Ivemark syndrome: prenatal diagnosis of an uncommon cystic renal lesion with heterogeneous associations. Pediatr Nephrol 1995; 9:594–8.
50. Brueton LA, Dillon MJ, Winter RM. Ellis–van creveld syndrome, Jeune syndrome, and renal–hepatic–pancreatic dysplasia: separate entities or disease spectrum? J Med Genet 1990; 27:252–5.
51. Kumar S, Rankin R. Renal insufficiency is a component of COACH syndrome. Am J Med Genet 1996; 61:122–6.
52. Pagon RA, Haas JE, Bunt AH, Rodaway KA. Hepatic involvement in the Bardet–Biedl syndrome. Am J Med Genet 1982; 13:373–81.
53. Habif DVJ, Berdon WE, Yeh MN. Infantile polycystic kidney disease: in utero sonographic diagnosis. Radiology 1982; 142:475–7.
54. Zerres K, Hansmann M, Mallmann R, Gembruch U. Autosomal recessive polycystic kidney disease. Problems of prenatal diagnosis. Prenat Diagn 1988; 8:215–29.
55. Lilford RJ, Irving HC, Allibone EB. A tale of two prior probabilities – avoiding the false positive antenatal diagnosis of autosomal recessive polycystic kidney disease. Br J Obstet Gynaecol 1992; 99:216–19.
56. Bronshtein M, Bar-Hava I, Blumenfeld Z. Clues and pitfalls in the early prenatal diagnosis of 'late onset' infantile polycystic kidney. Prenat Diagn 1992; 12:293–8.
57. Romero R, Bonal J, Campo E, Pelegri A, Palacin A. Glomerulocystic kidney disease: a single entity? Nephron 1993; 63:100–3.
58. Reuss A, Wladimiroff JW, Stewart PA, Niermeijer MF. Prenatal diagnosis by ultrasound in pregnancies at risk for autosomal recessive polycystic kidney disease. Ultrasound Med Biol 1990; 16:355–9.

59. Luthy DA, Hirsch JH. Infantile polycystic kidney disease: observations from attempts at prenatal diagnosis. Am J Med Genet 1985; 20:505–17.
60. Argubright KF, Wicks JD. Third trimester ultrasonic presentation of infantile polycystic kidney disease. Am J Perinatol 1987; 4:1–4.
61. Nasu K, Yoshimatsu J, Anai T et al. Magnetic resonance imaging of fetal autosomal recessive polycystic kidney disease. J Obstet Gynaecol Res 1998; 24:33–6.
62. Zerres K, Mucher G, Becker J et al. Prenatal diagnosis of autosomal recessive polycystic kidney disease (ARPKD): molecular genetics, clinical experience, and fetal morphology. Am J Med Genet 1998; 76:137–44.
63. Sumfest JM, Burns MW, Mitchell ME. Aggressive surgical and medical management of autosomal recessive polycystic kidney disease. Urology 1993; 42:309–12.
64. D'Amico G, Pagliaro L, Bosch J. The treatment of portal hypertension: a meta-analytic review. Hepatology 1995; 22:332–54.
65. McGonigle RJ, Mowat AP, Bewick M et al. Congenital hepatic fibrosis and polycystic kidney disease; role of porta-caval shunting and transplantation in three patients. Q J Med 1981; 50:269–78.
66. Consortium TEPKD. The polycystic kidney disease 1 gene encodes a 14 kb transcript and lies within a duplicated region on chromosome 16. Cell 1994; 77:881–94.
67. Mochizuki T, Wu G, Hayashi T et al. PKD2, a gene for polycystic kidney disease that encodes an integral membrane protein. Science 1996; 272:1339–42.
68. de Almeida S, de Almeida E, Peters D et al. Autosomal dominant polycystic kidney disease: evidence for the existence of a third locus in a Portuguese family. Hum Genet 1995; 96:83–8.
69. Daoust MC, Reynolds DM, Bichet DG, Somlo S. Evidence for a third genetic locus for autosomal dominant polycystic kidney disease. Genomics 1995; 25:733–6.
70. Turco AE, Clementi M, Rossetti S, Tenconi R, Pignatti PF. An Italian family with autosomal dominant polycystic kidney disease unlinked to either the PKD1 or PKD2 gene. Am J Kidney Dis 1996; 28:759–61.
71. Paterson AD, Pei Y. Is there a third gene for autosomal dominant polycystic kidney disease? Kidney Int 1998; 54:1759–61.
72. Harris PC, Ward CJ, Peral B, Hughes J. Polycystic kidney disease. 1: Identification and analysis of the primary defect. J Am Soc Nephrol 1995; 6:1125–33.
73. Qian F, Germino FJ, Cai Y et al. PKD1 interacts with PKD2 through a probable coiled-coil domain. Nat Genet 1997; 16:179–83.
74. Tsiokas L, Kim E, Arnould T, Sukhatme VP, Walz G. Homo- and heterodimeric interactions between the gene products of PKD1 and PKD2. Proc Natl Acad Sci USA 1997; 94:6965–70.
75. Ong AC, Wheatley DN. Polycystic kidney disease – the ciliary connection. Lancet 2003; 361:774–6.
76. Qian F, Watnick TJ, Onuchic LF, Germino GG. The molecular basis of focal cyst formation in human autosomal dominant polycystic kidney disease type I. Cell 1996; 87:979–87.
77. Brasier JL, Henske EP. Loss of the polycystic kidney disease (PKD1) region of chromosome 16p13 in renal cyst cells supports a loss-of-function model for cyst pathogenesis. J Clin Invest 1997; 99:194–9.
78. Koptides M, Hadjimichael C, Koupepidou P, Pierides A, Constantinou Deltas C. Germinal and somatic mutations in the PKD2 gene of renal cysts in autosomal dominant polycystic kidney disease. Hum Mol Genet 1999; 8:509–13.
79. Pei Y, Watnick T, He N et al. Somatic PKD2 mutations in individual kidney and liver cysts support a two-hit model of cystogenesis in type 2 autosomal dominant polycystic kidney disease. J Am Soc Nephrol 1999; 10:1524–9.
80. Hateboer N, v Dijk MA, Bogdanova N et al. Comparison of phenotypes of polycystic kidney disease types 1 and 2. European PKD1-PKD2 Study Group. Lancet 1999; 353:103–7.
81. Hateboer N, Veldhuisen B, Peters D et al. Location of mutations within the PKD2 gene influences clinical outcome. Kidney Int 2000; 57:1444–51.
82. Rossetti S, Burton S, Strmecki L et al. The position of the polycystic kidney disease 1 (PKD1) gene mutation correlates with the severity of renal disease. J Am Soc Nephrol 2002; 13:1230–7.
83. Magistroni R, He N, Wang K et al. Genotype–renal function correlation in type 2 autosomal dominant polycystic kidney disease. J Am Soc Nephrol 2003; 14:1164–74.
84. Guay-Woodford LM, Wright CJ, Walz G, Churchill GA. Quantitative trait loci modulate renal cystic disease severity in the mouse bpk model. J Am Soc Nephrol 2000; 11:1253–60.
85. Peters DJ, Breuning MH. Autosomal dominant polycystic kidney disease: modification of disease progression. Lancet 2001; 358:1439–44.
86. Persu A, Duyme M, Pirson Y et al. Comparison between siblings and twins supports a role for modifier genes in ADPKD. Kidney Int 2004; 66:2132–6.
87. Pérez-Oller L, Torra R, Badenas C, Milà M, Darnell A. Influence of the ACE gene polymorphism in the progression of renal failure in autosomal dominant polycystic kidney disease. Am J Kidney Dis 1999; 34:273–8.
88. Fryns JP, Vandenberghe K, Moerman F. Mid-trimester ultrasonographic diagnosis of early manifesting 'adult' form of polycystic kidney disease. Hum Genet 1986; 74:461.
89. Zerres K, Hansmann M, Knöpfle G, Stephan M. Prenatal diagnosis of genetically determined early manifestation of autosomal dominant polycystic kidney disease? Hum Genet 1985; 71:368–9.
90. Ross DG, Travers H. Infantile presentation of adult-type polycystic kidney disease in a large kindred. J Pediatr 1975; 87:760–3.
91. Kääriäinen H. Polycystic kidney disease in children: a genetic and epidemiological study of 82 Finnish patients. J Med Genet 1987; 24:474–81.
92. Taitz LS, Brown CB, Blank CE, Steiner GM. Screening for polycystic kidney disease: importance of clinical presentation in the newborn. Arch Dis Child 1987; 62:45–9.
93. Gal A, Wirth B, Kääriäinen H et al. Childhood manifestation of autosomal dominant polycystic kidney disease: no evidence for genetic heterogeneity. Clin Genet 1989; 35:13–19.

94. Fick GM, Johnson AM, Strain JD et al. Characteristics of very early onset autosomal dominant polycystic kidney disease. J Am Soc Nephrol 1993; 3:1863–70.
95. Tee JB, Acott PD, McLellan DH, Crocker JF. Phenotypic heterogeneity in pediatric autosomal dominant polycystic kidney disease at first presentation: a single-center, 20-year review. Am J Kidney Dis 2004; 43:296–303.
96. Gabow PA, Duley I, Johnson AM. Clinical profiles of gross hematuria in autosomal dominant polycystic kidney disease. Am J Kidney Dis 1992; 20:140–3.
97. Kaplan BS, Rabin I, Nogrady MB, Drummond KN. Autosomal dominant polycystic renal disease in children. J Pediatr 1977; 90:782–3.
98. Sedman A, Bell P, Manco-Johnson M et al. Autosomal dominant polycystic kidney disease in childhood: a longitudinal study. Kidney Int 1987; 31:1000–5.
99. Fick GM, Duley IT, Johnson AM et al. The spectrum of autosomal dominant polycystic kidney disease in children. J Am Soc Nephrol 1994; 4:1654–60.
100. Ivy DD, Shaffer EM, Johnson AM et al. Cardiovascular abnormalities in children with autosomal dominant polycystic kidney disease. J Am Soc Nephrol 1995; 5:2032–6.
101. Zeier M, Geberth S, Schmidt KG, Mandelbaum A, Ritz E. Elevated blood pressure profile and left ventricular mass in children and young adults with autosomal dominant polycystic kidney disease. J Am Soc Nephrol 1993; 3:1451–7.
102. Chapman AB, Johnson A, Gabow PA, Schrier RW. The renin–angiotensin–aldosterone system and autosomal dominant polycystic kidney disease. N Engl J Med 1990; 323:1091–6.
103. Sharp C, Johnson A, Gabow P. Factors relating to urinary protein excretion in children with autosomal dominant polycystic kidney disease. J Am Soc Nephrol 1998; 9:1908–14.
104. Torres VE, Wilson DM, Hattery RR, Segura JW. Renal stone disease in autosomal dominant polycystic kidney disease. Am J Kidney Dis 1993; 22:513–19.
105. Sklar AH, Caruana RJ, Lammers JE, Strauser GD. Renal infections in autosomal dominant polycystic kidney disease. Am J Kidney Dis 1987; 10:81–8.
106. Koslowe O, Frank R, Gauthier B, Vergara M, Trachtman H. Urinary tract infections, VUR, and autosomal dominant polycystic kidney disease. Pediatr Nephrol 2003; 18:823–5.
107. Hossack KF, Leddy CL, Johnson AM, Schrier RW, Gabow PA. Echocardiographic findings in autosomal dominant polycystic kidney disease. N Engl J Med 1988; 319:907–12.
108. Modi KB, Grant AC, Garret A, Rodger RS. Indirect inguinal hernia in CAPD patients with polycystic kidney disease. Adv Perit Dial 1989; 5:84–6.
109. Morris-Stiff G, Coles G, Moore R, Jurewicz A, Lord R. Abdominal wall hernia in autosomal dominant polycystic kidney disease. Br J Surg 1997; 84:615–17.
110. Milutinovic J, Fialkow PJ, Rudd TG et al. Liver cysts in patients with autosomal dominant polycystic kidney disease. Am J Med 1980; 68:741–4.
111. Gabow PA, Johnson AM, Kaehny WD et al. Risk factors for the development of hepatic cysts in autosomal dominant polycystic kidney disease. Hepatology 1990; 11:1033–7.
112. Everson GT, Scherzinger A, Berger-Leff N et al. Polycystic liver disease: quantitation of parenchymal and cyst volumes from computed tomography images and clinical correlates of hepatic cysts. Hepatology 1988; 8:1627–34.
113. Torres VE, Rastogi S, King BF et al. Hepatic venous outflow obstruction in autosomal dominant polycystic kidney disease. J Am Soc Nephrol 1994; 5:1186–92.
114. Telenti A, Torres VE, Gross JB Jr et al. Hepatic cyst infection in autosomal dominant polycystic kidney disease. Mayo Clin Proc 1990; 65:933–42.
115. Milutinovic J, Schabel SI, Ainsworth SK. Autosomal dominant polycystic kidney disease with liver and pancreatic involvement in early childhood. Am J Kidney Dis 1989; 13:340–4.
116. Main D, Mennuti MT, Cornfeld D, Coleman B. Prenatal diagnosis of adult polycystic kidney disease. Lancet 1983; 2:337–8.
117. Torra R, Nicolau C, Badenas C et al. Ultrasonographic study of pancreatic cysts in autosomal dominant polycystic kidney disease. Clin Nephrol 1997; 47:19–22.
118. Malka D, Hammel P, Vilgrain V et al. Chronic obstructive pancreatitis due to a pancreatic cyst in a patient with autosomal dominant polycystic kidney disease. Gut 1998; 42:131–4.
119. Stamm ER, Townsend RR, Johnson AM et al. Frequency of ovarian cysts in patients with autosomal dominant polycystic kidney disease. Am J Kidney Dis 1999; 34:120–4.
120. Gabow PA. Autosomal dominant polycystic kidney disease. N Engl J Med 1993; 329:332–42.
121. Fick GM, Johnson AM, Hammond WS, Gabow PA. Causes of death in autosomal dominant polycystic kidney disease. J Am Soc Nephrol 1995; 5:2048–56.
122. Chauveau D, Pirson Y, Verellen-Dumoulin C et al. Intracranial aneurysms in autosomal dominant polycystic kidney disease. Kidney Int 1994; 45:1140–6.
123. Proesmans W, Van Damme B, Casaer P, Marchal G. Autosomal dominant polycystic kidney disease in the neonatal period: association with a cerebral arteriovenous malformation. Pediatrics 1982; 70:971–5.
124. Anton PA, Abramowsky CR. Adult polycystic renal disease presenting in infancy: a report emphasizing the bilateral involvement. J Urol 1982; 128:1290–1.
125. Kubo S, Nakajima M, Fukuda K et al. A 4-year-old girl with autosomal dominant polycystic kidney disease complicated by a ruptured intracranial aneurysm. Eur J Pediatr 2004; 163:675–7.
126. Huston J 3rd, Torres VE, Sulivan PP, Offord KP, Wiebers DO. Value of magnetic resonance angiography for the detection of intracranial aneurysms in autosomal dominant polycystic kidney disease. J Am Soc Nephrol 1993; 3:1871–7.
127. Ruggieri PM, Poulos N, Masaryk TJ et al. Occult intracranial aneurysms in polycystic kidney disease: screening with MR angiography. Radiology 1994; 191:33–9.
128. van Dijk MA, Chang PC, Peters DJ, Breuning MH. Intracranial aneurysms in polycystic kidney disease linked to chromosome 4. J Am Soc Nephrol 1995; 6:1670–3.
129. Gabow PA, Johnson AM, Kaehny WD et al. Factors affecting the progression of renal disease in autosomal-

dominant polycystic kidney disease. Kidney Int 1992; 41:1311–19.

130. Fick-Brosnahan G, Johnson AM, Strain JD, Gabow PA. Renal asymmetry in children with autosomal dominant polycystic kidney disease. Am J Kidney Dis 1999; 34:639–45.
131. Zerres K, Weiss H, Bulla M, Roth B. Prenatal diagnosis of an early manifestation of autosomal dominant adult-type polycystic kidney disease. Lancet 1982; 2:988.
132. Reeders ST, Zerres K, Gal A et al. Prenatal diagnosis of autosomal dominant polycystic kidney disease with a DNA probe. Lancet 1986; 2:6–8.
133. Novelli G, Frontali M, Baldini D et al. Prenatal diagnosis of adult polycystic kidney disease with DNA markers on chromosome 16 and the genetic heterogeneity problem. Prenat Diagn 1989; 9:759–67.
134. Gabow PA, Kimberling WJ, Strain JD, Manco-Johnson ML, Johnson AM. Utility of ultrasonography in the diagnosis of autosomal dominant polycystic kidney disease in children. J Am Soc Nephrol 1997; 8:105–10.
135. Levine E, Grantham JJ. The role of computed tomography in the evaluation of adult polycystic kidney disease. Am J Kidney Dis 1981; 1:99–105.
136. Farrell TP, Boal DK, Wood BP, Dagen JE, Rabinowitz R. Unilateral abdominal mass: an unusual presentation of autosomal dominant polycystic kidney disease in children. Pediatr Radiol 1984; 14:349–52.
137. Porch P, Noe HN, Stapleton FB. Unilateral presentation of adult-type polycystic kidney disease in children. J Urol 1986; 135:744–6.
138. Ravine D, Gibson RN, Walker RG et al. Evaluation of ultrasonographic diagnostic criteria for autosomal dominant polycystic kidney disease 1. Lancet 1994; 343:824–7.
139. Sujansky E, Kreutzer SB, Johnson AM et al. Attitudes of at-risk and affected individuals regarding presymptomatic testing for autosomal dominant polycystic kidney disease. Am J Med Genet 1990; 35:510–15.
140. Zerres K, Rudnik-Schöneborn S, Deget F. Routine examination of children at risk of autosomal dominant polycystic kidney disease. Lancet 1992; 339:1356–7.
141. Golin CO, Johnson AM, Fick G, Gabow PA. Insurance for autosomal dominant polycystic kidney disease patients prior to end-stage renal disease. Am J Kidney Dis 1996; 27:220–3.
142. Torres VE, Wang X, Qian Q et al. Effective treatment of an orthologous model of autosomal dominant polycystic kidney disease. Nat Med 2004; 10:363–4.
143. Klahr S, Breyer JA, Beck GJ et al. Dietary protein restriction, blood pressure control, and the progression of polycystic kidney disease. Modification of Diet in Renal Disease Study Group. J Am Soc Nephrol 1995; 5:2037–47.
144. Schrier R, McFann K, Johnson A et al. Cardiac and renal effects of standard versus rigorous blood pressure control in autosomal-dominant polycystic kidney disease: results of a seven-year prospective randomized study. J Am Soc Nephrol 2002; 13:1733–9.
145. Lewis EJ, Hunsicker LG, Bain RP, Rohde RD. The effect of angiotensin-converting-enzyme inhibition on diabetic nephropathy. The Collaborative Study Group. N Engl J Med 1993; 329:1456–62.
146. Maschio G, Alberti D, Janin G et al. Effect of the angiotensin-converting-enzyme inhibitor benazepril on the progression of chronic renal insufficiency. The Angiotensin-Converting-Enzyme Inhibition in Progressive Renal Insufficiency Study Group. N Engl J Med 1996; 334:939–45.
147. Ecder T, Edelstein CL, Chapman AB et al. Reversal of left ventricular hypertrophy with angiotensin converting enzyme inhibition in hypertensive patients with autosomal dominant polycystic kidney disease. Nephrol Dial Transplant 1999; 14:1113–16.
148. Chapman AB, Gabow PA, Schrier RW. Reversible renal failure associated with angiotensin-converting enzyme inhibitors in polycystic kidney disease. Ann Intern Med 1991; 115:769–73.
149. Kanno Y, Suzuki H, Okada H, Takenaka T, Saruta T. Calcium channel blockers versus ACE inhibitors as antihypertensives in polycystic kidney disease. Q J Med 1996; 89:65–70.
150. National High Blood Pressure Education Program Working Group on Hypertension Control in Children and Adolescents. Update on the 1987 Task Force Report on High Blood Pressure in Children and Adolescents: a working group report from the National High Blood Pressure Education Program. National High Blood Pressure Education Program Working Group on Hypertension Control in Children and Adolescents. Pediatrics 1996; 98:649–58.
151. Elzinga LW, Golper TA, Rashad AL, Carr ME, Bennett WM. Trimethoprim–sulfamethoxazole in cyst fluid from autosomal dominant polycystic kidneys. Kidney Int 1987; 32:884–8.
152. Elzinga LW, Golper TA, Rashad AL, Carr ME, Bennett WM. Ciprofloxacin activity in cyst fluid from polycystic kidneys. Antimicrob Agents Chemother 1988; 32:844–7.
153. Chapman AB, Thickman D, Gabow PA. Percutaneous cyst puncture in the treatment of cyst infection in autosomal dominant polycystic kidney disease. Am J Kidney Dis 1990; 16:252–5.
154. Bennett WM, Elzinga L, Golper TA, Barry JM. Reduction of cyst volume for symptomatic management of autosomal dominant polycystic kidney disease. J Urol 1987; 137:620–2.
155. Chapuis O, Sockeel P, Pallas G, Pons F, Jancovici R. Thoracoscopic renal denervation for intractable autosomal dominant polycystic kidney disease-related pain. Am J Kidney Dis 2004; 43:161–3.
156. Butler WE, Barker FG 2nd, Crowell RM. Patients with polycystic kidney disease would benefit from routine magnetic resonance angiographic screening for intracerebral aneurysms: a decision analysis. Neurosurgery 1996; 38:506–15.
157. Chapman AB, Johnson AM, Gabow PA. Intracranial aneurysms in patients with autosomal dominant polycystic kidney disease: how to diagnose and who to screen. Am J Kidney Dis 1993; 22:526–31.
158. Wiebers DO, Torres VE. Screening for unruptured intracranial aneurysms in autosomal dominant polycystic kidney disease. N Engl J Med 1992; 327:953–5.
159. Pirson Y, Chauveau D, Torres V. Management of cerebral aneurysms in autosomal dominant polycystic kidney disease. J Am Soc Nephrol 2002; 13:269–76.

160. Schrier RW, Belz MM, Johnson AM et al. Repeat imaging for intracranial aneurysms in patients with autosomal dominant polycystic kidney disease with initially negative studies: a prospective ten-year follow-up. J Am Soc Nephrol 2004; 15:1023–8.
161. Gibbs GF, Huston J 3rd, Qian Q et al. Follow-up of intracranial aneurysms in autosomal-dominant polycystic kidney disease. Kidney Int 2004; 65:1621–7.
162. Chapman AB, Johnson AM, Gabow PA, Schrier RW. Overt proteinuria and microalbuminuria in autosomal dominant polycystic kidney disease. J Am Soc Nephrol 1994; 5:1349–54.
163. Fick-Brosnahan GM, Tran ZV, Johnson AM, Strain JD, Gabow PA. Progression of autosomal-dominant polycystic kidney disease in children. Kidney Int 2001; 59:1654–62.
164. Fivush BA, Jabs K, Neu AM et al. Chronic renal insufficiency in children and adolescents: the 1996 annual report of NAPRTCS. North American Pediatric Renal Transplant Cooperative Study. Pediatr Nephrol 1998; 12:328–37.
165. Mollet G, Salomon R, Gribouval O et al. The gene mutated in juvenile nephronophthisis type 4 encodes a novel protein that interacts with nephrocystin [erratum appears in Nat Genet 2002; 32(3):459]. Nat Genet 2002; 32:300–5.
166. Hildebrandt F, Otto E, Rensing C et al. A novel gene encoding an SH3 domain protein is mutated in nephronophthisis type 1. Nat Genet 1997; 17:149–53.
167. Saunier S, Calado J, Heilig R et al. A novel gene that encodes a protein with a putative src homology 3 domain is a candidate gene for familial juvenile nephronophthisis. Hum Mol Genet 1997; 6:2317–23.
168. Konrad M, Saunier S, Heidet L et al. Large homozygous deletions of the 2q13 region are a major cause of juvenile nephronophthisis. Hum Mol Genet 1996; 5:367–71.
169. Waldherr R, Lennert T, Weber HP, Födisch HJ, Schärer K. The nephronophthisis complex. A clinicopathologic study in children. Virchows Arch A Pathol Anat Histol 1982; 394:235–54.
170. van Collenburg JJ, Thompson MW, Huber J. Clinical, pathological and genetic aspects of a form of cystic disease of the renal medulla: familial juvenile nephronophthisis (FJN). Clin Nephrol 1978; 9:55–62.
171. Sherman FE, Studnicki FM, Fetterman G. Renal lesions of familial juvenile nephronophthisis examined by microdissection. Am J Clin Pathol 1971; 55:391–400.
172. Matsubara K, Suzuki K, Lin YW, Yamamoto T, Ohta S. Familial juvenile nephronophthisis in two siblings – histological findings at an early stage. Acta Paediatr Jpn 1991; 33:482–7.
173. Elzouki AY, al-Suhaibani H, Mirza K, al-Sowailem AM. Thin-section computed tomography scans detect medullary cysts in patients believed to have juvenile nephronophthisis. Am J Kidney Dis 1996; 27:216–19.
174. Clarke MP, Sullivan TJ, Francis C et al. Senior–Loken syndrome. Case reports of two siblings and association with sensorineural deafness. Br J Ophthalmol 1992; 76:171–2.
175. Tsukahara H, Kikuchi K, Mikawa H et al. Juvenile nephronophthisis diagnosed from glucosuria detected by urine screening at school. Acta Paediatr Jpn 1990; 32:548–51.
176. Hildebrandt F, Omram H. New insights: nephronophthisis-medullary cystic kidney disease. Pediatr Nephrol 2001; 16:168–76.
177. Chamberlin BC, Hagge WW, Stickler GB. Juvenile nephronophthisis and medullary cystic disease. Mayo Clin Proc 1977; 52:485–91.
178. Warady BA, Cibis G, Alon V, Blowey D, Hellerstein S. Senior–Loken syndrome: revisited. Pediatrics 1994; 94:111–12.
179. Ala-Mello S, Kivivuori SM, Rönnholm KA, Koskimies O, Siimes MA. Mechanism underlying early anaemia in children with familial juvenile nephronophthisis. Pediatr Nephrol 1996; 10:578–81.
180. Hildebrandt F, Strahm B, Nothwang HG et al. Molecular genetic identification of families with juvenile nephronophthisis type 1: rate of progression to renal failure. APN Study Group. Arbeitsgemeinschaft für Pädiatrische Nephrologie. Kidney Int 1997; 51:261–9.
181. Haider NB, Carmi R, Shalev H, Sheffield VC, Landau D. A Bedouin kindred with infantile nephronophthisis demonstrates linkage to chromosome 9 by homozygosity mapping. Am J Hum Genet 1998; 63:1404–10.
182. Otto EA, Schermer B, Obara T et al. Mutations in INVS encoding inversin cause nephronophthisis type 2, linking renal cystic disease to the function of primary cilia and left–right axis determination. Nat Genet 2003; 34:413–20.
183. Omran H, Haffner K, Burth S et al. Evidence for further genetic heterogeneity in nephronophthisis. Nephrol Dial Transplant 2001; 16:755–8.
184. Senior B, Friedmann AI, Braudo JL. Juvenile familial nephropathy with tapetoretinal degeneration: a new oculorenal dystrophy. Am J Ophthalmol 1961; 52: 625–33.
185. Løken AC, Hanssen O, Halvorsen S, Jolster NJ. Hereditary renal dysplasia and blindness. Acta Pediatrica 1961; 50:177–83.
186. Steele BT, Lirenman DS, Beattie CW. Nephronophthisis. Am J Med 1980; 68:531–8.
187. Caridi G, Murer L, Bellantuono R et al. Renal-retinal syndromes: association of retinal anomalies and recessive nephronophthisis in patients with homozygous deletion of the NPH1 locus. Am J Kidney Dis 1998; 32:1059–62.
188. Caridi G, Dagnino M, Gusmano R et al. Clinical and molecular heterogeneity of juvenile nephronophthisis in Italy: insights from molecular screening. Am J Kidney Dis 2000; 35:44–51.
189. Otto E, Hoefele J, Ruf R et al. A gene mutated in nephronophthisis and retinitis pigmentosa encodes a novel protein, nephroretinin, conserved in evolution. Am J Hum Genet 2002; 71:1161–7.
190. Olbrich H, Fliegauf M, Hoefele J et al. Mutations in a novel gene, NPHP3, cause adolescent nephronophthisis, tapeto-retinal degeneration and hepatic fibrosis. Nat Genet 2003; 34:455–9.
191. Stanescu B, Michiels J, Proesmans W, Van Damme B. Retinal involvement in a case of nephronophthisis associated with liver fibrosis Senior–Boichis syndrome. Birth Defects Orig Artic Ser 1976; 12:463–74.

192. Delaney V, Mullaney J, Bourke E. Juvenile nephronophthisis, congenital hepatic fibrosis and retinal hypoplasia in twins. Q J Med 1978; 47:281–90.
193. Giedion A. Phalangeal cone shaped epiphysis of the hands (PhCSEH) and chronic renal disease – the conorenal syndromes. Pediatr Radiol 1979; 8:32–8.
194. Fernández-Rodriguez R, Morales JM, Martínez R et al. Senior–Loken syndrome (nephronophthisis and pigmentary retinopathy) associated to liver fibrosis: a family study. Nephron 1990; 55:74–7.
195. Mainzer F, Saldino RM, Ozonoff MB, Minagi H. Familial nephropathy associated with retinitis pigmentosa, cerebellar ataxia and skeletal abnormalities. Am J Med 1970; 49:556–62.
196. Ellis DS, Heckenlively JR, Martin CL et al. Leber's congenital amaurosis associated with familial juvenile nephronophthisis and cone-shaped epiphyses of the hands (the Saldino–Mainzer syndrome). Am J Ophthalmol 1984; 97:233–9.
197. Di Rocco M, Picco P, Arslanian A et al. Retinitis pigmentosa, hypopituitarism, nephronophthisis, and mild skeletal dysplasia (RHYNS): a new syndrome? Am J Med Genet 1997; 73:1–4.
198. Mendley SR, Poznanski AK, Spargo BH, Langman CB. Hereditary sclerosing glomerulopathy in the conorenal syndrome. Am J Kidney Dis 1995; 25:792–7.
199. Parisi MA, Bennett CL, Eckert ML et al. The NPHP1 gene deletion associated with juvenile nephronophthisis is present in a subset of individuals with Joubert syndrome. Am J Hum Genet 2004; 75:82–91.
200. Betz R, Rensing C, Otto E et al. Children with ocular motor apraxia type Cogan carry deletions in the gene (NPHP1) for juvenile nephronophthisis. J Pediatr 2000; 136:828–31.
201. Takano K, Nakamoto T, Okajima M et al. Cerebellar and brainstem involvement in familial juvenile nephronophthisis type I. Pediatr Neurol 2003; 28:142–4.
202. Scolari F, Valzorio B, Vizzardi V et al. Nephronophthisis–medullary cystic kidney disease complex: a report on 24 patients from 5 families with Italian ancestry. Contrib Nephrol 1997; 122:61–3.
203. Garel LA, Habib R, Pariente D, Broyer M, Sauvegrain J. Juvenile nephronophthisis: sonographic appearance in children with severe uremia. Radiology 1984; 151:93–5.
204. Blowey DL, Querfeld U, Geary D, Warady BA, Alon U. Ultrasound findings in juvenile nephronophthisis. Pediatr Nephrol 1996; 10:22–4.
205. Ala-Mello S, Jaaskelainen J, Koskimies O. Familial juvenile nephronophthisis. An ultrasonographic follow-up of seven patients. Acta Radiol 1998; 39:84–9.
206. McGregor AR, Bailey RR. Nephronophthisis–cystic renal medulla complex: diagnosis by computerized tomography. Nephron 1989; 53:70–2.
207. Konrad M, Saunier S, Calado J et al. Familial juvenile nephronophthisis. J Mol Med 1998; 76:310–16.
208. Hildebrandt F, Rensing C, Betz R et al. Establishing an algorithm for molecular genetic diagnostics in 127 families with juvenile nephronophthisis. Kidney Int 2001; 59:434–45.
209. Valadez RA, Firlit CF. Renal transplantation in children with oculorenal syndrome. Urology 1987; 30:130–2.
210. D'Alton M, Romero R, Grannum P et al. Antenatal diagnosis of renal anomalies with ultrasound. IV. Bilateral multicystic kidney disease. Am J Obstet Gynecol 1986; 154:532–7.
211. Dillon E, Ryall A. A 10 year audit of antenatal ultrasound detection of renal disease. Br J Radiol 1998; 71:497–500.
212. Rabelo EA, Oliveira EA, Diniz JS et al. Natural history of multicystic kidney conservatively managed: a prospective study. Pediatr Nephrol 2004; 19:1102–7.
213. Kuwertz-Broeking E, Brinkmann OA, Von Lengerke HJ et al. Unilateral multicystic dysplastic kidney: experience in children. BJU Int 2004; 93:388–92.
214. van Eijk L, Cohen-Overbeek TE, den Hollander NS, Nijman JM, Wladimiroff JW. Unilateral multicystic dysplastic kidney: a combined pre- and postnatal assessment. Ultrasound Obstet Gynecol 2002; 19:180–3.
215. Belk RA, Thomas DF, Mueller RF et al. A family study and the natural history of prenatally detected unilateral multicystic dysplastic kidney. J Urol 2002; 167:666–9.
216. Srivastava T, Garola RE, Hellerstein S. Autosomal dominant inheritance of multicystic dysplastic kidney. Pediatr Nephrol 1999; 13:481–3.
217. Van Allen MI. Congenital disorders of the urinary tract. In: Rimoin DL, Connor JM, Pyeritz RE, eds. Emery and Rimoin's Principles and Practice of Medical Genetics. New York: Churchill Livingstone, 1997: 2611–41.
218. Beck AD. The effect of intra-uterine urinary obstruction upon the development of the fetal kidney. J Urol 1971; 105:784–9.
219. Matsell DG, Bennett T, Goodyer P, Goodyer C, Han VK. The pathogenesis of multicystic dysplastic kidney disease: insights from the study of fetal kidneys. Lab Invest 1996; 74:883–93.
220. Wacksman J. Multicystic dysplastic kidney. In: Ball TP, ed. AUA Update Series Houston: American Urological Association Office of Education, 1998: 66–71.
221. Kessler OJ, Ziv N, Livne PM, Merlob P. Involution rate of multicystic renal dysplasia. Pediatrics 1998; 102:E73.
222. Rottenberg GT, Gordon I, De Bruyn R. The natural history of the multicystic dysplastic kidney in children. Br J Radiol 1997; 70:347–50.
223. Triest JA, Bukowski TP. Multicystic dysplastic kidney as cause of gastric outlet obstruction and respiratory compromise. J Urol 1999; 161:1918–19.
224. Nakano M, Tada K, Takahashi Y et al. [Unilateral multicystic dysplastic kidney in an adult: report of a case]. Hinyokika Kiyo – Acta Urologica Japonica 1996; 42:373–6. [Japanese]
225. Ambrose SS. Unilateral multicystic renal disease in adults. Birth Defects Orig Artic Ser 1977; 13:349–53.
226. Singh I, Sharma D, Singh N, Jain BK, Minocha VR. Hydronephrotic obstructed kidney mimicking a congenital multicystic kidney: case report with review of literature. Int Urol Nephrol 2002; 34:179–82.
227. Sanders RC, Hartman DS. The sonographic distinction between neonatal multicystic kidney and hydronephrosis. Radiology 1984; 151:621–5.
228. Metcalfe PD, Wright JR Jr, Anderson PA. MCDK not excluded by virtue of function on renal scan. Can J Urol 2002; 9:1690–3.
229. Roach PJ, Paltiel HJ, Perez-Atayde A et al. Renal dyspla-

sia in infants: appearance on 99mTc DMSA scintigraphy. Pediatr Radiol 1995; 25:472–5.
230. Atiyeh B, Husmann D, Baum M. Contralateral renal abnormalities in multicystic-dysplastic kidney disease. J Pediatr 1992; 121:65–7.
231. John U, Rudnik-Schoneborn S, Zerres K, Misselwitz J. Kidney growth and renal function in unilateral multicystic dysplastic kidney disease. Pediatr Nephrol 1998; 12:567–71.
232. Mathiot A, Liard A, Eurin D, Dacher JN. [Prenatally detected multicystic renal dysplasia and associated anomalies of the genito-urinary tract]. J Radiol 2002; 83:731–5. [French]
233. Chen YH, Stapleton FB, Roy S 3rd, Noe HN. Neonatal hypertension from a unilateral multicystic dysplastic kidney. J Urol 1985; 133:664–5.
234. Webb NJ, Lewis MA, Bruce J et al. Unilateral multicystic dysplastic kidney: the case for nephrectomy. Arch Dis Child 1997; 76:31–4.
235. Wacksman J, Phipps L. Report of the Multicystic Kidney Registry: preliminary findings. J Urol 1993; 150:1870–2.
236. Homsy YL, Anderson JH, Oudjhane K, Russo P. Wilms tumor and multicystic dysplastic kidney disease. J Urol 1997; 158:2256–9.
237. Rackley RR, Angermeier KW, Levin H, Pontes JE, Kay R. Renal cell carcinoma arising in a regressed multicystic dysplastic kidney. J Urol 1994; 152:1543–5.
238. Beckwith JB. Wilms' tumor and multicystic dysplastic kidney disease. J Urol 1997; 158:2259–60.
239. Narchi H. Risk of Wilms' tumour with multicystic kidney disease: a systematic review. Arch Dis Child 2005; 90:147–9.
240. Perez LM, Naidu SI, Joseph DB. Outcome and cost analysis of operative versus nonoperative management of neonatal multicystic dysplastic kidneys. J Urol 1998; 160:1207–11.
241. Rudnik-Schoneborn S, John U, Deget F et al. Clinical features of unilateral multicystic renal dysplasia in children. Eur J Pediatr 1998; 157:666–72.
242. Eckoldt F, Woderich R, Wolke S et al. Follow-up of unilateral multicystic kidney dysplasia after prenatal diagnosis. J Matern Fetal Neonatal Med 2003; 14:177–86.
243. Feldenberg LR, Siegel NJ. Clinical course and outcome for children with multicystic dysplastic kidneys. Pediatr Nephrol 2000; 14:1098–101.
244. Strauss MB, Sommers SC. Medullary cystic disease and familial juvenile nephronophthisis. N Engl J Med 1967; 277:863–4.
245. Gardner KD Jr. Evolution of clinical signs in adult-onset cystic disease of the renal medulla. Ann Intern Med 1971; 74:47–54.
246. Dahan K, Fuchshuber A, Adamis S et al. Familial juvenile hyperuricemic nephropathy and autosomal dominant medullary cystic kidney disease type 2: two facets of the same disease? J Am Soc Nephrol 2001; 12:2348–57.
247. Christodoulou K, Tsingis M, Stavrou C et al. Chromosome 1 localization of a gene for autosomal dominant medullary cystic kidney disease. Hum Mol Genet 1998; 7:905–11.
248. Scolari F, Puzzer D, Amoroso A et al. Identification of a new locus for medullary cystic disease, on chromosome 16p12. Am J Hum Genet 1999; 64:1655–60.
249. Stavrou C, Pierides A, Zouvani I et al. Medullary cystic kidney disease with hyperuricemia and gout in a large Cypriot family: no allelism with nephronophthisis type 1. Am J Med Genet 1998; 77:149–54.
250. Auranen M, Ala-Mello S, Turunen JA, Jarvela I. Further evidence for linkage of autosomal-dominant medullary cystic kidney disease on chromosome 1q21. Kidney Int 2001; 60:1225–32.
251. Hateboer N, Gumbs C, Teare MD et al. Confirmation of a gene locus for medullary cystic kidney disease (MCKD2) on chromosome 16p12. Kidney Int 2001; 60:1233–9.
252. Scolari F, Ghiggeri GM, Casari G et al. Autosomal dominant medullary cystic disease: a disorder with variable clinical pictures and exclusion of linkage with the NPH1 locus. Nephrol Dial Transplant 1998; 13:2536–46.
253. Hart TC, Gorry MC, Hart PS et al. Mutations of the UMOD gene are responsible for medullary cystic kidney disease 2 and familial juvenile hyperuricaemic nephropathy. J Med Genet 2002; 39:882–92.
254. Turner JJ, Stacey JM, Harding B et al. UROMODULIN mutations cause familial juvenile hyperuricemic nephropathy. J Clin Endocrinol Metab 2003; 88: 1398–401.
255. Rampoldi L, Caridi G, Santon D et al. Allelism of MCKD, FJHN and GCKD caused by impairment of uromodulin export dynamics. Hum Mol Genet 2003; 12:3369–84.
256. Kroiss S, Huck K, Berthold S et al. Evidence of further genetic heterogeneity in autosomal dominant medullary cystic kidney disease. Nephrol Dial Transplant 2000; 15:818–21.
257. Snelling CE, Brown NM, Smythe CA. Medullary sponge kidney in a child. Can Med Assoc J 1970; 102:518–19.
258. Patriquin HB, O'Regan S. Medullary sponge kidney in childhood. AJR Am J Roentgenol 1985; 145:315–19.
259. Sluysmans T, Vanoverschelde JP, Malvaux P. Growth failure associated with medullary sponge kidney, due to incomplete renal tubular acidosis type 1. Eur J Pediatr 1987; 146:78–80.
260. Zawada ETJ, Sica DA. Differential diagnosis of medullary sponge kidney. S Med J 1984; 77:686–9.
261. Khoury Z, Brezis M, Mogle P. Familial medullary sponge kidney in association with congenital absence of teeth (anodontia). Nephron 1988; 48:231–3.
262. Glassberg KI, Hackett RE, Waterhouse K et al. Congenital anomalies of kidney, ureter and bladder. In: Kendall AR, Karafin L, eds. Harry S. Goldsmith's Practice of Surgery: Urology. Hagerstown, MD: Harper and Row, 1982: 1–82.
263. Palubinskas AJ. Renal pyramidal structure opacification in excretory urography and its relation to medullary sponge kidney. Radiology 1963; 81:963–70.
264. Ginalski JM, Schnyder P, Portmann L, Jaeger P. Medullary sponge kidney on axial computed tomography: comparison with excretory urography. Eur J Radiol 1991; 12:104–7.
265. Lang EK, Macchia RJ, Thomas R et al. Improved detection of renal pathologic features on multiphasic helical CT

compared with IVU in patients presenting with microscopic hematuria. Urology 2003; 61:528–32.
266. Green J, Szylman P, Sznajder II, Winaver J, Better OS. Renal tubular handling of potassium in patients with medullary sponge kidney. A model of renal papillectomy in humans. Arch Intern Med 1984; 144:2201–4.
267. Higashihara E, Nutahara K, Tago K, Ueno A, Niijima T. Medullary sponge kidney and renal acidification defect. Kidney Int 1984; 25:453–9.
268. Sage MR, Lawson AD, Marshall VR, Ryall RL. Medullary sponge kidney and urolithiasis. Clin Radiol 1982; 33:435–8.
269. Parks JH, Coe FL, Strauss AL. Calcium nephrolithiasis and medullary sponge kidney in women. N Engl J Med 1982; 306:1088–91.
270. Ginalski JM, Portmann L, Jaeger P. Does medullary sponge kidney cause nephrolithiasis? AJR Am J Roentgenol 1990; 155:299–302.
271. Higashihara E, Nutahara K, Niijima T. Renal hypercalciuria and metabolic acidosis associated with medullary sponge kidney: effect of alkali therapy. Urol Res 1988; 16:95–100.
272. Osther PJ, Hansen AB, Røhl HF. Renal acidification defects in medullary sponge kidney. Br J Urol 1988; 61:392–4.
273. Yagisawa T, Kobayashi C, Hayashi T, Yoshida A, Toma H. Contributory metabolic factors in the development of nephrolithiasis in patients with medullary sponge kidney. Am J Kidney Dis 2001; 37:1140–3.
274. Osther PJ, Mathiasen H, Hansen AB, Nissen HM. Urinary acidification and urinary excretion of calcium and citrate in women with bilateral medullary sponge kidney. Urol Int 1994; 52:126–30.
275. Higashihara E, Nutahara K, Tago K, Ueno A, Niijima T. Unilateral and segmental medullary sponge kidney: renal function and calcium excretion. J Urol 1984; 132:743–5.
276. Jayasinghe KS, Mendis BL, Mohideen R et al. Medullary sponge kidney presenting with hypokalaemic paralysis. Postgrad Med J 1984; 60:303–4.
277. Betts CD, O'Reilly PH. Profound haemorrhage causing acute obstruction in medullary sponge kidney. Br J Urol 1992; 70:449–50.
278. Levine E. Computed tomography of renal abscesses complicating medullary sponge kidney. J Comput Assist Tomogr 1989; 13:440–2.
279. Afonso DN, Oliveira AG. Medullary sponge kidney and congenital hemi-hypertrophy. Br J Urol 1988; 62:187–8.
280. Harris RE, Fuchs EF, Kaempf MJ. Medullary sponge kidney and congenital hemihypertrophy: case report and literature review. J Urol 1981; 126:676–8.
281. Indridason OS, Thomas L, Berkoben M. Medullary sponge kidney associated with congenital hemihypertrophy. J Am Soc Nephrol 1996; 7:1123–30.
282. Saypol DC, Laudone VP. Congenital hemihypertrophy with adrenal carcinoma and medullary sponge kidney. Urology 1983; 21:510–11.
283. Tomooka Y, Onitsuka H, Goya T et al. Congenital hemihypertrophy with adrenal adenoma and medullary sponge kidney. Br J Radiol 1988; 61:851–3.
284. Braga AC, Calheno A, Rocha H, Lourenço-Gomes J. Caroli's disease with congenital hepatic fibrosis and medullary sponge kidney. J Pediatr Gastroenterol Nutr 1994; 19:464–7.
285. Mrowka C, Adam G, Sieberth HG, Matern S. Caroli's syndrome associated with medullary sponge kidney and nephrocalcinosis. Nephrol Dial Transplant 1996; 11:1142–5.
286. Rao DS, Frame B, Block MA, Parfitt AM. Primary hyperparathyroidism. A cause of hypercalciuria and renal stones in patients with medullary sponge kidney. JAMA 1977; 237:1353–5.
287. Maschio G, Tessitore N, D'Angelo A et al. Medullary sponge kidney and hyperparathyroidism – a puzzling association. Am J Nephrol 1982; 2:77–84.
288. Schoeneman MJ, Plewinska M, Mucha M, Mieza M. Marfan syndrome and medullary sponge kidney: case report and speculation on pathogenesis. Int J Pediatr Nephrol 1984; 5:103–4.
289. Umeki S, Soejima R, Kawane H. Young's syndrome accompanied by medullary sponge kidney. Respiration 1989; 55:60–4.
290. Nakada SY, Erturk E, Monaghan J, Cockett AT. Role of extracorporeal shock-wave lithotripsy in treatment of urolithiasis in patients with medullary sponge kidney. Urology 1993; 41:331–3.
291. Higashihara E, Munakata A, Hara M et al. Medullary sponge kidney and hyperparathyroidism. Urology 1988; 31:155–8.
292. Colevas AD, Edwards JL, Hruban RH et al. Glutaric acidemia type II. Comparison of pathologic features in two infants. Arch Pathol Lab Med 1988; 112:1133–9.
293. Craver RD, Ortenberg J, Baliga R. Glomerulocystic disease: unilateral involvement of a horseshoe kidney and in trisomy 18. Pediatr Nephrol 1993; 7:375–8.
294. Kobayashi Y, Hiki Y, Shigematsu H, Tateno S, Mori K. Renal retinal dysplasia with diffuse glomerular cysts. Nephron 1985; 39:201–5.
295. Langer LO Jr, Nishino R, Yamaguchi A et al. Brachymesomelia-renal syndrome. Am J Med Genet 1983; 15:57–65.
296. Montemarano H, Bulas DI, Chandra R, Tifft C. Prenatal diagnosis of glomerulocystic kidney disease in short-rib polydactyly syndrome type II, Majewski type. Pediatr Radiol 1995; 25:469–71.
297. Saguem MH, Laarif M, Remadi S, Bozakoura C, Cox JN. Diffuse bilateral glomerulocystic disease of the kidneys and multiple cardiac rhabdomyomas in a newborn. Relationship with tuberous sclerosis and review of the literature. Pathol Res Pract 1992; 188:367–73.
298. Smith DW, Opitz JM, Inhorn SL. A syndrome of multiple developmental defects including polycystic kidneys and intrahepatic biliary dysgenesis in 2 siblings. J Pediatr 1965; 67:617–24.
299. Stapleton FB, Bernstein J, Koh G, Roy S 3rd, Wilroy RS. Cystic kidneys in a patient with oral–facial–digital syndrome type I. Am J Kidney Dis 1982; 1:288–93.
300. Fellows RA, Leonidas JC, Beatty EC Jr. Radiologic features of 'adult type' polycystic kidney disease in the neonate. Pediatr Radiol 1976; 4:87–92.
301. Edwards OP, Baldinger S. Prenatal onset of autosomal dominant polycystic kidney disease. Urology 1989; 34:265–70.

302. Dedeoglu IO, Fisher JE, Springate JE et al. Spectrum of glomerulocystic kidneys: a case report and review of the literature. Pediatr Pathol Lab Med 1996; 16:941–9.
303. Fredericks BJ, de Campo M, Chow CW, Powell HR. Glomerulocystic renal disease: ultrasound appearances. Pediatr Radiol 1989; 19:184–6.
304. Fitch SJ, Stapleton FB. Ultrasonographic features of glomerulocystic disease in infancy: similarity to infantile polycystic kidney disease. Pediatr Radiol 1986; 16:400–2.
305. Borges Oliva MR, Hsing J, Rybicki FJ et al. Glomerulocystic kidney disease: MRI findings. Abdom Imaging 2003; 28:889–92.
306. McAlister WH, Siegel MJ, Shackelford G, Askin F, Kissane JM. Glomerulocystic kidney. AJR Am J Roentgenol 1979; 133:536–8.
307. Cachero S, Montgomery P, Seidel FG et al. Glomerulocystic kidney disease: case report. Pediatr Radiol 1990; 20:491–3.
308. Dosa S, Thompson AM, Abraham A. Glomerulocystic kidney disease. Report of an adult case. Am J Clin Pathol 1984; 82:619–21.
309. Gonzalez JM, Lombardo ME, Truong LD, Brennan S, Suki WN. Unusual presentation of glomerulocystic kidney disease in an adult patient. Clin Nephrol 1994; 42:266–8.
310. Egashira K, Nakata H, Hashimoto O, Kaizu K. MR imaging of adult glomerulocystic kidney disease. A case report. Acta Radiol 1991; 32:251–3.
311. Oh Y, Onoyama K, Kobayashi K et al. Glomerulocystic kidneys. Report of an adult case. Nephron 1986; 43:299–302.
312. Rizzoni G, Loirat C, Levy M et al. Familial hypoplastic glomerulocystic kidney. A new entity? Clin Nephrol 1982; 18:263–8.
313. Kaplan BS, Gordon I, Pincott J, Barratt TM. Familial hypoplastic glomerulocystic kidney disease: a definite entity with dominant inheritance. Am J Med Genet 1989; 34:569–73.
314. Bingham C, Bulman MP, Ellard S et al. Mutations in the hepatocyte nuclear factor-1beta gene are associated with familial hypoplastic glomerulocystic kidney disease. Am J Hum Genet 2001; 68:219–24.
315. Kolatsi-Joannou M, Bingham C, Ellard S et al. Hepatocyte nuclear factor-1beta: a new kindred with renal cysts and diabetes and gene expression in normal human development. J Am Soc Nephrol 2001; 12:2175–80.
316. Mache CJ, Preisegger KH, Kopp S, Ratschek M, Ring E. De novo HNF-1 beta gene mutation in familial hypoplastic glomerulocystic kidney disease. Pediatr Nephrol 2002; 17:1021–6.
317. Carson RW, Bedi D, Cavallo T, DuBose TD Jr. Familial adult glomerulocystic kidney disease. Am J Kidney Dis 1987; 9:154–65.
318. Reznik VM, Griswold WT, Mendoza SA. Glomerulocystic disease – a case report with 10 year follow-up. Int J Pediatr Nephrol 1982; 3:321–3.
319. Melnick SC, Brewer DB, Oldham JS. Cortical microcystic disease of the kidney with dominant inheritance: a previously undescribed syndrome. J Clin Pathol 1984; 37:494–9.
320. Sharp CK, Bergman SM, Stockwin JM et al. Dominantly transmitted glomerulocystic kidney disease: a distinct genetic entity. J Am Soc Nephrol 1997; 8:77–84.
321. Yamagishi F, Kitahara N, Mogi W, Itoh S. Age-related occurrence of simple renal cysts studied by ultrasonography. Klin Wochenschr 1988; 66:385–7.
322. Caglioti A, Esposito C, Fuiano G et al. Prevalence of symptoms in patients with simple renal cysts. BMJ (Clin Res Ed) 1993; 306:430–1.
323. Tsugaya M, Kajita A, Hayashi Y et al. Detection and monitoring of simple renal cysts with computed tomography. Urol Int 1995; 54:128–31.
324. Terada N, Ichioka K, Matsuta Y et al. The natural history of simple renal cysts. J Urol 2002; 167:21–3.
325. McHugh K, Stringer DA, Hebert D, Babiak CA. Simple renal cysts in children: diagnosis and follow-up with US. Radiology 1991; 178:383–5.
326. Zinn HL, Rosberger ST, Haller JO, Schlesinger AE. Simple renal cysts in children with AIDS. Pediatr Radiol 1997; 27:827–8.
327. Blazer S, Zimmer EZ, Blumenfeld Z, Zelikovic I, Bronshtein M. Natural history of fetal simple renal cysts detected in early pregnancy. J Urol 1999; 162:812–14.
328. Holmberg G, Hietala SO, Karp K, Ohberg L. Significance of simple renal cysts and percutaneous cyst puncture on renal function. Scand J Urol Nephrol 1994; 28:35–8.
329. Singer AJ, Lee SK. Simple renal cysts causing loss of kidney function and hypertension. Urology 2001; 57:363–4.
330. Limjoco UR, Strauch AE. Infected solitary cyst of the kidney: report of a case and review of the literature. J Urol 1966; 96:625–30.
331. Churchill D, Kimoff R, Pinsky M, Gault MH. Solitary intrarenal cyst: correctable cause of hypertension. Urology 1975; 6:485–8.
332. Pedersen JF, Emamian SA, Nielsen MB. Significant association between simple renal cysts and arterial blood pressure. Br J Urol 1997; 79:688–91.
333. Reiner I, Donnell S, Jones M, Carty HL, Richwood AM. Percutaneous sclerotherapy for simple renal cysts in children. Br J Radiol 1992; 65:281–2.
334. Murthi GV, Azmy AF, Wilkinson AG. Management of simple renal cysts in children. J R Coll Surg Edinb 2001; 46:205–7.
335. Hanna RM, Dahniya MH. Aspiration and sclerotherapy of symptomatic simple renal cysts: value of two injections of a sclerosing agent. AJR Am J Roentgenol 1996; 167:781–3.
336. Fontana D, Porpiglia F, Morra I, Destefanis P. Treatment of simple renal cysts by percutaneous drainage with three repeated alcohol injection. Urology 1999; 53:904–7.
337. Steinhardt GF, Slovis TL, Perlmutter AD. Simple renal cysts in infants. Radiology 1985; 155:349–50.
338. Castillo OA, Boyle ET Jr, Kramer SA. Multilocular cysts of kidney. A study of 29 patients and review of literature. Urology 1991; 37:156–62.
339. Austin SR, Castellino RA. Multilocular cysts of kidney. Urology 1973; 1:546–9.
340. Chatten J, Bishop HC. Bilateral multilocular cysts of the kidneys. J Pediatr Surg 1977; 12:749–50.
341. Leichter HE, Dietrich R, Salusky IB et al. Acquired cystic kidney disease in children undergoing long-term dialysis. Pediatr Nephrol 1988; 2:8–11.

342. Kyushu Pediatric Nephrology Study Group. Acquired cystic kidney disease in children undergoing continuous ambulatory peritoneal dialysis. Am J Kidney Dis 1999; 34:242–6.
343. Querfeld U, Schneble F, Wradzidlo W et al. Acquired cystic kidney disease before and after renal transplantation. J Pediatr 1992; 121:61–4.
344. Hogg RJ. Acquired renal cystic disease in children prior to the start of dialysis. Pediatr Nephrol 1992; 6:176–8.
345. Mattoo TK, Greifer I, Geva P, Spitzer A. Acquired renal cystic disease in children and young adults on maintenance dialysis. Pediatr Nephrol 1997; 11:447–50.
346. Shepherd CW, Gomez MR, Lie JT, Crowson CS. Causes of death in patients with tuberous sclerosis. Mayo Clin Proc 1991; 66:792–6.
347. Torres VE, King BF, Holley KE, Blute ML, Gomez MR. The kidney in the tuberous sclerosis complex. Adv Nephrol Necker Hosp 1994; 23:43–70.
348. DiMario FJ Jr, Diana D, Leopold H, Chameides L. Evolution of cardiac rhabdomyoma in tuberous sclerosis complex. Clin Pediatr (Phila) 1996; 35:615–19.
349. Józwiak S, Schwartz RA, Janniger CK, Michalowicz R, Chmielik J. Skin lesions in children with tuberous sclerosis complex: their prevalence, natural course, and diagnostic significance. Int J Dermatol 1998; 37:911–17.
350. Al-Saleem T, Wessner LL, Scheithauer BW et al. Malignant tumors of the kidney, brain, and soft tissues in children and young adults with the tuberous sclerosis complex. Cancer 1998; 83:2208–16.
351. Verhoef S, van Diemen-Steenvoorde R, Akkersdijk WL et al. Malignant pancreatic tumour within the spectrum of tuberous sclerosis complex in childhood. Eur J Pediatr 1999; 158:284–7.
352. van Slegtenhorst M, de Hoogt R, Hermans C et al. Identification of the tuberous sclerosis gene TSC1 on chromosome 9q34. Science 1997; 277:805–8.
353. European Chromosome 16 Tuberous Sclerosis Consortium. Identification and characterization of the tuberous sclerosis gene on chromosome 16. Cell 1993; 75:1305–15.
354. Sepp T, Yates JR, Green AJ. Loss of heterozygosity in tuberous sclerosis hamartomas. J Med Genet 1996; 33:962–4.
355. Carbonara C, Longa L, Grosso E et al. Apparent preferential loss of heterozygosity at TSC2 over TSC1 chromosomal region in tuberous sclerosis hamartomas. Genes Chromosomes Cancer 1996; 15:18–25.
356. Jones AC, Daniells CE, Snell RG et al. Molecular genetic and phenotypic analysis reveals differences between TSC1 and TSC2 associated familial and sporadic tuberous sclerosis. Hum Mol Genet 1997; 6:2155–61.
357. Jones AC, Shyamsundar MM, Thomas MW et al. Comprehensive mutation analysis of TSC1 and TSC2 – and phenotypic correlations in 150 families with tuberous sclerosis. Am J Hum Genet 1999; 64:1305–15.
358. Torra R, Badenas C, Darnell A et al. Facilitated diagnosis of the contiguous gene syndrome: tuberous sclerosis and polycystic kidneys by means of haplotype studies. Am J Kidney Dis 1998; 31:1038–43.
359. Sampson JR, Maheshwar MM, Aspinwall R et al. Renal cystic disease in tuberous sclerosis: role of the polycystic kidney disease 1 gene. Am J Hum Genet 1997; 61:843–51.
360. Ewalt DH, Sheffield E, Sparagana SP, Delgado MR, Roach ES. Renal lesion growth in children with tuberous sclerosis complex. J Urol 1998; 160:141–5.
361. O'Hagan AR, Ellsworth R, Secic M, Rothner AD, Brouhard BH. Renal manifestations of tuberous sclerosis complex. Clin Pediatr (Phila) 1996; 35:483–9.
362. Stillwell TJ, Gomez MR, Kelalis PP. Renal lesions in tuberous sclerosis. J Urol 1987; 138:477–81.
363. Moolten SE. Hamartial nature of the tuberous sclerosis complex and its bearing on the tumor problem; report of a case with tumor anomaly of the kidney and adenoma sebaceum. Arch Intern Med 1942; 69:589–623.
364. Hendren WG, Monfort GJ. Symptomatic bilateral renal angiomyolipomas in a child. J Urol 1987; 137:256–7.
365. Clarke A, Hancock E, Kingswood C, Osborne JP. End-stage renal failure in adults with the tuberous sclerosis complex. Nephrol Dial Transplant 1999; 14:988–91.
366. Stapleton FB, Johnson D, Kaplan GW, Griswold W. The cystic renal lesion in tuberous sclerosis. J Pediatr 1980; 97:574–9.
367. Anderson D, Tannen RL. Tuberous sclerosis and chronic renal failure. Potential confusion with polycystic kidney disease. Am J Med 1969; 47:163–8.
368. Cree JE, Nash FW. Tuberous sclerosis with polycystic kidneys. Proc R Soc Med 1969; 62:327.
369. Baron Y, Barkovich AJ. MR imaging of tuberous sclerosis in neonates and young infants. AJNR Am J Neuroradiol 1999; 20:907–16.
370. Roach ES, DiMario FJ, Kandt RS, Northrup H. Tuberous Sclerosis Consensus Conference: recommendations for diagnostic evaluation. National Tuberous Sclerosis Association. J Child Neurol 1999; 14:401–7.
371. Balligand JL, Pirson Y, Squifflet JP et al. Outcome of patients with tuberous sclerosis after renal transplantation. Transplantation 1990; 49:515–18.
372. Fraser FC, Lytwyn A. Spectrum of anomalies in the Meckel syndrome, or: 'Maybe there is a malformation syndrome with at least one constant anomaly'. Am J Med Genet 1981; 9:67–73.
373. Salonen R. The Meckel syndrome: clinicopathological findings in 67 patients. Am J Med Genet 1984; 18:671–89.
374. Paavola P, Salonen R, Weissenbach J, Peltonen L. The locus for Meckel syndrome with multiple congenital anomalies maps to chromosome 17q21-q24. Nat Genet 1995; 11:213–15.
375. Morgan NV, Gissen P, Sharif SM et al. A novel locus for Meckel–Gruber syndrome, MKS3, maps to chromosome 8q24. Hum Genet 2002; 111:456–61.
376. Roume J, Genin E, Cormier-Daire V et al. A gene for Meckel syndrome maps to chromosome 11q13. Am J Hum Genet 1998; 63:1095–101.
377. Maddock IR, Moran A, Maher ER et al. A genetic register for von Hippel–Lindau disease. J Med Genet 1996; 33:120–7.
378. Maher ER, Yates JR, Harries R et al. Clinical features and natural history of von Hippel–Lindau disease. Q J Med 1990; 77:1151–63.
379. Latif F, Tory K, Gnarra J et al. Identification of the von Hippel–Lindau disease tumor suppressor gene. Science 1993; 260:1317–20.

Acute renal failure

23

Lawrence Copelovitch, Bernard S Kaplan, and Kevin EC Meyers

Introduction

Acute renal failure (ARF) is defined as a sudden decrease of normal kidney function that compromises the normal renal regulation of fluid, electrolyte, and acid–base homeostasis.[1] In practical terms ARF is characterized by a reduction in the glomerular filtration rate (GFR), which results in an abrupt increase in the concentrations of serum creatinine and blood urea nitrogen (BUN). The effect on urine volume in ARF is variable: patients may be anuric, oliguric, and, in some cases, polyuric. ARF develops over a period of hours to days, whereas chronic renal failure (CRF) progresses over months to years. In many circumstances there is little difficulty in discerning between ARF and CRF. Short stature, renal osteodystrophy, delayed puberty, normocytic anemia, and hyperparathyroidism all suggest CRF. However, it may be difficult to differentiate ARF from CRF without imaging studies and a kidney biopsy. Furthermore, at the time of presentation, a patient with CRF may have a superimposed ARF – this is referred to as acute on chronic renal failure. ARF is usually encountered in pediatric urologic patients as a complication of underlying chronic renal disease. The three most important contexts in pediatric urologic practice are acute pyelonephritis, aminoglycoside toxicity, and acute obstructive uropathy. Urologists must be alert to the possibility of ARF in any patient referred with macroscopic hematuria. The three most important contexts are urinary tract infection, glomerulonephritis, and myoglobinuria. Extracorporeal shock wave lithotripsy (ESWL) is the urologic treatment of choice for the majority of patients with renal or proximal ureteral stones.[2] Very rarely, bilateral or unilateral ESWL has been associated with ARF even in the absence of obstruction.[3] In order to diagnose the underlying cause of ARF and treat the metabolic complications, all patients should undergo a full evaluation by a pediatric nephrologist at the time of presentation.

Table 23.1 Causes of non-oliguric acute renal failure

Furosemide may convert oliguric renal failure to non-oliguric renal failure
Nephrotoxins
Non-fulminant acute viral hepatitis
Primary lymphoma of the kidney
Severe exertional rhabdomyolysis
Hemolytic uremic syndrome (HUS)

The likelihood of recovery from, and appropriate treatment of ARF, depends on the amount of urine output and the underlying cause. Quantifying the urine output is essential, because the amount of urine will often predict the clinical course and may aid in identifying the underlying renal insult. Patients with non-oliguric or high-output ARF (Table 23.1) have lower complication rates and higher survival rates than those with anuric or oliguric ARF.[4] Furthermore, children with acute interstitial nephritis or nephrotoxic renal insults, including aminoglycoside nephrotoxicity, are more likely to have ARF associated with either normal or increased urine output. In contrast, children with renal hypoperfusion injury, acute glomerulonephritis, hemolytic uremic syndrome (HUS), or other causes are more likely to have ARF associated with anuria or oliguria. The underlying cause of ARF may be classified as prerenal failure, intrinsic renal disease, or postrenal failure. It is important to note that many cases of ARF are multifactorial, especially in hospitalized children.

Prerenal failure

In prerenal ARF, renal function may be initially normal, but severe and/or prolonged renal hypoperfusion leads to renal injury and intrinsic ARF. Prerenal ARF results from renal hypoperfusion caused by intravascular volume contraction, decreased effective circulating blood volume, or from altered intrarenal hemodynamics. True intravascular volume contraction results from dehydration, acute blood loss, or extravascular accumulation of fluid – so-called third spacing of fluid. This is most often encountered in patients with the systemic inflammatory response syndrome or with hypoalbuminemia. Infants are particularly vulnerable to excessive volume loss. They have a proportionally higher percentage of insensible water losses and, in addition, cannot maximally concentrate their urine as a result of immature kidneys. Decreased effective blood circulation occurs when the true blood volume is normal or increased but renal perfusion is decreased. This occurs in left-sided heart failure, cardiac tamponade, or hepatorenal syndrome.[5] Intrarenal afferent arteriolar vasoconstriction occurs in hepatorenal syndrome, calcineurin toxicity, and non-steroidal anti-inflammatory drug (NSAID) use; intrarenal efferent arteriolar vasodilation occurs with the use of angiotensin-converting enzyme (ACE) inhibitors. Afferent arteriolar vasoconstriction or efferent arteriolar vasodilation decreases the glomerular filtration.

In prerenal ARF, the kidneys are intrinsically normal and the reduced GFR and urine output are appropriate physiologic responses to the reduced renal blood flow. In the early stages, restoration of renal perfusion results in a prompt return of renal function to normal. If the insult is prolonged, acute tubular necrosis (ATN) may develop and the ARF will not immediately correct with improved renal perfusion. This signifies the progression to intrinsic renal disease. The evolution from prerenal failure to intrinsic renal disease is a gradual process because there are a number of compensatory mechanisms that maintain adequate renal perfusion. The two primary mediators of the intrarenal compensatory mechanism are the prostaglandins (PGI_2, PGE_2, and PGD_2) and angiotensin II. The prostaglandins promote compensatory vasodilation of the glomerular afferent arterioles in an attempt to maintain adequate blood flow and preclude further deterioration of renal function.[6] Angiotensin II causes a preferential constriction of the glomerular efferent arterioles, which increases glomerular filtration pressure.[7] The dilation of the afferent arteriole and constriction of the efferent arteriole work in concert to promote an increased filtration fraction and thereby maintain the GFR. Furthermore, angiotensin II, through direct action on the proximal tubule and through the effect of aldosterone on the distal tubule, causes increased sodium and water reabsorption. This helps to maintain an appropriate intravascular volume at the expense of a decreased urine output.

Intrinsic renal disease

When ARF is the result of intrinsic renal pathology, attempts are made to define the location of the insult. Renal injury may occur at the level of the renal vasculature, tubules, interstitium, or glomeruli. The basic mechanisms of renal injury include hypoperfusion, ischemic cell damage, toxin-mediated cell injury, and inflammation. The inevitable outcome is varying degrees of cellular death as a result of necrosis or apoptosis.[8]

Vascular injury

Vascular injury may occur in large vessels, such as in renal artery thrombosis and renal vein thrombosis (RVT), or in the microvasculature, as in HUS and thrombotic thrombocytopenic purpura (TTP). Both renal artery thrombosis and RVT occur most commonly in newborn infants, whereas HUS is most common in young children. Conversely, TTP is rarely seen in pediatrics. Renal artery thrombosis is often associated with umbilical artery catheters and may result in hypertension. ARF rarely occurs unless there is a solitary kidney or the thrombosis is bilateral. In newborns, RVT is associated with maternal diabetes, polycythemia, and sepsis. Coagulation defects are increasingly being identified in neonates with RVT. In childhood, RVT is more closely associated with severe dehydration, nephrotic syndrome, and congenital hypercoagulable states.[9] RVT may present with large palpable kidneys, gross hematuria, hypertension, or oliguria. The neonate with RVT is usually very ill but the condition may also be clinically silent.

The classic triad seen in HUS is acute hemolytic anemia with fragmented erythrocytes, thrombocytopenia, and ARF. The illness is usually preceded by an episode of acute gastroenteritis, often accompanied by bloody diarrhea. Sudden onset of pallor usually develops several days after the diarrheal illness resolves. Oliguria is a common feature and one clue to making an early diagnosis is that the urine output remains decreased even with appropriate rehydration. The condition is usually caused by *Escherichia coli* O157:H7, a Shiga toxin-producing strain. The Shiga toxin is directly toxic to the glomerular vascular endothelium, where it initiates local coagulation (thrombotic microangiopathy), and to renal tubules, where it induces ATN. Several other strains of *E. coli*, as well as *Shigella dysenteriae* and *Aeromonas* produce similar toxins that cause HUS. Non-diarrhea-associated HUS is a much less common condition that is caused by *Streptococcus pneumoniae* infections. Additional causes include bone marrow transplantation, human immunodeficiency virus (HIV) infection, and medications. Inherited causes include deficiencies of factor H, factor I, and membrane cofactor protein (CD46).

Glomerular injury

Acute glomerulonephritis (AGN) is common in school-age children but rare in children under the age of 2 years. Postinfectious glomerulonephritis is the most common cause in childhood. Anti-GBM (glomerular basement membrane) antibody disease, ANCA (antineutrophil cytoplasmic autoantibody) positive (pauci-immune) glomerulonephritis, lupus nephritis, immunoglobulin A (IgA) nephropathy, Henoch–Schönlein purpura nephritis, and membranoproliferative glomerulonephritis all cause ARF.[8] The clinical features of AGN include hypertension, oliguria, painless cola-colored gross hematuria, and edema that is more often periorbital than pedal; laboratory findings include proteinuria, red blood cell (RBC) casts, an increased serum creatinine concentration, evidence of antecedent streptococcal infection, and a low serum complement C3 concentration. Glomerular hypercellularity and inflammation result in a decreased GFR, reduced urine output, retention of potassium, and signs of fluid overload. The tubules and interstitium are mostly spared during the inflammatory process. Each of the glomerulonephritides can lead to rapidly progressive glomerulonephritis (RPGN). This condition is characterized by oligoanuria, rapidly rising serum creatinine, and extensive crescent formation on renal biopsy. A diagnosis of RPGN must be made as soon as possible because treatment with corticosteroids, often used together with plasmapheresis, is essential in order to preserve renal function.

Tubular injury

Tubular injury is also known as acute tubular necrosis (ATN) and is the end result of either ischemic or toxin-mediated damage to the tubules. The tubular epithelial cells are particularly sensitive to anoxia and are vulnerable to toxins. The cells of the straight segment of the proximal tubule and the thick ascending limb of the loop of Henle are highly dependent on oxidative phosphorylation. This serves to maintain their high energy demand, which is required for their transport functions. As a result, they are particularly susceptible to ischemia and to nephrotoxins that disrupt energy supply or mitochondrial function.[10]

Ischemia-induced ATN is the result of renal hypoperfusion. If the insult is prolonged and severe, prerenal ARF may progress to ATN that is no longer immediately reversible with restoration of appropriate renal perfusion. Tubular epithelium damage results in the release of vasoactive compounds that increase afferent arteriolar resistance, thereby decreasing renal blood flow and perpetuating tubular injury. This process is known as tubuloglomerular feedback and plays an important role in the progression from renal hypoperfusion to tubular injury. The vasoconstriction is exacerbated by adrenergic stimulation, decreased intrarenal prostaglandin synthesis, and increased angiotensin II formation.[8] The decrease in GFR is further reduced by the intraluminal tubular obstruction caused by the debris formed from sloughing tubular cells as they undergo apoptosis. The denuded tubular epithelium allows tubular back-leak of glomerular filtrate into the medullary interstitium where it is returned to the systemic circulation. Tubuloglomerular feedback, intraluminal tubular obstruction, and tubular back-leak are all interrelated in the complex pathogenesis of ARF.[11] Several other vasoactive compounds, including endothelin and nitric oxide, are implicated in the progression of ARF but their roles are not fully elucidated.

The clinical course of ischemia-induced ATN comprises the anticipation phase, the initiating phase, the maintenance phase, and the recovery phase.[12] During the initiating phase, the only signs might be a slight decrease in urine output and a rise in serum creatinine concentration and BUN. The maintenance phase is characterized by oliguria, fluid overload, acidosis, hyperkalemia, and a more rapid decline in GFR (usually with oliguria or anuria). Polyuria in the context of increasing serum creatinine concentrations is known as non-oliguric ARF. The recovery phase is characterized by polyuria, kaliuresis, and hypokalemia, while the serum creatinine and BUN begin to return to normal. The recovery process may take weeks to months, and more subtle impairments of tubular function may persist for even longer. If the ATN is prolonged and severe, the child may develop cortical necrosis, which is often associated with only partial recovery of renal function.

Many medications, poisons, or endogenous toxins can cause toxin-mediated ATN. Common nephrotoxic medications are aminoglycosides, amphotericin,

Table 23.2 Nephrotoxins

Aminoglycosides	Amphotericin
Trimethoprim	Sulfinpyrazone
Acyclovir	Fluoroquinolones
Mefenamic acid	Cisplatin
NSAIDs	Acetaminophen
Ifosfamide	Calcineurins
Diethylene glycol	Paraquat

acyclovir, cisplatin, and radiocontrast agents (Table 23.2).[8]

Aminoglycoside nephrotoxicity occurs in 10–26% of patients[13] usually after 1 week of treatment, although the ARF may be delayed until after discontinuation of the medication. The renal injury usually presents with a decrease in urine concentrating capacity, and is usually transient, mild, and non-oliguric. Serum and urine electrolyte abnormalities range from combinations of hypokalemia, hypomagnesemia, and hypocalcemia to a complete acquired Fanconi syndrome or an acquired Bartter syndrome.[13,14] Accumulation of aminoglycosides in the lysosomes of the proximal tubules induces cell necrosis and the excretion of low molecular weight proteins (β_2-microglobulin) and brush border enzymes. Risk factors for aminoglycoside-induced ARF are extremes of age, hypovolemia, pre-existing renal insufficiency, multiple nephrotoxic agents, hypokalemia, hypomagnesemia, prolonged use, total lifetime exposure, and elevated peak and trough levels.[8,11] It is important to note that studies in humans are dogged by confounding variables of the critically ill and that the choice of an aminoglycoside should not be governed by nephrologic criteria; the dosing, however, must be adjusted for the level of GFR. In most cases there is full recovery, with no evidence of permanent injury or CRF.

Patients with amphotericin B-induced renal injury often present with non-oliguric ARF. Amphotericin B injures many different nephron segments as well as the collecting duct. In addition to toxin-mediated ARF, amphotericin B may also cause hypokalemia and hypomagnesemia. Distal renal tubular acidosis occurs as a result of back-leakage of hydrogen ions into the interstitium.[8] Risk factors for the development of ARF include maximal daily dose, duration of therapy, and concomitant use of cyclosporin A.

Acyclovir-induced ARF is usually non-oliguric and may present with microscopic hematuria. Acyclovir is relatively insoluble in urine and, by forming crystals within the renal tubule, causes intratubular obstruction and a reduced GFR. Risk factors for the development of ARF include high doses, rapid intravenous administration, hypovolemia, and pre-existing renal disease.[8]

Radiocontrast-induced nephropathy is uncommon in children and is usually mild and transient. The pathogenesis is unclear. Risk factors for contrast nephropathy include underlying renal disease, dehydration, large doses of contrast media, congestive heart failure, diabetes mellitus, NSAIDs, and ACE inhibitors.[11]

Poison-mediated ATN may occur from direct tubular toxicity, as in mercury poisoning, or from crystal formation, as in ethylene glycol and methanol poisoning. Both ethylene glycol and methanol are non-toxic until they are metabolized by alcohol dehydrogenase into their metabolites. Once their metabolites have been generated, crystals will form in the tubules, causing obstruction and ARF.[8]

Endogenous toxins that can cause ATN are myoglobin, hemoglobin, and uric acid. Pigment-induced ATN can be precipitated by either hemoglobinuria or myoglobinuria. Tubular injury results from the precipitation of pigment in the tubules and heme protein-induced oxidative stress.[11] Myoglobin- or hemoglobin-induced ARF is more likely to develop in the presence of dehydration, metabolic acidosis, severe muscle damage, or multiple organ failure. Rhabdomyolysis is caused by viral infections (influenza), medications (statins), seizures, prolonged exercise, or illicit drug use (Table 23.3). An elevated serum creatine phosphokinase level can confirm the diagnosis. The association between cocaine and rhabdomyolysis has been widely reported, whereas the association with amphetamines has only been described in case reports. Cocaine appears to have direct toxic effects on skeletal muscle as well as vasoconstrictive properties, which lead to muscle ischemia.[15] Several proposed mechanisms have been put forward to explain methamphet-

Table 23.3 Causes of rhabdomyolysis

Chronic and inflammatory myopathy
Metabolic myopathy
Non-ketotic hyperosmolar coma
Viral myositis
Malignant hyperthermia
Muscular dystrophy
Trauma
Exercise
Dystonia
Cocaine/methamphetamine ingestion

amine-induced rhabdomyolysis, although direct myocyte toxicity has never been demonstrated. Amphetamine users are often agitated and experience uncontrolled choreiform movements. The rhabdomyolysis might occur in a fashion similar to the exertional rhabdomyolysis after exhaustive physical exercise.[15,16] Hemolysis occurs in sickle cell disease, immune-mediated hemolysis, or glucose-6-phosphate dehydrogenase (G6PD) deficiency.[11]

Treatment of pigment-induced ARF includes volume expansion, forced diuresis with a loop diuretic, and alkalinization of the urine to increase pigment solubility.[8] An increasing serum creatinine concentration with fluid overload, despite adequate treatment, is an indication for hemodialysis.

Tumor lysis syndrome can be caused by excessive release of uric acid, phosphorus, and cell products, usually during treatment of acute lymphocytic leukemia or B-cell lymphoma. The probable mechanism of injury is related to precipitation of uric acid crystals in the tubules, with obstruction of urine flow. The highest risk for tumor lysis syndrome is with the most rapidly growing tumors or during induction chemotherapy.

Aggressive hydration, with the administration of allopurinol, helps to decrease the uric acid burden and the risk of tubular precipitation. Rasburicase (urate oxidase) is an effective alternative to allopurinol for rapidly reducing uric acid levels, improving patients' electrolyte status, and reversing renal insufficiency. Screening for G6PD deficiency is essential prior to rasburicase administration, as it may cause hemolytic anemia and methemoglobinemia in susceptible patients.[17] Dialysis may be necessary if the metabolic abnormalities cannot be controlled with the aforementioned medical management.

Interstitial injury

Interstitial nephritis most often occurs as a result of exposure to medications. It is also associated with infections, systemic diseases, tumor infiltrates, or genetic conditions. In many cases no cause is found. Medications commonly associated with interstitial nephritis include extended-spectrum penicillins, NSAIDs, sulfonamides, and rifampin. Almost every known medication has been implicated. The pathogenesis of medication-induced acute interstitial nephritis is thought to be a hypersensitivity-type or allergic reaction that causes an inflammatory reaction mainly in the medullary interstitium. Many patients are asymptomatic or have vague complaints. Typical symptoms include fever, rash, arthralgias, and flank pain. Urine output is usually increased or normal because this the most frequent cause of non-oliguric ARF. It is important to note interstitial nephritis does not present with gross hematuria or isolated microscopic hematuria and the urine may be bland or there may be combinations of microscopic hematuria, mild proteinuria, pyuria, white blood cell (WBC) casts, eosinophiluria, and peripheral eosinophilia. Acute pyelonephritis, Epstein–Barr virus (EBV), and cytomegalovirus (CMV) also cause interstitial nephritis. Sarcoidosis and tubulointerstitial nephritis and uveitis (TINU) are rare causes.

Postrenal failure

Congenital obstructive uropathies are among the most frequent causes of CRF in pediatrics; this is often erroneously referred to as ARF when the presentation is in the newborn child. ARF is rarely the result of postrenal obstruction, except when this occurs in solitary kidneys either from aplasia or transplantation. In pediatric individuals with two functioning kidneys, postrenal ARF will occur only with urethral obstruction, bladder neck obstruction, or bilateral ureteric obstruction, because a single normal kidney has sufficient ability to maintain a normal GFR. Most patients with acute obstruction leading to ARF have oliguric ARF, although non-oliguric ARF can occur with partial obstruction. Renal calculi, ureteral blood clots, retroperitoneal fibrosis, neurogenic bladder, bladder tumors and urethral strictures can cause an obstruction at different levels of the urinary tract and lead to ARF.[11] During acute obstruction a decreased GFR is the result of a rise in the intraluminal tubular pressure. A further decline in renal function is caused by arteriolar vasoconstriction. A prompt diagnosis is necessary to provide appropriate urologic intervention. Hydronephrosis detected by renal ultrasound is an important finding. All patients with suspected obstruction should undergo bladder catheterization, as it may be therapeutic as well as diagnostic. Percutaneous nephrostomy, lithotripsy, ureteral stenting, and urethral stenting are indicated when appropriate.

Diagnostic approach to acute renal failure

History and physical examination

The history and physical examination can provide invaluable clues that help determine whether the ARF is a result of a prerenal, renal, or postrenal event. A careful review of the patient's past medical history, family history, medication use, trauma, and recent febrile illnesses is essential. Furthermore, a careful assessment of fluid intake and urine output can help to narrow the differential diagnosis as well as dictate future management. A major purpose of the physical examination in a patient with ARF is to attempt to determine the effective circulating volume. The patient's weight, blood pressure (sitting and standing), and pulse rate provide important clues. On general examination the patient must be carefully assessed for edema, state of hydration, pallor, petechiae, rashes, and abdominal signs of tenderness, bladder fullness, and visceromegaly. Careful cardiac and pulmonary examinations are performed to determine the degree of fluid overload. Clues for systemic diseases such as rash, jaundice, arthritis, or uveitis must always be looked for.

Urine studies

The urinalysis, urinary sediment, and urine indices are the most important factors in determining the cause of ARF. But these parameters must never be interpreted on their own; each value must be interpreted in relation to clinical findings and serum chemistry results. A high urine specific gravity (SG), in the absence of proteinuria, is suggestive of decreased effective circulatory volume and prerenal ARF. An inappropriately dilute SG suggests tubular injury or interstitial nephritis. A dipstick test that is >3+ positive for protein indicates intrinsic ARF with glomerular damage. Less proteinuria (<2+) may be seen in prerenal ARF, ATN, and postrenal ARF. Protein excretion >2 g/24 hours suggests glomerular injury. A positive urine dipstick for blood usually indicates hematuria. However, if there are no red blood cells (RBCs) on microscopic examination, myoglobinuria or hemoglobinuria must be considered. RBCs with RBC casts strongly suggest a glomerular lesion, especially in conjunction with significant proteinuria. WBCs and WBC casts are seen in pyelonephritis, acute postinfectious glomerulonephritis, and acute interstitial nephritis. Pigmented casts, granular casts, tubule epithelial cells and casts, and cellular debris characterize the urinary sediment in ischemic ATN.

Urine diagnostic indices, which are particularly helpful in characterizing ARF, include urine sodium and creatinine concentrations. When used in conjunction with the serum sodium and creatinine, the fractional excretion of sodium (FENa) can be calculated:

$$\text{FENa} = \frac{\text{urine}_{\text{Na}} \times \text{plasma}_{\text{Cr}}}{\text{plasma}_{\text{Na}} \times \text{urine}_{\text{Cr}}} \times 100$$

The results of the FENa, urine sodium, and urine osmolality can be used to differentiate between prerenal and intrinsic ARF. A low urinary sodium (<10 mmol/L) and a low FENa (<1%) indicate avid sodium and water retention. This is characteristic of prerenal ARF in which the intact proximal and distal tubules are able to respond appropriately to renal hypoperfusion. Conversely, the damaged tubules in ATN are unable to reabsorb sodium efficiently and this results in a high urine sodium concentration (>10 mmol/L) and an FENa of >2%. Two important caveats when using the FENa to assess ARF are underlying renal disease and the concurrent use of diuretics. In postrenal obstruction the indices are more variable and not very helpful. Early in the course of the disease they may resemble those of prerenal ARF, but as tubular damage progresses the indices become more similar to those of intrinsic ARF.[8,11]

Blood studies

Evaluation of the BUN and serum creatinine concentration is essential in making a diagnosis of ARF, but the serum electrolyte concentrations are more important guides for morbidity and mortality. The serum potassium concentration must be monitored closely in a patient with oliguria and, even more so, anuria. Life-threatening hyperkalemia, particularly in association with a metabolic acidosis, must be treated immediately. Hemoglobin, hematocrit, platelet count, and serum concentration of calcium, phosphorus, bicarbonate, and albumin must be routinely evaluated in patients with ARF. Serologic tests for streptococcal infection and complement studies are indicated if there are signs of AGN. It has traditionally been taught that a serum BUN: creatinine ratio of >20 suggests prerenal ARF, whereas the ratio is about 10 in ATN. Unfortunately, this ratio is affected by many factors, including a catabolic state and gastrointestinal bleeding, which negates its value in critically ill patients.[11]

Diagnostic imaging

The two most helpful initial imaging studies in patients with ARF are a chest radiograph and a renal ultrasound. Chest radiographs can help define whether there is significant cardiomegaly or pulmonary edema as a result of fluid overload. Renal ultrasonography is extremely useful when either obstruction or RVT is suspected. Additionally, if it is unclear whether the patient has ARF or CRF, the ultrasound may be diagnostic. In patients with ARF, the kidneys are often large and swollen. Conversely, the kidneys in CRF are often small, scarred, or dysplastic. In both instances they lose the normal corticomedullary differentiation and are echogenic.

Renal biopsy

A percutaneous renal biopsy may be indicated in children with ARF if the cause is unknown or if there is any suspicion of a crescentic glomerulonephritis.

Complications of ARF

The major complications of ARF are either related to metabolic dysfunction or to fluid overload. Metabolic complications of ARF are hyperkalemia, metabolic acidosis, hypocalcemia, hyperphosphatemia, hyponatremia, and rarely uremia (Table 23.4). Hyperkalemia is the single most life-threatening complication of ARF. The hyperkalemia is the result of impaired tubular secretion, decreased filtration fraction, and extracellular shifts of potassium induced by acidosis. Peaked T waves are usually the first manifestation of cardiotoxicity followed by prolongation of the PR interval and widening of the QRS complex. Prompt treatment of hyperkalemia is required in order to prevent ventricular tachycardia or fibrillation. Uremia is characterized by mental status changes, evidence of serositis, and bleeding diathesis as a result of platelet dysfunction. It occurs when urea and other waste products build up in the tissues because the kidneys are unable to eliminate them adequately.

There are multiple causes for hypocalcemia in ARF, including hyperphosphatemia, decreased gastrointestinal calcium absorption, vitamin D deficiency, and parathyroid hormone (PTH) resistance. The most important acute reason is hyperphosphatemia. The hypocalcemia is usually mild and may cause tetany if markedly reduced. The hyperphosphatemia in ARF is the result of decreased renal excretion. Metabolic acidosis is very common in ARF. Declining renal function reduces the kidney's ability to excrete the net acids generated by the diet and to carry out normal metabolic function. Paradoxically, metabolic acidosis increases the fraction of serum calcium in the ionized form, which lessens the risk of hypocalcemia. Special attention must be paid to the serum ionized calcium concentration when correcting metabolic acidosis because tetany may ensue.

Table 23.4 Complications of acute renal failure

Complications
Fluid overload
Hypertension
Hyperkalemia
Hyponatremia
Metabolic acidosis
Hyperphosphatemia
Hypocalcemia
Hyperuricemia

Patients with oliguric or anuric ARF commonly present with hypervolemia and fluid overload. The hypertension is usually caused by fluid overload, but may also be the result of changes in vascular tone or activation of the renin–angiotensin system. If the fluid overload worsens, the patient may develop pulmonary edema and/or congestive heart failure.

Management of acute renal failure

There are five main principles in managing ARF:

1 Maintaining appropriate renal perfusion
2 Avoidance of nephrotoxic agents
3 Establishing fluid balance
4 Maintaining electrolyte and acid–base balance
5 Providing nutritional support

In almost all circumstances, with the important exception of glomerular nephritides, renal hypoperfusion is a predisposing factor to the development of ARF. Optimizing intravascular volume is a fundamental principle in preventing the development and progression of ARF. If children at risk for the development of ARF are adequately hydrated prior to a known incipient insult, the extent of the renal injury can often be decreased or even prevented. This is particularly important prior to the administration of contrast media, aminoglycosides, cisplatin, or amphotericin, and in preoperative patients. Additionally, it is important to stop or avoid medications that cause intrarenal afferent arteriole vasoconstriction (NSAIDs) or efferent arteriole vasodilation (ACE inhibitor). Even in well-hydrated patients, potential nephrotoxic agents should only be used when necessary and with special attention to dosing schedules and by monitoring serum concentrations.

Establishing fluid balance is perhaps the most challenging and critical step in managing ARF. Prerenal

ARF is the most common situation in which intrinsic renal damage can be prevented. Any hypovolemic patient who presents with oligoanuric ARF has a potential prerenal component. The first step in managing a patient with potential prerenal ARF is fluid resuscitation with one or more rapid infusions of normal saline, without any potassium, unless the patent is hypokalemic as a result of diarrhea or a tubulointerstitial disease. Maintenance fluids and replacement of ongoing losses should not be neglected during this period of initial rehydration. If the urine output does not increase after the patient is assessed to be euvolemic, intrinsic renal damage must be assumed. At this stage, in the absence of increased urine output, fluid restriction becomes essential to avoid hypertension, pulmonary edema, and congestive heart failure. During fluid restriction the patient should receive insensible losses (400 ml/m^2/24 hours of D5W) + urine output losses (milliliter per milliliter replacement with 0.45% NS). If the patient becomes hypervolemic after fluid resuscitation or requires large quantities of blood products or intravenous alimentation, a diuretic such as furosemide is administered in an attempt to increase urine output. Diuretics must be used with caution in the absence of good evidence of euvolemia or hypervolemia because they may worsen any prerenal component of the ARF. Patients who present with non-oliguric ARF (acute interstitial nephritis or the recovery phase of ATN) may actually be polyuric and require greater than normal volumes of fluid to avoid intravascular volume depletion.[12]

Maintaining the electrolyte and acid–base balance involves managing hyperkalemia, hypocalcemia, hyperphosphatemia, and metabolic acidosis. All potassium must be removed from the intravenous fluids in any patient with oligoanuric ARF. Treatment of hyperkalemia is indicated if electrocardiogram (ECG) abnormalities are noted or if serum concentrations are higher than 6–7 mEq/L. Treatment regimens are those that protect against hyperkalemia, those that redistribute potassium intracellularly, and those that remove potassium from the body.[8] Calcium gluconate, which is cardioprotective against the conduction abnormalities induced by hyperkalemia but does not remove potassium, is administered (0.5–1.0 mg/kg/dose) early in the course of treatment. Redistributive measures include albuterol, bicarbonate, and insulin + glucose infusions. All three interventions shift potassium intracellularly within 30 minutes; these are only temporizing measures and the serum potassium concentration may rise rapidly after they are discontinued. Potassium can be removed from the body via the gastrointestinal tract, the kidney, or by dialysis. Sodium polystyrene (Kayexalate), administered as 1 g/kg, exchanges sodium for potassium in the gastrointestinal tract and effects potassium removal. For every 1 g/kg of sodium polystyrene administered, the serum potassium decreases by 1 mmol/L. Hypernatremia is a side effect from excessive sodium absorption. If the patient is not anuric, loop diuretics are used to promote potassium losses by kaliuresis. Dialysis is the definitive therapy in patients who do not respond to these regimens.[8]

Hypocalcemia is usually mild and responds to correction of the hyperphosphatemia and dietary calcium supplementation. Intravenous calcium infusion is indicated if there is tetany or arrhythmia. Hyperphosphatemia is treated by dietary restriction and oral phosphate binders. Calcium carbonate and calcium acetate are well tolerated as phosphate binders when taken with meals. The treatment of the metabolic acidosis is important for maintaining a normal pH for optimal metabolism and for reducing the hyperkalemia. As previously mentioned, rapid correction of the acidosis can cause a precipitous decline in the serum concentration of ionized calcium. Oral sodium bicarbonate or sodium citrate tablets are given to correct the metabolic acidosis, but intravenous sodium bicarbonate is used for patients who have severe acidosis or who cannot take anything by mouth.

Nutritional support is essential because the patients are in a highly catabolic state. This is particularly challenging in oligoanuric patients who may be severely fluid restricted. Formula or parenteral nutrition should be concentrated whenever possible to provide maximum calories at a minimum volume. Children typically require only modest protein restriction (1–2 g/kg/day) and maintenance (or higher if catabolic) of non-protein calories. A low phosphorus and low potassium diet is also required. If adequate calories cannot be maintained because of fluid restriction, dialysis should be considered early in the course.[8]

Dialysis

The indications for initiating dialysis in ARF include:

1 Volume overload unresponsive to conservative management
2 Hyperkalemia, acidosis, or hypocalcemia unresponsive to medical therapy

3 Uremia (mental status changes, serositis, or bleeding diathesis)
4 Nutritional support

The patient's overall condition must be considered before making a decision to start dialysis. This is also important when selecting the appropriate type of dialysis. One important consideration is the patient's hemodynamic status. Hypotensive patients are poor candidates for hemodialysis but are often suitable for peritoneal dialysis or continuous renal replacement therapy (CRRT).[18] There are no precise criteria for selecting a particular dialysis modality, and practice patterns vary widely. However, CRRT is rapidly becoming the preferred modality for pediatric patients with ARF in the intensive care unit (ICU) setting.[19]

Conclusion

The prognosis for a child with ARF depends on the underlying cause, the length of insult, the number and type of other organs involved, the amount of residual urine output, and whether or not dialysis is required.[20] The major complications of ARF include fluid overload, hyperkalemia, metabolic acidosis, hyperphosphatemia, and hypocalcemia. Azotemia rarely produces uremic symptoms in the modern era. Judicious management of these complications can improve the morbidity and mortality associated with ARF in children. Immediate treatment of the underlying insult through fluid resuscitation in prerenal failure or relieving an acute obstruction in postrenal failure can prevent progression to intrinsic renal failure. Once intrinsic renal failure is established, it is essential to maintain adequate renal perfusion while avoiding further nephrotoxic insults whenever possible. If medical management fails to control the fluid and metabolic abnormalities, dialysis may be necessary. The choice of which dialysis modality to employ primarily depends on the hemodynamic status of the patient. Recovery from intrinsic renal disease also depends on the underlying cause of the ARF. Children with acute interstitial nephritis or ATN typically recover normal renal function and are at low risk for long-term morbidity. Conversely, children who lose a substantial number of nephrons, as occurs in HUS, cortical necrosis, or RPGN, are at risk for the development of CRF long after the initial insult. These children require lifelong monitoring of blood pressure, renal function, and urinalysis.

References

1. Thadhani R, Pascual M, Bonventre JV. Acute renal failure. N Engl J Med 1996; 334:1448–60.
2. Liguori G, Trombetta C, Bucci S et al. Reversible acute renal failure after unilateral extracorporeal shock-wave lithotripsy. Urol Res 2004; 32(1):25–7.
3. Treglia A, Moscoloni M. Irreversible acute renal failure after bilateral extracorporeal shock wave lithotripsy. J Nephrol 1999; 12(3):190–2.
4. Mogal NE, Brocklebank JT, Meadow SR. A review of acute renal failure in children: incidence, etiology, and outcome. Clin Nephrol 1998; 49:91–5.
5. Brady HR, Linger GG. Acute renal failure. Lancet 1995; 346:1533–40.
6. Whelton A. Nephrotoxicity of nonsteroidal anti-inflammatory drugs: physiologic foundations and clinical implications. Am J Med 1999; 106(5B):13–24S.
7. Wargo KA, Chong K, Chan EC. Acute renal failure secondary to angiotensin II receptor blockade in a patient with bilateral renal artery stenosis. Pharmacotherapy 2003; 23(9):1199–204.
8. Avner ED, Harmon WE, Niaudet P. Pediatric Nephrology, 5th edn. Philadelphia: Lippincott, Williams and Wilkins, 2004: 63–5, 1223–66.
9. Schmidt B, Andrew M. Neonatal thrombosis: report of a prospective Canadian and international registry. Pediatrics 1995; 96:939–43.
10. Cotran RS, Kumar V, Robbins SL. The kidney. In: Cotran RS, Kumar V, Robbins SL, eds. Pathologic Basis of Disease, 5th edn. Philadelphia: WB Saunders, 1994: 927–89.
11. Bhimma R, Kaplan BS. Acute renal failure. In: Hogg RJ. Kidney Disorders in Children and Adolescents: A Practical Handbook. London: Taylor and Francis, 2006.
12. Kaplan BS, Meyers KEC. Pediatric Nephrology and Urology: The Requisites in Pediatrics, 1st edn. Philadelphia: Elsevier Mosby, 2004: 241–9.
13. Gainza FJ, Minguela JI, Lampreabe I. Aminoglycoside-associated Fanconi's syndrome: an underrecognized entity. Nephron 1997; 77:205–11.
14. Landau D, Kher KK. Gentamicin-induced Bartter-like syndrome. Pediatr Nephrol 1997; 11:737–40.
15. Richards JR. Rhabdomyolysis and drugs of abuse. J Emerg Med 2000; 19(1):51–6.
16. Richards JR, Johnson EB, Stark RW, Derlet RW. Methamphetamine abuse and rhabdomyolysis in the ED: a 5-year study. Am J Emerg Med 1999; 7:681–5.
17. Browning LA, Kruse JA. Hemolysis and methemoglobinemia secondary to rasburicase administration. Ann Pharmacother 2005; 39:1932–5.
18. Maxvold NJ, Smoyer WE, Gardner JJ et al. Management of acute renal failure in the pediatric patient: hemofiltration vs hemodialysis. Am J Kidney Dis 1997; 30(S4):84–8.
19. Flynn JT. Choice of dialysis modality in pediatric acute renal failure. Pediatr Nephrol 2002; 17:61–9.
20. Arora P, Kher V, Rai PK et al. Prognosis of acute renal failure in children: a multivariate analysis. Pediatr Nephrol 1997; 11(2):153–5.

Renal transplantation

24

Nafisa Dharamsi, Curtis Sheldon, and Jens Goebel

Kidney transplantation is generally the therapy of choice for children with end-stage renal disease (ESRD) and has very few true contraindications (Table 24.1). For pediatric patients, this treatment modality offers special advantages with regards to growth and development,[1,2] in addition to the generally superior outcomes and cost-effectiveness of kidney transplantation as compared with chronic dialysis.[3,4] Patient as well as short- and mid-term graft survival have improved steadily over the past decades (Figure 24.1) due to ongoing advances in many areas related to transplantation, including the introduction of newer and more potent immunosuppressants. Accordingly, acute rejection rates within the first 12 months post-transplant are at an all-time low (Table 24.2). The improved graft survival has resulted in increasing recognition of several long-term complications affecting kidney transplant recipients, such as chronic allograft nephropathy (CAN), the high incidence of cardiovascular (CV) disease and malignancies, compared with the general population, post-transplant bone disease and non-compliance.[1,2] These complications, with special impact on pediatric patients because of their comparably longer life expectancy, represent the challenges faced by the transplant community in the years ahead.

Table 24.1 Contraindications to transplantation[a]

Malignancy
Chronic persistent infection
Recalcitrant non-compliance
Ongoing substance abuse
Severe irreversible extrarenal disease, including psychiatric illness
Absent insurance or equivalent coverage

[a] Contraindications are potentially modifiable – e.g. 'safe' time periods after curative treatment for malignancy are available in the literature; some centers offer kidney transplantation to certain patients infected with human immunodeficiency virus (HIV); non-compliance and substance abuse can be overcome in some instances; and financial coverage can eventually be established in many circumstances.

Based on Organ Procurement and Transplantation Network data from January 2005, approximately 5% of all kidney transplant recipients are <18 years old.

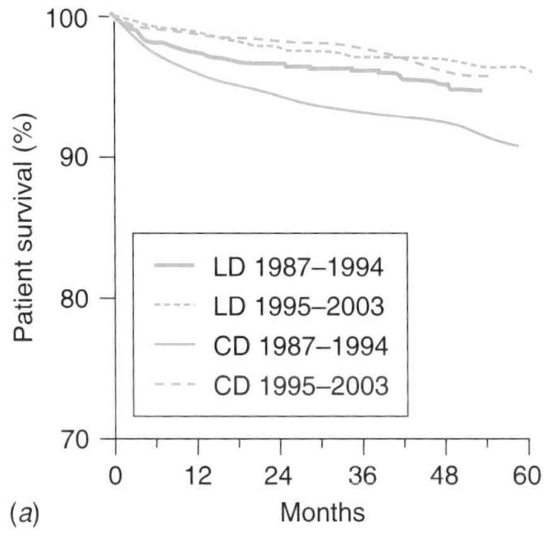

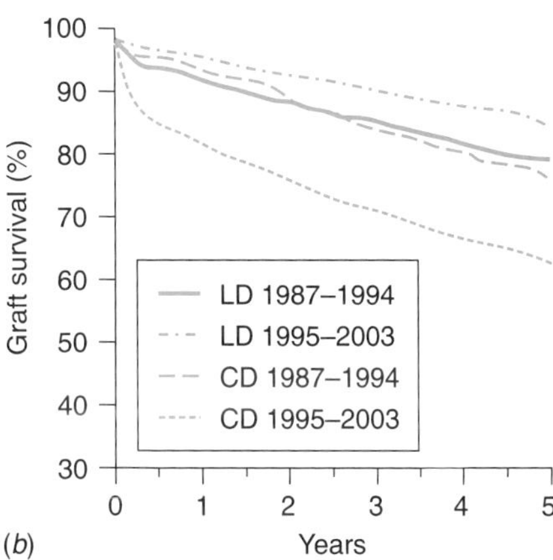

Figure 24.1 Patient (*a*) and graft (*b*) survival by era and allograft source in pediatric kidney transplantation. LD, living donor; CD, cadaveric/deceased donor. (Reproduced with permission from the NAPRTCS (North American Pediatric Renal Trials Collaborative Studies) 2004 Annual Report.)

Table 24.2 Acute rejection probability within the first post-transplant year by era in pediatric kidney transplantation

Transplant year	Living donor		Cadaver donor	
	%	SE	%	SE
1987–1990	54.2	1.7	69.0	1.5
1991–1994	45.0	1.5	60.8	1.6
1995–1998	34.0	1.4	41.0	1.7
1999–2003	24.8	1.6	28.8	2.1

From NAPRTCS 2004 Annual Report.

The causes of ESRD in these pediatric patients are substantially different from those in adults, as there is a preponderance of congenital obstructive and dysplastic conditions in pediatric patients and a virtual absence of diabetic or primary hypertensive nephropathy, the two most common causes of ESRD other than glomerular disease in adults (Table 24.3). Importantly, and as also shown in Table 24.3, failure of a previous renal allograft is the fourth most common indication for kidney transplantation both in children and adults. Lastly, there is an emerging additional group of individuals, including children, requiring treatment for chronic renal insufficiency (CRI) or ESRD: namely, recipients of non-kidney organ transplants who have developed renal dysfunction in large part related to chronic calcineurin inhibitor (CI) use.[5]

Urologic involvement in CRI care

The preponderance of primary urologic disease in children waiting for a kidney transplant explains why many of these patients will require pediatric urology services before, during, and after kidney transplantation. Early and aggressive management of CRI due to primary urologic disease may delay progression to ESRD and attenuate the adverse effects of uremia on growth and development. Elevated bladder pressures have specifically been shown to have a detrimental effect on upper tract function,[6] and upper tract deterioration in children with neurogenic bladders has been correlated with intravesical pressures >40 cmH_2O. This critical pressure threshold is associated with the onset of renal papillary morphologic distortion and intrarenal reflux of urine.[7–9] Such pressures can be documented using urodynamic studies with a focus on specific parameters, including compliance (pressure and volume), leak point pressures, voiding pressure, and postvoid residual urine (PVR).

The relationship between bladder dysfunction and deterioration of renal function is also illustrated in children with posterior urethral valves.[10] Figure 24.2 demonstrates the effect of age on bladder compliance in patients with ESRD that results from this disease. Urologic management of 'valve bladders' requires consideration of these maturational changes in function of these bladders. In young children, they tend to feature elevated pressures and low compliance, only to develop into larger-capacity, low-pressure reservoirs in older children. Medical management in this context is aimed at altering several parameters, including detrusor compliance and bladder emptying. Compliance can be altered by the administration of agents such as oxybutynin chloride or surgically by bladder augmentation. The detrusor pressure may be dramatically reduced for a given intravesical volume, but this may also result in an increase in PVR. In this persistently deleterious scenario, intermittent catheterization (IMC) will decrease PVR and lessen urinary stasis, thus reducing the risk for urinary tract infections (UTIs). In addition, IMC prevents pressure

Table 24.3 Most frequent indications for kidney transplantation in adults and children

Adults				Children	
Indication	*LD* (%)	*Non-ECDD* (%)	*ECDD* (%)	*Indication*	%
Glomerular disease	27.2	22.1	17.7	Obstructive uropathy	16.1
Diabetes	20.4	19.1	28.2	A-/hypo-/dysplasia	16.0
Hypertensive nephrosclerosis	10.5	16.1	22.2	Focal segmental glomerulosclerosis	11.4
Failed previous graft	9.7	13.4	6.3	Failed previous graft	8.0

LD, living donor; ECDD, extended criteria deceased donor.
From the 2003 Annual Report of the US Scientific Registry of Transplant Recipients and the Organ Procurement and Transplantation Network, NAPRTCS 2004 Annual Report.

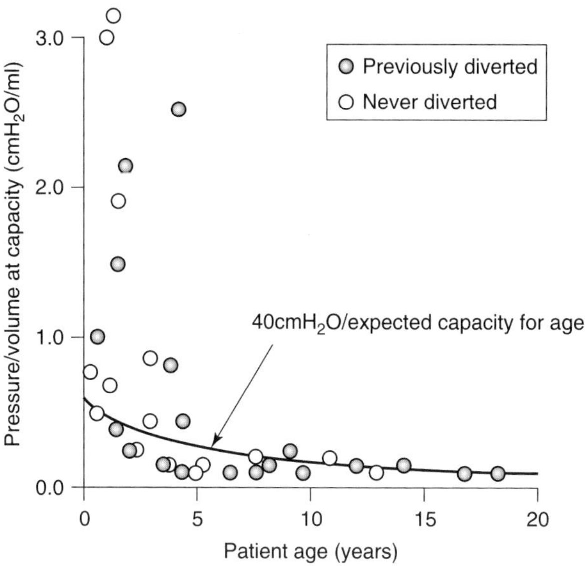

Figure 24.2 Relationship of valve bladder compliance characteristics versus patient's age. The line indicates the ratio of pressure (40 cmH_2O) divided by the expected bladder capacity for age.

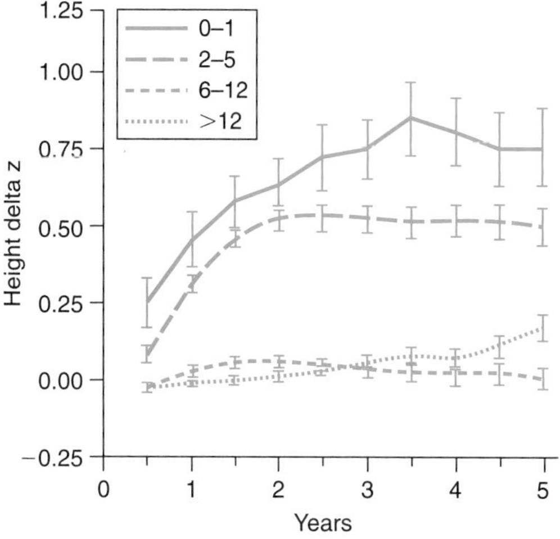

Sample sizes for height delta Z at follow-up months

Age group	12 months	36 months	60 months
0–1	272	215	141
2–5	853	628	442
6–12	1988	1432	1026
>13	2318	1258	502

Figure 24.3 Mean post-transplant change (with standard error) in standardized height scores of children with functioning kidney grafts by age groups, indicating substantial catch-up growth only in the younger recipients. (Reproduced with permission from the 2004 NAPRTCS Annual Report.)

increases during voiding. In older, and compliant, children, a less dramatic but often satisfactory improvement can also be obtained by frequent, e.g. 2 hourly, timed double voiding, with or without catheterization overnight.[11] A satisfactory working pressure range not only contributes to delaying the onset of ESRD but also ensures a safe receptacle for the allograft ureter if transplantation is needed.

Medical preparation of pediatric transplant recipients

The preparation of children for kidney transplantation is generally a multidisciplinary task shared by the patient's nephrology care team (e.g. nurses, dieticians, social workers, and nephrologists) and other services as needed (e.g. pediatric urology, surgery, psychiatry, anesthesiology, and critical care medicine). It cannot be emphasized enough how important it is to enable patients to enter the transplant procedure in as optimal a medical condition as possible. Specifically, children, like adults, with CRI or ESRD, should be encouraged to achieve and maintain physical fitness and weight control: CV fitness and absence of obesity will reduce surgical and anesthesthetic risks associated with the transplant operation and provide an advantage in the efforts to combat the increased risks for CV morbidity and excessive weight gain post-transplant.[12] Because transplanted children, especially once they are of school-age, do not uniformly display catch-up growth[1] (Figure 24.3), aggressive nutritional support is often required and, as indicated, growth hormone therapy needs to be considered before, and possibly after, transplantation.[13] Appropriate nutritional management pretransplant, frequently paired with the prescription of phosphate binders and active vitamin D and with regular monitoring of serum parathyroid hormone levels, will also attenuate post-transplant bone disease and thus increase the likelihood of appropriate growth.[14] Before transplantation, the recipients' up-to-date immunization status also needs to be ascertained, as no live vaccines can be given post-transplant and the response to other vaccines in the setting of immunosuppression may not be adequate.[15] Somewhat related, immunosuppressive therapy can lead to bothersome exacerbations of warts, and potential recipients should therefore have any warts dealt with as definitively as possible prior to transplantation.

In addition to these general principles, a number of issues need to be considered on an individual basis during preparation of the recipient. Psychosocial stability, both of the patient and the patient's family, is of tremendous importance for adherence to the relatively complex treatment regimen required for good long-term results.[16] Such stability is largely defined individually for each patient/family unit and, accordingly, requires case-by-case interventions ranging from counseling over more intense psychological interventions all the way to the involvement of authorities dealing with complicated custodial situations. Before transplantation, patients and families also need to be educated about the need for frequent and comprehensive follow-up, especially during the first few months after hospital discharge. This need can create significant logistical obstacles with regards to transportation and caregivers' time away from work, and a number of families will benefit from support in planning for this challenging period ahead of time. As part of this planning effort, it should also be ensured that the patients will have appropriate coverage for their post-transplant medications and that they or their caregivers know, in particular, how to obtain the required immunosuppressive drugs in the outpatient setting. Depending on the recipient's developmental and pre-transplant medical (e.g. dialysis) status, plans are also necessary regarding vascular and gastrointestinal (GI) tract access. A central line may be needed for a prolonged period of time post-transplant to facilitate frequent blood sampling in very young recipients, those with very limited peripheral venepuncture sites, in patients who may need pre- and post-transplant plasmapheresis for immunologic reasons (see below), or because they are considered to be at high risk for the recurrence of focal segmental glomerulosclerosis.[17] A gastrostomy tube is essential in patients who require supplementation of additional nutrition or fluid or are unable to take all their post-transplant medications by mouth. Lastly, there is a subgroup of patients at increased immunologic risk from a previous kidney or other organ transplant, from blood transfusions, or from other sensitizing events. These individuals will benefit from specialized immunologic characterization and consequently from consideration of desensitization strategies prior to transplantation to enhance their potential for long-term graft survival.[18,19]

Prior to actual transplantation, a risk assessment of the recipient for thrombotic complications is also important, as graft thrombosis is a significant cause of pediatric transplant loss.[20,21] Risk factors include hypercoagulopathy (e.g. as seen in chronic nephrotic states), antiphospholipid antibodies (seen in 30–50% of patients with systemic lupus erythematosus), prior thrombosis of a large vein postoperatively (e.g. a renal transplant vein), or thrombosis associated with vascular access (e.g. for dialysis).[22] Accordingly, hypercoagulability should be corrected before the actual transplant procedure whenever possible. Alternatively, consideration needs to be given to the prescription of anticoagulation during and after the transplant, although controversy exists regarding the routine use of heparin in the perioperative period to reduce the incidence of renal allograft thrombosis. A recent retrospective study showed that young recipient age, young donor age, and increased cold ischemia time were associated with a higher risk for graft thrombosis, but the administration of heparin did not decrease the incidence of early renal allograft thrombosis.[23]

Urologic pre-transplant interventions

Pediatric kidney transplant candidates with underlying urologic disease are assessed with special attention to optimization of the urinary bladder or its substitute, for urinary tract reconstruction, and for possible pre-transplant nephrectomy (see below). If a significant symptom complex or urodynamic abnormalities are present, an attempt is indicated to achieve bladder control with a voiding regimen, anticholinergic therapy, and/or IMC. If voiding cannot be evaluated because of urinary diversion, pretransplantation urinary undiversion can be an invaluable tool to help ensure adequate bladder function.[24] If a bladder cannot be adequately addressed because of oliguria or the presence of diversion, bladder cycling via IMC may help ensure transplant candidacy, and complex bladder pathology associated with ESRD may require extensive reconstruction, including augmentation. In general, however, an attempt is made to avoid this procedure in valve patients, although some younger patients with this diagnosis have required pretransplantation augmentation.

Structural bladder abnormalities may be further characterized pretransplant by cystourethroscopy to clarify whether surgical intervention e.g. lower urinary tract reconstruction, is required. Aggressive bladder management post-transplant may improve renal allograft survival and function,[25–27] as decreased allograft success may be secondary to urinary stasis and not simply due to a distorted bladder.[28]

Table 24.4 outlines the indications for pretransplant nephrectomy.[6,29–32] Persistent proteinuria originating from the native kidneys is considered an indication for native nephrectomies, not only because such proteinuria can cause diagnostic uncertainty post-transplant but also because significant, i.e.

Table 24.4 Indications for pretransplantation native nephrectomy

Chronic renal parenchymal infection
Infected urolithiasis
Heavy proteinuria
Intractable hypertension
Polycystic disease
Acquired renal cystic disease
Infected reflux
Infected hydronephrosis

nephrotic-range, proteinuria at the time of transplantation is associated with an increased risk for thrombotic and infectious complications. In children with congenital nephrotic syndrome, nephrectomies are oftentimes performed at some point during their CRI stage to eliminate substantial protein losses. Otherwise, the native nephrectomies can be carried out several weeks before transplantation to allow resolution of the nephrotic state.[10,31–33] A similar approach should be considered for older children with focal segmental glomerulosclerosis with persistent proteinuria. Malignant degeneration in the pediatric age range has also been reported,[34] but this possibility needs to be weighed against the risks associated with native nephrectomies when preparing children for kidney transplantation.

Several strategic considerations regarding nephrectomy are relevant. Even in advanced CRI and ESRD requiring dialysis, some native kidneys excrete substantial amounts of urine, often allowing easier blood pressure control and less day-to-day restrictions with regards to fluid intake. Consequently, if only one kidney requires removal, this can be done at the time of transplantation and possibly through the same incision as the transplant itself. If both kidneys need to be removed, differential function can be analyzed by isotope imaging and the worst kidney removed pretransplant, with the other being removed at the time of transplantation. Exceptions to this approach include the presence of renal-mediated diseases (e.g. intractable infection or hypertension), space-related issues (as seen with polycystic kidneys), or significantly surgically altered kidneys (e.g. diversion), all of which may make nephrectomy at the time of transplantation too difficult, requiring a more staged approach.

The nephrectomy incision should be positioned so as not to interfere with abdominal wall blood supply, as a subsequent transplant incision may result in sacrifice of the inferior epigastric vessels. If this has been performed bilaterally and previous ligation of the superior epigastric vessels has been done, compromised healing or even abdominal wall necrosis may therefore be encountered. Accordingly, transverse upper abdominal incisions (e.g. for bilateral native nephrectomies) should be avoided.

Bladder augmentation procedures may be necessary before renal transplantation to ensure a low-pressure urinary reservoir, because a relationship between high intravesical pressures and renal, including renal transplant, deterioration is well established (see above).[26,27,35–38] On the other hand, effective management of dysfunctional bladders is associated with long-term allograft survival comparable to that seen in recipients with normal bladders.[39,40] Since augmentation in the transplant setting can complicate the overall clinical course, it should only be performed in carefully selected patients with a clear need for this procedure. In Table 24.5, various types of bladder augmentation are reviewed. Although ileocystoplasty is the most prevalent procedure because of its ease of use, its disadvantages include significant mucus production, bladder calculus formation, and metabolic acidosis. These disadvantages are overcome by performing a gastrocystoplasty, but this approach is not a panacea either.[41]

In selected circumstances, bladder augmentation in the form of autoaugmentation or ureterocystoplasty can be performed extraperitoneally, as can the creation of a Mitrofanoff neourethra (Figure 24.4). If

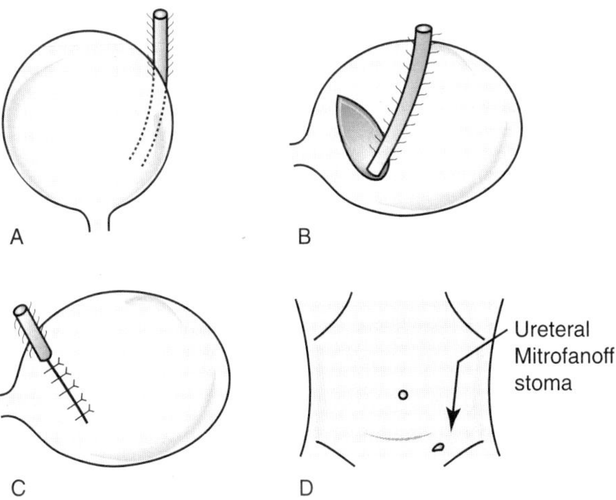

Figure 24.4 Retroperitoneal creation of a ureteral Mitrofanoff conduit. A, Ureter is mobilized with preservation of the adjacent vascular supply. Nephrectomy is performed (dorsal lumbotomy or flank incision). B, Detrusor incision is made and a mucosal trough developed. C, Detrusor flaps are approximated over the ureter. D, Final position of the Mitrofanoff stoma does not interfere with subsequent transplantation.

Table 24.5 Factors to consider in bladder augmentation

None	Low risk of complication	Renal injury if bladder non-compliant	Whenever possible
Autoaugmentation	No metabolic consequences May be performed extraperitoneally	Augmentation surface not amenable to ureteral or MNU implantation Risk of perforation Limited clinical experience	Sufficient native bladder surface for implantation Near-normal bladder capacity
Ureterocystoplasty	No metabolic consequences May be performed extraperitoneally	Augmentation surface not amenable to ureteral or MNU implantation Requires presence of large dilated ureter	Sufficient native bladder surface for implantation
Seromuscular augmentation	No metabolic consequences	Augmentation surface less amenable to ureteral or MNU implantation	Sufficient native bladder surface for implantation Near-normal bladder capacity
Ileocystoplasty	Technically simple	Augmentation surface less amenable to ureteral or MNU implantation Acidosis, mucus, or infection	Sufficient native bladder surface for implantation Stomach unavailable
Colocystoplasty	Technically simple Ureteral or MNU implantation possible	Acidosis, mucus, or infection	Stomach unavailable
Gastrocystoplasty	Avoids acidosis, mucus, or infection Ureteral or MNU implantation	Hematuria/dysuria syndrome readily performed Rare–alkalosis	Wide application

MNU, Mitrofanoff neourethra.

transperitoneal reconstruction is required before transplantation, this should be done when the patient is ready for listing or 6–12 weeks before scheduled living donor transplantation, with the patient maintained on hemodialysis in the interim.

The management of vesicoureteral reflux (VUR) in the native retained renal unit remains controversial. An increased incidence of acute symptomatic UTIs in patients with continued native VUR has been demonstrated compared with controls and with patients with previously corrected reflux,[42,43] although other studies have not confirmed this.[44] The consensus is that VUR associated with persistent or recurrent infection should be managed by ureteral reimplantation or nephroureterectomy. Reimplantation is preferable in order to preserve the native ureter, and is thus an additional option for the management of possible ureteral complications of future allografts. Additionally, higher-grade sterile reflux associated with ureteral dilation has been associated with sufficient morbidity to justify pretransplantation ureteral reimplantation,[42] with a pretransplant nephrectomy as an alternative.

In general, a key element in the surgical care of the transplant patient involves preservation of the peritoneal cavity whenever possible to allow effective peritoneal dialysis. An effort should therefore be made to avoid transperitoneal surgery, which may compromise effective exchange of dialysate secondary to postsurgical adhesions. In addition, even serosal changes can interfere with effective ultrafiltration and thus obviate peritoneal dialysis.

Timing of transplantation

Whereas the occurrence of an organ transplant from a deceased donor is largely unpredictable, transplantation can be scheduled in advance when a live donor is available. Once a transplant date is set, arrangements can also be made to initiate immunosuppressive therapy ahead of time, typically several days pretransplant at those centers choosing this approach, to facilitate therapeutic drug levels at the actual time of surgery. It should be noted, however, that data supporting this practice as a means to improve outcome are not available.[45]

Live donor transplantation allows the performance of a pre-emptive transplant, i.e. transplantation just before dialysis needs to be initiated. Pre-emptive transplantation has a number of advantages[46] and should thus be considered whenever possible. In the setting of pre-emptive transplantation, especially when an adult kidney is placed into a small child, caution with pretransplant immunosuppression should be exercised as these recipients can be quite uremic, and treatment with a CI for a number of days before transplantation may worsen this condition further. Under these circumstances, a grafted adult kidney that functions immediately can remove uremic toxins at a staggering rate and thus create a clinical scenario similar to the dysequilibrium syndrome seen in the setting of zealous, typically first-time, hemodialysis.

Renal allografts can either be obtained from a deceased donor or a living donor, and superior outcomes have been documented for the latter when adjusted for the degree of human leukocyte antigen (HLA) matching.[47,48] However, it should be noted that at least for the first several years post-transplant, North American first-time pediatric recipients of deceased donor kidneys now have essentially equivalent graft survival to those of live donor kidneys (Table 24.6). This phenomenon is probably multifactorial and, paired with the special advantages for pediatric patients with regards to growth and development associated with transplantation versus dialysis, supports the preferential waitlisting practices afforded to children as opposed to adults in North America and elsewhere, especially since children represent such a diminutively small fraction of the entire population of patients with ESRD. While efforts are ongoing to refine organ selection criteria for children, a useful rule of thumb is that the best kidney for a child is one from an otherwise healthy teenage or young adult donor and that a single kidney from a very young pediatric donor will not provide acceptable long-term function.[49] Under selected circumstances, however, consideration can be given to the transplantation of an en bloc pair of kidneys from such a very young donor into a pediatric recipient.[50] Similarly, the use of kidneys from deceased donors meeting expanded criteria or even from non-heart-beating donors, which is gaining increasing ground in adult kidney transplantation, is currently only indicated for children in extremely rare situations because these organs are unlikely to provide the very long graft survival desired especially for pediatric recipients.

Table 24.6 Similar 1-year graft survival rates in living and deceased donor kidney transplantation for pediatric recipients

Transplant year	Living donor	Cadaver
1987–1990	89.4%	75.2%
1991–1994	91.8%	85.0%
1995–1998	93.9%	90.4%
1999–2003	95.3%	92.3%

From NAPRTCS 2004 Annual Report.

The transplant

Deceased donor management

The optimal medical management of individuals who have died and become organ donors is evolving continuously, and a comprehensive review of this topic has recently been published.[51] Typically, specialized professionals from the local organ procurement organization are closely involved in this part of the donor care to ascertain optimal organ quality at the time of retrieval.

This retrieval is performed through a midline incision extending from the sternal notch to the pubis.[52,53] The intestines are mobilized and the distal aorta and inferior vena cava isolated. As necessary, the vascular anatomy of the liver, pancreas, and small intestine is defined and the aorta isolated at the level of its diaphragmatic hiatus. The distal aorta is cannulated, the supraceliac aorta clamped, venous drainage achieved (generally at the level of the right atrium), the aorta flushed with cold preservation solution, and the abdomen packed with sterile saline ice slush. Organs are sequentially removed, beginning with the heart, followed by the lungs, liver, small intestine, or pancreas, and finally, the kidneys. The kidneys are removed en bloc with the adjacent aorta and vena cava and the ureters divided at the level of the urinary bladder. Kidneys from very young donors are not separated until a decision has been made about whether or not they will be transplanted individually or en bloc. Otherwise, the kidneys are separated on the back table and cold-stored for distribution.

Table 24.7 Composition of cold storage solutions

Constituent	EuroCollins solution	University of Wisconsin solution
Na^+	9.3	
K^+	107	
Cl^-	14	
HCO_3^-	9.3	
PO_4^{2-}	93	
K^+ lactobionate		100
KH_2PO_4		25
$MgSO_4$		5
Glucose	182	
Raffinose		30
Hydroxyethyl starch (g/L)		50
Glutathione		3
Adenosine		3
Insulin (mg/L)		40
Dexamethasone	8	
pH	7	7.4
Osmolarity (mOsm/L)	325	320

From Ryckman.[52]

Organ preservation solutions are designed to minimize hypoxia- and hypothermia-induced injury. The active ingredients of the two most widely used solutions are outlined in Table 24.7.[52,53] A comparison of both solutions has revealed a significant benefit in graft function and survival favoring University of Wisconsin solution over EuroCollins solution.[54] The osmotic swelling and sodium pump paralysis associated with hypothermia are compensated by the elimination or reduction of chloride, whose intracellular shift facilitates osmotic edema, in favor of impermeable ionic agents such as phosphate, sulfate, and lactobionate. Lactobionate, raffinose, hydroxyethyl starch, and mannitol further contribute to reducing intercellular swelling. Intracellular acidosis is compensated by the avoidance of glucose and the addition of phosphate, which acts as a hydrogen ion buffer. Oxygen free radical-induced reperfusion injury is compensated by allopurinol and glutathione, and the depletion of high-energy phosphate compounds is countered by the addition of adenosine.

Live donor management

In part because of the ever-worsening relative shortage of deceased donors, the majority of pediatric recipients in North America currently receive a kidney from a live donor, and most live donors for these children are their parents (NAPRTCS 2004 Annual Report). This poses unique challenges and responsibilities on the centers caring for these families. Despite the now well-recognized short- and long-term risks associated with being a live donor,[55] parents may feel a special duty to donate one of their kidneys to their child, even if they jeopardize their own health. The issue of organ donation needs to be approached with sensitivity, and full disclosure and discussion of all relevant information in a family-centered setting is important. Specific strategies to consider include, but are not limited to, the provision of written educational material from center-independent resources like the United Network for Organ Sharing (http://www.unos.org), the performance of a parent's medical evaluation as a potential donor (Table 24.8) by an independent, critical physician otherwise dissociated from the transplant center, the facilitation of contacts between the potential donors and past donors who have had difficult experiences related to their donation, and possibly the identification of a donor advocate or the creation of a donor advocacy board somewhat similar to an ethics committee.

Furthermore, individuals who have been cleared for living donation need to be re-evaluated periodically for new or worsened conditions possibly jeopardizing their donor status if the planned transplant does not take place within a reasonable period of time, i.e. 6–12 months, either because of a stabilization in the recipient's health status or because of new medical or non-medical issues related to the recipient requiring postponement of the procedure.

This scrutiny in donor selection is particularly important when an individual who is not biologically, but emotionally, related to the potential recipient steps forward as a willing donor, or if an altruistic donor is found.[56] Local allocation practices of organs from such altruistic donors vary, but preference is sometimes given to children waitlisted for a deceased donor kidney. Generally, an in-depth psychological assessment of these donors is required to exclude hidden non-altruistic motives or other circumstances making donation unadvisable.

Another novel concept aiming to attenuate the deceased donor shortage and to specifically overcome the obstacles posed by blood type incompatibilities and presensitization is the creation of live donor exchange programs. Such programs have been established in several regions of the United States and are beginning to provide relief for recipients whose chances of receiving a suitable kidney graft would otherwise be slim.[56]

Table 24.8 Suggested evaluation of living donor candidates

Evaluation	Possible exclusion criteria
Initial screening	
History	Younger than legal age of consent, diabetes mellitus, marked obesity, significant cardiovascular or pulmonary disease, substance abuse, malignancy, transmissible infection
Blood typing	ABO incompatibility
Tissue typing and crossmatch	Positive crossmatch
Physical examination	see 'History' above
Psychological evaluation	Evidence of coercion, reluctance to donate
Pregnancy test in females	Positive test
Secondary screening	
Laboratory studies (complete blood count, coagulation studies, fasting glucose and cholesterol, electrolytes, liver enzymes, albumin/total protein, uric acid)	Significant uncorrectable abnormality
Renal assessment (urinalysis, serum creatinine and blood urea nitrogen, creatinine clearance, protein excretion, renal ultrasound, renal arteriography	Renal disease Complex abnormality of renal anatomy, e.g. vasculature
Chest radiograph	Significant pulmonary pathology
Screening for infection (cytomegalovirus, Epstein–Barr virus, and human immunodeficiency virus titers, hepatitis B and C serologies, purified protein derivative, urine culture)	Transmissible chronic infection
Pelvic examination with *Pap smear* and, if >40 years, *mammography* within 1 year in females	Malignancy
Rectal examination and, if >40 years, *prostate-specific antigen* in men	Malignancy
Tertiary screening	
For family history of diabetes or borderline fasting glucose: 2-hour postprandial glucose, glycosylated hemoglobin, oral glucose tolerance test	Diabetes mellitus
For older donor age, cardiac risk factors or symptoms: non-invasive stress testing, echocardiography	Significant cardiac disease
For pulmonary symptoms: pulmonary function tests	Significant pulmonary disease
Additional screening	
If scheduled transplant is postponed: Periodic re-evaluation for changes in donor health status	New significant medical problems

Living donor nephrectomy is performed simultaneously with the surgical exposure of the recipient. Antiembolism sequential compression stockings are used, and the patient is placed in a flank position. Traditionally, live donor nephrectomy has been performed through an extended 11th or 12th rib incision, which enables excellent retroperitoneal exposure of the renal hilar vessels and the ureter. The kidney is gently mobilized, taking care to avoid excessive dissection of the lower pole, so as to maintain ureteral blood supply. In addition, the ureter is mobilized with a generous cuff of retroperitoneal adipose tissue in order to maximize its vascularity. The hilar vessels are dissected to their junction with the aorta and vena cava.

When the recipient room is ready, the donor ureter is divided as far distally as possible and the distal ureteral stump ligated with absorbable suture material. Good urine output is documented from both the divided ureter and the indwelling urethral catheter. The renal artery and vein are clamped proximally, the vessels divided, and the kidney immediately flushed with cold preservation solution, placed in saline ice slush, and delivered to the adjacent recipient room, while the renal artery and vein stumps are oversewn with Prolene suture. Although significant morbidity and mortality have been low with this approach, postoperative discomfort, as well as length of recovery and associated time off work, may be significant and have in some instances served as a deterrent to donation.

Accordingly, encouraging early results have been reported with the use of laparoscopic live donor nephrectomies: e.g. decreased analgesic requirements, decreased length of hospital stay, and an earlier return to work.[57–61] However, recent data suggest that small pediatric recipients of adult kidneys removed laparoscopically may be at risk for inferior outcomes: i.e. delayed graft function and early rejection.[62] A relatively low threshold for open donor nephrectomy in these situations therefore seems advisable until more data are available.[63]

Recipient management

As mentioned above, recipients entering the operating room for a kidney transplant should be in their best possible medical condition. Moreover, children on dialysis may undergo hemodialysis on the day or peritoneal dialysis the night before their transplant for metabolic control (e.g. to reduce serum concentrations of potassium or blood urea nitrogen), but they should be relatively volume-loaded to facilitate adequate perfusion of the new allograft.[64] Therefore, dialysis immediately pretransplant should be performed with an adjusted ultrafiltration goal, possibly requiring an increase in antihypertensive drug therapy to compensate for this adjustment. If hemodialysis is required on the day of transplantation, anticoagulation should also be used sparingly or not at all to avoid an increased risk of bleeding during surgery.

The transplantation process in the recipient begins with the induction of general endotracheal anesthesia. The patient is positioned supine, a Foley catheter is placed, and the bladder is inflated with an antibacterial solution. Other potential lines include an arterial line, central venous access and, rarely, a pulmonary arterial catheter. A second-generation cephalosporin is administered and intravenous hydration undertaken. Red blood cell mass is expanded if indicated, but care should be taken to avoid possible sensitization.

The operation is performed through a 'hockey-stick' incision to give excellent retroperitoneal exposure. An attempt is made to place the kidney retroperitoneal in order to preserve the peritoneal cavity for future dialysis access if needed. Typically, grafts are readily placed retroperitoneal in recipients weighing >20 kg and in those weighing between 10 and 20 kg and receiving a pediatric or small adult kidney. Transabdominal placement through a midline incision is considered in recipients weighing <10 kg (Figure 24.5)[65] due to the limited volume of the retroperitoneum. However, these anatomic decisions need to be made on an individualized basis.

The venous and arterial trees for the anastomotic sites are carefully mobilized with division of the overlying lymphatic vessels between ligatures. In general,

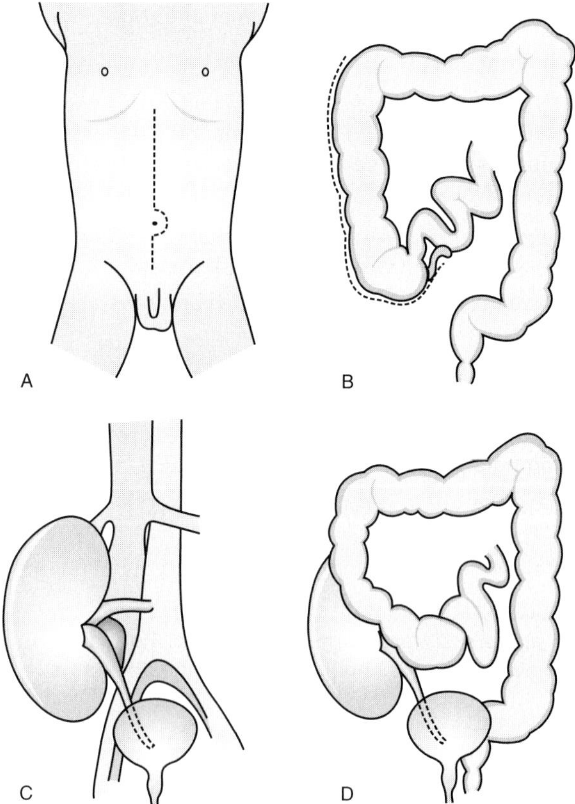

Figure 24.5 Transperitoneal approach to renal transplantation in the infant. A, Midline abdominal incision. B, Reflection of right colon to expose retroperitoneum. C, Renal vessels anastomosed to aorta and inferior vena cava; ureter reimplanted in bladder. D, Right colon repositioned to allow exposure of the lower pole of the graft. (Reproduced with permission from Sheldon et al.[66])

the anastomosis is placed at the level of the aorta or aortoiliac junction in infants and toddlers, in the common iliac artery in young children, and in the external iliac artery in adolescents and young adults. Once vascular control is achieved, the venotomy is made, the recipient vein injected with a heparin–saline solution, and the anastomosis is completed. The arteriotomy is then made, and the arterial anastomosis is then performed. If the aorta is to be occluded, the patient is treated with heparin. Mannitol (0.5 mg/kg) and furosemide (0.5–1 mg/kg) are administered before completing the anastomoses. The vascular clamps are removed, with gentle pressure applied to the renal artery to allow clearance of any debris or air pockets before kidney revascularization. An intraarterial injection of verapamil (0.1 mg/kg, not exceeding 5 mg, into the upstream recipient artery with the distal recipient artery still occluded) may be performed at this time.

Post-transplantation hypotension in the recipient is a major risk factor for allograft loss and must be aggressively avoided. Given this, the blood volume of the patient is expanded to a central venous pressure (CVP) of 12–16 cmH_2O, with the expectation that vascularization of an adult allograft will result in the acute sequestration of approximately 250–300 ml of blood from the general circulation. Failure to achieve adequate renal turgor may necessitate additional volume expansion or the addition of inotropic support, e.g. a low-dose dopamine infusion. Especially for small recipients of an adult kidney, the generous volume requirements to maintain a CVP sufficient for good blood flow to the transplant persist during and after the surgery, thus requiring special attention by anesthesia and by the management team providing recipient care immediately post-transplant.[64] Even long-term, generous fluid administration, possibly including night-time or bolus supplementations, e.g. via G-buttons, has been advocated.[64]

Variations in vascular anatomy may obviate the use of a kidney from a prospective living donor or may create reconstructive challenges in the cadaveric allograft.[66] As previously outlined, in cadaveric renal procurement, the kidneys are removed en bloc with the adjacent vena cava and aorta (Figure 24.6A). Here, the kidneys are visualized from a posterior perspective and the aorta opened in the midline posteriorly. This is followed by division of the anterior aorta and the vena cava, again in the midline. The kidney is thereby provided with an adjacent segment of both aorta and vena cava, which gives reconstructive flexibility. As demonstrated in Figure 24.6B, a renal vessel of good

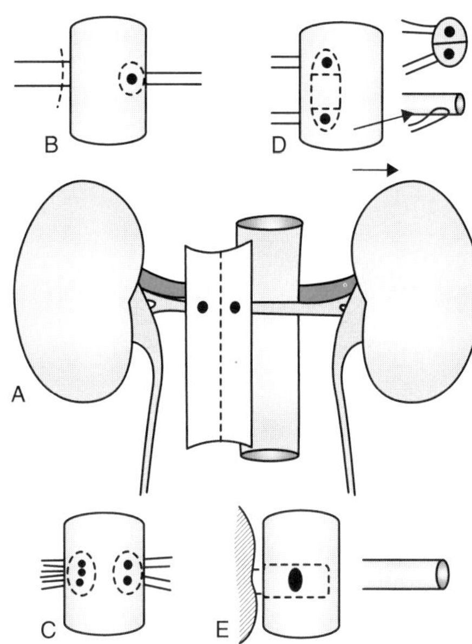

Figure 24.6 Management of variations in renal vascular anatomy. (Adapted with permission from Sheldon et al.[66])

dimension can be divided, spatulated, and anastomosed. If the vessel is small, it may be prepared with a small patch of adjacent aorta or vena cava to facilitate the anastomosis and minimize the risk of anastomotic stenosis or thrombosis. Multiple vessels entering the vena cava or aorta in a cluster may be prepared on a single large cuff of aorta or vena cava. If multiple vessels are encountered that enter the vena cava or aorta at sites remote from each other, reconstruction may be needed (see Figures 24.6C and D). If both vessels are particularly modest in size, two small patches may be anastomosed to create one larger cuff for anastomosis. If a dominant artery is encountered with a second smaller artery, an end-to-side anastomosis is undertaken. This type of vascular reconfiguration is enhanced by the use of an operative microscope.[67] Occasionally, an extremely short renal vein is encountered. Usually, generous mobilization of the recipient venous tree is sufficient to enable a tension-free anastomosis. When this is not possible or is insufficient, the renal vein may be extended by tubularizing adjacent flaps of vena cava (Fig. 24.6E).

Ureteral implantation is most commonly performed into the bladder. Recently, however, investigators have reported ureteroureteral anastomosis as another option in pediatric renal transplantation.[68] Ureterovesical reimplantation may be performed either transvesically (Paquin's method) or extravesically (detrusorrhaphy). Advantages of the extravesical approach (Figure 24.7)

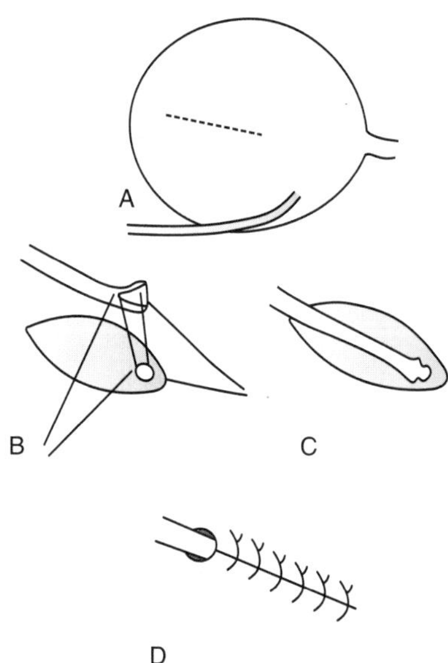

Figure 24.7 Technique for extravesical ureteral implantation.

include a shortened operating time, a very low incidence of anastomotic obstruction, and most importantly, a dramatic reduction of postoperative hematuria and urinary extravasation. This is particularly advantageous in the young recipient whose urethra only allows a small-caliber catheter. Ureteral implantation is considerably more critical in the child, as the incidence of dysfunctional voiding pathophysiology is particularly high in this age group. An attempt is made to place the anastomosis somewhat lateral on the bladder, where the bladder wall is less mobile, and a ureteral tunnel length-to-ureteral diameter ratio of 4:1 is sought (see Figure 24.7A). The detrusor is incised and a plane developed between the detrusor and the underlying bladder uroepithelium. A small defect is created distally in this mucosal trough, and a spatulated anastomosis is performed (Figure 24.7B). The ureter is advanced distally with the first suture placed (Figures 24.7C and D). Because ureteral obstruction (e.g. from anastomotic edema) or extravasation represent potentially devastating complications, an internal indwelling stent is often advantageous in the early postoperative period. This stent can then be removed several weeks post-transplant, oftentimes combined with removal of chronic dialysis access.

Postoperative care

In addition to general perioperative care, including circulatory, respiratory, and nutritional support, postoperative care of the pediatric transplant recipient includes immunosuppression and careful fluid and electrolyte management. The latter involves replacing insensible losses and urine output, initially on a volume-for-volume basis and with close attention to the patient's electrolyte status. The freshly transplanted kidney is often unable to concentrate the urine, so that urine output may be tremendous in the first several postoperative days.

Generally, immunosuppressive therapy is in constant evolution to achieve the best possible antirejection prophylaxis without an unacceptably high incidence of overimmunosuppression or other drug-related toxicities.[69] In this context, it has become quite clear that immunosuppressive protocols cannot be administered in a 'one size fits all' fashion: first-time Caucasian recipients of a live donor kidney who have no evidence of presensitization appear to require less powerful antirejection prophylaxis than recipients of a repeat transplant, especially one from a deceased donor, recipients with evidence of presensitization, or African-American recipients.[70] Additionally, the recent discovery of genetic polymorphisms and related phenomena affecting drug metabolism and exposure[71,72] and immunologic responsiveness[73] further undermines the concept of a unified immunosuppressive approach. It therefore likely behooves transplant programs to adapt flexible immunosuppression protocols that can be tailored to each recipient's perceived risk profile. Theoretically, the development of such protocols is augmented by sufficiently powered multicenter studies, but in view of the relatively small number of pediatric kidney transplants performed at any given time and given the increasing number of drugs and drug combinations available, such studies are quite difficult to set up and perform. Additional guidance in the selection of pediatric immunosuppressive regimens is therefore also derived from adult studies and from local practice and experience. A typical protocol to be used initially in pediatric kidney transplantation currently consists of triple therapy with a CI, an antiproliferative agent, and steroids, possibly paired with a course of induction with a non-depleting anti-T cell antibody (Table 24.9). The doses and target levels of these agents are geared towards the recipient's estimated risk for acute rejection, balanced against side effects and other potential disadvantages associated with the use of these agents. Of note, recent efforts by a variety of groups have further broadened the available choices for initial immunosuppression. They now include complete steroid avoidance, induction with alterna-

Table 24.9 Typical immunosuppression protocol for pediatric kidney transplant recipients

Induction[a]	Maintenance[b]
Consider non-depleting anti-T cell antibody	
High-dose steroids	Tapered steroids
Calcineurin inhibitor (CI), e.g. tacrolimus	Modest-dose CI
Antimetabolite, e.g. mycophenolate mofetil	Mycophenolate mofetil

[a] For first several weeks and months post-transplant.
[b] An inhibitor of the mammalian target of rapamycin (mTOR), such as sirolimus (rapamycin) or everolimus, can be added or substituted for any one of the three maintenance agents based on center practice.

tive antibody preparations, and introduction of a new class of maintenance immunosuppressants, the inhibitors of the mammalian target of rapamycin (mTOR), largely to reduce the use of CIs, which carries a substantial long-term risk of nephrotoxicity.[69,74]

Hypertension frequently occurs or, if pre-existing, worsens in the immediate post-transplant setting for several reasons, including liberal fluid management (see above) and treatment with high doses of corticosteroids. Whereas mild blood pressure elevations above the patient's pre-transplant range may even be temporarily desirable to enhance perfusion of the new allograft, more pronounced hypertension, especially if it is causing symptoms, should be treated expeditiously. In this setting, calcium channel antagonists are particularly safe and effective, although attention needs to be paid to the interference of some of these agents, particularly verapamil, diltiazem, amlodipine, and nicardipine, with CI metabolism.[70] Once transplant function has stabilized, the same group of agents may also be particularly beneficial,[75,76] although angiotensin-converting enzyme inhibitors (ACEIs) or angiotensin receptor blockers (ARBs) should also be considered, especially if there is evidence of CAN.[77,78]

Hypophosphatemia and hypomagnesemia can occur quickly post-transplant: the former is largely due to 'hungry bones' in the presence of a well-functioning kidney and frequently requires phosphorus supplementation for several months; the latter is associated with CI therapy especially tacrolimus, and may also require supplementation, especially if clinical symptoms of hypomagnesemia are present.

Infection prophylaxis against bacterial, viral, and fungal pathogens is part of essentially all routine post-transplant medication regimens. Antibiotic coverage is typically provided perioperatively to prevent wound infections and then transitioned to a prophylactic regimen against UTIs and *Pneumocystis carinii*. Specific guidelines have been developed for antiviral prophylaxis in the post-transplant setting.[79] This antiviral prophylaxis is largely directed against cytomegalovirus (CMV) and usually prescribed based on each patient's risk profile, as determined by the recipient's as well as the donor's history of CMV exposure and by the strength of immunosuppression used. Unfortunately, no convincingly effective prophylactic regimens are currently available for the prevention of Epstein–Barr virus (EBV) infection. Since many pediatric transplant recipients are EBV-naïve and many adult donors carry EBV, primary EBV infection of transplanted children via the graft is a considerable problem, especially because EBV can drive the development of post-transplant lymphoproliferative disorder (PTLD).[80] Lastly, antifungal prophylaxis is typically provided during the first several months post-transplant, i.e. while the degree of immunosuppression prescribed is considerable. Accordingly, a number of centers also 'recycle' the full spectrum of infection prophylaxis during and after episodes of acute rejection, requiring enhanced immunosuppressive therapy.

Gastrointestinal prophylaxis against steroid-associated gastritis and ulcer disease is typically given in the form of a histamine H_2 receptor blocker. At our center, recipients are tried off these agents once they are taking all their medicines by mouth and if they are free of gastrointestinal complaints.

Approach to early graft dysfunction and other complications

Graft dysfunction immediately post-transplant is suggested by lack or decrease of urine output and by absence of the expected decrease in serum creatinine. Initial non-function, i.e. the complete absence of urine production, is very concerning as it could be caused by thrombotic obstruction of arterial blood flow to the graft. Accordingly, initial non-function requires immediate diagnostic evaluation and subsequent correction if the transplant is to be salvaged. Many centers therefore perform a Doppler ultrasonographic evaluation or a nuclear scan of the transplant immediately after skin closure or upon arrival in the postoperative care unit, at least if there is no sufficient urine output attributable to the transplant. Along these lines, many recipients still have their native, oftentimes urine-producing, kidneys at the time of transplantation, making interpretation of urine output immediately post-transplant challenging at times. If blood flow to the transplant is adequate, acute tubular necrosis should be suspected as an alternative cause of initial non-function, especially in deceased donor transplants. In recipients who are not at particularly increased immunologic risk, hyperacute rejection is very unlikely. Lastly, the possibility of complete urinary tract obstruction needs to be excluded by ultrasound in this scenario.

In grafts with initially acceptable urine production but a subsequent decrease in output, additional possibilities need to be considered. These include low intravascular volume, rejection, and acute CI toxicity. Low intravascular volume can be diagnosed if a fluid challenge sufficient to raise CVP results in restitution of adequate diuresis, and acute CI toxicity is indicated by elevated trough levels, e.g. tacrolimus concentrations >20 ng/ml. Early rejection can be difficult to diagnose, as its recognition usually requires a kidney biopsy, which may be risky in a fresh transplant. Moreover, different types of rejection may need to be distinguished, as they require different therapeutic responses. Especially in presensitized recipients, acute rejection may not only be cellular- but also antibody-mediated, i.e. humoral, necessitating the initiation of plasmapheresis and potentially other specific therapeutic measures instead of treatment for cellular rejection, which consists of steroid pulses or the application of depleting anti-T cell antibody products. Moreover, cellular and humoral rejection can coexist, and the recognition of humoral rejection requires special studies both on the biopsy material, i.e. staining for C4d, and in the blood, i.e. identification of antidonor antibody.[81]

Additional complications resulting in early impairment of graft function are thrombosis of the renal vein or one of its major branches, obstruction of urine flow, e.g. by a blood clot, and urinary leakage, e.g. from an unsatisfactory ureteral anastomosis. Ultrasound and nuclear scan are useful tools to identify these problems.

Surgical/urologic complications of transplantation

A comprehensive review of surgical complications[82] of renal transplantation reveals technical problems in 13% of transplant operations, 35% of which resulted in graft loss. Urologic complications other than uncomplicated UTIs occurred in 5.6% and consisted primarily of urinary extravasation, ureteral anastomotic obstruction, ureteral necrosis, and symptomatic VUR. Urologic complications resulted in allograft loss in 31% of cases.

Renovascular complications were encountered in 5.5% of cases, with a 3.2% incidence of technical vascular problems consisting of renal artery stenosis or thrombosis and renal vein thrombosis. Of note, 86% of all vascular complications and 74% of technical vascular complications resulted in allograft loss. Renal artery and vein thromboses are associated with particularly high incidences of graft loss and may have a technical (e.g. anastomotic defect, vascular angulation, or compression) or a non-technical cause (e.g. a low-flow state, intimal injury from harvesting, cannulation, or existing donor vascular disease). Renovascular stenosis may be managed by percutaneous transluminal angioplasty,[83] although some centers have reported greater success with primary surgical reconstruction.[84]

Wound complications occurred in 4.2% of patients and consisted primarily of lymphocele, hemorrhage, and infection. Hemorrhage was associated with a 44% incidence of graft loss, and allograft rupture was reported in 2.4% of patients, generally associated with rejection. In several instances, hemorrhage was controlled and the kidney surgically salvaged, leaving a 57% incidence of acute graft loss. Long-term follow-up, however, has revealed a very poor prognosis regarding long-term function.[85,86]

Urolithiasis can complicate renal transplantation in approximately 6% of adult[87,88] and 5% of pediatric cases,[89–91] creating a particularly challenging situation because of the increased difficulty experienced with endoscopic stent placement and ureteroscopy in the post-transplant setting. A multifactorial etiology of urolithiasis has been demonstrated with low urine output, elevated calcium excretion, and possibly disturbances in uric acid metabolism secondary to CI therapy. Additional factors include increased frequency of UTIs, alkaline urinary pH, hypocitraturia, hypomagnesuria, hypophosphaturia, and hyperparathyroidism found in 36% of patients. A surgical cause for urolithiasis can also be retained suture material.[89] For stone management, extracorporeal shock wave lithotripsy (ESWL)[92] and/or endourological approaches[93] can be used.

The significance of VUR post-transplant has been the subject of intense discussion. When VUR was detected by routine post-transplantation screening, no statistical significance in the survival of patients or grafts has been demonstrated for adults[94] or children.[95] However, pathologic data from VUR-associated pyelonephritis in transplanted pediatric kidneys suggests that its occurrence reduces long-term survival of renal allografts.[96] Adult series have shown that no patient had greater than grade III reflux, whereas in the pediatric series all patients with greater than grade III reflux underwent antireflux surgery. More recently, endoscopic management of reflux has been attempted,[97] but this has shown little success. Most often, the underlying problem is occult or incompletely managed bladder dysfunction, and the reflux is controllable by management efforts directed at the bladder, which may require anticholinergics and/or IMC. Dilating reflux in the absence of a dysfunctional bladder should be considered for correction, because such reflux in young recipients is associated with a definite risk of pyelonephritis and subsequent allograft injury.[98] VUR has also been implicated as a significant etiologic factor for hypertension on long-term follow-up.[99]

Transition to outpatient management

After successful kidney transplantation, children typically spend at least a week in the hospital recovering from the procedure. During this time, their fluid, caloric, and medication intake is adjusted to their outpatient regimen, and central lines as well as bladder catheters are removed in most cases.

Transition to outpatient care occurs on an individualized basis, depending on medical as well as geographical aspects. Local patients will continue to be seen frequently at the transplant center, initially several times a week, whereas other patients, who may have been referred for transplantation from a nephrology care provider further away, may return rapidly to care rendered by that provider. Recipients with complex lower urinary tracts will also require long-term urologic follow-up.

Maintenance management, including immunosuppression

After hospital discharge, patient management is largely focused on maintaining graft function without overly toxic or complex treatment regimens, so as to facilitate maximal patient rehabilitation with regards to growth and development, allowing as 'normal' of a childhood as possible with regular school participation and sports or other extracurricular activities. Historically, maintenance of graft function largely consisted of the prevention or at least prompt recognition and treatment of acute rejection. With the application of the latest immunosuppressive strategies, however, the incidence of acute rejection in the first 6–12 post-transplant months should be less than 15%, and the most common reason for rehospitalization of pediatric kidney transplant recipients is now infection and not rejection.[100] These trends, paired with the almost inevitable development of CAN over time[69,74] and the considerable incidence of PTLD,[101] imply that a number of patients (probably excluding those at high immunologic risk) may currently be overimmunosuppressed. Discussions and efforts are therefore under way to develop more appropriate regimens for rejection prophylaxis, taking into consideration an individualized risk profile based on a variety of graft and recipient factors (see above). Generally, prudent combinations of several antirejection agents, adjusted based on various parameters as outlined above, will remain the mainstay of immunosuppressive therapy as long as the advent of protocols capable of inducing true immunologic tolerance remains uncertain. Of note, evidence is beginning to accrue in support of long-term administration of mycophenolate mofetil as antiproliferative immunosuppressant agent of choice as part of such a combination[102] (see Table 24.9).

Long-term aspects

Current survival statistics (see Figure 24.1 and Table 24.6) document excellent short- and mid-term patient and graft survival for children with kidney transplants, comparable with the outcomes of adult kidney transplantation. However, controversy exists regarding long-term outcomes, largely because of the propensity of the current immunosuppressive protocols to contribute to CAN, the leading actual cause of graft failure in adults after the first post-transplant year, and CV disease, the leading cause of death amongst adult kidney transplant recipients.[74,103] Therefore, and although half-lives of over 35 years for renal allografts from living donors have been predicted recently by some clinicians,[104] the challenge for the future is to develop better long-term care regimens for kidney transplant recipients with special emphasis on the problems of CAN and CV disease.[69]

Moreover, such optimistic half-life predictions are not shared by other clinicians,[105] and even a transplant half-life of 30 or 40 years would theoretically appear insufficient for children, as a substantial number of transplants would still be lost rather early during their adulthood. Accordingly, there is already a growing population of patients at especially high immunologic risk: namely, those who have lost a previous kidney transplant or are recipients of another organ transplant and have developed renal failure from chronic CI toxicity or for other reasons. These individuals not only compete with first-time transplant candidates for organs but they also have a high incidence of sensitization from their previous or ongoing alloexposure and are thus more difficult to transplant and to manage post-transplant.[18,19]

Another emerging challenge in the medical management of children with kidney transplants is the provision of a meaningful transition from teenage to adulthood, including transfer of their transplant-related care to providers for adults. In fact, teenage and the transition phase into adulthood are associated with an increased incidence of adverse outcomes, at least in part due to more frequent non-compliance.[16] Better strategies to enhance compliance during these critical stages in the life of pediatric transplant recipients are thus urgently needed.

Lastly, adequate living kidney donor follow-up is required because of the donor's increased risk of hypertension and proteinuria several decades after donation.[55] Along these lines, efforts to standardize this follow-up and to create a donor registry are under way in the United States. Some unfortunate former donors have even lost function of their remaining kidney, either because of trauma, malignancy, or kidney disease that was not apparent at the time they donated, and these individuals are given very high priority in the organ allocation algorithm currently in place via the United Network for Organ Sharing.

Summary

Renal transplantation is the treatment of choice for pediatric patients with ESRD and is associated with excellent short- and mid-term outcomes, at least in recipients without extraordinary immunologic or other risk factors. In many children receiving a kidney allograft, urologic issues are of special importance before, during, and after transplantation because of the comparably high incidence of urologic disease in this age group. Important current challenges revolve around optimal long-term outcome, specifically CAN, chronic CI nephrotoxicity, other complications of prolonged administration of immunosuppressive agents, and compliance.

References

1. Broyer M, Le Bihan C, Charbit M et al. Long-term social outcome of children after kidney transplantation. Transplantation 2004; 77(7):1033–7.
2. Groothoff JW, Cransberg K, Offringa M et al. Long-term follow-up of renal transplantation in children: a dutch cohort study. Transplantation 2004; 78(3):453–60.
3. Wolfe RA, Ashby VB, Milford EL et al. Comparison of mortality in all patients on dialysis, patients on dialysis awaiting transplantation, and recipients of a first cadaveric transplant. N Engl J Med 1999; 341(23):1725–30.
4. Eggers P. Comparison of treatment costs between dialysis and transplantation. Semin Nephrol 1992; 12(3): 284–9.
5. Ojo AO, Held PI, Port FK et al. Chronic renal failure after transplantation of a nonrenal organ. N Engl J Med 2003; 349(10):931–40.
6. Sheldon CA, Snyder III HM. Principles of urinary tract reconstruction. In: Gillenwater JY, Grayhack JT, Howards SS, Duckett JW, eds. Adult and Pediatric Urology, 3rd edn. St Louis: Mosby-Year Book, 1996: 2317–410.
7. McGuire EJ, Woodside JR, Borden TA, Weiss RM. Prognostic value of urodynamic testing in myelodysplastic patients. 1981. J Urol 2002; 167(2 Pt 2):1049–53, discussion 1054.
8. Churchill BM, Gilmour RF, Williot P et al. Urodynamics. Pediatr Clin North Am 1987; 34(5):1133–57.
9. Thomsen HS. Pyelorenal backflow. Clinical and experimental investigations. Radiologic, nuclear, medical and pathoanatomic studies. Dan Med Bull 1984; 31(6):438–57.
10. Lyon RP, Marshall S, Baskin LS. Normal growth with renal insufficiency owing to posterior urethral valves: value of long-term diversion. A twenty-year follow-up. Urol Int 1992; 48(2):125–9.
11. Nguyen MT, Pavlock CL, Zderic SA, Carr MC, Canning DA. Overnight catheter drainage in children with poorly compliant bladders improves post-obstructive diuresis and urinary incontinence. Presented at the American Academy of Pediatrics' Section on Urology scientific meeting, San Francisco, CA, October 2004 (abstract).
12. Hricik DE. Weight gain after kidney transplantation. Am J Kidney Dis 2001; 38(2):409–10.
13. Acott PD, Pernica JM. Growth hormone therapy before and after pediatric renal transplant. Pediatr Transplant 2003; 7(6):426–40.
14. Saland JM. Osseous complications of pediatric transplantation. Pediatr Transplant 2004; 8(4):400–15.
15. Neu AM, Fivush BA. Recommended immunization practices for pediatric renal transplant recipients. Pediatr Transplant 1998; 2(4):263–9.
16. Nevins TE. Non-compliance and its management in teenagers. Pediatr Transplant 2002; 6(6):475–9.

17. Bosch T, Wendler T. Extracorporeal plasma treatment in primary and recurrent focal segmental glomerular sclerosis: a review. Ther Apher 2001; 5(3):155–60.
18. Gebel HM, Bray RA, Nickerson P. Pre-transplant assessment of donor-reactive, HLA-specific antibodies in renal transplantation: contraindications vs. risk. Am J Transplant 2003; 3(12):1488–500.
19. Glotz D, Antoine C, Duboust A. Antidonor antibodies and transplantation: how to deal with them before and after transplantation. Transplantation 2005; 79(3):S30–2.
20. Singh A, Stablein D, Tejani A. Risk factors for vascular thrombosis in pediatric renal transplantation: a special report of the North American Pediatric Renal Transplant Cooperative Study. Transplantation 1997; 63(9):1263–7.
21. Wagenknecht DR, Becker DG, LeFor WM, McIntyre JA. Antiphospholipid antibodies are a risk factor for early renal allograft failure. Transplantation 1999; 68(2):241–6.
22. Manco-Johnson MJ. The infant and child with thrombosis. In: Goodnight SH, Hathaway WE, eds. Disorders of Hemostasis and Thrombosis, 2nd edn. New York: McGraw-Hill, 1999: 325–37.
23. Nagra A, Trompeter RS, Fernando ON et al. The effect of heparin on graft thrombosis in pediatric renal allografts. Pediatr Nephrol 2004; 19(5):531–5.
24. Gonzalez R, LaPointe S, Sheldon CA, Mauer MS. Undiversion in children with renal failure. J Pediatr Surg 1984; 19(6):632–6.
25. Rittenberg MH, Hulbert WC, Snyder HM 3rd, Duckett JW. Protective factors in posterior urethral valves. J Urol 1988; 140(5):993–6.
26. Churchill BM, Sheldon CA, McLorie GA, Arbus GS. Factors influencing patient and graft survival in 300 cadaveric pediatric renal transplants. J Urol 1988; 140(5 Pt 2):1129–33.
27. Reinberg Y, Gonzalez R, Fryd D, Mauer SM, Najarian JS. The outcome of renal transplantation in children with posterior urethral valves. J Urol 1988; 140(6):1491–3.
28. Reinberg Y, Nanvivel JC, Fryd D, Najarian JS, Gonzalez R. The outcome of renal transplantation in children with the prune belly syndrome. J Urol 1989; 142(6):1541–2.
29. Kasiske BL. Evaluation and management of prospective kidney recipients. In: Norman DJ, Turka LA, eds. Primer on Transplantation, 2nd edn. Mt Laurel, NJ: American Society of Transplantation, 2001: 414–20.
30. Guzzetta PC. Kidney. In: Oldham KT, Colombani PM, Foglia RP, eds. Surgery of Infants and Children: Scientific Principles and Practice. Philadelphia: Lippincott-Raven, 1997: 709–20.
31. Mahan J. Management of the child with congential nephrotic syndrome. In: Tejani AH, Fine RN, eds. Pediatric Renal Transplantation. New York: Wiley-Liss, 1994: 379–86.
32. Kim MS, Stablein D, Harmon WE. Renal transplantation in children with congenital nephrotic syndrome: a report of the North American Pediatric Renal Transplant Cooperative Study (NAPRTCS). Pediatr Transplant 1998; 2(4):305–8.
33. Harmon WE, Stablein D, Alexander SR, Tejani A. Graft thrombosis in pediatric renal transplant recipients. A report of the North American Pediatric Renal Transplant Cooperative Study. Transplantation 1991; 51(2):406–12.
34. Mattoo TK, Greifer I, Geva P, Spitzer A. Acquired renal cystic disease in children and young adults on maintenance dialysis. Pediatr Nephrol 1997; 11(4):447–50.
35. Bryant JE, Joseph DB, Kohaut EC, Diethelm AG. Renal transplantation in children with posterior urethral valves. J Urol 1991; 146(6):1585–7.
36. Mochon M, Kaiser BA, Dunn S et al. Urinary tract infections in children with posterior urethral valves after kidney transplantation. J Urol 1992; 148(6):1874–6.
37. Dewan PA, McMullin ND, Barker AP. Renal allograft survival in patients with congenital obstruction of the posterior urethra. Aust N Z J Surg 1995; 65(1):27–30.
38. Salomon L, Fontaine E, Gagnadoux MF, Broyer M, Buerton D. Posterior urethral valves: long-term renal function consequences after transplantation. J Urol 1997; 157(3):992–5.
39. Luke PP, Herz DB, Bellinger MA. Long-term results of pediatric renal transplantation into a dysfunctional lower urinary tract. Transplantation 2003; 76(11):1578–82.
40. Franc-Guimond J, Gonzalez R. Renal transplantation in children with reconstructed bladders. Transplantation 2004; 77(7):1116–20.
41. Leonard MP, Dharamsi N, Williot PE. Outcome of gastrocystoplasty in tertiary pediatric urology practice. J Urol 2000; 164(3 Pt 2):947–50.
42. Bouchot O, Guilloneau B, Cantarovich D et al. Vesicoureteral reflux in the renal transplantation candidate. Eur Urol 1991; 20(1):26–8.
43. Erturk E, Burzon DT, Orloff M, Rabinowitz R. Outcome of patients with vesicoureteral reflux after renal transplantation: the effect of pretransplantation surgery on posttransplant urinary tract infections. Urology 1998; 51(5A Suppl):27–30.
44. Sharifian M, Rees L, Trompeter RS. High incidence of bacteriuria following renal transplantation in children. Nephrol Dial Transplant 1998; 13(2):432–5.
45. Camara NO, Dias MF, Pacheco-Silva A. An open randomized study comparing immunosuppression therapy initiated before or after kidney transplantation in haploidentical living recipients. Clin Transplant 2004; 18(4):450–5.
46. Gill JS, Tonelli M, Johnson N, Pereira BJ. Why do preemptive kidney transplant recipients have an allograft survival advantage? Transplantation 2004; 78(6):873–9.
47. Terasaki PI, Cecka JM, Gjertson DW, Takemoto S. High survival rates of kidney transplants from spousal and living unrelated donors. N Engl J Med 1995; 333(6):333–6.
48. Gjertson DW, Cecka JM. Living unrelated donor kidney transplantation. Kidney Int 2000; 58(2):491–9.
49. Al-Akash SI, Ettenger RB. Kidney transplantation in children. In: Danovitch GM, ed. Handbook of Kidney Transplantation, 4th edn. Philadelphia: Lippincott, Williams and Wilkins, 2005: 414–50.
50. Schneider JR, Sutherland DE, Simmons RL, Fryd DS, Najarian JS. Long-term success with double pediatric cadaver donor renal transplants. Ann Surg 1983; 197(4):39–42.

51. Wood KE, Becker BN, McCartney JG, D'Alessandro AM, Coursin DB. Care of the potential organ donor. N Engl J Med 2004; 351(26):2730–9.
52. Ryckman FC. Organ donation, procurement and preservation. In: Oldham KT, Colombani PM, Foglia RP, eds. Surgery of Infants and Children: Scientific Principles and Practice. Philadelphia: Lippincott-Raven, 1997: 701–8.
53. Scantlebury VP. Cadaveric and living donation. In: Shapiro R, Simmons RL, Starzl TE, eds. Renal Transplantation. Stamford, CT: Appleton and Lange, 1997: 73–94.
54. Ploeg RJ, van Bockel JH, Langendijk PT et al. Effect of preservation solution on results of cadaveric kidney transplantation. The European Multicentre Study Group. Lancet 1992; 340(8812):129–37.
55. Davis CL. Evaluation of the living kidney donor: current perspectives. Am J Kidney Dis 2004; 43(3):508–30.
56. Abecassis M, Adams M, Adams P et al; Live Organ Donor Consensus Group. Consensus statement on the live organ donor. JAMA 2000; 284(22):2919–26.
57. Barry JM. Laparoscopic donor nephrectomy: con. Transplantation 2000; 70(10):1546–8.
58. Hiller J, Sroka M, Halochek MJ et al. Functional advantages of laparoscopic live-donor nephrectomy compared with conventional open-donor nephrectomy. J Transpl Coord 1997; 7(3):134–40.
59. Flowers JL, Jacobs S, Cho E et al. Comparison of open and laparoscopic live donor nephrectomy. Ann Surg 1997; 226(4):483–9, discussion 489–90.
60. Ratner LE, Kavoussi LR, Sroka M et al. Laparoscopic assisted live donor nephrectomy – a comparison with the open approach. Transplantation 1997; 63(2):229–33.
61. Nogueira JM, Cangro CB, Fink JC et al. A comparison of recipient renal outcomes with laparoscopic versus open live donor nephrectomy. Transplantation 1999; 67(5):722–8.
62. Troppmann C, McBride MA, Baker TJ, Perez RV. Laparoscopic live donor nephrectomy: a risk factor for delayed function and rejection in pediatric kidney recipients? A UNOS analysis. Am J Transplant 2005; 5:175–82.
63. Salvatierra O, Sarwal M. Vulnerability of small pediatric recipients to laparoscopic living donor kidneys. Am J Transplant 2005; 5:201–2.
64. Salvatierra O, Singh T, Shifrin R et al. Successful transplantation of adult-sized kidneys into infants requires maintenance of high aortic blood flow. Transplantation 1998; 66(7):819–23.
65. Sheldon CA, Najarian JS, Mauer SM. Pediatric renal transplantation. Surg Clin North Am 1985; 65(6):1589–621.
66. Sheldon CA, Martin LW, Churchill BM. Surgical perspectives of pediatric renal transplantation. In: Gillenwater JY, Grayhack JT, Howards SS, Duckett JW, eds. Adult and Pediatric Urology, 2nd edn. St Louis: Mosby-Year Book, 1991: 2301–42.
67. Brannen GE, Bush WH, Correa RJ Jr, Gibbons RP, Cumes DM. Microvascular management of multiple renal arteries in transplantation. J Urol 1982; 128(1):112–15.
68. Lapointe SP, Charbit M, Jan D et al. Urological complications after renal transplantation using ureteroureteral anastomosis in children. J Urol 2001; 166(3):1046–8.
69. Halloran PF. Immunosuppressive drugs for kidney transplantation. N Engl J Med 2004; 351(26):2715–29.
70. Danovitch GM. Immunosuppressive medications and protocols for kidney transplantation. In: Danovitch GM, ed. Handbook of Kidney Transplantation, 4th edn. Philadelphia: Lippincott, Williams and Wilkins, 2005: 72–134.
71. Cattaneo D, Perico N, Remuzzi G. From pharmcokinetics to pharmacogenomics: a new approach to tailor immunosuppressive therapy. Am J Transplant 2004; 4:299–310.
72. Anglicheau D, Legendre C, Thervet E. Pharmacogenetics in solid organ transplantation: present knowledge and future perspectives. Transplantation 2004; 78(3):311–15.
73. Akalin E, Murphy B. Gene polymorphisms and transplantation. Curr Opin Immunol 2001; 13(5):572–6.
74. Nankivell BJ, Borrows RJ, Fung CL et al. The natural history of chronic allograft nephropathy. N Engl J Med 2003; 349(24):2326–33.
75. Midtvedt K, Hartmann A, Foss A et al. Sustained improvement of renal graft function for two years in hypertensive renal transplant recipients treated with nifedipine as compared to lisinopril. Transplantation 2001; 72(11):1787–91.
76. Dudley CRK. Treatment of posttransplant hypertension: ACE is trumped? Transplantation 2001; 72(11):1728–9.
77. Bostom AD, Brown RS Jr, Chavers BM et al. Prevention of post-transplant cardiovascular disease – report and recommendations of an ad hoc group. Am J Transplant 2002; 2:491–500.
78. Artz MA, Hilbrands LB, Borm G, Assmann KJ, Wetzels JF. Blockade of the renin–angiotensin system increases graft survival in patients with chronic allograft nephropathy. Nephrol Dial Transplant 2004; 19(11):2852–7.
79. Jassal SV, Roscoe JM, Zaltzman JS et al. Clinical practice guidelines: prevention of cytomegalovirus disease after renal transplantation. J Am Soc Nephrol 1998; 9:1697–708.
80. Ellis D, Jaffe R, Green M et al. Epstein–Barr virus-related disorders in children undergoing renal transplantation with tacrolimus-based immunosuppression. Transplantation 1999; 68(7):997–1003.
81. Rifle G, Mousson C, Martin L, Guignier F, Hajji K. Donor-specific antibodies in allograft rejection: clinical and experimental data. Transplantation 2005; 79(3):S14–18.
82. Sheldon CA. Pediatric renal transplantation: surgical considerations. In: Gearhart JP, Rink RC, Mouriquand PDE, eds. Pediatric Urology. Philadelphia: WB Saunders, 2001: 801–27.
83. Rengel M, Gomez-Da-Silva G, Inchaustegui L et al. Renal artery stenosis after kidney transplantation: diagnostic and therapeutic approach. Kidney Int Suppl 1998; 68:S99–106.
84. Roberts JP, Ascher NL, Fryd DS et al. Transplant renal artery stenosis. Transplantation 1989; 48(4):580–3.
85. Sheldon CA, Churchill BM, Khoury AE, McLorie GA. Complications of surgical significance in pediatric renal transplantation. J Pediatr Surg 1992; 27(4):485–90.
86. Zaontz MR, Hatch DA, Firlit CF. Urological complica-

tions in pediatric renal transplantation: management and prevention. J Urol 1988; 140(5 Pt 2):1123–8.
87. Cho DK, Zackson DA, Cheiigh J, Stubenbord WT, Stnzel KH. Urinary calculi in renal transplant recipients. Transplantation 1988; 45(5):899–902.
88. Hayes JM, Streem SB, Graneto D et al. Renal transplant calculi. A reevaluation of risks and management. Transplantation 1989; 47(6):949–52.
89. Khositseth S, Gillingham KJ, Cook ME, Chavers BM. Urolithiasis after kidney transplantation in pediatric recipients: a single center report. Transplantation 2004; 78(9):1319–23.
90. Pena DR, Fennell RS, Iravani R, Neiberger RE, Richard GA. Renal calculi in pediatric renal transplant recipients. Child Nephrol Urol 1990; 10(1):58–60.
91. Guest G, Tete MJ, Beurton D, Broyer M. [Urinary lithiasis after kidney transplantation. Experience at a pediatric center]. Arch Fr Pediatr 1993; 50(1):15–19 [French].
92. Harper JM, Samuell CT, Hallson PC, Wood SM, Mansell MA. Risk factors for calculus formation in patients with renal transplants. Br J Urol 1994; 74(2):147–50.
93. Pardalidis NP, Waltzer WC, Tellis VA, Jarrett TW, Smith AD. Endourologic management of complications in renal allografts. J Endourol 1994; 8(5):321–7.
94. Vianello A, Pignata G, Caldato C et al. Vesicoureteral reflux after kidney transplantation: clinical significance in the medium to long-term. Clin Nephrol 1997; 47(6): 356–61.
95. Fontana I, Ginevri F, Arcuri V et al. Vesico-ureteral reflux in pediatric kidney transplants: clinical relevance to graft and patient outcome. Pediatr Transplant 1999; 3(3):206–9.
96. Ohba K, Matsuo M, Noguchi M et al. Clinicopathological study of vesicoureteral reflux (VUR)-associated pyelonephritis in renal transplantation. Clin Transplant 2004; 18(Suppl 11):34–8.
97. Latchamsetty KC, Mital D, Jensik S, Coogan CL. Use of collagen injections for vesicoureteral reflux in transplanted kidneys. Transplant Proc 2003; 35(4):1378–80.
98. Neuhaus TJ, Schwobel M, Schlumpf R et al. Pyelonephritis and vesicoureteral reflux after renal transplantation in young children. J Urol 1997; 157(4):1400–3.
99. Mastrosimone S, Pignata G, Maresca MC et al. Clinical significance of vesicoureteral reflux after kidney transplantation. Clin Nephrol 1993; 40(1):38–45.
100. Dharnidharka VR, Stablein DM, Harmon WE. Post-transplant infections now exceed acute rejection as cause for hospitalization: a report of the NAPRTCS. Am J Transplant 2004; 4:384–9.
101. Shroff R, Rees L. The post-transplant lymphoproliferative disorder – a literature review. Pediatr Nephrol 2004; 19(4):369–77.
102. Lang P, Pardon A, Audard V. Long-term benefit of mycophenolate mofetil in renal transplantation. Transplantation 2005; 79(3):S47–8.
103. Sahadevan M, Kasiske BL. Long-term posttransplant management and complications. In: Danovitch GM, ed. Handbook of Kidney Transplantation, 4th edn. Philadelphia: Lippincott, Williams and Wilkins, 2005: 234–78.
104. Hariharan S, Johnson CP, Bresnahan BA et al. Improved graft survival after renal transplantation in the United States, 1988 to 1996. N Engl J Med 2000; 342(9):605–12.
105. Meier-Kriesche H-U, Schold JD, Kaplan B. Long-term renal allograft survival: have we made significant progress or is it time to rethink our analytic and therapeutic strategies? Am J Transplant 2004; 4:1289–95.

Renal calculus disease

25

Pramod P Reddy and Eugene Minevich

Introduction

The purpose of this chapter is to review the current knowledge of pediatric urolithiasis, with the emphasis being on the pathophysiology, clinical presentation, evaluation, and medical management of this condition. The surgical management of urinary calculi will be addressed in Chapter 26.

It is well established that pediatric urolithiasis is a distinctly different condition and is not as common as adult urolithiasis; however, there are quite a few similarities in the presentation and evaluation of this condition regardless of the age of the patient. Urolithiasis is an important manifestation of disease conditions, with lifelong implications.

Epidemiology of pediatric urolithiasis

Children account for only 2–3% of all patients with calculous disease.[1,2] Pediatric urolithiasis is endemic to certain developing countries such as Turkey, India, and Thailand, and until recently was a relatively rare condition in the Western Hemisphere. The incidence in the USA has been increasing over the past decade, possibly due to changing dietary and physical activity patterns in our pediatric population. In the USA, urinary stone disease accounts for 1:1000 to 1:7600 hospital admissions, whereas in countries where stone disease is endemic the incidence is approx 1:1000 to 1:3000.[3] There has also been a shift in the pathophysiology of the stones encountered in the USA. Previously the majority of the stones were felt to be secondary to an identifiable underlying metabolic disorder.[4,5] Recent data, however, suggest that pediatric urolithiasis is evolving to a more adult-type pathophysiology, possibly due to changing dietary habits and lack of regular exercise in this age group.

Urinary calculus disease is more common in Caucasians, less commonly affecting those of African or Latin-American heritage.[1] Boys and girls appear to be affected equally, despite earlier data suggesting a male preponderance.

The mean age at presentation is 6.9 years for girls and 5.2 years for boys.[6] Infected stones tend to occur more frequently in children under 4 years of age. In the pediatric population the rate of recurrence of stones ranges from 3.6% to 68% and appears to be the highest for children with underlying metabolic risk factors.[7,8] It is the high recurrence rate that suggests that all children with stones should undergo a metabolic evaluation.

Classification

Several classifications have been proposed to organize pediatric stone disease. The schema proposed by Smith and Segura is one of the most comprehensive and useful systems that we have encountered (Table 25.1).

Pathophysiology of urolithiasis

Formation of a stone in the urinary tract is a consequence of complex physical processes and represents the end manifestation of a multitude of diseases. The stone is produced as the culmination of many interrelated anatomic and physiochemical processes.[10] The major factors are supersaturation of lithogenic ions and crystallization of compounds in the urine. The formation of stones is influenced by urinary volume, pH, and the presence of urinary ions or compounds that function as promoters or inhibitors of lithogenesis.

Table 25.1 Classification of urolithiasis in children

Enzyme disorders
Primary hyperoxaluria (deficiency of hepatic peroxisomal alanine–glyoxylate aminotransferase):
■ Type 1: glyoxylic aciduria
■ Type 2: glyceric aciduria
Xanthinuria (deficiency of xanthine dehydrogenase):
■ 1,8-Dihydroxyadeniuria
■ Lesch–Nyhan syndrome (hyperuricosuria due to deficiency of hypoxanthine–guanine phosphoribosyl transferase, HPRT)
Renal tubular syndromes
Cystinuria
Renal tubular acidosis (types 1–4)(calcium phosphate stones)
Hypercalcemic states
Hyperparathyroidism
Immobilization
Uric acid lithiasis
Enteric urolithiasis
Idiopathic calcium oxalate urolithiasis
Solute excess:
■ Hypercalciuria:
Absorptive (Dent disease, Bartter syndrome)
Renal
■ Hyperoxaluria
■ Hyperuricosuria
■ Hypocitraturia
■ Medications excreted into the urine (sulfadiazine, indinavir, etc.)
Endemic bladder stone formation
Secondary urolithiasis
Infection (struvite stones, secondary to UTI with bacteria that produce urease)
Obstruction (UPJ obstruction, UVJ obstruction, neurogenic bladder, exstrophy)
Structural abnormalities
Urinary diversion procedures
Foreign body (ureteral stent, suture, etc.)

UTI, urinary tract infection; UPJ, ureteropelvic junction; UVJ, ureterovesical junction.
Modified from Smith and Segura.[9]

The central event in calculus formation is supersaturation. If a urinary solute exceeds its solubility product (K_{sp} = a constant that is equal to the product of the concentrations of the pure chemical components at which the solid and the dissolved states are in equilibrium in water at standard conditions and temperature), crystallization of the solutes can occur. In normal individuals urine is undersaturated. When a solute is added to a solvent it dissolves in it until an equilibrium point is achieved [supersaturation (SS = 1)]. Beyond this point (i.e. between saturated and supersaturated states – metastable zone) no further dissolution is possible but new nuclei do not form spontaneously.[11]

In normal urine, the concentration of a component necessary to reach supersaturation is several times higher than would be expected from its solubility because of the presence of naturally occurring organic and inorganic inhibitors that raise the K_{sp} of the urinary solutes (i.e. magnesium, citrate, pyrophosphate, glycosaminoglycans, nephrocalcin, and Tamm–Horsfall protein).[12–16] Complexing agents are substances that form soluble complexes with specific crystals. Depending on the specific stone-forming substance, some chemicals such as citrate and magnesium may act as a complexor and/or an inhibitor.

Once urinary solutes exceed their K_{sp}, the solvent is said to be saturated (unstable zone) (Figure 25.1). Crystallization occurs via homogeneous nucleation (on itself) or heterogeneous nucleation (on top of particulate matter; i.e. other crystals, cells, and tubular casts). In vivo, heterogeneous nucleation is much more common. Once this process is initiated, growth of the stone is fostered by the nuclei coming in close contact and binding to each other (due to chemical and/or electrical forces), resulting in crystal aggregation (Figure 25.2).[11] Urinary pH influences the solubility of various lithogenic ions. Uric acid and cystine are more soluble in alkaline urine (pH >7.0).

Crystal retention and formation of calculi takes place initially in the papillary duct. Disorders of metabolism, or endocrine or urologic abnormalities may lead to the development of crystallized material in the urinary tract (Figure 25.3).

Any condition that results in urinary stasis – i.e. ureteropelvic junction (UPJ) obstruction, vesicoureteral reflux (VUR) – promotes growth of a stone by increasing excretion of stone-forming constituents, crystal aggregation and retention, and a decrease in the excretion of inhibitors or complexing agents. It is very important that in reality a combination of factors are involved in the genesis of urinary calculi.

Clinical presentation

The clinical manifestations of pediatric urinary stones are dependent upon a number of factors:

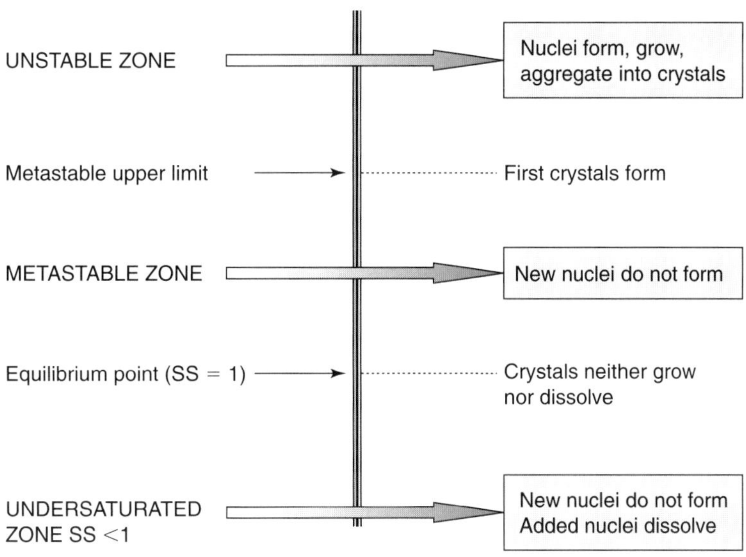

Figure 25.1 Supersaturation (SS) of urine.

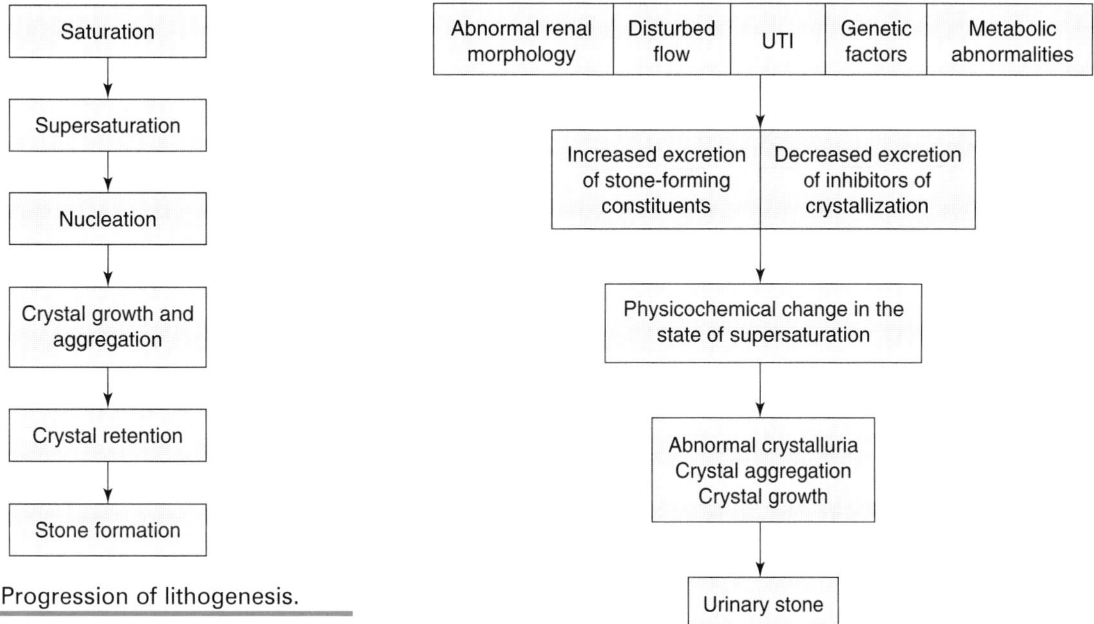

Figure 25.2 Progression of lithogenesis.

Figure 25.3 General aspects of lithogenesis. UTI, urinary tract infection.

- size of the stone
- location of the stone
- degree of obstruction to the flow of urine
- presence of infection
- presence or absence of a normal contralateral renal unit.

Presentation tends to be age-dependent, with symptoms such as flank pain and hematuria being more common in older children. Non-specific symptoms such as irritability and vomiting are more common in younger children.

Most symptoms related to urolithiasis occur when the calculus becomes lodged in the ureter, causing partial or complete obstruction. Typically, an obstructing calculus causes either renal colic and/or an infection. Renal colic, which occurs in approximately 40–75% of children with urolithiasis,[17,18] presents with a sudden onset of severe cramp-like flank, abdominal, or pelvic pain associated with gastrointestinal symptoms (nausea and vomiting). Irritative voiding symptoms (i.e. dysuria, urgency, and frequency) occur when the calculus is in the distal one-third of the ureter. In some patients the pain can present as diffuse abdominal pain and can obscure the clinical picture, delaying the correct diagnosis.[19]

Microscopic or macroscopic hematuria has been reported in 33–90% of children with urinary stones.[20]

Urinary tract infection (UTI) may complicate the clinical presentation, especially in an obstructed kidney, and may not be associated with acute renal colic, but rather persistent flank pain. The combination of flank pain and fever should immediately raise the suspicion for the presence of acute pyelonephritis occurring in the setting of an obstructed calculus, and this requires emergent intervention.

Children with urethral stones often present with terminal hematuria or the inability to void.

On physical examination, most children will be restless and costovertebral angle (CVA) tenderness may be elicited on the affected side. This presentation is less specific in younger children or renal transplant patients. Children under 5 years of age frequently present with symptoms suggestive of a UTI. Asymptomatic stones may be identified in children who are undergoing abdominal imaging for non-urologic diagnoses (i.e. acute appendicitis).

Evaluation of patient with urolithiasis

History and physical examination

The initial evaluation of a pediatric patient with urolithiasis may suggest the diagnosis through a complete history and physical examination. The evaluation should begin with a review of the history and include questions regarding:

- prematurity (especially with the use of furosemide), supplemental vitamin D, or enteral/parenteral nutrition formulas high in calcium and/or phosphorus
- current medications (i.e. steroids, chemotherapeutic agents, diuretics, protease inhibitors)
- concurrent illnesses (i.e. cystic fibrosis, neoplasms, seizures)
- recurrent skeletal fractures, which could indicate the presence of hyperparathyroidism or other bone disease
- nutritional habits (i.e. ketogenic diet, dietary excesses or deficiencies, type and amount of fluid intake)
- family history of nephrolithiasis, gout, or bowel disease.

A wide variety of medical conditions can be associated with urolithiasis in children. These include gastrointestinal (GI) disorders, resulting in malabsorption, chronic corticosteroid treatment, cystic fibrosis, myelodysplasia, and immobilization. The family history is helpful in patients with autosomal recessive disorders, such as cystinuria and primary hyperoxaluria, or with autosomal dominant diseases, such as renal tubular acidosis (RTA) or the syndrome of idiopathic calcium oxalate urolithiasis.

The physical examination should screen for chronic disease, including failure to thrive (distal RTA); hypertension as an indicator of underlying renal parenchymal injury; the characteristic bony deformities of rickets; photophobia due to band keratopathy (hypercalcemia-induced metastatic calcification); and evidence of UTI.

Imaging

The radiographic work-up of a child with suspected urolithiasis is relatively straightforward. Imaging modalities such as plain films of the abdomen [kidney, ureter, and bladder (KUB)] can be useful in detecting stones, and also suggesting the type of calculi (Table 25.2). Calcium oxalate stones are usually <2 cm in size, whereas struvite, uric acid, or cystine stones may fill the entire collecting system, i.e. staghorn calculi.

Renal and bladder ultrasound (US) and intravenous urography (IVP) are also useful in the diagnosis of urolithiasis and evaluating the degree of obstruction caused by the stone. The use of IVP is limited in the pediatric population because of concerns about the risks of cumulative radiation exposure. Currently, in both adult and pediatric stone

Table 25.2 Radiodensity of calculi on plain film imaging

Radiopaque calculi	Radiolucent calculi
Calcium oxalate	Uric acid
Calcium phosphate	2,8-Dihydroxyadenine
Struvite (carbonate apatite)	Triamterene
Cystine	Xanthine
	Silica

patients, the unenhanced, helical computeted tomography (CT scan) is the gold standard technique for radiologic evaluation of acute flank or abdominal pain. It allows for an accurate and timely diagnosis of obstructed urinary calculi and can also detect extraurinary lesions.[21,22] CT scanners are readily available in most pediatric institutions and have the advantages of the brevity of the scan and avoidance of intravenous contrast (and any associated adverse reactions), although concerns about radiation exposure also exist.

Voiding cystourethrogram (VCUG) and renal nuclear scintigraphy may be necessary to rule out associated anatomic abnormalities in some patients. Children with suspected neurogenic bladder and significant voiding dysfunction may benefit from urodynamic studies, to complete their evaluation when dealing with chronic or recurrent urolithiasis.

Laboratory evaluation

The evaluation of the patient may be divided into two phases – evaluation during an acute stone episode to direct therapy and subsequent evaluation to determine the underlying etiology of the stone. Owing to the high incidence of predisposing factors for urolithiasis in children (up to 75%) as well as the frequency of stone recurrences (up to 65%),[17] a complete evaluation of every child after the very first urinary stone is advisable.[23,24]

During the acute phase, the following tests are recommended:

1 Urine for urinalysis (UA) and culture and sensitivity (C&S). UA usually demonstrates hematuria, whereas pyuria may be a first sign of a UTI, which is confirmed with a urine culture.
2 Serum electrolytes, blood urea nitrogen (BUN), and creatinine. Determination of serum creatinine is helpful in grossly evaluating the renal function.
3 Complete blood count (CBC).
4 Serum for Ca^{2+}, phosphorus, magnesium, and parathyroid hormone (PTH) levels may be useful in determining the type of stone being treated.

After treating the acute stone episode, it is of critical importance to collect a 24-hour urine sample in order to determine a stone-risk profile and to rule out any subtle metabolic abnormalities. The urine collection is evaluated for volume, pH, calcium, uric acid, creatinine, sodium, oxalate, citrate, and cystine.

Supersaturation indices are felt to accurately predict stone composition and may be a more precise predictor of response to therapy.[25,26] We prefer two consecutive 24-hour urine samples as initial evaluation, ideally after the patient is free of stones. During the collection of 24-hour urine samples, patients should maintain their usual diet and fluid intake. We use urinary supersaturation values as the principal laboratory benchmark index of possible crystal formation. Adult reference ranges for urinary supersaturation indices do not accurately reflect the pathophysiology in children.[27] In a recently published study we have shown that there are significant differences in the normal ranges of urine chemistries of children and adults. Calcium, oxalate, and citrate levels are significantly higher in children than adults when referenced by creatinine (Table 25.3).[28] Chemical analysis and determination of the composition of the stone (with polarization microscopy, infrared imaging, or X-ray diffraction) should be performed whenever possible. The patient should be given a urine strainer to retrieve any stones that are passed in the urine.

In this next section we will discuss the pathophysiology and specific treatment of the various types of stones encountered in children.

Approximately 75% of all pediatric kidney stones in the USA are composed of calcium oxalate; these stones are usually mixed calculi with some component

Table 25.3 Mean pediatric and adult urine chemistry values

Parameter	Pediatric	Adult	*P*-value
Urine pH	6.44 ± 0.40	6.05 ± 0.41	<0.001
SS Uric acid	0.59 ± 0.53	1.14 ± 0.99	<0.001
SS Ca oxalate	7.88 ± 4.13	7.85 ± 6.30	1.00
SS Ca phosphate	2.48 ± 1.31	1.42 ± 1.19	<0.001
Citrate/Cr (mg/g)	592 ± 460	373 ± 216	0.01
Oxalate/Cr (mg/g)	41.2 ± 26.7	23.1 ± 15.0	<0.001
Ca/Cr (mg/g)	172 ± 99	113 ± 55	0.001
Uric acid/Cr (mg/g)	623 ± 390	396 ± 89	0.01

SS, supersaturation; Ca, calcium; Cr, creatinine.

of hydroxyapatite, or uric acid. The 10–20% of stones composed of struvite (magnesium ammonium phosphate) are usually encountered in the clinical setting of recurrent UTI;[29] 5% of stones are uric acid and 5% are composed mainly of brushite (calcium monohydrogen phosphate), whereas <1% are composed of cystine.[30]

Idiopathic calcium oxalate urolithiasis

Hypercalciuria

Hypercalciuria is the most common predisposing metabolic factor for stone formation in children. In general, children with a history of calcium oxalate urolithiasis excrete a higher fraction of dietary calcium in their urine than unaffected children.[17] Normal calcium excretion in children is <4 mg/kg/day. Hypercalciuria occurs in 53–81% of children with calcium stones.[31,32] Microscopic or gross hematuria may be encountered in children with hypercalciuria without urolithiasis, although up to 20% of them will develop stones within 5 years.[33,34] Hypercalciuria has also been reported in association with the urinary frequency-dysuria syndrome.[35] Hypercalciuria is seen with a higher prevalence than in the normal population in children with Beckwith–Wiedemann syndrome and cystic fibrosis.[36] Initial studies of idiopathic hypercalciuria suggested two relatively easily defined and genetically distinct subtypes of hypercalciuria, 'renal' and 'absorptive'.[37] Recent reports have postulated that absorptive and renal forms of hypercalciuria appear to represent a continuum of a single disease process.[38]

Absorptive hypercalciuria, by far the most common cause of excessive urinary calcium, results from an increased intestinal absorption of calcium, which is caused by either overly aggressive vitamin D supplementation or excessive ingestion of calcium-containing foods (milk-alkali syndrome). Increased intestinal calcium absorption produces a corresponding increase in serum calcium levels. Typically, serum PTH is in the low-normal range in absorptive hypercalciuria because of feedback from the high serum calcium level. Fasting urinary calcium levels are usually within the normal range in these patients.

Three types of absorptive hypercalciuria have been defined. In Type I, patients have hypercalciuria without calcium load, which is relatively uncommon and is the most severe type of absorptive hypercalciuria. In Type II, the most common variety, patients have hypercalciuria only, with a high calcium intake. In Type III, a relatively rare cause of hypercalciuria, the underlying etiology is a renal defect that causes excessive urinary phosphate excretion. This is suspected to result from inactivation of the renal epithelial sodium–phosphate cotransporter – NaPi2. The continuous urinary phosphate loss rapidly depletes the serum phosphate level, causing hypophosphatemia. This results in activation of vitamin D_3, which increases intestinal absorption of both phosphate and calcium. The absorbed calcium is ultimately excreted in the urine, causing the hypercalciuria.

Renal hypercalciuria results from a specific defect in the kidneys that allows excessive obligatory urinary calcium excretion, regardless of serum calcium levels, body stores, or calcium ingestion. The calcium:creatinine ratio is usually high (>0.20). The loss of serum calcium into the urine produces a mild hypocalcemia and secondary hyperparathyroidism, which is useful in diagnosing this condition. Renal leak hypercalciuria is far less common than absorptive hypercalciuria.

Hyperoxaluria

This condition is discussed in depth in a later section. Up to 20% of patients with idiopathic calcium oxalate urolithiasis will have hyperoxaluria.[17] Oxalate has a very strong chemical affinity for calcium, and calcium oxalate has a relatively low solubility. This is most frequently due to idiopathic hyperoxaluria, in which case urine oxalate values are only mildly elevated. It may be due to simple dietary excess of high-oxalate food sources or to an increased endogenous oxalate production. In patients with enteric hyperoxaluria, calcium stones develop because of fat malabsorption, which in turn results in colonic hyperabsorption of ingested oxalate. The latter occurs because malabsorbed fatty acids bind luminal calcium, which is then unavailable to precipitate and prevent the uptake of ingested oxalate.[39] Enteric hyperoxaluria is seen in patients with intestinal malabsorption or inflammatory bowel disease and may be treated with dietary adjustment and citrate supplementation.

Hyperuricosuria

Hyperuricosuria commonly occurs in patients with idiopathic calcium oxalate urolithiasis.[40,41] Hyperuricosuria may be the result of a diet high in purines, uricosuric drugs, or from tubular defects such as an isolated defect in renal tubular urate reabsorption, or from generalized tubular dysfunction. It can also occur in patients undergoing chemotherapy with rapid cell turnover, and in those who are in a negative nitrogen balance (catabolic state). Hyperuricosuria leads to calcium oxalate crystallization by heterogeneous nucleation and by reducing the levels of urinary inhibitors.[42,43]

Hypocitruria

Hypocitraturia is a risk factor for urinary stone formation in patients with idiopathic calcium oxalate urolithiasis.[44] Urinary citrate has a direct inhibitory effect on the crystallization and precipitation of calcium salts. It binds to calcium ions in the urine, reducing calcium ion activity, which results in a lowering of the supersaturation of calcium phosphate and calcium oxalate. It also increases the inhibitory activity of other urine macromolecules (e.g. Tamm–Horsfall protein) and may reduce the expression of urinary osteopontin, which is an important component of the protein matrix of urinary stones. In addition, urinary citrate excretion can increase urinary pH, which negatively influences uric acid crystallization and uric acid stone formation. Citrate excretion is impaired by acidosis, hypokalemia (causing intracellular acidosis), a high animal protein diet (with an elevated acid-ash content), and UTI. Acidosis reduces urinary citrate both by enhancing renal tubular reabsorption and reducing the synthesis of citrate. RTA is the most common cause of hypocitriuria in children.

Medical management

Since the single greatest risk factor of pediatric urinary stones is a low urinary flow rate,[45] the management of all patients with metabolic stones starts with maintaining an adequate level of oral fluid intake, even in young children. One should strive to maintain urine output greater than 2 L/day for adolescents and approximately 35 ml/kg/day for children.[46,47] Carbonated beverages are to be avoided and do not count as an appropriate oral fluid in these patients.

Calcium restriction in the growing infant, child, or adolescent should be avoided, as it only increases the risk for poorly mineralized bones. There appears to be widespread agreement that restriction of calcium intake contributes to the severity of a patient's osteopenia.[48,49] Individuals having elevated urine sodium:potassium ratios seem most responsive to the hypocalciuric effects of increased potassium intake in combination with a low-salt diet.[50] Dietary manipulations should initially be directed towards dietary excesses or deficiencies, and placing the child on a balanced and nutritious diet. The most frequently used medications to correct hypercalciuria are thiazide diuretics (1 mg/kg/day), which act to lower urinary calcium excretion by increasing the fractional calcium absorption by the distal nephron.[51] If RTA is suspected, potassium or sodium citrate is indicated, as it corrects the systemic acidosis, hypercalciuria, hypocitraturia, and hypocalcemia.[52] Children with type 3 absorptive hypercalciuria (phosphate leak) may benefit from treatment with orthophosphates.[3] Patients with urolithiasis secondary to a ketogenic diet need to be managed in close consultation with their neurologist, as these patients are on a very strictly regimented diet, in terms of volume and caloric intake (Table 25.4).

Hypercalcemic states

Hyperparathyroidism

Resorptive hypercalciuria results from the loss of calcium from the body's normal stores in the bony

Table 25.4 Dietary recommendations for pediatric patients with calcium urolithiasis

Nutrient	Dietary recommendation
Fluid intake	Maintain urine output >2 L/day for adolescents and >20 ml/kg/day for younger children
Dietary sodium	No added salt diet (maintain Na <2 g/day)
Dietary calcium	Recommended daily allowance of calcium for age; avoid calcium restriction in children
Dietary protein	Recommended daily allowance; avoid excessive animal protein intake
Dietary potassium	Five servings per day of high-potassium, low-oxalate foods
Dietary phosphorus	Recommended daily allowance
Dietary magnesium	Recommended daily allowance

skeleton and is typically diagnosed in children with hyperparathyroidism. Although primary hyperparathyroidism is not a common cause of hypercalcemic hypercalciuria in children, it must be considered in a patient with elevated serum calcium.[18] In this condition, calcium is released from bone in response to the increased activity of osteoclasts caused by excessive and inappropriate serum PTH levels. This causes significant hypercalcemia. Under normal conditions, PTH causes the kidney to limit calcium excretion, but, with the overwhelming serum calcium load produced with hyperparathyroidism, the kidneys are forced to excrete the extra calcium into the urine, resulting in hypercalciuria.

Immobilization

Immobilization of children is the most common cause in North America of secondary hypercalciuria.[6] The patients primarily at risk are those acutely immobilized for the management of fractures or postoperative management, as opposed to those with static neurologic disorders who are chronically bedridden (i.e. spastic quadriplegia).

Others

Gastrointestinal hyperabsorption can be secondary to symptomatic vitamin D intoxication characterized by failure to thrive, anorexia, polyuria, and dehydration, and variable degrees of renal insufficiency. The hypercalcemia of sarcoidosis is due to excessive 1,25-dihydroxyvitamin D_3 (1,25$(OH)_2D_3$) production by alveolar macrophages and in sarcoid granulomas. In the management of these conditions associated with hypercalcemia, it is critical to identify the underlying cause and correct it.

Uric acid lithiasis

Uric acid calculi are radiolucent and constitute up to 5% of the urinary calculi encountered in pediatric patients. These stones are usually white or orange. Uric acid crystals are orange and can often be mistaken for blood by the patient or their parents. A pH <5.8 promotes uric acid crystal precipitation, since they are poorly soluble in acidic urine. In the familial, or idiopathic, form of the disease, affected children have hyperuricosuria and normal uric acid serum concentration. Generalized dysfunction of tubular reabsorption, as seen in patients with Wilson's disease or various forms of the Fanconi syndrome, is associated with familial hyperuricosuria.

Disorders associated with overproduction of uric acid include inborn errors of metabolism such as Lesch–Nyhan syndrome and type I glycogen storage disease (glucose-6-phosphatase deficiency).[54] Uric acid overproduction can also occur secondary to myeloproliferative disorders (presenting acutely or in relapse), or other causes of cell breakdown (catabolic states induced by neoplasms or chemotherapy). Hyperuricosuria may be the result of a high purine intake or uricosuric drugs (such as probenecid, salicylate) or from tubular defects such as an isolated defect in renal tubular urate reabsorption, or from generalized tubular dysfunction.[55] Chronic diarrheal syndromes (e.g. ulcerative colitis, regional enteritis) or jejunoileal bypass surgery may cause uric acid lithiasis by inducing net alkali deficit and lowering urine volume (thereby reducing urinary pH and augmenting urinary concentration of uric acid, respectively).[56] The majority of patients with hyperuricosuria have coexistent hypercalciuria; therefore, calcium oxalate urolithiasis may be seen in these children as well.[40]

Since most of these patients have a low volume of chronically acidic urine throughout the day, increasing oral fluid intake and urinary alkalinization to a pH of 6.5–7.0 with potassium citrate or sodium bicarbonate are the primary goals of treatment. However, alkalinization of the urine above pH 7.0 can promote calcium phosphate stone formation. Patients with hyperuricemia secondary to myeloproliferative disorders may benefit from decreasing uric acid production with the xanthine oxidase inhibitor allopurinol. A rare complication of prolonged allopurinol therapy is the formation of xanthine stones.[57]

Renal tubular syndromes

Renal tubular acidosis

Renal tubular acidosis is a term applied to several clinical syndromes of metabolic acidosis that result from specific defects in renal tubular hydrogen ion secretion and urinary acidification. Three major types are currently recognized and are differentiated based on the nature of the tubular defect. Stones are composed principally of calcium phosphate (brushite), although calcium oxalate and struvite stones may be seen alone or in combinations.

In type 1 (distal) RTA, the primary functional abnormality is the inability of the distal nephron to establish and maintain a hydrogen ion gradient between the tubular fluid and the blood. As a result, the urine remains inappropriately alkaline regardless of the severity of the systemic acidemia. Type 1 RTA is associated with renal stone disease in up to 70% of cases. Factors contributing to stone formation include increased urinary pH, hypercalciuria, and hypocitraturia.[58,59] Obstructive uropathy is an example of an etiology of distal RTA.

In type 2 (proximal) RTA, the primary defect is a failure of bicarbonate reabsorption in the proximal tubule, leading to bicarbonate wasting. However, the kidney is able to acidify the urine appropriately and to excrete the daily load of acid, as distal tubular function is spared. Nephrolithiasis and nephrocalcinosis are not seen in proximal RTA.[58]

In type 4 RTA, chronic renal parenchymal damage, leading to moderate reductions in glomerular filtration rate (GFR), produces hyperkalemic, hyperchloremic metabolic acidosis in conjunction with bicarbonaturia, decreased ammonium excretion, and subnormal net acid excretion.[58] Nephrolithiasis and nephrocalcinosis are absent in type 4 RTA.

Type 1 RTA may present as an isolated entity or it may be the secondary manifestation of a variety of systemic and renal disorders, including Sjögren's syndrome, Wilson's disease, primary biliary cirrhosis, and in patients who have undergone a jejunoileal bypass. Children usually present early with familial (autosomal dominant) type 1 RTA. Infants generally present with vomiting and/or diarrhea (>33%) and failure to thrive (>50%), with subsequent growth retardation. Less than 10% have nephrolithiasis and nephrocalcinosis. Children present with metabolic bone disease (osteomalacia) or with signs and symptoms related to stone disease.

Patients with type 1 RTA will present with a hypokalemic, hyperchloremic metabolic acidosis. In these patients, the urinary pH will never fall below 5.5, no matter how low the serum bicarbonate level.[58] Hypocitraturia and hypercalciuria will only be found in type 1 RTA, but are not specific for this disorder. A diagnostic work-up for the presence of incomplete distal RTA is indicated when nephrocalcinosis or recurrent nephrolithiasis of unclear etiology occurs in the absence of spontaneous, non-anion gap acidosis. Although these patients do not have spontaneous metabolic acidosis, they are unable to acidify the urine appropriately when presented with an acid load.[60] This condition is diagnosed by means of an ammonium chloride loading test and monitoring the urine pH. If at any time the urinary pH falls below 5.5, the diagnosis of RTA can be excluded.

Cystinuria

Cystinuria is a complex autosomal recessive disorder, characterized by an abnormality in a specific transport system located in the brush-border membrane of the proximal straight renal tubule and the small intestine. The transporter (SLC3A1 dibasic amino acid transporter) is encoded on chromosome 2p21. Cystinuria results from an excessive urinary excretion of cystine (the disulfide dimer of cysteine) and the dibasic amino acids arginine, lysine, and ornithine.[61,62] Cystine has poor solubility in the normal urinary pH range and a pH below 7 causes cystine to precipitate. Cystine stones are usually very hard and resistant to fragmentation by extracorporeal shock wave lithotripsy (ESWL).

There are three subtypes of cystinuria, and it occurs with a frequency of 1 in 15 000 live births[63,64] and accounts for 1–3% of children with metabolic urolithiasis in industrialized countries.[6] Cystine crystals are characteristically flat, hexagonal, and colorless. Cystine crystals are diagnostic, but are detected in only 19–26% of homozygous cystinuric patients.[62] Cystinuria has been associated with hyperuricemia, uric acid urolithiasis, hemophilia, retinitis pigmentosa, muscular dystrophy, muscular hypotonia, mental retardation, trisomy 21, and hereditary pancreatitis.

The treatment goals of this condition include maintaining a high fluid intake to reduce cystine saturation (the goal is <300 mg cystine/L of urine) with urinary flow rates of up to 50 ml/kg/24 h.[65,66] Further reduction of cystine concentration can be achieved with a diet low in protein and sodium. Urinary alkalinization with potassium citrate at a pH of approximately 7.6 should be maintained in all patients. In children in whom hydration and alkalinization have failed, D-penicillamine (20–50 mg/kg/day) and/or *N*-(2-mercaptopropionyl)glycine (tiopronin; Thiola) (15 mg/kg/day) can be effective in decreasing the rate of stone formation. These drugs can be associated with serious side effects, and patients taking them must be monitored very closely for bone marrow suppression, nephrotic syndrome, and complications resembling systemic lupus erythematosus (SLE) and Goodpasture's syndrome. Thiola has been reported to be better tolerated by pediatric patients. Vitamin B_6 supplementation must be added to patients being treated with either medication. Captopril has also been shown to be effective in lowering the urinary cystine level in homozygous cystinuric patients, by forming a thiol–cysteine mixed disulfide compound that is more soluble in urine than cystine.[67] Patients with cystinuria are at a very high risk for recurrent urolithiasis.[68,69]

Enzymatic disorders

Primary hyperoxaluria

Primary hyperoxaluria is a very rare but serious disorder caused by a congenital defect resulting in very high levels (>200 mg/day) of endogenous oxalate production. Without treatment, the prognosis for these patients is poor. Renal failure occurs in 50% of patients by age 15 years and in 80% by age 30 years. Standard dialysis for uremia cannot remove enough serum oxalate to protect the kidneys and other organs from widespread calcium oxalate deposition (i.e. oxalosis) and calcium oxalate stone production.

Type I primary hyperoxaluria is the more common variety. It occurs in 1 in 120 000 live births and is transmitted as an autosomal recessive trait. It is caused by a deficiency of the peroxisomal liver-specific alanine–glyoxylate aminotransferase enzyme (i.e. AGT). Pyridoxine (vitamin B_6) is a cofactor in this chemical pathway, which normally converts glyoxylic acid ($C_2H_2O_3$) to glycine. Blocking of this pathway because of a deficiency or absence of AGT results in high levels of glycolic and oxalic acid, which are readily converted to oxalate, which is then excreted in the urine.

The median age for presentation of initial symptoms related to hyperoxaluria is 5 years. Oxalate deposition can occur in other organs (e.g. bones, joints, eyes, heart). In particular, bone tends to be the major repository of excess oxalate in patients with primary hyperoxaluria. Bone oxalate levels are negligible in healthy subjects. Oxalate deposition in the skeleton tends to increase bone resorption and decrease osteoblast activity. Because symptoms occur relatively late and are associated with very serious complications, screening all pediatric patients who have stones for hyperoxaluria is important. Discovering this condition may allow earlier testing, detection, diagnosis, and pre-emptive therapy in affected siblings.

Type II primary hyperoxaluria is much less common than type I primary hyperoxaluria and is caused by a deficiency of D-glycerate dehydrogenase (DGDH). This deficiency promotes the conversion of glyoxylate to oxalate. The degree of hyperoxaluria is approximately the same between the two types of primary hyperoxaluria. End-stage renal disease (ESRD) is slightly less common in patients with type II primary hyperoxaluria than in those with type I primary hyperoxaluria.

Primary hyperoxaluria requires vigorous management and careful follow-up. Therapy includes promoting a high urinary flow rate around the clock, and restricting dietary oxalate. Restriction of dietary calcium can result in increased oxalate absorption via the gastrointestinal tract and should be avoided.[20] Pyridoxine supplements (25–250 mg/day) have been shown to lower oxalate production and decrease the need for renal–liver transplantation.[70] Pyridoxine is generally not effective in patients with type II primary hyperoxaluria.

Curative treatment involves a combined kidney and liver transplantation. Renal transplantation alone is insufficient because the liver defect causing the hyperoxaluria is not corrected. In selected patients, an early liver transplantation prior to the development of overt renal failure may preserve the native kidneys, thus avoiding the need for renal transplantation.

Xanthinuria

Xanthinuria is a descriptive term for excessive urinary excretion of the purine base xanthine. The two inherited forms of xanthinuria result from a deficiency of the enzyme xanthine dehydrogenase, which is responsible for degrading hypoxanthine and xanthine to uric acid. The resultant increase in plasma levels and excess urinary excretion of the highly insoluble xanthine leads to urolithiasis, arthropathy, myopathy, crystal nephropathy, or renal failure.[71] More than 50% of the xanthine uroliths occur in children <10 years. Iatrogenic xanthinuria can occur during allopurinol therapy, which is used to reduce urine uric acid excretion in conditions with endogenous overproduction of uric acid. Inhibition of xanthine dehydrogenase by allopurinol may lead to accumulation and urinary excretion of xanthine. No specific therapies are available for classic xanthinuria

Lesch–Nyhan syndrome (hyperuricosuria)

The enzymatic defect associated with Lesch–Nyhan syndrome is a deficiency of the enzyme hypoxanthine–guanine phosphoribosyl transferase (HPRT). This enzyme normally plays a key role in the recycling of the purine bases hypoxanthine and guanine into the purine nucleotide pools. In the absence of HPRT, these purine bases are degraded and excreted, ultimately as uric acid. In addition to the failure of purine recycling, the rate of synthesis of purines is markedly increased, presumably to compensate for purines lost by the failure of the salvage process.

Lesch–Nyhan syndrome is a genetic disorder associated with overproduction of uric acid, neurologic disability, and behavioral problems. The overproduction of uric acid is associated with hyperuricemia. If left untreated, it can produce nephrolithiasis with renal failure, gouty arthritis, and solid subcutaneous deposits known as tophi. The neurologic disability encompasses a spectrum of extrapyramidal signs, including dystonia, choreoathetosis, and occasionally ballismus. The behavioral problems include cognitive dysfunction, aggressive and impulsive behaviors, and self-mutilation.[72]

The majority of patients present between 3 and 12 months of age with delayed motor development, most commonly hypotonia or failure to reach normal motor milestones. A smaller number of patients present with complications related to the overproduction of uric acid. Sometimes the parents give a history of 'orange sand' in the diapers, which is caused by uric acid crystalluria and microhematuria. Other patients may present with renal failure or frank hematuria, resulting from nephrolithiasis.

The control of uric acid requires allopurinol, which inhibits the metabolism of hypoxanthine and xanthine to uric acid by the enzyme xanthine oxidase.

Generous hydration is essential at all times. Hydration should be increased during periods of increased fluid loss, such as a febrile illness or recurrent emesis.

Infection stones

Infection-related stones constitute about 2–3% of the stones in pediatric patients and most commonly are seen in younger children (<6 years of age). Infection by urea-splitting bacteria results in increased urinary pH (large amount of NH_4) and increased urinary magnesium ammonium phosphate, conditions favoring the formation of struvite stones. Urinary pH of ≥6.8 results from the action of the bacterial enzyme urease on urinary urea. The resultant stones (which have a tendency to grow rapidly and form staghorn calculi) are intrinsically contaminated by bacteria, and the affected children all have findings of persistent pyuria, bacteriuria, and struvite crystalluria. Over 45 types of microorganisms are capable of urease production. *Proteus* spp are isolated in over 70% of all patients with infected stones, although *Pseudomonas, Klebsiella, Streptococcus* and *Mycoplasma* spp may also produce urease.[73]

To treat struvite stones successfully, the stone harboring the infection should be eliminated completely. In such cases, antibiotics alone cannot reach microorganisms and urinary infection recurs as soon as antibiotics are withdrawn. Select patients will benefit from hemiacidrin irrigation, which can dissolve some struvite stones. Acetohydroxamic acid (AHA), a urease inhibitor, is available for the management of stones caused by infection.[74] Genitourinary tract abnormalities predispose to the formation of infected stones (most frequently by obstruction); therefore, careful urologic evaluation of the patient with infected stones is mandatory. Findings of obstruction or a structurally anomalous urinary tract in these patients do not obviate the need for careful metabolic assessment. In one study of 66 patients with structural anomalies of the urinary tract, 36% had coexistent metabolic abnormalities. In the same study, of the 41 patients with infection-related stones, 56% had genitourinary anomalies and 29% had metabolic abnormalities.[17]

Miscellaneous stones

Triamterene stones

Triamterene is a potassium-sparing diuretic: 70% of the orally administered medication appears in the urine; 1 in 1500 patients on this medication will develop stones.[75]

Sulfadiazine stones

Sulfadiazine is a medication that is used to treat toxoplasmosis in patients with human immunodeficiency virus (HIV). Sulfadiazine crystalluria occurs in up to 49% of the patients treated with this medication, but the exact incidence of sulfadiazine causing stones is unknown. Most sulfadiazine stones are radiolucent. Treatment includes hyperhydration and alkalinization of the urine.[76]

Indinavir (Crixivan) stones

Indinavir is a protease inhibitor that is used as an antiviral drug in the treatment of HIV: 20% of the administered medication is excreted unchanged in the urine. Patients who do not maintain a urine output of >1.5 L/day while on this medication will often have crystalluria and occasionally develop indinavir stones.[77] Stone development occurs at higher urine pH (>6.0). These stones are typically radiolucent, and composed of a soft yellowish-brown gelatinous material. Unenhanced computed tomography (CT) imaging may fail to demonstrate these stones, and a high degree of suspicion should be maintained in patients at risk for these stones.[78] ESWL is often not useful in treating these stones, because of their soft nature, but they do respond to hyperhydration and mechanical removal of the stone (i.e. stone basketing).[79]

Summary

Urolithiasis in the pediatric population has diverse etiologies and presentations. With a careful and systematic evaluation of the patient and individualized management strategies, recurrent stones, renal injury, and patient morbidity can be minimized. Once again we would like to emphasize that the adult urinary values for the metabolic stone-risk profile are not accurate for their use in pediatric patients.

References

1. Kroovand RL. Pediatric urolithiasis. Urol Clin North Am 1997; 24:173–84.
2. Sinno K, Boyce WH, Resnick MI. Childhood urolithiasis. J Urol 1979; 121:662–4.
3. Stapleton FB. Nephrolithiasis in children. Pediatr Rev 1989; 11:21–30.
4. Parks JH, Coe FL. Pathogenesis and treatment of calcium stones. Semin Nephrol 1996; 16:398–411.
5. Laufer J, Boichis H. Urolithiasis in children: current medical management. Pediatr Nephrol 1989; 3:317–22.
6. Choi H, Snyder HM 3rd, Duckett JW. Urolithiasis in childhood: current management. J Pediatr Surg 1987; 22:158–64.
7. Husmann DA, Milliner DS, Segura JW. Ureteropelvic junction obstruction with concurrent renal pelvic calculi in the pediatric patient: a long-term followup. J Urol 1996; 156:741–3.
8. Segura JW, Preminger GM, Assimos DG et al. Ureteral Stones Clinical Guidelines Panel summary report on the management of ureteral calculi. The American Urological Association. J Urol 1997; 158:1915–21.
9. Smith L, Segura J. Urolithiasis. Philadelphia: WB Saunders, 1990: 1327–52.
10. Shetty S, Rivers K, Menon M. A practical approach to the evaluation and treatment of nephrolithiasis. AUA Update Series 2000; 19:234.
11. Balaji KC, Menon M. Mechanism of stone formation. Urol Clin North Am 1997; 24:1–11.
12. Ryall RL. Glycosaminoglycans, proteins, and stone formation: adult themes and child's play. Pediatr Nephrol 1996; 10:656–66.
13. Coe FL, Parks JH. Pathophysiology of kidney stones and strategies for treatment. Hosp Pract (Off Ed) 1988; 23:185–9.
14. Nakagawa Y. Urinary Tamm–Horsfall glycoprotein in patients with various renal diseases. Nippon Jinzo Gakkai Shi 1987; 29:529–34.
15. Nakagawa Y. Urinary Tamm–Horsfall glycoprotein in normal subjects. Nippon Jinzo Gakkai Shi 1987; 29:523–7.
16. Nakagawa Y, Ahmed M, Hall SL et al. Isolation from human calcium oxalate renal stones of nephrocalcin, a glycoprotein inhibitor of calcium oxalate crystal growth. Evidence that nephrocalcin from patients with calcium oxalate nephrolithiasis is deficient in gamma-carboxyglutamic acid. J Clin Invest 1987; 79:1782–7.
17. Milliner DS, Murphy ME. Urolithiasis in pediatric patients. Mayo Clin Proc 1993; 68:241–8.
18. Polinsky MS, Kaiser BA, Baluarte HJ. Urolithiasis in childhood. Pediatr Clin North Am 1987; 34:683–710.
19. Gearhart JP, Herzberg GZ, Jeffs RD. Childhood urolithiasis: experiences and advances. Pediatrics 1991; 87:445–50.
20. Stapleton FB. Current approaches to pediatric stone disease. AUA Update Ser 2000; 19:314.
21. Chen MY, Zagoria RJ. Can noncontrast helical computed tomography replace intravenous urography for evaluation of patients with acute urinary tract colic? J Emerg Med 1999; 17:299–303.
22. Chen MY, Zagoria RJ, Saunders HS et al. Trends in the use of unenhanced helical CT for acute urinary colic. AJR Am J Roentgenol 1999; 173:1447–50.
23. Tefekli A, Esen T, Ziylan O et al. Metabolic risk factors in pediatric and adult calcium oxalate urinary stone formers: is there any difference? Urol Int 2003; 70:273–7.
24. Erbagci A, Erbagci AB, Yilmaz M et al. Pediatric urolithiasis – evaluation of risk factors in 95 children. Scand J Urol Nephrol 2003; 37:129–33.
25. Asplin J, Parks J, Lingeman J et al. Supersaturation and stone composition in a network of dispersed treatment sites. J Urol 1998; 159:1821–5.
26. Parks JH, Coward M, Coe FL. Correspondence between stone composition and urine supersaturation in nephrolithiasis. Kidney Int 1997; 51:894–90.
27. Battino BS, DeFoor W, Coe F et al. Metabolic evaluation of children with urolithiasis: are adult references for supersaturation appropriate? J Urol 2002; 168: 2568–71.
28. DeFoor W, Asplin J, Jackson C et al. Results of a prospective trial to compare normal urine supersaturation in children and adults. J Urol 2005; 174:1708–10.
29. Coe F, Parks J. Nephrolithiasis, Pathogenesis and Treatment, 2nd edn. Chicago: Yearbook Medical, 1988: 1–37.
30. Millman S, Strauss AL, Parks JH, Coe FL. Pathogenesis and clinical course of mixed calcium oxalate and uric acid nephrolithiasis. Kidney Int 1982; 22:366–70.
31. Langman CB, Moore ES. Hypercalciuria in clinical pediatrics. A review. Clin Pediatr (Phila) 1984; 23:135–7.
32. Moore ES, Langman CB, Favus MJ, Schneider AB, Coe FL. Secondary hyperparathyroidism in children with symptomatic idiopathic hypercalciuria. J Pediatr 1983; 103:932–5.
33. Stapleton FB. Idiopathic hypercalciuria: association with isolated hematuria and risk for urolithiasis in children. The Southwest Pediatric Nephrology Study Group. Kidney Int 1990; 37:807–11.
34. Stapleton FB. What is the appropriate evaluation and therapy for children with hypercalciuria and hematuria? Semin Nephrol 1998; 18:359–60.
35. Alon U, Warady BA, Hellerstein S. Hypercalciuria in the frequency-dysuria syndrome of childhood. J Pediatr 1990; 116:103–5.
36. Goldman M, Shuman C, Weksberg R, Rosenblum ND. Hypercalciuria in Beckwith–Wiedemann syndrome. J Pediatr 2003; 142:206–8.
37. Coe FL, Parks JH, Moore ES. Familial idiopathic hypercalciuria. N Engl J Med 1979; 300:337–40.

38. Coe FL, Bushinsky DA. Pathophysiology of hypercalciuria. Am J Physiol 1984; 247:F1–13.
39. Dobbins JW. Nephrolithiasis and intestinal disease. J Clin Gastroenterol 1985; 7:21–4.
40. La Manna A, Polito C, Marte A, Iovene A, Di Toro R. Hyperuricosuria in children: clinical presentation and natural history. Pediatrics 2001; 107:86–90.
41. Polito C, La Manna A, Nappi B, Villani J, Di Toro R. Idiopathic hypercalciuria and hyperuricosuria: family prevalence of nephrolithiasis. Pediatr Nephrol 2000; 14:1102–4.
42. Coe FL. Uric acid and calcium oxalate nephrolithiasis. Kidney Int 1983; 24:392–403.
43. Deganello S, Chou C. The uric acid–whewellite association in human kidney stones. Scan Electron Microsc 1985; (Pt 4):1545–50.
44. Tekin A, Tekgul S, Atsu N et al. A study of the etiology of idiopathic calcium urolithiasis in children: hypocitruria is the most important risk factor. J Urol 2000; 164:162–5.
45. Miller LA, Stapleton FB. Urinary volume in children with urolithiasis. J Urol 1989; 141:918–20.
46. Borghi L, Meschi T, Amato F et al. Urinary volume, water and recurrences in idiopathic calcium nephrolithiasis: a 5-year randomized prospective study. J Urol 1996; 155:839–43.
47. Borghi L, Meschi T, Schianchi T et al. Urine volume: stone risk factor and preventive measure. Nephron 1999; 81 (Suppl 1):31–7.
48. Garcia-Nieto V, Ferrandez C, Monge M, de Sequera M, Rodrigo MD. Bone mineral density in pediatric patients with idiopathic hypercalciuria. Pediatr Nephrol 1997; 11:578–83.
49. Hess B. Low calcium diet in hypercalciuric calcium nephrolithiasis: first do no harm. Scanning Microsc 1996; 10:547–54, discussion 554–6.
50. Osorio AV, Alon US. The relationship between urinary calcium, sodium, and potassium excretion and the role of potassium in treating idiopathic hypercalciuria. Pediatrics 1997; 100:675–81.
51. Shimizu T, Nakamura M, Yoshitomi K et al. Interaction of trichlormethiazide or amiloride with PTH in stimulating Ca^{2+} absorption in rabbit CNT. Am J Physiol 1991; 261:F36–43.
52. Preminger GM, Sakhaee K, Pak CY. Alkali action on the urinary crystallization of calcium salts: contrasting responses to sodium citrate and potassium citrate. J Urol 1988; 139:240–2.
53. Blaszak R. Dietary advice for children with calcium urolithiasis. Dialog Pediatr Urol 2002; 25:14.
54. Morton WJ. Lesch–Nyhan syndrome. Urology 1982; 20:506–9.
55. Stapleton FB. Genetics of Urolithiasis. Boston: Kluwer Academic Publishers, 1990.
56. Riese RJ, Sakhaee K. Uric acid nephrolithiasis: pathogenesis and treatment. J Urol 1992; 148:765–71.
57. Greene ML, Fujimoto WY, Seegmiller JE. Urinary xanthine stones – a rare complication of allopurinol therapy. N Engl J Med 1969; 280:426–7.
58. Pohlman T, Hruska KA, Menon M. Renal tubular acidosis. J Urol 1984; 132:431–7.
59. Rothstein M, Obialo C, Hruska KA. Renal tubular acidosis. Endocrinol Metab Clin North Am 1990; 19:869–87.
60. Rocher LL, Tannen RL. The clinical spectrum of renal tubular acidosis. Annu Rev Med 1986; 37:319–31.
61. Singer A, Das S. Cystinuria: a review of the pathophysiology and management. J Urol 1989; 142:669–73.
62. Sakhaee K. Pathogenesis and medical management of cystinuria. Semin Nephrol 1996; 16:435–47.
63. Segal S. Inherited disorders of transport: aminoacidurias. Monogr Hum Genet 1978; 9:147–51.
64. Segal S. Genetics of renal transport disorders. Prog Clin Biol Res 1989; 305:101–9.
65. Dent CE, Friedman M, Green H, Watson LC. Treatment of cystinuria. Br Med J 1965; 5432:403–8.
66. Dent CE, Senior B. Studies on the treatment of cystinuria. Br J Urol 1955; 27:317–32.
67. Streem SB, Hall P. Effect of captopril on urinary cystine excretion in homozygous cystinuria. J Urol 1989; 142:1522–4.
68. Chow GK, Streem SB. Medical treatment of cystinuria: results of contemporary clinical practice. J Urol 1996; 156:1576–8.
69. Chow GK, Streem SB. Contemporary urological intervention for cystinuric patients: immediate and long-term impact and implications. J Urol 1998; 160:341–4, discussion 344–5.
70. Yendt ER, Cohanim M. Response to a physiologic dose of pyridoxine in type I primary hyperoxaluria. N Engl J Med 1985; 312:953–7.
71. Cameron JS, Moro F, Simmonds HA. Gout, uric acid and purine metabolism in paediatric nephrology. Pediatr Nephrol 1993; 7:105–18.
72. Watts RW, Spellacy E, Gibbs DA et al. Clinical, postmortem, biochemical and therapeutic observations on the Lesch–Nyhan syndrome with particular reference to the neurological manifestations. Q J Med 1982; 51:43–78.
73. Lerner SP, Gleeson MJ, Griffith DP. Infection stones. J Urol 1989; 141:753–8.
74. Rodman JS. Struvite stones. Nephron 1999; 81 (Suppl 1):50–9.
75. Ettinger B, Oldroyd NO, Sorgel F. Triamterene nephrolithiasis. JAMA 1980; 244:2443–5.
76. Catalano-Pons C, Bargy S, Schlecht D et al. Sulfadiazine-induced nephrolithiasis in children. Pediatr Nephrol 2004; 19:928–31.
77. Bruce RG, Munch LC, Hoven AD et al. Urolithiasis associated with the protease inhibitor indinavir. Urology 1997; 50:513–18.
78. Kohan AD, Armenakas NA, Fracchia JA. Indinavir urolithiasis: an emerging cause of renal colic in patients with human immunodeficiency virus. J Urol 1999; 161:1765–8.
79. Gentle DL, Stoller ML, Jarrett TW et al. Protease inhibitor-induced urolithiasis. Urology 1997; 50:508–11.

Endourology for stone disease

26

Aseem Shukla and Michael Erhard

Etiology/epidemiology

The incidence and prevalence of childhood urolithiasisis varies widely throughout the world. In Turkey and Southeast Asia, urolithiasis remains an endemic disease, with an estimated incidence in Turkish schoolchildren of 0.8%.[1] Bladder stones composed of ammonium urate and uric acid indicate dietary etiologies for the disproportionate incidence of urolithiasis in endemic areas. In contrast, pediatric renal stones are rare in North America, with nephrolithiasis accounting for 1 in 1000 to 1 in 7600 pediatric hospital admissions, depending on the geographical region.[2] The incidence of stone disease in children is only one-tenth of that in adults.[3,4] The southeast United States predominates in prevalence.

Only 50% of pediatric patients diagnosed with urolithiasis complain of flank pain.[2] Other presentations include gross or microscopic hematuria (25–40%), incidental finding on imaging examinations (15%), and urinary tract infection (10–30%).[2–5] Stones in infants are often discovered when investigating persistent symptoms of colic.

Spontaneous passage of pediatric urinary stones is common, and conservative management is preferred in the absence of obstructive uropathy, urosepsis, or uncontrolled pain and vomiting. The rate of spontaneous passage will vary according to both the size of the stone and its position within the ureter (Figure 26.1) Adult studies show an overall spontaneous passage of approximately 55% for all stones, with those <4 mm passing approximately 80% of the time.[6] The spontaneous passage rate in children is similarly high, at or near 66% among all pediatric age groups.[7] Other studies have shown that stones within the proximal collecting system pass approximately 22% of the time compared with 46% and 71% for those in the middle and distal third of the ureter, respectively.[8] Previous reports in the pediatric literature concluded that calculi <3 mm have a greater chance of passing spontaneously, whereas stones >4 mm most likely require surgical management.[9] It has been the authors' experience that even small stones that become symptomatic in the proximal ureter are often not likely to advance spontaneously. Furosemide administration in premature infants with bronchopulmonary disease, and the calcium and phosphorus content of premature infant formulas have resulted in a higher incidence of renal stones as compared with ureteral stones in that patient population.[10] In addition, these renal stones are often large and less likely to pass spontaneously. Whereas renal stones in infants are related to specialized medical therapy and systemic illness, urinary metabolic abnormalities commonly contribute to urolithiasis in older children.

If the clinical symptomatology suggests the presence of a urinary calculus, an algorithm similar to that

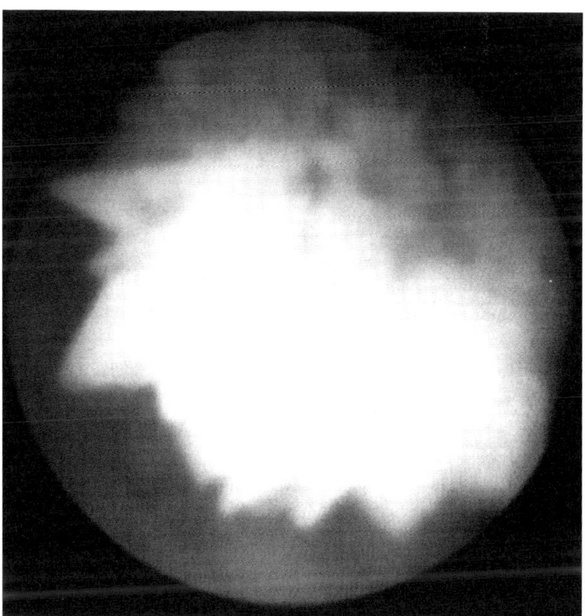

Figure 26.1 Even large stones with a smooth edge and a tapered leading edge may pass through the pediatric ureter; therefore, conservative management should be the first step unless symptoms warrant urgent intervention. Sharp 'spines' when present (as pictured here) may inhibit even a small stone from passing.

in adults, radiographic evaluation with a non-enhanced helical computed tomography (CT) scan of the abdomen and pelvis is most appropriate.[11,12] This will allow complete visualization of the collecting system and should identify all sizes and types of urinary calculi (Figure 26.2). If deemed necessary, intravenous contrast media may be administered after the non-contrast phase to evaluate for obstruction and focal changes in the kidney, providing more information than a traditional intravenous pyelogram (IVP). Most pediatric stones consist of calcium oxalate and may be radiopaque on plain X-ray. Although ultrasound is usually still performed to exclude large renal calculi, hydronephrosis, or perirenal collections, it has very low sensitivity for detecting ureteral calculi.[13] Total radiation exposure in children is a serious consideration, and CT protocols that image stones while reducing dosage are currently under evaluation.[12,14]

Metabolic and genitourinary anomalies that may predispose to urolithiasis often coexist in pediatric patients (Figure 26.3). Anatomic abnormalities, with ureteropelvic junction obstruction being the most common, are discovered in 10–40% of children evaluated for stones.[15] Metabolic abnormalities are exceedingly common and may exist in up to 90% of children with urinary stones, depending upon how strictly they are defined.[7,16,17] Common urine abnormalities include hypercalciuria, hypocitraturia, and hypomagnesuria. Urinary supersaturation indices are often elevated and may prove to be a more precise predictor of stone recurrence than traditional metabolic parameters.[18,19] Low urinary volume is also common and treatment should result in urine output of approximately 35 ml/kg/day.[20] Significant hypercalciuria and hypocitriuria should be aggressively treated in children with recurrent stone disease or multiple or bilateral calculi. Serum electrolyte evaluation is appropriate in children found to have significant urine metabolic abnormalities.

Conservative management is most appropriate for stones of relatively small size (<4 mm) without signs

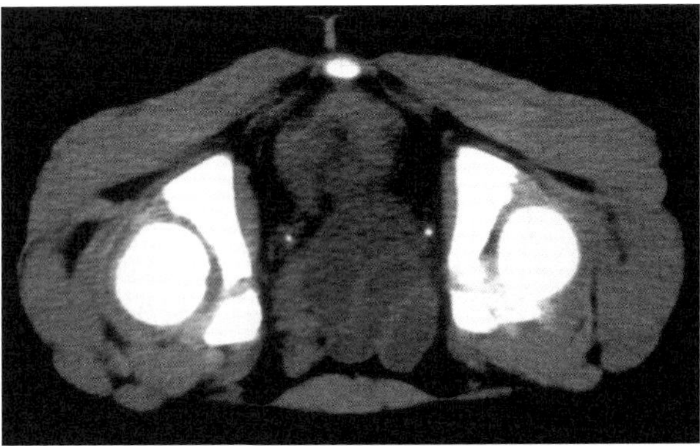

Figure 26.2 CT scan of the abdomen and pelvis allows for complete visualization and diagnosis of even small urinary calculi. This young boy had right-sided symptoms. On radiographic evaluation, he was found to have bilateral ureteral calculi and required subsequent bilateral therapy.

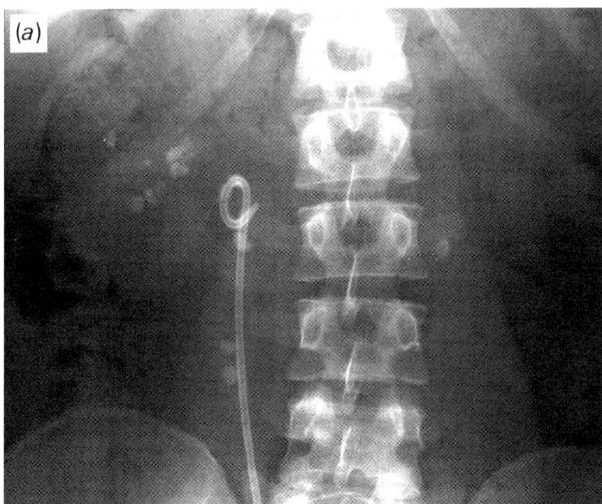

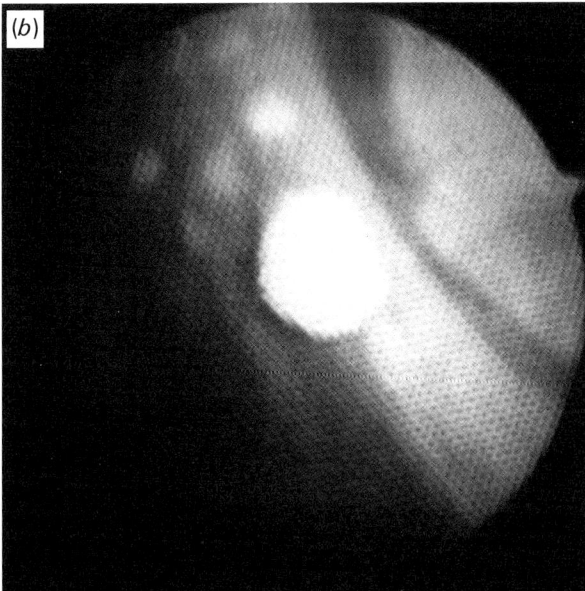

Figure 26.3 (*a*) A large stone burden is seen in both collecting systems in this teenage boy as well as encrustation of stone matter on the proximal portion of the pigtail stent. An underlying metabolic abnormality was suspected and, in fact, he had primary hyperparathyroidism. It is not uncommon to see papillary tip calculi (*b*) at the time of ureteroscopy for intrarenal calculi. These are seen as small areas of nephrocalcinosis on non-contrast CT scan. On metabolic urine evaluation, these children are more likely to show evidence of hypercalciuria.

of obstructive uropathy or urosepsis. It is important to have the child strain all urine so that calculus debris can be obtained and sent for stone analysis. This also gives an endpoint for conservative management, possibly eliminating the need for follow-up radiographic assessment.

Once the child has been cleared of any calculus disease, either through conservative management or surgical intervention, it is appropriate to obtain two consecutive 24-hour urine samples for metabolic stone analysis. These should include an internal creatinine standard to ensure completeness of urine sampling. Traditional urinary metabolic parameters include calcium, phosphate, magnesium, citrate, creatinine, uric acid, pH, and voided volume. For children not yet toilet trained, random urine measurements of creatinine, calcium, uric acid, and oxalate may be obtained, but preferably 2–4 hours after milk is ingested.[21] Pediatric reference ranges are now readily available and should be utilized.[2,21,22] Serum evaluation should be performed in children with stone recurrence or multiple calculi, and should include calcium, phosphate, uric acid, creatinine, sodium, and potassium. Surgical intervention is appropriate for any size stone with prolonged failure of spontaneous passage or unrelenting symptoms such as pain, nausea, vomiting, and gross hematuria. Proactive treatment of renal stones >5 mm should be considered, as a stone this size is likely to cause obstructive symptoms while passing through the urinary system. Treatment strategies should be based upon achieving the greatest stone-free rate for the particular situation, with the least morbidity and lowest risk for ancillary procedures. The most effective treatment plan may include multiple modalities.

Treatment options

Extracorporeal shock wave lithotripsy

Extracorporeal shock wave lithotripsy (ESWL) to treat pediatric stones was first reported in 1988.[23] Initial reports in animal models indicated evidence of significant renal damage following ESWL, which may have contributed to the delay in its use for children.[24,25]

Reported ESWL success rates after one session for mean stone sizes up to 2.5 cm are excellent, with a 75–98% stone-free rate at 3 months.[26–29] Ureteral stents are usually avoided after treatment for most stones, as children have an impressive ability to pass proportionately larger stone fragments than adults.[30,31] Initial experiences with ESWL monotherapy for staghorn calculi confirm the feasibility of this modality, with stone-free rates of approximately 75%.[32–34] These patients appear to benefit from pre-ESWL ureteral stent placement and often require ancillary procedures for complete stone clearance.[34]

Long-term functional studies on pediatric patients following ESWL now show no significant change in effective renal plasma flow or mean body height at least 4 years after treatment.[35–37] The safety and efficacy of ESWL have also been demonstrated in premature low birth weight infants.[10] Still, animal experimental studies demonstrating increased incidence and size of hematoma formation with increased number of administered shocks during ESWL require conservative use of this treatment modality.[38] Whereas extended long-term microvascular consequences and those on renal anatomy await elaboration in children, morphologic changes such as subcapsular or intrarenal hematomas have been infrequently noted. These findings usually resolve spontaneously within 1 week. It is not uncommon to see gross hematuria after ESWL, but this usually quickly resolves with increased fluid intake. Any child with significant abdominal or flank discomfort in the early postoperative period should be evaluated for possible hematoma or obstruction from calculus debris.

Hemoptysis has been reported postoperatively, particularly in children with significant orthopedic deformities.[39] Small stature and some skeletal deformities increase the risk of the pulmonary field being present within the shock wave path. Prevention of such a complication may be lessened through the use of styrofoam padding, and symptoms should resolve with conservative management.

Shock waves are generated and focused by a variety of mechanical systems. The original units are spark-gap generated, ellipsoid focused systems that are extremely powerful and have a wide focal point. The Dornier HM3 (Dornier MedTech, Kennesaw, Georgia) remains the gold standard in efficacy for stone fragmentation. However, the HM3 produces a wider area of shock wave effect and styrofoam sheets should be placed to protect the lungs, while gantry modification is required for smaller children.[10,40] Subsequent generations of lithotriptors have less scatter of energy, increased ease with which a child can be placed on the unit, and improved localization of radiolucent stones as a result of sonographic coordination. These improvements decrease the intensity of energy and exchange overall stone-free rates for potentially minimized renal trauma. Newer-generation ESWL units are portable and may be easily transported between operating room suites. In adults it is possible to perform ESWL under light anesthesia, although children generally require a deeper general anesthetic for successful completion. Localization of the stone during treatment is determined by fluoroscopy, sonography, or plain X-ray films. Sometimes it is necessary to position a child prone in order to access the stone for effective lithotripsy.

Similar principles are applied for children as for adults, and proper patient selection will help to improve treatment outcomes. Some relative contraindications for ESWL include morbid obesity, a large stone burden, increased stone density, congenital skeletal/renal anomalies, and previously failed ESWL. The number of shocks, and the maximum energy level should be tailored for each case, and periodic stone visualization during the procedure will demonstrate when adequate lithotripsy has occurred. The primary goal is always to use the least amount of energy necessary to accomplish successful treatment.

Ureteroscopy

Advances in fiberoptics and in the design of mini rigid, semirigid, and flexible ureteroscopes has allowed for miniaturization of endoscopes and a resurgence of interest in endoscopy for pediatric patients. Adequate visualization has not been significantly compromised despite the downsizing of endoscopes. Digital imaging as well as enhancements in video technology allow for clear visualization as well as instantaneous documentation of endourologic procedures. Digital chips incorporated into larger flexible endoscopes currently exist, but technologic limitations prevent their use in the smaller-caliber instruments.

Pediatric ureteroscopy was first reported in 1929 by Hugh Hampton Young.[41] The procedure was performed on a 2-month-old boy with massively dilated ureters secondary to posterior urethral valves. Young utilized a 9.5 Fr pediatric cystoscope and was able to visualize the ureter as well as the intrarenal collecting system. But ureteroscopy gained gradual widespread acceptance by pediatric urologists only after Ritchey and Shepherd independently published articles on the technique of pediatric ureteroscopy for treatment of urinary calculi in 1988.[42,43]

Two types of ureteroscopes are available to the pediatric urologist: the mini rigid fiberoptic ureteroscope and the flexible fiberoptic ureteroscope. The mini rigid fiberoptic (i.e. semirigid) ureteroscope has a metal outer casing, which is malleable enough to allow for limited bending without image distortion. These endoscopes are more durable than flexible ureteroscopes and most can be safely autoclaved for sterilization. Excellent visual fields, and two working channels that allow for simultaneous irrigation as well as placement of working instruments, make these endoscopes particularly useful in the distal ureter. However, passage into the proximal collecting system above the bony pelvis may be difficult. Varying lengths are available, and the authors use both a 15 cm and 33 cm endoscope tailored to the child's size and location of the stone (Figure 26.4) Although the distal tip is as small as 4.7 Fr, the gradual increase in the diameter of the malleable metal shaft proximally towards the eyepiece requires one to maintain vigilance to minimize the risk of meatal injury in the young male.

Flexible ureteroscopes are useful within the proximal and intrarenal collecting system due to their active as well as passive tip deflection. Some models have the capability of both primary and secondary active deflection (DUR-8 Elite, Circon ACMI, Southborough, MA) and others have 270° primary deflection in either direction (Flex-ex, Karl Storz, Tuttlingen, Germany). Most flexible ureteroscopes have a working channel of approximately 3.6 Fr, which is adequate for passage of instruments while maintaining space for irrigation. Rarely, however, is secondary passive tip deflection necessary for complete inspection of the intrarenal pediatric collecting system because the arc of deflection is adequate to access the lower pole in most pediatric kidneys. Many working instruments will decrease the ability to actively deflect the ureteroscope, and it is important to remember to straighten the distal tip of the ureteroscope prior to passage of any working instrument to help prevent damage to the working channel.

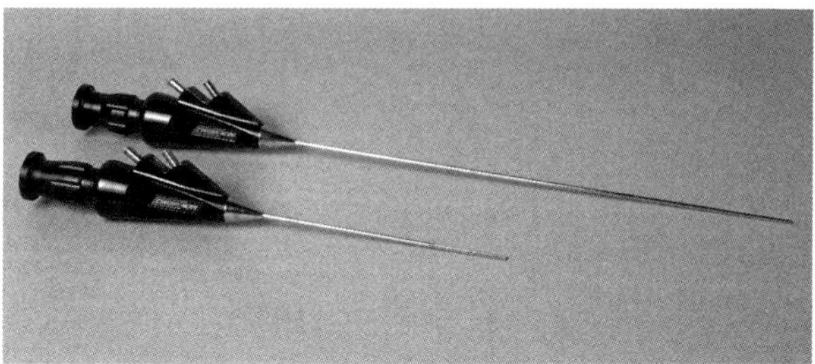

Figure 26.4 Semi-rigid ureteroscopes of varying lengths are most helpful for stone removal within the mid and distal ureter. The two separate lumens permit continuous irrigation through one port while performing tasks through the second port.

Resistance within the working channel may be decreased through the use of a silicone lubricant.

Recent technologic advancements have improved the durability of both the outside sheath, and deflecting mechanisms, but have resulted in an increased outer diameter. Because of their flexible design, these endoscopes are more prone to damage and need to be handled with care. Replacement of the fiberoptic bundles is necessary when the image becomes significantly distorted, and any perforation of the working channel will cause damage to the endoscopes. Flexible endoscopes can be safely soaked in cold sterilization solution or undergo gas sterilization, but cannot be autoclaved. The distal tip is approximately 7.4 Fr but gradually becomes 8.5 Fr or greater at the proximal shaft, which helps to strengthen the sheath and protect the inner bundle fibers. The authors prefer the use of three distinct lengths in children (35, 50, and 65 cm) in order to decrease the amount of redundant shaft outside of the body, which helps to prevent damage during use (Figure 26.5).

Working instruments

A variety of working instruments have been designed for use within miniaturized endoscopes. Guidewires are required as a platform for advanced ureteroscopy and are the most commonly used working instruments in endourology: not only do they aid in access to the ureter but also they help to prevent intraoperative complications by preventing loss of access to the collecting system. Most guidewires have an inner stainless steel core coated by polytetrafluoroethylene (PTFE) to reduce friction, and others have a superelastic nitinol (nickel–titanium) alloy core, which prevents kinking of the wire. There are varying diameters, but a 150 cm PTFE-coated guidewire with a 3 cm floppy distal tip is the most common type in our practice. The distal tip may be straight or angled and the length of its flexible floppy tip varies. A wire with a floppy tip on both ends is the safest choice for passage of a flexible ureteroscope because it minimizes potential damage to the working channel.

A hydrophilic-coated guidewire is helpful for negotiating a tortuous or narrowed ureter and for placement of a working wire proximal to an impacted ureteral calculus. These extremely slippery guidewires need to be kept moist and should not be used as safety wires, because of the ease with which they may be dislodged during an endoscopic procedure. Handling of the slippery hydrophilic wires is made easier through the use of a moistened gauze sponge. For straightening tortuous or reimplanted ureters, extra stiff guidewires may be used, and these should also be used for percutaneous tract dilatation. Importantly, these wires should not be used when placing a flexible ureteroscope because of the increased risk of damaging the delicate working channel.

Development of a wide spectrum of accessories, from stone baskets to grasping forceps, has significantly aided the extraction of stone debris from the collecting system. The instruments vary in diameter from 1.9 to 4.5 Fr and most are contained within a hydrophilic sheath (PTFE, polyimide) to facilitate passage.

A variety of designs of baskets exist, but the most significant improvement in basket design has been the tipless nitinol basket. The tipless design makes it particularly safe and useful for extraction of stones within a tight calyx (Figure 26.6) and, when deployed,

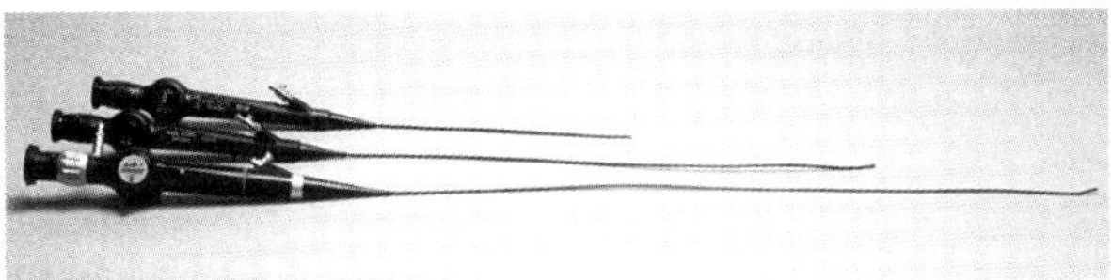

Figure 26.5 Flexible ureteroscopes are much more prone to damage because of their delicate design. To decrease this risk, it is helpful to have multiple lengths available, in order to eliminate redundancy of the endoscope outside of the body during the procedure.

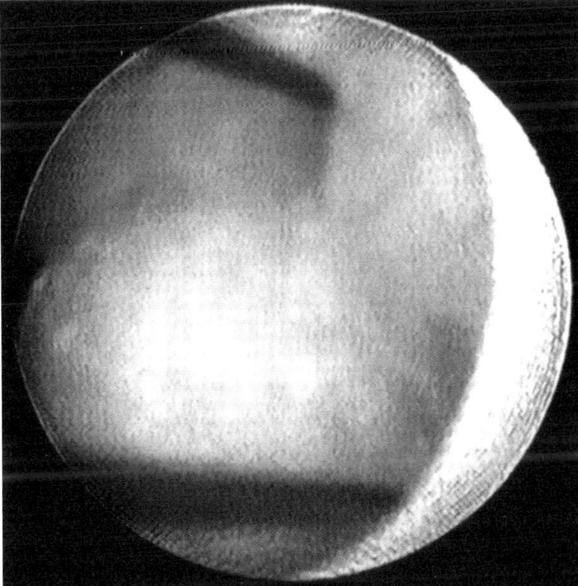

Figure 26.6 The small, tipless nitinol baskets enable removal of stones contained within tight calices with minimal trauma.

allows for more complete active deflection of the ureteroscope due its increased flexibility.[44] Some of the newer baskets have been designed to allow controlled active angulation of the baskets' wires (Dimension, Bard Urological Division, Covington, GA) and others enable a canopy to form that may engage multiple small calculi (Figure 26.7). Multi-sizing baskets omit the need for stocking multiple basket sizes, and some baskets have a central channel that allows for the simultaneous placement of electrohydraulic or laser lithotripsy probes once the stone is stabilized.

Grasping forceps are quite helpful during endoscopic stone extraction, particularly within the ureter, and, indeed, are the authors' preferred instruments in most cases (Figure 26.8). The most significant advantage is that a grasper will disengage from a stone if it becomes lodged within a relatively narrow ureteral segment. This helps to prevent trauma of the ureteral wall by eliminating entrapment during stone removal. The grasper should be opened only as wide as is needed to engage the stone, thus decreasing the risk of ureteral wall perforation (Figure 26.9). It is important to maintain contact with the stone while closing the graspers; therefore, slight advancement of the sheath is needed as the forceps are closed.

Proper selection of a stone retrieval device is important for the successful and timely completion of any endoscopic procedure. Several factors impact this decision – particularly, the size, position within the collecting system, and condition (i.e. impacted vs non-impacted) of the stone. Ptashnyk et al studied ex-vivo porcine kidneys and ureters to determine which stone retrieval devices were most effective in certain situations.[45] Their conclusions were that graspers are most efficient at the removal of a single ureteral stone (particularly impacted) with little mucosal damage,

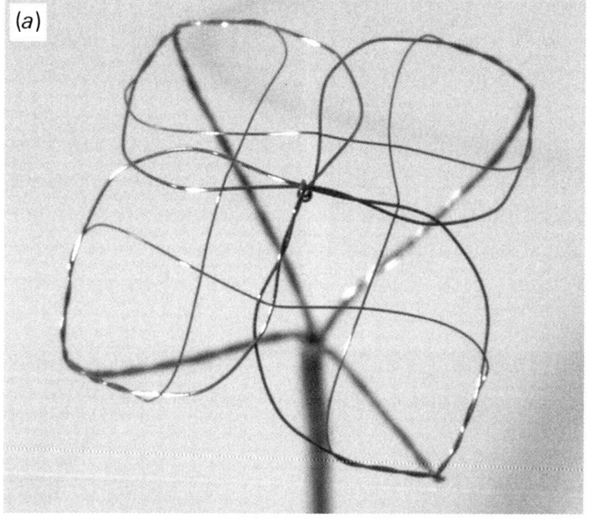

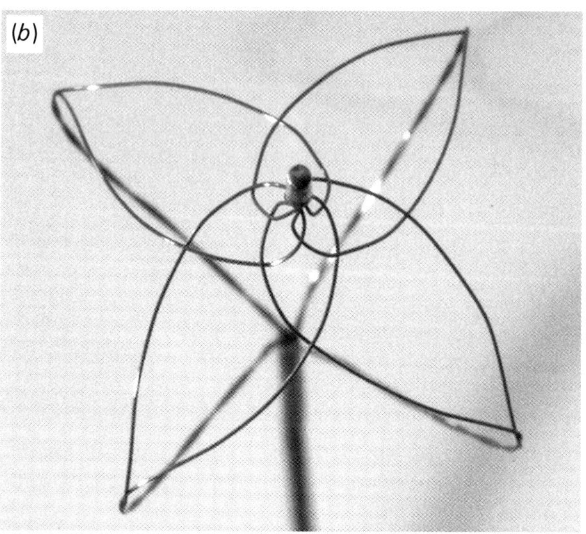

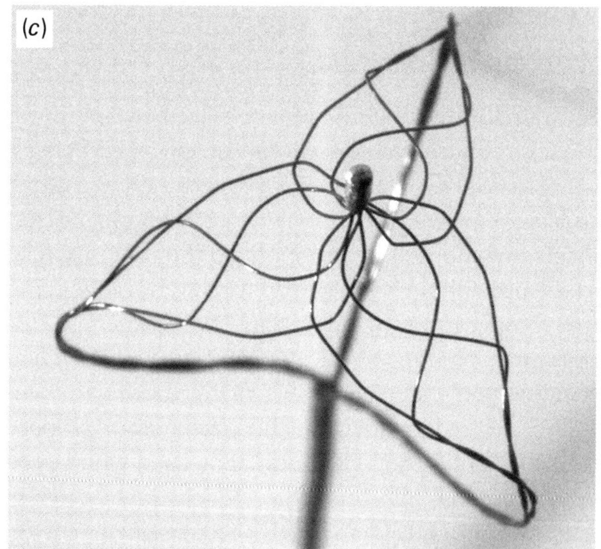

Figure 26.7 (*a–c*) The various configurations of other nitinol baskets enhance the retrieval of small particles remaining after laser lithotripsy. Some of these baskets have a central channel that allows for the placement of lithotripsy devices after stone entrapment. Always proceed cautiously when removing multiple stone fragments because the caliber of the ureteral lumen may be inadequate to allow for safe retrieval. (Courtesy of Cook Urological, Spencer, IN.)

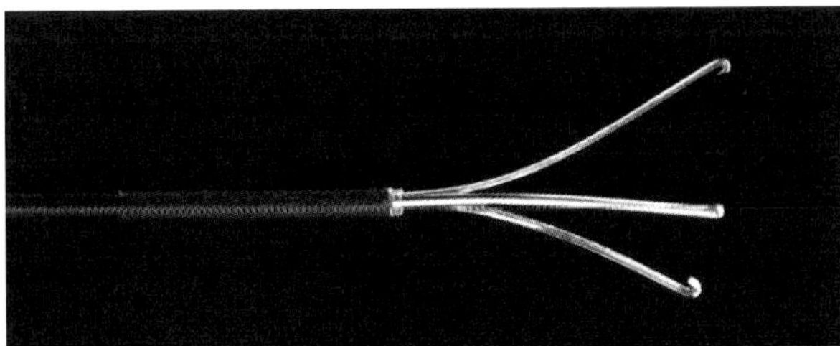

Figure 26.8 Grasping forceps are strong enough to dislodge embedded papillary calculi and delicate enough to disengage a stone if it becomes lodged within a narrow ureteral segment. (Courtesy of Cook Urological, Spencer, IN.)

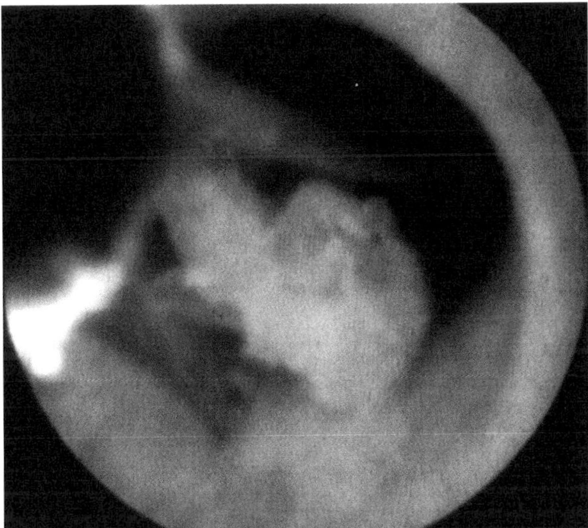

Figure 26.9 To prevent ureteral wall perforation, it is important to open the grasper only as far as needed to encompass the lateral aspects of the stone. This will also help to prevent the inadvertent grasping of the ureteral wall, which would probably result in ureteral trauma.

and that a helical basket was most effective for Steinstrasse. In another study, nitinol baskets have been shown to be most effective for caliceal stones and those in the lower pole.[46] The flexible nitinol component and the atraumatic tipless basket design allow complete deflection and produce minimal surrounding tissue trauma.

A newer instrument is the Dretler stone cone (Microvasive, Boston Scientific, Natick, MA), which is an 0.038 inch nitinol Teflon-coated wire that can be coiled proximal to the calculus acting as a backstop to prevent proximal migration. It has been shown to be effective in extracting stone fragments and more successful than flat-wire baskets in preventing stone migration.[47]

Intracorporeal lithotripsy

Historically there are four modes of intracorporeal lithotripsy:

- ultrasonic lithotripsy
- ballistic (i.e. pneumatic) lithotripsy
- electrohydraulic lithotripsy (EHL)
- laser lithotripsy.

Each has been extensively studied, and all have unique capabilities and limitations.

Ultrasonic lithotripsy was first described 1953.[48] The metal probe transmits vibrational energy to the tip, which, when in contact with the stone, results in disintegration due to cleavage of the crystal matrix. Small solid probes can be utilized through pediatric cystourethroscopes and large probes with a central suction channel are helpful for removal of stones during percutaneous procedures (Figure 26.10). These probes will lose energy transmission with any degree of bending, and, therefore are most effective when used in endoscopes with a straight working channel. Ultrasonic lithotripsy is safe and results in minimal tissue damage.[49] It is best suited for the percutaneous treatment of large renal stones.

Ballistic lithotripsy involves the pneumatic mechanical impaction of stones by a solid probe. There are no thermal or cavitation effects; therefore, risk of tissue injury is minimal. This modality has been effective in fragmenting all types of stones and smaller flexible probes are available.[50–53] Retrograde migration due to pneumatic impaction as well as loss of lithotripsy power, with significant deflection of the probe, are two significant shortcomings.

EHL was discovered by Yutkin in 1955 and

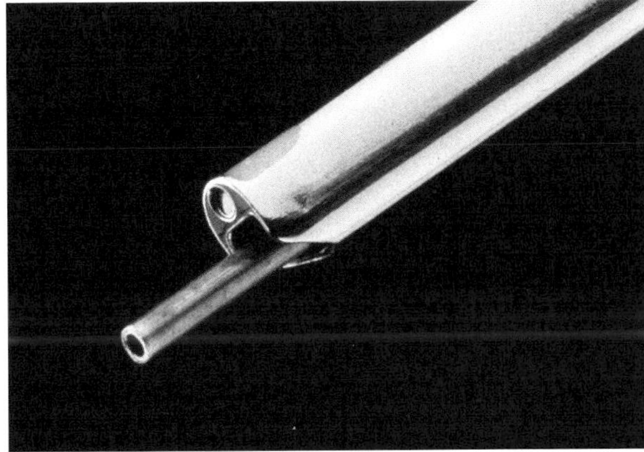

Figure 26.10 Ultrasonic lithotripsy probes can be used in straight-channel endoscopes and are most helpful during the percutaneous removal of staghorn calculi. (Courtesy of Circon ACMI, Southborough, MA.)

involves the generation of an electrical spark, which produces a cavitation bubble, providing sufficient energy to produce lithotripsy.[54] The energy is maximal at a distance of approximately 1 mm from the stone and therefore the tip of the probe should be kept just off the surface of the stone. Electrohydraulic lithotripsy may not fragment all stone compositions but is able to be used through both flexible and rigid endoscopes. One significant risk of EHL is lateral disbursement of the energy, which can increase injury to the surrounding soft tissues. Probes are as small as 1.9 Fr, which will allow access to lower pole calculi.

Holmium:yttrium–aluminum–garnet (Ho:YAG) laser lithotripsy is extremely effective at fragmenting all types of urinary calculi[55] and has become the preferred modality for stone fragmentation at our center (Figure 26.11). Holmium laser lithotripsy was first reported in 1992[56] and subsequent reports have shown it to be safe in adults and children.[57,58] Holmium lithotripsy involves direct stone absorption of laser energy, with subsequent disintegration.[59] Solid quartz fibers as small as 200 μm enable near complete deflection of a flexible ureteroscope, providing access to nearly all parts of the collecting system. The laser fiber is placed near the stone in order to result in fragmentation. Larger fibers are helpful in the disintegration of larger stones contained within the kidney or bladder. It is essential that the surgeon maintain direct visualization of the tip of the probe to prevent subsequent endoscope or tissue damage during use. Holmium laser lithotripsy results in dust particles and fragments <2 mm, which should be able to pass spontaneously.

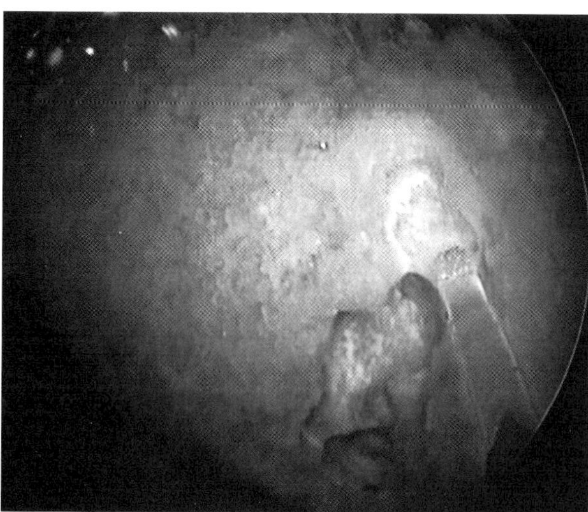

Figure 26.11 Holmium laser lithotripsy is safe and the most effective at breaking apart calculi. The precise delivery of energy allows the surgeon to smooth rough edges from a spiculated calculus, and to specifically cleave larger stones into distinct fragments for subsequent removal.

Ureteroscopy technique

Ureteroscopy in children requires general anesthesia. After being placed in the dorsal lithotomy position, the child is well padded to prevent excessive limb abduction or a compartment syndrome. The male urethral meatus is carefully inspected and gently dilated if necessary. Cystoscopy is performed to inspect the bladder and visualize the position of ureteral orifices. A urine sample is obtained at the time of the cystoscopy and sent for urine culture.

The authors first gauge the caliber of the ureteral orifice by using an 0.035 inch guidewire (Figure 26.12). The ureter has three physiologic areas of narrowing, with the narrowest portion being the orifice. These anatomic differences are age dependent, based on work by Cussen in 1971.[60] For practical purposes, if the orifice appears 'volcanic' and barely accepts an 0.035 inch guidewire, then either active dilatation or prestenting of the ureter is performed. It is sometimes helpful to gain access to the ureteral orifice using two guidewires, one inside the working channel and the other already independently placed in the ureter as a safety wire (Figure 26.13). This helps to control access

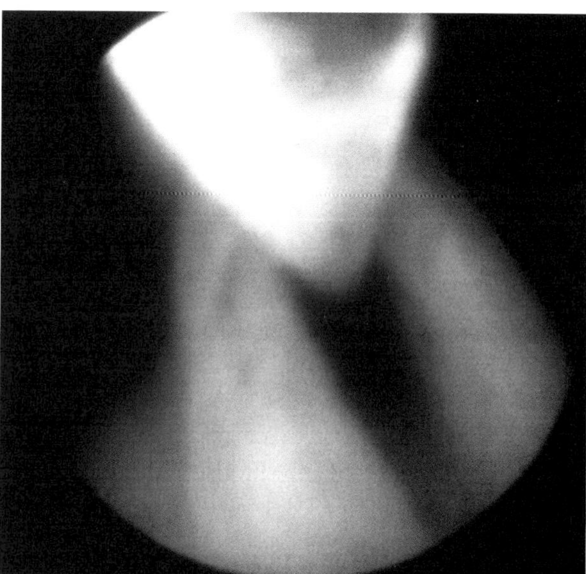

Figure 26.12 An 0.035 inch Teflon-coated guidewire is used to gauge the ureteral orifice at the beginning of a ureteroscopy procedure. If a gap is created with tenting up the ureteral lip, then a semirigid ureteroscope can usually be guided into the ureter without active dilatation. A volcanic-appearing orifice should be prestented to allow for subsequent passive dilatation.

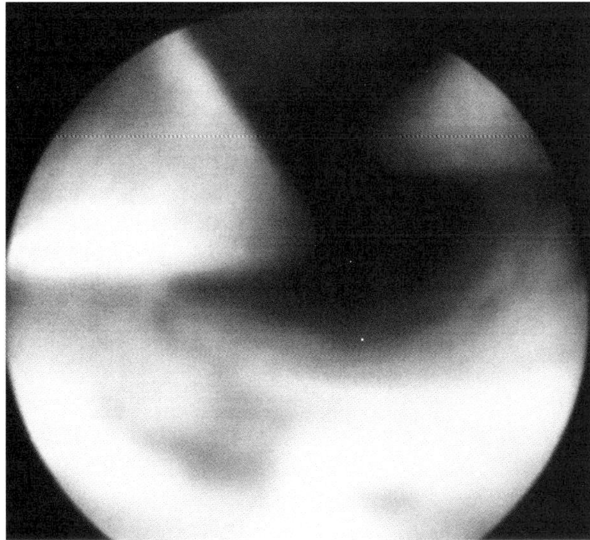

Figure 26.13 One helpful technique during difficult access is placing a second guidewire through the working channel of a semi-rigid ureteroscope after having placed a safety wire within the ureteral lumen. This will sometimes facilitate advancement of the ureteroscope by spreading the ureteral orifice.

and to increase the diameter by placing the endoscope directly between the two wires. If dilatation is needed, the authors' preference is to use a graduated single-shaft dilator, which ranges from 6 to 10 Fr (Figure 26.14). Dilatation to 2 Fr sizes greater than the diameter of the endoscope is usually needed for successful access (Figure 26.15). Dilatation can be facilitated by performing this over a stiff guidewire or through a 13 Fr cystoscope sheath in order to prevent buckling within the bladder. Reports of balloon dilatation to 15 Fr have previously shown no significant complications or reflux, but clearly produce more active dilatation than actually necessary. If these maneuvers do not allow easy dilatation or access of the ureter, the authors believe it is more prudent to place a ureteral stent to passively dilate the ureter rather than to perform significant active balloon dilatation. Dilatation of the ureter may be required in approximately 30% of children undergoing ureteroscopy.[61]

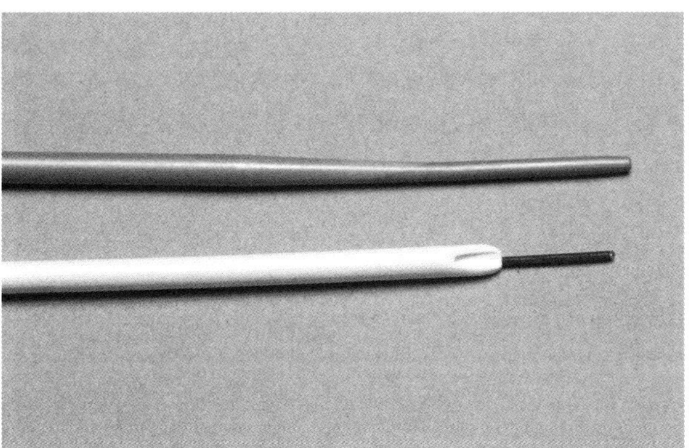

Figure 26.14 Controlled active dilatation can be performed using a soft graduated dilator (top) over a stiff guidewire. A dual-lumen catheter (bottom) is helpful when placing a second working wire and also for instillation of contrast material.

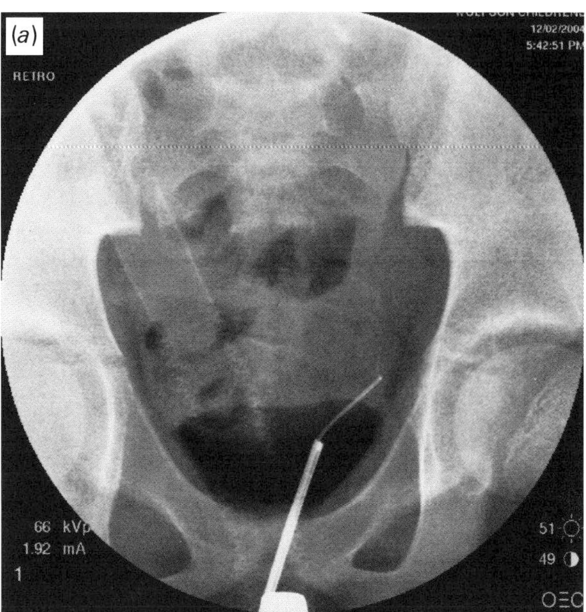

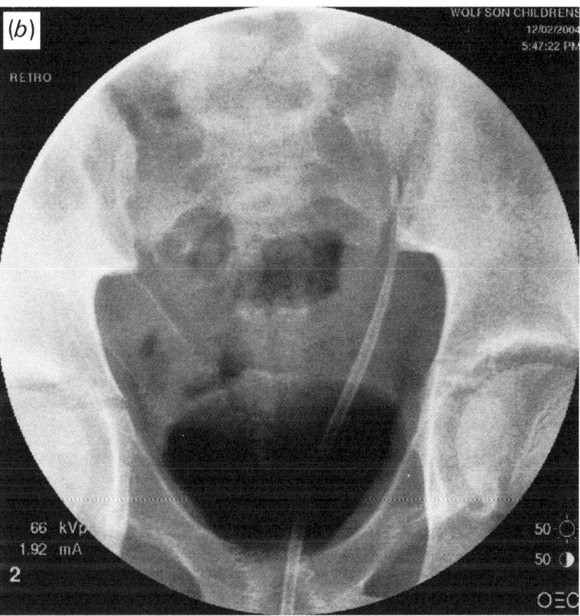

Figure 26.15 Dilatation is required if the semi-rigid endoscope cannot be placed directly into the ureteral orifice. If access is unsuccessful because of an impacted stone (*a*), dilatation will be needed (*b*) after establishing proximal control. In (*b*), the stiff guidewire has been removed and will be replaced with a standard Teflon-coated safety wire.

When therapeutic maneuvers are anticipated, it is important to maintain a safety guidewire within the ureter. As mentioned previously, a hydrophilic guidewire may aid in accessing a tortuous ureter or one with an impacted stone, but should not be used as a routine safety wire, because of the ease with which it may become dislodged. A flexible ureteroscope requires either the use of an access sheath or a second working guidewire for placement of the ureteroscope into the proximal collecting system (Figures 26.16 and 26.17). The smallest sheath that accepts flexible ureteroscopes is 9.5 Fr; therefore, in small children, prestenting of the ureter is often required in order to dilate the ureter to allow the safe use of an access sheath. Access sheaths should be used with caution and are most helpful when it will be necessary to traverse the ureteral orifice many times when treating large or multiple stones in the proximal collecting system. Fluoroscopic guidance is absolutely necessary during any ureteroscopic procedure.

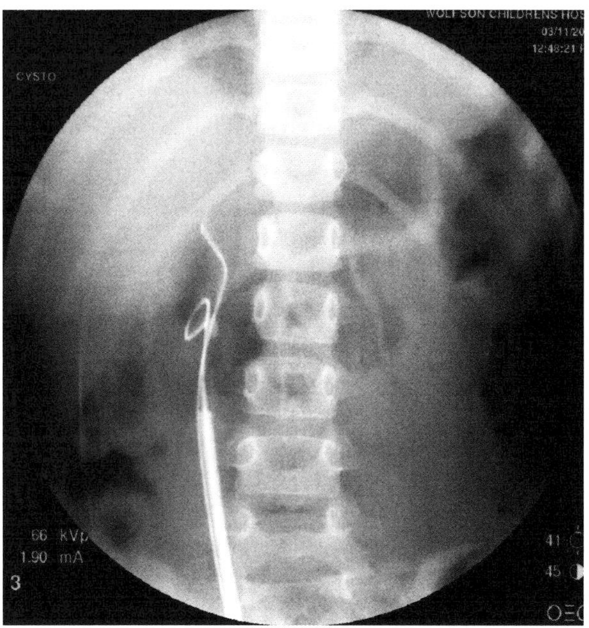

Figure 26.16 Placement of a flexible ureteroscope into the proximal collecting system is most often accomplished using a monorail technique, by guiding the scope over a wire. A second safety wire is necessary when therapeutic intervention is anticipated.

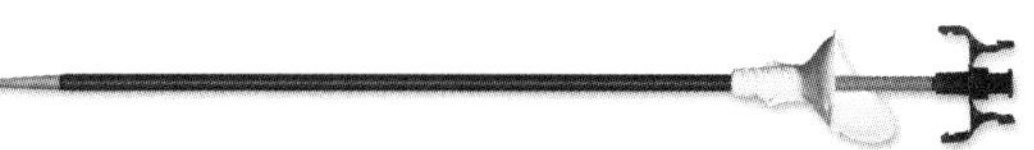

Figure 26.17 Access sheaths are quite helpful when removing large stone burdens from either the proximal ureter or the intrarenal collecting system. Placement of this sheath is made easier by prestenting the ureter or when working in a dilated collecting system. When removing stone fragments, it is important to make certain the ureteral mucosa does not get trapped between the stone and the proximal lip of the sheath. (Courtesy of Cook Urological, Spencer, IN.)

Previous urologic surgery involving either the bladder neck, ureter, urethra, or ureteropelvic junction is not necessarily a contraindication to ureteroscopy. Also, the authors have performed intrarenal ureteroscopy in an 11-month-old male infant with significant congenital ureteral 'valves'. A child who has undergone previous hypospadias surgery may require urethral dilatation prior to placement of the ureteroscope if there is meatal stenosis. It is important to use small-diameter endoscopes to avoid disruption of previous bladder neck reconstruction. Often, children who have had bladder neck reconstruction have had ureteral reimplantation at the time of their primary surgery, and care must be taken not to significantly distort the bladder neck when accessing the previously reimplanted ureter. Access to the ureter after previous reimplantation is clearly dependent upon the type of surgery performed. When either an advancement or extravesical procedure has been utilized, access is similar to the unoperated child. When a previous cross-trigonal reimplantation has been performed, access can be more difficult. In this instance, the ureteral orifice is usually laterally located and can be cannulated with an angled guidewire. If this maneuver is unsuccessful, an actively deflecting guidewire can be utilized. Once access has been gained, the initial wire should be replaced with a stiff guidewire, which then straightens the intramural portion of the ureter, allowing access for ureteroscopy. Dilatation of the tunnel is usually not necessary, although it is sometimes necessary to dilate the ureteral orifice. When the procedure is finished, the ureter will return to its preoperative cross-trigonal position. Recurrent reflux after ureteroscopy in the previously reimplanted ureter has not been demonstrated.

Intrarenal access after previous ureteropelvic junction (UPJ) repair is usually straightforward as long as there has been adequate healing and success of the previous surgery. The ureter remains supple at the site of previous repair and is at no greater risk of injury. Postoperative stenting is not always required after distal stone removal, or ureteroscopy in a prestented child, but should be performed after procedures requiring either extensive manipulation, significant active dilatation, or work within the proximal collecting system. If a stent is left in place, a 'dangler' string is used to facilitate removal without anesthesia in the office approximately 1 week after the procedure.

A semi-rigid ureteroscope should be used for distal and midureteral calculi (Figure 26.18). The instrument may be used for more proximal stones if it can be successfully passed above the pelvic brim. Flexible ureteroscopy is necessary most of the time for proximal ureteral calculi and should always be used for stones contained within the intrarenal collecting system (Figure 26.19). Complete access to the intrarenal system is usually accomplished through active deflection alone; rarely, is secondary passive deflection necessary in the smaller pediatric kidney. Installation of contrast during ureteroscopy will provide a guide during the complete inspection of the collecting system under fluoroscopy.

Once the stone is encountered, it is important to gauge the size of the stone versus the diameter of the ureter. Many ureteral stones can be removed intact through basket or grasper manipulation, provided the caliber of the distal ureter is adequate to allow atraumatic retrieval. For impacted stones, or those too large to remove intact, in-situ holmium laser lithotripsy is performed. For an impacted stone, attempts should be made to dislodge the stone into the proximally dilated portion of the ureter. This will allow more room for laser lithotripsy, and decrease the risk of complications. Once the stone is dislodged, the jagged surface is either precisely treated to smooth out rough edges or the entire stone can be cleaved into distinct fragments for subsequent removal. Stones that cannot be dislodged should be treated first on the periphery, which should help to disimpact the stone. It is desirable to retrieve at least one stone fragment for crystallographic analysis, and once this is achieved it is more efficient to deposit subsequent small fragments within the bladder to pass spontaneously. If a stone fragment becomes displaced outside the ureteral wall due to perforation, further attempts at extraction should be abandoned.

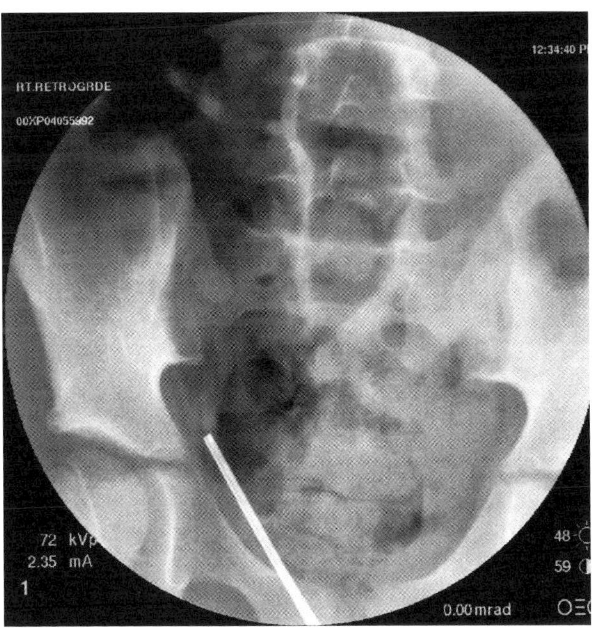

Figure 26.18 A semirigid ureteroscope is the instrument of choice for removal of distal and mid ureteral calculi. It can be utilized for proximal stones if the endoscope can be safely guided into the proximal collecting system. Care should be taken to ensure that the urethral meatus in young boys is not damaged by the increased diameter of the proximal shaft of any endoscope.

Percutaneous endourology

Thomas Hillier in 1865 is credited with the description of the first therapeutic percutaneous renal drainage of what was described as ureteropelvic junction obstruction.[62] Unfortunately, after 4 years of periodic percutaneous drainage, the young boy succumbed to septicemia at age 8. It wasn't until 1941 that Rupel described the removal of renal calculus debris through a nephrostomy tract using endoscopic equipment.[63] Percutaneous drainage of hydronephrosis was subsequently reported by Goodwin in 1955,

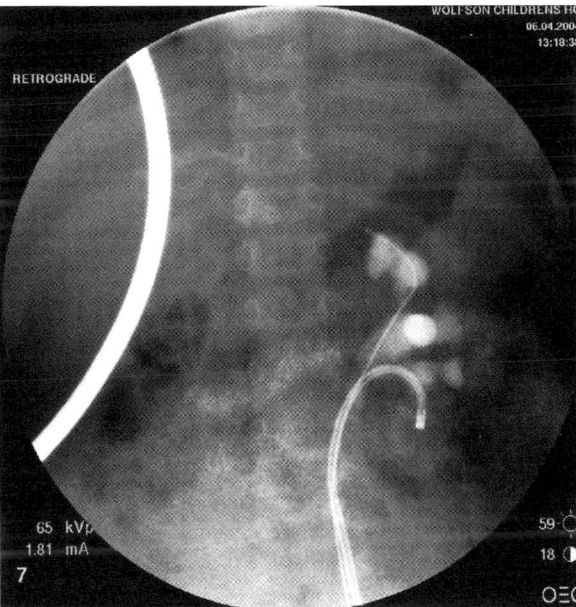

Figure 26.19 Flexible ureteroscopy is necessary for the removal of intrarenal calculi. Passive secondary deflection is rarely needed to gain access to the lower pole of the pediatric collecting system because of the arc of deflection.

but it wasn't until 1985 that Woodside et al presented a series of seven pediatric patients who had undergone a percutaneous procedure.[64]

In the early days of the procedure, percutaneous stone removal was limited to children ≥ 8 years old because of fears of significant blood loss and increased renal damage with large (>24 Fr) tract dilatation.[65] The defect created by a 24 Fr tract in a child's kidney corresponds to a 72 Fr defect in an adult kidney.[66] Increased tract size is directly correlated with increased complication rates, although no significant renal scarring or functional changes can be readily detected after large tract dilatation.[67,68] Subsequent reports have demonstrated that percutaneous procedures are technically feasible for children <8 years old, and that complications can be decreased by utilizing a tract <22 Fr.

Because of concerns regarding hematologic complications, the technique of a smaller-access percutaneous procedure has been developed. Helal et al presented their experience using a 15 Fr peel-away sheath in a 2-year-old child for percutaneous stone removal.[69] A smaller 11 Fr technique using a 'mini-perc' approach has also been reported, and a purpose-built access kit is available.[66] Access to the collecting system is thought to be less traumatic because of the smaller caliber site. There have been no reports of bleeding complications in uncomplicated procedures after mini-perc intervention, and the need for postoperative percutaneous nephrostomy drainage is often eliminated. Treatment of large (>3 cm) stones can be tedious; therefore, a larger peel-away sheath (15–22 Fr) is recommended to expedite stone fragment removal.

Most pediatric percutaneous procedures are performed for management of renal calculi. It is important that these procedures be performed in an institution where there is an endourologist and interventional radiologist experienced in the treatment of children. Needle access to the kidney is required for tract dilatation and therapeutic intervention, and there is some suggestion that obtaining early access (1 day prior to surgery) may decrease bleeding as well as operative time. This is particularly helpful for a mini-perc procedure because the smaller field of view becomes easily obscured by minimal bleeding. Nevertheless, it is possible to obtain access at the time of percutaneous intervention, which does in most cases result in safe completion of the procedure.

The proper site for percutaneous access should both allow a direct route to the stone and permit easy access to other areas of the collecting system. The optimal position is usually a posterior calyx with a wide, straight infundibulum. Multiple sites may be necessary, and should be utilized when there is a complete staghorn calculus or any intrarenal anomalies making it difficult to access all stone-containing calices through a single site. Bleeding requiring transfusion is not increased when multiple sites are utilized.[70] It is important to obtain the primary access site where it will be possible to maximally debulk the stone burden, and secondary sites where calices will be difficult to reach through the primary tract. If the stones are contained within a caliceal diverticulum or a calyx with a narrowed infundibulum, it is necessary to have direct access into that part of the collecting system. Upper pole access sites should be used with caution because of the increased risk of pneumo/hydrothorax. Consequently a chest X-ray should be obtained at the conclusion of any percutaneous procedure involving upper pole access.

Once needle access has been obtained, a wire is passed down the ureter into the bladder to allow a controlled tract dilatation and to avoid the accidental loss of access to the collecting system. Slippery hydrophilic guidewires should be exchanged for standard PTFE-coated wires prior to dilatation. The use of a stiff guidewire will facilitate dilation. If ureteral access is not possible or if access is obtained into an obstructed system or caliceal diverticulum, multiple coils of the wire should be placed within the contained collecting system prior to tract dilatation.

Once safe access has been confirmed, if mini-perc access is not to be used, the tract is dilated either using sequential graduated dilators (Amplatz) or active balloon dilatation (Figure 26.20). Both techniques have been proven safe and efficacious, but sequential dilatation of larger tracts may increase the risk of bleeding owing to the potential shearing effect of this technique. Constant vigilance under fluoroscopy is necessary to avoid disruption of the renal pelvis. The small non-dilated pediatric kidney is at greatest risk for this

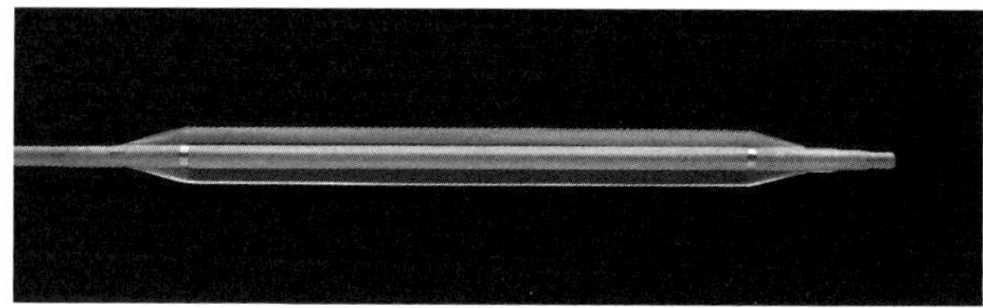

Figure 26.20 Percutaneous balloon dilators come in a variety of sizes. They need to maintain high radial pressures in order to dilate the fascia. The access is placed into the collecting system over the balloon after partial deflation. (Courtesy of Cook Urological, Spencer, IN.)

complication, and extreme caution must be undertaken to help prevent such occurrences. If there is significant disruption of the renal pelvis or UPJ, it may be necessary to abandon the procedure and to place a temporary nephrostomy or nephroureteral stent.

For balloon dilatation, the distal radiographic marker is placed into the renal pelvis, while the proximal portion of the balloon is located externally. The balloon is then inflated to its maximum pressure and then left fully inflated until there is no longer any evidence of fascial constriction (Figure 26.21). The balloon is kept inflated for several minutes to help aid in hemostasis. The access sheath can be placed into the pelvis over the balloon once it has been partially deflated. The balloon size should correlate with the size of the sheath to be used.

If there is any significant bleeding encountered after dilation, it may be necessary to temporarily place either a large Foley catheter or a tamponade balloon. If these techniques do not result in satisfactory hemostasis, it will be necessary to leave the catheter in place and perform the therapeutic intervention at another time. Uncontrolled hemorrhage requiring transfusion should be evaluated with angiography for possible vascular embolization.

After the working sheath has been placed, the planned procedure is undertaken. Both rigid as well as flexible instrumentation may be necessary and should be present in the operating room suite in case the need arises. If there is a large stone burden, the procedure will be facilitated through placement of a 22 Fr sheath. This allows access with an adult nephroscope, enabling the use of larger instruments, and the capability of removing large intact stone fragments. If a mini-perc procedure is performed through an 11 Fr peel-away sheath, then either an offset pediatric cystoscope with a straight working channel or a 9.5 Fr modified mini rigid ureteroscope will be necessary to access the kidney. The straight-channel offset lens endoscope will allow for the passage of ultrasonic and ballistic lithotripsy probes, whereas the in-line mini rigid cystoureteroscope will require the use of the holmium laser, electrohydraulic, or flexible ballistic lithotripsy devices for stone fragmentation. The authors like the in-line endoscope because it has two working channels, which facilitates simultaneous suction irrigation (5.4 Fr) and lithotripsy (2.3 Fr). (Figure 26.22) It also permits 360° rotation of the endoscope for maximum positioning of lithotripsy probes. The endoscope used should be several French

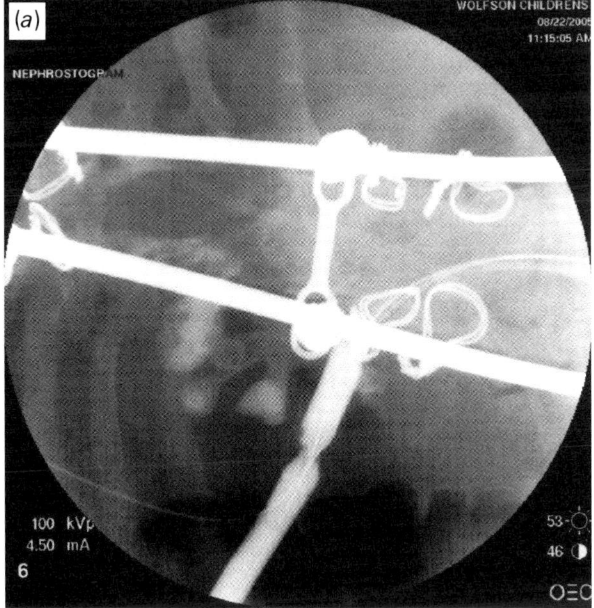

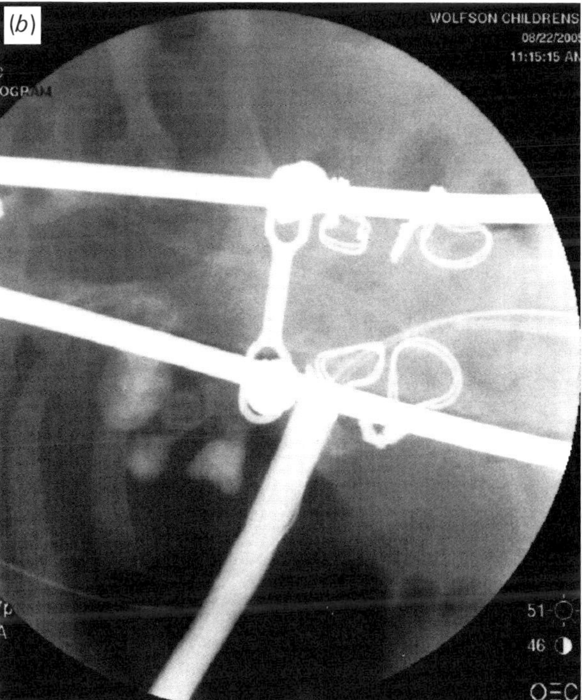

Figure 26.21 After proper positioning under fluoroscopy has been confirmed, contrast is used to expand the percutaneous balloon dilator under fluoroscopy. Initial fascial constriction (*a*) is noted, and the balloon is inflated to its maximum pressure until all constriction has been eliminated. (*b*) The size of the balloon should be slightly larger than the sheath to be utilized.

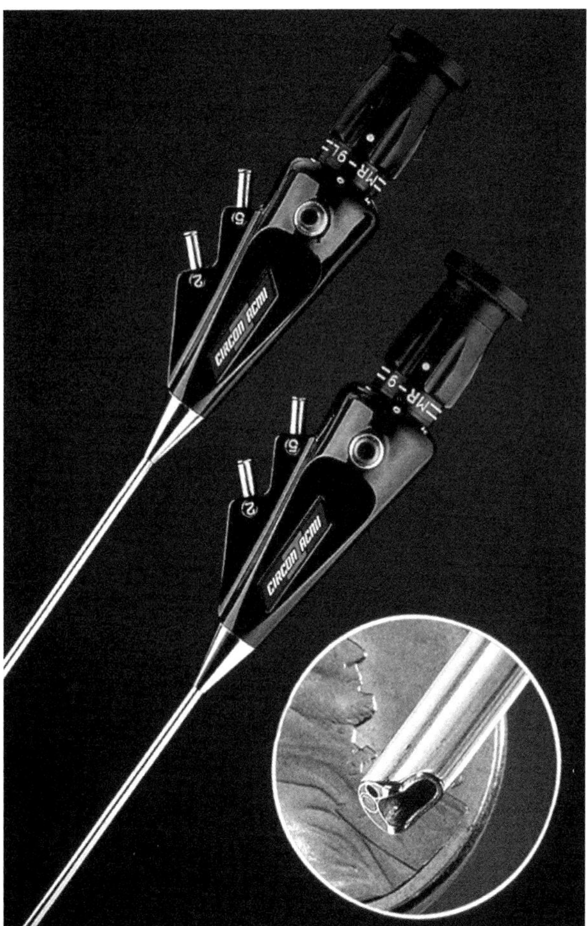

Figure 26.22 The mini-perc procedure requires the use of a small-caliber endoscope. A modified straight semirigid ureteroscope with two working channels is helpful because it allows for 360° rotation and also permits simultaneous lithotripsy and irrigation. (Courtesy of Circon ACMI, Southborough, MA.)

sizes less than the internal diameter of the sheath in order to allow continuous flow around the scope, which lessens the risk of significant extravasation. The use of warmed saline irrigant is encouraged, which will need to be changed to water or glycine if an electrosurgical procedure is planned. Note that this does not include EHL, which is effective in saline. The potential for dilutional hyponatremia in infants and children is significant, and therefore saline should be used whenever feasible. Levering of the nephroscope should be limited in order to avoid injury to the infundibulum, as well as the renal parenchyma, during the percutaneous procedure.

Endourologic instrumentation is similar to that used for other procedures. The holmium laser is particularly useful during small-caliber percutaneous access procedures in order to debulk large stone burdens. Extraction of stone fragments is facilitated by using a 4.5 Fr nitinol basket. Ultrasonic lithotripsy is quite safe and can be performed through the straight working channel of either a small-caliber offset cystourethroscope or an adult percutaneous nephroscope. Attempts should be made to remove all stone fragments >2 mm in order to limit a potential nidus for stone regrowth or obstruction with passage of a large fragment. Complete visualization of the intrarenal collecting system, as well as the ureter, should be undertaken. This usually requires the use of a flexible endoscope and should be undertaken prior to completion of the planned procedure. Complete inspection is sometimes hampered by limitations of the size of the pediatric kidney and the size of the percutaneous access sheath. Significant clots may obscure stone fragments; therefore, every attempt should be made to irrigate them free to allow complete visualization. Most of the time it is necessary to leave a percutaneous nephrostomy tube in place at the completion of the procedure, but it is possible to limit its use. Access to the kidney should be maintained until postoperative X-rays confirm that no second-look procedure will be needed.

Treatment strategies

Many factors need to be considered when deciding the proper treatment modalities for urinary tract calculi in children. Not only are the characteristics of the stone (size, shape, location, density, number, etc.) considered but also the characteristics of the child. Body habitus, as well as associated congenital and acquired conditions, need to be taken into consideration. Surgeon expertise and available technology may also guide treatment strategy. Each case needs to be individualized in order to choose the best form of treatment: shockwave lithotripsy vs retrograde ureteroscopy vs an antegrade percutaneous approach.

Renal calculi

ESWL is the least-invasive form of therapy, and offers reasonable stone-free rates of >80% with minimal complications.[71–77] Stones that are ≤1 cm are most efficaciously treated by this modality and often require a single treatment (Figure 26.23). Higher retreatment rates and the need for ancillary procedures are seen with large stone burdens and in children with renal or collecting system abnormalities.[77,78] Therefore, ESWL is not the best therapy when there is evidence of UPJ obstruction, caliceal diverticulum, or infundibular stenosis (Figure

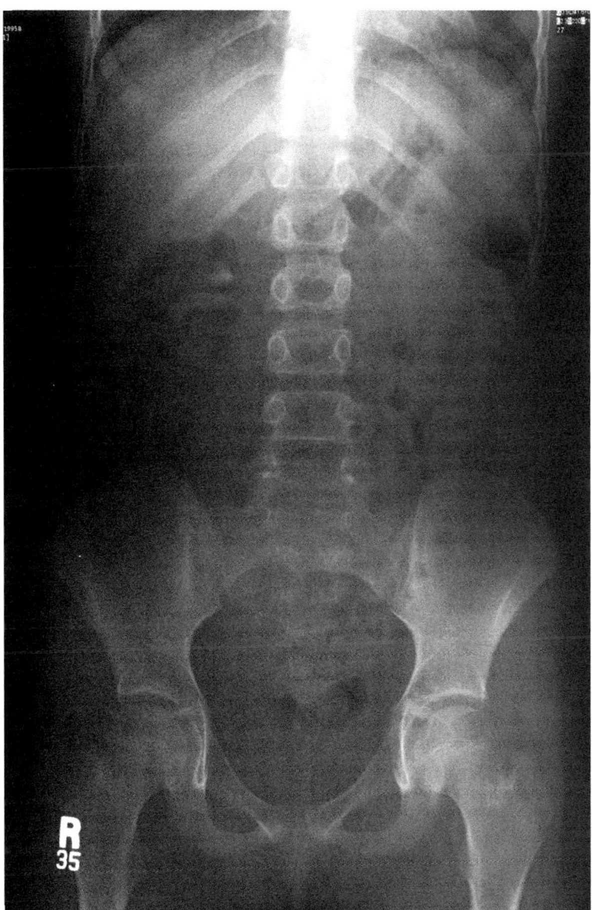

Figure 26.23 Stones that are ≤ 1.5 cm and do not appear extremely dense on X-ray, are best suited for ESWL.

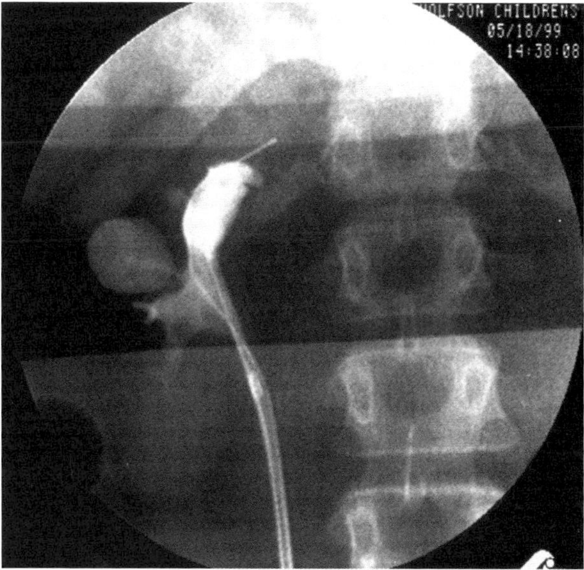

Figure 26.24 Renal stones associated with congenital urinary tract anomalies should be treated by either ureteroscopy or percutaneous access. Mid or upper pole caliceal diverticula with small stone burdens can be effectively treated using flexible ureteroscopy.

26.24). ESWL is also less effective for ectopic and horseshoe kidneys because of difficulties with precise energy delivery (increased surrounding bony and soft tissue structures) and the presence of an abnormally rotated collecting system which may prevent post-treatment stone clearance. In addition, alternative therapies to ESWL should be considered for extremely dense stones (brushite, cystine)[79] and those calculi within an abnormal lower pole (i.e. long, narrowed infundibulum). In these instances the energy may not be sufficient for adequate lithotripsy, and the abnormal intrarenal anatomy may promote fragment retention. Currently, it appears that ESWL is best suited for solitary renal stones ≤1.5 cm that are not contained within an abnormal lower pole calyx and are not associated with any congenital or acquired renal abnormalities. Nevertheless, ESWL monotherapy for the treatment of staghorn calculi has been shown to be effective, with stone-free rates of approximately 88% after multiple treatment sessions.

The role of ureteroscopy for the treatment of renal calculi in children remains to be defined. Several reports have demonstrated ureteroscopy to be an effective treatment for stones throughout the entire intrarenal collecting system. It has been successful for the treatment of stone-containing caliceal diverticula of the mid and upper pole.[80] Primary ureteropyeloscopy with stone removal should also be performed when ureteroscopy is being used to treat other ureteral stones. This enables easy access to the kidney for treatment and provides the greatest chance of success with one procedure. Residual fragments after ESWL, or failure of ESWL as the primary procedure, are two other reasons to perform ureteropyeloscopy for stone removal. As mentioned previously, placement of a ureteral access sheath in a prestented ureter may facilitate removal of large stones. Concomitant UPJ or intrarenal obstruction can also be treated endoscopically at the time of stone removal.

For intrarenal stones >1 cm, multiple large calculi, staghorn calculi, or children with urinary tract malformations or a previous reconstruction, a percutaneous approach may be preferable. Stone-free rates after a single percutaneous session range anywhere from 70 to 100%.[67,81–85] For large stones and staghorn calculi, combined 'sandwich' therapy (percutaneous stone removal followed by ESWL), provides stone-free rates >90% (Figure 26.25). A percutaneous procedure does carry the risk of bleeding

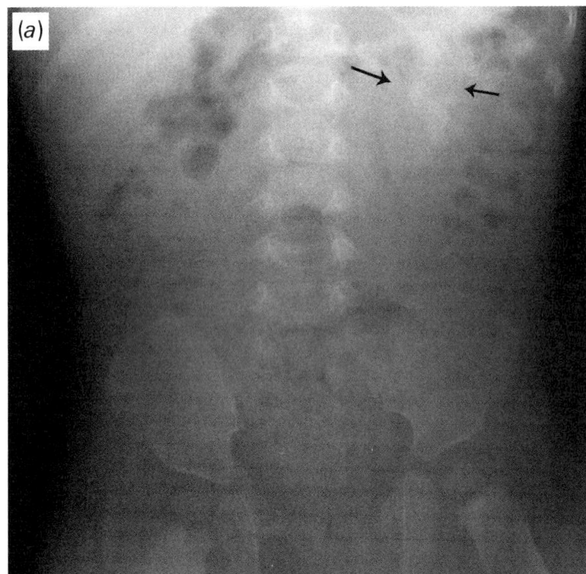

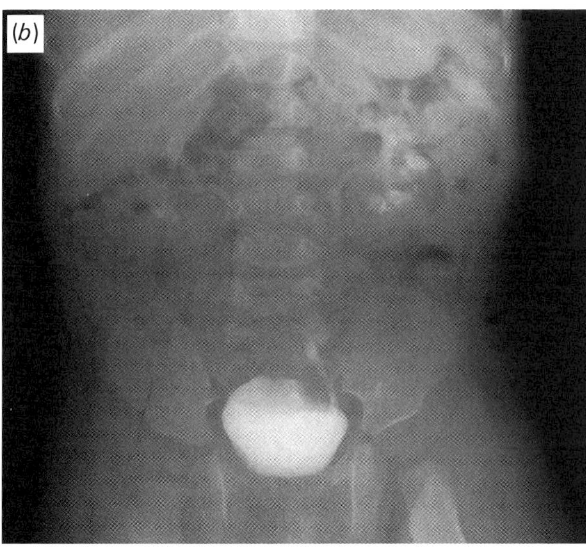

Figure 26.25 (*a*) A KUB in this 11-month-old girl who had been having recurring urinary tract infections reveals a mildly radiopaque left staghorn calculus (arrows). (*b*) A preoperative intravenous pyelogram was helpful in guiding surgical planning.

requiring transfusion, but several series have shown that utilization of a tract <22 Fr significantly limits this risk. Multiple percutaneous sites may be necessary for complete access to the stone, and have been shown not to increase the risk of transfusion. Long-term follow-up supports percutaneous procedures as being safe, with no significant damage to the pediatric kidney.

Laparoscopy in children has become more widespread and has recently been reported in the management of renal calculi.[86] Patient selection criteria included stones >2.5 cm, with failure of percutaneous renal access. Not only does laparoscopy provide a high stone-free rate but also it enables the repair of concomitant UPJ obstruction. Laparoscopy may also prove helpful in the management of large peripheral caliceal diverticula containing stones, by allowing surgical unroofing with ablation of the diverticular neck and lining. Further experience should better define the role of laparoscopy in the treatment of pediatric stone disease.

Ureteral calculi

Experience with ESWL for stones contained within the ureter has been shown to be effective 54–100% of the time. Retreatment for stones within the ureter is necessary in up to 23% of cases. Patient positioning may need to be modified for distal ureteral stones by placing the child in the prone position. Stones over the bony pelvis are difficult to treat using ESWL because of inadequate visualization and lack of adequate energy delivery.

A review of the literature shows that the stone-free rate after pediatric ureteroscopic lithotripsy is between 77 and 100%.[58,61,87–98] Advances in both endoscopic instrumentation as well as holmium laser lithotripsy have been the major reasons for increased success. In one study, use of holmium laser lithotripsy improved the stone-free rate, compared with pulsed-dye laser and EHL, and was associated with a lower complication rate.[99] In addition, a recent analysis of 65 ureteroscopic lithotripsies in a cohort with a mean age of 7.5 years showed that orifice dilatation is required in only one-third of cases and only one patient developed a ureteral stricture.[100]

One appealing aspect of the ureteroscopic removal of stones is that it offers an immediate stone-free condition at the completion of the procedure. The American Urological Association has issued guidelines to standardize the management of adult patients with stones, and Van Savage et al[95] have published their recommendations for the modification of these guidelines when applying it to the pediatric patient. The ureteroscopic removal of stones contained within the ureter is clearly safe and effective and should be considered the first-line treatment for most children.

The percutaneous removal of ureteral stones is

rarely indicated. It should be considered the primary form of therapy for children who have impacted stones with significant hydroureteronephrosis and urinary tract infection or urosepsis. The antegrade approach allows for prompt decompression of the obstructed collecting system with antegrade ureteroscopic access for subsequent removal. The technique for antegrade ureteroscopy is exactly the same as for the retrograde approach, and has been discussed previously. Flexible rather than mini rigid endoscopy should be utilized for antegrade ureteroscopy to limit potential complications.

Bladder

The term lithotomy was coined in 276 BC by the Greek surgeon Ammonious of Alexandria. It wasn't until the first century AD that the Roman Celsus provided a detailed description of the lithotomy procedure in a young child.[101] Virtually every ancient society has described the surgical removal of bladder calculi. Open cystolithotomy remains part of the practice of pediatric urology to this day (Figure 26.26). In most children, however, the endoscopic removal of such calculi is warranted. Bladder calculi in children are a well-known complication of bladder augmentation when using the large or small intestine.[101,102] They are related to both urinary stasis and mucus production, and occur rarely after gastrocystoplasty. The removal of all stone fragments in these cases is essential to prevent any nidus for stone regrowth, although no difference in stone recurrence is seen after removal of intact calculi or fragmentation techniques.

The cystoscopic removal of bladder calculi is somewhat limited by the caliber of the urethra in young children. All forms of intracorporeal lithotripsy have been proven effective for the management of bladder calculi.[103,104] The most potentially damaging devices to the wall of the augmented bladder include EHL and the holmium laser lithotriptor: it is important that neither of these energy sources come in near or direct contact with the bladder wall. EHL may result in perforation of the augmented bladder if the procedure is performed in a distended bladder or if a stone is wedged against the augmented portion. Other potential complications include gross hematuria from bladder wall irritation, which may necessitate catheterization postoperatively.

Percutaneous removal of bladder calculi has also been demonstrated to be an effective technique.[105–108] This is obviously a more invasive procedure in that it involves a percutaneous suprapubic puncture for direct visualization of the calculi as well as vacuum suction removal. If the urethra is not patent, a second suprapubic puncture is necessary for both visualization and removal of the calculi. This technique appears well suited for stones up to 1 cm in size, or multiple stones <1 cm (Figure 26.27).

The bladder is filled until it is palpable. A small-gauge needle is used to confirm both position and depth in order to percutaneously approach the bladder. A 14-gauge needle is then introduced, which

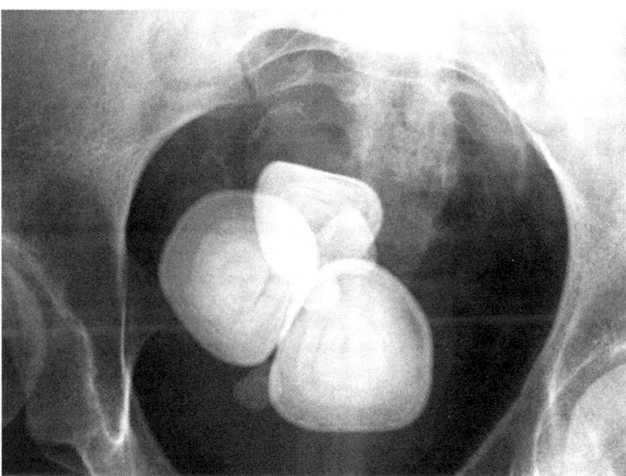

Figure 26.26 Large bladder calculi such as these require open surgical removal.

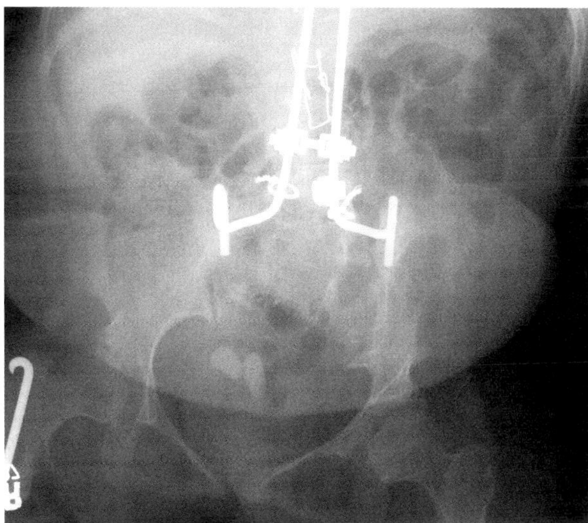

Figure 26.27 Small stones in a previously augmented bladder are well suited for either percutaneous or endoscopic removal. Endoscopic removal should not be performed in children who have had previous bladder neck procedures or in the small male urethra. It is imperative that all stone fragments be irrigated free from the bladder in order to help prevent stone recurrence.

allows placement of an 0.038 inch guidewire into the bladder. The tract is then dilated over the wire to a size equal to that of the largest stone in millimeters multiplied by 3 (i.e. an 8 mm stone requires at least a 24 Fr sheath). If intracorporeal lithotripsy is required, either EHL, ultrasonic ballistic, or laser has been proven suitable. The stones and any fragments are then removed using suction tubing attached to a vacuum device. Postoperative bladder drainage is necessary for 5–7 days.

References

1. Remzi D, Bakkaloglu MA, Erkan I, Ozen HAF. Pediatric urolithiasis. Turk J Pediatr 1984; 26:43–9.
2. Stapleton FB. Nephrolithiasis in children. Pediatr Rev 1989; 11:21–30.
3. Miliner DS, Murphy ME. Urolithiasis in pediatric patients. Mayo Clin Proc 1993; 68:241–8.
4. Diamond DA, Menon M, Lee PH, Rickwood AM, Johnston JH. Etiologic factors in pediatric stone recurrence. J Urol 1989; 142:606–8.
5. Choi H, Snyder HM 3rd, Duckett JW. Urolithiasis in childhood: current management. J Pediatr Surg 1987; 22:158–64.
6. Ueno A, Kawamura T, Ogawa A et al. Relation of spontaneous passage of calculi to size. Urology 1977; 19:544–6.
7. Pietrow PK, Pope JC IV, Adams MC, Shyr Y, Brock JW 3rd. Clinical outcome of pediatric stone disease. J Urol 2002; 167:670–3.
8. Morse R, Resnick M. Ureteral calculi: natural history and treatment in an era of advanced technology. J Urol 1991; 145:263–5.
9. Van Savage JG, Palanca LG, Andersen RD, Rao GS, Slaughenhoupt BL. Treatment of distal ureteral stones in children: similarities to the American Urological Association Guidelines in adults. J Urol 2000; 194 (3 Pt 2):1089–93.
10. Shukla AR, Hoover DL, Homsy YL et al. Urolithiasis in the low birth weight infant: the role and efficacy of extracorporeal shock wave lithotripsy. J Urol 2001; 165:2320–3.
11. Heidenreich A, Desgrandschamps F, Terrier F. Modern approach of diagnosis and management of acute flank pain: review of all imaging modalities. Eur Urol 2002; 41:351–62.
12. Strouse PJ, Bates DG, Bloom DA, Goodsitt MM. Noncontrast thin-section helical CT of urinary tract calculi in children. Pediatr Radiol 2002; 32:326–32.
13. Keir A, Fowler B, Locken JA et al. Ultrasound for detecting renal calculi with nonenhanced CT as a reference standard. Radiology 2002; 222:109–13.
14. Spielmann AL, Heneghan JP, Lee LJ et al. Decreasing the radiation dose for renal stone CT: a feasibility study of single- and multidetector CT. AJR Am J Roentgenol 2002; 178:10058–62.
15. Diamond DA, Menon M. Pediatric urolithiasis. AUA Update series 1991; 40:314–20.
16. Perrone HC, dos Santos DR, Santos MV et al. Urolithiasis in childhood: metabolic evaluation. Pediatr Nephrol 1992; 6:54–6.
17. Lim DJ, Walker RD 3rd, Ellsworth PI et al. Treatment of pediatric urolithiasis between 1984 and 1994. J Urol 1996; 156:702–5.
18. Parks JH, Coward M, Coe FL. Correspondence between stone composition and urine supersaturation in nephrolithiasis. Kidney Int 1997; 51:894–900.
19. Battino BS, DeFoor W, Coe F et al. Metabolic evaluation of children with urolithiaisis: are adult references for supersaturation appropriate? J Urol 2002; 168:2568–71.
20. Miller LA, Stapleton FB. Urinary volume in children with urolithiasis. J Urol 1989; 141:918–20.
21. Bartosh SM. Medical management of pediatric stone disease. Urol Clin North Am 2004; 31:575–87.
22. Polinsky MS, Kaiser KA, Balvarte HJ et al. Renal stones and hypercalciuria. Adv Pediatr 1993; 40:353–84.
23. Frick J, Kohle R, Kunit G. [Extracorporeal shock wave lithotripsy in childhood]. Padiatr Padol 1988; 23(1):47–52. [German]
24. Kaude JV, Williams CM, Miller MR, Scott KN, Finlayson B. Renal morphology and function immediately after extracorporeal shock-wave lithotripsy. AJR Am J Roentgenol 1985; 145:305–13.
25. Fuchs AM, Coulson W, Fuchs GJ. Effect of extra corporeally induced high-energy shock wave on rabbit kidney and ureter: a morphologic and functional study. J Endourol 1988; 4:341–3.
26. Demirkesen O, Tansu N, Yaycioglu O et al. Extracorporeal shock wave lithotripsy in the pediatric population. J Endourol 1998; 13:147–50.
27. Nazli O, Cal C, Ozyurt C et al. Results of extracorporeal shock wave lithotripsy in the pediatric group. Eur Urol 1998; 33:333–6.
28. Netto NR, Longo JA, Ikonomidis JA, Netto MR. Extracorporeal shock wave lithotripsy in children. J Urol 2002; 167:2164–6.
29. Sigman M, Laudone VP, Jenkins AD et al. Initial experience with extracorporeal shock wave lithotripsy in children. J Urol 1987;138:839–41.
30. Landau EH, Gofrit, ON, Shapiro A et al. Extracorporeal shock wave lithotripsy is highly effective for ureteral calculi in children. J Urol 2001; 165:2316–19.
31. Mobley TB, Myers DA, Jenkins JM, Grine WB, Jorden WR. Effects of stents on lithotripsy of ureteral calculi: treatment results with 18,825 calculi using the Lithostar lithotripter. J Urol 1989; 152:53–6.
32. Orsola A, Diaz I, Garat JM et al. Staghorn calculi in children: treatment with monotherapy extracorporeal shock wave lithotripsy. J Urol 1999; 162:1229–33.
33. Lottmann HB, Traxer O, Arhambaud F, Mercier-Pageyral B. Monotherapy extracorporeal shock wave lithotripsy for the treatment of staghorn calculi in children. J Urol 2001; 165:2324–7.
34. Al-Busaidy SS, Prem AR, Medhat M. Pediatric staghorn calculi: the role of extracorporeal shock wave lithotripsy monotherapy with special reference to ureteral stenting. J Urol 2003; 169:629–33.

35. Thomas R, Frentz JM, Harmon E. Effect of extracorporeal shock wave lithotripsy on renal function and body height in pediatric patients. J Urol 1992; 148:1064–6.
36. Brinkmann O, Griehl A, Kuwertz-Broking E et al. Extracorporeal shock wave lithotripsy in children. Eur Urol 2001; 39:591–7.
37. Vlajkovic M, Slavkovic A, Radovanovic M et al. Long-term functional outcome of kidneys in children after ESWL treatment. Eur J Pediatr Surg 2002; 12:118–23.
38. Rassweiler J, Kohrmann KU, Back W et al. Experimental basis of shockwave-induced renal trauma in the model of the canine kidney. World J Urol 1993; 11:43–53.
39. Tiede JM, Lumpkin EN, Wass CT, Long TR. Hemoptysis following extracorporeal shock wave lithotripsy: a case of lithotripsy-induced pulmonary contusion in a pediatric patient. J Clin Anesth 2003; 15:530–3.
40. Wu HY, Docimo SG. Surgical management of children with urolithiasis. Urol Clin North Am 2004; 31:589–94.
41. Young HH, McKay RW. Congenital valvular obstruction of the prostatic urethra. Surg Gynecol Obstet 1929; 48:509–11.
42. Ritchey M, Patterson DE, Kelalis PP, Segura JW. A case of pediatric ureteroscopic lasertripsy. J Urol 1988; 139:1272–4.
43. Shepherd P, Thomas R, Harmon EP. Urolithiasis in children: innovations in management. J Urol 1988; 140:790–2.
44. Kourambas J, Delvecchio FC, Munver R et al. Nitinol stone retrieval-assisted ureteroscopic management of lower pole renal calculi. Urology 2000; 56:935–9.
45. Ptashnyk T, Cueva-Maratinez A, Michel MS, Alken P, Kohrmann KU. Comparative investigations on the retrieval capabilities of various baskets and graspers in four ex vivo models. Eur Urol 2002; 41:406–10.
46. El-Gabry EA, Bagley DH. Retrieval capabilities of different stone basket designs in vitro. J Endourol 1999; 13:305–7.
47. Dretler SP. The stone cone: a new generation of basketry. J Urol 2001; 165:1593–6.
48. Mulvaney W. Attempted disintegration of calculi by ultrasonic vibration. J Urol 1953; 70:704–6.
49. Piergiovanni M, Desgrandclamps F, Cochand-Priollet B et al. Ureteral and bladder lesions after ballistic, ultrasonic, electrohydraulic or laser lithotripsy. J Endourol 1994; 8:293–9.
50. Schulze H, Haupt G, Piergiovanni M et al. The Swiss Lithoclast: a new device for endoscopic stone disintegration. J Urol 1993; 149:15–18.
51. Haupt G, Pannek J, Herde T et al. The Lithovac: new suction device for the Swiss Lithocast. J Endourol 1995; 9:375–7.
52. Ten CL, Fhong P, Preminger GM. Laboratory and clinical assessment of pneumatically driven intracorporeal lithotripsy. J Endourol 1998; 12:163–9.
53. Loisides P, Grasso M, Bagley DW. Mechanical impactor employing nitinol probes to fragment human calculi: fragmentation efficiency with flexible endoscope deflection. J Endourol 1995; 9: 371–4.
54. Yutkin L. Electrohydraulic Lithotripsy. English Translation for US Department of Commerce, Office of Technical Services, 1955: Dic 62–15184 MDL 1207/1-2.
55. Grasso M. Experience with the holmium laser as an endoscopic lithotrite. Urology 1996; 48:199–206.
56. Johnson DE, Cromeens DM, Price RE. Use of the holmium:YAG laser in urology. Lasers Surg Med 1992; 12:353–63.
57. Wollin TA, Teichman JM, Rogenes VJ et al. Holmium: YAG lithotripsy in children. J Urol 1999; 162:1717–20.
58. Reddy PP, Barrieras DJ, Bagli DJ et al. Initial experience with endoscopic holmium laser lithotripsy for pediatric urolithiasis. J Urol 1999; 162:1714–16.
59. Vassar GJ, Chan KF, Teichman JM et al. Holmium:YAG lithotripsy: photothermal mechanism. J Endourol 1999; 13:181–90.
60. Cussen LJ. The morphology of congenital dilatation of the ureter: intrinsic ureteral lesions. Aust N Z J Surg 1971; 41:185–94.
61. Minevich E, DeFoor W, Nishinaka K et al. Ureteroscopy is safe and effective in prepubertal children. J Urol 2004: 171:551A.
62. Bloom DA, Morgan RJ, Scardino PL. Thomas Hillier and the percutaneous nephrostomy. Urology 1999; 33:346–50.
63. Rupel E, Brown R. Nephrostomy in hydronephrosis. JAMA 1955; 157:891–4.
64. Woodside JR, Stevens GF, Stark GL et al. Percutaneous stone removal in children. J Urol 1985; 134:1166–7.
65. Hulbert JC, Reddy PK, Gonzalez R et al. Percutaneous nephrostolithotomy: an alternative approach to the management of pediatric calculus disease. Pediatrics 1985; 76:610–12.
66. Jackman SV, Hedican SP, Peters CA, Docimo SG. Percutaneous nephrolithotomy in infants and preschool age children: experience with a new technique. Urology 1998; 52:697–700.
67. Mor Y, Elmasry YE, Kellett MJ, Duffy PG. The role of percutaneous nephrolithotomy in the management of pediatric renal calculi. J Urol 1997; 158:1319–21.
68. Gunes A, Yahya Ugras M, Yilmaz U et al. Percutaneous nephrolithotomy for pediatric stone disease – our experience with adult-sized equipment. Scand J Urol Nephrol 2003; 37:477–81.
69. Helal M, Black T, Lockhart J, Figueroa TE. The Hickman peel-away sheath: alternative for pediatric percutaneous nephrolithotomy. J Endourol 1997; 11:171–2.
70. Desai MR, Kukreja RA, Patel SH, Bapat SD. Percutaneous nephrolithotomy for complex pediatric renal calculus disease. J Endourol 2004; 18:23–7.
71. Kroovand RL. Pediatric urolithiasis. Urol Clin North Am 1997; 12:173–84.
72. Marberger M, Turk C, Steikogler. Piezoelectric extracorporeal shockwave lithotripsy in children. J Urol 1989; 142:349–52.
73. Thornhill JA, Moran K, Moon EE et al. Extracorporeal shockwave lithotripsy monotherapy for paediatric urinary tract calculi. Br J Urol 1990; 65:638–40.
74. Picramenos D, Deliveliotis C, Alexopoulou K et al. Extracorporeal shockwave lithotripsy for renal stones in children. Urol Int 1966; 56:86–9.
75. Van Horn AC, Hollander JB, Kass EJ. First and second generation lithotripsy in children: results, comparison and followup. J Urol 1995; 153:1969–71.

76. Rizvi S, Naqvi SA, Hussain Z et al. Management of pediatric urolithiasis in Pakistan: experience with 1,440 children. J Urol 2003; 169:634–7.
77. Tan AH, Al-Omar M, Watterson JD et al. Results of shockwave lithotripsy for pediatric urolithiasis. J Endourol 2004; 18:527–30.
78. Al-Busaildy S, Prem A, Medhat M. Pediatric staghorn calculi: the role of extracorporeal shockwave lithotripsy monotherapy with special reference to ureteral stenting. J Urol 2003: 169:629–33.
79. Chuong CJ, Zhong P, Preminger GM. Acoustic and mechanical properties of renal calculi: implications in shockwave lithotripsy. J Endourol 1993; 7:437–44.
80. Erhard MJ. Pediatric endourology. In: Belman AB, King LR, Kramer SA, eds. Clinical Pediatric Urology, 4th edn. London: Martin Dunitz; 2002: 225–59.
81. Jayanthi VR, Arnold PM, Koff SA. Strategies for managing upper tract calculi in young children. J Urol 1999; 162:1234–7.
82. Badawy H, Salama A, Eissa M et al. Percutaneous management of renal calculi: experience with percutaneous nephrolithotomy in 60 children. J Urol 1999; 162:1710–13.
83. Al-Shammari AM, Al-Otaibi K, Leonard MP et al. Percutaneous nephrolithotomy in the pediatric population. J Urol 1999; 162:1721–4.
84. Zeren S, Satar N, Bayazit Y et al. Percutaneous nephrolithotomy in the management of pediataric renal calculi. J Endourol 2002; 16:75–8.
85. Desai MR, Kukreja RA, Patel SH et al. Percutaneous nephrolithotomy for complex pediatric renal calculus disease. J Endourol 2004; 18:23–7.
86. Casale P, Grady RW, Joyner BD et al. Transperitoneal laparoscopic pyelolithotomy after failed percutaneous access in the pediatric patient. J Urol 2004; 172:680–3.
87. Caione P, De Gennaro M, Capozza N et al. Endoscopic manipulation of ureteral calculi in children by rigid operative ureterorenoscopy. J Urol 1990; 144:492–3.
88. Thomas R, Ortenberg J, Lee BR et al. Safety and efficacy of pediatric ureteroscopy for management of calculous disease. J Urol 1993; 149:1082–4.
89. Shroff S, Watson GM. Experience with ureteroscopy in children. Br J Urol 1995; 75:395–400.
90. Scarpa RM, De Lisa A, Porru D, Canetto A, Usai E. Ureterolithotripsy in children. Urology 1995: 46:859–62.
91. Smith DP, Jerkins GR, Noe HN. Urethroscopy in small neonates with posterior urethral valves and ureteroscopy in children with ureteral calculi. Urology 1996: 47:908–10.
92. Kurzrock EA, Huffman JL, Hardy BE et al. Endoscopic treatment of pediatric urolithiasis. J Pediatr Surg 1996; 31:1413–16.
93. Minevich E, Rousseau MB, Wacksman J, Lewis AG, Sheldon CA. Pediatric ureteroscopy: technique and preliminary results. J Pediatr Surg 1977; 32:571–4.
94. Wollin TA, Teichman JM, Rogenes VJ et al. Holmium: YAG lithotripsy in children. J Urol 1999; 162:1717–20.
95. Van Savage JG, Palanca LG, Andersen RD, Rao GS, Slaughenhoupt BL. Treatment of distal ureteral stones in children: similarities to the American Urological Association guidelines in adults. J Urol 2000; 164:1089–93.
96. Schuster TG, Russell KY, Bloom DA et al. Ureteroscopy for the treatment of urolithiasis in children. J Urol 2002; 167:1813–15.
97. Bassiri A, Ahmadnia H, Darabi MR, Yonessi M. Transureteral lithotripsy in pediatric practice. J Endourol 2002; 16:257–260.
98. Satar N, Zeren S, Bayazit et al. Rigid ureteroscopy for the treatment of ureteral calculi in children. J Urol 2004; 172:298–300.
99. Raza A, Smith G, Moussa S et al. Ureteroscopy in the management of pediatric urinary tract calculi. J Endourol 2005; 19:151–8.
100. Minevich E, Defoor W, Reddy P et al. Ureteroscopy is safe and effective in prepubertal children. J Urol 2005; 174:276–9.
101. Wangensteen OH, Wangensteen SD. Lithotomy and lithotomies. In: The Rise of Surgery from Empiric Craft to Scientific Discipline. Minneapolis: University of Minnesota Press, 1978; 71–80.
102. Khoury AE, Saloman M, Doche R et al. Stone formation after augmentation cystoplasty: the role of intestinal mucus. J Urol 1997; 158:1133–7.
103. Kronner KM, Casale AJ, Cain MP et at. Bladder calculi in the pediatric augmented bladder. J Urol 1998; 160:1096–8.
104. Razvi HA, Song TY, Denstedt JD. Management of vesical calculi: comparison of lithotripsy devices. J Endourol 1996; 10:559–63.
105. Teichman JM, Rogenes VJ, McIver BJ, Harris JM. Holmium: yttrium–aluminum–garnet laser cystolithotripsy of large bladder calculi. Urology 1997; 50:44–8.
106. Cuellar D, Roberts WW, Docimo, SG. Minimally invasive treatment of bladder calculi. In: Docimo SG, ed. Minimally Invasive Approaches to Pediatric Urology. Abingdon: Taylor & Francis, 2005: 75–8.
107. Van Savage JG, Khoury AE, McLorie GA, Churchill BM. Percutaneous vacuum vesicolithotomy under direct vision: a new technique. J Urol 1996; 156:706–8.
108. Elder JS. Percutaneous cystolithotomy with endotracheal tube tract dilatation after urinary tract reconstruction. J Urol 1997: 157:2298–300.

Renal parenchymal imaging in children

27

J Michael Zerin

Increased renal cortical echogenicity and diffuse medical renal diseases

Renal cortical echogenicity in children and adults is normally less than that of the liver and spleen. However, in neonates the renal cortex is usually isoechoic, or even slightly more echogenic than the other solid organs.[1–6] Physiologically, increased renal cortical echogenicity in neonates is attributed to a higher cortical glomerulotubular ratio early in life and usually resolves by 6 months.[5–8] Abnormally increased renal parenchymal echogenicity is the sonographic hallmark of a large and clinically diverse group of glomerular, tubular, and interstitial disorders of the kidneys that are commonly referred to broadly in pediatric imaging as 'medical renal diseases.'[9–15] There is an imprecise relationship between the extent and intensity of the hyperechogenicity and the clinical severity of the renal disease as assessed by functional studies, although the correlation is not usually strong enough to reliably predict outcome. Diffuse renal cortical hyperechogenicity by itself is a non-specific finding requiring correlation with clinical and biochemical findings. The causes of the abnormally echogenic appearance of the cortex in renal parenchymal diseases are not well understood and may not be the same in different disorders. Any process that disrupts the normally well-organized, compact parenchymal architecture is likely to increase the number and reflectivity of the acoustic interfaces in tissue. Alterations in renal perfusion, cellular infiltration, and interstitial edema are all probably important in acute disorders. Fibrosis and histologic disorganization due to nephron disruption probably contribute to the appearance in chronic medical renal disorders.

The extent to which corticomedullary differentiation is affected in diffuse renal parenchymal disease varies widely.[5,11–13,16] In diseases that reduce glomerular perfusion or disrupt glomerular architecture, the pyramids often remain relatively hypoechoic and can even appear somewhat enlarged (Figure 27.1). On the other hand, in tubulointerstitial diseases and diseases that affect the parenchymal echo

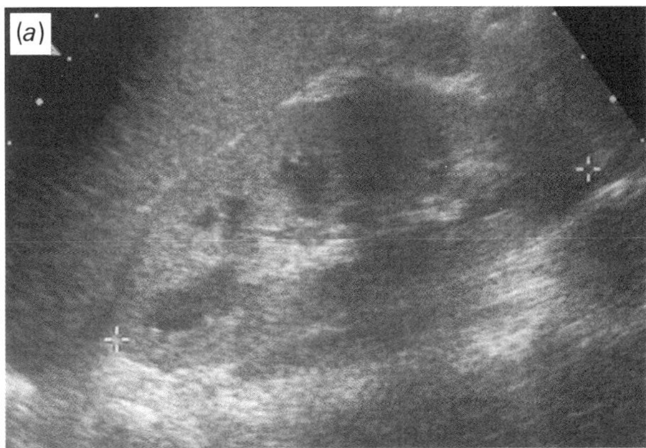

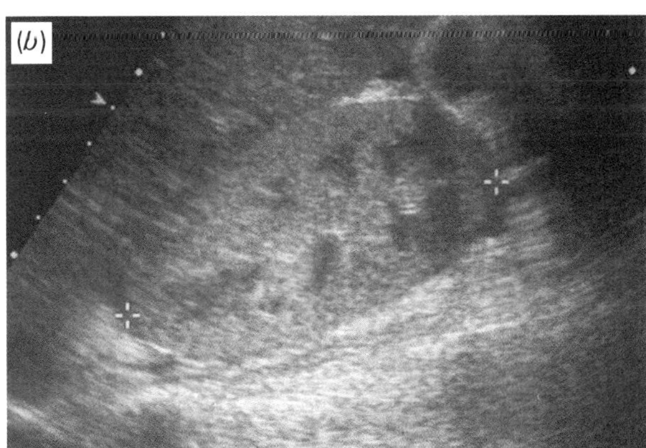

Figure 27.1 A 7-year-old boy with toxic shock syndrome presenting with scalded skin syndrome and acute oliguric renal failure. Ultrasound shows both kidneys are markedly enlarged with diffusely echogenic cortex. However, the pyramids remain hypoechoic and are easily identified. (*a*) Ultrasound: longitudinal view of the right kidney (length 9.3 cm). (*b*) Ultrasound: longitudinal view of the left kidney (length 9.3 cm).

texture more diffusely, both the cortex and the medulla are abnormal and corticomedullary differentiation is more likely to be reduced or absent.

Measurements of the sizes of the kidneys can also be very helpful.[5,11,17] Large, echogenic kidneys usually suggest an acute disorder in which there is edema or cellular infiltration of the renal interstitium. Conversely, small, echogenic kidneys indicate a chronic medical renal condition that is associated with renal atrophy (Figure 27.2). Serial evaluations of the renal sizes and parenchymal echogenicity generally correlate with the clinical course and renal functional assessment, but can also occasionally provide additional prognostic information. In acute medical renal disorders that are associated with generalized enlargement of the kidney, clinical recovery may be associated with return of the renal sizes toward normal, as well as improvement in the echo appearance of the renal cortex. On the other hand, persistence or intensification of the hyperechogenic appearance of the renal cortex is usually accompanied by further clinical and functional deterioration and can indicate a transition to a more chronic phase of the disorder, particularly when the renal sizes are decreasing.

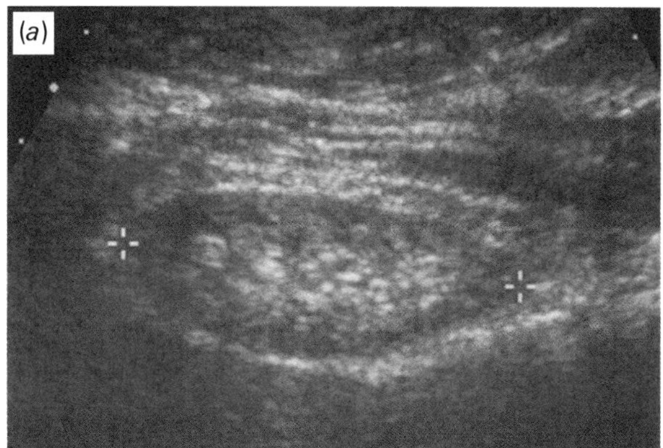

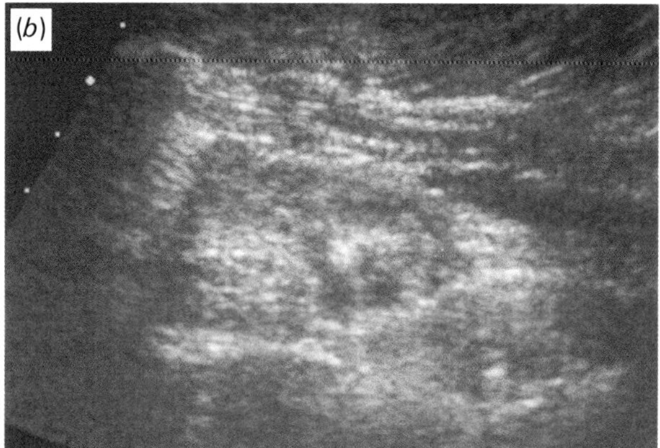

Figure 27.2 A 16-year-old boy with chronic medical renal disease and renal insufficiency on hemodialysis. Ultrasound of the kidneys shows that both kidneys are small with diffusely echogenic parenchyma and no visible corticomedullary differentiation. (*a*) Ultrasound: longitudinal view of the right kidney (length 6.7 cm). (*b*) Ultrasound: longitudinal view of the left kidney (length 6.8 cm).

The appearance of the Doppler waveforms in renal parenchymal diseases generally corresponds to the site of the involvement rather than the specific histopathologic features of the disease.[5,11,15,18] Elevation in the resistive index indicates an increase in the post-glomerular resistance. Hence, diseases that increase resistive index include those that cause obstruction at the level of renal veins, tubulointerstitial diseases, obstruction in the collecting system or ureter, and renal compression by disease in the perinephric space. Disorders that primarily cause a reduction in arterial inflow to the kidney and acute glomerular diseases are not typically associated with increased resistive index in the absence of secondary tubulointerstitial injury related to tissue infarction and edema.

Renal infections

Acute pyelonephritis

For several decades, ultrasound (US) has been the most widely used modality for imaging infants and children who have a urinary tract infection.[4,19–29] Inflammatory edema from pyelonephritis causes focal or generalized renal enlargement and bulging renal contours. Dramatic polar enlargement can occasionally mimic an echogenic mass. The walls of the collecting system may also be thickened. Infected parenchyma usually appears hyperechoic, with reduced corticomedullary differentiation (Figure 27.3a). However, severely hypovascular, partially necrotic areas can appear hypoechoic and can be difficult to distinguish from abscess. At power Doppler US, areas of acute pyelonephritis appear as wedge-shaped, hypovascular or avascular zones in the cortex, with the interlobar arteries following abnormally curvilinear courses around the edematous, infected segments.[27,28,30]

Unfortunately, both the sensitivity and specificity of the US findings are limited in acute pyelonephritis. Subtle changes in parenchymal echogenicity or the size and contours of the kidney are often difficult to differentiate prospectively from normal, even when they are easily seen in retrospect.[22,25,31,32] Transient pelvocaliectasis that results from endotoxin, urinary

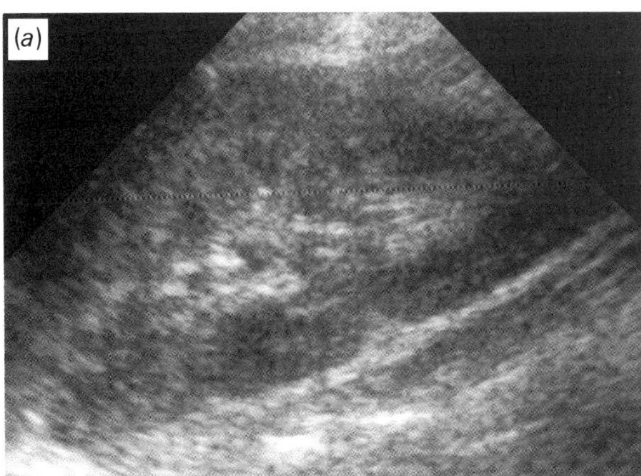

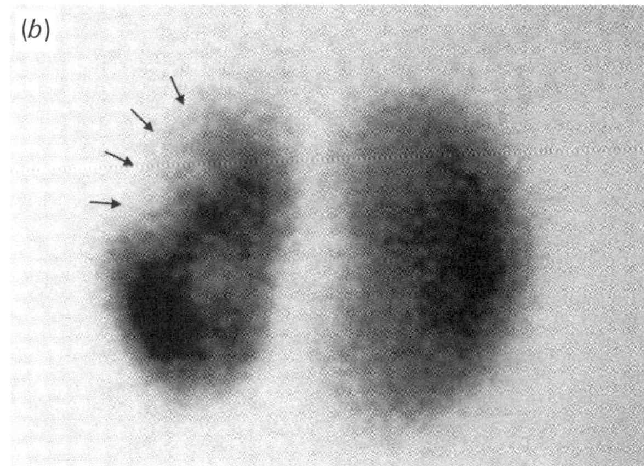

Figure 27.3 A 7-year-old girl with fever and left flank pain due to acute left pyelonephritis. (*a*) Ultrasound: longitudinal view of the left kidney (length 10.3 cm) shows that the upper half of the left kidney is enlarged and echogenic and appears somewhat bulbous compared with the lower pole. (*b*) ^{99m}Tc DMSA renal cortical scintigraphy (posterior view) confirms the presence of a large perfusion defect in the upper half of the left kidney (arrows).

retention, or vesicoureteral reflux (VUR) cannot be readily differentiated from obstructive hydronephrosis. Desquamated cellular and crystalline material in chronically obstructed, uninfected systems similarly cannot be reliably distinguished sonographically from purulent urine. Although power Doppler US is an excellent adjunct to the conventional gray-scale examination, it is less sensitive than renal cortical scintigraphy, computed tomography (CT), or magnetic resonance imaging (MRI).

At ^{99m}Tc DMSA (technetium 99m dimercaptosuccinic acid) renal cortical scintigraphy, acute pyelonephritis appears as wedge-shaped or triangular areas of diminished cortical uptake[25,27,33–36] (Figure 27.3b). Most defects occur in the renal poles and the adjacent renal contour often bulges outwardly. Rarely, diffuse pyelonephritis produces a globally enlarged, poorly functioning kidney. Acute defects resolve within 4–6 months after treatment, in the absence of scar formation. Dynamic planar diuretic ^{99m}Tc MAG3 (technetium 99m mercaptoacetyltriglycine) renal scintigraphy has also been used to diagnose acute pyelonephritis.[37,38] Functional defects caused by pyelonephritis show decreased early uptake and fill in slowly on static images, with prolonged late retention of activity. Fixed functional defects that persist on all phases can represent either acute pyelonephritis or scar.

At contrast-enhanced CT, acute pyelonephritis appears as segmental areas of decreased or striated parenchymal enhancement, with edematous, convex, rounded margins, most commonly in the renal poles[25,29,30,36,39,40] (Figure 27.4). The abnormal appearance can persist for several months before resolving or progressing to scar formation. Acute pyelonephritis is more difficult to detect on non-

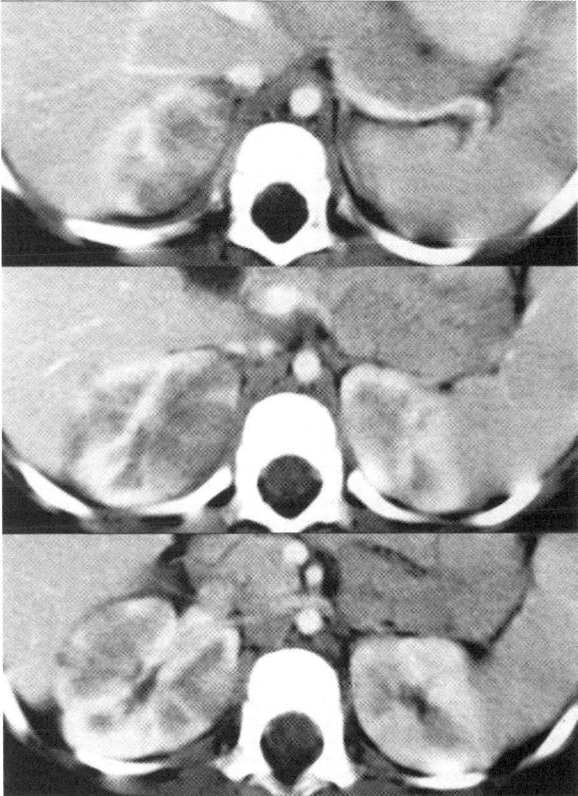

Figure 27.4 An 18-month-old girl with bilateral acute multifocal pyelonephritis, presenting with high fever and febrile seizure. Contrast-enhanced CT shows multiple wedge-shaped, low-attenuation, non-enhancing lesions in both kidneys.

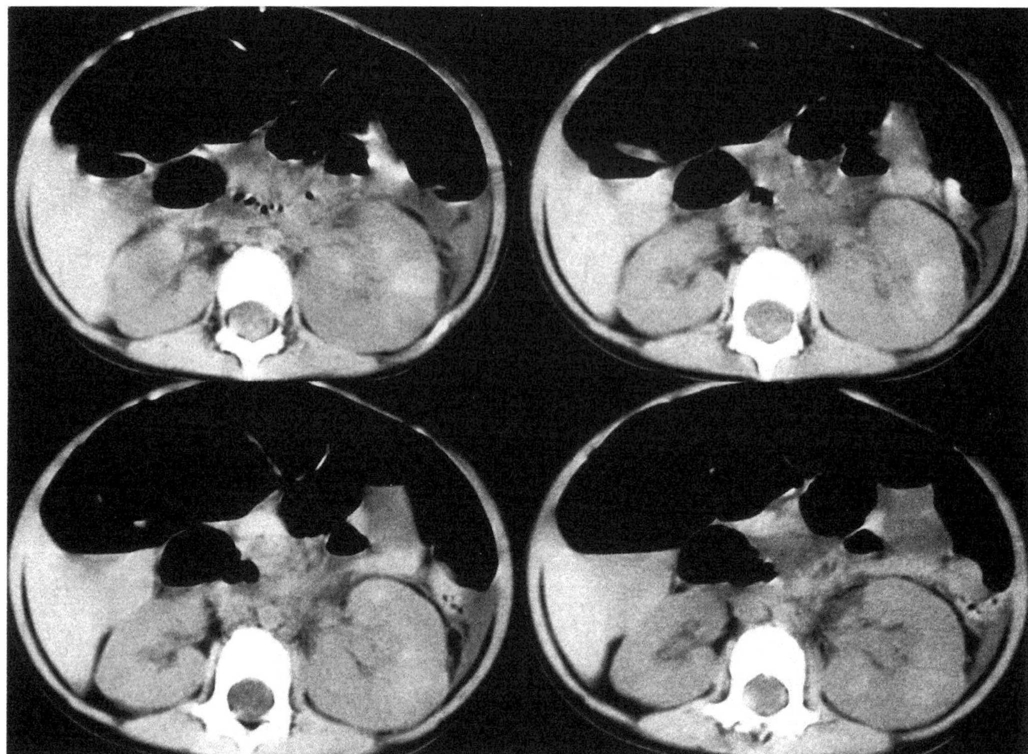

Figure 27.5 A 3-year-old girl with acute hemorrhagic pyelonephritis presenting with fever, gross hematuria, and *E. coli* bacteremia. Intravenous contrast material was not given for CT because of acute renal insufficiency requiring peritoneal dialysis. Non-enhanced CT shows that her left kidney is enlarged, with multiple slightly higher attenuation areas scattered throughout the parenchyma. Several similar, more subtle lesions are also present in the right kidney.

enhanced CT because the infected areas are isodense or only slightly hypodense in comparison with normal parenchyma. Increased attenuation within an area of acute pyelonephritis on non-enhanced CT may suggest parenchymal hemorrhage (Figure 27.5).

On postcontrast, fast spin-echo T2 and inversion recovery MRI sequences, gadolinium-related T1 and T2 shortening causes normally enhancing parenchyma to have markedly reduced signal intensity, whereas non-enhancing areas of acute pyelonephritis remain very bright.[29,35,36,40–43] Marked hyperintensity is also seen in both pyelonephritis and renal abscess on diffusion-weighted MRI.[44–46] Restricted diffusion in pyelonephritis is primarily due to cytotoxic edema, although intratubular inspissation of inflammatory cells is also probably important.

Published studies comparing these modalities[30,33,35,36] show no significant differences between DMSA, CT, and MRI, either in the diagnosis of pyelonephritis (sensitivity >90%) or in the localization of lesions. However, power Doppler US is less sensitive. Interobserver agreement is better for both CT and MRI than for DMSA. The ability to reliably differentiate scars from acute infection in the absence of a previous study is another important benefit of both CT and MRI. MRI also offers the advantages of multiplanar imaging and lack of ionizing radiation.

Fungal pyelonephritis

Fungal pyelonephritis is usually associated with fungal sepsis and occurs principally in neonates with indwelling central venous catheters and in children who are immunocompromised.[42,45–48] Hyperalimentation is another important risk factor. *Candida albicans* is the most common organism. In neonates with diffuse renal infection with *Candida*, US shows renal enlargement and diffuse parenchymal hyperechogenicity. Fungus balls (bezoars) appear as nonshadowing hyperechoic masses within the collecting system and can cause obstruction. Focal areas of fungal pyelonephritis appear hypoechoic and have low attenuation at CT[42,46,49,50] (Figure 27.6). Fungal abscesses have imaging features similar to those of bacterial abscesses.

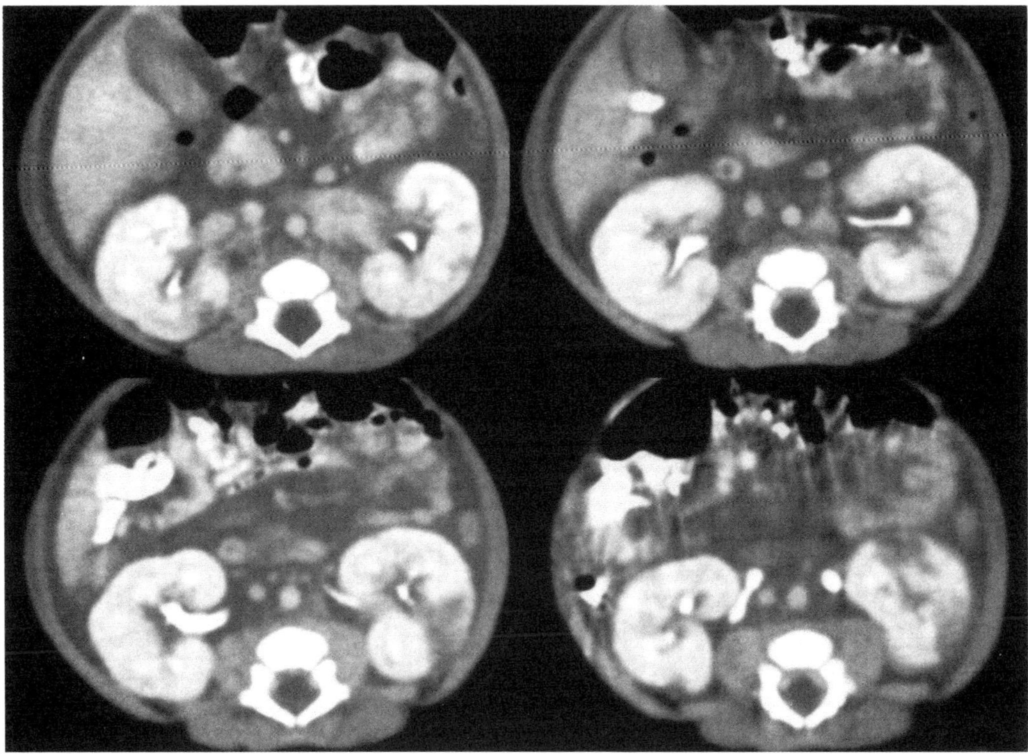

Figure 27.6 A 2-week-old boy with *Candida albicans* sepsis and bilateral fungal pyelonephritis. Contrast-enhanced CT shows both kidneys are enlarged and contain multiple scattered, peripheral, low-attenuation, non-enhancing parenchymal lesions.

Complications of acute pyelonephritis

At US, a renal abscess appears as a round, hypoechoic or anechoic, fluid-filled intraparenchymal mass with a thick, irregular wall.[9,10,25] Abscesses can be unilocular or multilocular and usually contain layering, echogenic debris. The appearance of adjacent parenchyma is usually consistent with acute pyelonephritis. Large perinephric abscesses are readily visualized with US. However, contrast-enhanced CT provides superior definition of both the intra- and extrarenal extent of the infection[39,42,46,51,52] (Figure 27.7). On a postcontrast CT, a renal abscess appears as a hypodense, cystic mass with an irregularly thickened, enhancing wall. Non-enhanced CT is generally less satisfactory. MRI is an excellent alternative to CT in patients in whom iodinated contrast media is contraindicated.

Pyonephrosis represents acute bacterial infection in a kidney with a dilated, obstructed collecting system. The sonographic appearance of a dilated collecting system filled with urine and floating or layering echogenic debris is suggestive of pyonephrosis.[25,42,46,51,52,53] Areas of pyelonephritis are often also evident and the kidney may be enlarged. Air bubbles in the collecting system appear as irregular, brightly echogenic, shadowing foci and usually float on top of the urine, a feature that distinguishes them from calculi, which tend to sink to more dependent locations. Hydronephrosis, with thickening and enhancement of the collecting system walls, is readily demonstrated at CT, as are associated areas of pyelonephritis. Calculi and air in the collecting system are also visible at CT. Although US provides superior definition of particulate debris in the collecting system, care should be taken not to mistake transient hydronephrosis that results from endotoxin-induced atony, urinary retention, or reflux for pyonephrosis. Debris may be present in children with uncomplicated pyelonephritis who have a non-obstructed system. Similarly, air that is introduced into the bladder during catheterization can also reach the collecting system in children with reflux. Mild dilatation is usually of little concern, particularly if the patient is otherwise healthy and responds rapidly to antibiotics. When the dilatation is more severe and a large amount of echogenic debris or air is present ('pseudo-pyonephrosis'), differentiation from pyonephrosis can be difficult.[25]

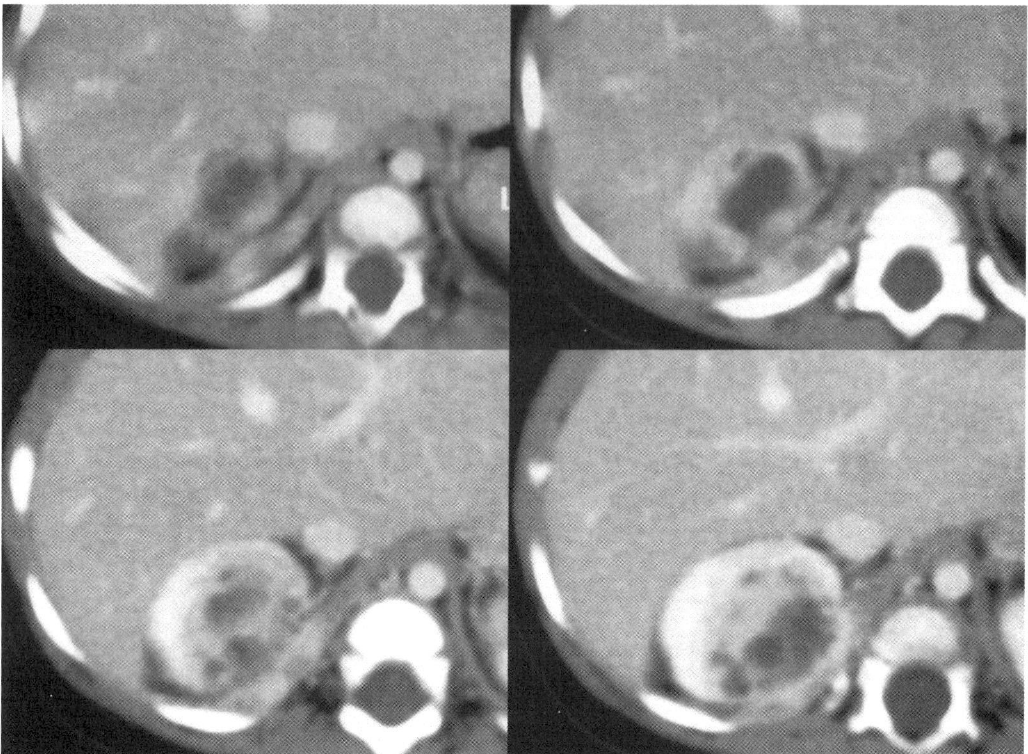

Figure 27.7 A 9-month-old boy with right acute pyelonephritis and intrarenal abscess. Contrast-enhanced CT shows a complex large-area abnormal enhancement with necrosis in the upper pole of the right kidney.

Xanthogranulomatous pyelonephritis is a rare form of chronic bacterial renal infection, usually caused by either *Escherichia coli* or *Proteus* spp., in which granulomatous infiltration of the kidney by lipid-laden macrophages leads to extensive parenchymal destruction.[25,42,54–57] Nephrolithiasis and chronic upper urinary tract obstruction are frequently present. The US appearance in diffuse xanthogranulomatous pyelonephritis is of a markedly enlarged, echogenic kidney in which the normal renal architecture is obliterated. Multiple hypoechoic, mass-like areas of parenchymal necrosis are visible throughout the kidney. Calculi are common, although the collecting system is usually not dilated. At postcontrast CT, the affected kidney is non-functioning and the parenchyma appears low in attenuation due to necrosis and infiltration by the lipid-laden macrophages ('foamy histiocytes'). One or more calculi are usually present. Perinephric and paranephric extension is better demonstrated at CT than US. Focal xanthogranulomatous pyelonephritis is quite rare and presents as a large, inflammatory, renal mass. The mass is hypoechoic at US and hypodense and non-enhancing at CT. Visualization of a calculus within the mass or in an adjacent calyx can be an important clue to the diagnosis.

Chronic atrophic pyelonephritis (reflux nephropathy)

Cortical scars and parenchymal atrophy in chronic pyelonephritis result from recurrent episodes of acute pyelonephritis.[23,27,29,34,58] Cortical scars are most common in the renal poles and typically become visible 4–6 months following infection. At excretory urography, cortical scarring appears as a deformed ('clubbed') calyx beneath an area of parenchymal thinning. The indentation in the surface of the kidney immediately overlying the affected calyx becomes more conspicuous over time as a result of fibrous retraction within the scar itself and continued growth of adjacent normal parenchyma. Although excretory urography was used extensively in the past, it has been entirely replaced by US for evaluating children with pyelonephritis.[4,19,20,21,23,27] The US findings of chronic pyelonephritis include a small poorly growing kidney with focal or diffuse cortical atrophy. Dilated, blunted calices are often present. Whereas larger cortical scars are usually easily identified, smaller scars are often not seen at US. Careful serial evaluation of renal measurements is critical, since poor renal growth and generalized parenchymal thinning may be present, even when focal scarring is not visible. In advanced cases, the kidney will appear small and irregular with diffusely echogenic parenchyma, indistinguishable from other forms of end-stage chronic medical renal disease.

Persistent fetal lobation (lobulation) and junctional parenchymal defect are two common, normal developmental variations in renal shape that should not be mistaken for cortical scarring at US.[5,6,29,59] Fetal lobation produces a smoothly undulating renal outline with evenly distributed superficial clefts between the fetal renal lobes. The indentations lie between the pyramids rather than over them, as in cortical scarring, and the adjacent calices are not dilated. Junctional parenchymal defect is a triangular, echogenic, cortical indentation along the anterolateral aspect of the junction of the mid and upper thirds of the kidney.[5,6,29,60] The defect extends inferomedially into the renal sinus and represents the anterior site of fusion of the superior and inferior renunculi.

The appearance of chronic pyelonephritis at ^{99m}Tc DMSA depends on the number, size, stage of maturation, and location of the scars.[27,29,34,61] Mature scars appear as sharply defined, wedge-shaped cortical defects. Renal volume is reduced and the renal contour is flattened due to fibrous retraction and loss of parenchymal substance. Cortical scars tend to appear more sharply defined than defects caused by acute pyelonephritis. However, the most reliable way to distinguish between acute and chronic cortical defects is to compare sequential examinations. Careful correlation with the clinical setting and with other imaging modalities, such as US, is also essential to assure that the defects are the result of pyelonephritis or scarring rather than of other lesions such as cysts, caliceal diverticula, or masses.

At MRI, chronic pyelonephritic scars appear as irregular cortical indentations that do not change in signal intensity between pre- and postcontrast inversion recovery sequences.[42,46,62,63] As scars mature, fibrous retraction leads to progressive loss of parenchymal volume. Although CT can also provide excellent anatomic and functional information in children with chronic pyelonephritis, this modality is rarely used for this application.

Renal vascular diseases

Renal vein thrombosis

Renal vein thrombosis presents with gross hematuria, hypertension, and an enlarged, palpable kidney.[5,11,42,64,65] Premature infants, infants of diabetic mothers, and neonates and infants with severe dehydration, hypotension, sepsis, or asphyxia are at greatest risk. Renal vein thrombosis also occurs in children with coagulopathies. Renal vein thrombosis is usually unilateral and the affected kidney functions poorly. Bilateral thrombosis causes severe renal insufficiency. In neonates and infants, thrombus formation begins in smaller intrarenal veins and the main renal vein and inferior vena cava are often patent. In neonates with adrenal hemorrhage, extension of thrombus into the kidney from the adrenal vein can lead to ipsilateral renal vein thrombosis. This is more common on the left, since the left adrenal vein drains directly into the left renal vein.

Renal vein thrombosis is usually diagnosed at US.[5,6,11,66–68] In the acute phase, the kidney is globally enlarged, and the parenchyma is diffusely echogenic with poor corticomedullary differentiation. Larger thrombi within interlobar and intralobular renal veins appear as linear, echogenic bands radiating peripherally between the renal lobes. Adjacent perivascular hemorrhage probably also contributes to this appearance. Thrombus can also be visible in the main renal vein and inferior vena cava. Even when the main renal vein is patent, the amplitude of flow is reduced at Doppler US. More importantly, renal artery Doppler US shows reduced or even retrograde flow during diastole, with markedly increased resistive index.[18] MAG3 renal scintigraphy shows a globally enlarged kidney, with markedly reduced or absent uptake and no excretion. With recovery, the affected kidney decreases in size as the edema recedes and there is variable restoration of function. Serial US examinations are required to document stabilization of the renal size and resumption of a normal rate of growth. Persistent cortical hyperechogenicity and diminished corticomedullary differentiation indicate parenchymal atrophy and are associated with poor functional recovery. With severe parenchymal infarction and parenchymal necrosis, severe atrophy and cyst formation can result in a small, echogenic, poorly functioning kidney.[5,6,11,42,66,67] In the chronic phase, punctate, linear, or branching calcifications can appear within the thrombosed intrarenal veins.[69,70] The presence of linear and punctate renal calcifications in a neonate with a small echogenic kidney is strongly suggestive of prenatal renal vein thrombosis.[71]

CT and MRI are rarely performed in children with renal vein thrombosis, since the diagnosis is readily established at US and MAG3 renal scintigraphy.[42,64,68] During the acute phase, the affected kidney is enlarged and edematous. Perfusion is diminished with inhomogeneous parenchymal attenuation and markedly reduced or no enhancement. Parenchymal infarction and hemorrhage are common. Associated adrenal hemorrhage and thrombosis of the inferior vena cava are also readily visualized. In the chronic phase, parenchymal atrophy ensues, with calcification of the residual thrombus in the renal veins and inferior vena cava.

Renal artery thrombosis

Non-traumatic renal artery thrombosis occurs primarily following umbilical or femoral artery catheterization, in infants of diabetic mothers, and in infants and children with sepsis, severe dehydration or hemoconcentration, coagulopathy, or vasculitis. The extent of parenchymal injury depends on the size of the occluded vessel. Complete occlusion of the main renal artery results in global renal infarction.[11,72,73] During the acute phase, the kidney may initially remain normal in size or even be slightly small and the cortex becomes hyperechoic, although the pyramids remain hypoechoic. Doppler imaging reveals reduced or absent flow in the main and segmental renal arteries with normal or low resistive index. Visualization of the echogenic intraluminal-filling defect representing the thrombus within the main renal artery is diagnostic. As parenchymal infarction and hemorrhage develop, the kidney swells and becomes increasingly echogenic and inhomogeneous, ultimately leading to complete disruption of the normal corticomedullary architecture. Functional evaluations such as renal scintigraphy show no uptake or excretion by the affected kidney. As in renal vein thrombosis, CT and MRI are rarely performed in neonates and infants with renal artery thrombosis. The anatomic and functional outcomes depend on the extent of parenchymal infarction and the timing and degree of revascularization. Chronic ischemia results in an atrophic, poorly or non-functioning echogenic kidney that is small with smooth, reniform contours. Small parenchymal calcifications and cysts can also be seen.

Segmental renal artery occlusion causes a wedge-shaped, avascular segmental defect with its apex at the renal hilum and its base at the renal capsule.[11,73] Doppler imaging can confirm the absence of flow in the infarct, although scar formation can be difficult to differentiate from that seen in chronic pyelonephritis. Intravascular sonographic contrast agents may improve visualization of cortical perfusion defects with power Doppler US, although this remains to be applied in clinical practice.[74,75]

Hemolytic uremic syndrome

Hemolytic uremic syndrome is a bacterial toxin-mediated vasculitis that is manifested clinically by acute renal failure, microangiopathic hemolytic anemia, fever, and thrombocytopenia. The disease primarily affects children <5 years of age and is frequently preceded by an episode of gastroenteritis associated with severe abdominal cramping and bloody diarrhea. Intimal inflammation with thrombosis of small intrarenal arteries and capillaries leads to acute renal failure with severe oliguria or anuria and hypertension. Spontaneous recovery usually occurs within 3–4 weeks, although dialysis is often necessary during the acute phase.

During the acute phase in hemolytic uremic syndrome, the kidneys are normal in size or slightly enlarged. The renal cortex is diffusely hyperechoic and the medullary pyramids are hypoechoic.[11,76,77] At Doppler US, the resistive index is elevated, with markedly reduced or absent forward diastolic flow in the renal arteries. Occasionally, flow can even be reversed during diastole, as in renal vein thrombosis. Normalization of the arterial waveform may precede the onset of diuresis during the recovery phase.[78] Cortical echogenicity also returns to normal in most children who experience complete recovery of renal function.

Nephrocalcinosis and other causes of renal medullary hyperechogenicity

Medullary nephrocalcinosis is the most common cause of renal medullary hyperechogenicity in infants and children.[11,42,79–81] Hypercalciuria, increased urinary phosphate excretion, and hypercalcemia are important predisposing factors. Dystrophic renal calcification can also form secondary to severe parenchymal injury from trauma, infection, or infarction.

Sonographically, nephrocalcinosis shows a characteristic periphery-to-center progression, with increased echogenicity first developing along the margins of the pyramids[11,42,82–84] (Figure 27.8). Over time, this peripheral echogenic rim gradually thickens, eventually filling in the centers of the pyramids. In the most severe cases, the pyramids are diffusely, intensely echogenic with posterior acoustic shadowing. Aggregates of extracellular calcium near the papillary tips (Randall's plaques) can perforate the caliceal epithelium, leading to extrusion of calculi into the collecting system (Anderson–Randall–Carr phenome-

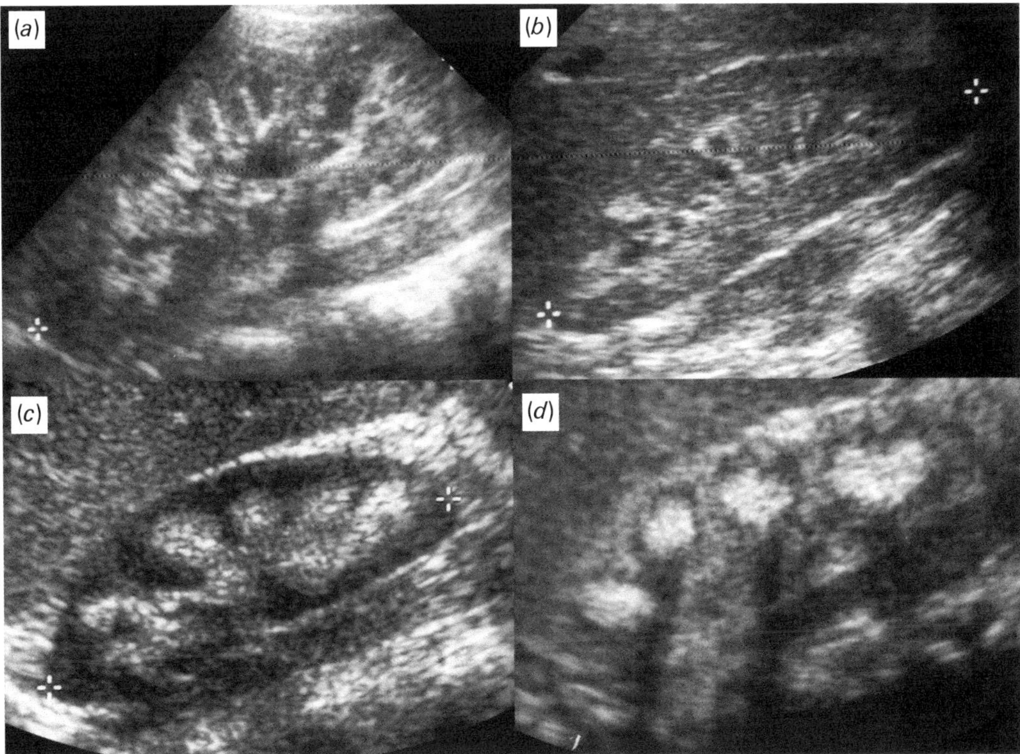

Figure 27.8 Sonographic patterns of medullary hyperechogenicity in nephrocalcinosis. (*a*) Longitudinal view of the left kidney in a 3-year-old girl with Williams syndrome shows thin, peripheral hyperechoic linear bands outlining the pyramids with the centers remaining hypoechoic. The cortex appears normal. (*b*) Longitudinal view of the right kidney in a 14-year-old boy with familial hypophosphatemic rickets shows thicker peripheral echogenic margins of the pyramids. Some pyramids appear almost uniformly hyperechoic. The cortex appears normal. (*c*) Longitudinal view of the right kidney in a 7-year-old boy with distal renal tubular acidosis shows diffusely and nearly homogeneously hyperechoic medullary pyramids. There is no posterior acoustic shadowing and the cortex appears normal. (*d*) Longitudinal view of the right kidney in a 7-week-old girl with severe idiopathic hypercalcemia shows very intense, diffuse medullary hyperechogenicity with posterior acoustic shadowing. The cortex is also thin and echogenic, consistent with cortical nephrocalcinosis.

non). Even in cases with marked medullary hyperechogenicity at US and increased medullary attenuation at non-enhanced CT, the calcification is not always visible on abdominal radiographs. Cortical calcification usually occurs only in the presence of advanced medullary nephrocalcinosis and is associated with marked hypercalcemia or severe generalized parenchymal injury, or both. Cortical nephrocalcinosis is manifested at sonography by generalized increase in cortical echogenicity, cortical acoustic shadowing, loss of the corticomedullary differentiation, and atrophy.

Renal medullary hyperechogenicity is also seen in a number of uncommon storage diseases, including glycogen storage disease, Lesch–Nyhan syndrome, and Wilson's disease, among others.[79,80,85–87] Both hypercalciuria and microscopic evidence of increased medullary calcium deposition have been reported in patients with these disorders. Hyperuricemia might also contribute in some patients, as it is known to produce hyperechoic pyramids in adults with gout and in children with leukemia. In some subtypes of glycogen storage disease, the kidneys are enlarged and become increasingly echogenic as a result of tubular and interstitial deposition of calcium, uric acid, and glycogen. The liver and spleen are also enlarged and echogenic. In Lesch–Nyhan syndrome, renal function is usually normal during childhood although the kidneys are small. Increased medullary echogenicity can be punctate or diffuse and is typically progressive and unaffected by therapy. Both nephrocalcinosis and renal calculi can develop.

Tamm–Horsfall proteinuria and other inspissation syndromes

Transient medullary hyperechogenicity as a result of intratubular inspissation of Tamm–Horsfall protein has been reported in 3–5% of otherwise healthy term neonates during the first week of life.[88,89] At US, the pyramids can appear diffusely speckled or the abnormality can appear as a splotchy hyperechoic focus involving the inner third of the pyramid, extending outward from the papillary tip. The abnormality can be unilateral or bilateral and is visible shortly after birth. Despite the fact that the deposits can be quite conspicuous at US, they are not visible at non-enhanced CT. Physiologically, decreased tubular flow during the first days of postnatal life is thought to be important. Tamm–Horsfall protein is known to precipitate and form intratubular aggregates when present in larger than normal quantity. Urinary excretion of Tamm–Horsfall protein is normally higher at birth and declines during the first week. Some authors have reported a temporal relationship between the disappearance of the hyperechogenicity and the establishment of a consistent pattern of micturition toward the end of the first week of life.

Similar sonographic appearances have been reported in children and adults with oliguric renal failure and persistently increased urinary Tamm–Horsfall excretion.[11] Medullary hyperechogenicity is also observed in patients with intratubular deposition of other large macromolecules, such as in rhabdomyolysis, myoglobinuria, toxic shock syndrome, and in children with leukemia and tumor lysis syndrome. The resistive index is usually increased at Doppler US examination and renal dysfunction is common. The reversibility of the US findings depends on re-establishment of a normal urine flow rate.

Renal tumors

Wilms' tumor

Wilms' tumor is a malignant neoplasm that arises from primitive, embryonal renal tissue and is the most common primary, solid, neoplasm in the pediatric abdomen, accounting for 95% of all malignant genitourinary neoplasms in children.[42,90,91] Most children with Wilms' tumor present between 1 and 4 years of age. Because Wilms' tumors grow rapidly, they are usually very large at diagnosis and present as a palpable abdominal mass. Hematuria, fever, abdominal pain, and hypertension are also common. Children with hemihypertrophy, sporadic aniridia, Beckwith–Wiedemann syndrome, Denys–Drash syndrome, and Perlman syndrome are predisposed to developing Wilms' tumor, but represent less than 5% of all cases.[92,93]

Wilms' tumor usually presents as a solitary renal mass and can occur anywhere in the kidney.[90–92,94,95] Multiple synchronous Wilms' tumors are present in 5% of patients at diagnosis and can be unilateral or bilateral (Figure 27.9). Metachronous contralateral tumors can also appear even many years after the nephrectomy for the original mass. The mass itself is surrounded by a well-defined pseudocapsule comprising tissue that has been compressed along the advancing surface of the enlarging mass. Histologically, Wilms' tumors are classified as either 'favorable' or anaplastic. Wilms' tumors with favorable histology account for more than 90% of cases. Children with anaplastic Wilms' tumors tend to be older and their tumors display a greater tendency to invade adjacent structures, as well as a higher frequency of distant metastases. Hematogenous metastasis is most common to the lungs, liver, and brain. Skeletal metastases are rare. Lymphatic spread to renal hilar and para-aortic lymph nodes can also occur. Intravascular extension into the renal vein and inferior vena cava occurs in 4% of children and in 1% the tumor thrombus propagates into the right atrium.

Ultrasound is the usually the first imaging study that is performed in an infant or young child who presents with a palpable abdominal mass.[5,11,42] At US, Wilms' tumor appears as a solid, intrarenal mass. The mass is often very large (>10 cm) and is usually primarily solid and hyperechoic. Cystic areas of necrosis

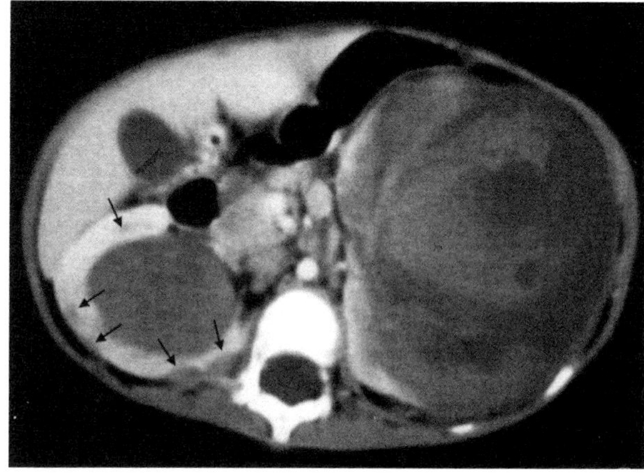

Figure 27.9 A 3-year-old girl with bilateral synchronous Wilms' tumors and right nephroblastomatosis. At contrast-enhanced CT, the left kidney is almost entirely replaced by a large, partially necrotic mass (Wilms' tumor) and there is a somewhat smaller mass (Wilms' tumor) distending the right renal sinus. Numerous tiny, low-attenuation perilobar nephrogenic rests (arrows) are visible in the residual enhancing right kidney.

and hemorrhage can be very extensive. However, primarily cystic Wilms' tumors are rare. At nonenhanced CT, Wilms' tumor presents as a low-attenuation, solid renal mass.[42,96] On postcontrast scans, the tumor generally appears more inhomogeneous, with variable enhancement of the solid components and no enhancement in cystic areas of hemorrhage and necrosis (Figures 27.9 and 27.10). Calcification is visible in less than 10% of cases. Wilms' tumors containing small amounts of fat have been reported rarely.[97] At MRI, the mass appears moderately inhomogeneous with relatively low signal intensity on T1-weighted sequences and has a bright signal on T2-weighted sequences.[42,98–100] Solid areas within the tumor enhance on postgadolinium sequences, although less than normal renal cortex. When present, calcification appears as very low signal foci, and is much less conspicuous at MRI than at either CT or US.[100,101] CT and MRI generally provide similar information regarding local tumor extent and regional adenopathy and are both superior to US for tumor staging.[91,102] In selected cases, direct multiplanar imaging with MRI can provide more detailed information, such as when direct invasion of adjacent structures is difficult to assess at CT. On all three modalities the contralateral kidney should be evaluated carefully for tumor or nephroblastomatosis. Although some clinicians have challenged routine intraoperative inspection and palpation of the contralateral kidney, this is still a widely accepted surgical practice, even when preoperative imaging studies show no contralateral renal abnormality.[95] Because of the propensity of Wilms' tumor to grow into the renal vein and inferior vena cava, these structures should be carefully evaluated.

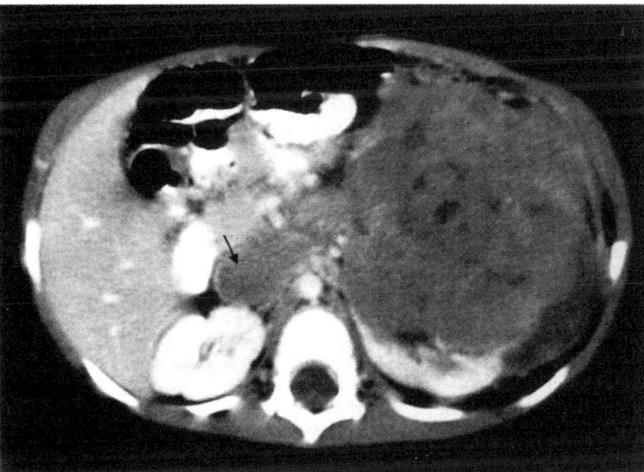

Figure 27.10 A 2-year-old girl with large left Wilms' tumor with extension into the left renal vein and inferior vena cava. Contrast-enhanced CT shows a large non-enhancing, solid left renal mass containing multiple small areas of necrosis and hemorrhage. Low-attenuation soft tissue is visible distending the left renal vein and inferior vena cava (arrow).

Identification of the superior extent of the thrombus is critical for presurgical planning[91,103,104] (see Figure 27.10). Gross intracaval tumor extension is usually readily visualized at Doppler US or with CT or MRI. However, both CT and MRI generally provide more detailed visualization of the vascular anatomy and can more readily demonstrate tumor extension into the adrenal or gonadal veins that may not be visible at US. Because the right renal vein is very short, sonographic evaluation of intravascular extension can also be more challenging in tumors that arise in the right kidney, particularly when they are very large. Large right renal tumors also often compress the inferior vena cava, even when there is no intravascular tumor. Congenital variations in the left renal vein (either retroaortic or circumaortic) can pose a challenge in patients with left renal tumors.

Ultrasound is generally used for postnephrectomy surveillance of both the nephrectomy bed and the contralateral kidney in children with Wilms' tumor.[11,42,105] Power Doppler US can aid in identifying smaller intrarenal masses that might not be as conspicuous on gray-scale imaging alone. Careful comparison with previous studies is critical and any unexplained change in the renal contour or focal enlargement of one portion of the kidney should be viewed with suspicion even when there is no clearly definable mass. CT or MRI should be performed when there is any question of a recurrent or contralateral mass.

Nephroblastomatosis

Nephroblastomatosis is the persistence of non-functioning, primitive, nephrogenic blastema in the kidney after birth.[94] Perilobar nephrogenic rests are positioned at the boundaries between the renal lobes and are more common than intralobar rests, which are located deep within the cortex or medulla. Panlobar nephroblastomatosis is a rare condition in which both kidneys are nearly entirely replaced by nephrogenic rest tissue (Figure 27.11). The clinical importance of nephroblastomatosis lies in the potential for malignant transformation of nephrogenic rests into Wilms' tumor.[94,106,107] Neoplastic transformation is more common with intralobar rests, although malignancy can develop within perilobar rests.

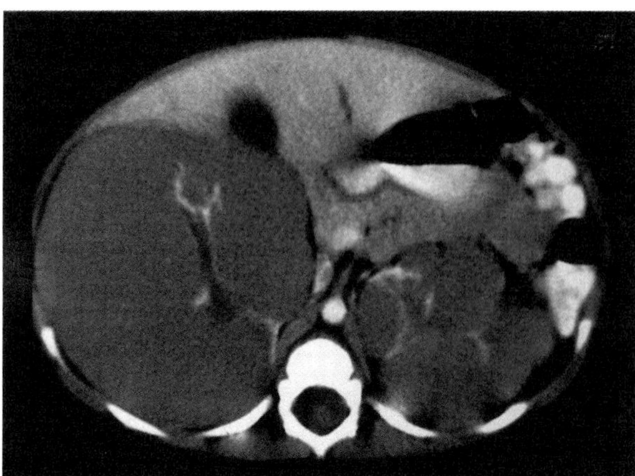

Figure 27.11 A 14-month-old boy with panlobar nephroblastomatosis, presenting with a markedly distended abdomen and bilateral palpable flank masses. Contrast-enhanced CT shows the kidneys are almost completely replaced by multiple low-attenuation, nonenhancing, solid masses. Residual compressed strands of functioning renal parenchyma are visible between the masses.

Macroscopic nephrogenic rests usually appear as hypoechoic solid masses at US.[107–110] At CT, nephrogenic rests have low attenuation and do not enhance (see Figure 27.10). CT is more sensitive than US in detecting nephroblastomatosis, although some lesions that are visible at US are not seen at CT and vice versa. Sclerosed perilobar rests can produce an irregularly flattened renal contour mimicking cortical scars from reflux nephropathy, whereas involuted intralobar rests can simulate renal cysts or caliceal diverticula. At MRI, nephrogenic rests do not enhance and appear homogeneously hypointense compared with cortex and isointense compared with the medulla on both T1- and T2-weighted sequences.

In children with Wilms' tumor, nephrogenic rests that are identified on prenephrectomy imaging studies should be carefully followed on subsequent examinations. Although some nephrogenic rests can be identified intraoperatively at the time of nephrectomy by inspection and palpation of the kidneys, many perilobar rests and most intralobar rests are not detectable in this fashion, including some that are identifiable at CT or MRI.[95] Microscopic nephrogenic rests are not detectable with any current imaging modality.

Patients who have syndromes that are associated with nephroblastomatosis and Wilms' tumor should have their kidneys screened periodically with US during infancy and early childhood.[90,92,93] Although the optimal frequency and duration of such US surveillance has not been well established, we follow patients every 3–6 months through infancy while progressively lengthening the interval between studies as the child gets older.[42,93,111] Just as is the case when following children with previous Wilms' tumor, careful comparison of the current examination with previous studies is critical and any unexplained change in the renal contour or focal or asymmetric enlargement should be viewed with suspicion even when there is no clearly definable mass or definite change in echo texture. Power Doppler US can also help to identify smaller intrarenal masses that might not be as conspicuous on gray-scale imaging alone. Whenever there is a question of a mass, CT or MRI should be performed without hesitation.

Clear cell sarcoma

Once thought to be a variant of Wilms' tumor, clear cell sarcoma accounts for 5% of primary pediatric renal tumors.[112–115] Children with clear cell sarcoma tend to be slightly older than those with Wilms' tumor and have a much poorer prognosis. The predilection for skeletal metastases in clear cell sarcoma also differentiates it from Wilms' tumor, in which skeletal metastases are rare. Clear cell sarcoma is also not associated with nephroblastomatosis. Ultrasound, CT, and MRI all demonstrate a predominantly solid, although usually complex renal mass with imaging characteristics that are usually indistinguishable from Wilms' tumor.[115] Well-defined cystic areas of necrosis and hemorrhage are common. Skeletal metastases can either be present at the time of initial diagnosis or can appear later and are usually osteolytic, although osteoblastic metastases also occur.[114] Both hot and cold defects can be seen on bone scan.

Malignant rhabdoid tumor

Malignant rhabdoid tumor is a very rare, aggressive, primary malignant pediatric renal neoplasm that frequently presents during the first year of life.[116] Malignant rhabdoid tumor is associated in up to half of patients with a histopathologically diverse group of primary central nervous system tumors, including primitive neuroectodermal tumor, ependymoma, and astrocytoma.[117] These tumors can be present when the renal mass is first detected or can appear later. At ultrasound, CT, and MRI, malignant rhabdoid tumor presents as a large, aggressive, infiltrating, solid renal mass.[118] The mass often arises centrally within or adjacent to the renal hilum and invades and compresses surrounding parenchyma as it enlarges. Linear calcifications are common. In some cases, the calcifications appear to outline distinct tumor lobules. Rapid enlargement of the mass can lead to necrosis and hemorrhage. Peritumoral hemorrhage can also occur, resulting in characteristic crescent-shaped fluid collections at the periphery of the mass. Because of the tumor's frequent association with both primary and metastatic neoplasms of the central nervous system, CT or MRI of the brain should be performed whenever the diagnosis of malignant rhabdoid tumor is suspected.

Renal cell carcinoma

The mean age at presentation in children with renal cell carcinoma is 11–12 years, although it has been reported as early as 6 months of age. Patients usually present with painless gross hematuria, abdominal pain, or a palpable mass. The histopathologic and imaging features of renal cell carcinoma in children are similar to adults. The tumor usually appears hyperechoic at US and hyperdense at CT, with variable tumor enhancement[119,120] (Figure 27.12). Necrosis and hemorrhage are common. Calcification is more common than in Wilms' tumor. Children with renal cell carcinoma have a relatively good prognosis if the entire tumor can be removed. However, if the primary resection is incomplete or there is distant metastatic spread, the prognosis is poor. Lung, bone, liver, or brain metastases are present in 20% of patients at diagnosis.

Renal medullary carcinoma

Renal medullary carcinoma is a very aggressive, malignant epithelial neoplasm that occurs almost exclusively in children and young adults with sickle cell trait or sickle cell disease.[120–123] In patients <25 years of age, males are affected three times as often as females. Gross hematuria, abdominal pain, and weight loss are common, although the mass itself is not always palpable. Renal medullary carcinoma arises along the urothelial margin of the renal medulla and grows quickly into the renal pelvis with early vascular and lymphatic invasion. Satellite parenchymal nodules are common and most patients have widely disseminated disease at diagnosis with metastases to the contralateral kidney, liver, lungs, and lymph nodes. Response to chemotherapy and radiotherapy is often poor. US shows a heterogeneous, centrally located, extensively infiltrative, solid intrarenal mass that frequently grows into the renal sinus. Smaller peripheral satellite nodules are common. At CT and MRI, the mass enhances heterogeneously.

Leukemia, lymphoma, and lymphoproliferative diseases

Despite the fact that many children who die with leukemia or lymphoma have histologic evidence of renal infiltration at postmortem examination, clinical and radiographic evidence of renal involvement is much less common during life.[11,124–126] Clinical signs of renal involvement, such as a palpable mass, hematuria, or reduced renal function, rarely precede other

(a)

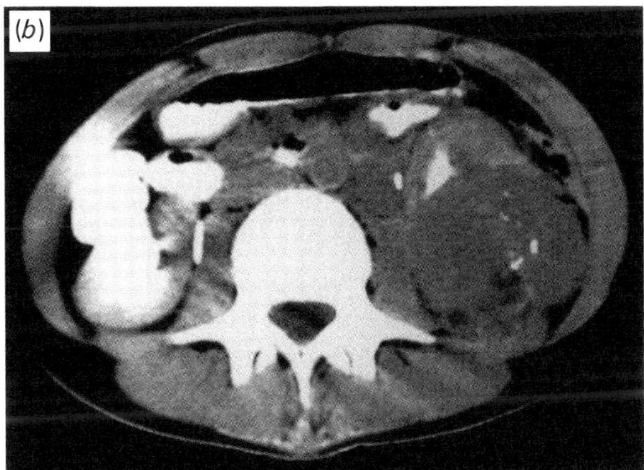

Figure 27.12 A 13-year-old girl with renal cell carcinoma of the lower pole of her left kidney, presenting with abdominal pain and a palpable left abdominal mass. (*a*) Ultrasound: longitudinal view of the left kidney shows a large, solid, slightly heterogeneous lower pole mass. Multiple small calcifications are visible within the mass. (*b*) Contrast-enhanced CT through the kidneys shows a large, solid mass in the lower pole of the left kidney posteriorly. Small calcifications are present within the mass. The residual functioning portion of the left kidney is visible anteriorly.

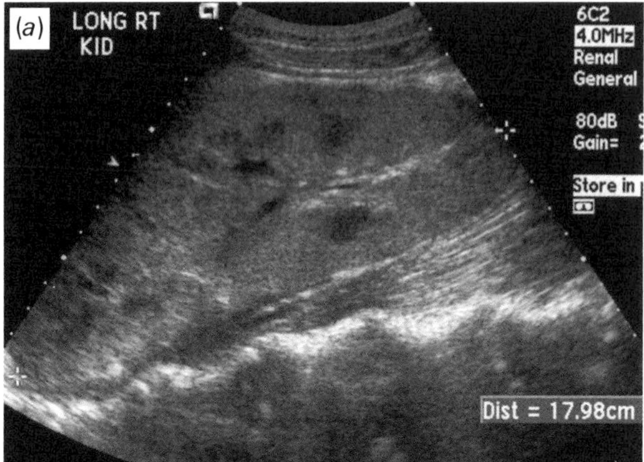

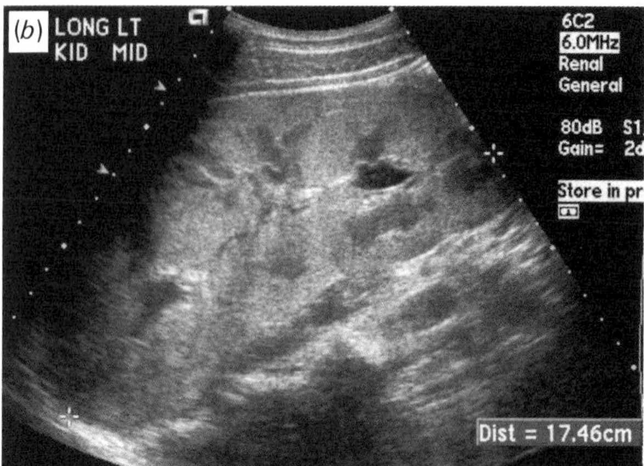

Figure 27.13 An 18-year-old boy with relapsed acute lymphocytic leukemia and diffuse bilateral leukemic renal infiltration. Ultrasound shows markedly enlarged, echogenic kidneys with multiple small, relatively hypoechoic, solid masses scattered throughout the parenchyma bilaterally. (*a*) Ultrasound: longitudinal view of the right kidney (length 18.0 cm). (*b*) Ultrasound: longitudinal view of the left kidney (length 17.5 cm).

manifestations of the disease. As a result, renal involvement is usually detected during staging or follow-up imaging studies in patients who are already known to have disease elsewhere.

Renal involvement is usually bilateral in both leukemia and lymphoma.[11,125,126] Leukemic infiltration of the kidneys causes diffuse renal enlargement, with disruption of the normal corticomedullary architecture (Figure 27.13). Discrete masses are less common in leukemia than in lymphoma. In lymphoma, neoplastic infiltration of the renal interstitium initially also causes non-specific renal enlargement, with diffuse increase in parenchymal echogenicity at US. As the infiltrating neoplastic cells coalesce to form larger, hypoechoic masses, the kidney enlarges and loses its reniform shape. The renal architecture is increasingly disrupted and the parenchyma becomes diffusely more inhomogeneous. At postcontrast CT, multiple coalescing low-attenuation, non-enhancing, solid masses are visible[124,126,127] (Figure 27.14). Perinephric extension and renal hilar and retroperitoneal lymph node involvement is better demonstrated at CT or MRI than at US. Follow-up imaging after successful treatment and regression of the masses often shows extensive cortical defects that can be indistinguishable from other causes of renal atrophy and cortical scarring. Dystrophic parenchymal calcifications are also occasionally seen following treatment for some forms of renal lymphoma (Figure 27.15).

Lymphoproliferative disorders are an important group of potentially life-threatening conditions that occur in patients who have severely impaired T-lymphocyte-mediated immunity. Lymphoproliferative disorders have been reported as a complication of immunosuppression for organ transplantation[128–130] in primary immunodeficiencies and in acquired immunodeficiency syndrome (AIDS).[50] Regardless of the cause

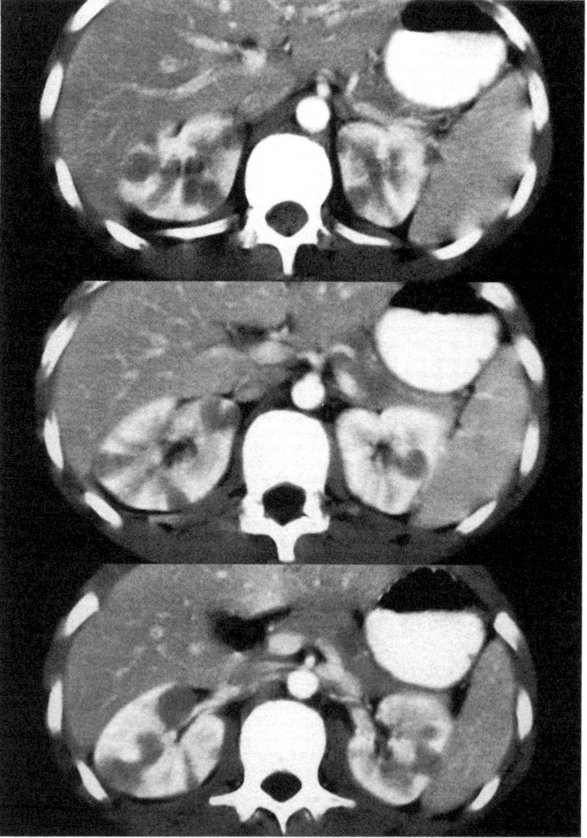

Figure 27.14 A 14-year-old boy with Burkitt's lymphoma of both kidneys. Contrast-enhanced CT shows multiple non-segmental, low-attenuation, non-enhancing solid masses scattered randomly throughout both kidneys.

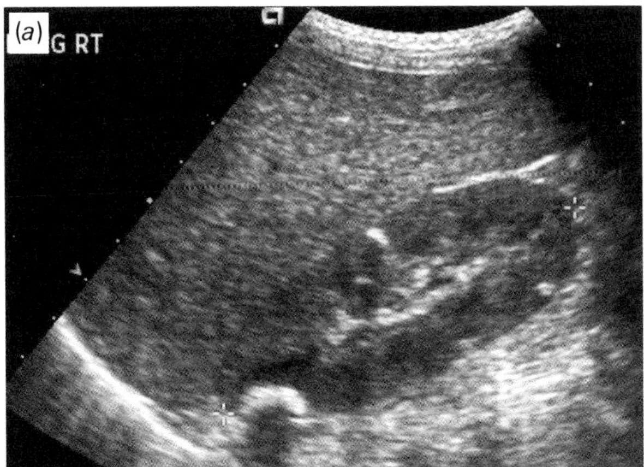

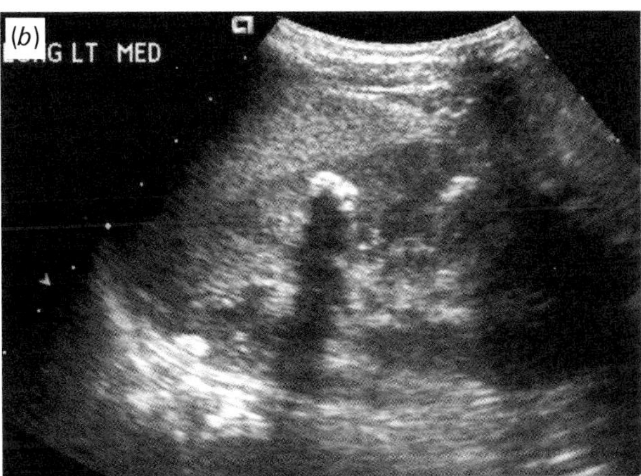

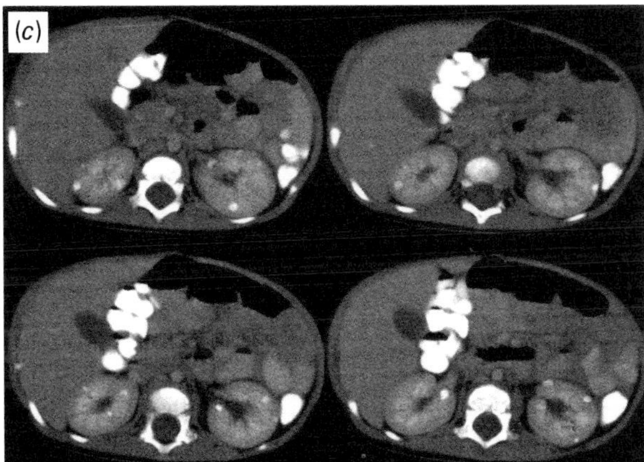

Figure 27.15 A young boy with bilateral dystrophic renal parenchymal calcifications 3 months after treatment for acute myelogenous leukemia. (*a*) Ultrasound: longitudinal view of the right kidney. (*b*) Ultrasound: longitudinal view of the left kidney. (*c*) Contrast-enhanced CT: four axial images through the kidneys.

of the immune defect, Epstein–Barr virus is critical in mediating the induction of polyclonal B-lymphocyte proliferation that leads to the development of lymphadenopathy, focal parenchymal masses, and diffuse infiltration of solid organs.[129,131] Involvement can be focal, multifocal, or widely disseminated, and any organ or body space can be involved. The gastrointestinal tract, solid abdominal organs, and abdominal lymph nodes are most often affected. Renal involvement occurs in 17–20% of cases and has imaging features similar to those of leukemia and lymphoma.

Congenital mesoblastic nephroma (fetal renal hamartoma)

Congenital mesoblastic nephroma (congenital fetal renal hamartoma) is the most common primary, renal tumor in the newborn and occurs almost exclusively in the first year of life.[132–135] Once believed to be a congenital form of Wilms' tumor, mesoblastic nephroma is distinguished by its younger presentation, its characteristically non-aggressive course and limited growth potential, its predominantly mesenchymal derivation, and its lack of a malignant epithelium. Recurrence is unusual as long as the entire mass is removed, although metastatic spread of mesoblastic nephroma to lung and brain has been reported very rarely.[136]

A mass is usually palpable at birth. However, mesoblastic nephroma is increasingly being detected at prenatal US. At US, mesoblastic nephroma appears as a large, solid, renal mass. The mass can be either homogeneous or complex. Cysts are present in 60% of cases and small, scattered calcifications can also occasionally be visible.[137] At CT the tumor presents as a non-enhancing, low-attenuation mass surrounded by enhancing residual normal parenchyma (Figure 27.16). Cystic areas of necrosis

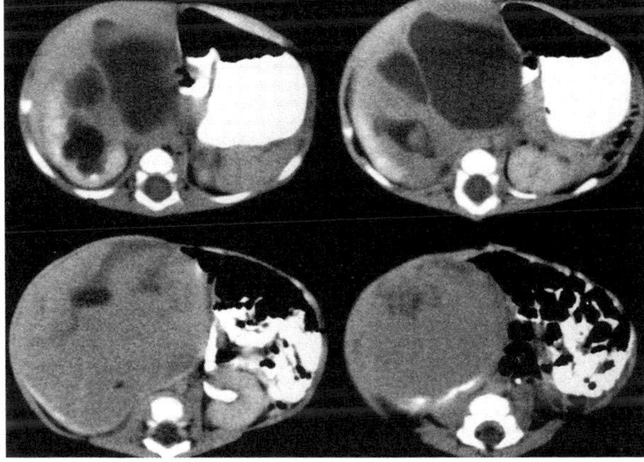

Figure 27.16 An 8-week-old girl with right congenital mesoblastic nephroma, presenting with a palpable right abdominal mass. Contrast-enhanced CT shows a large, solid, non-enhancing right renal mass that compresses the renal pelvis, resulting in obstruction and severe hydronephrosis.

and hemorrhage are readily demonstrated at CT, as are calcifications, when they occur.[133,134]

Multilocular cystic nephroma

Multilocular cystic nephroma is a benign, cystic renal tumor that is made up of non-communicating cysts of differing size separated by thin septa composed of fibrous tissue, tubular elements, and immature blastemal tissue.[138–140] The tumor can involve part or all of the kidney. Rarely, multiple discrete lesions are present. Although the cyst walls occasionally contain cellular elements that are histologically similar to Wilms' tumor, multilocular cystic nephroma has no malignant potential and local recurrence is rare after complete resection.

The imaging features of multilocular cystic nephroma are distinctive.[138,139] The tumor appears as a complex, multicystic mass with uniformly thin septa separating the cysts. The septa are usually more conspicuous at US than CT, although they can enhance somewhat after administration of contrast material. Thicker septa and septa that appear irregular or nodular are unusual in multilocular cystic nephroma and should raise concern that the lesion might instead represent a cystic Wilms' tumor.[140] Septal calcifications are occasionally present in adults, but are rarely seen in children. At MRI, the tumor capsule and septa appear hypointense on both T1- and T2-weighted images, with minimal enhancement after gadolinium.[141] The signal intensity of the fluid within the locules depends on their hemorrhagic and proteinaceous composition.

Angiomyolipoma

Angiomyolipoma is a benign, non-encapsulated, hamartoma of the kidney composed of blood vessels, smooth muscle, and fat.[142–144] In children, angiomyolipoma is very suggestive of tuberous sclerosis and is usually multiple and bilateral (Figure 27.17). Other clinical and imaging features of tuberous sclerosis are usually present. Less often, angiomyolipomas are detected in a child with undiagnosed tuberous sclerosis who presents with a palpable mass or hematuria. Renal cysts also occur in patients with tuberous sclerosis (Figure 27.18) and can coexist with angiomyolipomas.[143–145]

Visualization of fat within a renal mass in a child is highly suggestive of angiomyolipoma.[142–144] Rarely, the tumor has more vascular and muscular elements and contains little or no visible fat. Calcification is usually absent. Angiomyolipomas are usually very echogenic at US and have very low attenuation, similar to perinephric fat on non-enhanced CT scans. At MRI, the tumors are hyperintense on both T1- and T2-weighted images. Because angiomyolipomas are extremely vascular, they enhance very intensely at both CT and MRI. Larger angiomyolipomas tend to bleed, often profusely, resulting in intratumoral, subcapsular, and perinephric hemorrhage.

Renal lymphangioma and lymphangiomatosis

Renal lymphangioma is a rare, benign, cystic renal tumor with imaging features that are similar to multilocular cystic nephroma.[146,147] Renal lymphangioma

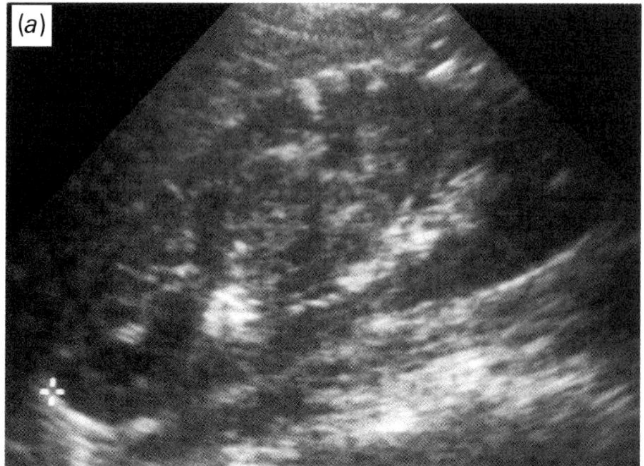

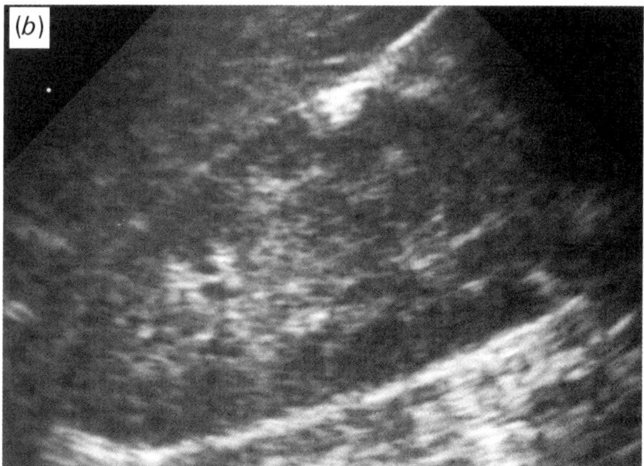

Figure 27.17 A 4-year-old girl with tuberous sclerosis and bilateral renal angiomyolipomas. Ultrasound shows multiple small, solid, non-shadowing echogenic masses scattered throughout both kidneys. (*a*) Ultrasound: longitudinal view of the right kidney (length 7.8 cm). (*b*) Ultrasound: longitudinal view of the left kidney (length 7.9 cm).

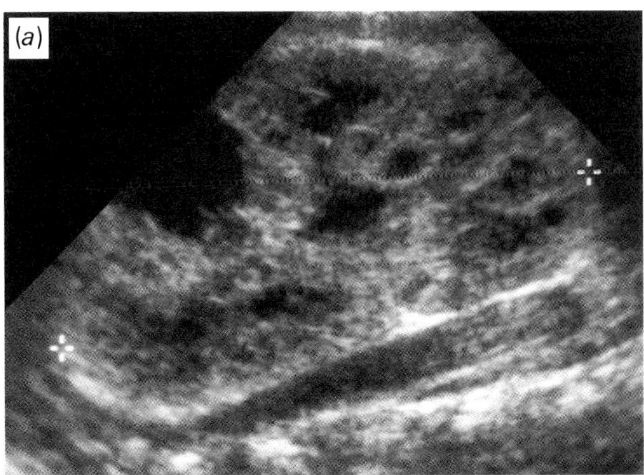

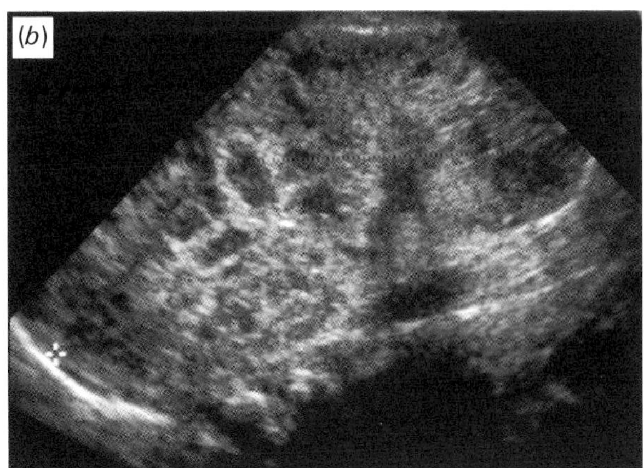

Figure 27.18 A 3-week-old boy with tuberous sclerosis and polycystic kidney disease. The kidneys are both enlarged and heterogeneous with numerous irregular cysts bilaterally. (*a*) Ultrasound: longitudinal view of the right kidney (length 7.0 cm). (*b*) Ultrasound: longitudinal view of the left kidney (length 7.9 cm).

can be either unilocular or multilocular and is usually solitary, although multiple lymphangiomas can occur. Renal lymphangiomatosis is a very rare disorder that is characterized by massive, bilateral nephromegaly with residual functioning islands of renal parenchyma appearing as irregular bands separating the innumerable cysts, simulating the appearance in advanced autosomal dominant polycystic kidney disease or tuberous sclerosis.[148] Lymphangiomatosis can be limited to the kidneys or can occur in association with more extensive retroperitoneal involvement. Cystic pulmonary lesions can also coexist.[149]

Renal cystic diseases

Ultrasound is the primary imaging modality that is used in renal cystic diseases.[5,6,11,150] CT and MRI are generally reserved for those cases in which either the sonographic appearances are uncertain or complications such cyst rupture, hemorrhage, or neoplasm are suspected.

Because isolated, simple renal cysts occur only very rarely in children,[5,6,151,152] the presence of renal cysts in a child should at least lead to consideration that these might be manifestations of an underlying renal disorder such as polycystic kidney disease or renal dysplasia. On the other hand, many cystic renal lesions that are identified at US in children are not cysts in the strict sense. Caliceal diverticula, dilated calices, and even very prominent and hypoechoic medullary pyramids are all very common and should not be mistaken for cysts.

At US, renal cysts appear as round or ovoid, thin-walled, fluid-filled structures.[11,50,150–152] The fluid within uncomplicated cysts is anechoic and the wall is thin and slightly hyperechoic. Cellular, purulent, or proteinaceous debris or blood clot in complicated cysts causes the fluid to appear more echogenic. Particular debris within the cyst fluid is best visualized at US. The fluid in uncomplicated cysts is of homogeneously low attenuation at CT and has low signal intensity on spin-echo and inversion recovery T1-weighted MRI images.[42,153,154] On spin-echo T2-weighted images, the signal intensity of the fluid increases and the wall of the cyst and the fluid may not be distinguishable. Although larger clots within cysts can often be identified at CT, differences in fluid composition and small particulate debris within the cyst fluid are more readily identified at MRI. The signal intensity in hemorrhagic cysts is generally brighter and more inhomogeneous on both T1- and T2-weighted images, but can vary considerably depending upon the age of the hemorrhage and the relative proportions of hemoglobin, deoxyhemoglobin, and hemosiderin. Mural calcification is rare in children in renal cysts, although it is well described in adults. Mural calcifications are best evaluated at CT or US, although larger calcifications are sometimes identifiable at MRI as a signal void within the cyst wall.

Caliceal diverticulum

Caliceal diverticulum is an urothelium-lined, saccular, outpouching of the collecting system that typically arises from one of the caliceal fornices.[42,88,155,156] Caliceal diverticula are believed to be congenital lesions. Rarely, a cyst, hematoma, or abscess that ruptures into a calyx will form a permanent communication with the collecting system and be can indistinguishable from a congenital diverticulum.

At US, caliceal diverticulum appears as a cystic lesion and is characteristically located centrally in the kidney, adjacent to the pyramids and collecting system.[42,88,155,156] Caliceal diverticula range in size from several millimeters to many centimeters. Individual diverticula can also vary considerably in size, depending upon the degree to which they are distended. Most diverticula communicate freely with the collecting system and will be opacified during either antegrade or retrograde urography as well as during postcontrast CT and MRI. However, when the neck of the diverticulum is stenotic, the fluid within the diverticulum will opacify only faintly or not at all. Comparison of the attenuation within the diverticulum on non-enhanced images with similar measurements on delayed postcontrast images may increase the chance of detecting faint opacification in a stenotic diverticulum. At non-enhanced CT and MRI, caliceal diverticula will similarly be difficult to differentiate from other centrally located cystic lesions.

Autosomal recessive polycystic kidney disease

Autosomal recessive polycystic disease is manifested by severe dilatation and ectasia of the interstitial portions of the collecting tubules.[157] At US, the kidneys are usually dramatically enlarged and inhomogeneously echogenic.[11,50,151,158,159] The echogenic appearance of the parenchyma relates to the abnormally increased reflectivity of the walls of the distended and ectatic tubules. The compressed renal cortex is studded with innumerable tiny cysts and appears as a relatively hypoechoic marginal halo around the kidney and occasionally around the individual renal lobes[158–160] (Figure 27.19). The same architectural changes are visible at CT, although the appearance is typically the video inverse of US, with relatively poorly enhancing ectatic tubules producing a peripherally radiating striated appearance to the enlarged central portions of the individual renal lobes surrounded by brightly enhancing compressed cortex studded with countless tiny cysts.[42]

Autosomal dominant polycystic kidney disease

When autosomal dominant polycystic disease presents in childhood the cysts are usually small and few in number early in life.[5,11,42,151] In neonates, the kidneys appear large and contain multiple small cysts, mimicking the appearance of the recessive form of the disease.[161] As the child becomes older, the cysts increase in size and number. Mural calcification is only rarely seen in children. Complications such as hemorrhage within a cyst can be visualized either at CT or MRI (Figure 27.20). MRI often shows striking differences in the signal intensity of the fluid in the cysts, reflecting differences in protein content of the fluid.[162]

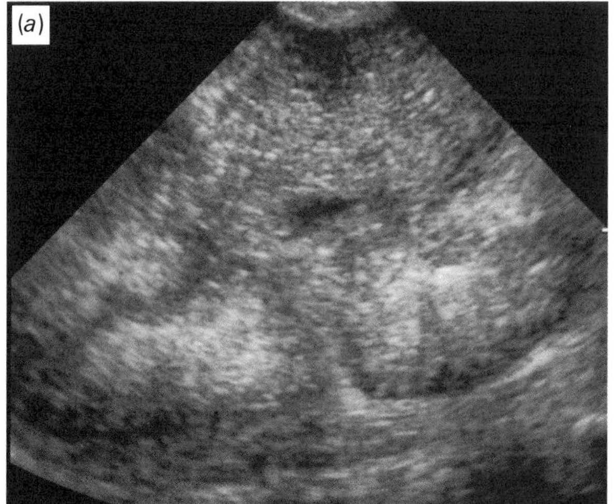

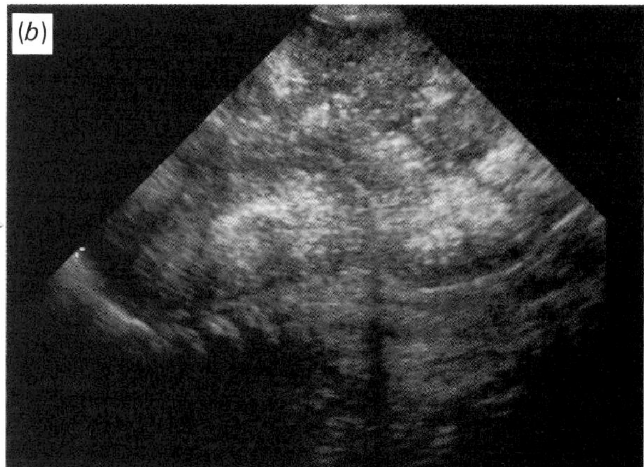

Figure 27.19 A newborn boy with autosomal recessive polycystic kidney disease. Ultrasound shows markedly enlarged kidneys, with accentuation of the renal lobar anatomy. The medullary portions of the renal lobes appear enlarged and very echogenic and are surrounded by a thin peripheral cortical halo. No larger macrocysts are visible. (*a*) Ultrasound: longitudinal view of the right kidney (length 12.7 cm). (*b*) Ultrasound: longitudinal view of the left kidney (length 13.2 cm).

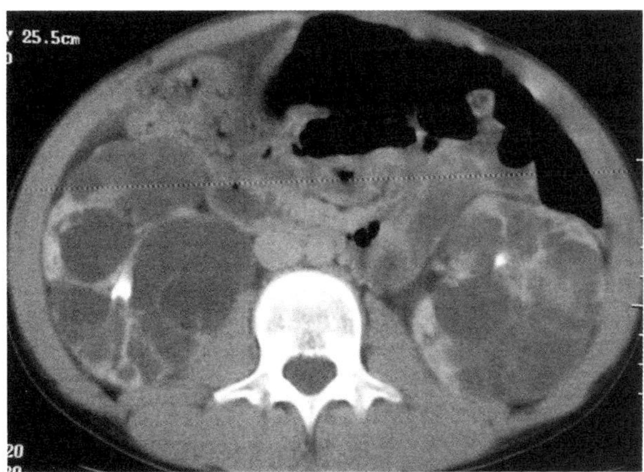

Figure 27.20 A 12-year-old girl with autosomal dominant polycystic kidney disease, presenting with abdominal pain and hematuria after a minor motor vehicle accident. Contrast-enhanced CT shows the kidneys to be almost entirely replaced by numerous large cysts, with strands of residual enhancing parenchyma visible between the cysts.

Glomerulocystic disease of the kidney

The characteristic histologic feature of glomerulocystic kidney disease is cystic dilatation of the space within Bowman's capsule surrounding the glomeruli.[11] Glomerulocystic kidney disease is a rare disorder that is frequently indistinguishable, based on its imaging and clinical features, from classic recessive polycystic disease in the neonate and from some cases of dominant polycystic kidney disease. Autosomal dominant transmission has been suggested in some lineages, with the parents of the affected infants presenting the classic imaging appearances of dominant polycystic disease. Liver disease similar to that in recessive polycystic disease can also occur. Glomerulocystic kidney disease also occurs in trisomy 13, oro–facial–digital syndrome, Zellweger syndrome, tuberous sclerosis, and Meckel–Gruber syndrome, and similar histologic changes are seen in some patients with renal dysplasia. Such widespread clinicopathologic overlap has led some clinicians to suggest that glomerulocystic kidney disease might in reality represent a non-specific histologic appearance rather than a specific disease.[163]

The imaging findings of countless small cysts in a predominantly cortical and subcapsular distribution suggests the diagnosis of glomerulocystic kidney disease.[11,159,164–167] The kidneys are often enlarged in neonates with this disorder, although often not as dramatically as in classic recessive polycystic disease, and the kidneys can decrease in size over time without apparent deterioration in renal function. In other cases, the appearance progresses over time to that typical of dominant polycystic disease. Because of the considerable overlap in the imaging appearances between this disorder and other more common forms of polycystic kidney disease, definitive diagnosis may ultimately require biopsy, where clinically justified.

Medullary cystic diseases

Juvenile nephronophthisis and adult-onset medullary cystic disease of the kidney are both familial forms of chronic tubulointerstitial nephritis that are associated with a urinary concentrating defect and progressive azotemia.[11,167–171] Medullary cysts are present in both diseases. However, the clinical manifestations and patterns of transmission are different. Juvenile nephronophthisis is an autosomal recessive disorder that primarily affects children and is characterized clinically by polyuria, growth failure, and progressive renal insufficiency, usually leading to death in later childhood. Juvenile nephronophthisis is frequently associated with a variety of extrarenal abnormalities, including retinitis pigmentosa, cone-shaped epiphyses, hepatic fibrosis, and cerebellar aplasia. Adult-onset medullary cystic disease is an autosomal dominant disorder with no extrarenal manifestations that typically presents in the third decade or later and is rarely diagnosed in children.

In juvenile nephronophthisis, the kidneys are small or normal in size at US, with diffusely increased parenchymal echogenicity and medullary cysts.[11,169–171] Although medullary cysts are regarded as a characteristic sonographic feature of juvenile nephronophthisis, increased parenchymal echogenicity with loss of corticomedullary differentiation can precede the development of visible macrocysts, resulting in a non-specific appearance in some patients. Very thin-section (1.5 mm) CT or MRI can confirm the presence of medullary cysts in children with atypical sonographic appearances.[167,168,170]

Medullary sponge kidney is a rare, non-hereditary disorder of unknown cause that is characterized by non-progressive medullary ductal ectasia, renal tubular acidosis, hypercalciuria, and nephrocalcinosis.[11] At excretory urography, the appearance reflects the severity of the ductal ectasia.[172] In very mild cases, the medulla has a thinly striated appearance. With more severe involvement, the linear medullary striations first become thicker and then cystic in appearance. Small calculi form within the tubules and the papillae enlarge as the calices become progressively more distorted. In the most advanced cases, abdominal radiographs reveal nephrocalcinosis, nephrolithiasis, or both. The appearance of multiple clusters of tiny calculi overlying the medullary pyramids is diagnostic of medullary sponge kidney. Calculi that have eroded into the collecting system are visible in the renal pelves, ureters, or bladder. At US, renal size is normal and the medullary pyramids appear hyperechoic as a result of intraluminal calcium deposition.[11,172,173] Shadowing intratubular calculi appear later in the disease. CT is generally inferior to excretory urography in detecting tubular ectasia in medullary sponge kidney and is invariably normal early in the disease. However, subsequently, non-enhanced CT may be better for identifying small intratubular calculi that would be obscured by contrast material at excretory urography.

Renal dysplasia and multicystic dysplastic kidney

Normal nephroureteral development entails a series of complex interactions between the ureteric bud and the developing metanephros, beginning in the 7th gestational week. Failure of these interactions to proceed normally can result in renal dysplasia. Although renal dysplasia is frequently associated with congenital obstructive uropathy,[174–176] it can also occur in the absence of detectable obstruction in patients with severe VUR and as an isolated anomaly.[7,177] Sonographically, dysplastic kidneys are usually small for age or body size and grow slowly. The renal parenchyma appears abnormally echogenic, with reduced or absent corticomedullary differentiation.[5,6,11,178,179] Cysts are present in 40–50% of cases. In cases of severe dysplasia associated with obstruction, the collecting system can be dysmorphic, with poor differentiation of the calices, infundibula, and renal pelvis.[6] When cysts or hydronephrosis are present, the renal measurements may underestimate the reduction in total renal parenchymal volume. At scintigraphy, dysplastic kidneys typically have reduced function, although complete absence of function is uncommon, a feature that is important in distinguishing typical renal dysplasia from multicystic dysplastic kidney (MCDK). Although the appearance at US of a small, echogenic kidney that functions poorly at scintigraphy is usually diagnostic of dysplasia in a neonate, this sonographic appearance is not specific. In an infant or child, a variety of chronic and atrophic renal parenchymal disorders, including interstitial nephritis, chronic glomerulonephritis, and severe reflux nephropathy, as well as renal infarction secondary to acute tubular or cortical necrosis, renal vein thrombosis, or renal arterial obstruction, can be sono-

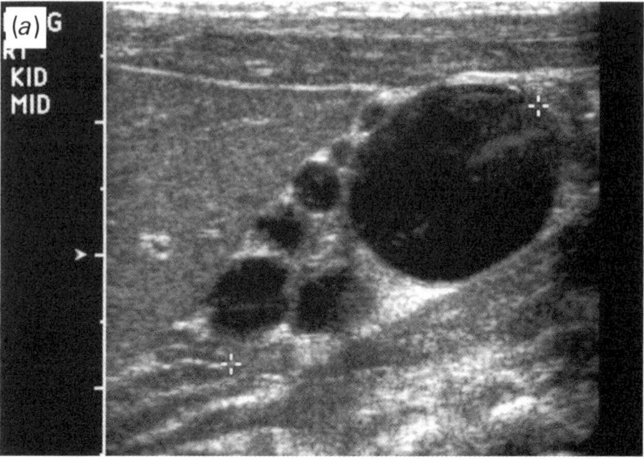

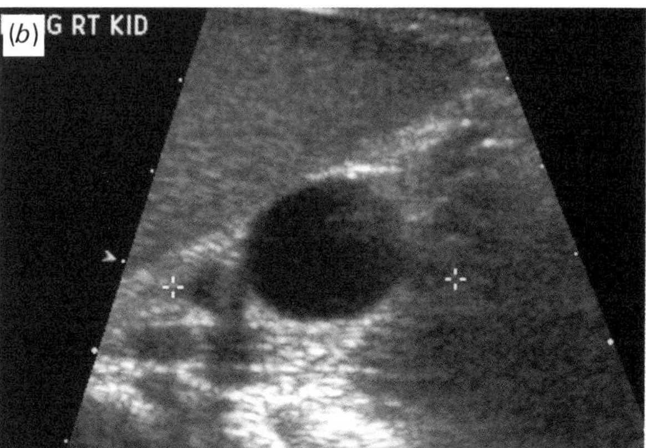

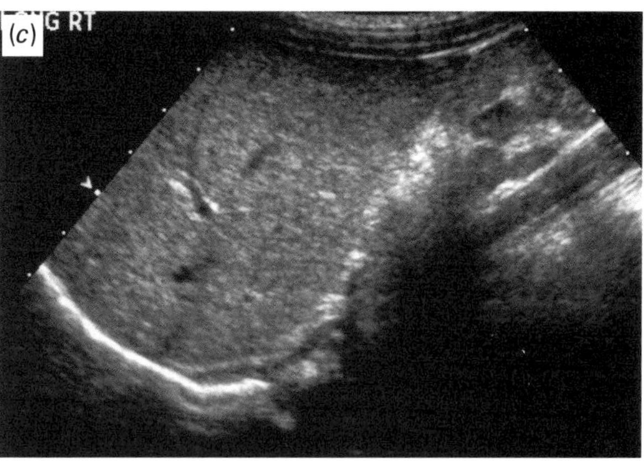

Figure 27.21 A newborn boy with right multicystic dysplastic kidney and subsequent involution. (*a*) Ultrasound: longitudinal view of the right kidney at 2 days old shows the right kidney (length 4.2 cm) is entirely replaced by multiple non-communicating cysts of different sizes separated by thin bands of echogenic, dysplastic parenchyma. (*b*) Ultrasound: longitudinal view of the right kidney at 8 months old shows all of the cysts have decreased in size and the kidney now measures 3.1 cm in length. (*c*) Ultrasound: longitudinal view of the right renal fossa at 18 months old shows no residual visible cysts or right kidney.

graphically indistinguishable from renal dysplasia in the absence of suggestive historical or biochemical information or previous imaging studies.[6,178,179]

In MCDK, atresia of the ureteral bud at or just below the ureteropelvic junction early in nephrogenesis results in a severely dysplastic, non-functioning, cystic kidney.[6,180–182] The diagnosis of MCDK is usually easily established based on characteristic imaging findings at US and renal diuretic or cortical scintigraphy of a non-functioning kidney that is replaced by multiple non-communicating cysts with no residual normal-appearing parenchyma.[6,182] At CT and MRI, the kidney is replaced by multiple cysts of different sizes that are separated by a small amount of non-functioning, dysplastic parenchyma (Figure 27.21). In the hydronephrotic variant of multicystic dysplasia, the kidney is non-functioning and contains one or more smaller peripheral cysts, with a large central cyst representing a rudimentary, dilated collecting system.[181] In segmental MCDK, the anomaly affects only one moiety of a partially or completely duplicated collecting system. When bilateral, MCDK is incompatible with extrauterine life and is usually accompanied by severe oligohydramnios, pulmonary hypoplasia, and other features of Potter's syndrome.

In most patients with MCDK, the fluid within the cysts is gradually absorbed and the kidney progressively decreases in size until it is no longer identifiable at US[183–186] (see Figure 27.21). Because the dysplastic renal remnant has no function, it will not be identifiable at renal scintigraphy. This process of 'involution' ultimately results in an appearance that is indistinguishable from unilateral renal agenesis.[187]

References

1. Einstein DM, Singer AA, Paushter DM, Nasif A, Nally JV Jr. Hypoechoic renal pyramids: sonographic visualization in older children and young adults. Urol Radiol 1992; 13:162–5.
2. Hricak H, Slovis TL, Callen CW, Callen PW, Romanski RN. Neonatal kidneys: sonographic anatomic correlation. Radiology 1983; 147:699–702.
3. McInnis AN, Felman AH, Kaude JV, Walker RD. Renal ultrasound in the neonatal period. Pediatr Radiol 1982; 12:15–20.
4. Leonidas JC, McCauley RG, Klauber GC, Fretzayas AM. Sonography as a substitute for excretory urography in children with urinary tract infection. AJR Am J Roentgenol 1985; 144:815–19.
5. Teele RL, Share JS. Renal screening. In: Teele RL, Share JS, eds. Ultrasonography in Infants and Children. Philadelphia, PA: WB Saunders, 1991: 137–92.
6. Zerin JM. Postnatal renal sonographic screening. In: Gearhart JP, Rink RC, Mouriquand PDE, eds. Pediatric Urology. Philadelphia: WB Saunders, 2001.
7. Marra G, Barbieri G, Dell'Agnola CA et al. Congenital renal damage associated with primary vesicoureteral reflux detected prenatally in male infants. J Pediatr 1994; 124(5 part 1):726–30.
8. Haller JO, Berdon WE, Friedman AP. Increased renal cortical echogenicity: a normal finding in neonates and infants. Radiology 1982; 142(1):173–4.
9. Vehmas T, Paivansalo M, Taavitsainen M, Suramo I. Ultrasound in renal pyogenic infection. Imaging and intervention. Acta Radiol 1988; 29(6):675–8.
10. Feeks EF, Maino TJ, Proctor JG, Bower EA. An abscess that wasn't: renal calyceal diverticulum in a student naval aviator. Aviat Space Environ Med 1998; 69(8):785–7.
11. Siegel MJ. The urinary tract. In: Siegel MJ, ed. Pediatric Sonography, 3rd edn. Philadelphia: Lippincott, Williams and Wilkins, 2001: 386–473.
12. Kraus RA, Gaisie G, Young LW. Increased renal parenchymal echogenicity: causes in pediatric patients. Radiographics 1990; 10:1009–18.
13. Brenbridge AN, Chevalier RL, Kaiser DL. Increased renal cortical echogenicity in pediatric renal disease: histopathologic correlations. J Clin Ultrasound 1986; 14(8):595–600.
14. Winkler P, Altrogge H. Sonographic signs of nephritis in children. A comparison of renal echography with clinical evaluation, laboratory data and biopsy. Pediatr Radiol 1985; 15(4):231–7.
15. Kraus SJ. Genitourinary imaging in children. Pediatr Clin North Am 2001; 48(6):1381–424.
16. Rochester D, Aronson AJ, Bowie JD, Kunzmann A. Ultrasonic appearance of acute poststreptococcal glomerulonephritis. J Clin Ultrasound 1978; 6(1):49–50.
17. Zerin JM, Blane CE. Sonographic assessment of renal length in children: a reappraisal. Pediatr Radiol 1994; 24:101–6.
18. Laplante S, Patriquin HB, Robitaille P et al. Renal vein thrombosis in children: evidence of early flow recovery with Doppler US. Radiology 1993; 189(1):37–42.
19. Kangarloo H, Gold RH, Fine RN, Diament MJ, Boechat MI. Urinary tract infection in infants and children evaluated by ultrasound. Radiology 1985; 154:367–73.
20. Johnson CE, DeBaz BP, Shurin PA, DeBartolomeo R. Renal ultrasound evaluation of urinary tract infections in children. Pediatrics 1986; 78:871–8.
21. Alon U, Pery M, Davidai G, Berant M. Ultrasonography in the radiologic evaluation of children with urinary tract infection. Pediatrics 1986; 78:58–64.
22. Dinkel E, Orth S, Dittrich M, Schulte-Wisserman H. Renal sonography in the differentiation of upper from lower urinary tract infection. AJR Am J Roentgenol 1986; 146:775–80.
23. Lebowitz RL, Mandell J. Urinary tract infection in children: putting radiology in its place. Radiology 1987; 165:1–9.
24. Klar A, Hurvitz H, Berkun Y et al. Focal bacterial nephritis (lobar nephronia) in children. J Pediatr 1996; 128:850–3.
25. Zerin JM. Uroradiologic emergencies in infants and children. Radiol Clin North Am 1997; 35:897–919.

26. American Academy of Pediatrics. Practice Guideline. The diagnosis, treatment, and evaluation of the initial urinary tract infections in febrile infants and young children (AC9830). Pediatrics 1999; 103:843–52.
27. Pennington DJ, Zerin JM. Imaging of the urinary tract infection in children. Pediatr Ann 1999; 28(11):678–86.
28. Dacher JN, Avni F, Francois A et al. Renal sinus hyperechogenicity in acute pyelonephritis: description and pathological correlation. Pediatr Radiol 1999; 29(3):179–82.
29. Zerin JM. Reflux nephropathy. In: Pollack HM, McClennan BL, eds. Clinical Urography. Philadelphia: WB Saunders, 2000.
30. Dacher JN, Pfister C, Monroc M, Eurin D, LeDosseur. Power Doppler sonographic pattern of acute pyelonephritis in children: comparison with CT. AJR Am J Roentgenol 1996; 166:1451–5.
31. Pickworth FE, Carlin JB, Ditchfield MR et al. Sonographic measurement of renal enlargement in children with acute pyelonephritis and time needed for resolution: implications for renal growth assessment. AJR Am J Roentgenol 1995; 165(2):405–8.
32. Johansson B, Troell S, Berg U. Renal parenchymal volume during and after acute pyelonephritis measured by ultrasonography. Arch Dis Child 1988; 63(11):1309–14.
33. Björgvinsson E, Majd M, Eggli KD. Diagnosis of acute pyelonephritis in children: comparison of sonography and ^{99m}Tc-DMSA scintigraphy. AJR Am J Roentgenol 1991; 157:539–43.
34. Rushton HG. The evaluation of acute pyelonephritis and renal scarring with technetium 99m-dimercaptosuccinic acid renal scintigraphy: evolving concepts and future directions. Pediatr Nephrol 1997; 11:108–20.
35. Lonergan GJ, Pennington DJ, Morrison JC et al. Childhood pyelonephritis: comparison of gadolinium-enhanced MR imaging and renal cortical scintigraphy for diagnosis. Radiology 1998; 207:377–84.
36. Majd M, Nussbaum Blask AR, Markle BM et al. Diagnosis of experimental pyelonephritis in piglets: comparison of 99m Tc DMSA SPECT, spiral CT, MRI and power Doppler US in an experimental pig model. Radiology 2001; 218(1):101–8.
37. Sfakianakis GN, Cavagnaro F, Zilleruelo G et al. Diuretic MAG3 scintigraphy (F0) in acute pyelonephritis: regional parenchymal dysfunction and comparison with DMSA. J Nucl Med 2000; 41(12):1955–63.
38. Sfakianakis GN, Georgiou MF. MAG3 SPECT: a rapid procedure to evaluate the renal parenchyma. J Nucl Med 1997; 38(3):478–83.
39. Lee JK, McClennan BL, Melson GL, Stanley RJ. Acute focal bacterial nephritis: emphasis on gray scale sonography and computed tomography. AJR Am J Roentgenol 1980; 135:87–92.
40. Dacher JN, Boillot B, Eurin D et al. Rational use of CT in acute pyelonephritis: findings and relationship with reflux. Pediatr Radiol 1993; 23:281–5.
41. Pennington DJ, Lonergan GJ, Flack CE, Waguespack RL, Jackson CB. Experimental pyelonephritis in piglets: diagnosis with MR imaging. Radiology 1996; 201:199–205.
42. Zerin JM. CT and MRI of the kidneys in children. In: Haaga JR, Lanzieri CF, Gilkeson RC, eds. Computed Tomography and Magnetic Resonance Imaging of the Whole Body, 4th edn. St Louis: Mosby, 2003.
43. Weiser AC, Amukele SA, Leonidas JC, Palmer LS. The role of gadolinium enhanced magnetic resonance imaging for children with suspected acute pyelonephritis. J Urol 2003; 169(6):2308–11.
44. Chan JH, Tsui EY, Luk SH et al. MR diffusion-weighted imaging of kidney: differentiation between hydronephrosis and pyonephrosis. Clin Imaging 2001; 25(2):110–13.
45. Verswijvel G, Vandecaveye V, Gelin G et al. Diffusion-weighted MR imaging in the evaluation of renal infection: preliminary results. JBR-BTR 2002; 85(2):100–3.
46. Altinok D, Zerin JM, Grattan-Smith JD. Magnetic resonance imaging of renal anomalies and pyelonephritis in infants and children. In: Morcos S, Cohan RH, eds. New Techniques in Uroradiology. London: Taylor & Francis, 2006.
47. Bryant K, Maxfield C, Rabalais G. Renal candidiasis in neonates with candiduria. Pediatr Infect Dis J 1999; 18(11):959–63.
48. Karlowicz MG. Candidal renal and urinary tract infection in neonates. Semin Perinatol 2003; 27(5):393–400.
49. Fung Y, Yeh HC. Renal aspergilloma mimicking a tumor on ultrasonography. J Ultrasound Med 1997; 16(8):555–7.
50. Zinn HL, Haller JO. Renal manifestations of AIDS in children. Pediatr Radiol 1999; 29:558–61.
51. Mendez G Jr, Ishikoff MB, Morillo G. The role of computed tomography in the diagnosis of renal and perirenal abscesses. J Urol 1979; 122:582–6.
52. Soulen MC, Fishman EK, Goldman SM. Sequelae of acute renal infections: CT evaluation. Radiology 1989; 173:423–6.
53. Jeffrey RB, Laing FC, Wing VW, Hoddick W. Sensitivity of sonography in pyonephrosis: a re-evaluation. AJR Am J Roentgenol 1985; 144(1):71–3.
54. Kim JC. US and CT findings of xanthogranulomatous pyelonephritis. Clin Imaging 2001; 25(2):118–21.
55. Quinn FM, Dick AC, Corbally MT, McDermott MB, Guiney EJ. Xanthogranulomatous pyelonephritis in childhood. Arch Dis Child 1999; 81(6):483–6.
56. Kim J. Ultrasonographic features of focal xanthogranulomatous pyelonephritis. J Ultrasound Med 2004; 23(3):409–16.
57. Tiu CM, Chou YH, Chiou HJ et al. Sonographic features of xanthogranulomatous pyelonephritis. J Clin Ultrasound 2001; 29(5):279–85.
58. Hodson CJ, Maling TM, McManamon PJ, Lewis MG. The pathogenesis of reflux nephropathy (chronic atrophic pyelonephritis). Br J Radiol 1975; (Suppl 13):1–26.
59. McInnis AN, Felman AH, Kaude JV, Walker RD. Renal ultrasound in the neonatal period. Pediatr Radiol 1982; 12:15–20.
60. Hoffer FA, Hanaberg AM, Teele RL. The interrenicular junction: a mimic of renal scarring on normal pediatric sonograms. AJR Am J Roentgenol 1985; 145:1075–8.
61. Rushton HG, Majd M, Jantausch B, Wiedermann BL, Belman AB. Renal scarring following reflux and nonreflux pyelonephritis in children: evaluation with 99m tech-

netium-dimercaptosuccinic acid scintigraphy. J Urol 1992; 147:1327–32.
62. Rodriguez LV, Spielman D, Herfkens RJ, Shortliffe LD. Magnetic resonance imaging for the evaluation of hydronephrosis, reflux and renal scarring in children. J Urol 2001; 166(3):1023–7.
63. Chan YL, Chan KW, Yeung CK et al. Potential utility of MRI in the evaluation of children at risk of renal scarring. Pediatr Radiol 1999; 29(11):856–62.
64. Brill PW, Jagannath A, Winchester P, Markisz JA, Zirinsky K. Adrenal hemorrhage and renal vein thrombosis in the newborn: MR imaging. Radiology 1989; 170(1 Pt 1):95–8.
65. Bennett WG, Wood BP. Radiological case of the month. Left renal vein thrombosis and left adrenal hemorrhage. Am J Dis Child 1991; 145:1299–300.
66. Metreweli C, Pearson R. Echographic diagnosis of neonatal renal venous thrombosis. Pediatr Radiol 1984; 14:105–8.
67. Hibbert J, Howlett DC, Greenwood KL, MacDonald LM, Saunders AJ. The ultrasound appearances of neonatal renal vein thrombosis. Br J Radiol 1997; 70(839):1191–4.
68. Argyropoulou MI, Giapros VI, Papadopoulou F et al. Renal venous thrombosis in an infant with predisposing thrombotic factors: color Doppler ultrasound and MR evaluation. Eur Radiol 2003; 13(8):2027–30.
69. Jayogapal S, Cohen HL, Brill PW, Winchester P, Eaton D. Calcified renal vein thrombosis demonstration by CT and US. Pediatr Radiol 1990; 20:160–2.
70. Rypens F, Avni F, Braude P et al. Calcified inferior vena cava thrombus in a fetus: perinatal imaging. J Ultrasound Med 1993; 12(1):55–8.
71. Wilkinson AG, Murphy AV, Stewart G. Renal venous thrombosis with calcification and preservation of renal function. Pediatr Radiol 2001; 31(3):140–3.
72. Helenon O, el Rody F, Correas JM et al. Color Doppler US of renovascular disease in native kidneys. Radiographics 1995; 15:833–54.
73. Martin KW, McAlister WH, Shackelford GD. Acute renal infarction: diagnosis by Doppler ultrasound. Pediatr Radiol 1988; 18:373–6.
74. Taylor GA, Ecklund K, Dunning PS. Renal cortical perfusion in rabbits: visualization with color amplitude imaging and experimental microbubble-based US contrast agent. Radiology 1996; 201:125–9.
75. Taylor GA. Potential pediatric applications for US contrast agents: lessons from the laboratory. Pediatr Radiol 2000; 30:101–9.
76. Choyke PL, Grant EG, Hoffer FA, Tina L, Korec S. Cortical echogenicity in the hemolytic uremic syndrome: clinical correlation. J Ultrasound Med 1988; 7(8):439–42.
77. Kenney PJ, Brinsko RE, Patel DV, Spitzer RE, Farrar FM. Sonography of the kidneys in hemolytic uremic syndrome. Invest Radiol 1986; 21(7):547–50.
78. Patriquin HB, O'Regan S, Robitaille P, Paltiel H. Hemolytic-uremic syndrome: intrarenal arterial Doppler patterns as a useful guide to therapy. Radiology 1989; 172(3):625–8.
79. Toyoda K, Miyamoto Y, Ida M, Tada S, Utsunomiya M. Hyperechoic medulla of the kidney. Radiology 1989; 173:431–4.
80. Jequier S, Kaplan BS. Echogenic renal pyramids in children. J Clin Ultrasound 1991; 19:85–92.
81. Schultz PK, Strife JL, Strife CF, McDaniel JD. Hyperechoic renal medullary pyramids in infants and children. Radiology 1991; 181:163–7.
82. Al-Murrani B, Cosgrove DO, Svensson WE, Blaszczyk M. Echogenic rings – an ultrasound sign of early nephrocalcinosis. Clin Radiol 1991; 44:49–51.
83. Paivansalo MJ, Kallioinen MJ, Merikanto JS, Jalovaara PK. Hyperechogenic 'rings' in the periphery of renal medullary pyramids as a sign of renal disease. J Clin Ultrasound 1991; 19:283–7.
84. Patriquin H, Robitaille P. Renal calcium deposition in children: sonographic demonstration of the Anderson–Carr progression. AJR Am J Roentgenol 1986; 146: 1253–6.
85. Fick JJA, Beek FJA. Echogenic kidneys and medullary calcium deposition in a young child with glycogen storage disease type 1a. Pediatr Radiol 1992; 22:72–3.
86. Rosenfeld DL, Preston MP, Salvaggi-Fadden K. Serial renal sonographic evaluation of patients with Lesch–Nyhan syndrome. Pediatr Radiol 1994; 24: 509–12.
87. Stevens SK, Parker BR. Renal oxypurine deposition in Lesch–Nyhan syndrome: sonographic evaluation. Pediatr Radiol 1989; 19:479–80.
88. Starinsky R, Vardi O, Batasch D, Goldberg M. Increased renal medullary echogenicity in neonates. Pediatr Radiol 1995; 25:S43–5.
89. Khoory BJ, Andreis IAB, Vino L, Fanos F. Transient hyperechogenicity of the renal medullary pyramids: incidence in the healthy term newborn. Am J Perinatol 1999; 16:463–7.
90. Breslow NR, Beckwith JB. Epidemiological features of Wilms' tumor: results of the National Wilms' Tumor Study. J Natl Cancer Inst 1982; 68:429–36.
91. D'Angio GJ, Beckwith JB, Breslow N et al. Wilms tumor: status report, 1990: By the National Wilms Tumor Study Committee. J Clin Oncol 1991; 9:877–87.
92. Beckwith JB. Children at increased risk for Wilms tumor: monitoring issues. J Pediatr 1998; 132:377–9.
93. DeBaun MR, Tucker MA. Risk of cancer during the first four years of life in children from the Beckwith–Wiedemann Syndrome Registry. J Pediatr 1998; 132:398–400.
94. Beckwith JB, Kiviat NB, Bonadio JF. Nephrogenic rests, nephroblastomatosis, and the pathogenesis of Wilms' tumor. Pediatr Pathol 1990; 10:1–36.
95. Ritchey ML, Green DM, Breslow NB, Moksness J, Norkool P. Accuracy of current imaging modalities in the diagnosis of synchronous bilateral Wilms' tumor. Cancer 1995; 75:600–4.
96. Fishman EK, Hartman DS, Goldman SM, Siegelman SS. The CT appearance of Wilms tumor. J Comput Assist Tomogr 1983; 7:659–65.
97. Parvey LS, Warner RM, Callihan TR, Magill HL. CT demonstration of fat tissue in malignant renal neoplasms: atypical Wilms' tumors. J Comput Assist Tomogr 1981; 5:851–4.
98. Belt TG, Cohen MD, Smith JA et al. MRI of Wilms' tumor: promise as the primary imaging method. AJR Am J Roentgenol 1986; 146:955–61.

99. Boechat MI. Magnetic resonance imaging of abdominal and pelvic masses in children. Top Magn Reson Imaging 1990; 3:25–41.
100. Bilal MM, Brown JJ. MR imaging of renal and adrenal masses in children. Magn Reson Imaging Clin N Am 1997; 5:179–97.
101. Bellin M, Maidenberg M, Raveau V et al. MR imaging of adult Wilms' tumor: correlation with US, CT, and pathology. Urol Radiol 1990; 12:148–50.
102. Reiman TAH, Siegel MJ, Shackelford GD. Wilms' tumor in children: abdominal CT and US evaluation. Radiology 1986; 160:501–5.
103. Nakayama DK, Norkool P, de Lorimier AA, O'Neill JA Jr, D'Angio GJ. Intracardiac extension of Wilms' tumor. A report of the National Wilms' Tumor Study. Ann Surg 1986; 204:693–7.
104. Weese DL, Appelbaum H, Taber P. Mapping intravascular extension of Wilms' tumor with magnetic resonance imaging. J Pediatr Surg 1991; 26:64–7.
105. Brasch RC, Randel SB, Gould RG. Follow-up of Wilms' tumor: comparison of CT with other imaging procedures. AJR Am J Roentgenol 1981; 137:1005–9.
106. Papadopoulou E, Efremidis SC, Gombakis N, Tsouris J, Kehagia T. Nephroblastomatosis: the whole spectrum of abnormalities in one case. Pediatr Radiol 1992; 22:598–9.
107. White KS, Kirks DR, Bove KE. Imaging of nephroblastomatosis: an overview. Radiology 1992; 182:1–5.
108. Rohrscheider WK, Weirch A, Rieden K et al. US, CT and MR imaging characteristics of nephroblastomatosis. Pediatr Radiol 1998; 28:435–43.
109. Fernbach SK, Feinstein KA, Donaldson JS, Baum ES. Nephroblastomatosis: comparison of CT with US and urography. Radiology 1988; 166:153–6.
110. Glylys-Morin VM, Hoffer FA, Kozkewich H, Shamberger RC. Wilms tumor and nephroblastomatosis: imaging characteristics. Radiology 1993; 188:517–21.
111. Andrews MW, Amparo EG. Wilms' tumor in a patient with Beckwith–Wiedemann syndrome: onset detected with 3-month serial sonography. AJR Am J Roentgenol 1993; 160:139–40.
112. Beckwith JB, Palmer NF. Histopathology and prognosis of Wilms' tumor: results from the first National Wilms' Tumor Study. Cancer 1978; 41:1937–48.
113. Morgan E, Kidd JM. Undifferentiated sarcoma of the kidney: a tumor of childhood with histopathologic and clinical characteristics distinct from Wilms' tumor. Cancer 1978; 42:1916–21.
114. Lamego CMB, Zerbini MCN. Bone-metastasizing primary renal tumors in children. Radiology 1983; 147:449–54.
115. Glass RBJ, Davidson AJ, Fernbach SK. Clear cell sarcoma of the kidney: CT, sonographic, and pathologic correlation. Radiology 1991; 180:715–17.
116. Weeks DA, Beckwith JB, Mierau GW, Luckey DW. Rhabdoid tumor of kidney: a report of 111 cases from the National Wilms' Tumor Study Pathology Center. Am J Surg Pathol 1989; 13:439–58.
117. Bonnin JM, Rubinstein LJ, Palmer NF, Beckwith JB. The association of embryonal tumors originating in the kidney and in the brain: a report of seven cases. Cancer 1984; 54:2137–46.
118. Sisler CL, Siegel MJ. Malignant rhabdoid tumor of the kidney: radiologic features. Radiology 1989; 172: 211–12.
119. Kabala JE, Shield J, Duncan A. Renal cell carcinoma in childhood. Pediatr Radiol 1992; 22:203–5.
120. Lowe LH, Isuani BH, Heller RM et al. Pediatric renal masses: Wilms tumor and beyond. Radiographics 2000; 20:1585–603.
121. Davidson AJ, Choyke PL, Hartman DS, Davis CJ Jr. Renal medullar carcinoma associated with sickle cell trait: radiologic findings. Radiology 1995; 195:83–5.
122. Wesche WA, Wilmas J, Khare V, Parham DM. Renal medullary carcinoma: a potential sickle cell nephropathy of children and adolescents. Pediatr Pathol Lab Med 1998; 18:97–113.
123. Davis CJ Jr, Mostofi FK, Sesterhenn IA. Renal medullary carcinoma: the seventh sickle cell nephropathy. Am J Surg Pathol 1995; 19:1–11.
124. Araki T. Leukemic involvement of the kidney in children: CT features. J Comput Assist Tomogr 1982; 6:781–4.
125. McGuire PM, Merritt CRB, Ducos RS. Ultrasonography of primary renal lymphoma in a child. J Ultrasound Med 1996; 15:479–81.
126. Weinberger E, Rosenbaum DM, Pendergrass TW. Renal involvement in children with lymphoma: a comparison of CT with sonography. AJR Am J Roentgenol 1990; 155:347–9.
127. Sheeran SR, Sussman SK. Renal lymphoma: spectrum of CT findings and potential mimics. AJR Am J Roentgenol 1998; 171:1067–72.
128. Donnelly LF, Frush DP, Marshall KW, White KS. Lymphoproliferative disorders: CT findings in immunocompromised children. AJR Am J Roentgenol 1998; 171:725–31.
129. Nalesnik MA, Makowka L, Starzl TE. The diagnosis and treatment of post-transplant lymphoproliferative disorders. Curr Prob Surg 1988; 25:370–472.
130. Pickhardt PJ, Siegel MJ. Post-transplantation lymphoproliferative disorder of the abdomen: CT evaluation in 51 patients. Radiology 1999; 213:73–8.
131. List AF, Greco FA, Vogler LB. Lymphoproliferative diseases in immunocompromised hosts: the role of Epstein–Barr virus. J Clin Oncol 1987; 5:1673–89.
132. Bolande RP. Congenital mesoblastic nephroma of infancy. Perspect Pediatr Pathol 1973; 1:227–50.
133. Chan HS, Cheng MY, Mancer K et al. Congenital mesoblastic nephroma: a clinicoradiologic study of 17 cases representing the pathologic spectrum of the disease. J Pediatr 1987; 111:64–70.
134. Hartman DS, Lesar MSL, Madewell JE, Lichtenstein JE, Davis CJ Jr. Mesoblastic nephroma: radiologic–pathologic correlation in 20 cases. AJR Am J Roentgenol 1981; 136:69–74.
135. Wooten SL, Rowen SJ, Griscom NT. Congenital mesoblastic nephroma. Radiographics 1991; 11:719–21.
136. Schlesinger AE, Rosenfield NS, Castle VP, Jasty R. Congenital mesoblastic nephroma metastatic to brain: a report of two cases. Pediatr Radiol 1995; 25(Suppl 1):S73–5.
137. Fernbach SK, Schlesinger AE, Gonzalez-Crussi F. Calcification and ossification in congenital mesoblastic nephroma. Urol Radiol 1985; 7:165–7.

138. Banner MP, Pollack HM, Chatten J, Witzleben C. Multilocular renal cysts: radiologic–pathologic correlation. AJR Am J Roentgenol 1981; 136:239–47.
139. Madewell JE, Goldman SM, Davis CJ Jr et al. Multilocular cystic nephroma: a radiographic–pathologic correlation of 58 patients. Radiology 1983; 146:309–21.
140. Joshi VV, Beckwith JB. Multilocular cyst of the kidney (cystic nephroma) and cystic, partially differentiated nephroblastoma: terminology and criteria for diagnosis. Cancer 1989; 64:466–79.
141. Dikengil A, Benson M, Sanders L, Newhouse JH. MRI of multilocular cystic nephroma. Urol Radiol 1988; 10:95–9.
142. Bell DG, King BF, Hattery RR et al. Imaging characteristics of tuberous sclerosis. AJR Am J Roentgenol 1991; 156:1081–6.
143. Narla LD, Slovis TL, Watts FB, Nigro M. The renal lesions of tuberosclerosis (cysts and angiomyolipoma) – screening with sonography and computerized tomography. Pediatr Radiol 1988; 18:205–9.
144. Stillwell TJ, Gomez MR, Kelalis PP. Renal lesions in tuberous sclerosis. J Urol 1987; 138:477–81.
145. Mitnick JS, Bosniak MA, Hilton S et al. Cystic renal disease in tuberous sclerosis. Radiology 1983; 147:85–7.
146. Laurent F, Joullie M, Biset JM et al. Cystic lymphangioma of the kidney: a rare cause of multiloculated renal masses. Eur J Radiol 1991; 12:67–8.
147. Pickering SP, Fletcher BD, Bryan PJ, Abramowsky CR. Renal lymphangioma: a cause of neonatal nephromegaly. Pediatr Radiol 1984; 14:445–8.
148. Davidson AJ, Hartman DS. Lymphangioma of the retroperitoneum: CT and sonographic characteristics. Radiology 1990; 175:507–10.
149. Graham JM Jr, Boyle W, Troxell J et al. Cystic hamartoma of lung and kidney: a spectrum of developmental abnormalities. Am J Med Genet 1976; 27:45–9.
150. Wood BP. Renal cystic disease in infants and children. Urol Radiol 1992; 14:284–95.
151. Hayden CK Jr, Swischuk LE, Smith TH, Armstrong EA. Renal cystic disease in childhood. RadioGraphics 1986; 6:97–116.
152. McHugh K, Stringer DA, Hebert D, Babiak CA. Simple renal cysts in children: diagnosis and follow-up with US. Radiology 1991; 178:383–5.
153. Hricak H, Crooks L, Sheldon P, Kaufman L. Nuclear magnetic resonance imaging of the kidney. Radiology 1983; 146:425–32.
154. Leung AWL, Bydder GM, Steiner RE et al. Magnetic resonance imaging of the kidneys. AJR Am J Roentgenol 1984; 143:1215–27.
155. Kavukcu S, Cakmakci H, Babayigit A. Diagnosis of caliceal diverticulum in two pediatric patients: a comparison of sonography, CT, and urography. J Clin Ultrasound 2003; 31(4):218–21.
156. Rathaus V, Konen O, Werner M et al. Pyelocalyceal diverticulum: the imaging spectrum with emphasis on the ultrasound features. Br J Radiol 2001; 74(883):595–601.
157. Madewell JE, Hartman DS, Lichtenstein JR. Radiologic–pathologic correlation in cystic diseases of the kidney. Radiol Clin North Am 1979; 17:261–79.
158. Hayden CK Jr, Swischuk LE. Renal cystic disease. Semin Ultrasound CT MR 1991; 12:361–73.
159. Jain M, LeQuesne GW, Bourne AJ et al. High-resolution sonography in the differential diagnosis of cystic diseases of the kidney in infancy and childhood: preliminary experience. J Ultrasound Med 1997; 16:235–40.
160. Currarino G, Stannard MW, Rutledge JC. The sonolucent cortical rim in infantile polycystic kidneys: histologic correlation. J Ultrasound Med 1989; 8:571–4.
161. Fellows RA, Leonidas JC, Beatty EC Jr. Radiologic features of 'adult type' polycystic disease in the neonate. Pediatr Radiol 1976; 4:87–92.
162. Dietrich RB, Kangarloo H. Kidneys in infants and children: evaluation with MR. Radiology 1986; 158:313–17.
163. Bernstein J, Slovis TL. Polycystic diseases of the kidney. In: Edelmann C Jr, ed. Pediatric Kidney Disease, 2nd edn. Boston: Little, Brown and Co., 1992: 1139–57.
164. Fitch SJ, Stapleton FB. Ultrasonographic features of glomerulocystic disease in infancy: similarity to infantile polycystic kidney disease. Pediatr Radiol 1986; 16:400–2.
165. Fredericks BJ, de Campo M, Chow CW, Powell HR. Glomerulocystic renal disease: ultrasound appearances. Pediatr Radiol 1989; 19:184–6.
166. Worthington JL, Shackelford GD, Cole BR, Tack ED, Kissane JM. Sonographically detectable cysts in polycystic kidney disease in newborn and young infants. Pediatr Radiol 1988; 18:287–93.
167. Elzouki AY, Al-Suhaibani H, Mirza K, Al-Sowailem AM. Thin-section computed tomography scans detect medullary cysts in patients believed to have juvenile nephronophthisis. Am J Kidney Dis 1996; 27(2): 216–19.
168. McGregor AR, Bailey RR. Nephronophthisis–cystic renal medulla complex: diagnosis by computerized tomography. Nephron 1989; 53:70–2.
169. Garel LA, Habib R, Pariente D, Broyer M, Sauregrain J. Juvenile nephronophthisis: sonographic appearance in children with severe uremia. Radiology 1984; 151:93–5.
170. Ala-Mello S, Jääskeläinen J, Koskimies O. Familial juvenile nephronophthisis. An ultrasonographic follow-up of seven patients. Acta Radiol 1998; 39:84–9.
171. Chuang Y-F, Tsai T-C. Sonographic findings in familial juvenile nephronophthisis–medullary cystic disease complex. J Clin Ultrasound 1998; 26:203–6.
172. Kawashima A, Goldman SM. Medullary sponge kidney. In: Pollack HM, McClennan BL, eds. Clinical Urography, 2nd edn, Volume 2. Philadelphia: WB Saunders, 2000; 1384–97.
173. Patriquin HB, O'Regan S. Medullary sponge kidney in childhood. AJR Am J Roentgenol 1985; 145(2):315–19.
174. Beck AD. The effect of intra-uterine urinary obstruction upon the development of the fetal kidney. J Urol 1971; 105(6):784–9.
175. Benacerraf BR, Peters CA, Mandell J. The prenatal evolution of a nonfunctioning kidney in the setting of obstructive hydronephrosis. J Clin Ultrasound 1991; 19:446–50.
176. Glazer GM, Filly RA, Callen PW. The varied sonographic appearance of the urinary tract in the fetus and newborn with urethral obstruction. Radiology 1982; 144 (3):563–8.

177. Blane CE, Koff AS, Bowerman RA, Barr M Jr. Non-obstructive fetal hydronephrosis: sonographic recognition and therapeutic implications. Radiology 1983; 147:95–9.
178. Mahoney BS, Filly RA, Callen PW et al. Fetal renal dysplasia: sonographic evaluation. Radiology 1984; 152(1):143–6.
179. Sanders RC, Nussbaum AR, Solez K. Renal dysplasia: sonographic findings. Radiology 1988; 167:623–6.
180. Felson B, Cussen LJ. The hydronephrotic type of congenital multicystic disease of the kidney. Semin Roentgenol 1975; 10:113–23.
181. Griscom NT, Vawter FG, Fellers FX. Pelvoinfundibular atresia: the usual form of multicystic kidney; 44 unilateral and two bilateral cases. Semin Roentgenol 1975; 10:125–31.
182. Bloom DA, Brosman S. The multicystic kidney. J Urol 1978; 120(2):211–15.
183. Avni EF, Thoua Y, Lalmand B et al. Multicystic dysplastic kidney: natural history from in utero diagnosis and postnatal follow-up. J Urol 1987; 138(6):1420–4.
184. Hashimoto BE, Filly RA, Callen PW. Multicystic dysplastic kidney in utero: changing appearance on US. Radiology 1986; 159(1):107–9.
185. Pedicelli G, Jequier S, Bowen AD, Boisvert J. Multicystic dysplastic kidneys: spontaneous regression demonstrated with US. Radiology 1986; 160:23–6.
186. Rottenberg GT, Gordon I, De Bruyn R. The natural history of the multicystic dysplastic kidney in children. Br J Radiol 1997; 70(832):347–50.
187. Hitchcock R, Burge DM. Renal agenesis: an acquired condition? J Pediatr Surg 1994; 29(3):454–5.

Assessment of renal obstructive disorders: ultrasound, nuclear medicine, and magnetic resonance imaging

28

James Elmore and Andrew J Kirsch

The widespread use of maternal sonography and the routine radiographic evaluation of children with febrile urinary tract infections have resulted in the increased diagnosis of both antenatal and postnatal hydronephrosis. Hydronephrosis is the most common abnormality detected by prenatal ultrasound (US) and is seen in an estimated 1 in 100 to 1 in 500 pregnancies.[1] One of the most important distinctions in the assessment of these children is determining which patients would benefit from surgery and which patients can be safely observed. This distinction is important since unnecessary intervention exposes patients needlessly to the morbidity of surgery, whereas inappropriate observation places patients at risk for infection and renal parenchymal loss.

The common pediatric renal obstructive disorders are listed in Table 28.1. Of these, ureteropelvic junction obstruction (UPJO) is the most common and accounts for nearly half of all prenatally detected uropathies.[1] Ureterovesical junction obstruction (UVJO), ureteroceles, and ectopic ureters are responsible for the majority of the remaining cases. The natural history of renal pelvic dilatation is largely related to the underlying diagnosis. For example, hydronephrosis secondary to an ectopic ureter is unlikely to resolve spontaneously, whereas patients with megaureter can often be followed for years without renal functional loss.[2] The outcome of patients with UPJO is more variable and, as a result, management is more controversial. Some clinicians recommend early surgery, whereas others advocate simple observation.[3–5] Regardless, most urologists will initially follow hydronephrotic kidneys conservatively and use decreasing differential renal function or worsening hydronephrosis as an indicator that surgery may be required.

Table 28.1 Causes of pediatric hydronephrosis

Obstructive causes
Ureteropelvic junction obstruction (UPJO)
Ureterovesical junction obstruction (UVJO)
Ectopic ureters
Ureteroceles
Posterior urethral valves
Urethral atresia
Anterior urethral valves
Congenital urethral stricture
Non-obstructive causes
Vesicoureteral reflux (VUR)
Primary non-obstructive megaureter
Megacalicosis
Fetal folds
Neurogenic bladder
Conditions mimicking hydronephrosis
Extrarenal pelves
Multicystic dysplastic kidney (MCDK)
Peripelvic cysts
Neonatal kidneys (sonolucent renal sinus)

Radiographic approaches to the diagnosis and assessment of renal obstructive disorders have evolved significantly over the past several decades. Intravenous urography (IVU) and the antegrade pressure–flow test, referred to as the Whitaker test, were once mainstays in the evaluation of these patients and are now only rarely used. Technologic advances have given way to US, diuretic renal scintigraphy (DRS), and, more recently, magnetic resonance imaging (MRI) for the evaluation of hydronephrosis. Voiding cystourethrography (VCUG) is frequently performed in conjunction with these studies to rule out

Table 28.2 Advantages and disadvantages of various diagnostic modalities for the assessment of renal obstructive disorders

Imaging study	Advantages	Disadvantages
Intravenous pyelography	Good anatomy if function is good	Inaccurate if poor function; nephrotoxic contrast; radiation exposure
Whitaker test	Only study that measures directly the pressure in the renal pelvis/bladder	Invasive; not reproducible; no functional information; radiation exposure
Ultrasound	Inexpensive, portable, no contrast or radiation exposure	No functional information; limited anatomy
Diuretic renal scintigraphy	Good functional and drainage information	Limited information in bilateral disease; no anatomic information; interpretative error; 15% false negative/positives
Gadolinium-enhanced MR urography	Superior anatomic and functional information even if poor function or bilateral disease; no radiation; contrast non-nephrotoxic	Expensive; not yet widely available; requires sedation and monitoring

vesicoureteral reflux (VUR) as the cause of hydronephrosis. Each of these diagnostic modalities has relative advantages and disadvantages (Table 28.2). In general, these studies provide either good anatomic or good functional information, whereas none of these studies, save MRI, provide both. Some tests are more invasive than others, which also influences test selection. Currently, no study is considered a gold standard for the evaluation of renal obstructive disorders and complete assessment typically involves a series of studies, including US, VCUG, and DRS. Consequently, a thoughtful diagnostic strategy is necessary to proceed with appropriate management at minimal cost and morbidity to the patient.

Ultrasonography

Ultrasonography (or ultrasound) constitutes a cornerstone in the radiologic evaluation of renal obstructive disorders. It is non-invasive, inexpensive, portable, does not require ionizing radiation or contrast media, and is not limited by renal failure. As a result, US is ideally suited as a screening study and for following patients with known abnormalities. A properly performed study provides information regarding renal size, cortical thickness and architecture, and the degree of dilatation of the collecting system. Nomographic charts are available that give 'normal' renal lengths for children of varying ages and body weights (Figure 28.1). The sonographic examination, however, is operator dependent and a skilled sonographer is essential for informative and reproducible studies. The US examination may be limited by body habitus, overlying bowel gas, and poor patient cooperation.

The hallmark finding of hydronephrosis on US is separation of the hyperechoic central renal sinus by anechoic branching structures that represent the dilated calices. With more chronic and severe forms of hydronephrosis, cortical thinning may be seen. Often, if the process is unilateral and leads to renal parenchymal loss, the contralateral kidney may undergo compensatory hypertrophy in young children. In moderate and severe UPJO, pronounced caliceal and renal pelvic dilatation may occur, giving the kidney a classic 'bear paw' appearance on US (Figure 28.2). The ureters can usually only be seen on US if they are dilated, and the presence of a dilated ureter lying posterior to the bladder helps distinguish megaureter from UPJO. When either diagnosis is a consideration, a VCUG to rule out VUR as the cause of dilatation should be performed. It should be kept in mind that VUR may coexist with UPJO in as many as 10% of children.[7]

The Society for Fetal Urology (SFU) has proposed a grading system for reporting hydronephrosis detected by US.[8] This system takes into consideration the appearance of the calices, renal pelvis, and parenchyma to grade the degree of hydronephrosis from I to IV (minimal to severe). SFU grades I and II represent mild to moderate degrees of pelviectasis and should not be considered hydronephrosis. Grades III and IV represent true hydronephrosis, grade IV being the most severe with cortical atrophy (Table

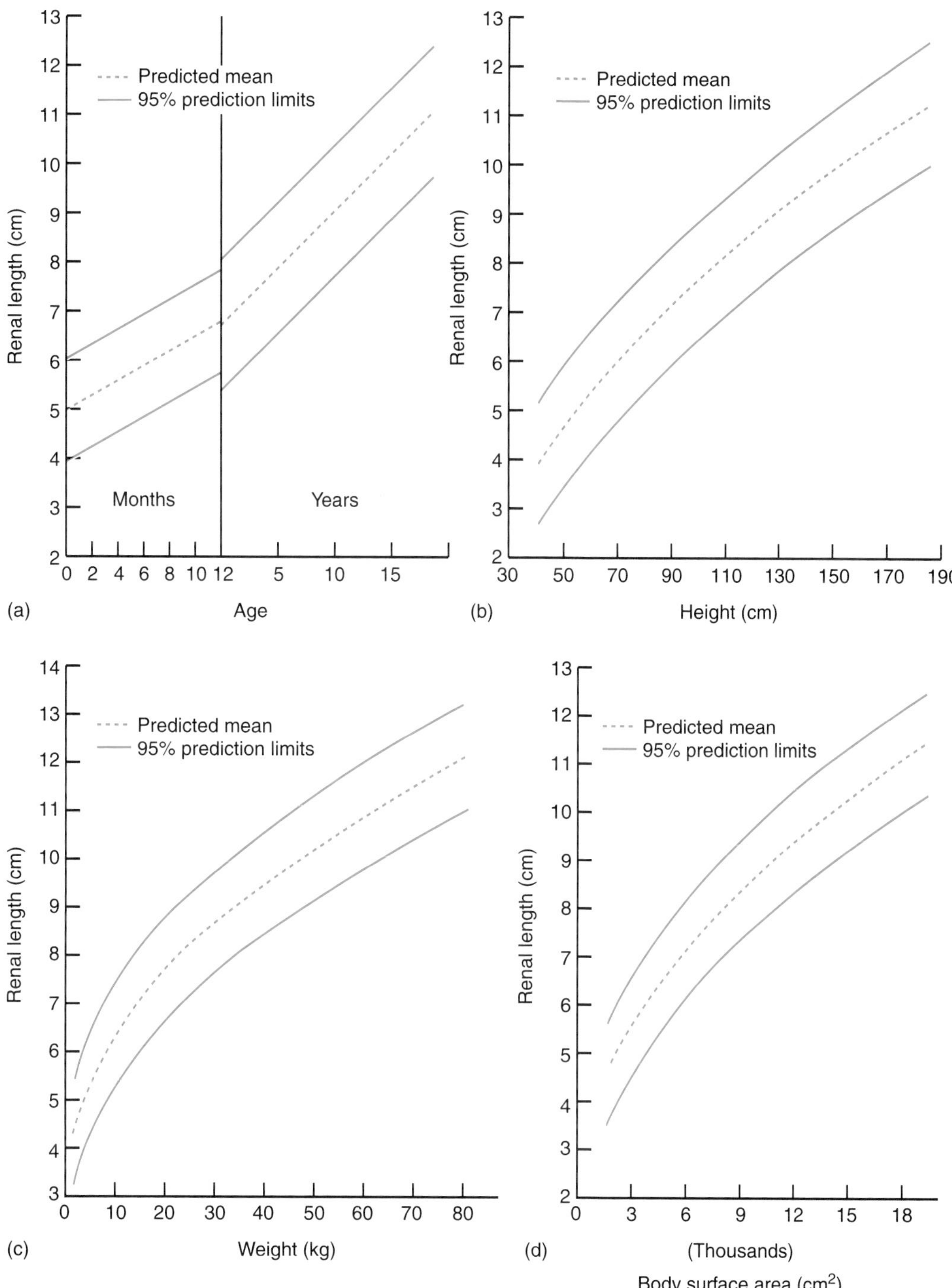

Figure 28.1 Renal nomographic chart. (Adapted from Han and Babcock.[6])

28.3). The degree of hydronephrosis is used to assist in decision making with regard to treatment and, additionally, provides some prognostic information. For example, SFU grades I and II hydronephrosis secondary to UPJO have a tendency to resolve with time and usually only require a VCUG to rule out VUR and sonographic re-evaluation. For SFU grades III and IV, some type of functional evaluation, in addition to a VCUG, is usually recommended since these patients are more likely to have significant urologic pathology and to require surgical intervention.

Although controversy exists over size cut-offs, there is a well-documented correlation between the anteroposterior diameter (APD) of the renal pelvis on prenatal ultrasound and the probability that a significant postnatal pathology will be present. Most authors use an upper limit of normal of 5 mm APD before 30 weeks of gestation, and up to 10 mm later in

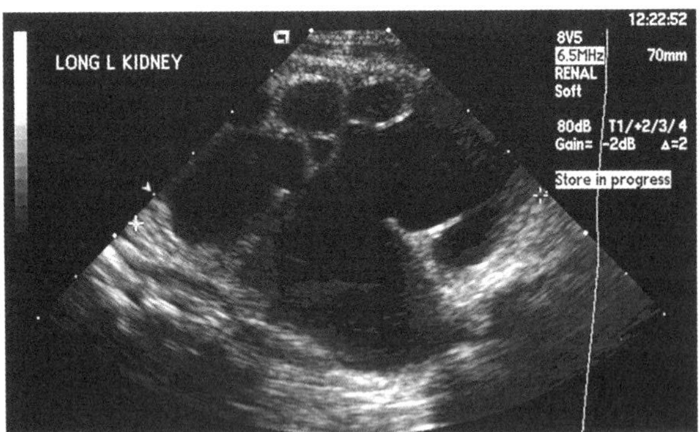

Figure 28.2 A 6-year-old boy with left ureteropelvic junction obstruction. Note the massive renal pelvic and caliceal hydronephrosis, giving the kidney the appearance of a 'bear paw' on ultrasound.

Table 28.3 SFU grading scale for hydronephrosis detected by US

Grade	Central renal complex (pelvis and calices)	Renal parenchyma
I	Slight splitting	Normal
II	Evident splitting; confined within renal border	Normal
III	Wide splitting; pelvis dilated outside renal border; calices dilated	Normal
IV	Wide splitting with pelvis dilated outside renal border; calices dilated and may appear convex	Atrophy

From Fernbach.[9]

Table 28.4 Correlation between anteroposterior diameter (APD) of the renal pelvis and requirement for surgical intervention

Maximal APD[a] of renal pelvis (mm)	Risk of requirement for surgical intervention (based on functional criteria) (%)
<15	2
15–20	7
20–30	29
30–40	61
40–50	67
>50	100

[a] The APD refers to the maximum size encountered at any stage on pre- or postnatal US. Findings derived from prospective studies undertaken at the Hospital for Sick Children, Great Ormond Street, London.[4]

pregnancy.[10] Bouzada et al found that an APD of >15 mm on postnatal US had a sensitivity of 100% and a specificity of 92.5% for identifying renal units that ultimately required pyeloplasty.[11] Similarly, Johnson et al found that 11 (79%) of 14 kidneys with an antenatal APD of >15 mm were obstructed or demonstrated VUR on postnatal evaluation.[12] Finally, a prospective trial undertaken at the Great Ormond Street Hospital demonstrated that the severity of renal pelvic dilatation is useful for predicting renal functional deterioration and the eventual need for surgery in the management of UPJO (Table 28.4).[13]

The term hydronephrosis implies obstruction, and exposes an important limitation of US. No functional information is obtained from conventional US, and obstruction cannot be diagnosed based solely on anatomic information. Therefore, although US is highly accurate in the diagnosis of renal dilatation, it is not reliable in predicting obstruction or providing information regarding renal function. Even in the presence of renal pelvic dilatation secondary to an obstructive process, the degree of dilatation does not necessarily reflect the degree of, or functional significance of, the obstruction. Indeed, numerous cases have been reported of mild dilatation with complete obstruction and marked dilatation when no obstruction is present. False-positive studies may result from an extrarenal pelvis, a peripelvic cyst, residual dilatation from previous obstruction, dilatation resulting from VUR, and pyelonephritis. The fetal and neonatal kidney may also appear hydronephrotic on US secondary to the sonolucent appearance of the medulla and pyramids (Figure 28.3). False-negative studies

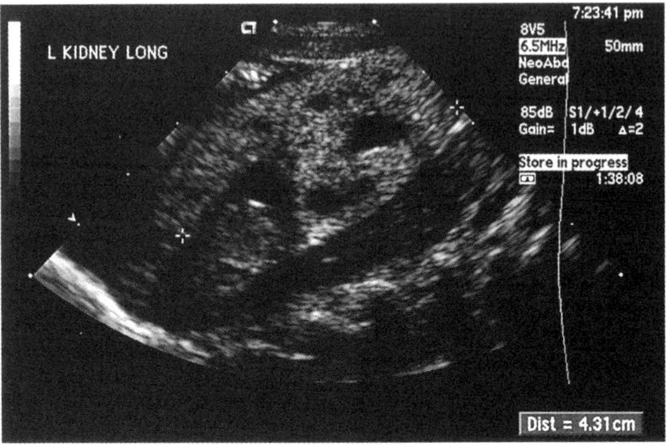

Figure 28.3 Left kidney of healthy neonate by ultrasonography. Note the relatively sonolucent renal sinus, which may be mistaken for hydronephrosis.

are less frequent, but obstruction may be present in the absence of dilatation in acute obstruction and in certain extrinsic processes such as metastases and retroperitoneal fibrosis. Oliguric states may also lead to false-negative studies. This is particularly true in the newborn, in whom renal sonography may underestimate or completely overlook renal dilatation because of the oliguric state of the healthy newborn. It is rare that this results in missing significant renal obstruction, however.

Duplex Doppler ultrasonography

Given the limitations of conventional US in distinguishing obstructive from non-obstructive causes of hydronephrosis, duplex Doppler US has recently been shown to have some value in the diagnosis of renal obstructive disorders. This adjunct to US is based on the fact that obstruction causes an increase in intrarenal arterial resistance, resulting in a relative reduction in diastolic flow compared with systolic flow. Renal arterial resistance is quantified using the formula:

$$\frac{\text{peak systolic velocity} - \text{minimum diastolic velocity}}{\text{peak systolic velocity}}$$

The result of this formula is referred to as the resistive index (RI) (Figure 28.4). Different criteria have been proposed to suggest obstruction, including an RI of >0.70, an inter-renal RI difference of >0.06–0.10 with unilateral dilatation, and an abnormal RI response to a diuretic challenge.[15] For children, and especially the neonate and infant, the RI tends to be elevated compared with adult standards. RIs of 0.7–1.0 can be normal in these populations and usually decrease to adult ranges by about 2–4 years of age.[16] Therefore, the latter two criteria appear most helpful in the pediatric age group.

Numerous studies have been performed evaluating the role of duplex Doppler US for the diagnosis of renal obstruction and with mixed results. Kessler et al evaluated the role of RI in distinguishing obstructive uropathy from non-obstructed dilatation in a group of children with unilateral hydronephrosis.[17] The kidneys were prospectively evaluated by using duplex Doppler US and obstruction was confirmed by either renography or at the time of surgery. Using an RI of ≥0.70 plus a difference in the RI between kidneys of ≥0.08 as the criteria for obstruction, they found duplex Doppler US had positive and negative predictive values of 95% and 100%, respectively. They concluded that the RI appears to be an effective parameter for both the evaluation and follow-up of obstructive or non-obstructive dilatation in children. Other clinicians have published less encouraging results. Gill et al studied the undilated urinary tracts of 47 children for the purpose of establishing a nomogram for RI values and to determine if an RI value of <0.7 reliably predicts an unobstructed collecting system.[18] They found that 37% of the normal renal units had an RI >0.70 and concluded that RI values in undilated (i.e. normal) kidneys vary significantly, and the routine use of this technique needs further evaluation. As indicated by these studies, the use of duplex Doppler US for the evaluation of renal obstructive disorders is currently controversial and, as a result, the modality is not widely utilized.

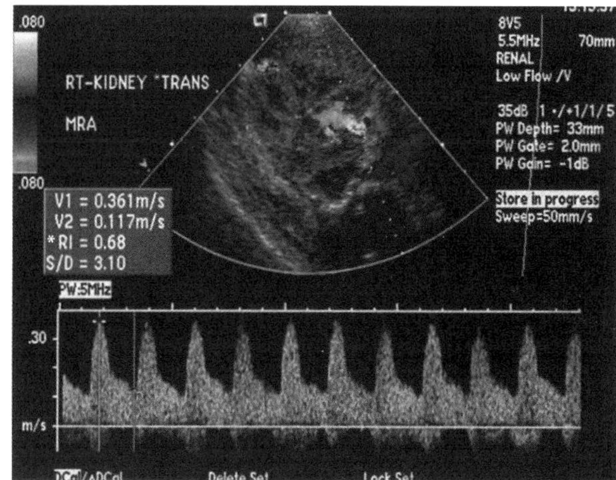

Figure 28.4 Duplex Doppler image taken from a 4-year-old boy. Note the arterial waveform and the normal resistive index (RI) of 0.68 (asterisk).

In summary, US is most commonly utilized as a screening method for the diagnosis of renal obstructive disorders. Although in theory duplex Doppler US can provide useful functional information, in practice other studies are used to better delineate the cause and functional significance of hydronephrosis once it is detected. Most commonly, after VUR has been ruled out by VCUG, the next study of choice is DRS.

Diuretic renal scintigraphy

DRS was developed in the late 1970s as a non-invasive method for evaluating patients with renal obstructive disorders. The introduction of better radiopharmaceuticals and gamma cameras has led to an increased use of nuclear imaging in pediatric urology. Once hydronephrosis is detected by other imaging methods, usually US, DRS is considered by many to be the pre-eminent method for estimating differential renal function and characterizing the severity of obstruction. Worsening renal function by DRS is often the impetus for pyeloplasty in patients being observed with UPJO. DRS also remains the most commonly used method for serial follow-up and postoperative assessment of patients with UPJO and megaureter.

The radiopharmaceuticals used for DRS comprise a radionuclide, most commonly technetium 99m (^{99m}Tc), bound to a carrier macromolecule. Renal handling of the various radiopharmaceuticals and, therefore, the information gained from DRS, is dictated solely by the biochemical properties of the carrier macromolecule. The ability to label these macromolecules, which have known physiologic destinations within the body, forms the basis of renal scintigraphy. The principal radiopharmaceuticals used for DRS are ^{99m}Tc mercaptoacetyltriglycine (Tc MAG3), ^{99m}Tc diethylenetriamine pentaacetic acid (Tc DTPA), and ^{99m}Tc dimercaptosuccinic acid (^{99m}Tc DMSA) (Table 28.5). ^{99m}Tc MAG3, one of the newest radiopharmaceuticals, is 90% bound to plasma proteins and is principally cleared by tubular secretion. It shows both the parenchyma and collecting system well and provides excellent functional quantification. These qualities and the fact that it requires lower radiation doses than other radiopharmaceuticals make it the current agent of choice for evaluating renal function and drainage. In contrast, ^{99m}Tc DTPA has little plasma protein binding and is cleared almost exclusively by glomerular filtration. It is rapidly filtered into the urine and therefore provides excellent visualization of the pelvicaliceal system, ureter, and bladder, but may not be retained in the renal parenchyma long enough for good visualization of parenchymal abnormalities. Also, since ^{99m}Tc DTPA relies principally on glomerular filtration, results are often suboptimal in infants with immature kidneys and a low glomerular filtration rate (GFR) or in patients with compromised renal function. In these scenarios ^{99m}Tc MAG3 is the preferred agent. ^{99m}Tc DMSA is unique among the other commonly used radiopharmaceuticals in that it tightly binds to the renal tubular cells and only a small amount is excreted into the urine. Therefore, it allows excellent visualization of the renal parenchyma and is primarily used for evaluating cortical lesions such as scars that occur as a result of pyelonephritis.

The basic principles of DRS are as follows. The radiopharmaceutical of choice is injected intravenously. Normally, during the first 2–3 minutes, renal parenchymal uptake occurs. The radionuclide emits gamma radiation that is detected by a gamma counter. This emitted radiation is temporally and spatially quantified with computer-assisted digital processing and represented morphologically and graphically as a scan (Figure 28.5). This information is analyzed and compared, allowing for the computation of differential renal function (DRF). It is generally accepted that the error in determining the DFR is ±5%. After about 20 minutes, furosemide is injected intravenously to promote diuresis and the velocity and pattern of drainage from the kidneys to the bladder are analyzed. In the absence of obstruction, half of the radionuclide is cleared from the renal pelvis within 10–15 minutes, termed the $T_{1/2}$. A $T_{1/2}$ of >20 minutes indicates obstruction, whereas a $T_{1/2}$ of <15 minutes is generally considered normal. Times between 15 and 20 minutes are indeterminate. Indications for surgical intervention based on DRS generally include DRF of <35–40% and a $T_{1/2}$ of >20 minutes, and US findings consistent with anatomic obstruction. Despite these parameters, neither should be used as an independent variable to determine if obstruction is present or absent.

Table 28.5 Common radiopharmaceuticals used in diuretic renal scintigraphy

Radiopharmaceutical	Renal handling	Application
^{99m}Tc Mercaptoacetyltriglycine (^{99m}Tc MAG3)	Principally cleared by tubular secretion	Renography
^{99m}Tc Dimercaptosuccinic acid (^{99m}Tc DMSA)	Localizes and binds to the proximal convoluted tubules	Renal parenchymal imaging
^{99m}Tc Diethylenetriamine pentaacetic acid (^{99m}Tc DTPA)	GFR dependent for clearance	Renography

GFR, glomerular filtration rate.

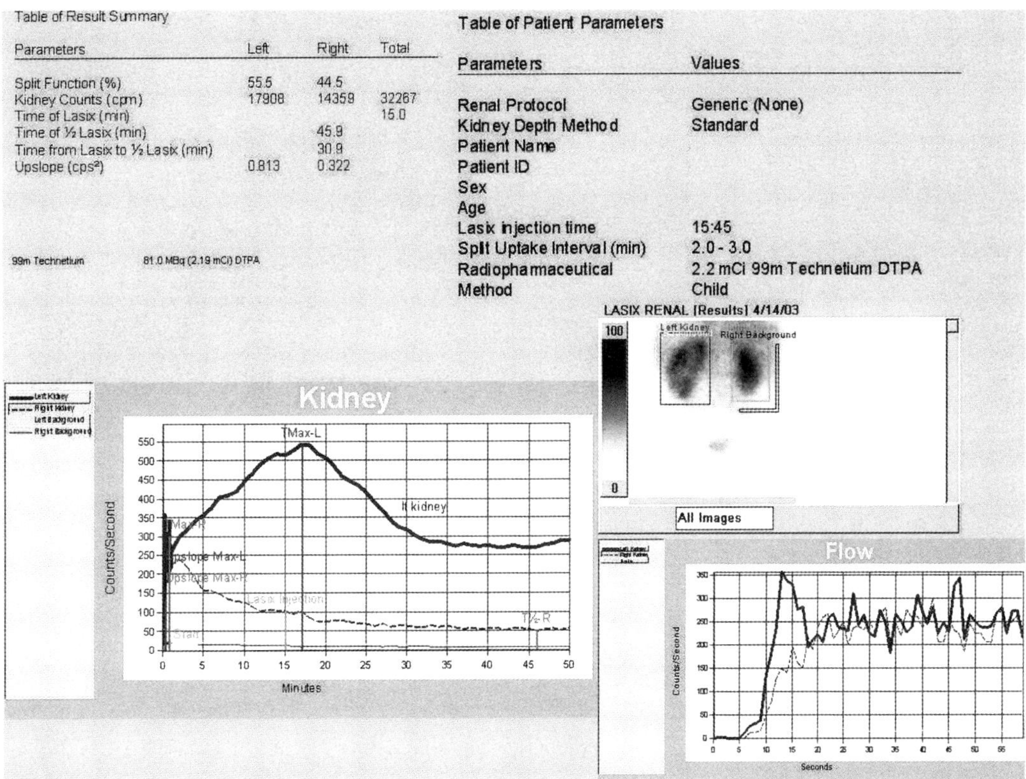

Figure 28.5 Diuretic renal scan (^{99m}Tc MAG3) taken from a 3-year-old boy with severe left ureteropelvic junction obstruction. Note that the $T_{1/2}$ of the left kidney is never reached.

Over the years a wide variety of protocols and techniques for diuretic renography have been used. Unfortunately, this has produced variability in interpretation among different institutions. In an attempt to promote standardization of the technique, the SFU and the Pediatric Nuclear Medicine Council (PNMC) of the Society for Nuclear Medicine published guidelines for the 'well-tempered' diuresis renogram in 1992.[19] Its purpose was to allow easy comparison between studies and institutions. The guidelines standardize many of the facets of the study, including intravenous hydration, bladder catheter placement, patient position, data acquisition and analysis, timing of diuretic administration, and regions of interest for which to monitor the diuretic effect. However, in practice, local protocols are still frequently used, which makes comparing results from different centers problematic.

Despite the widespread use of DRS, there are significant limitations with the technique. For example, DRS only provides differential renal function and, as a result, is less informative in patients with overall poor renal function or solitary kidneys. Caution must be taken when interpreting results in these scenarios. Very capacious collecting systems can also prove problematic, since radionuclide retained in the renal pelvis may be included in the region of interest (ROI) and falsely elevate differential function. Although debatable, this artifact may be responsible for the supranormal function (>55%) reported for some hydronephrotic kidneys.[20] Interpretation is also somewhat subjective and may lead to reporting error (Figure 28.6). Other disadvantages of DRS are its poor anatomic resolution and long examination times. Not infrequently, patients will fall into the equivocal category. These patients may require a repeat DRS, or less commonly, a Whitaker test, to further assess renal obstruction. Overall, DRS may fail to determine the presence or absence of obstruction in at least 15% of cases.[21]

Clearly, there are strengths and weaknesses associated with US and renal scintigraphy. Specifically, whereas US provides useful anatomic information, it provides no functional information. Conversely, renal scintigraphy provides functional information, but little anatomic information. Therefore, although these studies are highly informative in tandem, neither study alone is typically sufficient for making clinical

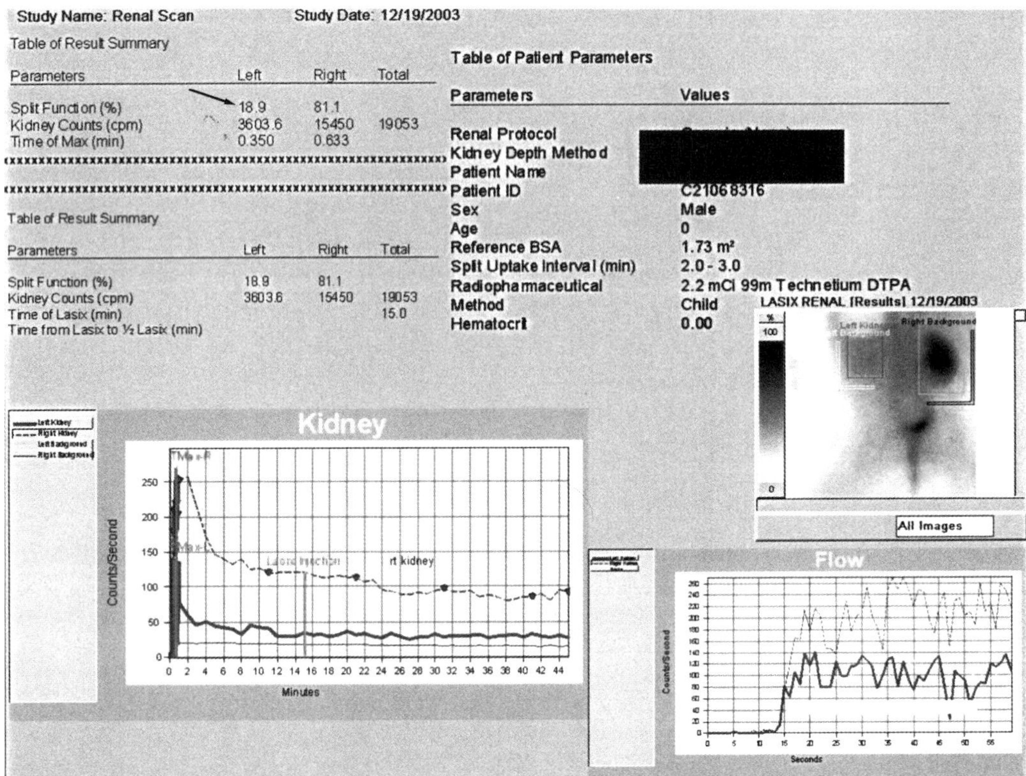

Figure 28.6 Diuretic renal scan from a 3-month-old boy. Note that the scan shows 18% differential left renal function. Further evaluation showed that the patient had a solitary right kidney, which highlights the interpretative error possible with scintigraphy.

decisions. Recently, contrast-enhanced MRI of the urinary tract, as a single study, has been shown to have promise in the investigation of renal obstructive disorders.

Magnetic resonance imaging

The use of magnetic resonance urography (MRU) in the diagnosis of pediatric renal obstructive disorders has increased dramatically since it was introduced in the late 1980s. This has been the result of a series of recent technologic advances that have enabled faster image acquisition, improved resolution, reduced motion artifact, and three-dimensional (3D) reconstruction. Even today, newer imaging sequences and shorter acquisition times are improving image quality and expanding the diagnostic capabilities of MRU. The advantages of MRU for evaluating renal tract anomalies in children are that it has multiplanar capabilities, offers excellent anatomic resolution and soft tissue contrast, and does not use ionizing radiation. Possibly, one of the most important developments occurred in the late 1990s when gadolinium-DTPA (Gd-DTPA) was first used in conjunction with MRU. Gd-DTPA and ^{99m}Tc DTPA share the same carrier macromolecule and are handled by the kidneys in an identical fashion. As a result, Gd-DTPA-enhanced MRU (Gd-MRU) measurements of renal perfusion, uptake, and excretion correlate with those obtained by ^{99m}Tc DTPA renal scintigraphy. Gd-MRU is the only study to date that has the capability of providing excellent morphologic detail typical of MRI as well as functional information that is equivalent or superior to DRS. Even at very low concentrations, Gd-DTPA has high signal intensity on MRI, giving Gd-MRU the ability to reliably detect hydronephrosis and transition in ureteral caliber even in non-functioning systems (Figure 28.7). The results of one study showed that Gd-MRU may be a useful tool for distinguishing an obstructed from a non-obstructed dilated system, even when ^{99m}Tc MAG3 renography results were compromised by reduced renal uptake in the affected kidney.[22] An added advantage is that gadolinium, unlike iodinated contrast agents, is not nephrotoxic and can be used safely in patients with impaired renal function.

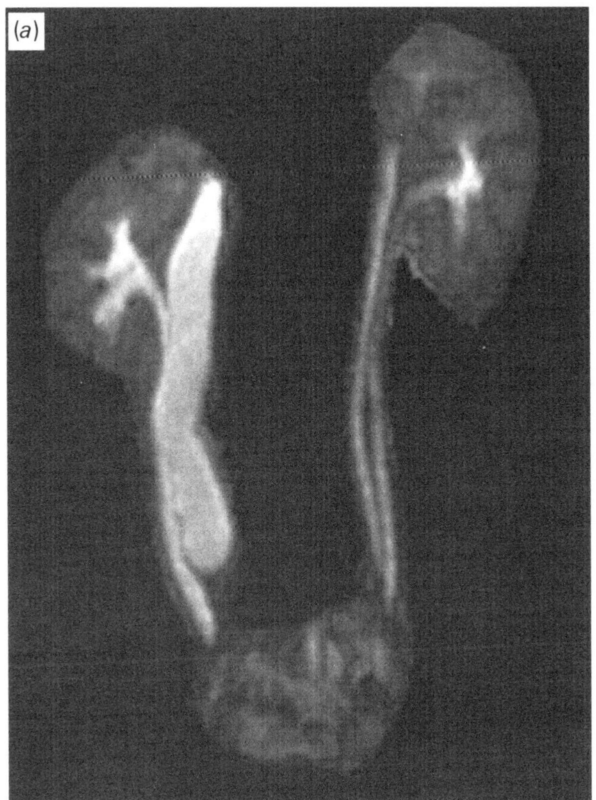

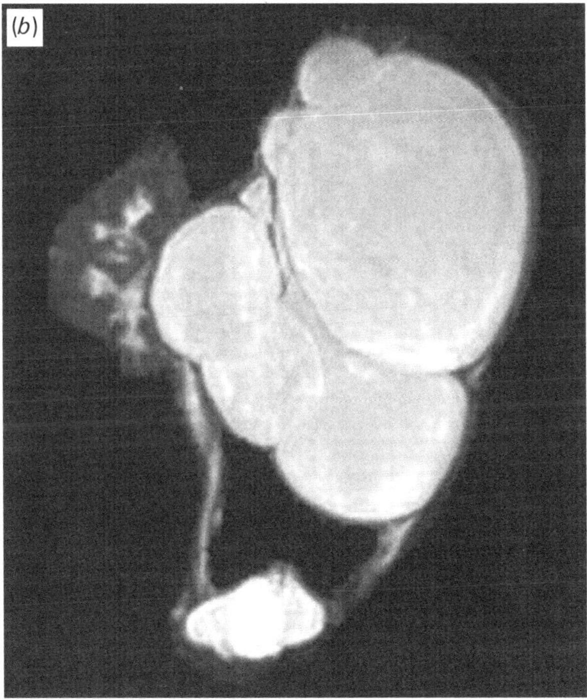

Figure 28.7 Gadolinium-enhanced MRU permits hydronephrosis and transition in ureteral caliber to be reliably detected even in non-functioning systems. (*a*) An 8-year-old patient with a dysmorphic right upper pole, with a dilated ureter down to the pelvis consistent with ureteral atresia. These findings could not be appreciated on either ultrasound or diuretic renal scintigraphy. (*b*) Left multicystic dysplastic kidney that had no function on diuretic renal scintigraphy.

Although protocols for Gd-MRU differ slightly among institutions, the basic principles are preserved. The study involves initial T1- and T2-weighted images through the kidneys, ureters, and bladder. Gd-DTPA is then administered intravenously and dynamic contrast-enhanced T1-weighted imaging using a volumetric gradient echo technique is performed over the entire urinary tract. In a fashion similar to IVU, the uptake, excretion, and drainage of Gd-DTPA can be visualized sequentially. The advantage of Gd-MRU is that, in addition to providing anatomic information which exceeds that of US, computer-assisted postprocessing techniques can be employed to objectively quantify function and the degree of obstruction, similar to DRS.

During postprocessing, image sequences are viewed as cinematic loops. This permits the assessment of renal perfusion and excretion and the generation of signal intensity vs. time curves. Following contrast administration, three distinct phases of enhancement are recognized (Figure 28.8). In the first phase, the renal cortex enhances vividly, differentiating renal cortex from medulla. This is followed by a medullary phase, where the medulla enhances greater than the cortex. The third phase consists of excretion of contrast medium into the collecting system and ureters. Gadolinium transit through these anatomic areas causes a variation in the MR signal intensity over time, which can be represented graphically by signal intensity vs time curves (Figure 28.9). When function is reduced in one kidney, signal intensity is reduced compared with the normal side. The 3D maximum intensity projection (MIP) images from delayed images of the renal pelvis and ureters that exhibit good contrast enhancement provide excellent anatomic resolution of the collecting system and ureters.

The diagnosis of obstruction on MRU is based morphologically on the findings of renal pelvic dilatation and ureteral narrowing. Functionally, obstruction is suggested by reduced enhancement, delayed excretion of contrast into the collecting system and ureter, swirling contrast, and fluid–fluid levels within the renal pelvis. With Gd-MRU, reduced enhancement and delayed excretion can be objectively quantified through the calculation of DRF and the renal transit time (RTT), which are tantamount to the split renal function and $T_{1/2}$ time obtained by DRS. Using a two-compartment mathematical model, referred to as the Rutland–Patlak plot, single kidney GFR can also be calculated with Gd-MRU. This technique enables MRU-based assessment of function in

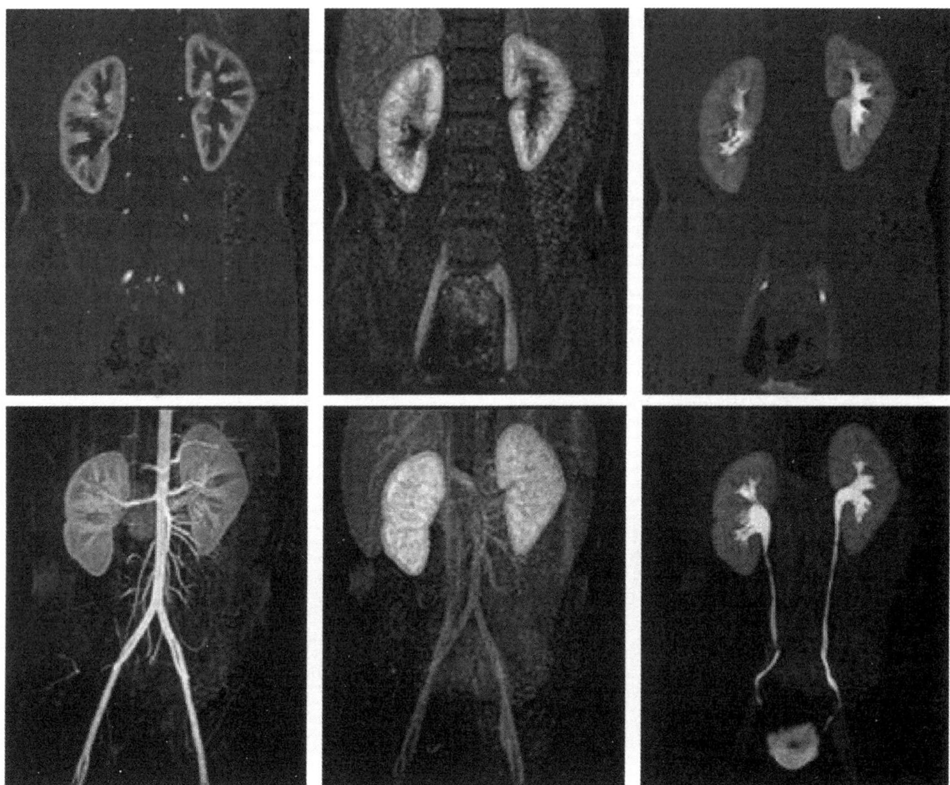

Figure 28.8 Following contrast administration, three distinct phases of renal enhancement can be recognized. Top row: left to right, cortical phase, medullary phase, and excretory phase. Bottom row shows the maximum intensity projections (MIPs) from which images were generated.

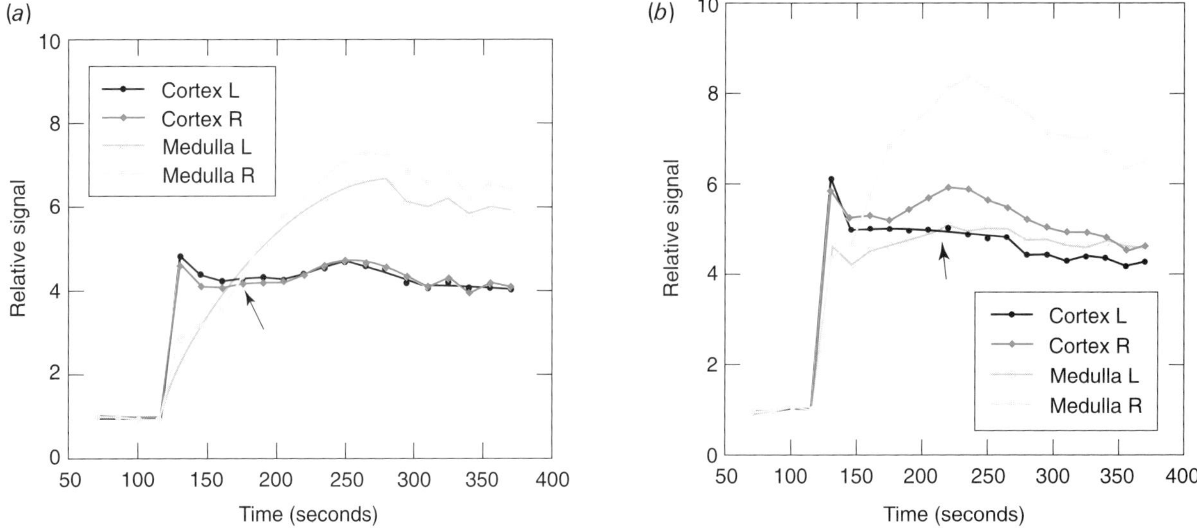

Figure 28.9 (*a*) Normal time–intensity graph. Parenchymal enhancement by MRU occurs in a predictable fashion. The corticomedullary crossover (CMC) point (arrow) is the time at which the medulla has a higher relative signal intensity than the cortex. (*b*) Time–intensity graph taken from a patient with left UPJO. Delayed corticomedullary crossover (arrow) indicates increased intratubular pressure, which is suggestive of obstruction.

patients with bilateral disease or solitary kidneys, a distinct advantage over DRS, which only provides differential information.

DRF is determined using images acquired at the time there is homogeneous enhancement within the kidney but prior to excretion of contrast into the collecting system. With 3D reconstruction, the volume of enhancing renal parenchyma is selected manually as an ROI. Vivid contrast enhancement of the renal parenchyma makes it possible to omit the collecting system and background. DRF is then calculated using the formula:

$$\text{percent renal function} = \frac{\text{individual kidney volume}}{\text{right kidney volume} + \text{left kidney volume}} \times 100.$$

Data published by the authors, as well as that of other clinicians, show a high correlation between DRF as determined by MRU and renal scintigraphy.[23–25] To better determine split renal function, and not volume, we have begun to use Patlak indices of GFR to compare the functional contribution of each kidney to overall renal function (AJ Kirsch and JD Grattan-Smith, unpublished work).

The RTT refers to the time between the appearance of the contrast in the kidney and its appearance in the ureter (below the UPJ) and is based on 3D sequences that allow the passage of contrast to be tracked though the kidneys. Based on the RTT, drainage can be classified as normal (RTT ≤4 minutes), equivocal (4 <RTT ≤8 minutes) or obstructed (RTT >8 minutes).[26] Receiver operating characteristic (ROC) analysis for comparison of results by MRU and DRS shows good agreement between the modalities for the diagnosis of renal obstruction. The unique ability of MRU to provide quantitative functional information such as DRF and RTT, in addition to excellent anatomic characterization of the parenchyma and collecting system, makes this the most comprehensive of currently available diagnostic studies.

Rohrschneider et al prospectively evaluated 62 patients with static–dynamic MRU and compared the results with DRS for split function and urinary excretion, which served as the reference standard.[24] DRF, by MRU, was determined by comparing right vs left parenchymal uptake and volume, and dynamic sequences were used to generate whole kidney ROIs, which were used to assess urinary excretion. Urinary excretion was classified similarly by MRU and DRS in 81% of the abnormal kidney–ureter units and in 100% of normal kidney units. Interestingly, in their study, MRU tended to overestimate the severity of obstruction compared with DRS. However, MRU never indicated sufficient urinary drainage when DRS indicated relevant obstruction. The higher sensitivity of Gd-MRU compared with DRS explains this finding.

One study, by Chu et al, offers limited evidence that Gd-MRU may also be more specific in the prognostication of renal deterioration than DRS.[22] In this study, 8 children with unilateral hydronephrosis were evaluated by both MRU and DRS. DRS showed drainage in 3 hydronephrotic kidneys and poor washout in 5. By contrast, Gd-MRU showed drainage in all but 1 of these patients. Four of the 5 hydronephrotic units labeled as obstructed on DRS, but that had drainage by MRU, had no evidence of worsening hydronephrosis or functional deterioration at a mean follow-up of 18 months. Furthermore, antegrade pyelography performed on 2 of these patients who were classified as obstructed by DRS, but not on MRU, showed no evidence of high-grade UPJO. The 1 patient with an obstructive pattern by both MRU and DRS was confirmed to have significant UPJO on antegrade pyelography, and this patient subsequently underwent dismembered pyeloplasty. In a prospective study at Children's Healthcare of Atlanta comparing US, DRS, and MRU in the evaluation of hydronephrosis, MRU provided equivalent information about renal function but superior information regarding morphology in a single study without ionizing radiation.[27] Gd-MRU has also been shown to have a higher sensitivity (100% vs 96%), positive predictive value (86% vs 76%), negative predictive value (100% vs 90%), and diagnostic efficiency (90% vs 79%) than DRS.[23]

At Children's Healthcare of Atlanta, we have used Gd-MRU to evaluate over 300 children with hydronephrosis. MRU has been found to be particularly useful for diagnosis and evaluation of a wide range of renal obstructive anomalies, including UPJO, megaureter, and ectopic ureters (Figure 28.10) and currently the technique is also used to evaluate surgical results in patients pre- and postoperatively. For example, kidneys following pyeloplasty have shown statistically significant improvements in GFR (Patlak), corticomedullary transit and renal transit times, and degree of hydronephrosis following dismembered pyeloplasty.[28] MRU has a sensitivity comparable with ^{99m}Tc DMSA renal scintigraphy for the detection of renal scars and has been combined with MR voiding cystourethrography to diagnose VUR.[25] Indeed, the availability of MRU has influenced our diagnostic strategy for the evaluation of

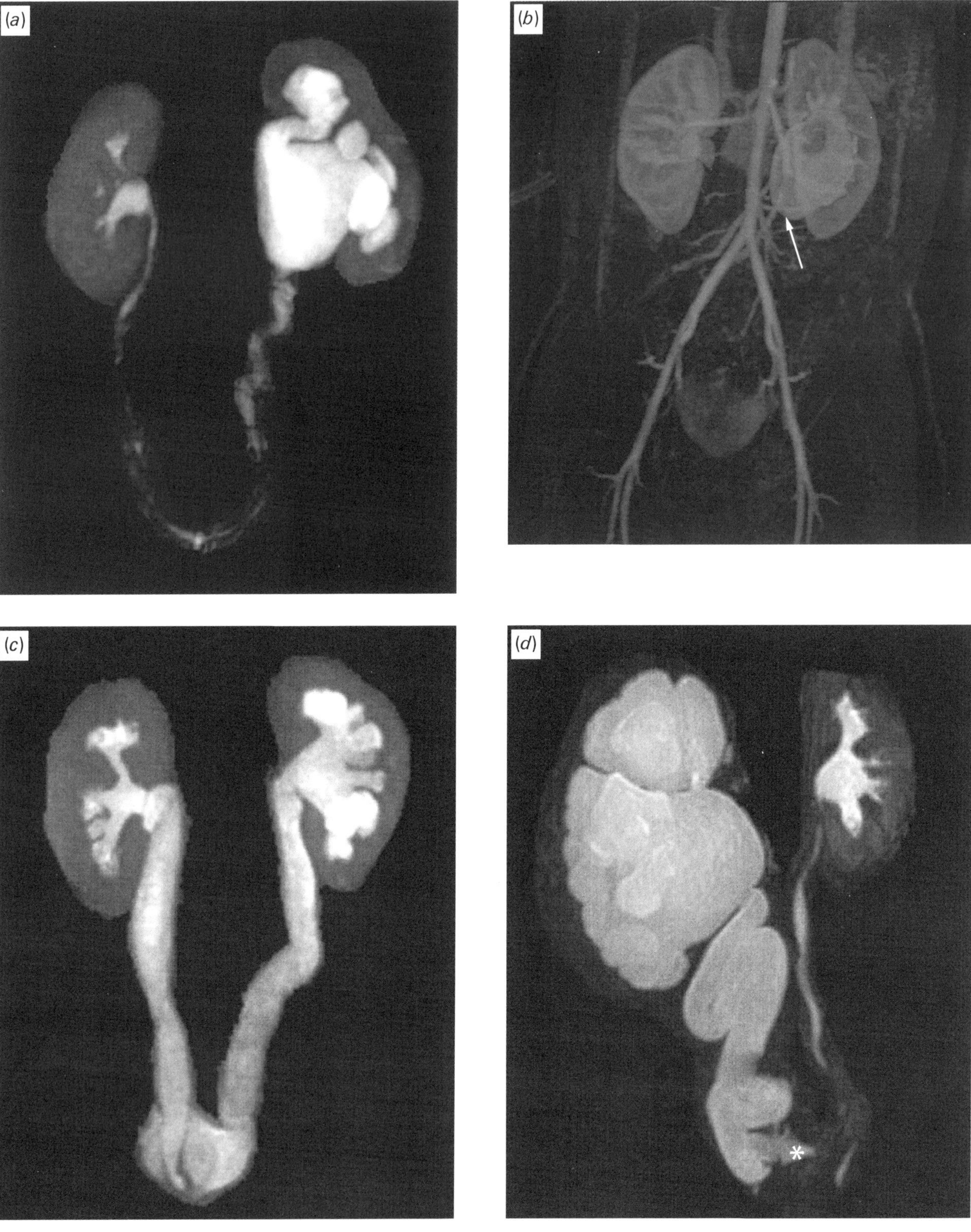

Figure 28.10 (*a*) A 6-year-old patient with left UPJO as seen by MRU. (*b*) On color enhanced images, a crossing vessel can be appreciated (arrow). (*c*) A 5-year-old child with bilateral non-obstructing megaureter. (*d*) A 9-year-old child with a right ectopic ureter, inserting below the bladder neck (asterisk), causing severe hydroureteronephrosis.

pediatric hydronephrosis. We have adapted our diagnostic algorithm to include MRU and currently use this modality in evaluation of most patients with SFU grades III and IV hydronephrosis on confirmatory sonography (Figure 28.11). Indications for surgical intervention based on Gd-MRU are more rigorous than DRS and include:

- DRF of <35–40%
- RTT of >8 minutes
- prolonged CMC times
- decreasing GFR, as indicated by the Patlak index
- anatomic findings

As for DRS, surgical decisions should not be based on isolated MRU criteria.

Despite the advantages of MRU, there are obstacles to its widespread acceptance. First, standardized equations and values used to determine function and classify drainage have not yet been wholly agreed upon. Larger studies with longer-term follow-up are still needed. Secondly, sedation is required for most children. Although techniques using phenobarbital or chloral hydrate have been shown to be safe, patients must be monitored throughout the study with oxygen saturation monitors. Lastly, there are increased costs associated with MRU and availability remains limited. Although MRU is currently more costly than renal scintigraphy, the comprehensive information obtained may justify its use, especially since it does not use ionizing radiation, and companion studies (e.g. retrograde urography), are no longer needed. Furthermore, cost and availability issues are likely to become less important in the future as use of this modality continues to increase. Indeed, over the next several years it is likely that MRU will replace renal scintigraphy in the evaluation of the pediatric urinary tract.

Conclusions

The accurate diagnosis and assessment of pediatric renal obstructive disorders is a principal task in pediatric urology. As a result of ongoing technologic advances, the diagnostic armamentarium available to clinicians for accomplishing this task has increased

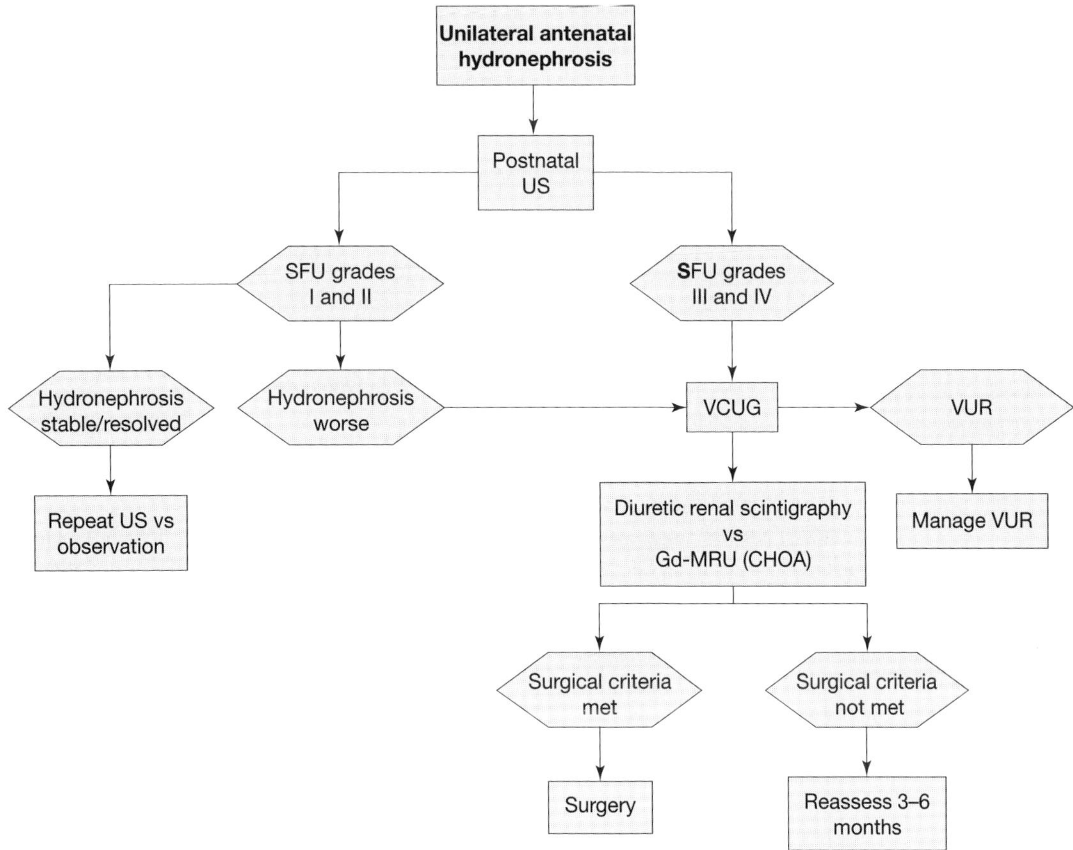

Figure 28.11 Algorithm for the evaluation of antenatal hydronephrosis. At Children's Healthcare of Atlanta (CHOA), gadolinium-enhanced MRU is used in preference to diuretic renal scintigraphy.

dramatically. Nevertheless, a series of radiologic studies, consisting of US, DRS, and VCUG, are still typically used to comprehensively evaluate many children. MRU has the potential to become a gold standard in the evaluation of these children. This single study, which does not require ionizing radiation, provides superior anatomic detail and, arguably, more accurate renal functional information than any other combination of studies. Cost and availability issues remain future challenges and may be the only factors preventing MRU from completely replacing renal scintigraphy.

References

1. Thomas D. Fetal uropathy. Br J Urol 1990; 66:225–31.
2. Baskin LS, Zderic SA, Snyder HM, Duckett JW. Primary dilated megaureter: long-term followup. J Urol 1994; 152(2 Pt 2):618–21.
3. Koff S, Campbell K. The nonoperative management of unilateral neonatal hydronephrosis: natural history of poorly functioning kidneys. J Urol 1994; 152:593–5.
4. Wen JG, Frokiaer J, Jorgensen TM, Djurhuus JC. Obstructive uropathy: an update of the experimental research. J Urol Res 1999; 27:29–39.
5. Houben CH, Wischermann A, Borner G, Slany E. Outcome analysis of pyeloplasty in children. Pediatr Surg Int 2000; 16:189–93.
6. Han BK, Babcock DS. Sonographic measurement and appearance of normal kidneys in children. AJR Am J Roentgenol 1986; 145:613.
7. Lebowitz RL, Blickman JG. The coexistence of ureteropelvic junction obstruction and reflux. AJR Am J Roentgenol 1983; 149(2):231–8.
8. Fernbach SK, Maizels M, Conway JJ. Ultrasound grading of hydronephrosis: introduction to the system used by the Society for Fetal Urology. Pediatr Radiol 1993; 23(6):478–80.
9. Fernbach SK, Maizels M, Conway JJ. Ultrasound grading of hydronephrosis: introduction to the system used by the Society for Fetal Urology. Pediatri Radiol 1993; 23(6):478–80.
10. Siemens DR, Prouse KA, MacNeily AE, Sauerbrei EE. Antenatal hydronephrosis: thresholds of renal pelvic diameter to predict insignificant postnatal pelviectasis. Tech Urol 1998; 4(4):198–210.
11. Bouzada MC, Oliveira EA, Pereira AK et al. Diagnostic accuracy of fetal renal pelvis anteroposterior diameter as a predictor of uropathy: a prospective study. Ultrasound Obstet Gynecol 2004; 24(7):745–9.
12. Johnson CE, Elder JS, Judge NE et al. The accuracy of antenatal ultrasonography in identifying renal abnormalities. Am J Dis Child 1992; 146(10):1181–4.
13. Dhillon HK. Prenatally diagnosed hydronephrosis: the Great Ormond Street experience. Br J Urol 1998; 81:39–44.
14. Dhillon HK. Data presented to the 9th Annual Meeting of the European Society of Pediatric Urology, Salzburg, 1998.
15. Platt JF. Urinary obstruction. Radiol Clin North Am 1996; 34(6):1113–29.
16. Bude RO, DiPietro MA, Platt JF et al. Age dependency of the renal resistive index in healthy children. Radiology 1992; 184(2):469–73.
17. Kessler RM, Quevedo H, Lankau CA et al. Obstructive vs nonobstructive dilatation of the renal collecting system in children: distinction with duplex sonography. AJR Am J Roentgenol 1993; 160(2):353–7.
18. Gill B, Palmer LS, Koenigsberg M, Laor E. Distribution and variability of resistive index values in undilated kidneys in children. Urology 1994; 44(6):897–901.
19. Conway JJ, Maizels M. The 'well tempered' diuretic renogram: a standard method to examine the asymptomatic neonate with hydronephrosis or hydroureteronephrosis. A report from combined meetings of The Society for Fetal Urology and members of The Pediatric Nuclear Medicine Council – The Society of Nuclear Medicine. J Nucl Med 1992; 33(11):2047–51.
20. Gluckman GR, Baskin LS, Bogaert GA et al. Contradictory renal function measured with mercaptoacetyltriglycine diuretic renography in unilateral hydronephrosis. J Urol 1995; 154:1486–9.
21. Dacher J, Pfister C, Thoumas D et al. Shortcomings of diuresis scintigraphy in evaluating urinary obstruction: comparision with pressure flow studies. Pediatr Radiol 1999; 29:742–7.
22. Chu WC, Lam WW, Chan KW et al. Dynamic gadolinium-enhanced magnetic resonance urography for assessing drainage in dilated pelvicalyceal systems with moderate renal function: preliminary results and comparison with diuresis renography. BJU Int 2004; 93(6):830–4.
23. Grattan-Smith JD, Perez-Brayfield MR, Jones RA et al. MR imaging of kidneys: functional evaluation using F-15 perfusion imaging. Pediatr Radiol 2003; 33:293–304.
24. Rohrschneider WK, Haufe S, Wiesel M et al. Functional and morphological evaluation of congenital urinary tract dilatation by using combined static–dynamic MR urography: findings in kidneys with a single collecting system. Radiology 2002; 224:683–94.
25. Rodriguez LV, Spielman D, Herfkens RJ, Shortliffe LD. Magnetic resonance imaging for the evaluation of hydronephrosis, reflux and renal scarring in children. J Urol 2001; 166(3):1023–7.
26. Jones RA, Perez-Brayfield MR, Kirsch AJ, Grattan-Smith JD. Renal transit time with MR urography in children. Radiology 2004; 233(1):41–50.
27. Perez-Brayfield MR, Kirsch AJ, Jones RA, Grattan-Smith JD. A prospective study comparing ultrasound, nuclear scintigraphy and dynamic contrast enhanced magnetic resonance imaging in the evaluation of hydronephrosis. J Urol 2003; 170(4 Pt 1):1330–4.
28. McMann L, Grattan-Smith J, Jones R et al. Dynamic contrast enhanced MRI in evaluating outcomes of pediatric pyeloplasty. Presented at the Southeastern Section of the AUA, March 3, 2005.

Assessment of renal obstructive disorders: urodynamics of the upper tract

29

Leo CT Fung* and Yegappan Lakshmanan

Introduction

Clinical presentation

Routine use of prenatal ultrasonography has resulted in the diagnosis of large numbers of fetuses with hydronephrosis, which occurs in approximately 1 in 800 pregnancies. Some of these asymptomatic congenitally hydronephrotic kidneys improve spontaneously, whereas others progressively deteriorate unless the obstruction is relieved. Clinical parameters used to evaluate hydronephrosis are not always helpful in differentiating between the two groups. The pediatric urologist is charged with the responsibility of distinguishing between ongoing significant obstruction and innocuous residual dilatation of the collecting system in order to institute the appropriate clinical management.

The distinction between true obstruction and mere residual dilatation can be challenging. Anatomic evaluation alone, by ultrasonography and other radiologic imaging, accurately delineates the degree of dilatation, but is insufficient to determine the degree of obstruction. Nuclear medicine renal scans provide functional information in the evaluation of hydronephrosis, but there is a lack of consensus in how these parameters should be used to guide management. In the absence of clear indications of obstruction or lack thereof, clinical decisions are usually based on serial assessments of the hydronephrotic, and possibly obstructed renal unit. The inherent risk in this approach is the possible loss of renal function, which may be sudden and irreversible, if surgical correction of the obstruction fails to be instituted before the loss of renal function occurs.

In situations where surgical intervention is clearly indicated, or if the risk of functional deterioration is minimal, the use of upper tract urodynamic studies is not necessary. When routine tests are insufficient, or unable to clarify the diagnosis, however, upper tract urodynamic studies can provide invaluable diagnostic information.

Role of upper tract urodynamics

Although hydronephrosis is a highly complex physiologic process, the source of the problem is essentially physical in nature. In any biologic fluid conduit system, the resistance of the conduit is directly proportional to pressure over flow (resistance ∞ pressure/flow), modified from the Poiseuille–Hagen law,[1] which was originally applied to the flow of Newtonian fluids through rigid tubes. Based on this principle, both pressure and flow must be taken into account simultaneously in order to derive a measurement of the resistance within the conduit. Without taking both pressure and flow parameters into account simultaneously, as is the case in ultrasonography and other purely image-based modalities, or in nuclear renography, results cannot be used to draw conclusions regarding the resistance within the collecting system. In contrast, upper tract urodynamics are designed to take into account both the pressure within the collecting system and the rate of fluid flow; hence the synonymous term percutaneous pressure–flow studies. Upper tract urodynamic studies are intrinsically different from imaging studies and nuclear renal scans in that they provide a measure of the resistance of the collecting system, which is fundamental in the evaluation of hydronephrosis and in the diagnosis of obstruction.

Percutaneous pressure–flow study

In performing pressure–flow studies in the assessment of upper tract urodynamics, direct access to the prox-

*Deceased December 2005

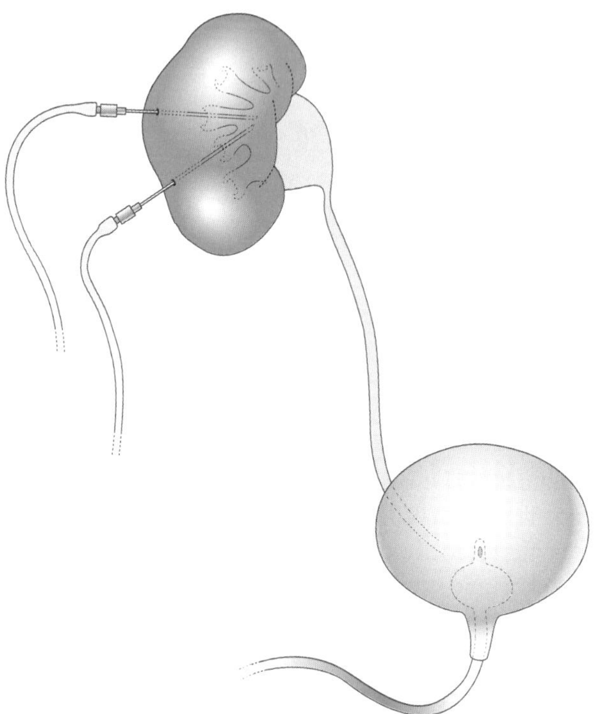

Figure 29.1 Whitaker pressure perfusion test. (Adapted from Wacksman,[2] with permission.)

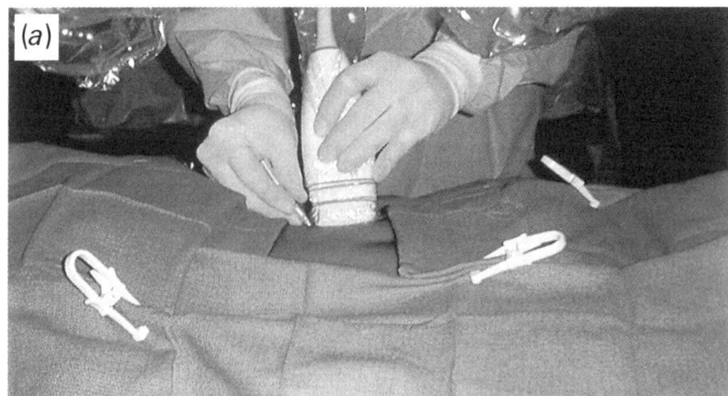

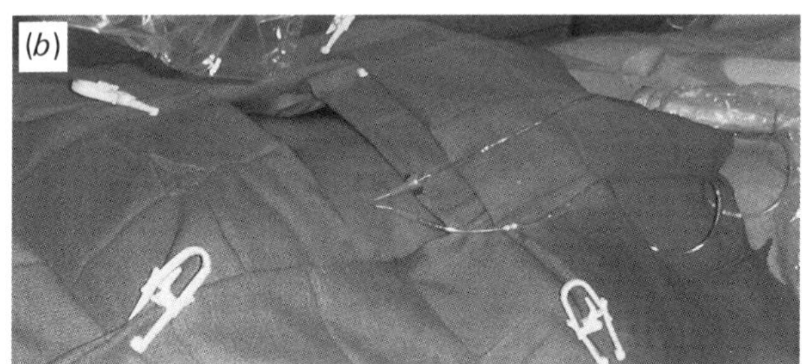

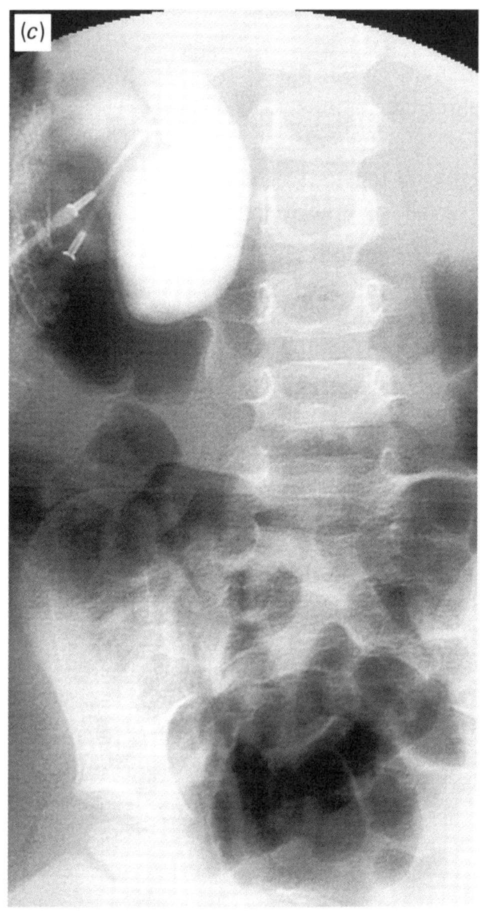

Figure 29.2 For the percutaneous pressure–flow studies performed in children at the authors' institution, all studies are performed under general anesthesia in the prone position. (*a*) and (*b*) Two 22 gauge angiocatheters are inserted into the collecting system percutaneously under ultrasonographic guidance. Infusion of contrast verifies satisfactory nephrostomy access. (*c*) Antegrade nephrostogram in prone position.

imal collecting system is necessary to measure the fluid pressure within the system (Figure 29.1). Insertion of two 22 gauge 2 inch angiocatheters under sonographic guidance and fluoroscopic monitoring has been found to be effective and safe in our experience (Figure 29.2). In children the study can be carried out under either heavy sedation or general anesthesia.

In performing upper tract urodynamic studies, or pressure–flow studies, as the name implies, there is a pressure component, and there is also a flow component. One therefore needs to establish what constitutes normal as opposed to abnormally elevated renal pelvic pressures. Secondly, one also needs to determine what constitutes appropriate flow rates that would optimally challenge the collecting system within physiologic limits. These considerations will now be described in turn.

Threshold for normal renal pelvic pressure

A number of experimental and clinical studies have attempted to define the upper limit of normal collecting system pressure. In the rat model, the proximal renal tubular pressure, intratubular and peritubular capillary pressures all remain constant until the collecting system pressure exceeds normal renal tubular pressure. In the rat, the normal proximal renal tubular pressure was established to be 14.1 ± 0.5 cmH_2O.[3] In the human, intrarenal arterial resistance increases acutely once the renal pelvic pressure rises above 14 cmH_2O.[4] Furthermore, Fichtner et al showed that in the congenitally hydronephrotic rat model, mean renal pelvic pressure was 14.1 ± 1.6 cmH_2O under very high urine output with an empty bladder.[5] The mean renal pelvic pressure increased further when the bladder was filled. In contrast, mean renal pelvic pressure in normal controls was below 14 cmH_2O under high urine output. Even with the bladder filled to capacity, the highest mean renal pelvic pressure recorded was only 13.2 ± 1.6 cmH_2O. These studies suggest that the upper limit of normal renal pelvic pressure is 14 cmH_2O, above which undesirable physiologic changes begin to occur.

Additional evidence indicates that continuous elevation in renal pelvic pressure leads to acute and irreversible renal injury within 24 hours. In a porcine model of constantly elevated renal pelvic pressure between 20 and 40 cmH_2O, the urinary level of *N*-acetyl-β-D-glucosaminidase (NAG) was found to be elevated, which is indicative of acute tubular cell membrane disruption.[6] Similar conditions also resulted in acute onset of apoptotic cell death, signifying irreversible injury.[7] These changes were associated with decreased renal blood flow, and up-regulated vascular endothelial growth factor (VEGF) mRNA levels, suggesting that decreased perfusion and tissue hypoxia play an important role when renal pelvic pressure is elevated.[6] Renal injury was significantly greater in the experimental group, with renal pelvic pressure ranging from 20 to 40 cmH_2O, compared with the control animals with renal pelvic pressure of 10 cmH_2O or less. Based on these results, the threshold for physiogically safe renal pelvic pressure seems to lie somewhere between 10 and 20 cmH_2O. Although the precise pressure threshold above which renal injury occurs remains undefined, these experiments are consistent with 14 cmH_2O as the upper limit of normal renal pelvic pressure, as established previously in both rat and human studies.

Optimal flow challenge to the collecting system

The normal renal collecting system handles a wide range of urinary flow rates, as urine output varies under a variety of normal physiologic conditions. A normal collecting system should be able to handle this normal range of flow rates without an undue rise in pressure. In an 'obstructed' collecting system, on the other hand, there is an abnormally high resistance, causing elevated pressures whenever the flow rate exceeds its limited capacity for fluid transport. The increase in pressure in an obstructed collecting system is directly proportional to the rate of flow and the degree of obstruction, according to the modified Poiseuille–Hagen law.[1] However, if the collecting system is presented with a flow challenge that is excessively high and unphysiologic, even normal collecting systems may potentially be overwhelmed and develop elevations in pressure beyond the physiologically normal limit. In performing upper tract urodynamic studies, the flow rate chosen to optimally challenge the collecting system should therefore reflect the maximum urine output that the kidney is capable of generating under normal physiologic conditions.

Individualized infusion pressure–flow study

The pioneering work in infusion pressure–flow studies was carried out by Whitaker,[8] and the initial form of pressure–flow study is referred to as the Whitaker test. Whitaker advocated using a standard external infusion rate of 10 ml/min, with lower infusion rates of 2–5 ml/min for smaller children. An even higher infusion rate of 15 ml/min can be used in adults for a more stringent flow challenge. Intrapelvic pressures <10 cmH_2O were interpreted as normal. Pressures >20 cmH_2O were abnormal and those between 10 and 20 cmH_2O were considered indeterminate. Although these concepts were sound in principle, there was no specific guideline to determine what infusion rate should be used for children of a given age and body size. Further work was therefore undertaken by Fung et al in an attempt to clarify the infusion rates used, to provide physiologically meaningful results.[9] Three patient parameters form the basis for the calculated estimate of the patient's maximum physiologic urine output:

- body surface area
- age-adjusted 90th percentile glomerular filtration rate (GFR)
- the maximum percentage of the GFR one can physiologically excrete as urine.

Both surface area[10] and 90th percentile GFR (ml/min/1.73 m^2) for the patient's age (Figure 29.3)[11] can be obtained from population nomograms. Since the renal tubules proximal to the segment sensitive to antidiuretic hormone reclaim about

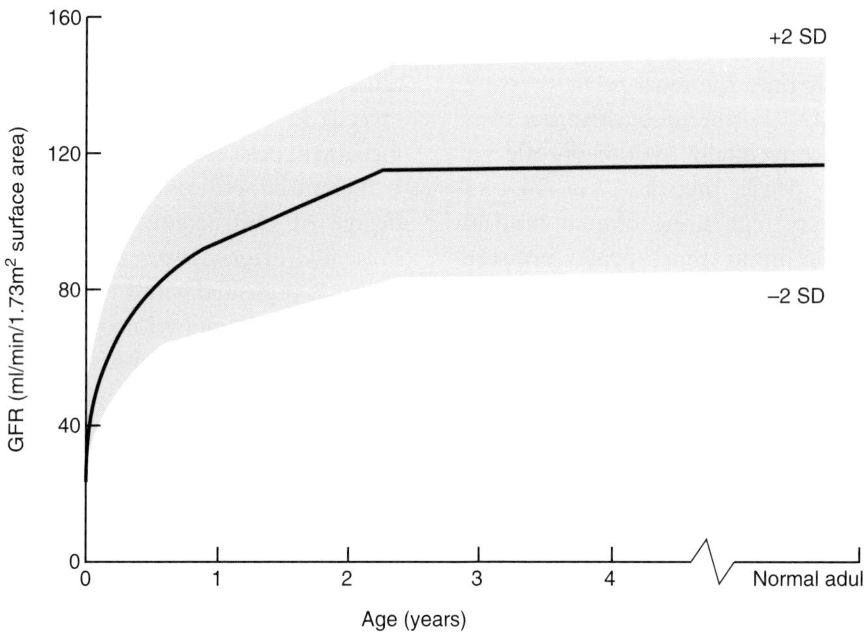

Figure 29.3 Age-adjusted glomerular filtration rate (GFR, in ml/min per 1.73 m^2) nomogram. (Adapted from McCrory.[11])

80% of the water in the glomerular ultrafiltrate, under non-pathologic conditions the maximum physiologic diuresis cannot exceed approximately 20% of the GFR, even in the complete absence of antidiuretic hormone.[12] The calculation can be summarized as:

$$\text{maximum physiologic urine output per kidney (ml/min)} = \frac{\text{surface area (m}^2) \times \text{age-adjusted GFR (ml/min/1.73 m}^2) \times 20\% \text{ of total GFR}}{1.73 \text{ m}^2 \times \text{number of kidneys}}$$

Since the pressure–flow study is applied to one kidney at a time, the flow rate employed is based on the maximum physiologic urine output per kidney: hence the correction factor 'number of kidneys'. For patients who have a solitary kidney, compensatory hypertrophy and hyperplasia need to be taken into account. This formula is directly applicable only if the GFR of the solitary kidney has compensated to a level similar to the population-normal total GFR.

For a patient whose total GFR and differential renal function are known, maximum physiologic urine output can be derived directly with this formula. Maximum physiologic urine output for the kidney of interest would then be 20% of the measured total GFR (ml/min) multiplied by the differential renal function for that kidney (%):

$$\text{maximum physiologic urine output per kidney (ml/min)} = \text{measured total GFR (ml/min)} \times 20\% \text{ of total GFR} \times \text{differential renal function (\%)}$$

When these calculations were performed for patients of different ages and body sizes, the appropriate infusion rate corresponding to the respective maximum physiologic urine output per kidney ranged from 0.85 ml/min (appropriate for a 4-week-old infant) to 16.31 ml/min (appropriate for a large ≥18-year-old patient) (Table 29.1). This tremendously wide range underscores the importance of individualizing the infusion rate used for each pediatric patient.[9]

As previously noted, a non-obstructed system should maintain a peak renal pelvic pressure no higher than the upper limit of normal physiologically – i.e. maintain a peak renal pelvic pressure of ≤14 cmH_2O. By contrast, a collecting system with significant obstruction can be expected to develop a peak renal pelvic pressure of >14 cmH_2O. If the renal pelvic pressure remains well below 14 cmH_2O at the individualized infusion rate, one can arbitrarily increase the infusion rate by 50% or 100% to challenge the collecting system drainage with a supraphysiologic flow rate to test the reserve capability of that collecting system. However, an elevated renal pelvic pressure (>14 cmH_2O) in this setting is not necessarily

Table 29.1 Height, weight, and glomerular filtration rate (GFR) values are obtained from population nomograms[a]

Age (years)	Height (cm)		Weight (kg)		Surface area (m^2)		GFR 90th percentile (ml/min/ 1.73 m^2)	Maximum physiologic urine output per kidney (ml/min)	
	10th percentile	90th percentile	10th percentile	90th percentile	10th percentile	90th percentile		10th percentile	90th percentile
4 weeks	50.5	56.5	3.3	4.8	0.210	0.260	70	0.85	1.05
8 weeks	53.0	60.0	3.9	5.6	0.225	0.290	80	1.04	1.34
12 weeks	55.5	63.0	4.6	6.6	0.250	0.320	90	1.30	1.66
16 weeks	58.0	66.0	5.3	7.5	0.275	0.350	98	1.56	1.98
20 weeks	60.0	68.0	5.9	8.3	0.295	0.375	105	1.79	2.28
0.5	62.5	71.0	6.6	9.4	0.320	0.405	108	2.00	2.53
0.6	64.5	73.0	7.1	10.0	0.340	0.430	111	2.18	2.76
0.7	66.5	75.0	7.5	10.5	0.355	0.445	114	2.34	2.93
0.8	68.0	76.5	7.8	10.9	0.360	0.460	116	2.41	3.08
0.9	69.5	78.5	8.1	11.3	0.380	0.480	118	2.59	3.27
1	74.0	80.0	8.4	11.7	0.400	0.490	120	2.77	3.40
2	80.0	90.0	10.5	14.5	0.470	0.630	138	3.75	5.03
3	88.0	99.0	12.5	17.0	0.540	0.660	144	4.49	5.49
4	94.5	107.0	13.0	19.0	0.560	0.730	144	4.66	6.08
5	101.0	114.5	14.5	21.5	0.630	0.810	144	5.24	6.74
6	107.0	121.0	17.0	24.5	0.700	0.890	144	5.83	7.41
7	112.0	128.0	19.0	28.0	0.760	0.980	144	6.33	8.16
8	117.5	133.5	21.0	31.0	0.820	1.050	144	6.83	8.74
9	123.0	139.0	23.0	35.0	0.870	1.150	144	7.24	9.57
10	128.0	144.5	25.0	40.0	0.930	1.260	144	7.74	10.49
11	133.5	150.0	27.5	44.5	1.000	1.360	144	8.32	11.32
12	138.5	157.0	30.0	51.0	1.070	1.480	144	8.91	12.32
13	143.5	164.0	32.5	59.5	1.140	1.640	144	9.49	13.65
14	152.0	169.0	39.5	64.5	1.300	1.740	144	10.82	14.48
15	154.0	177.0	47.0	68.0	1.420	1.830	144	11.82	15.23
16	154.5	181.0	48.5	71.5	1.450	1.900	144	12.07	15.82
17	154.5	182.5	48.5	73.5	1.450	1.940	144	12.07	16.15
18	154.5	183.0	49.0	74.5	1.460	1.960	144	12.15	16.31
19	154.5	183.0	49.0	75.0	1.460	1.970	144	12.15	16.40

[a] The calculated physiologically maximum urine outputs are provided as rough guidelines for the individualized pressure–flow study infusion rates.

Note: The maximum urine output estimates tabulated here are expressed as the infusion rate per kidney, representing half of the total calculated urine output estimate. For patients with a solitary kidney, the infusion rate may need to be increased in proportion to its compensatory increase in GFR.

indicative of significant obstruction, as the supraphysiologic infusion rate represents a flow rate that exceeds the urine output from the kidney under physiologic conditions; instead, it would be an indication that the collecting system being tested is borderline for a significant degree of obstruction, with little additional reserve capacity for handling higher urinary flow rates.

These modifications from Whitaker's original descriptions form the basis for the individualized infusion pressure–flow study. It is important to note that a urethral catheter is routinely used to keep the bladder empty during all pressure–flow studies to minimize the potential of renal pelvic pressure readings being artificially affected by a full bladder.

Diuresis pressure–flow study

Individualized adjusted infusion rates, as described in the individualized infusion pressure–flow study, help to ensure that the collecting systems being tested are challenged with appropriately infused flow rates. However, externally infused flow rates are, after all, from an extracorporeal source and are not physiologic. In order to render the flow challenge in upper tract urodynamics more physiologic, it is possible to eliminate the need for an external infusion during the pressure–flow study, and instead challenge the collecting system with a diuresis induced by pharmacologic means, such as the intravenous administration of furosemide.[13] Nephrostomy access is still necessary to measure renal pelvic pressure, as is urethral catheterization. Instead of an external infusion, the patient receives an intravenous bolus of 15 ml/kg of a crystalloid solution followed by 1 mg/kg of intravenous furosemide up to a maximum of 10 mg. Renal pelvic pressure is continuously monitored for 30 minutes after the furosemide administration (Figure 29.4), and urine output monitored every 5–10 minutes to ensure that an adequate diuresis has been induced. Similar to the individualized infusion pressure–flow study, a peak renal pelvic pressure of ≤14 cmH_2O is considered normal whereas a peak renal pelvic pressure of >14 cmH_2O is considered obstructed.

In a series of over 55 patients who received both the individualized infusion and the diuresis pressure–flow studies, peak renal pelvic pressures obtained from the two pressure–flow studies were found to be similar, agreeing in all but three cases. In these three patients, test results were either borderline positive or borderline negative, with the peak renal pelvic pressures differing by only 2–3 cmH_2O.[13]

The diuresis pressure–flow study differs from the individualized infusion pressure–flow study in more ways than just how the flow challenge to the collecting system is generated. The externally infused flow of an individualized infusion study challenges the collecting system, but cannot measure how the kidney may have responded to the obstruction present in the collecting system. Based on our current understanding of how the kidney responds to obstruction, however, the diuretic pressure–flow study not only provides information on the resistance present in the collecting system but also may help uncover compensatory physiologic changes present in kidneys in response to physiologically significant obstruction.

Based on our current understanding of renal obstruction, the collecting system pressure of a chronically obstructed kidney remains within the normal range.[14] In these obstructed kidneys, the normal collecting system pressure is a result of long-term compensatory changes occurring in the kidney, with reductions in renal blood flow and GFR proportional to the degree of outflow obstruction. In terms of the collecting system pressure at baseline conditions, a hydronephrotic kidney with a significantly obstructed collecting system is therefore indistinguishable from a non-obstructed kidney. However, the hydronephrotic kidney with ongoing significant obstruction maintains normal renal pelvic pressure because of a state of equilibrium from changes in renal blood flow and GFR compensating for the outflow obstruction.[14] In this compensated state of equilibrium, the renal blood flow and GFR decrease in the obstructed kidney just enough to compensate for the existing outflow obstruction at baseline conditions, and the collecting system has little or no reserve for handling any increase in urine flow. If such a kidney were to be challenged with a furosemide-induced diuresis, it is logical that an elevation in renal pelvic pressure would ensue. In a non-obstructed collecting system, by contrast, experimental animal studies have documented a significant reserve capacity for handling diuresis beyond baseline urine output, while maintaining renal pelvic pressures below the upper limit of normal.[5]

Furosemide-induced diuresis is therefore more than just a flow challenge to the collecting system; it is, in fact, also a means of 'agitating' the equilibrium established in the renal blood flow, GFR, and collecting system pressure of significantly obstructed kidneys. Thus, a positive diuresis pressure–flow study (peak renal pelvic pressure >14 cmH_2O) indicates not only a collecting system with an abnormally high resistance

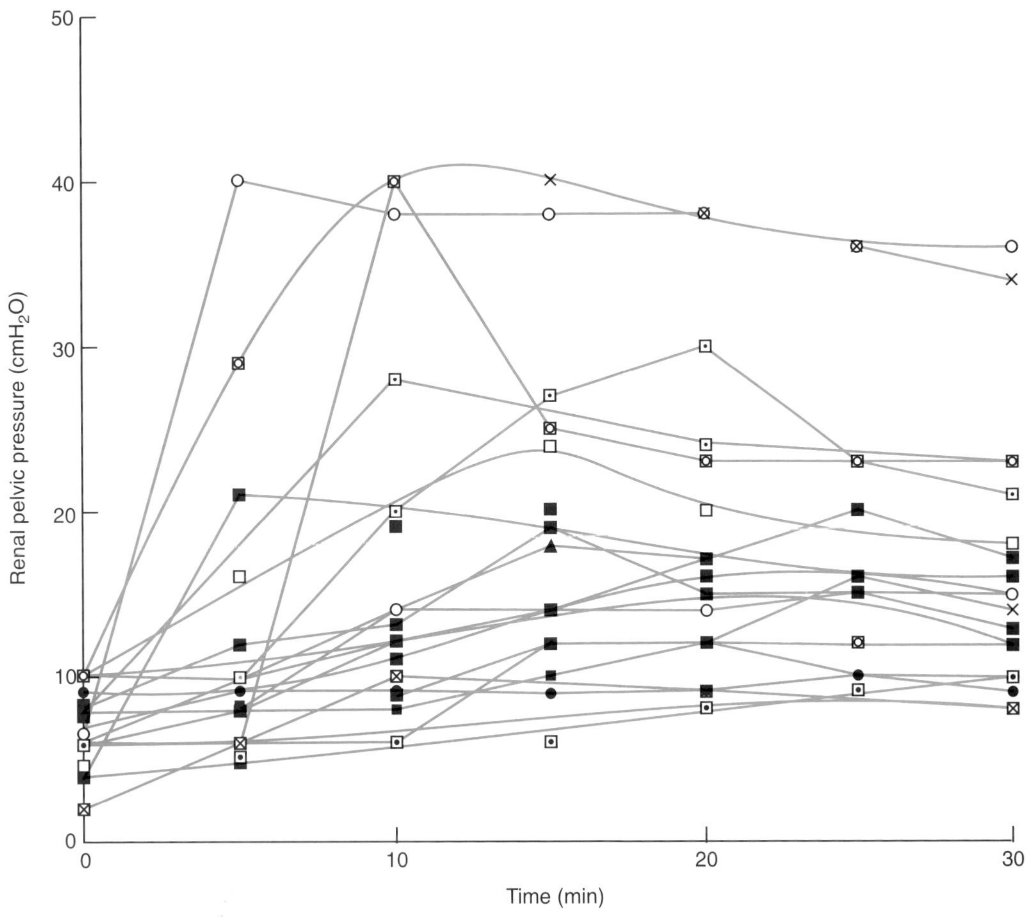

Figure 29.4 Composite graph of a representative group of patients with hydronephrosis undergoing diuresis pressure–flow studies, where renal pelvic pressure is plotted against time. Renal pelvic pressure at time 0 represents baseline pressure. Intravenous furosemide, 1 mg/kg, up to a maximum of 10 mg, was given at time 0, and renal pelvic pressure was monitored for 30 minutes. The furosemide-induced diuresis consitutes the sole form of fluid challenge, and no infusion of fluid takes place during these studies. In the authors' experience studying over 55 hydronephrotic kidneys to date (data not all plotted in this graph in order to maintain clarity), it has been consistently observed that the prediuresis baseline renal pelvic pressures remain relatively low, and do not exceed 10 cmH_2O. The highest renal pelvic pressure recorded to date is 63 cmH_2O, observed in a patient with ureteropelvic junction (UPJ) obstruction and no evidence of contrast draining across the UPJ throughout the entire pressure–flow study.

to flow but also that the kidney being tested is probably in a compensated state of equilibrium, precariously maintaining a normal renal pelvic pressure at baseline conditions at the expense of decreased renal blood flow and/or GFR.

In our current series of over 55 patients, positive studies correlate with those of patients who are symptomatic or show evidence of renal functional deterioration. These correlations suggest that a positive diuresis pressure–flow study is predictive of functionally significant obstruction. Conversely, those with negative diuresis pressure–flow studies have shown no evidence of deterioration or required surgical intervention for symptomatic complaints at a follow-up of 2 years (Figure 29.5).

Upper tract urodynamics and nuclear diuretic renography: similarities and differences

Because of the relatively invasive nature of establishing percutaneous nephrostomy access, it is important to clarify whether the pressure–flow studies reveal uniquely important diagnostic information as compared to the more commonly used diuretic renogram. The protocols for the diuresis pressure–flow study are similar to those for diuretic nuclear renography: both modalities share the use of a urethral catheter to keep the bladder empty, the infusion of an intravenous crystalloid solution to ensure adequate patient hydration, and the administration of 1 mg/kg of intra-

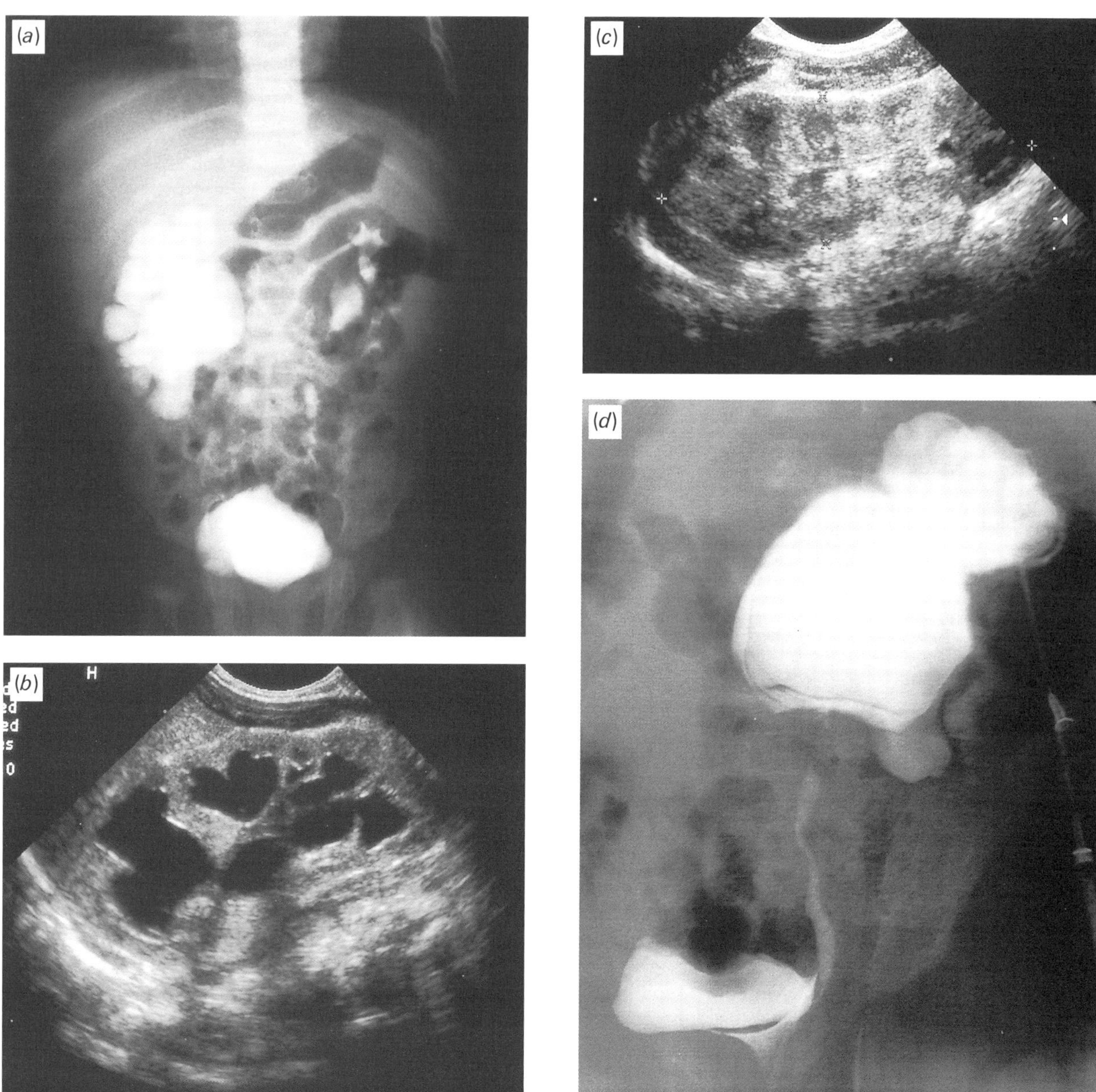

Figure 29.5 Male patient identified as having right hydronephrosis compatible with ureteropelvic junction (UPJ) obstruction, as shown by an intravenous pyelogram (*a*). Ultrasonography demonstrated marked right hydronephrosis with significant thinning of the renal cortex (*b*), and normal left kidney (*c*). A percutaneous pressure–flow study was performed when the patient was 7 weeks of age. (*d*) Right antegrade nephrostogram in the prone position. The pressure–flow study was negative for significant obstruction, where the peak renal pelvic pressure was only 5 cmH_2O, well below the upper limit of normal of 14 cmH_2O, under both furosemide-induced diuresis and a supraphysiologic infusion rate of 200%. Despite significant cortical thinning and pelvicaliectasis, the patient was managed with an observational approach in view of the negative pressure–flow study. From his initial right differential renal function of 30%, it spontaneously improved to 52% 1 year later, and further increased to 58% at his 2-year follow-up. It is unclear why his differential renal function increased to beyond 50%, but nevertheless the initial negative pressure–flow study appeared to be reliable in excluding significant UPJ obstruction.

venous furosemide to challenge the collecting system with a diuresis. However, the key parameters assessed by the two studies are fundamentally different: the diuresis pressure–flow study examines renal pelvic pressure changes as urine flow increases, whereas diuretic nuclear renography measures the washout $t_{1/2}$, a semiquantitative measure of the rate of flow of urine across the suspected site of obstruction. When

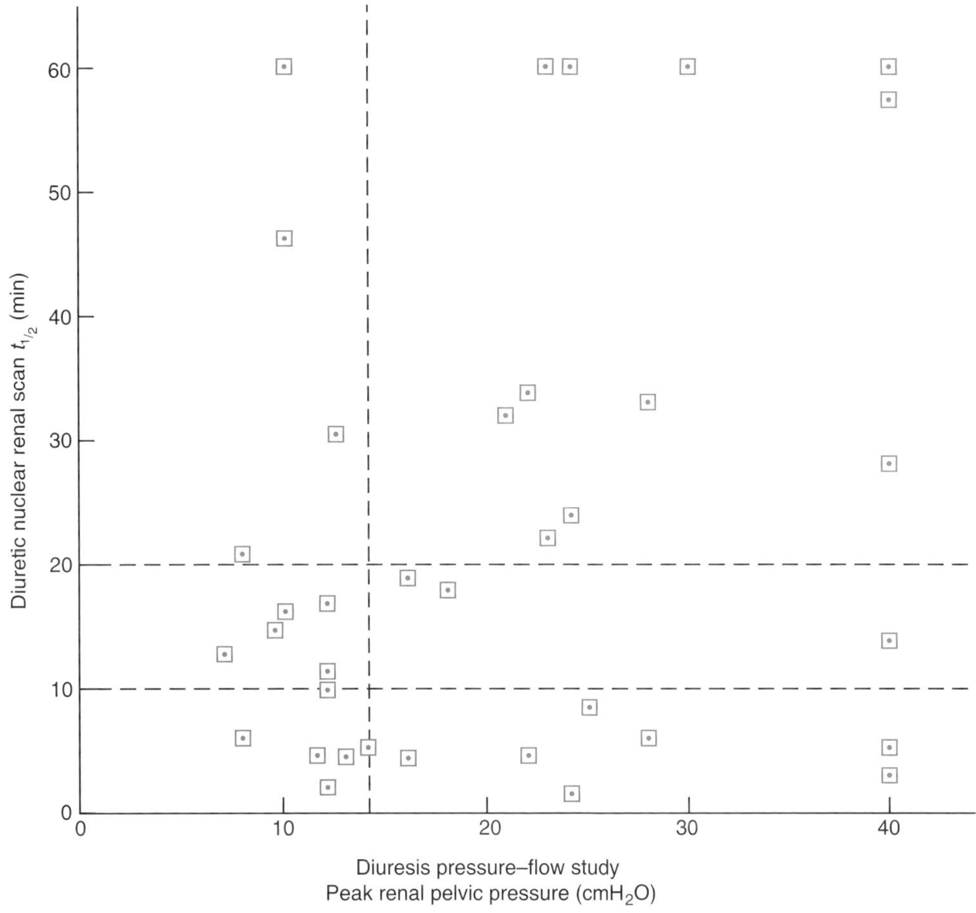

Figure 29.6 Correlation graph depicting diuretic nuclear renal scan $t_{1/2}$ against peak renal pelvic pressure recorded during diuresis pressure–flow studies. Whereas the basic protocols of the two forms of test appear similar, including similar intravenous hydration, furosemide administration, and the use of a bladder catheter, the results of the two tests have little correlation with each other, and these two variables are essentially independent of each other.

we studied 46 hydronephrotic kidneys with both the diuresis pressure–flow study and diuretic nuclear renography, it was found that renal pelvic pressure alterations had little correlation with the washout $t_{1/2}$, and that these two variables were essentially independent of each other (Figure 29.6). Some of the kidneys examined in this study showed evidence of significant obstruction, with markedly increased collecting system pressure on the diuresis pressure–flow study, yet the washout $t_{1/2}$ was normal. Conversely, some of the kidneys examined showed no evidence of significant obstruction, with normal renal pelvic pressure throughout, yet the washout $t_{1/2}$ was grossly elevated. A similar disparity between washout curve results and infusion pressure–flow study results was reported by Dacher et al;[15] however, those results that did not correlate were mostly from a specific group of postoperative patients with severely dilated collecting systems.

Resistance can be assessed only if both pressure and flow parameters are simultaneously taken into account. These differences observed between the washout $t_{1/2}$ and the diuresis pressure–flow study results support the concept that these parameters do not measure the same variables: namely, the washout $t_{1/2}$ provides a semiquantitative measure of flow across the suspected site of obstruction, whereas the pressure–flow study result reflects the resistance within the collecting system being tested. Further studies and long-term clinical follow-up will be required to clarify the clinical significance of these differences.

Fluoroscopic monitoring and ureteral opening pressure

At the beginning of a pressure–flow study, it is helpful to instill contrast into the renal pelvis to verify

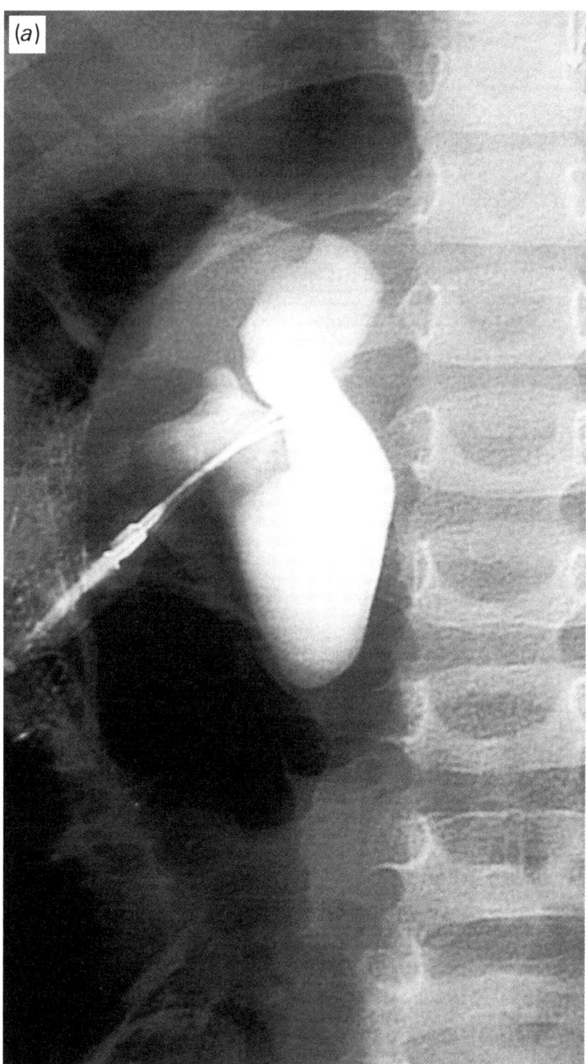

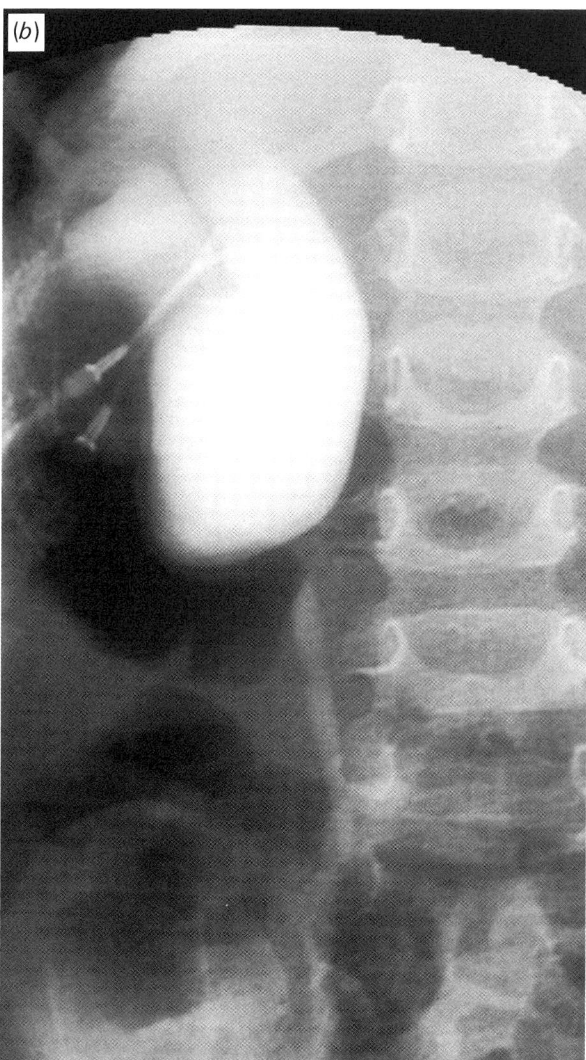

Figure 29.7 Ureteral opening pressure is defined as the pressure at which antegrade contrast is first seen distal to the suspected site of obstruction. In this 4-year-old boy with left hydronephrosis, no contrast was seen to enter the ureter ((*a*) left antegrade nephrostogram in the prone position) until his left renal pelvic pressure reached 17 cmH_2O (*b*). His ureteral opening pressure of 17 cmH_2O is compatible with significant ureteropelvic junction (UPJ) obstruction.

proper positioning of the nephrostomy access. Before the instillation of contrast, however, an equivalent volume of urine should first be aspirated out, so that the baseline pressure dynamics of the renal pelvis remain essentially unchanged. With contrast present in the renal pelvis, it has the added advantage that subsequent renal pelvic pressure changes can then be correlated with dynamic anatomic alterations seen by periodic fluoroscopic monitoring. For example, the pressure at which antegrade contrast is first seen distal to the suspected site of obstruction can be measured. This parameter is defined as the ureteral opening pressure[16] (Figure 29.7). In our study of 52 renal units in 43 patients, positive (obstructed) ureteral opening pressures (>14 cmH_2O) had a 100% association with a positive individualized infusion pressure–flow study. When the ureteral opening pressure was negative (<14 cmH_2O), however, it was predictive of a negative individualized infusion pressure–flow study in only 57%.[16]

Antegrade infusion of contrast media also delineates the anatomic site of obstruction, and defines the ureter distal to the site of obstruction, which is useful in surgical planning (Figure 29.8).

Finally, fluoroscopic monitoring may be helpful in assessing patients with intermittent obstruction secondary to kinking of the ureteropelvic junction (UPJ). On initial infusion, the drainage may be rela-

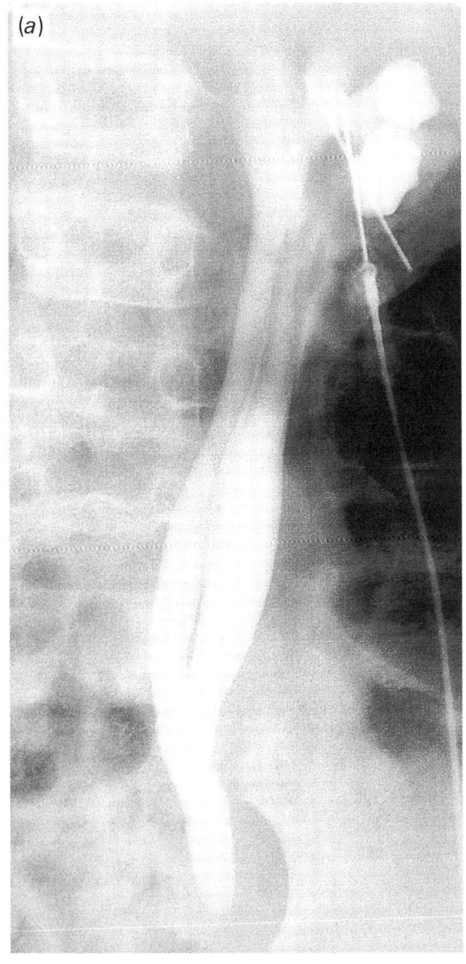

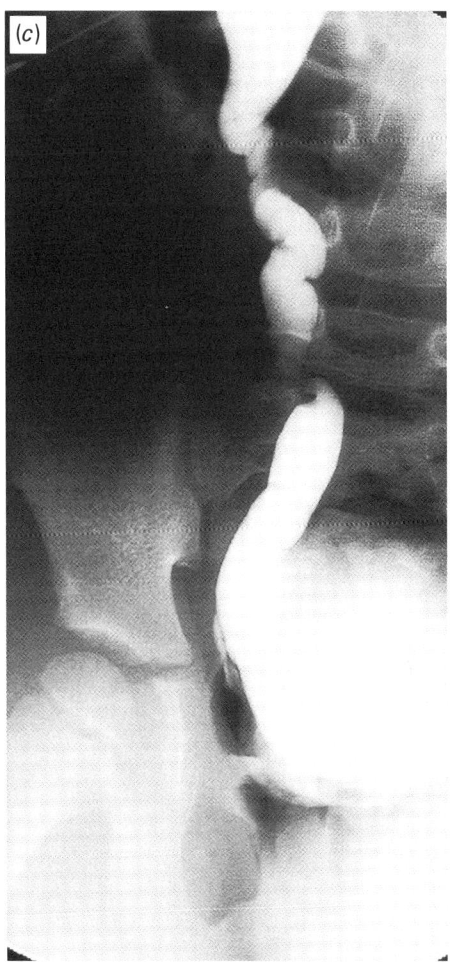

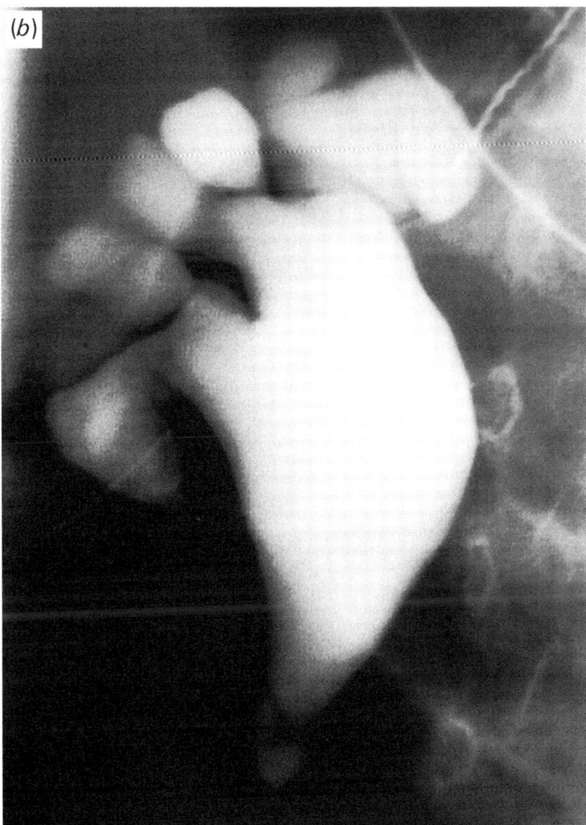

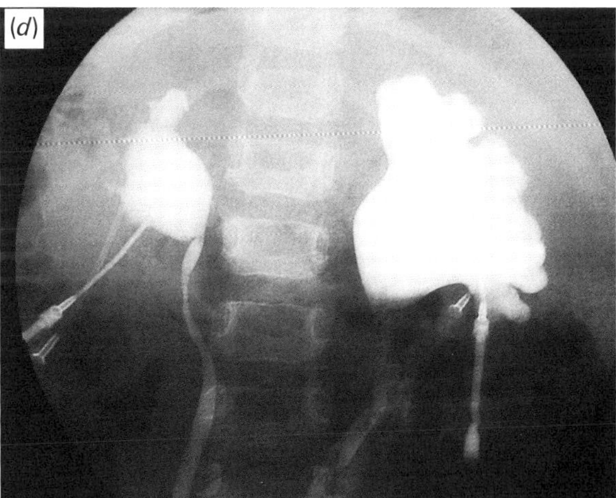

Figure 29.8 Antegrade infusion of contrast media can be an effective tool for delineating the anatomic site of obstruction. (*a*) In this 10-year-old girl, a partial ureteral duplication is well visualized with percutaneous nephrostomy access established to the lower moiety only. (*b*) Possible anomalies at the ureteropelvic junction (UPJ). (*c*) Possible anomalies at the UPJ, midureter, and ureterovesical can be seen in this 5.5-year-old boy with a history of posterior urethral valves. (*d*) Bilateral percutaneous pressure–flow studies can also be performed simultaneously.

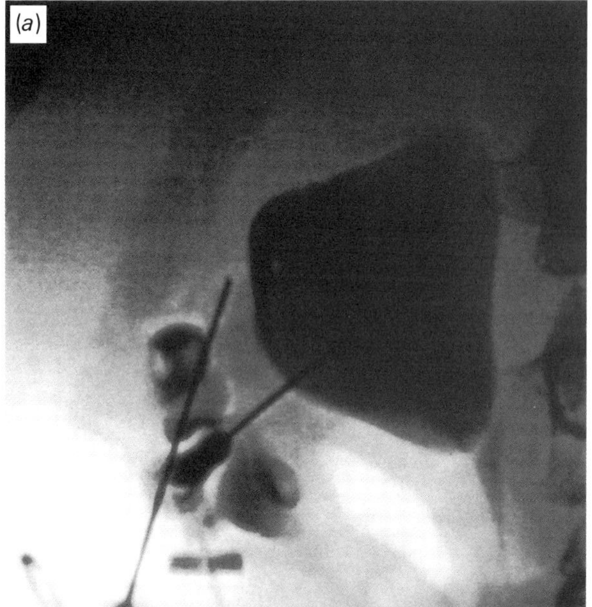

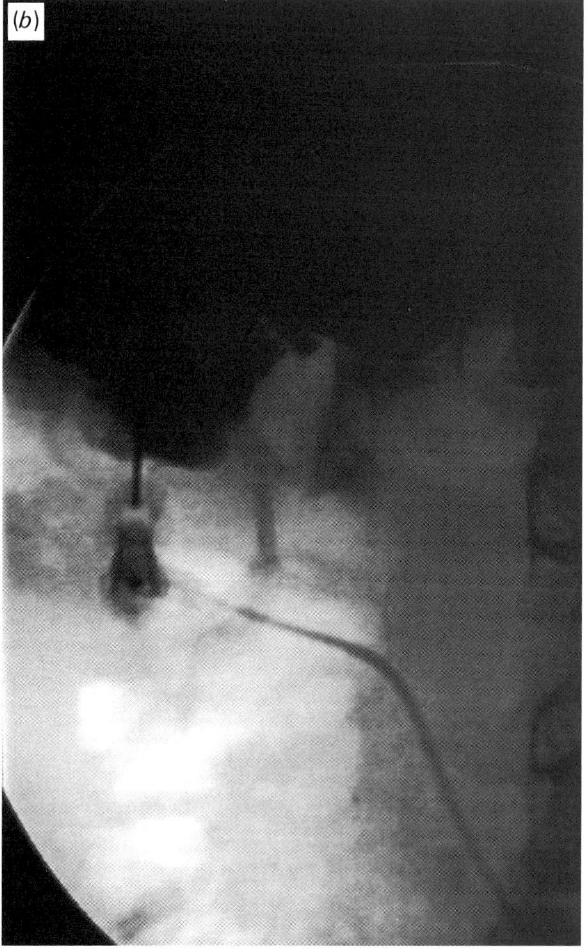

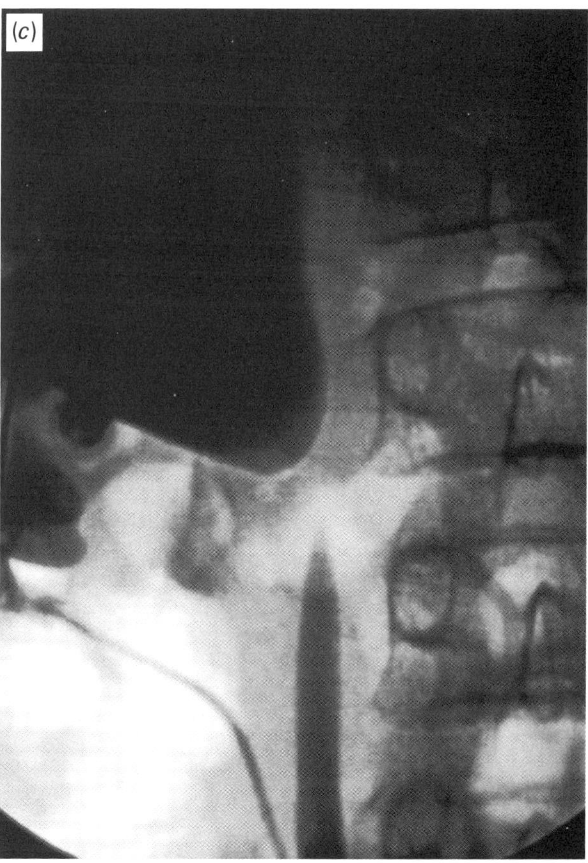

Figure 29.9 This 6-year-old girl was initially misdiagnosed as having chronic gastrointestinal disorder when she presented with recurrent abdominal pain, nausea, and vomiting. When she underwent a percutaneous pressure–flow study to evaluate her left hydronephrosis, contrast was seen to drain promptly across the ureteropelvic junction (UPJ) into the proximal ureter early in the study (*a*). As the renal pelvis became progressively more distended, the drainage of contrast across the UPJ ceased entirely (*b*). Renal pelvic pressure continued to rise sharply, and the pressure–flow study was terminated at 40 cmH_2O. No drainage of contrast was seen across the UPJ until fluid was aspirated out of the renal pelvis to decompress the grossly distended collecting system. When the renal pelvis dimensions returned towards their initial baseline, drainage across the UPJ resumed with a gush of contrast into the proximal ureter (*c*). This pattern of intermittent high-grade obstruction was presumed to be secondary to a kink at the UPJ that was accentuated by the renal pelvis becoming overdistended. Her recurrent abdominal pain, nausea, and vomiting episodes (Dietl's crisis) were successfully corrected by a dismembered pyeloplasty.

tively efficient. As the flow rate increases, however, the renal pelvis becomes increasingly dilated, progressively displacing the UPJ. In intermittently obstructing UPJs, this progressive dilation of the renal pelvis eventually causes the UPJ to kink, leading to an acute high-grade obstruction, with an ensuing progressive elevation in renal pelvic pressure. Little or no fluid moves through the UPJ. With cessation of infusion or

Table 29.2 Current percutaneous pressure–flow study protocol at University of Minnesota, Minneapolis, MN

- Patient is placed under general anesthesia with endotracheal intubation.
- With intravenous access established, antibiotic prophylaxis is given using 40 mg/kg of intravenous (i.v.) cefazolin up to a maximum of 1 g, provided that there is no history of allergic reaction, and hydration is begun with a minimum of 15 ml/kg of a crystalloid solution.
- In supine position, bladder catheter is inserted with the largest caliber catheter that the patient can accept.
- To facilitate placement of percutaneous nephrostomy needles, the bladder catheter may be plugged off at this stage to keep the bladder full and to maximize renal pelvic dilatation.
- The patient is turned to the prone position, and ultrasonographic examination is carried out to plan for nephrostomy access.
- The patient is sterilely prepared and draped. Under ultrasonographic guidance, two 22-gauge 2-inch angiocatheters (or other suitable catheters or needles) are inserted percutaneously into the renal pelvis to be examined. The bladder is emptied and the bladder catheter is connected to gravity drainage.
- To verify placement of the nephrostomy access and to establish a means to follow the progress of urine flow, radiographic contrast is injected into the renal pelvis via nephrostomy access. To preserve the baseline renal pelvic pressure dynamics, an equal volume of urine is first aspirated out before the injection of contrast.
- One of the nephrostomy accesses is capped off, and the other is connected to a pressure transducer with no flow going through the nephrostomy.
- The pressure transducer line is zeroed externally to the same level as the tip of the nephrostomy access within the renal pelvis. When connected to the nephrostomy access, the initial pressure reading represents the baseline renal pelvic pressure.
- Furosemide (1 mg/kg i.v., up to a maximum of 10 mg) is given to begin the *diuresis pressure–flow study* component.
- Renal pelvic pressure is continuously monitored for 30 minutes. Urine output is measured every 5 minutes to verify satisfactory overall response to i.v. hydration and furosemide. The peak renal pelvic pressure observed in this period determines whether the diuresis pressure–flow study is positive (peak renal pelvic pressure >14 cmH_2O) for significant obstruction.
- During this 30-minute interval, fluoroscopy is used intermittently. The renal pelvic pressure at which radiographic contrast is first seen distal to the suspected level of obstruction constitutes the *ureteral opening pressure*.
- If the diuresis pressure–flow study component is strongly positive for significant obstruction (peak renal pelvic pressure markedly above 14 cmH_2O), an antegrade nephrostogram is performed to obtain the anatomic details necessary for guiding surgical repair, and the percutaneous pressure–flow study is concluded at this point.
- If the diuresis pressure–flow study component peak renal pelvic pressure is close to or below 14 cmH_2O, the *individualized infusion pressure–flow study* is performed next. The other capped-off nephrostomy access is connected to an infusion pump, infusing a radiographic contrast solution. The rate of infusion is individually calculated based on patient's age, weight, and height (see Table 29.1) or calculated based on the GFR of the kidney being tested, if known.
- If the resulting renal pelvic pressure is positive for significant obstruction (>14 cmH_2O), an antegrade nephrostogram is performed to obtain the anatomic details necessary for guiding surgical repair, and the percutaneous pressure–flow study is concluded at this point.
- If the resulting renal pelvic pressure is negative for significant obstruction (≤ 14 cmH_2O), a supraphysiologic rate of infusion is then used (150–200% of the individualized infusion rate) as a measure of the reserve capability of the collecting system to handle additional urine flow.
  Note: Regardless of whether the renal pelvic pressure rises above 14 cmH_2O at this point, the pressure–flow study is still considered negative for significant obstruction.
- If a lower tract abnormality, which causes excessively high intravesical pressure, coexists with the upper tract obstructive site, an initially negative study for significant obstruction (diuresis pressure–flow study) can be further challenged with the bladder filled to the peak naturally occurring intravesical pressure. This is carried out by connecting an i.v. solution drip to the bladder catheter, and the drip chamber is raised to a level that is the same height (in cm) as the peak intravesical pressure (in cmH_2O). The desired intravesical pressure being simulated is reached when the drip slows to intermittent drops or stops altogether. The peak renal pelvic pressure recorded in this setting represents a combined effect of both the upper tract obstructive site and the lower tract anomaly on their corresponding upper tract urodynamics.
- Once all necessary urodynamic measurements have been completed, an antegrade nephrostogram is performed to obtain anatomic details necessary for guiding surgical repair. The renal pelvis is aspirated empty and the nephrostomy accesses are removed. The patient is turned back to supine position and awakened from anesthesia. The bladder catheter is removed once significant gross hematuria has been ruled out, and the patient is sufficiently awake to void.
- All patients who have percutaneous pressure–flow studies positive for significant obstruction are covered with oral antibiotic prophylaxis until successful surgical repairs have been achieved.

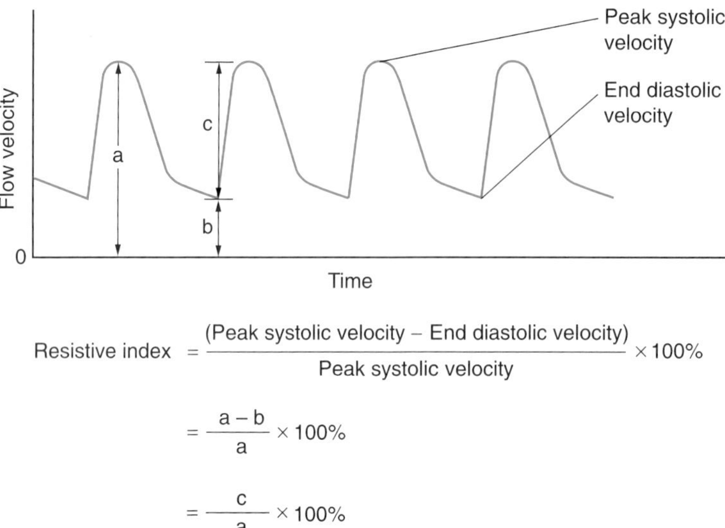

Figure 29.10 Schematic depiction of a typical intrarenal arterial waveform. Parameters and formula used for calculating intrarenal resistive index (RI) are shown. (After Fung et al.[4])

diuresis, the process eventually reverses itself. This may require drainage from the renal pelvic nephrostomy to speed up the decompression process. When intrapelvic volume reaches approximately the threshold at which the UPJ kinking initially occurred, the UPJ can be seen to suddenly open and renal pelvic pressure rapidly returns to normal thereafter (Figure 29.9).

Our current percutaneous pressure–flow study protocol, which represents our effort in combining the strengths of the various components of a pressure–flow study as discussed above, is presented in Table 29.2.

Diuretic Doppler sonography and intrarenal resistive index

The invasive nature of obtaining percutaneous access to the renal pelvis is one of the key factors preventing upper tract urodynamic studies from being performed on a more routine basis as part of the evaluation of hydronephrosis. Thus, it would be desirable to have a non-invasive method measuring parameters which reflect the collecting system pressure elevations in significantly obstructed renal units. The diuretic Doppler sonography study has the potential for being such a non-invasive study that is useful in upper tract urodynamic evaluations.

Diuretic Doppler sonography is a non-invasive test wherein the renal unit is stressed by a pharmacologically induced diuresis much like the diuretic pressure–flow study. Instead of monitoring renal pelvic pressure before and after the administration of furosemide, intrarenal resistive index (RI) is measured at regular intervals during a diuretic Doppler sonography study.[4] Resistive index is calculated based on an arterial Doppler waveform (Figure 29.10), and is defined as:

$$\text{resistive index} = \frac{\text{peak systolic velocity} - \text{end diastolic velocity}}{\text{peak systolic velocity}}$$

The resistive index is a measure of arterial resistance,[17] and is usually expressed as a percentage. Intrarenal RIs are generally recorded from the arcuate or interlobar arteries.[18]

Initial enthusiasm for using intrarenal RI to assess hydronephrosis stemmed from the observation that obstructed kidneys tend to be associated with elevated intrarenal RIs.[19] As obstructed kidneys are well documented to eventually develop a compensatory decrease in renal blood flow, it seemed promising that intrarenal RI might reflect this important physiologic compensation. Kidneys that developed acutely rising renal pelvic pressure were observed to also develop a progressive increase in intrarenal RIs.[4] This positive correlation suggested the possibility that instead of monitoring renal pelvic pressure during a relatively invasive diuresis pressure–flow study, intrarenal RIs could be monitored non-invasively instead (Figure 29.11).

However, using pressure–flow study results in 50 patients as the standard, there was no discernible

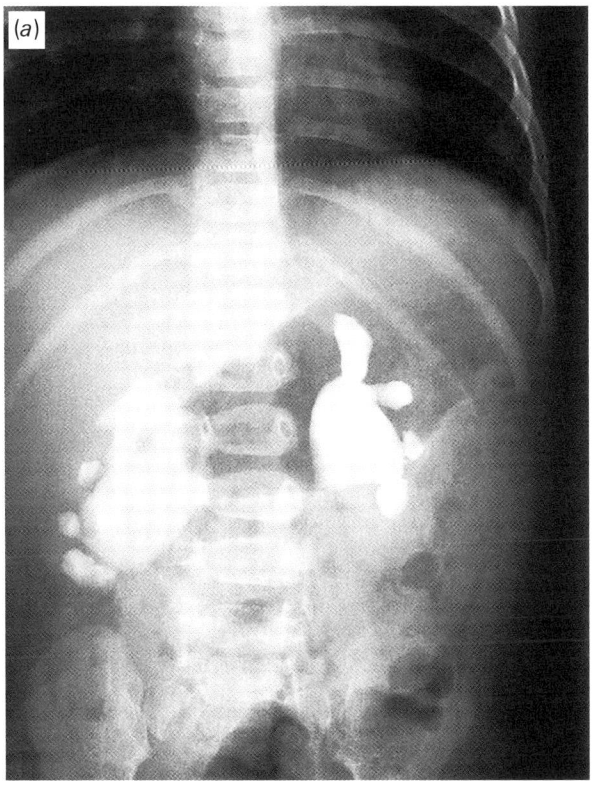

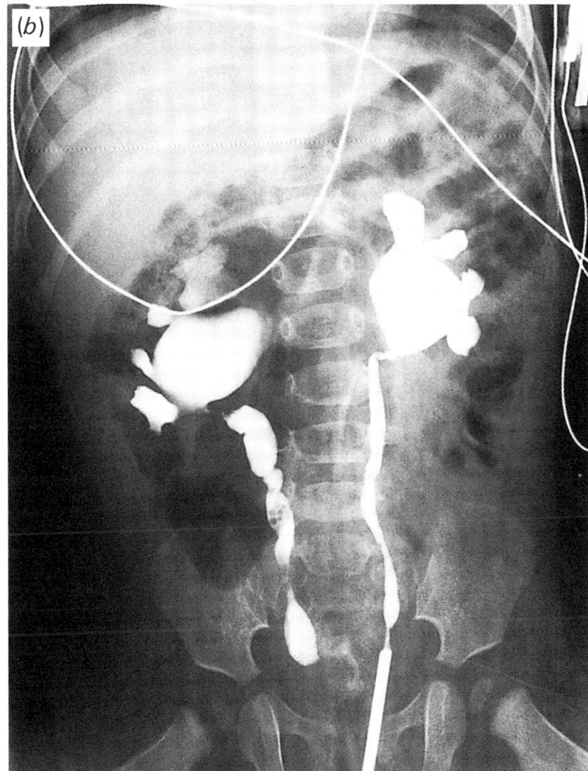

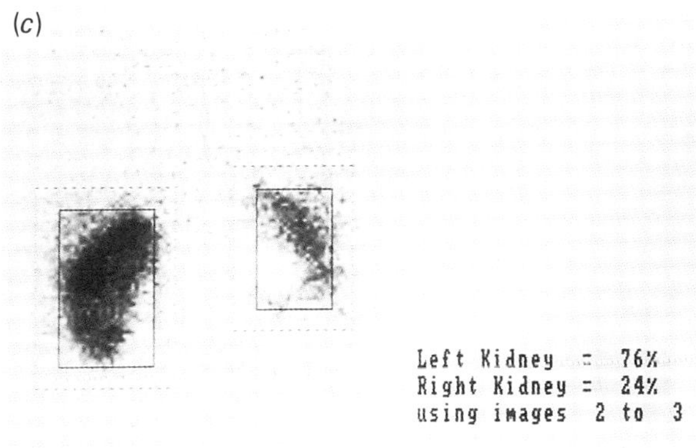

Figure 29.11 This male infant was diagnosed antenatally to have bilateral hydronephrosis. Configuration of the collecting systems are as shown by intravenous pyelography (IVP) at 5 minutes (*a*), and by bilateral retrograde pyelography (*b*). The right kidney had a differential renal function of 24% (*c*), and demonstrated a non-declining washout curve on furosemide nuclear renal scan (*d*) compatible with high-grade obstruction. The left kidney had a differential renal function of 76% (*c*) and $t_{1/2}$ of 3.2 minutes (*d*) compatible with normal non-obstructive drainage. *Continued overleaf.*

pattern that emerged from the diuretic Doppler sonogram. The reproducibility of any given RI reading was found to be poor, with widely variable measurements from one reading to the next.[20]

At present, there is no known diagnostic modality that can non-invasively and reliably demonstrate the changes in the upper tract urodynamics of obstructed as compared with normal collecting systems.

Summary

Prenatally detected hydronephrosis is a dynamic process, in which the initial presentation does not necessarily correlate with the ultimate outcome. There is currently no standard test that is uniformly successful at predicting the prognosis of hydronephrotic kidneys, or delineating whether surgical intervention is necessary for the prevention of deterioration in renal function. Of the available methods of assessment, upper tract urodynamics offers the most accurate, albeit more invasive, way of defining the mechanics of fluid handling by a hydronephrotic system. Of the parameters described, the resting or initial renal pelvic pressure, the maximum pressure obtained after induced diuresis, and the ureteral opening pressure appear to be of value in determining the resistance intrinsic to the collecting system, which in

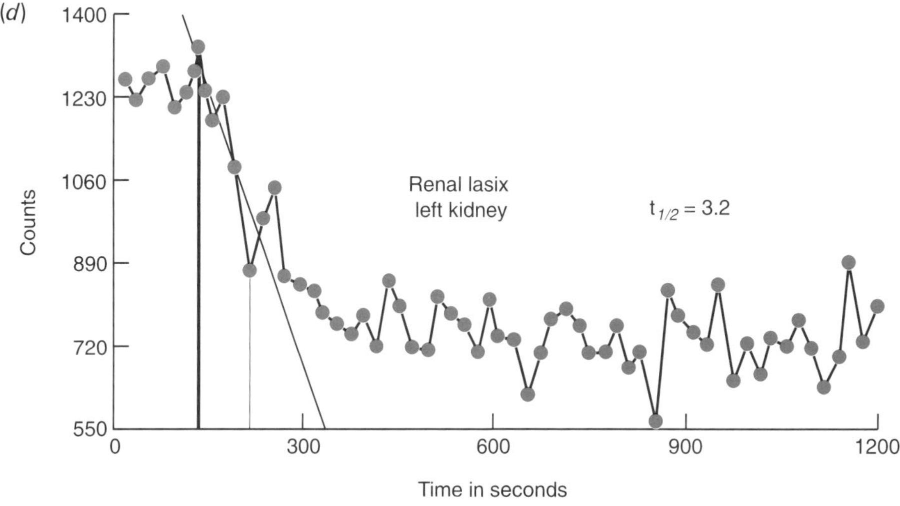

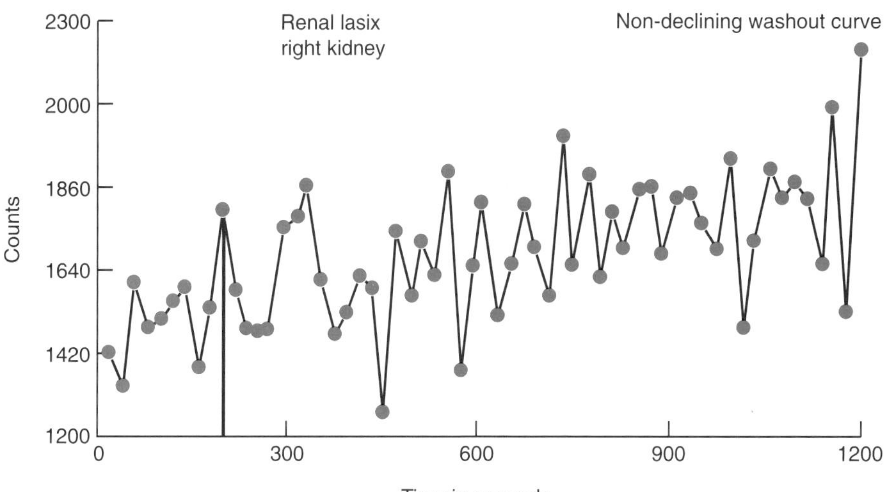

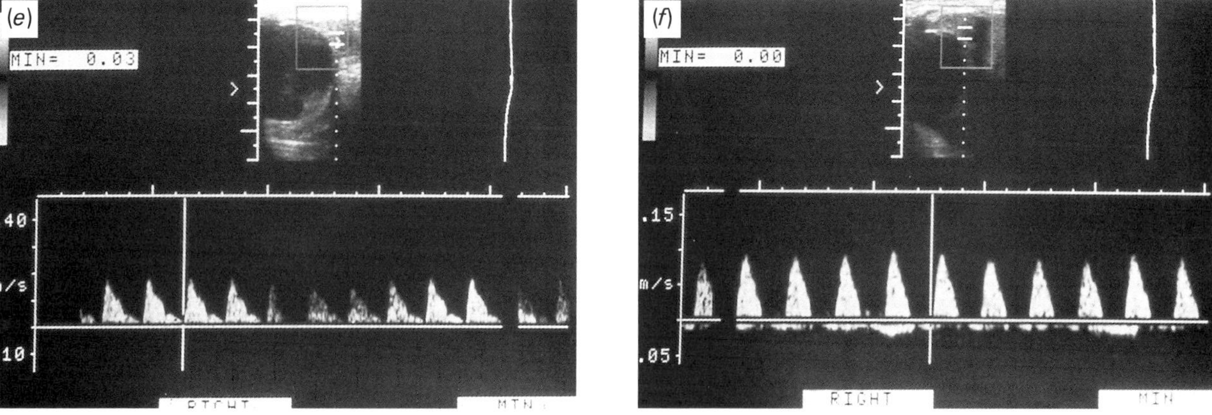

Figure 29.11 *Continued* Resistive index (RI) of the right kidney was 0.82 (82%) (*e*) at baseline, but rose to 1.00 (100%) with a complete cessation of diastolic flow after the administration of furosemide (*f*).

This dramatic increase in RI is presumably due to the furosemide-induced diuresis causing an increase in renal arterial blood flow as reflected by the elevation in RI. Although this case illustrates how changes in RI can non-invasively reflect important alterations in a hydronephrotic kidney with significant obstruction, we subsequently found that there are tremendous variabilities in RI measurements. This poor reproducibility of RI measurements renders the index unsuitable for reliably distinguishing non-obstructed from significantly obstructed hydronephrotic kidneys.

Pyeloplasty should be the best demonstration of the advantage of robot-assisted surgery in overcoming the difficulties encountered during laparoscopic suturing. Craig Peters[37–39] has presented the first preliminary results of robotic-assisted laparoscopic transperitoneal pyeloplasty in children. Olsen and Jorgensen have reported their unique experience on retroperitoneal robotic-assisted pyeloplasty.[40,41] They compared a group of 8 children operated on by the robotic-assisted procedures to a previous group of 15 children operated on by the standard procedure with laparoscopic instruments. The median operative time with the robotic-assisted procedures was lower than with standard equipment (172 minutes vs 210 minutes); the shortest operative time with robotic assistance was 110 minutes. The first impression is that robotic assistance makes suturing easier and may allow extending advanced laparoscopic reconstructive surgery to a larger number of surgeons without previous expertise in advanced laparoscopic surgery. However, in our experience, teaching laparoscopic pyeloplasty was not feasible when the surgeon did not already have an advanced experience in laparoscopy.[42]

Soulie et al[43] have compared retroperitoneal laparoscopic pyeloplasty vs open pyeloplasty with a minimal incision in 53 consecutive non-randomized adults. The mean operating time (165 minutes vs 145 minutes) was similar in both groups. Incidence of complications, hospital stay, and functional results were equivalent for both groups, but the return to painless activity was more rapid with laparoscopy in younger patients. Bauer et al[44] carried out a similar study, with no difference in the postoperative outcome between laparoscopic pyeloplasty and open pyeloplasty. In a recent review, we could not find any comparative study in children.[45] Recently, we have compared retroperitoneal laparoscopic pyeloplasty vs open pyeloplasty in 37 consecutive children.[36] The mean operative time was 96 minutes (range 50–150) and 219 minutes (range 140–310) for the open surgery and the laparoscopy groups, respectively ($p < 0.0001$). Mean hospital stay was 2.4 days (range 1–5) and 5 days (range 3–7) for the laparoscopy and the open surgery groups, respectively ($p < 0.0001$). The use of analgesics was less in the laparoscopy group, but this result needs to be confirmed in a randomized prospective study.

Midterm results confirm that dismembered retroperitoneal laparoscopic pyeloplasty is a safe and feasible approach in children. Although the technique is highly demanding, it has the advantage of duplicating the principles of the gold standard open approach. The transperitoneal approach may be better adapted in young infants, and some experienced laparoscopists prefer a transperitoneal approach in all children. Long operative times may be reduced with experience and possibly with robotic assistance.

Technique of laparoscopic retroperitoneal pyeloplasty[35]

The same access is used, as described for nephrectomy. Yeung et al[34] used different positioning according to the side of the kidney: semiprone for the right side and semilateral for the left side. We currently use a three-trocar technique (see Figure 31.1): the first trocar is 3 or 5 mm for the laparoscope (at the tip of the 12th rib); the second trocar of 3 mm is inserted in the costovertebral angle; and the third trocar of 3 mm is inserted in the top of the iliac crest. The kidney is approached posteriorly and the renal pelvis is first identified. The pyeloureteral junction is identified and a minimal dissection is done to free the junction from connective tissue. Small vessels are divided using bipolar electrocoagulation. Care is taken not to section ureteral blood vessels. A stay stitch is placed at the junction. Aberrant crossing vessels are identified. The renal pelvis is partially divided using scissors at the most dependent part and gentle traction on the stay suture helps to define this point. Keeping the traction, the ureter is partially divided and incised vertically for spatulation. The traction suture helps to mobilize the ureter, so the scissors can be in the axis of the ureter, usually introduced through the last trocar. The anterior surface of the kidney is left adherent to the peritoneum, so that the kidney is retracted medially without the need for individual kidney retraction. The ureteropelvic anastomosis begins using a 6–0 absorbable suture, with a tapered 3/8 circle needle, placed from the most dependent portion of the pelvis to the most inferior point or vertex of the ureteral spatulation. The suture is tied using the intracorporeal technique, with the knots placed outside the lumen. The same stitch is used to run the anterior wall of the anastomosis. The UPJ is kept intact for traction and stabilization of the suture line, and removed just before tying the last suture on the pelvis. This stay suture may be fixed to the psoas muscle to give stability and to facilitate the suturing. A double-pigtail stent is inserted through the costovertebral angle trocar, and if there is doubt, its position in the bladder is assured under fluoroscopy. The posterior ureteropelvic anastomosis is then performed. To avoid a second general anesthesia to remove the stent, we are currently inserting a transanastomotic pyelostomy stent. The stent is closed on the first postoperative day and removed at 1 week in the outpatient clinic. We still proceed with double-pigtail stent in the cases with intrarenal pelvis because of the technical difficulties associated with the pyelostomy stent in these cases. The pelvis is trimmed if needed. In cases of aberrant crossing vessels (see Figure 31.7), the technique is slightly different. After placement of the stay suture, the ureter is completely divided and the UPJ and the pelvis are delivered anterior to the vessels with the help of the stay suture; then the anastomosis is performed as described. A Foley catheter is left in the bladder for 24 hours postoperatively.

Technique of laparoscopic transperitoneal pyeloplasty

The same approach is used as described for the nephrectomy. Steps of the pyeloplasty are identical to the retroperitoneal approach. A traction suture may be inserted through the anterior abdominal wall to stabilize the suture line.

We have used the transperitoneal approach only in cases of UPJ obstruction in a horseshoe kidney. The anterior position of the UPJ in this specific anatomic variant makes it easier using the anterior transperitoneal approach.

References

1. Clayman RV, Kavoussi LR, Soper NJ et al. Laparoscopic nephrectomy: initial case report. J Urol 1991; 146:278–82.
2. Ehrlich RM, Gershman A, Mee S, Fuchs G. Laparoscopic nephrectomy in a child: expanding horizons for laparoscopy in pediatric urology. J Endourol 1992; 6:463.
3. Das S, Keizur JJ, Tashima M. Laparoscopic nephroureterectomy for end-stage reflux nephropathy in a child. Surg Laparosc Endosc 1993; 3:462–5.
4. Ehrlich RM, Gershman A, Fuchs G. Laparoscopic renal surgery in children. J Urol 1994; 151:735–9.
5. Roberts J. Retroperitoneal endoscopy. J Med Primatol 1976; 5:124–7.
6. Gaur D. Laparoscopic operative retroperitoneoscopy: use of a new devise. J Urol 1992; 148:1137–9.
7. Doublet JD, Barreto HS, Degremont AC, Gattegno B, Thibault P. Retroperitoneal nephrectomy: comparison of laparoscopy with open surgery. World J Surg 1996; 20:713–16.
8. Guilloneau B, Ballanger P, Lugagne PM, Valla JS, Vallancien G. Laparoscopic versus lumboscopic nephrectomy. Eur Urol 1996; 29:288–91.
9. Valla JS, Guilloneau B, Montupet P et al. Retroperitoneal laparoscopic nephrectomy in children. Preliminary report of 18 cases. Eur Urol 1996; 30:490–3.
10. Abbou C, Cicco A, Gasman D et al. Retroperitoneal laparoscopic versus open radical nephrectomy. J Urol 1999; 61:1776–80.
11. Hemal AK, Gupta NP, Wadhwa SN, Goel A, Kumar R. Retroperitoneoscopic nephrectomy and nephroureterectomy for benign nonfunctioning kidneys: a single-center experience. Urology 2001; 57:644–9.
12. El-Ghoneimi A, Valla JS, Steyaert H, Aigrain Y. Laparoscopic renal surgery via a retroperitoneal approach in children. J Urol 1998; 160:1138–41.
13. Borer JG, Cisek LJ, Atala A et al. Pediatric retroperitoneoscopic nephrectomy using 2 mm instrumentation. J Urol 1999; 162:1725–9.
14. Kobashi KC, Chamberlin DA, Rajpoot D, Shanberg AM. Retroperitoneal laparoscopic nephrectomy in children. J Urol 1998; 160:1142–4.
15. Shanberg AM, Sanderson K, Rajpoot D, Duel B. Laparoscopic retroperitoneal renal and adrenal surgery in children. BJU Int 2001; 87(6):521–4.
16. Kim HH, Kang J, Kwak C et al. Laparoscopy for definite localization and simultaneous treatment of ectopic ureter draining a dysplastic kidney in children. J Endourol 2002; 16:363–6.
17. El-Ghoneimi A. Renal dysplasia and cystic disease options. In: Docimo SG, ed. Minimally Invasive Approaches to Pediatric Urology, 1st edn. London: Taylor & Francis, 2005: 105–18.
18. El-Ghoneimi A, Sauty L, Maintenant J et al. Laparoscopic retroperitoneal nephrectomy in high risk children. J Urol 2000; 164:1076–9.
19. El-Ghoneimi A, Farhat W, Beckers G et al. Feasibility and outcomes of pediatric simultaneous retroperitoneal laparoscopic bilateral pretransplant nephrectomy. BJU Int 2003; 91:S1–74.
20. Fujisawa M, Kawabata G, Gotoh A et al. Posterior approach for retroperitoneal laparoscopic bilateral nephrectomy in a child. Urology 2002; 59(3):444.
21. Zuniga ZV, Ellis D, Moritz ML, Docimo SG. Bilateral laparoscopic transperitoneal nephrectomy with early peritoneal dialysis in an infant with the nephrotic syndrome. J Urol 2003; 170:1962.
22. Halachmi S, El-Ghoneimi A, Farhat W. Successful subcapsular laparoscopic nephrectomy in a child with xanthogranulomatous pyelonephritis. Pediatr Endosurg Innov Techn 2002; 6:269–72.
23. Peters C. Laparoendoscopic renal surgery in children. J Endourol 2000; 14:841–7.
24. Borzi P. A comparison of the lateral and posterior retroperitoneoscopic approach for complete and partial nephroureterectomy in children. BJU Int 2001; 87:517–20.
25. Adams JB, Micali S, Moore RG, Babayan RK, Kavoussi LR. Complications of extraperitoneal balloon dilation. J Endourol 1996; 10:375–8.
26. Capolicchio JP, Jednak R, Anidjar M, Pippi-Salle JL. A modified access technique for retroperitoneoscopic renal surgery in children. J Urol 2003; 170:204–6.

27. Micali S, Caione P, Virgili G et al. Retroperitoneal laparoscopic access in children using a direct vision technique. J Urol 2001; 165:229–32.
28. Halachmi S, El-Ghoneimi A, Bissonnette B et al. Hemodynamic and respiratory effect of pediatric urological laparoscopic surgery: a retrospective study. J Urol 2003; 170:1651–4.
29. Bernardo N, Smith AD. Endopyelotomy review. Arch Esp Urol 1999; 52:541–8.
30. Kavoussi LR, Peters CA. Laparoscopic pyeloplasty. J Urol 1993; 150:1891–4.
31. Schuessler WW, Grune MT, Tecuanhuey LV, Preminger GM. Laparoscopic dismembered pyeloplasty. J Urol 1993; 150:1795–9.
32. Ben Slama MR, Salomon L, Hoznek A et al. Extraperitoneal laparoscopic repair of ureteropelvic junction obstruction: initial experience in 15 cases. Urology 2000; 56:45–8.
33. Tan H. Laparoscopic Anderson–Hynes dismembered pyeloplasty in children. J Urol 1999; 162:1045–7.
34. Yeung CK, Tam YH, Sihoe JD, Lee KH, Liu KW. Retroperitoneoscopic dismembered pyeloplasty for pelviureteric junction obstruction in infants and children. BJU Int 2001; 87:509–13.
35. El-Ghoneimi A, Farhat W, Bolduc S et al. Laparoscopic dismembered pyeloplasty by a retroperitoneal approach in children. BJU Int 2003; 92:104–8.
36. Bonnard A, Fouquet V, Carricaburu E, Aigrain Y, El-Ghoneimi A. Retroperitoneal laparoscopic versus open pyeloplasty in children. J Urol 2005; 173:1710–13.
37. Peters C. Laparoscopic and robotic approach to genitourinary anomalies in children. Urol Clin North Am 2004; 31:595–605.
38. Peters C. Laparoscopy in pediatric urology. Curr Opin Urol 2004; 14:67–73.
39. Peters CA, Cilento BG, Borer JG, Retik AB. Robotically Assisted Laparoscopic Surgery in Pediatric Urology. Boston: Annual Meeting of AAP, 2002.
40. Olsen H, Jorgensen T. Robotic vs. standard retroperitoneoscopic pyeloplasty in children. BJU Int 2003; 91:S1–74.
41. Olsen LH, Jorgensen TM. Computer assisted pyeloplasty in children: the retroperitoneal approach. J Urol 2004; 171:2629–31.
42. Farhat W, Khoury A, Bagli D, McLorie G, El-Ghoneimi A. Mentored retroperitoneal laparoscopic renal surgery in children: a safe approach to learning. BJU Int 2003; 92:617–20.
43. Soulie M, Thoulouzan M, Seguin P et al. Retroperitoneal laparoscopic versus open pyeloplasty with a minimal incision: comparison of two surgical approaches. Urology 2001; 57:443–7.
44. Bauer JJ, Bishoff JT, Moore RG et al. Laparoscopic versus open pyeloplasty: assessment of objective and subjective outcome. J Urol 1999; 162:692–5.
45. El-Ghoneimi A. Paediatric laparoscopic surgery. Curr Opin Urol 2003; 13:329–35.

Wilms' tumor

32

Michael L Ritchey and Fernando A Ferrer

Introduction

Nephroblastoma, or Wilms' tumor, is an embryonal tumor that develops from remnants of immature kidney. It is the most common renal tumor of childhood. Current survival of children with Wilms' tumor is excellent, and emphasis is now on reducing the morbidity of treatment for low-risk patients. Unfortunately, there is still a subset of high-risk patients with poor survival for whom new treatment strategies are needed. This chapter reviews the epidemiology, pathology, and recent advances in the understanding of the biology of Wilms' tumor. The current management of children with all stages of nephroblastoma is discussed in detail.

Epidemiology

The overall annual incidence of Wilms' tumor is approximately 7.6 cases per million children under 15 years of age, or about 500 new cases annually in the United States. Wilms' tumor accounts for 6–7% of all childhood cancers.[1,2] It typically affects young children (median age 3.5 years), although older children and occasionally even adults can be affected. Wilms' tumor occurs at an earlier median age in children with bilateral tumors, 29.5 months for boys and 32.6 months for girls. The disease occurs nearly equally in girls and boys worldwide, but the frequency is slightly higher among girls in the United States.[3]

Children with Wilms' tumor frequently have associated congenital anomalies or recognizable syndromes. Syndromes associated with a predisposition to develop Wilms' tumor may be divided into those characterized by overgrowth and those lacking overgrowth. Syndromes with overgrowth features include hemihypertrophy, which may occur alone or as part of the Beckwith–Wiedemann syndrome (BWS). BWS is a rare disorder consisting of developmental anomalies characterized by excess growth at the cellular, organ (macroglossia, nephromegaly, hepatomegaly), or body segment (hemihypertrophy) levels.[4,5] The incidence of tumor development in BWS is 10–20%, including Wilms' tumor, adrenocortical neoplasms, and hepatoblastoma. The risk of Wilms' tumor development in patients with hemihypertrophy and BWS is estimated to be in the order of 4–10%,[5–8] with 21% of those children presenting with bilateral disease.[9] Data from the BWS registry suggest that nephromegaly is a strong risk factor for the subsequent development of Wilms' tumor.[10] The mean age at diagnosis of Wilms' tumor in hemihypertrophy patients is similar to that of the general Wilms' tumor population.[11] Other overgrowth syndromes, such as the Perlman and the Simpson–Golabi–Behmel syndromes, are also associated with the development of Wilms' tumor.[12,13]

Genitourinary anomalies (hypospadias, cryptorchidism, renal fusion anomalies) are present in 4.5% of patients with Wilms' tumor.[14] One specific association of male pseudohermaphroditism, renal mesangial sclerosis, and nephroblastoma is the Denys–Drash syndrome.[15,16] Although the classic presentation is that of ambiguous genitalia, up to 40% of children appear phenotypically female.[17] Genetic studies indicate that Denys–Drash syndrome is associated with mutations of the 11p13 Wilms' tumor gene.[16] Roughly 1% of Wilms' tumor patients are diagnosed with the WAGR (Wilms' tumor, aniridia, genital anomalies, and mental retardation) syndrome.[18] Most affected individuals have a constitutional deletion on chromosome 11 and the incidence of Wilms' tumor formation in these children is 42%. Children with WAGR present at an earlier age, have lower birth weights, and an increased incidence of bilateral disease.[19] Wilms' tumors have been reported in association with neurofibromatosis, Sotos's syndrome, and Klippel–Trénaunay–Weber syndrome.[20]

There is an increased risk of Müllerian duct anomalies in girls with Wilms' tumor.[21] Approximately 10% of girls will have abnormalities such as duplication of the cervix or uterus, or bicornuate uterus. Patients with horseshoe kidney have been noted to develop Wilms' tumor at a higher than expected rate.[22,23] Wilms' tumor has been reported in patients with multicystic dysplastic kidney, but there is not sufficient evidence that this occurs at an incidence greater than for children with two normal kidneys.[24,25]

Periodic imaging with renal ultrasound has been recommended in children with hemihypertrophy, BWS, and aniridia, with the hope that the tumor will be discovered at an earlier stage. A review of BWS patients reported to the National Wilms' Tumor Study Group (NWTSG) has found more stage I tumors,[9] and high-risk children undergoing periodic screening have more stage I tumors and small tumor diameters.[26] There were not enough patients in these retrospective reviews to determine if early detection had an impact on patient survival. Craft et al reported on 13 high-risk children undergoing screening with abdominal ultrasound and did not find any significant difference in stage distribution compared with children not undergoing screening.[27] The recommended screening interval is every 3–4 months.[28,29] Not all new lesions are Wilms' tumor, as there is an increased incidence of non-malignant renal lesions in children with BWS.[30,31] Nephrectomy has been performed for benign disease due to false-positive screening.

Biology and genetics

The role of genetic alterations in Wilms' tumor development has been intensely studied. Most Wilms' tumors arise from somatic mutations. These mutations are present in the tumor tissue only and cannot be transmitted to the progeny of the affected individual. A much smaller percentage of Wilms' tumors (~10%) appear to be the result of germline mutations. These mutations arise in the actual germ cells of the patient and can be inherited, although in some cases they can occur de novo. Patients with germ cell mutations are characterized by syndromic conditions, associated congenital anomalies, family history of tumor, and tumors that occur at an earlier age.[32] It was this group of patients that prompted Knudson to suggest that his 'two-hit' theory, originally developed by studying children with retinoblastoma, might also apply to Wilms' tumor.[33,34]

The Knudson model predicts that two genetic events are required for tumor formation.[33] Individuals with a genetic predisposition carry an initial lesion in their germline, either inherited from a parent or resulting from a de-novo germline mutation. In these individuals, all body cells have already been affected by the first event. Consequently, only one new event in any one cell is required for tumor development. By contrast, in individuals that are not genetically predisposed (sporadic cases), two relatively rare independent events are required in the same cell. Subsequent genetic studies in a number of tumors have confirmed the Knudson model, demonstrating that the two postulated 'genetic hits' constitute the inactivation of both alleles of a tumor suppressor gene.[35] The clearest example of tumorigenesis following the inactivation of both copies of a single tumor suppressor gene is the development of retinoblastoma following the inactivation of the retinoblastoma gene *RB1*. By contrast, the 'two-hit' theory which was so elegantly confirmed in patients with retinoblastoma, has not stood the test of time in Wilms' tumor. Today it is recognized that the biologic pathways leading to the development of the majority of Wilms' tumor are complex and probably involve several genetic loci.[32,34]

Observation that patients with aniridia, genital anomalies, and mental retardation were at a high risk for Wilms' tumor led to cytogenetic studies that identified a heterozygous deletion at band 11p13 of chromosome 11. Using cloning techniques, the *WT1* gene was identified.[36–38] Chromosome 11p13 encompasses various genes, including *PAX6*, abnormalities of which can be responsible for aniridia.[39] *WT1* is expressed in the normal developing kidney and abnormally expressed in some Wilms' tumor specimens. *WT1* encodes a zinc finger transcription factor that is thought to function as a classic tumor suppressor gene. A partial list of genes that are targets of *WT1* regulation include *EGFR*, *PDGF*, *IGF*, *N-Myc*, *PAX 2*, *MDR-1*, and *P-21*, all notable for their association with tumorgenesis.[40] *WT1* mutations have been shown to occur in human DNA from sporadic Wilms' tumor, as well as the germline of patients with a genetic predisposition to cancer.

Although at first, *WT1* was considered a classic tumor suppressor gene, i.e. loss of both copies of the gene are required for tumor development, it has now become clear that specific alterations in only one of the two *WT1* alleles may contribute to abnormal cell growth and associated genitourinary abnormalities.[35] Normal function of *WT1* is necessary for genitourinary development. Mutations at the *WT1* locus, particularly in males, may confer extensive genitourinary defects, most notably male pseudohermaphroditism.[16,41] The affected gonads and kidneys in patients with the Denys–Drash syndrome are heterozygous for germline mutations. Denys–Drash syndrome, characterized by pseudohermaphroditism, renal failure, and Wilms' tumor, is the result of point mutations in the binding domain of *WT1*.[16] The resulting phenotype is far more severe than that observed in children with a constitutional deletion of one *WT1* allele (i.e. WAGR patients) and suggests that the mutated protein can inhibit the activity of the wild-type protein, resulting in a 'dominant negative' effect.[42] A spectrum of phenotypes can be demonstrated by patients with the Denys–Drash syndrome, depending on the type of *WT1* mutation.[32] Interestingly, renal dysfunction once thought to be limited to those with Denys–Drash syndrome, is now known to occur years after treatment in patients with WAGR syndrome.[19]

In addition to WAGR and Denys–Drash patients, germline mutations have also been found in familial Wilms' tumor. Families harboring a constitutional *WT1* abnormality constitute only a small percentage of the reported affected pedigrees.[43] Germline *WT1* mutation has been correlated with a predominantly stromal pathology.[44] Constitutional mutations of *WT1* are rarely seen in patients with non-syndromic, unilateral tumors in the absence of genitourinary abnormalities.[43]

In summary, the majority of Wilms' tumors do not have genetic alterations at chromosome 11p13. Germline *WT1* mutations are associated with genitourinary anomalies. No increased risk of mutation is found in patients with nephrogenic rests, bilateral Wilms' tumor, or a family history of Wilms' tumor.[45]

A second potential Wilms' tumor gene, *WT2*, has been identified on chromosome 11p15, based on the observation of loss of heterozygosity at this site,[46,47] but the actual gene responsible remains to be determined. Much like the association between *WT1* at chromosome 11p13 and the WAGR syndrome, *WT2* has been linked to the BWS.[46,48] BWS is an overgrowth disorder that is associated with a 5–10% risk of Wilms' tumor.[46] Recent studies suggest that abnormal expression of embryonal growth factor encoded by the insulin-like growth factor-2 gene (*IGF2*) is involved in the pathophysiology of BWS.[49]

Loss of heterozygosity at chromosomes 16q (present in 20% of all Wilms' tumors) or 1p (seen in 10% of tumors) has been suggested to be a predictor of poor outcome in children with Wilms' tumor.[50–52] However, the prognostic significance of these features has been questioned.[53]

Abnormalities of chromosome 7p have been reported in patients with Wilms' tumor. Cytogenetic analysis of individuals with constitutional deletions in chromosome 7p who have demonstrated a loss of the second allele in tumor tissues suggests that this may be the site of another, as yet unidentified, tumor suppressor gene.[54] Alterations of the *p53* tumor suppressor gene located on chromosome 17p have been noted in approximately 75% of anaplastic tumors, suggesting an important role in the development of anaplasia.[55,56] By acting as a down-regulator of cell proliferation, and a positive regulator of cellular apoptosis, *p53* is known to play a significant role in tumor suppression. Malkin et al suggested that the absence of *p53* is an indicator of advanced disease in Wilms' tumor, regardless of the presence of anaplastic changes.[57] Monosomy at chromosome 22 has also been linked to the biology of Wilms' tumor. Bown et al have reported a significant decrease in tumor-free survival at 5 years in patients demonstrating monosomy of chromosome 22.[53]

Histopathology

Wilms' tumor usually compresses the adjacent normal renal parenchyma, forming a pseudocapsule composed of compressed, atrophic renal tissues. This intrarenal pseudocapsule can be helpful to distinguish Wilms' tumor from other renal tumors. Most tumors are soft and friable, with necrotic or hemorrhagic areas frequently noted. This consistency increases the chance of intraoperative tumor rupture that can predispose to local tumor recurrence. Wilms' tumor is characterized by tremendous histologic diversity. The classic triphasic pattern includes varying proportions of three cell types: blastemal, stromal, and epithelial. The proportion of each of these components varies, with some tumors consisting of only biphasic or even monomorphous patterns. These different components respond differently to treatment, which can have an impact on outcome (see below discussion under preoperative chemotherapy).[58] In addition to expressing a variety of cell types found in a normal developing kidney, Wilms' tumor often contains tissues such as skeletal muscle, cartilage, and squamous epithelium. These heterotopic cell types probably reflect the primitive developmental potentials of metanephric blastema that are not expressed in normal nephrogenesis. Most Wilms' tumors are unicentric, but 12% are multicentric unilateral tumors.[11] Extrarenal locations are rare and are thought to arise from displaced metanephric elements or mesonephric remnants.

One important observation was the identification of tumors with *unfavorable* histologic features that were associated with increased rates of relapse and death.[59] These unfavorable features occurred in approximately 10% of patients, but accounted for almost half of the tumor deaths in early NWTSG studies.[60] Anaplasia is defined by the presence of gigantic polyploid nuclei within the tumor sample. It is rare in the first 2 years of life but the incidence increases to 13% in children ≥ 5 years old.[61] Anaplasia is a feature of Wilms' tumor that is clearly associated with resistance to chemotherapy. There has been a similar incidence of anaplasia in the NWTSG study (5%) and in the International Society of Pediatric Oncology (SIOP) study (5.3%).[62] Anaplasia has been further divided into focal and diffuse patterns to reflect the different prognosis of anaplasia that is present throughout the kidney or in an extrarenal location. Focal anaplasia requires that cells with anaplastic nuclear changes be confined to sharply restricted foci within the primary tumor.[63] Diffuse anaplasia is diagnosed when anaplasia is present in more than one portion of the tumor or is found in any extrarenal or metastatic site. When the anaplastic component is completely removed (stage I), the outcome is generally excellent.[64] This suggests that anaplasia is more a marker of chemoresistance than inherent aggressiveness of the tumor. When anaplastic changes are not present, the tumor is referred to as being of favorable histology (FH) because of the generally good outcome for these patients.[65] Clear cell sarcoma of the kidney (CCSK) and rhabdoid tumor of the kidney (RTK) were previously grouped as unfavorable histology Wilms' tumors. They are now recognized as separate malignant entities (see below).[66,67]

More than one-third of kidneys resected for Wilms' tumor contain precursor lesions, known as nephrogenic rests.[68] Nephrogenic rests represent the abnormal persistence into postnatal life of embryonal cells that can produce a malignancy (Figure 32.1). Two distinct categories of nephrogenic rests exist, based on the position of these lesions within the renal lobe. Perilobar nephrogenic rests (PLNRs) are confined to the periphery of the renal lobe. Intralobar nephrogenic rests (ILNRs) occur anywhere in the kidney, including the renal sinus and collecting system. There are biologic differences distinguishing PLNR from ILNR (Table 32.1). Nephrogenic rests have a varied life and most do not form Wilms' tumor. A rest can undergo maturation, sclerosis, involution, and complete disappearance. PLNRs have been detected in 1% of kidneys in infants on postmortem examination; most of these rests apparently undergo involution.[69] ILNR can become cystic and be indistinguishable from renal dysplasia.

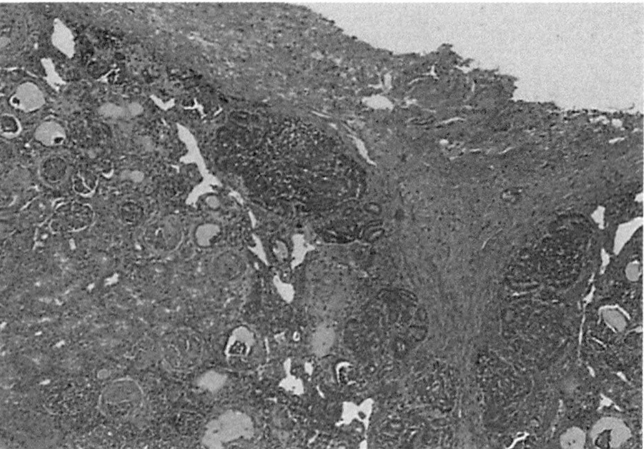

Figure 32.1 Perilobar nephrogenic rest composed of blastemal cells just beneath the renal capsule (hematoxylin and eosin, ×40).

Hyperplastic nephrogenic rests can produce a renal mass easily mistaken for a small Wilms' tumor.[69] Biopsy of a hyperplastic rest is of little value in distinguishing this lesion from a Wilms' tumor unless the interface between the rest and normal kidney is

Table 32.1 Clinical features of ILNR and PLNR

	ILNR	PLNR
Associated syndromes	WAGR Denys–Drash Genitourinary anomalies	BWS Hemihypertrophy Perlman
Median age of Wilms' tumor development	23 months	36 months
Wilms' tumor histology	Stroma predominant	Blastema, epithelial predominant

WAGR = Wilms' tumor, aniridia, genitourinary, and retardation; BWS = Beckwith–Wiedemann syndrome; ILNR = intralobar nephrogenic rest; PLNR = perilobar nephrogenic rest.

included. Wilms' tumor will have a pseudocapsule at the interface, with the normal parenchyma compressing the normal elements. Neoplastic induction of cells of a nephrogenic rest can produce Wilms' tumor and possibly other benign or malignant renal neoplasms. The Wilms' tumor will have a spherical shape, whereas hyperplasic rests will be more elliptical or lenticular in shape. Magnetic resonance imaging (MRI) may be of some value in distinguishing between the two lesions, but this needs to be confirmed prospectively in large numbers of patients.[70]

The presence of multiple or diffuse nephrogenic rests will lead to the diagnosis of nephroblastomatosis. The term nephroblastomatosis was originally used to describe massive bilateral nephromegaly in which the reniform shape was preserved.[71] Nephroblastomatosis can be subclassified according to the rest categories present: e.g. diffuse hyperplastic PLNRs, in which the majority of the cortical surface of one or both kidneys is composed of hyperplastic nephrogenic rests. The entire nephrogenic zone is involved, with a thick rind capping the entire kidney. These patients are prone to Wilms' tumor development and bilateral lesions are common. Perlman et al have reviewed 52 cases of diffuse hyperplastic PLNRs reported to the NWTSG pathology center.[72] Wilms' tumor developed in 23 patients at a median of 30 months. Of children receiving adjuvant therapy at diagnosis, 17/33 (52%) developed a Wilms' tumor.

Multiple rests in one kidney usually implies that nephrogenic rests are present in the other kidney.[68] Children younger than 12 months diagnosed with Wilms' tumor who also have nephrogenic rests have a markedly increased risk of developing contralateral disease.[73] They need regular imaging surveillance to detect contralateral recurrence.[74] The occurrence of metachronous Wilms' tumor in patients previously treated with conventional chemotherapeutic regimens suggests that nephrogenic rests are not always eradicated.

Presentation, preoperative evaluation, and staging

Most children with Wilms' tumor present with an asymptomatic abdominal mass. Other signs and symptoms at diagnosis are abdominal pain, gross hematuria, and fever. Occasionally, a child will present with an acute abdomen due to tumor rupture, with hemorrhage into the peritoneal cavity. Other atypical presentations may result from compression or invasion of adjacent structures: e.g. extension of the tumor into the renal vein and inferior vena cava (IVC). Varicocele, hepatomegaly due to hepatic vein obstruction, ascites, and congestive heart failure are found in fewer than 10% of patients with intracaval or atrial tumor extension.[75] Hypertension is present in 25% of cases and has been attributed to elevated plasma renin levels.[76] During the physical examination, it is important to note any physical findings of associated Wilms' tumor syndromes such as aniridia, hemihypertrophy, and genitourinary anomalies.

The preoperative evaluation can generally be completed in 48 hours. Emergent operation is not necessary unless there is evidence of active bleeding or tumor rupture. Laboratory evaluation should include a complete peripheral blood count, platelet count, renal function tests, liver function tests, serum calcium, and urinalysis. Elevation of the serum calcium can occur in children with congenital mesoblastic nephroma and RTK. Acquired von Willebrand's disease has been found in 8% of newly diagnosed Wilms' tumor patients.[77]

The preoperative imaging evaluation of children with a solid abdominal mass has evolved over the years. The first study obtained is often a renal ultrasound that can determine if the mass is predominantly solid or cystic. Contrast-enhanced computed tomography (CT) or MRI of the abdomen is obtained next. All of the solid renal tumors of childhood have similar radiographic features. However, defining the exact histology is not as important as establishing that there is a solid renal tumor present, which will help the surgeon plan for a major cancer operation.[78] Another important role of imaging studies is to establish the presence of a functioning contralateral kidney prior to nephrectomy.

The radiologist should exclude intracaval tumor extension, which occurs in 4% of Wilms' tumor patients (Figure 32.2).[75] This can usually be excluded on ultrasound, but MRI is the study of choice if extension of tumor into the IVC cannot be excluded by ultrasound.[79]

There is some controversy regarding the utility of preoperative imaging for tumor staging.[74,80,81] Accurate staging of children with Wilms' tumors is essential to define tumor extent prior to initiating treatment, as outcome is highly correlated with stage.[82] However, the staging system used in NWTSG studies relies on surgical findings and pathologic examination (Table 32.2). It would be a great asset if imaging provided reliable information regarding local extension of tumor beyond the renal capsule

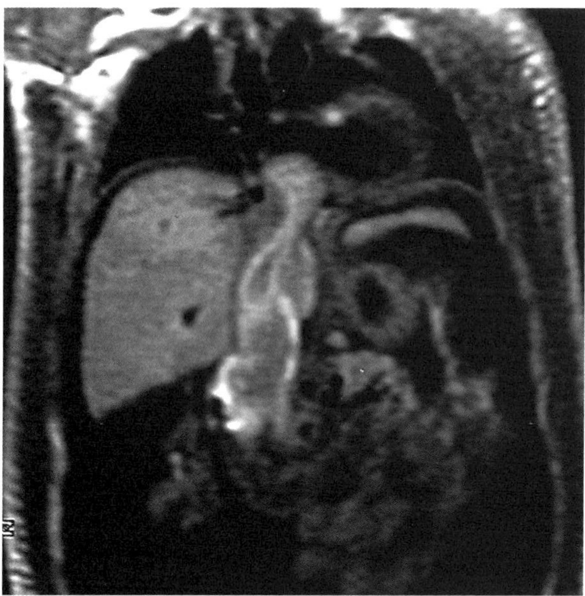

Figure 32.2 Magnetic resonance imaging scan demonstrating tumor extension into the inferior vena cava.

or into regional lymph nodes. The local tumor burden (e.g. regional lymph node involvement) determines the intensity of the chemotherapy regimen and whether a child receives abdominal irradiation. However, prospective correlation with pathologic findings has not been done. Preoperative CT can certainly identify regional adenopathy, but enlarged benign retroperitoneal lymph nodes are common in children. Correlation between pathologic findings and lymph node evaluation at surgical exploration in Wilms' tumor patients has found high false-positive and false-negative error rates.[83] It is unlikely that CT or MRI will be more accurate than surgical inspection of the regional lymph nodes.

Detection of extrarenal tumor extension into the perirenal fat and into adjacent structures is also problematic. Most children identified as having possible invasion of the liver on CT are found at the time of surgical exploration to have hepatic compression, rather than hepatic invasion.[84] Therefore, determination of inoperability must be made at surgical exploration. Non-opacification of the kidney on CT may result from tumor obstruction of the collecting system,[85] complete replacement of the renal parenchyma with neoplasm, or intravascular tumor extension.[75] Plain chest radiographs may be obtained to determine whether pulmonary metastases are present. However, most centers obtain a CT of the chest in the initial evaluation of children with Wilms' tumor. This can detect small lesions missed on chest

Table 32.2 NWTS-5 staging system for Wilms' tumor

Stage I: The tumor is limited to the kidney and was completely excised. The renal capsule has an intact outer surface. The tumor was not ruptured or biopsied prior to removal (fine-needle aspiration biopsies are excluded from this restriction). The vessels of the renal sinus are not involved. There is no evidence of tumor at or beyond the margins of resection.

Stage II: The tumor extends beyond the kidney, but was completely excised. There may be regional extension of tumor (i.e. penetration of the renal capsule or extensive invasion of the renal sinus). The blood vessels outside the renal parenchyma, including those of the renal sinus, may contain tumor. The tumor was biopsied (except for fine-needle aspiration), or there was spillage of tumor before or during surgery that is confined to the flank, and does not involve the peritoneal surface. There must be no evidence of tumor at or beyond the margins of resection.

Stage III: Residual non-hematogenous tumor is present, and confined to the abdomen. Any one of the following may occur: (1) Lymph nodes within the abdomen or pelvis are found to be involved by tumor (renal hilar, para-aortic, or beyond). (Lymph node involvement in the thorax, or other extra-abdominal sites would be a criterion for stage IV.) (2) The tumor has penetrated through the peritoneal surface. (3) Tumor implants are found on the peritoneal surface. (4) Gross or microscopic tumor remains postoperatively (e.g. tumor cells are found at the margin of surgical resection on microscopic examination). (5) The tumor is not completely resectable because of local infiltration into vital structures. (6) Tumor spill not confined to the flank occurred either before or during surgery.

Stage IV: Hematogenous metastases (lung, liver, bone, brain, etc.), or lymph node metastases outside the abdominopelvic region are present.

Stage V: Bilateral renal involvement is present at diagnosis. An attempt should be made to stage each side according to the above criteria on the basis of the extent of disease prior to biopsy or treatment.

X-ray, although the management of such lesions is debated.[86,87] Additional imaging studies are helpful under specific conditions. For example, a radionuclide bone scan and X-ray skeletal survey should be obtained postoperatively on all children with CCSK.[88] Brain imaging, using MRI or CT, should be obtained on all children with CCSK or with RTK, as both are associated with intracranial metastases.[89]

The NWTSG has long recommended formal exploration of the contralateral kidney in all children undergoing nephrectomy for presumed unilateral Wilms' tumor. This has been considered necessary to identify lesions that might be missed on preoperative imaging. If lesions are identified intraoperatively, biopsy alone of the lesions is advised and definitive surgical resection is deferred (for both kidneys). Review of NWTS-4 patients with bilateral Wilms' tumor found that 7% of lesions were missed on preoperative imaging studies.[90] Most lesions were managed with biopsy alone, yet extended follow-up of the children has not demonstrated any relapses.[91] The majority of these children had nephrectomy of the more involved kidney at diagnosis before exploration of the contralateral kidney. This was also noted in a recent report of NWTS-5 patients.[92] The conclusion of the latest report was that routine exploration is not necessary, provided that preoperative imaging with thin slices on multidetector helical CT scanners or MRI is performed.[91]

Surgery

The surgeon has an important role in the management of a child with Wilms' tumor. Careful removal of the tumor without rupture or spill is mandatory to decrease the risk of local abdominal relapse.[93] Complete tumor resection also improves patient survival. Another important surgical objective is determining tumor extent. As noted above, staging of the tumor is surgical. A transperitoneal approach is preferred to allow thorough exploration of the abdominal cavity. Exploration of the contralateral kidney is no longer mandated prior to nephrectomy if the preoperative CT or MRI demonstrate a normal kidney.[91] If exploration is needed, the colon is reflected and Gerota's fascia opened so that the kidney can be inspected on all surfaces. Any abnormalities of the kidney should be biopsied to exclude Wilms' tumor or nephrogenic rests.

Palpation of the renal vein and IVC should be performed to exclude intravascular tumor extension prior to vessel ligation. Radical nephrectomy is performed with partial ureterectomy. Formal lymph node dissection is not required but lymph node sampling is an integral step during surgery for Wilms' tumor.[83] Lymph node metastases (stage III) have an adverse outcome on survival. Failure to sample lymph nodes has been identified as a risk factor for local relapse in stage I patients, suggesting inadequate staging.[93]

One should not overlook the morbidity of surgery that can produce both acute and late complications. A review of NWTS-4 patients undergoing primary nephrectomy found an 11% incidence of surgical complications.[94] The most common complications were hemorrhage and small bowel obstruction. Risk factors associated with increased surgical complications are higher local tumor stage, intravascular extension, en bloc resection of other visceral organs, and incorrect preoperative diagnosis.[78]

Treatment and outcome

The development of effective systemic chemotherapy in the 1960s rapidly changed the outcome and approach to treatment of Wilms' tumor.[95] Randomized clinical trials have been conducted by NWTSG, SIOP, and the United Kingdom Children's Cancer Study Group (UKCCSG) to determine the appropriate role for each of the therapeutic modalities available. Patients are stratified into different treatment groups based on extent of disease and histopathologic features. The goals of these trials are to allow a reduction in the intensity of therapy for most patients, while maintaining overall survival, and to decrease potential late sequelae. For example, radiation therapy (XRT), once administered routinely to all children, is now reserved for those with advanced stage disease or specific adverse prognostic features.

National Wilms' Tumor Study Group

The first two NWTSG studies, NWTS-1 (1969–1973) and NWTS-2 (1974–1978), showed that postoperative local irradiation was unnecessary for group I patients.[96,97] The combination of vincristine (VCR) and dactinomycin (AMD) was noted to be more effective than the use of either drug alone, and the addition of doxorubicin (DOX) improved survival for higher-stage patients. Important findings of NWTS-1 and -2 were identification of unfavorable histologic features and other prognostic factors that allowed refinement of the staging system, stratifying patients into high-risk and low-risk treatment groups.[98] It was recognized that the presence of lymph node metastases had an adverse outcome on survival.[96,97] Children with lymph node metastases as well as those with diffuse tumor spill were found to be at increased risk of abdominal relapse. Therefore, such patients were from then on classified as having stage III disease and given whole abdominal irradiation.[82] These findings were incorporated into the design of NWTS-3 to try and decrease the intensity of therapy for the majority of low-risk patients.

In NWTS-3 (1979–1986), patients with stage I, FH Wilms' tumor were treated successfully with either a 10- or 18-week regimen of VCR and AMD.[82] This considerably decreased the amount of chemotherapy administered and the total duration of treatment. The 4-year relapse-free survival was 89%, and the overall survival was 95.6%. Stage II FH patients treated with AMD and VCR without postoperative XRT had an equivalent survival (4-year overall survival of 91.1%) to patients who received the same treatment plus DOX with or without XRT. This demonstrated that the cardiotoxic drug DOX is not necessary for the successful treatment of this group of patients. This also demonstrated that XRT could now be omitted for the majority of children with Wilms' tumor. For stage III FH patients, 10.8 Gy of abdominal irradiation was shown to be as effective as 20 Gy in preventing abdominal relapse if DOX was added to VCR and AMD. The 4-year relapse-free survival for stage III patients was 82% in NWTS-3 and the 4-year overall survival was 90.9%. Patients with stage IV FH tumors received abdominal (local) irradiation based on the local tumor stage. In addition, they all received 12 Gy to both lungs. In combination with VCR, AMD, and DOX, the 4-year relapse-free survival was 79% and the overall survival was 80.9%. There was no statistically significant improvement in survival when cyclophosphamide was added to the three-drug regimen.

The goals of NWTS-4 (1986–1994) were to continue improving treatment results while decreasing the cost of therapy through modification of the schedule of drug administration. 'Pulse-intensive' chemotherapy regimens, employing single doses of AMD and DOX, were compared with regimens using divided doses of the drugs. Pulse-intensive regimens utilized simultaneous administration of agents at less frequent intervals to decrease the number of clinic visits and hence the cost of cancer treatment. In addition, treatment durations of approximately 6 and 15 months were compared in patients with stages II–IV FH tumors. NWTS-4 demonstrated that, while the administered drug dose–intensity was greater on pulse-intensive regimens, these regimens produce less hematologic toxicity than the standard regimens.[99] Patients treated with pulse-intensive regimens achieved equivalent survival compared with those treated with standard chemotherapy regimens.[100] Treatment with 6 months of chemotherapy was as effective as 15 months.

Children with anaplastic Wilms' tumors were randomized in NWTS-3 and NWTS-4 to receive VCR, AMD, DOX, or those three drugs with the addition of cyclophosphamide. The results were analyzed after the tumors were reclassified using the criteria of Faria et al.[63] There was no difference in outcome between the regimens for children with focal anaplasia, who had a prognosis similar to that for favorable histology patients.[101] For stage II–IV diffuse anaplasia, the addition of cyclophosphamide to the three-drug regimen improved the 4-year relapse-free survival (27.2% vs 54.8%).

Treatment recommendations used in NWTS-5 (1995–2003) are outlined in Table 32.3. Treatment of patients with stage I or II FH tumors, and stage I anaplastic Wilms' tumor was the same. They received a pulse-intensive regimen of VCR and AMD for 18 weeks. Patients with stage III FH and stage II–III focal anaplasia were treated with AMD, VCR, and DOX, and 10.8 Gy XRT. Patients with stage IV FH tumors received abdominal irradiation based on the local tumor stage and 12 Gy to both lungs.

NWTS-5 was a single-arm therapeutic trial without any randomization for therapy. Prospective collection of information regarding biologic features of the tumors was part of this study. A collection of banked tumor specimens is available to evaluate new prognostic factors that may be identified in the future. Most importantly, the clinical outcome is available for patients for whom there are banked specimens. One of the primary goals of the study was to verify the preliminary findings that loss of heterozygosity (LOH) for chromosomes 16q and 1p is useful in identifying patients at increased risk for relapse and death.[51] Among patients with stage I–II FH tumors, the relative risk (RR) of relapse and death were increased for LOH 1p only (RR = 2.2 for relapse; RR = 4.0 for death), for LOH 16q only (RR = 1.9 and RR = 1.4), and for LOH for both regions (RR = 2.9 and RR = 4.3) in comparison with patients lacking LOH at either locus.[52] The risks of relapse and death for patients with stage III–IV FH tumors were increased only with LOH for both regions (RR = 2.4 and RR = 2.7). These results demonstrate that LOH for these chromosomal regions can now be used as an independent prognostic factor, together with disease stage, to target intensity of treatment to risk of treatment failure.

A unique aspect of the NWTS-5 trial was that a select group of patients <2 years of age with stage I

Table 32.3 Treatment schema used in National Wilms' Tumor Study-5

	Radiotherapy	Chemotherapy[a]
Stage I and II, favorable histology	None	Regimen EE-4A
Stage I focal or diffuse anaplasia		
Stage I, favorable histology, age <2 years, tumor weight <550 g	None	Regimen EE-4A
Stage III and IV, favorable histology	Yes	Regimen DD-4A
Stage II–IV, focal anaplasia		
Stage II–IV, diffuse anaplasia	Yes	Regimen I
Stage I–IV clear cell sarcoma of the kidney		
Stage I–IV rhabdoid tumor of the kidney	Yes	Regimen RTK

[a] 1998 modification to original protocol:
- Regimen EE-4A: pulse-intensive dactinomycin, vincristine (18 weeks)
- Regimen DD-4A: pulse-intensive dactinomycin, vincristine, doxorubicin (24 weeks)
- Regimen I: dactinomycin, vincristine, doxorubicin, cyclophosphamide, and etoposide (24 weeks)
- Regimen RTK: carboplatin, etoposide and cyclophosphamide (24 weeks)
- Stage IV/FH patients are given radiation based on the local tumor stage.

FH tumors, weighing <550 g, were managed with surgery alone. This was based on preliminary observation of favorable outcomes on small numbers of such patients when postoperative adjuvant therapy had been omitted.[102] Also a review of NWTSG patients had found excellent outcomes for such patients, albeit with postoperative chemotherapy.[103] This portion of the study was closed when the number of tumor relapses exceeded the limit allowed by the design of the study. However, the 2-year overall survival of this cohort was 100% due to the high rate of retrieval of the relapsed patients.[104] These results suggest that such an approach should continue to be evaluated in future trials.

International Society of Pediatric Oncology

The clinical protocols conducted by SIOP differ from the NWTSG in that therapy is given before surgery. This approach usually results in tumor shrinkage, reducing the risk of intraoperative rupture or spill.[105] It is also postulated that the neoadjuvant therapy will treat micrometastases, leading to a more favorable stage distribution at the time of surgery. A greater number of patients have 'postchemotherapy stage I' tumors. This postchemotherapy stage is used to stratify patients for treatment.

The first two SIOP studies answered questions with regard to the use of prenephrectomy XRT.[105] The third SIOP study, SIOP-5, showed that 4 weeks of AMD and VCR was as effective as prenephrectomy XRT in avoiding surgical tumor rupture and increasing the proportion of patients with low-stage disease.[106] SIOP-6, the fourth SIOP study on Wilms' tumor, demonstrated that patients with postnephrectomy stage I disease can safely be treated with 18 weeks of AMD and VCR.[107] Those patients with stage II lymph node-negative disease, however, were shown to have a higher rate of relapse if postoperative abdominal irradiation was omitted. It was concluded that these children require more intensive postnephrectomy chemotherapy, including the use of an anthracycline.[107] Finally, SIOP-6 confirmed the need for a three-drug chemotherapy regimen following nephrectomy for those with more advanced stage disease, i.e. stage II lymph node positive and stage III.

The fifth SIOP Wilms' tumor trial, SIOP-9 (1987–1991), evaluated the duration of prenephrectomy chemotherapy. The number of postchemotherapy stage I was similar after either 4 or 8 weeks of therapy (64% vs 62%) and 2-year event-free survival (EFS) was equivalent.[108] Also, there was no significant additional tumor shrinkage benefit after 4 weeks of preoperative chemotherapy.[108] Children with stage IIN0 disease were treated with VCR, AMD, and an anthracycline for 27 weeks without XRT, whereas children with IIN1 and III disease were given the same regimen and abdominal irradiation. The 2-year EFS and overall survival (OS) for stage IIN0 was

84% and 88% and for stage IINI and III was 71% and 85%, respectively. There were 59 children with stage I–IV tumors who had complete tumor necrosis induced by chemotherapy, and 98% of these children had no evidence of disease at 5 years.[109] The latest SIOP study on Wilms' tumor, SIOP 93–01 (1993–2000), evaluated a reduction in postoperative therapy for patients with stage I intermediate risk and anaplastic Wilms' tumor.[110] Patients were randomized to receive either 4 or 18 weeks of postoperative chemotherapy with AMD and VCR. Two-year EFS was 91.4% after 4 weeks and 88.8% after 18 weeks of therapy, demonstrating that survival can be maintained while shortening the duration of postnephrectomy therapy. The current SIOP 2001 study is evaluating the ability to stratify patients for treatment based on postchemotherapy histologic findings.[58]

United Kingdom Children's Cancer Study Group

The UKCCSG has also conducted trials of children with Wilms' tumor.[111–113] The UK approach is to biopsy the tumor prior to treatment. They have noted a 12% incidence of non-Wilms' tumors in patients with the typical features of Wilms' tumor on imaging study.[114] Overall, there was 1% of benign lesions on biopsy, similar to rates found in SIOP studies.[108] The UKW1 and UKW2 studies evaluated the single-agent vincristine for treatment of stage I FH tumors.[111,112] The OS of 96% compares well with two-drug chemotherapy, but age >4 years was considered an adverse prognostic factor.[113]

Preoperative chemotherapy vs immediate nephrectomy

In summary, there is a different philosophical approach between the pediatric cancer cooperative groups. Both the NWTSG and SIOP tumor staging systems are designed to stratify patients into low-risk and high-risk groups. The goal is to select out high-risk patients for more intense therapy, while minimizing treatment and thus morbidity for low-risk patients. Both groups want to reduce the number of patients receiving irradiation and doxorubicin to avoid the late effects of treatment (see below). Currently, approximately 50% of SIOP patients are treated with an anthracycline and 17% undergo irradiation, whereas approximately 35% of NWTSG patients have received both therapies.[115,116] The NWTSG trials have relied on surgical and pathologic staging following immediate nephrectomy. Preoperative treatment can produce dramatic reduction in the size of the primary tumor, decreasing the morbidity of surgery (Figure 32.3).[117] However, the staging information obtained following prenephrectomy chemotherapy may inadequately define the risk of relapse.[107] The current SIOP and UK approach is using the histologic response of the tumor to preoperative therapy to decide postoperative treatment. The current strategy in North America will be to use biologic prognostic factors to stratify patients for therapy.

There are situations where preoperative chemotherapy is routinely recommended. This includes children with bilateral Wilms' tumors,[119,120] tumors inoper-

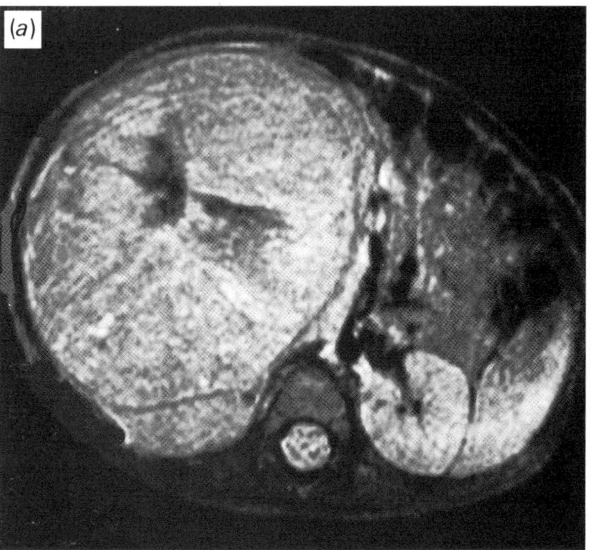

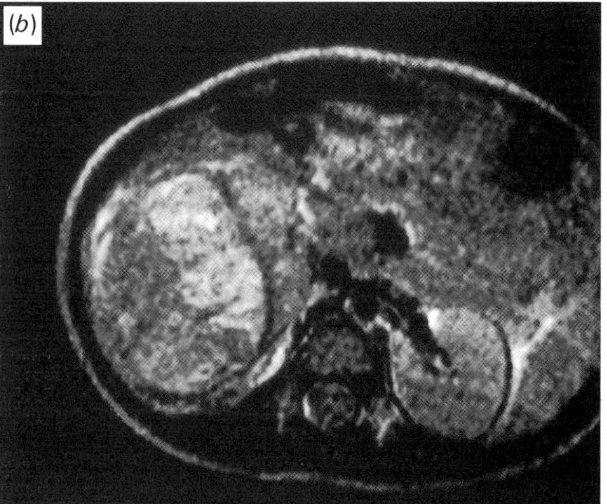

Figure 32.3 (*a*) Magnetic resonance imaging scan of a large inoperable Wilms' tumor. (*b*) After 6 weeks of chemotherapy, the same tumor has dramatically decreased in size. (Reproduced with permission from Richey et al.[118])

able at surgical exploration,[121] and tumor extension into IVC above the hepatic veins.[122–124] The latter two conditions are associated with an increased risk for surgical complications if primary nephrectomy is undertaken.[78] The rationale for preoperative chemotherapy in patients with bilateral tumors is to preserve renal parenchyma. This is important because renal failure is a significant risk in patients with bilateral disease.[125,126]

Vascular extension

For vena caval involvement below the level of the hepatic veins, the caval thrombus can be removed via cavotomy after proximal and distal vascular control is obtained. Generally, the thrombus will be free-floating, but if there is adherence of the thrombus to the caval wall, the thrombus can often be delivered with the passage of a Fogarty or Foley balloon catheter. If the thrombus extends above the level of the hepatic veins, preoperative chemotherapy can shrink the tumor and thrombus, facilitating complete removal.[122,127]

Inoperable tumor

A tumor should not be judged inoperable based on imaging studies alone. Preoperative imaging can overestimate local tumor extension and inoperability should only be determined on surgical exploration. It is also important to remember that the misdiagnosis rate of renal masses after assessment by diagnostic imaging is still 5%.[108,114] If the tumor is found to be unresectable, pretreatment with chemotherapy almost always reduces the bulk of the tumor, and renders it resectable[121,128] (see Figure 32.3). Patients who are staged by imaging studies alone are also at risk for understaging.[108] A patient determined to have an inoperable tumor should be considered stage III and treated accordingly.[121]

Repeat imaging is performed after 6 weeks of chemotherapy. Experience in SIOP has shown that maximal reduction in tumor volume occurs in the first 8 weeks.[108] After there has been adequate shrinkage of the tumor, definitive resection can be completed. A clinically good response (by imaging) is usually associated with a pathologically good response in terms of regressive histologic changes.[58,129] The converse is not always true. The distribution of histologic subtypes is different following preoperative chemotherapy compared with primary surgery, with differentiation of the tumor occurring after chemotherapy. Stromal and epithelial predominant tumors are found more often after preoperative chemotherapy.[58,129] These histologic subtypes may demonstrate a poor clinical response to therapy but have an excellent prognosis if the tumor is completely excised. Patients with progressive disease have a very poor prognosis and these patients will require treatment with a different chemotherapeutic regimen.[121]

Bilateral disease

Synchronous bilateral nephroblastoma occurs in about 5% of children with Wilms' tumor, with metachronous lesions developing in only 1% (Figure 32.4).[119,130,131] Therapy of children with bilateral Wilms' tumor (BWT) is directed towards preservation of renal parenchyma to avoid renal insufficiency. A review of NWTSG patients with BWT found that 9.1% of synchronous bilateral tumors and 18.8% of metachronous bilateral tumors have developed renal failure.[125] The most common etiology for renal failure was the need for bilateral nephrectomy for persistent or recurrent tumor in the remaining kidney after initial nephrectomy. NWTSG investigators noted that

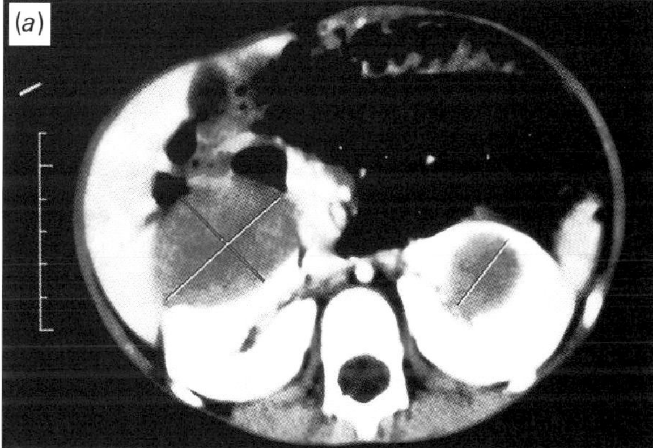

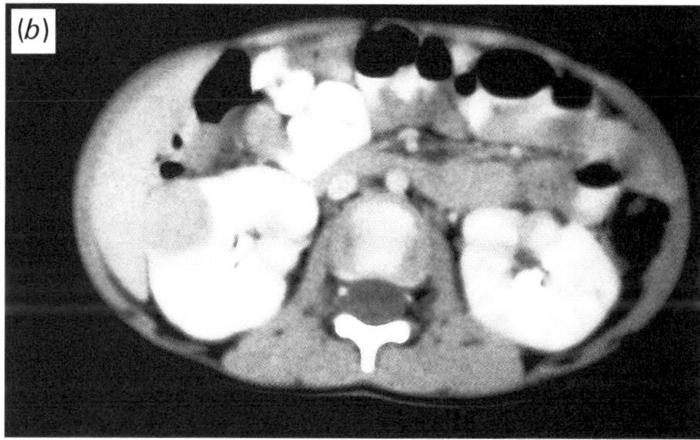

Figure 32.4 Computed tomography scan demonstrating bilateral Wilms' tumor: (*a*) before chemotherapy; (*b*) 6 weeks after chemotherapy, showing a marked reduction in the size of the masses.

nephrectomy could be avoided entirely in almost 50% of the group of patients undergoing initial biopsy followed by chemotherapy.

The initial management, therefore, is chemotherapy. Repeat imaging is done 6 weeks later to assess response of the tumors. Experience in SIOP has shown that maximal shrinkage occurs after 4–6 weeks of chemotherapy. As noted above, one cannot predict the histology of the tumor by response (on imaging) to the chemotherapy.[58,129] Differentiated tumors may show a poor clinical response to therapy, but have an excellent prognosis if the tumor is completely excised. Tumors with complete necrosis and predominantly regressive changes can also increase in size during therapy.[58] Tumors not responding to therapy require open biopsy to exclude anaplasia.

At the time of the second-look procedure, partial nephrectomy or wedge excision of the tumor should be considered, but only if complete tumor resection with negative margins can be obtained and part of either or both of the kidneys can be salvaged. If the tumors are not amenable to partial resections, patients with persistent viable tumor are then treated with a different chemotherapeutic regimen. The patient should be reassessed after an additional 12 weeks of chemotherapy to determine the feasibility of resection. If it appears that either or both of the kidneys can be salvaged, partial nephrectomies or wedge excisions of the tumors are performed. Radical nephrectomy is performed to remove the kidney with too extensive tumor involvement when only one of two can be preserved. Bilateral nephrectomies and dialysis may rarely be required when the tumors fail to respond to chemotherapy and radiation therapy. The recommended interval between successful completion of treatment of the Wilms' tumor and renal transplantation varies. Some clinicians advocate a waiting period of 2 years to ensure that the patient does not develop metastatic disease; others have found that a 1-year interval is sufficient.[132] SIOP investigators have noted that late relapses have occurred in patients with BWT more than 4 years post-treatment and recommended long-term follow-up.[131]

Partial nephrectomy in unilateral tumors

The success of renal preservation in BWT has prompted some centers to recommend renal sparing surgery for unilateral tumors.[133–135] They cite concern about the late occurrence of renal dysfunction in children who have undergone unilateral nephrectomy. There is both clinical and experimental evidence of hyperfiltration damage of remnant nephrons after a loss of renal mass. Following treatment for unilateral Wilms' tumor, some patients develop proteinuria and a decrease in creatinine clearance.[136,137] However, other investigators have failed to confirm these findings.[138,139] A review of NWTSG patients found that the incidence of renal failure in children with unilateral tumors is 0.25%.[125] Most of those patients had the Denys–Drash syndrome with intrinsic renal disease, which often progresses to end-stage disease even in the absence of tumor. More recently, other subgroups of patients at increased risk for renal insufficiency have been identified.[126] Patients with the WAGR syndrome have a markedly increased risk of renal failure. Breslow et al[126] found a 38% risk of renal failure that occurred at a median of 14 years from diagnosis. They also noted an increased risk for renal failure in children presenting with genitourinary anomalies and Wilms' tumor. In summary, the risk of developing renal failure following treatment appears to be quite low for most children with unilateral Wilms' tumor, although continued long-term follow-up of this cohort of children is necessary.

Screening of patients at an increased risk for the development of Wilms' tumor (e.g. BWS, hemihypertrophy, aniridia) will occasionally detect a small lesion inviting the possibility of a renal sparing procedure.[29] There is an increased incidence of metachronous Wilms' tumor development in patients undergoing unilateral nephrectomy if nephrogenic rests are found in the kidney adjacent to the tumor.[73] Children with BWS, hemihypertrophy, and aniridia do have an increased incidence of nephrogenic rests in comparison to patients with unilateral Wilms' tumor not associated with congenital anomalies.[69]

The majority of Wilms' tumors are too large for a partial nephrectomy at initial presentation. Therefore, pretreatment with chemotherapy is usually necessary if renal sparing surgery is to be considered.[133–135] Staging of the patient after chemotherapy could lead to inaccuracy, as discussed above. Some clinicians advocate enucleation of the tumor to allow parenchymal sparing procedures for even centrally located tumors where partial nephrectomy with a rim of renal tissue would be inadvisable.[134] However, anaplastic histology must be excluded before consideration of enucleation. The possible benefits of renal parenchymal conserving surgery must be evaluated against the potential risks of such procedures. Partial nephrectomy and enucleation increase the risk for positive surgical margins. A review of children with BWT enrolled in NWTS-4 found that the incidence of local recurrence was 7.5% following partial nephrectomy and 14% after enucleation.[140] Although OS was comparable, patients with residual disease and recurrences required additional therapy to attain a similar outcome.

In summary, parenchymal sparing procedures for patients with unilateral Wilms' tumor are controversial. It seems reasonable to consider partial nephrectomy for patients with BWT, tumor in a solitary kidney, and renal insufficiency. For other children, this option should be approached with caution. The data reviewed above suggest a fivefold increase or 5% incidence of the development of metachronous Wilms' tumor in children in these high-risk categories. Does this risk justify the routine use of preoperative chemotherapy to facilitate partial nephrectomies in all patients with BWS, hemihypertrophy, or aniridia found to have unilateral tumors? As noted in the discussion above, there is a risk for undertreatment and potentially increased risk of local recurrence. These risks must be weighed against the possible benefit of decreasing the incidence of renal failure.

Late effects of treatment

Each therapeutic modality used in the management of Wilms' tumor can result in both acute and delayed toxicities. Numerous organ systems are subject to the late sequelae of anticancer therapy. Late effects of cancer therapy are predictable, based on treatment modalities used, age of patient at treatment, and time elapsed since therapy. Clinicians must now become familiar with the spectrum of problems that face these children as they grow into adulthood. Long-term follow-up of treatment-related complications has been an integral role of the NWTSG. One of the major objectives of the pediatric cancer cooperative groups has been to reduce the intensity of treatment in order to prevent or lower the morbidity of multimodal therapy without reducing efficacy.[141]

Children treated for Wilms' tumor are at increased risk for second malignant neoplasms (SMNs). NWTSG investigators reported that 15 years after initial (Wilms' tumor) diagnosis, the cumulative incidence of an SMN is 1.6% and increasing steadily.[142] This is more than eight times the expected incidence. The risk of developing leukemia or lymphoma is greatest in the first 8 years after treatment. The risk of developing a solid tumor continues to increase over time. Most tumors occur in previously irradiated areas, but prior treatment for relapse, and use of DOX were also associated with an increased incidence of SMNs.

Congestive heart failure is a known complication of treatment with an anthracycline.[143] The frequency is directly proportional to the cumulative dose of DOX received. In addition to the acute cardiotoxicity, reports are surfacing of cardiac failure up to 20 years after treatment.[144] In a preliminary review of patients entered on NWTS-1, -2, and -3, the frequency of congestive heart failure was 1.7% among DOX-treated patients.[145] The risk was increased if the patient received whole lung irradiation. In light of these findings, all children who undergo treatment with these modalities should undergo periodic re-evaluation.

Growth disturbances are known complications of cancer therapy in children. Spinal irradiation can result in severe reduction in spinal growth.[146] Similarly, chemotherapeutic agents can have a direct effect on chondrocytes, resulting in resistance to endogenous growth hormone and subsequent growth impairment.[147] Hogeboom et al studied the impact of treatment on stature in Wilms' tumor patients.[148] They concluded that while reductions in stature directly correlated to total radiation dose and age at treatment, currently recommended radiation doses should not result in a clinically significant impact.

Damage to reproductive systems can lead to problems with hormonal dysfunction and/or infertility. Gonadal radiation in males can result in temporary azoospermia and hyogonadism.[149] The effect on the testis is dose related, and the prepubertal germ cells also appear to be radiosensitive. In a follow-up of 10 men treated for Wilms' tumor in childhood, oligospermia or azoospermia was found in 8.[150] The Leydig cells are more radioresistant than the germ cells, but higher doses can produce damage resulting in inadequate production of testosterone. This can result in delayed sexual maturation.

Chemotherapeutic agents can interfere with testicular function, particularly alkylating agents. Acute toxicity with germ cell depletion occurs in all age groups. Some long-term studies suggested that prepubertal testes are resistant to chronic toxicity.[151] However, recent studies have indicated that prepubertal testes are not protected from chemotherapy-induced damage.[152,153] One report found that 12 of 19 prepubertal males treated for a variety of solid tumors were sterile as a result of treatment.[153]

Female Wilms' tumor patients who received abdominal radiation have a 12% incidence of ovarian failure.[154] Of 16 women who received whole abdominal irradiation, all had evidence of ovarian failure and 75% were amenorrheic.[155] As with the testis, the effect on the ovaries is dose dependent. Chemotherapy-induced damage to the ovaries is most often associated with alkylating agents. A decrease in the number of follicles is seen in prepubertal girls treated with chemotherapy.[156] Premature menopause is a common complication of female childhood cancer survivors.[157] It is usually associated with radiation therapy and/or treatment with alkylating agents. Byrne et al demonstrated that women receiving alkylating agents were 9.2 times more likely to enter premature menopause.[157] Although further studies are needed to assess the extent of the problem, it appears prudent to counsel survivors at risk that a delay in first pregnancy may preclude having children.[158] In the future, cryopreservation and reimplantation of oocytes may be a viable alternative for these patients.

Several studies have addressed the risk of pregnancy in survivors after childhood cancer therapy. As noted above, girls with Wilms' tumor appear to have a higher incidence of Müllerian anomalies, causing some authors to suggest postpubertal level 2 ultrasound evaluation to detect these abnormalities prior to pregnancy.[21] Women with prior abdominal radiation have the greatest potential for adverse pregnancy outcomes. In a study of patients treated for Wilms' tumor, an adverse outcome occurred in 3% among non-irradiated women compared with 30% of women who received abdominal irradiation.[159] Perinatal mortality rates are higher, and infants are more likely to have low birth weights. The potential mutagenic effects of anticancer therapy are of concern. Most studies have found no increase in the incidence of congenital anomalies and no cases of Wilms' tumor in the offspring of survivors.[159,160]

Most children treated for Wilms' tumor undergo unilateral nephrectomy as part of the initial treatment. As noted above, there is risk of dysfunction of the solitary remaining kidney. Impairment of renal function may be related to irradiation, administration of nephrotoxic chemotherapeutic agents, or hyperfiltration of the remaining nephrons. Initially, there is compensatory hypertrophy that develops in this kidney.[161,162] The data are conflicting regarding renal compensatory hypertrophy in patients who receive whole abdominal irradiation. Walker et al found no difference in renal lengths between patients treated with chemotherapy and radiation vs chemotherapy alone.[161] However, a more recent report used ultrasound to calculate renal lengths and found that patients receiving radiation had poor compensatory growth.[162]

The kidney is sensitive to the effects of radiation. Radiation doses to the kidney should be limited to 12–15 Gy. Mitus and colleagues correlated functional impairment with the renal radiation dose in a review of 100 children treated for Wilms' tumor.[163] The incidence of impaired creatinine clearance was significantly greater for children receiving >12 Gy to the remaining kidney and all cases of overt renal failure occurred in patients who had received >23 Gy. Clinical signs of radiation nephritis may occur very acutely or begin months or years after therapy is discontinued.[163] Direct radiation nephrotoxicity is the usual cause, with injury to the intrarenal vasculature. Nephrotoxicity related to chemotherapy is well documented. Studies in children have demonstrated that alkylating agents in particular are associated with renal tubular dysfunction related to drug metabolites.[164] Unfortunately, Mesna has not been protective against these effects. A recent study by Bardi et al has suggested that high-risk Wilms' patients receiving agents such as cyclophosphamide may be at risk for early, subclinical, renal dysfunction, as evidenced by elevated levels of cystatin C, a measure of glomerular function, and elevated *N*-acetyl-β-D-glucosaminidase along with microalbuminuria.[165] The latter are both indicators of proximal tubular dysfunction. The long-term significance of these findings remains to be determined.

Other renal tumors of childhood

Cystic partially differentiated nephroblastoma

Cysts are common in Wilms' tumor and range in size from microscopic to several centimeters in diameter. Tumors composed of only cysts with immature nephrogenic elements and blastema within the delicate septa are designated cystic partially differentiated nephroblastoma. The majority of these lesions occur in the first year of life.[166] These lesions are indistinguishable radiographically from solitary multilocular cyst described below. Surgery is curative in almost all patients, with recurrence the result of incomplete resection.[167,168]

Multilocular cystic nephroma

Multilocular cystic nephroma, also known as solitary multilocular cyst, is an uncommon, benign renal tumor with a bimodal incidence. This tumor is distinguished by the finding of only mature cell types within the septa of the cyst wall. Fifty percent of the multilocular cysts reported in the literature have been found in children younger than 4 years; boys predominate in a ratio of 2:1. The second peak incidence occurs in adults, and, unlike the pediatric cases, are usually in women.[169]

Cystic nephromas are commonly found incidentally on radiographic studies, but may present as an abdominal mass found on routine physical examination. Whereas the majority of cases of multilocular cystic renal disease have been unilateral, there are rare reports of bilateral cases.[170] The gross appearance of the tumor is its most distinguishing feature. The cut surfaces reveal a well-circumscribed multilocular tumor composed of cysts ranging from several millimeters to several centimeters in greatest diameter. The tumor is well encapsulated, compressing the surrounding renal parenchyma.

Multilocular cystic nephroma is a benign lesion which is cured by nephrectomy. Recurrence has occurred following incomplete excision by partial nephrectomy. If partial nephrectomy is considered, frozen section is indicated to exclude cystic, partially differentiated nephroblastoma.[166]

Congenital mesoblastic nephroma

Congenital mesoblastic nephroma (CMN) is the most common renal tumor in infants, with a mean age at diagnosis of 3.5 months.[171] The typical presentation is a newborn with an abdominal mass, but in recent years a number of cases have been recognized prenatally, with polyhydramnios a frequent prenatal finding.[172,173] Tumor induction is postulated to occur at a time when the multipotent blastema is predominately stromagenic.[174] The neoplasm is distinct from Wilms' tumor and has three histologic subtypes: classic, cellular, and mixed (showing areas of both classical and cellular).The classic subtype, 24% of cases, is characterized by interlacing sheets of bland spindle cells. Classic CMN resembles infantile fibromatosis. The cellular variant, 66% of cases, has a solid sheet-like growth pattern and cells with little cytoplasm and frequent mitoses.[175–177] The cellular variant is virtually identical histologically to congenital fibrosarcoma. Molecular studies have found a similar translocation in both tumors that fuses the *ETV6* (*TEL*) gene from chromosome 12p13 with the chromosome 15q25 neurotrophin-3 receptor gene, *NTRK3*.[178]

Imaging studies cannot reliably distinguish CMN from other renal mass lesions. Abdominal CT shows a heterogeneous solid mass arising from the kidney (Figure 32.5). Complete excision is curative for most patients with CMN.[171] Local recurrence and metastasis can occur, particularly with the cellular variant of CMN.[175,176] The pathology specimen will often identify extension of tumor into the hilar or perirenal soft tissue; therefore, complete surgical resection is important.[177] The risk of recurrence is thought to be less in children under 3 months of age at diagnosis, but metastases have been reported in a few infants.[179] Neither chemotherapy nor radiation therapy is routinely recommended,[171] but consideration for adjuvant treatment should be given to patients with cellular variants that are incompletely resected.[176] There are reports demonstrating response of both inoperable and recurrent tumors to chemotherapy.[180,181]

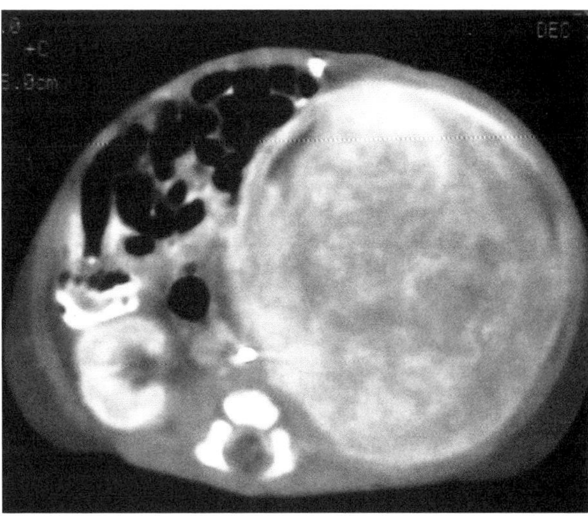

Figure 32.5 Computed tomography scan of an infant with congenital mesoblastic nephroma.

Clear cell sarcoma of the kidney

This tumor is also known as the 'bone-metastasizing renal tumour of childhood' because of its predilection for these sites.[59,182] There are also an increased number of brain metastases with this entity.[183] CCSK accounts for 3% of renal tumors reported to the NWTSG. Unlike anaplastic Wilms' tumor, even stage I CCSK lesions are associated with increased rates of relapse. There are no reports of children with bilateral CCSK. Studies have demonstrated that the use of DOX is associated with a significant improvement in outcome for these children.[82,184] Patients with CCSK were treated on NWTS-5 with a regimen combining VCR, DOX, cyclophosphamide, and etoposide in an attempt to further improve the survival of this high-risk group, but results of that trial are pending. All patients with CCSK require irradiation to the tumor bed.

Rhabdoid tumor of the kidney

RTK was first identified by NWTSG pathologists in 1978.[59] This is a highly malignant tumor of the kidney and accounts for 2% of renal tumors registered to the NWTSG.[82,89] The tumor derives its name from the resemblance to rhabdomyoblasts, but it is not derived from myogenic cells; the cell of origin is unknown. This tumor is typically seen in infants and very young children, with a median age of 13 months. Infants with RTK often have concurrent brain tumors. It is difficult to ascertain if these are metastases or two distinct primary tumors.[185] Recent studies suggest that there is a common genetic basis for renal and extrarenal rhabdoid tumors in infants.[186] There is a deletion or mutation in the tumor suppressor gene *INI-1* on chromosome 22 that predisposes to the development of this tumor. Staining for the products of the *INI-1* gene can be useful, as RTK is consistently negative.[187] The prognosis of patients with rhabdoid tumor remains dismal with conventional chemotherapeutic regimens, with over 80% of children dying within 1 year of diagnosis.[188] In NWTS-5, children with all stages of rhabdoid tumor were treated with carboplatin, cyclophosphamide, and etoposide; they also received abdominal irradiation, but results of that trial are pending.

Renal cell carcinoma

Only 5% of renal cell carcinomas occur in children.[189] These patients generally present after age 5 years, and it is the most common renal malignancy in the second decade of life.[190] Survival of children with renal cell carcinoma is dependent on the ability to completely resect the tumor. Raney et al found that all children with stage I lesions survived;[191] OS was about 50%. Age is also a prognostic factor, with improved survival in children younger than 11 years.[191] A recent report suggested that local lymph node involvement does not predict a poor outcome compared with adult renal cell carcinoma.[192] Renal cell carcinomas in children also differ in their morphology and molecular characterization. There is a higher percentage of *TFE3* (transcription factor micro E3 binding protein) 'translocation' carcinomas and 'unclassified' carcinomas in the first two decades of life.[193] There is also a lower frequency of clear cell carcinomas and *VHL* (von Hippel–Lindau gene) alterations compared with adults. These tumors do not appear responsive to chemotherapy or radiation therapy.

References

1. Breslow N, Olshan A, Beckwith JB, Green DM. Epidemiology of Wilms' tumor. Med Pediatr Oncol 1993; 21:172–81
2. Bernstein L, Linet M, Smith MA, Olshan AF. Renal tumors. In: Ries LAG, Smith MA, Gurney JG et al, eds. Cancer Incidence and Survival among Children and Adolescents: United States SEER program 1975–1995, National Cancer Institute, SEER Program. Bethesda, MD: National Institutes of Health, Pub. No. 99–4649; 1999: 79–90.
3. Breslow N, Olshan A, Beckwith JB et al. Ethnic variation in the incidence, diagnosis, prognosis and follow-up of children with Wilms' tumor. J Natl Cancer Inst 1994; 86:49–51.
4. Beckwith JB. Macroglossia, omphalocele, adrenal cytomegaly, gigantism and hyperplastic visceromegaly. Birth Def Orig Art Ser 1969; 5:188–96.
5. Sotelo-Avila C, Gonzalez-Crussi F, Fowler JW. Complete and incomplete forms of Beckwith–Wiedemann syndrome: their oncogenic potential. J Pediatr 1980; 96:47–50.
6. Debaun MR, Tucker MA. Risk of cancer during the first four years of life in children from The Beckwith–Wiedemann Syndrome Registry. J Pediatr 1998; 132:377–9.
7. Beckwith JB. Certain conditions have an increased incidence of Wilms' tumor. AJR Am J Roentgenol 1996; 164:1294–5.
8. Wiedemann H. Tumors and hemihypertrophy associated with the Wiedemann–Beckwith syndrome. Eur J Pediatr 1983; 141:129.
9. Porteus MH, Norkool P, Neuberg D et al. Characteristics and outcome of children with Beckwith–Weidemann syndrome and Wilms' tumor: a report from the National Wilms' Tumor Study Group. J Clin Oncol 2000; 18:2026–31.
10. Debaun MR, Siegel MJ, Choyke PL. Nephromegaly in infancy and early childhood: a risk factor for Wilms tumor in Beckwith–Wiedemann syndrome. J Pediatr 1998; 132:401–4.
11. Breslow N, Beckwith JB, Ciol M, Sharples K. Age distribution of Wilms' tumor: report from the National Wilms' Tumor Study. Cancer Res 1988; 48:1653–7.
12. Perlman M, Levin M, Wittels B. Syndrome of fetal gigantism, renal hamartomas, and nephroblastomatosis with Wilms' tumor. Cancer 1975; 35:1212–17.
13. Neri G, Gurrieri F, Zanni G, Lin A. Clinical and molecular aspects of the Simpson–Golabi–Behmel syndrome. Am J Med Genet 1998; 79:279–83.
14. Breslow NE, Beckwith JB. Epidemiological features of Wilms' tumor: results of the National Wilms' Tumor Study. J Natl Cancer Inst 1982; 68:429–36.
15. Drash A, Sherman F, Hartmann WH, Blizzard RM. A syndrome of pseudohermaphroditism, Wilms' tumor, hypertension and degenerative renal disease. J Pediatr 1970; 76:585–93.

16. Coppes MJ, Huff V, Pelletier J. Denys–Drash syndrome: relating a clinical disorder to genetic alterations in the tumor suppressor gene WT1. J Pediatr 1993; 123:673–8.
17. McTaggart SJ, Algar E, Chow CW, Powell HR, Jones CL. Clinical spectrum of Denys–Drash and Frasier syndrome. Pediatr Nephrol 2001; 16:335–9.
18. Hittner HM, Riccardi VM, Ferrell RE et al. Genetic heterogeneity of aniridia: negative linkage data. Metab Pediatr Ophthalmol 1980; 4:179–82.
19. Breslow NE, Norris R, Norkool PA et al. Characteristics and outcomes of children with the Wilms' tumor–Aniridia syndrome: a report from the National Wilms' Tumor Study Group. J Clin Oncol 2003; 21:4579–85.
20. Clericuzio CL. Clinical phenotypes and Wilms tumor. Med Pediatr Oncol 1993; 21:182–7.
21. Byrne J, Nicholson HS. Excess risk for Mullerian duct anomalies in girls with Wilms tumor. Med Pediatr Oncol 2002; 38:258–9.
22. Mesrobian HG, Kelalis PP, Hrabovsky E et al. Wilms tumor in horseshoe kidneys: a report from the National Wilms Tumor Study. J Urol 1985; 133:1002–3.
23. Neville H, Ritchey ML, Shamberger RC et al. Wilms tumor occurring in a horseshoe kidney. Report from the NWTSG. J Pediatr Surg 2002; 37:1134–7.
24. Beckwith JB. Wilms tumor in multicystic dysplastic kidneys: What is the risk? Dial Pediatr Urol 1996; 19:3–5.
25. Narchi H. Risk of Wilms tumour with multicystic kidney disease: a systematic review. Arch Dis Child 2005; 90:147–9.
26. Green DM, Breslow NE, Beckwith JB, Norkool P. Screening of children with hemihypertrophy, aniridia, and Beckwith–Wiedemann syndrome in patients with Wilms' tumor: a report from the National Wilms' Tumor Study. Med Pediatr Oncol 1993; 21:188–92.
27. Craft AW, Parker L, Stiller C, Cole M. Screening for Wilms' tumour in patients with aniridia, Beckwith syndrome, or hemihypertrophy. Med Pediatr Oncol 1995; 24:231–4.
28. Choyke PL, Siegel MJ, Craft AW, Green DM, DeBaun MR. Screening for Wilms tumor in children with Beckwith–Wiedemann syndrome or idiopathic hemihypertrophy. Med Pediatr Oncol 1999; 32:196–200.
29. McNeil DE, Brown M, Ching A, DeBaun MR. Screening for Wilms tumor and hepatoblastoma in children with Beckwith–Wiedemann syndromes: a cost-effective model. Med Pediatr Oncol 2001; 37:349–56.
30. Choyke PL, Siegel MJ, Oz O, Sotelo-Avila C, DeBaun MR. Nonmalignant renal disease in pediatric patients with Beckwith–Wiedemann syndrome. AJR Am J Roentgenol 1998; 171:733–7.
31. Borer JG, Kaefer M, Barnewolt CE et al. Renal findings on radiological followup of patients with Beckwith–Wiedemann syndrome. J Urol 1999; 161:235–9.
32. Dome JS, Coppes MJ. Recent advances in Wilms tumor genetics. Curr Opin Pediatr 2002; 14:5–11.
33. Knudson AG, Strong LC. Mutation and cancer: a model for Wilms' tumor of the kidney. J Natl Cancer Inst 1972; 48:313–24.
34. Strong LC. The two-hit model for Wilms' tumor: where are we 30 years later? Genes Chromosomes Cancer 2003; 38:294–9.
35. Coppes MJ, Haber DA, Grundy PE. Genetic events in the development of Wilms' tumor. N Engl J Med 1994; 331:586–90.
36. Call KM, Glaser T, Ito CY et al. Isolation and characterization of a zinc finger polypeptide gene at the human chromosome 11 Wilms' tumor locus. Cell 1990; 60:509–20.
37. Gessler M, Poustka A, Cavenee W et al. Homozygous deletion in Wilms' tumours of a zinc-finger gene identified by chromosome jumping. Nature 1990; 343:774–8.
38. Bonetta L, Kuehn SE, Huang A et al. Wilms tumor locus on 11p13 defined by multiple CpG island-associated transcripts. Science 1990; 250:994–7.
39. Ton CC, Hirvonen H, Miwa H et al. Positional cloning and characterization of a paired box- and homeobox-containing gene from the aniridia region. Cell 1991; 67:1059–74.
40. Lee SB, Haber DA. Wilms tumor and the WT1 gene. Exp Cell Res 2001; 264:74–99.
41. Pelletier J, Bruening W, Kashtan CE et al. Germline mutations in the Wilms' tumor suppressor gene are associated with abnormal urogenital development in Denys–Drash syndrome. Cell 1991; 67:437–47.
42. Little MH, Williamson KA. Evidence that WT1 mutations in Denys–Drash syndrome patients may act in a dominant-negative fashion. Hum Mol Genet 1993; 2:259–64.
43. Little SE, Hanks SP, King-Underwood L et al. Frequency and heritability of WT1 mutations in nonsyndromic Wilms' tumor patients: a UK Children's Cancer Study Group Study. J Clin Oncol 2004; 22:4140–6.
44. Schumacher V, Schneider S, Figge A et al. Correlation of germ-line mutations and two-hit inactivation of the WT1 gene with Wilms tumors of stromal-predominant histology. Proc Natl Acad Sci USA 1997; 94:3972–7.
45. Diller L, Ghahremani M, Morgan J et al. Constitutional WT1 mutations in Wilms' tumor patients. J Clin Oncol 1998; 16:3634–40.
46. Koufos A, Grundy P, Morgan K et al. Familial Wiedemann–Beckwith syndrome and a second Wilms tumor locus both map to 11p15.5. Am J Hum Genet 1989; 44:711–19.
47. Mannens M, Devilee P, Bliek J et al. Loss of heterozygosity in Wilms' tumors, studied for six putative tumor suppressor regions, is limited to chromosome 11. Cancer Res 1990; 50:3279–83.
48. Ping AJ, Reeve AE, Law DJ et al. Genetic linkage of Beckwith–Wiedemann syndrome to 11p15. Am J Hum Genet 1989; 44:720–3.
49. Sparago A, Cerrato F, Vernucci M et al. Microdeletions in the human H19 DMR result in loss of IGF2 imprinting and Beckwith–Wiedemann syndrome. Nat Genet 2004; 36:958–60.
50. Maw MA, Grundy PE, Millow LJ et al. A third Wilms' tumor locus on chromosome 16q. Cancer Res 1992; 52:3094–8.
51. Grundy PE, Telzerow PE, Breslow N et al. Loss of heterozygosity for chromosomes 16q and 1p in Wilms' tumors predicts an adverse outcome. Cancer Res 1994; 54:2331–3.
52. Grundy PE, Breslow NE, Li S et al. Loss of heterozygos-

ity for chromosomes 1p and 16q is an adverse prognostic factor in favorable histology Wilms tumor. A report from the National Wilms Tumor Study Group. J Clin Oncol 2005; 23:7312–21.
53. Bown N, Cotterill SJ, Roberts P et al. Cytogenetic abnormalities and clinical outcome in Wilms tumor: a study by the U.K. cancer cytogenetics group and the U.K. Children's Cancer Study Group. Med Pediatr Oncol 2002; 38:11–21.
54. Wilmore HP, White GF, Howell RT et al. Germline and somatic abnormalities of chromosome 7 in Wilms' tumor. Cancer Genet Cytogenet 1994; 77:93–8.
55. Bardeesy N, Falkoff D, Petruzzi MJ et al. Anaplastic Wilms' tumour, a subtype displaying poor prognosis, harbours p53 gene mutations. Nat Genet 1994; 7:91–7.
56. Beniers AJ, Efferth T, Fuzesi L et al. p53 expression in Wilms' tumor: a possible role as prognostic factor. Int J Oncol 2001; 18:133–9.
57. Malkin D, Sexsmith E, Yeger H et al. Mutations of the p53 tumor suppressor gene occur infrequently in Wilms' tumor. Cancer Res 1994; 54:2077–9.
58. Weirich A, Leuschner I, Harms D et al. Clinical impact of histologic subtypes in localized non-anaplastic nephroblastoma treated according to the trial and study SIOP-9/GPOH. Ann Oncol 2001; 12:311–19.
59. Beckwith JB, Palmer NF. Histopathology and prognosis of Wilms' tumor. Results from the National Wilms' Tumor Study. Cancer 1978; 41:1937–48.
60. Breslow NB, Churchill G, Beckwith JB et al. Prognosis for Wilms' tumor patients with nonmetatastic disease at diagnosis – Results of the Second National Wilms' Tumor Study. J Clin Oncol 1985; 3:521–31.
61. Bonadio JF, Storer B, Norkool P et al. Anaplastic Wilms' tumor: clinical and pathological studies. J Clin Oncol 1985; 3:513–20.
62. Schmidt D, Beckwith JB. Histopathology of childhood renal tumors. Hematol Oncol Clin North Am 1995; 9:1179–200.
63. Faria P, Beckwith JB, Mishra K et al. Focal versus diffuse anaplasia in Wilms' tumor – new definitions with prognostic significance: a report from the National Wilms' Tumor Study Group. Am J Surg Pathol 1996; 20:909–20.
64. Zuppan CW, Beckwith JB, Luckey DW. Anaplasia in unilateral Wilms' tumor: a report from the National Wilms' Tumor Study Pathology Center. Hum Pathol 1988; 19:1199–209.
65. Beckwith JB, Palmer NF. Histopathology and prognosis of Wilms' tumors: results from the First National Wilms' Tumor Study. Cancer 1978; 41:1937–48.
66. Argani P, Perlman EJ, Breslow NE et al. Clear cell sarcoma of the kidney: a review of 351 cases from the National Wilms' Tumor Study Group Pathology Center. Am J Surg Pathol 2000; 24:4–18.
67. Schuster AE, Schneider DT, Fritsch MK, Grundy P, Perlman EJ. Genetic and genetic expression analyses of clear cell sarcoma of the kidney. Lab Invest 2003; 83:1293–9.
68. Beckwith JB, Kiviat NB, Bonadio JF. Nephrogenic rests, nephroblastomatosis, and the pathogenesis of Wilms' tumor. Pediatr Pathol 1990; 10:1–36.
69. Beckwith JB. Nephrogenic rests and the pathogenesis of Wilms tumor: developmental and clinical considerations. Am J Med Genet 1998; 79:268–73.
70. Gylys-Morin V, Hoffer FA, Kozakewich H, Shamberger RC. Wilms tumor and nephroblastomatosis: imaging characteristics at gadolinium-enhanced MR imaging. Radiology 1993; 188:517–21.
71. Hou LT, Holman RL. Bilateral nephroblastomatosis in a premature infant. J Pathol Bacteriol 1961; 82:249–55.
72. Perlman EJ, Faria P, Soares A et al. Hyperplastic perilobar nephroblastomatosis. Long-term survival of 52 patients. Pediatr Blood Cancer 2005; 46:203–21.
73. Coppes MJ, Arnold M, Beckwith JB et al. Factors affecting the risk of contralateral Wilms' tumor development: a report from the National Wilms' Tumor Study Group. Cancer 1999; 85:1616–25.
74. D'Angio GJ, Rosenberg H, Sharples K et al. Position paper: imaging methods for primary renal tumors of childhood: cost versus benefits. Med Pediatr Oncol 1993; 21:205–12.
75. Ritchey ML, Kelalis PP, Breslow N et al. Intracaval and atrial involvement with nephroblastoma: review of National Wilms' Tumor Study-3. J Urol 1988; 140:1113–18.
76. Voute PA, Van Der Meer J, Staugaard-Kloosterziel W. Plasma renin activity in Wilms' tumour. Acta Endocrinol (Copenh) 1971; 67:197–202.
77. Coppes MJ, Zandvoort SWH, Sparling CR et al. Acquired von Willebrand disease in Wilms' tumor patients. J Clin Oncol 1993; 10:1–7.
78. Ritchey ML, Kelalis PP, Breslow N et al. Surgical complications following nephrectomy for Wilms' tumor: a report of National Wilms' Tumor Study-3. Surg Gynecol Obstet 1992; 175:507–14.
79. Weese DL, Applebaum H, Taber P. Mapping intravascular extension of Wilms' tumor with magnetic resonance imaging. J Pediatr Surg 1991; 26:64–7.
80. Cohen MD. Staging of Wilms' tumor. Clin Radiol 1993; 47:77–81.
81. Ditchfield MR, DeCampo JF, Waters KD, Nolan TM. Wilms' tumor: a rational use of preoperative imaging. Med Pediatr Oncol 1995; 24:93–6.
82. D'Angio GJ, Breslow N, Beckwith JB et al. Treatment of Wilms' tumor: results of the Third National Wilms' Tumor Study. Cancer 1989; 64:349–60.
83. Othersen HB Jr, DeLorimer A, Hrabovsky E et al. Surgical evaluation of lymph node metastases in Wilms' tumor. J Pediatr Surg 1990; 25:1–2.
84. Ng YY, Hall-Craggs MA, Dicks-Mireaux C et al. Wilms' tumour: pre- and post-chemotherapy CT appearances. Clin Radiol 1991; 43: 255–9.
85. Nakayama DK, Ortega W, D'Angio GJ, O'Neill JA. The nonopacified kidney with Wilms' tumor. J Pediatr Surg 1988; 23:152–5.
86. Meisel JA, Guthrie KA, Breslow NE, Donaldson SS, Green DM. Significance and management of computed tomography detected pulmonary nodules: a report from the National Wilms' Tumor Study Group. Int J Radiat Oncol Biol Phys 1999; 44:579–85.
87. Owens CM, Veys PA, Pritchard J et al. Role of chest computed tomography at diagnosis in the management of Wilms tumor: a study by the United Kingdom Children's Cancer Study Group. J Clin Oncol 2002; 20:2768–73.

88. Feusner JH, Beckwith JB, D'Angio GJ. Clear cell sarcoma of the kidney: accuracy of imaging methods for detecting bone metastases. Report from the National Wilms' Tumor Study. Med Pediatr Oncol 1990; 18: 225–7.
89. Weeks DA, Beckwith JB, Mierau G, Luckey DW. Rhabdoid tumor of kidney. A report of 111 cases from the National Wilms' Tumor Study Pathology Center. Am J Surg Pathol 1989; 13:439–58.
90. Ritchey ML, Green DM, Breslow NE, Monksness J, Norkool P. Accuracy of current imaging modalities in the diagnosis of synchronous bilateral Wilms' tumor. A report from the National Wilms' Tumor Study Group. Cancer 1995; 75:600–4.
91. Ritchey ML, Shamberger RC, Hamilton TE et al. Fate of bilateral lesions missed on preoperative imaging: a report from the National Wilms' Tumor Study Group. J Urol 2005; 174:1519–21.
92. Ehrlich PF, Ritchey ML, Hamilton TE et al. Quality assessment for Wilms tumor: a report from the National Wilms Tumor Study Group-5. J Pediatr Surg 2005; 40:208–13.
93. Shamberger RC, Guthrie KA, Ritchey ML et al. Surgery-related factors and local recurrence of Wilms' tumor in National Wilms' Tumor Study 4. Ann Surg 1999; 229:292–7.
94. Ritchey ML, Shamberger RC, Haase G et al. Surgical complications after nephrectomy for Wilms' tumor: report from the National Wilms' Tumor Study Group. J Am Coll Surg 2001; 192:63–8.
95. Farber S. Chemotherapy in the treatment of leukemia and Wilms' tumor. JAMA 1966; 198: 826–36.
96. D'Angio GJ, Evans AE, Breslow N et al. The treatment of Wilms' tumor: results of the National Wilms' tumor study. Cancer 1976; 38: 633–46.
97. D'Angio GJ, Evans A, Breslow N et al. The treatment of Wilms' tumor: results of the Second National Wilms' Tumor Study. Cancer 1981; 47: 2302–311.
98. Farewell VT, D'Angio GJ, Breslow N, Norkool P. Retrospective validation of a new staging system for Wilms' tumor. Cancer Clin Trials 1981; 4:167–71.
99. Green DM, Breslow NE, Beckwith JB et al. Comparison between single-dose and divided-dose administration of dactinomycin and doxorubicin for patients with Wilms' tumor: a report from the National Wilms' Tumor Study Group. J Clin Oncol 1998; 16: 237–45.
100. Green DM, Breslow NE, Beckwith JB et al. Effect of duration of treatment on treatment outcomes and cost of treatment for Wilms' tumor: a report from the National Wilms' Tumor Study Group. J Clin Oncol 1998; 16:3744–51.
101. Green DM, Beckwith JB, Breslow NE et al. Treatment of children with stages II to IV anaplastic Wilms' tumor: a report from the National Wilms' Tumor Study Group. J Clin Oncol 1994; 12:2126–31.
102. Larsen E, Perez-Atayde A, Green DM et al. Surgery only for the treatment of patients with stage I (Cassady) Wilms' tumor. Cancer 1990; 66:264–6.
103. Green DM, Beckwith JB, Weeks DA et al. The relationship between microsubstaging variables, age at diagnosis, and tumor weight of children with stage I/favorable histology Wilms' tumor. A report from the National Wilms' Tumor Study. Cancer 1994; 74:1817–20.
104. Green DM, Breslow NE, Beckwith JB, et al. Treatment with nephrectomy only for small, stage I/favorable histology Wilms' tumor: a report from the National Wilms' Tumor Study Group. J Clin Oncol 2001; 19:3719–24.
105. Lemerle J, Voute PA, Tournade MF et al. Preoperative versus postoperative radiotherapy, single versus multiple courses of actinomycin D, in the treatment of Wilms' tumor. Preliminary results of a controlled clinical trial conducted by the International Society of Paediatric Oncology (S.I.O.P.). Cancer 1976; 38: 647–54.
106. Lemerle J, Voute PA, Tournade MF et al. Effectiveness of preoperative chemotherapy in Wilms' tumor: results of an International Society of Paediatric Oncology (SIOP) clinical trial. J Clin Oncol 1983; 1:604–9.
107. Tournade MF, Com-Nougue C, Voute PA et al. Results of the Sixth International Society of Pediatric Oncology Wilms' Tumor Trial and Study: a risk-adapted therapeutic approach in Wilms' tumor. J Clin Oncol 1993; 11:1014–23.
108. Tournade MF, Com-Nougue C, de Kraker J et al. Optimal duration of preoperative therapy in unilateral nonmetastatic Wilms' tumor in children older than 6 months: results of the Ninth International Society of Pediatric Oncology Wilms' Tumor Trial and Study. J Clin Oncol 2001; 19:488–500.
109. Boccon-Gibod L, Rey A, Sandstedt B et al. Complete necrosis induced by preoperative chemotherapy in Wilms tumor as an indicator of low risk: report of the International Society of Pediatric Oncology (SIOP) nephroblastoma trial and study 9. Med Pediatr Oncol 2000; 34:183–190.
110. de Kraker J, Graf N, van Tinteren H et al. Reduction of postoperative chemotherapy in children with stage I intermediate-risk and anaplastic Wilms' tumour (SIOP 93–01 trial): a randomised controlled trial. Lancet 2004; 364:1229–35.
111. Pritchard J, Imeson J, Barnes J et al. Results of the United Kingdom Children's Cancer Study Group (UKCCSG) first Wilms' Tumour Study (UKW1). J Clin Oncol 1995; 13:124–33.
112. Mitchell C, Jones PM, Kelsey A et al. The treatment of Wilms' tumour: results of the United Kingdom Children's Cancer Study Group (UKCCSG) second Wilms' tumour study. Br J Cancer 2000; 83:602–8.
113. Pritchard-Jones K, Kelsey A, Vujanic G et al. Older age is an adverse prognostic factor in stage I, favorable histology Wilms' tumor treated with vincristine monochemotherapy: a study by the United Kingdom Children's Cancer Study Group, Wilms' Tumor Working Group. J Clin Oncol 2003; 21:3269–75.
114. Vujanic GM, Kelsey A, Mitchell C, Shannon RS, Gornall P. The role of biopsy in the diagnosis of renal tumors of childhood: results of the UKCCSG Wilms' tumor study 3. Med Pediatr Oncol 2003; 40:18–22.
115. Pritchard Jones K. Controversies and advances in the management of Wilms' tumour. Arch Dis Child 2002; 87:241–4.
116. D'Angio GJ. Pre- or post-operative treatment for Wilms tumor? Who, what, when, where, how, why – and which. Med Pediatr Oncol 2003; 41:545–9.
117. Godzinski J, Tournade MF, deKraker J et al. Rarity of

surgical complications after postchemotherapy nephrectomy for nephroblastoma. Experience of the International Society of Paediatric Oncology-Trial and Study 'SIOP-9'. International Society of Paediatric Oncology Nephroblastoma Trial and Study Committee. Eur J Pediatr Surg 1998; 8:83–6.

118. Ritchey ML, Andrassy R, Kelalis PP et al. Pediatric urologic oncology. In: Gillenwater J, Howards S, Duckett J, eds. Adult and Pediatric Urology. Chicago: Mosby Year Book, 1996: 2675–720.
119. Blute ML, Kelalis PP, Offord KP et al. Bilateral Wilms tumor. J Urol 1987; 138:968–73.
120. Ritchey ML, Coppes M. The management of synchronous bilateral Wilms tumor. Hematol Oncol Clin North Am 1995; 9:1303–16.
121. Ritchey ML, Pringle K, Breslow N et al. Management and outcome of inoperable Wilms tumor. A report of National Wilms' Tumor Study-3. Ann Surg 1994; 220: 683–90.
122. Ritchey ML, Kelalis PP, Haase GM et al. Preoperative therapy for intracaval and atrial extension of Wilms' tumor. Cancer 1993; 71:4104–10.
123. Shamberger RC, Ritchey ML, Haase GM, Bergemann TL. Intravascular extension of Wilms tumor. Ann Surg 2001; 234:116–21.
124. Szavay P, Luithle T, Semler O, Graf N, Fuchs J. Surgery of cavoatrial tumor thrombus in nephroblastoma: a report of the SIOP/GPOH study. Pediatr Blood Cancer 2004; 43:40–5.
125. Ritchey ML, Green DM, Thomas P et al. Renal failure in Wilms' tumor patients: a report from the National Wilms' Tumor Study Group. Med Pediatr Oncol 1996; 26:75–80.
126. Breslow NE, Takashima JR, Ritchey ML, Strong LC, Green DM. Renal failure in the Denys–Drash and Wilms' tumor–aniridia syndromes. Cancer Res 2000; 60: 4030–2.
127. Dykes EH, Marwaha RK, Dicks-Mireaux C et al. Risks and benefits of percutaneous biopsy and primary chemotherapy in advanced Wilms' tumour. J Pediatr Surg 1991; 26:610–12.
128. Grundy RG, Hutton C, Middleton H et al. Outcome of patients with stage III or inoperable WT treated on the second United Kingdom WT protocol (UKWT2); a United Kingdom Children's Cancer Study Group (UKCCSG) study. Pediatr Blood Cancer 2004; 42: 311–19.
129. Zuppan CW, Beckwith JB, Weeks DA, Luckey DW, Pringle KC. The effect of preoperative therapy on the histologic features of Wilms' tumor. An analysis of cases from the Third National Wilms' Tumor Study. Cancer 1991; 68:385–94.
130. Montgomery BT, Kelalis PP, Blute ML et al. Extended follow-up of bilateral Wilms' tumor: results of the National Wilms' Tumor Study. J Urol 1991; 146:514–18.
131. Coppes MJ, de Kraker J, van Dijken PJ et al. Bilateral Wilms' tumor: long-term survival and some epidemiological features. J Clin Oncol 1989; 7:310–15.
132. Penn I. Renal transplantation for Wilms' tumor: report of 20 cases. J Urol 1979; 122:793–4.
133. McLorie GA, McKenna PH, Greenberg M et al. Reduction in tumor burden allowing partial nephrectomy following preoperative chemotherapy in biopsy proved Wilms' tumor. J Urol 1991; 146:509–13.
134. Zani A, Schiavetti A, Gambino M et al. Long-term outcome of nephron sparing surgery and simple nephrectomy for unilateral localized Wilms tumor. J Urol 2005; 173:946–8.
135. Moorman-Voestermans CG, Aronson DC, Staalman CR, Delemarre JF, de Kraker J. Is partial nephrectomy appropriate treatment for unilateral Wilms tumor? J Pediatr Surg 1998; 33:165–70.
136. Bertolone SJ, Patel CC, Harrison HL et al. Long term renal function in patients with Wilms' tumor. Proc Am Soc Clin Oncol 1987; 6:265 (abstract 1040).
137. Robitaille P, Mongeau JG, Lortie L et al. Long-term follow-up of patients who underwent nephrectomy in childhood. Lancet 1985; 1:1297–9.
138. Barrera M, Roy LP, Stevens M. Long-term follow-up after unilateral nephrectomy and radiotherapy for Wilms' tumor. Pediatr Nephrol 1989; 3:430–2.
139. Bhisitkul DM, Morgan ER, Vozar MA et al. Renal functional reserve in long-term survivors of unilateral Wilms tumor. J Pediatr 1990; 118:698–702.
140. Horwitz J, Ritchey ML, Moksness J et al. Renal salvage procedures in patients with synchronous bilateral Wilms tumors: a report from the National Wilms' Tumor Study Group. J Pediatr Surg 1996; 31:1020–5.
141. Evans AE, Norkool P, Evans I et al. Late effects of treatment for Wilms' tumor. A report from the National Wilms' Tumor Study Group. Cancer 1991; 67: 331–6.
142. Breslow NE, Takashima JR, Whitton JA et al. Second malignant neoplasms following treatment for Wilms' tumor: a report from the National Wilms' Tumor Study Group. J Clin Oncol 1995; 13:1851–9.
143. Gilladoga AC, Manuel C, Tan CT et al. The cardiotoxicity of adriamycin and daunomycin in children. Cancer 1976; 37:1070–8.
144. Steinherz LJ, Steinherz PG, Tan CTC et al. Cardiac toxicity 4 to 20 years after anthracycline therapy. JAMA 1991; 266:1672–7.
145. Green DM, Breslow NE, Moksness J, D'Angio GJ. Congestive failure following initial therapy for Wilms tumor. A report from the National Wilms Tumor Study. Pediatr Res 1994; 35:161A (abstract).
146. Shalet SM, Gibson B, Swindell R, Pearson D. Effect of spinal irradiation on growth. Arch Dis Child 1987; 62:461–4.
147. van Leeuwen BL, Kamps WA, Jansen HW, Hoekstra HJ. The effect of chemotherapy on the growing skeleton. Cancer Treat Rev 2000; 26:363–76.
148. Hogeboom CJ, Grosser SC, Guthrie KA et al. Stature loss following treatment for Wilms tumor. Med Pediatr Oncol 2001; 36:295–304.
149. Kinsella TJ, Trivette G, Rowland J et al. Long-term follow-up of testicular function following radiation for early-stage Hodgkin's disease. J Clin Oncol 1989; 7:718–24.
150. Shalet SM, Beardwell CG, Jacobs HS, Pearson D. Testicular function following irradiation of the human prepubertal testis. Clin Endocrinol (Oxf) 1978; 9:483–90.
151. Lentz RD, Berstein J, Steffens MW et al. Postpubertal

evaluation of gonadal function following cyclophosphamide therapy before and during puberty. J Pediatr 1977; 91:385–94.
152. Mustieles C, Munoz A, Alonso M et al. Male gonadal function after chemotherapy in survivors of childhood malignancies. Med Pediatr Oncol 1995; 24:347–51.
153. Aubier F, Flamant F, Brauner R et al. Male gonadal function after chemotherapy for solid tumors in childhood. J Clin Oncol 1989; 7:304–9.
154. Stillman RJ, Schinfeld JS, Schiff I et al. Ovarian failure in long term survivors of childhood malignancy. Am J Obstet Gynecol 1987; 139:62–6.
155. Shalet SM, Beardwell CG, Morris-Jones PH et al. Ovarian failure following abdominal irradiation in childhood. Br J Cancer 1976; 33:655–8.
156. Nicosia SV, Matus-Ridley M, Meadows AT. Gonadal effects of cancer therapy in girls. Cancer 1985; 55:2364–72.
157. Byrne J, Fears TR, Gail MH et al. Early menopause in long-term survivors of cancer during adolescence. Am J Obstet Gynecol 1992; 166:788–93.
158. Meacham L. Endocrine late effects of childhood cancer therapy. Curr Probl Pediatr Adolesc Health Care 2003; 33:217–42.
159. Li FP, Gimbrere K, Gelber RD et al. Outcome of pregnancy in survivors of Wilms' tumor. JAMA 1987; 257:216–19.
160. Green DM, Fine NE, Li FP. Offspring of patients treated for unilateral Wilms' tumor in childhood. Cancer 1982; 49:2285–8.
161. Walker RD, Reid CF, Richard GA et al. Compensatory renal growth and function in postnephrectomized patients with Wilms tumor. Urology 1982; 19:127–30.
162. Levitt GA, Yeomans E, Dicks Mireaux C et al. Renal size and function after cure of Wilms' tumor. Br J Cancer 1992; 66:877–82.
163. Mitus A, Tefft M, Feller FX. Long-term follow-up of renal function of 108 children who underwent nephrectomy for malignant disease. Pediatrics 1969; 44:912–21.
164. Aleksa K, Woodland C, Koren G. Young age and the risk for ifosfamide-induced nephrotoxicity: a critical review of two opposing studies. Pediatr Nephrol 2001; 16:1153–8.
165. Bardi E, Olah AV, Bartyik K et al. Late effects on renal glomerular and tubular function in childhood cancer survivors. Pediatr Blood Cancer 2004; 43(6):668–73.
166. Joshi VV, Beckwith JB. Multilocular cyst of the kidney (cystic nephroma) and cystic, partially differentiated nephroblastoma. Terminology and criteria for diagnosis. Cancer 1989; 64:466–79.
167. Eble JN, Bonsib SM. Extensively cystic renal neoplasms: cystic nephroma, cystic partially differentiated nephroblastoma, multilocular cystic renal cell carcinoma, and cystic hamartoma of renal pelvis. Semin Diag Pathol 1998; 15:2–20.
168. Blakely ML, Shamberger RC, Norkool P, Beckwith JB. Outcome of children with cystic partially differentiated nephroblastoma treated with or without chemotherapy. J Pediatr Surg 2003; 38:897–900.
169. Banner MP, Pollack HM, Chatten J, Witzleben C. Multilocular renal cysts: radiologic–pathologic correlation. AJR Am J Roentgenol 1981; 136:239–47.
170. Ferrer FA, McKenna PH. Partial nephrectomy in a metachronous multilocular cyst of the kidney (cystic nephroma). J Urol 1994; 151(5):1358–60.
171. Howell CJ, Othersen HB, Kiviat NE et al. Therapy and outcome in 51 children with mesoblastic nephroma: a report of the National Wilms' Tumor Study. J Pediatr Surg 1982; 17:826–30.
172. Ohmichi M, Tasaka K, Sugita N et al. Hydramnios associated with congenital mesoblastic nephroma: a case report. Obstet Gynecol 1989; 74:469–71.
173. Leclair MD, El-Ghoneimi A, Audry G, Ravasse P. The outcome of prenatally diagnosed renal tumors. J Urol 2005; 173:186–9.
174. Tomlinson GE, Argyle JC, Velasco S, Nisen PD. Molecular characterization of congenital mesoblastic nephroma and its distinction from Wilms tumor. Cancer 1992; 70:2358–61.
175. Joshi VJ, Kasznica J, Walters TR. Atypical mesoblastic nephroma: pathologic characterization of a potentially aggressive variant of conventional congenital mesoblastic nephroma. Arch Pathol Lab Med 1986; 110:100–6.
176. Gormley TS, Skoog SJ, Jones RV, Maybee D. Cellular congenital mesoblastic nephroma: what are the options? J Urol 1989; 142:479–83.
177. Beckwith JB. Congenital mesoblastic nephroma. When should we worry? Arch Pathol Lab Med 1986; 110:98–9.
178. Argani P, Fritsch M, Kadkol SS et al. ETV6-NTRK3 Gene fusions and trisomy 11 establish a histogenetic link between mesoblastic nephroma and congenital fibrosarcoma. Cancer Res 1998; 58:5046–8.
179. Heidelberger KP, Ritchey ML, Dauser RC, McKeever PE, Beckwith JB. Congenital mesoblastic nephroma metastatic to the brain. Cancer 1993; 72:2499–502.
180. Loeb DM, Hill DA, Dome JS. Complete response of recurrent cellular congenital mesoblastic nephroma to chemotherapy. J Pediatr Hematol Oncol 2002; 24:478–81.
181. McCahon E, Sorensen PH, Davis JH, Rogers PC, Schultz KR. Non-resectable congenital tumors with the ETV6-NTRK3 gene fusion are highly responsive to chemotherapy. Med Pediatr Oncol 2003; 40:288–92.
182. Marsden HB, Lawler W. Bone metastasizing renal tumour of childhood. Histopathological and clinical review of 38 cases. Virchows Arch A Pathol Anat Histol 1980; 387:341–51.
183. Green DM, Breslow NE, Beckwith JB et al. The treatment of children with clear cell sarcoma of the kidney. A report from the National Wilms Tumor Study Group. J Clin Oncol 1994; 12:2132–7.
184. Seibel NL, Li S, Breslow NE et al. Effect of duration of treatment on treatment outcome for patients with clear-cell sarcoma of the kidney: a report from the National Wilms' Tumor Study Group. J Clin Oncol 2004; 22:468–73.
185. Burger PC, Yu IT, Tihan T et al. Atypical teratoid/rhabdoid tumor of the central nervous system: a highly malignant tumor of infancy and childhood frequently mistaken for medulloblastoma: a Pediatric Oncology Group study. Am J Surg Pathol 1998; 22:1083–92.
186. Biegel JA, Zhou J, Rorke LB et al. Germ-line and acquired mutations of INI1 in atypical teratoid and rhabdoid tumors. Cancer Res 1999; 59:74–9.

187. Hoot AC, Russo P, Judkins AR, Perlman EJ, Biegel JA. Immunohistochemical analysis of hSNF5/INI1 distinguishes renal and extra-renal malignant rhabdoid tumors from other pediatric soft tissue tumors. Am J Surg Pathol 2004; 28:1485–91.

188. Vujanic GM, Sandstedt B, Harms D, Boccon-Gibod L, Delemarre JF. Rhabdoid tumour of the kidney: a clinicopathological study of 22 patients from the International Society of Paediatric Oncology (SIOP) nephroblastoma file. Histopathology 1996; 28:333–40.

189. Broecker B. Renal cell carcinoma in children. Urology 1991; 38:54–6.

190. Hartman D, Davis C, Madewell J, Friedman A. Primary malignant tumors in the second decade of life: Wilms tumor versus renal cell carcinoma. J Urol 1982; 127:888–91.

191. Raney RB Jr, Palmer N, Sutow WW et al. Renal cell carcinoma in children. Med Pediatr Oncol 1983; 11:91–8.

192. Geller JI, Dome JS. Local lymph node involvement does not predict poor outcome in pediatric renal cell carcinoma. Cancer 2004; 101:1575–83.

193. Bruder E, Passera O, Harms D, Leuschner I. Morphologic and molecular characterization of renal cell carcinoma in children and young adults. Am J Surg Pathol 2004; 28:1117–32.

Surgical approaches for renal tumors

33

Joao Luiz Pippi Salle and Roman Jednak

The diagnosis of a renal tumor in children is always accompanied by great apprehension in the family and caregivers. Preoperative management has been extensively described in the previous chapter. The surgeon is an important member of the team managing such patients. A detailed and well-organized surgical plan not only facilitates complete tumor removal without spillage but also ensures accurate staging and improves patient survival. Surgical approaches can differ depending on the suspected diagnosis and patient age.[1] In order to decide on the best surgical strategy, several anatomic and physiologic points should be considered and deserve further discussion.

Anatomic relationships

Adjacent organs

The kidneys are located in the lumbar fossa surrounded by a layer of perinephric fat, which is covered by a thin fascial layer called Gerota's fascia. Organs and structures adjacent to the kidneys are:

- Posteriorly: diaphragm, psoas major, and quadratus lumborum muscles.
- Anteriorly:
  - Right kidney: liver, hepatic flexure of the colon, second portion of the duodenum, adrenal gland.
  - Left kidney: spleen, body of the pancreas, stomach, splenic flexure of the colon, adrenal gland.

Renal vasculature

The kidney has four vascular segments, termed apical, anterior, posterior, and basilar. A relative avascular plane exists between the junction of the anterior and posterior segments. This is the preferred line of incision whenever parenchymal incisions are necessary.

Arterial blood supply

Each segment is supplied by one or more arterial branches. Ligation of one of these branches results in devascularization of the corresponding renal segment since they are end arteries without collateral circulation. Multiple renal arteries occur unilaterally in 23% and bilaterally in 10% of the population.[2]

The kidney is susceptible to ischemia due to a very active aerobic metabolism. Experimental studies indicate that a warm ischemic time of up to 30 minutes can be sustained without significant functional loss.[3] Renal proximal tubular cells are the most sensitive to ischemia during arterial occlusion and may be damaged transiently or permanently depending on the duration and severity of the injury. When a long surgical period of ischemia is expected, external surface cooling or perfusion of the kidneys with cold solution instilled into the renal artery is required. External surface cooling is the more practical and less invasive of the two methods. It is preferable to keep the entire kidney covered with ice for 10–15 minutes after arterial occlusion. Temperatures of 20–25°C can be maintained using this method and animal and humans studies have shown that hypothermia to this degree allows for complete renal protection from arterial occlusion for up to 3 hours.[4] Generous preoperative and intraoperative hydration and the avoidance of unnecessary renal artery manipulation or traction are additional measures to protect against ischemic renal injury. The administration of mannitol 10–15 minutes prior to arterial occlusion is also beneficial, since it increases renal plasma flow, decreases intrarenal vascular resistance, minimizes cellular edema, and promotes an osmotic diuresis when renal circulation is re-established.[5,6] When renal ischemia is necessary for surgery, it is preferable to occlude the artery alone since the simultaneous occlusion of the artery and vein seems to produce additional venous congestion and more renal damage.[5]

Venous drainage

Multiple renal veins are less common than multiple renal arteries. The right renal vein is shorter than the left and has no tributaries. The left renal vein is longer and has a thicker muscular layer. Injuries to the right renal vein occur more easily, given its thinner wall. Both renal veins enter the inferior vena cava (IVC) laterally. The left adrenal and gonadal veins are significant branches, draining into the left renal vein, and their presence has important implications for extensive vascular resections. Occlusion of the left renal vein at the level of the IVC will not significantly impair venous drainage of the left kidney, since collateral venous drainage can develop via the tributaries of the left renal vein. Involvement of the IVC by tumor thrombus has variable clinical repercussion, depending on the side as well as the level of involvement. Lower extremity edema, a varicocele, dilated superficial abdominal veins, proteinuria, pulmonary embolism, a right atrial mass or non-function of the involved kidney are all clinical signs suggestive of intravascular tumor extension.[7] Transabdominal color Doppler ultrasonography and magnetic resonance imaging (MRI) are the preferred studies when evaluating for intravascular tumor extension.[8] Tumor thrombus extending to the IVC is variable, and the more cephalad the extension the more difficult the surgical resection will be. Fortunately, the tumor thrombus does not usually invade the wall of the IVC and can be removed with the affected kidney using a simple venotomy. When the thrombus does involve the wall of the IVC, resection of the involved segment is required. Resection of the infrarenal segment of the IVC can usually be done safely, since a rich collateral circulation develops in most cases. With right-sided renal tumors, the suprarenal portion of the IVC can also be safely removed since venous drainage from the left kidney can occur via the gonadal and adrenal tributaries. A similar resection cannot be performed for left renal tumors, since there is no significant collateral venous circulation for the right renal vein once drainage to the IVC is interrupted. Knowledge of these anatomic particularities has great importance when planning the surgical strategy for renal tumors with vascular involvement.

Collecting system

Each renal segment contains one or more major calices draining the corresponding portion of the kidney. In total, 8–10 major calices open into the renal pelvis. An understanding of the caliceal anatomy is required when performing partial nephrectomy if one is to adequately repair the collecting system if it is entered during tumor resection.

Preoperative evaluation

Laboratory investigations

All children should have a preoperative hemoglobin level, a white blood cell (WBC) count with differential, and a platelet count. Acquired von Willebrand's disease can occur in up to 8% of patients, and consideration may be given to performing a bleeding time.[9] Renal function should be assessed with serum electrolytes, along with a serum creatinine and blood urea nitrogen (BUN) level. Liver function testing should include serum aspartate aminotransferase (AST), serum alanine aminotransferase (ALT), total bilirubin, and alkaline phosphatase. The serum calcium level should be checked, since it may be elevated in children with congenital mesoblastic nephroma and rhabdoid tumor of the kidney.[9] Urinalysis and urine culture complete the laboratory investigations. Patients with suspected or proven urinary tract infection should receive 48 hours of antibiotic therapy since severe bacteremia can occur following manipulation of an infected kidney.

Radiologic imaging

The goal of preoperative imaging is to evaluate local extension of the mass, assess for possible contralateral lesions, confirm adequate contralateral renal function, and evaluate for possible vascular invasion. Ultrasonography can confirm the organ of origin and the solid nature of the lesion. Doppler assessment of the renal vein and IVC is essential when evaluating for intravascular tumor extension.[7] Computer tomography (CT) can assess the degree of local involvement and regional extension. The contralateral kidney should also be carefully assessed for additional masses and adequate function. Three-dimensional reconstruction of CT images is important when a partial nephrectomy is planned.[10] MRI is excellent for mapping intravascular tumor extension and can be used when the ultrasound results are inconclusive.[8] Chest radiographs and a chest CT are performed to identify pulmonary lesions.

Certain investigations are necessary only with specific types of tumors. Renal cell carcinoma and clear cell carcinoma tend to metastasize to bone. Consequently, patients should undergo a bone scan and skeletal survey.[11] Brain metastases can occur with both clear cell sarcoma and rhabdoid tumor of the kidney; therefore, a head MRI or CT scan should be performed in these patients.[12]

The surgical management of Wilms' tumor

Patient preparation

Proper patient preparation and positioning is essential for an optimal surgical outcome. The incision should allow for unhindered access to the tumor mass, enable the surgeon to accurately assess the abdomen for staging purposes, and allow the surgeon to deal appropriately with potential complications should they develop. The typical incision is transverse, extending from the tip of the 12th rib on the affected side to the lateral margin of the opposite rectus muscle. Some surgeons prefer to extend the incision further, by taking it to the tip of the 12th rib on the opposite side.

The placement of intravenous (IV) lines in the lower extremities should be avoided. This is particularly important when tumor thrombus extends into the renal vein or vena cava and surgical management is anticipated. The placement of an arterial line is recommended to accurately measure mean arterial blood pressure. This is especially important in patients with large tumors or vascular involvement.

Most solid renal tumors in children are malignant. The most prevalent diagnosis in younger patients is Wilms' tumor. Renal cell carcinoma occurs more commonly in older children and adolescents. Patient age therefore has potential implications when planning the surgical strategy. Preoperative management, as well as the timing for surgical intervention in children with Wilms' tumor, has been discussed earlier.

Surgical principles

Adequate exposure is essential and is usually achieved via a transabdominal, transperitoneal incision. Prior to nephrectomy, a complete abdominal exploration should be performed and the kidneys palpated and inspected completely to exclude bilateral pathology. The entire abdominal cavity is inspected in order to rule out macroscopic metastatic disease and to provide surgical staging. Gerota's fascia of the contralateral kidney should be opened, and both the anterior and posterior renal surfaces inspected. This must be performed routinely, since preoperative imaging may miss approximately 6% of bilateral Wilms' tumors (although the necessity for contralateral exploration is controversial, as survival rates are not different in those with contralateral metachronous tumor). Most of these missed tumors are <2 cm, and their removal has an excellent outcome.[13,14] Suspicious areas within the kidney parenchyma noted on preoperative imaging should be biopsied. Chemotherapy should be the initial approach when bilateral Wilms' tumor is encountered. Suspected residual tumor is removed following chemotherapy.[15,16] Similarly, areas suspicious for abdominal metastases should be biopsied and marked with small titanium clips. At the time of surgical resection, clipping is recommended to mark areas of possible residual tumor and resection margins. Biopsy of the tumor prior to nephrectomy should be avoided in order to prevent tumor spillage.

Nephrectomy

The left colon is reflected to achieve adequate renal exposure and access to the great vessels. Division of the splenocolic ligament facilitates colonic mobilization and avoids excessive traction and possible splenic injury. On the right side, the colon and duodenum are mobilized in order to get adequate access to the IVC and aorta.

Exposure and ligation of the renal vessels should be attempted, if technically feasible, prior to mobilizing the kidney, in order to reduce the risk of hematogenous tumor dissemination. As previously mentioned, the renal vein is shorter on the right, and care must be taken to avoid injury to the IVC. The right renal artery can be dissected either lateral to the vena cava or between the vena cava and aorta. The latter approach can be helpful with large tumors that extend medially. The renal vein is longer on the left and passes over the aorta. Tributaries of the left renal vein include the gonadal, adrenal, and lumbar veins, and care must be taken to avoid their inadvertent injury. The left renal artery is located by retracting the renal vein. Early ligation of the renal vessels may not be possible with large tumors, and a technically difficult or dangerous dissection should not be attempted.

Biopsies should not be taken prior to tumor resection in order to avoid tumor spillage. Rupture of the renal capsule or tumor spillage into the peritoneum will upgrade the tumor stage. Gerota's fascia should be removed with the kidney, since extension into the perinephic fat can occur and is an important factor when staging the disease. The adrenal gland may be preserved if it is not adjacent to the tumor mass. The presence of an upper pole tumor usually requires removal of the ipsilateral adrenal gland. Ureteral ligature is performed as distal as convenient, but complete resection of the ureter is not necessary.

Radical resection of involved organs should be undertaken only if complete resection of tumor is possible. If complete resection is not technically possible, a tumor biopsy should be performed. Since tumor often adheres to and compresses surrounding organs without actual invasion, chemotherapy can be used to shrink the tumor and subsequently allow resection with preservation of adjacent structures. Titanium clips should be used to mark suspicious areas, resection margins, and residual tumor in order to guide future radiologic investigation or radiation planning. Clips should not be used for hemostasis, and the number used should be kept to a minimum.

Inoperable tumors

Occasionally a tumor is found involving vital structures and is considered inoperable. It is important to keep in mind that large tumors may give the misleading appearance of extension into adjacent organs. They often compress or adhere to these structures without true invasion and are amenable to complete resection. This notwithstanding, consideration on the part of the surgeon should include the feasibility of safe removal of these large tumors. Intraoperative rupture and peritoneal spillage upstage the disease when they occur and necessitate postoperative radiation. This is usually worse for prognosis than biopsy, chemotherapy, and eventual resection. Unresectable tumors should be considered stage III and treated accordingly.[17]

Lymph node sampling

A formal lymph node dissection is not required.[18] In addition to assessing for hilar lymph node involvement, routine lymph node sampling should be performed from the iliac, para-aortic, and celiac regions. All suspicious lymph nodes require excision.

Intravascular invasion

Careful palpation of the renal vein and IVC can reveal evidence of intravascular invasion. Intracaval tumor extension occurs in 4% of patients.[7] This is particularly important to keep in mind when patients present with lower extremity edema, varicocele, dilated superficial abdominal veins, proteinuria, pulmonary embolism, a right atrial mass, or non-function of the involved kidney.

Intravascular tumor extension should be removed en bloc with the kidney if possible. Left-sided renal tumors with IVC involvement present a greater technical challenge than similar right-sided tumors. The right renal vein lacks significant tributaries to provide collateral venous drainage in the absence of the IVC. Tumor extension above the hepatic veins can be treated with preoperative chemotherapy. Tumor thrombus unresponsive to chemotherapy and involving the vena cava above the hepatic veins should be resected with the assistance of the cardiac surgery team, especially if atrial involvement is present. A midline thoracoabdominal incision is required in such cases. A chevron transabdominal incision is preferred when there is renal vein or infrahepatic vena caval involvement. The renal artery and ureter are ligated and divided, and the entire kidney is mobilized outside Gerota's fascia. The kidney is left attached only by the involved renal vein. It is important to avoid excessive mobilization of the renal vein and IVC in order to avoid displacement of the tumor thrombus. The IVC is dissected and controlled above and below the renal veins and any additional small tributaries are also controlled and ligated. The contralateral renal vein is controlled as well. The anterior surface of the renal vein is incised over the thrombus and the incision is then continued posteriorly beneath the thrombus. In the majority of cases there is no attachment of the thrombus to the wall of the vena cava, and gentle traction on the kidney extracts the thrombus. At this point it is important to release the suprarenal vena cava and apply positive pulmonary pressure. This maneuver ensures that small remaining fragments of the thrombus are flushed from the vena cava, which is then repaired.[2]

When the thrombus is invading the wall of the vena cava, an en bloc resection is mandatory. Resection of the infrarenal portion of the vena cava can usually be performed safely because of the rich collateral circulation that develops in most cases. Resection of the suprarenal portion of the vena cava is also possible, but some important principles must be taken into consideration. For right-sided tumors, this resection can be accomplished provided ligation of the left renal vein is performed adjacent to the vena cava. This allows collateral circulation from the gonadal and adrenal veins to drain the left kidney. For left-sided tumors, a similar resection cannot be performed since right-sided renal venous drainage lacks a similar collateral network.

Tumor spillage and rupture

Peritoneal soiling during resection classifies the patient as stage III. It is important to define whether soiling is diffuse or local. Percutaneous needle biopsy is considered local spillage. An incisional biopsy at the time of surgery is considered local spillage unless the operating surgeon considers peritoneal soiling to have occurred. Tumor spillage is considered when the primary tumor capsule is violated or tumor is cut across during the dissection of adherent organs, lymph nodes, or intravascular tumor thrombus. Tumor rupture disseminates tumor cells throughout the peritoneal cavity. Bloody peritoneal fluid is a sign of major spillage. It is also important to describe if an intraoperative hematoma develops, since the hematogenous spread of tumor cells is presumed to occur in this case and necessitates a stage III classification. Finally, when tumor penetrates the renal capsule such that the free surface communicates with the peritoneum, major spillage is considered. It is very important to describe precisely how spillage occurs and to define it as local or diffuse.

Partial nephrectomy

Partial nephrectomy is not routinely indicated for Wilms' tumor except in the presence of bilateral disease or tumors in a solitary kidney. Partial nephrectomy in these situations is performed following an initial biopsy and course of chemotherapy to reduce tumor size. Partial nephrectomy can also play a role in the management of patients with underlying conditions predisposing to Wilms' tumor such as Beckwith–Wiedemann syndrome or WAGR syndrome.[19] Children with a solitary kidney or renal failure are also candidates.[13] The surgical principles for performing partial nephrectomy are described in detail later.

Pathology specimen

All surgical specimens should be submitted fresh and intact. Fixing the specimen in formalin should be avoided. The specimen should not be bivalved, since the capsule may retract and compromise the accuracy of staging on the basis of capsular invasion (i.e. distinguishing stage I from stage II disease).

Surgical outcome

The surgical outcome following nephrectomy for Wilms' tumor is very good. Despite the resection of large tumors approached primarily without preoperative reductive chemotherapy, the complication rate is 9.8%. Intestinal obstruction is the most common complication and occurs more commonly in patients undergoing preoperative chemotherapy. Not surprisingly, surgeons accustomed to regularly performing nephrectomies generate the lowest complication rates.[20]

Renal cell carcinoma

Wilms' tumor typically presents between 1 and 5 years of age, with 90% of tumors being diagnosed before age 7. Adolescent and adult Wilms' tumor does occur but is uncommon. Renal cell carcinoma (RCC) occurs infrequently in children and presents at a mean age of 9–10 years.[21] Notably, in children between the ages of 10 and 20, the incidence of RCC has been shown to be similar to the incidence of Wilms' tumor.[22]

No consensus has been reached as to the definitive form of therapy for RCC, but radical nephrectomy has been the main surgical approach. Primary treatment with partial nephrectomy has been reported in one pediatric case.[23] The adult form is aggressive and responds poorly to chemotherapy. Some authors have suggested a less aggressive course for the pediatric form of the disease, even when associated with positive lymph nodes. Like the adult form, however, disseminated disease predicts a poor outcome.[21,24]

Nephrectomy

When an RCC is suspected, a subcostal transperitoneal or extraperitoneal flank incision may be considered and does not appear to influence survival rates.[25] Should a Wilms' tumor be encountered, adequate staging including lymph node sampling and perhaps inspection of the contralateral kidney is necessary. A subcostal incision can be easily extended in this case. Certain anatomic variables, such as a narrow subcostal angle, may make a midline transperitoneal approach more appropriate. Certainly, any case potentially requiring vascular access to the superior vena cava or right atrium should be approached via a midline approach, since the incision can be extended as a median sternotomy. A transverse transperitoneal or chevron incision gives good exposure to the lateral and superior aspects of the kidney in addition to the great vessels.[2]

Radical nephrectomy for RCC is performed following the same principles as described for Wilms' tumor. This also applies to the surgical approaches for tumors with vascular invasion. An important difference in the tumor biology of these two lesions has important implications on the surgical approach to RCC, however. RCC responds poorly to both chemotherapy and external beam radiation. As a consequence, complete surgical resection is mandatory in order to optimize chances for a long-term cure.[26] Quek et al[27] reviewed their experience with 99 adult patients having intravascular tumor extension. The tumor extended to the renal vein in 31 patients, infrahepatic vena cava in 22 patients, intrahepatic vena cava in 34 patients, and right atrium in 12 patients. Overall 2- and 5-year survival rates following extensive resection were 54% and 33%, respectively. They advocated an aggressive surgical approach for those patients with clinically confined tumors with isolated venous tumor thrombus extension.[27] There are no similar studies in pediatric patients.

Partial nephrectomy

The main difference in the initial surgical approach to RCC in comparison to Wilms' tumor lies in the application of partial nephrectomy: partial nephrectomy for Wilms' tumor is deferred until completion of an initial course of chemotherapy, whereas partial nephrectomy for RCC can be used as the primary surgical approach in appropriately selected cases. An adequate resection should leave 1 cm margins of normal parenchyma surrounding the tumor.[2] It is important to remember that data on the success of partial nephrectomy for RCC have been collected from series in adults. Nevertheless the 90–100% cancer-specific survival obtained in adults with lesions of <4 cm is encouraging.[10]

Most cases of partial nephrectomy necessitate transient ischemia to the kidney. Certain points are important to understand before proceeding with the surgery. Renal tolerance to warm ischemia is approximately 30 minutes, as derived from canine studies.[3] Cold ischemia is tolerated for up to 3 hours.[28] Prior to partial nephrectomy, the core temperature of the kidney should therefore be lowered by placing it on ice for 10–15 minutes after clamping the artery.[4] Immediately after renal artery occlusion, there is an accumulation of monophosphate nucleotides produced by ATP degradation within the kidney. Progressive loss of ATP depletes cellular energy reserves, causing dysfunction of the cellular membrane, influx of water and salt, cellular edema, and ultimately cellular death. Proximal tubular cells are the most predisposed to injury during ischemia, whereas glomeruli and blood vessels are more resistant.[29] When the renal artery and vein are occluded simultaneously, renal damage is more pronounced.[30] Solitary kidneys and kidneys with extensive collateral circulation seem to better tolerate longer periods of renal ischemia.[31,32] Experimental studies indicate that manual renal compression to control intraoperative hemorrhage seems to cause more renal injury than simple arterial occlusion.[5] Protective factors that can be used to reduce ischemic damage include adequate hydration, avoiding hypotension, minimizing arterial manipulation, and the administration of mannitol 5–15 minutes prior to arterial occlusion.[6]

Advances in renal imaging can allow for detailed reconstruction of renal anatomy when preparing for partial nephrectomy. Specific indications for partial nephrectomy for RCC include solitary kidney, compromised renal function, the presence of a benign disease that could compromise future renal function, or bilateral tumors.[33] Further studies clarified success of partial nephrectomy in patients with localized disease <4 cm and a normal contralateral kidney.[34,35] The major disadvantage of partial nephrectomy for RCC is the risk of missing multifocal disease predisposing to local tumor recurrence. This can occur in 4–6% of patients.[33,36,37] The technical success rate is excellent, and operative morbidity and mortality is low. Long-term cancer-free survival for low-stage disease is comparable to radical nephrectomy. The overall incidence of local recurrence is low, at 0–10%. For tumors ≤4 cm, local recurrence rates are even less, at 0–3%. The risk of local recurrence depends primarily on the initial local pathologic tumor stage. The reported incidence of multifocal renal cell carcinoma is approximately 15%, but it also depends on tumor size, histology, and stage. The pathologic risk of multifocal disease is <5% when the maximal diameter of the primary tumor is ≤4 cm.[10]

An extraperitoneal flank incision is preferred for partial nephrectomy. Optimal exposure is accomplished without the need to remove a rib in most children. The kidney is mobilized, leaving Gerota's fascia intact. Arterial control is not necessary for small peripheral lesions. Temporary arterial occlusion is recommended for larger lesions. Occlusion of both the renal vein and artery can further minimize bleeding for large lesions or for those that are centrally located. After occluding the renal vessels, the kidney should be surface-cooled in ice slush for 10–15 minutes. It is not advisable to perfuse the renal artery with cold solutions, because of the risk of tumor dissemination.[2] Depending on the characteristics of the lesion, partial nephrectomy can be performed using simple enucleation, polar segmental nephrectomy, wedge resection, transverse resection, or extracorporeal partial nephrectomy. In every case, regardless of the technique used, it is essential to remove the tumor completely, leaving a small surrounding margin of grossly normal renal parenchyma. Intraoperative ultrasonography can be helpful in delineating tumor margins and enabling a complete safe resection. This is especially helpful in central or poorly defined lesions. As the resection is carried through the renal parenchyma, arterial and venous branches are identified and suture ligated to minimize excessive bleeding following vascular unclamping. The collecting system should be repaired with absorbable sutures if entered. Frozen section biopsies of the tumor bed should be obtained following resection. Further resection is required if tumor is identified in the biopsy specimens.

Segmental polar nephrectomy

Segmental polar nephrectomy is performed in patients with a tumor mass confined to the upper or lower pole of the kidney. The arterial and venous branches supplying the corresponding pole are first ligated and divided. An ischemic line of demarcation generally appears, outlining the limits of the segment to be excised. For obvious reasons it is not possible to spare the renal capsule, as it overlies the tumor area. Simple, interrupted 2–0 or 3–0 chromic sutures are placed in the renal edges and perirenal fat or Oxycel secured within the defect.

Wedge resection

Wedge resections are necessary for non-polar, peripheral lesions. As significant bleeding can occur during

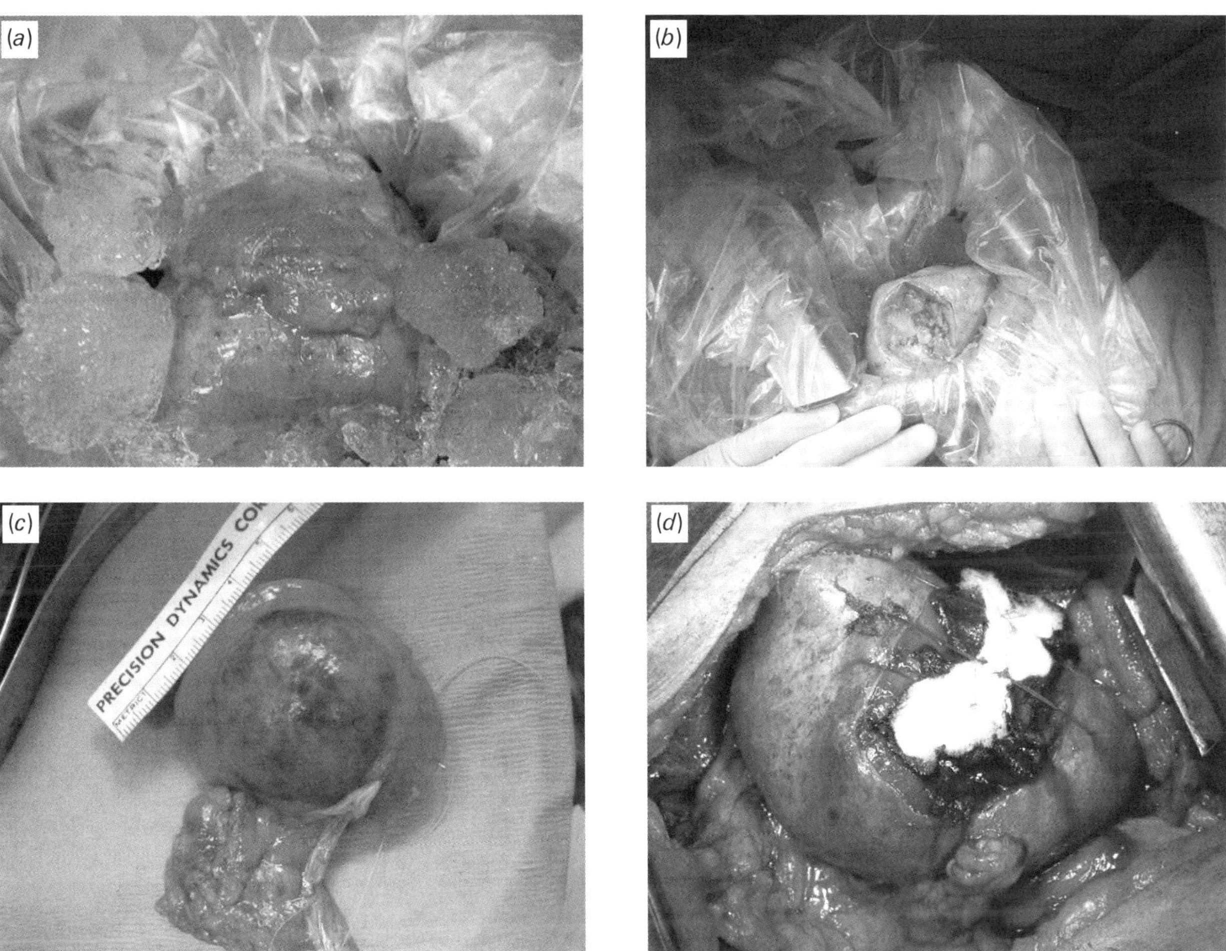

Figure 33.1 (*a*) Renal cell carcinoma in a 12-year-old child with tuberous sclerosis. The renal artery has been temporarily occluded and the kidney cooled with ice slush. Note that perinephric fat is left attached to the tumor. (*b*) A wedge partial nephrectomy performed in the midpole of the kidney. The arterial and venous branches suture ligated during the excision of the tumor. (*c*) The tumor is removed with a margin of normal parenchyma around the periphery of the lesion. (*d*) The renal artery has been unclamped and the kidney revascularized. Oxycel has been placed in the renal defect.

this procedure, it is advisable to control the renal artery with the application of surface hypothermia. The procedure is then carried out in a fashion similar to that described above for segmental nephrectomy (Figure 33.1).

Transverse resection

Transverse resection is used for large tumors involving the upper or lower renal pole. It is important to identify the major arterial and venous branches close to the hilum in this situation. Following ligation and division of the vessels, the ischemic portion of the kidney along with the tumor and a margin of normal tissue are removed.

Central tumors

Central tumors present a technically more challenging problem. Preoperative imaging with three-dimensional CT reconstruction is mandatory to outline the vascular anatomy. The dissection is carried out close to the central renal vessels and, consequently, significant arterial and venous bleeding may occur. Both the renal artery and vein need to be transiently occluded.[2] Only the smaller arterial branches providing blood supply to the tumor area should be clamped and divided. Arteries supplying the normal parenchyma should be carefully spared, since they are end arteries and their division will permanently devascularize the corresponding normal renal segment. Intraoperative ultrasonography can be a valuable tool in identifying central tumors, which are not easily palpable and consequently difficult to localize.

Simple enucleation

Simple enucleation is sometimes indicated in patients having received preoperative chemotherapy for bilateral Wilms' tumor or patients with von Hippel–Lindau disease and multiple low-stage encapsulated tumors.[38–40]

Extracorporeal partial nephrectomy

Extracorporeal partial nephrectomy and renal autotransplantation is a good option for tumors involving the renal hilum. Although this procedure has the advantage of providing a bloodless surgical field and allowing for a precise dissection, the surgical time is increased since a vascular anastomosis is required. It is preferable to leave the ureter attached during surgery if possible, but if necessary it can be divided. Care must be taken to avoid injury to the vascular supply of the ureter and pelvis during removal of tumors close to the hilum or those involving the lower pole.

Complications of partial nephrectomy

Complications of partial nephrectomy include hemorrhage, urinary fistula formation, ureteral obstruction, renal insufficiency, and infection.

Congenital mesoblastic nephroma

Nephrectomy for infants with congenital mesoblastic nephroma (CMN) should be performed with great care to avoid leaving behind residual tumor. This is particularly important for cellular variants of CMN and infants older than 3 months of age. Special attention should be given to the dissection of the renal hilum, which is the most common location for invasion and local recurrence.[41,42]

References

1. Nethercliffe J, Wood DN, Andrich DE, Greenwell TJ, Mundy AR. Retroperitoneal and transthoracic anatomy and surgical approaches. BJU Int 2004; 94:705–18.
2. Novick AC. Surgery of the kidney. In: Walsh PC, Retik AB, Vaughan ED Jr, Wein AJ, eds. Campbell's Urology, 8th edn, Vol 4. Philadelphia: WB Saunders, 2002: 3570–643.
3. Ward J. Determination of the optimum temperature for regional renal hypothermia during temporary renal ischemia. Br J Urol 1975; 47:17–24.
4. Stubbs AJ, Resnick MI, Boyce WH. Anatrophic nephrolithotomy in the solitary kidney. J Urol 1978; 119:457–60.
5. Neely WA, Turner MD. The effect of arterial, venous, and arteriovenous occlusion on renal blood flow. Surg Gynecol Obstet 1959; 108:669–72.
6. Collins GM, Green RD, Boyer D, Halasz NA. Protection of kidneys from warm ischemic injury. Dosage and timing of mannitol administration. Transplantation 1980; 29:83–4.
7. Ritchey ML, Kelalis PP, Breslow N et al. Intracaval and atrial involvement with nephroblastoma: review of the National Wilm's Tumor Study-3. J Urol 1988; 140:1113–18.
8. Weese DL, Applebaum H, Taber P. Mapping intravascular extension of Wilms' tumor with magnetic resonance imaging. J Pediatr Surg 1991; 26:64–7.
9. Coppes MJ, Zandvoort SW, Sparling CR et al. Acquired Von Willebrand disease in Wilms' tumor patients. J Clin Oncol 1993; 10:422–7.
10. Uzzo RG, Novick AC. Nephron sparing surgery for renal tumors: indications, techniques and outcomes. J Urol 2001; 166(1):6–18.
11. D'Angio GJ, Rosenberg H, Sharples K et al. Position paper: imaging methods for primary renal tumors of

childhood: cost versus benefits. Med Pediatr Oncol 1993; 21:205–12.
12. White KS, Grassman H. Wilms' and associated renal tumors of childhood. Pediatr Radiol 1991; 21:81–8.
13. Ritchey ML. Wilms' Tumor. In: Belman AB, King LR, Kramer SA, eds., Clincial Pediatric Urology, 4th edn. London: Martin Dunitz, 2002: 1269–89.
14. Ritchey ML, Shamberger RC, Hamilton T et al. Fate of bilateral lesions missed on preoperative imaging: a report from the National Wilms Tumor Study Group. San Francisco: American Academy of Pediatrics, Urology Section, 2004.
15. Blute ML, Kelatis PP, Offord KP et al. Bilateral Wilms tumor. J Urol 1987; 138:968–73.
16. Ritchey ML, Coppes MJ. The management of synchronous bilateral Wilms tumor. Hematol Oncol Clin North Am 1995; 9:1303–15.
17. Ritchey ML, Pringle KC, Breslow N et al. Management and outcome of inoperable Wilms tumor. A report of the National Wilms Tumor Study-3. Ann Surg 1994; 220:683–90.
18. Othersen HB Jr, Delorimer A, Hrabovsky E et al. Surgical evaluation of lymph node metastases in Wilms tumor. J Pediatr Surg 1990; 25:330–1.
19. McNeil DE, Langer JC, Choyke P, DeBaun MR. Feasibility of partial nephrectomy for Wilms' tumor in children with Beckwith–Wiedemann syndrome who have been screened with abdominal ultrasonography. J Pediatr Surg 2002; 37(1):57–60.
20. Ritchey ML, Shamberger RC, Haase G et al. Surgical complications following nephrectomy for Wilms tumor: a prospective study from the National Wilms Tumor Study Group (NWTSG) and International Society of Pediatric Oncology (SIOP). San Francisco: American Academy of Pediatrics, Urology Section, 2004.
21. Carcao MD, Taylor GP, Greenberg ML et al. Renal-cell carcinoma in children: a different disorder from its adult counterpart. Med Pediatr Oncol 1998; 31:153–8.
22. Hartman DS, Davis CJ Jr, Madewell JE, Friedman AC. Primary malignant renal tumors in the second decade of life: Wilms' tumor versus renal cell carcinoma. J Urol 1982; 127:888–91.
23. Manion S, Hayani A, Husain A, Rink R, Hatch D. Partial nephrectomy for pediatric renal cell carcinoma: an unusual case presentation. Urology 1997; 49:465–8.
24. Barros LR, Glina S, Melo LF. Renal cell carcinoma in childhood. Int Braz J Urol 2004; 30:227–9.
25. Sugao H, Matsuda M, Nakano E et al. Comparison of lumbar flank approach and transperitoneal approach for radical nephrectomy. Urol Int 1991; 46(1):43–5.
26. Aronson DC, Medary I, Finlay JL et al. Renal cell carcinoma in childhood and adolescence: a retrospective survey for prognostic factors in 22 cases. J Pediatr Surg 1996; 31:183–6.
27. Quek ML, Stein JP, Skinner DG. Surgical approaches to venous tumor thrombus. Semin Urol Oncol 2001; 19(2):88–97.
28. Marberger M, Georgi M, Guenther R, Hohenfellner R. Simultaneous balloon occlusion of the renal artery and hypothermic perfusion in in situ surgery of the kidney. J Urol 1978; 119:463–7.
29. Collins GM, Taft P, Green RD, Ruprecht R, Halasz NA. Adenine nucleotide levels in preserved and ischemically injured canine kidneys. World J Surg 1977; 1:237–43.
30. Schirmer HKA, Taft JL, Scott WW. Renal metabolism after occlusion of the renal artery and after occlusion of the renal artery and vein. J Urol 1966; 96:136.
31. Askari A, Novick AC, Stewart BH, Staffron RA. Surgical treatment of renovascular disease in the solitary kidney: results in 43 cases. J Urol 1982; 127:20–2.
32. Schefft P, Novick AC, Stewart BH, Staffron RA. Renal revascularization in patients with total occlusion of the renal artery. J Urol 1980; 124:184–6.
33. Licht MR, Novick AC, Goormastic M. Nephron sparing surgery in incidental versus suspected renal cell carcinoma. J Urol 1994; 152:39–42.
34. Butler BP, Novick AC, Miller DP, Campbell SA, Licht MR. Management of small unilateral renal cell carcinomas: radical versus nephron-sparing surgery. Urology 1995; 45:34–40.
35. Lerner SE, Hawkins CA, Blute ML et al. Disease outcome in patients with low stage renal cell carcinoma treated with nephron sparing or radical surgery. 1996. J Urol 2002: 155(Pt 2):884–9.
36. Morgan WR, Zincke H. Progression and survival after renal-conserving surgery for renal cell carcinoma: experience in 104 patients and extended followup. J Urol 1990; 144:852–7.
37. Steinbach F, Stockle M, Muller SC et al. Conservative surgery of renal tumors in 140 patients: 21 years of experience. J Urol 1992; 148:24–9.
38. Rosenthal CL, Kraft R, Zingg EJ. Organ-preserving surgery in renal cell carcinoma: tumor enucleation versus partial kidney resection. Eur Urol 1984; 10:222–8.
39. Marshall FF, Taxy JB, Fishman EK, Chang R. The feasibility of surgical enucleation for renal cell carcinoma. J Urol 1986; 135:231–4.
40. Blackley SK, Ladaga L, Woolfitt RA, Schellhammer PF. Ex situ study of the effectiveness of enucleation in patients with renal cell carcinoma. J Urol 1988; 140:6–10.
41. Joshi V, Kasznica J, Walters TR. Atypical mesoblastic nephroma. Pathologic characterization of a potentially aggressive variant of conventional congenital mesoblastic nephroma. Arch Pathol Lab Med 1986; 110:100–6.
42. Gormley TS, Skoog SJ, Jones RV, Maybee D. Cellular congenital mesoblastic nephroma: what are the options? J Urol 1989; 142:479–83.

Upper urinary tract trauma

34

Douglas A Husmann

Similarities and differences in evaluating pediatric versus adult traumatic injuries

General comments

Whether the incidence of renal injury following blunt abdominal trauma is increased in the pediatric compared with the adult patient population is controversial.[1–4] Hypothetically, the pediatric kidney is believed to be more susceptible to trauma due to a decrease in the physical renal protective mechanisms found in childhood: i.e. a slightly lower renal position in the abdomen, an immature thoracic cage, and weaker abdominal musculature. Statistical evaluations to confirm that children have an increased risk of renal injury have revealed mixed results and the question remains unresolved.[1–5] What is known, however, is that pre-existing congenital renal abnormalities are found 3–5-fold more commonly in pediatric patients undergoing a screening computed tomography (CT) scan for trauma than the adult population.[2–4,6] Classically, patients with a pre-existing genitourinary (GU) abnormality present with a history of hematuria disproportionate to the severity of trauma. In the pediatric population the most common pre-existing GU anomalies found, listed in decreasing frequency, are: ureteropelvic junction (UPJ) obstruction, hydroureteronephrosis secondary to reflux, horseshoe kidney, non-obstructing, non-refluxing hydronephrosis/hydroureteronephrosis, and primary obstructing megaureter.[2–4]

Traumatic induced hematuria

In children, hematuria is unreliable for determining the extent of renal injury; indeed, some studies have failed to find any evidence of either gross or microscopic hematuria in up to 70% of children sustaining grade 2 or higher renal injuries (Table 34.1). In essence, post-traumatic hematuria cannot be used as the sole determinant in deciding whether or not to screen the child for the presence of a GU injury.[7,8]

Indications for imaging the genitourinary tract following trauma

In the adult, radiographic assessment of the GU tract is recommended following all penetrating trauma, as well as blunt trauma, victims that have one of four criteria:

1 A significant deceleration (motor vehicle accident (MVA), fall from >15 feet) or high-velocity injury (strike to the back or flank with a high-velocity foreign object, i.e. football helmet, baseball bat, etc.).
2 Significant external trauma resulting in fractures of thoracic bony structures, spine, pelvis, and femur, bruising of the torso/perineum and/or signs of peritoneal irritation.
3 Gross hematuria.
4 Microscopic hematuria (>50 red blood cells per high-power field (RBCs/HPF)) associated with shock (systolic blood pressure <90 mmHg).[4,9–12]

Clinicians debate about whether the adult screening criteria outlined above apply to children.[7,10,13–17] This controversy is based on three separate concerns. First, hypotension in children is not a reliable indicator of the severity of the injury. Children often have normal blood pressure in spite of significant blood loss. In children, a fall in serial hemoglobin or hematocrit value is a better determinant of blood loss than hypotension.[14] Secondly, there is not a consensus opinion in the literature regarding the definition of an associated injury in the child. For example, does an isolated closed head injury indicate the need for a screening abdominal CT?[7] Finally, there is no standard definition of a deceleration or high-velocity injury with some authors neglecting to include the latter criteria in their list of indications for abdominal three-dimensional imaging.

To help end this controversy, in 2004 Santucci and

associates reviewed all of the previous data regarding traumatic renal injuries in children.[10] In this excellent review article, they found that use of adult screening criteria is highly accurate and applicable in children. We currently recommend the same radiographic screening criteria noted in the first paragraph of this section be used in both children and adults.

Radiographic and endoscopic assessment and treatment of genitourinary injuries

Abdominal and pelvic computed tomography and single-shot intravenous pyelography

The patient's hemodynamic stability determines whether, when, and occasionally what type of imaging studies should be done. In the clinically stable patient, a triphasic abdominal and pelvic CT scan (precontrast study, followed by a study immediately after injection of contrast, and then a 15–20 minute delayed study) is the most sensitive method for diagnosis and classification of GU trauma (see Table 34.1 for classification of renal trauma[4,7,8,10,11,15,16]).

In the clinically unstable patient, a single-phase CT scan is frequently obtained, with the images taken immediately following injection of contrast. In our experience, this test is beneficial in determining renal perfusion and the presence of major renal fractures, but will be unable to accurately determine the presence of urinary extravasation and will miss the majority of the isolated ureteral injuries.[2,18,19] In the unstable patient requiring emergent laparotomy, with no preoperative imaging studies obtained, once the patient is stabilized in the operating room, a single-shot intravenous pyelogram (IVP) (2 ml/kg intravenous bolus of contrast), with the X-ray taken 10–15 minutes following injection of contrast, may be of benefit. In our experience, this study frequently results in a poor imaging of the urinary tract. These unstable patients usually have a history of profound hypotension, associated with poor renal perfusion and subsequently poor excretion and visualization of contrast. The main benefit of a single-shot IVP may be to detect a normally functioning contralateral kidney if unilateral nephrectomy is a consideration. As an alternative to the single-shot IVP, the patient can be resuscitated and a delayed CT evaluation is obtained. If necessary, a definitive surgical repair of any GU injury is subsequently deferred for 12–24 hours.[4,20]

Table 34.1 Grading of renal injuries

Grade of renal injury	Description
1	Renal contusion or subcapsular hematoma
2	Non-expanding perirenal hematoma, <1 cm parenchymal laceration, no urinary extravasation, all renal fragments viable
3	Non-expanding perirenal hematoma, >1 cm parenchymal laceration, no urinary extravasation, renal fragments may be viable or devitalized
4	Laceration extending into the collecting system with urinary extravasation, renal fragments may be viable or devitalized or Injury to the main renal vasculature with contained hemorrhage
5	Completely shattered kidney, by definition multiple major lacerations of >1 cm associated with multiple devitalized fragments or Injury to the main renal vasculature with uncontrolled hemorrhage, renal hilar avulsion

Indications and use of arteriography

Up to 25% of grade 3–4 renal trauma managed by non-operative protocols will require angiography and selective angioinfarction of bleeding vessels for persistent or delayed renal hemorrhage.[21,22] Clinical signs of persistent bleeding are hematuria associated with blood clots in the voided or catheterized bladder and a falling serial hemoglobin. Orthostatic blood pressure alterations are a late finding in the pediatric patient population.[4,21,23–25] Delayed hemorrhage classically develops 10–14 days post injury, but may occur up to 1 month following the traumatic insult. Delayed hemorrhage usually arises from the development of arteriovenous (AV) or pseudoaneurysm malformations.[4,23–25] Unlike AV malformations arising from a renal biopsy, AV malformations following renal fractures rarely, if ever, resolve spontaneously: nearly all require active intervention.[4,23–25]

Superselective angiographic embolization of isolated renal artery branches for persistent or delayed hemorrhage has a success rate approaching 80%. This is the preferred treatment method for persistent or delayed bleeding. Surgical exploration is reserved for angiographic embolization failure.[4,23–25] Occasionally, angiographic embolization is used to treat persistent urinary fistulas. In this clinical scenario, a functionally transected renal fragment following a grade 3, 4, or 5 renal injury is completely separated from the renal collecting system, and a persistent urinary fistula develops despite management by a double-J stent and/or a percutaneous nephrostomy tube. In these unusual patients, selective angiographic embolization can be performed to resolve the urinary fistula by necrosing the isolated functional renal fragment.[4,26]

Postembolization syndrome (fever, flank pain, and an adynamic ileus) is a well-recognized and self-limiting condition that occurs after angiographic embolization. Symptoms usually resolve by the 5th postembolization day.[4,27–30] Bacterial seeding of either the necrotic renal tissue or the hematoma from the angiographic intervention must be ruled out in patients with postembolization fever. It is therefore mandatory to obtain blood and urine cultures if a febrile response develops postembolization. If the fever persists for ≥5 days following angiographic infarction or if a patient becomes clinically labile, the clinician should consider a repeat CT scan with possible aspiration and culture of the hematoma/urinoma.[4,30]

Indications and use of retrograde pyelography and percutaneous drainage

In patients with a history of trauma, two indications exist for performing retrograde pyelography. First, to rule out the presence of a partial/total ureteral disruption and secondly to aid in placement of a double-J ureteral stent for the management of a symptomatic urinoma.[2–6,18,31] Most post-traumatic urinomas are asymptomatic. Approximately 75% of the urinomas spontaneously resolve.[4,31–34] Occasionally, the urine collection is associated with persistent flank pain, adynamic ileus, and/or low-grade temperature. In these cases we manage these patients with endoscopic intervention with cystoscopy, retrograde pyelography, and placement of a ureteral stent.[31] Although percutaneous drainage and internal stenting are both efficacious, the major advantages to internal drainage include improvements in quality of life during convalescence, specifically avoidance of external catheter care, and the reduced risk of inadvertent tube dislodgment.[4,31,32,35] A disadvantage of internal drainage is that stent placement and removal requires general anesthesia in the child. In addition, smaller ureteral stents (4–5 Fr) placed in young children occasionally become blocked with debris and blood clot from the dissolving hematoma. We recommend placement of percutanous nephrostomy tubes to manage urinomas in one of three situations:

1 Patients who have failed attempts at endoscopic management.
2 Patients who are unstable and therefore not candidates for general anesthesia.
3 Patients with persistent gross hematuria in whom we are afraid that the small-caliber ureteral stent will become occluded.[31,32]

Indications and use of DMSA and follow-up radiographic imaging following renal trauma

We do not recommend follow-up renal imaging for grade 1–2 renal injuries. In patients with grade 3, 4, and 5 renal injuries, a repeat CT scan with delayed images should be obtained 2–3 days after the traumatic insult. This study assesses the extent of the hematoma/urinoma and functions as a baseline evaluation in case delayed hemorrhage occurs.[4,6] Additional repeat CT scans are considered if fever, flank pain, and hematuria persist or increase.[6] A 3-month follow-up CT scan is ordered in all grade 3, 4, and 5 renal injuries. This latter study is used to verify resolution of a perinephric hematoma/urinoma and to define the anatomic configuration of the residual functioning renal parenchyma.[8]

Nuclear renal scanning using technetium 99m dimercaptosuccinic acid (^{99m}Tc DMSA) allows the physician to determine renal cortical function and differential renal function. Serial DMSA scans obtained post trauma have revealed that little if any renal parenchyma recovers function 7 days following injury; therefore, a DMSA scan obtained more than 1 week after the injury provides a valid estimate of subsequent renal function.[36,37] We suggest that all patients with grade 3 injuries with devitalized fragments, all grade 4 and 5 renal injuries, and all patients with persistent post-traumatic hypertension should be evaluated with a quantitative radionuclide scintigraphy, preferably DMSA. The study should be performed at least 1 week after the traumatic insult.[4,36] Provided the serum creatinine is normal, a differential renal function exceeding 30% suggests satisfactory function that would prevent renal failure in the event that the uninjured kidney is lost.[4,34,37]

Effect of etiology on the management of traumatic genitourinary injuries

Blunt versus penetrating genitourinary trauma

The etiology of the traumatic injury plays an important role in determining the management of the patient. In North America, blunt trauma, usually high-velocity, or sudden deceleration injury causes approximately 90% of renal injuries in children. Fewer than 2% of the children with blunt renal trauma will require radiographic or surgical intervention.[4,6,8,33]

Approximately 10% of traumatic pediatric renal injuries result from penetrating trauma. In the presence of penetrating trauma, the physician should immediately triage the patient into one of two groups, depending on the source of the penetrating trauma: either a stab/low-velocity penetrating-wound group or a high-velocity penetrating-wound group.[4,6,8] Although penetrating trauma results in the risk of wound contamination by outside material, several studies have shown that a selective non-operative approach to the management of patients with stab wounds and, in very select cases, low-velocity gunshot wounds, can be safely implemented.[4,23,38] In hemodynamically stable patients with a penetrating wound posterior to the anterior axillary line, intravenous antibiotics are initiated and a screening triphasic abdominal and pelvic CT is obtained. In these patients surgical exploration/laparoscopy is indicated for persistent blood loss, the presence of air in the peritoneum, signs of developing peritonitis, or radiographic findings consistent with a ureteral injury.[4,23,38–41]

Gunshot wounds to the trunk are associated with a GU injury approximately 15% of the time.[39] In patients with GU trauma secondary to a gunshot wound, the kidney is the site of injury in approximately 60% of the patients, the bladder in 20%, the urethra in 5%, the ureter in 2%, and 13% will have two or more GU injuries.[39,42] If a GU structure is traumatically damaged as a result of a gunshot wound, the likelihood of associated organ injury is approximately 90%.[21,39,42] Although the majority of blunt renal trauma and the majority of penetrating renal trauma from stab wounds are amenable to complete radiographic staging and non-operative management, rarely are gunshot wounds to the kidney amenable to non-operative management. In most cases, gunshot wounds to the abdomen result in a hemodynamically unstable patient with multiple associated organ injuries that require urgent laparotomy. The need for emergent surgery excludes the ability to adequately stage the renal injury.[21,22,39] If the patients with a gunshot wound can undergo adequate radiographic staging, isolated grade 1 or 2 renal injuries can be managed successfully with a non-operative approach, with minimal complications[21] (Table 34.2).

Gunshot wounds caused by high-velocity missiles (>350 m/s) deserve special consideration. The kinetic energy of a high-velocity bullet creates a surrounding energy wave 30–40 times the missile diameter. In addition, the missile will frequently yaw or tumble during penetration; the combination of blast injury and missile tumbling results in extensive damage to the surrounding tissues at a large distance from its path.[6] With high-velocity gunshot wounds to the torso, radiographic and/or surgical evaluation at the time of the assault may not reveal the presence of a GU injury. In some patients with a high-velocity injury, the renal pelvis and/or ureter will appear intact or perhaps only slightly contused at the time of the radiographic examination and/or surgical exploration. As the high-velocity blast injury matures, necrosis of the ureter or portions of the renal pelvis may develop, the extent of the GU injury finally coming to attention as urinary extravasation develops as a result of delayed necrosis. Blast injuries to the urinary drainage system may only be apparent 3–5 days after the injury, when an increase in urine output from surgically placed drains is recorded.[4,43,44]

Management of renal trauma

Multiple studies have found that the nephrectomy rate in patients with traumatic renal injuries was higher with surgical exploration than with non-operative management.[34,38,45–47] These reports hypothesize that hemorrhage from the severely injured kidney is tamponaded (controlled) by an intact Gerota's fascia. Surgical exploration would disrupt the fascia, resulting in uncontrollable renal bleeding thereby increasing the need for emergency nephrectomy. This hypothesis is controversial. Current studies using the

Table 34.2 Consensus recommendations for management of renal trauma

Clinical findings and/or grade of renal injury	Recommended treatment
Grade 1 or 2 renal injury, irrespective of traumatic etiology	Non-operative
Isolated grade 3, 4, and hemodynamically stable grade 5 renal injuries	Non-operative
Uncontrollable renal hemorrhage/vascular instability (usually grade 4 vascular or the vast majority of grade 5 injuries)	Absolute requirement for surgical intervention
Persistent or delayed hemorrhage not responding to angiographic embolization	Absolute requirement for surgical intervention
Expanding pulsatile retroperitoneal mass found on surgical exploration for coexisting intra-abdominal injuries	Absolute requirement for surgical intervention (verify contralateral renal function prior to exploration)
Penetrating trauma; inadequate preoperative radiographic staging resulting from vascular instability of patient; retroperitoneal hemorrhage found on exploration	Retroperitoneal (renal) exploration strongly recommended (verify contralateral renal function)
Blunt trauma; inadequate preoperative radiographic staging resulting from vascular instability of patient; coexisting intra-abdominal injuries, especially stomach, duodenum, pancreas and colon; retroperitoneal hemorrhage found on exploration	Retroperitoneal (renal) exploration recommended (verify contralateral renal function)
Blunt trauma; radiographic screening studies reveal grade 3, grade 4, or 5 renal injury; coexisting intra-abdominal injuries, especially stomach, duodenum, pancreas, and colon	Retroperitoneal (renal) exploration recommended

combination of CT staging of renal injuries combined with the application of trauma-related severity scores, have revealed that emergency nephrectomy during renal exploration for trauma is directly related to the severity of the initial renal injury, and the presence of multiple coexisting injuries, not due to the disruption of Gerota's fascia and the release of a confined tamponade.[4,32,48–51]

Based on the hypothesis that Gerota's fascia would contain renal hemorrhage, three different concepts regarding the management of renal injuries exist:

1 Observation of all grades of renal injury, unless there is an absolute indication for renal exploration.[34,38,52]
2 If a laparotomy is to be performed for a coexisting intra-abdominal injury (especially stomach, duodenal, pancreatic and colonic injuries), renal exploration and renorrhapy of all renal injuries ≥ grade 3 should be simultaneously performed: grades 1 and 2 can be observed. At the time of surgery control of the renal vessels medial to Gerota's fascia should be obtained prior to renal exploration. The surgeon should repair the GU injury and provide drainage of the GU injury separate from the site of the coexisting injuries.[4,6,32,53] In this setting, control of the renal vessels prior to opening Gerota's fascia may prevent life-threatening hemorrhage. It should be noted that with the passage of time, even the need for vascular control before renal exploration has become controversial, with some studies revealing the incidence of nephrectomy being equivalent whether or not prior vascular control is used.[4,6,49,53]
3 In patients with concurrent intra-abdominal injuries, the trauma surgeon should separate the enteric injury from the urinary tract injury with omentum or other alternative tissue and places perioperative drains. All stages of renal injury can be observed if this situation it is hypothesized that the separation of the enteric or pancreatic injury from the GU injury by the omentum, along with the placement of perioperative drains, will prevent breakdown of enteric repairs by leaking urine and/or help prevent the development of urinary tract complications by removal of excess contaminating bacteria or pancreatic enzymes from the site of GU injury.[6,32,48,54,55]

Current recommendations for operative intervention on renal injuries are based on three findings: the hemodynamic stability of the patient, an accurate radiographic staging of the renal trauma, and the presence of associated organ injury.[4,6,21,31,32] Absolute indications for renal exploration include life-threatening hemorrhage from a renal source (usually grade 4 vascular and the vast majority of grade 5 renal injuries), a pulsatile expanding retroperitoneal hematoma found at emergency laparotomy, and persistent or delayed renal bleeding not responding to angioinfarction.[4,6] It is also strongly recommended that patients with penetrating trauma found to have a retroperitoneal hematoma in the absence of adequate preoperative imaging should be explored once contralateral renal function is verified by an intraoperative single-shot IVP.[4,6]

The ideal candidate for non-operative management is the hemodynamically stable patient sustaining either blunt or penetrating trauma, with or without associated intra-abdominal injuries, that has a grade 1–2 renal injury. GU complications in this subset of patients are minimal.[4,6,21] Patients with isolated grade 3, 4 and hemodynamically stable grade 5 renal injuries are also candidates for non-operative treatment. Even identification of a large perinephric hematoma or urinoma is not an absolute indication for operative management, provided the distal ureter is documented to be intact. Angiographic, endoscopic, or percutaneous intervention will eventually be required in up to 55% of the patients. Intervention is necessary for delayed bleeding in approximately 25%, and for symptomatic urinomas in approximately 25%. Surgical exploration to control complications not amenable to non-operative techniques will develop in approximately 5%. In essence, conservative management of isolated grade 3, 4 and hemodynamically stable grade 5 renal injuries will avoid the need for open surgical intervention in approximately 95% of renal injuries.[4,6,8,21,31,32,54,56]

Controversy regarding the management of blunt renal trauma currently involves two different patient populations:

1 Patients with inadequate radiographic staging found to have a non-expanding and non-pulsatile retroperitoneal hematoma found on surgical exploration.
2 Patients with a ≥ grade 3 renal injury undergoing laparotomy for associated intra-abdominal trauma especially if injuries to the stomach and colon are noted. In these situations the urologist should be aware of the relationship between GU morbidity, associated organ injury, and the grade of the renal injury. For example, if a colonic injury and a retroperitoneal hematoma are simultaneously present, approximately 10% of patients will be found to have a grade 1–2 renal injury, and 90% will have a grade 3 or higher renal injury.[4,6,21] In addition, if a colonic or pancreatic injury is concurrently present with devitalized renal tissue, non-operative management of the renal injury is associated with a 3–4-fold higher incidence of complications compared with renal exploration and renorrhaphy. In addition, renal exploration in this latter group of patients does not appear to result in increased risk of nephrectomy.[8,32,48,51] Knowledge of these facts has resulted in the consensus that patients with a known grade 3 or higher renal injury undergoing exploratory laparotomy for multiorgan injury should simultaneously undergo renal exploration with renorrhaphy and the placement of retroperitoneal drains. It is also accepted that patients undergoing emergent laparatomy without adequate preoperative radiographic studies who are found to have stomach, duodenal, colonic or pancreatic injuries and a coexisting retroperitoneal hematoma, should have a single-shot IVP obtained, to verify contralateral renal function, and proceed with renal exploration[4,6,8] (see Table 34.2).

Non-operative therapy for renal trauma

Non-operative therapy consists of bedrest, close monitoring of the vital signs and urine output, serial abdominal examinations, serial hemoglobin/hematocrit determinations, and transfusion as indicated for decreasing hematocrit or hypotension. In the patient with a ≥ grade 3 renal injury, massive blood loss and vascular instability may rapidly appear. The patient managed in this fashion should have blood immediately available.[4,6] Repeat CT imaging of the kidney 2–3 days following trauma is recommended in patients with grade 3, 4, and 5 renal injuries. CT imaging should be pursued earlier if prompted by clinical indications (see earlier section on DMSA and follow-up radiographic imaging following renal trauma). If the child remains hemodynamically stable with or without transfusions, and CT verifies a stable or resolving urinoma and/or hematoma, observation can continue. If the child becomes hemodynamically unstable or continues to have a falling hemoglobin/hematocrit despite transfusions, renal angiography with selective angioinfarction of the bleeding site should be performed. Children with a urinoma who complain of chronic or increasing flank pain, or have a persistent low-grade fever and/or a persistent ileus, should be considered for endoscopic or percutaneous management of the urinoma. They should be allowed to walk as soon as gross hematuria has resolved. Resumption of strenuous physical activity is prohibited for 6 weeks.[4,6,8,21,22]

We recommend intravenous broad-spectrum antibiotics in patients with a renal injury secondary to penetrating trauma on a non-operative protocol, due to the high risk of wound contamination from outside material. In renal injuries following blunt trauma, antibiotics may be considered if a large retroperitoneal hematoma or urinary extravasation exist. In this latter situation, the presence of an indwelling urethral catheter and/or multiple intravascular catheters may cause bacteremic colonization of the hematoma or urinoma.[4,6,8,21,22]

Operative intervention for renal trauma

Renal salvage by renorrhaphy or partial nephrectomy requires complete exposure of the injured kidney, debridement of non-viable tissue, suture ligation of bleeding arterial vessels, and repair of the collecting system injury. Defects in the renal parenchyma may be closed primarily with renal capsule. For larger defects, we prefer the placement of gel foam and Surgicel pack (small pieces of gel foam wrapped in Surgicel) into the parenchymal defect and closure of the renal capsule defect with woven polyglycolic acid mesh. Alternatively, perinephric fat, omentum, or thrombin-soaked gel foam may be used to pack the parenchymal defect. Watertight closure of the collecting system is not always possible, and may be inadvisable. If the renal pelvis or ureter is closed with tension, tissue ischemia and delayed resolution of urinary leakage may occur. If a major violation of the urinary drainage system is present, placement of intraoperative ureteral stents and/or a nephrostomy tube should be considered. Adequate drainage of the perinephric area following repair is vital. In the presence of concurrent stomach, duodenal, pancreatic, and colonic injuries, interposition of omentum or peritoneum between the site of the major renal injury and the site of the coexisting intra-abdominal injury is usually necessary. Nephrectomy should be considered in irreparable grade 4–5 renal injuries and in the hemodynamically unstable patient with multiorgan trauma.[4,6]

Renal vascular injuries

In terms of arterial renal blood flow the kidney is an end organ, and only rarely is collateral blood flow sufficient to maintain renal function if a segmental or main renal artery is damaged. In a patient sustaining renal arterial trauma, the clinical triad of decreased/absent renal arterial blood flow, inadequate collateral blood flow, and warm ischemic time almost invariably results in the loss of renal function.[4,6] Therefore, no attempt to repair injuries to segmental renal vessels should be considered, and repair of the traumatically injured main renal artery is rarely indicated. In essence, reconstruction of the main renal artery following trauma should only be considered in patients that are hemodynamically stable with an injury to a solitary kidney or in patients with bilateral renal injuries; otherwise, nephrectomy is the most expeditious and least-moribund treatment.[4,6] The infrequent exception to this rule is the presence of an incomplete renal arterial injury where perfusion to the kidney has been maintained by flow of blood through either the partially occluded main renal artery or via collateral vessels.[4,6]

Traumatic induced renal vascular hypertension

The most common causes of post-traumatic renal hypertension are

- renal ischemia from segmental arterial occlusion
- main renal artery occlusion with intact peripheral blood flow to the kidney
- a traumatically induced AV malformation or
- on rare occasion, compression of the renal parenchyma by hematoma/fibrosis (the Page kidney model).

The presence of hypertension immediately following the traumatic insult may be secondary to pain; however, persistent hypertension 30 days post injury could result from a renal source and the diagnosis of traumatically induced renal vascular hypertension should be considered. The incidence of traumatically induced hypertension is almost nonexistent after grade 1 and 2 renal injuries and will be found in approximately 5% of patients with ≥ grade 3 renal injuries.[4,6]

Hypertension from renovascular trauma will usually develop within 36 months following the injury.[4,6] If sustained hypertension develops, an evaluation with a DMSA scan to determine differential renal function and radiographic studies – magnetic resonance imaging (MRI) or CT angiography – to rule out development of an AV fistula as the source of the hypertension should be performed. Hypertension related to an AV malformation should initially be treated with angiographic embolization. If consideration for surgical intervention is entertained, renal vein renin sampling for split renin ratios should be considered. This ratio is especially helpful in the presence of segmental renal scarring where partial nephrectomy is a consideration for surgical management. In this situation, hypertension related to segmental renal ischemia is treated with a partial nephrectomy. The most common clinical finding in post-traumatic-induced hypertension, however, is a small poorly functioning kidney (<30% differential renal function), associated with scarring. Most authorities believe that a differential renal function of <30% would not prevent the onset of renal failure in the event that the uninjured kidney is lost.[4,6,34,37] Nephrectomy or partial nephrectomy is therefore the treatment of choice for post-traumatic hypertension. Rarely is renal revascularization of any benefit, since hypertension is almost invariably the result of increased renin production from intrarenal or subcapsular fibrosis.[4,6] Surgical treatment of hypertension by decortication of subcapsular fibrosis in patients with a Page kidney-induced hypertension has been published; however, the long-term results of this surgical treatment modality are extremely controversial.[4,6]

Ureteropelvic junction disruption

If the screening CT evaluation reveals the presence of medial and perirenal contrast extravasation with no visualization of the ipsilateral distal ureter on delayed images, the diagnosis of either a large laceration of the renal pelvis or avulsion of the UPJ is entertained and further investigation mandated with either a retrograde pyelogram or surgical exploration.[4,6,18] Disruption of the UPJ is most commonly caused by acceleration–deceleration injuries (fall from >15 feet) or by a sudden extreme hyperextension of the trunk (pedestrian MVA, patient thrown from the vehicle during an MVA). The mechanism of injury results from a sudden displacement of the more mobile kidney associated with a relatively fixed ureter, with force vectors from the traumatic impact interacting at the UPJ.[2,3,18]

Although some reports suggest that a large extrarenal pelvis or a congenital UPJ obstruction renders the patient more susceptible to disruptions of the UPJ, this is controversial. The vast majority of patients with a congenital UPJ or congenital hydronephrosis with a traumatic injury will be found to have a rupture of the renal pelvis or a major laceration through a thinned renal cortex, not a UPJ disruption.[2,3,5,18] Generally, a laceration of an enlarged renal pelvis will appear as an isolated renal injury, whereas a UPJ disruption tends to occur in association with life-threatening injuries. The majority of patients sustaining a UPJ disruption will present with vascular instability, requiring emergency laparatomy, with the patient unable to undergo preoperative imaging. Urinalysis on presentation will have some degree of hematuria present in 70% of patients; however, 30% of patients with a UPJ disruption will have a completely normal urinalysis. In patients undergoing exploratory laparatomy for a coexisting intra-abdominal injury, a retroperitoneal hematoma is rarely revealed.[2,3,18,19] Because of the frequent association of this injury with life-threatening trauma, inadequate preoperative radiographic staging studies, and the absence of a retroperitoneal hematoma, the diagnosis of a UPJ disruption is delayed for >36 hours in more than 50% of patients.[18,19] Patients will eventually come to attention, as a result of persistent post-operative fever flank pain, continued ileus, or sepsis.[2,3,18,19]

Three classic findings on a triphasic CT scan are associated with UPJ disruption:

- good renal contrast excretion, with extravasation around the upper ureter into the medial perirenal space
- absence of parenchymal lacerations and intact renal calices
- non-visualization of the ipsilateral ureter.

When a diagnosis of a possible disruption of the UPJ is entertained, careful evaluation of the delayed CT images is necessary. This diagnosis may be difficult, even if suspected. Specifically, the severely injured patient usually has a history of volume depletion; contrast excretion resulting from the coexistence of hypovolemia, acute tubular necrosis, or renal contusion may be minimal. To definitively rule out the presence of a UPJ disruption, it is necessary to confirm the presence of contrast material in both distal ureters. This can be especially difficult in patients where this injury may be associated with a type 3 renal injury where contrast material may be preferentially accumulating in the retroperitoneum. If the results of the CT scan remain inconclusive, a retrograde pyelogram should be performed.[2–4,6,18,19]

Children with pre-existing hydronephosis from a UPJ obstruction frequently have, at the site of injury, a major laceration through the thinned renal cortex (grade 3 renal injury) or laceration of the renal pelvis and not disruption of the UPJ. These patients should have a retrograde pyelogram to confirm continuity of the UPJ and, if not suspicious for disruption, they can be safely managed with either a percutaneous nephrostomy or a double-J stent placement with delayed pyeloplasty performed after stabilization of the patient.[3,5,31,55]

In patients with a disruption of the UPJ, a delay in diagnosis may significantly increase the risk of nephrectomy.[5,18,19] In the clinically stable patient where the diagnosis is made within 5 days after the traumatic insult, we prefer to proceed to surgical repair, with debridement of any devitilized ureteral tissure, spatulation, and reanastomosis of the ureter over a stent, with concurrent placement of an intra-operative nephrostomy tube and retroperitoneal drain. Since the area of ureteral necrosis may extend for 2–3 cm, mobilization and downward displacement of the kidney may be necessary to obtain a tension-free ureteral anastomosis.[18,19] In patients with a delayed diagnosis of a UPJ disruption ≥ 6 days post-traumatic insult, we prefer to place a nephrostomy tube and allow the injury to stabilize for 6–8 weeks. Differential renal function is then obtained via a DMSA renal scan, and the length of the ureteral injury ascertained by a combined antegrade and retrograde pyelogram. The combination of known percent renal function and length of the ureteral defect will allow the surgeon to make the proper surgical planning. Surgical alternatives in this situation include primary ureteroureterostomy, ileal ureter, autotransplantation, and nephrectomy (renal function <30% in the presence of a normal serum creatinine and renal clearance).[4,6,18,19]

References

1. Brown S, Elder J, Spirnak J. Are pediatric patients more susceptible to major renal injury from blunt trauma? A comparative study. J Urol 1998; 160:138–41.
2. Chopra P, St-Vil D, Yazbeck S. Blunt renal trauma-blessing in disguise? J Pediatr Surg 2002; 37:779–82.
3. McAleer I, Kaplan G, LoSasso B. Congenital urinary tract anomalies in pediatric renal trauma patients. J Urol 2002; 168:1808–10.
4. Heyns C. Renal trauma: indications for imaging and surgical exploration. BJU Int 2004; 93:1165–70.
5. Smith M, Johnston B, Wessells H, Tainer L. Trauma cases from Harborview Medical Center. Rupture of a uteropelvic junction-obstructed kidney in a 15 year old football player. AJR Am J Roentgenol 2003; 180:504.
6. Santucci R, Wessells H, Bartsch G et al. Evaluation and management of renal injuries: consensus statement of the renal trauma subcommittee. BJU Int 2004; 93:937–54.
7. Morey A, Bruce J, McAninch J. Efficacy of radiographic imaging in pediatric blunt renal trauma. J Urol 1996; 156:2014–18.
8. Buckley J, McAninch J. Pediatric renal injuries: management guidelines from a 25-year experience. J Urol 2004; 172:687–90.
9. Hardeman S, Husmann D, Chinn H, Peters P. Blunt urinary trauma: identifying those patients who require radiographic studies. J Urol 1987; 138:99–101.
10. Santucci R, Langenburg S, Zachareas M. Traumatic hematuria in children can be evaluated as in adults. J Urol 2004; 171:822–5.
11. Mee S, McAninch J. Indications for radiographic assessment in renal trauma. Urol Clin North Am 1989; 16:187–95.
12. Herschorn S, Radomski S, Shoskes D et al. Evaluation and treatment of blunt renal trauma. J Uol 1991; 146:274–7.
13. Levy J, Bellah R, Baskin L et al. Non-operative management of blunt pediatric major renal trauma. Urology 1993; 42:418–24.
14. Quinlan D, Gearhart JJ. Blunt renal trauma in childhood. Features indicating severe injury. Br J Urol 1990; 66:526–9.
15. Brown S, Haas C, Dinchman KH, Elder J, Spirnak J. Radiologic evaluation of pediatric blunt renal trauma in patients with microscopic hematuria. World J Surg 2001; 25:1557–9.
16. Stein J, Kaji DM, Eastham J et al. Blunt renal trauma in the pediatric population: indications for radiographic evaluation. Urology 1994; 44:406–9.
17. Mee SL, McAninch J, Robinson AL, Auerbach P, Carroll P. Radiographic assessment of renal trauma: a 10-year prospective study of patient selection. J Urol 1989; 141:1095–8.
18. Boone T, Gilling P, Husmann D. Ureteropelvic junction disruption following blunt abdominal trauma. J Urol 1993; 150:33–6.
19. Kattan S. Traumatic pelvi-ureteric junction disruption. How can we avoid the delayed diagnosis? Injury 2001; 32:797–800.
20. Azimuddin K, Ivatury R, Porter J, Allman DB. Damage control in a trauma patient with ureteric injury. J Trauma 1997; 43:977–9.
21. Wessells H, McAninch JW, Meyer A, Bruce J. Criteria for nonoperative treatment of significant penetrating renal lacerations. J Urol 1997; 157:24–7.
22. Kansas BT, Eddy MJ, Mydlo JH, Uzzo RG. Incidence and management of penetrating renal trauma in patients with multiorgan injury: extended experience at an inner city trauma center. J Urol 2004; 172:1355–60.
23. Heyns CF, Van Vollenhoven P. Selective surgical man-

agement of renal stab wounds. Br J Urol 1992; 69:351–7.
24. Dinkel HP, Danuser H, Triller J. Blunt renal trauma: minimally invasive management with microcatheter embolization experience in nine patients. Radiology 2002; 223:723–30.
25. Goffette PP, Laterre PF. Traumatic injuries: imaging and intervention in post-traumatic complications (delayed intervention). Eur Radiol 2002; 12:994–1021.
26. Pinto IT, Chimeno PC. Treatment of a urinoma and a post-traumatic pseudoaneurysm using selective arterial embolization. Cardiovasc Intervent Radiol 1998; 21:506–8.
27. Oesterling JE, Fishman EK, Goldman SM, Marshall FF. The management of renal angiomyolipoma. J Urol 1986; 135:1121–4.
28. Kehagias D, Mourikis D, Kousaris M, Chatziioannou A, Vlahos L. Management of renal angiomyolipoma by selective arterial embolization. Urol Int 1998; 60:113–17.
29. Kalman D, Varenhorst E. The role of arterial embolization in renal cell carcinoma. Scand J Urol Nephrol 1999; 33:162–70.
30. Mitra K, Prabhudesai V, James R et al. Renal artery embolization: a first line treatment option for end-stage hydronephrosis. Cardiovasc Intervent Radiol 2004; 27:204–7.
31. Husmann DA, Morris JS. Attempted nonoperative management of blunt renal lacerations extending through the corticomedullary junction: the short-term and long-term sequelae. J Urol 1990; 143:682–4.
32. Husmann DA, Gilling PJ, Perry MO, Morris JS, Boone TB. Major renal lacerations with a devitalized fragment following blunt abdominal trauma: a comparison between nonoperative (expectant) versus surgical management. J Urol 1993; 150:1774–7.
33. Bozeman C, Carver B, Zabari G, Caldito G, Venable D. Selective operative management of major blunt renal trauma. J Trauma 2004; 57:305–9.
34. Keller MS, Coln CE, Garza JJ et al. Functional outcome of nonoperatively managed renal injuries in children. J Trauma 2004; 57:108–10.
35. Philpott JM, Nance ML, Carr MC, Canning DA, Stafford PW. Ureteral stenting in the management of urinoma after severe blunt renal trauma in children. J Pediatr Surg 2003; 38:1096–8.
36. Moog R, Becmeur F, Dutson E, Chevalier-Kauffmann I, Sauvage P, Brunot B. Functional evaluation by quantitative dimercaptosuccinic acid scintigraphy after kidney trauma in children. J Urol 2003; 169:641–4.
37. Wessels H, Deirmenjian J, McAninch J. Preservation of renal function after reconstruction for trauma: quantitative assessment with radionuclide scintigraphy. J Urol 1997; 157:1583–6.
38. Hammer C, Santucci R. Effect of an institutional policy of nonoperative treatment of grade 1–4 renal injuries. J Urol 2003; 169:1751–3.
39. Velmahos GC, Degiannis E. The management of urinary tract injuries after gunshot wounds of the anterior and posterior abdomen. Injury 1997; 28:535–8.
40. Velmahos GC, Demetriades D. Is nonoperative management of abdominal gunshot wounds reasonable? Adv Surg 2002; 36:123–40.
41. Pryor JP, Reilly PM, Dabrowski GP, Grossman MD, Schwab CW. Nonoperative management of abdominal gunshot wounds. Ann Emerg Med 2004; 43:344–53.
42. Hudolin T, Hudolin I. Surgical management of urogenital injuries at a war hospital in Bosnia-Hrzegovina, 1992 to 1995. J Urol 2003; 169:1357–9.
43. al-Ali M, Haddad L. The late treatment of 63 overlooked or complicated ureteral missile injuries: the promise of nephrostomy and role of autotransplantation. J Urol 1996; 156:1918–21.
44. Perez-Brayfield MR, Keane TE, Krishnan A et al. Gunshot wounds to the ureter: a 40-year experience at Grady Memorial Hospital. J Urol 2001; 166:119–21.
45. Cass A, Ireland G. Comparison of the conservative and surgical management of the more severe degrees of renal trauma in multiple injured patients. J Urol 1973; 109:8–11.
46. Cass AS, Luxenberg M, Gleich P, Smith C. Long-term results of conservative and surgical management of blunt renal lacerations. Br J Urol 1987; 59:17–20.
47. Kristjanson A, Pederson J. Management of blunt renal trauma. Br J Urol 1993; 72:692–6.
48. Wessells H, McAninch J. Effect of colon injury on the management of simultaneous renal trauma. J Urol 1996; 155:1852–6.
49. Gonzalez RP, Falimirski M, Holevar MR, Evankovich C. Surgical management of renal trauma: is vascular control necessary? J Trauma 1999; 47:1039–42.
50. Santucci RA, McAninch JW, Safir MA et al. Validation of the American Association for the Surgery of Trauma organ injury severity scale for the kidney. J Trauma 2001; 50:195–200.
51. Santucci RA, McAninch J. Grade IV renal injuries: evaluation, treatment, and outcome. World J Surg 2001; 25:1565–72.
52. Altman AL, Haas C, Dinchmann KH, Spirnak JP. Selective nonoperative management of blunt grade 5 renal injury. J Urol 2000; 164:27–31.
53. Corriere JJ, McAndrew J, Benson G. Intraoperative decision making in urology. J Trauma 1991; 31:1390–2.
54. el Khader K, Mhidia A, Ziade J et al. [Conservative treatment of stage III kidney injuries]. Acta Urol Belg 1998; 66:25–8. [French]
55. Matthews LA, Smith EM, Spirnak JP. Nonoperative treatment of major blunt renal lacerations with urinary extravasation. J Urol 1997; 157:2056–8.
56. El-Sherbiny MT, Aboul-Ghar ME, Hafez AT, Hammad AA, Bazeed MA. Late renal functional and morphological evaluation after non-operative treatment of high-grade renal injuries in children. BJU Int 2004; 93:1053–6.

Section IV

The Ureter

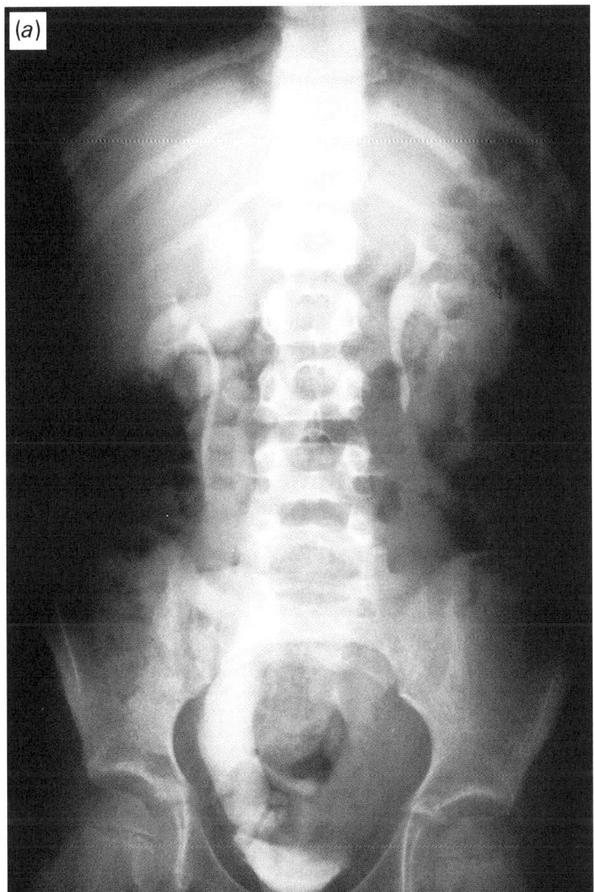

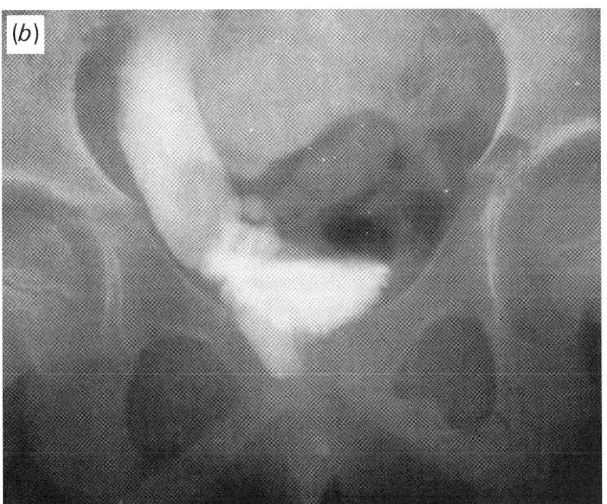

Figure 37.9 An intravenous pyelogram (IVP) showing a right duplex kidney and with an obstructed ectopic upper pole ureter. (*a*) An image from an IVP demonstrates right upper pole moderate, hydroureteronephrosis. The right lower pole and left kidney and collecting systems appear normal. (*b*) The right upper pole has a low ectopic ureteral insertion, below the bladder neck into the vagina.

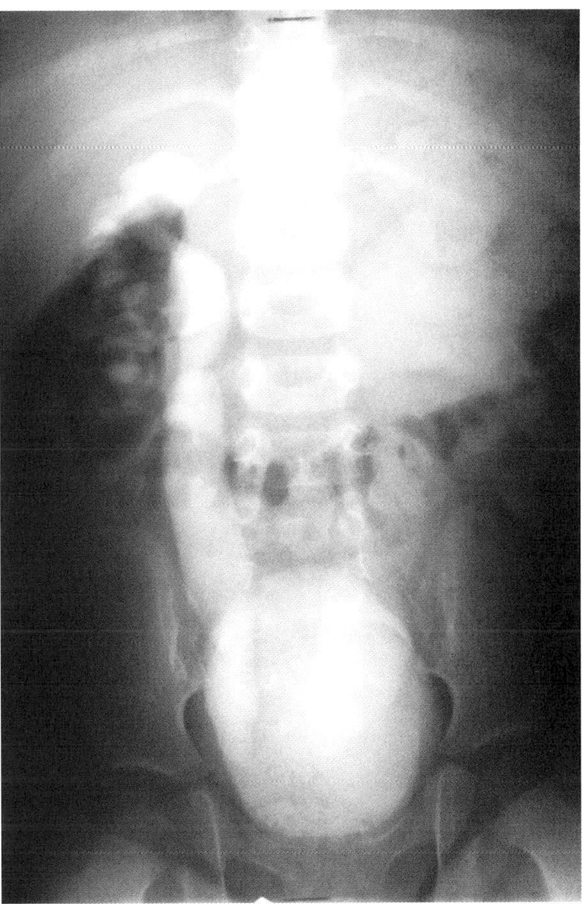

Figure 37.10 A bilateral primary megaureter. An intravenous pyelogram at 2 hours demonstrates left greater than right moderate to severe hydroureteronephrosis. There is marked delayed excretion bilaterally, especially on the left. The sites of ureteral insertion are normal.

should be treated surgically without delay. The IVP with delayed images may allow one to visualize the distal ureter in order to make this important distinction, whereas ultrasound cannot.

Postoperative assessment

For many patients who undergo repair of an UPJ or UVJ obstruction, the hydronephrosis or hydroureteronephrosis does not resolve dramatically on early (1–3 month) postoperative ultrasound imaging. In this setting, an IVP may be invaluable in demonstrating signs of improved excretion and drainage relative to preoperative studies that confirm that a good result is evolving. Alternatively, the IVP is an excellent study for demonstrating a technically poor surgical result, if one fails to see a dependent, funneled anastomosis.

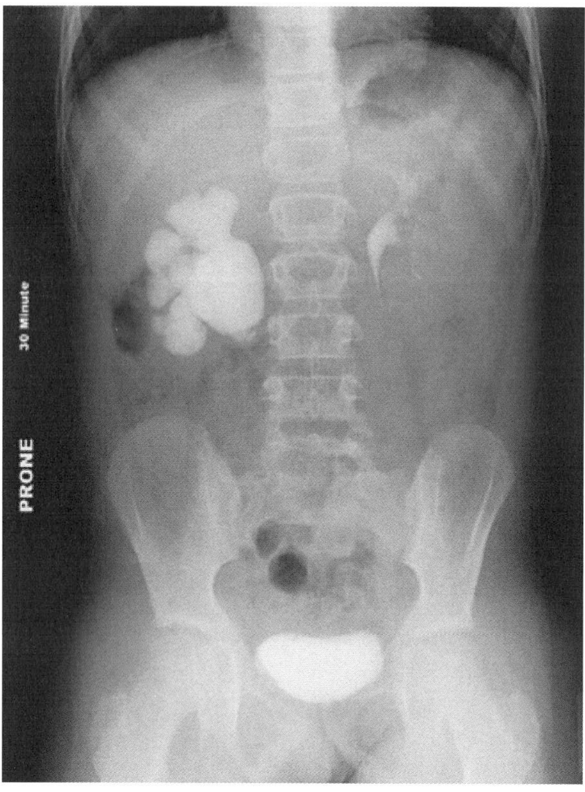

Figure 37.11 An intravenous pyelogram of an 8-year-old boy demonstrating ureteropelvic junction obstruction associated with a crossing lower pole vessel. Note the linear filling defect at the inferior aspect of the renal pelvis.

A setting in which IVP is particularly valuable is in looking for an anterior crossing vessel that may produce intermittent kinking at the UPJ and, as a result, intermittent renal colic. Such a vessel may present as a proximal ureteral filling defect that disappears after surgically transposing the pelvis and ureter anterior to the crossing lower pole artery (Figure 37.11).

MAG3 renal scan

Introduction

During dynamic renal scintigraphy, the activity of intravenously injected ^{99m}Tc MAG is imaged and measured to assess the form and function of the kidney and ureters. ^{99m}Tc DTPA (diethylenetriamine penta-acetic acid) is a less preferred agent. These agents show excellent images of the functioning renal cortex and the collecting system. The time–activity curve, or time for uptake and excretion of the radiotracer, is measured and compared with normal values.

Diuresis renography is performed to distinguish urinary obstruction from a dilated non-obstructed renal collecting system. After initial imaging during a dynamic renal scan, a diuretic, typically furosemide, is injected intravenously. The kidney's ability to drain the radiopharmaceutical over time is measured. In significantly obstructed kidneys, radiotracer fails to be excreted normally.

The Society for Fetal Urology and the Pediatric Nuclear Medicine Council developed the 'well-tempered' diuretic renogram to standardize the evaluation of asymptomatic neonates with hydronephrosis or hydroureteronephrosis.[25] Patients need to be well hydrated prior to the examination. Guidelines are specified within the 'well-tempered' diuretic renogram protocol.

Several patient factors can confound the interpretation of the diuretic renograms. The appearance of refluxed contrast in the collecting system may mimic normal function in a patient with impaired function. Thus, the bladder should be drained by catheter in children with reflux who cannot void spontaneously. Infants, especially those younger than 1 month of age, have functionally immature kidneys, and do not concentrate the radiopharmaceutical into the urine well.[26,27] Studies performed in the first month of life need to interpreted with this in mind. Similarly, kidneys with impaired function may not respond to diuresis. As a result, intravenous urography, renal angiography, and other tests using contrast agents eliminated by the kidneys may have reduced renal uptake and prolong the time for examination.

Hydronephrosis, hydroureteronephrosis, and obstruction

For the assessment of a hydronephrotic kidney or hydroureteronephrotic collecting system the MAG3 renal scan provides quantitative information regarding renal function and drainage of the dilated system. Based on the results of the MAG3 scan, one can determine whether or not relative renal function appears to have been compromised and whether drainage is in the normal, intermediate or obstructive range: clearance time of half of tracer ($T_{1/2}$) <15 minutes is normal, 15–20 minutes intermediate, and >20 minutes obstructive.[28] This information is particularly crucial for the postnatal assessment of prenatal hydronephrosis in healthy, asymptomatic babies. Typically, one waits until 1 month of age prior to performing the MAG3 scan in order to assure adequate renal maturity; then, the severity of an apparent UPJ or UVJ obstruction can be accurately assessed. These functional results, in conjunction with postnatal ultra-

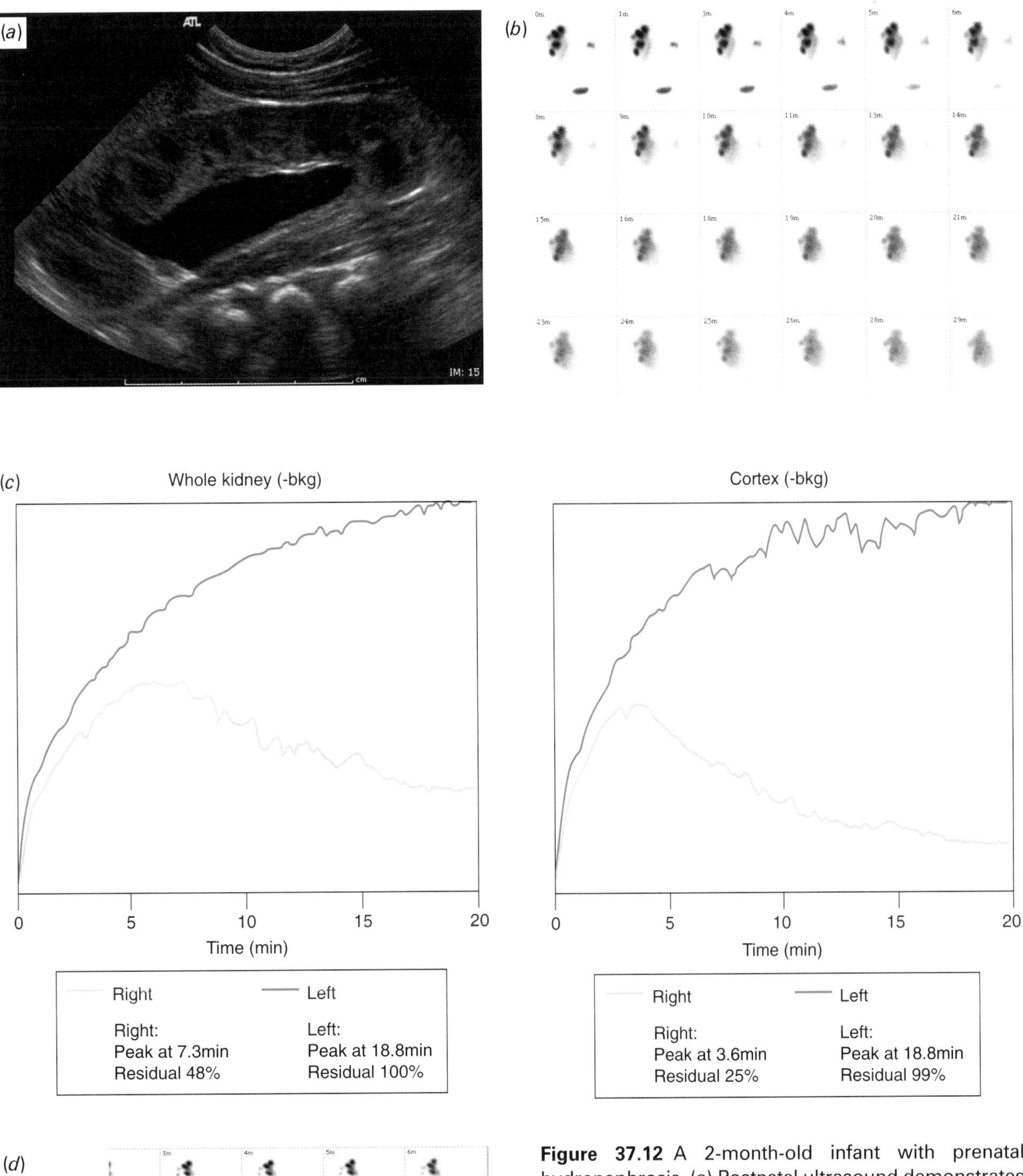

Figure 37.12 A 2-month-old infant with prenatal hydronephrosis. (*a*) Postnatal ultrasound demonstrates unilateral moderate hydronephrosis. (*b* and *c*) Initial MAG3 study with lasix demonstrates delayed drainage of the left kidney as a result of a ureteropelvic junction obstruction. The time–activity curve demonstrates delayed excretion of contrast in the obstructive range. (*d*) Postoperative MAG3 examination demonstrates improvement.

sound findings (Figure 37.12), should enable one to develop a rational management plan – rarely for immediate surgery, and usually for follow-up imaging, entailing serial ultrasound or MAG3 studies, depending upon the initial findings.

Computed tomography/computed axial tomography

Introduction

Computed tomography, also known as computerized axial tomography (CAT), is a widely used modality for pediatric ureteral imaging because of its applicability to stone disease, trauma, and the evaluation of renal masses.

Early CT scans acquired one 'slice' or axial cross section of information at a time. With spiral or helical scanners, X-rays are emitted and detected as the patient moves continuously through the scanner, creating a volume of information. Multislice or multidetector CT (MDCT) scanners have multiple detectors rotating simultaneously around the patient with the effect of increasing spatial resolution and decreasing the time to perform a study over standard spiral scanners.

With a volume of information created, images can be reconstructed in many planes and reformatted to enhance the conspicuity of ureters. The ease and speed of obtaining large quantities of information by CT scan needs to be weighed against the radiation risk and financial cost of the examination. The absorbed radiation dose of a single CT scan of the abdomen is eight times that of an abdominal radiograph. The rapidly growing tissues of children are very susceptible to the deleterious effects of radiation.

Contrast- and non-contrast-enhanced CT scans are used in the evaluation of the ureter. Non-contrast-enhanced CT is used for the evaluation of nephroureterolithiasis and resulting obstruction. Contrast-enhanced CT, especially timed during the excretory phase, is useful for showing the opacified ureters. Multiphase CT scans evaluate the genitourinary system without contrast, then with contrast, timed to the cortical and excretory phases of contrast enhancement. Multiphase CT scans should be used sparingly in children because of their high radiation doses.

Methods used to enhance ureteral opacification after contrast administration include abdominal compression with bellows,[29] intravenous (IV) hydration during the examination,[30] prone and supine imaging,[31] multiplanar reformatting, and virtual endoscopy. The angiographic phase of contrast enhancement is useful in clarifying vascular anatomy in the cases of trauma or UPJ obstruction.[32–34]

Nephroureterolithiasis

The spiral CT scan, without contrast, can rapidly assess the upper tract for a calculus. On the basis of Hounsfield units (Hu), it has the advantage, relative to ultrasound, of distinguishing a stone from an air bubble or intraluminal polyp. Its disadvantage is the ionizing radiation entailed. For patients with VUR, air bubbles may be introduced at the time of a VCUG, producing an upper tract echogenic lesion and mimicking stone on renal ultrasound. Radiolucent filling defects on IVP, which may represent uric acid calculi, can be confirmed as such with CT scan.

Two methods, non-contrast-enhanced CT scan and the combination of ultrasound and plain film, have largely replaced IVP for the initial evaluation of stone disease (Figure 37.13). Non-contrast CT and ultrasound with plain films are more sensitive examinations than IVP,[35–37] have no risk of contrast reaction, and often find alternative diagnoses. Low-dose CT methods for detecting urolithiasis confer approximately double the radiation dose of an IVP.[38]

Although non-contrast CT has greater sensitivity, negative predictive value, and accuracy than the combination of ultrasound and plain films, both methods yield comparable results without causing significant differences in clinical management.[39] Given the often

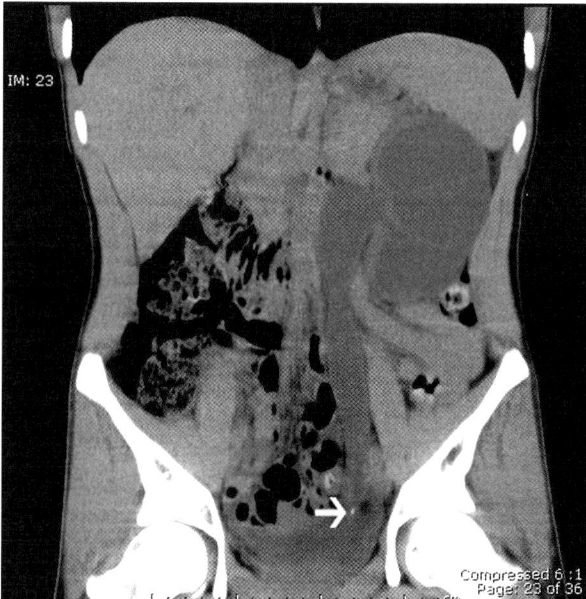

Figure 37.13 Computed tomography with coronal reformatting showing a left ureterovesical junction calculus (arrow) in a patient with a primary megaureter.

lower test cost and absence of ionizing radiation, ultrasound is often the first modality of choice[40] in children.

Ureteral trauma

In the assessment of urologic trauma, the CT scan with contrast is invaluable. Images performed during the excretory phase of contrast enhancement are the best for the evaluation of the ureter.[41–43] Computed tomography is capable of demonstrating extravasation as a result of pelviureteric disruption of the UPJ secondary to hyperextension injuries or ureteral disruption (Figure 37.14) from penetrating trauma. It also affords one the capability of assessing injuries to associated organs such as the spleen or liver.

Other ureteral anomalies

Computed tomography has a wide range of uses, including the assessment of an abnormal course of the ureter such as a retrocaval ureter,[44] ectopic ureteral insertion,[45] or ureteral obstruction. The CT scan with contrast is also valuable in assessing the solid retroperitoneal mass, such as Wilms' tumor or neuroblastoma, and its effect on ureteral anatomy.

Specialized opacification techniques

Introduction

The specialized opacification techniques enable one to visualize the ureter precisely in complex anatomic or operative clinical settings.

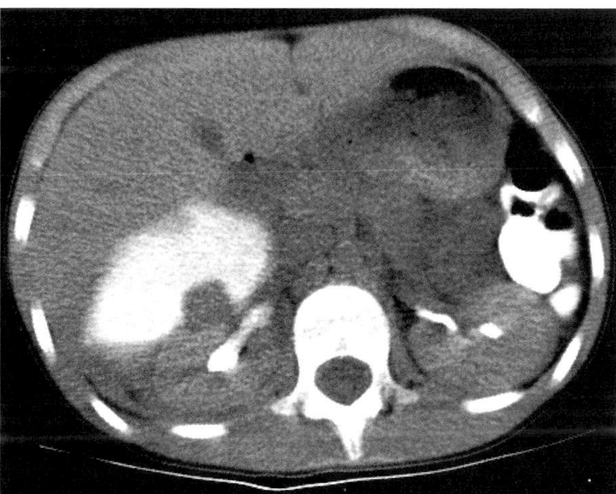

Figure 37.14 Axial computed tomography image performed during the excretory phase of contrast enhancement demonstrates right perinephric contrast extravasation resulting from a ureteral tear at the ureteropelvic junction.

Retrograde ureterography and pyelography

Retrograde ureterography and pyelography is performed cystoscopically in the anesthetized child through a ureteral catheter using one-half strength Cystograffin. It is used to opacify the distal ureter prior to pyeloplasty, to ensure normal distal ureteral anatomy, and to confirm the level of ureteral obstruction. It can be invaluable in distinguishing a typical UPJ obstruction from rare lesions such as fibroepithelial polyps of the UPJ and mid-ureteral strictures.[46] Retrograde pyelography is also useful in the assessment of ureteral trauma and evaluation of the stone patient prior to ureteral stone basketing or lithotripsy. In difficult diagnostic situations, such as unusual duplication anomalies or ectopic ureters, retrograde ureterography and pyelography can be extremely valuable in defining the anatomy (Figure 37.15).

Antegrade pyelography and ureterography

Antegrade pyelography and ureterography are uncommon studies, utilized to define unusual anatomy, often in conjunction with the goal of draining a hydronephrotic collecting system. The antegrade study can be extremely valuable in defining postsurgical complications such as obstruction or urinary extravasation. It is particularly useful in defining the anatomy of duplex collecting systems, dilated ureters draining ectopically, and collecting systems associated with poorly functioning kidneys that do not excrete contrast well.

Whitaker test

The Whitaker test is a physiologic study combined with the anatomic benefit of antegrade pyelography that is used to assess upper tract obstruction.[47] The Whitaker test is performed with percutaneous access to the kidney and catheter drainage of the bladder. Pressures within the renal pelvis and bladder are measured during a constant infusion of contrast into the renal pelvis. Pressure differentials between kidney and bladder of <15 cmH_2O are considered normal, whereas pressure differentials >20 cmH_2O are consistent with obstruction. During the course of the study, imaging of the ureter clearly demonstrates the level of obstruction (Figure 37.16). This test is particularly valuable in assessing a postoperative result when hydronephrosis persists and renal function is so impaired that nuclear renography is non-diagnostic.

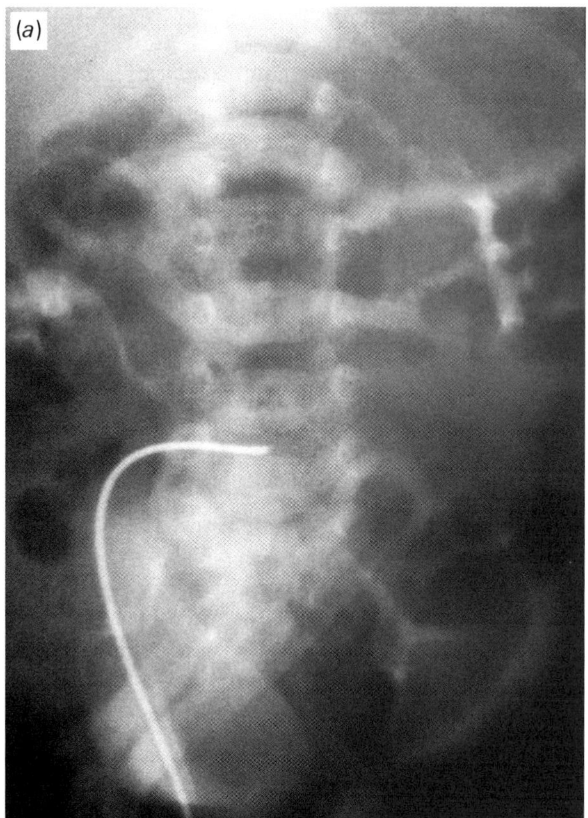

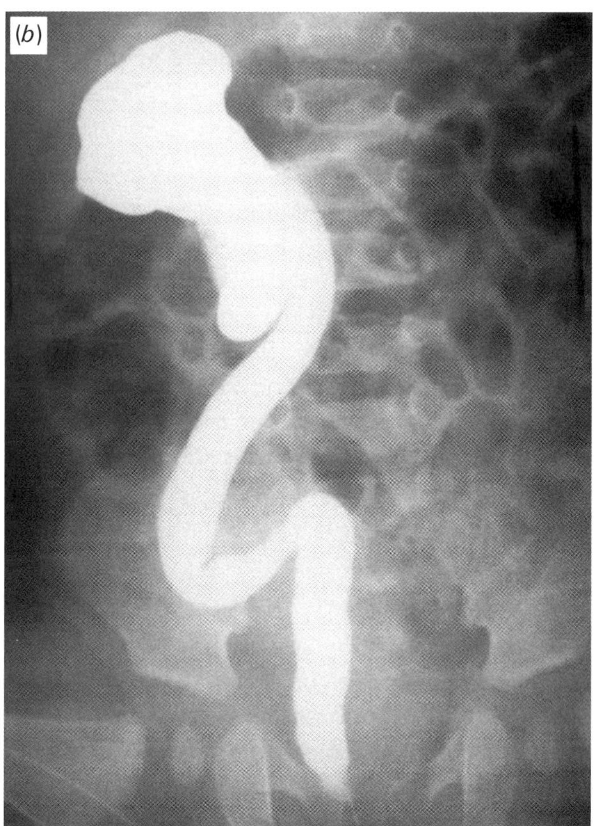

Figure 37.15 An intravenous pyelogram (IVP) and a retrograde ureterogram of a patient with a right upper pole ectopic ureter. (*a*) An IVP of a newborn infant demonstrates lateral deviation of the right lower pole collecting system. The left kidney appears normal. (*b*) A retrograde ureterogram demonstrates the ectopic upper pole ureter and pelvis.

Magnetic resonance urography

Magnetic resonance urography (MRU) offers the combination of high-resolution anatomic imaging and functional information of the genitourinary system without radiation. In children, MRU is used to evaluate urinary tract dilatation[22] and differentiate it from obstruction,[48,49] evaluate complex genitourinary anatomy,[50] and assess the ureters.[51]

MRU is more accurate than ultrasound[52] and IVP[51] in assessing renal anatomy and can provide functional imaging comparable with renal diuretic scintigraphy.[49,53] Unlike IVP and scintigraphy, visualization of the ureters and kidneys is not dependent on renal function. MRU is especially useful in children with poorly functioning kidneys and obstruction (Figure 37.17) or

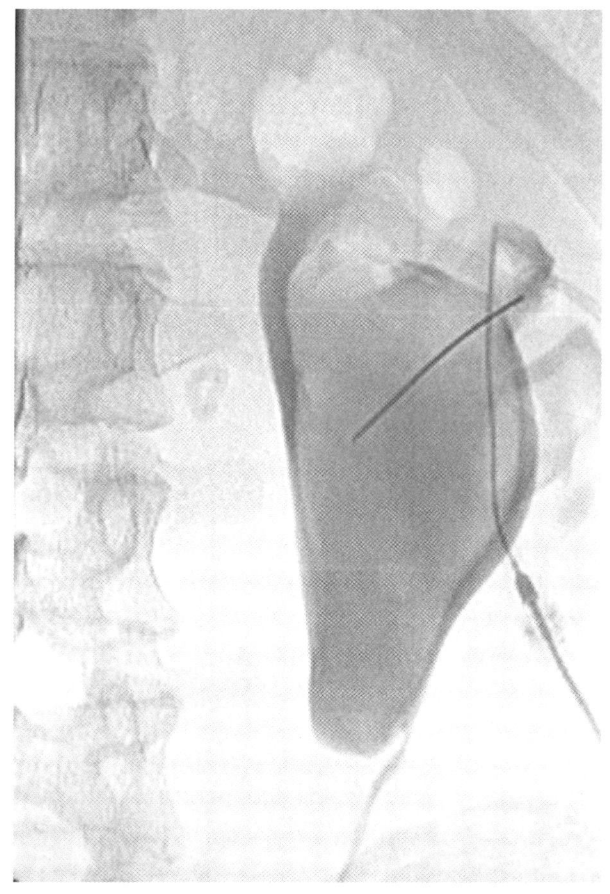

Figure 37.16 Whitaker test in 17-year-old boy following left pyeloplasty, having intermittent flank pain, consistent with slightly high insertion of ureter, but no obstruction.

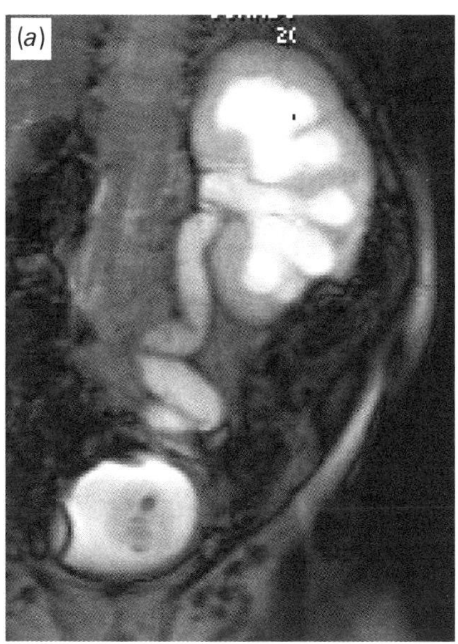

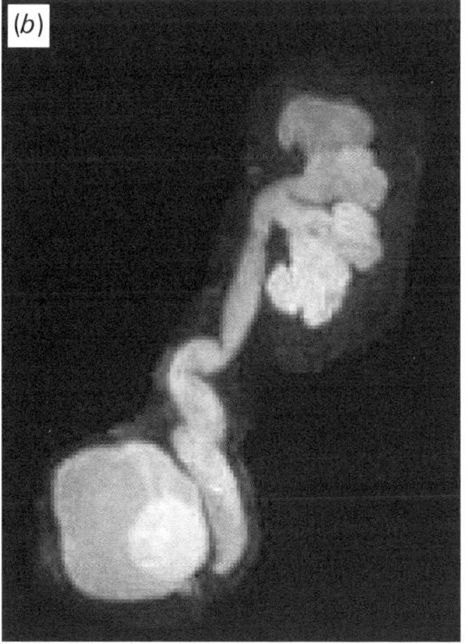

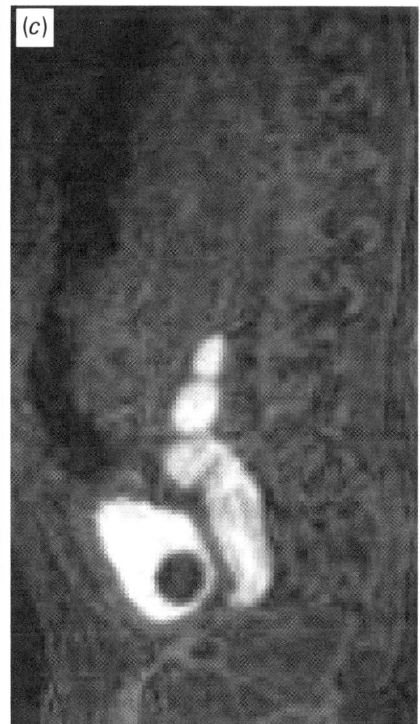

Figure 37.17 (*a–c*) Magnetic resonance urograms show an ectopically inserting obstructed solitary left ureter.

complex anatomy. Some clinicians advocate this method to replace ultrasound and renal diuretic scintigraphy in the evaluation of hydronephrosis.[49]

Many protocols are widely available.[48,49,54–56] Modern MR techniques and improved coils allow for improved spatial and temporal resolution and faster acquisition time. The fast-imaging MR techniques allow evaluation of parenchymal perfusion, glomerular filtration rate,[57] renal excretory function, and urinary drainage.[58] The main limitation of MRU is the relatively long duration of the examination (approximately 30–45 minutes), which often necessitates sedation in young or uncooperative children.

Key points

1 Ultrasound is the initial imaging modality for most forms of ureteral pathology.
2 Nuclear medicine or contrast studies remain essential for the evaluation of VUR.
3 Opacification techniques and MRI are both valuable for imaging of more complex pathology.
4 A CT scan is valuable for stone, trauma, and tumor evaluation.

References

1. Paltiel HJ, Rupich RC, Kiruluta HG. Enhanced detection of vesicoureteral reflux in infants and children with use of cyclic voiding cystourethrography. Radiology 1992; 184:753–5.
2. Koff SA. Estimating bladder capacity in children. Urology 1983; 21:248.
3. Berger RM, Maizels M, Moran GC, Conway JJ, Firlit CF. Bladder capacity (ounces) equals age (years) plus 2 predicts normal bladder capacity and aids in diagnosis of abnormal voiding patterns. J Urol 1983; 129:347–9.
4. Diamond DA, Kleinman PK, Spevak M et al. The tailored low dose fluoroscopic voiding cystogram for familial reflux screening. J Urol 1996; 155:681–2.
5. Kleinman PK, Diamond DA, Karellas A et al. Tailored low-dose fluoroscopic voiding cystourethrography for the reevaluation of vesicoureteral reflux in girls. AJR Am J Roentgenol 1994; 162:1151–4; discussion 1155–6.
6. Mooney RB, McKinstry J. Paediatric dose reduction with the introduction of digital fluorography. Radiat Prot Dosimetry 2001; 94:117–20.
7. Persliden J, Helmrot E, Hjort P, Resjo M. Dose and image quality in the comparison of analogue and digital techniques in paediatric urology examinations. Eur Radiol 2004; 14:638–44.
8. Hernandez RJ, Goodsitt MM. Reduction of radiation dose in pediatric patients using pulsed fluoroscopy. AJR Am J Roentgenol 1996; 167:1247–53.
9. Boland GW, Murphy B, Arellano R, Niklason L, Mueller PR. Dose reduction in gastrointestinal and genitourinary fluoroscopy: use of grid-controlled pulsed fluoroscopy. AJR Am J Roentgenol 2000; 175:1453–7.
10. Bazopoulos EV, Prassopoulos PK, Damilakis JE et al. A comparison between digital fluoroscopic hard copies and 105-mm spot films in evaluating vesicoureteric reflux in children. Pediatr Radiol 1998; 28:162–6.
11. Ward V, Barnewolt C, Strauss K et al. Radiation exposure and image quality: preliminary results of a comparison of viable-rate pulsed fluoroscopy with continuous

fluoroscopy in a swine model of pediatric genitourinary abnormalities. Miami, FL: Annual Meeting of Association of University Radiologists, 2003: 8–54.

12. Darge K, Troeger J. Vesicoureteral reflux grading in contrast-enhanced voiding urosonography. Eur J Radiol 2002; 43:122–8.
13. Mentzel HJ, Vogt S, Patzer L et al. Contrast-enhanced sonography of vesicoureterorenal reflux in children: preliminary results. AJR Am J Roentgenol 1999; 173: 737–40.
14. Darge K, Troeger J, Duetting T et al. Reflux in young patients: comparison of voiding US of the bladder and retrovesical space with echo enhancement versus voiding cystourethrography for diagnosis. Radiology 1999; 210:201–7.
15. Valentini AL, Salvaggio E, Manzoni C et al. Contrast-enhanced gray-scale and color Doppler voiding urosonography versus voiding cystourethrography in the diagnosis and grading of vesicoureteral reflux. J Clin Ultrasound 2001; 29:65–71.
16. Galia M, Midiri M, Pennisi F et al. Vesicoureteral reflux in young patients: comparison of voiding color Doppler US with echo enhancement versus voiding cystourethrography for diagnosis or exclusion. Abdom Imaging 2004; 29:303–8.
17. Galloy MA, Mandry D, Pecastaings M, Mainard-Simard L, Claudon M. [Sonocystography: a new method for the diagnosis and follow-up of vesico-ureteric reflux in children]. J Radiol 2003; 84:2055–61.
18. Mate A, Bargiela A, Mosteiro S, Diaz A, Bello MJ. Contrast ultrasound of the urethra in children. Eur Radiol 2003; 13:1534–7.
19. McGee K. The role of a child life specialist in a pediatric radiology department. Pediatr Radiol 2003; 33:467–74.
20. Elder JS, Longenecker R. Premedication with oral midazolam for voiding cystourethrography in children: safety and efficacy. AJR Am J Roentgenol 1995; 164:1229–32.
21. Practice parameter: the diagnosis, treatment, and evaluation of the initial urinary tract infection in febrile infants and young children. American Academy of Pediatrics. Committee on Quality Improvement. Subcommittee on Urinary Tract Infection. Pediatrics 1999; 103:843–52.
22. Riccabona M. Potential of modern sonographic techniques in paediatric uroradiology. Eur J Radiol 2002; 43:110–21.
23. Kenney IJ, Negus AS, Miller FN. Is sonographically demonstrated mild distal ureteric dilatation predictive of vesicoureteric reflux as seen on micturating cystourethrography? Pediatr Radiol 2002; 32:175–8.
24. Cvitkovic Kuzmic A, Brkljacic B, Rados M, Galesic K. Doppler visualization of ureteric jets in unilateral hydronephrosis in children and adolescents. Eur J Radiol 2001; 39:209–14.
25. Conway JJ, Maizels M. The 'well tempered' diuretic renogram: a standard method to examine the asymptomatic neonate with hydronephrosis or hydroureteronephrosis. A report from combined meetings of The Society for Fetal Urology and members of The Pediatric Nuclear Medicine Council – The Society of Nuclear Medicine. J Nucl Med 1992; 33:2047–51.
26. Treves S, Majid M, Kuruc A et al. In: Treves ST, ed. Pediatric Nuclear Medicine, 2nd ed. New York: Springer-Verlag, 1995: 339–99.
27. Schofer O, Konig G, Bartels U et al. Technetium–99m mercaptoacetyltriglycine clearance: reference values for infants and children. Eur J Nucl Med 1995; 22:1278–81.
28. Kass EJ, Fink-Bennett D. Contemporary techniques for the radioisotopic evaluation of the dilated urinary tract. Urol Clin North Am 1990; 17:273–89.
29. Caoili EM, Cohan RH, Korobkin M et al. Effectiveness of abdominal compression during helical renal CT. Acad Radiol 2001; 8:1100–6.
30. McTavish JD, Jinzaki M, Zou KH, Nawfel RD, Silverman SG. Multi-detector row CT urography: comparison of strategies for depicting the normal urinary collecting system. Radiology 2002; 225:783–90.
31. Levine J, Neitlich J, Smith RC. The value of prone scanning to distinguish ureterovesical junction stones from ureteral stones that have passed into the bladder: leave no stone unturned. AJR Am J Roentgenol 1999; 172:977–81.
32. Rabah D, Soderdahl DW, McAdams PD et al. Ureteropelvic junction obstruction: does CT angiography allow better selection of therapeutic modalities and better patient outcome? J Endourol 2004; 18:427–30.
33. Mitsumori A, Yasui K, Akaki S et al. Evaluation of crossing vessels in patients with ureteropelvic junction obstruction by means of helical CT. Radiographics 2000; 20:1383–93, discussion 1393–5.
34. Rouviere O, Lyonnet D, Berger P et al. Ureteropelvic junction obstruction: use of helical CT for preoperative assessment – comparison with intraarterial angiography. Radiology 1999; 213:668–73.
35. Shokeir AA, Abdulmaaboud M. Prospective comparison of nonenhanced helical computerized tomography and Doppler ultrasonography for the diagnosis of renal colic. J Urol 2001; 165:1082–4.
36. Miller OF, Rineer SK, Reichard SR et al. Prospective comparison of unenhanced spiral computed tomography and intravenous urogram in the evaluation of acute flank pain. Urology 1998; 52:982–7.
37. Fielding JR, Silverman SG, Samuel S, Zou KH, Loughlin KR. Unenhanced helical CT of ureteral stones: a replacement for excretory urography in planning treatment. AJR Am J Roentgenol 1998; 171:1051–3.
38. Liu W, Esler SJ, Kenny BJ et al. Low-dose nonenhanced helical CT of renal colic: assessment of ureteric stone detection and measurement of effective dose equivalent. Radiology 2000; 215:51–4.
39. Catalano O, Nunziata A, Altei F, Siani A. Suspected ureteral colic: primary helical CT versus selective helical CT after unenhanced radiography and sonography. AJR Am J Roentgenol 2002; 178:379–87.
40. Patlas M, Farkas A, Fisher D, Zaghal I, Hadas-Halpern I. Ultrasound vs CT for the detection of ureteric stones in patients with renal colic. Br J Radiol 2001; 74:901–4.
41. McNicholas MM, Raptopoulos VD, Schwartz RK et al. Excretory phase CT urography for opacification of the urinary collecting system. AJR Am J Roentgenol 1998; 170:1261–7.
42. Siegel MJ, Balfe DM. Blunt renal and ureteral trauma in childhood: CT patterns of fluid collections. AJR Am J Roentgenol 1989; 152:1043–7.

43. Templeton PA, Mirvis SE, Whitley NO. Traumatic avulsion of the ureter: computed tomography correlation. J Comput Tomogr 1988; 12:159–60.
44. Lautin EM, Haramati N, Frager D et al. CT diagnosis of circumcaval ureter. AJR Am J Roentgenol 1988; 150:591–4.
45. Schwartz ML, Kenney PJ, Bueschen AJ. Computed tomographic diagnosis of ectopic ureter with seminal vesicle cyst. Urology 1988; 31:55–6.
46. Cockrell SN, Hendren WH. The importance of visualizing the ureter before performing a pyeloplasty. J Urol 1990; 144:588–92, discussion 593–4.
47. Whitaker RH. Methods of assessing obstruction in dilated ureters. Br J Urol 1973; 45:15–22.
48. Jones RA, Perez-Brayfield MR, Kirsch AJ, Grattan-Smith JD. Renal transit time with MR urography in children. Radiology 2004; 233:41–50.
49. Grattan-Smith JD, Perez-Bayfield MR, Jones RA et al. MR imaging of kidneys: functional evaluation using F-15 perfusion imaging. Pediatr Radiol 2003; 33:293–304.
50. Avni FE, Nicaise N, Hall M et al. The role of MR imaging for the assessment of complicated duplex kidneys in children: preliminary report. Pediatr Radiol 2001; 31:215–23.
51. Leppert A, Nadalin S, Schirg E et al. Impact of magnetic resonance urography on preoperative diagnostic workup in children affected by hydronephrosis: should IVU be replaced? J Pediatr Surg 2002; 37:1441–5.
52. Riccabona M, Ruppert-Kohlmayr A, Ring E et al. Potential impact of pediatric MR urography on the imaging algorithm in patients with a functional single kidney. AJR Am J Roentgenol 2004; 183:795–800.
53. Rohrschneider WK, Haufe S, Wiesel M et al. Functional and morphologic evaluation of congenital urinary tract dilatation by using combined static-dynamic MR urography: findings in kidneys with a single collecting system. Radiology 2002; 224:683–94.
54. Riccabona M, Simbrunner J, Ring E et al. Feasibility of MR urography in neonates and infants with anomalies of the upper urinary tract. Eur Radiol 2002; 12:1442–50.
55. Borthne AS, Pierre-Jerome C, Gjesdal KI et al. Pediatric excretory MR urography: comparative study of enhanced and non-enhanced techniques. Eur Radiol 2003; 13:1423–7.
56. Staatz G, Nolte-Ernsting CC, Adam GB et al. Feasibility and utility of respiratory-gated, gadolinium-enhanced T1-weighted magnetic resonance urography in children. Invest Radiol 2000; 35:504–12.
57. Hackstein N, Heckrodt J, Rau WS. Measurement of single-kidney glomerular filtration rate using a contrast-enhanced dynamic gradient-echo sequence and the Rutland–Patlak plot technique. J Magn Reson Imaging 2003; 18:714–25.
58. Rohrschneider WK, Becker K, Hoffend J et al. Combined static-dynamic MR urography for the simultaneous evaluation of morphology and function in urinary tract obstruction. II. Findings in experimentally induced ureteric stenosis. Pediatr Radiol 2000; 30:523–32.

Ureteral anomalies and their surgical management

38

Christopher S Cooper

Introduction

Aside from ureteropelvic junction (UPJ) or ureterovesical junction (UVJ) obstruction, the pediatric urologist is occasionally confronted with relatively rare causes of ureteral obstruction. These causes include the retrocaval ureter, ureteral strictures or valves, as well as ureteral polyps. The diagnosis of these conditions may follow clinical symptoms of obstruction such as pain, hematuria, or urinary tract infection. Increasingly, the diagnosis of these entities occurs as an incidental finding with anatomic imaging for non-urologic symptoms. This chapter provides a basic description of these rare conditions and management options.

Surgical technique

Ureteral obstruction often dictates operative intervention. Ureteral operations by open or laparoscopic techniques require adherence to certain basic principles. The blood supply to the mid ureter is more tenuous than that of the proximal and distal ureter. The abdominal segment of the ureter receives its blood supply from the renal and gonadal arteries. The pelvic segment of the ureter receives branches from the vesical and middle rectal vessels and, at times, from the common or internal iliac arteries. The adventitia supports multiple blood vessels and nerve fibers. The vessels of the ureter penetrate first through the muscular layers, where they supply the ureter with capillaries, and then form a plexus in the deep aspect of the mucosa.[1] To preserve the adventitia and blood supply, the ureter is usually mobilized with as much surrounding soft tissue as possible. Ischemic injury resulting from indelicate tissue handling will result in ureteral stricture. Delicate handling is, therefore, a requirement for successful ureteral reconstruction and often requires a 'no-touch' technique utilizing ureteral traction sutures.

Critical to the success of ureteral reconstruction is the creation of a tension-free anastomosis. Data from experimental studies demonstrate that accurate tissue approximation without tension optimizes wound healing and decreases the amount of fibrotic tissue. At times, renal mobilization may be necessary to permit additional ureteral length. Since wound contracture constitutes a routine phase of healing, a spatulated anastomosis, when possible, helps maintain an adequate luminal diameter. Absorbable sutures are used in the anastomosis, with the knot tied outside the lumen. Stents are frequently used and serve to promote urinary flow through the ureter and diminish extravasation of urine. Extravasation is thought to result in a localized tissue reaction that inhibits regular ureteral regeneration.[2] Drains placed near the anastomosis are also frequently employed to permit evacuation of any extravasated urine from the site of repair.

Retrocaval ureter

The reported incidence of retrocaval ureter is about 1 in 1000 and occurs three times more frequently in males.[3] The retrocaval ureter almost always involves the right ureter; however, rare cases involving the left side have been reported. The retrocaval ureter is a result of anomalous vascular development and is associated with increased cardiovascular or genitourinary tract abnormalities.[4,5] In the fetus, the supracardinal vein lies dorsal to the ureter and usually forms most of the infrarenal segment of the inferior vena cava. The subcardinal, or posterior cardinal vein lies ventral to the ureter; if the subcardinal vein persists, it becomes the infrarenal segment of the vena cava. In this situation, the ureter must pass around and behind the vena cava – retrocaval ureter.[6] Most patients with a retrocaval ureter are asymptomatic; however, this anomaly may result in ureteric obstruction, presenting with pain, hematuria, urinary tract infections (UTIs), or stones. In these cases, the retrocaval segment of the ureter is often stenotic. Children are frequently diagnosed after evaluation for UTI.[4]

In the past, most cases of retrocaval ureter were found incidentally on intravenous pyelography (IVP). Two types of retrocaval ureters have been described, based on the radiographic criteria. Type I (low-loop) retrocaval ureter is more common and is associated with moderate or severe hydronephrosis, with significant medial deviation of the ureter toward the midline at the L3 level. This has been described as an S-shape or fishhook deformity (Figure 38.1). Type II (high-loop) retrocaval ureter is seen less frequently, and is associated with mild hydronephrosis and less medial deviation.[6] The widespread use of ultrasonography has resulted in more cases of retrocaval ureter being diagnosed following identification of hydronephrosis. Computed tomography (CT) and magnetic resonance imaging (MRI) scans have also been reported as excellent modalities for confirming the diagnosis.[4,7] A nuclear renal scan provides an estimate of relative renal function as well as the degree of obstruction.

Surgical treatment involves resection of the retrocaval segment and anastomosis anterior to the inferior vena cava (IVC). Frequently, redundant proximal ureter is also excised. The operative approach may be performed through the abdomen or the retroperitoneum using an open incision or via the laparoscope (Figure 38.2).[7–9]

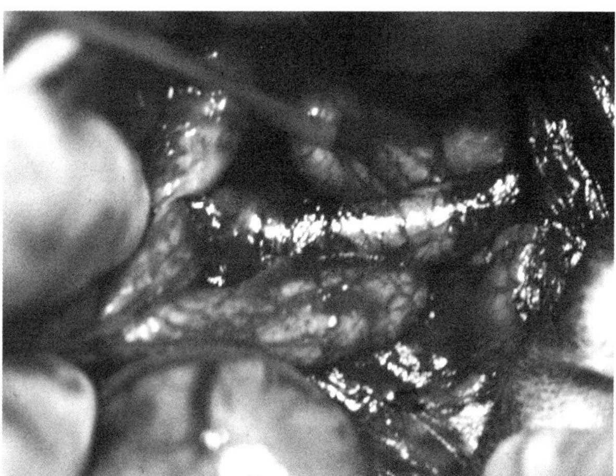

Figure 38.2 Intraoperative view of the retrocaval ureter.

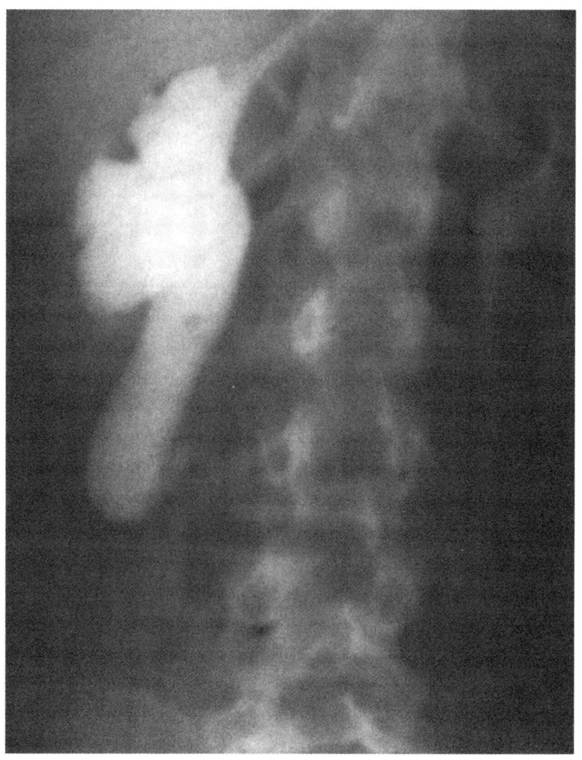

Figure 38.1 Intravenous pyelogram of a patient with a retrocaval ureter, demonstrating dilated proximal ureter with significant medial deviation at the L3 level.

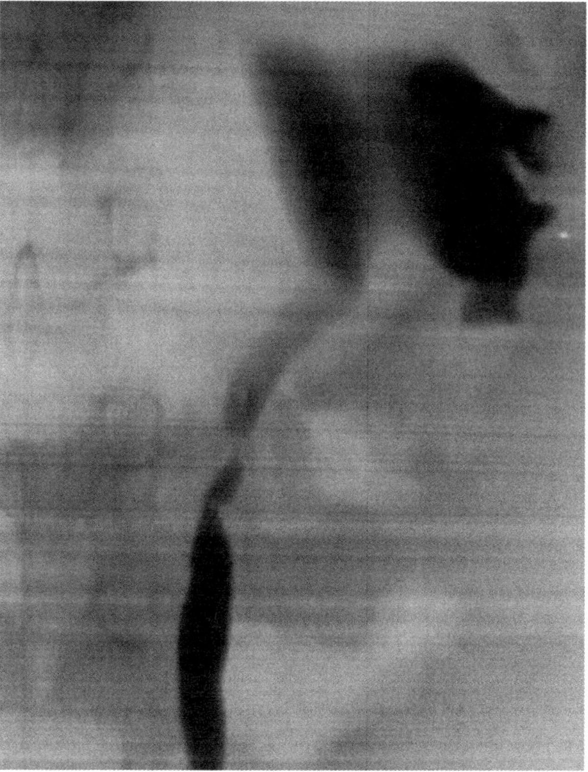

Figure 38.3 A retrograde ureteropyelogram demonstrating a short mid-proximal ureteral stenosis.

Congenital ureteral stenosis and valves

Although ureteral stenosis or strictures most commonly occur in the distal ureter and are associated with megaureters, these segments may also occur in the mid ureter (Figure 38.3). The etiology of congenital ureteral strictures is unknown; however, the location of congenital strictures is predominantly at regions of ureteral development associated with another structure or a change in form such as the junction with the bladder or renal pelvis. In children with a congenital mid ureteral stricture, an association with contralateral renal agenesis or atrophy has been reported, suggesting possible bilateral aberrant ureteral development. Aside from a narrowed lumen lined by the usual transitional epithelium, histologic findings at the site of the stenosis vary from that of thickened muscle to those with a near absence of muscle.[10,11] The symptoms of congenital ureteral strictures are variable and depend upon the degree of obstruction and renal function. The pathologic changes proximal to the stricture are a reflection of the severity and duration of the obstruction. Pyelonephritis, complicating obstruction, may lead to decreased renal function.[12]

With widespread use of prenatal ultrasonography, an increased number of children investigated for antenatal hydronephrosis are found to have congenital mid ureteral strictures. Although asymptomatic, the natural history of these strictures may require a more aggressive approach than other causes of antenatal hydronephrosis.[10] Following the identification of hydronephrosis by renal ultrasonography, a retrograde ureteropyelogram offers the most accurate method of localizing the strictured area and determining the length of the obstruction as well as providing the opportunity to catheterize or stent the ureter. The presentation of a mid ureteral stricture may mimic a classic UPJ obstruction, underscoring the importance of a retrograde ureteropyelogram if the location of the obstruction is in question.

Dilation or endoscopic incision of the ureteral stricture may be considered, but these techniques have a lower chance of success than an ureteroureterostomy or ureteral reimplant. Similar to the retrocaval ureter, treatment may require excision of redundant or kinked segments of the ureter.[12] Mobilization of the kidney may also be required to facilitate a tension-free primary ureteroureterostomy. If the narrowed segment is several centimeters, it may be best to divide the strictured segment in the middle and then spatulate through the narrowed segment in both directions as opposed to performing a complete resection of this segment. This permits use of the entire ureter and may help to avoid tension.[11]

Ureteral valves are also rare and often reported along with ureteral strictures. Valves consist of a transverse fold of tissue lined on both sides by uroepithelium and contains smooth muscle fibers that extend from the wall of the ureter and narrow the ureteral lumen.[11] They have been reported more commonly in boys and on the left side, although others have not demonstrated these associations.[13] During fetal development multiple transverse non-obstructing folds (Ostling's folds) occur and normally disappear with postnatal growth as the ureter loses its tortuosity (Figure 38.4).[12] On occasion, a fold

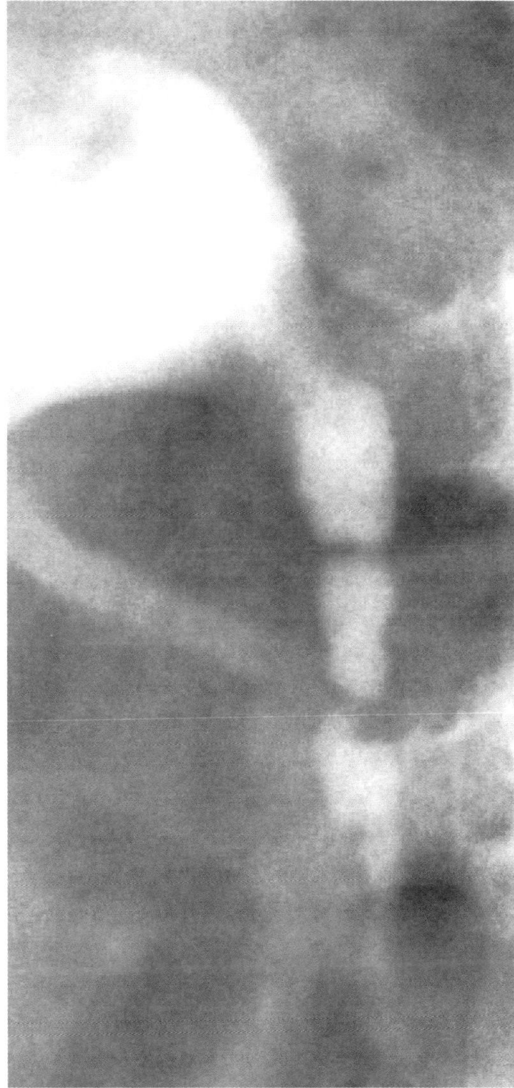

Figure 38.4 An intravenous pyelogram demonstrating non-obstructive Ostling's folds in the proximal ureter of a 5-month-old infant.

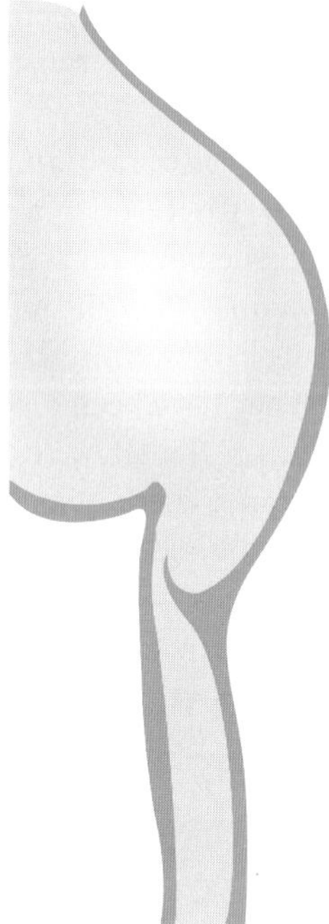

Figure 38.5 Schematic configuration of a ureteral valve with the long axis of the dilated proximal ureteral lumen eccentric to the axis of the non-dilated distal ureter.

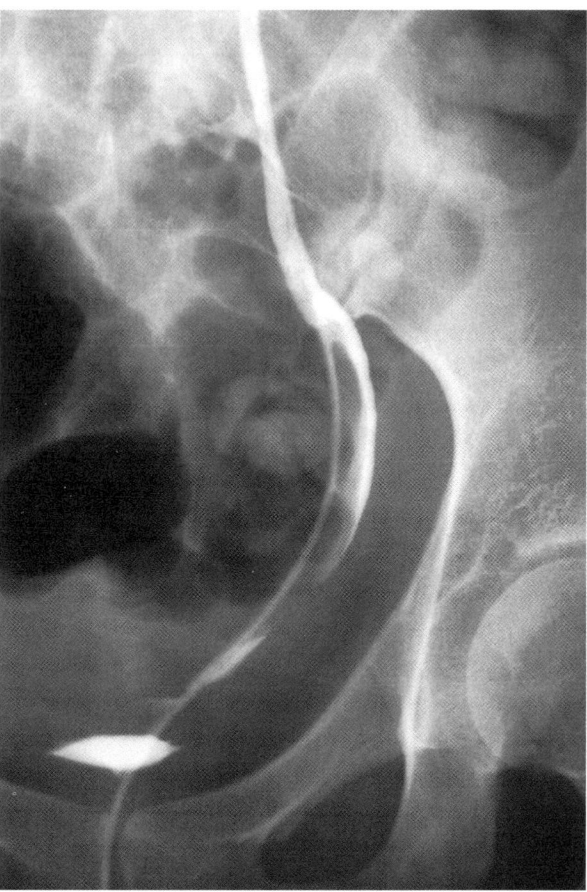

Figure 38.6 Retrograde ureteropyelogram demonstrating a long, smooth filling defect in the distal ureter of a patient with a fibroepithelial polyp.

remains and there is frequently redundancy and kinking of the ureter proximal to an apparent obstruction.

Two subtypes of ureteral valves have been described: one with ureteral stenosis at and distal to the site of the valve, and one that involves a distal ureter of normal caliber. Both types of valves have the orifice and long axis of the distal ureter eccentrically located with respect to the long axis and lumen of the more proximal dilated ureter (Figure 38.5). This configuration inhibits antegrade flow, but retrograde flow in patients with a normal distal ureter is unimpeded. Whether the ureteral valve is the cause of obstruction or a secondary change that occurs as a result of obstruction with proximal dilation has not been completely resolved. Treatment of the valves depends on location and may involve resection, with subsequent ureteropyelostomy, ureteroureterostomy, or ureteroneocystostomy.

Ureteral polyps

Fibroepithelial polyps are the most common benign neoplasm of the ureter.[14] These lesions occur in all age groups and commonly present with hematuria or flank pain. An intravenous ureteropyelogram usually reveals a cylindrical ureteral filling defect that may prolapse into the bladder (Figure 38.6). Ureteroscopy allows identification of the smooth-surfaced fibroepithelial polyp. Endoscopic resection may permit complete removal of the polyp; however, if it is not completely removed, regrowth may occur.[14] With large polyps, complete endoscopic excision may be facilitated by an antegrade approach via percutaneous nephroureteroscopy. Alternatively, ureterotomy and complete excision of the polyp at its base is curative.

References

1. Velardo JT. Histology of the ureter. In: Bergman H, ed. The Ureter, 2nd edn. New York: Springer-Verlag, 1981: 13–54.
2. Hinman F. Ureteral reconstitution. In: Bergman H, ed. The Ureter, 2nd edn. New York: Springer-Verlag, 1981: 179–85.
3. Soundappan SVS, Barker AP. Retrocaval ureter in children: a report of two cases. Pediatr Surg Int 2004; 20:158–60.

4. Perimenis P, Gyftopoulos, Athanasopoulos A, Pastromas V, Barbalias G. Retrocaval ureter and associated abnormalities. Int Urol Nephrol 2002; 33:19–22.
5. Kumeda K, Takamatsu M, Sone M et al. Horseshoe kidney with retrocaval ureter: a case report. J Urol 1982; 128:361–2.
6. Carrion H. Retrocaval ureter: diagnosis and management. In: Bergman H, ed. The Ureter, 2nd edn. New York: Springer-Verlag, 1981: 647–53.
7. Lin HY, Chou YH, Huang SP, et al. Retrocaval ureter: report of two cases and literature review. Kaohsiung J Med Sci 2003; 19:127–31.
8. Polascik T, Chen RN. Laparoscopic ureteroureterostomy for retrocaval ureter. J Urol 1998; 160:121–2.
9. Miyazato M, Kimura T, Ohyama C et al. Retroperitoneoscopic ureteroureterostomy for retrocaval ureter. Acta Urol Jpn 2002; 48:25–8.
10. Smigh BG, Metwalli AR, Leach J, Cheng EY, Kropp BP. Congenital midureteral stricture in children diagnosed with antenatal hydronephrosis. Urology 2004; 64:1014–19.
11. Stephens FD, Smith ED, Hutson JM. Primary obstructed megaureter. In: Congenital Anomalies of the Urinary and Genital Tracts. Oxford: Isis Medical Media, 2002: 212–19.
12. Culp DA. Congenital anomalies of the ureter. In: Bergman H, ed. The Ureter, 2nd edn. New York: Springer-Verlag, 1981: 625–47.
13. Maizels M, Stephens FD. Valves of the ureter as a cause of primary obstruction of the ureter: anatomic, embryologic and clinical aspects. J Urol 1980; 123:742–7.
14. Cooper CS, Hawtrey CE. Fibroepithelial polyp of the ureter. Urology 1997; 50:280–1.

Megaureter

39

David B Joseph

Introduction

The word megaureter conveys the image of a grossly dilated ureter. The term is non-specific and does not provide insight into the pathophysiology. Our knowledge of the megaureter has changed greatly over the past 15 years, primarily due to fetal sonography, which has allowed us to follow the natural history of the megaureter and gain a better insight into treatment (Figure 39.1).

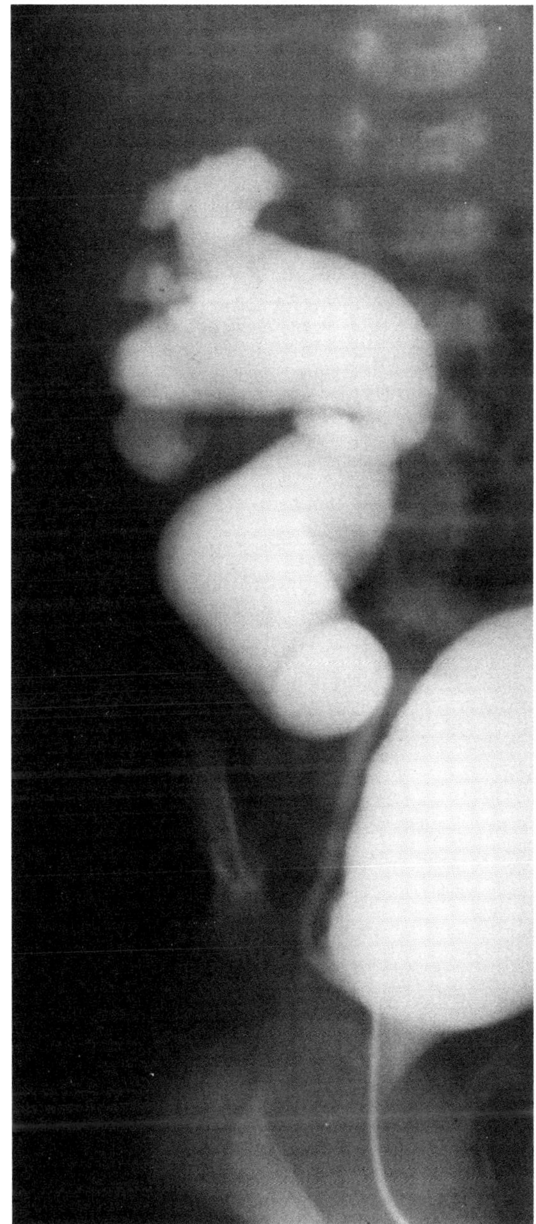

Figure 39.1 An obstructed refluxing megaureter with an unusually long obstructing distal ureterovesical segment. (Reproduced from Joseph,[1] with permission.)

Historic perspective

Classification

Megaureter is synonymous with a dilated ureter, megaloureter, wide ureter, big ureter, hydroureter – all descriptive terms that lack true meaning.[2] Cussen in 1971 reported on autopsy findings of the urinary system in infants and children. He found a child's ureter consistently measured less than 5 mm.[3] This was supported by the work of Hellstrom and coworkers who reviewed excretory urograms in 100 boys and 94 girls. They directly measured ureteral size from the imaging studies and uniformly found the ureter to be less than 6 mm.[4] By definition, a megaureter equates to a ureter of >8 mm in diameter. In 1977 Smith[5] reported on a classification system developed by a working party of pediatric urologists.[6] The group presented their findings and recommendations at an international pediatric urologic seminar in Philadelphia in 1976. An agreement was made to standardize the nomenclature and classification of the megaureter. The megaureter was classified as primary, referring to a lesion intrinsic to the ureter, and secondary, denoting a reaction of the ureter to a process elsewhere. They went on to create the 'ABC' subclassification, 'A' representing a refluxing megaureter, 'B'

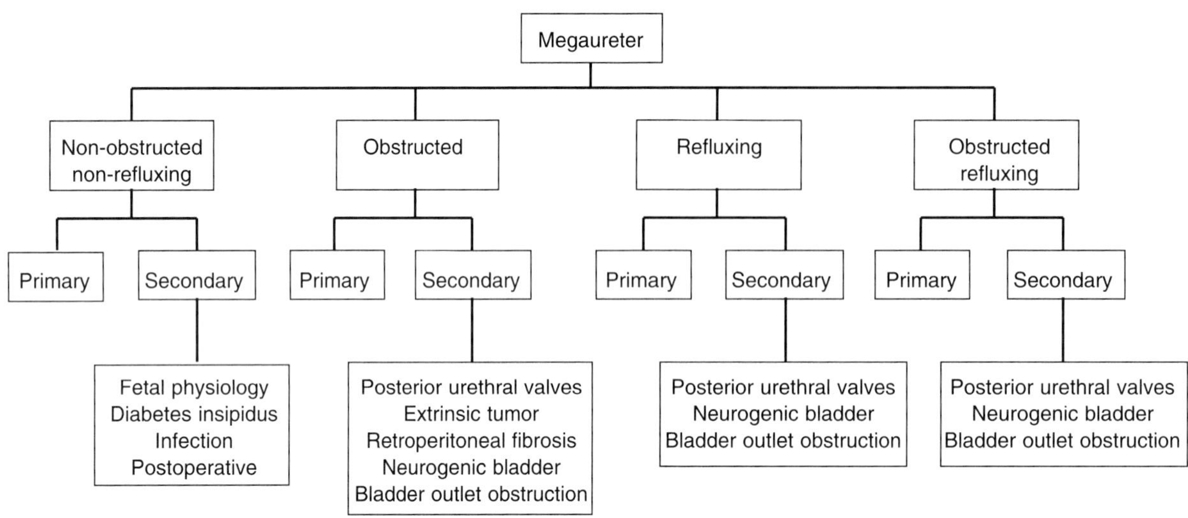

Figure 39.2 Classification of the ureter. (Adapted from King.[7])

an obstructed megaureter, and 'C' a non-refluxing non-obstructed megaureter. King modified this classification in 1980, adding a fourth subclassification consisting of the refluxing obstructed megaureter.[7] King's classification is used most often when describing the megaureter (Figure 39.2).

Anatomy

In order to understand pathophysiology, it is important to have a framework of normal anatomy. The ureter is divided into three distinct regions:

- the ureteropelvic junction
- the middle spindle
- the ureterovesical junction.

The ureterovesical junction is subsequently divided into the juxtavesicoureter and terminal ureter. The terminal ureter then separates into intramural and submucosal segments.[8]

The ureter is enclosed in a loose, ill-defined sheath within the retroperitoneum. This sheath is a protective barrier for the adventitia, particularly when confronted with neoplastic or inflammatory retroperitoneal processes. Proximally, the ureteral sheath and the ureteral adventitia become continuous with the renal pelvis. Distally, the sheath and ureteral adventitia join to form Waldeyer's sheath, which extends into the bladder wall as a portion of the deep trigone.[8]

The ureter consists of three layers: adventitia, muscularis, and mucosa. The adventitia is composed of longitudinally running collagen[9] loosely attached to the underlying muscularis, allowing for free peristaltic activity. The muscularis is made up of smooth muscle cells interspersed with collagen. The inner muscle bundles are arranged longitudinally, the middle circumferentially, and the outer longitudinally.[10] This configuration changes into longitudinally oriented muscle fibers in each layer with sparse collagen as the ureter enters the bladder and intramural region.[11,12] The mucosa consists of multiple layers of transitional epithelium lying directly on the lamina propria.

The ureter is supplied by a rich anastomotic arterial network. The proximal ureter is vascularized predominantly by an artery originating from the renal artery. The middle spindle receives a branch from the aorta and gonadal artery. The distal ureter is supported by arteries from the internal iliac, superior and inferior vesical arteries.[13] A periureteral arterial plexus courses the full extent of the ureter through the adventitia.

The proximal ureter receives neuronal input via the renal and aortic plexus. Unmyelinated nerves travel throughout the adventitial layer.[9] The middle spindle is innervated by the superior hypogastric plexus and the ureterovesical segment by the pelvic plexus.[14] Both adrenergic and cholinergic nerves have been identified within the ureter.[15] It is interesting that ureteral peristalsis is modulated by but not dependent on neuronal input.

Pathophysiology

Obstructed megaureter

The primary obstructed megaureter has generated the greatest interest and investigation. The primary obstructed megaureter has been reported in approximately 25% of children with obstructive uropathy.[16] It is bilateral in 25% and occurs four times more often in boys.[17] The left ureter is more frequently affected, and the contralateral kidney may be dysplastic or obstructed in 10–15% of children.[2,17] Endoscopically, the obstructed ureteral orifice can have a normal appearance and insert appropriately on the trigone. Caulk[18] and Swensen et al[19] proposed that the obstructed megaureter was similar to the megacolon seen in Hirschsprung's disease. However, this proposition has been refuted based on histologic evidence showing ganglia present in the distal primarily obstructed megaureter in a similar distribution to that of a normal ureter.[20]

Several different histologic abnormalities have been associated with the primary obstructed megaureter, indicating a spectrum of pathologic events. A localized deficiency of muscle fibers within the ureterovesical ureter, with hypertrophy of circular muscle bundles immediately proximal to the deficiency, has been described as an adynamic distal segment resulting in obstruction[21–23] (Figure 39.3). The degree of obstruction may be correlated with the percentage of circular fibers. Gregoir and Debled found three histologic variants of obstructed megaureters:

- dense collagen infiltration of the terminal ureter
- distal circular muscular hypertrophy
- varying degrees of distal muscular dysplasia.[24]

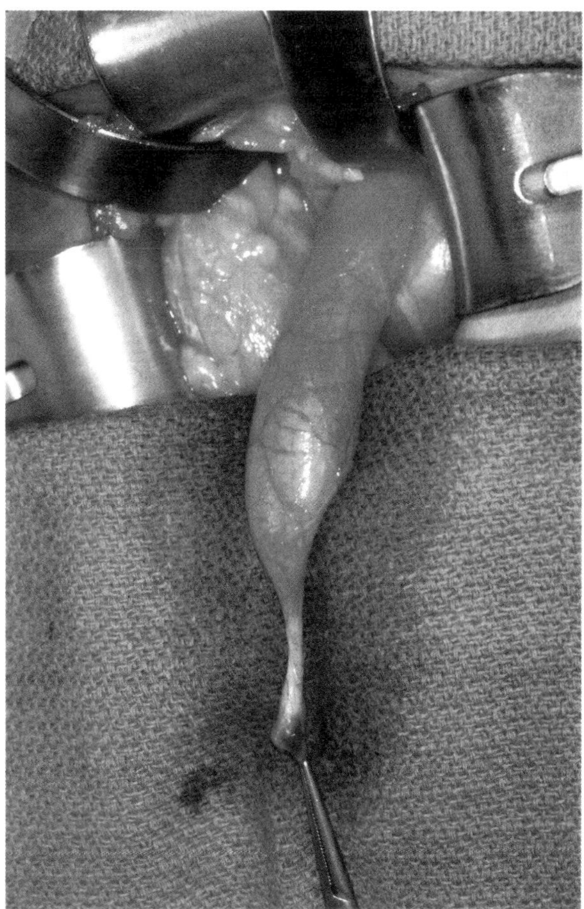

Figure 39.3 Obstruction due to an adynamic distal segment. (Reproduced from Joseph,[1] with permission.)

Increase in collagen deposition between the lamina propria and muscle bundles of the distal ureter has been seen with electron microscopy.[25–27] These pathologic changes result in muscular derangement and increased interstitial connective tissue within the ureterovesical junction. The middle spindle and ureteropelvic junction segments are spared.[28]

Dixon and associates assessed the histologic structure of the ectopic obstructed ureter and found the terminal ureter was encircled by an additional thick collar of smooth muscle.[29] Normally oriented muscle layers were also present but had a diminished diameter. They speculate this embryologic malformation does not spontaneously resolve and becomes the subgroup of obstructed megaureter that requires early intervention.

Other clinicians have suggested abnormal acetylcholinesterase activity in the juxtavesical segment, a tonic response to norepinephrine, and increased intracellular calcium as etiologies of the obstructed megaureter.[30,31]

Some forms of the megaureter improve with time.[16,32–36] Spontaneous improvement may result from segmental maturation of the obstructed distal ureter. Nicotina and associates postulate segmental hypoplasia of the inner longitudinal muscle layer and the possible pathogenic involvement of transforming growth factor-β (TGF-β), which has been shown to effect maturation of smooth muscle cells.[32] TGF-β delays muscle cell differentiation and is detectable in the 11–21-week-old fetus but diminishes thereafter. TGF-β has been found in the distal ureters of children >2 years old with obstructive uropathy, but not in children >2 years old who had repair of a non-obstructed megaureter.[32] The spontaneous improvement in the obstructed megaureter may correlate with TGF-β depletion within the first 2 years of life.[32]

Refluxing megaureter

The refluxing megaureter is endoscopically characterized by a gaping lateral ureteral orifice. Bladder filling and cyclic voiding can transmit pressure into the ureter, resulting in mechanical enlargement (Figure

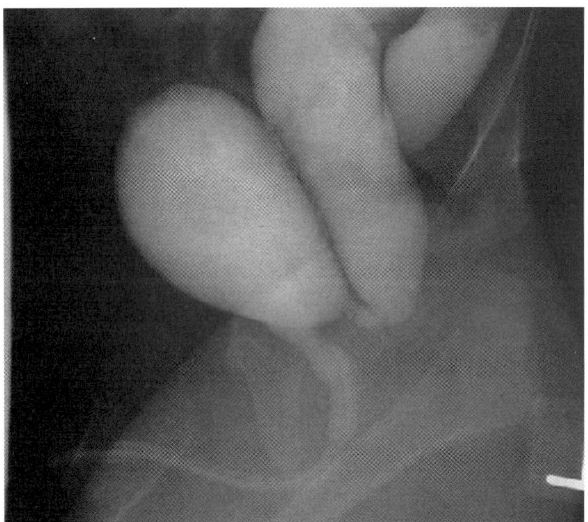

Figure 39.4 Vesicoureteral reflux in a male neonate with elevated voiding pressure.

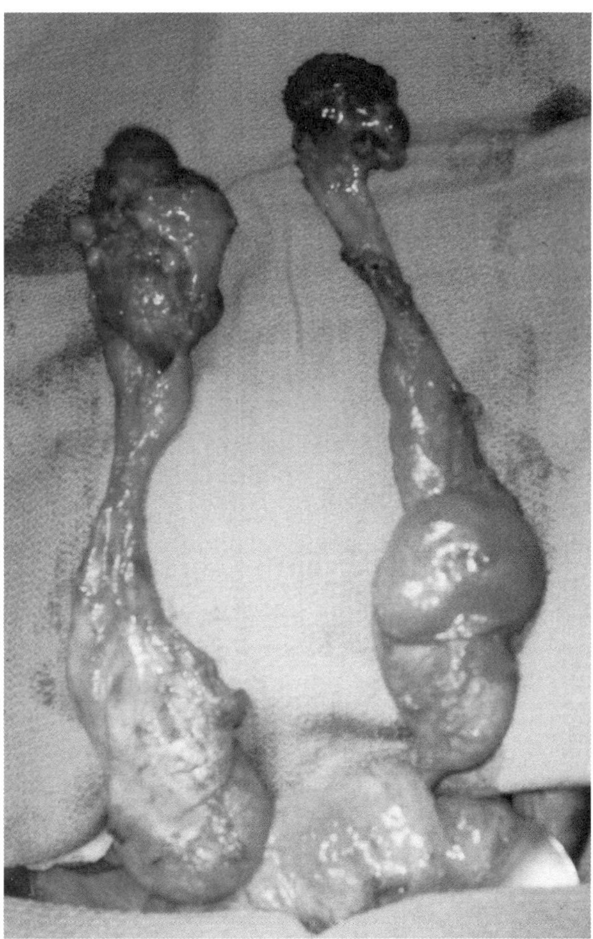

Figure 39.5 The gross appearance of the ureter in prune belly syndrome. These ureters are elongated, tortuous, and dilated. There is often ureteral asymmetry, with the distal ureter showing significant ectasia. (Reproduced from Joseph,[39] with permission.)

39.4). Lee and associates have found a twofold increase in the ratio of collagen fibers to smooth muscle fibers in the refluxing megaureter compared with the obstructed megaureter and control ureter.[37,38] They defined collagen fiber types and have shown an increase in collagen types I and III for both obstructed and refluxing megaureters. However, the refluxing megaureter contains a significantly greater percentage of type III collagen than other megaureters. Type III collagen is a less-distensible fiber, raising speculation that this intrinsic characteristic stiffens the ureter. This may play an important role in the failure rate after operative correction of refluxing megaureters compared with the success noted in other forms of megaureters.[37]

The refluxing megaureter associated with prune belly syndrome represents a unique abnormality.[39] In gross appearance, these ureters are elongated, tortuous, and dilated (Figure 39.5). Endoscopically, the ureteral orifices are lateral, golf hole in appearance, and frequently associated with diverticulum. The distal ureter is characterized by asymmetric ectasia and is more often involved than the proximal ureter. Secondary obstruction may occur from kinking and folding of the redundant ureter. Primary obstruction has been reported at the ureterovesical junction in a select group.[39] Histologically, there is an increase in fibrous tissue at the expense of normally developed ureteric muscle. Children with prune belly syndrome and vesicoureteral reflux have been reported to have an increased ratio of collagen to smooth muscle fibers in the muscularis.[40] This may help explain the poor dynamic characteristics of the ureter, resulting in ineffective peristalsis and urinary stagnation.[39] Degeneration of non-myelinated Schwann fibers and a decreased number of nerve plexi may also contribute to decreased ureteral peristalsis.[41] Ureteric abnormalities tend to predominate in the distal portion of the ureter, an important concept to consider during operative intervention.

Non-refluxing non-obstructed megaureter

The non-refluxing non-obstructed megaureter is most often encountered in the neonate with the antenatal diagnosis of hydronephrosis. Whereas the etiology remains in question, fetal renal physiology may play a role. Rapid changes in renal vascular resistance, glomerular filtration rate (GFR), and urinary concentration result in a 4–6 times increase in urine production prior to birth. This increase in urine output may surpass the dynamic ability of the ureter to transmit the increased volume to the bladder, resulting in transient ureteral dilation.

McLellan et al report resolution of the non-refluxing megaureter in the majority of children, with the time to resolution based on the initial grade of hydronephrosis. Children with grades 1–3 hydronephrosis resolved at a median age of 13, 24, and 35 months, respectively, and children with grade 4 and 5 hydronephrosis resolved at a median age of 48 months.[42]

Refluxing obstructed mgaureter

The refluxing obstructed megaureter results from ectopic insertion of the ureteral orifice in the region of the bladder neck. During bladder filling, the bladder neck is closed, acting as a distal obstruction. With voiding, the bladder neck opens and allows for reflux. A cyclic voiding cystourethrogram may be required for diagnosis in suspected cases.

Diagnosis

The routine use of fetal sonography has dramatically increased the diagnosis of the megaureter. Brown et al delineated the impact that fetal sonography has on identification of the megaureter.[43] Prior to fetal sonography, the diagnosis of a megaureter was preceded by clinically significant symptoms, particularly infection, hematuria, and pain.[2] In the presonography era, clinically significant megaureters accounted for 8% of children found to have hydroureteronephrosis (ureteropelvic junction obstruction was noted in 22%, posterior urethral valves in 19%, and the ectopic ureterocele in 14%).[43] With fetal sonography now routine, the megaureter is noted to occur in 23% of asymptomatic neonates, surpassed only by hydronephrosis, which is seen in 41%.[43] The increased incidence of the megaureter can be explained by a more liberal use of fetal sonography and improved technology.

An unknown percentage of infants identified as having an asymptomatic megaureter will subsequently go on to have clinical symptomatology. This places a greater burden on imaging technology and our ability to assess the true clinical significance of the megaureter's pathologic state.

Evaluation

Ultrasonography

Ultrasonography is the primary imaging modality in the assessment of antenatal hydronephrosis and the initial imaging study obtained for symptomatic genitourinary abnormalities. Sonography plays a key role in the assessment of the megaureter. Evaluating the size, shape, tortuosity, and bulbar appearance of the ureter in conjunction with similar findings of the renal pelvis can often give the impression of an obstructive process. The course of the ureter may be traced from the renal pelvis to its distal insertion. Careful pelvic sonography assists in the differential diagnosis of the megaureter. The ureter may enter an obstructed ureterocele or end in an ectopic location within the bladder neck or posterior urethra. An obstructed distal segment may be recognized when a peristaltic wave of urine abruptly stops a few centimeters from the bladder and rebounds into the dilated proximal ureter (Figure 39.6). The echogenicity of the kidney is a helpful parameter used to distinguish between an obstructive and a non-obstructive process, with increased echogenicity supporting obstruction.[44] A renal resistance index (RI) >0.70 has been suggested to correlate with obstruction. However, the utility of RI in the pediatric population may be limited in the absence of normal standards based on age.[45,46] In addition, sonography lacks the ability to quantify a dynamic process, and the true significance of any abnormal megaureter must be determined by a functional imaging study.

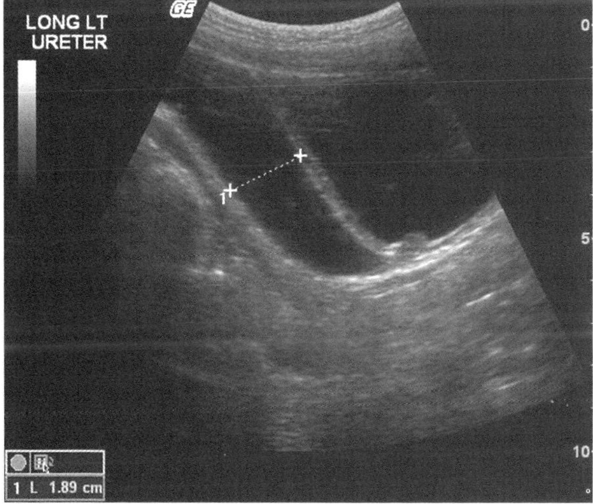

Figure 39.6 Sonographic appearance of the distal megaureter with a diminutive terminal segment.

Voiding cystourethrography

Voiding cystourethrography is essential to rule out vesicoureteral reflux. A conventional fluoroscopic cystogram is preferred over a nuclear cystogram in that the anatomic appearance of the bladder, bladder neck, urethra, and ureters is necessary for precise diagnosis and treatment. The cyclic voiding cystourethrogram is beneficial when an ectopic, sphincteric ureter is suspected. In this scenario, the ureter can be obstructed when the bladder is at rest and refluxes only during the voiding phase. Blickman and Lebowitz characterize the obstructed refluxing megaureter as having a markedly enlarged proximal ureter with a normal-appearing ureterovesical segment.[47]

Excretory urography

Excretory urography is waning as a diagnostic modality in the evaluation of pediatric uropathy. Even with tomography, only limited information is gained. Stool, bowel gas, and immaturity of the neonatal kidney limit its utility. In addition, the degree of hydronephrosis noted does not equate to severity of obstruction. On a rare occasion, excretory uropathy may play a role when anatomic definition is required.[48]

Renography

Diuresis renal scintigraphy provides the greatest quantitative information of functional and dynamic data. The degree of obstruction can be determined by evaluating multiple parameters, including renal uptake, excretion, time to peak activity, and $T_{1/2}$ following lasix washout. Two of the more common radiotracers used to evaluate obstruction are technetium 99m (^{99m}Tc) DTPA (diethylene triamine-penta-acetic acid) and ^{99m}Tc MAG3 (mercapto-acetyltriglycine).[49,50] DTPA is a glomerular agent and provides limited information during the first month of life because of a low neonatal GFR. MAG3 is extracted by the kidney and dependent on effective renal plasma flow not GFR. This results in less background artifact. These factors make MAG3 a more attractive agent during the neonatal period.[49]

Multiple variables affect data acquisition and interpretation. Consequently, renal scintigraphy must be performed in a standardized fashion, using a protocol that optimizes hydration state, administration of diuretic, and acquisition of time–activity curves.[51] It is important to have a separate activity curve generated for the kidney and the ureter when assessing for an obstructive pattern. Isolating simply over the kidney can produce deceiving results that show an acceptable washout of the radiotracer from the kidney only to be washed into an obstructed ureter (Figure 39.7). Obtaining activity curves over the ureter will help confirm distal ureteral obstruction. The timing of diuretic administration can play a role in assessing $T_{1/2}$, with benefits attributed to administration at a standard time either before or after radiopharmaceutical administration.[52] Regardless of the protocol used, it is most important that a consistent methodology is maintained in order to compare successive studies in the same individual.

Magnetic resonance urography

Magnetic resonance urography (MRU) may play a future role in the evaluation of the megaureter. MRU with gadolinium has less nephrotoxic effects than contrast agents used for intravenous urography and conventional computed tomography (CT) imaging. This imaging modality may become the anatomic study of choice, particularly when renal compromise is present.[53–55]

Percutaneous perfusion studies

Upper urinary tract urodynamic assessment can be helpful in difficult cases. The Whitaker test has traditionally been the procedure of choice.[56] However, the Whitaker test has limitations in the pediatric population. It is invasive and requires sedation for placement of a percutaneous renal catheter and bladder catheter. Whitaker described the test using a constant infusion of 10 ml/min, with obstruction defined as an elevation in renal pressure >22 cmH_2O of water pressure over baseline.[56] The rate of infusion accommodated by the normal infant ureter is unknown. Infusing the renal pelvis at a rate of 10 ml/min may overcome the peristaltic flow potential of the normal infant or child's ureter. A constant perfusion of testing medium while recording the renal pelvic pressure may be a more appropriate test.[57,58]

Fung and associates explored ureteral opening pressure as a novel parameter for evaluating the obstructive nature of pediatric hydroureteronephrosis.[58] Renal pelvic pressure was assessed while simultaneously documenting the passage of contrast material from the distal ureter into the bladder. The infusion rate was individually calculated for each patient and maintained within a physiologically relevant range. A pressure increase of 14 cmH_2O within the renal pelvis was deemed consistent with distal ureteral obstruc-

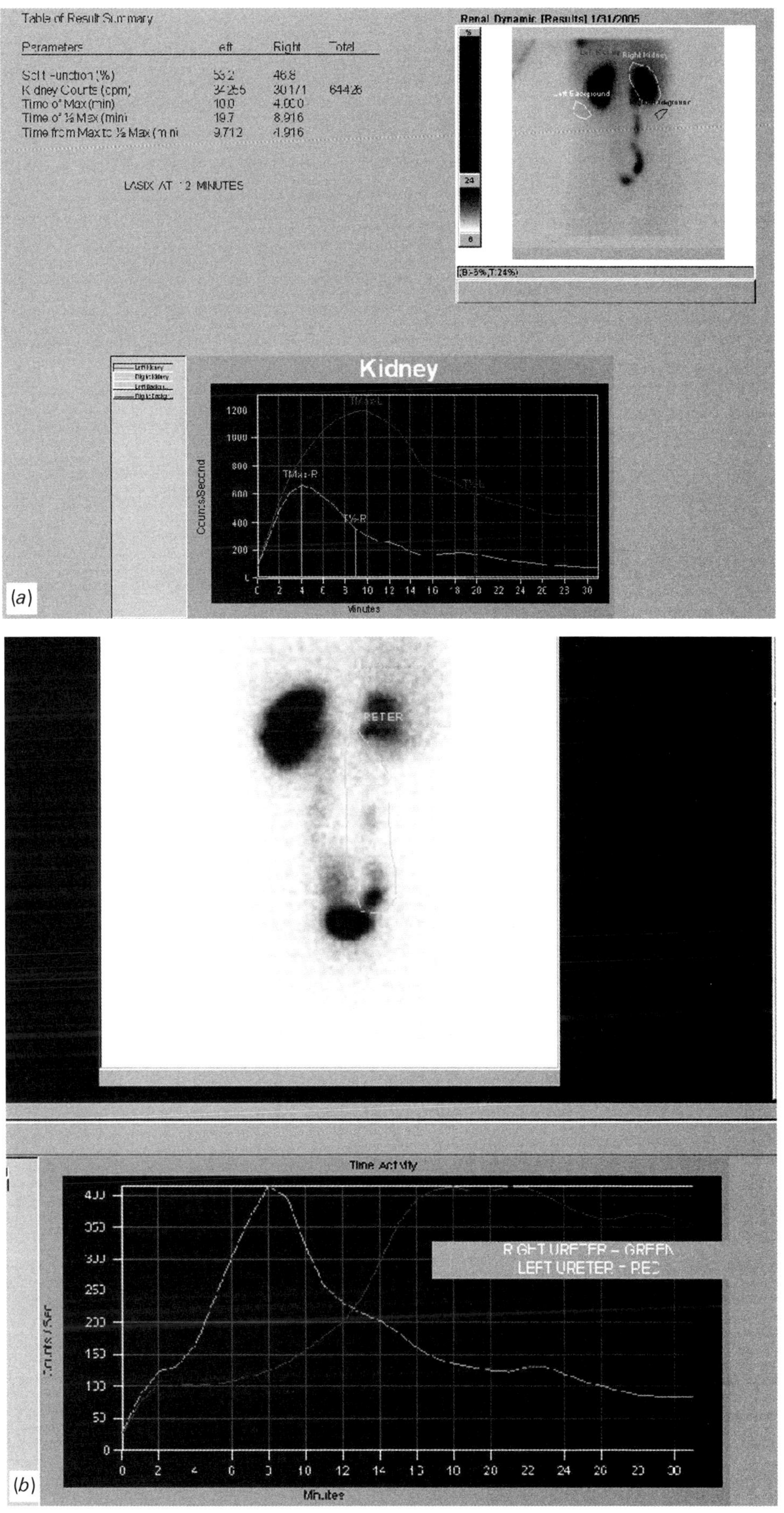

Figure 39.7 (*a*) A MAG3 renal scan, showing a composite pixel image and computer generated kidney washout curve. There is a relatively equal function with a delay in peak activity of the left system with $T_{1/2}$ washout of both kidneys <20 minutes. (*b*) A right ureteral pixel image and curve (**1**), indicating normal time–activity washout. A left ureteral time–activity curve (**2**), shows an obstructive pattern with progressive accumulation and no washout.

tion. Although this approach is invasive, it eliminates the problems of the infusion rate noted in the classic Whitaker study.[58]

Differential treatment

Therapeutic intervention of the megaureter is dependent on accurate classification. Secondary causes of a megaureter justify treatment of the primary problem, whether it is due to a neurogenic bladder, posterior urethral membrane, ureterocele, diabetes insipidus, or a retroperitoneal process. Treatment of those problems is described elsewhere.

Refluxing megaureter

Traditionally, grade IV/V and V/V vesicoureteral reflux (International Study Classification) has prompted operative intervention.[59] That approach may be appropriate for older children presenting with symptomatic urinary infections; however, there is growing evidence that operative intervention is not required in all neonates with refluxing megaureters, especially when identified during the work-up of asymptomatic antenatal hydronephrosis. High-grade vesicoureteral reflux in neonates occurs more often in males than females, and improvement can occur during the first year of life.[59] There is little reason to proceed with early intervention, particularly when an infant has remained symptom-free on prophylactic medical management.

The association of megacystis–megaureter was first described by Williams in 1954[60] and is now well understood.[61] By definition, megacystis–megaureter is a large-capacity, thin-walled bladder with massive primary vesicoureteral reflux.[60,61] Megacystis–megaureter occurs in approximately 80% of boys diagnosed antenatally with bilateral reflux and found to have renal impairment.[62] The etiology of the male predominance is unknown and does not appear to be due to bladder outlet obstruction. It is speculated that higher voiding pressure occurs in the male neonate. Children with megacystis–megaureter show progressive upper tract hydroureteronephrosis and bladder enlargement as a result of recurrent cycling of urine into the upper tract during a detrusor contraction followed by rapid refilling of the bladder upon relaxation of the detrusor after voiding. Over time, this cyclic event continually increases bladder volume and hydroureteronephrosis. Double voiding can temporize this process in children who are toilet trained: 10–15 minutes after the initial void, the child is encouraged to void again, allowing for an overall decrease in volume of retained urine. Positive effects of this technique occur first with stabilization of bladder volume, followed by reduction in bladder size and improvement of hydroureteronephrosis. Intermittent bladder catheterization can be an effective technique of eliminating residual urine in neonates and toddlers who are not toilet trained, allowing the child to reach an age where operative reconstruction would be beneficial. Ultimately, children with a megacystis–megaureter are best served by operative correction of the reflux.[61]

Non-refluxing, non-obstructed megaureter

Approximately 6–10% of neonates diagnosed with fetal sonography will have a non-refluxing non-obstructed megaureter.[63] A functional study is required to confirm adequate ureteral drainage. The initial medical management will be prophylactic antibiotics. Children with a non-refluxing non-obstructed megaureter maintain normal renal function and the megaureter often reverts to normal.

Obstructed refluxing megaureter

The obstructed refluxing megaureter occurs as a result of either a laterally positioned aperistaltic distal segment or ectopic insertion of the ureter into the bladder neck/posterior urethra. Although the condition is not an emergency, operative correction is required in order to diminish the risk of upper urinary tract deterioration and reduce risks of urinary tract infections, particularly those associated with the obstruction component.

Obstructed megaureter

The indication for treatment of the obstructed megaureter prior to fetal sonography was relatively straightforward. Most children presented with a symptomatic urinary tract infection, abdominal pain, nausea, or vomiting and underwent repair.[2] Fetal sonography has identified a substantial number of neonates with an obstructed megaureter, many of whom will not have clinical symptoms. Current management of the obstructed megaureter is controversial.[16,64–67] Medical management, based on prophylactic antibiotics and watchful waiting, allows for potential spontaneous regression of the obstructed megaureter. Renal parenchymal thickness and function must be objectively followed with sonography and renography in order to identify renal compromise.

Repair of the infant megaureter is technically feasible but remains a challenge even in experienced hands. Secondary operative procedures have been reported as high as 10% when correcting an obstructed megaureter in an infant <8 months of age.[68] It is best to temper the initial urge to repair a megaureter until the child is older than 12 months of age, at which time technical hurdles are not as great.[69]

Occasionally, a neonate with an obstructed megaureter will present with severe renal compromise. In this situation, a distal cutaneous ureterostomy can provide temporary relief,[63] adequately draining the upper urinary tract and decreasing the risk of infection. The decompressed ureter may regain tone and a more normal caliber as the child grows and develops.[63]

Operative approach

Temporary diversion

A percutaneous nephrostomy is helpful when rapid drainage is required. But small nephrostomy tubes are difficult to maintain longer than a few weeks. When prolonged drainage is required, a distal ureterostomy is appropriate. A pyelostomy can be undertaken, but this results in unnecessary proximal diversion when the pathology exists at the bladder level.

A cutaneous ureterostomy is practical for the severely obstructed neonatal megaureter. The procedure carries minimal morbidity, allows for rapid continuous decompression, and can often be performed in the outpatient setting. The ureter is approached through a 2 cm incision placed within an ipsilateral low inguinal skin crease. The muscles are separated and the space of Retzius entered. Identification of the ureter is facilitated when the bladder is partially full and it is usually easily visualized on account of its size. Caution should be taken before opening the ureter, because bowel can be mistaken for a distended ureter, particularly in the infant. When there is doubt, a 21-gauge needle should be used to aspirate the contents and confirm urine. If the ureter is not easily identified, the obliterated umbilical artery provides a suitable landmark for initiating the search. The ureter will often be found just beneath the transected obliterated umbilical artery. Once mobilized, a cutaneous loop ureterostomy provides adequate drainage. The ureter is secured to the anterior rectus fascia with 4–0 or 5–0 absorbable suture and to the skin with the same. The size of the ureter prevents postoperative stenosis.

Definitive reconstruction

The approach to the ureter for definitive urinary reconstruction can be either intravesical, extravesical, or combined. The dilated ureter is redundant and tortuous. Straightening and tapering the ureter without devascularization is required. The functional ability of the ureter to transmit urine into the bladder via peristalsis is inversely related to the size of the megaureter. The ureter is tapered to achieve a ureteral diameter that will allow for a 4–5:1 ratio of tunnel length to ureteral diameter necessary for an antirefluxing repair. Enough ureter is mobilized in order to taper the intravesical ureter and a short portion of extravesical ureter. There should be a gradual transition from the tapered to dilated ureter to prevent a sharp gradient, which can act as a pseudo-obstruction. Multiple tailoring techniques exist for ureteral tapering and include ureteral imbrication and formal ureteral excision.[70–73]

Imbrication

Ureteral imbrication is appropriate for marginally dilated ureters. Two common imbricating techniques are the Starr and Kalicinski plications.[70,71] In the Starr plication, a Lembert technique with 6–0 absorbable suture is used to 'fold in' the redundant ureter over a 10 or 12 Fr catheter[70] (Figure 39.8). Kalicinski established a plication technique that excludes the redundant ureter from the urinary system[71] (Figure 39.9). A 10 or 12 Fr catheter is used for a template and an avascular segment of excess ureter is isolated. A running 5–0 or 6–0 absorbable suture follows the course of the ureter, separating it from the redundant segment. The redundant segment is then folded over the ureter and secured with a second absorbable suture layer (Figure 39.10). Regardless of the imbrication technique, the plicated ureter is brought into the bladder and secured to the floor either in a cross trigonal or a Politano–Leadbetter fashion.

Ureteral stents may be placed for 3–7 days, but are often unnecessary. The advantage of ureteral plication relates to preservation of the blood supply, decreased incidence of devascularization, minimal risk of urinary leak, and infrequent obstruction. When massive ureteral dilation is present, imbrication will add unwanted bulk, making the ureter difficult to reimplant particularly if a bilateral procedure is performed.

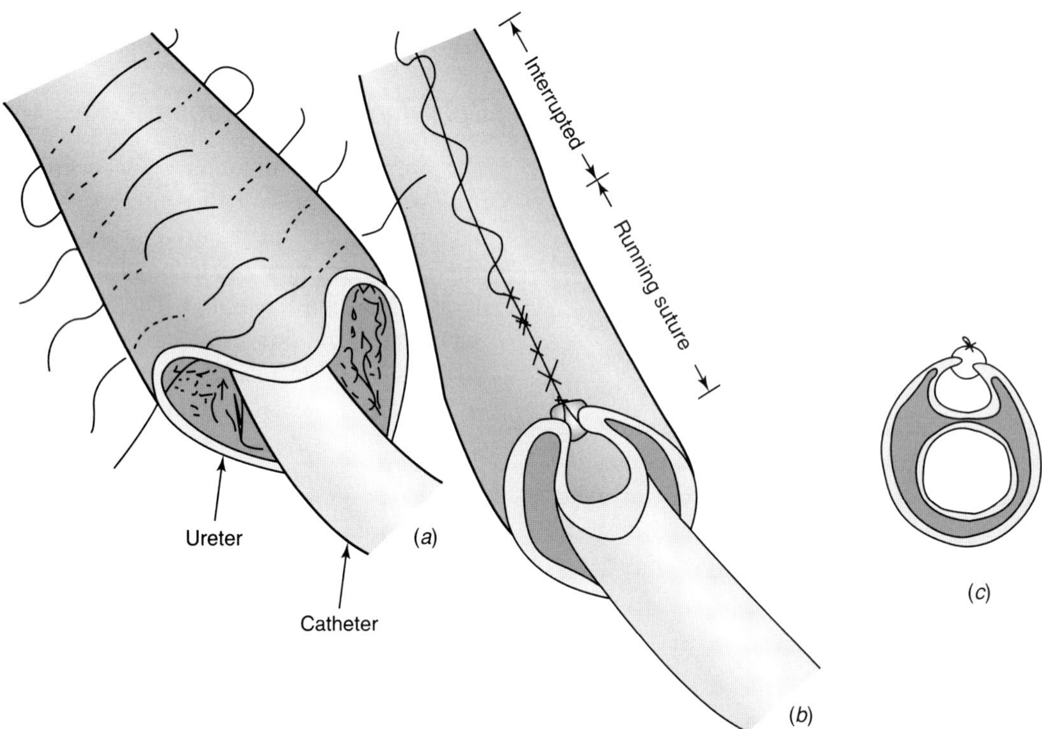

Figure 39.8 Starr technique of ureteral imbrication. (*a*) The ureter is folded inward over a 10 or 12 Fr catheter as a guide. (*b*) The distal portion is secured with interrupted sutures to allow for transection without compromising the running suture line. (c) Cross section of (b).

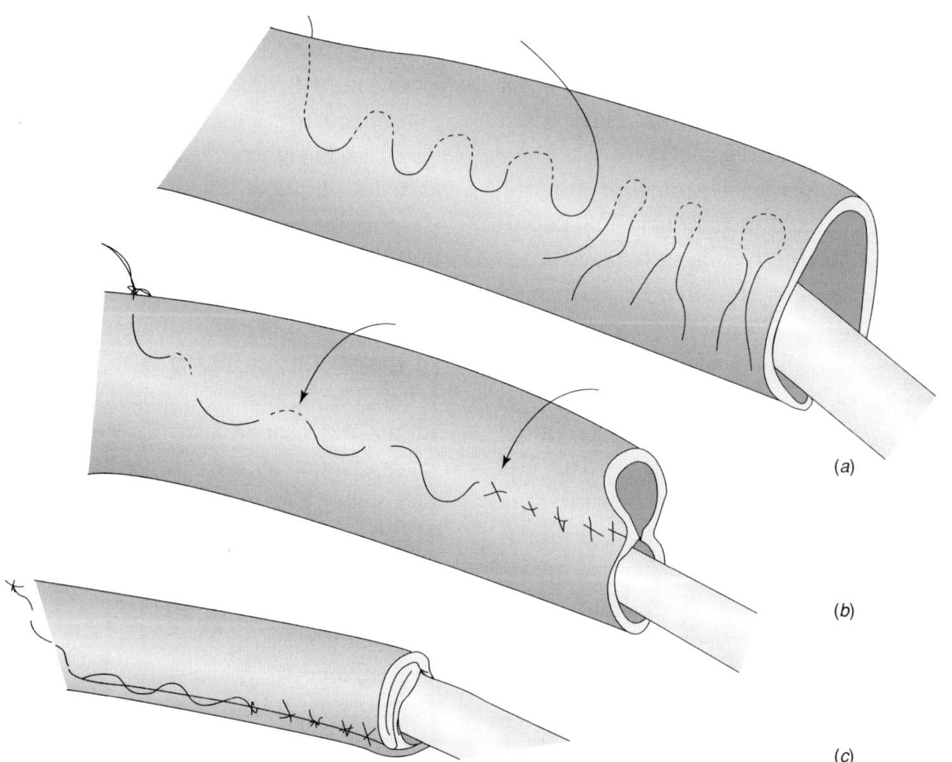

Figure 39.9 The Kalicinski technique of ureteral imbrication. (*a*) The excess segment of ureter is excluded from the flow of urine. (*b*) It is then folded over the ureter using a 10 or 12 Fr catheter as a guide. (*c*) The distal portion is secured with interrupted sutures to allow for transection.

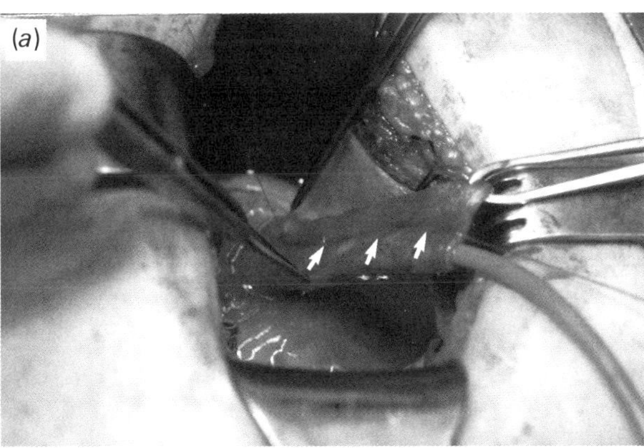

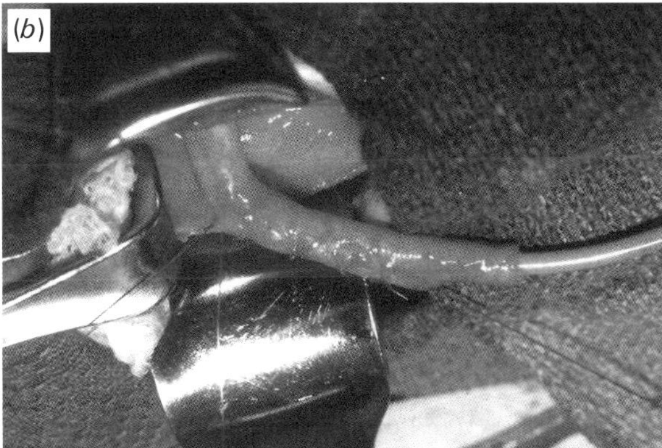

Figure 39.10 (*a*) Kalicinski plication technique isolating the redundant ureter from the distal flow of urine (arrows). (*b*) The excluded segment has been folded and secured to the distal ureter. (Reproduced from Joseph,[1] with permission.)

Excisional tapering

Formal excisional tapering of the ureter is required for extremely bulky ureters or a bilateral process. Hendren pioneered ureteral remodeling and the technique has stood the test of time.[72] The ureter is loosely tapered over a 10 or 12 Fr catheter, depending on the child's age and size. Straight Allis clamps are placed longitudinally along the ureter in a region of least vascularity. Angled Allis clamps are then placed over the ureter, securing the internal 10–12 Fr catheter (Figure 39.11). Care is taken to prevent the temptation of excluding too much redundant ureter, which results in excessive tapering around the catheter. The ureter is closed in two layers: first a running, locking 5–0 or 6–0 absorbable suture directly opposes the mucosa and the muscularis of the ureter – the locking technique limits ureteral reefing and decreases extravasation; a second running adventitial layer of absorbable suture decreases leaking. Both running layers stop a few centimeters from the distal end of the ureter. The very distal portion of the ureter is closed in two layers with interrupted sutures. This allows for excision of the distal ureter, if required, without interruption of the running suture line. A ureteral stent can be placed:

- to decrease urinary extravasation
- to provide a scaffold for the ureter to conform to during the postoperative period
- to prevent kinking
- to bypass the tapered region, which initially may act as an obstruction as a result of postoperative edema.

The ureter may be stented for 7–14 days. The necessity for a Penrose drain is variable, depending on the technique used for ureteral tailoring and the presence of a

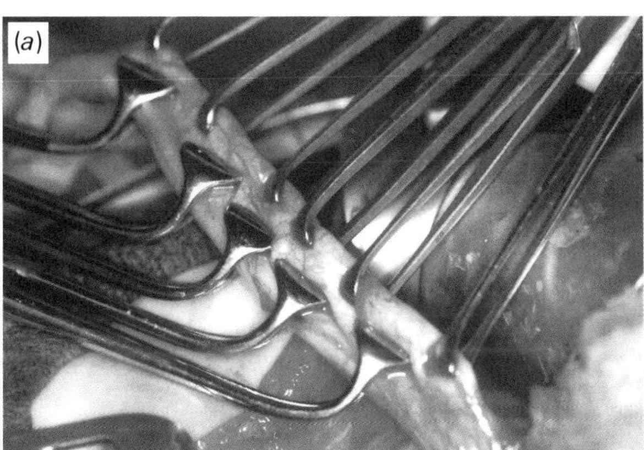

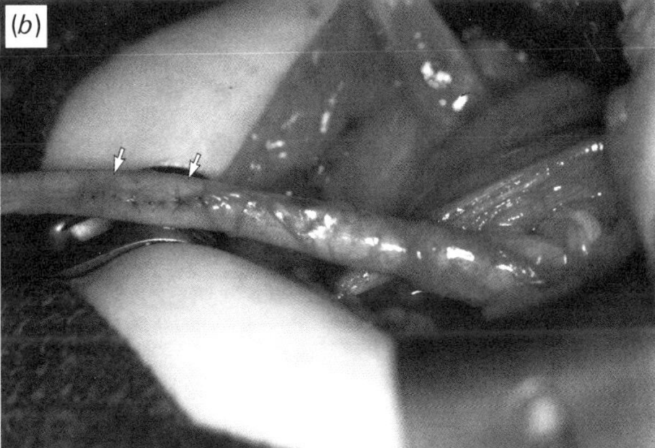

Figure 39.11 (*a*) Angled Hendren clamps placed loosely over a 10 or 12 Fr catheter securing the retained portion of the distal ureter. Straight Allis clamps isolate the segment to be excised. (*b*) A two-layer technique is used to close the ureter, interrupting the distal most portion and allowing for excision, as needed. The arrows indicate the interrupted portion. (Reproduced from Joseph,[1] with permission.)

ureteral stent. A Penrose drain may be helpful when a ureteral stent has not been placed and a substantial portion of tapered distal ureter remains extravesical.

In most situations, only the portion of the distal ureter which is going to be placed within the bladder and 1 or 2 cm beyond needs to be tapered. There should be a gentle transition from the ureteral hiatus at the bladder to the non-tapered ureter. Proximal ureteral tapering is rarely required and limited to children with persisting proximal hydroureteronephrosis, with an obstructed pattern in the face of a patent distal ureter.[73] In complex reconstructive cases, consideration should be given to a transureteroureterostomy and a unilateral tapered reimplant, particularly when there is small bladder.

Postoperative management

Removal of the ureteral stent is dependent on the procedure performed. The stent can be removed 3–7 days after imbrication, and 7–14 days following an excisional repair. Ureterograms at the time of stent removal are not necessarily beneficial. Postoperative edema can limit drainage, giving the appearance of a high-grade obstruction, when, in fact, removal of the stent is all that is required. Administration of a broad-spectrum antibiotic prior to removing a stent decreases the possibility of urosepsis even when the child has been maintained on prophylactic antibiotics.

Postoperative ureteral edema can persist for 6 weeks. Imaging studies, either sonography or renal scintigraphy, should be avoided during that time. The initial images on sonography may show increased hydronephrosis and proximal hydroureter when compared with preoperative sonographic imaging, particularly when repairing a refluxing megaureter (Figure 39.12). This is because of the compliant proximal ureter and relative resistance to flow through the tapered segment. It is important to review the ureteral size on the preoperative cystogram to help determine the significance of postoperative sonographic dilatation. Renal scintigraphy should be used to assess for postoperative obstruction in troublesome cases.

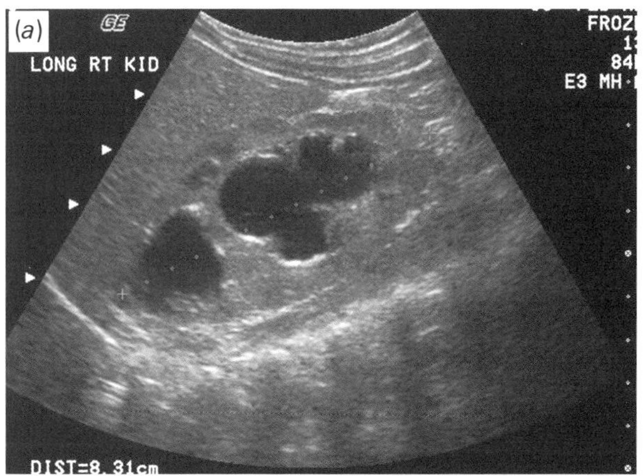

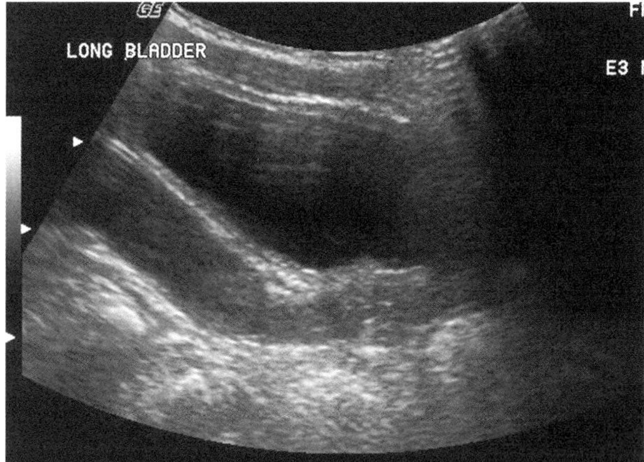

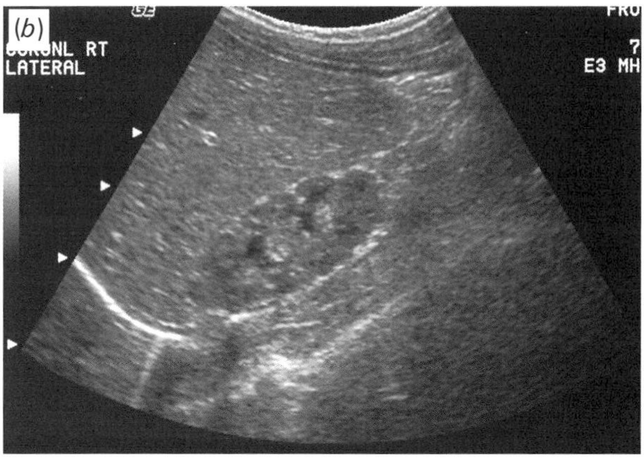

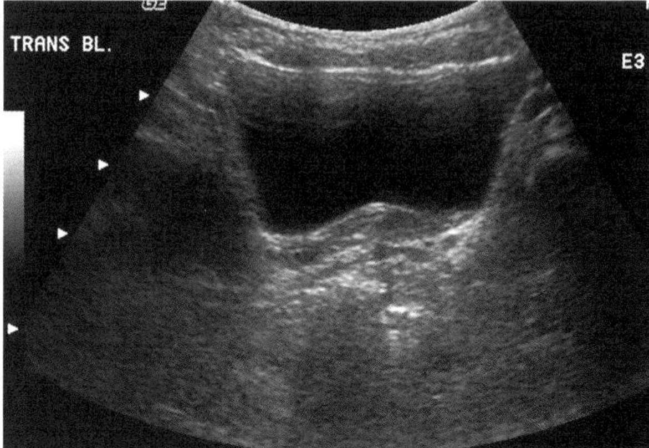

Figure 39.12 (*a*) A 6-week postoperative ultrasound, showing hydronephrosis (left) and a hydroureter (right). The preoperative ultrasound was normal. (*b*) A 3-month postoperative ultrasound. The hydronephrosis (left) and hydroureter (right) has resolved.

A postoperative voiding cystourethrogram at 6 months is performed to confirm the absence of vesicoureteral reflux. Prophylactic antibiotics can be discontinued with resolution of the reflux.

Complications

Successful operative outcome of megaureter reconstruction has been reported to be 93–95% for imbrication,[68,71,74–78] and 74–90% for excisional tapering.[68,74,76,79–82] However, the complication rate and morbidity is greater than when performing a non-tapered ureteroneocystostomy. The two most common complications are obstruction and persisting reflux.

Postoperative complications are not simply due to technical error; inherent ureteral characteristics and bladder dysfunction affect a successful outcome. Increased collagen deposition and altered smooth muscle may be the etiology for a higher rate of persisting vesicoureteral reflux following repair.[29,37]

Postoperative edema can lead to obstruction that requires temporary percutaneous nephrostomy diversion. Physician patience is prudent to allow for the operative edema to subside, which might take 2–3 months. Persistent obstruction is probably the result of ureteral ischemia and will ultimately require revision.

Persisting vesicoureteral reflux has been reported to occur in approximately 5% of tapered reimplants.[68,71,74–84] Transient mild reflux noted at 6 months can resolve with further time. Reflux persisting greater than 3 years is unlikely to improve:[68] when it is significant and symptomatic, secondary corrective intervention is required. A formal reoperative procedure is undertaken, with attention paid to preserving the ureteral blood supply and maximizing the ratio of ureteral tunnel length to diameter of at least 5:1. In-situ ureteral tailoring is an appealing alternative to a formal excisional repair. It achieves a gradual decrease in intraluminal diameter without compromising vascularity and avoids the difficult ureteral dissection. This should be considered in cases when the ureteral tunnel length had been maximized at the first encounter.[83] Contralateral reflux may occur more following repair of the refluxing megaureter compared with the obstructed megaureter. It has been suggested that the functional anatomy of the trigone is impaired in reflux but not in obstruction.[85]

Summary

The asymptomatic megaureter is commonly encountered as a result of the routine use of fetal sonography. The natural history of the megaureter supports observation and non-operative management of most infants. When operative management is required, precise classification of the pathophysiology, along with intervention by a pediatric specialist, should result in a successful outcome.

References

1. Joseph DB. Ureterovesical junction anomalies – megaureters. In: Gearhart JP, Rink RC, Mouriquand PDE, eds. Pediatric Urology. Philadelphia: WB Saunders, 2000.
2. Kass EJ. Megaureter in clinical pediatric urology. In: Kelalis PP, King LR, Belman AB, eds. Philadelphia: WB Saunders, 1992: 781–821.
3. Cussen LJ. The morphology of congenital dilatation of the ureter: Intrinsic ureteral lesions. Aust NZ J Surg 1971; 41:185.
4. Hellstrom M, Hjalmas K, Jacobsson B, Jodal U, Oden A. Normal ureteral diameter in infancy and childhood. Acta Radiol (Diagn) (Stockh) 1985; 26:433–9.
5. Smith ED, Cussen LJ, Glenn J et al. Report of working party to establish an international nomenclature for the large ureter. Birth Defects Orig Artic Ser 1977; 13:3.
6. Stephens FD, Smith ED, Hutson JM. Megaureters in congenital anomalies of the urinary and genital tracts. Oxford: Isis Medical, 1996: 187–92.
7. King LR. Megaloureter: definition, diagnosis and management (guest editorial). J Urol 1980; 123:222–3.
8. Hinman F. Atlas of Urosurgical Anatomy. The Ureter. Philadelphia: WB Saunders, 1993:284–9.
9. Notley RG. The innervation of the upper ureter in man and in the rat: an ultrastructural study. J Anat 1969; 105:393–402.
10. Notley RG. The musculature of the human ureter. Br J Urol 1970; 42:724–7.
11. Tanagho EA, Pugh RC. The anatomy and function of the ureterovesical junction. Br J Urol 1963; 35:151–65.
12. Hanna MK, Jeffs RD, Sturgess JM et al. Ureteral structure and ultrastructure. Part 1. The normal human ureter. J Urol 1976; 116:725.
13. McCormack LU, Anson BJ. The arterial supply of the ureter. Q Bull Northwest Univ Med School 1950; 24:1.
14. Mitchell GAG. The innervation of the kidney, ureter, testicle and epididymis. J Anat 1935; 70:10.
15. Schulman CC. Innervation of the ureter. Anat Clin 1981; 3:127.
16. Keating MA, Escala J, Snyder H et al. Changing concepts in management of primary obstructive megaureter. J Urol 1989; 142:636–40.
17. Shokeir AA, Nijman RJM. Primary megaureter: current trends in diagnosis and treatment. BJU Int 2000; 86:861–8.

18. Caulk JR. Megaloureter: the importance of the ureterovesical valve. J Urol 1923; 9:315.
19. Swenson O, MacMahon E, Jaques WE, Campbell JS. A new concept of the etiology of megaloureters. N Engl J Med 1952; 246:41–6.
20. Leibowitz S, Bodian M. A study of the vesical ganglia in children and the relationship to the megaureter megacystis syndrome and Hirschsprung's disease. J Clin Pathol 1963; 16:342–50.
21. MacKinnon KJ, Foote JW, Wiglesworth FW, Blennerhasse JB. The pathology of the adynamic distal ureteral segment. J Urol 1970; 103:134–7.
22. Kretschmer HL, Hibbs WG. A study of the vesical end of the ureter in hydronephrosis. Surg Gynecol Obstet 1933; 57:170.
23. Tanagho EJ, Smith DR, Guthrie TH. Pathophysiology of functional ureteral obstruction. J Urol 1970; 104:73.
24. Gregoir W, Debled G. [The etiology of congenital reflux and primary megaureter]. Urol Int 1969; 24:119–34. [French]
25. Notley RG. Electron microscopy of the primary obstructive megaureter. Br J Urol 1972; 44:229–34.
26. Medel R Jr, Quesada EM. Ultrastructural characteristics of collagen tissue in normal and congenitally dilated ureter. Eur Urol 1985; 11:324–9.
27. Hanna MK, Jeffs RD, Sturgess JM, Barkin M. Ureteral structure and ultrastructure: Part II. Congenital ureteropelvic junction obstruction and primary obstructive megaureter. J Urol 1976; 116:725–30.
28. Tokunaka S, Gotoh T, Koyanagi T, Miyabe N. Muscle dysplasia in megaureters. J Urol 1984; 131:383–90.
29. Dixon JS, Jen PYP, Yeung CK, Gosling JA. The vesicoureteric junction in three cases of primary obstructive megaureter associated with ectopic ureteric insertion. Br J Urol 1998; 81:580–4.
30. Hofman J, Friedrich U, Hofmann B et al. Acetylcholinesterase activities in association with congenital malformation of the terminal ureter in infants and children. Z Kinderchir 1986; 41:32.
31. Hertle L, Nawrath H. In vitro studies on human primary obstructed megaureters. J Urol 1985; 133:884–7.
32. Nicotina PA, Romeo C, Arena F, Romeo G. Segmental up-regulation of transforming growth factor-β in the pathogenesis of primary megaureter. An immunocytochemical study. Br J Urol 1997; 80:946–9.
33. Keating MA, Retik AB. Management of the dilated obstructed ureter. In: Retik AB, ed. Pediatric Urinary Obstruction. Urol Clin North Am 1990; 17(Suppl): 291–306.
34. Belloli G, Campobasso P, Cappelari F, Mercurella A. Management of primary non-refluxing upper urinary tract dilation: an analysis of 219 paediatric patients. Pediatr Surg Int 1993; 8:229–35.
35. Cozzi F, Madonna L, Maggi E et al. Management of primary megaureter in infancy. J Pediatr Surg 1993; 8:1031–3.
36. Liu HYA, Dhillon HK, Yeoung CK et al. Clinical outcome and management of prenatally diagnosed primary megaureters. J Urol 1994; 152:614–17.
37. Lee BR, Silver RI, Partin AW, Epstein JI, Gearhart JP. A quantitative histologic analysis of collagen subtypes: the primary obstructed and refluxing megaureter of childhood. Urology 1998; 51:820–3.
38. Lee BR, Partin AW, Epstein JI et al. A quantitative histological analysis of the dilated ureter of childhood. J Urol 1992; 148:1482–6.
39. Joseph DB. Triad syndrome and other disorders of abnormal detrusor development. In: Gonzales ET, Bauer SB, eds. Pediatric Urology Practice. Philadelphia: Lippincott, Williams and Wilkins, 1999: 323–37.
40. Gearhart JP, Lee BR, Partin AW et al. Quantitative histological evaluation of the dilated ureter of childhood, II: Ectopia, posterior urethral valves and the prune belly syndrome. J Urol 1995; 153:172–6.
41. Ehrlich RM, Brown WJ. Ultrastructural anatomic observations of the ureter in the prune belly syndrome. Birth Defects Orig Artic Ser 1977; 13:101–3.
42. McLellan DL, Retik AB, Bauer SB et al. Rate and predictors of spontaneous resolution of prenatally diagnosed primary nonrefluxing megaureter. J Urol 2002; 168(5):2177–80.
43. Brown T, Mandell J, Lebowitz RL. Neonatal hydronephrosis in the era of sonography. AJR Am J Roentgenol 1987; 148:959–63.
44. Estroff JA, Mandell J, Benacerraf BR. Increased renal parenchymal echogenicity in the fetus: importance and clinical outcome. Radiology 1991; 181:135–9.
45. Shokeir AA, Provoost AP, el-Azab M, Dawaba M, Nijman RJ. Renal Doppler ultrasound in children with normal upper urinary tracts: effect of fasting, hydration with normal saline, and furosemide administration. Urology 1996; 47:740–4.
46. Shokeir AA, Provoost AP, el-Azab M, Dawaba M, Nijman RJ. Renal Doppler ultrasound in children with obstructive uropathy: effect of intravenous normal saline fluid load and furosemide. J Urol 1996; 156: 1455–8.
47. Blickman JG, Lebowitz RL. The coexistence of primary megaureter and reflux. AJR Am J Roentgenol 1984; 143:1053–7.
48. Carrico C, Lebowitz RL. Incontinence due to an infrasphincteric ectopic ureter: why the delay in diagnosis and what the radiologist can do about it. Pediatr Radiol 1998; 28:942–9.
49. Erbas B, Royal S, Joseph D. Scintigraphic evaluation of obstructing primary megaureter with Tc-99m MAG3. Clin Nucl Med 1997; 22:355–8.
50. Anton-Pacheco Sanchez J, Gomez Fraile A, Aransay Brantot A, Lopez Vazquez F, Encinas Goenechen A. Diuresis renography in the diagnosis and follow-up of unobstructive primary megaureter. Eur J Pediatr Surg 1995; 5:338–41.
51. The Society for Fetal Urology and Members of the Pediatric Nuclear Medicine Council: The 'well tempered' diuretic renogram: standard method to examine the asymptomatic neonate with hydronephrosis or hydroureteronephrosis. J Nucl Med 1992; 33:2047.
52. English PJ, Testa HJ, Lawson RS, Carroll RN, Edwards EC. Modified method of diuresis renography for the assessment of equivocal pelviureteric junction obstruction. Br J Urol 1987; 59:10–14.
53. Willie S, von Knobloch R, Klose KJ, Heidenreich A,

Hofmann R. Magnetic resonance urography in pediatric urology. Scand J Urol Nephrol 2003; 37(1):16.
54. Berrocal T, Lopez-Pereira P, Arjonilla A, Gutierrez J. Anomalies of the distal ureter, bladder, and urethra in children: embryologic, radiologic, and pathologic features. Radiographics 2002; 22(5):1139–64.
55. Riccabona M, Simbrunner J, Ring E et al. Feasibility of MR urography in neonates and infants with anomalies of the upper urinary tract. Eur Radiol 2002; 12(6):1442–50.
56. Whitaker RH. Methods of assessing obstruction in dilated ureters. Br J Urol 1973; 45:15–22.
57. Joseph DB. Imaging of the megaureter. In: Brock JW, guest ed. Dialogues in Pediatric Urology 1993; 16:2.
58. Fung LCT, Churchill BM, McLorie GA, Chait PG, Khoury AE. Ureteral opening pressure: a novel parameter for the evaluation of pediatric hydronephrosis. J Urol 1998; 159:1326–30.
59. Special Communications. Elder JS, Peters CA, Arant BS, Ewalt DH et al. Pediatric vesicoureteral reflux guidelines panel summary report on the management of primary vesicoureteral reflux in children. J Urol 1997; 157:1846–51.
60. Williams DI. The chronically dilated ureter: Hunterian Lecture. Ann R Coll Surg 1954; 14:107.
61. Burbige KA, Lebowitz RL, Colodny AH, Bauer SB, Retik AB. The megacystis–megaureter syndrome. J Urol 1984; 131:1133–6.
62. Mandell J, Lebowitz RL, Peters CA et al. Prenatal diagnosis of the megacystis–megaureter association. J Urol 1992; 148:1487–9.
63. Lettgen B, Kropfl D, Bonzel KE et al. Primary obstructed megaureter in neonates. Treatment by temporary ureterocutaneostomy. Br J Urol 1993; 72:826–9.
64. Arena F, Baldari S, Proietto F et al. Conservative treatment in primary neonatal megaureter. Eur J Pediatr Surg 1998; 8:347–51.
65. Sheu JC, Chang PY, Wang NL, Tsai TC, Huang FY. Is surgery necessary for primary non-refluxing megaureter? Pediatr Surg Int 1998; 13:501–3.
66. Mollard P, Foray P, de Godoy JL. Management of primary obstructive megaureter without reflux in neonates. Eur Urol 1993; 24:505–10.
67. Stehr M, Metzger R, Schuster T, Porn U, Dietz HG. Management of the primary obstructed megaureter (POM) and indication for operative treatment. Eur J Pediatr Surg 2002; 12(1):32–7.
68. Peters CA, Mandell J, Lebowitz RL et al. Congenital obstructed megaureters in early infancy: diagnosis and treatment. J Urol 1989; 142:641–5.
69. Atala A, Keating MA. Vesicoureteral reflux and megaureter. In: Walsh PC, Retik AB, Vaughan ED, Wein AJ, eds. Campbell's Urology, 7th edn, vol 3. Philadelphia: WB Saunders, 1998.
70. Starr A. Ureteral plication. A new concept in ureteral tapering for megaureter. Invest Urol 1979; 17:153–8.
71. Kalicinski ZH, Kansy J, Kotarbinska B, Joszt W. Surgery of megaureters – modification of Hendren's operation. J Pediatr Surg 1977; 12:183–8.
72. Hendren WH. Operative repair of megaureter in children. J Urol 1969; 101:491–507.
73. Hanna MK. New surgical method for one-stage total remodeling of massively dilated and tortuous ureter: tapering in situ technique. Urology 1979; 14:453–64.
74. Perdzynski W, Kalicinski ZH. Long-term results after megaureter folding in children. J Pediatr Surg 1996; 31:1211–17.
75. Ehrlich RM. The ureteral folding technique for megaureter surgery. J Urol 1985; 134:668–70.
76. Parrot TS, Woodard JR, Wolpert JJ. Ureteral tailoring: a comparison of wedge resection with infolding. J Urol 1990; 144:328–9.
77. Fretz PC, Austin JC, Cooper CS, Hawtrey CE. Long-term outcome analysis of Starr plication for primary obstructive megaureters. J Urol 2004; 172(2): 703–5.
78. Daher P, Diab N, Ghorayeb Z, Korkmaz G. The Kalicinski ureteral folding technique for megaureter in children. Experience in 23 cases. Eur J Pediatr Surg 1999; 9(3):163–6.
79. Bjordal RI, Eek S, Knutrud O. Early reconstruction of wide ureter in children. Urology 1978; 11:325–37.
80. Bjordal RI, Stake G, Knutrud O. Surgical treatment of megaureters in the first few months of life. Ann Chir Gynaecol 1980; 69:10–14.
81. Hendren WH. Complications of megaureter repair in children. J Urol 1975; 113:238–54.
82. Sripathi V, King PA, Thompson MR et al. Primary obstructive megaureter. J Pediatr Surg 1991; 26:826–9.
83. Diamond DA, Parulkar BG. Ureteral tailoring in situ: a practical approach to persistent reflux in the dilated reimplanted ureter. J Urol 1998; 160:998–1000.
84. Coleman JW, McGovern JH. A 20-year experience with pediatric ureteral reimplantation: surgical results in 701 children. In: Hodson J, Kincaid-Smith P, eds. Reflux Nephropathy. New York: Masson, 1979: 299–305.
85. Caione P, Capozza N, Asili L, Lais A, Matarazzo E. Is primary obstructive megaureter repair at risk for contralateral reflux? J Urol 2000; 164(3 Pt 2):1061–3.

Ureteral duplication anomalies: ectopic ureters and ureteroceles

40

Michael A Keating

Introduction

Ureteral duplication is one of the most common anomalies affecting the genitourinary tract. Variants, including incomplete ureteral duplication and complete duplications with normally developed renal moieties, constitute the vast majority. As such, they represent no more than radiologic curiosities. Anomalies with clinical significance, including ectopic ureters and ureteroceles, are much less common. Historically, the majority of these were probably clinically silent.[1] A smaller portion became evident as a consequence of hydronephrosis, vesicoureteral reflux (VUR), or incontinence, either in combination or alone. More recently, antenatal diagnosis has uncovered many urologic anomalies, including different variants of ureteral duplications, which are asymptomatic. Antenatal detection enables the preservation of renal function and the avoidance of illness for some children. For others, perinatal identification creates controversy by introducing a large group of abnormalities that may have gone harmlessly undetected in the past.

Despite these decision-making dilemmas, it seems prudent to institute pre-emptive therapy for urinary tract anomalies that pose risk to a child, until those characteristics that typify their spontaneous resolution or a lifetime free of urologic problems are better defined. Spontaneous resolution seems unlikely for most ectopic ureters and uretereoceles. As a consequence, pediatric urologic surgeons must remain familiar with the natural history of duplication anomalies, well versed in the evolving recommendations for their management, and familiar with the variety of surgical techniques available for their reconstruction.

Embryologic considerations

Normal development

A review of normal development provides the basis for understanding the pathophysiology of anomalies of the ureter and, in some cases, aids in their diagnosis and clinical management.

Ureteral development coincides with that of the kidney between 4 and 8 weeks of gestation. The ureteral bud (metanephric duct) projects from the wolffian (mesonephric) duct just proximal to its junction with the cloaca (Figure 40.1). As the ureteral

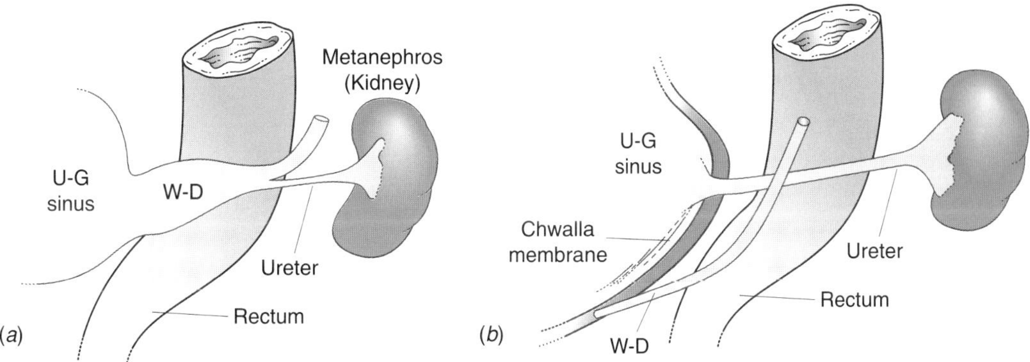

Figure 40.1 (*a* and *b*) Relationships of ureteral bud, wolffian (mesonephric) duct (W-D) and urogenital sinus (U-G). The segment of wolffian duct between urogenital sinus and ureteral bud represents the common excretory duct.

bud elongates in a cephalad direction, it penetrates the adjacent metanephric tissue and divides into the calices and collecting ducts. Proper fusion of the bud and the nephrogenic blastema is critical to tubular maturation within the renal anlage and ultimate function of the kidney. Mesenchymal–epithelial interactions, perhaps under the influence of local paracrine factors acting via receptors on the ducts, help pattern normal formation.[2]

The segment of wolffian duct between the cloaca and takeoff of the ureteral bud (the future ureteral orifice) is called the common excretory duct. The migration of tissue that occurs during the excretory duct's incorporation into the urogenital sinus helps to explain the variable relationships that sometimes occur between the ureter(s) and the trigone of the bladder, urethra, and genital ducts. Conceptually, these events represent some of the most difficult to understand in urinary tract embryology.

In brief, as the common excretory duct is absorbed into the bladder, the ureteral orifice migrates in a cranial and lateral direction. While this occurs, the excretory duct migrates to the midline and fuses with its contralateral partner to form the primitive trigone. This would explain the presumed mesodermal origin of the trigone, although recent studies have suggested that the tissue may instead be endodermal in origin.[3] The orifice of the wolffian duct ends in a caudal and medial position at the utricle. The wolffian (mesonephric)) duct ultimately differentiates into the prostate, seminal vesicles, vas deferens, and epididymis in males. In females, the wolffian ducts guide the müllerian ducts into position in the midline, where the latter fuse to form the uterus, proximal vagina, and fallopian tubes. After their involution, wolffian remnants persist in as many as 25% of women as Gartner's duct lying along the anterolateral vaginal wall and uterus, and the epoophoron and oophoron within the broad ligament supporting the fallopian tubes.

Explanations for the variety of anomalies that affect the ureter have their basis in this developmental progression, although the causes of the initial insult remain unclear.[4] An alteration in timing seems key.

Abnormal development

Lateral orifice ectopia occurs when the ureteral bud originates from a more caudal position than usual on the mesonephric duct. As a result, the ureteral orifice has more time to be absorbed within the bladder and begin its cranial and lateral migration. As the degree of laterality becomes more exaggerated, the length of submucosal ureter is progressively shortened. In addition, because the common excretory duct is shortened by the premature takeoff of the ureteral bud, its mesenchymal contribution to the trigone is blunted. This results in muscular deficiency of the trigonal–ureteral complex. Primary reflux becomes a common consequence of lateral ectopia and is thoroughly discussed elsewhere (see Chapters 42–46).

Caudal ectopia of the ureter results from an abnormally high takeoff of the ureteral bud. This allows less time for the orifice to be absorbed into the bladder. Now more closely positioned to ductal tissue typically destined to become wolffian, the ureter arrives in a medial trigonal or urethral location or extravesically positioned along the path of wolffian duct structures or remnants. The location of wolffian remnants helps explain an important difference in presentation of ectopic ureters between males and females (Figure 40.2). Ectopic ureters in males are connected to structures that continue to drain into the bladder proximal to the urinary sphincter. Urinary control should be normal. In contrast, ectopic ureters in females potentially vent into remnants adjacent to the fallopian tube (epoophoron), body of the uterus (paroophoron), and vagina (Gartner's duct), where they presumably rupture or are absorbed. Since the urinary sphincter is bypassed, incontinence results.

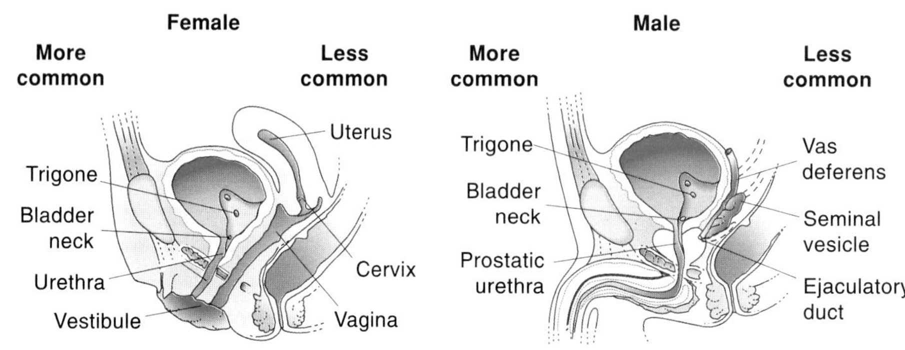

Figure 40.2 Anatomic locations of ectopic ureters.

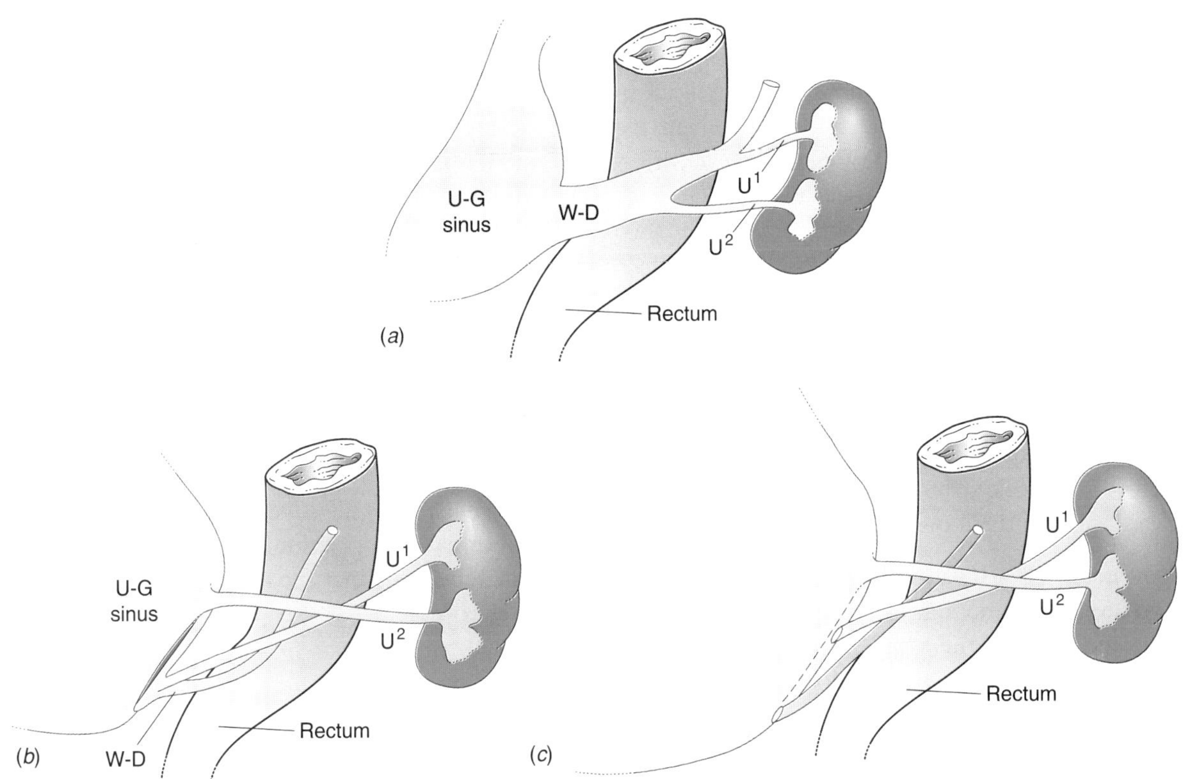

Figure 40.3 (*a–c*) Complete ureteral duplication. Caudal ectopia (U^1) results from abnormally high takeoff of ureteral bud, which remains positioned near wolffian duct tissue. Lateral ectopia (U^2) results from more caudal position, allowing more time for intravesical migration.

Ureteral duplication occurs when a single ureteral bud branches prematurely during its ascent or when two distinct ureteral buds arise from the wolffian (mesonephric) duct (Figure 40.3). The clinical significance of these anomalies depends on the location of the buds and their interplay with the developing kidney.

Branching of a single bud after its takeoff from the mesonephric duct results in incomplete ureteral duplication. The configurations that can occur range from anomalies as mild as a bifid renal pelvis (late branching) to nearly complete duplications having a common intravesical stem (early branching). The location of the ureteral orifice with incomplete duplications depends upon the takeoff of the ureteral bud in the sequence cited above. Bifurcations can occur at any level from the bladder to the renal pelvis but begin in the lower third of the ureter.[5] Most buds are normally positioned along the mesonephric duct and, as a consequence, incomplete duplications are usually radiologic curiosities having little clinical significance.

Complete ureteral duplication occurs when two ureteral buds project from the mesonephric duct, each having a separate interaction with the metanephric blastema. During their early takeoff, the buds interact with the primordial kidney in logical fashion. The most superior/cephalad bud induces the upper portion of the blastema (upper pole), while the lower bud joins the lower pole moiety. However, the ultimate positions of the ureteral orifices are governed by the same enigmatic rules of tissue migration and incorporation into the bladder described for singlets above.

When both buds are close together and project from a normal position along the mesonephric duct, both ureters will have normally positioned orifices. When the buds are more widely separated, one or both will be ectopic. If the superior/upper pole bud projects from an abnormally high position along the mesonephric duct, caudal ectopia is the outcome. If the bud to the lower pole originates from a more caudal position along the duct, lateral ectopia results. To achieve their ultimate positions, the ureters and their orifices complete a 180° clockwise rotation along their longitudinal axes. These relationships, defined by the Weigert–Meyer law, are unusually consistent.[6,7] Exceptions have been described but are rare.[8,9]

Recent studies using angiotensin type 2 receptor (*AGTR2*) gene mutant animals have demonstrated features similar to those of humans with duplication anomalies.[10,11] Similarities in renal development to the relationships defined by the Weigert–Meyer principle and the theories proposed by Mackie and Stephens (below) have been correlated with this genetic abnormality. There is a high likelihood that *AGTR2* plays a part in the polygenic mode of inheritance of ureteral abnormalities in humans.

Ureteroceles

Several theories have been proposed for the development of ureteroceles, though their etiology remains unclear. Some of the more popular theories are:

1 Persistence of Chwalla's membrane, which is a two-layered membrane that transiently separates the caudal end of the wolffian duct from the urogenital sinus (37 days' gestation),[12] is possible. Incomplete dissolution of the membrane could account for the cystic dilatation of the terminal ureter and stenosis of the orifice found with ureteroceles.
2 Abnormal muscular development of the terminal ureter has been implicated by a number of studies.[13] Ballooning of the distal ureter could be explained by a deficiency or an absence of its muscular investing layers, a finding shown in over 90% of specimens in one study.[14] By comparison, the distal segments of ectopic ureters consistently have musculature that is better developed than ureteroceles.[15] The ureterocele itself is covered with vesical mucosa, whereas the internal lining is made up of ureteral mucosa. Varying degrees of attenuated smooth muscle and connective tissue are sandwiched between. An element of meatal or perisphincteric obstruction,[16] may also contribute to the dilatation. However, some ureteroceles present without a functioning kidney, suggesting to some clinicians that urinary output is an unnecessary impetus to distal ureteral ectasia.[17] It is also plausible that the kidneys associated with these so-called 'blind ureteroceles' produce urine during an early critical stage in development but subsequently involute.[18]
3 Abnormal widening of the mesonephric duct may occur in the segment between its insertion at the urogenital sinus and the ureteral bud. This area normally dilates in concert with an undefined stimulus for vesical and urethral expansion. Ureteral migration is presumably completed before this expansion occurs. Proximal extension of the widening process into the distal ureter could result in ureterocele development.[4] This explanation seems plausible for intravesical ureteroceles, the ureter and orifice of which have migrated appropriately. Late incorporation of the ureteral bud from an abnormally proximal position within this dilated segment is another possibility. This explanation is more compatible with extravesical ureteroceles accompanied by ectopic orifices. Notably, ectopic ureters associated with even more proximal buds that insert into wolffian remnants are rarely ectatic at their distal ends. They are presumably unaffected by the stimulus that alters the urogenital sinus.[13] As discussed below, the concept of abnormal bud position may also account for the renal dysplasia that accompanies many extravesical ureteroceles.

Ureteral–renal interactions

The ultimate maturation of the renal blastema is dictated by its interaction with the ureteral bud. When this interplay is experimentally altered, the expected transformation of blastema to normal nephron does not occur.[19,20] Mackie and Stephens[21] proposed the mid-region of the elongate metanephric blastema as being most conducive to becoming normal renal parenchyma. Ureteral buds that originate from abnormally cephalic or caudal positions along the wolffian duct are destined to induce polar blastema, which results in cystic dysplasia (Figure 40.4). This theory offers a ready explanation for the dysplasia and scars found within kidneys with associated VUR where urinary tract infections (UTIs) have never occurred. It could explain why ectopic ureters with urinary insertions (GU-ectopy) are more likely to be associated with functioning renal parenchyma than ectopic ureters having wolffian or gynecologic (GYN-ectopy) insertions, where dysplasia is often present.[22] Ureteral bud takeoff could also explain the difference between the salvageable renal function usually seen with intravesical ureteroceles, and the poor function that occurs with extravesical ureteroceles.

Clinical correlates offer only guarded support of this theory, despite its attractiveness. Most studies generally cite poor renal function in the presence of severe reflux or marked ureteral ectopia,[23] though the difference between GU- and GYN-ectopy has come into question.[24] In addition, antenatal detection has added some new twists. In one review of specimens from 50 consecutive patients undergoing hemi-

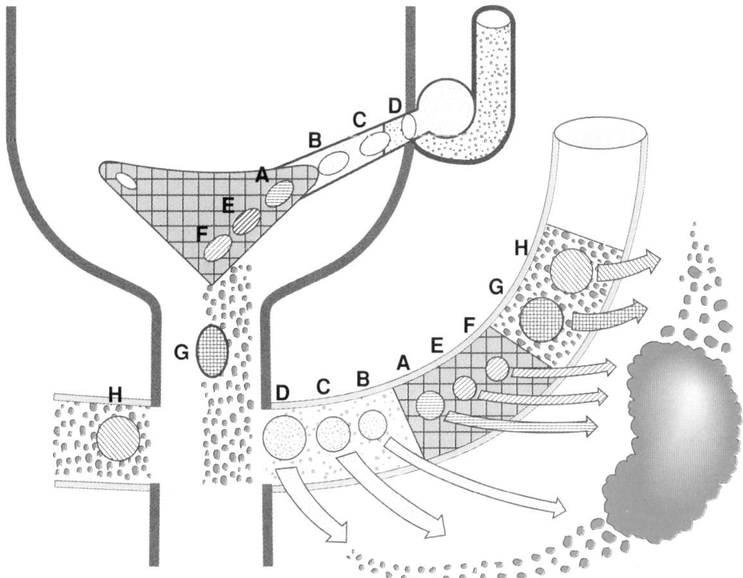

Figure 40.4 In theory, the position of the ureteral bud on the wolffian (mesonephric) duct corresponds to the final position of the ureteral orifice and differentiation of the metanephric blastema. Lateral and caudal ectopia can both result in renal dysplasia.

nephrectomies, dysplasia was seen in 70% from ureteroceles and 30% from ectopic ureters.[25] Each had been diagnosed antenatally, yet none were felt to have histologic changes that may have benefited from renal preservation surgery. By contrast, in a similar series of 40 consecutive antenatally diagnosed duplication anomalies, only six required heminephrectomy because of poor function and none of these showed evidence of dyplasia.[26]

Most historical reports cite salvageable renal function in only 20–30% of patients with ureteroceles. This pales next to the yield of contemporary series, whose numbers are inflated by the addition of antenatally diagnosed anomalies and the sensitivity of better diagnostics. The clinical implications are obvious (see Recommendations). Are these renal moieties that were previously destined to lose renal function as a consequence of progressive obstruction? Do they truly benefit from being surgically diverted or endoscopically decompressed? Or is renal parenchyma being preserved that has an intrinsic developmental insult? Nodular renal blastema has been reported in upper pole heminephrectomy specimens removed with ectopic ureteroceles.[27] Dysplasia is also a common finding.[28] The study by Arena et al[29] failed to show any evidence of reversible histologic changes in heminephrectomy specimens of patients whose ureteroceles had been prenatally diagnosed. It is unclear as to whether this is cause for concern. To date, no chronic complications of renal salvage unrelated to the surgery itself (e.g. hypertension or tumor formation) have been reported.

Nomenclature and classification

Ectopic ureters

The term ectopic ureter refers to a ureter that has migrated with the wolffian duct structures and is more caudally positioned than a normal ureter. Such ureters drain into the urethra, wolffian, or müllerian structures. The ureter to the lower pole of a duplication, which is often laterally displaced and ectopic in the purest sense, is regarded as orthotopic. Single-system ureters, that are laterally misplaced and reflux as a consequence, are discussed elsewhere (see Chapters 42–46).

Ureteroceles

Historically, ureteroceles associated with single systems were regarded as orthotopic or simple and considered adult type, despite the fact that some such variants are clearly ectopic and are found in children (Figures 40.5–40.9). Ureteroceles subtending the upper pole ureter of a duplex system have been described as ectopic and pediatric, although exceptions to both descriptions also commonly occur.[30] Gonzalez[31] felt it simplest to describe the anomaly based on the location of its orifice. Other than their

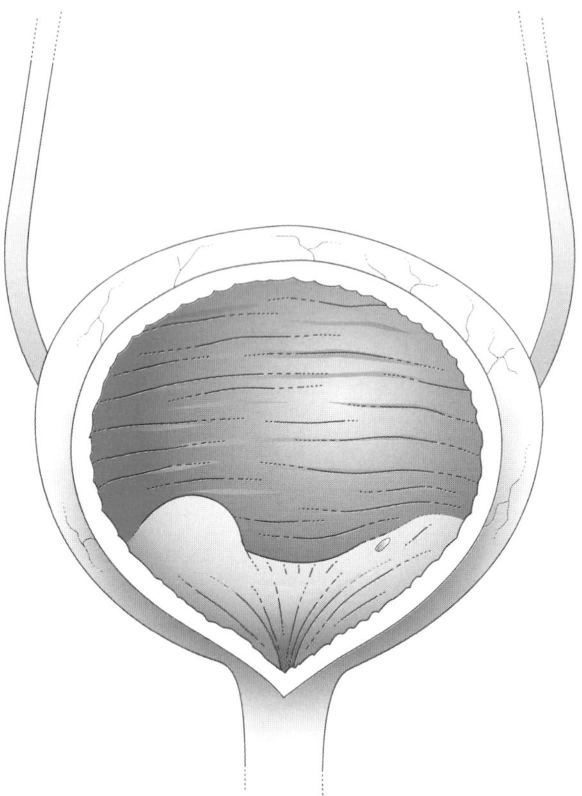

Figure 40.5 Intravesical ureterocele subtending a single ureter. This can also be classified as orthotopic or simple.

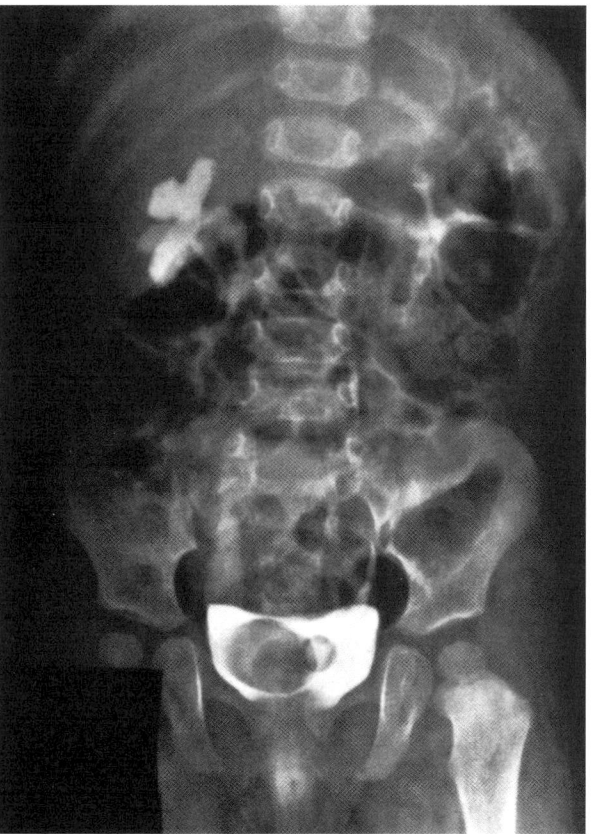

Figure 40.6 Excretory urogram shows bilateral single-system intravesical ureteroceles, right larger than left. Renal function is typically preserved.

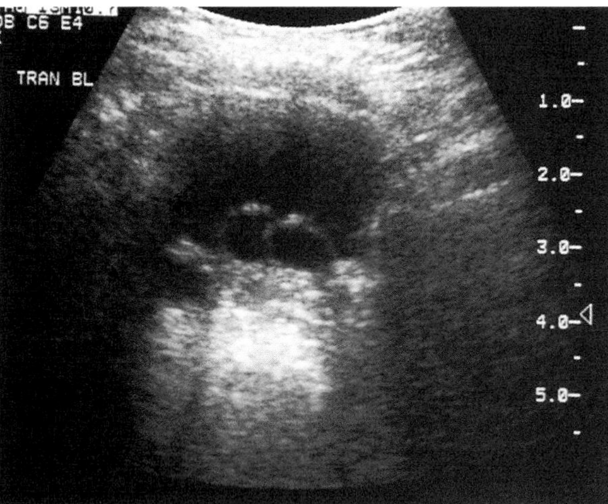

Figure 40.7 Ultrasonic appearance of a similar patient with bilateral intravesical ureteroceles.

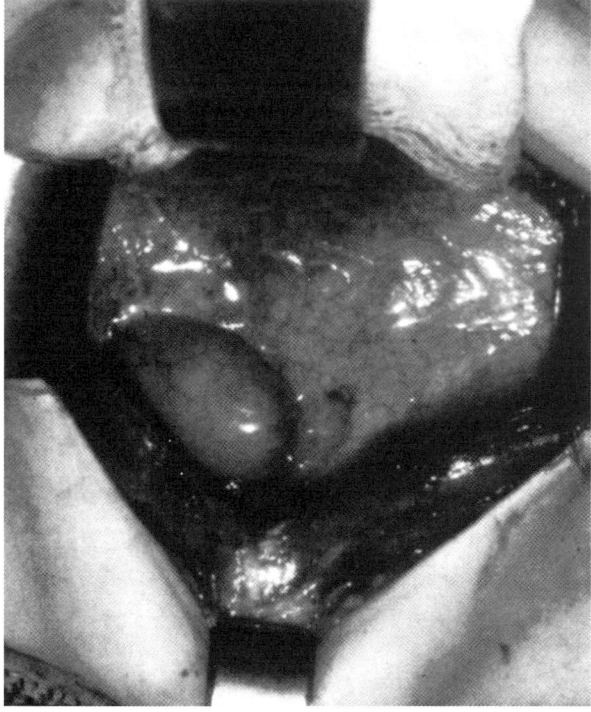

Figure 40.8 Intraoperative photograph of bilateral intravesical single-system ureteroceles.

association with a single or duplex system, two types of ureteroceles exist: intravesical or extravesical. This definition avoids the confusion associated with the terms ectopic and orthotopic. In addition, such nomenclature reflects the embryologic importance of

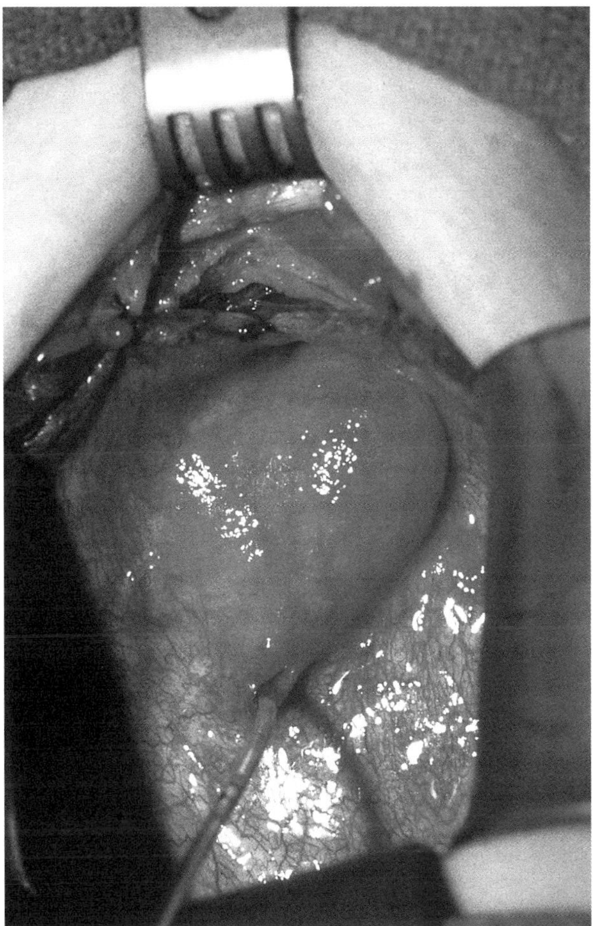

Figure 40.9 Large ureterocele extending towards the bladder neck (top). There is a catheter in the lower pole ureter, which is displaced and freely refluxes.

the ureteral bud/orifice to renal development and distortion of the bladder neck. However, this form of categorization potentially mislabels ureteroceles with an intravesical orifice but an extension into the bladder neck or urethra. Anatomically, these could also be considered extravesical.

A variety of other classification schemes have been proposed for ureteroceles, although no system has been adopted universally. Stephens' categorization[16] can be used to provide additional information about the location and configuration of the orifice of the ureterocele. These factors presumably account for the degree of distortion of the bladder neck and urethra, as well as the extensiveness of the renal dysplasia accompanying the anomaly (Table 40.1; Figures 40.10 and 40.11).

Characteristics

Ureteral duplications

Duplication is the most common congenital anomaly in the urinary tract: a 0.7% incidence was found in one series of more than 50 000 autopsies.[32] Intravenous urograms demonstrate duplications in 4% of studies, and hydronephrosis and scarring is seen in 27% of these.[33] Females are affected two to four times more commonly than males. The right and left collecting systems are affected equally. Bilateral duplications occur in 17–33% of cases.

The anomaly is an inheritable defect transmitted in an autosomal fashion having variable penetrance.[34]

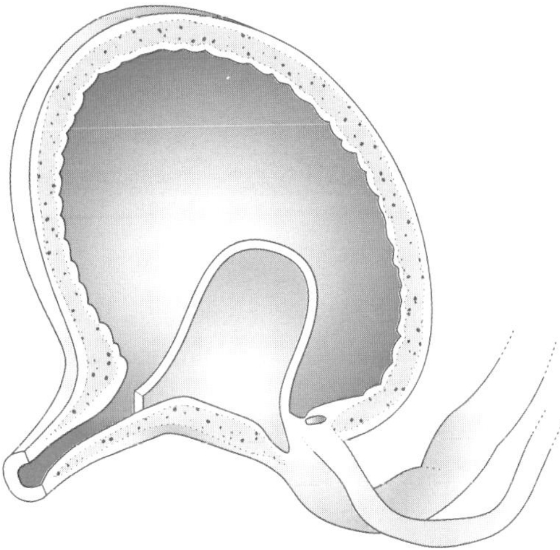

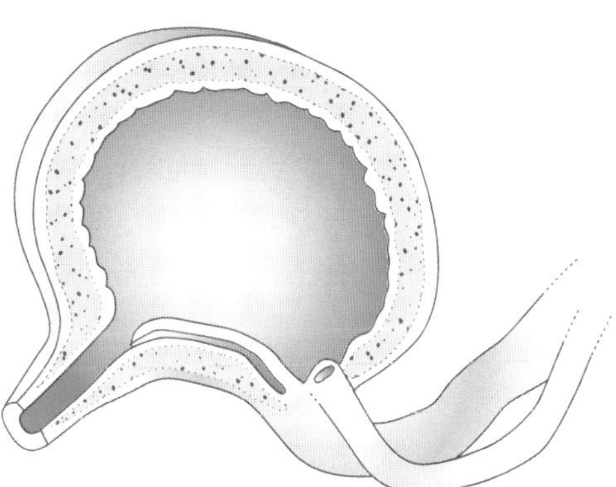

Figure 40.10 Sphincteric variant of extravesical ureterocele subtending upper pole ureter of duplex system. The orifice opens proximal to the external sphincter. Normal contraction of the bladder neck may contribute to ureteral obstruction.

Table 40.1 Classification of duplex ureteroceles

Ureterocele	Frequency (%)	Features
Intravesical		
Stenotic	40	Involve a congenitally small ureteral orifice adding an element of obstruction for the upper pole
Non-obstructed	5	The ureteral orifice is large and balloons open without any ureteral obstruction
Extravesical		
Sphincteric	40	The orifice opens outside the bladder and the ureterocele extends into the bladder neck and urethra. The orifice is normal or large and usually opens proximal to the external sphincter. In females, the meatus may open distal to the sphincter. At rest, the bladder neck and sphincter contract on the ureter and orifice, causing obstruction
Sphincterostenotic	5	Similar to sphincteric, but the ureteral orifice is stenotic
Cecoureteroceles	5	A large orifice opens in the bladder but a blind pouch or cecum extends into the submucosa of the urethra. When the cecum distends with urine, urethral obstruction can result
Blind ectopic	5	Similar to sphincteric, with no ureteral orifice

From Stephens.[13]

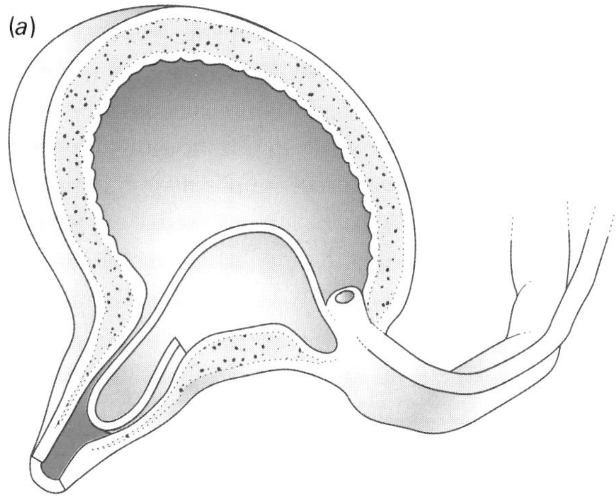

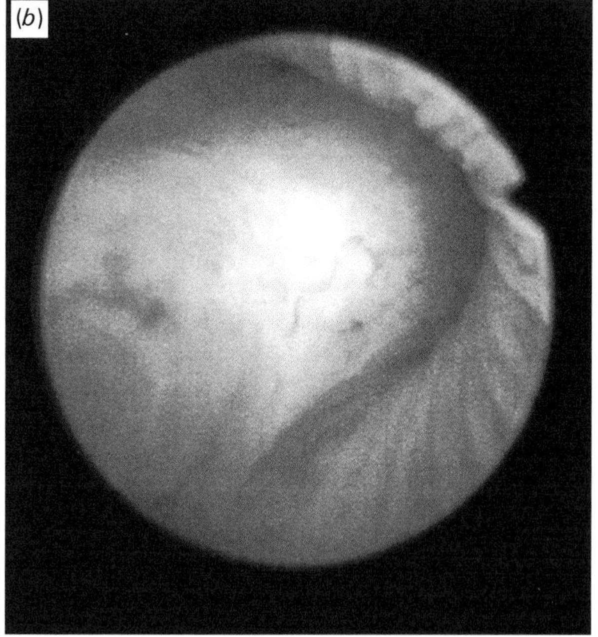

Figure 40.11 (*a*) Cecoureterocele variant of an extravesical ureterocele. Blind-ending extension beneath submucosa of urethra can prolapse and/or cause bladder outlet obstruction. (*b*) Cystoscopic appearance of the urethral extension of the cecoureterocele.

The parents or siblings of a child with a duplex ureter have as much as a one in eight chance of having a similarly affected child.[35]

Ectopic ureters

The incidence of ureteral ectopia was approximately 1 in 2000 in one series of autopsies in children. Many remain asymptomatic and a true incidence is difficult to determine.[36] Ectopic ureters occur in females two to three times more commonly than males,[37,38] although as high as 12-fold increases have been cited.[39] More than 80% of females with ectopic ureters have duplex systems. The majority (75%) in males are singlets.[40,41] Between 70 and 80% of ectopic ureters are associated with complete duplications. Nearly 20% of patients with ureteral ectopy have bilateral involvement.[37] In one report of nearly 500 ectopic ureters, the posterior urethra and prostatic urethra (57%) were the most common sites of drainage in males. The seminal vesicle (33%) was also commonly involved. More remote terminations at the ejaculatory duct and vas were rare (10%). The urethra and vestibule were the most common drainage sites for 69% of females. Vaginal ectopy occurred in another 25%.[37]

Ureteroceles

The incidence of ureteroceles was as high as 1 in 500 in one autopsy study. They occur in females four times more commonly than in males.[42,43] Ureteroceles in girls are associated with duplex systems 95% of the time. By contrast, up to 66% of boys have single-system anomalies.[44] Nearly all appear in Caucasians.

Eighty percent of ureteroceles are associated with the upper pole of a duplex system; the remainder are single-system ureteroceles. Bilateral involvement occurs in 15% of cases.[45] A genetic predisposition has been shown.[46]

Presentation

Antenatal ultrasonography has dramatically increased the detection of urinary anomalies and, in some cases, has altered our understanding of their natural history. The yield from routine screening is significant. Abnormalities of the urinary system are detected in approximately 1 in 500 studies, second only to those of the nervous system. The breakdown of diagnoses in a typical series is shown in Table 40.2. Notably, ectopic ureters, duplications, and ureteroceles can all be detected antenatally. Further evaluation after birth is warranted, even in instances where the anomaly was present earlier in gestation and has presumably resolved.[48] In many cases, the exact etiology of hydronephrosis, the most common antenatal finding, cannot be determined until after delivery. Prenatal cases of bladder outlet obstruction have been reported.[49] Antenatal intervention has been described for rare cases of bladder outlet obstruction caused by ureteroceles.[50,51] Because of the tendency for urinary infections with hydronephrosis, it seems reasonable to keep newborns on prophylactic antibiotics (amoxicillin) until their anatomy is better defined (see Evaluation below).

After delivery, an extravesical ureterocele represents the most common cause of bladder outlet obstruction in newborn girls and the second most common cause in boys, after posterior urethral valves (PUVs). A true pediatric urologic emergency can result, depending on the degree of obstruction. The diagnosis of an obstructing ureterocele should be considered in any infant, especially a girl, with bladder distention, anuria, or ascites.[52] When full-blown prolapse occurs, clinicians will encounter a congested, ecchymotic interlabial mass (Figures 40.12–40.15). The mass may have varying

Table 40.2 Prenatal diagnosis of hydronephrosis and the breakdown of prenatally diagnosed duplex systems

Prenatal diagnosis of hydronephrosis (177 cases)[a]	
Hydronephrosis:	154
Bilateral hydronephrosis	73
Unilateral hydronephrosis	61
Bladder outlet obstruction	9
Duplex/hydronephrosis	9
Prune belly syndrome	2
Multicystic dysplastic kidney	10
Autosomal recessive kidney	5
Other	8
Breakdown of prenatally diagnosed duplex systems (39 cases)[b]	
Ureterocele	15
Ectopic ureter	15
Lower pole reflux	6
Lower pole UPJ obstruction	2
Yo-yo reflux	1

[a]Adapted from Mandell et al.[47]
[b]Adapted from Jee et al.[23]

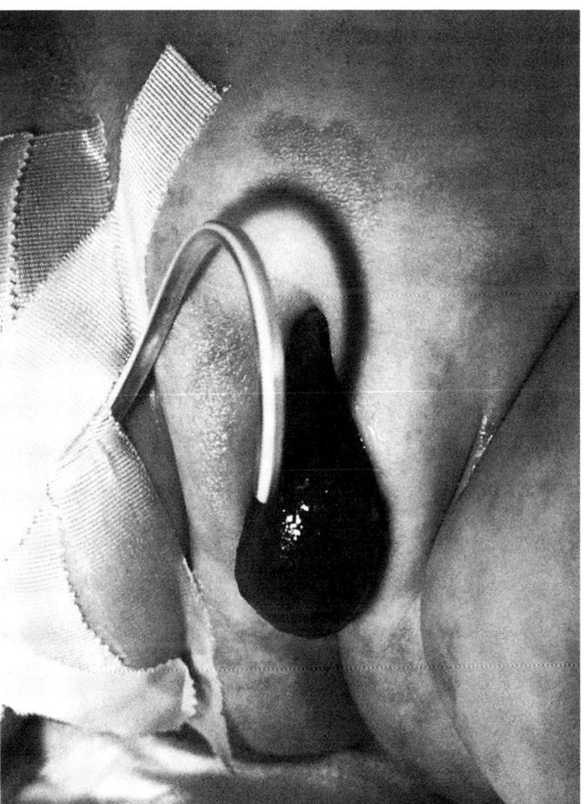

Figure 40.12 Congested and ecchymotic prolapsed ureterocele presenting as an interlabial mass.

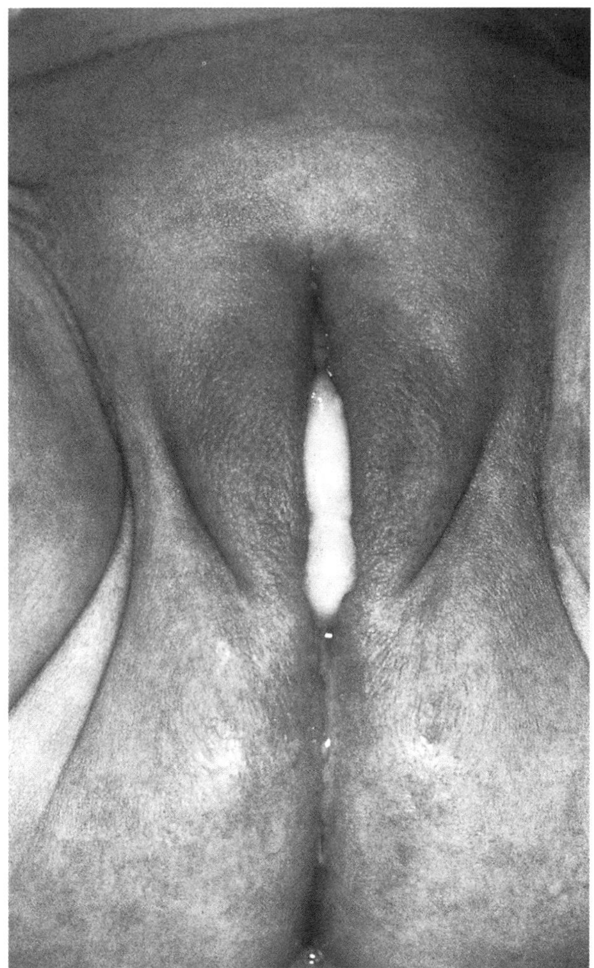

Figure 40.18 Gross pus from the vagina of an infant with an ectopic ureter.

Flank pain, fever, and abdominal mass are common presentations of ectopic ureters left undetected until a later age.[55] Ureteroceles can cause irritative voiding symptoms by obstruction or infection but voiding abnormalities accompany ectopic ureters far more commonly. In addition, the distal segment of ectopic ureters inserting at the verumontanum can elevate the bladder neck, causing outlet obstruction in boys of any age.[56] It is important to remember that ectopic ureters always insert proximal to the urinary sphincter in males. As a result, incontinence does not usually occur in boys with the anomaly. Bilateral single ectopic ureters, associated with bladder neck maldevelopment and lack of sphincter control, are one exception (see below). Another is the frequency and urgency that sometimes results from the trickle of urine into the posterior urethra.[37] However, the more usual proximal insertions into structures of wolffian origin (seminal vesical, vas, epididymis) present their own problems, and ureteral ectopia should be suspected in any infant or child who presents with a culture-proven case of bacterial epididymo-orchitis.

Clinicians should also be wary of any girl who reportedly has never been fully toilet trained. These patients must be approached with an open mind, and the possibility of ureteral ectopia entertained, especially when damp underwear is found on examination. In many cases, a cadre of physicians has treated the patient for presumed bladder dysfunction or psychosocial problems. When the ureter exits along the urethra, the voiding pattern often includes bladder control and spontaneous emptying (from the other ureters having normal bladder insertion) followed by an uncontrollable loss of urine as the obstructed system vents secondarily (Figure 40.19). With vaginal ectopy, continuous wetting in a girl having an otherwise normal micturition pattern and control (in contrast to bladder dysfunction) is a classic presentation[57] (Figures 40.20 and 40.21). The degree of incontinence depends on the urinary output from the affected kidney. In some cases, small amounts of urine cause sporadic incontinence that occurs only while standing. The latter is commonly mistaken for vaginal voiding or stress incontinence. Table 40.3 summa-

Table 40.3 Clinical presentations

Gender	Features
Ectopic ureters	
Both	Acute or recurrent urinary infection Abdominal mass/pain Failure to thrive
Females	Continuous dampness with otherwise normal voiding pattern after toilet training Vaginal discharge Orifice evident along the urethrovaginal septum
Males	Epididymo-orchitis Urgency and frequency Constipation, pelvic pain, painful ejaculation, epididymitis
Ureteroceles	
Both	Acute or recurrent urinary tract infections Hematuria Failure to thrive, abdominal or pelvic pain Abdominal mass
Females	Prolapsed interlabial mass Bladder outlet obstruction
Males	Bladder outlet obstruction

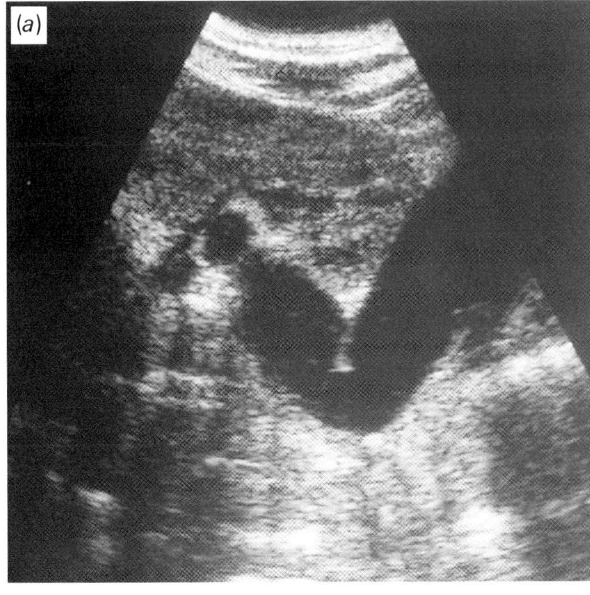

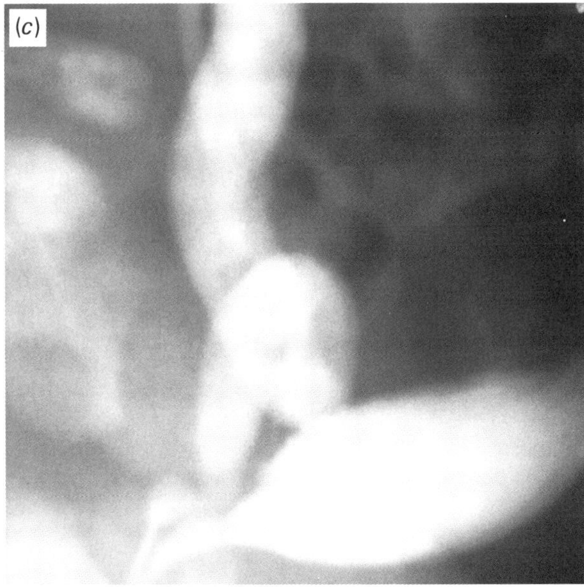

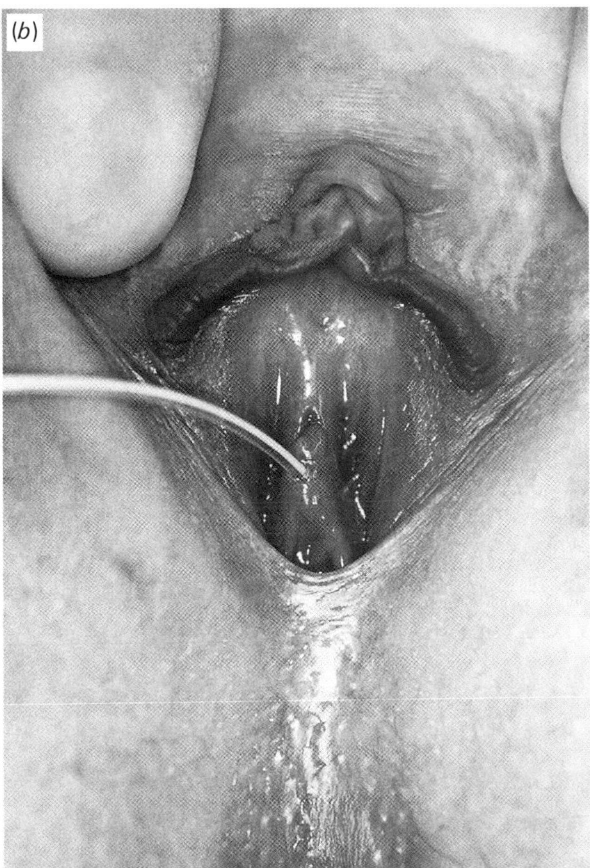

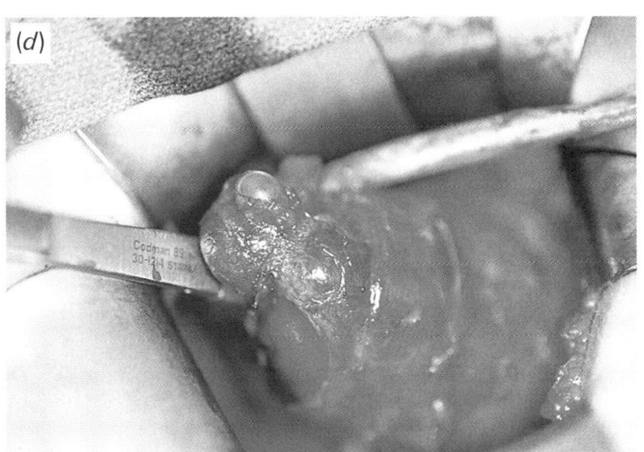

Figure 40.19 Ectopic ureter in a 7-year-old-girl with incontinence. (*a*) Ultrasound provides useful screening of such patients and often makes the diagnosis. Shown here is the dilated upper ureter with duplex kidney. Lower pole differentiation is preserved. (*b*) Close physical examination revealed pinpoint opening (cannulated with a feeding tube). (*c*) Retrograde study of the ectopic ureter. (*d*) At exploration, the megaureter is shown entering the cap of the cystic dysplastic upper pole moiety.

rizes the clinical manifestations of these two ureteral anomalies.

Both anomalies sometimes remain undetected until adulthood.[58,59] Ectopic ureters in girls that pass through the urinary sphincter but are positioned proximal to the meatus can maintain continence during development. Multiparity can unmask the anomaly, which is often mistaken for stress incontinence. With cases of ectopic ureters that terminate in the male genital tract, prostatitis, seminal vesiculitis, and epididymitis can all occur. Most do not become apparent until the onset of sexual activity. Historically, single-system ureteroceles usually presented during adulthood. An intravesical location, coupled with preserved renal function, allows most to go unnoticed until later age (Figure 40.22). This accounted for their prior designation as 'adult type', a label since dropped with the advent of antenatal diagnosis. Common presentations still include stones, milk of calcium, and recurrent UTIs.[60]

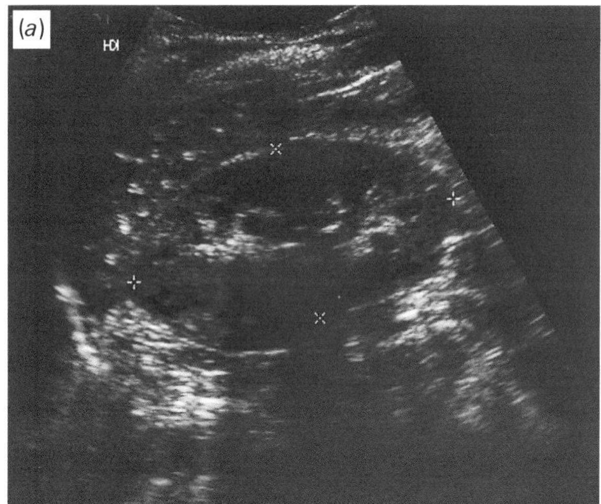

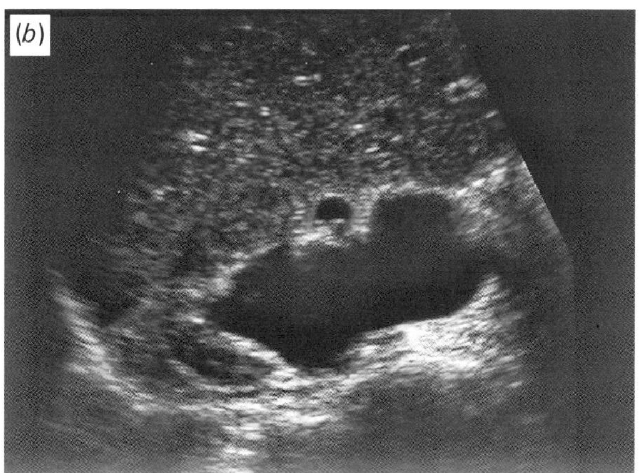

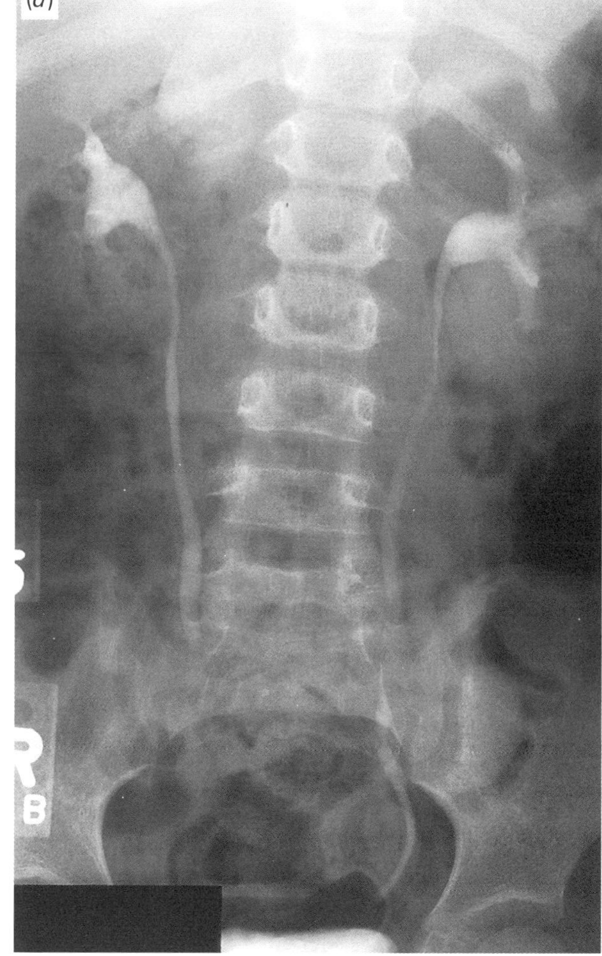

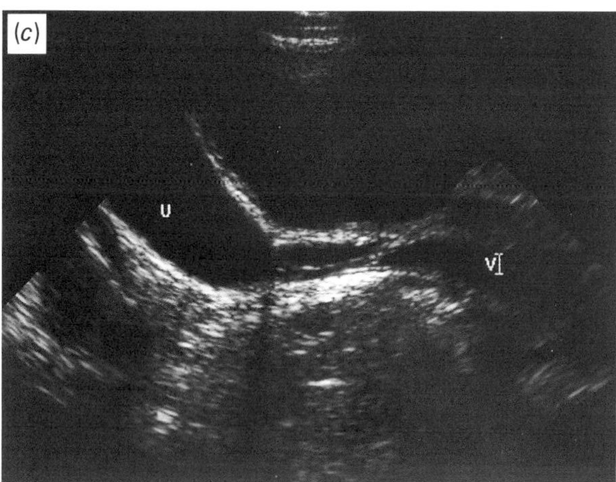

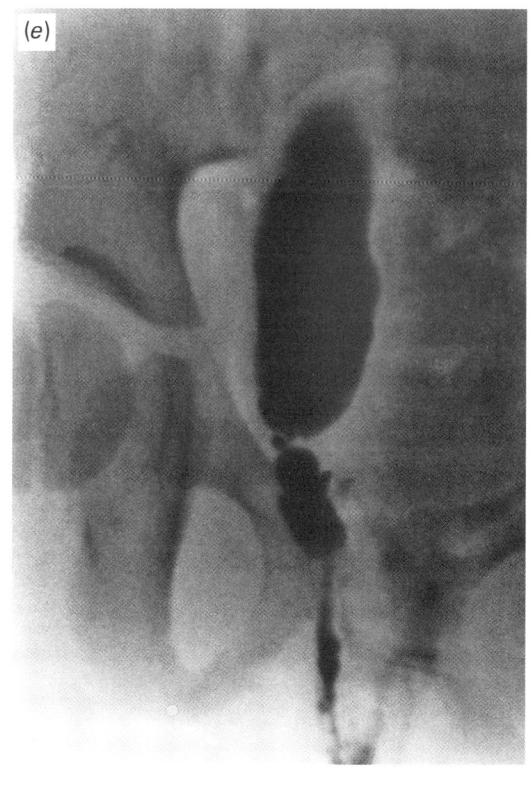

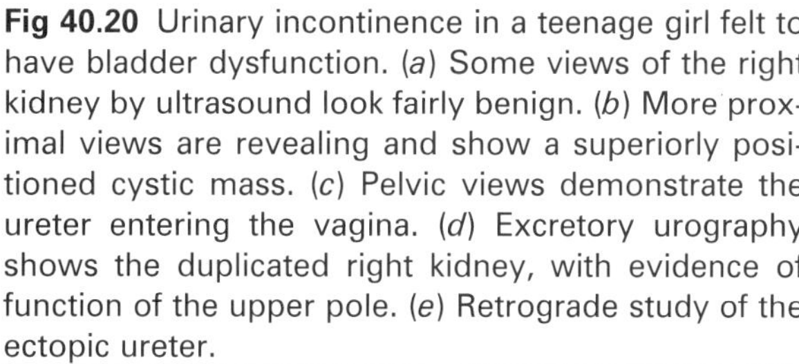

Fig 40.20 Urinary incontinence in a teenage girl felt to have bladder dysfunction. (*a*) Some views of the right kidney by ultrasound look fairly benign. (*b*) More proximal views are revealing and show a superiorly positioned cystic mass. (*c*) Pelvic views demonstrate the ureter entering the vagina. (*d*) Excretory urography shows the duplicated right kidney, with evidence of function of the upper pole. (*e*) Retrograde study of the ectopic ureter.

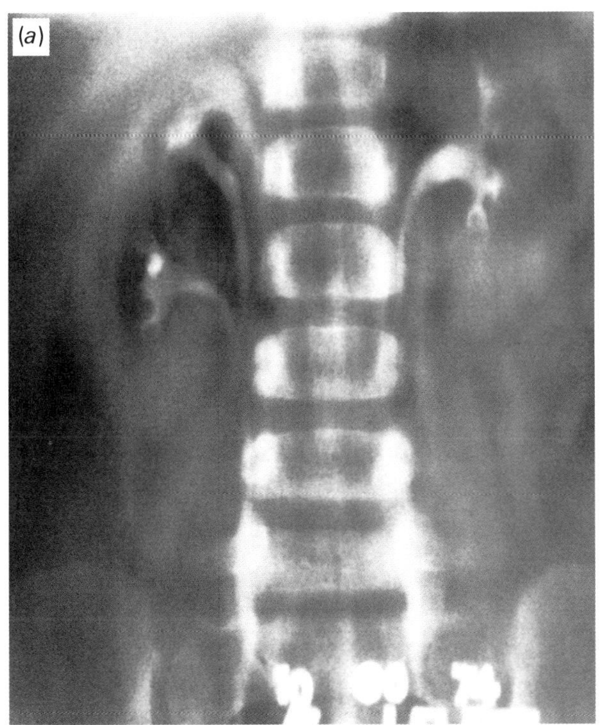

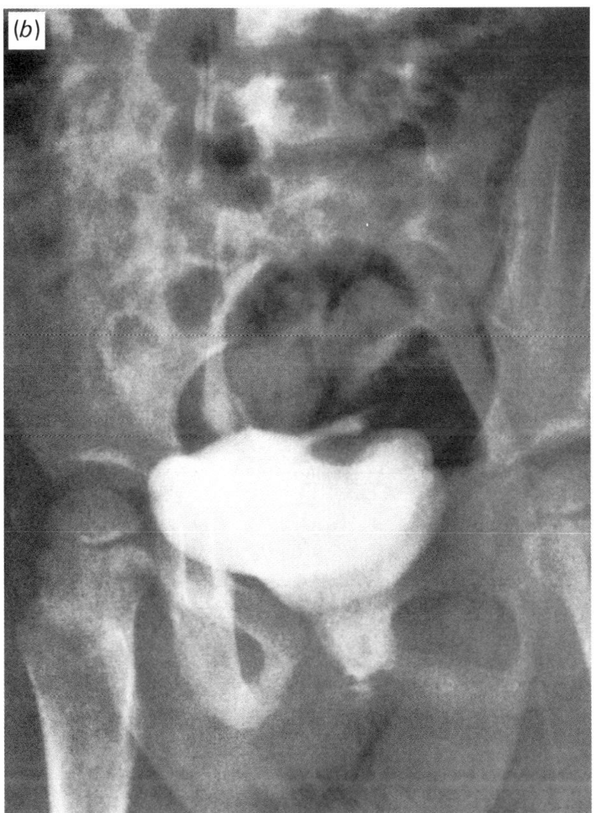

Figure 40.21 Ectopic ureter in a 4-year-old girl with incontinence, demonstrated by excretory urograms. (*a*) Duplication on the right. (*b*) Pooling of contrast into the vagina from the ectopic ureter.

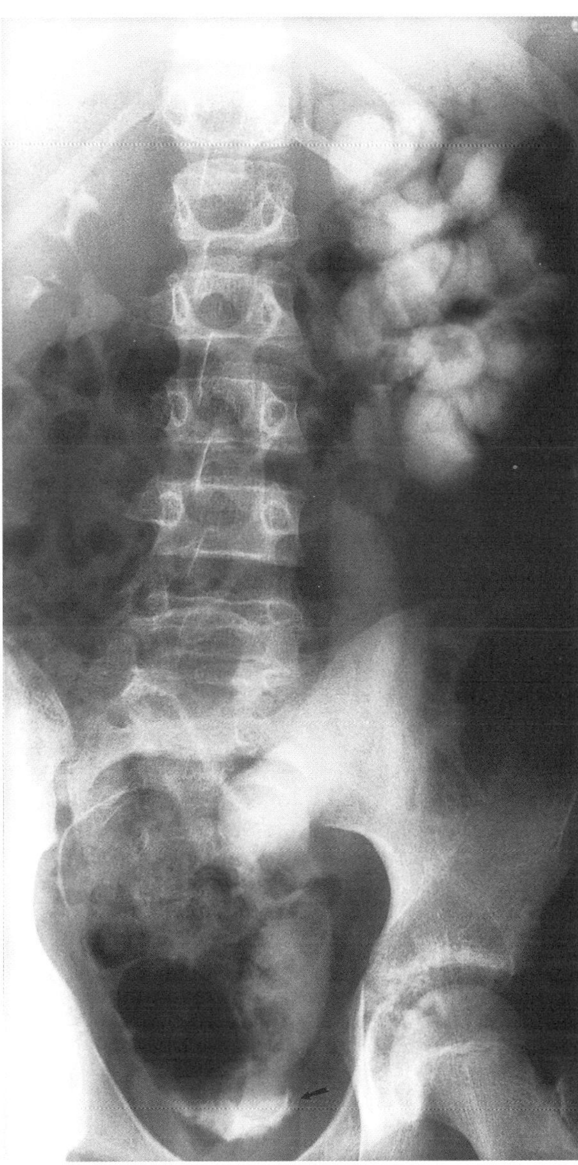

Figure 40.22 Single-system intravesical ureterocele presenting as a urinary tract infection in a 16-year-old. If the impressive dilatation above the small ureterocele represents a progressive change, questions are raised about the natural history of the anomaly and the validity of the expectant treatment of antenatally diagnosed ureteroceles.

Evaluation and diagnosis

Ectopic ureters and ureteroceles present diagnostic dilemmas when it is difficult to determine from which renal moiety they arise. They can also mimic one another at the bladder level, which has implications for treatment. A sonogram (also called ultrasonography, ultrasound, or US) and voiding cystourethrography (VCUG) are indicated in the initial evaluation of any child suspected of having a ureteral anomaly. Once detected, a functional test (radionuclide renal scan) becomes necessary to the decision-making process when considering the different options in management. Additional studies – e.g. excretory urography (EU) and computed tomography (CT) – are also sometimes necessary. Cystoscopy, sometimes in concert with retrograde ureteropyelography (RUP), completes the evaluation.

Ultrasonography

During initial screening, the differentiation of single from duplex systems is usually possible by ultrasound evaluation. The renal manifestations of ureteroceles and ectopic ureters can be identical. Variable degrees of hydronephrosis of the affected kidney or upper pole moiety depend on the severity of ureteral obstruction (Figure 40.23). Hyperechoic parenchyma is sugges-

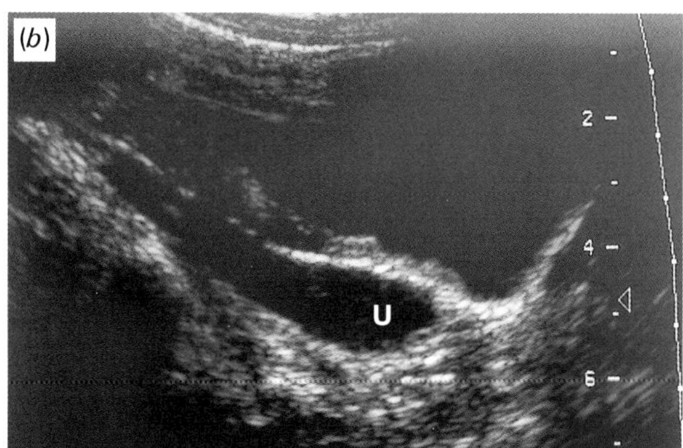

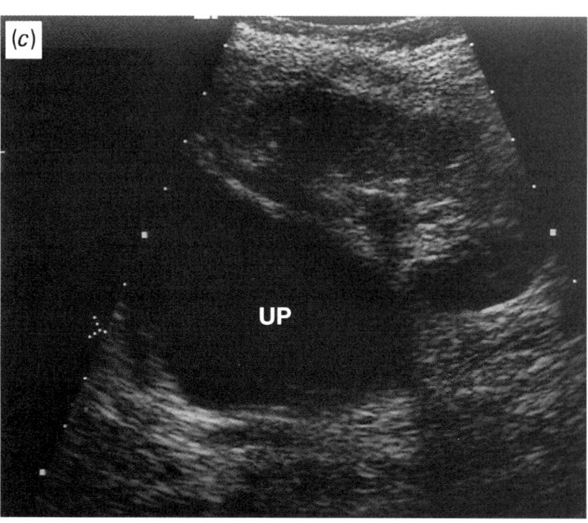

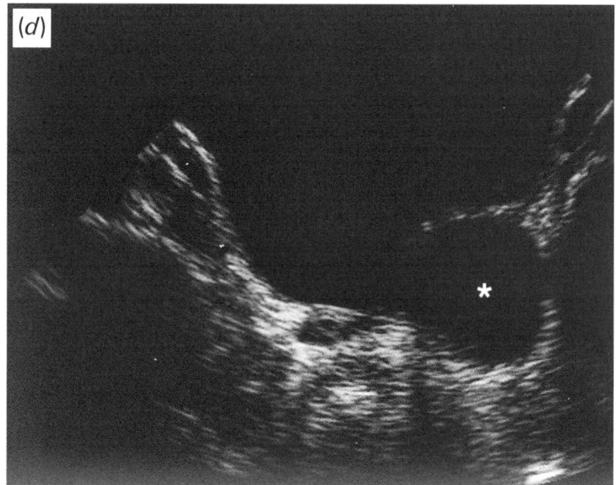

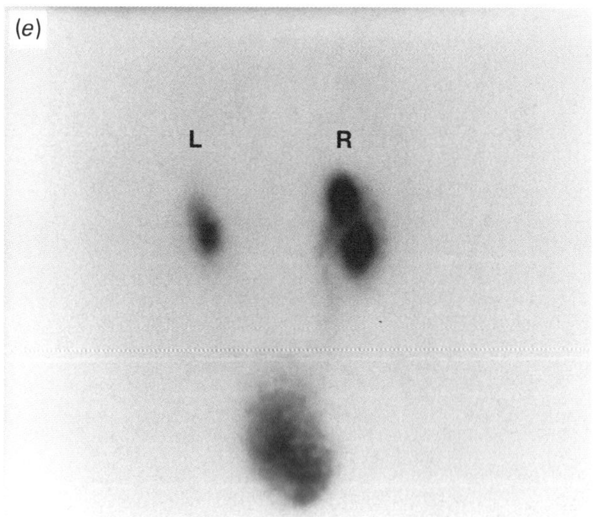

Figure 40.23 Variable appearance of hydronephrosis with duplications. (*a*) Subtle suggestion of obstructed duplication (arrow) of the upper pole in a 10-year-old girl with persistent urinary incontinence. (*b*) Dilated ureter shown behind bladder (U). Urethral ectopy was found to be the cause of wetness. (*c*) Second adolescent girl with similar presentation and vaginal ureteral ectopy. Ultrasound shows markedly dilated upper pole moiety (UP) of the left kidney. (*d*) Transverse view of bladder shows impingement by dilated ureter and pseudoureterocele appearance (*). (*e*) Renal scintigraphy shows deviated axis of the left lower pole and no function of the upper pole.

tive of dysplasia. With duplication, the adjacent lower pole moiety can also be hydronephrotic. Reflux (because of lateral ectopia) or obstruction caused by the dilated upper pole ureter must be considered. Hydronephrosis of the lower pole moiety and contralateral kidney can also result from bladder outlet obstruction or direct compression by a ureterocele.

Ultrasonography should always include a survey of the bladder, where the two anomalies can often be differentiated. Ultrasound is probably the best study for making the diagnosis of ureteroceles, which usually appear as thin-walled cystic protrusions from the posterolateral side of the bladder (Figure 40.24). The ureter can then be followed proximally into the bony pelvis and, in some cases, up to the kidney.[61,62] The degree of bladder fullness, however, can reduce the sensitivity of the study. Overdistention causes some ureteroceles to collapse, whereas an empty bladder can allow a large ureterocele to completely fill the bladder. This gives the impression of a partially full but normal bladder. Ectopic ureters will sometimes displace the bladder and mimic a ureterocele, resulting in a so-called pseudoureterocele[63] (Figures 40.25 and 40.26) The muscle wall of the bladder gives a thicker line of demarcation between its lumen and that of an ectopic ureter than the thin wall of a ureterocele. More typically, the dilated ectopic ureter will taper and terminate into an abnormally inferior position beneath the bladder base. Occasionally, the ureter associated with either anomaly is so tortuous and dilated that it mimics a cystic abdominal mass with multiple septae.

Rarely, these ureteral abnormalities do not result in dilatation of the renal moieties they subserve. Instead,

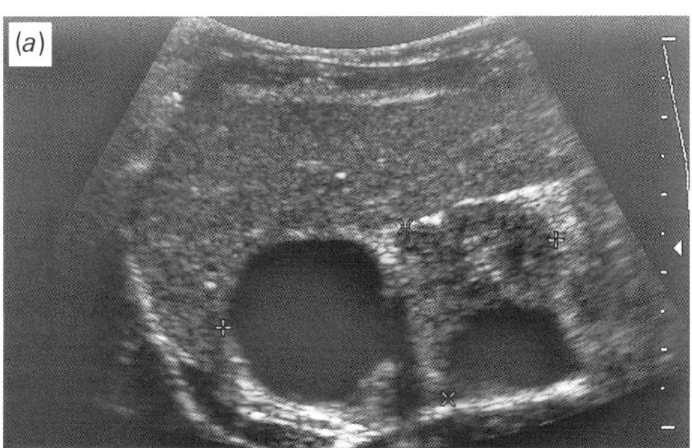

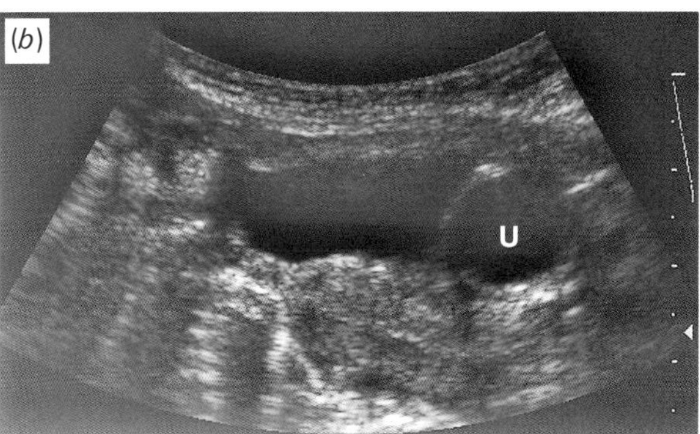

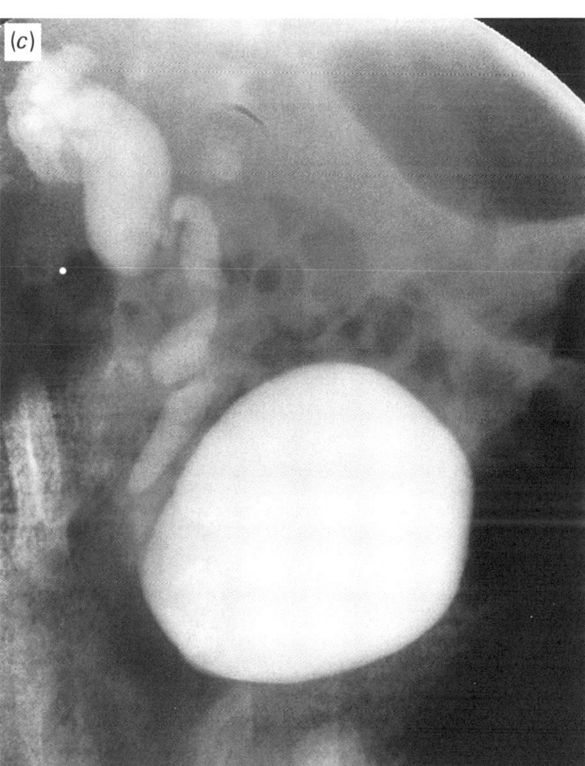

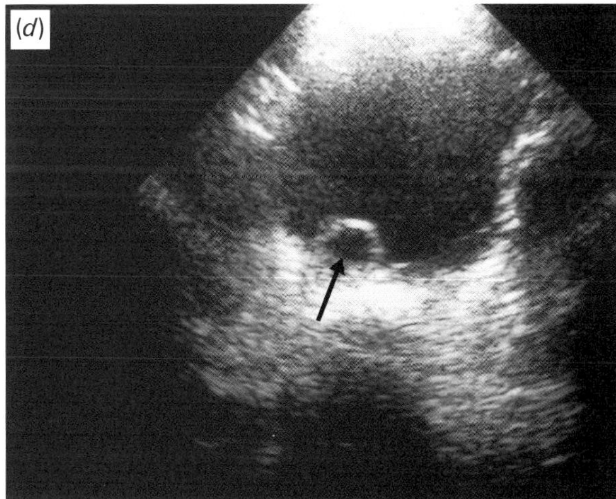

Figure 40.24 Antenatally diagnosed ureterocele in a newborn girl. (*a*) Ultrasonogram shows hydronephrosis of both segments of the right kidney, strongly suggesting a ureterocele. (*b*) Intravesical ureterocele (U) shown on sagittal view of the pelvis. (*c*) Reflux into the lower pole ureter on the right as cause of hydronephrosis. (*d*) Ultrasonic appearance of a small, intravesical, single-system ureterocele in a different patient (arrow).

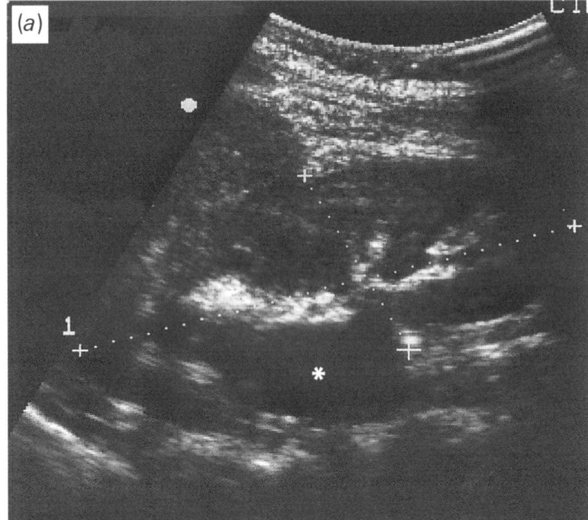

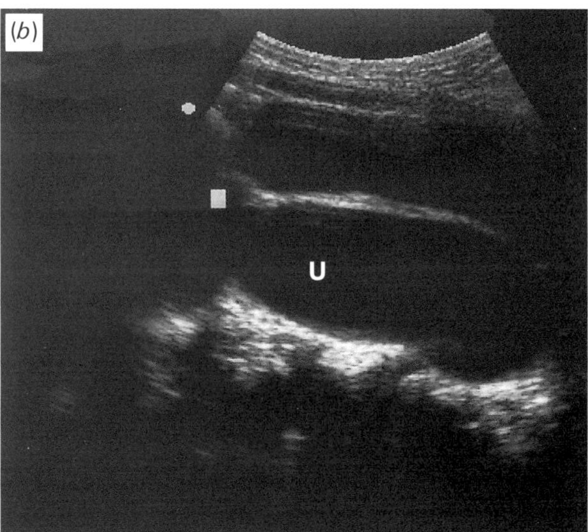

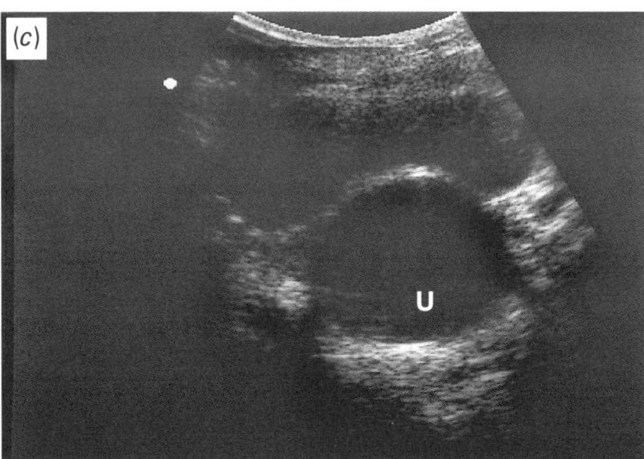

Figure 40.25 Pseudoureterocele appearance of ureter ectopic to the vagina. Ultrasonography in a newborn female with antenatally diagnosed hydronephrosis. (*a*) Upper pole hydronephrosis (*) with preservation of the lower pole parenchyma. (*b*) Sagittal view of the ureter in the pelvis behind the bladder. (*c*) Pseudoureterocele mimicking a ureterocele on transverse view. Differentiation can usually be made at cystoscopy. Incision is to be avoided with indeterminant cases (U = ureter).

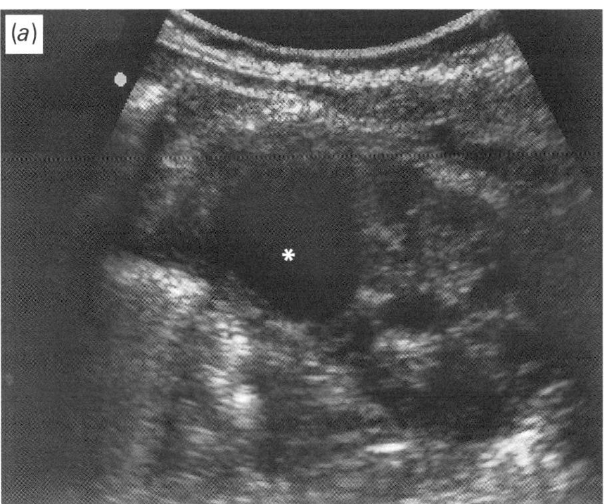

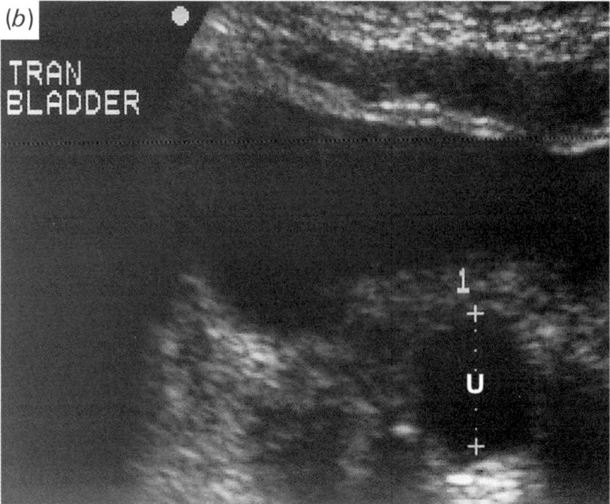

Figure 40.26 Ultrasonic evaluation of antenatally diagnosed hydronephrosis in a newborn girl. (*a*) Markedly hydronephrotic upper pole moiety surrounded by virtually no parenchyma (*). (*b*) More typical appearance of ectopic ureter (U) en route to the vagina, where the detrusor separating bladder lumen from the ureter is well developed.

the kidneys associated with single-system anomalies are sometimes small and abnormally positioned, making them difficult to localize (ureterocele disproportion)[64] (Figure 40.27). In similar fashion, the upper pole variants accompanying duplex variants can be tiny dysplastic remnants crowning otherwise normal kidneys. In both instances, a dilated ureter or ureterocele is still often visualized at the level of the bladder. Additional diagnostics become necessary to define the anatomy more fully.

Voiding cystourethrography

Infant feeding tubes are used to perform this test. These allow for spontaneous voiding and avoid any confusion or distortion offered by the balloons of Foley catheters. Ureteroceles appear as smooth, broad-based filling defects positioned near the trigone. Some ureteroceles evert into the ureter with the bladder full and appear as a diverticulum.[65] This is especially true of single-system ureteroceles, where mimics of periureteral diverticula were seen in nearly one-half of VCUG in one series.[66] Other ureteroceles efface during the latter stages of bladder filling and cannot be appreciated. Obtaining early images during the filling phase avoids these problems. An eccentric position may help define the involved side, although many ureteroceles appear centrally located. When laterality cannot be determined and cystoscopy is inconclusive, a cyst puncture with retrograde injection may become necessary.

The presence of VUR plays an important role in the management of ureteroceles. Reflux can occur into the ipsilateral lower pole, since the backing required of an effective flap valve is presumably lost with the posteriorly positioned ureterocele (Figure 40.28). Lateral ectopia, trigonal distortion, and ever-

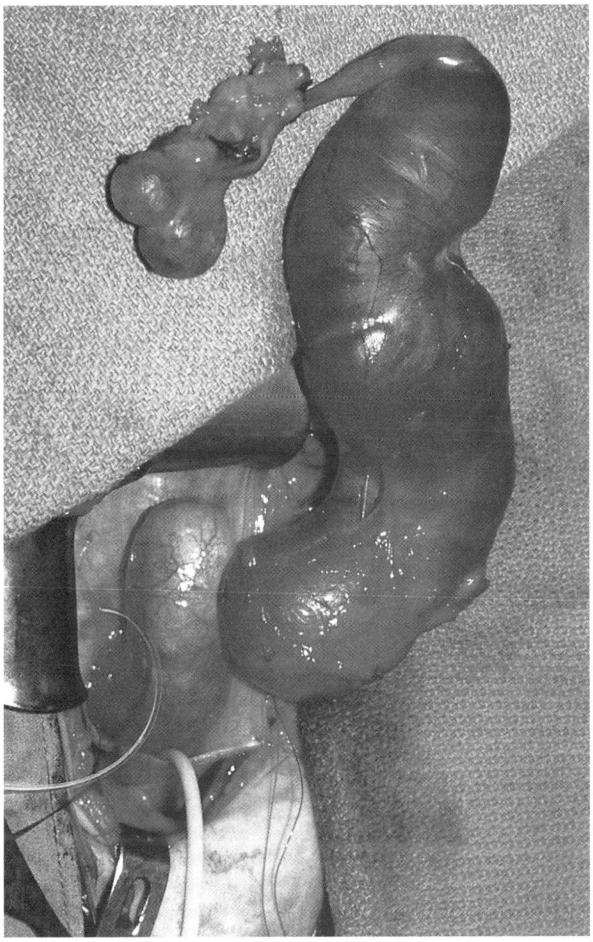

Figure 40.27 Gross example of ureterocele disproportion. Remant dysplastic cap of tissue as shown are typically associated with massively dilated ureteroceles and ectopic ureters whose renal moiety cannot be appreciated diagnostically.

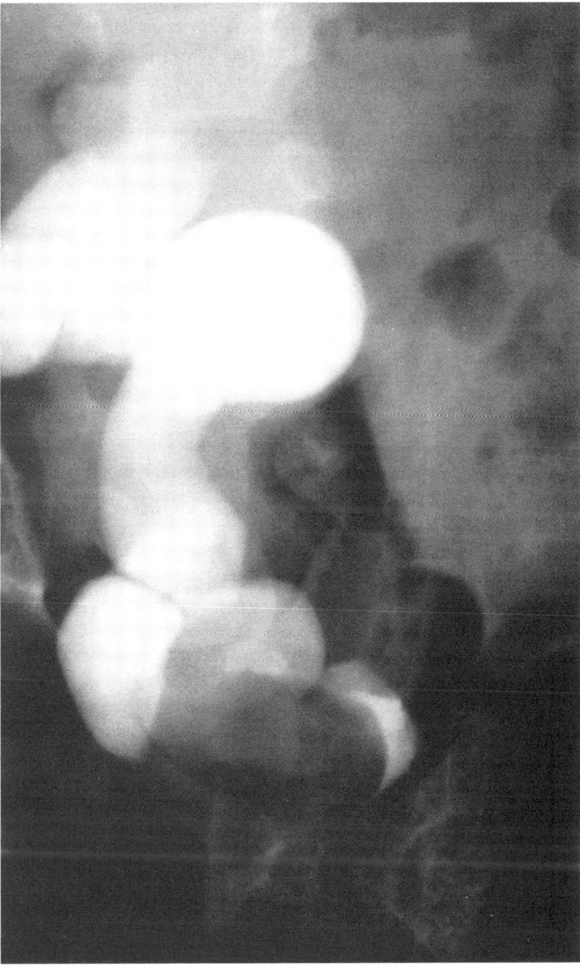

Figure 40.28 Massive reflux into the lower pole ureter. An element of obstruction from the significantly enlarged ureterocele can also contribute to the dilatation.

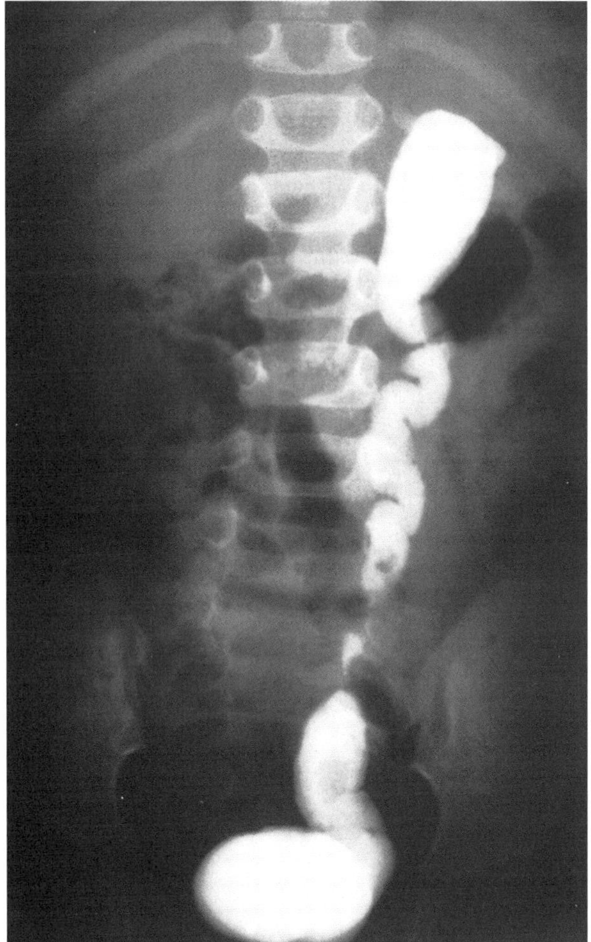

Figure 40.29 Reflux into the ureterocele and upper pole system of the left kidney.

sion of the ureterocele can also contribute. At times, the ipsilateral reflux is severe enough that the ureterocele and its duplex kidney are not detected until the time of surgery.[67] Reflux is also seen in the contralateral system if the anomaly is large enough to distort the trigone and opposing submucosal ureteral tunnel. In one series of 148 ureteroceles, ipsilateral VUR was seen in 80 (54%), whereas contralateral VUR was appreciated in 28%.[68] Smaller series have documented similar incidences.[69,70] Reflux into the ureterocele itself is uncommon but can also occur (Figure 40.29).

VUR is also a common finding with ectopic ureters (Figure 40.30). The ipsilateral lower pole ureter refluxes in at least 50% of cases. Upper pole VUR can also be appreciated, depending on the position of the ectopic orifice. Ectopic ureters whose distal extent is positioned within the bladder neck can both reflux and obstruct. Obstruction is intermittent and emptying occurs during voiding, in concert with relaxation of

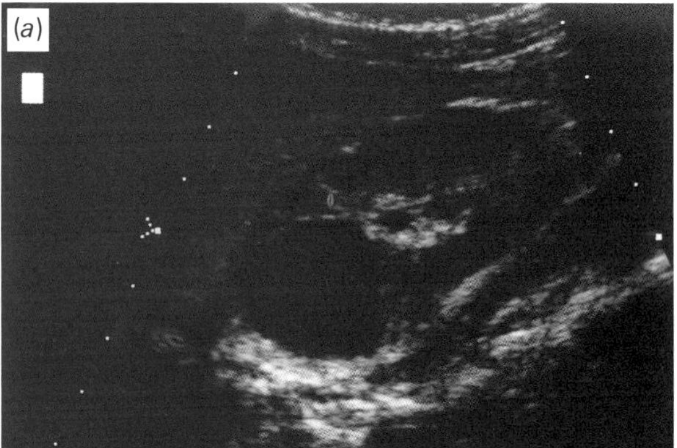

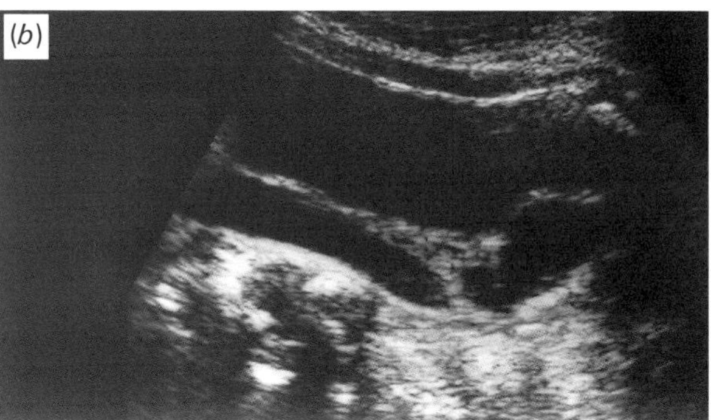

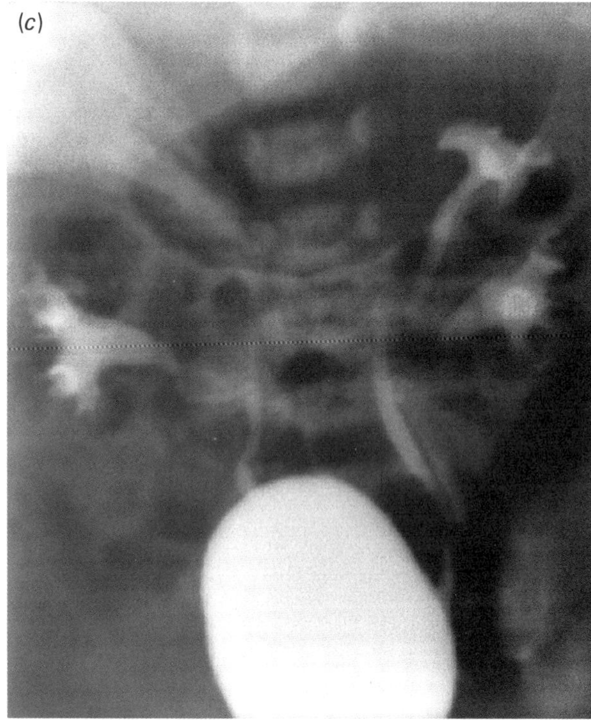

Figure 40.30 Vesicoureteral reflux associated with ectopic ureter to the urethra. (*a*) Duplex right kidney with hydronephrotic upper pole. (*b*) Ectopic ureter behind the bladder could be confused with a ureterocele. (*c*) Voiding cystourethrogram shows reflux into duplicated ureters on the left and lower pole on the right.

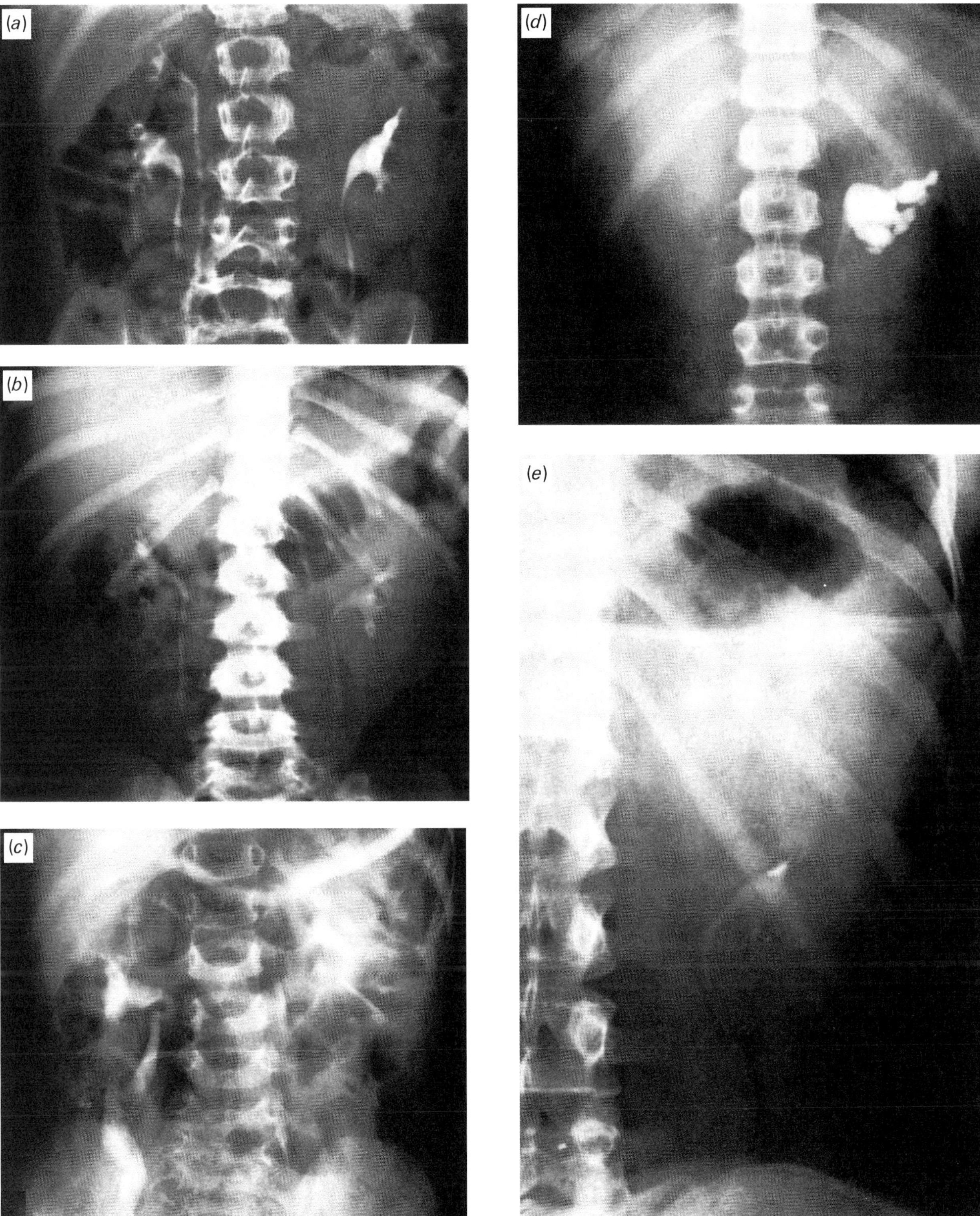

Figure 40.31 Examples of characteristic lateral and downward displacement of lower segment when the functionless upper pole is dilated. (*a*) Functionless upper left segment. (*b*) Poorly functioning upper right segment and functionless upper left segment. (*c*) Functionless upper right segment and displacement of the lower segment. (*d*) Reflux into displaced lower pole segment of the left kidney. (*e*) Minimally functioning upper left segment simulating mass effect of the upper pole.

the surrounding musculature. Reflux occurs once the ureter is somewhat emptied. This phenomenon may only be appreciated by performing cyclic (repeated) voiding studies.[71] Orifices proximal to the bladder neck can reflux freely with or without voiding.

Excretory urography

Despite its declining role in the routine evaluation of children with UTIs, excretory urography remains a useful tool in the work-up of certain ureteral anomalies (Figures 40.31 and 40.32). This is occasionally the case with ureteroceles, when the anatomy is undefinable with ultrasound and renal scintigraphy alone, and is especially true of ectopic ureters. Some clinicians remain steadfast in their belief that EU remains the definitive diagnostic study for the latter. For girls with infrasphincteric ectopia, who arrive with the classic history of constant urinary dribbling despite being successfully toilet-trained, EU is often the only imaging study necessary to make the diagnosis.[72] (Figures 40.33 and 40.34). Radiographic signs of the non-functioning, occult duplications found with ectopic ureters are shown in Table 40.4.

Ureteroceles with minimally functioning upper pole moieties can cause identical upper tract findings. The ureterocele appears as a filling defect within the bladder that gradually fills with contrast from the other functioning kidney. When ureteroceles are associated with a functioning kidney, they appear as a contrast-filled 'cobra head' at the ureterovesical junction.

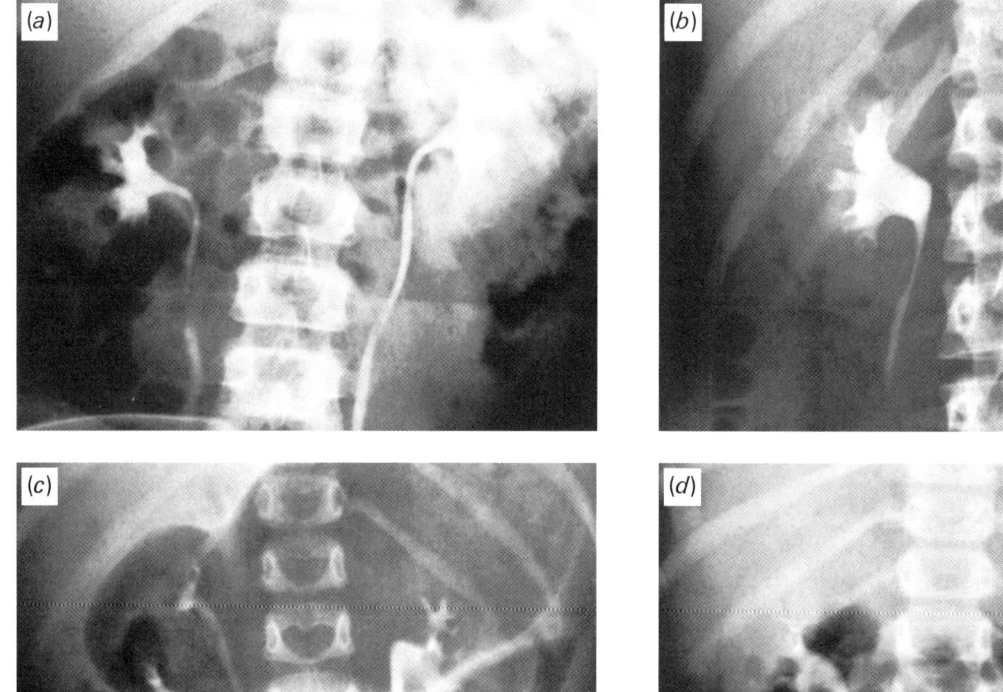

Figure 40.32 Appearance of lower pole pelvis when the upper pole is functionless and non-dilated. (*a*) Functionless upper right segment. The caliceal system of the lower segment is smaller but relatively normal. (*b*) Functionless upper pole on left, with decreased number of calices of the lower segment. (*c*) Functionless upper left segment, with apparent increase in renal substance of upper pole. The presence of a duplication of the contralateral kidney is often a key to diagnosis. (*d*) Functionless upper right segment, with apparent increase in renal thickness on the medial side of the upper pole.

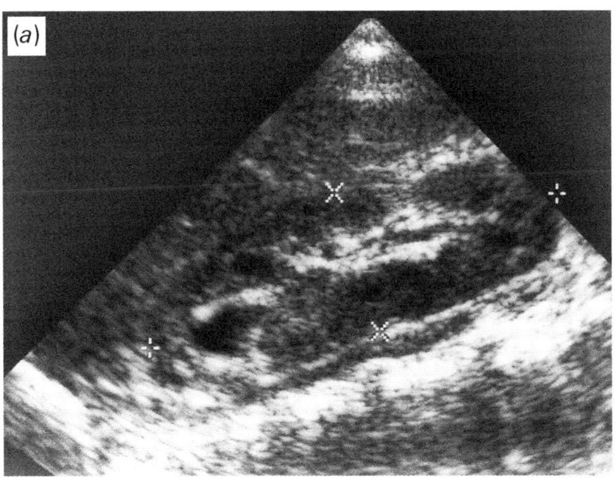

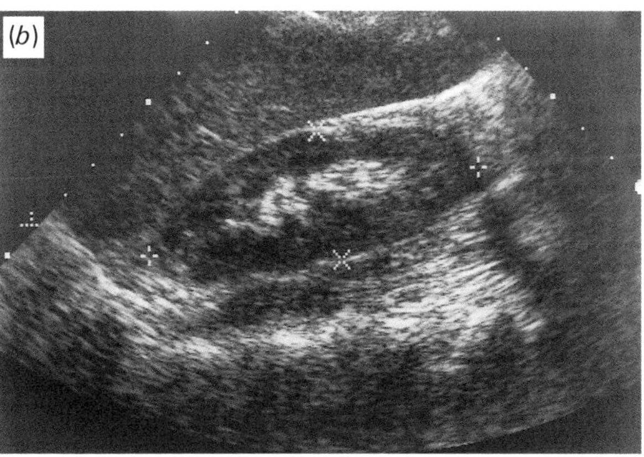

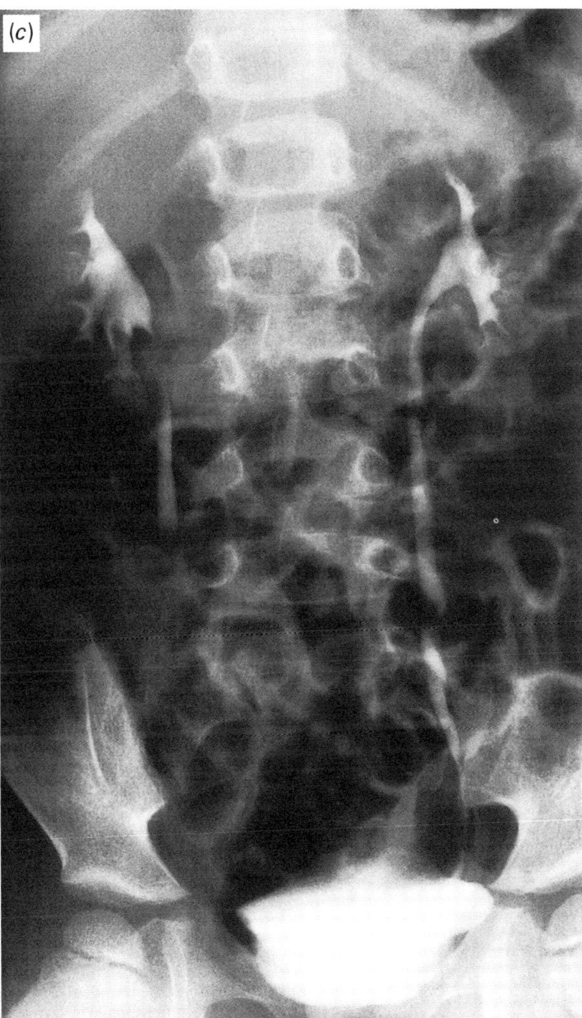

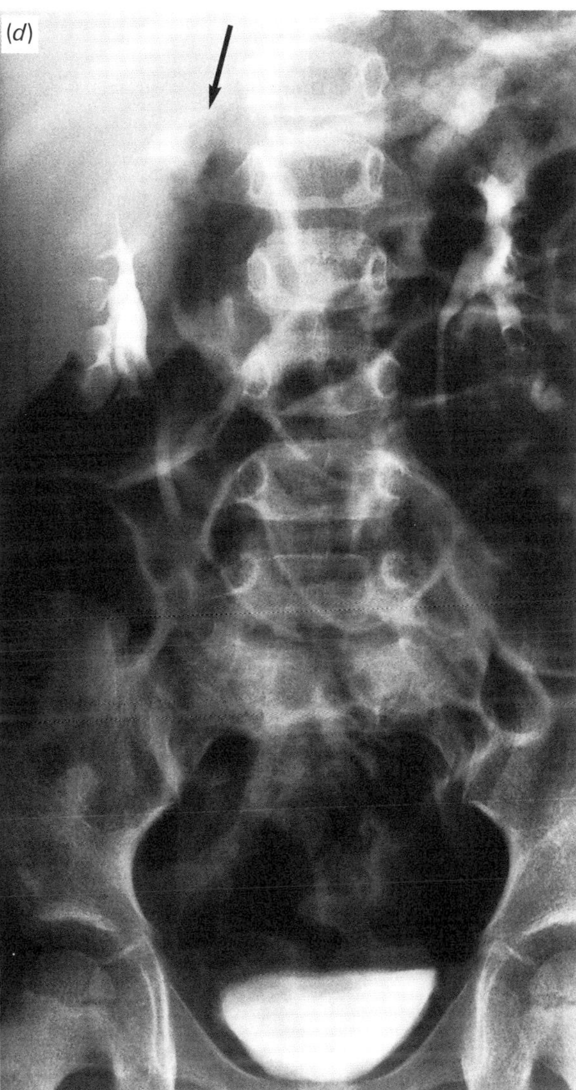

Figure 40.33 Utility of excretory urography. Studies in a 13-year-old girl with continuous wetting were strongly suggestive of an ectopic ureter. Sonograms for the past 7 years read as normal. (*a*) Initial ultrasound at 6 years old suggests mild upper pole dilatation. (*b*) Current ultrasound is essentially unremarkable. Retrieval and review of early excretory urogram confirms the clinical impression. (*c*) Note the deviated axis of the right kidney and ureteral displacement on early sequence of excretory urogram. (*d*) A later film shows delayed uptake of contrast in the upper pole (arrow).

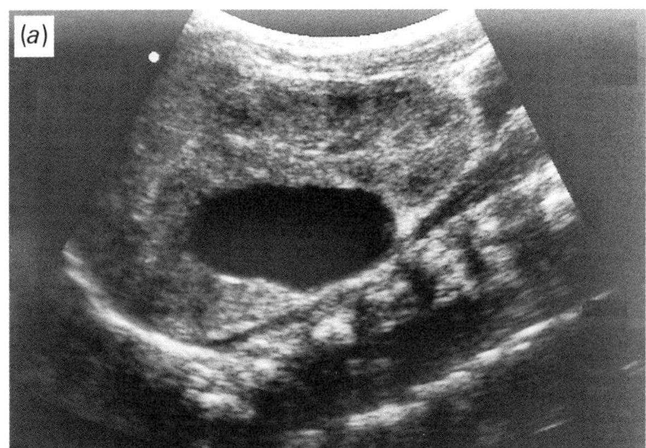

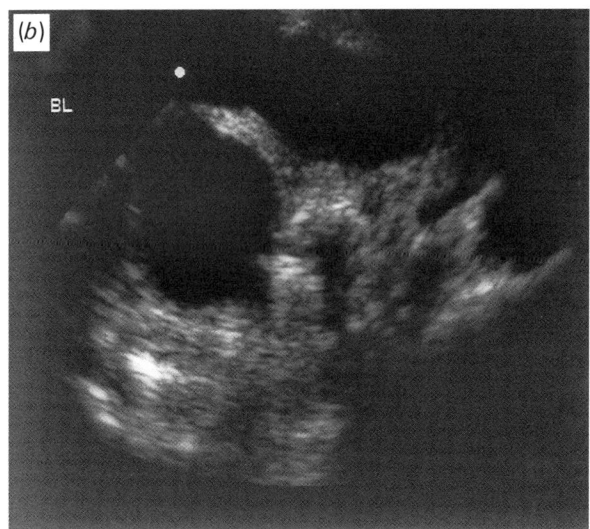

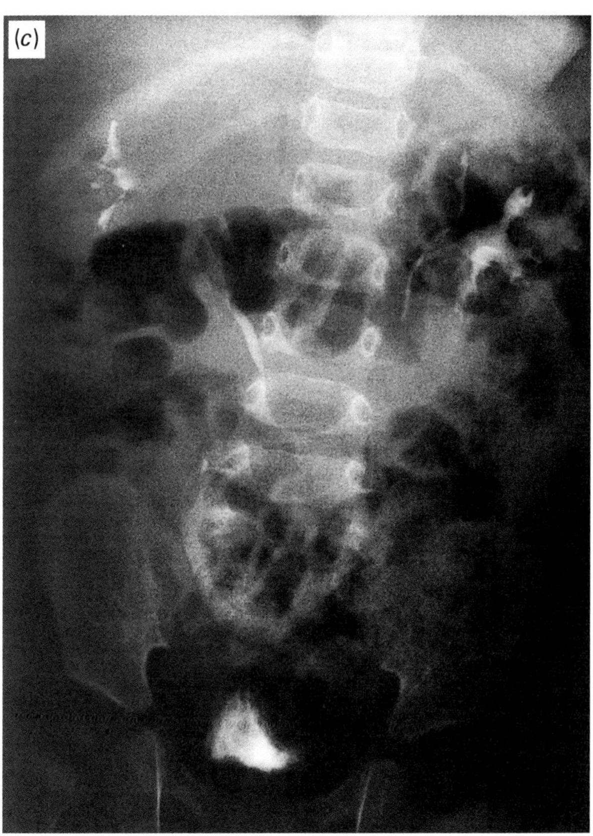

Figure 40.34 An infant boy with urinary tract infection. The role of excretory urography. (*a*) Ultrasonogram initially felt to represent single-system hydronephrotic right kidney. (*b*) Pelvic sonogram demonstrates a markedly dilated right ureter behind the bladder. (*c*) Excretory urography shows displaced lower pole of the right kidney.

Table 40.4 Excretory urography: findings suggesting occult duplex kidney with ectopic ureter

Finding	Features
'Drooping lily sign'	Inferior and lateral displacement of lower pole by minimally or non-functioning upper pole. Delayed films may show function, but most are 'silent'. Axes of the kidneys should normally cross the body of the 10th thoracic vertebra
Lateral displacement of lower pole ureter	Compared with contralateral ureter, differences in the distance from an adjacent vertebral pedicle
'Missing calyx'	Incomplete compliment of calices with absence of system draining upper pole. A shortened or cut-off infundibulum to the upper pole calyx, which is normally the longest
More upper pole parenchyma than expected with increased renal length	
Duplex kidney on the contralateral side	
Dilated, ectopic ureter appreciated on postvoid film	

Renal scintigraphy

Radionuclide scans help to quantify the amount of functioning renal parenchyma. This is crucial information when renal salvage is being considered. The degree of obstruction is also assessed, although most ectopic ureters and ureteroceles, by default, exhibit delayed drainage because of ureteral dilatation. Technetium 99m (^{99m}Tc) diethylenetriamine penta-acetic acid (DTPA) and mercaptoacetyltriglycine (MAG3) scans provide reasonable assessments of function and obstruction. Since ^{99m}Tc dimercaptosuccinic acid (DMSA) scans result in renal tubular labeling and are unaffected by obstruction, they are more sensitive to low levels of renal function and are sometimes helpful in detecting occult duplex anomalies and small kidneys associated with ureteral anomalies that are not identified by other techniques,[73,74] DMSA scintigraphy can also detect subclinical cortical defects and functional impairment in lower pole moieties that show no ultrasonic evidence of parenchymal damage.[75]

Some clinicians believe that the transitional physiology of the newborn may affect the perinatal kidney's handling of radionuclides and contrast. This could contribute to the lower yield of functioning kidneys in historical series when EU was obtained in newborns and provided the measure of function. It could also result in overestimates of the recovery of function after procedures done to alleviate obstructed newborn kidneys, when early scans are compared with studies performed when the physiology is more conducive to scanning. As a consequence, scans performed early after delivery may not provide an accurate assessment of renal function and should probably be deferred for 4–6 weeks after delivery to allow for some maturation of renal function.

Other diagnostic modalities

CT scans may help define the anatomy of kidneys with collecting systems of bizarre appearance. Duplications in which both ureters and renal pelves are dilated are one example. CT can also be considered for patients suspected of having ureteral ectopia or ureterocele disproportion but whose poorly functioning renal moiety cannot be defined by other modalities[76,77] (Figure 40.35). Magnetic resonance imaging (MRI) is becoming increasingly useful in cases where conventional imaging studies fail to delineate occult dysplastic renal moieties, ectopic ureters, and ureteroceles.[78,79] Respiratory gated excretory and static fluid MR urography appear to complement each other well in evaluating such systems.[80] Percutaneous drainage can also be used to vent obstructed kidneys or renal segments that appear salvageable by ultrasound but function poorly. However, recoverability of function is rare when renal scintigraphy demonstrates little function.

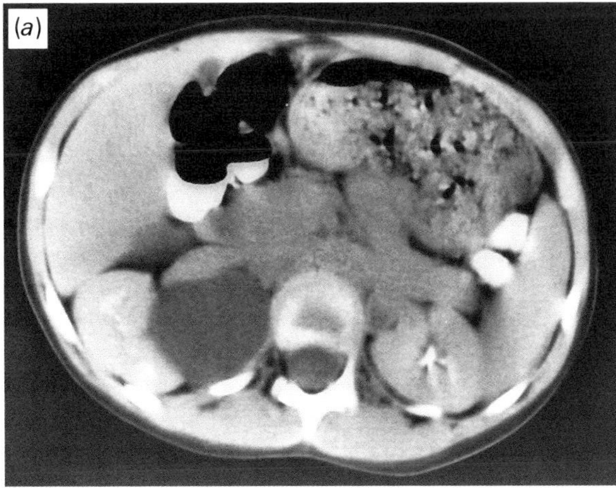

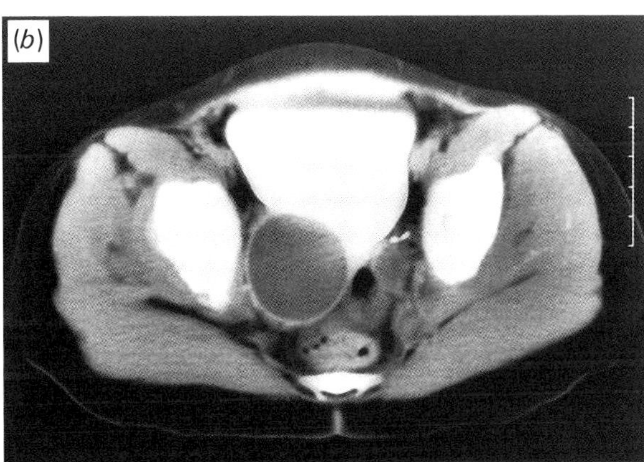

Figure 40.35 Computed tomography in a female toddler with abdominal pain and palpable mass. (*a*) Markedly dilated ureter displacing the right kidney associated with duplication. (*b*) The ureter is shown behind the bladder.

A variety of dye tests have been used clinically to diagnose ectopic ureters. For example, indigo carmine or methylene blue can be instilled in the bladder with a catheter, which is then removed. Continued evidence of dampness and leakage of clear urine implicates ureteral ectopia. Another test involves placing a dental roll in the vagina. After indigo carmine is given intravenously, the roll will appear blue, provided there is some function in the affected kidney and the child has not stained the roll by spontaneously voiding. The relative invasiveness of such tests, coupled with the increased sensitivities of today's diagnostics, has reduced their utility in most cases.

Cystoscopy

Examples of the cystoscopic appearance of ureteroceles are shown in Figure 40.47. With smaller intravesical ureteroceles, the cystic dilatation expands with each peristalsis, then shrinks as urine drains through its orifice. Not all variants are as easy to appreciate, however. Extravesical variants have ill-defined borders that can undermine the bladder neck and urethra. If the bladder is overfilled, they efface and can even appear to be a diverticulum. The orifice of the ureterocele may be difficult to appreciate but is often positioned distal to the bladder neck and, with cecoureterocele and sphincteric variants, will balloon open with the efflux of irrigant. With larger ureteroceles, the adjacent ureteral orifices are also difficult to appreciate because of displacement.

Cystoscopy is less helpful for ectopic ureters. The ectopic orifice cannot be appreciated in more than half of cases. Bladder neck and urethral ectopy offer a higher yield. Prostatic ectopy sometimes presents as a widened ejaculatory duct that allows easy retrograde study.[40] Examining the vaginal vault along its anterior/lateral aspect for GYN-ectopy is less fruitful. In rare cases, a small cystic structure is identified that can be unroofed and cannulated for retrograde study.[31] Intravenous indigo carmine is sometimes excreted by even minimally functioning kidneys and can aid in identification. Within the bladder, the hemitrigone on the affected side is often underdeveloped and may be elevated from behind by the dilated ureter. In some cases, the dilated ureter can be palpated on rectal examination. Failure to identify the ectopic orifice rarely changes management. In cases where a lower tract approach is planned, the ectopic ureter can be identified outside the bladder or transvesically after incising the trigone on the affected side (see Management, below).

Management considerations

Once the work-up is complete and the diagnosis made, the management of ectopic ureters and ureteroceles is defined by the answers to the following questions:

1 Is the affected ureter(s) a singlet or portion of a duplex system?
2 Is the affected ureter(s) obstructed, refluxing, or both?
3 Are the contralateral and/or ipsilateral ureter(s) and/or the bladder affected by the primary anomaly?
4 What is the status of the kidney or portion of kidney associated with the ureter(s) in question?
5 What is the age and clinical status of the patient?

A description of the experience with various techniques and their technical nuances follows. Simply put, the algorithms in management of these two anomalies historically branched with two main decisions: whether to save or discard the involved kidney and whether or not there is a need to reconstruct the bladder. These remain the mainstays of management for ectopic ureters.

The recommendations for ureteroceles have become controversial, however, with the inclusion in the treatment armamentarium of selective puncture. A minimally invasive and seemingly simple solution, the benefits of cystoscopically decompressing ureteroceles must be weighed against the risks of creating reflux in the involved ureter.

Until recently, the two main areas of contention with ureteroceles dealt with the salvage of functioning upper pole moieties and the need, if any, for removal of ureteroceles subtending upper pole segments after heminephrectomy or proximal ureteral diversion (ureteroureterostomy or ureteropyelostomy) caused by their collapse (Figure 40.36). The introduction of selective puncture offers the obvious third controversy of which ureteroceles to decompress. The answers to these questions continue to be modified by contemporary clinical studies.

A 'cookbook approach' should be avoided when composing algorithms for the management of any urinary abnormality. Each patient requires individualized treatment, since there is often no uniform solution to every urologic anomaly. Nevertheless, trends become apparent in reviewing the literature that allow certain recommendations to be applied to most cases, which give the highest likelihood of a favorable outcome.

Recommendations for management

Ectopic ureters

Single system – minimal or non-functioning kidney

Most kidneys (90%) that accompany single-system ectopic ureters do not function appreciably. Nephrectomy is the treatment of choice. In some cases, the question of renal salvage is raised by the appearance of marginal function on nuclear scintigraphy. How much function is enough to warrant ureteral reconstruction rather than ablation of its associated kidney? Nephrectomy is indicated when the creatinine clear-

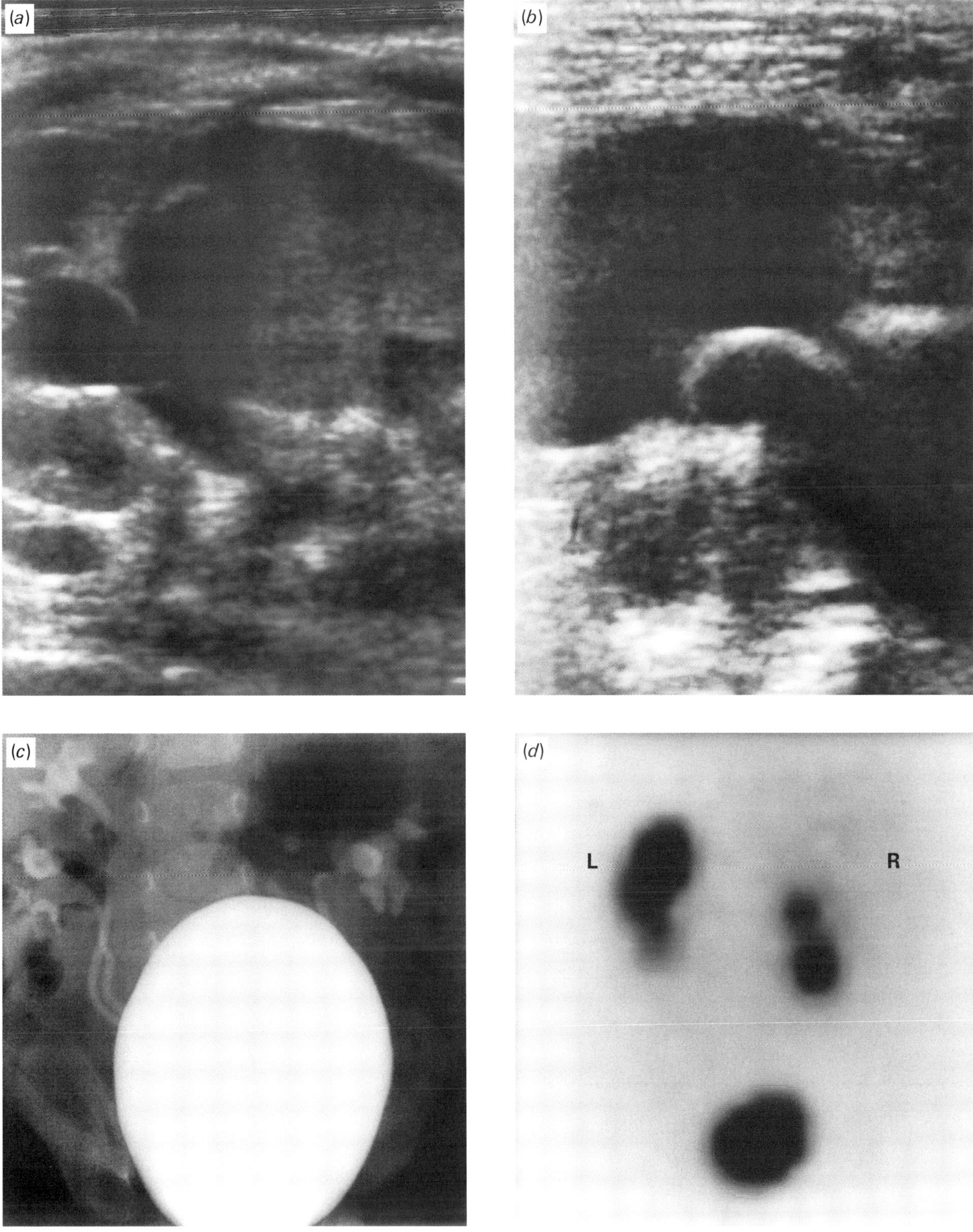

Figure 40.36 Antenatally diagnosed ureterocele in a newborn girl. (*a*) The sonogram shows a dilated upper pole segment of the duplex left kidney. (*b*) Pelvic view of the ureterocele projecting within the bladder. (*c*) Cystogram demonstrates reflux into the contralateral duplex ureters and lower pole ureter on the left. (*d*) Renal scan shows preservation of function and hydronephrosis of the left upper pole moiety.

ance provided by the affected kidney, if it were isolated, would not eliminate the need for dialysis. Using percent function as a cut-off, like the commonly cited standard of 10 or 15%, may have little meaning, especially if the contralateral kidney also exhibits impaired function. In addition, kidneys that function marginally in infancy sometimes assume a progressively smaller portion of overall renal function with interval growth of the affected child. An intrinsic developmental insult and/or the rules governing renal hypertrophy, where healthy kidneys do not relinquish the additional renal function they are asked to assume, can be implicated when this occurs.

One area of controversy for some ectopic ureters involves the management of the lower ureteral segment. In cases of wolffian or GYN-ectopy, where an element of obstruction is the rule, the lower ureter need not be removed. Once decompressed, ascending infections of these dry, isolated segments are uncommon and the need for secondary ureterectomies after subtotal ureterectomy is rare. The obstructed ureters found with GU-ectopy typically enter the bladder neck or urethra. These can also remain, although a small number will predispose to recurrent urinary infections that ultimately necessitate their removal. It may be that such systems begin to reflux after the outflow of urine ceases from above (see Voiding cystourethrography, above).

Refluxing lower ureters have typically been removed in concert with nephrectomy. An extravesical approach through a second lower transverse muscle-splitting (Gibson) incision adds little additional morbidity. However, the necessity for a simultaneous approach for these variants has been questioned. In a study by Plaire et al,[81] secondary surgery for removal of the distal ureter was required in only 4 of 38 such patients. Subsequent series have drawn similar conclusions. Long ureteric stumps or those in patients with dysfunctional voiding appear to pose the most risk.[82] In cases where a ureteral stump is left, be it refluxing or obstructed, it should be taken as distal as possible, ligated with absorbable sutures, and urine should be aspirated from its distal end. Urinary fistulas have occurred when presumably obstructed ureteral stumps have been left open and unappreciated reflux commences.

Duplex system – minimal or non-functioning upper pole

Heminephrectomy is recommended for the affected upper pole.[83] The case made for salvage is similar to that in singlets and depends on relative function. Developmentally, the upper 'half' of a normal duplex kidney typically contributes only one-third of that kidney's glomeruli, or, at most, 16% of overall renal function. The lack of an optimal inductive influence during fetal development combined with an element of obstruction significantly reduces the contribution of most upper pole moieties drained by ectopic ureters. As in single systems, a subtotal ureterectomy is usually sufficient, taking the ectopic ureter as far distal as possible through a flank incision. When there is reflux into the upper pole and concerns about the ureteral stump persist, it can be removed through a second incision.

Single system – salvageable function

Reimplantation of the affected ureter is the treatment of choice. It helps to initially identify the ureter outside the bladder, especially when the insertion of the ectopic meatus cannot be localized cystoscopically. Once the ureter is mobilized, a transvesical or an extravesical approach to ureteroneocystostomy can be successfully applied. The distal-most segment that enters the bladder neck/urethra should be disregarded with these and other ectopic ureters. The tedious dissection required for their removal risks damaging the urinary sphincter complex. Ureteral tailoring is often necessary and can be done using any one of a variety of techniques (see Chapter 39 Megaureters).

Duplex system – salvageable function

In cases where the upper pole is obstructed, yet provides salvageable function, its ureter can be anastomosed to the adjacent lower pole renal pelvis (ureteropyelostomy) or ureter (ureteroureterostomy). The lower ureteral segment can be mobilized to the pelvic brim and excised, and the remainder left alone. Concerns about discrepancy in size between the ectopic and recipient ureter are usually unfounded.[84] These operations are usually no more challenging than the dismembered pyeloplasties required of infants with ureteropelvic junction (UPJ) obstructions. Rates of success should be similar. When technical concerns persist or if the upper pole moiety exhibits signs of cystic dysplasia, a heminephrectomy is recommended. Visualization of the upper pole moiety in assessment of dysplasia is one advantage of this approach. Renal sparing surgeries could probably be utilized more frequently in this setting. In one study, normal histology was found in 57% of upper pole heminephrectomy specimens removed from ectopic ureters.[83]

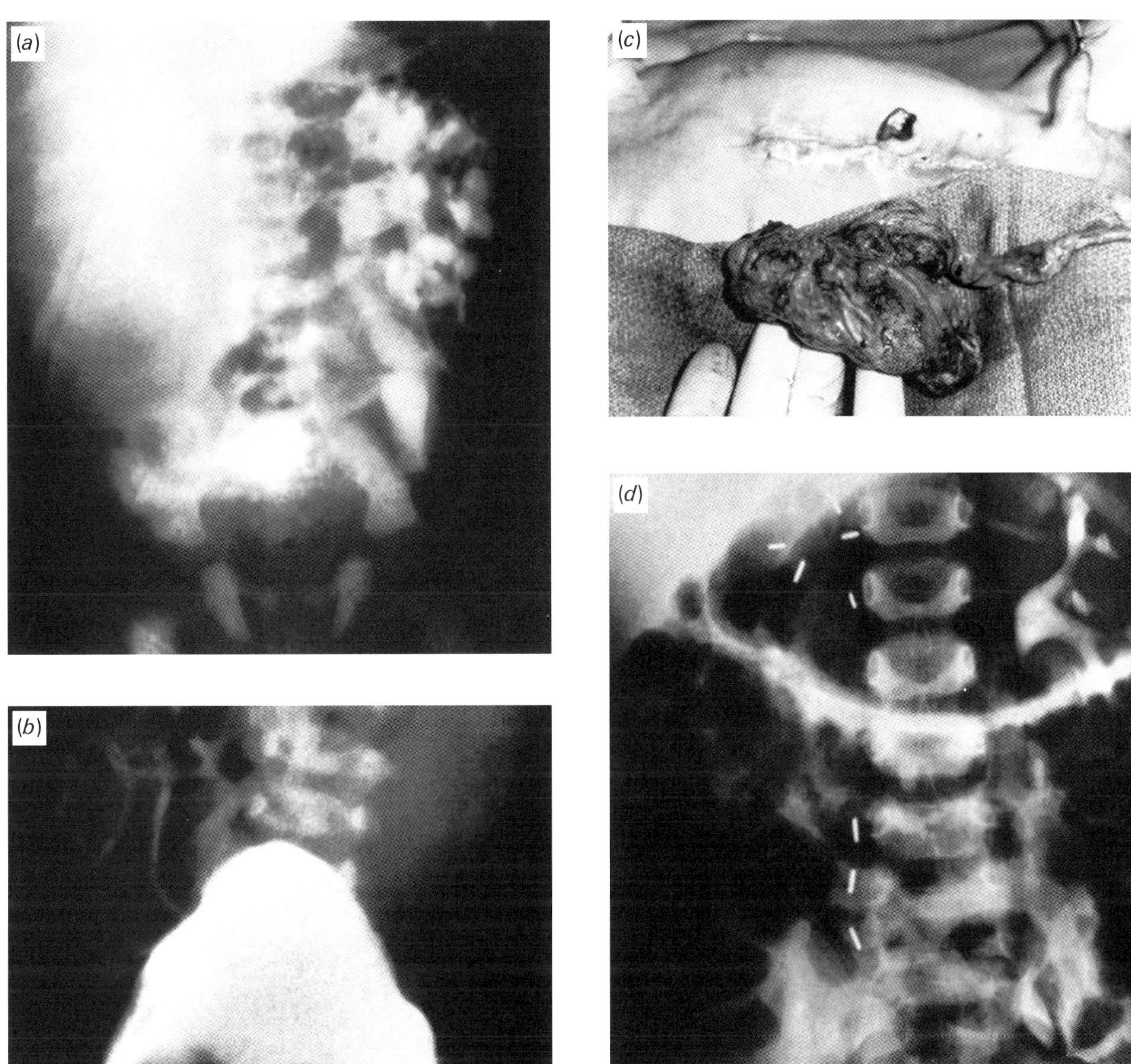

Figure 40.37 Newborn male with large, single-system ureterocele on the right side. (*a*) Excretory urogram shows poor visualization of the right collecting system and hydronephrosis of the left. (*b*) Cystogram shows a large ureterocele filling the bladder and extending through the bladder neck. (*c*) At surgery, the grossly dysplastic hydronephrotic kidney was removed and extravesical dissection of the ureterocele was completed. (*d*) A postoperative excretory urogram shows significant improvement of the left-sided hydronephrosis and collapse of the ureterocele.

Another option for obstructed systems is to approach the duplication from below. When reflux is present into one or both ureters, a common sheath ureteral reimplantation is the preferred method of treatment.[85] The repair can be technically challenging, especially in smaller infants. Tailoring of the upper pole ureter usually becomes necessary to achieve the desired length/diameter ratio required of successful ureteroneocystostomy. Revisions are made along the length of ureter opposite the common wall where vascularity is shared by the duplication. When folding techniques cause excessive bulk with larger ureters, excisional tapering is preferred. A psoas hitch is sometimes necessary to gain additional length for the reimplantation. Another option for duplications with an obstructed upper pole ureter and refluxing lower pole ureter is to perform a proximal diversion of the upper pole ureter (ureteropyelostomy), discard its remainder, and reimplant the lower pole ureter alone. Although two incisions are required for this approach, it avoids the problems that accompany ureteroneocystotomy of duplex ureters, where one or both may be dilated.

Ureteroceles

Single system – minimal or non-functioning kidney

Nephrectomy is the treatment of choice. Ordinarily, the ureterocele remains collapsed after aspiration and any element of obstruction to the bladder neck or contralateral ureter resolves (Figure 40.37). The latter may unmask reflux into the contralateral, now solitary, kidney. With larger ureteroceles a significant reservoir for lower UTIs remains, despite their decompression. Although not well defined in the literature, some of these eventually require secondary surgery for their removal. Cystoscopic evidence of the open meatus typically accompanying sphincteric or cecoureteroceles may identify those variants particularly at risk for future problems. Simultaneous excision of the ureterocele with bladder reconstruction is not unreasonable, if the age of the patient permits. Otherwise, the patient can be followed medically after nephrectomy and repair of the bladder deferred to a later age, if indicated.

Whether antenatal diagnosis alters the long-term implications of such anomalies is unclear. A non-operative approach has been taken in a small group of infants whose ureteroceles subtended multicystic dysplastic kidneys. In limited follow-up, the ureterocele collapsed or remained stable in each case, whereas affected kidneys uniformly involuted. None required surgery.[18]

Selective cystoscopic puncture is not an option for obstructed ureteroceles associated with a non-functioning kidney. This risks converting the anomaly from one that can be potentially addressed solely from above to one requiring another incision to correct a refluxing ureterocele. Non-selective cystoscopic 'unroofing', as advocated by Tank,[86] remains an option for decompressing obstructed ureteroceles in children who are extremely ill and unable to tolerate open surgery. Interestingly, 50% of renal moieties that showed no function on EU subsequently demonstrated excretion of contrast after their decompression. These data suggest that some kidneys may recover function after being vented, but may also point to the shortcomings of EU compared with radionuclide studies in infants with obstructed kidneys. Reflux is an expected sequela of this predecessor of selective puncture.[87] Decompression can also be achieved with percutaneous drainage, which is the current preferred method of temporizing until the ureterocele can be definitively addressed.[88]

Single system – functioning kidney

The experience with selective incisions and puncture of these ureterocele variants has been encouraging enough that it should be considered the procedure of choice[69,89] (Figure 40.38). In one series, for example, endoscopic decompression was successful in 22 of 25 patients (88%) with single-system intravesical ureteroceles.[90] Reflux tends to appear into larger ureteroceles whose detrusor defects result in very little backing to the anomaly. Ureterocele excision, ureteral reimplantation, and correction of any detrusor defects usually become necessary when reflux appears, although a trial of medical management, similar to that used with primary VUR, can be reasonable, especially in younger children.

Duplex system – minimal or non-functioning upper pole

An upper pole heminephrectomy is indicated but may not finalize the problem (Figures 40.39 and 40.40). This upper tract approach effectively decompresses the ureterocele, potentially restores trigonal anatomy, and may be the only treatment needed for some patients.[91,92] In the series reported by Caldamone et al,[15] seven of 36 patients (19%) ultimately required secondary procedures for persistent reflux (three patients) or bladder outlet obstruction (four patients). VUR appeared in 10 cases after decompression, where none was present beforehand. The reflux resolved in three patients. Long-term outcomes into adulthood are unavailable in the literature. Other clinicians report similar rates (about 20%) of persistent reflux into ipsilateral lower pole or contralateral ureters after heminephrectomy alone.[43,93] In another series of 19 patients reported by Scherz et al,[94] 9 patients (47%) required intravesical surgery for urinary infection or reflux (Figure 40.41).

These types of data have led some clinicians to advocate a combined approach where heminephrec-

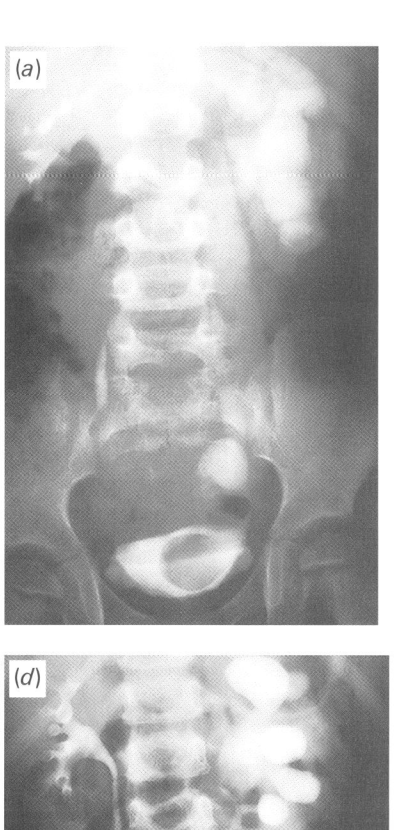

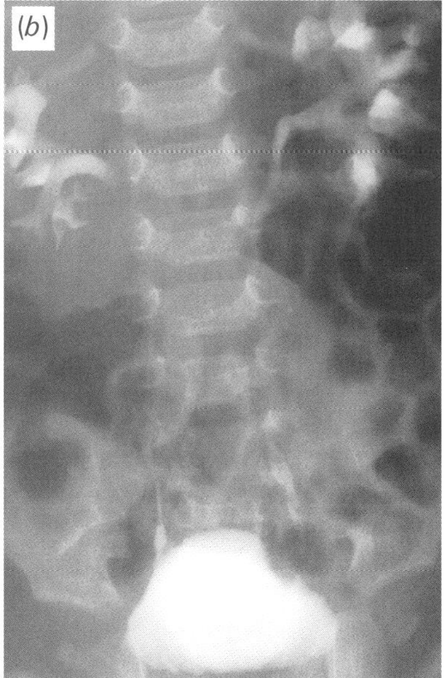

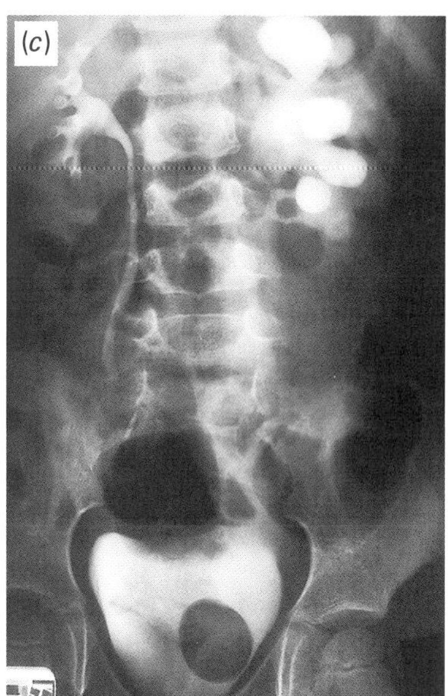

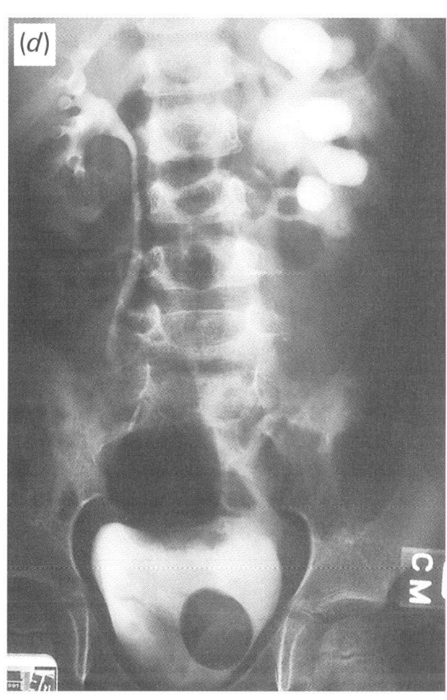

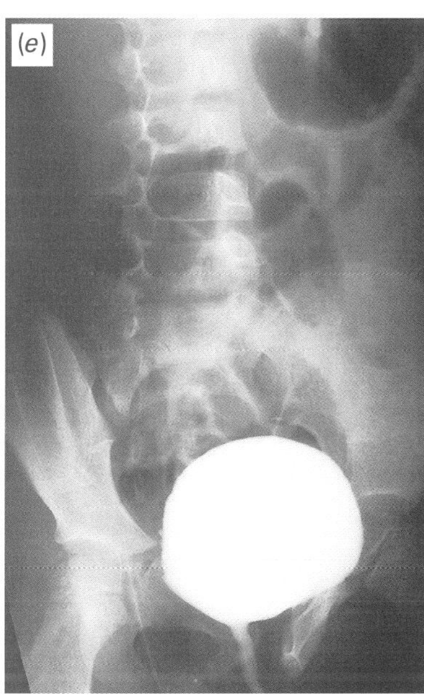

Figure 40.38 (*a*) Single-system intravesical ureterocele causing significant hydroureteronephrosis of the left collecting system. (*b*) After incision, a marked improvement in the degree of dilatation is seen. No reflux was present before or after surgery. (*c*) A similar variant with hydronephrosis of the left kidney treated with selective incision. (*d*) Significant improvement is shown after surgery. (*e*) Voiding cystourethrogram is unremarkable.

tomy, ureterocele excision, and ureteral reimplantation are completed with one surgery.[44,95] The need for secondary surgeries is far less common with the combined approach. For example, only 14% of patients in the Scherz series[94] required reoperations for persistent reflux after the combined approach. To its detriment, ureterocele excision and duplex ureteral reimplantation can present a technical tour-de-force in smaller infants. In addition, intravesical repairs are unnecessary in perhaps half of these patients. The characteristics of ureteroceles that ultimately require excision and bladder reconstruction remain to be fully defined. Such selection criteria would help identify patients whose problem would be best finalized by the upper tract approach alone and limit the combined approach to those that truly need it.

The review by Husmann et al[96] has been revealing in this regard. Of 87 patients with a ureterocele and nonfunctioning upper pole treated by heminephrectomy, subtotal ureterectomy, and observation (initial upper tract alone approach), 54 (62%) required additional surgery to correct reflux. Notably, the need for additional surgery was directly related to the number of renal moieties that originally had VUR present. When a ureterocele alone was present, 21 of 21 patients required no further surgery. If low-grade reflux (less than III/V) was present into only one ureter, eight of 15 patients (53%) did well with the upper tract alone

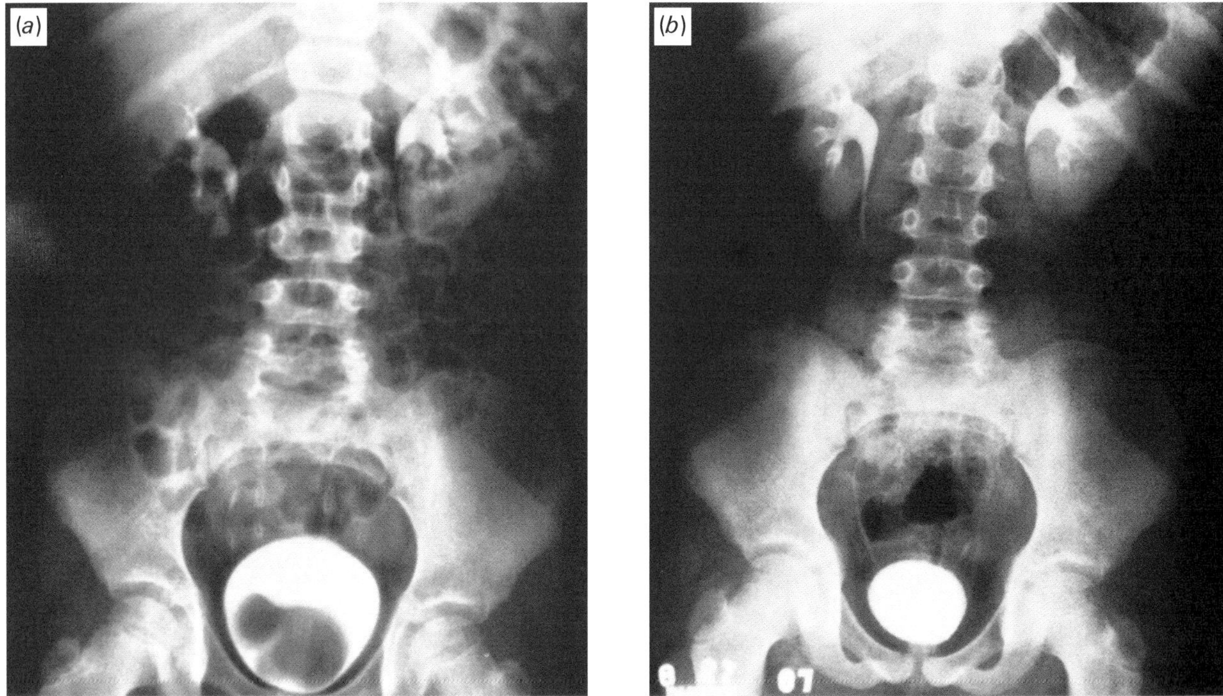

Figure 40.39 (*a*) Preoperative view shows minimally functioning upper pole moiety of the right kidney. (*b*) Postoperative view shows decompression of the ureterocele and an essentially normal right kidney.

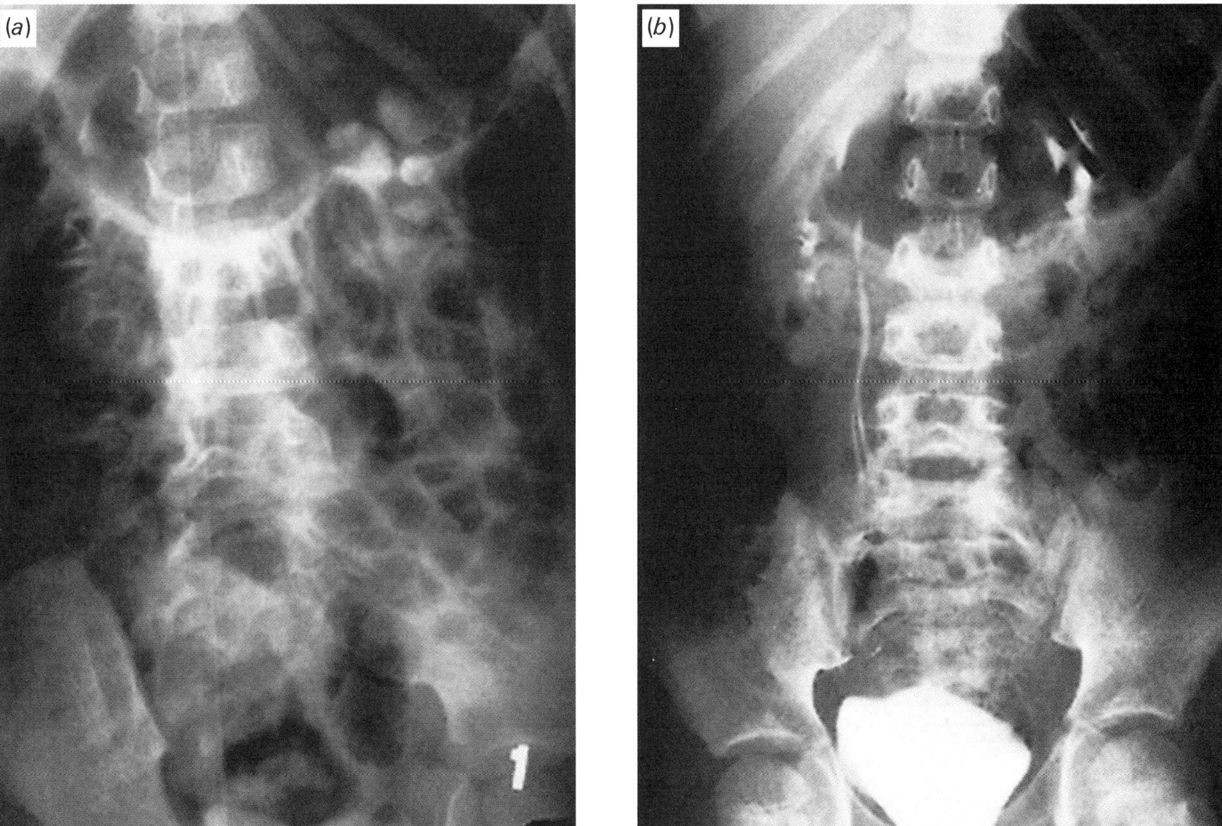

Figure 40.40 Extravesical ureterocele treated by heminephrectomy and subtotal ureterectomy. (*a*) Preoperative excretory urogram shows a left-sided anomaly and a markedly hydronephrotic lower pole. (*b*) Postoperative view. Preservation of function and appearance of remaining kidney are often surprisingly good. The ureterocele is fully decompressed.

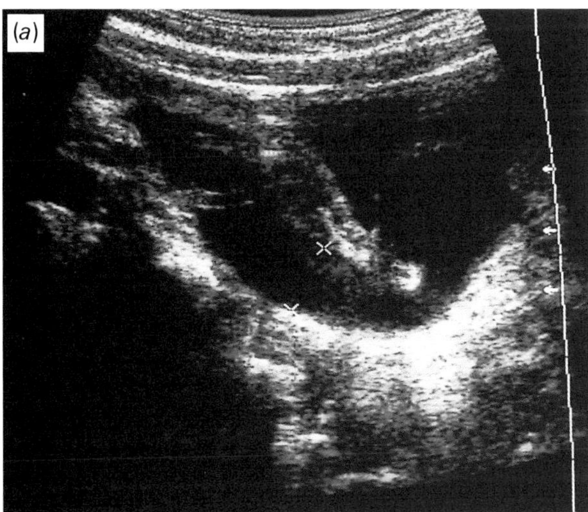

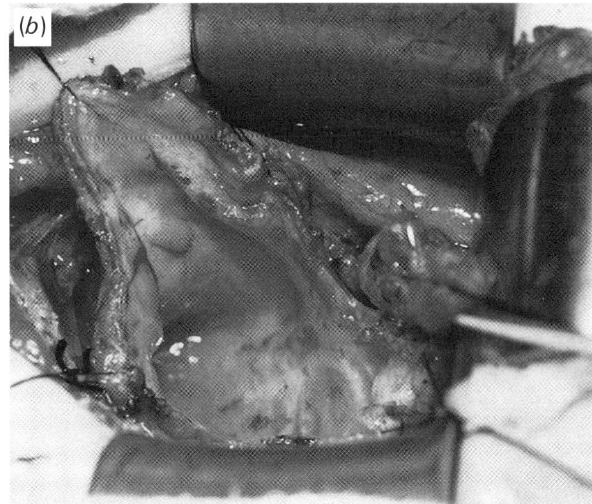

Figure 40.41 (*a*) The stump of residual ureter and ureterocele remain after heminephrectomy. The patient presented with recurrent urinary infections. (*b*) Large ureterocele opened at surgery.

approach. Finally, and most significantly, when high-grade reflux was seen in one ureter or reflux was associated with more than one moiety, regardless of grade, surgery became inevitable for 48 of 50 (96%) patients. A more recent review by DeFoor et al[97] echoed similar findings. Ureteroceles that involve other renal segments are more likely to require secondary surgery. Ureterocele prolapse is another finding that inevitably portends bladder reconstruction.[98] In addition, the occasional ureterocele that itself refluxes at presentation will, by default, require a combined 'up-and- down' approach for management.

Given these data, families and patients can be better informed as to the likelihood of needing lower urinary tract surgery if an upper tract approach is initially used. In addition, strong consideration can be given to a complete urinary tract reconstruction if the preoperative work-up returns such ominous prognosticators and the patient's size permits. Finally, and while it might seem an anathema to some, unroofing the ureterocele becomes an option in newborns and small infants who appear destined to require 'up-and-down' surgery regardless because of the 'clinical staging' of their anomaly. Eliminating obstruction significantly lessens the threat of urinary infections and decompression of the ureterocele simplifies the bladder repair (Figure 40.42). Most children can be effectively managed with antibiotic prophylaxis until they are old enough to have definitive reconstructive surgery. However, infections can still occur. In one series of 15 neonates with a ureterocele, eight developed infections during the first few days of life, including three who were receiving prophylactic antibiotics.[99] Assessment, with considerations to surgery, should be done at an early age to optimize the advantage given children whose anomalies have been discovered antenatally.[100]

The report of Gran et al[101] offers a different solution to the long-term follow-up required of residual ureteroceles that remain after the upper tract alone approach has been used. Rather than remove a non-functioning moiety, reconstruction of its ureter and the bladder was successfully completed in 16 patients. No morbidity has yet (mean 5 years follow-up) been associated with the non-functioning kidneys that remain. Detractors, concerned about preserving possibly dysplastic tissue, will explain that families are now offered extended follow-up of such kidneys in exchange for that of the bladder. However, if parallels are drawn with the relative benefits of removing multicystic dysplastic kidneys, the argument may ultimately prove to be a weak one. Future management may see many children with ureteroceles initially punctured and decompressed during the newborn period until they are old enough for bladder reconstruction, if reflux persists or appears, regardless of the status of their kidneys.

Finally, on the far end of the spectrum, an expectant approach has been used with success in some children with a non-functioning upper pole moiety and a low-grade lower pole VUR. In a group of 52 patients, whose anomalies were detected antenatally, 14 (27%) have done well, with a median of 8 years of follow-up.[102] Each was kept on prophylactic antibi-

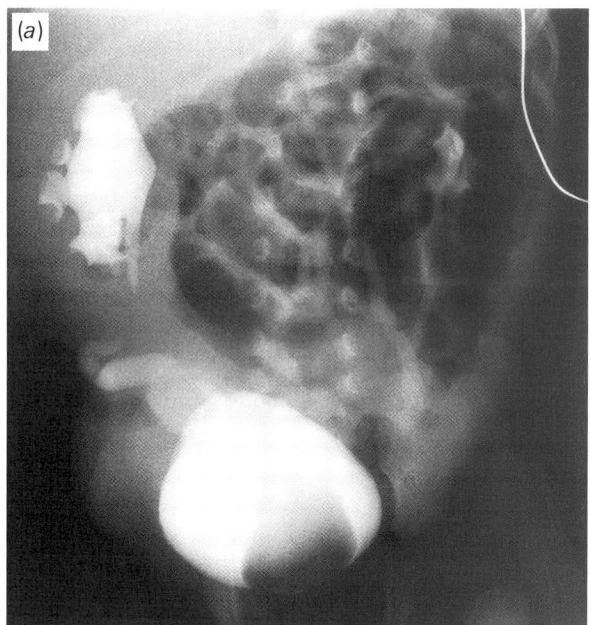

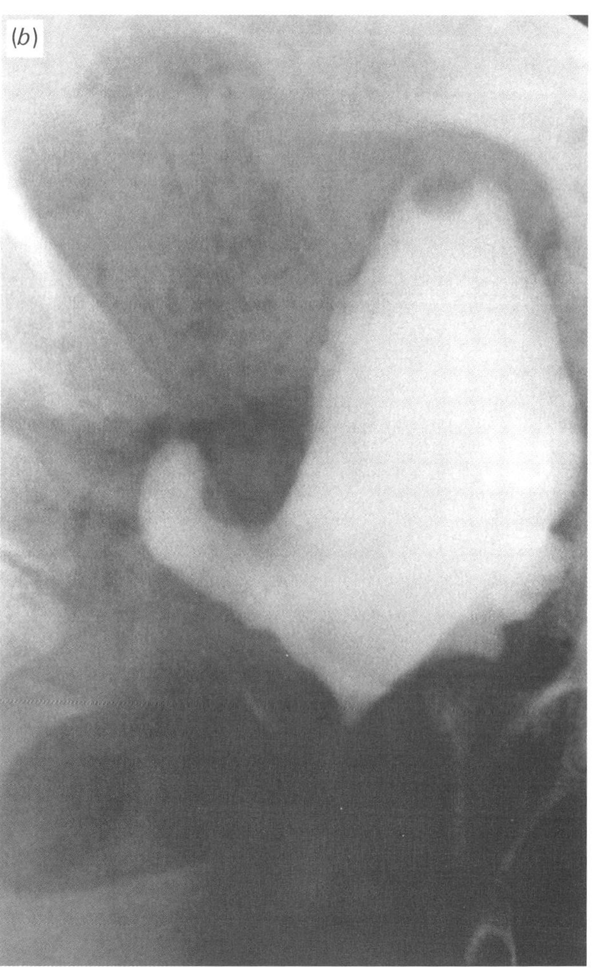

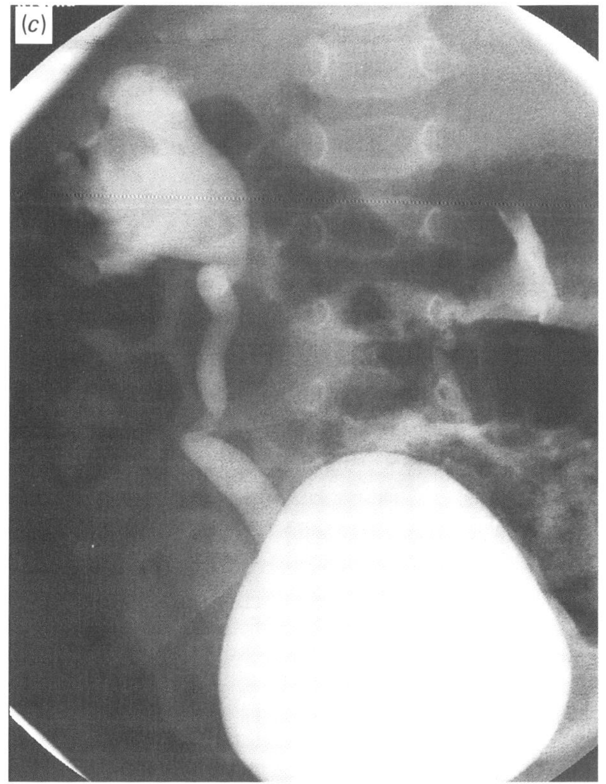

Figure 40.42 A newborn female with urinary tract infection needing a combined approach in the management of a ureterocele. (*a*) Excretory urogram shows a large ureterocele filling the base of the bladder, and a non-functioning upper pole of the right kidney. (*b*) Preoperative cystogram demonstrates eversion of the ureterocele forming a diverticulum, an indication of a significant detrusor defect. No reflux was seen. (*c*) Postincision cystogram shows bilateral vesicoureteral reflux but decompressed ureterocele. Heminephrectomy and ureterocelectomy were deferred until 1 year of age, since the child remained infection free.

otics until the completion of toilet training and none required surgery. These findings raise more questions than they answer.

Duplex system – functioning upper pole

Like their non-functioning partners, these conditions too can be addressed with an 'upper tract alone' approach. It should be remembered that upper pole duplications optimally contribute perhaps 16% of overall renal function. Because of this somewhat marginal contribution, some clinicians recommend heminephrectomies for the majority of duplications, whether they function or not. This avoids the potential complications of the reconstruction, risks to the lower pole, and the unknown long-term implications of upper pole retention.[31] The other option is salvage of the upper pole by creating a ureteropyelostomy or ureteroureterostomy in combination with a subtotal

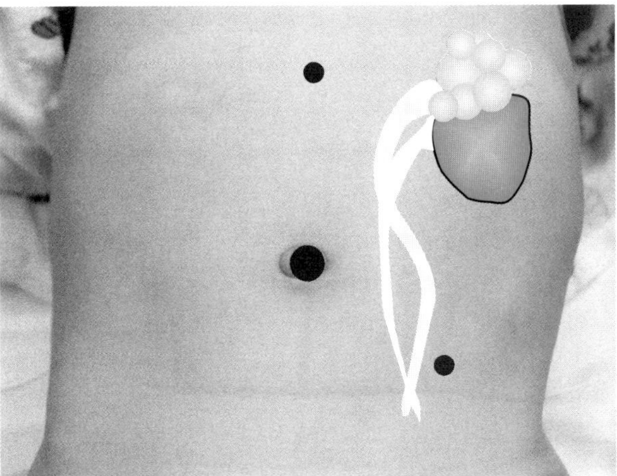

Figure 41.4 Port placement for the transperitoneal approach to the kidney, which provides excellent access to the distal ureter when this must be resected.

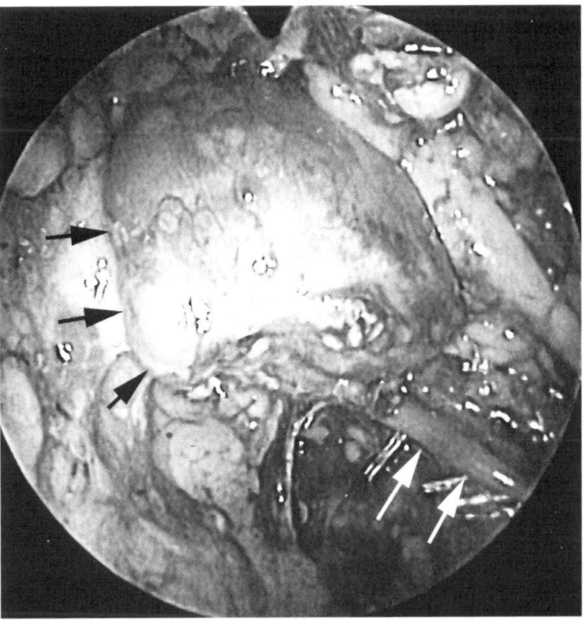

Figure 41.5 Appearance of the remnant upper pole of a left kidney following lower pole nephrectomy. The lateral edge of the upper pole is marked by the dark arrows and the upper pole ureter is marked by the white arrows.

monic scalpel or with the bipolar cautery.[9] The remainder of the ureter is then dissected away from the remaining ureter, with care taken to avoid devascularizing it, which is best done by staying very close to the ureter being removed. The distal ureteral stump should be suture-ligated when reflux is present. In the ectopic ureter with both obstruction and reflux, usually those entering the bladder neck, the entire ureter should be removed and the defect closed with sutures. The specimen is removed from the largest port incision. Large cysts in dysplastic upper poles may need to be aspirated before the specimen can be removed.

The typical indication for lower pole heminephrectomy in duplicated anomalies is a severely compromised lower pole as a result of high-grade vesicoureteral reflux (VUR). The procedure can be undertaken, transperitoneal or retroperitoneal, and prone or lateral, in a similar fashion to an upper pole partial nephrectomy. It is best to expose the entire hilum first in order to positively identify the lower pole vessels. In lower pole partial nephrectomy, the plane between the upper and lower pole pelves is not as distinct and may be difficult to develop. Also, the calices of the dilated lower pole often protrude into the upper pole and may be entered during separation of the two moieties. All remnants of the calices and parenchyma must be removed in order to prevent formation of a urinoma (Figure 41.5). If the upper pole collecting system is inadvertently entered, suture closure is recommended as well as drainage.[1] Removal of the lower pole through the initial incision may require morcellation.

Results of laparoscopic partial nephrectomy

Table 41.1 shows the results of several series of pediatric laparoscopic partial nephrectomy. In general, the operative times are acceptable and the conversion rate to open surgery is low. In comparative studies of transperitoneal and retroperitoneal approaches, there is minimal difference in times or outcomes. In a study from this institution with age-matched open surgical controls, operative times were identical at 3.2 hours, hospital stay was significantly reduced (1.7 vs 4.7 days ($p = 0.001$), and analgesic requirements were significantly less in the retroperitoneal partial nephrectomy group. Even in the infant, laparoscopic approaches for complex renal surgery are both safe and efficient, perhaps even more so than open surgery.

Complications

Possible complications of laparoscopic partial nephrectomy include bowel, liver, and spleen injuries, abdominal wall vessel injuries, and vascular injuries.[16] On the right side, the duodenum can be injured while exposing the upper pole. It is important to recognize that what looks like the renal vein may in fact be the

Table 41.1 Summary data for laparoscopic partial nephrectomy in children, with conversion rates to open surgery

First author	Year	No. of patients	Operative time (hours)	Length of stay (days)	Conversion rate	Conversion rate (% of total)	Comment
Janetschek[10]	1997	14	3.75	4.4	0	0	Transperitoneal
Yao[11]	2000	6	3.75	1	0	0	Transperitoneal
Horowitz[12]	2001	14	1.66	2.6	0	0	Transperitoneal
El-Ghoneimi[3]	2003	15	2.5	1.4	1	6.7	Retroperitoneal
Robinson[13]	2003	11	3.33	1.0	0	0	Transperitoneal
Valla[14]	2003	24	2.66	3.4	3	12.5	Retroperitoneal
Lee[15]	2005	14	3.2	1.7	0	0	Retroperitoneal
Total		**98**	**2.98**	**2.21**	**4**	**4.1**	

vena cava if proper orientation of the camera is lost. It is important to briefly reorient oneself prior to any definitive clip placement. Arterial injuries require prompt control of bleeding and repair. Conversion to open surgery may be necessary, depending upon the severity of the injury and the experience of the surgeon. Although there is less need to manipulate the remnant pole during a laparoscopic partial nephrectomy, the possibility of arterial spasm in the remnant pole must be recognized and anticipated. This is more likely in infants, but can occur at any age. Any tension on the remnant pole vessels should be released and a syringe of papaverine prepared. If the affected pole does not 'pink-up', 0.5 ml of papaverine should be forcefully squirted at the affected artery. If no effect is seen, a second bolus of 0.5 ml should then be instilled. Alternatively, lidocaine (without epinephrine) may be useful to correct the vasospasm.

Postoperative complications have been limited to urinoma formation, although none have been clinically significant. Simple aspiration is usually associated with rapid recurrence. If there is concern about a remnant pole leak, a double-J stent may be placed for several weeks. We have not seen any long-term problems with these and have usually simply observed them without untoward outcomes.

Ureteral surgery associated with duplication anomalies

Laparoscopic vesicoureteral reimplant has limited indications in duplication anomalies. Isolated VUR of the lower pole is best managed by ureteroureterostomy. If the upper pole is also refluxing, typically as a result of previous incision of a UC, a common sheath reimplant is appropriate. An isolated lower pole reimplant is considered when the upper moiety had been previously removed.

In unilateral cases, simple or common sheath reimplant can be accomplished laparoscopically with a Lich–Gregoire extravesical reimplantation.[17–19] The patient is positioned supine, and ports are placed at the umbilicus and symmetrically in the midclavicular lines, 2–3 cm below the umbilicus. The ureter is exposed by incising the peritoneum and a detrusor incision of 2.5–3 cm is made with the hook cautery. A hitch stitch is placed to hold the bladder upwards to aid exposure. The muscle is then brought around the ureter with interrupted sutures. No ureteral stenting is required. In bilateral cases, a laparoscopic intravesical approach has been described by Olsen et al.[20] Laparoscopic ureterocele excision has also been described, including extravesical reimplantation of the remnant ureter.

Associated lower pole ureteropelvic junction (UPJ) obstruction is best treated by creating a wide anastomosis between the lower pole pelvis and the upper pole ureter (pyeloureterostomy). On occasion, however, an isolated lower pole dismembered pyeloplasty can be considered. This is one of the most challenging laparoscopic procedures in pediatric urology, and can be performed transperitoneally or retroperitoneally.[21–23] Ports are placed as in a transabdominal partial nephrectomy, but the retroperitoneal space can be exposed through a transmesenteric incision. The operation is carried out as an open dismembered pyeloplasty, with resection of the stenotic segment, spatulation of the ureter, and reanastomosis. A double-J internal stent is left in the repaired ureter. This operation requires significant skill in laparoscopic suturing and knot tying. For this reason, it can be more efficiently accomplished by those without the requisite experience by using the da Vinci robotic surgical system (Intuitive Surgical, Sunnyvale, CA).[24–26]

Robotic laparoscopy for duplication anomalies

The use of robotics potentially expands the number of laparoscopic cases, enabling surgeons with limited laparoscopic experience to perform complex laparoscopic reconstructions requiring extended suturing skills. Of the different available devices, the da Vinci robotic surgical system seems the more appropriate to pediatric urologic needs. It is composed of three main parts: the robotic unit, with three (or four) robotic arms that hold camera and instruments; the video–insufflation–light source unit, as in conventional laparoscopy; and the remote console from where the surgeon controls the robotic arms.[25] It is equipped with a double camera that facilitates an optimal three-dimensional view. The instruments presently available are 8 and 5 mm in diameter, the larger ones permitting the greatest maneuverability.[27] Whereas robotic laparoscopy presents enormous advantages in terms of visual and fine suturing capabilities, accuracy, and speed of surgery over freehand laparoscopy, it also carries the limitation that once the robot is engaged no further adjustment to patient position is possible without disengaging the robot. Therefore, care must be taken in terms of patient preparation and positioning, set-up, and port placement. A dedicated nursing team is advisable and all members should have had laboratory training on the system.

Extravesical ureteral reimplants, pyeloplasties, and partial nephrectomies have been performed robotically.[25] In pyeloplasties and partial nephrectomies, the approach is currently transperitoneal, whereas retroperitoneal approaches are being investigated.

To perform a ureteral reimplant, the robot is brought in from the feet of the patient and a 30° up-angled camera is used. For renal surgery, the robot is brought in from the side and angled from the shoulder, with care being taken to engage it perpendicular to the major longitudinal axis of the kidney. An important point in all robotic laparoscopic procedures is that once the robot is engaged, any adjustment of robot position requires disengaging the system. While the surgeon sits at the console, the assistant will remain scrubbed at the patient's side, taking care of instrument changes. With the da Vinci robot, current instruments include a hook cautery, scissors, DeBakey forceps, larger grasping forceps, and two sizes of needle holder. These instruments are integrated with conventional laparoscopic clip appliers, irrigation/aspiration devices, scissors, and graspers. Dissection is carried out mostly with the hook cautery, as is the parenchymal resection in a partial nephrectomy. Vessels are clipped with a traditional clip applier maneuvered by the assistant. The operations are carried out as previously described. Operation times are usually reduced, compared with conventional freehand laparoscopy, although overall time may be equal due to the set-up time required with the robot. With the use of the da Vinci robotic surgical system, laparoscopic nephrectomies, partial nephrectomies, pyeloplasties, and reimplants may become accessible to a larger number of surgeons with limited experience in conventional laparoscopy.

References

1. Peters CA. Laparoendoscopic renal surgery in children. J Endourol 2000; 14(10):841–17, discussion 847–8.
2. Borer JG, Peters CA. Pediatric retroperitoneoscopic nephrectomy. J Endourol 2000; 14(5):413–16, discussion 417.
3. El-Ghoneimi A, Farhat W, Bolduc S et al. Retroperitoneal laparoscopic vs open partial nephroureterectomy in children. BJU Int 2003; 91(6):532–5.
4. Borer JG, Cisek LJ, Atala A et al. Pediatric retroperitoneoscopic nephrectomy using 2 mm instrumentation. J Urol 1999; 162(5):1725–9, discussion 1730.
5. Borzi PA. A comparison of the lateral and posterior retroperitoneoscopic approach for complete and partial nephroureterectomy in children. BJU Int 2001; 87(6):517–20.
6. El-Ghoneimi A, Valla JS, Steyaert H, Aigrain Y. Laparoscopic renal surgery via a retroperitoneal approach in children. J Urol 1998; 160(3 Pt 2):1138–41.
7. Kobashi KC, Chamberlin DA, Rajpoot D, Shanberg AM. Retroperitoneal laparoscopic nephrectomy in children. J Urol 1998; 160(3 Pt 2):1142–4.
8. Guillonneau B, Ballanger P, Lugagne PM, Valla JS, Vallancien G. Laparoscopic versus lumboscopic nephrectomy. Eur Urol 1996; 29(3):288–91.
9. Jackman SV, Cadeddu JA, Chen RN et al. Utility of the harmonic scalpel for laparoscopic partial nephrectomy. J Endourol 1998; 12(5):441–4.
10. Janetschek G, Seibold J, Radmayr C, Bartsch G. Laparoscopic heminephroureterectomy in pediatric patients. J Urol 1997; 158(5):1928–30.
11. Yao D, Poppas DP. A clinical series of laparoscopic nephrectomy, nephroureterectomy and heminephroureterectomy in the pediatric population. J Urol 2000; 163(5):1531–5.

12. Horowitz M, Shah SM, Ferzli G, Syad PI, Glassberg KI. Laparoscopic partial upper pole nephrectomy in infants and children. BJU Int 2001; 87(6):514–16.
13. Robinson BC, Snow BW, Cartwright PC et al. Comparison of laparoscopic versus open partial nephrectomy in a pediatric series. J Urol 2003; 169(2):638–40.
14. Valla JS, Breaud J, Carfagna L, Tursini S, Steyaert H. Treatment of ureterocele on duplex ureter: upper pole nephrectomy by retroperitoneoscopy in children based on a series of 24 cases. Eur Urol 2003; 43(4):426–9.
15. Lee RS, Retik AB, Borer JG, Diamond DA, Peters CA. Pediatric retroperitoneal laparoscopic partial nephrectomy: comparison with an age matched cohort of open surgery. J Urol 2005; 174(2):708–11, discussion 712.
16. Peters CA. Complications of retroperitoneal laparoscopy in pediatric urology: prevention, recognition and management. In: Caione P, Kavoussi LR, Micali F, eds. Retroperitoneoscopy and Extraperitoneal Laparoscopy in Pediatric and Adult Urology. Milan: Springer-Verlag 2003: 203–10.
17. Atala A, Kavoussi LR, Goldstein DS, Retik AB, Peters CA. Laparoscopic correction of vesicoureteral reflux. J Urol 1993; 150:748–51.
18. Peters CA. Robotic assisted surgery in pediatric urology. Pediatr Endosurg Innov Techn 2003; 7(4):403–13.
19. Lakshmanan Y, Fung LC. Laparoscopic extravesicular ureteral reimplantation for vesicoureteral reflux: recent technical advances. J Endourol 2000; 14(7):589–93, discussion 593–4.
20. Olsen LH, Deding D, Yeung CK, Jorgensen TM. Computer assisted laparoscopic pneumovesical ureter reimplantation a.m. Cohen: initial experience in a pig model. APMIS Suppl 2003; 109:23–5.
21. El-Ghoneimi A, Farhat W, Bolduc S et al. Laparoscopic dismembered pyeloplasty by a retroperitoneal approach in children. BJU Int 2003; 92(1):104–8, discussion 108.
22. Tan HL. Laparoscopic Anderson–Hynes dismembered pyeloplasty in children. J Urol 1999; 162(3 Pt 2):1045–7, discussion 1048.
23. Yeung CK, Tam YH, Sihoe JD, Lee KH, Liu KW. Retroperitoneoscopic dismembered pyeloplasty for pelvi-ureteric junction obstruction in infants and children. BJU Int 2001; 87(6):509–13.
24. Peters CA. Robotically assisted paediatric pyeloplasty: cutting edge or expensive toy? BJU Int 2004; 94(9):1214–15.
25. Peters CA. Robotically assisted surgery in pediatric urology. Urol Clin North Am 2004; 31(4):743–52.
26. Olsen LH, Jorgensen TM. Computer assisted pyeloplasty in children: the retroperitoneal approach. J Urol 2004; 171(6 Pt 2):2629–31.
27. Camarillo DB, Krummel TM, Salisbury JK Jr. Robotic technology in surgery: past, present, and future. Am J Surg 2004; 188(4A Suppl):2–15S.

Vesicoureteral reflux: anatomic and functional basis of etiology

42

John M Park

Vesicoureteral reflux (VUR), a retrograde flow of bladder urine into the upper urinary tract, is one of the most commonly encountered pediatric urologic anomalies. It occurs normally in many animal species but is generally considered abnormal in humans. Traditionally, VUR has been categorized etiologically into primary and secondary. Primary VUR is thought to represent an abnormal anatomy and function of the ureterovesical junction (UVJ), whereas secondary VUR implies an acquired condition as a result of increased intravesical pressure in the setting of neurogenic bladder dysfunction, non-neurogenic bladder dysfunction, or outlet obstruction. The clinical association of VUR and urinary tract infection (UTI) that leads to pyelonephritis, renal scarring, hypertension, and chronic renal insufficiency (reflux nephropathy) has been the primary impetus for diagnostic and therapeutic interventions for VUR during the last three decades. However, various clinical and experimental studies seeking to establish a causal relationship between the pathophysiologic components of VUR, UTI, and other clinical sequelae have led to many contentious debates rather than a unifying consensus. In fact, most pediatric urologists and nephrologists now consider VUR not as a disease in and of itself but rather as a marker of heterogeneous condition of the whole urinary tract. It includes congenital renal hypoplasia and dysplasia (in addition to acquired pyelonephritic renal damage), primary reflux caused by incompetent UVJ, altered lower urinary tract function, and inherent predisposition to UTI. In this chapter, the etiologic components of VUR – both anatomic and functional – are discussed to establish the conceptual framework within which clinical management issues are presented in the subsequent chapters.

Historical perspective

Galen and Leonardo da Vinci were the first to propose that normal UVJ allowed unidirectional flow of urine into the bladder and that VUR might be abnormal in humans.[1,2] In 1893, Pozzi reported that VUR could occur in humans after noting an unexpected urine leakage from the accidentally severed ureter during a pelvic gynecologic procedure.[3] The systematic identification of VUR came as the result of technologic advances in contrast radiography – voiding cystourethrography (VCUG). Initially, VUR was not thought to be a significant clinical problem for humans, although Bumpus speculated in 1924 that VUR was related to UTI and that in children, unlike adults, VUR was not associated with other urinary tract pathology.[4] In 1930, Campbell found VUR in 12% of over 700 VCUGs but assumed that there was other underlying pathology as the cause of VUR.[5] In 1944, Prather proposed that VUR was abnormal in children,[6] and this notion gained increasing acceptance, after accumulating evidence suggested that VUR was typically absent in normal neonates and children. The modern era of clinical VUR management was ushered in by Hutch's observation that VUR and pyelonephritis might be causally related in paraplegic patients.[7] Hodson, applying Hutch's concept to children, noted that VUR was more common in children with UTI and renal parenchymal abnormality.[8,9] Other clinical and experimental observations soon followed, providing the anatomic and functional basis for the UVJ mechanism and the etiology of VUR.

Anatomic features of ureterovesical junction

The UVJ is anatomically and functionally adapted to allow intermittent passage of a urinary bolus from the ureter into the bladder, while preventing the retrograde flow of bladder urine back toward the kidney during storage and micturition. To achieve these functions, the ureter enters the bladder wall with an oblique intramural path (intramural ureter) and

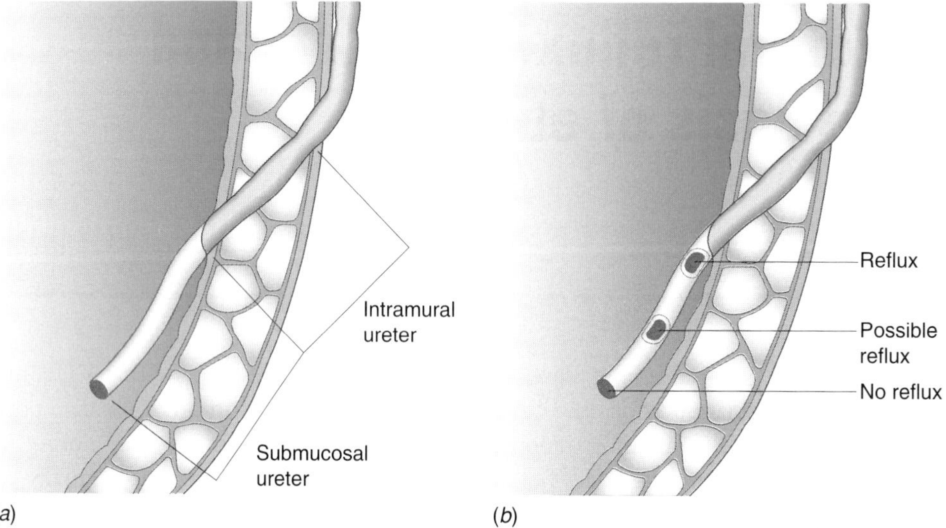

Figure 42.1 (*a*) Normal ureterovesical junction (UVJ): demonstration of the intravesical ureter (intramural + submucosal). (*b*) Refluxing UVJ: unlike a non-refluxing orifice, there is an inadequate length of the intravesical ureter, compromising the 'flap-valve' mechanism. (Modified from Politano,[10] with permission.)

extends through a submucosal tunnel of appropriate length (submucosal ureter) to open onto the trigone in a correct location. This 'flap-valve' configuration causes the intramural and submucosal ureter to be compressed with progressive bladder filling against the detrusor muscle backing, as if one were stepping on compressible straw on the ground (Figure 42.1).

The UVJ mechanism, however, is not entirely passive. It is also active, requiring a functional integration with bladder and trigone. The functional components of the UVJ were first appreciated in 1812 when Bell noted that extension of the ureteral longitudinal muscle fibers into the trigone (Bell's muscle) was important in the preservation of intramural ureter obliquity.[11] Tanagho and Pugh provided an anatomic description of the ureteral muscle fiber extension intravesically.[12] The inner longitudinal ureteral fibers form the superficial trigone, down to the level of verumontanum in males and the dorsal surface of the urethra in females. At the trigone, the muscle fibers extend fanwise, and at the midline of the trigone, they intermingle with those of the contralateral ureter. The middle circular ureteral muscle is not seen beyond the level of the ureteral hiatus. The adventitia of the distal ureter just outside the bladder wall fuses with the fibromuscular sheath that encircles the ureter (known as Waldeyer's sheath). Waldeyer's sheath is thought to anchor the ureter within the hiatus while allowing the intramural ureter to slide freely within the hiatus during bladder filling and emptying (Figure 42.2). In 1972 Elbadawi[14] (later

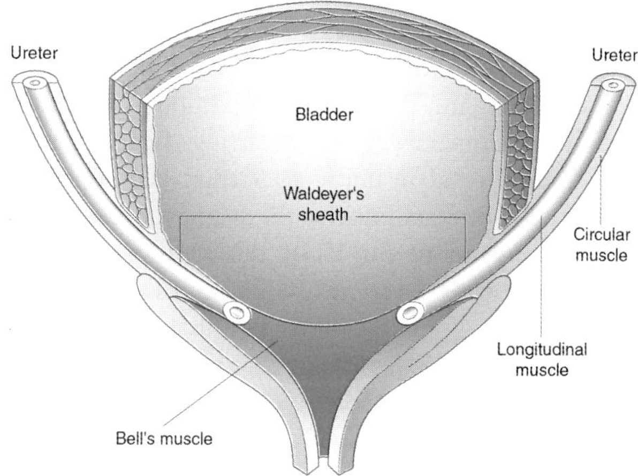

Figure 42.2 Passage of the distal ureter through the ureteral hiatus in the bladder wall. Ureteral inner longitudinal muscle fibers extend into the trigone to form the Bell's muscle. The Waldeyer's sheath anchors the distal ureter at the hiatus. (Modified from Mathisen,[13] with permission.)

confirmed by Stephens[15]) identified a separate intermediate layer extending from the ureter into the deep trigone.

Immunohistochemical studies using antibodies that differentiate the ureteral and bladder embryologic origins have also confirmed these ureteral muscle extensions into the deep trigone, richly innervated by noradrenergic receptors, similar to vas deferens.[16] This intermediate layer may be important in the overall development of ureter and trigone. The ureteral maldevelopment may be tied together with an abnormal trigonal development, which derives from the common nephric duct (the segment of mesonephric duct distal to the origin of ureteric bud). A recent study of vitamin A signaling-deficient mice demonstrated an abnormal development of trigone, thereby resulting in a high incidence of distal ureteral anomalies.[17]

Despite somewhat conflicting opinions about the precise anatomic details of the ureter–trigone relationship, there is sound physiologic evidence to suggest that a functional integration of ureter and trigone is important in the normal UVJ mechanism. Tanagho et al's series of elegant experiments in dogs defined their roles in preventing VUR.[18] Unilateral sympathectomy at L3–5 uniformly induced reflux. These findings were consistent with earlier observations by Langworthy in 1938, where unilateral sympathectomy in cats induced a unilateral dilated ureter with ipsilateral widening of the ureteric orifice. Additional experiments demonstrated that increasing the trigonal tone and contractility using electrical stimulation, epinephrine injection, bladder distention, and micturition all resulted in functional occlusion of the ureteric orifices. Finally, surgical incision of ureter–trigone continuity below the ureteric orifice resulted in VUR, which then disappeared after healing of the incision.

The anatomic mechanisms of the UVJ can be then summarized as follows. The natural tone of ureteral muscle provides a mild passive closure of the intramural ureter except during the efflux of the urinary bolus. As the bladder fills and becomes distended, there is a progressive obliquity of the intramural and submucosal ureter, creating a 'flap-valve' mechanism, provided that there is a sturdy back-wall support of the detrusor muscle. The tone and contractility of the trigone increases steadily during bladder filling as it becomes stretched, and it provides a secure anchoring of the ureteric orifices, further augmenting the flap-valve mechanism. Micturition also stimulates the trigonal tone, anchoring the ureter and preventing the lateral displacement of the orifice. The critical factor of this flap-valve mechanism is the effective occlusion of the intramural and submucosal ureter as the rising intravesical pressure compresses it against the detrusor muscle. The anatomic and functional integration of ureter and trigone is a remarkable piece of bioengineering that allows an unimpeded unidirectional flow of urine at the UVJ.

In addition to the experimental observations noted above, clinical findings lend further support to the importance of the flap-valve mechanism in preventing VUR. The intravesical ureter (the intramural segment plus the submucosal tunnel) has been estimated to lengthen with age, providing rationale for spontaneous VUR resolution with maturation. In neonates, the average length of the intravesical ureter was 0.5 cm, whereas in adults it was 1.3 cm.[19,20] The mature length was thought to be achieved by 10–12 years of age. In examining other animal species, the variability of VUR incidence was also associated with the length of intravesical ureter. Trigonal competency plays a critical role in maintaining the adequate length and obliquity of the intravesical ureter during bladder distention and micturition. Inadequate trigonal function allows the ureteric orifice to displace laterally and migrate away from the bladder neck during bladder filling, leading to reduction of the intravesical ureteral length.

The lateral displacement of the ureteric orifice and its abnormal appearance in association with VUR are well established (Figure 42.3). The classic explanation proposed by Mackie and Stephens suggests that the lateral displacement may occur as the result of abnormal ureteric bud origin along the developing mesonephric duct.[22] They found a correlation between the lateral displacement of the ureteric orifice and the degree of renal dysplasia and hypoplasia, and postulated that the ectopic origin of the ureteric bud during metanephric development was the primary embryologic error leading to anomalous renal differentiation and an abnormally located ureteric orifice.

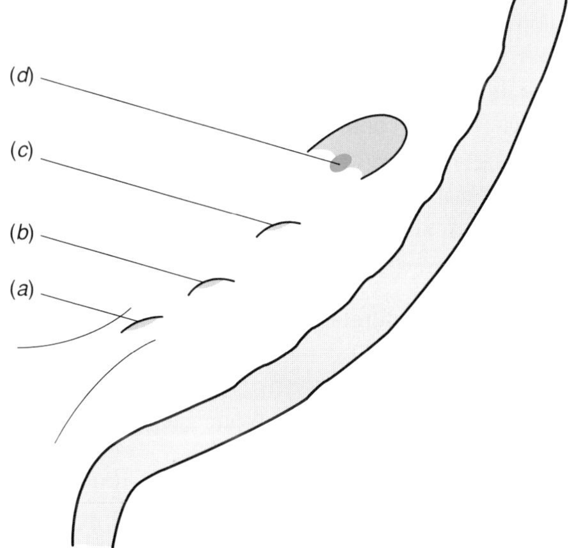

Figure 42.3 Four different ureteric orifice positions: (*a*) normal; (*b*) moderately lateral; (*c*) very lateral; and (*d*) orifice at the mouth of a diverticulum. (Reproduced from Glassberg et al,[21] with permission.)

This view is most plausible when applied to duplex system anomalies but may also be pertinent to the congenital renal anomalies associated with VUR. An alternative embryologic view of VUR may be the concept of primary trigonal disorder. The trigone develops as a result of a common nephric duct and the distal ureter incorporation into the developing bladder, and it is reasonable to postulate that the lateral displacement and the abnormal ureteral anchoring may occur as a result of functional disorganization of the trigone during development.[17]

Endoscopic observations confirm the importance of the flap-valve mechanism in preventing VUR. Specifically, the ratio of the submucosal tunnel length to the ureteral diameter appears to be a critical factor that determines the effectiveness of UVJ function.[19,20] Paquin noted that in children without VUR, the ratio of tunnel length to ureteral diameter was 5 to 1, whereas in children with VUR, the ratio was 1.4 to 1.[19] Cussen documented the relationship among intravesical ureteral length, submucosal ureteral length, and ureteral diameters in normal infants and children[20] (Table 42.1). The relative position and shape of the ureteric orifice also seem to correlate with the length of the intravesical ureter. Orifices that are placed laterally, away from the bladder neck, are associated with a higher incidence of VUR and probably reflect poor trigonal anchoring and short intravesical ureteral length. Lyon and colleagues described four basic orifice shapes that reflect the competency of the UVJ anatomy: cone, stadium, horseshoe, and golf-hole.[23] VUR was seen in 4% of patients with a normal cone configuration, 28% in those with a stadium orifice, 83% in those with a horseshoe orifice, and 100% in those with a golf-hole orifice. Heale confirmed Lyon's observations by reporting a higher prevalence and grade of VUR as well as renal scarring in patients with more laterally placed and abnormal ureteric orifices.[24] Stephens

Table 42.1 Mean ureteral tunnel lengths and diameters in children

Age (years)	Intravesical ureteral length (mm)	Submucosal ureteral length (mm)	Ureteral diameter (mm)
1–3	7	3	1.4
3–6	7	3	1.7
6–9	9	4	2.0
9–12	12	6	1.9

Adapted from Cussen,[20] with permission.

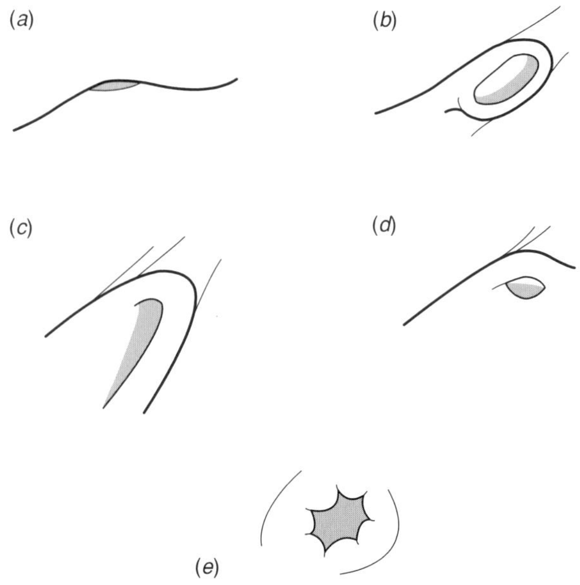

(a) (b) (c) (d) (e)

Figure 42.4 Orifice morphology (endoscopic view): (*a*) normal cone-shaped orifice; (*b*) stadium orifice; (*c*) horseshoe orifice; (*d*) lateral pillar defect; and (*e*) golf-hole orifice. (Reproduced from Glassberg et al,[21] with permission.)

described another orifice configuration – the lateral pillar defect – which probably represents a type of ureter–trigone abnormality between horseshoe and golf-hole orifices.[25] Although endoscopic appearances of ureteric orifices are no longer considered particularly reliable clinical indicators of VUR (especially in low- to moderate-grade situations), these observations provide insight into the overall mechanism of competence of the UVJ (Figure 42.4).

Demographic features of vesicoureteral reflux

In most cases, VUR is discovered clinically after investigation of either UTI or antenatal hydronephrosis. In children without UTI or any other urologic problems, the true incidence of VUR is difficult to ascertain but may be in the order of 0.4–1.8% of the overall pediatric population.[26,27] In contrast, the incidence of VUR in children with UTI is typically around 30–50%, with an even higher incidence in infants.[28–30] Hydronephrosis is identified antenatally in about 1 of every 500–1200 live births, and VUR is identified in about 25% of these infants undergoing postnatal evaluation.[31,32] Infants with antenatally detected VUR show a male preponderance in contrast to older children who are diagnosed with VUR after presenting with UTI, in which females predominate. Boys tend to present at a younger age, and they tend to have more severe degrees of VUR, especially if diagnosed in infancy.[33] A transient urethral obstruction causing high intravesical pressures has been proposed to explain this phenomenon. Urodynamic studies of infants with VUR suggested that high voiding pressures and small functional capacity are more common in boys.[34]

VUR appears to be an heritable disorder. Identical twins have been observed to have a higher incidence of VUR.[35] It occurs in siblings of affected children at a significantly higher rate than that in the general population. The sibling VUR rate has been estimated to be as high as 40–50%.[36–38] Various studies suggest a dominant inheritance pattern with a variable penetrance. These include an approximately 50% incidence of sibling VUR in the first 2 years of life and a high incidence (about 60%) of parent-to-child transmission.[39] Evidence of genetic heterogeneity has been published, suggesting that different genes act on different families.[40] Furthermore, the incidence of VUR varies among races. Children of Asian and African ancestry have a lower rate of VUR than those of Caucasian genetic background (ratio of 3.4 to 1).[41,42]

Primary versus secondary vesicoureteral reflux

The distinction between primary and secondary VUR is important in the conceptualization of contributing pathophysiology and relevant anatomic/functional etiologies that need to be addressed clinically. In certain cases, the distinction is not entirely clear in that some forms of 'primary' VUR may be associated with bladder anomalies which contribute to the progression of the underlying UVJ malfunction. The clinical reality is that in all patients presenting with VUR, the proper management must include a global view of the entire urinary tract, including UVJ mechanism, bladder dysfunction, predisposition to UTI, and renal anomalies. A short intravesical ureter or a marginally competent ureter–trigone complex may increase the likelihood of VUR in unfavorable conditions such as bladder hypertonicity, high pressure voiding, and UTIs. On the other hand, an extremely competent UVJ may resist VUR even in cases of challenges by an abnormal bladder until there is an irreversible deformation of the UVJ structures.

The concept of 'secondary' VUR is critical in that understanding the dynamic process of reflux will be incomplete without considering the effect of the bladder. In a normal, mature urinary tract, increasing the intravesical pressure alone does not necessarily induce VUR. The clinical association of bladder abnormalities and VUR is well recognized. It is known that VUR can be acquired secondary to bladder anomalies such as neurogenic bladder disorders and various types of bladder outlet obstruction (as in boys with posterior urethral valves). Elevated voiding pressures may have a role in VUR pathophysiology, especially in infants. A higher incidence of high-grade VUR in infant males has been attributed to high voiding pressures caused by transient urethral obstruction, especially when intravesical ureteral tunnels are not fully mature. The chronic elevation of bladder storage pressure and the subsequent distortion of the bladder wall at the UVJ (such as paraureteral diverticulum) may be critical in the formation of secondary VUR. The structural and neurologic perturbation of the trigone in the abnormal bladder is likely to be important as well.

The most common anatomic cause of secondary VUR is seen in boys with posterior urethral valves, which are associated with VUR in over 50% of patients.[43] Anatomic obstructions causing VUR in girls are rare and may occur in the setting of an obstructing ureterocele. Any child with an altered bladder function is at risk for secondary VUR. A poorly compliant bladder, along with its abnormal interaction with dyssynergic urinary sphincters, can lead to increased intravesical pressures, which then weakens and alters the UVJ to cause VUR. A strong correlation was established by McGuire that if the bladder pressures exceed 40 cmH_2O, the incidence of VUR is seen in over 80% of patients with myelodysplasia and neurogenic bladders.[44,45]

Role of urinary tract infection in vesicoureteral reflux

Tanagho and colleagues proposed that lower urinary tract inflammation might affect the mildly deficient UVJ and induce VUR.[18] New VUR was reportedly acquired in 6 out of 7 experimental piglets after *Escherichia coli* infection and bladder inflammation.[46] Some *E. coli* strains have been implicated as affecting the activity of urinary tract smooth muscle directly, rather than via an inflammatory reaction. Bacterial endotoxin was found to inhibit α-adrenergic receptors of trigonal musculature in cats.[47] Similarly, UTI may cause human ureteral dilatation.[48,49] Such a direct effect of bacterial infection on ureteral smooth muscle function could conceivably induce ureter–trigonal dysfunction, thereby facilitating VUR. Since UTI is also known to induce bladder hypercontractility and lower compliance, a combined challenge of both ureter and bladder muscle dysfunction by UTI may well cause VUR in patients with marginally competent UVJ.

Clinically, it had been suggested that VCUG performed at the time of ongoing UTI might 'falsely' demonstrate VUR, which was not present when the urine was sterile. Gross and Lebowitz surveyed over 600 children undergoing cystographic evaluation for VUR and found no evidence of increased VUR in the setting of positive urine cultures.[50] In other words, their data did not support the notion that VUR was caused by UTI.

Role of lower urinary tract function in vesicoureteral reflux

In infants and children, abnormal lower urinary tract function often coexists with VUR without any apparent neurogenic or anatomic pathology. These observations suggest a possible role for lower urinary tract function in the pathogenesis of VUR and its implication in the clinical management of VUR.

Infantile bladder has been shown to have a higher voiding pressure. Urodynamic studies have shown that this may be the result of imperfect coordination between detrusor contraction and sphincter relaxation.[51,52] This pattern of immaturity typically disappears after 2 years, and is thought to result from lack of integration between the bladder, the external urethral sphincter, the brainstem, and the higher cortical centers. Compared with normal infants, those with VUR have even higher voiding pressure and abnormal bladder function, even in the absence of UTI.[51] A discoordinated pattern of voiding was the most common urodynamic abnormality in both male and female infants with VUR. Another urodynamic abnormality – abnormally high voiding pressure with small functional bladder capacity or poor bladder contractility with inadequate emptying – was seen primarily in boys. Other clinicians have also noted an increased incidence of bladder 'hypercontractility' in infant boys with VUR.[53] In a fetal sheep model of VUR, defunctionalization of UVJ (surgical unroofing of the submucosal ureter) was insufficient to produce VUR reliably in females, who also required a partial ligation of the urethra in order to reproduce a similar degree of VUR as seen in males with UVJ unroofing only.[54] Such experimental observation, along with VUR-associated urodynamic abnormality analogous to that seen in boys with posterior urethral valves, led to speculation that transient urethral obstruction may be the cause of infantile VUR in some cases.

The abnormal urodynamics seen in infants with VUR may also imply a global maldevelopment of the trigone and proximal urethral mechanism, which need to funnel open in coordination with detrusor contraction in order to induce efficient, low-pressure emptying. Godley and colleagues studied the clinical outcome of infants with VUR in relation to overall renal status and bladder function and found that those infants with abnormal kidneys were more likely to have abnormal bladder function as well as failure of VUR resolution.[55] These observations further support the notion that the entire spectrum of VUR disorder – reflux, renal anomaly, and bladder dysfunction – may result from the primary maldevelopment of the ureter–trigonal complex.[17,22]

Symptoms of pediatric voiding dysfunction – frequency, urgency, and enuresis – are a manifestation of detrusor instability (DI) and/or detrusor–sphincter dyssynergia (DSD), and they are often found in patients with UTI and VUR. A study of over 360 children with dysfunctional voiding found that 60% of children had UTI and 20% had VUR.[56] The European branch of the International Reflux Study found the presence of dysfunctional voiding in 18% of over 300 children with VUR and UTI.[57] Urodynamic investigation showed that detrusor instability may be found in up to 60% of children with VUR.[58,59] Despite these well-documented associations, it is unlikely that VUR is directly initiated by DI in most cases. Many more children have DI than VUR. There are also reports showing no statistical causal association between DI and VUR.[60] However, in patients with marginally competent UVJ, DI may exaggerate the VUR. It is generally accepted that unrecognized DI can delay the resolution of VUR, and there are reports that the treatment of DI with anticholinergics can facilitate VUR resolution.[58,61] Some studies, however, have not shown any beneficial effect of anticholinergic therapy in the elimination of VUR.[62] Although DI may not induce VUR directly, it plays an important role in the overall pathophysiology of the VUR–UTI–nephropathy complex. The presence and severity of dysfunctional voiding symptoms correlated significantly with the persistence of VUR during medical management and further correlated with UTI recurrence regardless of surgical correction of VUR.[57] In fact, the mutual association of DI and VUR to UTI may explain its clinical coexistence in many clinical scenarios. Whether the combined challenge of UTI and abnormal bladder dynamics leads to the secondary (or acquired) VUR or merely discloses pre-existent primary VUR, it is clear that they are critical cofactors to contend with in the overall management of patients with VUR.

Concluding remarks

Although VUR remains a significant and commonly encountered clinical problem in pediatric urology, it may be a normal transitory phenomenon in many species and in some humans. It is a dynamic process that involves an anatomic and functional anomaly and maldevelopment of the ureter–trigone complex and the UVJ, as well as the effects of UTI and lower urinary tract dysfunction. The clinical significance of VUR must be interpreted in the context of global urinary tract anomalies, including bladder dysfunction, inherent predisposition to UTI, and congenital/acquired reflux nephropathy.

References

1. Lines D. 15th century ureteric reflux. Lancet 1982; 2:1473.
2. Polk HC Jr. Notes on Galenic urology. Urol Surv 1965; 15:2–6.
3. Pozzi S. Ureteroverletzung bei Laparotomie. Zentrlbl Gynacol 1893; 17:97.
4. Bumpus HCJ. Urinary reflux. J Urol 1924; 12:341–6.
5. Campbell MF. Cystography in infancy and childhood. Am J Dis Child 1930; 39:386–402.
6. Prather GC. Vesicoureteral reflux: report of a case cured by operation. J Urol 1944; 52:437–47.
7. Hutch JA, Miller ER, Hinman F Jr. Vesicoureteral reflux. Role in pyelonephritis. Am J Med 1963; 34:338–49.
8. Hodson CJ, Edwards D. Chronic pyelonephritis and vesico-ureteric reflex. Clin Radiol 1960; 11:219–31.
9. Hodson CJ. The radiology of chronic pyelonephritis. Postgrad Med J 1965; 41:477–80.
10. Politano VA. Vesicoureteral reflux. In: Glenn JF, ed. Urologic Surgery, 2nd edn. New York: Harper & Row, 1975: 272–93.
11. Bell C. Account of the muscles of the ureter, and their effects in the irritable states of the bladder. Med Chir Trans 1812; 3:171–90.
12. Tanagho EA, Pugh RCB. The anatomy and function of the ureterovesical junction. Br J Urol 1963; 35:151–65.
13. Mathisen W. Vesicoureteral reflux and its surgical correction. Surg Gynecol Obstet 1964; 118:965–71.
14. Elbadawi A. Anatomy and function of ureteral sheath. J Urol 1972; 107:224–9.
15. Stephens FD. The vesicoureteral hiatus and paraureteral diverticula. J Urol 1979; 121:786–91.
16. Gearhart JP, Canning DA, Gilpin SA, Lam EE, Gosling JA. Histological and histochemical study of the vesicoureteric junction in infancy and childhood. Br J Urol 1993; 72:648–54.
17. Batourina E, Choi C, Paragas N et al. Distal ureter morphogenesis depends on epithelial cell remodeling mediated by vitamin A and Ret. [erratum appears in Nat Genet 2002; 32(2):331]. Nat Genet 2002; 32:109–15.
18. Tanagho EA, Hutch JA, Meyers FH, Rambo ON Jr. Primary vesicoureteral reflux: experimental studies of its etiology. J Urol 1965; 93:165–76.
19. Paquin AJJ. Ureterovesical anastomosis: the description and evaluation of a technique. J Urol 1959; 82:573–83.
20. Cussen LJ. Dimensions of the normal ureter in infancy and childhood. Invest Urol 1967; 5:164–78.
21. Glassberg KI, Hackett RE, Waterhouse K. Congenital anomalies of the kidney, ureter, and bladder. In: Kendall AR, Karafin L, Goldsmith HS, eds. Urology, Volume 1. Philadelphia: Harper & Row, 1987.
22. Mackie GG, Stephens FD. Duplex kidneys: a correlation of renal dysplasia with position of the ureteral orifice. J Urol 1975; 114:274–80.
23. Lyon RP, Marshall S, Tanagho EA. The ureteral orifice: its configuration and competency. J Urol 1969; 102:504–9.
24. Heale WF. Age of presentation and pathogenesis of reflux nephropathy. In: Hodson CJ, Kincaid-Smith P, eds. Reflux Nephropathy. New York: Masson, 1979: 140–6.
25. Stephens FD. Ureteric configurations and cystoscopy schema. Soc Pediatr Urol Newslett 1980; Jan 23:2.
26. Ransley PG. Vesicoureteric reflux: continuing surgical dilemma. Urology 1978; 12:246–55.
27. Bailey RR. Vesicoureteral reflux in healthy infants and children. In: Hodson CJ, Kincaid-Smith P, eds. Reflux Nephropathy. New York: Masson, 1979: 59–61.
28. Smellie JM, Normand IC. Clinical features and significance of urinary tract infection in children. Proc R Soc Med 1966; 59:415–16.
29. Savage DC, Wilson MI, McHardy M, Dewar DA, Fee WM. Covert bacteriuria of childhood. A clinical and epidemiological study. Arch Dis Child 1973; 48:8–20.
30. Wein AJ, Schoenberg HW. A review of 402 girls with recurrent urinary tract infection. J Urol 1972; 107:329–31.
31. Burge DM, Griffiths MD, Malone PS, Atwell JD. Fetal vesicoureteral reflux: outcome following conservative postnatal management. J Urol 1992; 148:1743–5.
32. Zerin JM, Ritchey ML, Chang AC. Incidental vesicoureteral reflux in neonates with antenatally detected hydronephrosis and other renal abnormalities. Radiology 1993; 187:157–60.
33. Yeung CK, Godley ML, Dhillon HK et al. The characteristics of primary vesico-ureteric reflux in male and female infants with pre-natal hydronephrosis. Br J Urol 1997; 80:319–27.
34. Sillen U, Hellstrom AL, Hermanson G, Abrahamson K. Comparison of urodynamic and free voiding pattern in infants with dilating reflux. J Urol 1999; 161:1928–33.

35. Kaefer M, Curran M, Treves ST et al. Sibling vesicoureteral reflux in multiple gestation births. Pediatrics 2000; 105:800–4.
36. Kenda RB, Fettich JJ. Vesicoureteric reflux and renal scars in asymptomatic siblings of children with reflux. Arch Dis Child 1992; 67:506–8.
37. Jerkins GR, Noe HN. Familial vesicoureteral reflux: a prospective study. J Urol 1982; 128:774–8.
38. Wan J, Greenfield SP, Ng M et al. Sibling reflux: a dual center retrospective study. J Urol 1996; 156:677–9.
39. Noe HN, Wyatt RJ, Peeden JN Jr, Rivas ML. The transmission of vesicoureteral reflux from parent to child. J Urol 1992; 148:1869–71.
40. Feather SA, Malcolm S, Woolf AS et al. Primary, nonsyndromic vesicoureteric reflux and its nephropathy is genetically heterogeneous, with a locus on chromosome 1. Am J Human Genet 2000; 66:1420–5.
41. Arant BS Jr. Medical management of mild and moderate vesicoureteral reflux: followup studies of infants and young children. A preliminary report of the Southwest Pediatric Nephrology Study Group. J Urol 1992; 148:1683–7.
42. Askari A, Belman AB. Vesicoureteral reflux in black girls. J Urol 1982; 127:747–8.
43. Hassan JM, Pope JC 4th, Brock JW 3rd, Adams MC. Vesicoureteral reflux in patients with posterior urethral valves. J Urol 2003; 170:1677–80, discussion 1680.
44. Flood HD, Ritchey ML, Bloom DA, Huang C, McGuire EJ. Outcome of reflux in children with myelodysplasia managed by bladder pressure monitoring. J Urol 1994; 152:1574–7.
45. McGuire EJ, Woodside JR, Borden TA, Weiss RM. Prognostic value of urodynamic testing in myelodysplastic patients. J Urol 1981; 126:205–9.
46. Arnold AJ, Sunderland D, Hart CA, Rickwood AM. Reconsideration of the roles of urinary infection and vesicoureteric reflux in the pathogenesis of renal scarring. Br J Urol 1993; 72:554–6.
47. Nergardh A, Boreus LO, Holme T. The inhibitory effect of coli-endotoxin on alpha-adrenergic receptor functions in the lower urinary tract. An in vitro study in cats. Scand J Urol Nephrol 1977; 11:219–24.
48. Marild S, Hellstrom M, Jacobsson B, Jodal U, Svanborg Eden C. Influence of bacterial adhesion on ureteral width in children with acute pyelonephritis. J Pediatr 1989; 115:265–8.
49. Hellstrom M, Jodal U, Marild S, Wettergren B. Ureteral dilatation in children with febrile urinary tract infection or bacteriuria. AJR Am J Roentgenol 1987; 148:483–6.
50. Gross GW, Lebowitz RL. Infection does not cause reflux. AJR Am J Roentgenol 1981; 137:929–32.
51. Yeung CK, Godley ML, Dhillon HK, Duffy PG, Ransley PG. Urodynamic patterns in infants with normal lower urinary tracts or primary vesico-ureteric reflux. Br J Urol 1998; 81:461–7.
52. Bachelard M, Sillen U, Hansson S et al. Urodynamic pattern in asymptomatic infants: siblings of children with vesicoureteral reflux. J Urol 1999; 162:1733–7.
53. Sillen U. Vesicoureteral reflux in infants. Pediatr Nephrol 1999; 13:355–61.
54. Gobet R, Cisek LJ, Zotti P, Peters CA. Experimental vesicoureteral reflux in the fetus depends on bladder function and causes renal fibrosis. J Urol 1998; 160:1058–62.
55. Godley ML, Desai D, Yeung CK et al. The relationship between early renal status, and the resolution of vesicoureteric reflux and bladder function at 16 months. BJU Int 2001; 87:457–62.
56. Schulman SL, Quinn CK, Plachter N, Kodman-Jones C. Comprehensive management of dysfunctional voiding. Pediatrics 1999; 103:E31.
57. van Gool JD, Hjalmas K, Tamminen-Mobius T, Olbing H. Historical clues to the complex of dysfunctional voiding, urinary tract infection and vesicoureteral reflux. The International Reflux Study in Children. J Urol 1992; 148:1699–702.
58. Scholtmeijer RJ, Nijman RJ. Vesicoureteric reflux and videourodynamic studies: results of a prospective study after three years of follow-up. Urology 1994; 43:714–18.
59. Nielsen JB. Lower urinary tract function in vesicoureteral reflux. Scand J Urol Nephrol Suppl 1989; 125:15–21.
60. Griffiths DJ, Scholtmeijer RJ. Vesicoureteral reflux and lower urinary tract dysfunction: evidence for 2 different reflux/dysfunction complexes. J Urol 1987; 137:240–4.
61. Koff SA, Murtagh D. The uninhibited bladder in children: effect of treatment on vesicoureteral reflux resolution. Contrib Nephrol 1984; 39:211–20.
62. Taylor CM, Corkery JJ, White RH. Micturition symptoms and unstable bladder activity in girls with primary vesicoureteric reflux. Br J Urol 1982; 54:494–8.

Non-surgical management of vesicoureteral reflux

43

Jack S Elder

In a child with vesicoureteral reflux (VUR), the primary goal of therapy is to prevent pyelonephritis, because repeated upper urinary tract infection (UTI) can lead to renal scarring, hypertension, reduced somatic growth, renal insufficiency, and end-stage renal disease. In addition, reflux-related complications during pregnancy may occur. If a child already has reduced renal function, then additional treatment may be necessary to preserve existing renal function as the child grows.

Non-surgical therapy is based on the principle that reflux often resolves over time, and that sterile reflux is not harmful to the kidneys and has no significant effect on renal function. In addition, the morbidity or complications of reflux can be prevented by preventing infection. In contrast, the principle of surgical therapy is that the complications of reflux and non-surgical therapy can be prevented with surgical correction of reflux. The benefits and risks of these two approaches must be considered when deciding on a course of therapy.

Non-surgical therapy consists of:

1 Antibiotic prophylaxis:
   - daily
   - intermittent (i.e. treatment of UTIs as they are diagnosed).
2 Bladder training.
3 Treatment of voiding dysfunction:
   - anticholinergic
   - α-blocker
   - treatment of constipation
   - biofeedback.
4 Periodic assessment of reflux and child well-being:
   - serial urinalysis/urine culture
   - serial voiding cystourethrogram (VCUG) or radionuclide cystogram
   - serial upper urinary tract studies
   - serial assessment of blood pressure and renal function.

The approach to each child is individualized and takes into account the child's gender, reflux grade, age, presentation (UTI, sibling screening, antenatal diagnosis), renal status at the beginning of therapy, compliance with treatment, likelihood of reflux resolution, as well as parent and child preferences.

Reflux resolution

The decision to choose non-surgical management in a child with reflux is based on the fact that reflux often resolves, and when it resolves, the risk of upper tract infection is less. The reason that reflux resolves spontaneously is uncertain. Presumably it occurs with bladder growth and with bladder functional maturation. Whether the intramural tunnel length increases is unproved.

There are several difficulties in analyzing reported rates of reflux resolution:

1 The reflux grading scale has been modified over time and has increased from three to five different grades.
2 Some series only report ureteral resolution, whereas others only report patient resolution, which is more relevant.
3 Some centers utilize radionuclide cystography for grading rather than contrast VCUG.
4 Some series combine children with single and duplicated collecting systems, although reflux in the latter may be less likely to resolve spontaneously.
5 Reflux may be intermittent, and show resolution, only to reappear if a VCUG is repeated 1 year later.[1]
6 Follow-up among various case series has been variable, and a significant number are lost to follow-up.

The best data on reflux resolution come from the few randomized prospective trials and a few retrospective

Table 43.1 Reflux resolution of children, by grade

Series	No. of patients	Grade I (%)	Grade II (%)	Grade III (%)	Grade IV (%)
Bellinger and Duckett, 1984[10]	269[a]	87	63	53	33
Goldraich and Goldraich, 1992[2]	202	80(I/II)		50(III/IV)	
Huang et al, 1995[11]	214	92	76	62	32
Greenfield et al, 1997[12]	601	69	56	49	
Smellie et al, 2001[6]	149			73[b]	44[b]
Schwab et al, 2002[13]	214	83	77	68	36

[a] Renal units, not patients.
[b] 10-year data: results disparate for unilateral vs bilateral reflux.

case series from centers with a commitment to nonsurgical management.[1–9]

It is impossible to predict whether a specific child will show spontaneous reflux resolution. In the past, cystoscopy was performed at some centers to try to measure ureteral tunnel length, but in most children cystoscopic findings failed to correlate with likelihood of resolution. The exception, however, was that if the ureteral orifice was patulous or hydrodistended significantly, resolution was uncommon.[10]

Reflux resolution is most likely in younger children and those with lower reflux grades (Table 43.1). The American Urological Association (AUA) Vesicoureteral Reflux Practice Guidelines Committee analyzed the raw data from the series published by Skoog et al,[3] Arant,[1] and the International Reflux Study, European Arm[4] to develop the curves in Figure 43.1.[14,15] In their analysis, at 5 years, approximately 92% with grade I and 81% with grade II showed reflux resolution, irrespective of age at presentation or whether the reflux was unilateral or bilateral. In contrast, in grade III, resolution was highest for unilateral grade III reflux in children <2 years (70%) and lowest for children with bilateral grade III reflux >5 years at diagnosis (12.5%). The data for grade III reflux in children >5 years at diagnosis were based on 27 children. In the series by Greenfield et al, for children with grade III reflux, resolution was similar irrespective of age at presentation.[12] In the combined series, unilateral grade IV reflux resolved in 58% at 5 years, whereas only 10% of those with bilateral grade IV reflux resolved. For grade IV reflux, age was not stratified because of small patient numbers.

Beyond 5 years, few data are available. Reflux can resolve during adolescence, but there are no predictable features. For example, in the series by Lenaghan, reflux resolution was reported in 20%, but their patients were not studied systematically.[16] In a long-term follow-up of the International Reflux Study, at 10 years following study entry, in the children randomized to medical therapy, 73% of those with unilateral grade III or IV reflux had resolved.[6] In

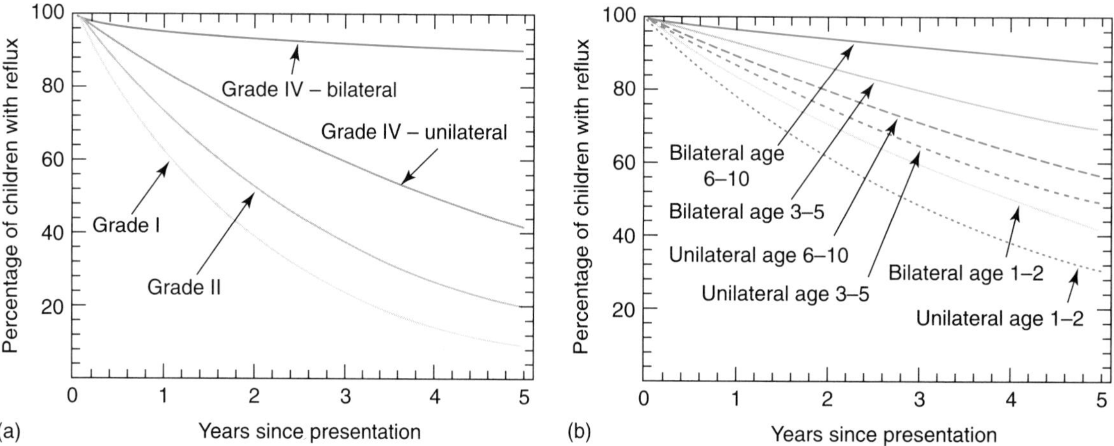

Figure 43.1 Likelihood of spontaneous reflux resolution. The percent chance of reflux persistence for 1–5 years following presentation.[10,12,15] A, grades I, II and IV reflux. B, grade III reflux by patient age at presentation. (Reproduced from Elder.[14])

children with grade III/IV reflux on one side and grade I/II on the other, 49% had resolved, and in those who presented with bilateral grade III/IV reflux, only 39% resolved.

Antibiotic prophylaxis

The cornerstone of UTI prevention is daily antimicrobial prophylaxis. The basis for prophylaxis is that, in the 1960s and 1970s, children with reflux were managed by treating each UTI as it occurred. Lenaghan et al reported that in children with pre-existing scars, 66% developed new scars, and in children who had normal kidneys, 21% developed new scars.[16] The average age of boys was 1 year and of girls was 7 years. Most new scars were observed in girls. Lenaghan concluded that intermittent therapy of UTI was associated with an unacceptably high rate of new scar formation in children with reflux. Govan et al reported that 50% of girls with reflux had a UTI during the observation period and 20% had febrile UTI.[17] Scarring was most likely to occur in those with dilating reflux, but 23% with grade I reflux developed new scarring. In a non-randomized study, O'Donnell et al found that 35% of refluxing children followed without prophylaxis developed new scars, compared with 9% who were placed on prophylaxis.[18] From these studies, it was concluded that girls with reflux were more likely to develop renal scars than boys, that scars could occur at any age, children with mild reflux were susceptible to scar formation, and that scarring could occur in normal kidneys.

In contrast, there is a generous body of literature supporting the effectiveness of continuous prophylaxis. In a prospective evaluation of 203 children with all grades of reflux, Goldraich and Goldraich found that only 3% developed new scars, and these were associated with UTI.[2] None of the new scars occurred in children over 4 years. Consequently, they recommended discontinuing prophylaxis after age 5 years. In contrast, in a prospective multicenter trial of children <5 years of age with grades I, II, or III reflux, Arant found that 34% developed a breakthrough UTI and 8% developed new scars.[1] In this series, compliance with the antibiotic regimen was highly variable, ranging from 12% to 75%. Skoog et al retrospectively evalutated 545 children with grades I through IV reflux from 6 months to 10 years on continuous prophylaxis.[3] Overall, only three children (0.5%) developed a new scar and two of the three children had a documented breakthrough UTI.

Although there is general agreement that antibiotic prophylaxis is effective in preventing UTI in children with reflux,[19] the ideal antimicrobial for prophylaxis is uncertain. Typical medications include nitrofurantoin, trimethoprim–sulfamethoxazole, and trimethroprim alone. Generally a dosage that is one-quarter to one-half of the full dose is prescribed and administration at bedtime theoretically yields the optimal benefit. Potential adverse effects of nitrofurantoin suspension include gastric upset, nausea, and a very poor taste to the medication. Use of nitrofurantoin macrocrystals in a capsule can obviate these problems. In young children the capsule may be opened and the macrocrystals can be mixed with food or formula. More serious side effects are rare, with one study documenting only 40 reports out of 8.6 million uses.[20] Trimethoprim–sulfamethoxazole is generally well tolerated, although Uhari et al reported that the medication was changed because of adverse effects in 15% of children receiving sulfonamides and 8% receiving trimethoprim.[21] The most common adverse effect is allergic skin reaction, usually from the sulfa component. This problem may occur following several weeks or months of therapy, but anaphylaxis is rare. Although neutropenia, thrombocytopenia, and/or eosinophilia occur in 12–34% of children receiving full-dose trimethoprim–sulfamethoxazole for only 10 days,[22] the incidence of these side effects in children receiving prophylactic dosages for as long as 1 year is quite low.[23] Photosensitivity is another concern with sulfa-based antimicrobials. Another potential problem is dental caries secondary to the fructose in the liquid preparation, but this problem can be prevented by having the children brush their teeth after taking the drug. The most serious potential side effect is Stevens–Johnson syndrome, but this reaction is extremely rare.

In babies up to 2 months of age, amoxicillin or cephalexin (50–75 mg once or twice daily) should be prescribed instead of a sulfa-based antibiotic, because of potential hepatic toxicity. Nitrofurantoin is also contraindicated in infants <2 months old.

Some have questioned whether antibiotic prophylaxis is necessary. Garin et al recently performed a randomized prospective trial comparing prophylaxis with no prophylaxis in children with vesicoureteral reflux diagnosed following pyelonephritis.[24] The study showed no clinical advantage to administering prophylaxis. However, there were only 45 patients in each treatment group, making it impossible to develop sufficient study power. In addition, patients were only studied for one year. The National Institutes of Health has sponsored a new protocol comparing the outcomes in children with and without prophylaxis in Cleveland. Children 6 months to 6 years with grades I through IV will be studied; half will be assigned to antibiotic prophylaxis and half to no prophylaxis.

Breakthrough urinary tract infection

In girls who are receiving antibiotic prophylaxis for recurrent UTI, those with reflux and those with voiding dysfunction are most likely to develop a breakthrough UTI.[25] In boys with reflux, those who are uncircumcised are most likely to develop a breakthrough UTI.[26] In both sexes, children with scarring on a dimercaptosuccinic acid (DMSA) scan are at greatest risk for breakthrough UTI. If the child has a febrile UTI, consideration should be given to obtaining a DMSA renal scan to determine whether there is acute pyelonephritis, which was found in 17% of refluxing children.[27] Children with acute pyelonephritis are at risk of developing new renal scarring, and prompt treatment of these children is necessary.

A breakthrough UTI is an indication of failure of non-surgical management, and surgical therapy should be considered, particularly if the UTI was febrile. In children with a breakthrough UTI with symptoms of cystitis, an alternative is to prescribe an antibiotic to which the breakthrough organism is sensitive, or to use 'double prophylaxis', in which both trimethoprim–sulfamethoxazole and nitrofurantoin are administered daily.[24]

Discontinuing antibiotic prophylaxis (expectant management)

UTI in girls occurs most commonly in those between birth and 5 years and in adulthood. In uncircumcised boys the risk of UTI is greatest in those up to 6 months of age[28] and then it drops off considerably, corresponding to the time of spontaneous retraction of the prepuce. Thereafter, the risk of UTI in uncircumcised boys is slightly higher than in circumcised boys. The risk of UTI in circumcised boys with reflux has not been studied systematically but appears to be lower than in uncircumcised boys.[25]

In selected patients it seems reasonable to discontinue prophylaxis. Cooper et al retrospectively evaluated 51 children, selected from their practice over a period of 14 years, with grades I–IV VUR in whom prophylaxis had been discontinued.[29] All children had a normal voiding pattern and began expectant management at a mean age of 8.6 years. All had an annual renal sonogram and a biannual radionuclide cystogram. These children were followed for a mean of 3.7 years. A UTI occurred in 5/40 girls and 1/11 boys. All of the UTIs in the girls were febrile, and these children underwent ureteral reimplantation. All of the children with UTI had grade III VUR at presentation and four of the six who developed a UTI still had bilateral VUR when the prophylaxis was discontinued. The reflux resolution rate was 20%, and no children developed evidence of new renal scarring on follow-up sonography or underwent DMSA renal scintigraphy. In a similar study, Al Sayyad et al retrospectively reviewed 78 children with VUR (94% grade I or II), in whom prophylaxis was discontinued.[30] All had a normal voiding pattern. The mean age at discontinuation of prophylaxis was 5.7 years. Of the 67 girls, nine developed a UTI, but only one had a febrile UTI. All had a normal renal sonogram on follow-up. Taken together, these two studies suggest that prophylaxis may be unnecessary in some children with VUR, if their voiding pattern is normal. In addition, boys with VUR seem to be at significantly lower risk for febrile UTI, particularly those with lower grades of VUR. It is unresolved whether children with VUR who were detected by sibling screening or screening following detection of a multicystic kidney or renal agenesis have a lower risk of reflux-related complications than children who were diagnosed with reflux following a UTI.

Although antibiotic prophylaxis may be unnecessary in the short term, female patients and their families should understand that if there is ongoing VUR into adulthood, then these women may be at increased risk of clinical pyelonephritis, particularly in association with pregnancy and onset of sexual activity. For example, Smellie et al studied 226 adults with a history of UTI and VUR as children.[5] Of the group, 23% had VUR at most recent follow-up. Overall, 39% of the adults without VUR had UTI in adulthood, compared with 38% of adults who still had VUR. No new scars were observed after age 4 years. However, clinical pyelonephritis occurred in 8/168 (5%) of those without reflux compared with 9/53 (17%) of those who were still refluxing. In a similar study, Martinell et al reported on 107 girls with clinical pyelonephritis at a mean age of 7.1 years and followed for 13–38 years.[31] Using excretory urography, 18 girls developed new scars in previously normal kidneys, and 28 kidneys with scarring developed progressive scarring. The highest risk factors for new or progressive scarring were UTI and clinical pyelonephritis. VUR can be discovered in adult women with a febrile UTI. Kohler

Table 43.2 Disfunctional voiding scoring system

Date:
Patient Name:
Hospital Number:
Reason for Referral:

Over the last month	Almost never	Less than half the time	About half the time	Almost every time	Not available
1 I have had wet clothes or wet underwear during the day	0	1	2	3	NA
2 When I wet myself, my underwear is soaked	0	1	2	3	NA
3 I miss having a bowel movement every day	0	1	2	3	NA
4 I have to push for my bowel movements to come out	0	1	2	3	NA
5 I only go to the bathroom one or two times each day	0	1	2	3	NA
6 I can hold onto my pee by crossing my legs, squatting, or doing the 'pee dance'	0	1	2	3	NA
7 When I have to pee, I cannot wait					
8 I have to push to pee	0	1	2	3	NA
9 When I pee it hurts	0	1	2	3	NA
10 Parents to answer. Has your child experienced something stressful like the example below?		No (0)		Yes (3)	
Total					

Reproduced from Farhat et al,[40] with permission.

reported on 115 adult women with VUR discovered after 16 years of age;[32] 73% of the refluxing kidneys had evidence of reflux nephropathy, even though the reflux grade was I or II in most cases. This group has also reported that adult women with a history of clinical pyelonephritis and VUR who underwent surgical reflux correction had significantly fewer febrile UTIs than those women who had persistent VUR.[33] Several other studies have demonstrated that women with VUR have a higher risk of febrile UTI compared with those without VUR.[34–36] In most of these cases the reflux grade was low. Taken together, these studies suggest that if there is persistent VUR in a female child, open surgical or endoscopic correction should be considered, even though the child may be doing well on expectant management.

Bladder training

Bladder training refers to regular, volitional, complete emptying of the bladder through behavioral conditioning to achieve balanced, low-pressure voiding with coordinated relaxation of the external sphincter and pelvic floor during voiding. The goal of bladder training is to reduce the likelihood of developing UTI and reduce voiding pressure. Infrequent voiding, detrusor–sphincter dyssynergia, and constipation can increase the likelihood of bacteriuria.[24] Measures include a voiding schedule every 2–3 hours, complete bladder emptying during micturition, re-education in proper voiding dynamics if voiding dysfunction is present, and elimination of constipation. The practice also includes genital and perineal hygiene. Although these recommendations are practical, no firm evidence exists that a specific regimen is beneficial.

Voiding dysfunction

Voiding dysfunction refers to disturbances in normal bladder or bowel function. Many children with VUR and UTI have elements of voiding dysfunction.[37–39] The spinning top deformity of the urethra seen on the voiding film of the VCUG in some girls, and a similar appearance of a dilated prostatic urethra in boys (although the latter could be secondary to posterior urethral valves), may be suggestive signs of voiding dysfunction. Typically, some degree of bladder trabeculation is observed in these children also. 'Dysfunctional elimination' refers to children who have constipation as well as infrequent voiding or difficulty with overactive bladder contractions. Children with VUR and dysfunctional elimination have a higher rate of breakthrough UTI compared with those without dysfunctional elimination.[39,40] For example, Snodgrass reported 128 children with VUR identified prospectively who answered a questionnaire pertaining to voiding dysfunction.[38] Of the girls, 43% with voiding dysfunction had breakthrough UTI compared with 11% with a normal voiding pattern. Similarly, Koff et al retrospectively studied 143 children with VUR who were old enough to be toilet trained.[39] Breakthrough UTIs were four times more common in children with dysfunctional elimination, and there was a longer time to spontaneous resolution of VUR in affected children. Furthermore, unsuccessful surgical outcomes were observed only in children with voiding dysfunction.

To help assess whether voiding dysfunction is present, Farhat et al reported a validated Dysfunctional Voiding Scoring System (DVSS), which consisted of 10 questions pertaining to urinary and bowel habits (Table 43.2).[40] Subsequently, this group applied the DVSS to children with reflux in a retrospective study. In children with a high symptom score managed with behavioral modification, those with a significant reduction in symptom score were most likely to show reflux resolution or improvement, whereas those with only a minor reduction in symptom score tended to have persistent reflux.[41] Prospective trials of this type of scoring system are necessary.

Anticholinergic therapy

Children with an overactive bladder typically have urgency, frequency, and/or urge incontinence. When girls with this condition sense a sudden bladder contraction, they often cross their legs or squat down on their foot to try to prevent incontinence. In these children, a combination of anticholinergic therapy and timed voiding may be beneficial.[42] The anticholinergic is administered according to the incontinence pattern of the specific child. Most children with an overactive bladder experience incontinence throughout the day and night, and these children should receive the medication so that the effect lasts for 24 hours. Other children may be incontinent only during the day, and these children do not need night-time medication. Typically, oxybutynin chloride 2.5–5 mg tid is prescribed. The medication is available as a tablet or suspension. Typical side effects include xerostomia (dry mouth), facial flushing, reduced sweating, constipation, and, less commonly, blurred vision and drowsiness. Side effects are dose related and may be eliminated with dose reduction. Other antimuscarinics include hyoscyamine, which is available as a sublingual tablet, 0.125–0.25 mg qid or as a capsule taken twice daily; tolterodine, 1–2 mg bid; and trospium, 10–25 mg daily in two doses.[43] These medications have the same potential for side effects as oxybutynin, but their incidence and severity are less. These medications are also available as long-acting tablets taken once daily or as a patch applied twice weekly, and these formulations may be more effective than the shorter-acting drugs.[44] Although these medications are not specifically approved for use in children, they are utilized in many centers, but their dosage and timing of administration need to be individualized and closely monitored. Other antimuscarinics being studied include darifenacin and solifenacin. On the other hand, a recent meta-analysis of the few randomized controlled trials of anticholinergic therapy in children found that there is no evidence that they are beneficial in the treatment of overactive bladder.[45] The beneficial effect attributed to anticholinergic medications may be due in part to a placebo effect.

Anticholinergic therapy may be a beneficial therapeutic modality in children with reflux and an overactive bladder, in that there is an increased likelihood of spontaneous reflux resolution in children treated with anticholinergics.[46,47]

α-blocker therapy

Some children with voiding dysfunction have pelvic floor overactivity and have significant postvoid residual urine volumes. These children may benefit from α-blocker therapy. In a prospective randomized double-blind trial of 38 children, Kramer et al found that doxazosin 0.5 mg resulted in a reduction in incontinence episodes, compared with no change in the placebo group.[48] The differences were not statistically significant, because of small patient numbers. There was significant subjective improvement, however, in the children receiving doxazosin. A larger trial is necessary to determine whether α-blocker therapy is beneficial.

Treatment of constipation

Dysfunctional elimination syndrome is a common component of children with UTIs and reflux.[39] Treatment of constipation is an important component of therapy. Numerous bowel regimens are available. Polyethylene glycol 3350 is a tasteless powder that can be mixed with any liquid and is useful as a single-agent laxative. In a retrospective study of 46 children with voiding dysfunction and constipation treated with this laxative, 39% became dry and 57% had improved urinary continence.[49] Voided volume increased significantly and postvoid residual urine volume decreased significantly.

Biofeedback

In children with dysfunctional voiding, typically there is inconsistent relaxation of the external sphincter during voiding. This pattern may occur because of repeated unstable bladder contractions that cause the child to tighten his or her sphincter, as opposed to a normal pattern in which the sphincter is relaxed during a detrusor contraction. Many of these children demonstrate a staccato voiding pattern on a uroflow study. Biofeedback may be useful, not only to establish a normal pattern of sphincteric relaxation during voiding but also to reduce or eliminate the need for anticholinergic medication for the overactive bladder. A typical treatment session might include a uroflow study, sonographic evaluation of postvoid residual urine volume, and a 1-hour session with perineal patch electrodes for electromyography (EMG). The child watches the sphincter activity on a television screen, and learns to contract and relax the external sphincter, which are essentially Kegel exercises. In addition to this simple office setup, video games have been developed that help the child coordinate sphincter tone.[50] An alternative is to simply teach the child pelvic floor exercises without using sophisticated urodynamic equipment.[51]

The concept of biofeedback is that children may have difficulty isolating their external sphincter, and biofeedback sessions allow them to learn sphincteric relaxation, which is necessary as a prerequisite to normal bladder emptying. In addition, these pelvic floor exercises may also ameliorate unstable bladder contractions. It is important that children perform these exercises daily, although no definite regimen is used. Several monthly sessions are necessary to reinforce the importance of the treatment, as well as determine whether voiding patterns are improving and whether residual urine volumes are decreasing. Subsequently, the sessions can be spaced further apart.

Most reports of biofeedback for the management of voiding dysfunction have been favorable.[50–55] Some treatments utilize biofeedback in children with symptoms of an overactive bladder that do not respond to anticholinergic therapy and timed voiding, whereas other treatments use it as an alternative to anticholinergic medication. However, it is uncertain how often anticholinergic therapy can be reduced or eliminated in children with an overactive bladder. Some centers have reported that the need for antireflux surgery was eliminated in many cases[50] and that the likelihood of reflux resolution was higher in children submitted to biofeedback.[56]

Follow-up assessment

Screening for urinary tract infection

In a child with VUR, periodic surveillance is generally recommended to monitor for UTI, because the complications of reflux often occur when infection is present. However, no guidelines exist for frequency of monitoring (e.g. monthly, every 3 months), or type of surveillance (urine dipstick, dipstick with microscopy, urine culture, or a combination).[14] Most children with a UTI are symptomatic, with fever and abdominal/flank pain for an upper tract infection, or they experience dysuria, urgency, frequency, and possibly incontinence and malodorous urine with a lower tract infection. There is no evidence that periodic screening of asymptomatic children with VUR for a UTI is beneficial. Consequently, if the child is suspected of having a UTI, a urine culture should be obtained. If the child has symptoms of upper tract infection, approximately 17% will have evidence of acute pyelonephritis on a DMSA renal scan.[27]

Follow-up cystography

In a child receiving medical therapy, follow-up cystography is generally performed every 12–18 months. Some prefer a radionuclide cystogram, because the radiation dose to the gonads is significantly less than with a standard contrast cystogram.[57] Unfavorable prognostic factors include demonstration of reflux at less than 60% of bladder capacity and reflux volume >2% of bladder capacity.[58,59] Demonstration of intermittent reflux is common. However, the assessment of reflux grade or severity is not entirely comparable with a contrast cystogram. With digital fluoroscopy equipment and a tailored contrast cystogram performed by a pediatric radiologist, the radiation exposure can be kept to a minimum.[60]

Non-compliance with follow-up visits is common; in one large study it was 33%.[61] Seeing the patient at least annually allows the clinician to reassess the child's voiding and bowel habits, dosage of medication, and status of the kidneys and reflux. One reason for non-compliance in children who are doing well on antibiotic prophylaxis is the trauma of the VCUG.[62,63] There are several other potential strategies to consider.

First, a children's hospital is more likely to provide the support services, such as Child Life, as well as radiologic personnel who recognize a child's special needs.[64] Zelikovsky et al found that coping skills training and parent coaching were beneficial.[65]

One option is to reduce the frequency of VCUG in children with reflux. In 1992, the AUA Vesicoureteral Practice Guidelines Committee reported a survey of various specialists in their practice patterns pertaining to reflux, and found that general urologists recommended performing a VCUG as often as every 6 months.[66] However, the likelihood that grade II reflux will resolve is only 18% per year, and for unilateral grade IV reflux the chance is only 8% per year. Thompson et al used the AUA Reflux Guidelines data for reflux resolution and proposed that a VCUG be performed every other year for children with mild reflux and every 3 years for children with moderate or severe reflux.[67] This practice would significantly reduce the number of VCUGs and medical costs of treatment. Whether long-term compliance would be maintained is questionable.

An alternative to the standard VCUG is to administer either oral or nasal midazolam in selected children undergoing a VCUG, because it provides anxiolysis and anterograde amnesia. The medication takes effect in 10–20 minutes, and no anesthesiologist or anesthetist is present. A registered nurse checks vital signs every 10–15 minutes. In this author's initial report, 60% remembered none of the study, whereas 31% remembered part or all of the procedure but did not have a negative experience.[68] No child had a change in vital signs or oxygen saturation. More recently, the benefit of midazolam before VCUG was demonstrated in prospective randomized trials.[69,70]

Several other options include the use of lidocaine jelly to lubricate the catheter,[71] the use of continuous-flow 50% nitrous oxide before catheterization,[72] and self-hypnosis.[73]

Upper tract imaging

Regular upper tract imaging with sonography or a DMSA renal scan allow the clinician to assess renal size and development of renal scarring. There are no standards regarding the timing of follow-up or type of imaging. However, if there has not been a symptomatic UTI, it is highly unlikely that a new scar will develop. In a retrospective study of 64 consecutive children with low- and medium-grade reflux and a normal renal sonogram, Lowe et al found that all 128 renal units remained normal in follow-up.[74] In contrast, with a febrile UTI, in a prospective trial, Szlyk et al reported that 17% had changes of acute pyelonephritis on a DMSA renal scan,[27] and these patients are those at risk for developing new renal scars.

Other assessment

The AUA Practice Guidelines Committee recommended that follow-up evaluation be performed at least annually, at which time the patient's height and weight should be recorded. If the child has renal scarring, the blood pressure should also be monitored.[14,15] There are no guidelines regarding measurement of renal function, but if there is significant reflux nephropathy, serum creatinine should be assessed regularly.

References

1. Arant BS Jr. Medical management of mild and moderate vesicoureteral reflux: followup studies of infants and young children. A preliminary report of the Southwest Pediatric Nephrology Study Group. J Urol 1992; 148:1683–7.
2. Goldraich NP, Goldraich IH. Followup of conservatively treated children with high and low grade vesicoureteral reflux: a prospective study. J Urol 1992; 148:1688–92.
3. Skoog SJ, Belman AB, Majd M. A nonsurgical approach to the management of primary vesicoureteral reflux. J Urol 1987; 138:941–6.
4. Smellie JM, Tamminen-Mobius T, Olbing H et al. Five-year study of medical or surgical treatment in children with severe reflux: radiological renal findings. The International Reflux Study in Children. Pediatr Nephrol 1992; 6:223–30.
5. Smellie JM, Prescod NP, Shaw PJ, Risdon RA, Bryant TN. Childhood reflux and urinary infection: a follow-up of 10–41 years in 226 adults. Pediatr Nephrol 1998; 12:727–36.
6. Smellie JM, Jodal U, Lax H et al. Outcome at 10 years of severe vesicoureteric reflux managed medically: report of the International Reflux Study in Children. J Pediatr 2001; 139:656–63.
7. Weiss R, Duckett J, Spitzer A. Results of a randomized clinical trial of medical versus surgical management of infants and children with grades III and IV primary vesicoureteral reflux (United States). The International Reflux Study in Children. J Urol 1992; 148:1667–73.
8. Prospective trial of operative versus non-operative treatment of severe vesicoureteric reflux in children: 5 years' observation. Birmingham Reflux Study Group. Br Med J (Clin Res Ed) 1987; 295:237–41.
9. Elo J, Tallgren LG, Alfthan O et al. Character of urinary

tract infections and pyelonephritic renal scarring after antireflux surgery. J Urol 1983; 129:343–6.
10. Bellinger MF, Duckett JW. Vesicoureteral reflux: a comparison of non-surgical and surgical management. Contrib Nephrol 1984; 39:81–93.
11. Huang FY, Tsai TC. Resolution of vesicoureteral reflux during medical management in children. Pediatr Nephrol 1995; 9:715–17.
12. Greenfield SP, Ng M, Wan J. Resolution rates of low grade vesicoureteral reflux stratified by patient age at presentation. J Urol 1997; 157:1410–13.
13. Schwab CW Jr, Wu HY, Selman H et al. Spontaneous resolution of vesicoureteral reflux: a 15-year perspective. J Urol 2002; 168:2594–9.
14. Elder JS, Peters CA, Arant BS Jr et al. Pediatric Vesicoureteral Reflux Guidelines Panel summary report on the management of primary vesicoureteral reflux in children. J Urol 1997; 157:1846–51.
15. American Urological Association Pediatric Vesicoureteral Reflux Clinical Guidelines Panel. Report on The Management of Primary Vesicoureteral Reflux in Children. Baltimore: American Urological Association, Inc., 1997.
16. Lenaghan D, Whitaker JG, Jensen F et al. The natural history of reflux and long-term effects of reflux on the kidney. J Urol 1976; 115:728–30.
17. Govan DE, Fair WR, Friedland GW, Filly RA. Urinary tract infections in children. Part III – Treatment of ureterovesical reflux. West J Med 1974; 121:382–9.
18. O'Donnell B, Moloney MA, Lynch V. Vesico-ureteric reflux in infants and children: results of 'supervision', chemotherapy and surgery. Br J Urol 1969; 41:6–13.
19. Williams JG, Lee A, Craig JC. Long-term antibiotics for preventing recurrent urinary tract infection in children. Cochrane Database Syst Rev 2001; 4:CD001534.
20. Coraggio MJ, Gross TP, Roscelli JD. Nitrofurantoin toxicity in children. Pediatr Infect Dis J 1989; 8:163–6.
21. Uhari M, Nuutinen M, Turtinen J. Adverse reactions in children during long-term antimicrobial therapy. Pediatr Infect Dis J 1996; 15:404–8.
22. Asmar BI, Mapbool S, Dajani AS. Hematologic abnormalities after oral trimethoprim–sulfamethoxazole therapy in children. Am J Dis Child 1981; 135:1100–3.
23. Smellie JM, Gruneberg RN, Bantock HM et al. Prophylactic co-trimoxazole and trimethoprim in the management of urinary tract infection in children. Pediatr Nephrol 1988; 2:12–17.
24. Garin EH, Olavarria F, Nieto VG, et al. Clinical significance of primary vesicoureteral reflux and urinary antibiotic prophylaxis after acute pyelonephritis: a multicenter, randomized, controlled study. Pediatrics 2006; 117:626–32.
25. Smith EM, Elder JS. Double antimicrobial prophylaxis for breakthrough urinary tract infections in girls. Urology 1994; 43:708–13.
26. Singh-Grewal D, MacDessi J, Craig J. Circumcision for the prevention of urinary tract infection in boys: a systematic review of randomised trials and observational studies. Arch Dis Child 2005; 90:853–8.
27. Szlyk GR, Willliams SB, Majd M, Belman AB, Rushton HG. Incidence of new renal parenchymal inflammatory changes following breakthrough urinary tract infection in patients with vesicoureteral reflux treated with antibiotic prophylaxis: evaluation by 99mtechnetium dimercaptosuccinic acid renal scan. J Urol 2003; 170:1566–8.
28. Wiswell TE. Prepuce presence portends prevalence of potentially perilous periurethral pathogens. J Urol 1992; 148:739–42.
29. Cooper CS, Chung BI, Kirsch AJ et al. The outcome of stopping prophylactic antibiotics in older children with vesicoureteral reflux. J Urol 2000; 163:269–72.
30. Al-Sayyad AJ, Pike JG, Leonard MP. Can prophylactic antibiotics safely be discontinued in children with vesicoureteric reflux? J Urol 2005; 174:1587–9, discussion 1589.
31. Martinell J, Hansson S, Claesson I et al. Detection of urographic scars in girls with pyelonephritis followed for 13–38 years. Pediatr Nephrol 2000; 14:1006–10.
32. Kohler J, Tencer J, Thysell H et al. Vesicoureteral reflux diagnosed in adulthood. Incidence of urinary tract infections, hypertension, proteinuria, back pain and renal calculi. Nephrol Dial Transplant 1997; 12:2580–7.
33. Kohler J, Thysell H, Tencer J, Forsberg L, Hellstrom M. Conservative treatment and anti-reflux surgery in adults with vesico-ureteral reflux: effect on urinary-tract infections, renal function and loin pain in a long-term follow-up study. Nephrol Dial Transplant 2001; 16:52–60.
34. Williams GL, Davies DKL, Evans KT et al. Vesicoureteric reflux in patients with bacteriuria in pregnancy. Lancet 1968; 4:1202–5.
35. Heidrick WP, Mattingly RF, Amberg JR. Vesicoureteral reflux in pregnancy. Obstet Gynecol 1967; 29:571–8.
36. Martinell J, Jodal U, Lidin-Janson G. Pregnancies in women with and without renal scarring after urinary infection in childhood. BMJ 1990; 300:840–4.
37. Koff S. Relationship between dysfunctional voiding and reflux. J Urol 1992; 148:1703–5.
38. Snodgrass W. The impact of treated dysfunctional voiding on the nonsurgical management of vesicoureteral reflux. J Urol 1998; 160:1823–5.
39. Koff SA, Wagner TT, Jayanthi VR. The relationship among dysfunctional elimination syndromes, primary vesicoureteral reflux and urinary tract infections in children. J Urol 1998; 160:1019–22.
40. Farhat W, Bagli DJ, Capolicchio G et al. The dysfunctional voiding scoring system: quantitative standardization of dysfunctional voiding symptoms in children. J Urol 2000; 164:1011–15.
41. Upadhyay J, Bolduc S, Bagli DJ et al. Use of the dysfunctional voiding symptom score to predict resolution of vesicoureteral reflux in children with voiding dysfunction. J Urol 2003; 169:1842–6.
42. Humphreys MR, Reinberg YE. Contemporary and emerging drug treatments for urinary incontinence in children. Paediatr Drugs 2005; 7:151–62.
43. Pereira PL, Miguelez C, Caffarati J et al. Trospium chloride for the treatment of detrusor instability in children. J Urol 2003; 170:1978–81.
44. Reinberg Y, Crocker J, Wolpert J et al. Therapeutic efficacy of extended release oxybutynin chloride, and immediate release and long acting tolterodine tartrate in children with diurnal urinary incontinence. J Urol 2003; 169:317–19.

45. Sureshkumar P, Bower W, Craig JC et al. Treatment of daytime urinary incontinence in children: a systematic review of randomized controlled trials. J Urol 2003; 170:196–200.
46. Koff SA, Murtagh DS. The uninhibited bladder in children: effect of treatment on recurrence of urinary infection and on vesicoureteral reflux resolution. J Urol 1983; 130:1138–41
47. Seruca H. Vesicoureteral reflux and voiding dysfunction: a prospective study. J Urol 1989; 142:494–8.
48. Kramer SA, Rathbun SR, Elkins D, Karnes RJ, Husmann DA. Double-blind placebo controlled study of alpha-adrenergic receptor antagonists (doxazosin) for treatment of voiding dysfunction in the pediatric population. J Urol 2005; 173:2121–4, discussion 2124.
49. Erickson BA, Austin JC, Cooper CS et al. Polyethylene glycol 3350 for constipation in children with dysfunctional elimination. J Urol 2003; 170:1518–20.
50. Herndon CD, Decambre M, McKenna PH. Interactive computer games for treatment of pelvic floor dysfunction. J Urol 2001; 166:1893–8.
51. Wiener JS, Scales MT, Hampton J et al. Long-term efficacy of simple behavioral therapy for daytime wetting in children. J Urol 2000; 164:786–90.
52. De Paepe H, Hoebeke P, Resnon C et al. Pelvic-floor therapy in girls with recurrent urinary tract infections and dysfunctional voiding. Br J Urol 1998; 81 (Suppl 3):109–13.
53. Schulman SL, Von Zuben FC, Plachter N et al. Biofeedback methodology: does it matter how we teach children how to relax the pelvic floor during voiding? J Urol 2001; 166:2423–6.
54. Chin-Peuckert L, Salle JL. A modified biofeedback program for children with detrusor–sphincter dyssynergia: 5-year experience. J Urol 2001; 166:1470–5.
55. Duel BP. Biofeedback therapy and dysfunctional voiding in children. Curr Urol Rep 2003; 4:142–5.
56. Palmer LS, Franco I, Rotario P et al. Biofeedback therapy expedites the resolution of reflux in older children. J Urol 2002; 168:1699–702.
57. Conway JJ, Belman AB, King LR et al. Direct and indirect radionuclide cystography. J Urol 1975; 113:689–93.
58. Mozley PD, Heyman S, Duckett JW et al. Direct vesicoureteral scintigraphy: quantifying early outcome predictors in children with primary reflux. J Nucl Med 1994; 35: 1602–8.
59. Barthold JS, Martin-Crespo R, Kryger JV et al. Quantitative nuclear cystography does not predict outcome in patients with primary vesicoureteral reflux. J Urol 1999; 162:1193–6.
60. Kleinman PK, Diamond DA, Karellas A et al. Tailored low-dose fluoroscopic voiding cystourethrography for the reevaluation of vesicoureteral reflux in girls. AJR Am J Roentgenol 1994; 162:1151–4.
61. Wan J, Greenfield SP, Talley M et al. An analysis of social and economic factors associated with followup of patients with vesicoureteral reflux. J Urol 1996; 156:668–72.
62. Stashinko EE, Goldberger J. Test or trauma? The voiding cystourethrogram experience of young children. Issues Compr Pediatr Nurs 1998; 21:85–96.
63. Quas JA, Goodman GS, Bidrose S et al. Emotion and memory: children's long-term remembering, forgetting, and suggestibility. J Exp Child Psychol 1999; 72:235–70.
64. American Academy of Pediatrics. Committee on Hospital Care. Child life services. Pediatrics 2000; 106:1156–9.
65. Zelikovsky N, Rodrigue JR, Gidycz CA et al. Cognitive behavioral and behavioral interventions help young children cope during a voiding cystourethrogram. J Pediatr Psychol 2000; 25:535–43.
66. Elder JS, Snyder HM, Peters C et al. Variations in practice among urologists and nephrologists treating children with vesicoureteral reflux. J Urol 1992; 148:714–17.
67. Thompson M, Simon SD, Sharma V et al. Timing of follow-up voiding cystourethrogram in children with primary vesicoureteral reflux: development and application of a clinical algorithm. Pediatrics 2005; 115:426–34.
68. Elder JS, Longenecker R. Premedication with oral midazolam for voiding cystourethrography in children: safety and efficacy. AJR Am J Roentgenol 1995; 164:1229–32.
69. Stokland E, Andreasson S, Jacobsson B et al. Sedation with midazolam for voiding cystourethrography in children: a randomised double-blind study. Pediatr Radiol 2003; 33:247–9.
70. Akil I, Ozkol M, Ikozoglu OY et al. Premedication during micturating cystourethrogram to achieve sedation and anxiolysis. Pediatr Nephrol 2005; 20:1106–10.
71. Gerard LL, Cooper CS, Duethman KS et al. Effectiveness of lidocaine lubricant for discomfort during pediatric urethral catheterization. J Urol 2003; 170:564–7.
72. Keidan I, Zaslansky R, Weinberg M et al. Sedation during voiding cystourethrography: comparison of the efficacy and safety of using oral midazolam and continuous-flow nitrous oxide. J Urol 2005; 174: 1598–600, discussion 1601.
73. Butler LD, Symons BK, Henderson SL, Shortliffe LD, Spiegel D. Hypnosis reduces distress and duration of an invasive medical procedure for children. Pediatrics 2005; 115:e77–85.
74. Lowe LH, Patel MN, Gatti JM et al. Utility of follow-up renal sonography in children with vesicoureteral reflux and normal initial sonogram. Pediatrics 2004; 113:548–50.

Surgery for vesicoureteral reflux

44

John W Brock III and Romano T DeMarco

Introduction

Multiple techniques for the open surgical repair of vesicoureteral reflux (VUR) have been described since Hutch first reported the successful correction of VUR in 1952.[1] Although many methods have been proposed, most of these techniques have become footnotes in the evolution of the surgical management of VUR. Today, most surgeons employ only a handful of the previously described repairs.

The surgical correction of VUR has as its goal, the restoration of the flap-valve mechanism absent in children with reflux. Success using any of the described open techniques involves the general surgical principles of tissue handling with the preservation of tissue vascularity. Specific surgical tenets of ureteral reimplantation surgery include the establishment of an adequate submucosal tunnel, a smooth course for the intravesical ureter, and an adequate posterior bladder wall for submucosal tunnel backing. Whereas newer, less-invasive, and novel alternatives to antireflux surgery exist, open surgical repair of VUR remains the gold standard against which all other methods are measured.

Historical background

The earliest descriptions of ureteral reimplantation surgery appeared in the medical literature near the turn of the 20th century. The first reported ureteroneocystostomy is credited to Tauffer in 1877 by Bovee in a review article on ureteral surgery in 1900.[2] Bovee described 80 cases of ureteral reimplant surgeries, the vast majority performed following accidental division of the ureter at the time of laparotomy for ureteral fistulae resulting from prolonged labor or forceps delivery. Subsequently, other innovative procedures for reimplanting the ureter were described in the early part of the 20th century unrelated to the treatment of VUR.[3–9]

In 1952, Hutch reported the successful correction of VUR in 7 out of 9 paraplegic patients with a combined extravesical and intravesical dissection.[1] Hodson followed with his findings that VUR was more common in children with urinary tract infections (UTIs), and that there was a high correlation between VUR and chronic pyelonephritis on intravenous pyelography (IVP).[10] These landmark papers led to further investigations into the treatment of VUR and played a pivotal role in the development of pediatric urology as a separate subspecialty.

Following Hutch's seminal paper, many surgical techniques were described. Landmark refinements of Hutch's operation included Politano and Leadbetter's technique of intravesical mobilization of the terminal ureter, with subsequent reimplantation through a new vesical hiatus and submucosal tunnel.[11] Paquin's method summarized several fundamental requirements of successful VUR surgery, including the creation of a tension-free ureteral anastomosis and a submucosal tunnel length five times longer than the diameter of the ureter.[12] An extravesical approach soon followed, with almost simultaneously reported techniques described by Lich and colleagues in the United States and Grégoir and Van Regemorter in France in the early 1960s.[13,14] Glenn and Anderson reported success using their modified ureteral advancement technique without creating a new muscular hiatus in the mid-1960s.[15] Cohen subsequently modified the ureteral advancement procedure and achieved adequate submucosal tunnel length by using the posterior aspect of the bladder for cross-trigonal tunneling.[16] These descriptions, in addition to contributions by other surgeons over the past 50 years, have made open surgical correction of VUR an effective and durable surgical treatment.

Indications

The surgical indications for VUR should be tailored to the individual patient. Absolute indications for surgery include breakthrough UTIs despite prophylactic antibiotics or because of medical non-compliance. Relative indications for reimplant surgery include the following: persistent grade IV or V reflux; VUR associated with congenital abnormalities at the ureterovesical junction; renal growth retardation or the presence of new renal scars; and dilating reflux persisting in girls who have reached full somatic growth potential.

At Vanderbilt Children's Hospital (VCH), counseling is initiated at the first clinic visit for those patients referred to our office with UTIs and VUR. Good voiding mechanics, adherence to daily antibiotic suppression, and avoidance of dysfunctional elimination issues are repeatedly stressed to both the patient and parents. If indications for surgical intervention are present, other complicating factors, including the nature of the infections while on medical therapy, possible neurologic or non-neurologic bladder dysfunction, and the presence of dysfunctional elimination, are taken into account. Informed operative consent and expectations following surgery are explained in detail to both parents and child.

Presurgical techniques

Cystoscopy

Cystoscopy can be performed prior to open ureteral reimplantation surgery following induction of general anesthesia. Cystoscopy should take only a few minutes from positioning to completion. It alerts the surgeon to unexpected anatomic findings not found on preoperative imaging studies. Duplication anomalies, the presence of small ureteroceles, or evidence of posterior urethral valves or other urethral abnormalities may be found. Bladder trabeculae are seen well during cystoscopy and may be related to voiding dysfunction. Additionally, acute cystitis (if found during endoscopy) delays open surgery until an appropriate course of antibiotic therapy has been completed.

However, cystoscopy is not mandatory in all patients and, with the improvement in diagnostic imaging techniques, typically adds little information. Male patients, those with unclear radiographic findings, or patients with anatomic abnormalities found on preoperative imaging studies are a few of the select group of patients who may benefit from endoscopy.

Positioning

If cystoscopy is performed, the bladder is left moderately distended. The child is then positioned supine with either a rolled towel placed at the level of the upper sacrum or a slight break in the table used to raise the lower pelvis and hips (Figure 44.1). All pressure points are appropriately padded and a wide surgical prep is performed with the perineum draped and exposed within the surgical field.

Intravesical techniques

Exposure/initial dissection

Exposure for all of the intravesical repairs involves a series of similar steps before the individual techniques diverge during ureteral reimplantation. A Pfannenstiel skin incision is made along an appropriate skin crease about one finger breadth above the pubic symphysis (Figure 44.2a). The subcutaneous tissue and Scarpa's fascia are incised the length of the skin incision. The anterior rectus sheath is then opened in a horizontal fashion with superior and inferior rectus flaps created (Figure 44.2b). The rectus muscle bellies are then incised in the midline through the linea alba, separating the rectus and the pyramidalis muscle. Alternatively, the anterior rectus fascia can be opened in a vertical fashion, extending the incision posteriorly through the linea alba (Figure 44.2c).

Following the fascial incision, the space of Retzius is entered bluntly. The peritoneal reflection is displaced superiorly, the bladder is visualized, and full-thickness bladder wall stay sutures are placed on either side of the midline of the bladder. The Denis

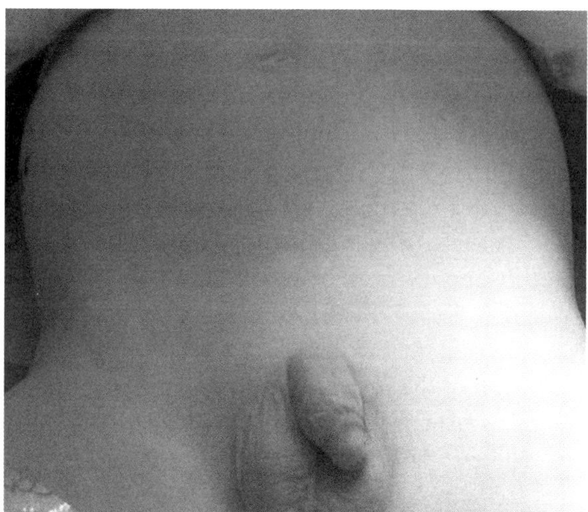

Figure 44.1 A child positioned for ureteral reimplant. The legs are gently abducted. A towel placed under the sacrum provides a slight rise of the pelvis.

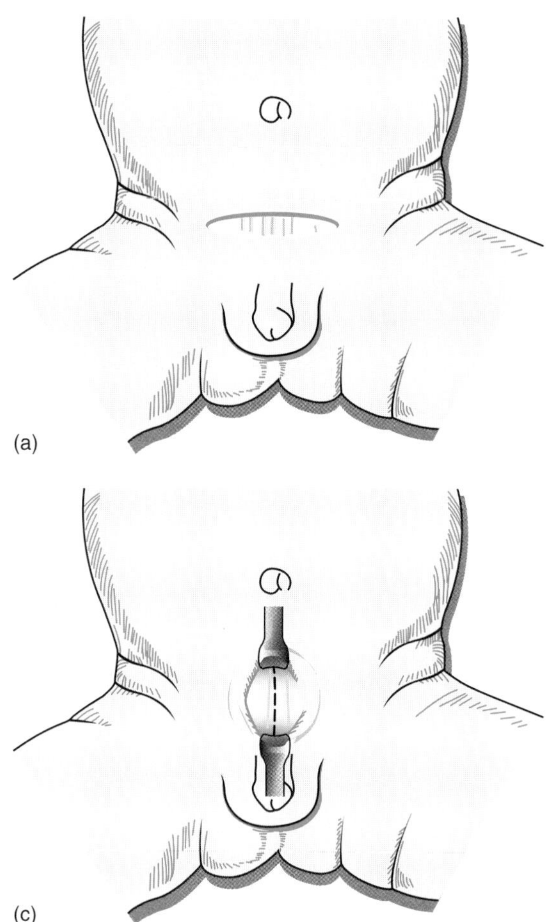

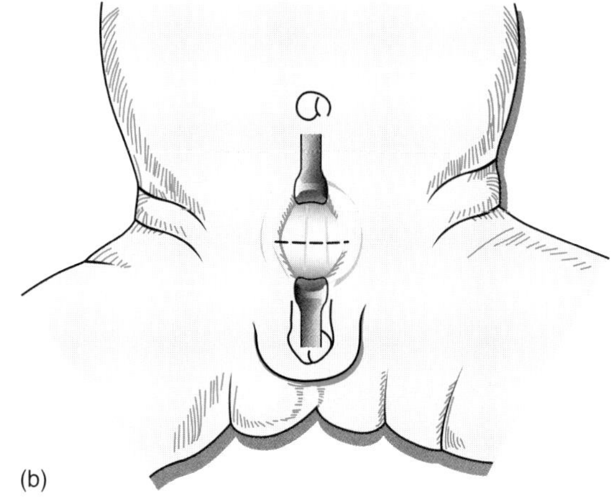

Figure 44.2 (*a*) A Pfannenstiel skin incision is made approximately one finger-breadth above the pubic symphysis. (*b*) The anterior rectus sheath can be opened transversely. Superior and inferior rectus flaps are then created, and allow for excellent exposure. (*c*) Alternatively, the fascia can be incised longitudinally and the rectus bellies separated in the midline.

Brown retractor is a helpful aid in allowing for sustained exposure. The anterior bladder wall is then incised longitudinally, and the inferior edges of the bladder wall are sewn to the lower abdominal skin edges, immobilizing the inferior aspect of the bladder. Moist sponges are packed in the dome of the bladder behind the cephalad blade retractor to flatten the posterior bladder wall and elevate the entire bladder in the pelvis, bringing the ureteral orifices into the middle of the operative field. Lateral blades are secured to the Denis Brown retractor to obtain further exposure. These maneuvers ensure optimal exposure of the posterior aspect of the bladder and trigone. Care must be taken during positioning of the Denis Brown retractor to prevent tearing of the bladder incision through the bladder neck region. Also, excessive touching, suctioning, or rubbing of the bladder mucosa are avoided to prevent edema or inflammation of the mucosa, which can lead to bleeding and difficult mucosal dissection.

Ureteral dissection begins with intubation of the ureter with either a 5 or 3 Fr feeding tube, depending on the size of the ureteral orifice. The tube is secured to the ureter with a 4–0 silk suture placed in a transverse fashion just inferior to the ureteral orifice, and then through the feeding tube which maintains orientation of the ureter throughout mobilization (Figure 44.3a). The mucosa is then circumferentially incised around the ureteral orifice with an electrocautery device in the cutting mode, leaving a several-millimeter cuff of bladder mucosa (Figure 44.3b). The muscular attachments of the ureter to the bladder are then carefully divided with the electrocautery device, using the coagulation mode. This dissection involves gentle countertraction of the ureter away from the periureteral tissue using the feeding tube, in concert with judicious use of the cautery device (Figure 44.3c). Care is taken to avoid both devascularization and injury to the continuity of the ureter. The appropriate plane of dissection is achieved if the shiny, reflective ureteral wall in Waldeyer's sheath is seen. As dissection proceeds proximally, division of the ureteral attachments is taken down further from the ureter to avoid devascularization. Ureteral dissection is completed after an adequate distance of the ureter has been mobilized. A good measure of this distance is for the ureter to have enough length to reach the contralateral bladder wall. An additional clue is the subtle feel-

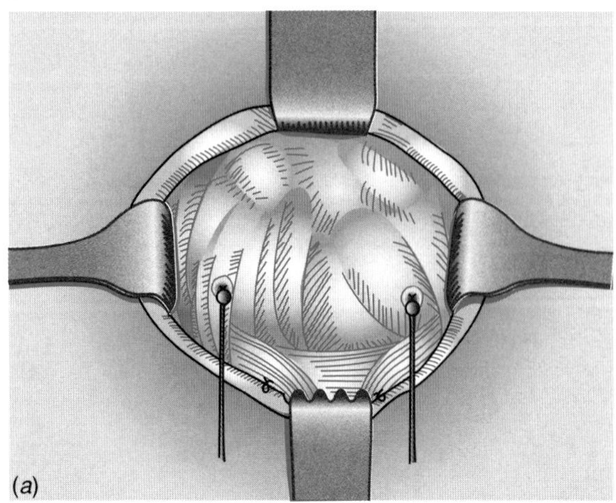

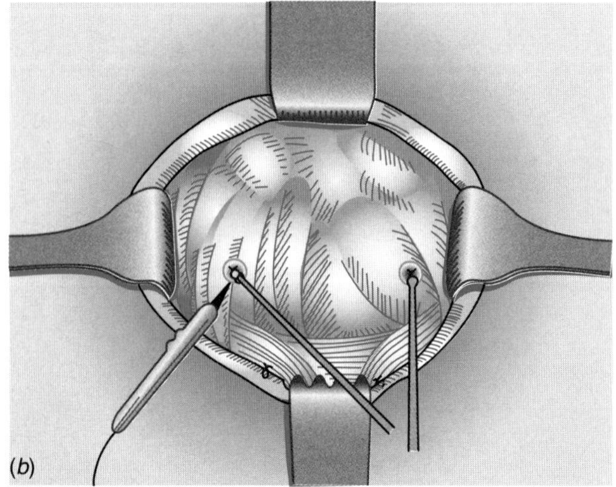

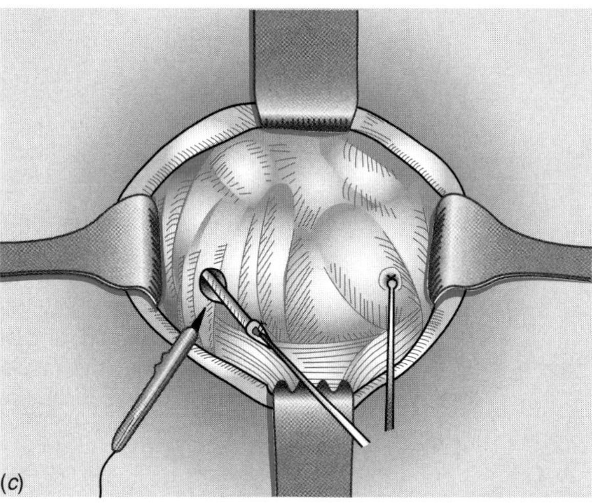

Figure 44.3 (*a*) The refluxing ureter(s) are intubated with an appropriate-sized feeding tube. The feeding tube is secured with a silk stay suture. (*b*) The mucosa is incised circumferentially around the ureteral orifice with an electrocautery device. (*c*) The ureteral attachments are carefully divided, and an adequate ureteral length for reimplant is obtained.

ing of ureteral release the experienced surgeon is alert to, which allows the redundant ureter to easily slide back and forth in the muscular hiatus (Figure 44.4).

Politano–Leadbetter repair

The original Politano–Leadbetter technique described in 1958 involved the blind creation of a new suprahiatal muscular location for the ureter.[11] Following adequate ureteral mobilization as described above, the peritoneum is reflected superiorly away from the posterior aspect of the bladder using the original muscular hiatus as a window in which to work through (Figure 44.5a). If the muscular opening is not adequate for exposure, the posterior bladder wall may be incised superiorly to allow for better visualization. Perivesical crossing vessels, when encountered during

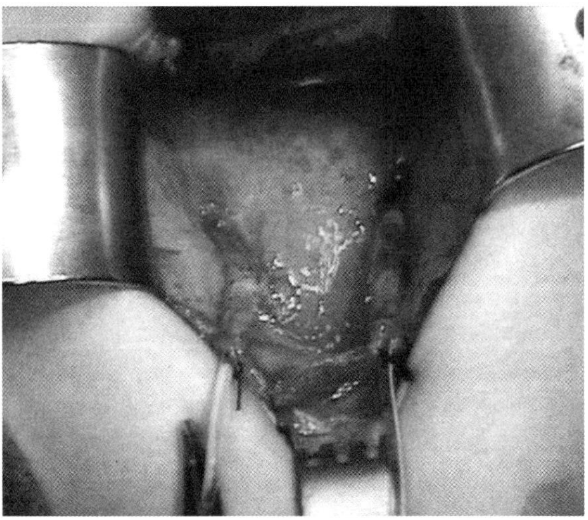

Figure 44.4 Following ureteral dissection, adequate mobilization of the ureters for reimplantation is demonstrated.

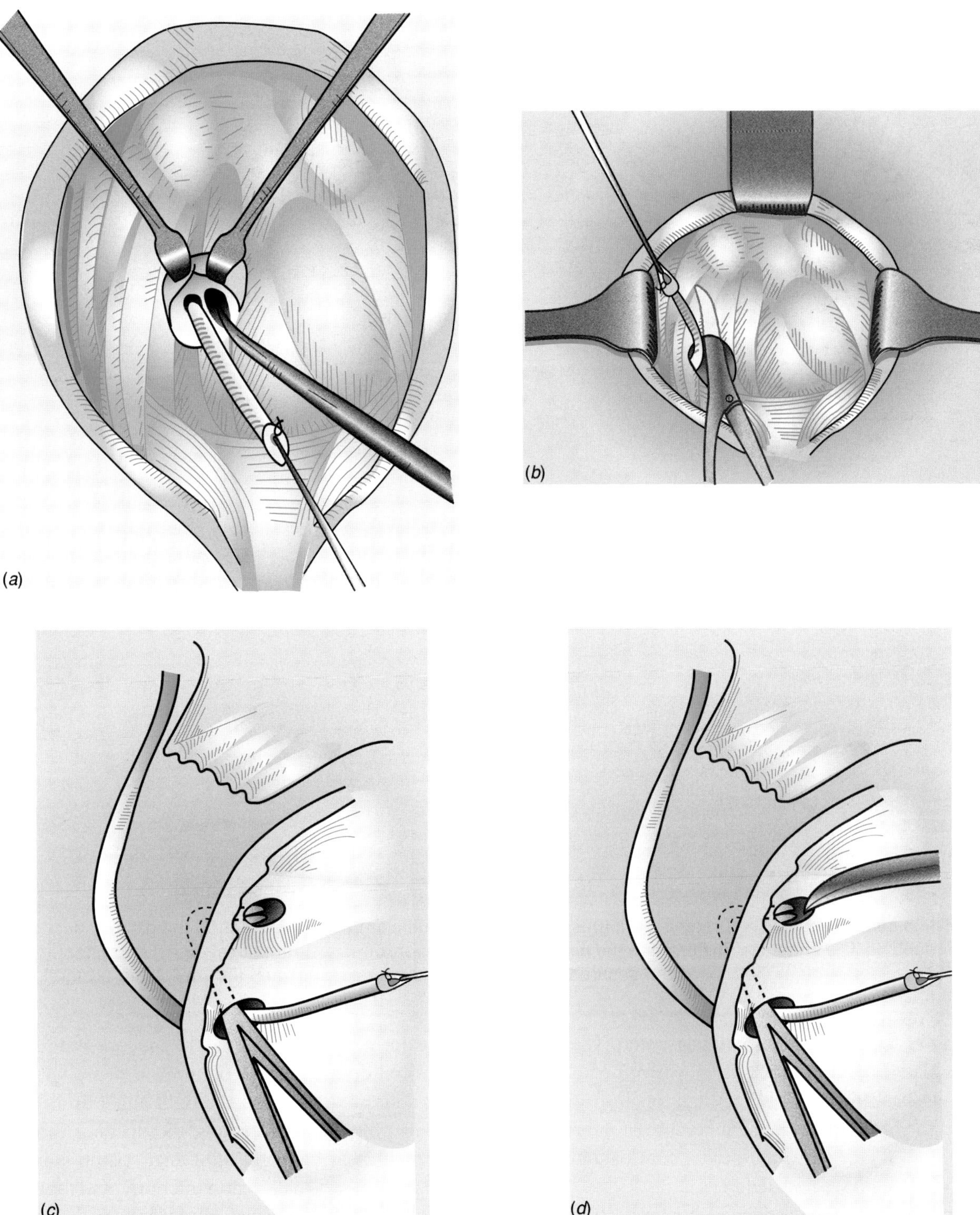

Figure 44.5 (*a*) Following adequate ureteral mobilization, the peritoneum and other structures (vas deferens or vagina) are displaced under direct vision. The posterior aspect of the bladder may be opened to allow for better visualization during this dissection. (*b*) Once the peritoneum is swept away, a right angle clamp is passed from the original hiatus, indenting a region superior and medial to the native hiatus. The electrocautery device incises the bladder tissue indented by the clamp. (*c*) The new hiatus is opened widely with the tip of the right angle clamp to allow for accommodation of the ureter. (*d*) A second right angle clamp is passed from the new hiatus down through the original hiatus.

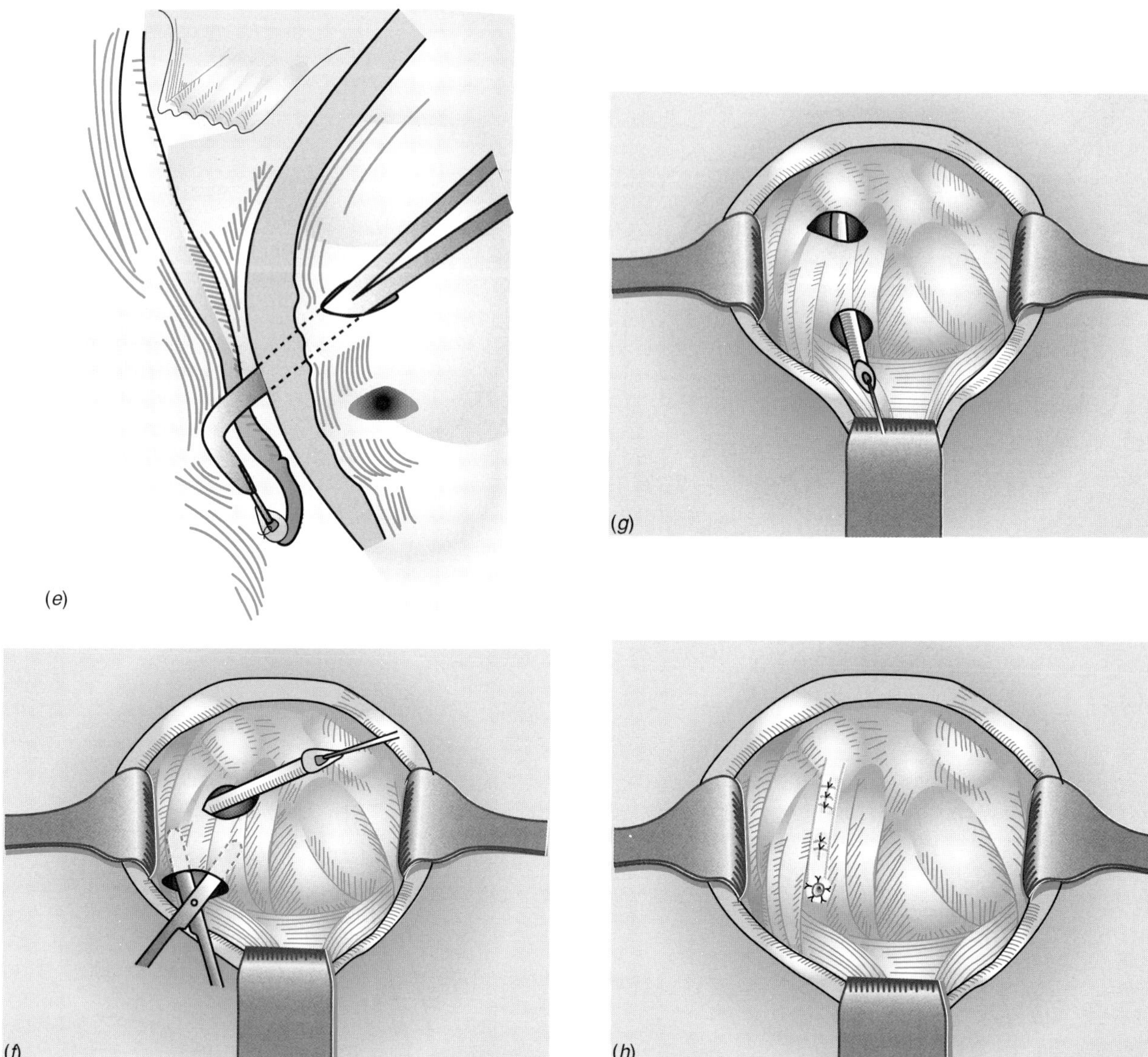

Figure 44.5 *continued* (*e*) The ureter is then grasped by the second clamp after amputating the distal aspect of the feeding tube. (*f*) The ureter is transferred to the new hiatus and an appropriate submucosal tunnel is created. (*g*) The ureter is brought through the tunnel and secured distally to the new mucosal hiatus. (*h*) Completed ureteral reimplant.

division of the bladder wall, are fulgurated. The posterior bladder wall dissection is performed under direct visualization. Blind passage of instruments behind the bladder is forbidden because of the risk of unrecognized entry into the peritoneum or injury to the bowel, vagina, or vas deferens.

Once the posterior bladder wall is freed from the peritoneal reflection, a right angle clamp is passed through the original hiatus superiorly under direct vision, hugging the posterior wall and indenting the bladder wall superiorly, marking the new muscular entrance for the ureter (Figure 44.5b). The location of the new hiatus is slightly medial and cephalad, typically 2–3 cm above the original hiatus. Excessive lateral placement allows for potential kinking and J-hooking of the ureter during bladder filling. The mucosa and muscle are incised directly on the right angle clamp with the electrocautery device, and the right angle tip is delivered into the bladder, dilating the opening carefully (Figure 44.5c). A second right angle clamp is passed through the newly made hiatus inferiorly, and the ureter is then transferred to its new muscular hiatus, using the amputated feeding tube as a handle (Figure 44.5c–f). Careful relocation of the ureter involves ensuring a relatively smooth entrance of the ureter without acute angulations or kinks. The original muscular opening is then closed with 3–0 interrupted chromic sutures in a buried fashion. Adequate room for the ureter to emerge through the new hiatus is measured by the gentle insertion of the tip of a Schnidt clamp.

A submucosal tunnel or mucosal flaps are created from the new entrance of the ureter inferomedially towards the bladder neck, which is marked with the electrocautery device. A modification of Politano and Leadbetter's original method involves increasing the submucosal tunnel length by extending the tunnel past the native ureteral orifice toward the bladder neck. Submucosal dissection is performed carefully with tenotomy scissors or the electrocautery device, and should proceed with ease through a bloodless field if in the correct plane (Figure 44.5f). Once an adequate submucosal tunnel has been made, the ureter is transferred through the tunnel (Figure 44.5g). The feeding tube is then removed, and the ureter is spatulated if needed. If excessive ureteral redundancy is present, the distal tip of the ureter may be excised. Three 6–0 Vicryl sutures are placed through the posterior apex of the distal ureter and through both bladder mucosa and muscle to secure the ureter distally and prevent it from retracting back into the tunnel. Then, 6–0 Vicryl mucosal sutures are placed circumferentially around the ureteral orifice, completing the mucosal anastomosis. The original mucosal opening is closed with a fine absorbable suture, and if mucosal flaps were created they are approximated with a running fine absorbable suture (Figure 44h). The bladder is then closed in two layers with 3–0 chromic suture in a running fashion.

Cohen's cross-trigonal repair

Arguably, today's most popular open technique for ureteral reimplantation is the cross-trigonal repair described by Cohen in 1975.[16] Ureteral dissection is performed as described above; however, this method typically requires less ureteral mobilization than the Politano–Leadbetter technique. The submucosal tunnel is created along the posterior bladder wall without transferring the ureter to a new muscular hiatus, virtually eliminating kinking of the distal ureter. The major drawback to this operation is the subsequent difficult intubation of the ureteral orifices related to their transtrigonal location.

Following ureteral mobilization, the muscular hiatus may need approximation if a patulous opening is present. Cinching of the hiatus with a 3–0 chromic suture should bring the muscle together tightly but allow for the tip of a Schnidt clamp to pass between the bladder and ureter. Aggressive closure of the muscular hiatus can cause kinking with angulation of the ureter and possible distal ureteral obstruction. In contrast, too lax of a muscular approximation may lead to diverticulum formation.

During unilateral ureteral reimplantation, a submucosal tunnel is developed across the posterior bladder wall in a cross-trigonal fashion. The new mucosal hiatus is created above the contralateral ureteral orifice. This ureteral position allows for an adequate submucosal tunnel. Once the submucosal tunnel is created, the ureter is transferred through the tunnel using the shortened feeding tube and stay suture as a handle. The feeding tube is then removed from the ureter. The ureter is spatulated, as indicated, and three fine absorbable sutures are placed through the lateral, posterior apex of the ureter and the bladder mucosa and muscle. Placement of these tacking sutures in the correct position creates an appropriate lateral vector force on the ureter, preventing medial regression of the ureter and loss of the effective submucosal tunnel. The newly created ureteral orifice is then matured with circumferential fine absorbable sutures. The mucosal defect from the old ureteral orifice is then closed with interrupted fine absorbable sutures (Figure 44.6a and b). Prior to closing the bladder, the free, smooth passage of a small feeding tube rules out excessive ureteral kinking.

When both ureters are reimplanted, the submucosal tunnel for the most superior ureter is made with the mucosal hiatus located just above the contralateral ureter. Subsequently, the other ureter is brought across the posterior bladder wall, with the new ureteral orifice positioned close to the inferior portion of the old contralateral hiatus. Visual inspection of the anatomy of the trigone and posterior bladder wall aids the surgeon in deciding how to orient the ureters with regard to superior and inferior location. At times, proper positioning of the submucosal tunnels dictates carefully incising the posterior bladder wall following peritoneal displacement in a superolateral fashion (Figure 44.6b). This leads to a cephalad shift of the ureter at the muscular hiatus, and allows for a smoother course across the posterior bladder wall for the superior-most ureter. Additionally, a lateral, muscular incision may be performed to recess the ureter laterally and can be used to increase the tunnel length in small bladders. Following ureteral reimplantation, the bladder is closed in two layers using 3–0 chromic suture.

Glenn–Anderson repair

In 1967, Glenn and Anderson refined and popularized the intravesical ureteral advancement procedure

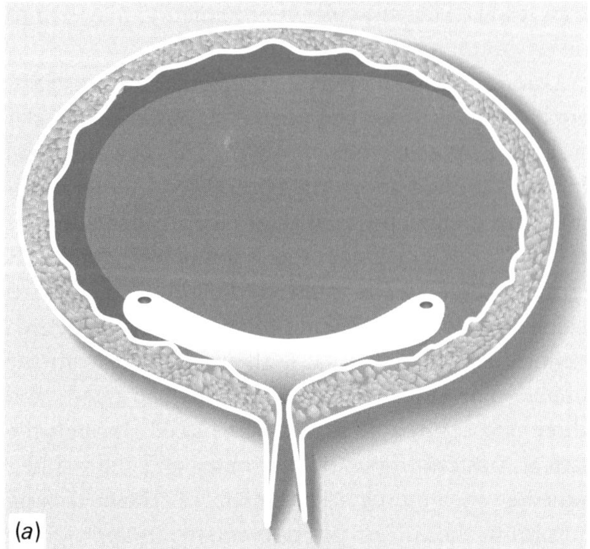

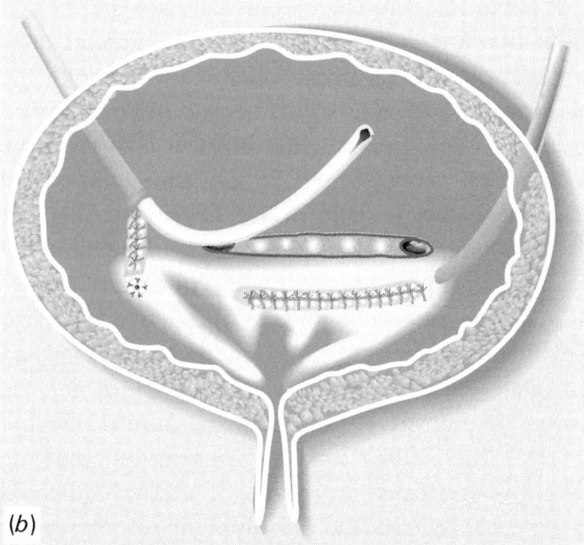

Figure 44.6 (*a*) Laterally displaced, refluxing ureteral orifices with an adequate posterior bladder wall for cross-trigonal reimplantation. (*b*) The left ureter was reimplanted using this technique. The native right ureteral orifice becomes the new left orifice after reimplant. The right ureteral muscular hiatus is incised superiorly to shift the ureter in a cephalad fashion, allowing a smooth tunnel for cross-trigonal reimplant.

that had been reported by several other authors.[15,17,18] Patients in whom this technique is used are selected based upon the location of their refluxing ureteral orifice(s) (Figure 44.7a). Those patients with laterally displaced ureters and a sufficient posterior bladder wall are good candidates for this procedure.

Ureteral dissection is performed in a fashion as described previously. If the muscular hiatus is gaping, the muscle edges are approximated with a buried, 3–0 chromic suture allowing for an adequate, smooth entrance for the ureter (Figure 44.7b). Following ureteral mobilization, a mucosal tunnel or mucosal flaps are developed from the original mucosal hiatus and extended in a caudal fashion to a point marked superior to the bladder neck. Once the tunnel or flaps are created, the ureter is transferred either through the tunnel or placed in the mucosal trough. The ureter is then secured distally to the newly created mucosal hiatus in a manner similar to the Poli-

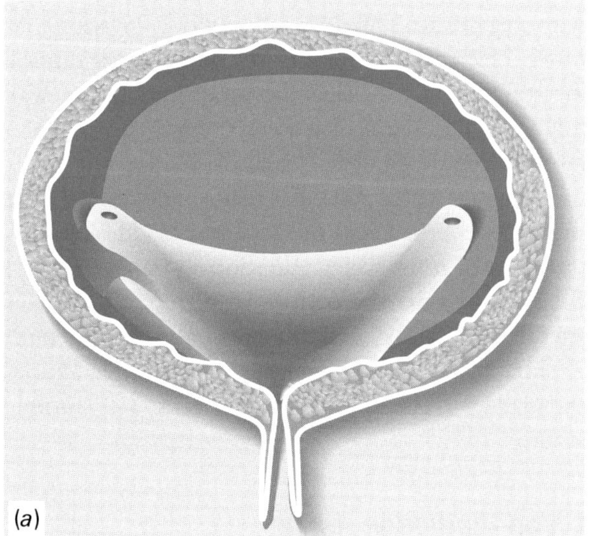

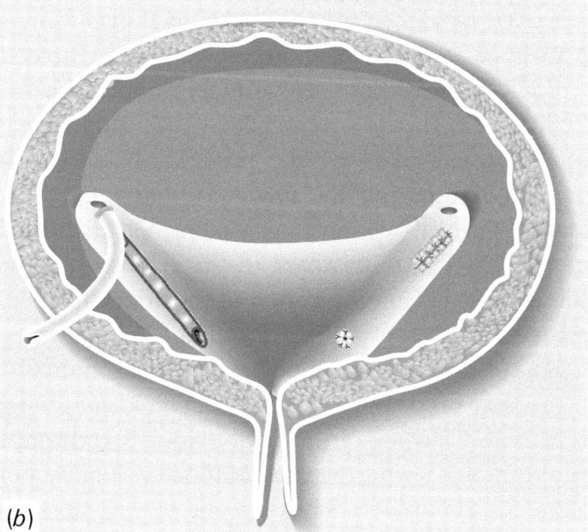

Figure 44.7 (*a*) Lateral and cephalad ureteral orifices that are ideal for the Glenn–Anderson advancement technique. (*b*) The ureters are advanced to an area superior to the bladder neck with an adequate submucosal tunnel.

tano–Leadbetter technique. The mucosal hiatus is then matured circumferentially with interrupted absorbable sutures or the mucosal trough is closed with a running fine, absorbable suture (Figure 44.7b). The bladder is then closed in a similar fashion to the other repairs.

Gil-Vernet repair

A simple, advancement technique for those patients with lateral ectopia and a widened, 'mega-trigone' was described by Gil-Vernet in 1984.[19] Exposure of the ureters is similar as in the other open procedures; however, minimal ureteral dissection is needed. A traction suture is placed at the medial aspect of the ureteral orifice and adequate mobility of the distal ureter and intrinsic muscular fibers of the terminal ureter is demonstrated by the ability of the ureter to be pulled towards the midline (Figure 44.8a and b).

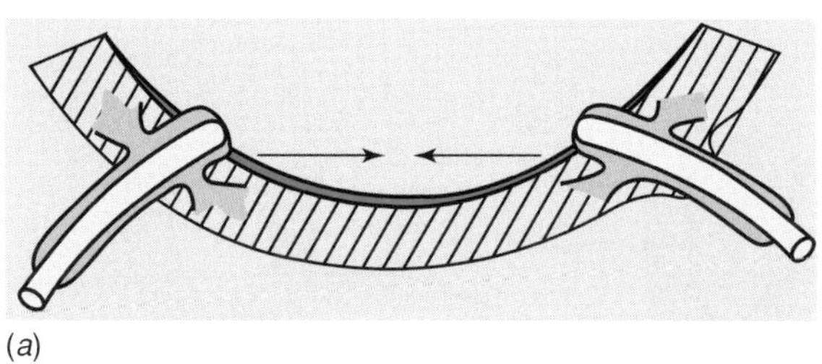

(*a*)

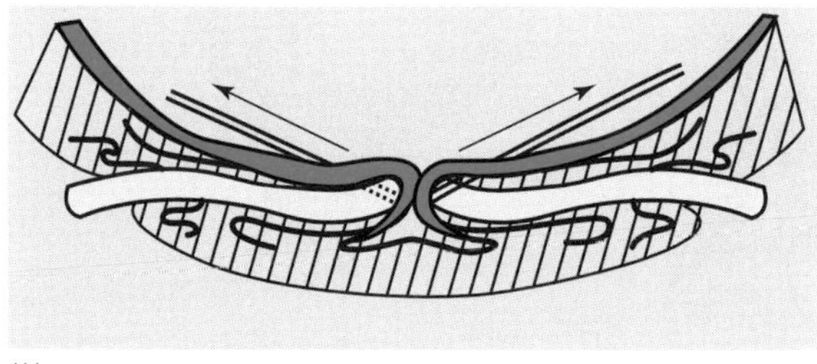

(*b*)

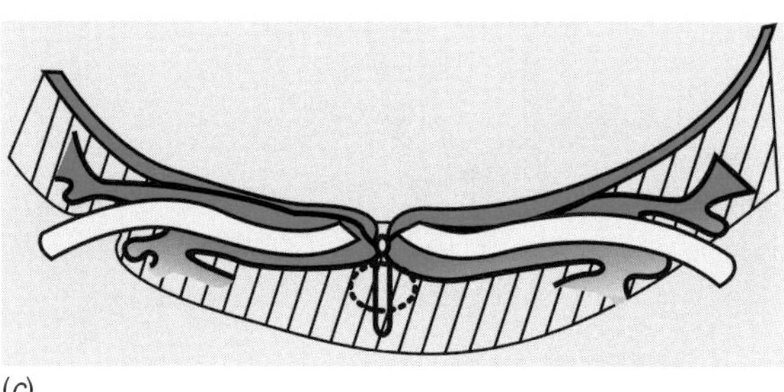

(*c*)

Figure 44.8 (*a*) The Gil-Vernet technique of advancing mobile ureters across the trigone. (*b*) Traction sutures are placed at the medial aspect of the ureteral orifices to test mobility. (*c*) Mattress sutures advance the ureters towards the midline, increasing their submucosal tunnel length. (Modified from Gil-Vernet,[19] with permission.)

If mobility of the distal ureter is found to be adequate, a transverse incision is made through the mucosa across the superior aspect of the trigone between the ureteral orifices. The mucosa is then elevated off the bladder wall muscle. The classic description by Gil-Vernet uses a single 3–0 nylon or Prolene suture placed in a mattress fashion at the base of each ureter encompassing the periureteral sheath and muscle. This suture advances the ureters toward the midline, increasing their intramural length. The permanent suture is then buried by approximating the bladder muscle with 3–0 chromic sutures. The mucosa is then closed vertically with interrupted, fine absorbable sutures (Figure 44.8c). A modification of this technique using absorbable suture for the medial advancement has been described, and that is our practice at VCH.[20] The bladder and the overlying incision are then closed in a routine fashion.

Extravesical techniques

Lich–Grégoir repair

An extravesical approach to the correction of VUR was almost simultaneously described here in the United States and in Europe by Lich and colleagues and Grégoir and Van Regemorter in the early 1960s.[13,14] This technique, commonly referred to as Lich–Grégoir, is similar to previous methods published by other surgeons around the turn of the 20th century.[4,21] Despite its popularity in Europe, US surgeons were less enthused following Hendren's disappointing initial results using a modification of this repair.[22] Subsequent studies with minor modifications have found this technique to be both durable and reliable.[23,24]

Because the bladder is not opened during the repair, cystoscopy is performed following induction of anesthesia to rule out any bladder abnormalities. Once cystoscopy is complete, a Foley catheter is placed, clamped, and the bladder is left moderately full. Bladder exposure is obtained in a fashion similar to the intravesical repairs. The bladder volume is then emptied, and the bladder is retracted medially to expose the refluxing ureter. The peritoneum is reflected superiorly away from the posterior bladder wall, and the obliterated hypogastric artery is identified and ligated. The ureter is then found, mobilized, and freed of attachments distally to the posterior aspect of the bladder (Figure 44.9a) A network of small vessels typically congregates near the ureterovesical junction, and they need to be divided carefully with an electrocautery device.

Following ureteral mobilization, the serosal and muscular layers of the detrusor are incised superiorly for a distance of 4–5 cm to create a trough for the ureter. The bulging bladder mucosa is seen following muscular division and ensures adequate mucosal exposure. Distention of the bladder during this step makes this dissection easier. Mucosal rents made during this step are closed with fine absorbable suture. The muscular division continues in a caudal direction 1–2 cm past the ureterovesical junction. The ureterovesical junction is freed circumferentially. Mobility of the ureterovesical junction is needed for ureteral advancement. Two or three 4–0 chromic vest-type sutures are placed through the bladder wall and ureter to advance and anchor the ureter to the distal aspect of the trough (Figure 44.9b–d). The ureter is then placed in the trough, and the detrusor is closed over it with interrupted 3–0 chromic sutures (Figure 44.9e). Approximation of the muscle edges proximally should be loose, and able to accommodate the tip of a Schnidt clamp at the muscular hiatus. Although no perivesical drain is typically used, an indwelling Foley catheter is left overnight and removed on postoperative day 1. If bilateral extravesical reimplants are performed, a voiding trial is initiated prior to discharge because of the risk of transient postoperative urinary retention.

Postoperative evaluation

The majority of children following simple ureteroneocystostomy are managed without indwelling urethral catheterization or perivesical drainage at VCH. Surgical repair of VUR via a catheterless ureteroneocystostomy at our institution was found to reduce hospital stay for patients when compared with those patients undergoing ureteral reimplantation with a

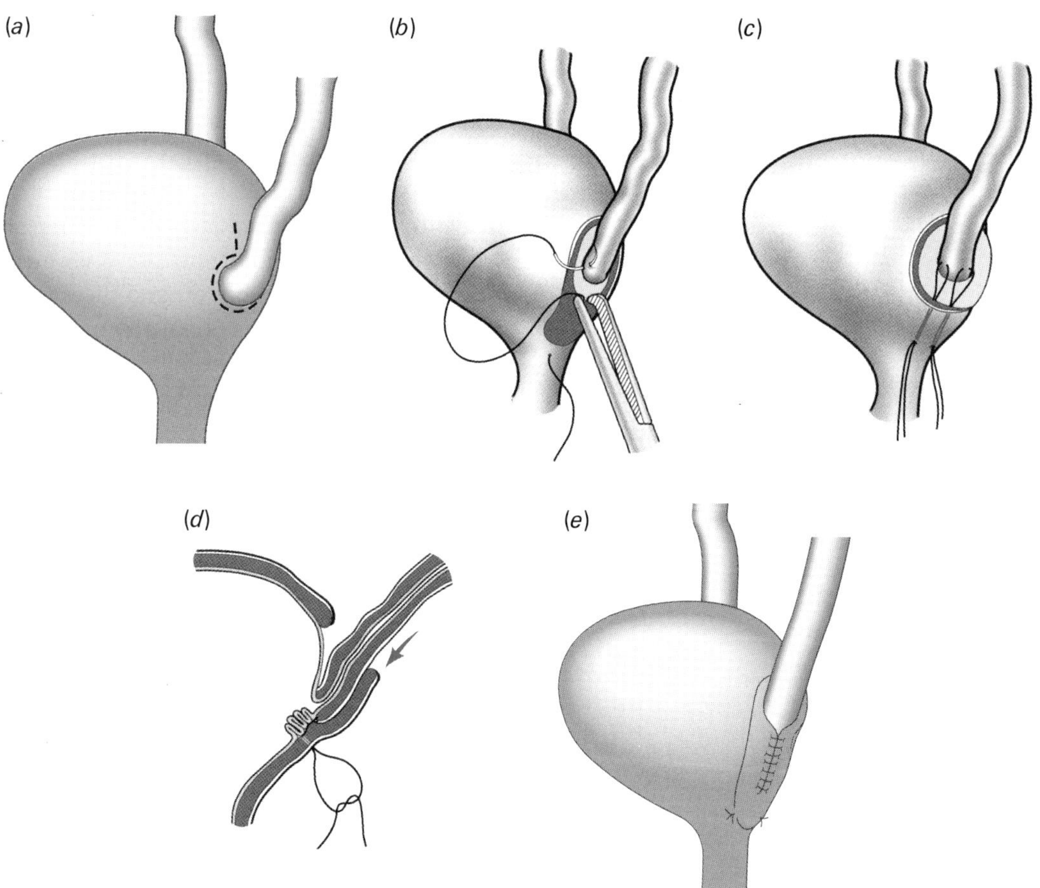

Figure 44.9 (*a*) The extravesical approach begins with ureteral mobilization followed by detrusorrhaphy. (*b*) After mobilization of the mucosa off the bladder muscle, two or three vest sutures are placed in an appropriate fashion. (*c*) Tying of the sutures advances the ureter down toward the inferior aspect of the trough. (*d*) A sagittal view following ureteral advancement. (*e*) The detrusor is loosely closed over the ureter once secured in the trough.

urethral catheter, without increasing complication rates.[25] Most children are discharged on postoperative day 1: i.e. once the child demonstrates adequate oral intake and postoperative pain is controlled with oral medications.

Standard postsurgical management includes a renal ultrasound at the first postoperative visit at 1 month to assess for the presence of hydronephrosis. Mild, transient hydronephrosis is commonly seen and usually resolves within the first several postoperative months. Management of persistent severe hydronephrosis will be discussed later in the chapter.

Voiding and stooling habits are reviewed during all postoperative clinic visits, and dysfunctional elimination issues are treated aggressively with educational reinforcement and medications. Suppressive antibiotic therapy is continued for 3–6 months following surgery. The child's preventive antibiotics are discontinued on an individual basis. Factors considered in the cessation of antimicrobial therapy include the demonstration of good elimination habits, a consistent UTI-free state, and evidence of resolved hydronephrosis. Routine voiding cystourethrography (VCUG) in patients undergoing simple ureteroneocystostomy is not performed at our institution, and this approach has been supported by others.[26,27] Following the early postoperative clinic visits, annual or semi-annual appointments are made to follow the child's voiding history and check the blood pressure, urine (with a urinalysis), and kidneys (with ultrasonography). Later in adult life, periodic evaluation should continue as indicated.

Results

The open surgical treatment of VUR has a long record of impressive correction rates. Initial and follow-up series of accepted surgical methods have success rates of 94–99%. The American Urological Association (AUA) Pediatric Vesicoureteral Reflux Guidelines Panel, released in 1997, analyzed 86 publications with respect to failure rate after ureteroneocystostomy, and found an overall success rate of 95.9% in 8061 open surgically treated ureters.[28] Reimplanted ureters with grade I–IV VUR had surgical correction rates of 98–99%, independent of technique, and these findings hold true at VCH.[29] However, patients with grade V VUR were found to have a persistent but lower grade of VUR 19% of the time following surgery.[28] With improvements in instrumentation and suture material, modifications of techniques, proper performance, and appropriate selection of patients, success nears 99% in those patients undergoing simple ureteral reimplantation with low to moderate grade reflux.

Complications

Ureteral obstruction

Postoperative complications are rare following ureteroneocystostomy. Mild hydronephrosis is not unusual in the early recovery period. In our series of patients who underwent ureteral reimplantation surgery, 8% of patients had grade I hydronephrosis that resolved over a period of several months.[26] Severe, persistent hydronephrosis is uncommon and is probably related to ureteral obstruction. Fortunately, ureteral obstruction is rare, with an occurrence rate of around 1%.[26,27,30] In cases of ureteral obstruction, initial management includes the placement of a percutaneous nephrostomy tube or indwelling stent in the hope that the obstruction is transient and will resolve over time. In patients with persistent ureteral obstruction, a repeat ureteral reimplant is required. This procedure may necessitate significantly more ureteral mobilization than the initial surgery, requiring both an intravesical and extravesical approach. A viable ureter is identified and the distal fibrotic ureter is discarded. A psoas hitch or Boari flap may be required if a significant length of distal ureter is lost. In rare instances, a transureteroureterostomy or ileal ureter is required for reconstruction.

Persistent reflux

Persistent reflux following ureteroneocystostomy is rare. The success rate, as noted previously, exceeds 98% in those patients with a non-dilating VUR. Poor selection of patients for specific operative techniques may have led to early reports of persistent reflux following surgery using specific methods.[22] The creation of an adequate submucosal tunnel in children with severe, dilating VUR is challenging. Ureteral tapering is often required; this increases the complexity of the surgery and the risk for postoperative morbidity and is discussed in detail in Chapter 39. Fortunately, in most patients with persistent VUR, their reflux is downgraded substantially following surgery and may resolve with growth and good voiding mechanics. One unusual cause of persistent VUR is the development of a ureterovesical fistula postoperatively. This complication does not typically resolve with expectant management. If problematic, surgical correction is indicated.

New contralateral reflux

The development of new contralateral VUR following unilateral ureteral reimplantation is uncommon. Occurrence rates vary from 1 to 18%.[31,32] Possible factors associated with de-novo contralateral VUR include a prior history of resolved contralateral reflux, correction of grade V VUR, or VUR into a duplicated system.[31,33] Contralateral VUR is usually low grade, causes no sequelae, and resolves within 1–2 years if the child adheres to a good voiding regimen. The need for surgical correction of new-onset, contralateral VUR following surgery is a rare event.

Conclusions

The open surgical repair for the correction of VUR is both a safe and effective management option. Classically described methods, such as the Politano–Leadbetter and the Cohen cross-trigonal techniques, are successful, durable repairs and continue to be used today. Whereas laparoscopic and endourologic techniques are being performed in greater numbers, the ease and success of the open surgical repair is the standard by which all other repairs should continue to be judged.

Key points

1 The open surgical correction of vesicoureteral reflux is highly effective, has few complications, and is the current gold standard of treatment.
2 The appropriate intravesical surgical technique is determined by trigonal anatomy.
3 The modified Politano–Leadbetter repair involves the creation of a new suprahiatal location of the ureter under direct vision.
4 When creating a new suprahiatal location for the ureter during the modified Politano–Leadbetter repair, it is important to avoid lateral placement to prevent J-hooking of the ureter.
5 The cross-trigonal method of ureteral reimplantation results in less potential for kinking because of its use of the original muscular hiatus.
6 The major drawback to the cross-trigonal method is the subsequent difficult intubation of the ureteral orifice due to its position following surgery.
7 The Glenn–Anderson technique is highly successful when used in those patients with laterally displaced ureters, allowing for sufficient ureteral advancement and tunnel length.
8 For experienced surgeons, routine postoperative VCUG is not mandatory in all patients following reimplant surgery.

References

1. Hutch JA. Vesicoureteral reflux in the paraplegic: cause and correction: J Urol 1952; 68:457–69.
2. Bovee JW. A critical survey of ureteral implantation. Ann Surg 1900; 32:165–93.
3. Payne RL. Ureteral-vesical implantation. A new method of anastomosis. JAMA 1908; 51:1321–5.
4. Coffey RC. Physiologic implantation of the severed ureter or common bile-duct into the intestine. JAMA 1911; 56:397–403.
5. Peterson A. The effect on the kidney of ureterovesical anastomosis. JAMA 1918; 71:1885–91.
6. Vermooten V, Neuswanger CH. Effects on the upper urinary tract in dogs of an incompetent ureterovesical valve. J Urol 1934; 32:330–4.
7. Stevens AR, Marshall VR. Reimplantation of the ureter into the bladder. Surg Gynecol Obstet 1943; 77:585–94.
8. Prather GC. Vesicoureteral reflux. Report of a case cured by operation. J Urol 1944; 52:437–47.
9. Dodson AI. Some improvements in the technique of ureterocystostomy. J Urol 1946; 55:225–37.
10. Hodson CJ. The radiologic diagnosis of pyelonephritis. Proc R Soc Med 1959; 52:669–72.
11. Politano VA, Leadbetter WF. An operative technique for the correction of vesicoureteral reflux. J Urol 1958; 79:932–41.
12. Paquin AJ Jr. Ureterovesical anastomosis: the description and evaluation of a technique. J Urol 1959; 82:573–83.
13. Lich R Jr, Howerton LW, Davis LA. Recurrent urosepsis in children. J Urol 1961; 86:554–8.
14. Grégoir W, Van Regemorter GV. Le reflux vésicourétéral congénital. Urol Int 1964; 18:122–36.
15. Glenn JF, Anderson EE. Distal tunnel ureteral reimplantation. J Urol 1967; 97:623–6.
16. Cohen SJ. Ureterozystoneostomie: Eine neue antirefluxtechnik. Aktuelle Urologie 1975; 6:1–8.
17. Williams DI, Scott J, Turner-Warwick RT. Reflux and recurrent infection. Br J Urol 1961; 33:435–41.
18. Hutch JA. Ureteric advancement operation: anatomy, technique and early results. J Urol 1963; 89:180–4.
19. Gil-Vernet JM. A new technique for surgical correction of vesicoureteral reflux. J Urol 1984; 131:456–8.
20. Carini M, Selli C, Lenzi R, Barbagli G, Costantini A. Surgical treatment of vesicoureteral reflux with bilateral medialization of the ureteral orifices. Eur Urol 1985; 11:181–3.
21. Witzel O. Extraperitoneale Ureterocystostomie mit Schrägkanalbildung. Centrablatt für Gynakologie 1896; 20:289–93.
22. Hendren WH. Reoperation for the failed ureteral reimplantation. J Urol 1974; 111:403–11.
23. Zaontz MR, Maizels M, Sugar EC, Firlit CF. Detrussorrhaphy: extravesical ureteral advancement to correct vesicoureteral reflux in children. J Urol 1987; 138:947–9.

24. Wacksman J, Gilbert A, Sheldon CA. Results of the renewed extravesical reimplant for surgical correction of vesicoureteral reflux. J Urol 1992; 148:359–61.
25. Duong DT, Parekh DJ, Pope JC 4th, Adams MC, Brock JW 3rd. Ureteroneocystostomy without ureteral catheterization shortens hospital stay without compromising postoperative success. J Urol 2003; 170:1570–3.
26. Grossklaus DJ, Pope JC, Adams MC, Brock JW. Is postoperative cystography necessary after ureteral reimplantation? Urology 2001; 58:1041–5.
27. Lavine MA, Siddiq FM, Chan DJ et al. Vesicoureteral reflux after ureteroneocystostomy: indications for postoperative voiding cystography. Tech Urol 2001; 7:50–4.
28. Elder JS, Peters CA, Arant BS Jr et al. Pediatric Vesicoureteral Reflux Guidelines Panel summary report on the management of primary vesicoureteral reflux in children. J Urol 1997; 157:1856–51.
29. Flicklinger JE, Trusler L, Brock JW III. Clinical care pathway for the management of ureteroneocystostomy in the pediatric population. J Urol 1997; 158:1221–5.
30. Steffens J, Langen PH, Haben B et al. Politano–Leadbetter ureteroneocystostomy: a 30-year experience. Urol Int 2000; 65:9–14.
31. Diamond DA, Rabinowitz R, Hoenig D, Caldamone AA. The mechanism of new onset contralateral reflux following unilateral ureteroneocystostomy. J Urol 1996; 156:665–7.
32. McCool AC, Perez LM, Joseph DB. Contralateral vesicoureteral reflux after simple and tapered unilateral ureteroneocystostomy revisited. J Urol 1997; 158:1219–20.
33. Ross JH, Kay R, Nasrallah P. Contralateral reflux after unilateral ureteral reimplantation in patients with a history of resolved contralateral reflux. J Urol 1995; 154:1171–2.

Minimally invasive approaches to correct vesicoureteral reflux

45

Patrick Cartwright and Brent W Snow

The narrow bony pelvis of the child leads to the bladder occupying a more intra-abdominal position than in the adult. This creates relatively easy access to the bladder and perivesical space. Percutaneous bladder access is quite familiar to pediatric urologists, with suprapubic aspiration for culture being a standard practice for many years. In addition, placing a needle or port directly into the distended bladder may allow access for other procedures, including:

- placement of a suprapubic catheter
- antegrade ablation of a posterior urethral valve
- injection of bulking agents at the bladder neck
- catheterization of ureteral orifices with an unusual orientation (such as after Cohen's reimplant).

This background and a growing expertise with transperitoneal laparoscopy has inevitably led pediatric urologists to approach the common problem of vesicoureteral reflux laparoscopically; both intravesical and extravesical approaches have been reported and continue to be pursued.

Extravesical laparoscopic ureteral reimplantation

To assess the feasibility of this approach, early research work included creating reflux in a porcine model by incising the roof of the ureteral tunnel intravesically and subsequently creating a new submucosal tunnel via a transperitoneal, laparoscopic extravesical approach similar to the Lich–Grégoir repair.[1] Repair proved to be achievable with good reflux resolution rates but involved 1–2 hours per reimplant with bladder perforation and ureteral obstruction noted among the complications.[2–4] The procedure described involved splitting detrusor fibers superolaterally from the ureteral hiatus to expose urothelium, laying the ureter into this trough, and then closing detrusor edges together over the ureter to create a longer submucosal tunnel. This basic surgical approach is very similar to what has been undertaken clinically.

In 1994, the initial clinical report of transperitoneal, extravesical laparoscopic reflux correction was made and included patients aged 2 and 5 years with successful outcomes and long but acceptable operating times.[5] Janetschek and coworkers followed this shortly with a report on six patients, one of whom required ureteral stenting for 6 weeks.[6] These authors were impressed that the procedure was unwieldy and seemed to offer little recovery advantage to patients. While some surgeons may have been dissuaded by these reports, others have continued to pursue improvements.

Four significant series of transperitoneal, laparoscopic extravesical reimplantation studies have been reported over the past several years. In 2000, Lakshmanan and Fung reported on 26 patients (36 ureters), utilizing a technique with four ports, having an operative time of 1.5 hours/ureter and resulting in only one failure (follow-up of 3 months).[7] This series was updated in 2001 with 53 patients (83 ureters) accumulated in a period 'beyond the learning curve'. In these patients, there was failure of resolution in only one ureter (1.1%) and obstruction in another (1.1%), with each requiring open revision.[8] Shu et al have taken a similar approach, using four ports, and have recently documented excellent results and recovery, particularly in postpubertal patients.[9] Finally, Peters and associates have recently (2005) applied robotic technology to reimplantation in 24 children. Their initial results at 19.5 months mean follow-up include no obstruction in any patient, with resolution of reflux in 18/20 patients (90%) undergoing cystography. Mean operative times were 2.5 hours for unilateral and 3.5 hours for bilateral cases, with variable catheter usage and hospital stays of 0.25–3 days.[10] It is unclear whether a robotic approach will allow for reduction in the problematic postoperative voiding dysfunction sometimes seen in open bilateral extravesical reimplantation. Of interest, this group has pursued and reported robotic reimplant approaches both intravesically and extravesically; they suspect that the greatest benefit may lie with extravesical approaches. To summarize all these reports, creating good exposure of the posterior bladder wall and avoiding injury to both the ureter and urothelium seem to be crucial advantages of this transperitoneal, extravesical approach.

Intravesical (transvesical) laparoscopic ureteral reimplantation

It has been shown by many groups that the intravesical space can be accessed with percutaneous laparoscopic ports and that carbon dioxide insufflation can create a 'pneumovesicum' appropriate for surgical procedures. With such an approach, authors differ as to how many ports they place, which port holds the camera, and whether there is a working instrument via the urethra or just a balloon catheter to prevent desufflation.

Initial attempts at intravesical reimplantation were reported by Okamura, Tsuji, and coworkers, replicating the Gil-Vernet technique of medial orifice advancement.[11] This innovative group accessed the bladder with two ports and used the urethra as a third access site to perform 'endoscopic trigonoplasty'. They were able to make an incision along the trigonal ridge and draw the ureters medially to the midline with sequential suturing. Their original experience (mostly adults), published in 1997, documented resolution in 95% of patients at 1–3 months, but this fell to 79% at 12 months.[12] They concluded from follow-up evaluation that progressive separation or splitting of the trigone, with lateral drift of the orifices to their original position, was often the cause of failure.[13] Cartwright et al reported on a variation of this same concept (percutaneous endoscopic trigonoplasty) shortly after this initial report[14] (Figure 45.1). This series of 23 children had reasonable initial resolution rates that fell significantly, with long-term follow-up of 30–37 months, to an unimpressive 47%.

The Japanese group has continued to assess technical changes to their procedure. In 2003, they reported on a procedure involving incision around the orifice in a U-shaped fashion, thus making a more significant flap of ureter and bladder muscle.[15] This flap is

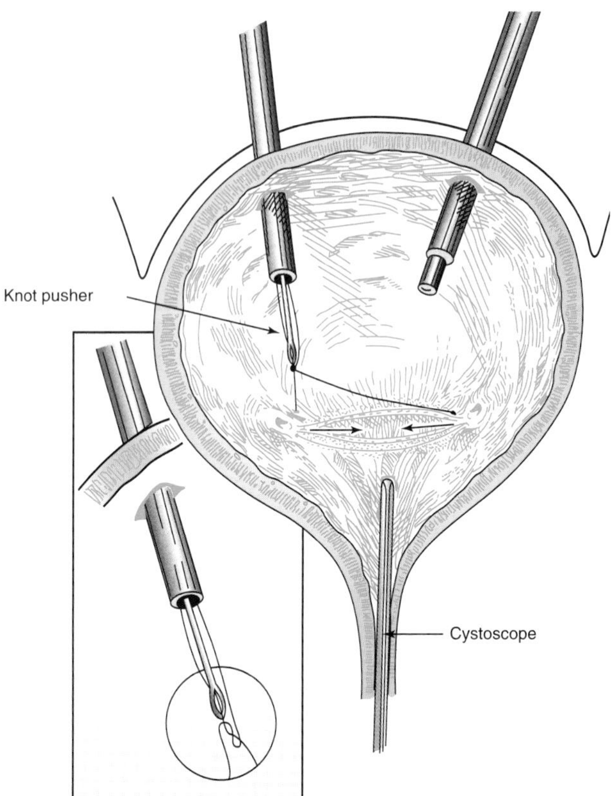

Figure 45.1 Percutaneous endoscopic trigonoplasty (PET): note the two working ports placed through the bladder wall superolaterally, and the cystoscope being used to assist and suction. Urothelium has been dissected, creating a muscular trough between the orifices; the suture being tied will advance each orifice toward the midline.

advanced distally onto the dissected trigone after the muscular hiatus is repaired to be certain that effective tunnel length is maximized. Reflux resolved in 12/14 ureters (86%) operated upon with mean operative time of 4 hours. We (Cartwright and Snow) also changed our original approach seeking better results. In 1999, we reported an intravesical cross-trigonal (Cohen) reimplant performed with the same two transvesical ports and a cystoscope[16] (Figure 45.2). This was performed in eight patients, with 83% long-term resolution. These results were more encouraging but are still significantly inferior to open approaches.

More recently, there have been three reports on intravesical laparoscopic approaches to reimplantation. Gill et al documented a cross-trigonal reimplant technique in three patients with operative times of 2.5–4.5 hours and no reflux postoperatively in two of the three patients.[17] Yeung and colleagues, as well, have reported on a laparoscopic Cohen reimplant done inside the bladder in 16 children (23 ureters).[18]

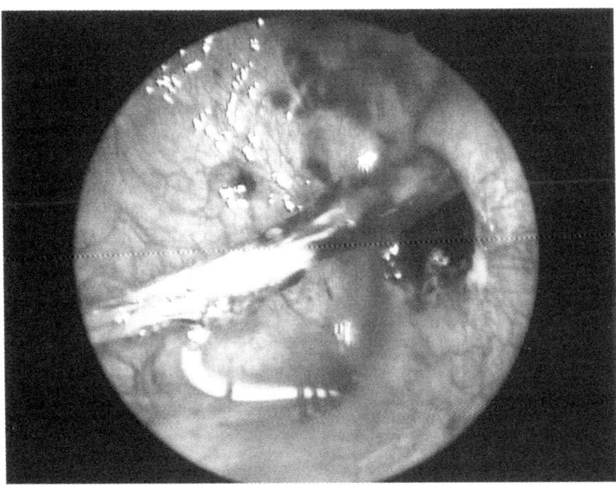

Figure 45.2 Intravesical view of a ureter mobilized via transvesical ports. The stent is coming through the bladder neck to enter the ureteral orifice; 3–4 cm of ureteral mobility can be achieved.

They report operative times of 1.9–3 hours for bilateral cases and had one conversion to open for trocar displacement from the bladder. They found minimal long-term complications, and patients had a mean hospital stay of 1.9 days, with a Foley catheter in place for 1–2 days.[19] The resolution rate was 96% at 3–4 month follow-up cystogram. Peters and Woo very recently added their experience with the da Vinci surgical robot in performing intravesical reimplantation. The ports required are 10–12 mm, with the sites dissected enough to place a suture into the bladder wall to prevent perivesical insufflation and to facilitate closure once the port is removed. Operating on 6 children with no open conversion, 2–4 day hospital stay, and 24-hour catheterization, they had 1 bladder leak from a port-site closure, and 5/6 with resolved reflux on early follow-up and no ureteral obstruction. For many of these authors, one challenge was getting secure closure at the bladder wall level once a port was removed; this was probably the cause for at least overnight catheter drainage in many cases. Another challenge noted by two of the authors was eventual accumulation of carbon dioxide within the perivesical space and a resultant decrease in intravesical working space as bladder walls were forced inward.

Future direction

Optics, instruments, and our own understanding and technical abilities with laparoscopic ureteral reimplantation will all undoubtedly improve over time. Smaller scars, less pain, and quicker recovery are all potential benefits of laparoscopic reimplantation, but these seem most pronounced in older children, adolescents, and adults and may be less apparent in younger children. Our own recent experience with open, unilateral, extravesical reimplantation is that 93% of children can be managed as outpatients, with a mean total hospital stay of just over 6 hours.[20] It seems likely that laparoscopic reimplants will need to be routinely achievable on an outpatient basis and without stents or catheters if they are to become mainstream in our management of reflux for the younger group of children that we most commonly treat.

References

1. Lich RH Jr, Howerton LW, Davis LA. Recurrent urosepsis in children. J Urol 1961; 86:554–8.
2. Atala A, Kavoussi LR, Goldstein DS, Retik AB, Peters CA. Laparoscopic correction of vesicoureteral reflux. J Urol 1993; 150:748–51.
3. Schimberg W, Wacksman J, Rudd R, Lewis AG, Sheldon CA. Laparoscopic correction of vesicoureteral reflux in the pig. J Urol 1994; 151:1664–7.
4. McDougall EM, Urban DA, Kerbl K et al. Laparoscopic repair of vesicoureteral reflux utilizing the Lich–Grégoir technique in the pig model. J Urol 1995; 153:497–500.
5. Ehrlich RM, Gershman A, Fuchs G. Laparoscopic vesicoureteroplasty in children: initial case reports. Urology 1994; 43:255–61.
6. Janetschek G, Radmayr C, Bartsch G. Laparoscopic ureteral anti-reflux plasty reimplantation. First clinical experience. Ann Urol (Paris) 1995; 29:101–5.
7. Lakshmanan Y, Fung LC. Laparoscopic extravesicular ureteral reimplantation for vesicoureteral reflux: recent technical advances. J Endourol 2000; 14:589–93, discussion, 593–4.
8. Fung LCT. Laparoscopic ureteral reimplantation: an extravesical approach. Dialog Pediatr Urol 2001; 24(10): 4–6.
9. Shu T, Cisek LJ Jr, Moore RG. Laparoscopic extravesical reimplantation for postpubertal vesicoureteral reflux. J Endourol 2004; 18:441–6.
10. Peters CA, Borer JG, Bauer SB. Robotically assisted laparoscopic antireflux surgery in children. Abstract 562, AUA National Meeting, May 2005.
11. Gil-Vernet JM. A new technique for surgical correction of vesicoureteral reflux. J Urol 1984; 131:456–8.
12. Okamura K, Ono Y, Yamada Y et al. Endoscopic trigonoplasty for primary vesico-ureteric reflux. Br J Urol 1995; 75:390–4.
13. Okamura K, Kato N, Takamura S et al. Trigonal splitting is a major complication of endoscopic trigonoplasty at 1-year followup. J Urol 1997; 157:1423–5.
14. Cartwright PC, Snow BW, Mansfield J, Hamilton BD. Percutaneous endoscopic trigonoplasty: a minimally

invasive approach to correct vesicoureteral reflux. J Urol 1996; 156:661–4.
15. Tsuji Y, Okamura K, Nishimura T et al. A new endoscopic ureteral reimplantation for primary vesicoureteral reflux (endoscopic trigonoplasty II). J Urol 2003; 169:1020–2.
16. Gatti J, Cartwright PC, Hamilton BD, Snow BW. Percutaneous endoscopic trigonoplasty in children: long-term outcomes and modifications in technique. J Endourol 1999; 13:581–4.
17. Gill IS, Ponsky LE, Desai M, Kay R, Ross JH. Laparoscopic cross-trigonal Cohen ureteroneocystostomy: novel technique. J Urol 2001; 166:1811–14.
18. Yeung CK, Sihoe JD, Borzi PA. Endoscopic cross-trigonal ureteral reimplantation under carbon dioxide bladder insufflation: a novel technique. J Endourol 2005; 19:295–9.
19. Peters CA, Woo R. Intravesical robotically assisted bilateral ureteral reimplantation. J Endourol 2005; 19: 618–21, discussion 621–2.
20. Putman S, Wicher C, Wayment R et al. Unilateral extravesical ureteral reimplantation in children performed on an outpatient basis. J Urol 2005; 174:1987–90.

Injection therapy for vesicoureteral reflux

46

Anthony A Caldamone

Introduction

Vesicoureteral reflux (VUR), the most common urologic abnormality in children, occurs in 0.4–1% of the general population and in 30–50% of those children who present with urinary tract infections (UTIs).[1] When correction of VUR is determined to be necessary, historically open ureteral reimplantation by a variety of techniques has been the mainstay of treatment. This approach is justified because surgical correction affords a very high success rate, approaching 99% in experienced hands, and a low complication rate.[2]

The search for a less-invasive approach to the correction of reflux, however, dates back to 1981 when Matouschek[3] first described the injection of polytetrafluoroethylene (PTFE) at the ureteral orifice to correct VUR. Reports then followed by McDonald and McDonald.[4] Following reports of the use of PTFE for incontinence, Politano reported on its use in VUR.[5–8] Puri and O'Donnell brought this clinical concept to the laboratory and demonstrated the successful correction of experimentally produced VUR in a piglet model by the intravesical injection of PTFE.[9] In their classic article in 1986, they reported on the successful endoscopic correction of primary VUR in 103 ureters, achieving a success rate of 75% after a single injection.[10] They termed this technique the STING.

This approach earned widespread international acceptance but only sporadic usage in the United States because of the lack of Food and Drug Administration (FDA) approval. It was quite apparent, however, that the potential for revolutionizing the management of children with VUR was real. Although the procedure requires general anesthesia and possible repeat injections, the ease of treatment, lack of open surgery, and minimal hospitalization were extremely attractive in the pediatric population. However, the lack of demonstrated long-term safety and concerns raised in experimental and clinical settings on the potential migration of PTFE particles prohibited its widespread acceptance in the United States. It was quite clear, however, that while the material had its drawbacks, the technique itself was reproducible and reliable. The search was on, therefore, for a substance that would fulfill the following characteristics: ease of injection, maintenance of injected volume, minimal host response, no evidence of distant migration of material particles, maintenance of the injected mound without shifting, and biocompatibility. The mechanism for the endoscopic correction of VUR involves one or more of the following effects: (1) improved backing of the intramural ureter, (2) fixation of the ureterovesical junction (UVJ) to the trigone by spot welding, or (3) decreased caliber of the distal ureter.

In this chapter we will review the substances that have been used both experimentally and clinically for the endoscopic correction of reflux. In addition to the use of this technique for primary VUR, the applicability of the endoscopic correction technique to other reflux variations will also be discussed. Finally, as with any new technology, one must address the issue of whether this new technology changes the indications for surgical correction of VUR.

Technique of endoscopic injection

The technique of endoscopic injection for correction of VUR has changed little since it was first described by O'Donnell and Puri.[11] The technique is relatively independent of the material used, although variations in material properties do exist, which result in minor modifications in technique, as will be described. The technique is often referred to as the STING, an acronym for subtrigonal injection (Figure 46.1).

Under cystoscopic control, the orifices and bladder mucosa are inspected. Whereas the type of cystoscope

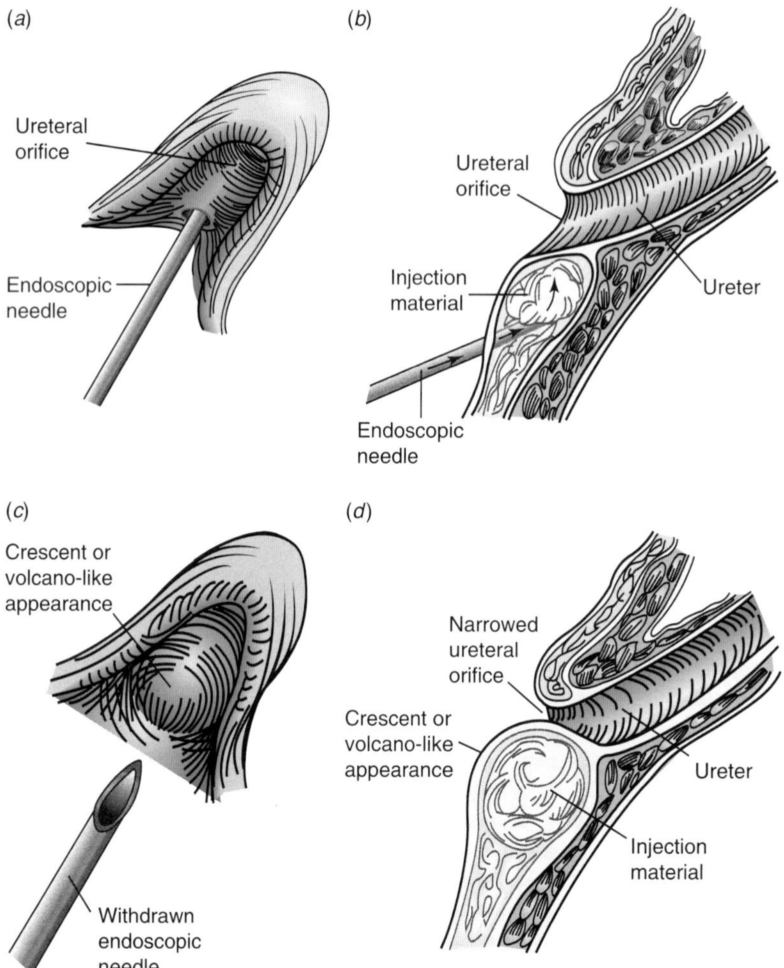

Figure 46.1 (*a*) Needle placed at 6 o'clock position, bevel upward. (*b*) Slow injection in subureteric space. (*c*) Postinjection appearance. (*d*) Appropriate position of injected material. (Reproduced from Russinko and Tackett,[12] with permission.)

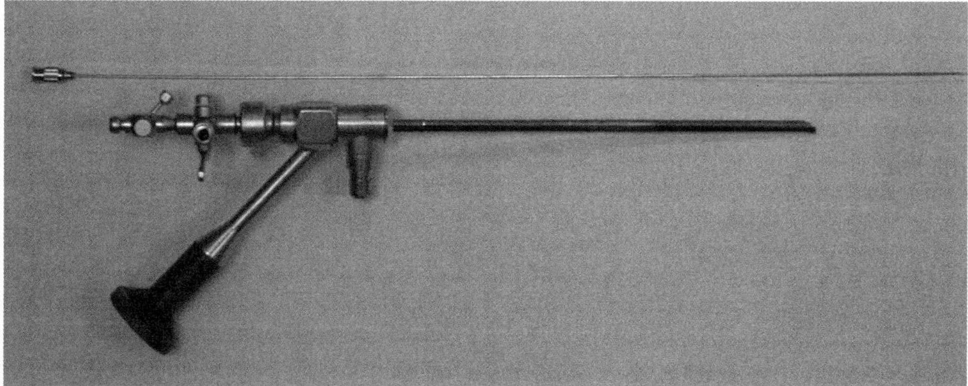

Figure 46.2 Offset lens 'STINGER' scope, allowing for a straight 4 Fr channel to pass a rigid or flexible needle for injection of material.

is not critical, an offset lens system allows for a straight route for the needle through the scope, which is helpful if using a metal needle (Figure 46.2). The degree of bladder filling is critical, as a full bladder may make it more difficult to accurately place the material behind the ureter and still be in the wall of

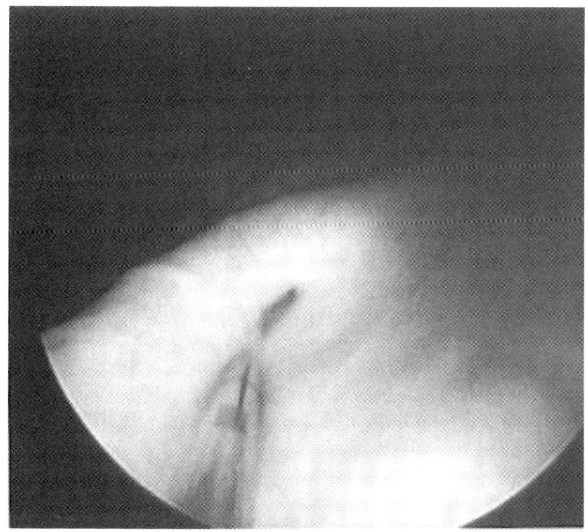

Figure 46.3 Needle in 6 o'clock position at left ureteral orifice.

the bladder. Either a rigid metal needle or a malleable needle may be used, most commonly 3.7–4 Fr in size. A syringe of material is fixed to the needle and, depending on the thickness of the material, a ratcheted metal syringe holder may be needed. This is necessary for PTFE and silicone, in particular. The needle is introduced through a cystoscope using a 0° or 30° lens. Under direct vision the needle is advanced bevel-up and introduced submucosally at the 6 o'clock position of the UVJ (Figure 46.3). Puri and O'Donnell originally reported piercing the mucosa 2–3 mm distal to the UVJ and advancing the needle 4–5 mm into the lamina propria of the submucosal portion of the ureter. Alternatively, for more gaping orifices, the needle can be placed directly through the mucosa at the UVJ. This can be facilitated by hydrodistention of the ureter, by having irrigation flowing through the cystoscope at the time of the injection and thus dilat-

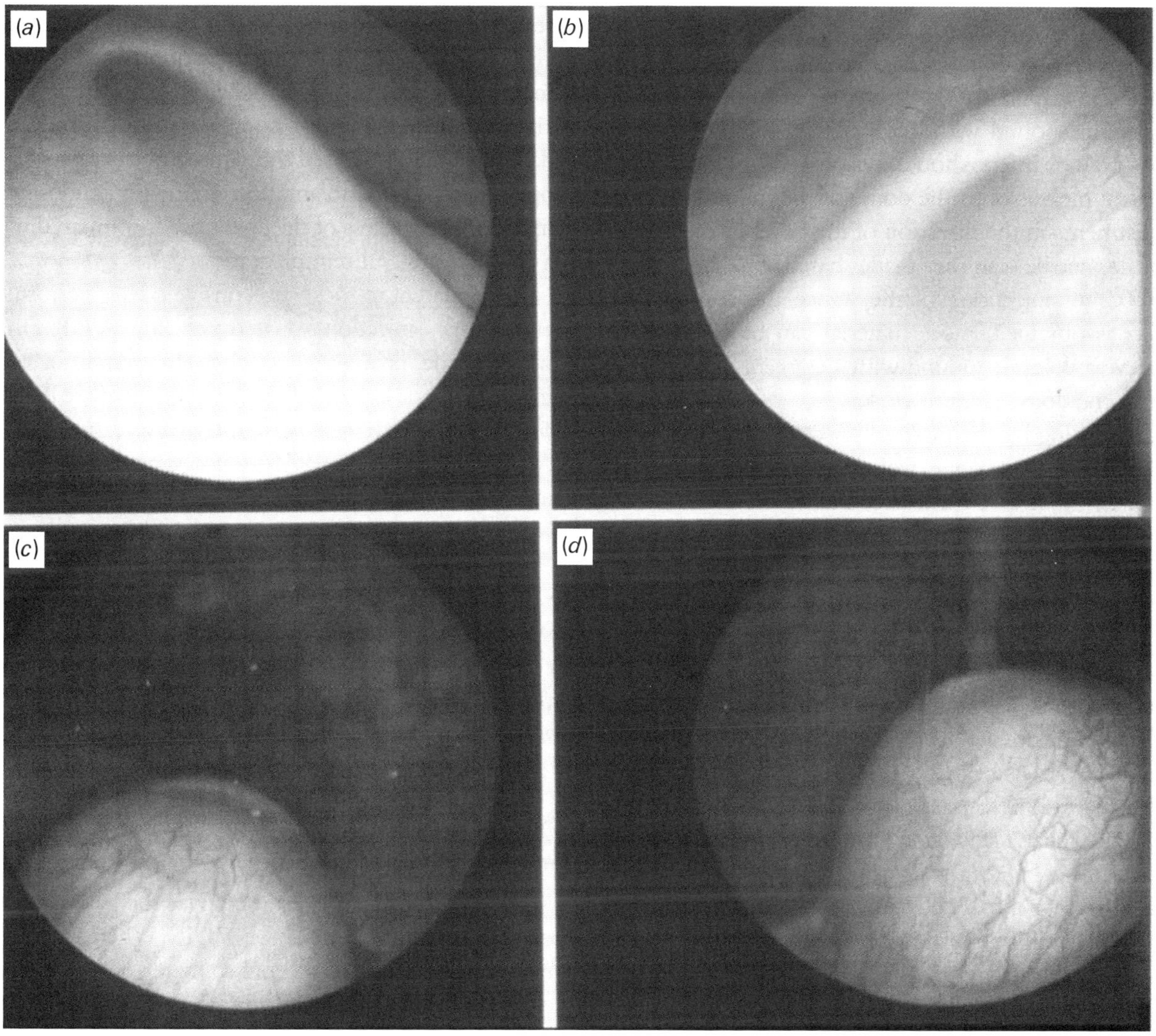

Figure 46.4 Endoscopic injection of calcium hydroxyl apatite. (*a* and *b*) Preinjection appearance of left and right orifice with bladder minimally filled, on top. (*c* and *d*) Left and right orifice postinjection, demonstrating a crescent appearance of orifice a top a mound of material.

years.[23,24] In this multicentered study the overall success rate in 6216 ureters and 4166 children treated at 18 European centers demonstrated a cure rate of 86% after 1–4 injections, with an obstruction rate of 0.0003%. In a 17-year follow-up of 247 patients treated with PTFE, Chertin et al demonstrated a sustained 95% success rate after 1–4 injections and a 5% recurrence rate, with 1.8% requiring open surgery.[25] In the meta-analysis review by Elder et al of 33 studies reporting on the results of PTFE, the overall success rate after a single injection was 67%.[26]

Experimental studies done shortly after the introduction of PTFE in clinical reports demonstrated the migratory property of PTFE as a result of a significant percentage of particles being <80 μm.[27,28] These particles become phagocytized and carried to regional lymph nodes or enter into capillaries directly upon injection. Experimental studies by Malizia et al have found particles in lymph nodes and distant organs.[29,30] Particle migration has also been reported in humans,[28,31–33] including, in a speculative report, to a child's cerebral microcirculation and associated with an ischemic stroke.[34] Some clinicians have argued that particle migration is at least partially related to the volume of injection; however, clinical reports indicate that particle migration has occurred with small volumes of 0.5 ml of PTFE.[35]

The potential of carcinogenesis with PTFE and other non-autologous substances has been of concern. Although there has not been direct evidence of carcinogenesis with PTFE in an experimental model,[36] there has been experimental evidence linking injected foreign substances of large particulate size to potential carcinogenesis.[37]

Cross-linked bovine collagen

Cross-linked bovine collagen has been used for multiple medical purposes such as cardiac valves, hemostatic agents, sutures, and as a soft tissue substitute. It is harvested from bovine hide and treated with pepsin to reduce its antigenicity associated with the telopeptides of the collagen helix. It is composed of 95% type I collagen and 5% type III collagen. It is cross-linked with glutaraldehyde to reduce breakdown after implantation by human collagenases. For human implantation, several products have become available (Contigen, Zyplast, Zyderm, GAX 35, GAX 65).

Upon injection, collagen causes very little local tissue reaction and no granuloma formation. To variable degrees, there is an ingrowth of fibroblasts and eventual replacement with native collagen.[38–40] The degree to which native collagen ingrowth occurs is thought to determine the potential for long-term cure.

Table 46.2 Results of endoscopic treatment of vesicoureteral reflux with collagen

Authors	No. of ureters treated	Percent success, after one injection
Lipsky and Würnschimmel[41]	79	68
Frey et al[42]	204	63
Reunanen et al[43]	197	84
Capozza et al[44]	184	78
Leonard et al[45]	45	75
Polito et al[46]	76	74
Haferkamp et al[47]	21	95
Haferkamp et al[48]	26	92
De Grazia and Cimador 2000[49]	129	74
Tsuboi et al[50]	8	–

Modified from Läckgren et al.[53]

Collagen is injected easily with finger pressure, with no special device required. However, as a result of this relatively low viscosity, precise injection may be more difficult. Preinjection skin testing is necessary, as 3% have a hypersensitivity reaction to collagen, although a negative reaction does not completely eliminate the risk of an allergic reaction.[41] As noted in Table 46.2, the initial success with the endoscopic injection of collagen is similar to that of other materials. However, several reports indicate poor sustained results. Haferkamp et al reported an initial success of 92% after a single injection in 36 children, with a recurrence of reflux in 91% after 37 months.[47] In a similar study, the recurrence rate was 63%.[48] The use of a more concentrated mixture of 65 mg collagen/ml (GAX 65) has shown promise of a more sustained cure in a report by Frey et al, where a 6-month evaluation postinjection demonstrated more retained volume, 26.9% vs 0.1% for GAX 35.[52] Reunanen et al reported on 197 ureters treated with endoscopically implanted collagen in which 84% remained without reflux at 4 years follow-up.[43] De Grazia and Cimador reported a 16.8% recurrence rate in 129 refluxing ureters injected, with higher rates of recurrence in the higher initial grades of VUR.[49]

Polydimethylsiloxane

This bulking agent is composed of particulate silicone in an injectable mixture of fully vulcanized polydimethylsiloxane (40%) suspended in a water-soluble polyvinylpyrrolidone (60%). The particulate size ranges from 35 to 540 μm (average 209 μm) with 28% <80 μm and 7% <50 μm.[53] It is not surprising, therefore, that studies by Buckley et al[54,55] and Henly et al[56] found particle migration to the lungs, kidneys, brain, and lymph nodes after injection in animal models. It has been shown that particulate size <80 μm facilitates particle migration.[29] Shedding of silicone particles with migration has been reported from implanted medical devices.[57] The advantage of particulate silicone is there appears to be less inflammatory response and granuloma formation, although those findings have not been consistent. Silicone is non-biodegradable and, therefore, should be permanent once injected at the UVJ. Similar to PTFE, a ratcheted mechanism is required for injection. The injection of silicone induces an inflammatory response with macrophages and fibroblasts and later ingrowth of collagen.[58]

Silicone has been implicated in autoimmune reactions[27,56] and associated with a possible risk of malignancy,[38,59–61] although the data for the latter have been inconsistent.[62] Multiple studies have demonstrated the reproduced effectiveness of injected particulate silicone to correct reflux.[53] Herz et al demonstrated a success rate of 81% after a single injection and 90% of ureters after repeated injection with a 12-month follow-up.[63] In a 1-year follow-up study from two centers, van Capelle et al reported success with the endoscopic implantation of silicone in 155/195 children treated, representing 82.3% of ureters injected one or more times.[64] Aboutaleb et al compared particulate silicone injection versus extravesical ureteral reimplantation for primary low-grade reflux (grades I–III) in 180 patients, 74 silicone injections and 106 extravesical reimplantations.[65] Of the injected group, 81% were cured at 3 months and 92% at last follow-up compared with 96% at 3 months and 99% at 1 year in the reimplantation group. There were no complications in the injected population, whereas 7% of the reimplanted group had postoperative complications, including 3.3% (2 patients) with transient urinary retention. In summary, silicone appears to be an effective agent for the treatment of VUR. Concerns remain regarding its particle size, and, therefore, its migratory potential, as noted in experimental studies.

Dextranomer/hyaluronic acid copolymer

Dextranomer microspheres were first introduced by Stenberg and Lackgren in experimental models in which 1 ml was placed into the abdominal wall of rats and into the bladder wall of piglets.[66] At 3 months, the implants became encapsulated, with a 23% reduction of the injected volume. Repeat studies performed with radiolabeled dextranomer spheres demonstrated no evidence of distant migration, lymphadenopathy, mutagenic effect, DNA changes, or tumor development.[67] The larger particulate size of the dextranomer/hyaluronic acid (Dx/HA) copolymer compared with PTFE and silicone is thought to account for the fact that it is not phagocytized, and, therefore, its lack of particulate migration to distant organs.

The Dx/HA copolymer is a solution of cross-linked dextranomer microspheres (80–250 μm in diameter) suspended in a carrier gel of stabilized sodium hyaluronate.[51] Dextranomers have found previous uses in medicine for wound healing, and sodium hyaluronate has been used for eye surgery and joint injection. The Dx/HA copolymer differs from other non-autologous materials such as PTFE and silicone in that it is biodegradable. Its volume stability over time results from fibroblast migration and collagen ingrowth between the dextranomer microspheres (Figure 46.7), as the hyaluronate dissipates 12 weeks after implantation.[68] It is injected with a standard syringe mounted on an endoscopic needle with finger pressure. In animal studies, carried out for 3 years, the durability of the spheres has been demonstrated without granuloma formation or calcification.[66,69]

The overall results with Dx/HA copolymer compare favorably with that of PTFE and silicone, as

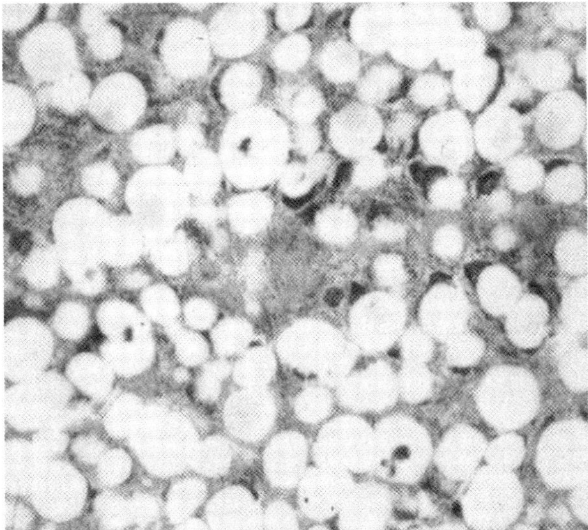

Figure 46.7 Ingrowth of native fibroblasts around dextranomer microspheres. (Reproduced from Stenberg et al,[68] with permission.)

Table 46.3 Results of the endoscopic treatment of vesicoureteral reflux with the dextranomer/hyaluronic acid (Dx/HA) copolymer

Authors	No. of ureters treated	Percent success, after one injection
Stenberg and Läckgren[66]	115	69
Capozza et al[70]	52	71
Oswald[71]	55	77
Läckgren et al[14]	334	75[a]
Puri[72]	166	>86
Kirsch[15]	134	72
Capozza et al[46]	1050	82[a]

[a] Reported only after multiple injections.

noted in Table 46.3, which lists the results after a single injection. In a long-term follow-up study by Läckgren et al of 221 children followed for a mean of 5 years, 68% of patients (75% ureters) maintained grade 1 VUR or less and 81% (85% ureters) grade 2 VUR or less at the last VCUG done. Of 49 patients who had a VCUG at 3–12 months, reflux recurred in 13%, 4% of which were grade 3 or greater.[14] No long-term adverse effects were noted, with 2% developing postoperative UTIs, and early mild postoperative hydronephrosis occurring in 4 patients, none of whom developed signs of ureteral obstruction. In a study comparing Dx/HA copolymer and silicone, Oswald et al reported a slightly higher success rate with silicone, but the difference was not statistically significant.[71]

Coaptite

Calcium hydroxylapatite is composed of calcium hydroxylapatite spheres suspended in a water and glycerin mixture with 3% methylcellulose gel. Calcium hydroxylapatite particles are synthetic, and, therefore, a uniform spherical shape with a narrow range of 75–125 μm. This material represents synthetic bone, and, therefore, as a subureteric bulking agent, theoretically it should have a limited local reaction and a very durable long-term effect. A clinical trial by Mevorach et al on 98 patients and 155 ureters with grade II–IV reflux demonstrated reflux resolution in 67% of patients and 75% of ureters, and improvement was noted in 77% of patients and 84% of ureters.[73] Interestingly 5 patients in this particular subgroup demonstrated progression, from improvement in reflux grade postinjection at 1 year to reflux resolution when evaluated with a VCUG at 2 years. The procedure was tolerated well by all patients and there were no significant safety issues disclosed. Calcium hydroxylapatite, therefore, is determined to be a safe, durable, and effective material for the endoscopic treatment of reflux, although at this time clinical trials are still being evaluated by the FDA.

Autologous materials

Autologous materials have the appeal of not having the concern of a foreign body reaction to the injected mound. The disadvantage, however, is the need for a harvesting step, which, with all materials tried to date in the pediatric population, requires an additional anesthetic. These autologous materials must behave as free grafts, and, therefore, are subject to the physiology of graft survival. To date, the autologous materials that have been tried are chondrocytes, collagen, and fat.

Chondrocytes

Following demonstration that the harvesting and subsequent implantation of autologous chondrocytes resulted in viable chondrocytes, first in the mouse model and later in the pig model by Atala,[74,75] Diamond and Caldamone used harvested chondrocytes in the human model.[76,77] Chondrocytes were harvested from the posterior auricular cartilage, grown in culture for 6 weeks, suspended in an aqueous mixture of alginate and calcium salts, and subsequently injected at the UVJ. Long-term results of 47 ureters with grade II–IV VUR demonstrated an 80% cure rate at 3 months and an 86% cure rate at 1 year following one or more implantations. In those children requiring a subsequent open ureteral reimplantation, no viable chondrocytes were identified, however. It was unclear whether the failure to correct the reflux was attributed to a failure of chondrocytes survival, or whether this was a more universal effect. In those children who underwent a second injection or open reimplantation after a failed injection, the most common findings were shifting of the materials and a loss of material volume.[77]

Fat

Autologous fat has been used as an implant for correction of reflux. It was initially reported in an experimental model by Matthews in 1994, followed by clinical reports by Palma and Chancellor.[78–80] In

Table 46.4 Overall resolution rate after single injection based on ureter and material

Agent	Number in studies	Sample	Percent resolution
Poly/tetrafluoroethylene	33	3616	66.9
Collagen	10	947	56.9
Dextranomer	3	385	68.7
Polydimethylsiloxane	8	347	76.5
Chondrocytes	1	47	50.5
Blood	1	13	5.0

From Elder et al.[26]

Table 46.5 Overall resolution rate after single injection based on reflux grade by ureters for all materials

Grade	Number in studies	Sample	Percent resolution
1	16	117	78.5
2	18	444	78.5
3	22	477	72.3
4	17	172	62.6[a]
5	9	25	50.9[a]

[a] Grade 4 and 5 significantly decreased with respect to grades 1 and 2.
From Elder et al.[26]

follow-up studies at 3 months postimplantation, reflux persisted in 70% of Chancellor's study group and 83% of Palma's group. Viability appears to rely on vascular ingrowth to the injected cells and, therefore, small volumes injected appear to be more effective in survival. In the rabbit model by Matthews, there was a 25–100% loss of volume postinjection in 47% of sites injected.[78]

Collagen

Cendron et al reported on the use of autologous collagen as an injectable material for correction of VUR.[81] The rationale for the use of autologous collagen is to improve on the longevity of bovine collagen preparations, as well as to avoid the hypersensitivity potential. Collagen fibers were isolated by centrifuge from the dermis. In an experimental study, collagen integrity was demonstrated at 50 days.

Muscle

Autologous bladder muscle cells have been used in an experimental study to correct reflux.[82] Muscle cells were harvested from the bladder, coupled with an alginate mixture, and reinjected through a 21-gauge needle. Cell survival was demonstrated in a short-duration study.

Cumulative results

Endoscopic treatment for VUR in children has a high success rate (Table 46.4). The success rate is universally proportional to the grade of reflux treated (Table 46.5). Multiple injections are advantageous in increasing the success rate and prior endoscopic material implantation does not appear to significantly alter the open surgical success rate.

Special considerations

Neuropathic bladder

A significant number of patients, upwards of 50%, with spina bifida have associated VUR. This can be a cause of significant morbidity and renal damage in this population. The mainstay of management of VUR in association with a neurogenic bladder has been modulation of bladder pressures and frequent complete emptying. This is usually accomplished by a combination of intermittent catheterization with or without the addition of anticholinergic therapy and/or suppressive antibiotics. When children fail this regimen, treatment has been bladder augmentation with or without ureteral reimplantation. Some articles

Table 46.6 Results of reported series of the endoscopic treatment of vesicoureteral reflux in children with neuropathic bladder

Authors	Material	No. of ureters	Success rate after one or more injections	Recurrence rate per corrected ureter
Haferkamp et al[48]	Collagen	26	24/26	15%
Granata et al[83]	Polytetrafluoroethylene	40	72.5%	2/29
Engel et al[84]	Polytetrafluoroethylene	60	56.7%	–
Misra et al[85]	Polydimethylsiloxane	69	82%	4/57
Yokoyama et al[86]	Collagen	13	100%	5/13
Sugiyama et al[87]	Polytetrafluoroethylene	4	75%	–
Kaminetsky and Hanna[88]	Polytetrafluoroethylene	20	70%	–
Dewan and Guiney[89]	Polytetrafluoroethylene	29	23/29	4/23
Puri and Guiney[90]	Polytetrafluoroethylene	15	12/15	–
Perez-Brayfield et al[91]	Dextranomer	9	78%	–

have advocated the addition of endoscopic correction of reflux to the armamentarium for management of VUR in the setting of the neurogenic bladder (Table 46.6). Technically, this can be more difficult to perform because of the trabeculation of the bladder, and a ureteral catheter in the orifice at the time may facilitate injection. However, in spite of these difficulties, success has been reported in up to 90% of cases after multiple injections.[85,90,92,93] Engel et al reported success in 57% of reflux in ureters after a single injection of PTFE and 62% after a second injection.[84] They compared this to their open surgical population, in which they were able to achieve an 84% success rate in 30 patients undergoing ureteral reimplantation. Haferkamp et al found that the long-term success rate using collagen (GAX 35) was only 15% of treated units after 24 months.[48] Part of that fall off in success rate could be a result of the degeneration of collagen, but also may result from the inherent neuropathic disorder. It is imperative that, once these children are treated endoscopically or with open surgery, continued bladder management is carried out in order to prevent long-term complications such as the recurrence of reflux or functional UVJ obstruction. Similarly, Dewan and Guiney reported 4 of 23 successfully treated ureters recurred after initial treatment was successful.[89] Granata et al reported a comparative study on surgical and endoscopic correction of reflux in children with a neuropathic bladder.[83] They found an overall success rate of 72.5% using PTFE, compared with 95.5% when a Cohen cross-trigonal ureteroneocystotomy was performed. They found that 2 of their 29 ureters that were cured with the endoscopic approach reccurred with VUR; however, both were treated successfully by a repeat endoscopic procedure. There were no recurrences observed in the patients cured by open reimplantation. In a meta-analysis recorded by Elder et al of 10 articles, there was a significantly lower rate of success of the endoscopic approach in the neuropathic bladder (53.5%) vs the non-neuropathic bladder (74.2%).[26]

Dysfunctional voiding

Studies by Frey,[38] Trsinar,[94] and Capozza[44,95] have implicated undisclosed dysfunctional voiding as a cause of failure of endoscopic correction of VUR. In each of these cases the authors found displacement of the mound, a common occurrence using either collagen or dextranomer microspheres. In each of these studies, however, the diagnosis of dysfunctional voiding was based on clinical history and not urodynamic findings, representing some limitation to their conclusion. The implication from these studies, therefore, would be to control or at least stabilize the dysfunctional voiding prior to the endoscopic correction of the reflux. Several studies have pointed out that management of dysfunctional voiding in refluxers improves the spontaneous resolution rate and decreases the need for ureteral reimplantation.[96,97] Lackgren and Stenberg noted, however, that when the endoscopic correction of reflux in children with dysfunctional elimination syndrome was undertaken, they found an overall cure rate of 65% across all grades of reflux, indicating no particular difference as to whether or not preinjection bladder retraining had been undertaken.[98] Of 35 patients that were cured of their reflux on a single injection, 8 continued to have evidence of minor bladder dysfunction, whereas 27 appeared to have completely resolved their symptoms of bladder dysfunction. This may indicate a potential role of the reflux in either the causation or the promotion of bladder dysfunction in this particular population.

Duplicated systems

More experience is being gained in the use of injectable materials for duplicated systems. At one time, a duplicated system was considered to be a relative contraindication to the use of injectable material;[99] however, several reports have now indicated that, with experience, the success rate for the endoscopic correction of reflux in the duplicated system approaches that of a single system. Miyakita et al[101] reported on their results with the use of PTFE in both partial and complete duplication. Their success rates were 87% in partial duplication and 59% in complete duplication. Similarly, Steinbrecher et al reported a cure rate of 68% in completely duplicated systems using PTFE.[101] Dewan and O'Donnell reported on 32 children with duplex systems and VUR treated endoscopically with PTFE.[102] They were able to cure VUR in 21/32 patients. In the meta-analysis by Elder et al, the success rate of endoscopic correction for duplicated systems was 50% compared with 73% for non-duplicated systems.[26] Perez-Brayfield et al reported a 73% success rate in using dextranomer microspheres for the endoscopic correction of reflux and completely duplicated systems.[91] Lackgren et al reported on the use of Dx/HA copolymer and duplicated systems, and found a 63% success rate, defined by improvement to grade 0–1.[103]

It should be pointed out, however, that the technique of the injection varies with the anatomy. For those completely duplicated systems in which there is wide separation of the ureteral orifices, and, therefore, more likely to reflux just to the lower pole, separate injections under each orifice are recommended. However, for those duplicated systems where the orifices are closely approximated, a single injection may suffice (Figure 46.8).

Aboutaleb et al compared the results with polydimethylsiloxane injection vs open surgery for the treatment of VUR in duplex systems.[104] The open surgical approach for reflux in this study was extravesical common sheath ureteral reimplantation. The endoscopic injection of polydimethylsiloxane was performed in 15 patients with 22 refluxing units. The success rate for the endoscopic correction was 68% at

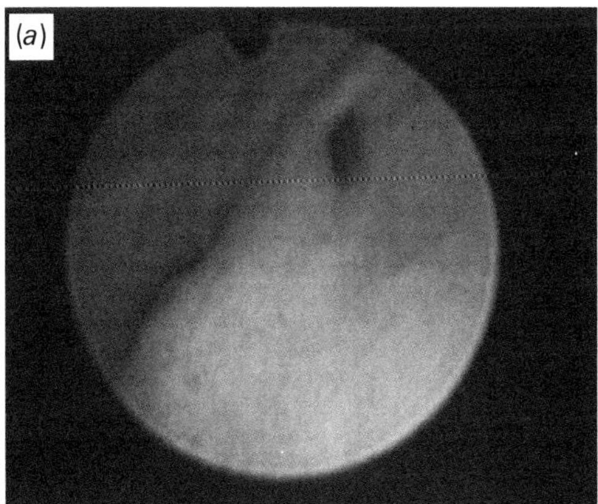

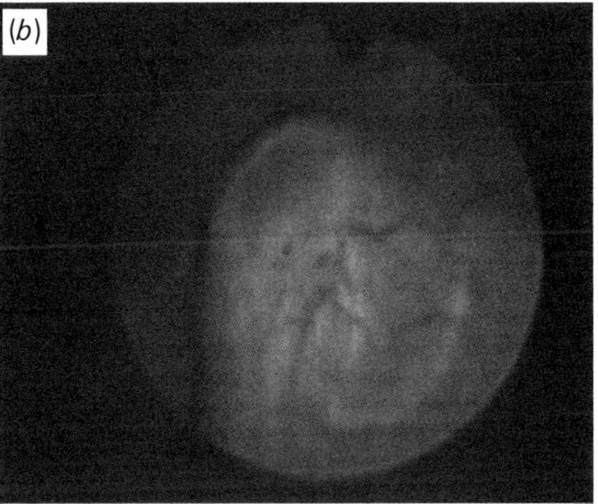

Figure 46.8 (*a*) Duplicated left ureters with lower pole reflux. (*b*) Mound under lower pole refluxing orifice.

3 months, 82% at 12 months, with 1 patient developing contralateral VUR. There were no cases of de-novo hydronephrosis or UTIs postoperatively. This compared with the success rate of extravesical common sheath ureteral reimplantation of 96% at 3 months and 97% at 15 months. The authors concluded that whereas injection therapy was highly successful in patients with low-grade VUR in duplex systems, it still fell short of the open surgical cure rate.

Paraureteric diverticulum with VUR

Bladder diverticulum can be found in association with VUR. Whereas those diverticulae which are small have a similar spontaneous resolution rate as primary VUR, moderate to large diverticulae, which usually lie lateral and cephalad to the ureteric orifice, will often drag the orifice into the diverticula on filling or voiding. This relationship portends a poor spontaneous resolution rate. The presence of a paraureteric diverticulum that is associated with reflux presents a significant challenge to the accurate placement of material at the UVJ endoscopically. Perez-Brayfield et al[91] report on six such cases, with a respectable success rate of 67% using the Dx/HA copolymer. It appears that with experience, therefore, the presence of a paraureteric diverticulum represents only a relative contraindication to endoscopic treatment. Puri and Lackgren (pers comm) have stated that a modified technique to this anatomy is needed, in which the material is injected beneath the ureteric orifice for a longer length into the diverticulum.

The refluxing ureteral stump

There have been isolated reports of success using the endoscopic approach for the refluxing ectopic ureter, refluxing ureteral stump, and reflux after transurethral ureterocele incision.[91,105,106] The results in the ectopic ureter, however, have been very disappointing to date.[92] This may also be true for the refluxing stump, which is often ectopic at or below the bladder neck, although there have only been a few reported cases.[106,107]

Failed ureteral reimplantation

From the report of the American Urological Association Pediatric Vesicoureteral Reflux Guidelines Panel, the success rate for correction of reflux by open ureteral reimplantation ranges from 80 to 99%, based on the grade of reflux.[107] Overall, the incidence of persistent reflux is generally 2% and the incidence of ureteral obstruction is 2%. Reoperation for the failed ureteral reimplantation can be a difficult procedure, with a significant complication rate.[108] There have been reports on the use of the endoscopic approach to reflux correction for the failed ureteral reimplantation.[91,109–111]

Kumar and Puri reported on 31 children with persistent reflux with 40 persistently refluxing units after failed ureteral reimplantation.[109] These patients represented a diverse group of refluxers, including primary refluxers, duplicated systems, reflux secondary to neuropathic bladder, posterior urethral valves, ureterocele, bladder exstrophy, and UVJ obstruction. Twenty-seven of 40 persistently refluxing units were cured after a single injection of PTFE, 7 refluxing units required two injections, and 4 required three injections for correction of the reflux. Failure to correct reflux by endoscopic correction was noted in 2 ureters of one patient with bladder exstrophy. In the report by Gaschignard et al, 1 of 12 patients developed a late meatal stricture, occurring 2 years after endoscopic correction following a failed ureteral reimplantation.[111] Perez-Brayfield et al reported on 17 patients who had failed open surgical correction of reflux. The success rate with endoscopic correction in this group was 88%.[91] Capozza et al reported success in 12 of 18 ureters with endoscopic treatment after failed ureteral reimplantation.[44] In a review of 9 studies and 80 ureters, Elder et al reported a cumulative success rate of 65% for endoscopic injection after failed ureteral reimplantation, compared with 74% in the non-reimplanted ureter.[26]

Complications

The risk/benefit ratio for endoscopic correction of reflux remains very low. Specific complications related to inherent material properties have been mentioned, such as particle migration with PTFE and with polydimethylsiloxane. Other specific concerns have been raised, such as malignant degeneration with PTFE or the development of connective tissue disorders with polydimethylsiloxane.[61,112–115]

More generic complications, such as ureteric obstruction, have been reported infrequently. Engel et al reported obstruction in a single ureter after the endoscopic implantation of PTFE in their series of 60 injected ureters.[84] In the reported series by Capozza et al of 1244 patients injected with a variety of materials, 8 (0.006%) developed temporary obstruction, 2 requiring a double-J stent.[44] In their meta-analysis, Elder et al noted a very low incidence of post-injection hydronephrosis (Table 46.7).[26] Other outcomes such as UTIs, febrile or not, do not appear to occur with an increased frequency over that seen with open ureteral reimplantations: 6.4% in a meta-analysis of 11 studies, 0.7% for febrile UTI, and 6% for cystitis.[26]

The development of contralateral denovo VUR following reflux correction may be troublesome.[116] Studies by Ross et al indicate a 35% risk of contralateral VUR after unilateral open correction if there has been a remote history of contralateral VUR.[117] Hoenig et al reported an incidence of contralateral VUR occurring in 17% of cases after unilateral open correction similar to that reported by other surgeons.[116,118–120] Following the endoscopic correction of reflux with PTFE, Kumar and Puri reported the contralateral denovo VUR rate to be much lower, at 7%.[121] Similarly, Kirsch et al reported its occurrence in 4.5% with Dx/HA copolymer.[15] This would led credence to the theory of trigonal distortion during open reimplantation rather than a pop-off mechanism theory as the etiology for denovo postoperative VUR.[122]

Table 46.7 De-novo postinjection hydronephrosis based on material used: a meta-analysis

Material	Denovo hydronephrosis/total number[a]	No. requiring intervention[a]
Polytetrafluoroethylene	34/3616	19
Collagen	2/947	0
Polydimethylsiloxane	4/347	3
Dextranomer	2/385	2

[a] From Elder et al.[26]

Recurrence of vesicoureteral reflux

Recurrence after proven correction of reflux remains an issue with certain materials. The difficulty is determining a firm and reliable figure for this, as only selected series have performed a VCUG beyond the initial negative study. In addition, one must distinguish between a maintained clinical cure (i.e. no febrile UTIs) and a proven long-term cure by a negative VCUG. Chertin et al reported on 247 patients who were treated for VUR with PTFE and followed for 17 years.[25] They reported a recurrence rate of 5%, with 1.8% requiring open ureteral reimplantation. Capozza et al reported on their long-term experiences with bulking agents – specifically PTFE, collagen, and dextranomer – in 1244 patients, all of whom had a VCUG at 3 and 12 months postinjection. They found that a significant percentage of those patients who relapsed had evidence of voiding dysfunction by micturation questionnaire.[44] Lackgren et al reported their long-term results with the use of Dx/HA copolymer in 221 children who had a VCUG at 3 and 12 months postinjection.[14] In addition, a later VCUG was performed in 49 patients 2–5 years after initial treatment. Reflux on the late VCUG occurred in 13% of those previously cured. It is unclear how many, if any, of those late recurrences were symptomatic.

Haferkamp et al reported on the use of a second collagen injection in 16 children with 21 ureters, with a failed first injection.[48] They found that the reflux was cured after a second injection in 17/21 ureters. Of those cured with a second injection, a repeat VCUG was performed every 6 months, with a mean follow-up of 11 months. Of these patients, 8 ureters remained reflux free, whereas in 9 units the reflux recurred. The authors noted that the interval to recurrence of reflux was longer after the second injection compared with the first injection. In a similar report, Haferkamp et al found that of 55 renal units successfully treated with collagen, only 5 (9%) remained reflux free after 37 months of follow-up.[48] Other studies have shown a more modest recurrence rate of 11–16%.[49] In a report of 132 children, Frey et al reported late reflux recurrence in 11.3% of 204 renal units treated with GAX 35 collagen.[42] In the meta-analysis study by Elder et al, the probability of recurrence for all agents used was 8%.[26] Overall, it appears that collagen carries a higher recurrence rate than other bulking agents that have been followed with a VCUG beyond 1 year postinjection, with the lowest recurrence rate from PTFE.

Reasons for failure of endoscopic treatment

Whereas most series have demonstrated a high success rate for the endoscopic subureteric injection for the treatment of VUR, very few have discussed the reasons for failure. The mechanisms of failure of endoscopic correction of reflux can be divided into three categories:

- technical factors
- bladder dynamics issues
- individual physical properties of the particular material used.

Technical factors include anatomic abnormalities of the UVJ or bladder, including duplicated systems, paraureteric diverticulum, a trabeculated bladder, either from neuropathic origin, or obstructive origin, be it functional or anatomic, or a previously reimplanted ureter. In addition, the position of the orifice can certainly be influenced by the degree of fullness of the bladder, making the injection zone for the material larger or smaller. It is also theoretically possible that – with the bladder relatively empty at the time of the injection, as is the standard recommendation – when the bladder fills, the mound and orifice may not have the same relationship to each other.

Factors relative to bladder dynamics include scenarios where elevated bladder pressure is present, such as seen in the neuropathic bladder, the previously obstructed bladder, or in dysfunctional voiding. It is theoretically possible that in the face of elevated bladder pressures from whatever etiology, the shifting of the mound may be possible from the pressure itself. Capozza et al implied that voiding dysfunction could contribute to endoscopic injection failure.[44] They theorized that elevated intravesical pressures could displace or shift the injection mound or cause migration from the original site of implantation. They found, in retrospect, that a high percentage of those patients that had failed initial endoscopic treatment had evidence of voiding dysfunction on clinical evaluation. Therefore they advocated that voiding dysfunction be addressed prior to undertaking the endoscopic treatment for reflux. Trsinar et al also observed displacement of failed injection mounds and theorized that this was due to voiding dysfunction, although there were no urodynamic studies or voiding diaries presented.[94]

Specific material properties may also play a role in the failure of endoscopic correction of reflux. Materials that have been utilized have a variable degree of longevity. Loss of material can occur either by absorption of the carrier substance that is used for the specific material, as seen with glycerol for PTFE, hyaluronic acid with dextranomer particles, alginate solution with chondrocytes, or aqueous gel with calcium hydroxylapatite. These materials will be absorbed in a variable amount of time from the implant site, decrease the site of the injection mound, and, therefore, possibly hinder the mechanism for ureteral closure or insufficient support of the intramural ureter. In addition, there is an intrinsic material biodegradability that plays a role with certain substances. Collagen is known to have a significant loss of volume over time and its long-term success is thought to be due to the development of natural collagen to replace the resorbed injected collagen. Haferkamp et al[49] demonstrated a low rate of long-term success with collagen in that after 37 months only 5 out of 57 ureters previously corrected with a single injection remained cured. Similarly, dextranomer microspheres have some degree of biodegradability, which eventually should be replaced by the ingrowth of native fibroblasts.

The ability of a particular material to weld at the injection site may be a factor in the long-term success as well. Materials that tend to create an inflammatory response may be more likely to stick to the site of the injection. The viscosity of the material may also be a factor that may or may not allow it to easily leak through the needle track of the injection site.

When dealing with autologous materials, as previously mentioned, free graft issues come into play. The ability of fat, collagen, muscle, or chondrocytes to grow in their new location may require some of the same principles of imbibition and inosculation as with larger tissue graft physiology. This was shown in the report by Diamond et al on autologous chondrocytes in which those mounds that were explanted at the time of ureteral reimplantation failed to demonstrate viable chondrocytes.[123]

Several studies have documented that in those cases where observation of the injection site was possible after a failed implantation, displacement appeared to occur quite frequently (Figure 46.9). In a series reported by Diamond et al on cystoscopic examina-

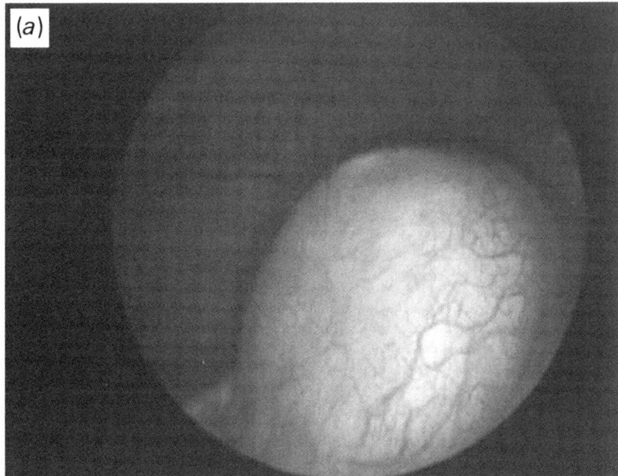

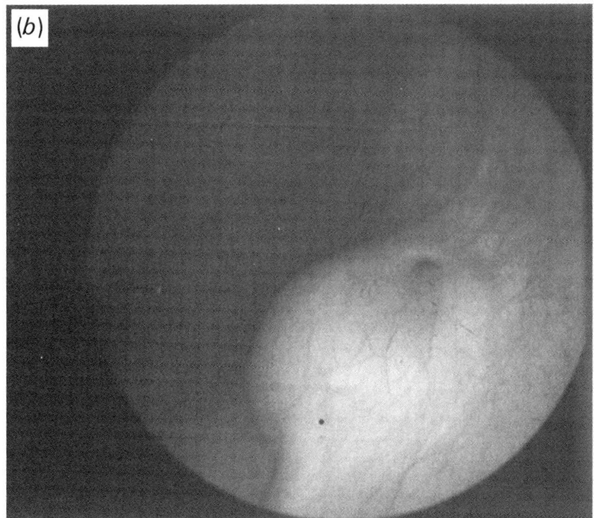

Figure 46.9 Mound shifting or displacement. (*a*) Appearance of mound and left ureteral orifice at time of initial injection. (*b*) Appearance at time of reinspection for persistent VUR on VCUG.

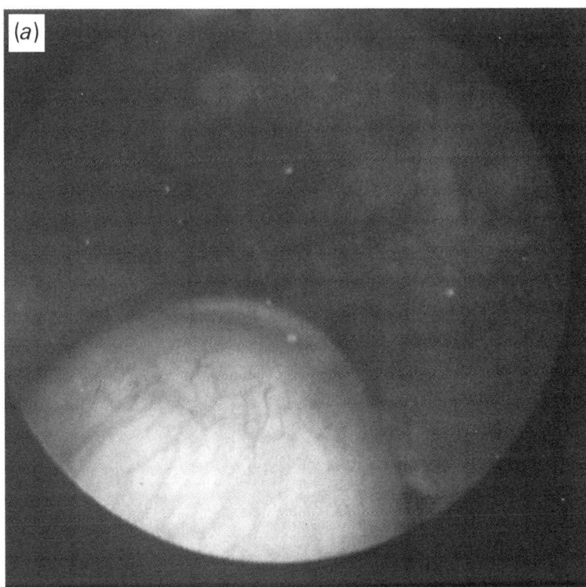

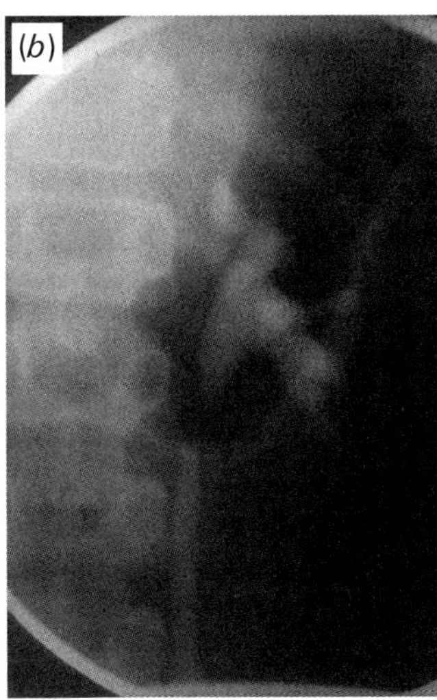

Figure 46.10 Perfectly injected mound with persistent VUR on VCUG classified as an indeterminate failure. (*a*) Mound on recystoscopy. (*b*) VCUG demonstrating left VUR.

tion of patients who had failed subureteric injection with autologous chondrocytes, it was noted that 35% had mound shifting, 25% had shifting and volume loss, and 13% had isolated volume loss. It appeared that the most frequent direction of mound shifting was distally and medially towards the bladder neck from the original injection site.[123] Eleven percent of their population, however, were classified as indeterminate: i.e. there was failure on postoperative VCUG to resolve the reflux but the appearance of the mound on cystoscopic or intraoperative inspection was perfectly normal (Figure 46.10). Other studies also found that either mound displacement or absence of a mound were the most common causes of failures on reinspection either cystoscopically or by open surgery of failed primary injections.[63,124–126]

Few studies have focused on failures from the injection of the dextranomer microspheres. Capozza et al reported on 45 failures with Dx/HA copolymer, and found 60% had mound displacement and 33% had absence of the mound on reinspection.[127] They reported a high percentage of their cases with failed dextranomer microspheres and suspected high intravesical pressures noted by voiding diaries. In 2 cases, however, there was a unilateral cure and contralateral mound displacement. It is uncertain as to whether this represented a technical failure or an anatomic failure. However, it is unlikely that they represented abnormal bladder physiology. Kirsch et al[15] reported on 18 patients who underwent reinjection for primary failures, and found that 61% had shifting of the mound away from the injection site. In the remainder of patients, the mound was either absent or present, and, therefore, indeterminate.

Conclusion

With a technology that is reproducible and at least a single agent that is widely available for endoscopic correction of reflux that appears safe, the obvious question that is raised is where does this fit in the management of children with VUR? This question must be addressed in light of the present day concerns for the use of long-term antibiotics with growing patterns of resistance. Studies have questioned the effectiveness of long-term antibiotic prophylaxis,[128] and the potential for long-term complications.[129] In this regard, Stenberg et al have proposed an algorithm which includes a shorter term of antibiotic prophylaxis, based on the child's age and grade of VUR, with endoscopic treatment with Dx/HA copolymer, as seen in Figure 46.11.[130] The use of Dx/HA copolymer has been shown to be a cost-effective alternative to open surgery for persistent VUR in children on a prophylactic antibiotic program.[131]

The effectiveness of endoscopic therapy requires that its approach be presented to parents as an upfront treatment in lieu of antibiotics. However, there has been a paucity of studies looking at long-term outcomes in a comparative analysis between antibiotic therapy and endoscopic correction. Studies

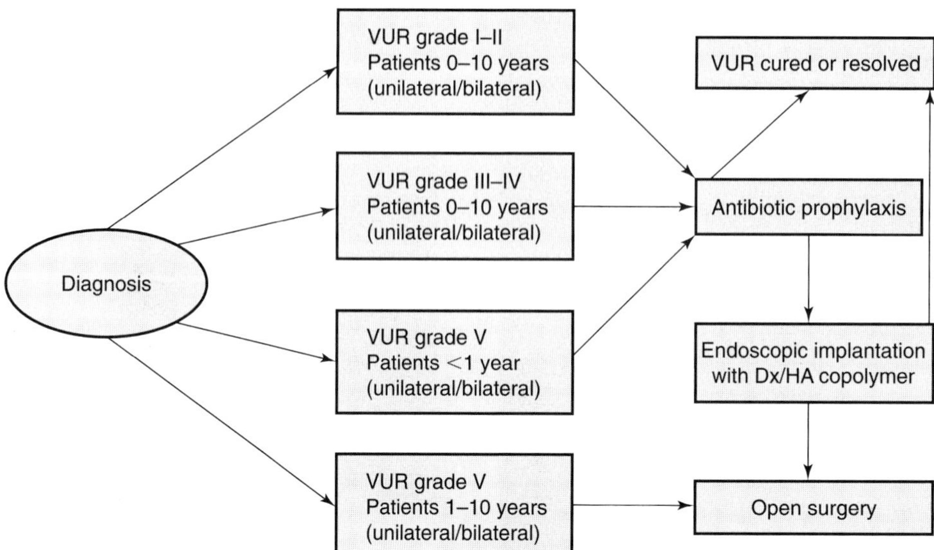

Figure 46.11 Algorithm proposed by Läckgren et al for the management of VUR in children, incorporating an endoscopic correction into the treatment plan. (Reproduced from Läckgren et al,[51] with permission.)

which have shown endoscopic treatment with Dx/HA copolymer to be more effective than antibiotic prophylaxis have often been of relatively short duration, raising the criticism of an adequate clinical trial. Additionally, is the outcome of VUR resolution the only outcome we should be concerned with? These questions will only be answered with multivariant prospective trials, which are difficult to perform in children. It is possible that endoscopic correction may change our approach to children with secondary reflux as well. Traditionally, children with neurogenic bladders or dysfunctional voiding and VUR are approached by managing the bladder dysfunction initially and reserving correction of VUR for those children with upper tract deterioration or breakthrough pyelonephritis. One could argue, however, as this population has a high rate of breakthrough UTIs and renal scarring,[132] for correcting the VUR endoscopically while ongoing and often tedious efforts at bladder rehabilitation are undertaken, thus protecting the upper tracts from pyelonephritis and potential scarring. This approach may have merit in light of the observation of Läckgren and Stenberg on the improvement in dysfunctional voiding in children treated primarily with endoscopic injection of Dx/HA copolymer without bladder management, implying that the reflux itself may contribute in some way to the abnormal bladder function.[98] Clinical trials in these scenarios would be most valuable.

In the integration of new technology and new concerns in the management of children with VUR, it would be helpful if we were better able to identify groups at high and low risk for renal scarring and tailor our management accordingly. With further progress in clinical research of VUR, we may be able to withhold therapy for certain low-risk groups, while taking a very aggressive approach, by either endoscopic correction or open ureteral reimplantation, for patients at high risk of renal scarring from VUR and infection.

Key points

1 Technique of endoscopic injection:
   - an incompletely filled bladder improves the accuracy of the injection
   - the needle is introduced with the bevel up
   - the assessment of the mound position should be made after an injection of 0.1–0.2 ml.
2 Key characteristics of commonly used materials:
   - polytetrafluoroethylene demonstrated a high success rate, with tendency for particular migration and foreign body reaction
   - cross-linked bovine collagen demonstrated an early success rate, with lack of durability
   - polydimethylsiloxane demonstrated an excellent success rate, with the potential for particulate migration
   - dextranomer microspheres demonstrated excellent success rate, with no evidence of migration.
3 Complications:
   - malignant degeneration or the development of connective tissue disorders is material dependent

- ureteral obstruction has been reported infrequently with most materials
- development of contralateral denovo VUR occurs less commonly with injection therapy than with ureteral reimplantation.

4 Reasons for failure of endoscopic treatment:
- specific material properties play a significant role in the failure rate of endoscopic correction as well as durability
- bladder dynamic factors may play a role in success rate insofar as they may result in mounds shifting within the bladder
- the most common finding in failed endoscopic correction has been mound shifting towards the bladder neck.

References

1. Bailey RR, Maling TMJ, Swainson CP. Vesicoureteral reflux and reflux nephropathy. In: Schrier RW, Gottschalk CW, eds. Diseases of the Kidney, 5th edn. Boston: Little, Brown, 1993: 689–727.
2. Weiss R, Duckett J, Spitzer A. Results of a randomized clinical trial of medical versus surgical management of infants and children with grades III and IV primary vesicoureteral reflux (United States). The International Reflux Study in Children. J Urol 1992; 148:1667–73.
3. Matouschek E. Die Behandlund des Vesikorenalen refluxes durch transurethrael einspritzung von teflonpaste. Urologe A 1981; 20:263.
4. McDonald H Jr, McDonald H Sr. Treatment of vesical ureteral reflux using endoscopic teflon paste in section. Presented at the 78th annual meeting of the American Urological Association, Las Vegas, April 1983.
5. Politano VA, Small MP, Harper JM, Lynne CM. Periurethral Teflon injection for urinary incontinence. J Urol 1974; 111:180–3.
6. Politano VA. Periurethral polytetrafluoroethylene injection for urinary incontinence. J Urol 1982; 127:439–42.
7. Politano VA, Molina L, Lynne CM. Endoscopic correction of vesicoureteral reflux with Polytef paste. Presented at the 83rd annual meeting of the American Urological Association, Boston, June 1988.
8. Vorstman B, Lockhart J, Kaufman MR, Politano V. Polytetrafluoroethylene injection for urinary incontinence in children. J Urol 1985; 133:248–50.
9. Puri P, O'Donnell B. Correction of experimentally produced vesicoureteral reflux in the piglet by the intravesical injection of Teflon. Br Med J (Clin Res Ed) 1984; 289:5–7.
10. O'Donnell B, Puri P. Endoscopic correction of primary vesicoureteral reflux. Br J Urol 1986; 58:601–4.
11. O'Donnell B, Puri P. Treatment of vesicoureteric reflux by endoscopic injection of Teflon. Br Med J (Clin Res Ed) 1984; 289:7–9.
12. Russinko PJ, Tackett LD. Endoscopic correction of reflux. In: Caldamone AA, ed. Pediatric Surgical Procedures. Atlas Urol Clin 2004; 12:55–63.
13. Kirsch AJ, Perez-Brayfield MR, Smith EA, Scherz HC. The modified STING procedure to correct vesicoureteral reflux: improved results with submucosal implantation within the intramural ureter. J Urol 2004; 171:2413–16.
14. Läckgren G, Wahlin N, Skoldenberg E, Stenberg A. Long-term followup of children treated with dextranomer/hyaluronic acid copolymer for vesicoureteral reflux. J Urol 2001; 166:1887–92.
15. Kirsch AJ, Perez-Brayfield MR, Scherz HC. Minimally invasive treatment of vesicoureteral reflux with endoscopic injection of dextranomer/hyaluronic acid copolymer: the Children's Hospital of Atlanta experience. J Urol 2003; 170:211–15.
16. Berg S. Polytef augmentation urethroplasty. Correction of surgically incurable urinary incontinence by injection technique. Arch Surg 1973; 107:379–81.
17. O'Donnell B, Puri P. Endoscopic correction of primary vesicoureteral reflux: results in 94 ureters. Br Med J 1986; 293:1404–6.
18. Ruenanen MS, Toikkanen S, Viljanto J. Long term follow-up of tissue reactions caused by Teflon and cross-linked collagen in rats. Pediatr Surg Int 1991; 6:241–4.
19. Vandenbossche M, Delhove O, Dumortier P et al. Endoscopic treatment of reflux: experimental study and review of Teflon and collagen. Eur Urol 1993; 23(3):386–93.
20. Aragona F, D'Urso L, Scremin E, Salmaso R, Glazel GP. Polytetrafluoroethylene giant granuloma and adenopathy: long-term complications following subureteral polytetrafluoroethylene injection for the treatment of vesicoureteral reflux in children. J Urol 1997; 158:1539–42.
21. Läckgren G, Wahlin N, Stenberg A. Endoscopic treatment of children with vesicoureteral reflux. Acta Pediatr Scand Suppl 1999; 431:62–71.
22. Schulman CC, Sassine AM. Endoscopic treatment of vesicoureteral reflux. Eur J Paediatr Surg 1992; 2:32–4.
23. Puri P, Ninan GK, Surana R. Subureteric Teflon injection (STING). Results of a European Survey. Eur Urol 1995; 27:71–5.
24. Puri P. Ten year experience with subureteric Teflon (polytetrafluoroethylene) injection (STING) in the treatment of vesico-ureteric reflux. Br J Urol 1995; 75: 126–31.
25. Chertin B, Colhoun E, Velayudham M, Puri P. Endoscopic treatment of vesicoureteral reflux: 11 to 17 years of followup. J Urol 2002; 167(3):1443, discussion 1445.
26. Elder JS, Diaz M, Caldamone AA et al. Endoscopic therapy for vesicoureteral reflux: a meta-analysis. I. Reflux resolution and urinary tract infection. J Urol 2006; 175:716–22.
27. Aaronson IA. Current status of the 'STING': an American perspective. Br J Urol 1995; 75(2):121–5.
28. Aaronson IA, Rames RA, Greene WB et al. Endoscopic treatment of reflux: migration of Teflon to the lungs and brain. Eur Urol 1993; 23:394–9.
29. Malizia AA, Reinman HM, Myers RP et al. Migration and granulomatous reaction after periurethral injection of polytef (Teflon). JAMA 1984; 251:3277–81.
30. Malizia AA, Rushton HG, Woodard JR et al. Migration and granulomatous reaction after periurethral injection of Polytef. J Urol 1987; 137 (Part 2):122A. [abstract 74]

31. Dewan PA, Fraundorfer M. Skin migration following periurethral polytetrafluoroethylene injection for urinary incontinence. Aust N Z J Surg 1996; 66(1):57–9.
32. Rames RA, Aaronson IA. Migration of polytef paste to the lung and brain following intravesical injection for the correction of reflux. Pediatr Surg Int 1991; 6:239.
33. Claes H, Stroobants D, van Meerbeck J et al. Pulmonary migration following periurethral polytetrafluoroethylene injection for urinary incontinence. J Urol 1989; 142:821–2.
34. Borgatti R, Tettamanti A, Piccinelli P. Brain injury in a healthy child one year after periureteral injection of Teflon. Pediatrics 1996; 98:290–1.
35. Steyaert H, Sattonnet C, Bloch C et al. Migration of PTFE paste particles to the kidney after treatment for vesico-ureteral reflux. BJU Int 2000; 85:168–9.
36. Dewan PA. Is injected polytetrafluoroethylene (Polytef) carcinogenic? Br J Urol 1992; 69(1):29–33.
37. Dewan PA, Owen AJ, Byard RW. Long-term histological response to subcutaneously injected Polytef and Bioplastique in a rat model. Br J Urol 1995; 76(2):161–4.
38. Frey P, Berger D, Jenny P, Herzog B. Subureteral collagen injection for the endoscopic treatment of vesicoureteral reflux using cross-linked bovine dermal collagen. Pediatr Surg Int 1992; 6:295–300.
39. Leonard MP, Canning DA, Epstein JI et al. Local tissue reaction to the subureteral injection of glutaraldehyde cross-linked bovine collagen in humans. J Urol 1990; 143(6):1209–12.
40. Cendron M, Leonard M, Gearhart JP, Jeffs RD. Endoscopic treatment of vesico-ureteric reflux using cross-linked bovine dermal collagen. Pediatr Surg Int 1991; 6:295–300.
41. Lipsky H, Würnschimmel E. Endoscopic treatment of vesicoureteric reflux with collagen. Five years' experience. Br J Urol 1993; 72(6):965–8.
42. Frey P, Lutz N, Jenny P, Herzog B. Endoscopic subureteral collagen injection for the treatment of vesicoureteral reflux in infants and children. J Urol 1995; 154:804–7.
43. Reunanen M. Correction of vesicoureteral reflux in children by endoscopic collagen injection: a prospective study. J Urol 1995; 154:2156–8.
44. Capozza N, Lais A, Nappo S, Caione P. The role of endoscopic treatment of vesicoureteral reflux: a 17-year experience. J Urol 2004; 172:1626–8, discussion 1629.
45. Leonard MP, Decter A, Mix LW et al. Endoscopic treatment of vesicoureteral reflux with collagen: preliminary report and cost analysis. J Urol 1996; 155:1716–20.
46. Polito M, Muzzonigro G, Caraceni E, Azizi B. Il trattamento endoscopico del reflusso vescico-ureteral nell adulto mediante collagene bovino. Arch It Urol Androl 1997; 69:55–9.
47. Haferkamp A, Mohring K, Staehler G, Dorsam J. Pitfalls of repeat subureteral bovine collagen injection for the endoscopic treatment of vesicoureteral reflux. J Urol 2000; 163:1919–21.
48. Haferkamp A, Mohring K, Staehler G, Gerner HJ, Dorsam J. Long-term efficacy of subureteral collagen injection for endoscopic treatment of vesicoureteral reflux in neurogenic bladder cases. J Urol 2000; 163:274–7.
49. De Grazia E, Cimador M. Long-term follow-up results of vesico-ureteric reflux treated with subureteral collagen injection (SCIN). Minerva Pediatr 2000; 52:7–14.
50. Tsuboi N, Horiuchi K, Osawa S, et al. Endoscopic treatment of vesicoureteral reflux in children with glutaraldehyde cross-linked bovine dermal collagen. Short-term results. J Nippon Med Sch 2000; 67(1):9–12.
51. Läckgren G, Lottmann H, Hensle TW, Stenberg A. Endoscopic treatment of vesicoureteral reflux and urinary incontinence in children. AUA Update Lesson 37, Volume XXII, 2003.
52. Frey P, Gudinchet F, Jenny P. GAX 65: a new injectable cross-linked collagen for the endoscopic treatment of vesicoureteral reflux: a double-blind study evaluating its efficiency in children. J Urol 1997; 158:1210–12.
53. Smith DP, Kaplan WE, Oyasu R. Evaluation of polydimethylsiloxane as an alternative in the endoscopic treatment of vesicoureteral reflux. J Urol 1994; 152:1221–4.
54. Buckley JF, Azmy AA, Fyfe A et al. Endoscopic correction of vesicoureteral reflux with injectable silicone microparticles. J Urol 1993; 149:259A
55. Buckley JF, Scott R, Aitchison M et al. Periurethral microparticulate silicone injection for stress incontinence and vesicoureteral reflux. Minim Invasive Ther 1991; 1(Suppl 1): 72.
56. Henly DR, Barrett DM, Weiland TL et al. Particulate silicone for use in periurethral injections. Local tissue effects and search for migration. J Urol 1995; 153:2039–43.
57. Barrett DM, O'Sullivan DC, Malizia AA, Reiman HM, Abel-Aleff PC. Particle shedding and migration from silicone genitourinary prosthetic devices. J Urol 1991; 146:319–22.
58. Smith DP, Beegle BE, Noe HN, Wilson EA. Does technique or material used affect bladder tissue reactions when injecting teflon or silicone paste? Urology 1996; 48(1):119–23.
59. Dewan PA, Byard RW. Histological response to injected Polytef and Bioplastique in a rat model. Br J Urol 1994; 73:370–6.
60. Dewan PA, Stefanek W, Byard RW. Long-term histological response to intravenous Teflon and Silicone in a rat model. Pediatr Surg Int 1995; 10:129–33.
61. Hatanaka S, Oneda S, Okazaki K et al. Induction of malignant fibrous histiocytoma in female Fisher rats by implantation of cyanoacrylate, zirconia, polyvinyl chloride or silicone. In Vivo 1993; 7(2):111–15.
62. Janowsky EC, Kupper LL, Hulka BS. Meta-analyses of the relation between silicone breast implants and the risk of connective-tissue diseases. N Engl J Med 2000; 342:781–90.
63. Herz D, Hafez A, Bagli D et al. Efficacy of endoscopic subureteral polydimethylsiloxane injection for treatment of vesicoureteral reflux in children: a North American clinical report. J Urol 2001; 166:1880–6.
64. van Capelle JW, de Haan T, El Sayed W, Azmy A. The long-term outcome of the endoscopic subureteric implantation of polydimethylsiloxane for treating vesico-ureteric reflux in children: a retrospective analysis of the first 195 consecutive patients in two European centres. BJU Int 2004; 94: 1348–51.
65. Aboutaleb H, Bolduc S, Upadhyay J et al. Subureteral

polydimethylsiloxane injection versus extravesical reimplantation for primary low grade vesicoureteral reflux in children: a comparative study. J Urol 2003; 169:313–16.
66. Stenberg A, Läckgren G. A new bioimplant for the endoscopic treatment of vesicoureteral reflux: experimental and clinical results. J Urol 1995; 154(2):800–3.
67. Stenberg AM, Sundin A, Larsson BS, Läckgren G, Stenberg A. Lack of distant migration after injection of a ^{125}iodine labeled dextranomer based implant into the rabbit bladder. J Urol 1997; 158:1937–41.
68. Stenberg A, Larsson E, Lindholm A et al. Experimental studies of an injectable dextranomer-based implant. Histopathology, volume changes and DNA analysis. Postmenopausal disorders with special reference to urinary continence. Acta Universitatis Uppsalienis 1998; 1–15.
69. Stenberg A, Larsson E, Lindholm A et al. Injectable dextranomer-based implant: histopathology, volume changes and DNA-analysis. Scand J Urol Nephrol 1999; 33:355–61.
70. Capozza N, Caione P. Dextranomer/hyaluronic acid copolymer implantation for vesico-ureteral reflux: a randomized comparison with antibiotic prophylaxis. J Pediatr 2002; 140: 230–4.
71. Oswald J, Lusuardi M, Riccabona M et al. A comparison of endoscopic subureteric polydimethylsiloxane versus dextranomer/hyaluronic copolymer injection to treat VUR in children. BJU Int 2002: 89(Suppl 2):16.
72. Puri P, Chertin B, Velaydham M et al. Treatment of vesicoureteral reflux by endoscopic injection of dextranomer/hyaluronic acid copolymer: preliminary results. J Urol 2003; 170:1541–4.
73. Mevorach R, Rabinowitz R, Beck C et al. Endoscopic treatment of vesicoureteral reflux with Coaptite: the first 50 patients. Presented at the American Urology Association meeting, Orlando, Florida, May 5, 2002 [abstract 429].
74. Atala A, Cima LG, Kim W et al. Injectable alginate seeded with chondrocytes as a potential treatment for vesicoureteral reflux. J Urol 1993; 150:745–7.
75. Atala A, Kim W, Paige K et al. Endoscopic treatment of vesicoureteral reflux with a chondrocyte-alginate suspension. J Urol 1994; 152: 641–3.
76. Caldamone AA, Diamond DA. Long-term results of the endoscopic correction of vesicoureteral reflux in children using autologous chondrocytes. J Urol 2001; 165:2224–7.
77. Diamond DA, Caldamone AA. Endoscopic correction of vesicoureteral reflux in children using autologous chondrocytes: preliminary results. J Urol 1999; 162:1185–8.
78. Matthews RD, Christensen JP, Canning DA. Persistence of autologous free fat transplant in bladder submucosa of rats. J Urol 1994; 152:819–21.
79. Palma PC, Ferreira U, Ikari O et al. Subureteric lipoinjection for vesicoureteral reflux in renal transplant candidates. Urology 1994; 43:174–7.
80. Chancellor MB, Rivas DA, Liberman SN et al. Cystoscopic autogenous fat injection treatment of vesicoureteral reflux in spinal cord injury. J Am Paraplegia Soc 1994; 17(2):50–4.
81. Cendron M, DeVore DP, Connolly R et al. The biological behavior of autologous collagen injected into the rabbit bladder. J Urol 1995; 154:808–11.
82. Cilento BG, Atala A. Use of autologous transplantable tissue for endoscopic correction of vesicoureteral reflux in children. Dial Pediatr Urol 1995; 18:11.
83. Granata C, Buffa P, Di Rovasenda E et al. Treatment of vesicoureteral reflux in children with neuropathic bladder. A comparison of surgical and endoscopic correction. J Pediatr Surg 1999; 34:1836–8.
84. Engel JD, Palmer LS, Cheng EY, Kaplan WE. Surgical versus endoscopic correction of vesicoureteral reflux in children with neurogenic bladder dysfunction. J Urol 1997; 157:2291–4.
85. Misra D, Potts SR, Brown S, Boston VE. Endoscopic treatment of vesico-ureteric reflux in neurogenic bladder – 8 years' experience. J Pediatr Surg 1996; 31:1262–4.
86. Yokoyama O, Ishiura Y, Seto C et al. Endoscopic treatment of vesicoureteral reflux in patients with myelodysplasia. J Urol 1996; 155:1882–6.
87. Sugiyama T, Hashimoto K, Kiwamoto H et al. Endoscopic correction of vesicoureteral reflux in patients with neurogenic bladder dysfunction. Int Urol Nephrol 1995; 27:527–31.
88. Kaminetsky JC, Hanna MK. Endoscopic treatment of vesicoureteral reflux in children with neurogenic bladders. Urology 1991; 37:244–7.
89. Dewan PA, Guiney EJ. Endoscopic correction of vesicoureteral reflux in children with spina bifida. Br J Urol 1990; 65:646–9.
90. Puri P, Guiney EJ. Endoscopic correction of vesicoureteral reflux secondary to neuropathic bladder. Br J Urol 1986; 58:504–8.
91. Perez-Brayfield M, Kirsch AJ, Hensle TW et al. Endoscopic treatment with dextranomer/hyaluronic acid for complex cases of vesicoureteral reflux. J Urol 2004; 172:1614–16.
92. Quinn FMJ, Diamond T, Boston VE. Endoscopic correction of vesicoureteral reflux secondary to neuropathic bladder due to myelomeningocele. Z Kinder 1988; 43:43–5.
93. Aubert D, Zoupanos G, Destuynder O, Hurez F. 'Sting' procedure in the treatment of secondary reflux in children. Eur Urol 1990; 17:307–9.
94. Trsinar B, Cotic D, Oblak C. Possible causes of unsuccessful endoscopic collagen treatment of vesicoureteral reflux in children. Eur Urol 1999; 36: 635–9.
95. Capozza N, Caione P, De Gennaro M, Nappo S, Patricolo M. Endoscopic treatment of vesico-ureteric reflux and urinary incontinence: technical problems in the pediatric patient. Br J Urol 1995; 75:538–42.
96. Koff SA, Wagner TT, Jayanthi VR. The relationship among dysfunctional elimination syndromes, primary vesicoureteral reflux and urinary tract infections in children. J Urol 1998; 160:1019–22.
97. Snodgrass W. The impact of treated dysfunctional voiding on the nonsurgical management of vesicoureteral reflux. J Urol 1998; 160(5):1823–5.
98. Läckgren G, Stenberg A. Endoscopic treatment of children with bladder dysfunction and vesicoureteral reflux: preliminary results. In press.

99. Reunanen M. Endoscopic collagen injection: its limits in correcting vesico-ureteral reflux in duplicated ureters. Eur Urol 1997; 31:243–5.
100. Miyakita H, Ninan GK, Puri P. Endoscopic correction of vesico-ureteric reflux in duplex systems. Eur Urol 1993; 24:111–15.
101. Steinbrecher HA, Edwards B, Malone PS. The STING in the refluxing duplex system. Br J Urol 1995; 76:165–8.
102. Dewan PA, O'Donnell B. Polytef paste injection of refluxing duplex ureters. Eur Urol 1991; 19:35–8.
103. Läckgren G, Wahlin N, Skoldenberg E et al. Endoscopic treatment correction of vesicoureteral reflux with dextranomer/hyaluronic acid copolymer in either double ureters or a small kidney. J Urol 2003; 170:1551–5.
104. Aboutaleb H, Bolduc S, Khoury AE et al. Polydimethylsiloxane injection versus open surgery for the treatment of vesicoureteral reflux in complete duplex systems. J Urol 2003; 170:1563–5.
105. De Caluwe D, Chertin B, Puri P. Long-term outcome of the retained ureteral stump after lower pole heminephrectomy in duplex kidneys. Eur Urol 2002; 42:63–6.
106. De Caluwe D, Chertin B, Puri P. Fate of the retained ureteral stump after upper pole heminephrectomy in duplex kidneys. J Urol 2002; 168(2):679–80.
107. Elder JS, Peters CA, Arant BS Jr et al. Pediatric Vesicoureteral Reflux Guidelines Panel summary report on the management of primary vesicoureteral reflux in children. J Urol 1997; 157:1846–51.
108. Mesrobian HG, Kramer SA, Kelalis PP. Reoperative ureteroneocystostomy: review of 69 patients. J Urol 1985; 133:388–90.
109. Kumar R, Puri P. Endoscopic correction of vesicoureteral reflux in failed reimplanted ureters. Eur Urol 1998; 33:98–100.
110. Cloix P, Dawahra M, Choukair M et al. Endoscopic treatment of vesico-ureteric reflux after reimplantation of the ureter. Prog Urol 1992; 2:66–71.
111. Gaschignard N, Plattner V, Boullanger P, Heloury Y. Endoscopic treatment of residual vesico-ureteral reflux after reimplantation in children: twelve cases. Prog Urol 1997; 7(4):618–21.
112. Hakky M, Kolbusz R, Reyes CV. Chondrosarcoma of the larynx. Ear Nose Throat J 1989; 68:60–2.
113. Montgomery R. Polytetrafluorethylene. Pattys Indust Hygiene Toxicol 2C 1982; 4308–10.
114. Lewy RB. Experience with vocal cord injection. Ann Otol Rhinol Laryngol 1976; 85:440–50.
115. Lockhart JL, Walker RD, Vorstman B, Politano VA. Periurethral polytetrafluoroethylene injection following urethral reconstruction in female patients with urinary incontinence. J Urol 1988; 140:51–2.
116. Parrot TS, Woodard JR. Reflux in the opposite ureter after successful correction of unilateral vesico-ureteric reflux. Urology 1976; 7:266–79.
117. Ross JH, Kay R, Nasarallah P. Contralateral reflux after unilateral ureteral reimplantation in patients with a history of resolved contralateral reflux. J Urol 1995; 154:1171–5.
118. Hoenig DM, Diamond DA, Rabinowitz R et al. Contralateral reflux after unilateral ureteral reimplantation. J Urol 1996; 156:196–7.
119. Warren MM, Kelalis PP, Stickler GB. Unilateral ureteroneocystostomy: the fate of the contralateral ureter. J Urol 1972; 107:466–8.
120. Quinlan D, O'Donnell B. Unilateral ureteric reimplantation for primary vesico-ureteric reflux in children. A policy revisted. Br J Urol 1985; 57:406–7.
121. Kumar R, Puri R. Newly diagnosed contralateral reflux following successful unilateral endoscopic correction. Is it due to a 'pop off' mechanism? J Urol 1997; 158:1213–15.
122. Diamond DA, Rabinowitz R, Hoening DM, Caldamone AA. The mechanism of new onset contralateral reflux following unilateral ureteroneocystostomy. J Urol 1996; 145:665–7.
123. Diamond DA, Caldamone AA, Bauer SB et al. Mechanism of failure of endoscopic treatment of vesicoureteral reflux based on endoscopic anatomy. J Urol 2003; 170:1556–9.
124. Tabatowski K, Elson CE, Johnston WW. Silicone lymphadenopathy in a patient with a mammary prosthesis. Fine needle aspiration cytology, histology and analytical electron microscopy. Acta Cytol 1990; 34:10.
125. Bhatti HA, Khattak H, Boston VE. Efficacy and causes of failure of endoscopic subureteric injection of Teflon in the treatment of primary vesicoureteral reflux. Br J Urol 1993: 71:221–5.
126. Dewan PA, Higgs MJ. Correlation of the endoscopic appearance with clinical outcome for submucous Polytef paste injection in vesico-ureteric reflux. Aust N Z J Surg 1995; 65:642–4.
127. Capozza N, Lais A, Matarazzo E et al. Influence of voiding dysfunction on the outcome of endoscopic treatment for vesicoureteral reflux. J Urol 2002; 168:1695–8.
128. Pomeranz A, El-Khayam A, Korzets Z et al. A bioassay evaluation of the urinary antibacterial efficacy of low dose prophylactic antibiotics in children with vesicoureteral reflux. J Urol 2000; 164:1070–3.
129. Velicer CM, Heckbert SR, Lampe JW et al. Antibiotic use in relation to the risk of breast cancer. JAMA 2004; 291(7):827–35.
130. Stenberg A, Hensle TW, Läckgren G. Vesicoureteral reflux: a new treatment algorithm. Curr Urol Rep 2002; 3(2):107–14.
131. Kobelt G, Canning DA, Hensle TW, Läckgren G. The cost-effectiveness of endoscopic injection of dextranomer/hyaluronic acid copolymer for vesicoureteral reflux. J Urol 2003; 169:1480–4; discussion 1484–5.
132. Naseer SR, Steinhardt GF. New renal scars in children with urinary tract infections, vesicoureteral reflux and voiding dysfunction: a prospective evaluation. J Urol 1997; 158:566–8.

Section V

The Bladder and Prostate

Basic science of the urinary bladder

47

Armando J Lorenzo and Darius J Bägli

Introduction

The urinary bladder is a unique organ. As a hollow structure, it demonstrates a remarkable integration of neuromuscular, mechanical, and physical properties that are crucial for its normal function. No other organ is evolutionarily programmed to fill with fluid over hours at low pressures, and then contract on demand to evacuate its contents. The bladder is the only autonomic organ under voluntary control. Indeed, the sociobiologic etiology and reasons for the existence of this unique behavior have been argued for decades. Although the ability to accommodate a fluid volume (filling) is thought to represent largely a passive phenomenon, this is not entirely the case. Recruitment of active neuromechanical properties is crucial for maintenance of low intravesical pressures during filling, and to this end the character of the surrounding cellular elements and extracellular matrix (ECM) can either facilitate or compromise this function. Bladder contraction (emptying), on the other hand, is largely an active neuromuscular process, although it is also influenced by the physicochemical nature of the ECM, and obviously depends on the overall mass and optimal functional status of bladder smooth muscle cells (bSMCs). This chapter reviews some of the biologic concepts related to normal bladder development and function, a complex orchestration of events that, if disturbed, can lead to a significant functional disharmony that places both continence and renal function at risk.

Bladder development

The urogenital sinus develops to form the bulk of the urinary bladder, with its endoderm giving rise to the urothelium and the surrounding mesenchyme to the lamina propria and smooth muscle layer. A smaller, albeit crucial, part of this organ – the trigone – originates from the gradual incorporation of the mesonephric ducts and ureteric buds into the caudal aspect of the bladder wall.[1] Early in gestation the undifferentiated mesenchymal cells are highly proliferative[2] and differentiate into smooth muscle cells with ample spatiotemporal opportunity for interaction with the surrounding primitive urothelium.[3] As differentiation occurs, fetal bSMCs begin to express markers that will come to signify their smooth muscle lineage – α-smooth muscle actin, desmin, and smooth muscle myosin[4] – in a process that coincides with changes in expression of specific ECM proteins such as collagen, fibronectin, and laminin.[5] Although the significance of these temporal associations is still not completely understood, they highlight the early molecular interactions between different developing cell types and their surrounding environment. Evidence to date indicates that specific epithelial–mesenchymal–ECM interactions are necessary for orderly differentiation and development. For example, laminins and fibronectin have been found in the basal lamina during development, and are probably important in mediating interactions between the developing urothelium and its underlying mesenchyme.[1] Other ECM molecules, such as the structural collagens, whose different types are expressed differently between the lamina propria and detrusor muscle fibers,[6] interact with adjacent cells via specific cell-surface receptors, the most important of which are believed to be the integrins.[7] The cell–matrix transduction of different stimuli through different mechanoreceptors (integrins, cell adhesion molecules, and selectins) probably regulates cellular proliferation and differentiation, as well as modulates ECM synthesis.[7] Consequently, normal prenatal bladder development not only results from a complex interaction of ECM and developing cells but also depends on appropriate mechanical stimulation. As gestation progresses, this type of stimulation varies as a result of the multiple factors regulating the mechanical distention stimulus. Compliance appears to increase gradually,[8] the bladder wall thickness and composition changes,[9] and urine production increases as the fetus grows. Later, the bladder acquires a pattern of cyclical emptying.

Contraction and relaxation

As storage and emptying alternate, the complex function of the detrusor muscle demands integrated control of perhaps its most important cellular component, the smooth muscle cell. During filling, bSMCs must relax and elongate over a considerable length of time (hours) to accommodate the urine volume at low pressures. Conversely, during micturition a rapid change occurs, leading to coordinated and synchronized force generation and cell shortening. By means of dense innervation and abundant intercellular communications (gap junctions), these activities – contraction and relaxation – respond to various transmitters and modulators that activate different cellular pathways.[10]

Contraction of bSMCs is mainly the result of interaction between the contractile proteins actin and myosin, in a similar manner to other muscle cells in the body. In an energy-dependent process, a multistep enzymatic reaction allows for the cross-bridging and attachment of these two proteins in a cyclical fashion, following the same general scheme proposed for skeletal muscle. ATP is the immediate energy substrate, and is crucial for membrane pump Ca^{2+} handling, phosphorylation events, and cross-bridge cycling. The cellular concentration of ATP is therefore essential, and is maintained by mitochondrial respiration, glycolysis, and conversion of the high-energy compound phosphocreatine. Successful regulation of free Ca^{2+} in the cytosol is a highly energy-dependent process. Activation of the contractile apparatus by phosphorylation of the myosin light-chain kinase is modulated by cytosolic Ca^{2+}, whose concentration is regulated by Ca^{2+} channel pumps in the sarcoplasmic reticulum and plasma membrane. Thus, significant energy expenditures are required to maintain these Ca^{2+} gradients. Therefore, mitochondrial function is yet another factor essential for the normal generation of the contractile force by bSMCs.[11]

Even though different isoforms have been described for both actin and myosin, their functional significance remains unclear. Smooth muscle myosin is composed of a pair of heavy chains and two pairs of myosin light chains. Through alternative splicing, the mRNA that encodes vertebrate smooth muscle myosin heavy chains can produce two C-terminal isoforms (SM1 and SM2) and two N-terminal isoforms (SMA and SMB). Some studies suggest that the SM1 isoform forms better contractile filaments than SM2, and that SMB is associated with increased ATPase activity, increased shortening velocity, and more phasic contractions than the SMA isoform.[12–14] Although it remains possible that the presence and relative concentrations of actin and myosin vary with developmental state and in response to obstruction or other pathologic processes,[14,15] their function not only supports the contractile apparatus but also helps to define the cytoskeleton.[16] Indeed, the cytoskeletal framework of the bSMC forms a dynamic structure, with linkages to the ECM. At the same time, these points of linkage, or adhesion complexes with the ECM, mediate intracellular signaling that leads to gene expression, cell migration, cell growth, apoptosis, and adaptation.[10,17,18] Although a relatively novel finding in urology, this paradigm has been appreciated in other biologic systems where it governs cell–matrix relationships in a multitude of ways. Nevertheless, it should be pointed out that, at this time, a coherent picture of the molecular nature of bladder outlet obstruction remains elusive. The question is a difficult one, as bladder outlet obstruction seems to be remarkably heterogeneous.

Mechanotransduction

Cycling between filling and emptying continually exposes the bladder to mechanical stimulation, with force transduction to the cells and their surrounding environment. As a conditioning and modifying process, forcible changes in cell shape induced by various combinations of stretching, contraction, pressure, and membrane and cytoskeletal deformation eventually lead to alterations in gene expression (Figure 47.1). The macroscopic changes often appreciated in the bladder wall are thus the result of genetically mediated tissue remodeling and activation of different molecular pathways. The process of converting physical forces into biochemical signals and integrating these signals into a cellular response, also known as mechanotransduction,[19] is an important concept in bladder development and response to different pathologic stimuli. The bladder, among other mechanosensitive organs, derives essential mitogenic stimuli from mechanical stimulation through the activation of members of the mitogen-activated protein kinase (MAPK) family – the c-Jun N-terminal kinase

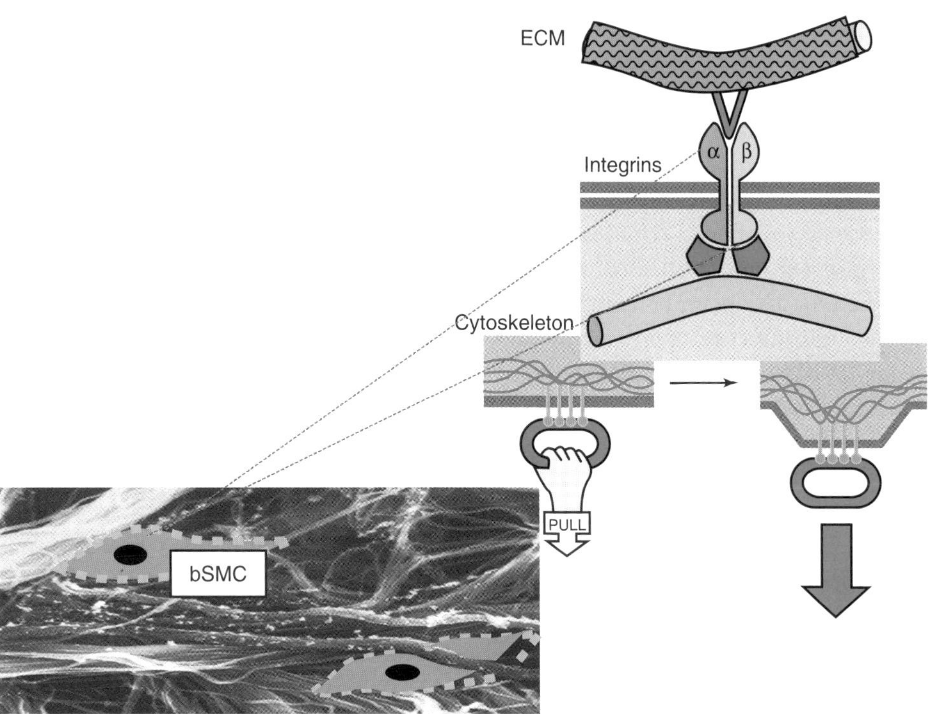

Figure 47.1 Mechanotransduction: schematic representation of conditioning forces (depicted as action over handle on the cytoskeleton), leading to changes in cell shape. This can be induced by various combinations of stretching, contraction, pressure, and membrane and cytoskeletal deformation, eventually leading to alterations in gene expression. Note that the integrins are shown as important mediators of such a process. ECM, extracellular matrix; bSMC, bladder smooth muscle cells.

(JNK), p38, and extracellular signal-regulated kinase (ERK)[20,21] – and other pathways (such as the phosphoinositide 3-kinase (PI3K)/Akt pathway),[22] that in turn up-regulate and activate transcription factors responsible for cell growth and survival.

A key factor in this process is the signaling system that mediates this mechanotransduction. It is probable that the pathways are multiple and perhaps redundant; however, it is currently believed that the integrin receptors, along with stretch-activated ion channels, play an important role in these series of events.[23] These linkage molecules are almost ubiquitous, acting as a relay between the matrix and different cells. Individual tissues thus display different complex responses to mechanical stimulation, the eventual response modulated by the type of mechanical stimulation as well as the signaling molecules and transcription factors expressed by that particular tissue.[19] As a group, these ECM receptor molecules provide a physical link between cell membranes and surrounding structural ECM proteins, such as collagen, laminins, vitronectin, and fibronectin. In particular, the integrins represent a large and versatile family of heterodimeric transmembrane mechanoreceptors capable of transducing a wide range of alterations in the cell microenvironment.[24] Growth factors can further stimulate cell responses through integrins by either mutual interaction, or integrin clustering with growth factor receptors. This process is tightly regulated and expression of different integrin subunits may be specifically modulated by different growth factors and/or ECM molecules under different developmental and pathologic situations. Even though much of the current knowledge about these molecules remains to be revealed in relation to the bladder, their importance in response to bladder distention and dynamic alterations in ECM expression has been demonstrated.[7]

Smooth muscle growth

The generation of contractile force is one of the principal roles for bSMC. Beyond the immediate effect of recruitment and longer contraction times, bladder response to increased work demand (i.e. increased outlet resistance) results in an increase in bSMC mass through hypertrophy (increase in cell number) and hyperplasia (increase in cell size). Bladder SMC growth is mediated by growth factors such as basic fibroblast growth factor (bFGF), platelet-derived growth factor-BB (PDGF-BB),[25] and heparin-binding EGF-like growth factor (HBEGF),[26] along with other mitogenic signals. In many instances, the transcription of specific genes eventually leads to increase in cell mass and/or number, and is mediated through MAPKs,[27] as previously mentioned, although other kinase signaling families are probably involved (Figure 47.2). These bioactive peptides contribute to tissue expansion through autocrine and paracrine signaling mechanisms. It has become increasingly clear that diverse signals can participate in a number of positive and negative feedback loops which may amplify or reduce the initial stimulus, differentially contributing to specific DNA transcription, protein synthesis, and inactivation of proapoptotic pathways. There exists considerable interest in the modulation of the bSMC mitogenic response, as it is believed that progressive increase in smooth muscle mass is a key component of bladder dysfunction. Currently, management of bladder wall thickening is based on the use of anticholinergics, such as oxybutynin and tolterodine. Interestingly, besides its well-described antimuscarinic effect, oxybutynin appears to inhibit bSMC proliferation and gene expression in vitro, giving us another potential explanation for its proven clinical efficacy.[29] Once the pathways mediating a mitogenic response are better elucidated, specific inhibitors may lead to clinical trials. As an example, a recent area of interest has been regulating compensatory bladder hypertrophy with calcineurin inhibitors such as cyclosporine and FK506 (tacrolimus). Initial evidence suggesting modulation of cardiac muscle hypertrophy has been described in a transgenic model of murine cardiac hypertrophy,[30] and more recently in a bladder outlet obstruction animal model.[31] Ideally, translational research would be the venue for new pharmacologic therapies to be developed; however, molecules such as botulinum toxin have appeared in experimental clinical use based

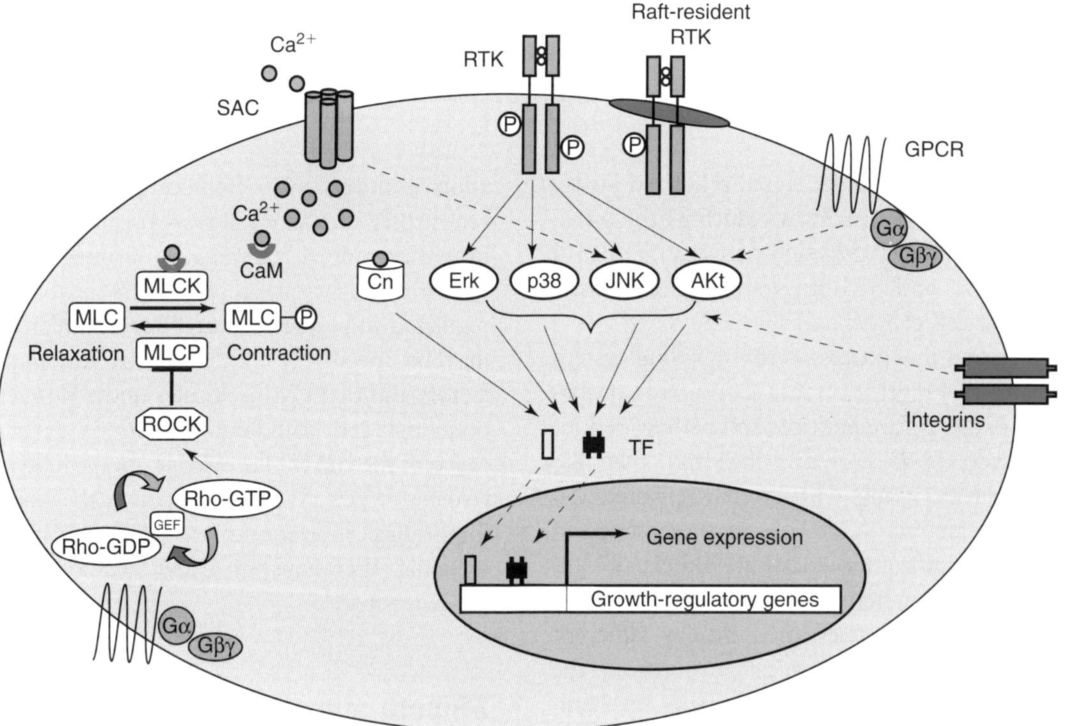

Figure 47.2 Signaling cascades in bladder smooth muscle cells: external stimuli are transduced by stretch-activated ion channels (SAC), receptor tyrosine kinases (RTK), G-protein coupled receptors (GPCR), and integrin subunits. SAC-mediated calcium (Ca^{2+}) entry promotes calmodulin (CaM) binding and activation of myosin light-chain kinase (MLCK), leading to MLC phosphorylation and initiation of smooth muscle contraction. MLC phosphatase (MLCP)-induced relaxation is inhibited by Rho-associated kinase (ROCK). Ca^{2+} influx also activates calcineurin (Cn), leading to dephosphorylation and nuclear translocation of transcription factors (TF). RTK activation promotes activation of the mitogen-activated protein kinases (MAPKs) Erk, p38 stress-activated protein kinase 2 (SAPK2), and c-Jun N-terminal kinase (JNK), and Akt. These signaling intermediates in turn promote activation and nuclear translocation of TF, and alterations in gene expression. (Adapted from Adam,[28] with permission.)

on an acceptable clinical response in other conditions.[32–34] Known to have a chemodenervating effect based on skeletal muscle studies, the different toxin serotypes (BTX A-G) target different proteins involved in the SNARE [soluble N-ethylmaleimide-sensitive factor attachment protein (SNAP) receptor] proteins complex[32] (Figure 47.3). The mechanism of action in smooth muscle, however, may be more complex, as new evidence suggest an antinociceptive and neuromodulating effect.[34]

Even though several elegant studies have suggested that different growth factors contribute to bladder impedance pathology, these proteins are by no means the exclusive mediators of bSMC mechanical responses. For instance, studies of the cyclooxygenase (COX) pathway have suggested that COX-2 expression – active during bladder development[36] – is re-expressed during bladder distention[37] (making COX-2 inhibitors potential pharmacologic inhibitors of stretch-induced bSMC proliferation). These observations suggest that obstruction responses may reactivate mechanisms employed during development itself. Teleologically, this may represent an effort to restore the function originally intended during development. Convergence of these protein and enzymatic pathways in the regulation of bladder obstruction has yet to be demonstrated.

Extracellular matrix remodeling

As the bladder develops, or adapts to different stimuli, the extracellular matrix also remodels in concert with the changes described for bSMCs. An important group of enzymes – the matrix metalloproteinases (MMPs) – are crucial in this process of altering the ECM structure and function. They are multifunctional proteases that degrade ECM proteins, liberate or modulate the bioactivity of growth factors, cytokines or other proteases, as well as alter the bio-

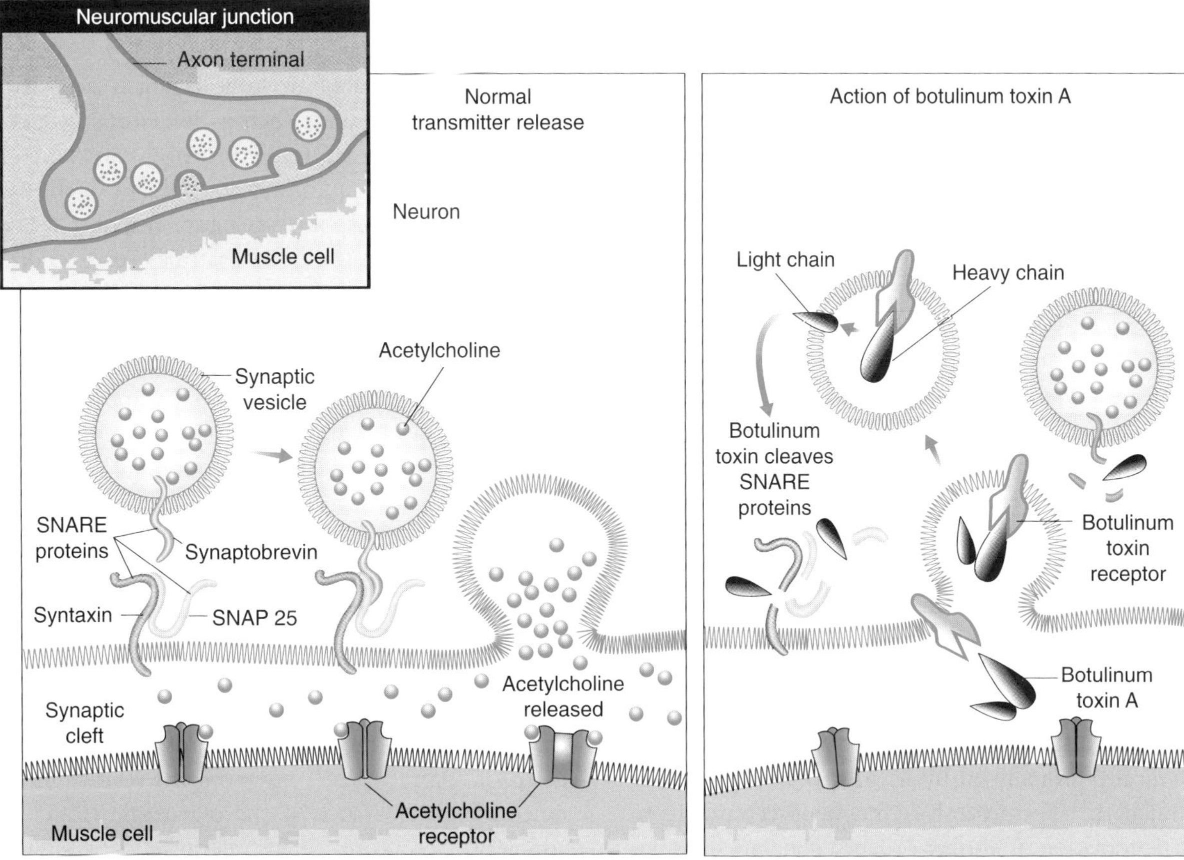

Figure 47.3 Under normal conditions, acetylcholine is packaged in vesicles that fuse with those of the nerve terminals, releasing the transmitter into the synaptic cleft. This process is mediated by a series of proteins, collectively called the SNARE proteins. Botulinum toxin cleaves the SNARE proteins, preventing assembly of the fusion complex and thus blocking the release of acetylcholine (Adapted from Rowland,[35] with permission.)

physical characteristics of the matrix. A cascade of events is initiated in the setting of excessive distention or high-pressure emptying, grossly resulting in thickening of the bladder wall. In conjunction with bSMC hyperplasia and hypertrophy, there is an increase in collagen synthesis, with deposition of collagens I and III,[38] associated with increased expression of MMP-2 and MMP-9, which are MMPs known to have an active role in matrix turnover in animal models.[39]

While the bladder matrix contributes to the physicomechanical characteristics of bladder dysfunction, it is proving to directly orchestrate bSMC biologic responses as well. The prototypical matrix protein in the bladder is fibrillar collagen. Stretching bSMCs promotes collagen production, and bladder obstruction models have demonstrated the new expression of both protein and collagen mRNA within the muscle bundles. Mostly, type I and type III are associated with the detrusor, although 19 different collagen types have been identified so far in other tissues, some with structural roles and others that associate with the structural types. For example, type XII collagen contributes to cross-linking type I fibrils during fiber assembly and may contribute to stiffness of tissues. Furthermore, type XII mRNA expression increases during mechanical distention of the whole bladder.[40] Diverse matrix alterations (accumulation, breakdown, redistribution, and structural rearrangements) are all occurring when tissues are remodeled during development as well as during response-to-injury or wound repair. In fact, many biologic mechanisms in development are recapitulated during repair. MMPs are substances with the ability to edit matrix collagen as well as many of the other ECM proteins. Although MMPs are now known to perform a variety of functions, they are best known for their originally described ability to break down (proteolyse) the ECM during morphogenesis, cell (tumor) invasion, and wound repair. Increased MMP activity or production has been described during bladder development and bladder obstruction in animal models. However, it now appears that the alterations in collagen may directly stimulate bSMC growth. When collagen is denatured experimentally, it elicits a strong proliferative response in bSMCs. Similarly, when collagen is chemically proteolysed by MMPs, bSMC growth is stimulated.[41] The proteolytic fragments released from the degradation of fibrillar collagen generate different signals than intact collagen, and potentially modulate bladder remodeling and bSMC growth by differential signaling pathways.[42]

It is likely that the receptors on the surface of all cells, including bSMCs, which permit cell-matrix attachment, are recognizing new epitopes in ECM macromolecules exposed as a result of protease activity. Inhibition of matrix receptors, such as the integrins, can potentially prevent bSMC proliferation in response to proteolysed matrix. Since bSMCs themselves are producing the enzymes (MMPs) responsible for matrix rearrangement, a powerful dynamic reciprocity is being revealed wherein bSMCs cause matrix alterations, which can then directly stimulate bSMC growth. Since natural regulators or inhibitors of these molecules also exist in the bladder (tissue inhibitors of MMPs, or TIMPs), we begin to appreciate a complex set of balanced mechanisms that depend on cell–matrix interactions. These processes are probably disturbed during bladder obstruction responses.

Finally, an integral, yet poorly understood and sometimes overlooked, part of the ECM is composed of proteoglycans and glycosaminoglycans. For instance, they may serve as ligands for some of the collagens present in the bladder wall and mediate response to injury or hyperdistention.[40] Most of the current research regarding these molecules has been directed towards the urothelium and the protection of this layer against noxious stimuli, which is probably disrupted in conditions such as interstitial cystitis.[43] The accumulation of ECM proteoglycans and glycosaminoglycans is a known integral part of the early phases of tissue response to injury response, conditioning changes in the ECM that may serve to direct the later deposition of the structural collagens. Evidence for a role in bladder wall remodeling comes from studies on the receptors for the ubiquitous glycosaminoglycan hyaluronic acid, a molecule that appears to play a role in bSMC collagen gene expression and regulation during distention.[40,44]

Neurotransmitters and modulators

Bladder function is tightly regulated, mainly under the influence of nervous and hormonal control systems. To date, the muscarinic receptors seem to be the most important ones in regards to activation of detrusor contractions;[45] however, the relative importance of others – such as the purinergic (P2X) and adrenergic receptors – gains relevance, depending on the species studied and the presence of a pathologic process. The human bladder can express all of the known cholinergic muscarinic receptors (M_1–M_5),[46] with well-described predominance of the M_2 and M_3

subtypes.[47] Even though the M_3 receptor has been clearly linked to detrusor contraction stimulation through activation of phosphoinositide hydrolysis and generation of inositol triphosphate, it is the M_2 receptor that predominates in the human bladder by a ratio of at least 3:1 over the M_3 subtype. Notwithstanding the unclear functional role of the M_2 receptor, it is interesting to note that its expression further increases in experimental pathologic states, potentially facilitating bladder contractions and muscle hypertrophy.[48,49] Beyond the evidence for adenylyl cyclase inhibition after M_2 or M_4 activation, other ill-defined signaling pathways may be involved, such as modulation of purine-evoked relaxation and activation of non-specific cation channels.[10,45,50,51] Interest in this topic has been rekindled after the recent introduction of subtype selective pharmacologic agents: i.e. M_3 specific antagonists solifenacin and darifenacin.[52]

In regard to congenital disorders, the issue is compounded by the limited understanding of neural control and maturation during development. Fetal human studies have shown variation in some receptor subtype expression when compared with adults, as is the case for P2X receptors.[53] In contrast, most reports describe little difference in cholinergic innervation or response to stimulation of muscarinic receptors, suggesting functional capacity early in life.[54] Abnormalities in receptor expression and function are probable in disorders that affect the bladder during its organogenesis. However, the role of these receptors in terms of detrusor functional alterations remains to be established.

Posterior urethral valves as a model of congenital bladder outflow obstruction

How the underlying molecular signaling cascades mediate survival and cell death can help lay the foundations for understanding how extrinsic pathologies mediate intrinsic bladder responses. Posterior urethral valves (PUV) represent an archetypical form of increased resistance to urinary flow in humans. In the pediatric sphere, this is somewhat analogous to the impedance generated by benign prostatic enlargement in the adult male. Whereas similar clinical bladder responses are noted between these two pathologies, multiple factors probably differentiate childhood from adult obstructive uropathies. PUV bladder trabeculation and altered function represents a spectrum of pathology which may derive as much from its timing during gestation as it does from the degree of impedance. Experimental observations on extrinsic manipulation of the bladder neck would suggest that while extrinsic obstruction models do reproduce some of the structural and functional consequences seen in clinical PUV bladders, they may also unwittingly distract from the true nature of the problem at the molecular level.

The 'valve' bladder has long been viewed as the bladder's response to a mechanical problem. Bladder SMCs must simply work harder to expel urine. They must mount an increased contraction effort. In doing so, the bladder phenotype (structure and function) changes. Finely tuned neurosensory perception of pressure/stretch, which accompanies higher than expected voiding pressure, is relayed through reflex arcs and may increase efferent motor demands on the detrusor. Furthermore, abnormalities in the outlet region of the bladder neck and sphincter areas, which harbor the valves themselves, may give rise to neurodevelopmental changes that directly influence bSMC function. Nevertheless, the apparent normalization of PUV bladder morphology and function that can occur when valves are ablated suggests that bSMCs can retain the capacity for normal function despite the creation of an outlet defect during gestation. This is in contrast to bSMCs from neurogenic bladders, which appear to harbor more permanent phenotypic changes, as demonstrated by in-vitro culture experiments.[55] It would seem then, that bSMCs themselves are sensing the presence of impedance to flow, whatever the etiology of the obstruction itself.

During development and during the brief periods of normal unobstructed emptying, bSMCs are being programmed to accept and work against a range of elevated intravesical pressures. However, the resistance afforded by the PUV increases this pressure. Whether indirectly through a stretch/tension neural receptor mechanism and/or directly via SMC stretch/mechanoreceptors, alterations in muscle membrane ion channels, or changes in SMC shape, bladder SMCs contract more forcefully. As inefficient emptying progresses, the excessive bladder storage may actually overstretch the detrusor muscle to excess degree and duration; indeed, this may become a dominant insult that erodes bladder function.

Clearly, the role of physical stretch and tension in bSMC biology is more complex and difficult to sort out from a mechanistic point of view than it first appears. We now appreciate that stretch operates under different conditions in different pathologies, and may contribute to bladder alterations at different points in natural history of any given obstructive uropathy. The paradox is that although mechanical stretching of bSMCs in vitro may generate clinically familiar responses generated by hypercontracting or excessively stretched bSMCs in vivo, it may do so through physiologically irrelevant or unrelated molecular mechanisms. Nonetheless, to determine whether the physical stimulus of stretch per se can predict and elucidate relevant changes in bSMC phenotype, cultured bSMCs have been subjected to controlled mechanical stretching in vitro. Studies of this nature have provided compelling information and suggest that bSMCs alone may be a primary cellular recipient of relevant stretch (mechanical) stimuli in vivo.

Limitations of research tools: in-vivo, ex-vivo, and in-vitro models

The study of any biologic problem is often dependent on the availability of appropriate models. More importantly, investigation may be guided by a series of appropriately framed segments or aspects of the problem. As previously mentioned, these emerging segments include proteins and molecules which affect SMC growth and phenotype, the influence of mechanical and neural stimuli, and the role and regulation of the bladder ECM components. Clearly, these areas of investigation will intersect, and new segments of the problem are to be anticipated. Although none of the molecules currently reported to influence bSMC growth and behavior in the context of bladder obstruction have affected clinical practice as yet, they may hold keys to appreciating how bSMCs truly work. There are, however, conceptual shortcomings to the use of in-vitro, ex-vivo, and in-vivo animal models as a means of deciphering the intricacies behind normal and pathologic bladder function and development. Experimental conditions differ in timing, reversibility, stretching parameters, and cyclicity, as well as the nature (extrinsic vs intrinsic) of the obstructive stimuli. Therefore, the results observed are potentially not the same as the ones elicited by the detrusor in congenital anomalies.

The promise of tissue engineering

As the full potentials of molecular mechanisms and therapeutics, prenatal diagnosis, and sheer curiosity about bladder disease are awakened and converge in the coming decade, we can expect new and frankly unexpected approaches to emerge for the treatment and even prevention of obstructive bladder pathologies. Increasingly, intense research has focused on the fields of regenerative medicine and tissue engineering, as the principles of bioengineering, biomaterials, and cell transplantation are applied to construct biologic substitutes that would restore function in diseased urologic tissues.[56] This process has uncovered that, perhaps not unexpectedly, the biology of the bladder is every bit as complex and enigmatic as the other vital body systems. It has proven difficult to regenerate all the functional layers of the bladder as the engineered tissue needs to have optimal mechanical and structural characteristics while being biocompatible and capable of eliciting enough neovascularization to survive once implanted.[57] Most of the available data are based on in-vitro and promising animal models.[58]

Conclusion

The past decades have witnessed a changing view of the bladder, from a simple organ that contracts in order to volitionally eliminate urine, to a complex unit responsive to fine neuromodulation and smooth muscle–ECM interaction.[1,41,59,60] As such, the approach to bladder dysfunction is shifting from a symptomatic basis (based solely on treating urinary tract symptoms and incontinence) to measures aimed at preventing overdistention and high intravesical pressures. In this manner, the tendency is to prevent end-stage damage to affected organs (requiring aggressive and morbid interventions such as augmentation cystoplasty or renal transplantation) by modulating the fibroproliferative response and its consequent loss of compliance, contraction inefficiency, and hyperdistention.[61] Even though great advances have been made in the past few decades, understanding the molecular mechanisms behind bladder development and response to abnormal stretch and dysfunction remains a fertile area for research and development.

References

1. McCarthy LS, Smeulders N, Wilcox DT. Cell biology of bladder development and the role of the extracellular matrix. Nephron Exp Nephrol 2003; 95:e129–33.
2. Smeulders N, Woolf AS, Wilcox DT. Smooth muscle differentiation and cell turnover in mouse detrusor development. J Urol 2002; 167:385–90.
3. Baskin LS, Hayward SW, Young P, Cunha GR. Role of mesenchymal–epithelial interactions in normal bladder development. J Urol 1996; 156:1820–7.

4. Baskin LS, Hayward SW, Young PF, Cunha GR. Ontogeny of the rat bladder: smooth muscle and epithelial differentiation. Acta Anat (Basel) 1996; 155:163–71.
5. Smeulders N, Woolf AS, Wilcox DT. Extracellular matrix protein expression during mouse detrusor development. J Pediatr Surg 2003; 38:1–12.
6. Koo HP, Howard PS, Chang SL et al. Developmental expression of interstitial collagen genes in fetal bladders. J Urol 1997; 158:954–61.
7. Upadhyay J, Aitken KJ, Damdar C, Bolduc S, Bagli DJ. Integrins expressed with bladder extracellular matrix after stretch injury in vivo mediate bladder smooth muscle cell growth in vitro. J Urol 2003; 169:750–5.
8. Baskin L, Meaney D, Landsman A, Zderic SA, Macarak E. Bovine bladder compliance increases with normal fetal development. J Urol 1994; 152:692–5; discussion 696–7.
9. Kim KM, Kogan BA, Massad CA, Huang YC. Collagen and elastin in the normal fetal bladder. J Urol 1991; 146:524–7.
10. Andersson KE, Arner A. Urinary bladder contraction and relaxation: physiology and pathophysiology. Physiol Rev 2004; 84:935–86.
11. Zderic SA, Wein A, Rohrman D et al. Mechanisms of bladder smooth-muscle hypertrophy and decompensation: lessons from normal development and the response to outlet obstruction. World J Urol 1998; 16:350–8.
12. Hypolite JA, DiSanto ME, Zheng Y et al. Regional variation in myosin isoforms and phosphorylation at the resting tone in urinary bladder smooth muscle. Am J Physiol Cell Physiol 2001; 280:C254–64.
13. Rovner AS, Fagnant PM, Lowey S, Trybus KM. The carboxyl-terminal isoforms of smooth muscle myosin heavy chain determine thick filament assembly properties. J Cell Biol 2002; 156:113–23.
14. DiSanto ME, Stein R, Chang S et al. Alteration in expression of myosin isoforms in detrusor smooth muscle following bladder outlet obstruction. Am J Physiol Cell Physiol 2003; 285:C1397–410.
15. Mannikarottu AS, Hypolite JA, Zderic SA et al. Regional alterations in the expression of smooth muscle myosin isoforms in response to partial bladder outlet obstruction. J Urol 2005; 173:302–8.
16. Arner A, Lofgren M, Morano I. Smooth, slow and smart muscle motors. J Muscle Res Cell Motil 2003; 24:165–73.
17. Zamir E, Geiger B. Molecular complexity and dynamics of cell-matrix adhesions. J Cell Sci 2001; 114:3583–90.
18. Ingber DE. Mechanical signaling and the cellular response to extracellular matrix in angiogenesis and cardiovascular physiology. Circ Res 2002; 91:877–87.
19. Iqbal J, Zaidi M. Molecular regulation of mechanotransduction. Biochem Biophys Res Commun 2005; 328:751–5.
20. Aitken K, Bägli DJ. Stretch-induced bladder smooth muscle cell (SMC) proliferation is mediated by RHAMM-dependent extracellular-regulated kinase (erk) signaling. Urology 2001; 57:109.
21. Nguyen HT, Adam RM, Bride SH et al. Cyclic stretch activates p38 SAPK2-, ErbB2-, and AT1-dependent signaling in bladder smooth muscle cells. Am J Physiol Cell Physiol 2000; 279:C1155–67.
22. Adam RM, Roth JA, Cheng HL et al. Signaling through PI3K/Akt mediates stretch and PDGF-BB-dependent DNA synthesis in bladder smooth muscle cells. J Urol 2003; 169:2388–93.
23. Yamaguchi O. Response of bladder smooth muscle cells to obstruction: signal transduction and the role of mechanosensors. Urology 2004; 63:11–16.
24. Wallner EI, Yang Q, Peterson DR, Wada J, Kanwar YS. Relevance of extracellular matrix, its receptors, and cell adhesion molecules in mammalian nephrogenesis. Am J Physiol 1998; 275:F467–77.
25. Adam RM, Roth JA, Cheng HL et al. Signaling through PI3K/Akt mediates stretch and PDGF-BB-dependent DNA synthesis in bladder smooth muscle cells. J Urol 2003; 169:2394–6.
26. Borer JG, Park JM, Atala A et al. Heparin-binding EGF-like growth factor expression increases selectively in bladder smooth muscle in response to lower urinary tract obstruction. Lab Invest 1999; 79:1335–45.
27. Schaeffer HJ, Weber MJ. Mitogen-activated protein kinases: specific messages from ubiquitous messengers. Mol Cell Biol 1999; 19:2435–44.
28. Adam RM. Recent insights into the cell biology of bladder smooth muscle. Nephron Exp Nephrol 2006; 102:e1–7. Epub 2005 Sep 19.
29. Park JM, Bauer SB, Freeman MR, Peters CA. Oxybutynin chloride inhibits proliferation and suppresses gene expression in bladder smooth muscle cells. J Urol 1999; 162:1110–14.
30. Wilkins BJ, Molkentin JD. Calcium–calcineurin signaling in the regulation of cardiac hypertrophy. Biochem Biophys Res Commun 2004; 322:1178–91.
31. Nozaki K, Tomizawa K, Yokoyama T, Kumon H, Matsui H. Calcineurin mediates bladder smooth muscle hypertrophy after bladder outlet obstruction. J Urol 2003; 170:2077–81.
32. Frenkl TL, Rackley RR. Injectable neuromodulatory agents: botulinum toxin therapy. Urol Clin North Am 2005; 32:89–99.
33. Smith CP, Chancellor MB. Emerging role of botulinum toxin in the management of voiding dysfunction. J Urol 2004; 171:2128–37.
34. Schurch B, Corcos J. Botulinum toxin injections for paediatric incontinence. Curr Opin Urol 2005; 15:264–7.
35. Rowland LP. Stroke, spasticity, and botulinum toxin. N Engl J Med 2002; 347:382–3.
36. Park JM, Yang T, Arend LJ et al. Cyclooxygenase-2 is expressed in bladder during fetal development and stimulated by outlet obstruction. Am J Physiol 1997; 273:F538–44.
37. Park JM, Yang T, Arend LJ et al. Obstruction stimulates COX-2 expression in bladder smooth muscle cells via increased mechanical stretch. Am J Physiol 1999; 276:F129–36.
38. Tekgul S, Yoshino K, Bägli D et al. Collagen types I and III localization by in situ hybridization and immunohistochemistry in the partially obstructed young rabbit bladder. J Urol 1996; 156:582–6.
39. Sutherland RS, Baskin LS, Elfman F, Hayward SW, Cunha GR. The role of type IV collagenases in rat blad-

der development and obstruction. Pediatr Res 1997; 41:430–4.
40. Capolicchio G, Aitken KJ, Gu JX, Reddy P, Bägli DJ. Extracellular matrix gene responses in a novel ex vivo model of bladder stretch injury. J Urol 2001; 165:2235–40.
41. Aitken KJ, Block G, Lorenzo A et al. Mechanotransduction of extracellular signal-related kinases 1 and 2 mitogen-activated protein kinase activity in smooth muscle is dependent on the extracellular matrix and regulated by matrix metalloproteinases. Am J Pathol 2006; 169:459–70.
42. Herz DB, Aitken K, Bägli DJ. Collagen directly stimulates bladder smooth muscle cell growth in vitro: regulation by extracellular regulated mitogen activated protein kinase. J Urol 2003; 170:2072–6.
43. Lokeshwar VB, Selzer MG, Cerwinka WH et al. Urinary uronate and sulfated glycosaminoglycan levels: markers for interstitial cystitis severity. J Urol 2005; 174:344–9.
44. Bägli DJ, Joyner BD, Mahoney SR, McCulloch L. The hyaluronic acid receptor RHAMM is induced by stretch injury of rat bladder in vivo and influences smooth muscle cell contraction in vitro [corrected]. J Urol 1999; 162:832–40.
45. Andersson KE. Detrusor contraction – focus on muscarinic receptors. Scand J Urol Nephrol Suppl 2004; 215:54–7.
46. Sigala S, Mirabella G, Peroni A et al. Differential gene expression of cholinergic muscarinic receptor subtypes in male and female normal human urinary bladder. Urology 2002; 60:719–25.
47. Hegde SS. Muscarinic receptors in the bladder: from basic research to therapeutics. Br J Pharmacol 2006; 147(Suppl 2):580–7.
48. Braverman AS, Ruggieri MR Sr. Hypertrophy changes the muscarinic receptor subtype mediating bladder contraction from M3 toward M2. Am J Physiol Regul Integr Comp Physiol 2003; 285:R701–8.
49. Pontari MA, Braverman AS, Ruggieri MR Sr. The M2 muscarinic receptor mediates in vitro bladder contractions from patients with neurogenic bladder dysfunction. Am J Physiol Regul Integr Comp Physiol 2004; 286:R874–80.
50. Giglio D, Delbro DS, Tobin G. On the functional role of muscarinic M2 receptors in cholinergic and purinergic responses in the rat urinary bladder. Eur J Pharmacol 2001; 428:357–64.
51. Kotlikoff MI, Dhulipala P, Wang YX. M2 signaling in smooth muscle cells. Life Sci 1999; 64:437–42.
52. Nijman RJ. Role of antimuscarinics in the treatment of nonneurogenic daytime urinary incontinence in children. Urology 2004; 63:45–50.
53. O'Reilly BA, Kosaka AH, Chang TK et al. A quantitative analysis of purinoceptor expression in human fetal and adult bladders. J Urol 2001; 165:1730–4.
54. Longhurst P. Developmental aspects of bladder function. Scand J Urol Nephrol Suppl 2004; 215:11–19.
55. Lin HK, Cowan R, Moore P et al. Characterization of neuropathic bladder smooth muscle cells in culture. J Urol 2004; 171:1348–52.
56. Atala A. Regeneration of urologic tissues and organs. Adv Biochem Eng Biotechnol 2005; 94:181–210.
57. Atala A, Bauer S, Soker S et al. Tissue-engineered autologous bladders for patients needing cystoplasty. Lancet 2006; 367:1241–6.
58. Oberpenning F, Meng J, Yoo JJ, Atala A. De novo reconstitution of a functional mammalian urinary bladder by tissue engineering. Nat Biotechnol 1999; 17:149–55.
59. Levin RM, Wein AJ, Buttyan R, Monson FC, Longhurst PA. Update on bladder smooth-muscle physiology. World J Urol 1994; 12:226–32.
60. Levin RM. Overview of nerves and pharmacology in the bladder. Adv Exp Med Biol 1999; 462:237–40.
61. Holmdahl G, Sillen U, Hellstrom AL, Sixt R, Solsnes E. Does treatment with clean intermittent catheterization in boys with posterior urethral valves affect bladder and renal function? J Urol 2003; 170:1681–5, discussion 1685.

Basic science of prostatic development

48

Ellen Shapiro and Hongying Huang

The fetal prostate is the most proliferative state of the prostate gland and represents an excellent model for the study of morphogenesis, hormonal imprinting, and epithelial–mesenchymal interactions in the genitourinary (GU) tract. Events associated with fetal prostate development and in-utero influences which may alter growth in adulthood will probably provide insights into the mechanisms giving rise to benign and malignant aberrant growth of the prostate.

Embryology of the prostate

The prostate develops from the endodermal urogenital sinus (UGS), which is derived from the terminal end of the hindgut or 'cloaca' (Latin for sewer). Septation of the cloaca by the urorectal septum begins at about 28 days of gestation.[1] The rectum and primitive UGS form by the 44th day. The primitive UGS proximal to the mesonephric duct develops into the vesicourethral canal, whereas the region distal of the mesonephric duct becomes the definitive UGS. The UGS adjacent to the bladder (pelvic urethra) differentiates into the lower portion of the prostatic and membranous urethra.[2]

Prostate growth and development are dependent on androgen production by the fetal testes, which begins at about the 8th week of gestation.[3] Unlike development of the wolffian duct (WD) derivatives, which are dependent solely on testosterone, the differentiation of the UGS is dependent on the 5α reduced form of testosterone, dihydrotestosterone (DHT). DHT is essential for the growth and development of the prostate.[3–6] By 10 weeks, the prostatic ductal network develops from solid epithelial outgrowths, or prostatic buds, which evaginate from the endodermal UGS immediately below the bladder and penetrate into the surrounding urogenital mesenchyme (UGM).[7] The prostatic ducts rapidly lengthen, arborize, and canalize. By 13 weeks, at the peak of testosterone production, 70 primary ducts are present and exhibit secretory cytodifferentiation.[7]

Within the fetal prostate lies the utricle. Although the embryologic origin of the utricle is thought to be a remnant of the fused caudal ends of the müllerian ducts (MDs), compelling evidence from Shapiro et al indicates that the utricle forms as an ingrowth of specialized urothelium lining the dorsal wall of the UGS.[8] This is occurring during complete caudal MD regression (Figure 48.1). Since utricular development from the UGS is similar to that of the vagina in the female fetus, it has been appropriately referred to as the 'sinus vagina'. Testosterone inhibits the formation of the lower vagina in the female, and therefore formation of an enlarged utricle in some males with severe hypospadias may be caused by inadequate virilization of this region of the UGS at a critical time during early gestation.[9]

Prostate morphology

In 1912, Lowsley studied the human fetal prostate and noted that the branching ductal system consisted of five distinct groups.[7] These lobes were termed the posterior, lateral (two), anterior, and middle lobes. The ducts of the posterior lobes originate from the floor of the prostatic urethra distal to the openings of the ejaculatory ducts (EDS) and grow posteriorly. The epithelial buds of the two lateral lobes branch lateral to the verumontanum. The ducts of the middle lobe originate on the posterior urethra proximal to the openings to the EDs. The anterior lobe buds branch anterior to the verumontanum.

Xia et al qualitatively examined prostate growth, histogenesis, and secretory activity in normal fetuses ranging in age from 20 weeks gestation to 1 month

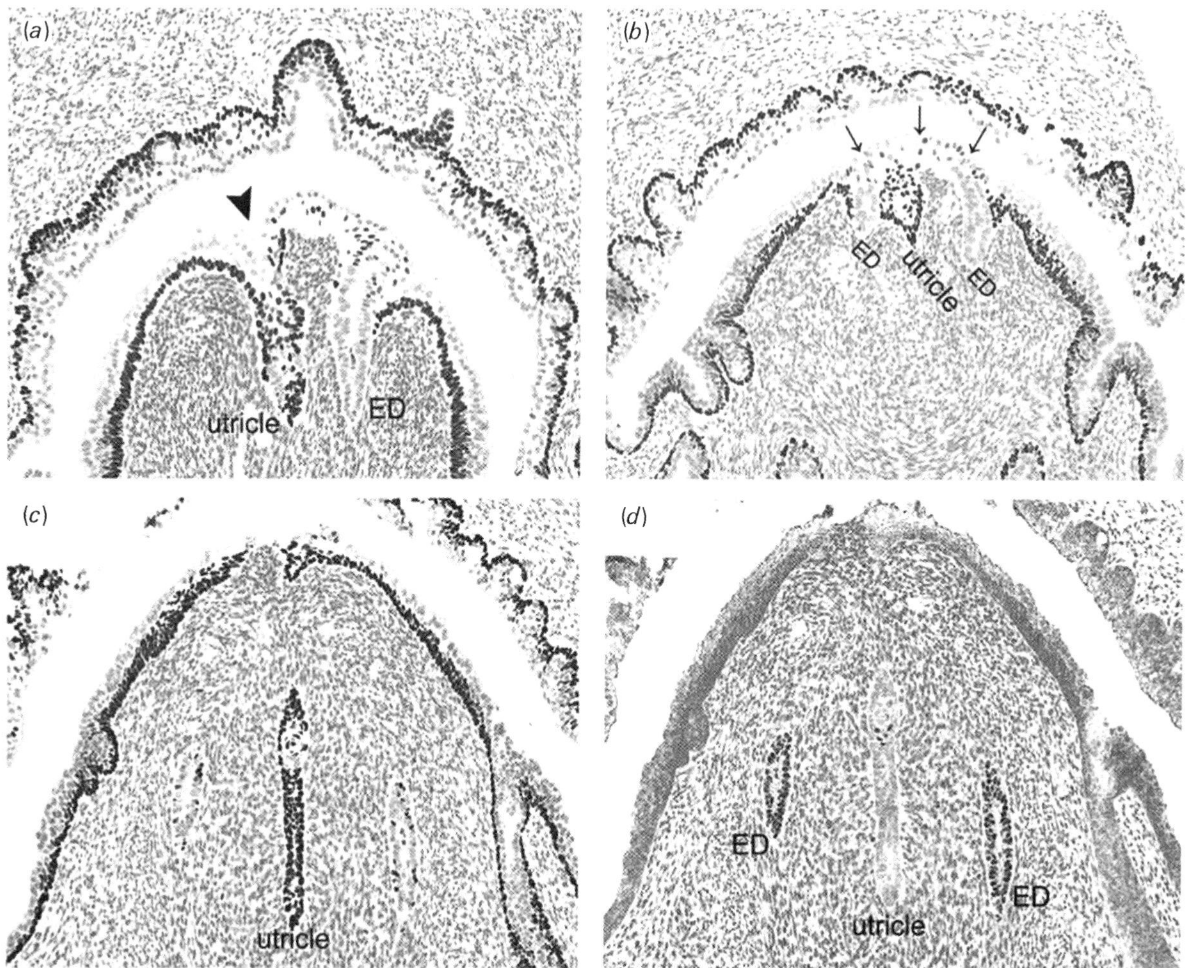

Figure 48.1 Cross section of a human fetal prostate, aged 15 weeks. (*a* and *b*) Two different specimens showing the evaginated p63 (basal cell marker) positive cells that form the utricle (arrowhead) and only weakly staining basal cells in the urogenital sinus (UGS) between the ejaculatory ducts (EDs; arrows). (*c*) The p63 positive cells of the utricle continue to grow into the midline of the mesenchyme and surround the small solid remnants of the müllerian ducts (MDs) in its path, which (*d*) also express Pax-2 (marker for MD and wolffian ducts). The EDs are also Pax-2 positive (×200).

(postnatal).[10] No sharply delineated 'lobules' were recognized. Two zones were identified: the inner submucosal zone (IZ) and the peripheral zone (PZ). The IZ was characterized by a concentric mass of fibromuscular connective tissue containing ducts at various stages of development. The PZ contained less concentrically organized fibromuscular connective tissue, with secondary ducts, gland buds, and groups of acinar glands. Lowsley's work, together with Xia et al's observations, lends support to the current concept of the morphology of the adult prostate gland, which exhibits three zones – central, transition, and peripheral zones – corresponding to three distinct sets of ducts. This is important as prostatic diseases are region-specific, with prostate adenocarcinoma developing primarily in the peripheral zone and benign prostatic hyperplasia (BPH) developing primarily in the transition zone. The development of BPH is important to understand, because growth of new acini in this condition deviates from the normal development of most organs.[11] The prostate is the only organ to demonstrate new growth as part of the aging process. However, the new acinar architecture is unlike that of the fetus, since the ducts of the fetal prostate branch parallel and away from each other rather than toward each other, as seen in BPH nodules.

Endocrinology of prostatic development

Development of the prostate is androgen dependent and DHT is the active intracellular androgen.[3,12] The

5α-reductase deficiency syndrome is a form of autosomal recessive male pseudohermaphroditism characterized by severe penoscrotal hypospadias, a blind vaginal pouch, and normal testes with normal epididymes, vasa deferentia, and seminal vesicles.[13] The EDs terminate in the blind-ending vagina, and the prostate is small or undetectable. The selective effects of testosterone and DHT are defined since the defect in virilization during embryogenesis is limited to the UGS and the anlagen of the external genitalia.

Although there is no compelling molecular evidence for homology between specific rodent prostatic lobes and human prostatic zones, the rodent has been extensively studied to further our understanding of prostatic development. Imperato-McGinley and coworkers demonstrated prostatic bud formation in the rat model of 5α-reductase deficiency,[5] a finding that was unexpected since finasteride, a 5α-reductase inhibitor, did not completely abolish prostatic differentiation, which suggested that budding may have different thresholds of response for DHT. Further studies showed that flutamide, a non-steroidal antiandrogen, in high enough doses to feminize the external genitalia of the male rat, failed to inhibit prostatic development whereas cyproterone acetate (CA), a steroidal antiandrogen, inhibited prostatic bud development and external genitalia development. Low-dose DHT could induce prostatic buds in female fetuses. The WDs could not be abolished in males with CA, and high-dose antitestosterone treatment failed to inhibit prostatic buds. Although DHT is important for prostatic growth, the developing prostate may be responsive to exceedingly low levels of DHT or other androgens.[5]

Also, some aspects of postnatal prostatic growth may be independent of androgens, as castration in the rat during this period does not completely inhibit prostate development,[14,15] which suggests that other non-androgen growth factors such as peptide growth factors are capable of mediating arborization and growth of prostatic ducts.[6] These findings suggest that varying phenotypes occur and are species dependent.

This concept is supported by the observations of Mahendroo and colleagues, where unexpected virilization in male mice lacking steroid 5α-reductase enzymes was observed.[16] These mice had normal external and internal genitalia and were fertile but had smaller prostates and seminal vesicles than controls. As expected, high testosterone levels were found in target tissues. DHT administration led to an increase in seminal vesicles and coagulating gland wet weights in the 5α-reductase type 2 deficient mouse and an increase in the prostate size, seminal vesicle, and coagulating gland in both the 5α-reductase type 1 and 2 deficient mouse. When DHT was administered to the mouse deficient in only 5α-reductase type 2, no increase in prostatic size occurred, whereas DHT administered to the 5α-reductase type 1 and 2 deficient mouse resulted in an increase in prostatic size. Androgen-dependent gene expression was decreased in the seminal vesicles lacking one or more of the 5α-reductase enzymes, but was restored with testosterone or DHT. These studies show that only testosterone is needed for differentiation of the male UGS in the mouse, and synthesis of DHT serves largely as a signal amplification mechanism.

Using immunohistochemistry, we studied human fetal prostates, with gestational ages of 7–22 weeks. Representative tissue sections were stained with antibodies for the androgen receptor (AR) and 5α-reductase. At 7 weeks, we demonstrated AR and 5α-reductase expression in the peripheral stroma, above the ejaculatory ducts (EDs) while only AR is seen in the UGS luminal epithelium. By 9 weeks, AR expression was ubiquitous in the stroma and suprabasal cells of the UGS but was observed in the basal cells of only the central dorsal UGS below the EDs. Stromal 5α-reductase expression was significantly increased and was observed throughout the UGS. By 11–13 weeks, AR expression increased in the stroma especially in the periphery. Epithelial AR increased from the base to the apex with AR observed in all cell layers of the UGS, ducts and acini except for the basal cells of the UGS and ducts above the EDs which remained negative. 5α-reductase expression was observed throughout the stroma except in the ventral SM, ventral periurethral stroma, and the posterior periphery where expression is diminished. Epithelial 5α-reductase expression increased from the base to the apex, with no expression in the ductal epithelium of the posterior lobe (Figure 48.2). The lateral lobes showed only distal duct and acini expression whereas the ducts emanating from above the EDs expressed 5α-reductase throughout their epithelium. By 22 weeks, AR expression is ubiquitous with greatest staining in the epithelium and the posterior and posterolateral peripheral stroma, while 5α-reductase is almost undetectable.

We concluded that epithelial AR expression is significantly greater below the EDs than above the EDs at each gestational age up to 22 weeks, when no difference in the AR expression pattern is observed in the gland and 5α-reductase is almost absent. In contrast, UGS and ductal epithelial 5α-reductase was

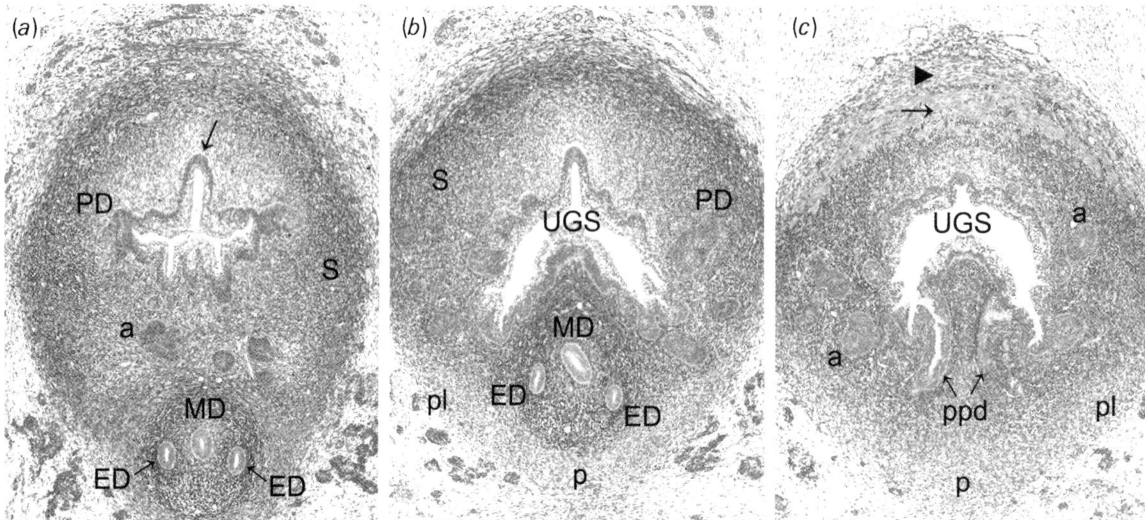

Figure 48.2 Cross section of a human fetal prostate, aged 11 weeks. (*a*) Bladder neck region with significant 5α-reductase expression throughout the prostatic stroma (S) and the stroma surrounding the ejaculatory ducts (EDs) and müllerian duct (MD). Expression is noted in the basal epithelium of the urogenital sinus (UGS) (arrow) and in the prostatic ducts (PD) and acini (a). (*b*) Region between the bladder neck and the entrance of the EDs into the UGS, with similar stromal 5α-reductase expression, except posteriorly (p) and posterolaterally (pl) and much less UGS, prostatic ductal (PD), and acinar expression. (*c*) Region below the entrance of the EDs into the UGS, with no 5α-reductase expression in the UGS epithelium, posterior prostatic ducts (ppd), or lateral acini (a). There is no 5α-reductase in the posterior (p) and posterolateral stroma (pl) or in the smooth (arrow) or skeletal muscle (arrowhead) in the anterior stroma (×100).

expressed in a gradient fashion from the apex to the base/bladder neck. This suggests a regional, reciprocal relationship between select areas of stromal and epithelial AR and 5α-reductase expression. This detailed localization study supports other investigations which have suggested that DHT serves largely as a hormonal signal amplification during prostate development.[16,17]

Stromal–epithelial interactions

Stromal and epithelial interactions that occur in the developing prostate are androgen dependent.[14] Lasnitzki et al performed tissue recombinant experiments by combining mesenchyme isolated from fetal rat or mouse UGS with fragments of prostate or bladder epithelium. These tissue recombinants are grafted under the renal capsule of recipient animals and form prostatic ductal tissue. Lasnitzki has utilized testicular feminization (Tfm) syndrome in mice to elucidate the roles of epithelial vs mesenchymal androgen receptor (ARs) in prostatic development.[18] The Tfm syndrome results in complete failure of the prostate to develop[19] due to defective or absent ARs. The WDs undergo degeneration and the external genitalia are feminized despite normal testosterone levels. Therefore, Tfm mice have deficient AR and fail to develop prostates. When tissue recombinants constructed of wild-type (WT) mesenchyme (UGM) and Tfm epithelium are exposed to androgen as a result of grafting of the recombinants into intact male hosts, normal prostatic morphogenesis ensues.[18,20–23] When the Tfm mesenchyme is combined with either the Tfm or the wild-type epithelium, the prostate does not form. From these studies, it is concluded that there is a critical role for mesenchymal AR in prostate development and that many androgen effects on prostatic epithelium do not require epithelial AR but are elicited by the paracrine action of AR + mesenchyme. It is interesting to note though that mouse prostatic epithelial ARs are not expressed until postnatal day 1, whereas human prostatic epithelial ARs are present in the urogenital epithelium as early as 7 weeks' gestational age.[17,24,25] Prostatic epithelial ARs are required for the expression of AR-dependent secretory proteins during postnatal development.

Tissue recombinant experiments have also been used to examine epithelial–mesenchymal interactions in the differentiation and organization of prostatic smooth muscle (SM).[26] Experiments combined adult prostatic epithelium (PRE) with UGM or seminal vesicle mesenchyme (SVM) or bladder epithelium (BLE) with UGM or SVM. Prostatic ducts developed in all tissue recombinants when UGM was used with either epithelium. SM cells also organized into sheets that resembled prostate. When SVM was combined with either epithelium, the prostatic ducts were surrounded by thick SM cells, resembling seminal vesicle. The SM was unorganized in grafts of SVM or UGM. These experiments suggest that male UGM dictates spatial organization, but SM differentiation is induced by epithelium. Urothelium may also direct the organization of SM tissue, since urothelium is thought to be a potent inducer of SM differentiation. Cunha has shown that the proximal segments of prostatic ducts near the urethra express urothelial membrane antigen and have associated thick layers of SM cells surrounding them.[12] All of these tissue recombinant experiments show that interactions between the mesenchyme and epithelium are reciprocal.

Hormonal imprinting

For more than 50 years, the role of natural and synthetic estrogens in prostate development and the effects of hormonal imprinting have been studied.[27–29] Estrogens alter the hypothalamic–pituitary–gonadal axis, resulting in decreased androgen levels and subsequent regression of the prostatic epithelium.[30,31] Investigations have focused on the correlation between estradiol and prostatic development in fetal mice depending on their intrauterine position, the effects of experimental increases in estradiol in mouse fetuses, the inhibition of prostate development following administration of high-dose estrogens, and the opposing effects of high- and low-dose estrogen on prostatic development.[32]

It has been postulated in humans that the early testosterone surge at 30–60 days of life may be a critically important 'imprinting' event that may have an impact on the gland's propensity for future abnormal prostatic growth and disease. Hormonal imprinting has been studied in the rat.[33] Naslund and Coffey showed that early hormonal surges are requisite for normal adult prostate growth in the rat, and that an alteration in the normal endocrine events that occurs shortly after birth can have significant and permanent effects on the androgen sensitivity and growth of the adult prostate.[34] These hormonal surges are thought to affect prostatic growth by altering the properties of the prostatic stem cells. Recently, Tsujimura et al have shown that the proximal region of the mouse prostatic ducts is enriched in a subpopulation of epithelial cells that have a number of properties of stem cells: they are slow-cycling, possess high in-vitro proliferative potential, and single cells are able to reconstitute complex highly branched glandular structures in vitro that contain basal and luminal cells.[35] The absolute number of these stem cells is important because it ultimately determines the size of the gland. Therefore, hormonal events occurring before puberty can imprint or program the prostatic size, androgen sensitivity, and function and maintenance of the stem cells.

Prins and others have shown that brief exposure of rodents to estrogens during the neonatal period leads to permanent irreversible and dose-dependent effects of the prostate gland's morphology, cellular organization, and function.[2,3,36,37] If estrogenic exposure is high, the permanent imprints include reduced prostatic growth, epithelial differentiation defects, altered secretory function, and aging-associated dysplasia similar to prostatic intraepithelial neoplasia or (PIN). This process, referred to as estrogenic imprinting or developmental estrogenization, is used as a model to evaluate the role of exogenous and endogenous estrogens as a potential predisposing factor for prostate diseases later in life.[36,37]

Prins' study also examined the effects of neonatal estrogen exposure on the development of the AR.[37,38] Estrogen receptors (ERs) have been shown to be strongly expressed in the mouse prostate mesenchyme.[22] While the stroma is strongly ER positive (ER+ve), the prostate SM is weakly to negatively staining after differentiating from mesenchyme. Fibroblasts remain strongly ER+ve. There are no ERs in the epithelium of the prostate. Brief exposure to neonatal estrogen down-regulates AR and permanently alters its expression, as well as retarding ductal development.[37,38] SM development is generally unaffected, as is the development of basal cells. Estrogenization does not inhibit epithelial cell differentiation (determined by the appearance of luminal cell cytokeratins) completely, indicating that initiation of cytodifferentiation precedes elevated AR expression rather than increasing AR-triggering cytodifferentiation. These experiments suggest that functional differentiation is dependent on AR expression in epithelial cells.

Although this response is mediated through alterations in steroid receptor expression, other downstream mechanisms in the signaling cascade that mediate prostate ductal morphogenesis may be involved. The Sonic hedgehog gene (*Shh*) encodes a secreted glycoprotein that is expressed at many sites in the vertebrate embryo and participates in the molecular signaling for the development of the notochord, limb, hindgut, and GU tract.[39,40] Loss of *Shh* function results in severe defects in neural and skeletal development, growth inhibition, and embryonic lethality. Using a murine model, *Shh* is expressed in the prostatic anlage of the UGS, and that expression is stimulated by testosterone. Pu et al showed that highly localized *Shh*-patched *gli* expression along with regulation of downstream morphogens participate in dichotomous branching during prostate morphogenesis.[40] Neonatal exposure to high-dose estradiol suppressed *Shh*-patched *gli* and blocked ductal branching in the dorsal and lateral prostate lobes.

Barnett et al studied *Shh* expression in the human fetal prostate at 9.5–20 weeks' gestation.[41] *Shh* expression was present in the prostatic urothelium, prostatic ducts, and glandular epithelium at 9.5, 11.5, 13, and 16 weeks and in the prostatic buds by 11.5 weeks. Staining was observed in the EDs, MDs, and anterior SM and SKM. Staining intensity diminished after 16 weeks as testosterone levels declined to baseline and was almost absent by 18 and 20 weeks, suggesting a direct relationship between testosterone levels and *Shh* expression.

Other studies of the effects of estrogen on the prostate have used the induction of squamous metaplasia (SQM) as a reliable marker for estrogen action on the gland.[31,42] Risbridger et al studied this transformation of the epithelium and showed proliferation of basal cells and the expression of K10.[31] They also showed that mice lacking the stroma and/or epithelial estrogen receptor α (ERα) did not develop SQM.[43] These studies suggest that stroma and epithelial ERα are required for the induction of SQM in the prostate gland.

Shapiro et al examined the immunolocalization of ERα and estrogen receptor β (ERβ) in the human fetal prostate (Figure 48.3). ERα expression was not detected until 15 weeks, with sparse staining in the utricle.[23] By 19 weeks, increased ERα expression is seen within luminal cells of the ventral urogenital epithelium (UGE), basal cells of the dorsal UGE, the utricle, distal periurethral ducts, peripheral stroma, and posterior prostatic duct. K14 is detected in basal cells of the UGE and in several posterior acini. At 22 weeks, ERα expression is more intense in all of these areas. ERβ is expressed throughout the UGE, EDs, MDs, and entire stroma at 7 weeks. Intense ERβ staining is observed in these areas and the prostatic buds by 8 weeks, with persistent intense staining through 22 weeks. The work of Shapiro and associates shows the earliest expression of ERα (15 weeks) and ERβ (7 weeks) and that the induction of SQM in the UGE, distal periurethral ducts, and utricle is associated with ERα expression in these areas, whereas the induction of SQM in peripheral prostatic acini is associated with peripheral stromal ERα expression. This suggests important estrogen signaling pathways in the human fetal prostate via ERα that involve epithelial–epithelial and epithelial–stromal interaction. Also, the timing of the appearance of SQM is thought to be associated with the decline in testosterone levels after 18 weeks when the Leydig cells are known to regress.[44] This results in an imbalance of the hormone milieu, with a predominance of estrogens, which may then induce metaplastic changes

The role of ERα and ERβ in prostatic development has been further elucidated in studies of the estrogen receptor α knockout (ERKOα) and estrogen receptor β knockout (ERKOβ) mouse, respectively.[45,46] Couse and Korach studied neonatal diethylstilbestrol (DES) exposure in males using both ERKOα and ERKOβ knockout cell lines.[46] The ERKOα males were completely resistant to the effects of neonatal DES exposure and the ERKOβ response was similar to the wild type, with significant decreases in the AR levels and seminal vesicle size, increased stromal mass, marked epithelial hyperplasia and dysplasia, and lymphocytic infiltration. It was concluded that the initial effect of DES, resulting in the down-regulation of AR levels, is mediated by ERα. Therefore, the ERKOα males did not show any of the effects of neonatal DES, but, unlike the wild-type, the AR levels recover in the adult ERKOβ males.

Other investigators have suggested an involvement of ERβ in the pathogenesis of prostate cancer, since ERβ expression is down-regulated in prostate cancer, supporting its role in prostatic cellular homeostasis.[47] We have shown that ERβ expression is intense during the early period of prostatic ductal morphogenesis and may be critical in maintaining normal glandular growth and proliferation.

Prostate morphometry

Shapiro et al developed a technique for quantifying the cellular elements of the prostate that involves double immunoenzymatic staining and computer-assisted color image analysis.[48,49] The only comprehensive study of prostatic morphometry in the prepubertal male has been reported by Shapiro et al.[50]

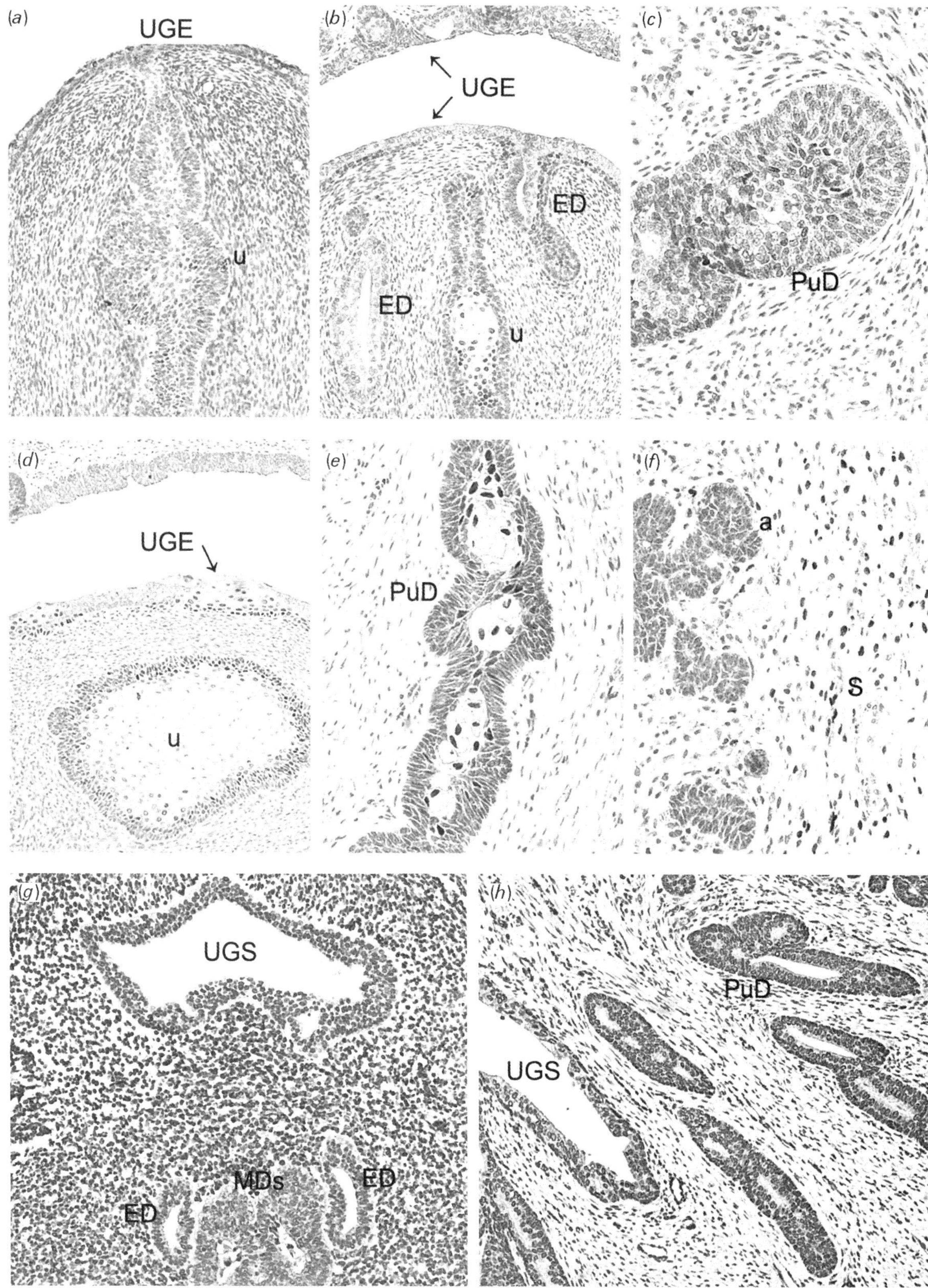

Figure 48.3 Cross section of a human fetal prostate. (*a*) Estrogen receptor α (ERα) expression at 15 weeks in the ventral urogenital epithelium (UGE) and utricle (u) (×200). (*b*) At 21 weeks, ERα expression in the UGE (arrows), utricle, and ejaculatory ducts (EDs) (×200), and (*c*) periurethral ducts (PuD) (×400). (*d*) ERα expression at 22 weeks in the UGE (arrows) and utricle (×200), (*e*) periurethral ducts (×400), and (*f*) peripheral stroma (S), with no staining of the peripheral acini (a) (×400). (*g*) ERβ expression throughout the epithelium and stroma at 7 weeks (MDs, müllerian ducts; UGS, urogenital sinus) and (*h*) at 24 weeks (×200).

Quantitative morphometric studies were performed on pediatric and other non-hyperplastic prostate specimens obtained from 45 males ranging in age from 2 days to 40 years. The entire group was stratified, based upon age, into categories reflecting the neonatal, childhood, peripubertal, adolescent, and young adult period. Double immunoenzymatic staining using antiactin and anti-PSAP was used to label the tissue components.[49] Color image analysis demonstrated age-related changes in the density of SM that appear to parallel serum testosterone levels, which vary as a result of the postnatal testosterone surge and the increased level of testosterone at the onset of puberty.[3,51]

A progressive decrease in SM area density throughout childhood, prepuberty, and puberty was observed. The density of SM significantly increased following puberty and throughout adolescence and early adulthood. There was a concomitant increase in connective tissue (CT) from the neonatal period throughout childhood, prepuberty and puberty, and a decrease after puberty and throughout adolescence and early adulthood. Since the changes in SM and CT were inversely related, the percent contribution of the stromal compartment to the total gland remained constant. No significant changes were seen in the epithelium or glandular lumen during these periods. The stromal to epithelial ratio remains constant from birth to age 40 in non-hyperplastic glands and is similar to those in asymptomatic and symptomatic BPH tissues. These morphometric observations suggest that BPH is not a unique stromal process.[50] These studies demonstrate that the stromal compartment is a dynamic structure, and the relationship between changes in cellular content and hormone milieu may be important to our understanding of growth of the prostate from birth to age 40 and the subsequent development of BPH.

Shapiro et al compared prostate development in normal human male fetuses and those with myelomeningocele (MMC) at 20 weeks' gestational age.[51] Immunohistochemical staining was performed using Masson's trichrome and antibodies to smooth muscle (SM) and skeletal muscle (SKM) actin. S-100 protein for Schwann cell localization and neurofilament protein was also performed. These studies demonstrated a marked decrease in the peripheral innervation to the prostate in MMC. Trichrome and SM actin staining also showed that SM in MMC specimens was less well differentiated. Prostatic size, ductal morphogenesis, and SM were decreased when compared with controls. At the level where the EDs enter into the prostatic urethra, the mean cross-sectional area was 6.79 mm^2 and 11.91 mm^2 in the MMC and normal prostate, respectively. Control prostates showed posterior peripheral SM surrounding acini, which subsequently become cannulated, as well as SM surrounding the EDs and along the periphery. In MMC prostates, SM was absent in the periphery, where ductal branching and formation of acini normally occur. The other areas of SM were also poorly formed. It was concluded that there is a global defect in the development of SM in MMC prostate at 20 weeks' gestation. Since the peripheral nerve density was diminished in the MMC prostate, an intact nervous system may be important in the SM and ductal morphogenesis of the developing prostate.

Summary

The foundation for our understanding of the development of the human prostate was derived from human fetal studies reported by Lowsley and by unraveling the biochemical basis for the 5α-reductase deficiency syndrome. Tissue recombinant studies, genetic knockout studies in nude mice, and meticulous step sectioning of fetal prostates with immunohistochemical staining gestation has greatly enhanced our understanding of prostatic development. Additional studies in animal models have provided insights into the impact of hormonal perturbations on prostatic development. It is likely that future studies extending our understanding of prostatic development in man will provide important insights into the mechanism of benign and malignant prostatic growth in aging.

References

1. Stephens FD. Congenital Malformations of the Urinary Tract. New York: Praeger, 1993.
2. Hamilton WJ, Mossman HW. The urogenital system. In: Human Embryology: Prenatal Development of Form and Function, 4th edn. New York: Macmillan, 1976: 201.
3. Siiteri PK, Wilson JD. Testosterone formation and metabolism during male sexual differentiation in the human embryo. J Clin Endocrinol Metab 1974; 38:113–25.
4. Cunha GR. Epithelio–mesenchymal interactions in primordial gland structures which become responsive to androgenic stimulation. Anat Rec 1972; 172:179–95.
5. Imperato-McGinley J, Binienda Z, Arthur A et al. The development of a male pseudohermaphroditic rat using an inhibitor of the enzyme 5α-reductase. Endocrinology 1985; 116:807–12.

6. Raghow S, Shapiro E, Steiner MS. Immunohistochemical localization of transforming growth factor-alpha and transforming growth factor-beta during early human fetal prostate development. J Urol 1999; 162:509–13.
7. Lowsley OS. The development of the human prostate gland with reference to the development of other structures at the neck of the urinary bladder. Am J Anat 1912; 13:299–346.
8. Shapiro E, Huang H, McFadden DE et al. The prostatic utricle is not a Mullerian duct remnant: immunohistochemical evidence for a distinct urogenital sinus origin. J Urol 2004; 172 (pt 2): 1753–6; discussion 1756.
9. Shapiro E, Huang H, Wu XR. Uroplakin and androgen receptor expression in the human fetal genital tract: insights into the development of the vagina. J Urol 2000; 164:1048–51.
10. Xia T, Blackburn WR, Gardner WA Jr. Fetal prostate growth and development. Pediatr Pathol 1990; 10:527–37.
11. McNeal JE. The prostate gland: morphology and pathobiology. Monogr Urol 1988; 9:3.
12. Cunha GR, Donjacour AA, Cooke PS et al. The endocrinology and developmental biology of the prostate. Endocr Rev 1987; 8(3):388–62.
13. Imperato-McGinley J, Guerrero L, Gautieer T, Peterson RE. Steroid 5α-reductase deficiency in man: an inherited form of pseudohermaphroditism. Science 1974; 186:1213–15.
14. Donjacour AA, Cunha GR. The effect of androgen deprivation on branching morphogenesis in the mouse prostate. Dev Biol 1988; 128:1–14.
15. Price D. Normal development of the prostate and seminal vesicles of the rat with a study of experimental postnatal modifications. Am J Anat 1936; 60:79.
16. Mahendroo MS, Cala KM, Hess DL, Russell DW. Unexpected virilization in male mice lacking steroid 5α-reductase enzymes. Endocrinology 2001; 142(11):4652–62.
17. Shapiro E, Huang H, Masch RJ et al. Regional expression of the androgen receptor and 5α-reductase type 2 in the human fetal prostate. J Urol 2006; 175: 464.
18. Lasnitzki I, Mizuno T. Prostatic induction: interaction of epithelium and mesenchyme from normal wild-type and androgen-insensitive mice with testicular feminization. J Endocrinol 1980; 85:423–8.
19. Griffin JE, Wilson JD. Disorders of sexual differentiation. In: Walsh PC, Gittes RF, Perlmutter AD et al, eds. Campbell's Urology 5th edn, Philadelphia: WB Saunders, 1986: 1819.
20. Cunha GR, Lung B. The possible influence of temporal factors in androgenic responsiveness of urogenital tissue recombinants from wild-type and androgen-insensitive (Tfm) mice. J Exp Zool 1978; 205:183–93.
21. Cunha GR, Cooke PS, Kurita T. Role of stromal–epithelial interactions in hormonal responses. Arch Histol Cytol 2004; 67(5):417–34.
22. Cooke PS, Young P, Hess RA, Cunha GR. Estrogen receptor expression in developing epididymis, efferent ductules, and other male reproductive organs. Endocrinology 1991; 128(6):2874–9.
23. Shapiro E, Huang H, Masch RJ et al. Immunolocalization of estrogen receptor α and β in human fetal prostate. J Urol 2005; 174:2051–3.
24. Cooke PS, Young P, Cunha GR. Androgen receptor expression in developing male reproductive organs. Endocrinology 1991; 128(6):2867–73.
25. Prins G, Cooke P, Birch L et al. Androgen receptor expression and 5a-reductase activity along the proximal–distal axis of the rat prostatic duct. Endocrinology 1992; 130:3066–73.
26. Cunha GR, Battle E, Young P et al. Role of epithelial–mesenchymal interactions in the differentiation and spatial organization of visceral smooth muscle. Epithelial Cell Biol 1992; 1:76–83.
27. Huang L, Pu Y, Alam S, Birch L, Prins GS. Estrogenic regulation of signaling pathways and homeobox genes during rat prostate development. J Androl 2004; 25(3):330–7.
28. Weniger JP, Zeis A. Sur la secretion precoce de testosterone par le testicule embryonnaire de souris. Comp Rend Acad Sci Paris 1972; 275:1431.
29. Winter JSD, Faiman C, Reyes F. Sexual endocrinology of fetal and perinatal life. In: Austin CR, Edward RG, eds. Mechanisms of Sex Differentiation in Animal and Man. New York: Academic Press, 1981: 205.
30. Jarred RA, Cancilla B, Prins GS et al. Evidence that estrogens directly alter androgen-regulated prostate development. Endocrinology 2000; 141(9):3471–7.
31. Risbridger G, Wang H, Young P et al. Evidence that epithelial and mesenchymal estrogen receptor-α mediates effects of estrogen on prostatic epithelium. Dev Biol 2001; 229:432–42.
32. Timms BG, Petersen SL, vom Saal FS. Prostate gland growth during development is stimulated in both male and female rat fetuses by intrauterine proximity to female fetuses. J Urol 1999; 161(5):1694–701.
33. Rajfer J, Coffey DS. Sex steroid imprinting of the immature prostate: long-term effects. Invest Urol 1978; 16:186–90.
34. Naslund MJ, Coffey DS. The differential effects of neonatal androgen, estrogen, and progesterone on adult rat prostate growth. J Urol 1986; 136:1136–40.
35. Tsujimura A, Koikawa Y, Salm, S et al. Proximal location of mouse prostate epithelial stem cells: a model of prostatic homeostasis. J Cell Biol 2002; 157:1257–65.
36. Prins GS, Woodham C, Lepinske M, Birch L. Effects of neonatal estrogen exposure on prostatic secretory genes and their correlation with androgen receptor expression in the separate prostate lobes of the adult rat. Endocrinology 1993; 132:2387–98.
37. Prins GS, Birch L. The developmental pattern of androgen receptor expression in rat prostate lobes is altered after neonatal exposure to estrogen. Endocrinology 1995; 136:1303–14.
38. Prins G. Neonatal estrogen exposure induces lobe-specific alterations in adult rat prostate and androgen receptor expression. Endocrinology 1992; 130:3703–14.
39. Ingham PW, McMahon AP. Hedgehog signaling in animal development: paradigms and principles. Genes Dev 2001; 15:3059–87.
40. Pu Y, Huang L, Prins GS. Sonic hedgehog-patched Gli signaling in the developing rat prostate gland: lobe-specific suppression by neonatal estrogens reduces ductal growth and branching. Dev Biol 2004; 273(2):257–75.

41. Barnett DH, Huang HY, Wu XR et al. The human prostate expresses *sonic hedgehog* during fetal development. J Urol 2002; 168:2206–10.
42. Zondek T, Zondek LH. The fetal and neonatal prostate. In: Goland M, ed. Normal and Abnormal Growth of the Prostate. Springfield, Illinois: CC Thomas, 1975: 5–28.
43. Risbridger G, Wang H, Young P et al. Evidence that epithelial and mesenchymal estrogen receptor-α mediates effects of estrogen on prostatic epithelium. Dev Biol 2001; 229:432–42.
44. Codesal J, Regadera J, Nistal M, Regadera-Sejas J, Paniagua R. Involution of human fetal Leydig cells. An immunohistochemical, ultrastructural and quantitative study. J Anat 1990; 172:103–14.
45. Prins GS, Birch L, Couse JF et al. Estrogen imprinting of the developing prostate gland is mediated through stromal estrogen receptor α: studies with αERKO and βERKO. Cancer Res 2001; 61:6089–97.
46. Couse JF, Korach KS. Estrogen receptor-α mediates the detrimental effects of neonatal diethylstilbestrol (DES) exposure in the murine reproductive tract. Toxicology 2004; 205(1–2):55–63.
47. Horvath LG, Henshall SM, Lee CS et al. Frequent loss of estrogen receptor-beta expression in prostate cancer. Cancer Res 2001; 61(14):5331–5.
48. Shapiro E, Becich MJ, Hartanto V, Lepor H. The relative proportion of stromal and epithelial hyperplasia is related to the development of symptomatic benign prostate hyperplasia. J Urol 1992; 147:1293–7.
49. Shapiro E, Hartanto V, Lepor H. Quantifying the smooth muscle content of the prostate using double-immunoenzymatic staining and color assisted image analysis. J Urol 1992; 147:1167–70.
50. Shapiro E, Perlman E, Hartanto V et al. Morphometric analysis of pediatric and nonhyperplastic prostate glands: evidence that BPH is not a unique stromal process. Prostate 1997; 33:177–82.
51. Shapiro E, Seller MJ, Lepor H et al. Altered smooth muscle development and innervation of the lower genitourinary and gastrointestinal tract of the human male fetus with myelomeningocele. J Urol 1998; 160:1047–53, discussion 1079.

Embryology of the anterior abdominal wall, bladder, and proximal urethra

49

Steven E Lerman, Irene M McAleer, and George W Kaplan

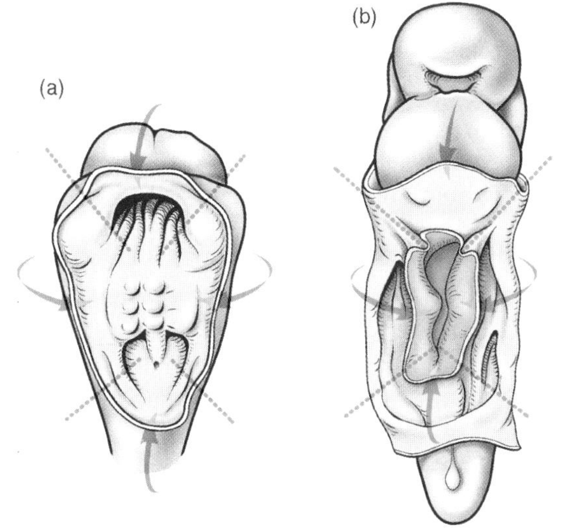

Figure 49.1 Ventral views of human embryos of 2 and 3 mm. The body stalk has been cut distal to the site of the future umbilical ring. Arrows show the direction of infolding; dotted lines indicate the arbitrary boundaries of the four infoldings. (Reproduced from Gray and Skandalakis,[1] with permission.)

Anterior abdominal wall

During the first 3 weeks of development, the embryo is a plate of cells, the embryonic disk, whose ventral surface is a membrane called the somatopleure. The anterior abdominal wall is at first represented by the somatopleure of the overhanging head and tail folds. The somatopleure closes concentrically from the cranial, caudal, and lateral margins, centering on the future umbilical ring (Figure 49.1).

In the 6th week of development, the midgut closes and the body stalk reduces in relative size. The somatopleure is invaded by mesoderm from myotomes on either side of the vertebral column. This mesoderm migrates laterally and ventrally as a sheet (Figure 49.2).

The primordia of the two rectus abdominis muscles form laterally and begin to move toward the midline during the 7th week. At that time, the mesoderm laterally splits into three sheets, eventually producing the external oblique muscle, the internal oblique muscle,

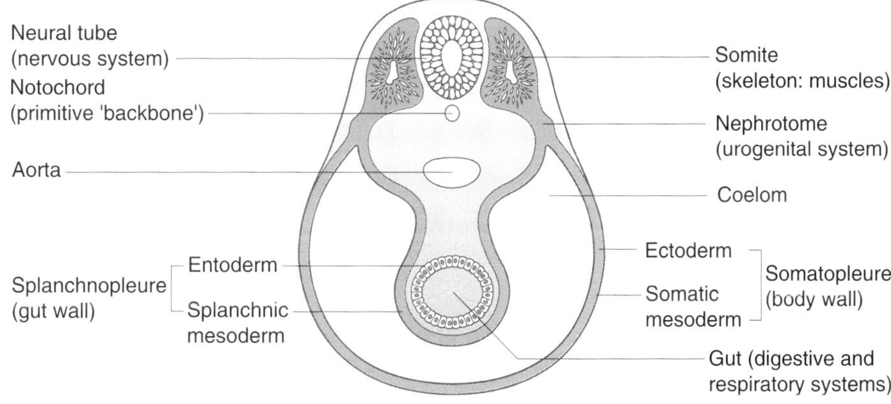

Figure 49.2 Diagrammatic transverse section of a vertebrate embryo. (Reproduced from Arey,[2] with permission.)

and the transversus abdominis muscle. These layers are all recognizable during the 7th week (Figure 49.3). In the infraumbilical area, the formation of three muscle layers is preceded by invasion of secondary mesoderm that arises from the primitive streak just behind the cloaca. This secondary mesoderm then surrounds the cloaca and invades the body wall caudal to the body stalk, providing primary closure to the body wall between the phallus and the body stalk and forming part of the anterior bladder musculature as well (Figure 49.4).[3]

Between the 7th and 12th weeks of development, the rectus abdominis muscles meet in the midline except around the umbilicus. During this same time the secondary mesoderm forming the lower abdominal wall is reinforced externally by invading somatic mesoderm that forms the muscular layers of the lower abdominal wall.

The important urologic anomalies resulting from faulty embryogenesis of the abdominal wall are the Eagle–Barrett (prune belly) syndrome, exstrophy of the bladder or cloacal exstrophy. None of these is an arrested stage of normal embryogenesis. The Eagle–Barrett syndrome seems most likely to be due to faulty mesodermal development during the 6th to the 12th week, as several mesodermal elements (abdominal wall, ureter, bladder, and testes) are usually involved.[4] Another theory states that the Eagle–Barrett syndrome is a deformation of the abdominal wall produced by distended viscera or increased intra-abdominal pressure.[5] A third theory

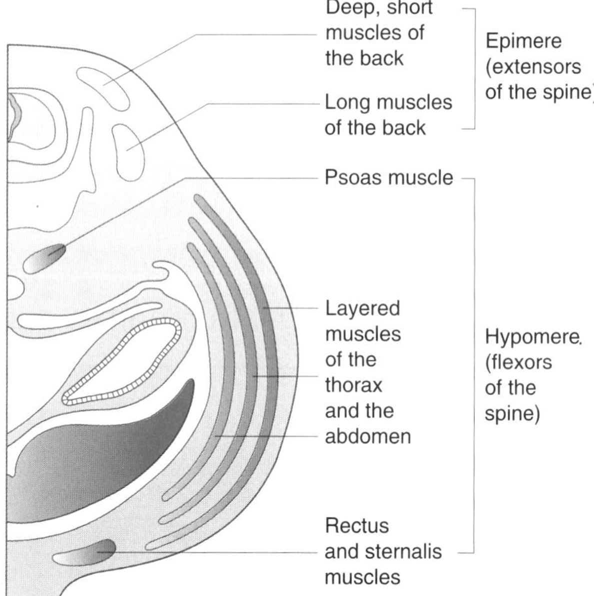

Figure 49.3 Diagrammatic transverse hemisection through the abdomen or thorax of a 7-week human embryo. (From Arey,[2] with permission.)

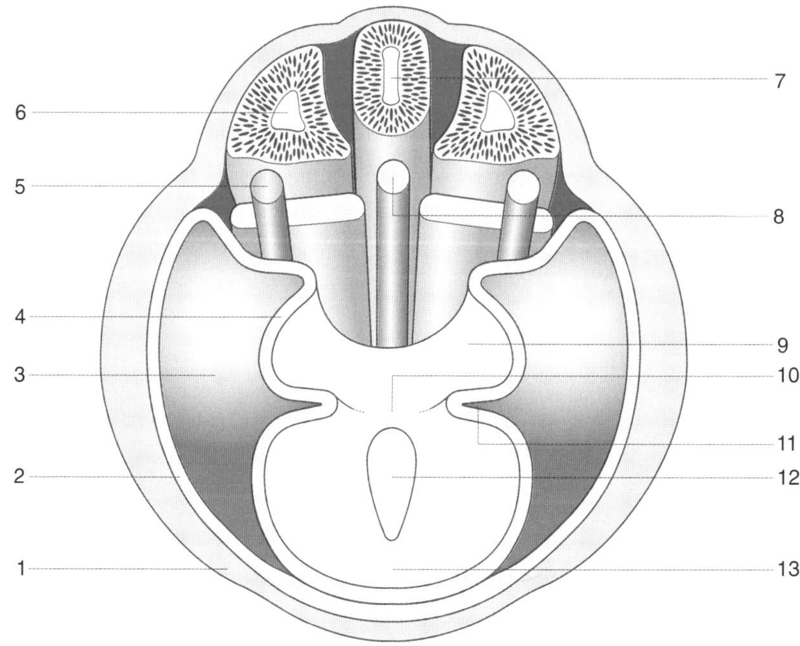

Figure 49.4 Disposition of mesoderm at the caudal end of a somite embryo as viewed working down from inside the caudal end of the embryo: (1) surface epithelium; (2) somatic layer of the lateral plate mesoderm; (3) coelomic cavity; (4) visceral layer of the lateral plate mesoderm; (5) nephrogenic cord; (6) somite; (7) neural tube; (8) notochord; (9) unsegmented paraxial mesoderm; (10) primitive streak; (11) site of developing urorectal septum; (12) site of cloacal membrane; (13) infraumbilical abdominal wall. (Reproduced from Glenister,[3] with permission.)

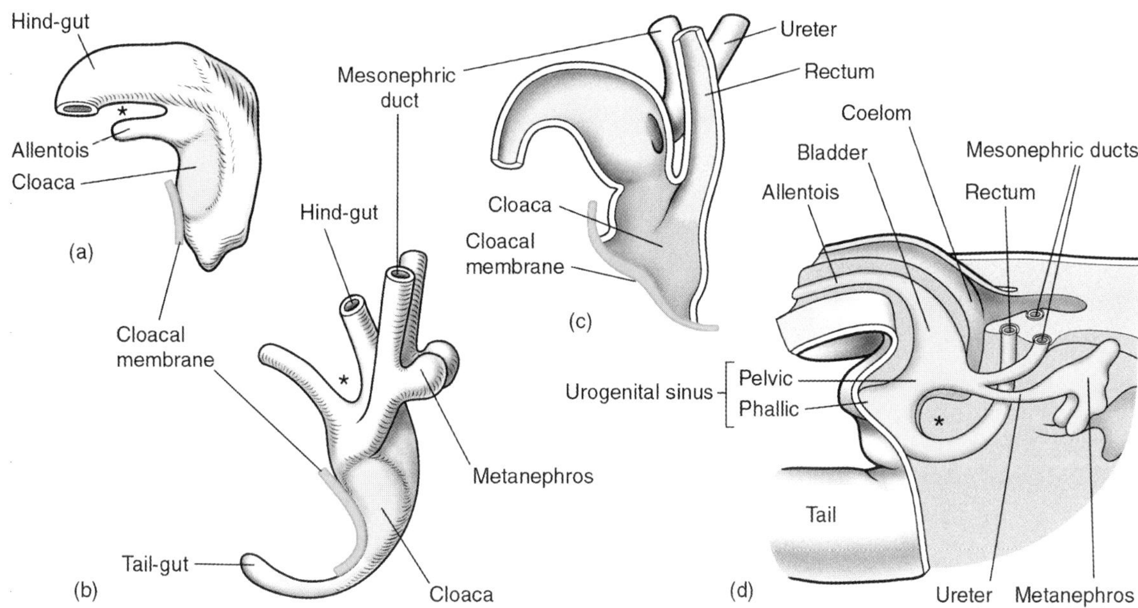

Figure 49.5 Division of the human cloaca: (*a*) 3.5 mm stage; (*b*) 4 mm stage; (*c*) 8 mm stage; (*d*) 1 mm stage. The asterisks in (*a*), (*b*) and (*d*) indicate the cloacal septum. (Reproduced from Arey,[2] with permission.)

attributes the urinary abnormalities to a primary abdominal wall defect resulting in decreased intra-abdominal pressure.[6]

Exstrophy may result from a failure of the secondary mesoderm to cover the infraumbilical abdominal wall. Rupture of the cloacal membrane prematurely could also produce such a failure. Should this occur in the 5th week, cloacal exstrophy could result.[7] If this does not occur until the 7th week, so that some of the secondary mesoderm is in place, classical bladder exstrophy might result. Still later (the 10th or 11th week), failure of invasion by somatic mesoderm might result in superior vesical fissure or epispadias.

Lower urinary tract

The development of the lower urinary tract is closely interrelated with that of the genital tract and the hindgut, but for clarity the genital tract is not discussed here but covered in Chapter 58.

During the first 3 weeks the cloaca develops from endoderm as a blind caudal expansion of the hindgut (Figure 49.5). The hindgut meets the ectoderm of the body wall at the cloacal membrane. This membrane extends caudally from the primitive streak and is turned under by the tailfold. It extends from the tailbud to the body stalk. As the mesoderm grows, the area of the cloacal membrane is decreased. The cloaca gives off a ventrally directed allantoic stalk and receives the mesonephric duct laterally and extends caudally as the tailgut.

The cloaca, during the 5th week, is divided by opposing walls of the hindgut in the allantois, meeting in a saddle-shaped notch with its apex pointing caudally. This notch fills in with mesenchyme to form the urorectal septum. This septum pushes caudally as a fold and advances, dividing the cloaca into the primitive rectum posteriorly and a urogenital sinus anteriorly (Figure 49.6).

Various regions of the urogenital sinus are recognizable in the 6th week: the allantois, bladder, pelvic, and phallic portions of the urogenital sinus. The pelvic portion of the urogenital sinus lies cephalad to the entrance of the mesonephric duct but below the bladder, whereas the phallic portion of the urogenital sinus lies caudad to the entrance of the mesonephric duct and extends distally toward the genital tubercle.

By the 7th week the ureters empty into the bladder by a process in which nephric ducts, after the ureteral buds have appeared, are absorbed into the urogenital sinus and acquire four separate openings into the sinus (Figure 49.7). The mesonephric ducts are shifted further caudad in the sinus and come to lie close to each other at Müller's tubercle, while the ureters shift cephalad and laterally into the bladder. It is then that the trigone is formed. The trigone is temporarily mesodermal but fills in with urogenital sinus epithelium, so that it, too, is eventually endodermal.

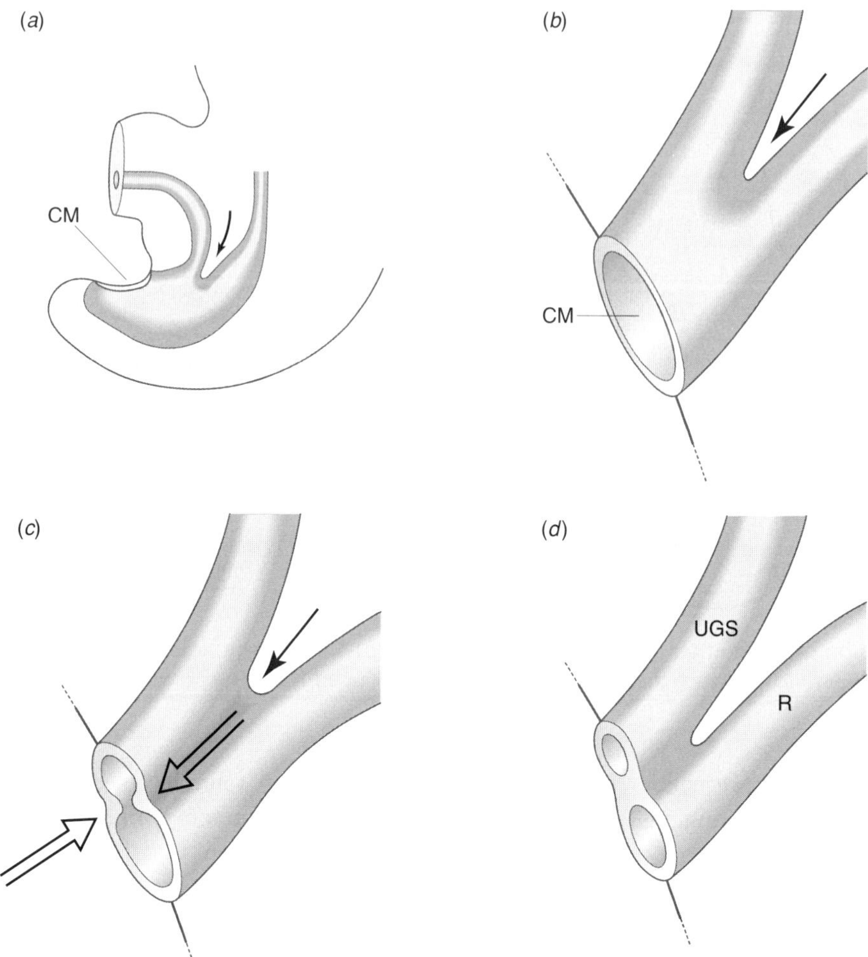

Figure 49.6 Septation of the cloaca. (*a*) Lateral view of caudal embryo (CM, cloacal membrane). Septation of the cloaca occurs in a coronal plane as Tourneux's fold (*b*) extends to the cloacal membrane from above, and (*c*) as Rathke's plicae extend towards each other from the sides. (*d*) Septation establishes the primitive urogenital sinus (UGS) and rectum (R). (Reproduced from Stephens and Smith,[8] with permission.)

The bladder epithelium at this time consists of a single layer.

The urorectal septum reaches the cloacal membrane and divides the cloaca into the urogenital sinus and the rectum; the cloacal membrane then ruptures (see Figure 49.6). The caudal edge of the urorectal septum, which is covered with endoderm, is exposed as the perineal body. It merges with lateral folds flanking this fissure and becomes covered with ectoderm. It is eventually marked by a median raphe and becomes the perineum. Hillocks behind the anus encircle this area and form the anal canal, which eventually becomes lined with ectoderm.

In the 8th week the bladder muscle begins to appear as a longitudinal layer on the dorsal surface of the bladder. By the 9th week the bladder cavity begins to expand into a sac, the apex of which (the urachus) is elongated. The urachus is continuous with the allantoic stalk at the umbilicus. The bladder and urachus elongate as the infraumbilical body wall forms from the somatic mesoderm.

In the 12th week the bladder epithelium becomes transitional, and its muscular wall is formed from mesenchyme. The smooth muscle of the urinary tract is acquired in an ascending fashion from bladder to intrarenal collecting system.[10] The bladder epithelium over the ureteral orifice forms Chwalla's membrane, which temporarily covers and occludes the ureteral orifice. Chwalla's membrane perforates and the ureter becomes continuous with the bladder. By the 16th week the bladder is completely muscularized and the urachus is closed.

Agenesis of the bladder is a rare anomaly that may arise because the allantoic stalk fails to develop.[11]

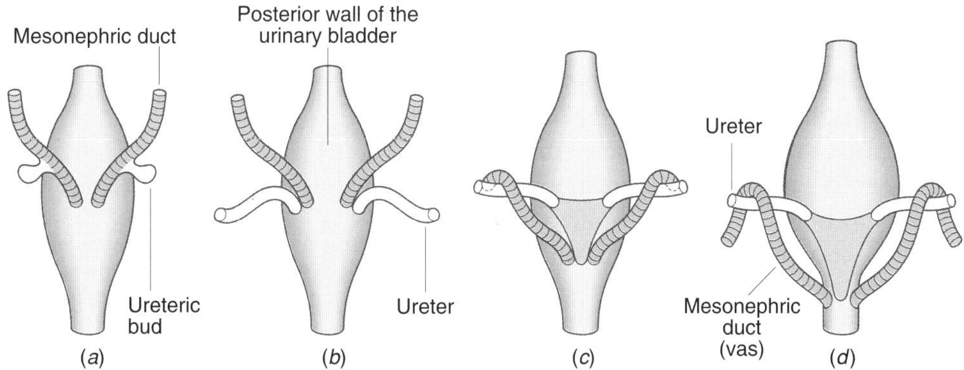

Figure 49.7 (*a–d*) Dorsal views of the bladder to show the relationship of the ureters and mesonephric ducts during development. Initially, the ureters are formed by an outgrowth of the mesonephric duct, but with time they assume a separate entrance into the urinary bladder. Note the trigone of the bladder formed by incorporation of the mesonephric ducts. (Reproduced from Sadler,[9] with permission.)

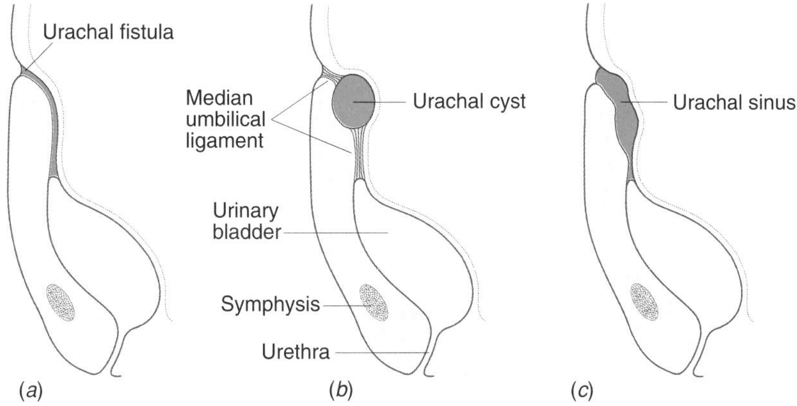

Figure 49.8 Diagrams of (*a*) urachal fistula, (*b*) urachal cyst, and (*c*) urachal sinus. The sinus may or may not be in open communication with the urinary bladder. (Reproduced from Sadler,[9] with permission.)

However, if migration of the ureters and formation of the trigone are the events that induce enlargement of the allantoic stalk, then bilateral failure of ureteral migration with resultant ureteral ectopia would result in the same anomaly.

Urachal anomalies (patent urachus, urachal cyst, urachal sinus, and urachal diverticula) may be encountered clinically (Figure 47.8). Some anomalies result from a general mesodermal failure (the urachal diverticulum of the Eagle–Barrett syndrome);[14] however, most seem to result from delayed closure of the urachus. Lower urinary tract obstruction <12 weeks of age (by virtue of bladder distention) could prevent closure.[12] There is, in addition, a definite association of patent urachus with upper tract problems, and therefore the entire urinary tract should be investigated.[13] Urachal cysts and sinuses presumably result from incomplete closure of the urachus.

Duplications of the bladder and urethra are usually associated with other hindgut and lower spinal cord duplications. Hence, it would appear that these result from a splitting of the hind end of the embryo at a very early stage of development, distinct from the lower abdominal wall defect resulting in exstrophy.

Ureteral ectopia, vesicoureteral reflux (VUR), and paraureteral diverticula appear to arise because the ureteral bud appears at a locus on the mesonephric duct more craniad or caudad than normal. As the ureter is incorporated into the urogenital sinus, its final site would be more craniad and lateral or caudad, respectively. The former results in VUR and diverticula, whereas the latter results in ureteral ectopia.[14]

Ectopic ureteroceles probably result from abnormalities of the ureteral bud in addition to ectopia and are often associated with renal dysplasia.[14] Intravesical (simple) ureteroceles are thought to be due to persistence of Chwalla's membrane beyond the time when urine flow begins.[15]

Posterior urethral valves (type 1) may result from persistence of the path of migration of the mesonephric ducts distal to Müller's tubercle so that they cross the urogenital sinus and enter anteriorly. Persistence of this portion coupled with anterior fusion might then produce the diaphragm known as valves.[16] Another type of valves (type 3) seems to result from persistence of the cloacal membrance at the junction of the end of the phallic portion of the urogenital sinus and the bulbomembranous urethra.[17]

References

1. Gray SW, Skandalakis JE. Embryology for Surgeons. Philadelphia: WB Saunders, 1972: 496.
2. Arey LB. Developmental Anatomy, 6th edn. Philadelphia: WB Saunders, 1974.
3. Glenister TW. A correlation of the normal and abnormal development of the penile urethra and of the infra-umbilical abdominal wall. Br J Urol 1958; 30:117–26.
4. Spence HM, Allen T. Congenital absence of the abdominal musculature. Urologic aspects. JAMA 1964; 187:814–18.
5. Pagon RA, Smith DW, Shepard TH. Urethral obstruction malformation complex: a cause of abdominal muscle deficiency and the 'prune belly'. J Pediatr 1979; 94: 900–6.
6. Osler W. Congenital absence of abdominal muscles with distended and hypertrophied urinary bladder. Bull Johns Hopkins 1901; 12:311.
7. Muecke EC. The role of the cloacal membrane in exstrophy: the first successful experimental study. J Urol 1964; 92:659–67.
8. Stephens FD, Smith ED. Anorectal Malformations in Children. Chicago: Year Book, 1971.
9. Sadler TW. Longman's Medical Embryology, 7th edn. Philadelphia: Williams & Wilkins, 1996.
10. Baker LA, Gomez RA. Embryonic development of the ureter and bladder: acquisition of smooth muscle. J Urol 1998; 160:545–50.
11. Glenn JF. Agenesis of the bladder. JAMA 1959; 169: 2016–8.
12. Javadpour N, Graziano MF, Terrill R. Experimental induction of patent allantoic duct by intrauterine bladder outlet obstruction. J Surg Res 1974; 17:341–5.
13. Rich RH, Hardy BE, Filler RM. Surgery for anomalies of the urachus. J Pediatr Surg 1983; 18:370–2.
14. Mackie GC, Stephens FD. Duplex kidneys: a correlation of renal dysplasia with position of the ureteral orifice. J Urol 1975; 114:274–80.
15. Tanagho EA. Anatomy and management of ureteroceles. J Urol 1972; 107:729–36.
16. Stephens FD. Congenital Malformations of the Urinary Tract. New York: Praeger, 1983: 96.
17. Field PL, Stephens FD. Congenital urethral membranes causing urethral obstruction. J Urol 1974; 111:250–5.

Radiologic assessment of bladder disorders

50

Douglas E Coplen

Introduction

Congenital anomalies and abnormalities of the urinary bladder can be a significant cause of morbidity in infants and children. The function of the bladder may adversely affect the upper urinary tract and may have an effect on urinary continence. Radiologic evaluation of the bladder and adjacent structures gives useful diagnostic information to direct therapeutic intervention. In children, ultrasonography (ultrasound) is usually the initial diagnostic study. Fluoroscopic imaging (voiding cystourethrogram or VCUG) is frequently obtained as indicated by the clinical history and ultrasound findings. Cross-sectional imaging – computed tomography (CT) and magnetic resonance imaging (MRI) – is often used in complex cases where other imaging does not clearly define the anatomy.

Ultrasound is ideally suited for the evaluation of children with symptoms suggestive of a bladder or lower urinary tract abnormality because it is painless, associated with no radiation exposure, and provides excellent anatomic definition of the bladder. For this study a partially distended bladder is preferable. The clear differentiation between the anechoic urine and the bladder wall and surrounding structures enhances the diagnostic utility of ultrasound (Figure 50.1).

If upper urinary tract dilatation is identified during an examination, the ultrasound should also include imaging after bladder emptying, since the degree of bladder distention may affect the upper tract findings. Doppler ultrasound can be used to identify ureteral jets (urine flow into the bladder) that are evidence of antegrade flow into the bladder.[1] Postvoid views can be obtained to assess bladder emptying and bladder wall thickening. Bladder volume can be estimated by ultrasound using the empirical equation:[2]

$$\text{bladder volume} = 0.7 \times \text{width} \times \text{length} \times \text{depth}$$

The VCUG is the best method of fluoroscopic bladder imaging. The study consists of direct opacification of the bladder with iodinated contrast medium that is usually instilled through a urethral catheter. Preferably both filling and voiding views are obtained during the study. Dynamic visualization of the bladder may give

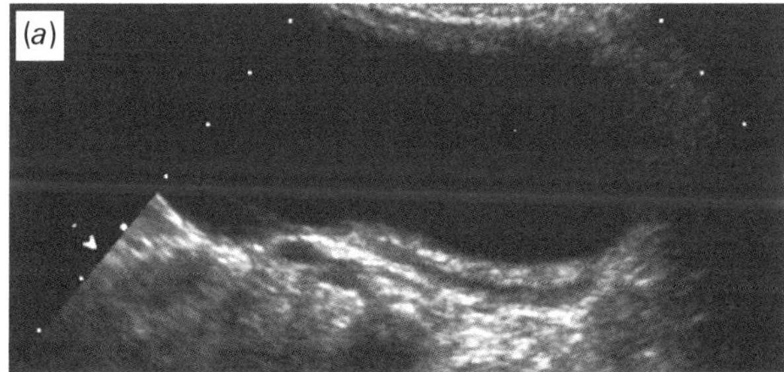

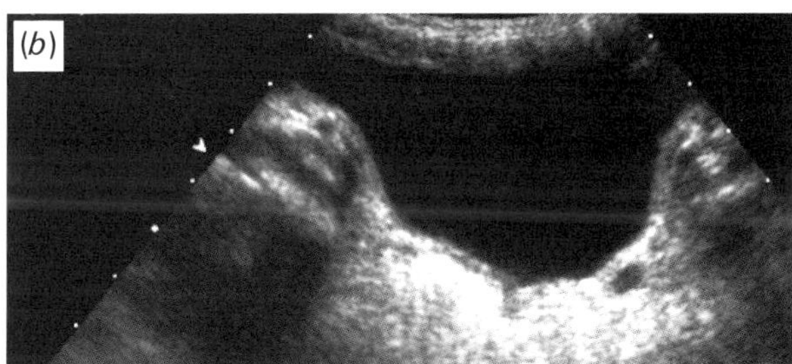

Figure 50.1 Bladder ultrasound obtained in a male with isolated bladder distention identified prenatally. Note the clear definition of the lumen and bladder wall on ultrasound. Longitudinal (*a*) and transverse (*b*) views show a dilated left ureter is seen posterior to the bladder. The child had bilateral grade V reflux but no infravesical obstruction.

very useful information regarding bladder function and disordered elimination. Voiding views are especially important in the male, since abnormalities of the bladder outlet and urethra greatly impact the bladder.

Intravenous pyelography (IVP) is rarely used as a primary bladder imaging modality. The excreted contrast gives passively filled bladder images. This modality may be preferable in older males who are reluctant to undergo urethral catheterization, but the contrast is dilute and opacification of the bladder and urethra is not as good, perhaps resulting in a non-diagnostic study.

CT and MRI give improved spatial resolution when compared with more commonly utilized imaging modalities. Images are obtained in an axial mode, but can be reformatted in both the sagittal and coronal planes. With current software, both planar reconstructions and three-dimensional reconstructions give excellent resolution.[3]

Superior soft-tissue resolution is an advantage of MRI over CT. On T1-weighted images the bladder wall may be indistinguishable from the urine, but on T2-weighted studies fluid-filled structures like the bladder are very well defined (Figure 50.2).[4] Because of prolonged acquisition times, sedation is required in younger children. MRI is very expensive when compared with ultrasound and fluoroscopy and should probably be reserved for complex cases where anatomy is not well-defined using other modalities.

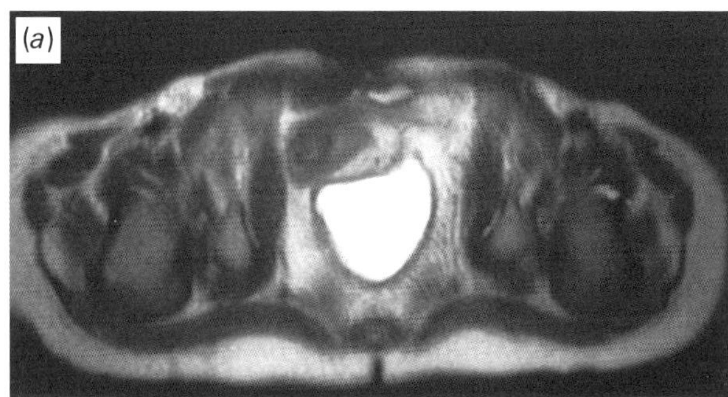

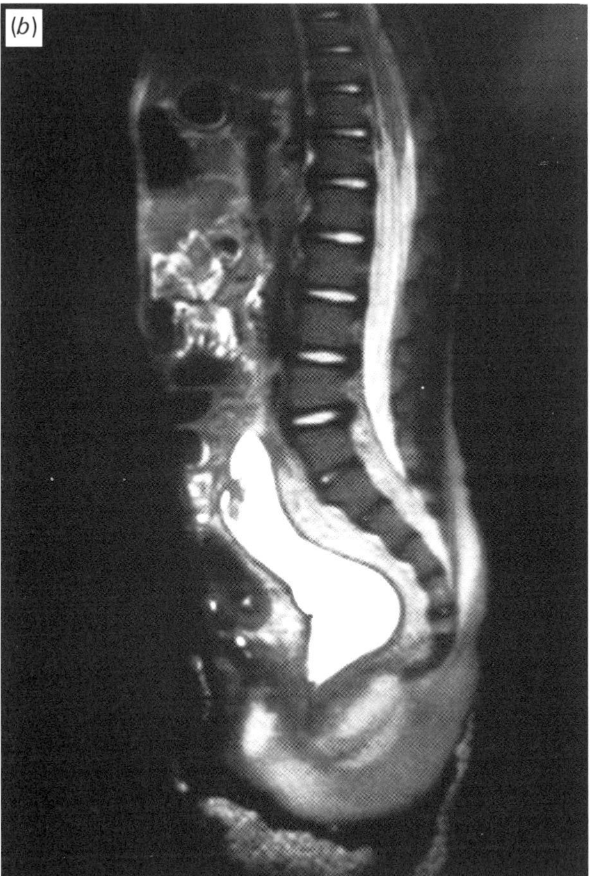

Figure 50.2 MRI obtained on a 6-year-old adopted male with an apparent history of bladder exstrophy based on physical examination. He is incontinent of both urine and stool per 'rectum' but these do not appear to be mixed. The study clearly defines the lower tract anatomy. On coronal section (*a*) the rectum is visualized anterior to the sigmoid 'bladder', which has been pulled through posterior to the rectum. The ureters are reimplanted into a sigmoid segment as seen in sagittal section (*b*) (filling defect in sigmoid 'bladder').

Bladder enlargement

An enlarged bladder may be identified on physical examination. Whereas bladder distention may be a normal finding prior to voiding, it may be indicative of significant bladder or urethral pathology. Congenital anomalies such as spinal dysraphism and prune belly syndrome should be evident on examination and help with the differential diagnosis. A thickened bladder wall on ultrasound is suggestive of bladder outlet obstruction, although, when the bladder is markedly distended, wall thickening may not be readily apparent (Figure 50.3).[5] Concomitant ureteral dilatation in the presence of bladder distention and a thin bladder wall is suspicious for high-grade vesicoureteral reflux (see Figure 50.1).

A VCUG gives both the anatomic detail and functional information that defines the etiology of bladder distention. Views of the urethra are essential in the evaluation of these children. Bladder trabeculation and cellules are commonly identified in children with posterior urethral valves or neurogenic bladder. Children with prune belly syndrome or megacystis/microcolon usually have large smooth-walled bladders (Figure 50.4).

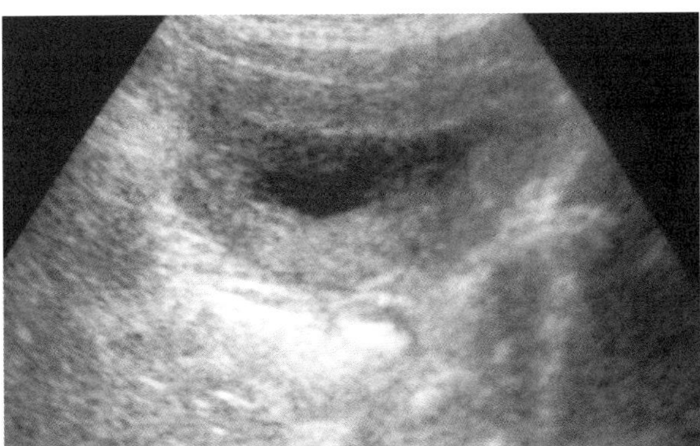

Figure 50.3 Postvoid ultrasound in a boy with posterior urethral valves. He empties completely, and marked bladder wall thickening is clearly apparent.

Urachal abnormalities

The urachus, sometimes called the median umbilical ligament, has usually obliterated by the 12th week of gestation. In theory, a patent urachus may occur in the presence of bladder outlet obstruction, but no evidence of obstruction is identified in the majority of cases.[6] Occasionally, a patent urachus is identified at birth when there is free discharge of urine through the umbilicus. More commonly, only a tiny fistula is present and the umbilicus is enlarged or edematous. In these situations, the differential diagnosis includes omphalitis, 'normal' hypertrophic granulation tissue, and a patent omphalomesenteric duct. Ultrasound may identify an inflamed tract, but a fistulogram with radiopaque contrast is often diagnostic (Figure 50.5). Voiding cystourethrography is helpful in fully evaluating the lesion and any associated bladder outlet obstruction.

Partial obliteration of the urachus results in a urachal cyst. These cysts are usually asymptomatic but occasionally become infected and are identified during the evaluation of lower abdominal pain, fever, and voiding symptoms. The diagnosis can be made by ultrasound. CT may be useful in defining the extent of the cyst and evaluating adjacent structures (Figure 50.6).

A urachal diverticulum is often an incidental finding on VCUG that does not require treatment. A large diverticulum is commonly identified in prune

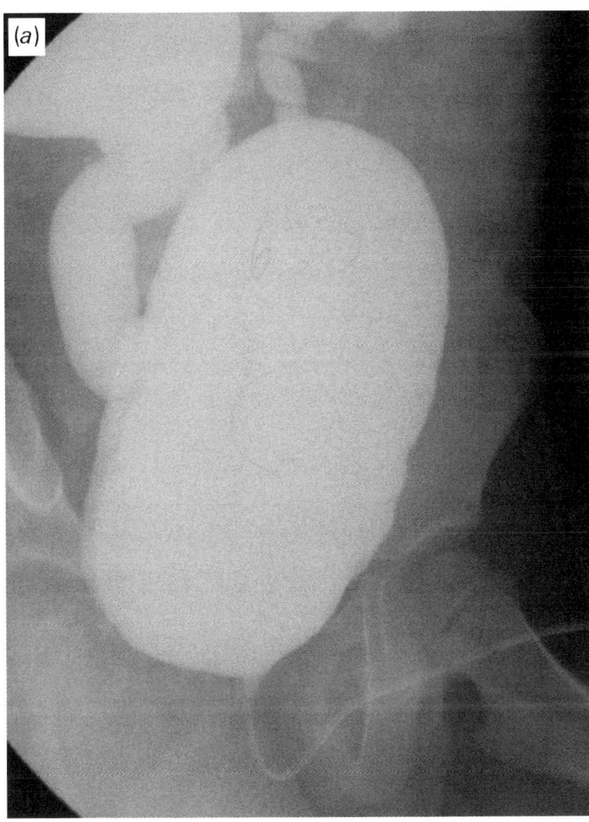

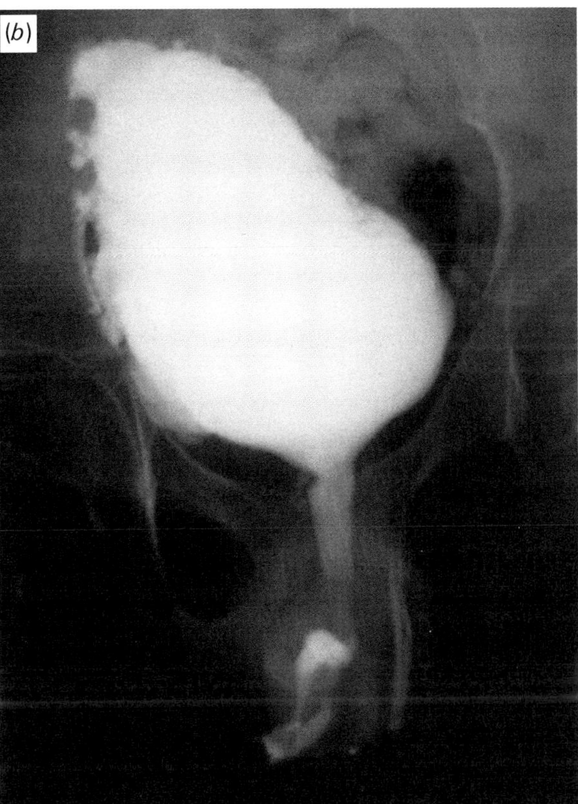

Figure 50.4 VCUG in two boys with bladder enlargement: (*a*) bilateral high-grade reflux with a smooth bladder wall and no outlet obstruction; (*b*) marked bladder trabeculation and 'Christmas tree' deformity in a boy with spinal dysraphism.

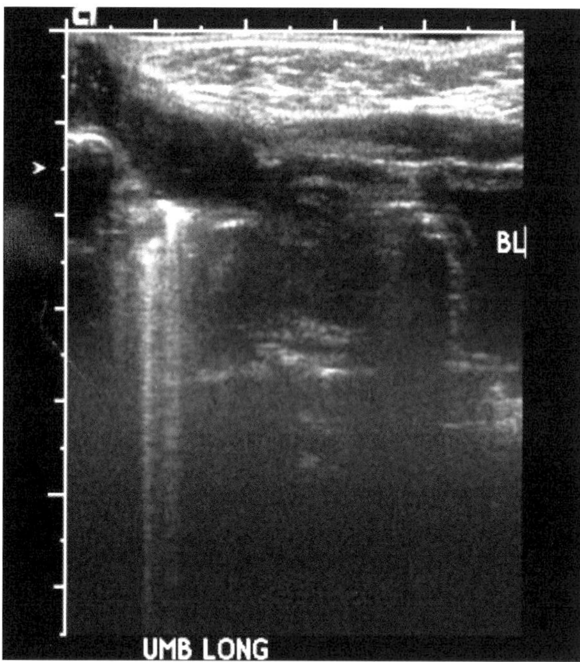

Figure 50.5 A 1-month-old male with a moist umbilicus. The ultrasound shows a well-defined tract from the umbilicus down to the dome of the bladder (BL). The tract expanded during a bladder contraction (real-time imaging), documenting a communication with the bladder.

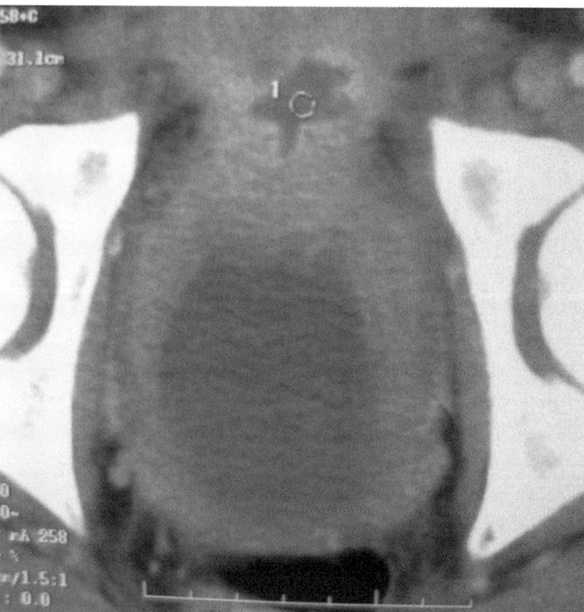

Figure 50.6 A 14-year-old male with lower abdominal pain, pyuria, and an infected urachus. CT shows an inhomogeneous mass cephalad to the bladder. Anterior bladder wall inflammation and thickening can be seen.

belly syndrome and rarely may require excision if it is a source of significant urinary stasis (Figure 50.7).

Bladder diverticulum

A bladder diverticulum is the result of a weakening in the muscular layer of the bladder wall. This may be congenital, but it can be acquired in the presence of bladder outlet obstruction or dysfunctional voiding. In children, the diverticulum is most commonly periureteral. Diverticuli are most commonly identified during the evaluation of urinary tract infections and they may, theoretically, be a significant source of urinary stasis. The fluid-filled extravesical structure identified on ultrasound is definitively differentiated from a dilated ureter on VCUG (Figure 50.8). The oblique bladder views localize the location of the diverticulum and whether or not it is broad based.

Bladder masses

Bladder masses are distinctly unusual in children. Presenting symptoms are usually related to outflow obstruction (strangury). Occasionally, gross hematuria is identified by the parents, but most children with gross hematuria have no identifiable anatomic abnormality and have a nephrologic source of bleeding. Ultrasound is the initial test of choice in children, because it is non-invasive and will usually identify an intravesical or infravesical abnormality. If an abnormality is identified, cross-sectional imaging is usually

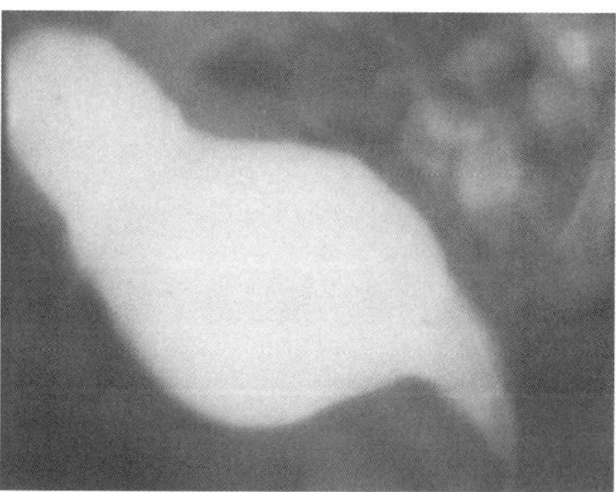

Figure 50.7 A VCUG in a boy with an abnormal abdominal wall shows a wide-mouthed urachal diverticulum. Typical bladder neck and urethral findings confirm the diagnosis of prune belly syndrome.

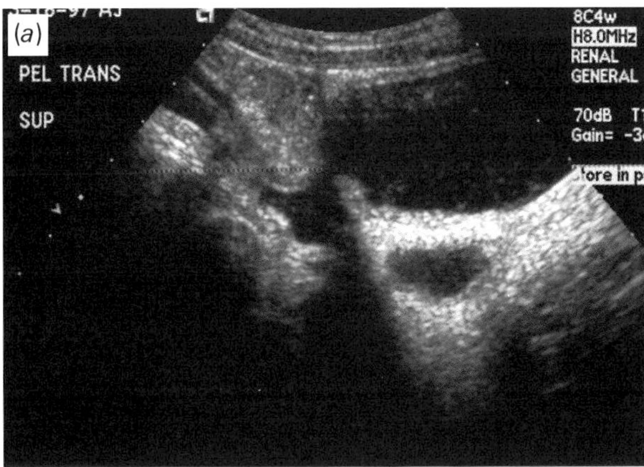

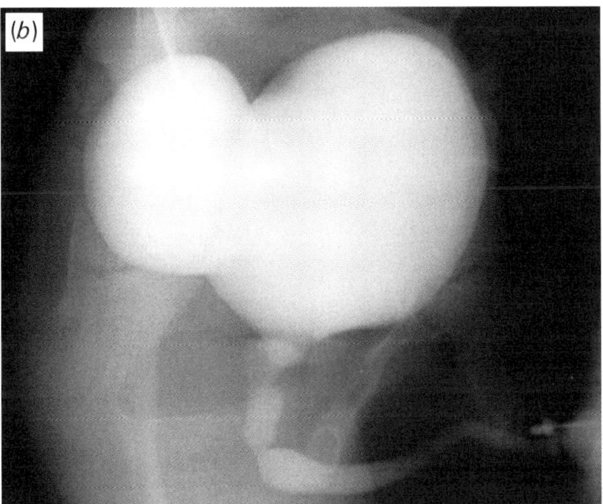

Figure 50.8 Bladder diverticulum in a 7-year-old male with recurrent staphylococcal cystitis. (a) On ultrasound, it is evident that the tubular structure does not extend cephalad and is not a ureter. (*b*) On VCUG, the lateral view confirms an origin low on the bladder base, which is consistent with a congenital periureteral diverticulum.

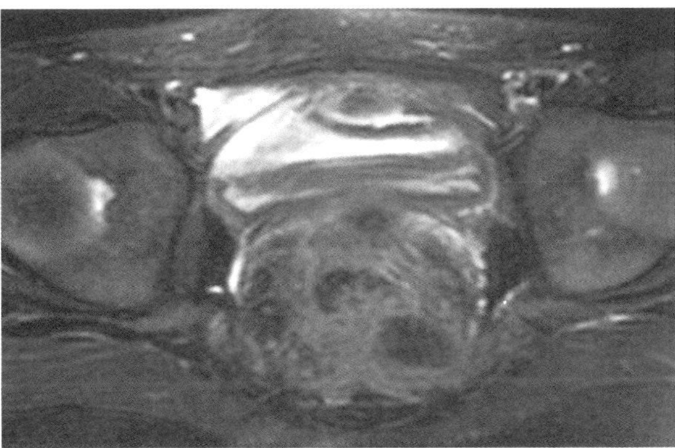

Figure 50.9 Rhabdomyosarcoma detected during evaluation of a febrile urinary tract infection. T2-weighted imaging reveals thickening of the bladder base and lateral walls. There is bladder wall bulging, with no evidence of perivesical involvement.

obtained, although in some clinical situations an endoscopic evaluation is the next best step.

Rhabdomyosarcoma is the most common bladder malignancy in children: most present with obstruction and a palpably distended bladder and/or lower abdominal mass. An ultrasound usually reveals a mass at the base of the bladder. MRI offers the best detail in relation to other pelvic organs and is the preferred study for radiologic staging (local and metastatic) (Figure 50.9).

Transitional cell carcinomas of the bladder and fibroepithelial polyps are very rare in children. They are usually well visualized on ultrasound because they usually have a narrow stalk and project into the lumen of the bladder (Figure 50.10).

Bladder calculi

Historically, bladder calculi were related to dietary intake. However, stones are now identified in up to 50% of children after bladder augmentation.[7] They are often identified during routine follow-up imaging. On ultrasound, stones are echogenic foci, with associated shadowing (Figure 50.11). They are usually mobile on the dependent portion of the bladder. Images are better if the bladder is partly distended, since stones may be in some mucosal folds and confused with echogenic stool that is often present in the true pelvis of these children. A KUB (kidney, ureter, and bladder abdominal X-ray) helps define the number of calculi.

Although ultrasound is not the best imaging study for upper tract stones, it can be useful in the evaluation of distal ureteral calculi that are not readily apparent on plain films. A dilated distal ureter is easily visualized behind the bladder and a shadowing and echogenic focus at the ureterovesical junction confirms the presence of a stone. If the ureter is not dilated or the stone is proximal to the bladder, ultrasound is usually not useful.

Bladder rupture

Bladder perforation may occur with blunt abdominal trauma and/or pelvic fractures. Children with a history of bladder augmentation may have spontaneous perforation in the absence of any identifiable trauma. A high index of suspicion is required in the evaluation of children with a history of bladder augmentation and abdominal pain. A VCUG is diagnostic in most cases, but thorough technique, including

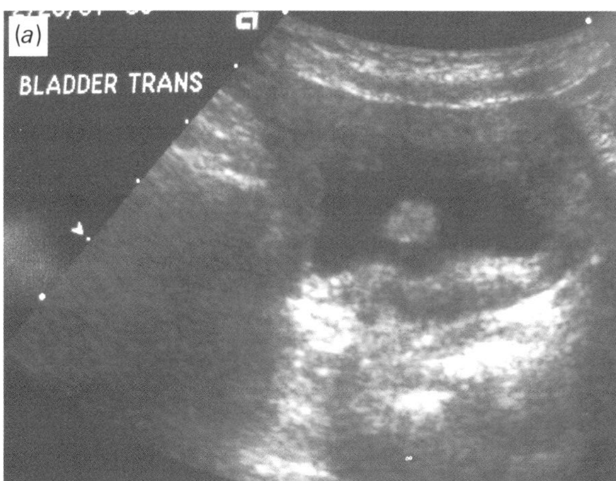

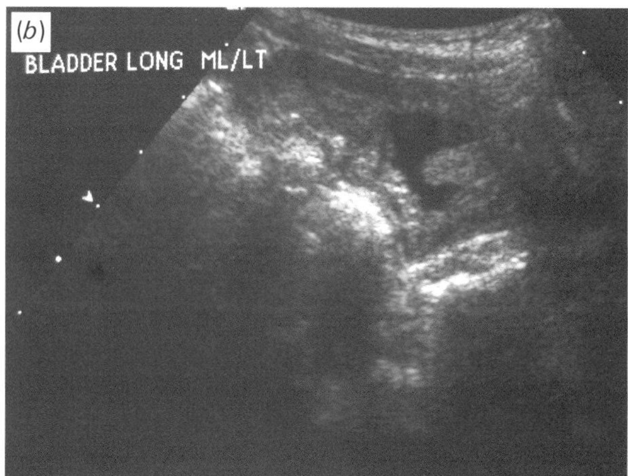

Figure 50.10 A fibroepithelial polyp identified in a 2-year-old male with intermittent urinary retention. Transverse views (*a*) show a 'free-floating' mass that extends across the bladder neck on longitudinal views (*b*) of the bladder. The bladder wall is thickened, which is consistent with intermittent obstruction.

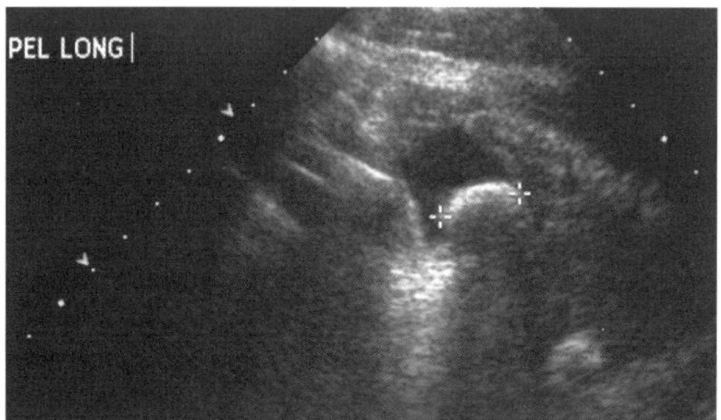

Figure 50.11 Bladder calculus in an augmented bladder. A curvilinear shadowing defect is evident on the bladder base.

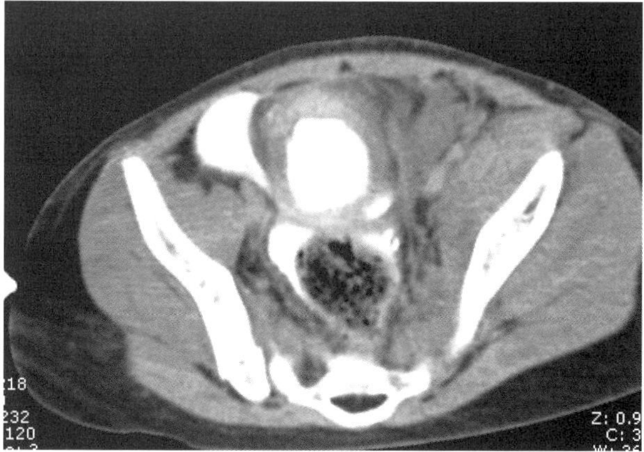

Figure 50.12 Intraperitoneal bladder perforation after blunt abdominal trauma. The CT scan reveals contrast in the bladder but it is also evident in the peritoneal cavity and perirectally in the pouch of Douglas.

postdrainage films, is required to identify smaller perforations. The irregularities normally present in the augmented bladder increase the chance of a false-negative study and a CT scan improves the diagnostic accuracy. Passive bladder distention is inadequate. Retrograde distention with diluted (4–5%) contrast is necessary to appropriately evaluate for perforation using CT cystography (Figure 50.12).[8] A CT cystogram should be obtained when a perforation is suspected and a VCUG is normal.

Ureteral abnormalities

Anomalies of the distal ureter are frequently identified during bladder imaging. The normal ureter should not be visualized on ultrasound imaging. When a dilated ureter is identified, it may be indicative of urethral, bladder, or ureterovesical junction pathology.

Megaureter is a generic term applied to an enlarged ureter. Ultrasound easily identifies the presence of these dilated ureters (Figure 50.13). The megaureter can be obstructed or non-obstructed, and refluxing or non-refluxing. While ultrasound identifies the dilation, a VCUG and renal scintigraphy are required to classify the megaureter.

Ectopic insertion of the ureter occurs most commonly in the setting of renal duplication. The duplication is usually easily identified on ultrasound evaluation of the upper tract because the lower pole of the kidney is not associated with a dilated ureter. Longitudinal ultrasonic bladder views frequently demon-

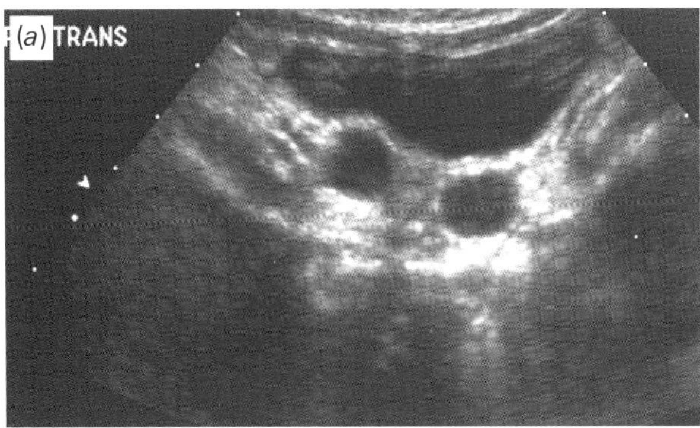

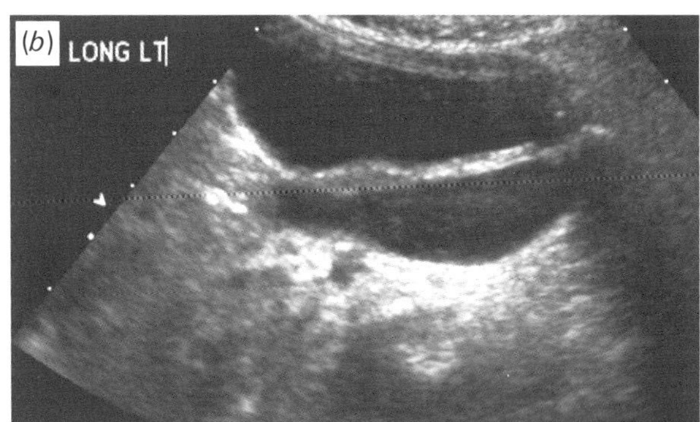

Figure 50.13 Bladder ultrasound in a female with recurrent febrile urinary tract infections. (*a*) A Transverse view reveals dilation of the distal ureters bilaterally. (*b*) A longitudinal view shows the dilated ureter coursing distal to the bladder neck. The child had bilateral duplications, with upper pole ectopia.

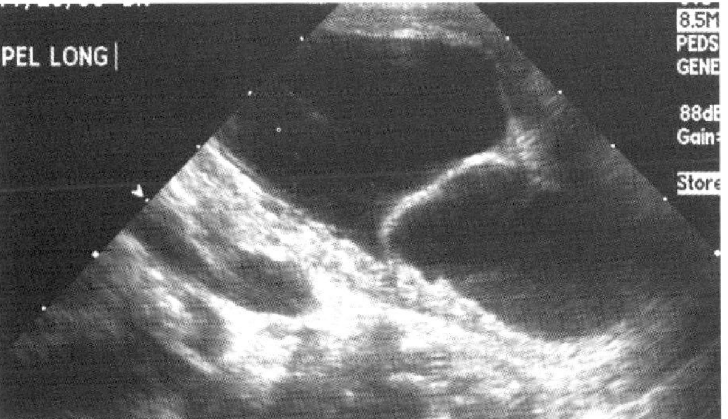

Figure 50.14 Bladder ultrasound images in a male with an ectopic ureterocele that obstructs the bladder outlet. The ureterocele extends down into a dilated prostatic urethra. Note the bladder wall thickening and trabeculation secondary to the outlet obstruction.

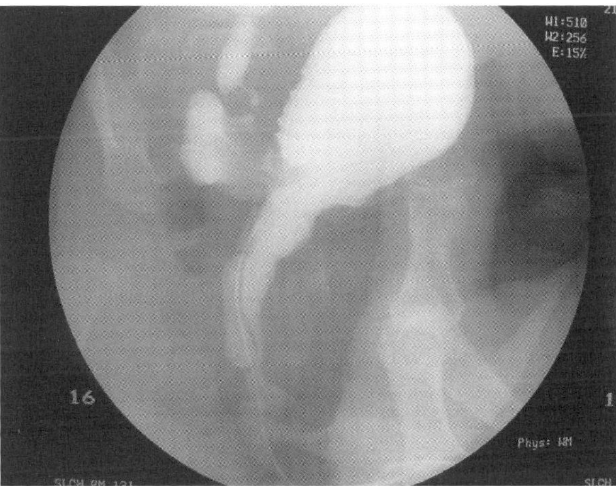

Figure 50.15 Cystogram in a female with a ureterocele. The filling defect in the urethra confirms its ectopic position. The ureterocele also everts during voiding because of the muscular deficiency in the right hemitrigone.

strate a ureteral insertion distal to the bladder neck. Occasionally, the dilated ureter deforms the posterior bladder wall and can be confused with a ureterocele. This pseudoureterocele can be differentiated by noting that the anterior wall is the same thickness as the rest of the bladder wall.[9]

Ureteroceles are cystic dilations of the intravesical segment of the ureter. Ureteroceles have a unique appearance on ultrasound: they are thin-walled cystic masses at the bladder base (Figure 50.14). Ureteroceles are usually simple, but are occasionally bilobed or lobulated. In the presence of infection, they may contain echogenic debris. Occasionally, a large ureterocele is not identified if the child has just voided because the apparent bladder urine is actually within the ureterocele, with no urine outside the ureterocele in the bladder. Ureteroceles are usually associated with a dilated ureter posterior to the bladder wall. Intravenous urography and cystography usually reveal a non-opacified filling defect in the bladder. There may be a significant detrusor defect and the ureterocele often everts during bladder filling on VCUG, resembling a diverticulum (Figure 50.15).[10]

References

1. Burge HJ, Middleton WD, McClennan BL, Hildebolt CF. Ureteral jets in healthy subjects and in patients with unilateral ureteral calculi: comparison with color Doppler US. Radiology 1991; 180:437–42.
2. Huang YH, Bih LI, Chen SL, Tsai SJ, Teng CH. The accuracy of ultrasonic estimation of bladder volume: a comparison of portable and stationary equipment. Arch Phys Med Rehabil 2004; 85(1):138–41.

3. Johnson PT, Halpern EJ, Kuszyk BS et al. Renal artery stenosis: CT angiography – comparison of real-time volume-rendering and maximum intensity projection algorithms. Radiology 1999; 211:337–43.
4. Teeger S, Sica GT. MR imaging of bladder diseases. Magn Reson Imaging Clin N Am 1996; 4:565–81.
5. Kaefer M, Barnewolt C, Retik AB, Peters CA. The sonographic diagnosis of infravesical obstruction in children: evaluation of bladder wall thickness indexed to bladder filling. J Urol 1997; 157(3):989–91.
6. Cilento BG Jr, Bauer SB, Retik AB, Peters CA, Atala A. Urachal abnormalities: defining the best diagnostic modality. Urology 1998; 52:120–2.
7. Palmer LS, Franco I, Koan SJ et al. Urolithiasis in children following augmentation cystoplasty. J Urol 1993; 150:726–9.
8. Deck AJ, Shaves S, Talner L, Porter JR. Computerized tomography cystography for the diagnosis of traumatic bladder rupture. J Urol 2000; 164:43–6.
9. Sumfest JM, Burns MW, Mitchell ME. Pseudoureterocele: potential for misdiagnosis of an ectopic ureter as a ureterocele. Br J Urol 1995; 75(3):401–5.
10. Bellah RD, Long FR, Canning DA. Ureterocele eversion with vesicoureteral reflux in duplex kidneys: findings at voiding cystourethrography. AJR Am J Roentgenol 1995; 165(2):409–13.

Urodynamics of the lower and upper urinary tract

51

William E Kaplan

Introduction

Many of the patients evaluated by a pediatric urologist have urinary tract dysfunction requiring urodynamic studies. Although the majority of urodynamics performed involve the assessment of lower tract function, there are select patients who need upper tract urodynamic studies.

Most children referred for urodynamic studies already have a specific pathologic diagnosis (spinal dysraphism, spinal cord injury, cerebral pathology, etc.) but require a more definitive neurologic classification for appropriate therapy. Many patients with voiding dysfunction require urodynamics to determine whether their urinary problems are neurologic or functional in origin. In addition, patients are referred for urodynamics when other diagnostic studies, e.g. radiographic or isotopic, are equivocal.

The expansion of pediatric urodynamics in the late 1970s and early 1980s came about because of the need to understand the volume–pressure relationships of the urinary tract. The introduction of clean intermittent catheterization in the 1970s[1] opened the creative gates for the management of children with dysfunctional storing and emptying of their urinary tracts. However, correct characterization of the pathology by urodynamics was critical.

Adult diagnostic techniques needed modification for children, and what began with work on flow rates by Gierup et al,[2] progressed to sophisticated flow and electromyographic (EMG) studies by Blaivis et al,[3] and to the introduction of surface monitoring of the pelvic floor by Maizels and Firlit.[4] An additional valuable contribution of correct filling rates by Joseph in 1992,[5] and sedation techniques, emphasized the importance of a more focused approach to children.

There is still controversy regarding the diagnostic methodology best suited for upper tract pathology. The child with idiopathic hydronephrosis with preservation of renal function and no symptoms creates the greatest diagnostic dilemma. Standard imaging techniques are usually adequate for patients with normal renal function. However, when renal function becomes impaired, renal perfusion studies may offer a more useful diagnostic role. It is clear that the physiology of the upper tract does not exist in isolation. Therefore, although pure upper tract obstruction – e.g. well-defined ureteropelvic junction (UPJ) obstruction – is associated with pressure elevation with less dependence on lower tract function, the surgeon must always be aware of the equilibrium between lower and upper tract pressures. The fact that bladder pressure must be 'in the loop' in any diagnostic study emphasizes how important bladder dynamics has become in modern pediatric urology. The ability to assess and manage bladder function and pressure has contributed to the increase in surgical, pharmacologic, and neuromodulating techniques used to manage the child with neurourologic dysfunction.

This chapter focuses on pediatric urodynamic studies that best categorize neuropathology and help to define the best treatment modalities.

Historical features

The basics of pediatric urodynamics are founded on the principles of good medicine. A thorough history and physical examination must precede any diagnostic study (Table 51.1). In patients in whom the diagnosis is clear, e.g. spinal cord trauma or myelomeningocele, eliciting a diagnostic history will not usually be challenging. However, patients with urinary tract dysfunction with no obvious neurologic abnormality will challenge the diagnostic skill of even the experienced pediatric urologist.

Table 51.1 Evaluation of children who wet

History	Prenatal, congenital history Voiding characteristics Bladder and bowel function
Physical examination	Abdomen and perineum Spine Lower extremities: Reflexes Gait Physical structure
Laboratory	Urinalysis/culture Chemistry: urine/serum
Radiography	Ultrasonography: renal/bladder Voiding cystography Flat plate abdomen/spine (AP and lateral)
Urodynamics	Flow/bladder capacity Cystometry Pelvic muscle evaluation: pads/needle Compliance: LPP/VLPP and PSBV

AP = anteroposterior; LPP = leak point pressure; VLPP = Valsalva leak point pressure; PSBV = pressure-specific bladder volume.

An accurate voiding history is most important. The patient's age and expectations of urinary control may dictate the concerns about voiding habits. However, even in infants, the pattern of wet and dry diapers may be important to discovering the diagnosis. Newborns with constant dribbling or signs of overflow incontinence may have undergone a traumatic delivery, e.g. hyperextension injury to the cervical spinal cord. Infants of diabetic mothers have an increased risk of neural tube defects. Infants of mothers with substance abuse are at increased risk for hydronephrosis. These are only a few examples that illustrate the importance of a thorough prenatal and obstetric history before scheduling and tailoring the type of urodynamics study.[6–8] Historic information, such as prematurity or global delay in physical or mental capabilities, is important. Although this information may not aid in therapy, it may help to explain to parents how delays in gaining urinary control occur. Infants with irregular bowel habits (diarrhea or constipation) in association with urinary symptomatology should prompt careful evaluation.

As the child matures, urinary tract infections (UTIs) or incontinence may become the primary symptoms. Van Gool et al[9] proposed the use of a standardized questionnaire that addressses common themes in the child with dysfunctional voiding. Frequency of wetting, voiding characteristics, and the presence of urgency are the focus of the questionnaire. The concept of a standardized approach is valid, although in a large practice, the similarity of the patients in any given day may ensure a routine history.

The use of a voiding diary or 12-hour home pad test may also be helpful.[10,11] In practice, the clinician may easily misinterpret the results if less than fastidious notes are kept, or if the pads are not changed promptly. The quality of the flow rate and whether a child is always wet despite effective voiding are important historic features. The boy with a poor flow rate would be suspicious for having posterior urethral valves, whereas the girl with paradoxical incontinence (continuously damp while voiding normally) might have an ectopic ureter. In the older child, the history must include details on bowel habits, because it is clear that constipation has a direct relationship to urinary control, as well as urinary infections.[12,13]

Physical examination

Before planning a urodynamic study, a thorough physical examination is essential. Children may exhibit evidence of delayed gross motor development or abnormal fine motor skills consistent with global abnormalities from in utero or birthing issues. In these children, a complete neurologic examination by a pediatric neurologist, including muscle tests and nerve conduction velocity, may be indicated.

A routine systematic approach, including having the child completely undressed from head to toe (although covered with a warm blanket and with a nurse and parent in attendance), will help to reveal general congenital defects that might contribute to syndromes that involve the urinary tract. Following the general assessment, most of the pertinent pathology is found below the umbilicus. The abdomen should be palpated for stool, although significant fecal retention can exist with a soft abdomen and an empty rectal vault.

The back, perineum, and lower extremities should be examined critically. During examination of the back, all midline abnormalities should be cause for concern. However, there is less importance if a simple dimple can be grasped with the tip of the coccyx. Obvious or subtle midline skin tags, tufts of hair, or

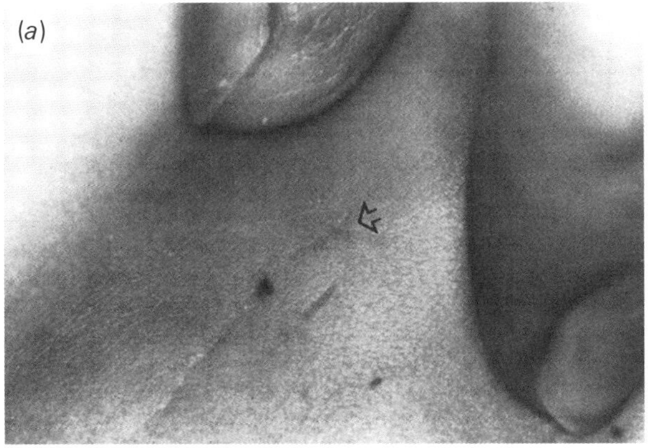

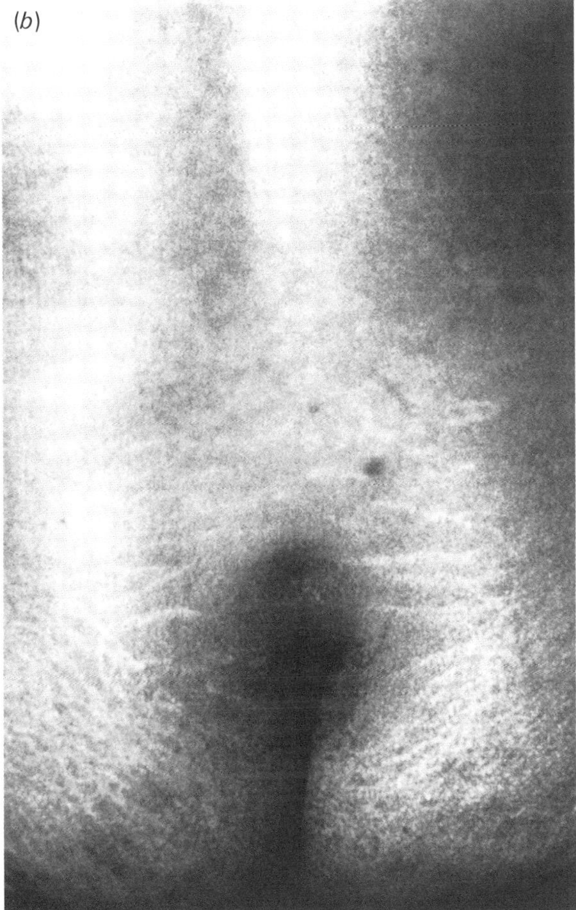

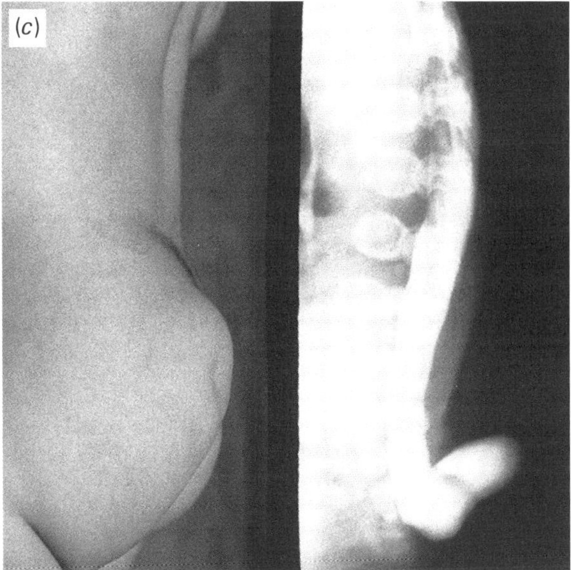

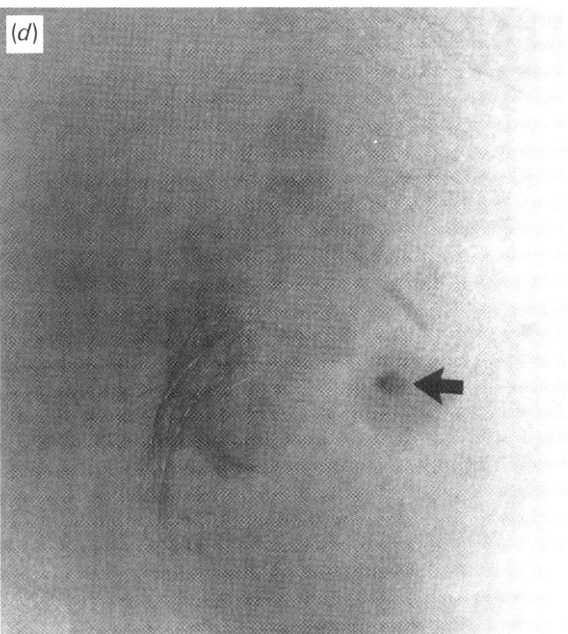

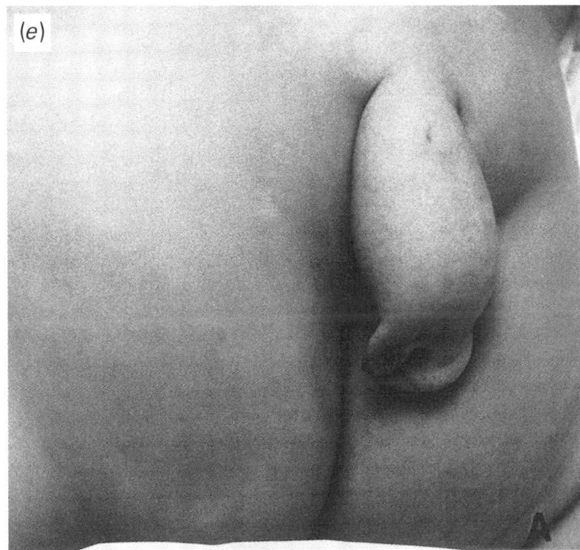

Figure 51.1 Cutaneous lesions discovered on midline spinal examination: (*a*) dermal sinus tract (open arrow) in infant who developed meningitis shortly after birth; (*b*) a subtle fullness of one buttock and mild scoliosis in a child with incontinence and subsequently discovered to have a lipoma; (*c*) an obvious sinus tract and lipoma in infant with lipomeningocele; (*d*) a sinus (arrow) and associated hairy patch characteristically associated with a flat capillary hemangioma; (*e*) an unusual appendage and dermal sinus tract.

vascular malformations may indicate underlying spinal malformations, e.g. lipomas, and spinal magnetic resonance imaging (MRI) is then indicated. A short or abnormal gluteal cleft may indicate an underlying sacral dysgenesis or agenesis. A flattened buttock suggests deficient gluteal muscle tone, consistent with an anorectal malformation or caudal regression syndrome (Figure 51.1).

Rectal tone, perianal sensation, and the presence or absence of a bulbocavernosus reflex should be noted. A digital rectal examination confirms the presence of stool and rules out rare prostatic lesions. The vaginal introitus should be inspected to rule out significant labial adherence or urethrovaginal abnormalities. In the boy, the meatus should be observed, and if uncircumcised, the foreskin either retracted gently or pulled forward, so that the meatus can be inspected through the tunnel of foreskin.

The lower musculoskeletal system should be examined and any discrepancy in muscle tone or muscle mass should be noted. It is essential to remove the shoes and socks to discover a high arched foot or hammer claw digits, consistent with a true neurologic abnormality (Figure 51.2). A gait disturbance is noted easily in barefoot children as they walk up and down the corridor. The author recently saw an incontinent child who was a star rollerblader, but on barefoot gait analysis was noted to have severe ankle weakness and intoeing. This was masked by the above-the-ankle rollerblades. Subsequent MRI revealed a tethered spinal cord. Finally, the deep tendon reflexes should be evaluated. Exaggerated reflexes are consistent with cerebral palsy.

At the first office visit, a urinalysis (glucose and specific gravity), flow rate, and postvoid residual measured by ultrasound should be accomplished. In children with a normal renal/bladder sonogram, and no history of significant UTIs, the majority of patients will be started on a timed voiding program, with attention to bowel habits, and a brief course of anticholinergic medication. In the remaining patients, a more thorough work-up, including radiographic evaluation and urodynamic studies, is indicated.

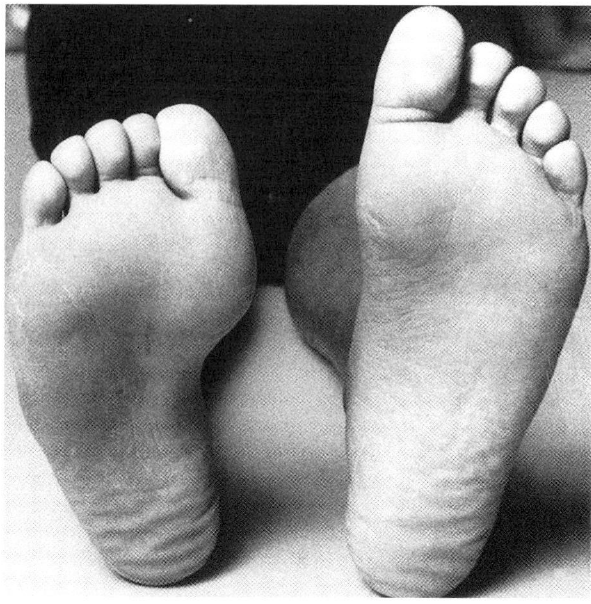

Figure 51.2 Leg length and foot asymmetry in a 10-year-old child with spina bifida.

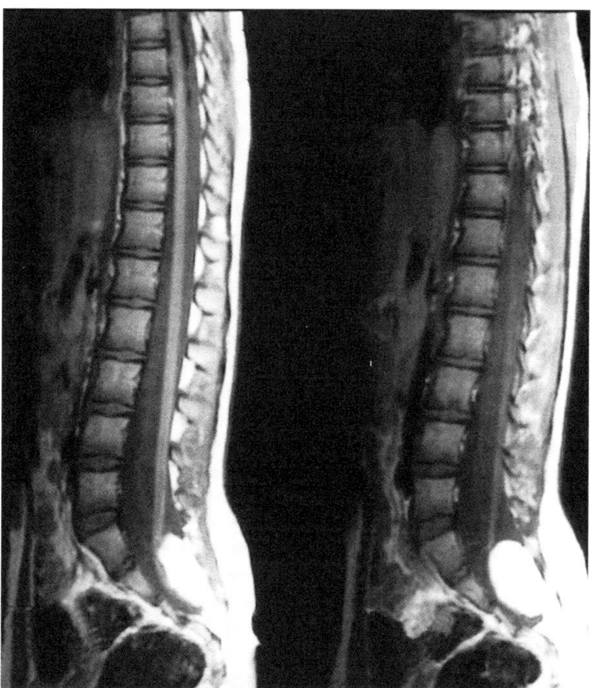

Figure 51.3 Lumbosacral MRI. T1-weighted image indicates a long tethered spinal cord. The elongated (bowstring) cord ends in the lipoma rather than at L3.

Radiographic evaluation

Radiographic examination is used selectively. All children undergo a renal and bladder sonogram with postvoid imaging to evaluate bladder emptying and the effects of bladder fullness on upper tract dilatation. If UTIs are an issue, a conventional X-ray voiding cystourethrogram (VCUG) is performed to evaluate the bladder, outlet, and urethra. This study can document whether there is significant stool in the colon. Children with both fecal and urinary incontinence should have lumbosacral images. In patients with clearly abnormal studies, spinal MRI is performed (Figure 51.3).

Lower urinary tract urodynamics

A complete voiding history should precede urodynamic evaluation. A parental questionnaire includes the details of the foregoing discussion. This can be accomplished at the time of the examination, but the study can be best modified to the needs of the child if the staff is made aware of significant problems by telephone or mail consultation before the office appointment. All outside studies should accompany the family to the laboratory.

In the majority of cases, the child with a non-neurogenic voiding abnormality will be old enough to cooperate, tolerating a precystometrogram flow study followed by a cystometrogram with patch electrodes and a postvoid study. Typically, the child with neurogenic disease comes to the laboratory on a clean intermittent catheterization program and is being evaluated because of increasing dysfunction (tethered cord, shunt malfunction). Voiding studies become less important and needle electrode myography may be more important. In all instances, a relatively clean rectum will result in a more accurate study.

It is most important that the child is comfortable, and that the laboratory is child friendly (posters, movies, books, stickers, etc.) and temperature controlled. All voidings should be as private as possible. For the older child, a separate room with a flowmeter and a one-way mirror to observe voidings can be helpful. Given enough time and patience, most studies can be completed successfully with reproducible results. Meperidine, 1 mg/kg, can be given to an extremely anxious child, although this is not common practice (Table 51.2).[14]

Table 51.2 Urodynamic studies

Urodynamic study	Purpose: to evaluate:
Uroflow/residual urine	Voiding function sensation, storage, emptying of the bladder
Cystometry	Coordination/function of muscular outlet
Pelvic floor/external sphincter EMG	Bladder/outlet function
Leak point pressure:	
Bladder	Storage pressure
Stress (VLPP)	Competence of bladder neck/proximal urethra
Videourodynamics	Anatomy and function of bladder and outlet (simultaneously)

EMG = electromyogram; VLPP = Valsalva leak point pressure.

Urinary flow rate and bladder capacity

The urinary flow rate measurement is a simple non-invasive study that is defined as the voided volume per unit time (ml/s) (Figures 51.4 and 51.5). This study can evaluate incontinence secondary to problems in storage or emptying. Reliability comes from repeated studies (at least two) and is related to voided volume. Bladder capacity (BC) should be based on age rather than body surface. Although the linear formula of Berger et al[16] and Koff:[17]

BC (ounces) = age + 2

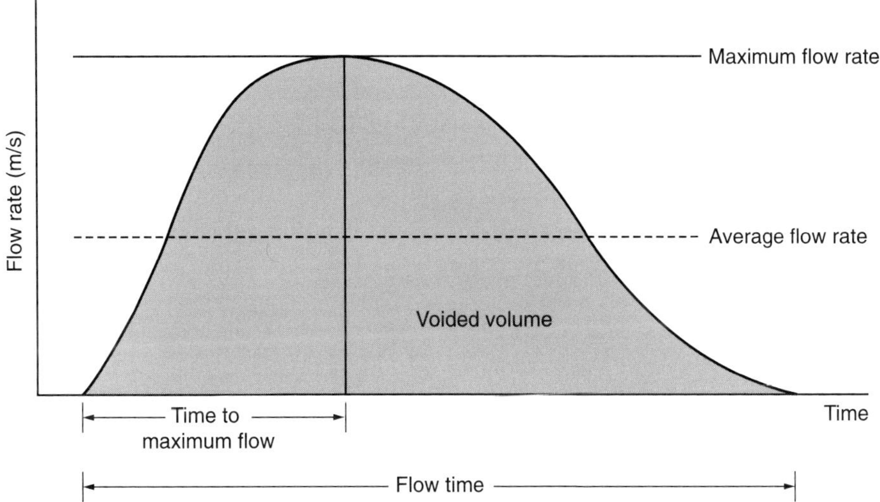

Figure 51.4 Idealized diagram of urine flow. (Modified with permission from Blaivas and Chancellor.[15])

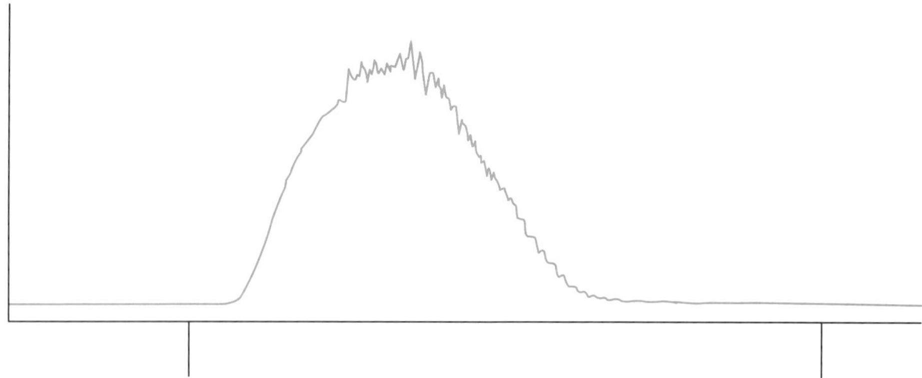

Figure 51.5 Normal uroflow in a 12-year-old male: maximum = 38 ml/s, average = 17 ml/s, volume = 222 ml.

has been the most frequently used to estimate bladder capacity, it is clear that bladder growth from a newborn (especially in the first years) to 13 years is not linear. Kaefer et al[18] responded to the challenge of modifying this equation with their non-linear equation:

$$2 \times \text{age (years)} + 2 = \text{capacity (ounces)}$$

for children <2 years old and

$$\frac{\text{age (years)}}{2} + 6 = \text{capacity (ounces)}$$

for children ≥2 years old. In all of these studies, data were based on findings in normal children. Children <14 years of age with spina bifida and neuropathic bladders do not exhibit similar growth rates to normal children. In fact, on comparing bladder growth in a small group of patients with spina bifida to the linear formula of Berger, bladders of patients with spina bifida grew half as well as those without neurologic abnormalities.[19] Thus, in order to calculate normal flow patterns and rates, one must first know the expected bladder capacity in order to determine whether the voiding volume is within the expected range. Accurate determination of the flow rate/voided volume is a common problem, particularly in the anxious child or in the child who voids frequently in small volumes. In general, voided volumes of <50% expected capacity should be suspect.[20,21] I recommend filling the bladder by forcing oral fluids on the way into the laboratory or by intravenous hydration. Multiple voids can be spontaneous, but furosemide administration can be helpful to ensure repeated measurements.

Critical features of the flow rate include the shape of the curve, maximum flow rate, and average flow rate. In a study of 180 schoolchildren aged 7–16 years, 98% had a bell-shaped flow pattern[20] (see Figure 51.4). The shape of the curve had no relationship to voided volume, but the other parameters were volume dependent. Although the maximum flow, average flow, and time to maximum flow can be of diagnostic interest, the shape of the flow appears to be the best screening parameter. Repeated deviations from the bell-shaped curve should prompt further studies (Figure 51.6). Estimation of residual urine can be an important clue to overall bladder function. Except in infants, the child's bladder should empty to completion with each void. There are multiple pitfalls when evaluating for retained urine. An anxious child in a foreign setting will not void efficiently. Furthermore, children with significant reflux may often harbor residual urine just after voiding. Thus, whereas complete evacuation can be helpful to know, an elevated postvoid residual may not signify important pathology. A bladder scan with ultrasound or placement of a catheter just prior to the cystometrogram will determine the residual urine.

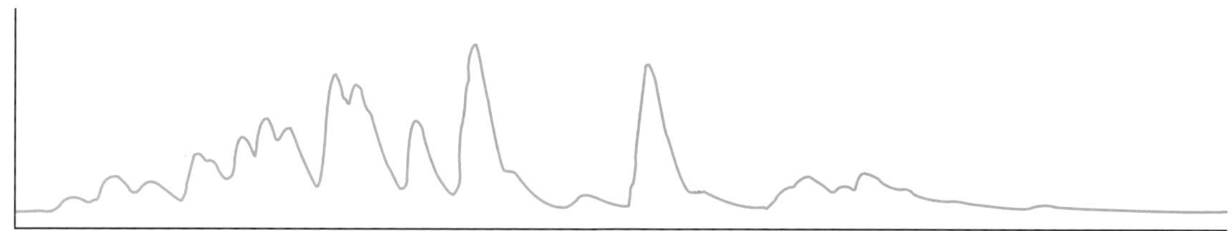

Figure 51.6 Abnormal uroflow in an 8-year-old male with abdominal straining and no detrusor activity.

Cystometry

Cystometry is the pressure–volume study of the bladder that examines both the storage and the voiding phase of micturition (Figures 51.7 and 51.8). Both parameters are instrumental in the assessment of bladder health in relationship to upper tract drainage. An accurate assessment of bladder storage must begin in a calm laboratory setting with the necessary techniques and props to decrease patient anxiety. The technician then passes an age-appropriate catheter. Male newborns usually require a 5 Fr feeding tube connected to a three-way stopcock that allows for both measuring pressure and fluid instillation. We try to take care to avoid an overly large catheter in newborns, which can obstruct the urethra and produce an abnormally high leak point pressure, as the fluid tries to leak around the catheter.[24] In older children, we use a 7–10 Fr catheter. Latex-free materials are essential for individuals with spina bifida, as they are prone to severe latex allergy and reactions.

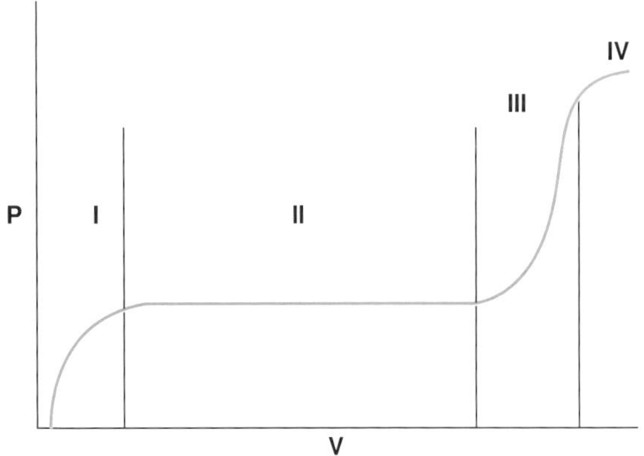

Figure 51.7 Cystometrogram indicating four phases and filling and detrusor activity: I, initial vesical pressure with early filling; II, stable tonus limb; III, increase in tonus at full vesicoelastic expansion; IV, voiding. (Modified with permission from Dmochowski.[22])

We record both intravesical and abdominal pressures. The abdominal pressure is obtained by inserting a pressure catheter into the rectum. These readings are easily made by tying a latex-free finger cot to a small plastic tube connected to a pressure monitor. The software from the urodynamics system then

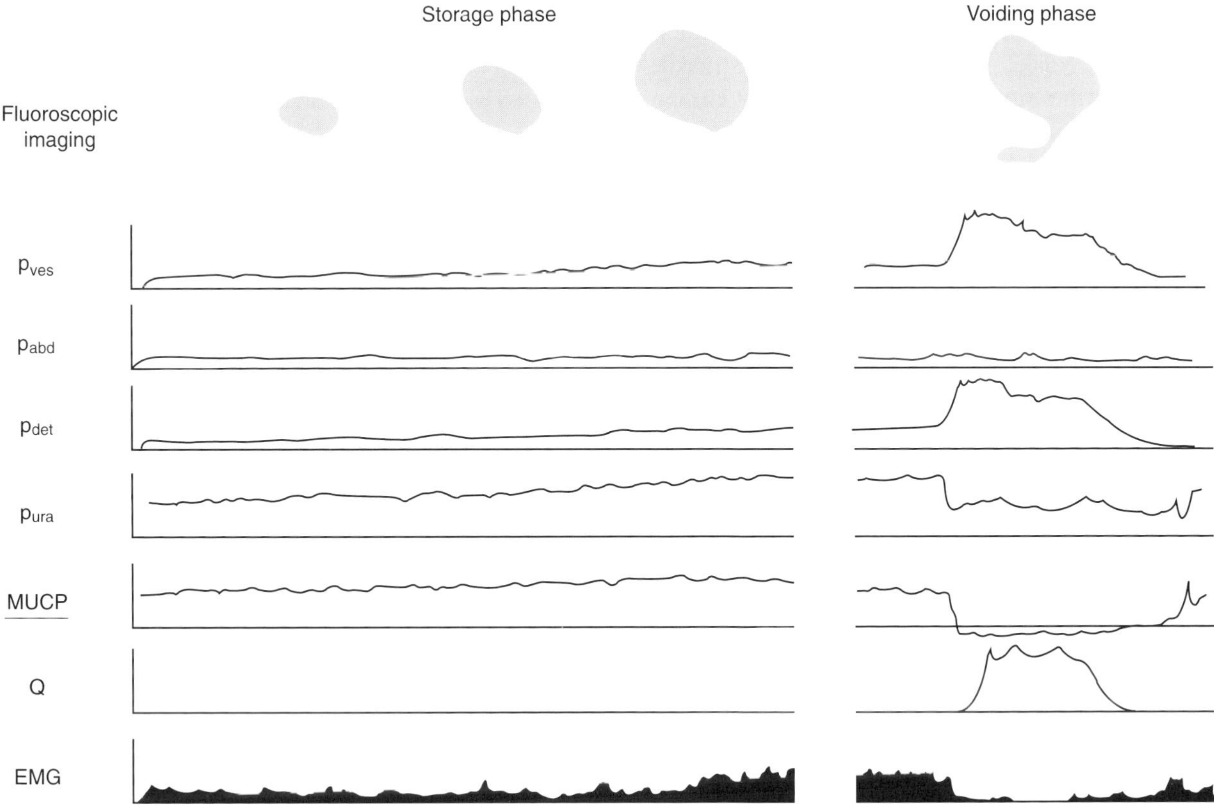

Figure 51.8 Idealized urodynamic tracing with accompanying fluoroscopic images. p_{ves} = intravesical pressure; p_{abd} = abdominal pressure; p_{det} = detrusor pressure; i.e. the $p_{ves} - p_{abd}$; p_{ura} = urethral pressure; MUCP = maximal urethral closure pressure; Q = urinary flow; EMG = surface electromyography. (Modified with permission from Abrams et al.[23])

subtracts the rectal (abdominal) pressure from the intravesical pressure to obtain a true detrusor pressure. These are basic measurements taken with a two-channel recorder. Membrane or microtip transducer catheters and multichannel recorders are readily available if so desired. The equipment varies; however, direct, hands-on, expert observation is probably more important than the size and complexity of the equipment. Straining, crying, and gross movements need to be noted and subtracted to obtain accurate detrusor pressures. The pressure transducer should be level with the symphysis pubis.

We use warm saline from a range of body to room temperature. We don't recommend carbon dioxide. Joseph[5] noted that a change in detrusor pressure, as well as maximum detrusor pressure, was adversely affected by increasing the rate of filling from slow (approximately 2% of estimated bladder capacity, 0–10 ml/min) to medium fill (approximately 20% of estimated bladder capacity, 10–100 ml/min). In general, we recommend filling at less than 10 ml/min in children.

An EMG should be performed at the same time as detrusor pressure evaluation. The electrodes can be surface pads, wires, or concentric needles. In children with neurogenic disease and lack of perineal sensation, we record from the external sphincter/perineal floor. In the male, we place a concentric needle directly into the bulbocavernosus muscle by aiming towards the bulb of the urethra. For the external sphincter, the needle is placed through the perineal skin just below the bulb of the urethra. A finger in the rectum will help to guide the needle. In females the external sphincter is identified by a needle placed just lateral to the urethral meatus and advanced <1 cm. To capture individual motor action potentials correctly, both an audio channel and oscilloscope are needed. A trained neurophysiologist best performs this study. This technique is the most accurate method of diagnosing the degree of denervation of the urethral sphincter and establishing the diagnosis of detrusor–sphincter dyssynergia (Figure 51.9). It should be noted, however, that in the majority of children, surface pad electrodes give excellent information about a composite view of muscle activity.

In select circumstances, a urethral pressure profile is helpful. Saline is infused at a rate of 2 ml/min while the catheter is slowly withdrawn at 2 mm/s. The urethral pressure profile measures the passive resistance of a particular point in the urethra. To obtain dynamic information of the outlet during voiding, we use micturition urethral pressure profilometry. This study is done in mid-voiding cycle to help eliminate the transient responses of the bladder neck and external sphincter during micturition. In some sophisticated laboratories, microtipped transducer catheters are used rather than saline infusion.

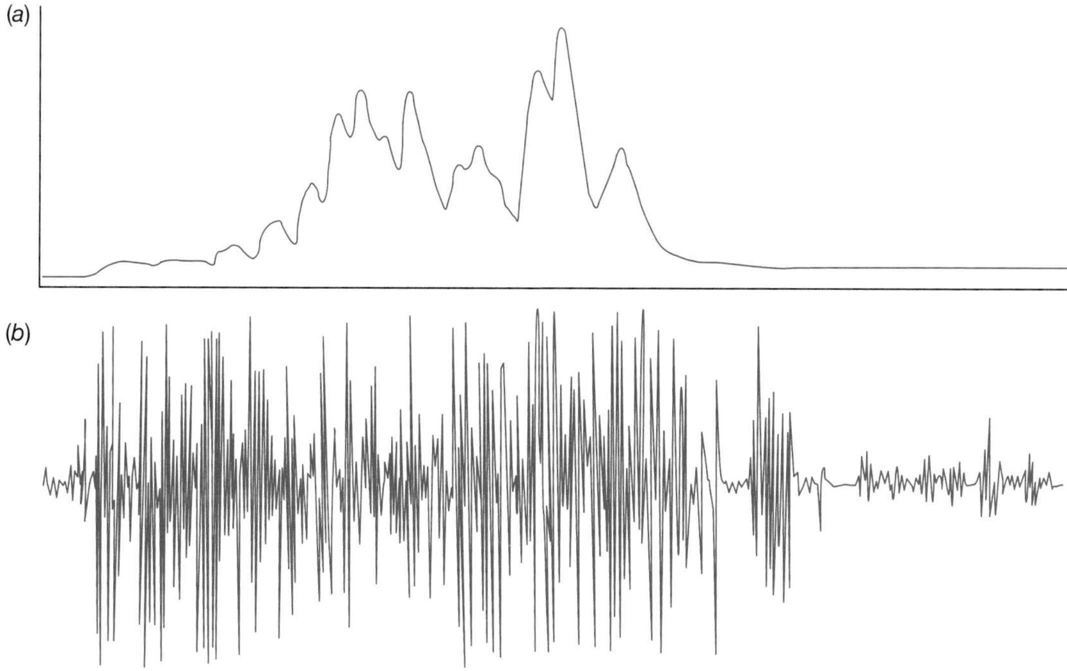

Figure 51.9 Urodynamics tracing in incontinent child with vesicosphincter dyssynergia: (*a*) uroflow; (*b*) electromyogram.

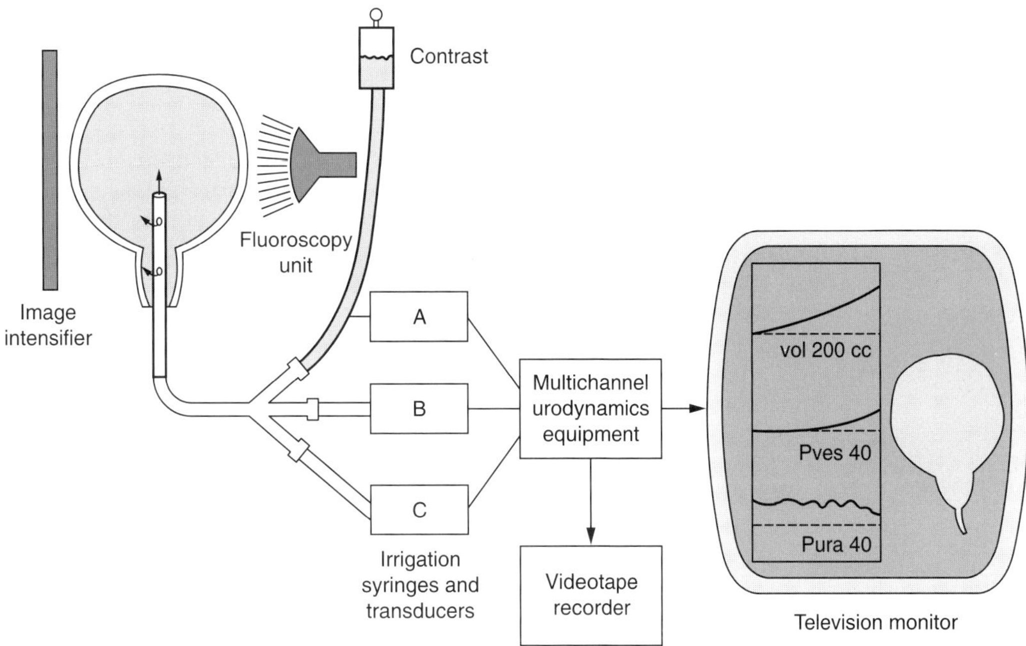

Figure 51.10 Videourodynamic equipment. (Modified with permission from McGuire et al.[25])

Videourodynamics is a technique that simultaneously combines the evaluation of the anatomy of the lower tract with recorded urodynamic studies (Figure 51.10). In the last 10 years, compact video recording equipment and computer technology have advanced this once research tool into an accessible clinical modality. As cost containment becomes more essential, portable urodynamic equipment can be brought into the fluoroscopy suite, to help share costs with the radiology team. Some investigators have found that real-time ultrasonography can be a suitable alternative to fluoroscopy. The disadvantage of ultrasonography is the less than ideal anatomic resolution.

In our facility, computer-generated digital images are stored and urodynamic parameters are superimposed on the image. Hard copies of the storage and voiding phase are also obtained and results in a radiologic interpretation component. Regardless of the imaging technology, videourodynamics is especially useful in delineating the bladder outlet during storage and voiding and identifying the causes of incontinence. When assessing the incontinent patient without uninhibited contractions noted on the cystometrogram, the urologist may evaluate the position and function of the bladder neck and proximal urethra under fluoroscopy to determine whether the urethra's incompetence or mobility is the etiology of the wetting. Videofluoroscopy may also be used to evaluate bladder compliance in relation to vesicoureteral reflux (VUR): i.e. reflux may act as a 'pop-off' valve for elevation in detrusor pressure, and knowledge of the time of reflux relative to bladder pressure can be important for proper management with clean intermittent catheterization and anticholinergics (Figures 51.11 and 51.12).

The urodynamic portion of videourodynamics is conducted in the routine fashion, by having the child arrive at the urodynamic suite in as a relaxed state as possible. Prestudy rituals include detailed discussions with the family about expectation and methods to alleviate the child's fears during the procedures. A scout film before placement of EMG patches or catheter probes helps to assess bowel status and guides future management of constipation if present. Severe constipation adversely affects vesicosphincter activity. If the child arrives with a full bladder, we perform a non-invasive flow study with patch electrodes. For the cystometry portion of the examination, the technique is the same, except that the infusant is radiographic contrast. A triple-lumen urethral catheter is slowly withdrawn and a urethral pressure profile is obtained. We position a radiopaque marker that identifies the urethral port at the point of highest urethral pressure.

The study can be performed initially with the patient supine on a fluoroscopy table, imaged with a C-arm that eliminates the need for an expensive table, or seated in a multipositional, radiolucent micturition seat. The standing position can help delineate the bladder neck and urethrovaginal component more

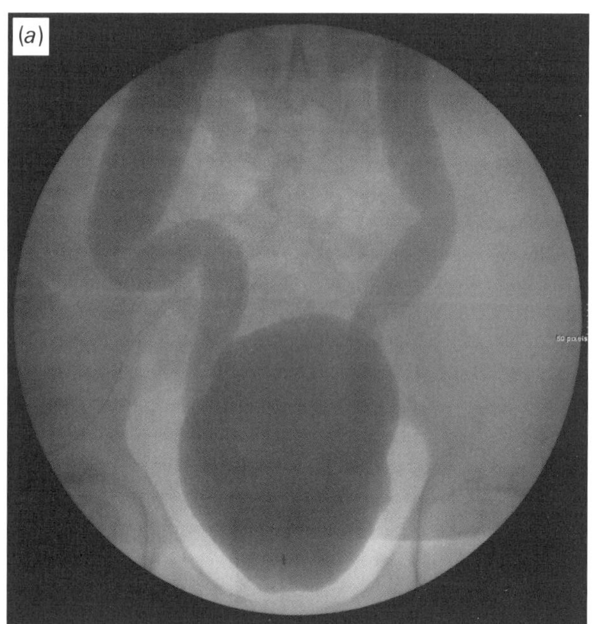

Figure 51.11 A 14-year-old male with imperforate anus, tethered spinal cord, and neurogenic bladder. He presents with recurrent urinary tract infection and incontinence despite clean intermittent catheterization and pharmacotherapy. (*a*) Videourodynamics were performed to evaluate the incidence of reflux and the bladder dynamics prior to further management. (*b*) Videourodynamics revealed a bladder capacity of 760 ml and low-pressure (19 cmH_2O) bilateral VUR. The bladder outlet was competent. Surgical options include augmentation cystoplasty with antireflux surgery. A Mitrofanoff and Malone antegrade colonic enema (MACE) procedure would be an option.

V_{infus} = volume of infusete; P_{ves} = intravesical pressure; P_{abd} = abdominal pressure; P_{det} = detrusor pressure; Qura = urinary flow.

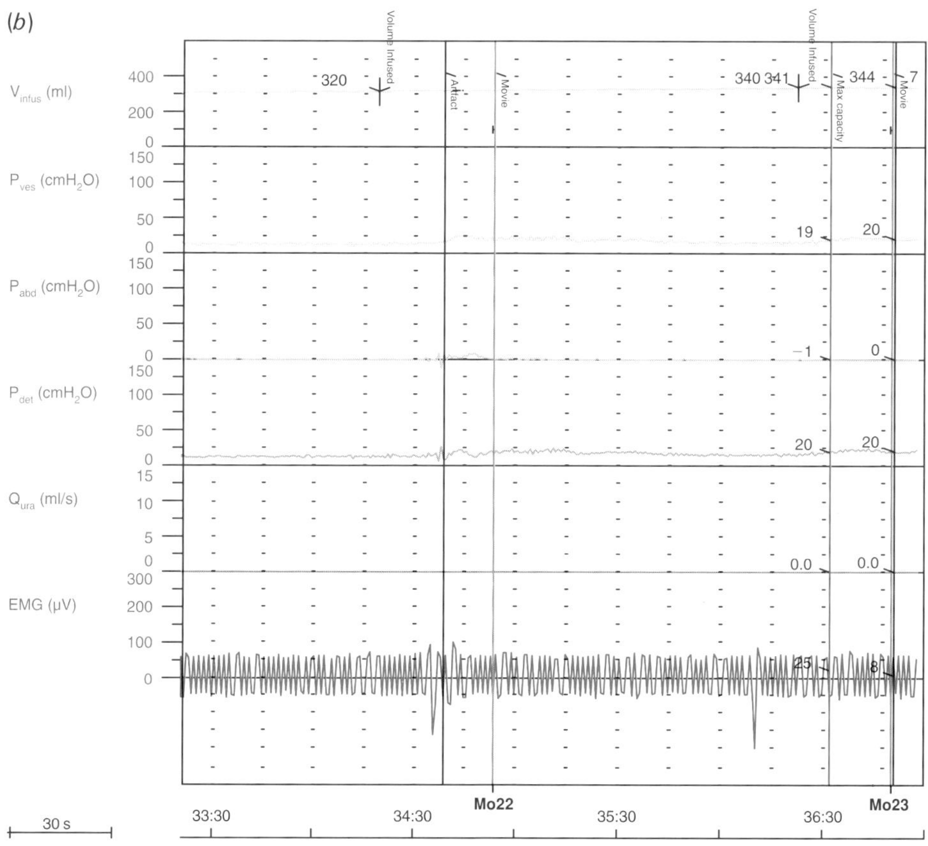

readily; however, many adolescent and young adult females may not easily initiate a void in the unusual standing position. In the standing position, the right posterior oblique projection provides the best image of the bladder neck. Under fluoroscopic control, the bladder, bladder neck, and urethra are visualized while the pressure is recorded.

Bladder filling is accomplished at 10% of expected bladder capacity. Valsalva and requests for repeated coughing are utilized to provoke the patient's incontinence symptoms. We examine the bladder base and urethra fluoroscopically for mobility and leakage, respectively. A postvoid residual is calculated and compared with the prestudy non-invasive residual. The

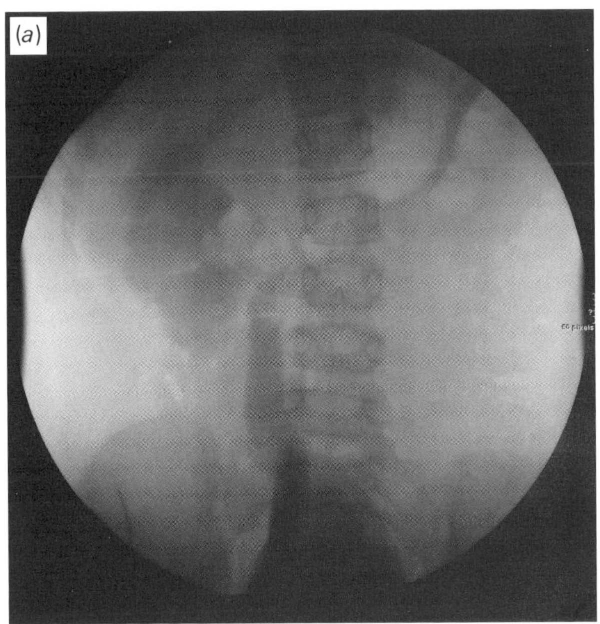

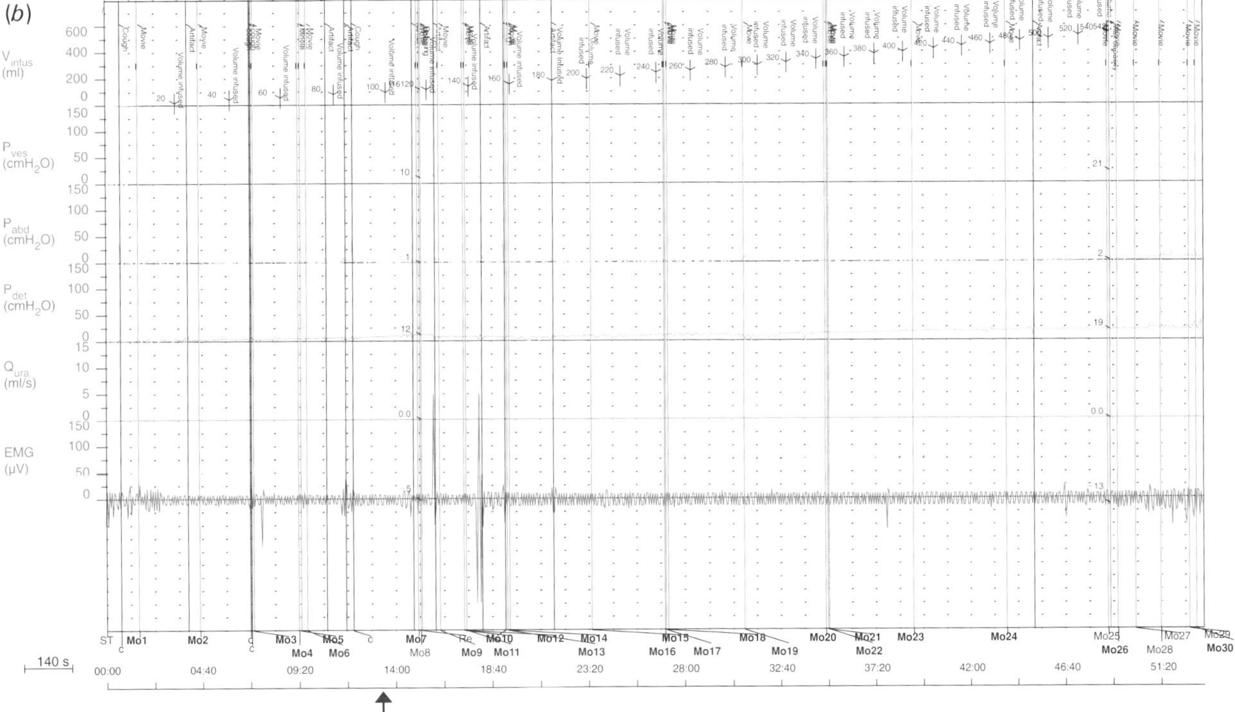

Figure 51.12 A 9-year-old female with dysfunctional elimination syndrome with recurrent febrile urinary tract infections. Videourodynamics revealed a bladder capacity of 875 ml, with no leakage. Her capacity pressure was 20 cmH_2O and she revealed grade 4 reflux at 117 ml (arrow) with a pressure of 10 cmH_2O. Her management included bowel management, biofeedback, and a subsequent successful subureteric injection of Deflux paste. (Key, see Figure 51.11.)

videourodynamic study accurately detects detrusor leak point pressure with straining. The importance of this finding relates to bladder compliance. If the outlet is open fluoroscopically, incontinence occurs with no change in bladder compliance. On the other hand, if the outlet is closed during a detrusor contraction (detrusor–sphincter dyssynergia), incontinence may still occur, but only with elevated detrusor pressures (compliance).

The first leak through the bladder neck is recorded. McGuire used videourodynamics and the abdominal leak point pressure (ALPP), also called the stress leak point pressure, to correctly diagnose the incontinent older patient with detrusor instability/ineffective outlet, as well as the pediatric patient with complex causes of incontinence (Figure 51.13). Videourodynamics easily evaluates the neurologically normal child with pseudosphincter dyssynergia and helps in the diagnostic dilemma of the child with neurogenic disease and decreased compliance, detrusor–sphincter dyssynergia, and areflexic emptying[25] (Figure 51.14).

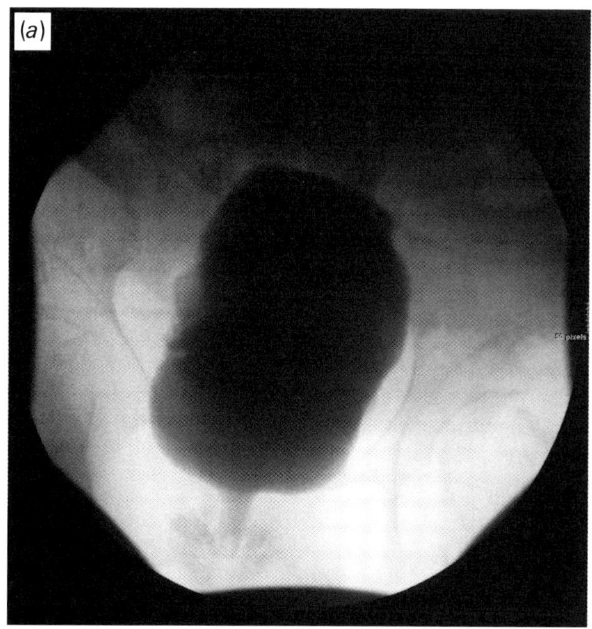

Figure 51.13 A 16-year-old male with L3–4 myelomeningocele had previous augmentation cystoplasty, Mitrofanoff and MACE procedure. He presented with continued incontinence, despite adequate anticholinergic therapy and clean intermittent catheterization (CIC) every 3–4 hours. His videourodynamic study revealed a bladder capacity of 810 ml. Radiographically, reflux occurred at 353 ml, (arrow) and the urethra was visible at his first leak point of 4 cmH_2O at 418 ml. His therapy included a sling procedure and a suburetric injection of Deflux paste. (Key, see Figure 51.11).

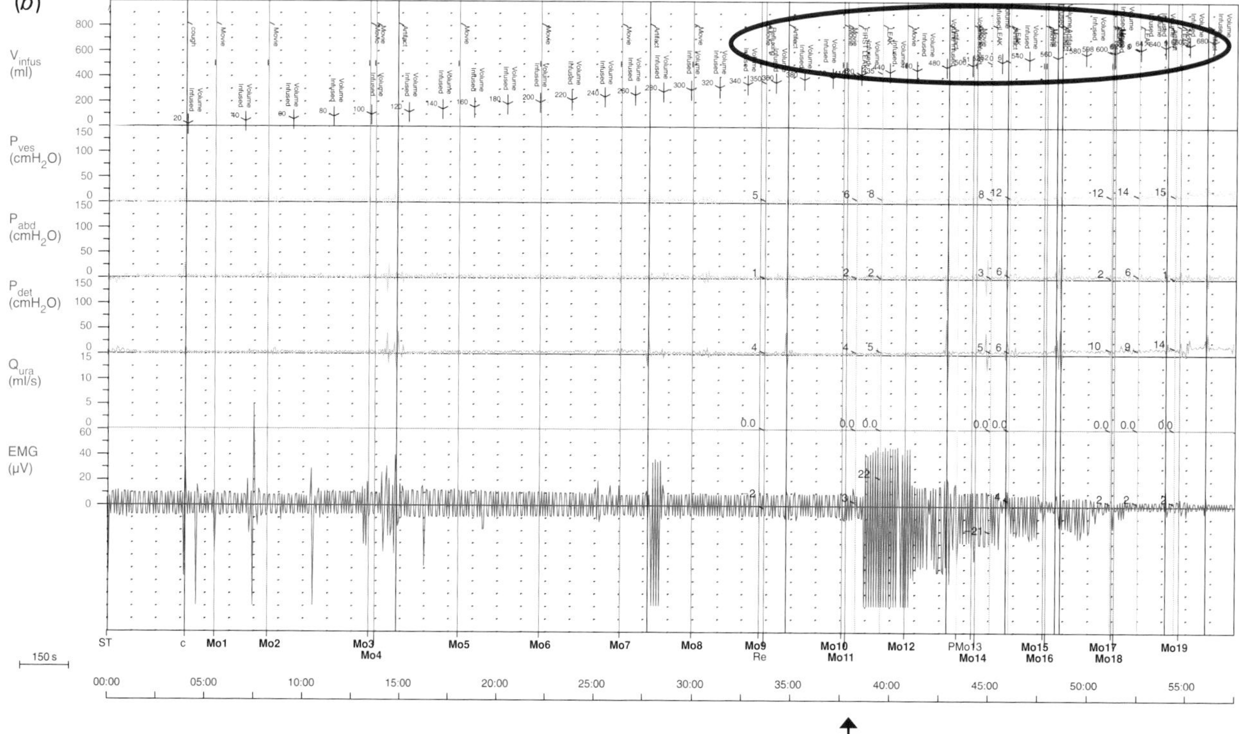

Compliance

Since the late 1970s, great advances in pediatric urology have occurred in the field of bladder management. A firm grasp of the importance of bladder health or 'safe' compliance became evident coincident with the introduction of clean intermittent catheterization by Lapides. The interest in neurourology blossomed with non-surgical as well as reconstructive techniques introduced to reconfigure bladder compliance. McGuire[26], Houle et al,[27] and McGuire et al[25] (1996) described two complementary studies to evaluate lower tract function and health.

McGuire popularized the concept of the leak point pressure. The leak point pressure is the detrusor pressure at which leakage occurs through the outlet. It is dependent on the resistance to flow. Without fluoroscopy the point of resistance will not be evident. It

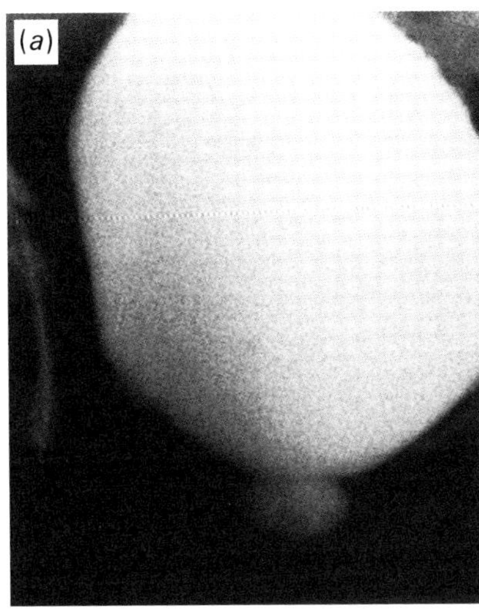

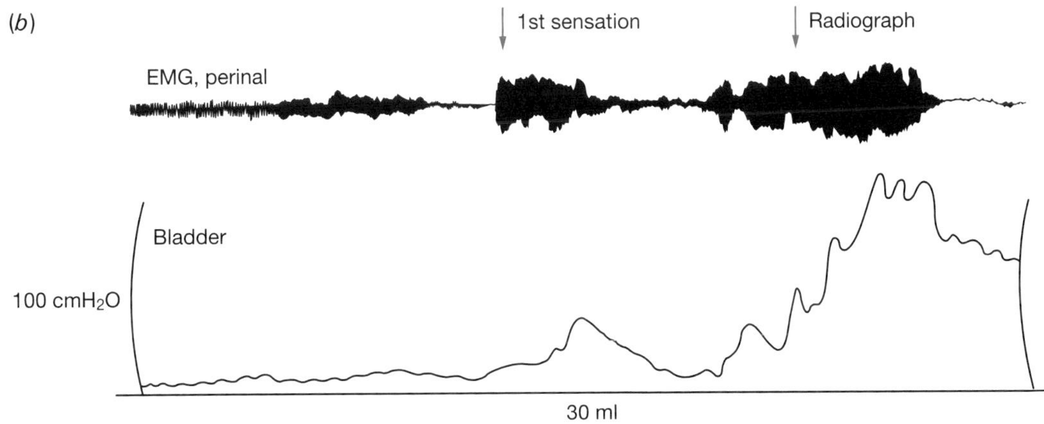

Figure 51.14 Videourodynamic study to indicate detrusor external sphincter dyssynergia. Note: detrusor contraction and simultaneous perineal EMG activity. The video indicates the dysfunctional void.

is measured by performing a slow fill cystometrogram, noting the pressure at which the leak occurs around the catheter per urethra. It has been shown in several centers that in the myelodysplastic population, children with leak point pressures of >40 cmH_2O are at greater risk for upper tract damage (hydronephrosis and reflux) than patients who have leak point pressures <40 cmH_2O.[27,28] Although many groups base their treatment program on this 'magic number' of 40, the limitations of a single leak point pressure are considerable.

Despite its relationship to outlet resistance, measurement of leak point pressure can be misleading when used to evaluate continence capability. Specifically, a high leak point pressure implies a good chance for continence. However, in the myelodysplastic population, the leak point pressure may be high but still not correlate with significant continence in the presence of a fixed but open bladder outlet.

The stress leak point pressure measurement was an innovation to help in the assessment of continence capability. The stress leak point pressure is slightly different from the simple bladder leak point pressure and can be determined without fluoroscopy. This value is obtained by slowly filling the bladder and having the child strain as if to have a bowel movement. The lowest pressure is then noted during which leakage first occurs. We ask the child to cough vigorously while the pressure is measured. This marker helps evaluate the capability of the outlet in both the open and poorly functioning state (e.g. the myelodysplastic child). The stress leak point pressure helps to determine whether outlet reconstructive procedures are needed to achieve urinary continence.[29]

The leak point pressure is an accurate measure of bladder storage pressure. However, Houle proposed that observing the volume at which a child can safely store urine, i.e. pressure-specific bladder volume, might better assess bladder storage characteristics. Houle indicated that in normal children, 99% of bladder capacity can be stored at <30 cmH_2O. Thus, a safe pressure of 20–30 cmH_2O was chosen and the volume noted which kept the pressure in that range.[26,30] This may be a most useful judge of compliance. Therapeutic interventions can be implemented based on this safe storage pressure. Voiding

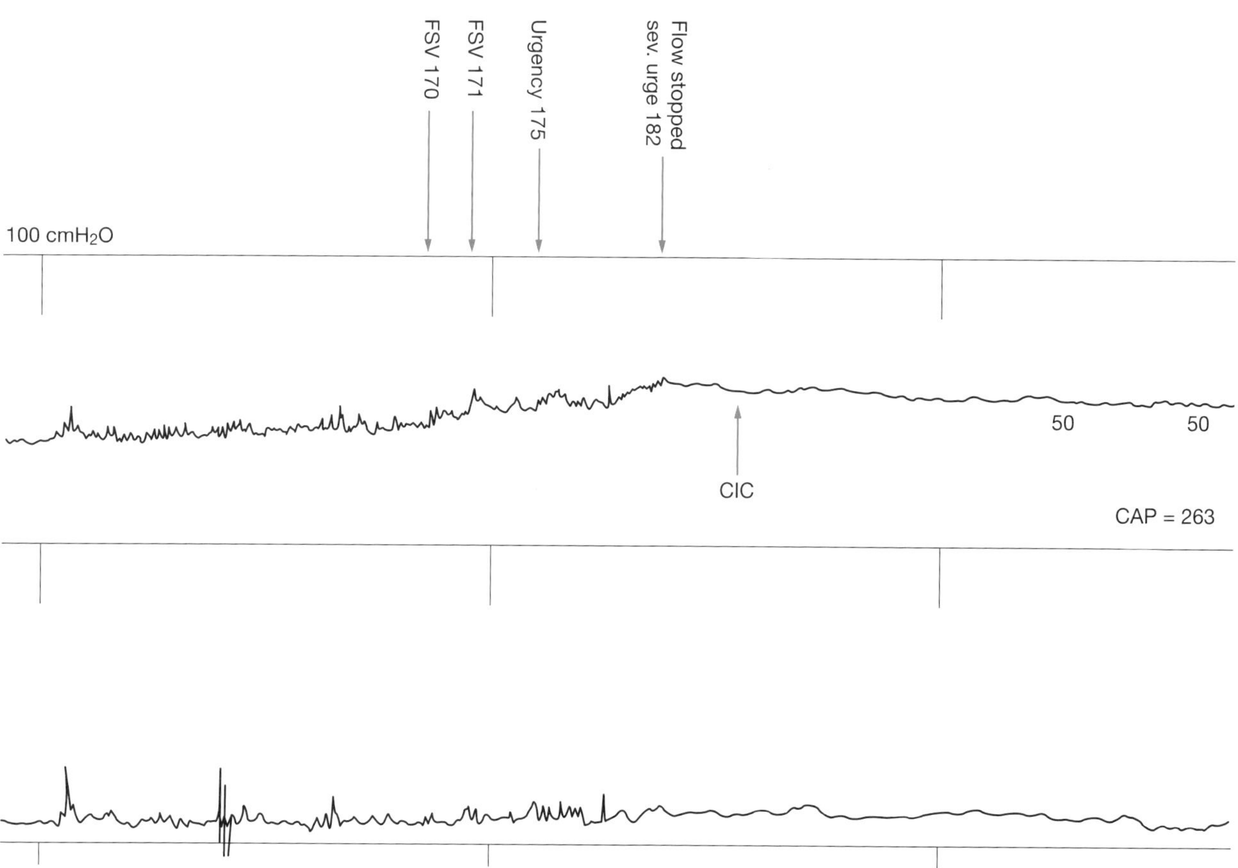

Figure 51.15 Urodynamic study to show poorly compliant neuropathic bladder pressure at capacity is 62 cmH_2O and patient-recorded typical catheterization volumes (CIC) that were at elevated pressures (70 cmH_2O). Failure at conservative management resulted in augmentation.

and catheterization diaries for patients may be obtained, and evacuation schedules or additions of medications (anticholinergics) adjusted accordingly. If conservative measures do not consistently allow the bladder to store in a safe zone, augmentation or neuromodulation procedures are used (Figure 51.15). It seems prudent and it is easy to obtain the leak point pressures, both simple and stress, as well as the pressure-specific bladder volume. However, it is unclear whether these data alone should be used as a basis to intervene prophylactically or must be interpreted in conjunction with imaging (e.g. renal and bladder sonography). Both programs have their staunch advocates. Accurate studies performed in a consistent and timely manner can only benefit the current population of children and give guidance for future cost-effective management.

Upper tract urodynamics

The issue of flow and pressure extends to the upper urinary tract. There is a variety of modalities to evaluate the functional patency of the upper tract. As in most aspects of medicine, the more tests that are available to evaluate a single subject, the more likely it is that no one test is the gold standard. At both ends of the spectrum, one would hope that clear-cut obstruction versus non-obstruction would be evident by studies including serial ultrasonography, diuretic excretory urography, retrograde pyelography, or diuretic renography. Urodynamics of the upper tract may be helpful when any or all of these studies become equivocable. Although the invasive Whitaker study (as originally described) would have promise as being the gold standard, it is also fraught with interpretive error. However, as in the case of the static leak point pressure, stress leak point pressure, and pressure-specific bladder volume, a variety of methods exist to evaluate the response of the upper urinary tract to flow and pressure.

The classic antegrade perfusion test as applied by Whitaker,[31] based on the work of Kiil[32] and Backlund and Reuterskold,[33] is well known. Simply, the test requires the infusion of saline into the renal pelvis at a constant flow rate, and pressure transducers placed

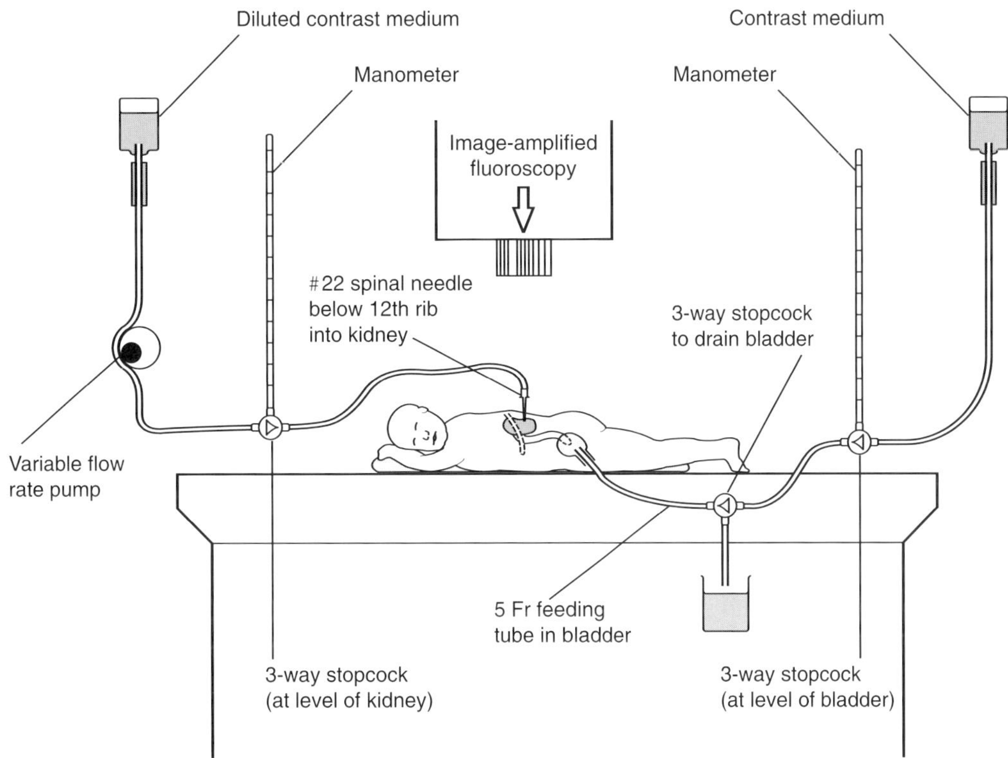

Figure 51.16 Whitaker test. Percutaneous puncture of renal pelvis and measurement of renal and bladder pressure. (Modified with permission from King and Levitt.[34])

in the renal pelvis and the bladder simultaneously to record the relative pressures. The access to the pelvis is typically percutaneously (in the preoperative evaluation); however, open access is certainly possible (Figure 51.16).

Why would one feel compelled to go to the bother and expense of this invasive test? There is a select group of patients and circumstances where diuretic renography will not be diagnostic: i.e. in the child in whom renal function is so compromised that the renal parenchyma cannot adequately handle the introduced isotope, technetium 99 m diethylenetriamine pentaacetic acid (^{99m}Tc DTPA).[35] The technique of the renogram, as well as the timing of the diuretic administration and the upper tract compliance can also influence the results. The diuretic renogram, even under ideal conditions, cannot evaluate renal pelvic pressure. Thus, in the proper setting, the effort involved in a urodynamic evaluation of the upper tract is indicated.

The patient is sedated and often anesthetized, and a catheter is inserted into the bladder and attached to a three-way stopcock. We place the patient prone, but before renal pelvic access, the 22-gauge access catheter is infused at 10 ml/min to determine the resistance of the catheter itself. Both the infusion and bladder catheters are connected to pressure transducers and leveled to the renal pelvis and superior border of the symphysis pubis, respectively. For the classic Whitaker pressure–flow study; a motor-driven syringe pump infuses fluid at a constant rate of 10 ml/min. The study can be repeated at 5 and 2 ml/min. If there is a sudden and rapid rise in renal pressure, the catheter may be abutting against the wall of the pelvis, and needs adjustment. If the bladder pressure rises significantly, the stopcock is opened and the bladder drained. The issue of bladder fullness is critical, because as the bladder fills and its pressure elevates, it can result in greater emptying pressure of the ureter and pelvis. The bladder pressure, as well as the infusion pressure through the infusant catheter and tubing, needs to be subtracted from the pelvic pressure.[36] The pelvic or absolute pressure, minus the bladder and tubing pressure, equals the relative pressure.

During the analysis of the pressure data, two groups of patients emerge: those with relative pressures <15 cmH_2O and those with relative pressures >22 cmH_2O. In the ideal, the test can indicate obstruction (>22 cmH_2O), no obstruction (<15 cmH_2O), and the general site of obstruction. That is, if the renal pelvic pressure and bladder pressure drop by emptying the bladder, elevated bladder

Table 51.3 Summary of the Whitaker test

Kidney pressure	Normal	Raised	Raised	Raised
Relative pressure (cmH_2O) (Pelvic–tubing–bladder)	<15	>22	<15	>22
Bladder pressure	Normal	Normal	Raised	Raised
Result	Unobstructed	Obstructed	Non-compliant bladder	Non-compliant bladder and obstruction

pressure is causing the poor emptying of the renal pelvis and bladder management is needed, i.e. to improve bladder compliance by surgical or non-surgical means. If the relative pressure differential is subtracted from the absolute renal pelvic pressure and the result is >12–15 cmH_2O, there is some degree of ureteral obstruction[37] (Table 51.3). There are several concerns regarding the accuracy and predictability of Whitaker's relative pressure. In the original description, Whitaker noted that the fullness of pelvis and ureter could be noted if radiopaque contrast is used for the infusant. This equilibrium/fullness factor, however, may be somewhat arbitrary. To assess the pressure correctly, the system needs to be full. The infusion rate has also come under question. Fung et al[38] adjusted the nomogram, by suggesting that the original Whitaker test may be made more accurate by infusing a volume more individualized for patient size and glomerular function rather than the standard rate of 10 ml/min. Mortensen et al[39] found, in the pig, large enough overlaps in the relative pressure to call into question the concern over a 12–15 cmH_2O pressure. Forthcoming were debates over constant flow versus constant pressure studies. The constant pressure technique is compared with the pressure-specific bladder volume work: i.e. it may be important to know the pressure required to produce flow across the system, as the pressure should be the final determinate of upper tract health. In the human one-kidney model, keeping pressure constant by elevating the infusant solution to known levels and measuring flow can be assessed. However, in the child with two kidneys, measuring output from the studied kidney only is still a challenge.[40,41] Finally, a variety of influences on the urinary tract can significantly alter the renal pelvis emptying pressure, e.g. pharmacotherapy (principally anticholinergics), infections, and reflux.[42–44]

The expanded subject of the pressure–flow study, renogram, prediction of pathology, and prediction of renal salvage is beyond the scope of this technical chapter. Complex diagnostic dilemmas may not be solved by the use of urodynamics of the upper tract (however one chooses to execute the study). In the select patient with poor renal function and a dilated system, however, a carefully planned diagnostic attack should also include the capability to perform a reproducible evaluation of the pressure–flow characteristics of the system.

References

1. Lapides J, Diokno AC, Silber SJ, Lowe BS. Clean intermittent self catheterization in the treatment of urinary tract disease. J Urol 1972; 107:458–61.
2. Gierup J, Ericksson NO, Okmain L. Micturition studies in infants and children: technique. Scand J Urol Nephrol 1969; 3:1–8.
3. Blaivas JG, Labib KB, Bauer SB, Retik AB. Changing concepts in the urodynamic evaluation of children. J Urol 1977; 117:778–81.
4. Maizels M, Firlit CF. Pediatric urodynamics: clinical comparison of surface versus needle pelvic floor/external sphincter electromyography. J Urol 1979; 122:518–22.
5. Joseph DB. The effect of medium-fill and slow-fill saline cystometry on detrusor pressure in infants and children with myelodysplasia. J Urol 1992; 147:444–6.
6. Mahalik MP, Gautieri RF, Mann DE Jr. Teratogenic potential of cocaine hydrochloride in CF–1 mice. J Pharm Sci 1980; 69:703–6.
7. Chasnoff IJ, Chisum GM, Kaplan WE. Maternal cocaine use and genitourinary tract malfunctions. Teratology 1988; 37:201–4.
8. Phelan SA, Mariko I, Loeken MR. Neural tube defects in embryos of diabetic mice. Role of the Pax-3 genes and apoptosis. Diabetes 1997; 46:1189–97.
9. van Gool JD, Hjälmås K, Tamminen-Möbius T, Olbing H. Historical clues to the complex of dysfunctional voiding, urinary tract infection and vesicoureteral reflux. The International Reflux Study in Children. J Urol 1992; 148:1699–702.
10. Hellstrom A-L, Andersson K, Hjälmås K, Jodal U. Pad tests in children with incontinence. Scand J Urol Nephrol 1986; 20:47–50.
11. Mattsson SH. Voiding frequency, volumes and intervals in healthy schoolchildren. Scand J Urol Nephrol 1994; 28:1–11.
12. Loening-Baucke V. Urinary incontinence and urinary

tract infection and their resolution with treatment of chronic constipation of childhood. Pediatrics 1997; 100:228–32.

13. Koff SA, Wagner TT, Jayanthi VR. The relationship among dysfunctional elimination syndromes, primary vesicoureteral reflux and urinary tract infections in children. J Urol 1998; 160:1019–22.
14. Ericsson NO, Hellstrom B, Negardth A, Rudhe U. Micturition urocystography in children with myelomeningocele. Acta Radiol Diagn 1971; 11:321–36.
15. Blaivas J, Chancellor M (eds). Atlas of Urodynamics. Baltimore: Williams and Wilkins, 1996.
16. Berger RM, Maizels M, Moran GC et al. Bladder capacity (ounces) equals age (years) plus 2 predicts normal bladder capacity and aids in diagnosis of abnormal voiding patterns. J Urol 1983; 129:347–9.
17. Koff SA. Estimating bladder capacity in children. Urology 1983; 21:248.
18. Kaefer M, Zurakowski D, Bauer SB et al. Estimating normal bladder capacity in children. J Urol 1997; 158:2261–4.
19. Kaplan WE, Richards TW, Richards I. Intravesical transurethral bladder stimulation to increase bladder capacity. J Urol 1989; 142:600–2.
20. Mattsson S, Spångberg A. Urinary flow in healthy school children. Neurourol Urodyn 1994; 13:281–96.
21. Szabo L, Fegyverneki S. Maximum and average urine flow rates in normal children – the Miskolc nomograms. Br J Urol 1995; 76:16–20.
22. Dmochowski R. Cystometry. Urol Clin North Am 1996; 23:243–51.
23. Abrams P, Khoury S, Wein A. WHO Publication. Geneva: World Health Organization, 1998:353–401.
24. Decter R, Harpster L. Pitfalls in determination of leak point pressure. J Urol 1992; 148:588–91.
25. McGuire EJ, Cespedes RD, O'Connell HE. Leak point pressures. Urol Clin N Am 1996; 23:253–62.
26. McGuire EJ, Woodside JR, Barden TA, Weiss RM. Prognostic value of urodynamic testing in myelodysplastic patients. J Urol 1981; 126:205–9.
27. Houle A, Gilmour RF, Churchill BM et al. What volume can a child normally store in the bladder at a safe pressure. J Urol 1993; 149:561–4.
28. Bauer SB, Hallett N, Khoshbin et al. Predictive value of urodynamic evaluation in newborns with myelodysplasia. JAMA 1984; 252:650–2.
29. Wan J, McGuire EJ, Bloom DA, Ritchie ML. Stress leak point pressure: a diagnostic tool for incontinent children. J Urol 1993; 150:700–2.
30. Landau EH, Churchill BM, Jayanthi VR et al. The sensitivity of pressure specific bladder volume versus total bladder capacity as a measure of bladder storage dysfunction. J Urol 1994; 152:1578–81.
31. Whitaker RH. The Whitaker test. Urol Clin North Am 1979; 6:529–39.
32. Kiil F. The Function of the Ureter and Renal Pelvis. Oslo: Oslo University Press, 1957.
33. Backlund L, Reuterskold AG. The abnormal ureter in children. I. Perfusion studies of the wide non-refluxing ureter. Scand J Urol Nephrol 1969; 3:219–28.
34. King LR, Levitt SB. Vesicoureteral reflux, megaureter and ureteral reimplantation. In: Walsh PC, Gittes RF, Perlmutter AD et al, eds. Campbell's Urology, 5th edn. Philadelphia: WB Saunders, 1986: 2031–88.
35. O'Reilly PH, Lawson RS, Shields RA. Ideopathic hydronephrosis. J Urol 1979; 121:153–5.
36. Smyth TB, Shortliffe LMD, Constantinou CE. The effect of urinary flow and bladder fullness on renal pelvic pressure in a rat model. J Urol 1991; 146:592–6.
37. Whitaker RH. An evaluation of 170 diagnostic pressure flow studies on the upper urinary tract. J Urol 1979; 121:602–4.
38. Fung LCT, Khoury AE, McLorie GA et al. Evaluation of pediatric hydronephrosis using individualized pressure flow criteria. J Urol 1995; 154:671–6.
39. Mortensen J, Kjurhuus JD, Laursen H, Bisballe S. The relationship between pressure and flow in the normal pig renal pelvis. Scand J Urol Nephrol 1983; 17:369–72.
40. Ripley SH, Somerville JJF. Whitaker revisited. Br J Urol 1982; 54:594–8.
41. Woodbury PW, Mitchell ME, Scheidler DM et al. Constant pressure perfusion: a method to determine obstruction in the upper urinary tract. J Urol 1989; 142:632–5.
42. Fichtner J, Boinlau FG, Lewy JE, Shortliffe LMD. Oxybutynin lowers elevated renal pelvic pressures in a rat with congenital unilateral hydronephrosis. J Urol 1998; 160:887–91.
43. Cowan BF, Shortliffe LMD. Oxybutynin decreases renal pelvic pressures in normal and infected rat urinary tract. J Urol 1998; 160:882–6.
44. Angell SK, Pruthi RS, Shortliffe LMD. The urodynamic relationship of renal pelvic and bladder pressures, and urinary flow rate in rats with congenital vesicoureteral reflux. J Urol 1998; 160:150–6.

Neurologic control of storage and voiding

52

Julian Wan and John M Park

Introduction

The body controls storage and emptying of urine by a series of neurologic pathways. These pathways are similar to electrical circuits that help control and coordinate the activities of a complex machine. They grant the ability to rapidly shift the lower urinary tract between two different modes of function: storage and emptying. In infants, the switching process between these two functions acts in a reflex manner to produce involuntary voiding. In older children, urine storage and emptying are under voluntary control. This degree of control is unique in the body. Autonomic or involuntary reflex mechanisms almost exclusively control other visceral structures, such as the heart, bowels, and lungs. They react to volitional activity but are not under volitional control. Yogis have been able to consciously slow their heart rate and rhythm and elite athletes such as Olympic target shooters can delay the onset of their QRS complex as seen on an electrocardiogram (ECG) to allow them to fire between ventricular contractions. Yet, neither of these groups exhibits the degree of volitional control exerted over an autonomic system as experienced routinely by children over their bladder and urethra.[1–3]

In over a century of study, the physiology and neurology of the bladder and urethra have been fruitful areas of research. Clinical observation of patients, laboratory studies of human tissue, and animal models have helped to contribute to this knowledge. For pediatric urologists, an understanding of the normal process of urine storage and drainage provides the foundation for the evaluation and treatment of congenital and acquired abnormalities of storage and emptying. This chapter reviews what is currently understood about these neurologic pathways, their interaction with the target organs, and their clinical relevance to pediatric urology. We use specific disease entities as examples to further our discussion, but these conditions (e.g. neurogenic bladder dysfunction) are discussed elsewhere in detail. We begin by reviewing the various components of bladder physiology and follow in each case with a description of the reflex pathways that contribute to coordination of bladder filling and emptying. We also discuss the role of higher centers and the plasticity of neurologic control.

Overview summary

The lower urinary tract, which comprises the bladder, urethra, and urinary sphincter, has two principal functions: storage of urine and emptying of urine. A complex neural control system involving the brain, spinal cord, and autonomic and somatic nerves governs these actions. This system performs as a series of circuits that overlay each other. At the most basic level, it works as a simple switch to maintain a reciprocal relationship between the reservoir (bladder) and the outlet (urethra, urinary sphincter). The circuits also interconnect and create a complex sequence of coordinated selective excitation and inhibition of the bladder, urethra, and sphincter (Figure 52.1). A variety of neurotransmitters play significant roles in these pathways, and may provide opportunities for pharmacologic intervention.

During bladder filling, the viscoelastic properties of the bladder wall and an absence of an excitatory input from the parasympathetic ganglia to the bladder smooth wall musculature allow the bladder to accommodate more urine while keeping pressures low. As the bladder continues to fill, an increase in outlet resistance occurs by means of a rhabdosphincter somatic reflex called the guarding reflex. In humans

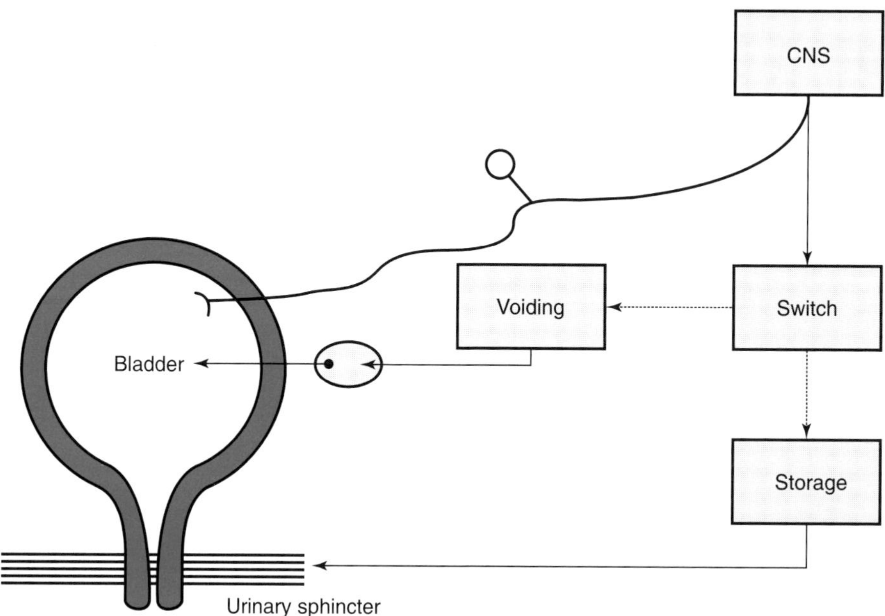

Figure 52.1 The relationship between the anatomy of the lower urinary tract and the switch function of the micturition pathways. During urine storage, a low level of afferent activity activates efferent input to the urethral sphincter. A high level of afferent activity caused by bladder filling activates the switch in the central nervous system (CNS). This causes firing of the efferent pathways, inhibition of the efferent pathway to the urinary sphincter, leading to relaxation, and excitation to the bladder, causing contraction and emptying.

and many mammalian species, a sympathetic reflex also aids this process by increasing outlet resistance. This is achieved by increasing tension on the smooth muscle component of the sphincter and by inhibiting bladder contractility through an inhibitory effect on the parasympathetic ganglia. Finally, the sympathetic output also decreases the tension of bladder smooth muscle. The intrinsic competence of the bladder outlet, with some reflex help from the rhabdosphincter, maintains continence during increases in intra-abdominal pressure.

Bladder emptying can be volitional or involuntary and involves an inhibition of the spinal somatic and sympathetic reflexes and activation of the parasympathetic pathways leading to the bladder. The coordinating center lies in the pons region of the brainstem. Initially there is relaxation of the bladder neck and sphincter muscle, which is controlled by the cessation of somatic and sympathetic spinal reflexes as well as local factors such as nitric oxide (NO) released by parasympathetic stimulation. Subsequently, a coordinated synchronized contraction of the bladder smooth muscle occurs. The bladder neck or outlet develops a funnel shape that is due in part to the continuity of the bladder base and proximal urethra. There is modulation of this process from other peripheral reflexes and from supraspinal sources. The bladder then empties and drains normally to completion.

The ability to control and modulate between these two states develops with maturation. In neonates, the switch between the two modes of storage and emptying occurs on a reflex level once the bladder reaches a threshold volume. With maturation, the ability to modulate this action develops volitionally. This change occurs because a layer of modulating and inhibitory controls that originate above the sacral spine and are mediated by the cerebral cortex and other higher centers is overlaid to modify the primitive set of pathways that function initially. These pathways remain malleable throughout life. Injury and disease can cause these suprasacral inhibitory and modulating pathways to become lost or diminished. Earlier reflex pathways are then unmasked and can re-emerge. Plasticity and re-emergence of earlier more primitive pathways may help to explain the nature of many conditions caused by neurogenic dysfunction.

Target organs: bladder, urethra, and urinary sphincter

A multilayer weave of smooth muscle surrounds the bladder and urethra. The bladder and urethra form one anatomic unit with two distinct functional regions: the body or fundus, and the base and proximal urethra. The demarcation between these two areas roughly coincides with the division between the bladder body and the trigone.[4–6] The bladder and urethra receive different types of autonomic innervation. Muscarinic cholinergic receptors are found throughout the smooth muscle but are most numerous in the fundus. Preganglionic cholinergic receptors in the sympathetic and parasympathetic ganglia are nicotinic, as are the cholinergic receptors of the striated muscle component of the urinary sphincter, the rhabdosphincter. α-Adrenergic receptors are more numerous in the smooth muscle of the posterior urethra and bladder base.[4,7,8] This cluster of α-adrenergic receptors is more concentrated in boys than in girls and many contribute to the tight bladder neck closure seen during ejaculation.[9] Beta-adrenergic receptors are found in the fundus and act to help relax the bladder during filling.[10] Human fetal studies have shown that β-adrenergic and cholinergic receptors are present as early as 3 months' gestation.[11] α-Adrenergic receptors appear in the trigone and urethra after 6 months' gestation.[6] These observations suggest that even very early in infancy a complex system is already at work. Pharmacologists have exploited the differences in receptor distribution to create drugs that target specific receptors. This distribution may change as a result of injury or disease.

The organization of the bladder smooth muscle affects its normal function. Smooth muscles are organized into fascicles of 4–12 cells. Extracellular matrix (ECM), consisting of collagen, elastin, and rare fibroblasts, surrounds each fascicle.[12] These bundles collectively form circumferential and longitudinal patterns around the bladder and proximal urethra; they are interwoven, with no distinct layers. In males, the smooth muscle forms part of the prostatic capsule. The rhabdosphincter consists of circumferential fibers of striated muscle that surround the smooth muscle from the bladder base to the urogenital diaphragm.[13] It appears that the rhabdosphincter is distinct and separate from the urogenital diaphragm and pelvic-supporting striated muscles in both males and females.[14,15] The striated muscles are both fast and slow twitch. The fast-twitch, more easily fatigued fibers fire during voluntary attempts to stop micturition or during acts of active suppression of voiding. The slow-twitch fatigue-resistant fibers contract during bladder filling as part of the guarding reflex. The rhabdosphincter initially contracts as a reflex. With maturation, it comes under volitional control from the higher cortical centers. In addition to somatic and sensory connections, the urinary sphincter also receives parasympathetic and sympathetic fibers from the pelvic plexus, making it 'triple innervated.'[16] Clinically, this concept is important, as α blockers are useful in treating urinary obstruction and dysfunctional voiding. This combination of sympathetic, parasympathetic, and somatic innervation is present in the cat; the sympathetic component is present in humans. The full functional significance of the autonomic innervation of the striated sphincter in humans is not yet known. Urinary physiologists have identified autonomic innervation of the striated sphincter in patients with lower motor neuron lesions but not in patients with detrusor–sphincter dyssynergia (DSD) – suggesting that the degree of autonomic innervation changes as a response to injury or disease.[4,17]

Nerve endings do not innervate each individual smooth muscle cell of the human bladder. Electron microscopy shows that normal muscle cells are about 0.2 nm apart without intercellular links.[4] Direct cell-to-cell excitation has not been shown. Electromechanical coupling rather than direct neuronal excitation propagates efficient coordinated detrusor contractions. A few muscle cells are directly triggered, which in turn contract and pull on their neighboring cells, thereby triggering further excitation. Some researchers believe that changes at a myogenic level may be responsible for urge and urge incontinence seen with overactive bladder.[18,19]

The normal bladder exhibits excellent compliance and viscoelasticity. The parameters are influenced by the properties of the ECM, which (as stated previously) is a mixture of collagen, elastin, and occasional fibroblasts. In many pathologic states, there are changes in the ECM that affect the mechanical function of the bladder. The type of collagen that is present appears to play an important role.[20] Type I and type III collagen predominate in the ECM: type I is thicker and stiffer, whereas type III is thinner and more pliable. As the human fetus matures, the ratio between types I and type III decreases, with an associated rise in bladder compliance and increase in elastin. A normal fetal bladder becomes more compliant as gestation progresses. Fibroblasts in the interstitium are the source of most of the connective tissue. Normally there is little fibroblast activity in the bladder. Denervation experiments show that increases in ECM may be in part due to a slowing of collagen degradation and decrease of activity of local proteases. Increases in ECM come not only from the fibroblasts but also from the smooth muscles themselves.[21] Dedifferentiation of smooth muscle cells under repetitive stress leads to more elaboration of collagen and elastin in the interstitium. This resembles the process seen in stressed walls of vasculature, wherein an injury or disease can initiate a spiraling cascade of pathology. A neurogenic bladder, for example, may lose the neurologic modulation that maintains compliance, which in turn leads to higher storage pressure, which causes higher stress, which promotes dedifferentiation of smooth muscles and greater deposits of elastin and collagen, which further decreases elasticity and compliance, and so on. Removal or alteration of normal innervation may result, therefore, in lasting changes to the histology of the bladder.

Neurotransmitters

The basic autonomic neurotransmitters are well known. The sympathetic nerves are adrenergic and use norepinephrine as a neurotransmitter in postganglionic synapses. Preganglionic sympathetic and all parasympathetic nerves are cholinergic and use acetylcholine. Less well known is a third system, the purinergic or peptidergic system. Found in animals and humans, it comprises a wide variety of molecules, including vasoactive intestinal peptide (VIP), neuropeptide Y, adenosine triphosphate (ATP), substance P, somatostatin, and calcitonin gene-related peptide (CGRP).[4,22,23] This third pathway acts as a modulator of overall autonomic activity. Neuropeptides are present throughout the smooth and striated muscle of the lower urinary tract. In addition, observations in some pathologic states of autonomic denervation suggest that the effects are clinically more significant. The existence of this third pathway of the autonomic system was inferred when muscarinic blockade with atropine did not completely ablate in-vitro bladder muscle contraction.[7] Atropine is also less effective in blocking bladder muscle contractions from specimens taken from neurogenic bladders, suggesting that there is an enhanced purinergic factor in these pathologic bladders.

Several purinergic transmitters are inhibitory: opioid peptides (enkephalins), inhibitory amino acids [glycine, γ-aminobutyric acid (GABA)], serotonin, dopamine, and non-opioid peptides such as neuropeptide Y and corticotropin-releasing factor. All of these can inhibit the micturition reflex when applied to the central nervous system (CNS). Excitatory purinergic transmitters include glutamic acid, neuropeptides such as substance P and VIP, NO, and norepinephrine.[24,25] These neurotransmitters affect the vascular smooth muscle, may alter local blood flow, and can appear in increased concentration in obstructed or neurogenic bladders. VIP is lower in concentration in biopsy specimens of hypercontractile bladders.[26] Because of elevated levels of VIP and neuropeptide Y in the urethras of patients with spinal cord injury, a compensatory role for them has been suspected.[27] ATP levels are higher than normal in the bladder muscle of spina bifida patients and interact with two families of receptors: P2X receptors and the G protein-coupled P2Y receptors.[6] Therefore, it has been speculated that hyperactivity observed in neurogenic and obstructed bladders might be the result of abnormal purinergic influences mediated by these neurotransmitters.[28]

Cholinergic receptors found throughout the smooth muscle of the lower urinary tract are numerous in the body of the bladder but are distributed with subtle variations depending on the anatomic location.[8] At least five subtypes of muscarinic receptors exist (M1–M5). Types M1, M2, and M3 are found in the human bladder.[29] Types M2 and M3 may act synergistically, with M2 enhancing the effect of M3-mediated contractions. Types M2 and M4 together may play a role in the prejunctional inhibition of acetylcholine release.[30] The identification of subtypes make possible the development of specific agents that act not only to crudely block the postjunctional receptor but also may be able to modulate prejunctional release. The preganglionic cholinergic receptors in the sympathetic and parasympathetic ganglia in contrast are nicotinic, as are the cholinergic receptors in the rhabdosphincter. Pancuronium, an anesthetic, and botulinum toxin, both nicotinic blocking agents, may be used to paralyze the rhabdosphincter, but total incontinence does not result because the smooth muscle component of the sphincter and bladder neck remains unaffected.[31]

As noted earlier, α-adrenergic receptors are concentrated in the posterior urethra and trigone bladder neck and are more numerous in boys than in girls.[8] Stimulation of β-adrenergic receptors in the detrusor leads to relaxation of the smooth muscle. Adenylylcyclase mediates the effect, which leads to accumulation of cyclic adenosine monophosphate (cAMP). This observation led to speculation that β blockers could be used directly or that phosphodiesterase (PDE) inhibitors, which slow the breakdown of cAMP, could be adapted as drugs for treating bladder instability.[32] Hypogastric nerve stimulation and α-adrenergic agonists produce a rise in intraurethral pressure that is blocked by α antagonists.[33] This supports the role for α-agonist agents in treating some forms of incontinence and α blockers in relaxing the bladder neck and urethra.

Nitric oxide is a major inhibitory transmitter mediating relaxation of the urethral smooth muscle during micturition.[34] Parasympathetic postganglionic nerves release NO. Inhibitors of nitric oxide synthase block relaxation. NO is also involved with bladder afferent modulation. In situations of bladder irritation, NO inhibitors help decrease or eliminate bladder instability. NO-mediated smooth muscle relaxation results from increased intracellular accumulation of cyclic guanosine monophosphate (cGMP). PDE inactivates cGMP, as it does cAMP, and therefore cGMP may be a target for PDE inhibitors.

Neuropeptides such as substance P, neurokinin A, CGRP, VIP, pituitary adenylate cyclase-activating peptide (PACAP), and enkephalins play a role in modulating afferent sensory nerves. The actions of these purinergic transmitters have led to the recognition that the bladder urothelium may act as a large sensory organ, and the urothelium as an integral part of the afferent pathway in the same way the detrusor or rhabdosphincter act as distinct components.[35,36] Their actions help shape and form the type of afferent signal that enters the micturition reflex. This concept has led to novel approaches to treating conditions such as overactive bladder and interstitial cystitis. Rather than focusing on the efferent pathways, new treatments and therapies aim to dampen or alter the afferent signals from the urothelium.[35–37] For example, neuropeptides are active in capsaicin-sensitive C-fiber bladder afferents. These afferents are of particular interest because they are normally quiescent but become very sensitive when faced with major bladder inflammation or other noxious intravesical events.[38–40] Agents directed against vanilloid receptors can desensitize them. Capsaicin and its analogue resiniferatoxin have attracted recent interest because of their potent ability to affect the vanilloid receptors and desensitize these C fibers.

Peripheral innervation

The peripheral innervation of the lower urinary tract includes components of the sympathetic, parasympathetic, and somatic nervous systems. They connect to the target organs of the bladder, urethra, and urinary sphincter by the pelvic, hypogastric, and pudendal nerves. There are also modulating influences from the sympathetic ganglia chain and intramural ganglia.

The pelvic nerves are parasympathetic and originate from the sacral spinal cord. They excite the bladder and relax the urethra and urinary sphincter. The efferent nerves originate from the upper and middle sacral spinal cord segments S2–S4 and course outward as the pelvic nerves. Parasympathetic preganglionic neurons are located in the lateral part of the sacral intermediate gray matter in the region termed the sacral parasympathetic nucleus (SPN) and the axons exit the ventral roots to reach the peripheral ganglia. In humans, parasympathetic postganglionic neurons are located in the detrusor wall layer as well as in the pelvic plexus. Patients with cauda equina or pelvic plexus injury may be neurologically decentralized but are not completely denervated. Afferent and efferent neuronal interconnection at the level of the intramural ganglia is still possible.[39]

The hypogastric nerves are sympathetic and arise from the lumbar spinal cord. They excite the bladder base, urethra, and urinary sphincter. The efferent sympathetic nerves originate from spinal cord segments T11–L2. These nerves pass from the cord to the lumbar chain ganglia and then to the superior hypogastric plexus. Nerves from the plexus coalesce to form the right and left hypogastric nerve. Sympathetic pathways arise from the rostral lumbar spinal cord and provide noradrenergic excitatory and inhibitory stimuli to the bladder and urethra.[37] Activation of the sympathetic nerves causes relaxation of the bladder body and contraction of the bladder outlet and urethra, which facilitates storage of urine in the bladder.

The pelvic and hypogastric nerves meet to form the inferior hypogastric plexus. Nerves from this plexus then travel to the lower ureter, bladder, urethra, and urinary sphincter. The preganglionic nerves of the hypogastric plexi are closely associated with the ganglia close to or within these target organs. Intramural ganglia are present in the adventitia, muscle, and suburothelium of the bladder and urethra. Postganglionic nerves from the intramural ganglion then travel the final distance to directly innervate the smooth muscle lining these organs. This last group of ganglia and nerves comprise the so-called urogenital short neuron system.[5,31]

The pudendal nerves excite the rhabdosphincter. They are somatic and arise from the sacral cord segments S1–S4. The nucleus of these nerves resides in the lateral border of the ventral horn of the sacral cord and is called Onuf's nucleus (after Wladislaus

Onufrowicz, Swiss anatomist, 1836–1900): found in cats, dogs, and humans, it also innervates the bulbocavernosus and ischiocavernosus muscles. The rhabdosphincter initially behaves reflexively and later comes under voluntary control from the higher cortical centers with maturation. The sphincter motor neurons have dendrites that project laterally to the lateral funiculus, dorsally to the intermediate gray matter, and dorsomedially to the central canal. These connections with interneurons allow for a complex pattern and reflexes to be created.

The ability to sense fullness is important to both the storage and emptying of urine. Afferent activity that occurs during bladder contraction has an important reflex function and appears to reinforce the central drive that maintains detrusor contraction. All of these named nerves also carry afferent sensory information back to the spinal cord.[39] Afferent nerves travel along the hypogastric and pelvic nerves to link the urogenital smooth muscle to the hypogastric plexus and further upward to the lumbar and sacral dorsal root ganglia (DRG). Afferent sensory nerves also travel along the pudendal nerve to the sacral spinal cord. These nerves conduct information from the bladder suburothelium and muscle, the sense of fullness, urgency, and pain. The primary afferent nuclei of the pelvic and pudendal nerves are contained in the sacral DRG, whereas the afferent innervation of the hypogastric nerves come from the rostral lumbar DRG. The central axons of these DRG neurons carry the sensory information to the second-order neurons within the spinal cord.[39,41] Visceral afferent fibers of the pelvic nerve and pudendal nerve enter the cord and move within the portion of the dorsal cord called Lissauer's tract[41,42] (after Heinrich Lissauer, German neurologist, 1861–1891). This is a longitudinal bundle of thin, unmyelinated, and poorly myelinated fibers capping the apex of the posterior horn of the spinal gray matter composed of posterior root fibers and short association fibers that interconnect neighboring segments of the posterior horn. Pelvic nerve afferents monitor bladder volume and degree of contraction and are carried on both myelinated and unmyelinated axons. The myelinated axons are Aδ fibers and the unmyelinated axons are C fibers. Neuropathic conditions and possibly inflammatory conditions can lead to recruitment of C fibers which can form new functional afferent pathways which are believed to cause urge incontinence and possibly increased bladder pain. Aδ fibers carry information from smooth muscle and sense wall tension: when inflamed, there is increased discharge at a lower threshold pressure. The C fibers carry stretch and bladder fullness sensation from urothelium and smooth muscle and act as nociceptors for overdistention. Usually quiet, when irritated C fibers discharge at lower threshold, become more sensitive, and unmask new afferent pathways during inflammation. This has formed the basis for several lines of treatment that act against the sensory end (e.g. capsaicin, resiniferatoxin). Current theory holds that several different types of afferents are present: stretch, volume, tension, and silent (nociceptors). Irritation intravesically can lower the pressure threshold. Most C fibers are insensitive to normal distention but can become mechanosensitive and active when irritated or inflamed.

Reflex pathways

Several reflex pathways help mediate urinary storage and emptying. The central pathways that control the lower urinary tract function are organized as simple on–off switching circuits. Some reflexes promote urine storage and others facilitate voiding. These reflexes can become interlinked to create complex feedback mechanisms. The guarding reflex, which links bladder distention to external sphincter activity during filling, activates sphincter afferents that inhibit the parasympathetic excitatory inputs to the bladder; this explains how bladder to rhabdosphincter activity could lead to decreased bladder activity during storage. The disruption or discoordination of these interactions may be the underlying cause in forms of neurogenic bladder dysfunction (Figures 52.2 and 52.3).

There are four types of pathways in the spinal cord that link together to form the reflex pathways:

1 Spinal efferent nerves, which include autonomic preganglionic neurons and somatic motor neurons.
2 Spinal interneurons, which are located between the dorsal and ventral horns.
3 Primary afferent neurons.
4 Central neurons from the brain and brainstem, which modulate spinal reflexes.[40]

These pathways were elucidated using intracellular labeling, pseudorabies virus tracing, and measurement of gene product expression.[43]

Urine storage, guarding, and sphincter-to-bladder reflex

During the storage of urine, distention of the bladder stimulates afferent nerves. These in turn stimulate

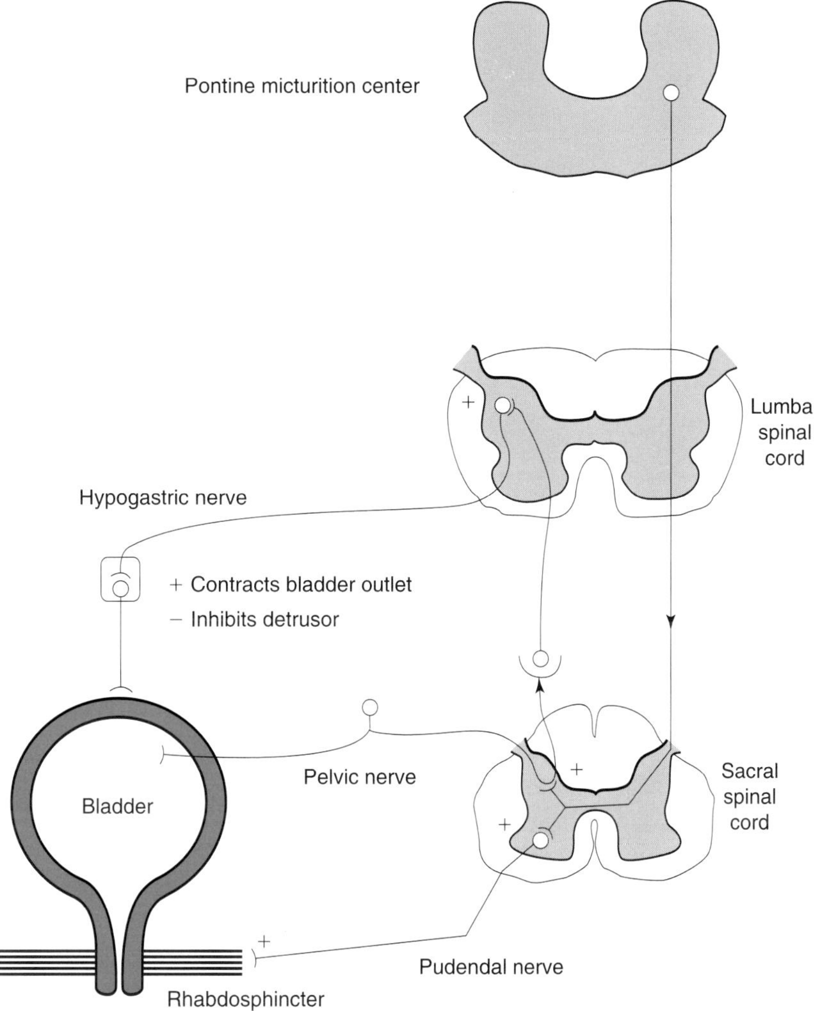

Figure 52.2 During storage, distention of the bladder causes low-level bladder afferent activity, which in turn activates the sympathetic outflow to the bladder and urethra, and increases pudendal nerve activity to the rhabdosphincter. These effects constitute the guarding reflex. Sympathetic activity also inhibits detrusor activity and transmission in the bladder ganglia.

sympathetic excitatory outflow to the bladder trigone and urethra, and pudendal outflow to the rhabdosphincter. These responses together are collectively known as the guarding reflex. Sympathetic stimulation also inhibits detrusor muscle and bladder ganglia transmission. The guarding reflex in turn diminishes during the start of micturition.[39,44] This sequence of reflex activity is demonstrable clinically. During bladder distention with urodynamic measurement, an involuntary increase in the activity of the rhabdosphincter is measurable with either an intraluminal pressure transducer placed at the highest-pressure zone of urethral pressure or by a perineal electromyogram (EMG) (Figure 52.4). The EMG of the urinary sphincter will show increased activity, reflecting the increase in the efferent firing in the pudendal nerve and an increase in outlet resistance that contributes to the maintenance of continence. The external urethral sphincter activity reaches a peak just before the onset of micturition. At low bladder volume, the reflex is involuntary, but as the bladder volume reaches the sensory threshold of fullness, the external urethral sphincter activity increases and becomes a conscious and voluntary phenomenon. Whereas bladder afferent stimulation is the primary activation of pudendal motor neuron activity, urethral and perineal afferents may contribute.[44,45] This part of the guarding reflex links proprioceptive afferents from the pelvic floor to induce closure of the urethral outlet.

How is this clinically important? It was originally theorized that the reflex increase might be a mechanism that protects against stress incontinence.[46] This

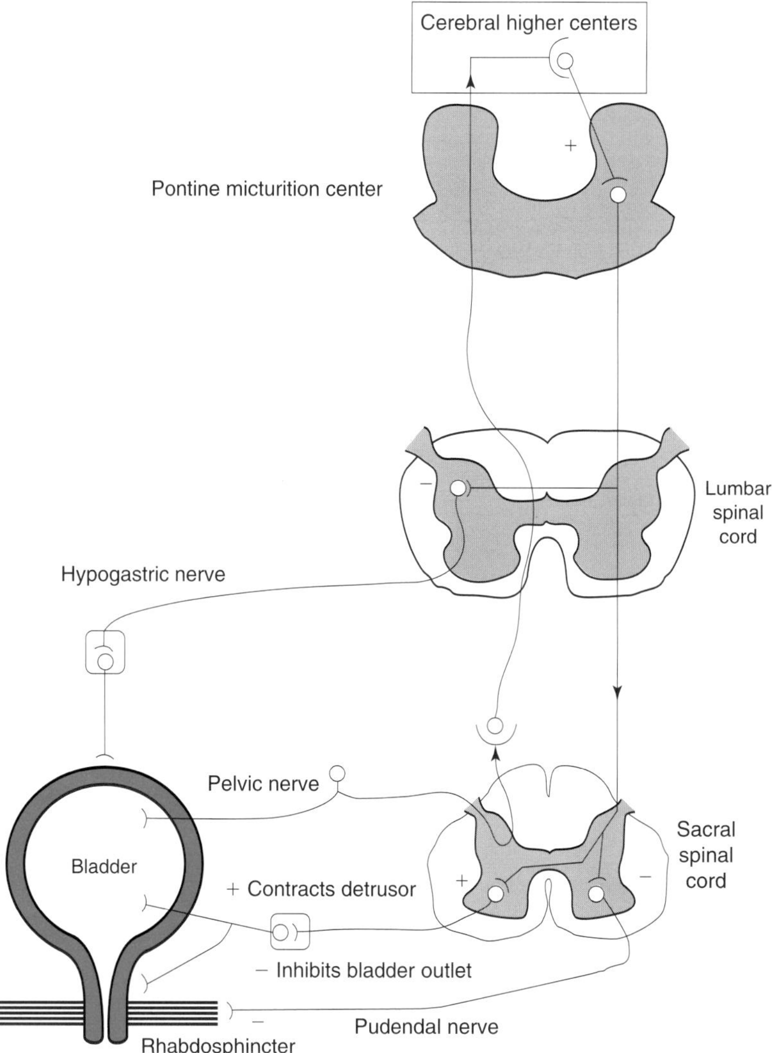

Figure 52.3 At the initiation of voiding, bladder afferent activity increases, which activates the pontine micturition center. This inhibits the spinal guarding reflexes, which are conducted via the pudendal nerve. It also stimulates the parasympathetic outflow to the bladder and bladder neck. Ascending afferents complete the reflex loop by bringing feedback input to the cerebral cortex and higher centers.

mechanism explains how certain avoidance maneuvers, such as vigorously crossing the legs repeatedly and 'squirming' (doing the 'potty dance') or tucking the heel into the perineum (Vincent's curtsy), are used by children who are infrequent voiders to reduce feelings of urgency, thereby allowing them to continue to hold urine for prolonged periods. The fact that stimulation of the somatic afferent pathways of the pudendal nerve to the caudal lumbosacral spinal cord can inhibit voiding further supports this observation. Afferent input can come from a variety of sites, such as the penis, vagina, rectum, perineum, urethral sphincter, and anal sphincter. This pathway has been termed the sphincter-to-bladder reflex pathway. Studies in cats suggest that this is mediated by suppression of the interneuronal pathways in the sacral spinal cord and by direct inhibition of the parasympathetic preganglionic neurons.[47] The sacrolumbar intersegmental spinal reflex pathway, which is triggered by vesical afferent activity in the pelvic nerves, initiates sympathetic firing at least in part. The vesicosympathetic reflex represents a negative feedback mechanism whereby an increase in bladder pressure triggers an increase in inhibitory input to the bladder, thus allowing the bladder to accommodate larger volumes of urine. The reflex pathway is inhibited during voiding, and this inhibition is in turn abolished by transection of the spinal cord at the thoracic level, which suggests that it originates at a supraspinal site, probably at the pontine micturition center.

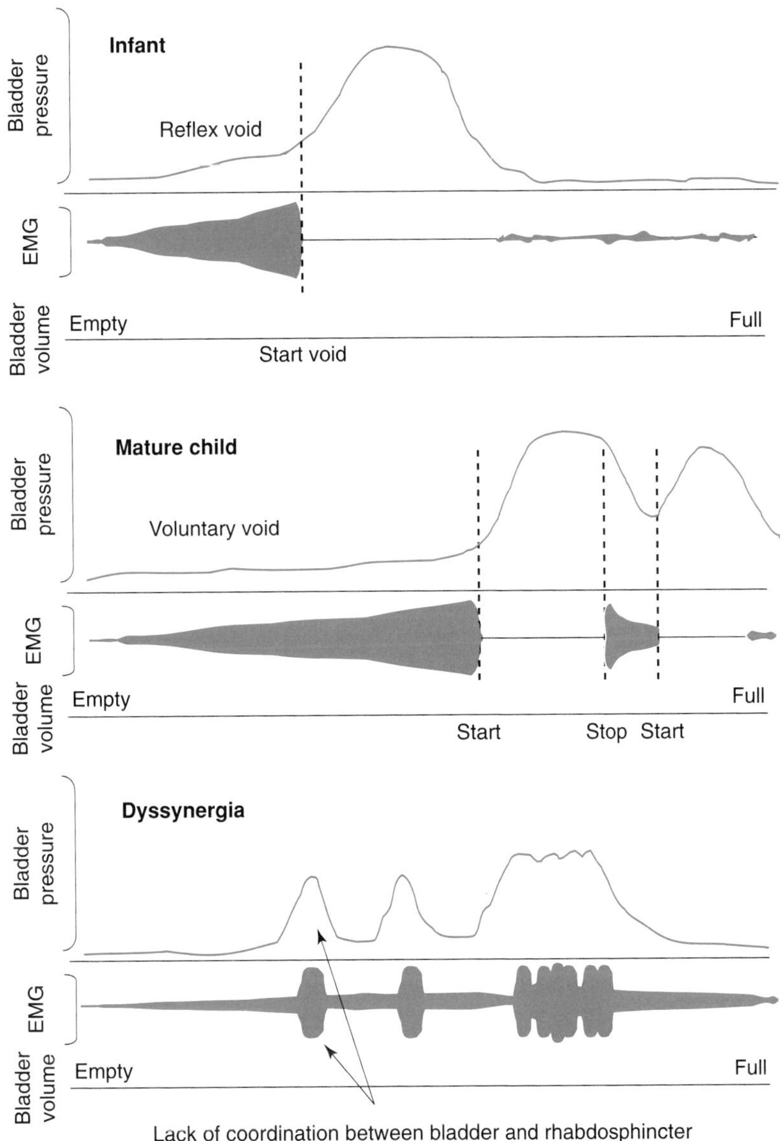

Figure 52.4 The differences between infantile, mature child, and dyssynergic voiding, where there is a loss of coordination between the bladder and sphincter. The latter condition is often seen as a result of injury or disease to the central nervous system. Note that in both the infantile and mature child there is coordination between bladder and the sphincter, so that the sphincter relaxes before the onset of bladder contraction; the EMG becomes quiet. In the mature child and adult there also exists the ability to interrupt voiding volitionally. When this occurs, note that the sphincter activity precedes the cessation of bladder contractions and, when voiding is restarted, relaxation of the sphincter occurs before voiding is resumed. In contrast, in dyssynergia, the detrusor and sphincter contract out of sequence, thereby working against each other.

Voiding or micturition reflex

The switch from storage to voiding phase can occur voluntarily or reflexively. Infants and patients with neuropathic bladder demonstrate the former, when the volume of urine exceeds the threshold volume beyond which micturition occurs (see Figure 52.3 and 52.4). At that point, increased afferent firing from the tension receptors in the bladder leads to a shift in the efferent activity. Sympathetic and somatic pathways are inhibited; sacral parasympathetic activity increases. There is an initial relaxation of the urethral sphincter, followed within a few seconds by the contraction of the bladder, an increase in bladder pressure, and a flow of urine. Relaxation of the urethral smooth muscle during micturition is mediated by a parasympathetic stimulation to the urethra that triggers the release of NO, which acts as an inhibitory transmitter, and by removal of excitatory inputs to the urethra. The parasympathetic outflow to the detrusor and urethra has a more complicated central organization that involves spinal and spinobulbospinal pathways passing through the pontine micturition center (PMC). When this coordination is disrupted by injury or disease, simultaneous contraction of the bladder and rhabdosphincter can occur, leading clinically to DSD (see Figure 52.4).[48]

Voiding is mediated by activation of the sacral parasympathetic efferent pathway to the bladder and the urethra, along with reciprocal inhibition of the somatic pathway to the urinary sphincter. Cat studies reveal that the neurons in the brainstem have an essential role in the control of the parasympathetic component of voiding. Removal of the areas of the brain above the pons usually facilitates voiding by removing inhibitory inputs from higher centers. Transection at any point below abolishes micturition. The region thereby isolated is located in the pontine region and is termed the pontine micturition center. Physiologic and anatomic experiments show that the PMC is the key switch in the voiding pathway. Chemical and electrical stimulation of the PMC in cats and dogs causes suppression of the urethral sphincter EMG activity, firing of the sacral preganglionic neurons, bladder contractions, and release of urine. These regions have a regulatory role, as shown by injections of inhibitory transmitter, GABA, into the PMC of cats, which can increase the volume threshold for inducing micturition and, in high-enough doses, completely block reflex voiding. In contrast, administration of a GABA inhibitor, such as bicuculline, can lower micturition volume threshold. Injuries above the lumbosacral area but beneath the PMC lead initially to an areflexic bladder and complete retention (similar to the spinal shock seen in human spinal cord injury patients) and later with automatic micturition but with bladder hyperactivity and DSD.[39,49]

The voiding reflex analogy to the guarding reflex is the urethra-to-bladder reflex. Barrington first noted that flow of urine or mechanical stimulation of the urethra with a catheter would excite afferent nerves, which can lead to bladder contractions in anesthetized cats.[50,51] It was thought that the urethral-to-bladder reflex helps to promote emptying. Two pathways have been identified: one pathway is activated by somatic afferents in the pudendal nerve and needs facilitation from the PMC; the other pathway uses afferents in the pelvic nerves to facilitate other spinal reflex mechanisms. Desensitizing the urethral afferents by capsaicin decreases this reflex. This pathway may explain why stress and urge incontinence can occur together. The leakage of urine into the urethra triggers the reflex, leading to urgency. Similarly, correction of stress incontinence seems to paradoxically improve detrusor instability.[43,52]

Spinal and supraspinal pathways

In the spinal cord, afferent pathways terminate and connect with second-order interneurons that relay information to the brain and to other regions of the spinal cord, including the preganglionic and motor nuclei at other levels. These are polysynaptic processes and interlink the various bladder, urethral, and sphincter reflexes. These interneuronal mechanisms play an important role in modulating lower urinary tract function.[53] The lower tract interneurons also receive afferent inputs from the bladder. Glutamic acid is the excitatory transmitter of these pathways.[52] About 15% of interneurons located medial to the sacral parasympathetic nuclei have inhibitory connections to the parasympathetic preganglionic nuclei (PGN). These inhibitory neurons use GABA and glycine.[52] Reflex pathways, which control the external sphincter muscles, also use glutamic excitatory and GABA or glycine inhibitory interneurons. Afferents from the cutaneous and striated muscle sources modulate the micturition reflex at the spinal cord level. Stimulation of afferent fibers inhibits the firing of sacral interneurons evoked by bladder distention that occurs as a result of presynaptic inhibition of primary afferents or due to direct postsynaptic inhibition of second-order neurons. Direct postsynaptic inhibition of bladder PGN occurs by somatic afferent stimulation in the pudendal nerves. Suppression of bladder hyperactivity in patients with sacral root stimulation reflects in part activation of the afferent limb of these inhibitory reflexes. Urologists have used this mechanism to artificially modulate bladder behavior by sacral nerve stimulation.[54]

Control of the bladder function starts in the higher cortical centers through the brainstem pons regions in the PMC. These impulses are mediated through the spinal cord nuclei to the efferent and afferent peripheral pathways. The micturition reflex is normally controlled and mediated by the pathway linking the brain with the reflexes described above. This pathway is termed the spinobulbospinal reflex pathway. Animal brain lesion studies show that the neurons in the brainstem at the level of the inferior colliculus have an essential role in the control of the parasympathetic component of micturition.[39] Decerebration above the colliculus facilitates micturition by eliminating inhibitory inputs from more cephalad centers. Transections below the colliculi abolish micturition. The essential control center thus isolated was found in the dorsal pontine tegmentum. First described in 1921, this center is commonly referred to as the pontine micturition center or medial location.[55] The medial and lateral region of the pons is responsible for the micturition reflex. The medial region controls detrusor contraction via the reticulospinal tracts, which synapse with the preganglionic parasympathetic neurons in the sacral micturition center. Electrical stimulation of the medial region causes relaxation and opening of the urethral sphincter, followed within milliseconds by a contraction of the detrusor muscles.[56] The lateral regions of the PMC are connected via the corticospinal tracts to Onuf's nucleus. Electrical stimulation of this area leads to contraction of the rhabdosphincter. Voluntary control is via a link with the frontal cortex.[57,58] Neurons from the PMC project to the periaqueductal gray matter, thalamic nuclei, and limbic system. Neurons from the PMC communicate with supraspinal neuronal clusters that coordinate micturition with other functions. The location is of note because of two interesting neural topographic findings. First, the facial nerve nucleus is very near the PMC. Patients with Ochoa's syndrome (urofacial syndrome) exhibit a combination of voiding dysfunction and a characteristic inversion of facial expression. Researchers have failed to show an obvious structural lesion on imaging studies, but speculation suggests that there could be subtle synaptic or interneuron abnormalities.[59] Secondly, the nucleus locus ceruleus within the brainstem is a close neighbor of the PMC. The locus ceruleus in animals is activated by colonic stimulation. The PMC has been shown to affect the afferent signals from the pelvic viscera that reach the locus ceruleus. This has led to speculation that there may be bilateral interaction. Clinically, constipation and bowel dysfunction are associated with bladder dysfunction. A local phenomenon such as rectal distention impinging on the trigone or the pelvic nerves may be responsible. However, this concept fails to explain why women seem to be equally affected yet have the uterus and vagina 'shielding' the bladder from the rectum. Perhaps the problem is at the central level and results from interaction between the PMC and the locus ceruleus.[60,61]

The PMC has important direct synaptic inputs to the sacral PGN and to the GABAnergic neurons. The former carry excitatory outflow to the detrusor, whereas the latter act as an inhibitor on rhabdosphincter motor neurons. These reciprocal connections results in promoting bladder urethral sphincter synergy. Studies in rats indicate that inotropic glutamate receptor antagonists block activation of bladder PGN from the PMC, suggesting that neurons in the PMC utilize glutamate as a neurotransmitter.[48,62–64]

Central cerebral pathways

Voluntary control of voiding is dependent on the connections between the frontal cortex and the septal/preoptic region of the hypothalamus as well as connections between the paracentral lobule and the brainstem.[39] Lesions to those areas of cortex appear to directly increase bladder activity by removing cortical inhibitory control. Brain imaging by positron emission tomography (PET) has implicated the frontal cortex and anterior cingulated gyrus in the control of micturition and that it is predominantly a right-sided function.[65,66] Since sacral parasympathetic pathways to the bladder form a predominantly positive feedback system, further inhibitory modulation is required to store urine and prevent early voiding. Higher centers such as the cerebral cortex, cerebellum, basal ganglia, thalamus, and hypothalamus thus play an inhibitory role, modulating the activity of the PMC.[67]

Studies in humans indicate that voluntary control of micturition is dependent on connections between the frontal cortex and septal preoptic region of the hypothalamus, and the paracentral lobule, brainstem, and spinal cord. Lesions in these areas as a result of trauma, tumors, or cerebrovascular disease appear to indirectly increase bladder activity by removing cortical inhibitory control. In cats, removal of the cortex lowers the functional bladder capacity. If the rest of the neuraxis is intact, removal of the cerebrum lowers the inhibitory input from the cortex. The hypothalamus plays a role in activating the sacral parasympathetic excitatory pathways, thereby inducing bladder contraction and voiding. It is thought to act through direct inputs to the PMC and sacral micturition center or indirectly. This is not a unidirectional process. The hypothalamus receives modulating afferent inputs from the bladder. The gene *c-fos* has been identified as a marker for subsets of second-order neurons. Expression of the *c-fos* gene is increased in these neurons.[68,69]

Plasticity, maturation, and re-emergence

The neonatal bladder is not an effective storage organ. At birth, there is little cerebral input and the bladder reflexively empties. In modern urodynamic parlance, a newborn through infancy and early toddler years has bladder instability. This is also seen in neonatal animals, whose bladders show early spontaneous repetitive contractions. These early pathways become incorporated into more mature pathways by active inhibition from increasing cerebral maturation. Inhibition rather than cessation of these infantile reflexes is the important observation. Much as a layer of inhibition from the cerebrum modulates the spinal reflexes, a layer of inhibitory control is overlaid atop the neonatal reflexes. In newborn kittens and rats, a primitive reflex, the exteroceptive perineal-to-bladder reflex, is the principal voiding reflex until the mature spinobulbar or PMC-based reflex begins functioning at several weeks of life.[70] During the subsequent weeks, the adult-type voiding mediated by the micturition center and spinobulbospinal pathway becomes active and the perineal–bladder reflex becomes progressively weaker and ultimately vanishes. Studies using pseudorabies virus tracing, cellular labeling, and CNS transection preparations in animals demonstrate that there is prominent reorganization of synaptic connections in the bladder reflex pathways.[71] At this time, the bulbospinal pathways that connect to the PMC are fewer and weaker. But as the neonate matures, there is pruning of the interneu-

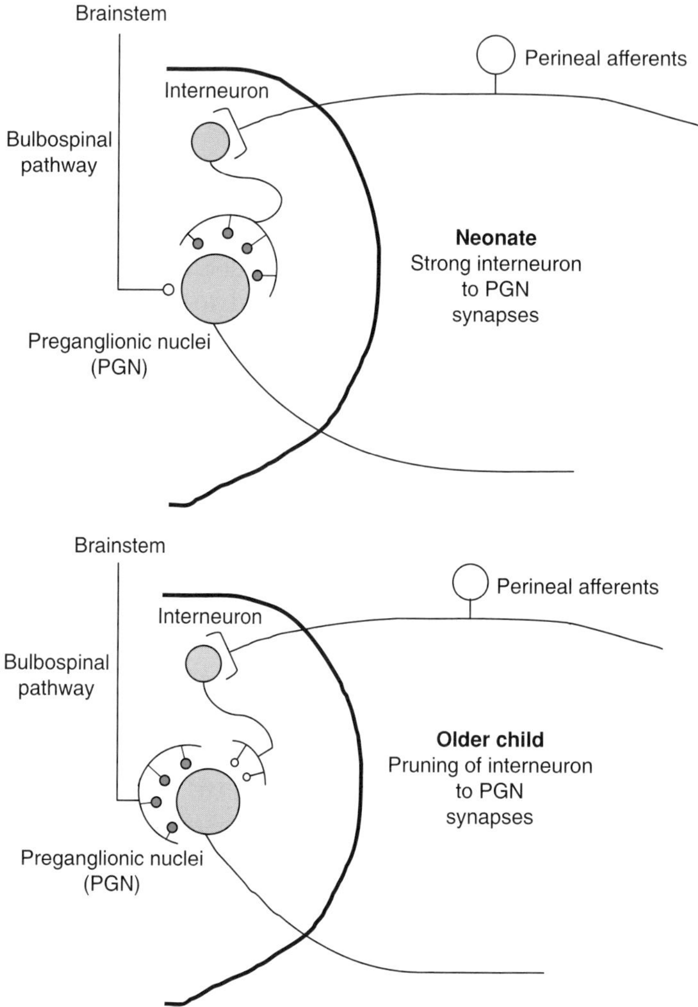

Figure 52.5 Schematic diagram shows possible anatomic changes at the synapses of the preganglionic nuclei in the sacral spinal cord of neonatal mammals (rats and kittens) and presumably humans as well, that explain the changes which occur during the first few weeks of life. Early in life, the interneurons bring greater active input (●) from the perineal afferents; but with maturation, these connections become pruned and become down-regulated (○). Input from the bulbospinal pathways then predominates.

ron to preganglionic synapses from the afferents and increased synapses from the bulbospinal pathways[71,72] (Figure 52.5).

Interestingly, the higher pathways seem to be present and organized but inactive at birth. In animal studies, decerebration unmasks reflex bladder activity that responds to bladder distention, and is mediated by a supraspinal pathway. This indicates that supraspinal bladder-to-bladder reflexes are organized early after birth but are suppressed by inhibitory mechanisms within the brain. Postnatal development is associated with a marked reorganization of the circuitry of the CNS affecting micturition.

The mechanism underlying the developmental suppression of the perineal-to-bladder reflex and the later re-emergence after spinal cord injury appears to be similar to the maturation process. Down-regulation occurs in the interneuronal to preganglionic neuron excitatory synapses, possibly by synapse elimination as a result of competition for synaptic space between the boutons of the interneurons and the descending axons. Injury that causes degeneration of the descending axons, such as transection of the spinal cord, blocks this reorganization and maintains the primitive neonatal reflex. A similar degeneration of the descending axons in mature animals could stimulate axonal sprouting in interneuronal pathways and cause re-emergence of the neonatal perineal-to-bladder reflex. Although the exact details are not known, it is certain that remodeling of the interneuron to preganglionic synapses in the sacral parasympathetic nuclei has a prominent role. This synaptic plasticity and rearrangement leads to the down-regulation of primitive spinal reflexes and the appearance of mature supraspinal control of voiding.[71]

Plasticity is therefore not a one-way process. Where inhibitory controls can be overlaid, they can also be removed. Disease processes can decrease or eliminate inhibitory influences, thereby unmasking the primitive neonatal reflexes. The urologic sequelae of injury and disease, therefore, may not be a 'new' change as much as an old reflex pathway that has re-emerged. The classic example is the chilled water bladder test. Infants will develop involuntary bladder contractions when saline cooled to 4°C is instilled rapidly into the bladder. Mature children and adults can sense the cold but are able to maintain control. Patients with neuropathic bladders are not able to do so. The cold receptors are mediated by C fibers, and the chilled fluid response reflects unmasking of the neuropathology. It is positive until about age 4.[73,74] Further studies have shown that unmasking of reflexes can lead to structural changes that are not limited to the CNS and can occur in the periphery as well. In chronic spinal cord transected cats, the afferent limb of the micturition reflex consists primarily of C-fiber afferents, whereas in intact cats the pathways are myelinated Aδ afferents.[75]

In the human fetus before maturation of the nervous system, urine is presumably eliminated by non-neural mechanisms. Later, primitive reflex pathways organized in the spinal cord regulate voiding. As the CNS matures, this reflex voiding is eventually brought under voluntary control that originates in the higher centers of the brain. Like the animal models, a hierarchical control system overlays the more primitive components that are intrinsic to the target organs and spinal cord as well as more complex components of the cerebral cortex. In adults, injuries and diseases of the CNS can lead to the re-emergence of primitive functions that were suppressed during maturation.[76]

How do these observations correlate with the development of micturition control in humans? It appears that the process in humans does not occur suddenly. The process of maturation is not a simple switch from a primitive voiding reflex to the mature model, but rather a gradual transition. Several observations support this viewpoint. First, small infants wake up to void when asleep.[77] By age 6 months, 90% of infants show signs of waking or arousal with voiding.[78] Another observation is that if an infant is disturbed while voiding, micturition halts or becomes interrupted. Longitudinal studies show increasing percentages of infants who arouse when voiding at night. This correlates with the degree of activation of cortical areas of the voiding reflex and the degree of maturation.[77,78] The infant may also have variable bladder volumes, which puts doubt that threshold volume alone triggers voiding.[77–79] Interrupted voiding has been noted. This is defined as being two voids within 10 minutes: seen in two-thirds of preterm and only one-third of full-term infants, it decreases over the first year and is not seen at all in the fully toilet-trained child. This may be due to a form of DSD. Studies suggest that this dyssynergia may be a normal part of development.[80,81] There seem to be more interrupted voids in patients with posterior urethral valves (PUV) and high-grade vesicoureteral reflux (VUR). Whether there is a more severe form of dyssynergia than the normal physiologic form or an increase in hyperactivity of the neonatal detrusor is unclear. It is also unknown if this observation has any relationship to bladder problems that can be associated with these conditions later in life (e.g. detrusor instability with VUR, myogenic detrusor failure with PUV).[81,82] Increasing bladder capacity with age has been observed, and leads to speculation that the stimulus for increasing bladder capacity is when the child begins to hold more urine at night, contrary to the conventional notion that daytime continence is a prerequisite for night-time dryness.[79,80] Finally, during the first few months, increased hyperactivity on cystometry may be present, and may be a response to filling that is faster than normal and/or stimulus by the catheter. This fades as the neonate matures.[81] Increased reactivity of the detrusor may be responsible also for high voiding pressures. Voiding pressures of up to 100 cm H_2O have been measured in infants, which decreases by age 3 years, down to 70 cm H_2O, and continue to drop thereafter.[83]

These observations together suggest that the first few years of life mark an important transition period for infants and toddlers as they begin to shift over from a more primitive to a more mature micturition process. This transition seems to progress through a period where neither reflex pathway is clearly preeminent; hence, the higher voiding pressure, hyperactive detrusor, and the period of physiologically normal DSD. Therefore, the transition in infants is not as abrupt and rapid as seen in animals, which accomplish this change over weeks rather than months. These findings, and the earlier observation of the plastic nature of the micturition pathways and the re-emergence of primitive pathways, suggest that perhaps voiding dysfunction seen in childhood may have its roots in an incomplete transition to a more mature micturition pathway or the re-emergence of the more primitive pathway.

References

1. Helin P, Sihvonen T, Hanninen O. Timing of the triggering action of shooting in relation to the heart cycle. Br J Sports Med 1987; 21:33–6.
2. Konttinen N, Lyytinen H, Konttinen R. Brain slow potentials reflecting successful shooting performance. Res Q Exerc Sport 1995; 66:64–72.
3. Hatfield BD, Landers DM, Ray WJ. Cardiovascular–CNS interactions during a self-paced, intentional attentive state: elite marksmanship performance. Psychophysiology 1987; 24:542–9.
4. Elbadawi A. Pathology and pathophysiology of detrusor in incontinence. Urol Clin North Am 1995; 22:499–512.
5. Elbadawi A. Functional pathology of urinary bladder muscularis: the new frontier in diagnostic uropathology. Semin Diagn Pathol 1993; 10:314–54.
6. Levin RM, Longhurst PA, Monson FC, Kato K, Wein A. Effect of bladder outlet obstruction on the morphology, physiology, and pharmacology of the bladder. Prostate 1990; S3:9–26.
7. Saito M, Kondo A, Kato T, Levin RM. Response of isolated human neurogenic detrusor smooth muscle to intramural nerve stimulation. Br J Urol 1993; 72:723–7.
8. Ek A, Alm P, Andersson KE, Persson CG. Adrenergic and cholinergic nerves to the human urethra and urinary bladder. A histochemical study. Acta Physiol Scand 1977; 99:345–52.
9. Gosling JA, Dixon JS, Lendon RG. The autonomic innervation of the human male and female bladder neck and proximal urethra. J Urol 1977; 118:302–5.
10. Benson G, McConnell JA, Wood JG. Adrenergic innervation of the human bladder body. J Urol 1979; 122:189–91.
11. Mitolo-Chieppa D, Schonauer S, Grasso G, Cicinelli E, Carratu MR. Ontogenesis of autonomic receptors in detrusor muscle and bladder sphincter in human fetus. Urology 1983; 221:599–603.
12. Elbadawi A. Microstructural basis of detrusor contractility: the MIN approach to its understanding and study. Neurourol Urodyn 1991; 10:77–85.
13. DeLancey JO. Correlative study of paraurethral anatomy. Obstet Gynecol 1986; 68:91–7.
14. DeLancey JO. Pubovesical ligament: a separate structure from the urethra supports ('pubo-urethral ligaments'). Neurourol Urodyn 1989; 8:53–61.
15. Gosling JA, Dixon JS, Critchley HOD, Thompson SA. A comparative study of the human external sphincter and periurethral levator ani muscles. Br J Urol 1981; 53:35–41.
16. Elbadawi A, Schenck EA. A new theory of the innervation of the bladder musculature. Innervation of the vesicourethral junction and external sphincter. J Urol 1974; 111 (Pt 4):613–15.
17. Crowe R, Burnstock G, Light JK. Adrenergic innervation of the striated muscle of the intrinsic external urethral sphincter from patients with lower motor spinal cord lesion. J Urol 1989; 141:47–9.
18. Brading AF. A myogenic basis for the overactive bladder. Urology 1997; 50(6A Suppl):57–67, discussion 68–73.
19. de Groat WC. A neurologic basis for the overactive bladder. Urology 1997; 50(6A Suppl):36–52, discussion 53–6.
20. Kim KM, Kogan BA, Massad CA, Huang Yi-C. Collagen and elastin in the normal fetal bladder. J Urol 1991; 146:524–7.
21. Ewalt DH, Howard PS, Blyth B et al. Is lamina propria matrix responsible for normal bladder compliance? J Urol 1992; 148:544–9.
22. Milner P, Crowe R, Burnstock G, Light JK. Neuropeptide Y- and vasoactive intestinal polypeptide-containing nerves in the intrinsic external urethral sphincter in the areflexic bladder compared to detrusor-sphincter dyssynergia in patients with spinal cord injury. J Urol 1987; 135:888–92.
23. Elbadawi A. Functional anatomy of the organs of micturition. Urol Clin North Am 1996; 23:177–210.
24. de Groat WC. Neuropeptides in pelvic afferent pathways. Experientia 1987; 43:801–12.

25. Keast JR, de Groat WC. Segmental distribution and peptide content of primary afferent neurons innervating the urogenital organs and colon of male rats. J Comp Neurol 1992; 319:615–23.
26. Gu J, Restorick JM, Blank MA et al. Vasoactive intestinal polypeptide in the normal and unstable bladder. Br J Urol 1983; 55:645–7.
27. Crowe R, Burnstock G, Light JK. Spinal cord lesions at different levels affect either the adrenergic or vasoactive intestinal polypeptide-immunoreactive nerves in the human urethra. J Urol 1988; 140:1412–14.
28. Saito M, Kondo A, Kato T, Hasegaw S, Miyake K. Response of the human neurogenic bladder to KCl, carbachol, ATP, and $CaCl_2$. Br J Urol 1993; 72:298–302.
29. Kondo S, Morita T, Tashima Y. Muscarinic cholinergic receptor subtypes in human detrusor muscle studied by labeled and nonlabeled pirenzepine, AFDX-116 and 4DAMP. Urol Int 1995; 54:150–3.
30. Braverman AS, Kohn IJ, Luthin GR, Ruggieri MR. Prejunctional M1 facilitory and M2 inhibitory muscarinic receptors mediate rat bladder contractility. Am J Physiol 1998; 274(2 Pt 2):R517–23.
31. Crowe R, Burnstock G, Light JK. Intramural ganglia in the human urethra. J Urol 1988; 140:183–7.
32. Longhurst PA, Briscoe JA, Rosenberg DJ, Leggett RE. The role of cyclic nucleotides in guinea-pig bladder contractility. Br J Pharmacol 1997; 121:1665–72.
33. Yalla SB, Rossier AB, Fam BA et al. Functional contribution of autonomic innervation to urethral striated sphincter: studies with parasympathomimetic, parasympatholytic and alpha-adrenergic blocking agents in spinal cord injury and control male subjects. J Urol 1977; 117:494–9.
34. Bennett BC, Kruse MN, Roppolo JR et al. Neural control of urethral outlet activity in vivo: role of nitric oxide. J Urol 1995; 153:2004–9.
35. Birder LA. Involvement of the urinary bladder urothelium in signaling in the lower urinary tract. Proc West Pharmacol Soc 2001; 44:85–6.
36. Birder LA, Nealen ML, Kiss S et al. Beta-adrenoceptor agonists stimulate endothelial nitric oxide synthase in rat urinary bladder urothelial cells. J Neurosci 2002; 22:8063–70.
37. Birder LA, Apodaca G, De Groat WC, Kanai AJ. Adrenergic- and capsaicin-evoked nitric oxide release from urothelium and afferent nerves in urinary bladder. Am J Physiol 1998; 275(2 Pt 2):F226–9.
38. Chancellor MB, de Groat WC. Intravesical capsaicin and resiniferatoxin therapy: spicing up the ways to treat the overactive bladder. J Urol 1999; 162:3–11.
39. de Groat WC, Booth AM. Synaptic transmission in pelvic ganglia. In: Maggi CA, ed. The Autonomic Nervous System, Vol 3, Nervous Control of the Urogenital System. London: Harwood Academic, 1993: 291–347.
40. Andersson KE, Wein AJ. Pharmacology of the lower urinary tract: basis for current and future treatments of urinary incontinence. Pharmacol Rev 2004; 56:581–631.
41. Morgan C, Nadelhaft I, de Groat WC. The distribution of visceral primary afferents from the pelvic nerve to Lissauer's tract and the spinal gray matter and its relationship to the sacral parasympathetic nucleus. J Comp Neurol 1981; 201:415–40.
42. Thor KB, Morgan C, Nadelhaft I, Houston M, De Groat WC. Organization of afferent and efferent pathways in the pudendal nerve of the female cat. J Comp Neurol 1989; 288:263–79.
43. de Groat WC. Central nervous system control of micturition. In: O'Donnell PD, ed. Urinary Incontinence. Mosby: St Louis, 1997: 33–47.
44. Park JM, Bloom DA, McGuire EJ. The guarding reflex revisited. Br J Urol 1997; 80:940–5.
45. Fedirchuk B, Hochman S, Shefchyk SJ. An intracellular study of perineal and hindlimb afferent inputs onto sphincter motorneurons in the decerebrate cat. Exp Brain Res 1992; 89:511–16.
46. Garry RC, Roberts TDM, Todd JK. Reflexes involving the external urethral sphincter in the cat. J Physiol 1959; 149:653–65.
47. de Groat WC, Booth AM, Milne RJ, Roppolo JR. Parasympathetic preganglionic neurons in the sacral spinal cord. J Auton Nerv Sys 1982; 5:23–43.
48. Blaivas JG. The neurophysiology of micturition: a clinical study of 550 patients. J Urol 1982; 127:958–63.
49. Yoshimura N, de Groat WC. Neural control of the lower urinary tract. Int J Urol 1997; 4:111–25.
50. Barrington FJF. The component reflexes of micturition in the cat: I and II. Brain 1931; 54:177–88.
51. Barrington FJF. The component reflexes of micturition in the cat: III. Brain 1941; 64:239–43.
52. Chancellor MB, Yoshimura N. Physiology and pharmacology of the bladder and urethra. In: Walsh PC, Retik AB, Vaughan ED Jr, Wein AJ, eds. Campbell's Urology, 8th edn. Philadelphia: WB Saunders, 2002: 831–86.
53. Araki I, de Groat WC. Developmental synaptic depression underlying reorganization of visceral reflex pathways in the spinal cord. J Neurosci 1997; 17:8402–7.
54. Chartier-Kastler EJ, Ruud Bosch JL, Perrigot M et al. Long-term results of sacral nerve stimulation (S3) for the treatment of neurogenic refractory urge incontinence related to detrusor hyperreflexia. J Urol 2000; 164:1476–80.
55. Tang PC. Levels of the brainstem and diencephalons controlling the micturition reflex. J Neurophysiol 1955; 18:583–95.
56. Fletcher TF, Bradley WE. Neuroanatomy of the bladder-urethra. J Urol 1978; 119:153–60.
57. Andrew J, Nathan PW, Spanos NC. Disturbances of micturition and defaecation due to aneurysms of anterior communicating or anterior cerebral arteries. J Neurosurg 1966; 24:1–10.
58. Andrew J, Nathan PW. Lesions of the frontal lobes and disturbances of micturition and defaecation. Brain 1964; 87:233–62.
59. Ochoa B. Can a congenital dysfunctional bladder be diagnosed from a smile? The Ochoa's syndrome updated. Pediatr Nephrol 2004; 19:6–12.
60. Rouzade-Dominguez ML, Miselis R, Valentino RJ. Central representation of bladder and colon revealed by dual transsynaptic tracing in the rat: substrates for pelvic visceral coordination. Eur J Neurosci 2003; 18:3311–24.
61. Rouzade-Dominguez ML, Pernar L, Beck S, Valentino RJ. Convergent responses of Barrington's nucleus neu-

rons to pelvic visceral stimuli in the rat: a juxtacellular labelling study. Eur J Neurosci 2003; 18:3325–34.
62. Matsumoto G, Hisamitsu T, de Groat WC. Non-NMDA glutamatergic excitatory transmission in the descending limb of the spinobulbospinal micturition reflex pathway of the rat. Brain Res 1995; 693:246–50.
63. Lindstrom S, Fall M, Carlsson CA, Erlandson BE. The neurophysiological basis of bladder inhibition in response to intravaginal electrical stimulation. J Urol 1983; 129:405–10.
64. Fall M, Erlandson BE, Carlsson CA, Lindstrom S. The effect of intravaginal electrical stimulation on the feline urethra and urinary bladder. Neuronal mechanisms. Scand J Urol Nephrol Suppl 1977; 44:19–30.
65. Blok BFM, Holstege G. The central control of micturition and continence: implications for urology. BJU Int 1999; 83(Suppl 2):1–6.
66. Blok BF, Willemsen AT, Holstege G. A PET study on brain control of micturition in humans. Brain 1997; 120(Pt 1):111–21.
67. Gjone R, Setekleiv J. Excitatory and inhibitory bladder responses to stimulation in the cerebral cortex in the cat. Acta Physiol Scand 1963; 59:337–48.
68. Birder LA, Roppolo JR, Erickson VL, de Groat WC. Increased c-fos expression in spinal lumbosacral projection neurons and preganglionic neurons after irritation of the lower urinary tract in the rat. Brain Res 1999; 834:55–65.
69. Birder LA, Roppolo JR, Iadarola MJ, de Groat WC. Electrical stimulation of visceral afferent pathways in the pelvic nerve increases c-fos in the rat lumbosacral spinal cord. Neurosci Lett 1991; 129:193–6.
70. de Groat WC, Douglas JW, Glass J et al. Changes in somato-vesical reflexes during postnatal development in the kitten. Brain Res 1975; 94:150–4.
71. de Groat WC. Plasticity of bladder reflex pathways during postnatal development. Physiol Behav 2002; 77: 689–692.
72. Sugaya K, Roppolo JR, Yoshimura N, Card JP, de Groat WC. The central neural pathways involved in micturition in the neonatal rat as revealed by the injection of pseudorabies virus into the urinary bladder. Neurosci Lett 1997; 223:197–200.
73. Geirsson G, Lindstrom S, Fall M. The bladder cooling reflex in man: characteristics and sensitivity to temperature. Br J Urol 1993; 71:675–80.
74. Geirsson G, Fall M, Lindstrom S. The ice-water test: a simple and valuable supplement to routine cystometry. Br J Urol 1993; 71:681–5.
75. de Groat WC, Kawatani M, Hisamitsu T et al. Mechanisms underlying the recovery of urinary bladder function following spinal cord injury. J Auton Nerv Syst 1990; 30(Suppl):S71–7.
76. de Groat WC, Araki I, Vizzard MA et al. Developmental and injury induced plasticity in the micturition reflex pathway. Behav Brain Res 1998; 92:127–40.
77. Yeung CK, Godley ML, Ho CK et al. Some new insights into bladder function in infancy. Br J Urol 1995; 76:235–40.
78. Jansson UB, Hanson M, Hanson E, Hellstrom AL, Sillen U. Voiding pattern in healthy children 0 to 3 years old: a longitudinal study. J Urol 2000; 164:2050–4.
79. Sillen U. Bladder function in healthy neonates and its development during infancy. J Urol 2001; 166:2376–81.
80. Sillen U, Solsnes E, Hellstrom AL, Sandberg K. The voiding pattern of healthy preterm neonates. J Urol 2000; 163:278–81.
81. Bachelard M, Sillen U, Hansson S et al. Urodynamic pattern in asymptomatic infants: siblings of children with vesicoureteral reflux. J Urol 1999; 162:1733–7, discussion 1737–8.
82. Holmdahl G, Hanson E, Hanson M et al. Four-hour voiding observation in young boys with posterior urethral valves. J Urol 1998; 160:1477–81.
83. Bachelard, Hjalmas K. Urodynamics in normal infants and children. Scand J Urol Nephrol Suppl 1988; 114:20–7.

Neurogenic voiding dysfunction and non-surgical management

53

Stuart B Bauer

Introduction

Neurologic lesions that affect lower urinary tract function cause at least 25% of the more severe clinical problems in pediatric urology. The advent of clean intermittent catheterization (CIC), introduced in the early 1970s by Lapides,[1] and the refinements in the techniques of urodynamic studies in children,[2–4] dramatically changed the way these children were managed.[5] As a result, a greater understanding of the pathophysiology of the many diseases that primarily affect children coupled with improved functional assessment of the lower urinary tract has changed the thinking regarding treatment options.[6,7] Once it was realized that urodynamic studies could define children at risk for urinary tract deterioration, early aggressive and even proactive therapy became the mainstay of management. Urodynamic testing is discussed in Chapter 51.

Assessment

Initially, all children with overt or suspected neuropathic bladder dysfunction should undergo a thorough evaluation:

1 History:
   - prenatal health
   - birth and development
   - perinatal complications
   - bowel and bladder habits
   - pattern of incontinence
   - bowel emptying regimen:
     frequency, soiling.

2 Physical examination:
   - spine
   - lower extremities
     reflexes
     muscle mass and strength
     sensation
     gait
     perineal sensation/tone/reflexes
   - central nervous system
     handedness
     fine/gross motor coordination.

3 Laboratory:
   - urine analysis/culture
   - urine specific gravity
   - serum creatinine level.

4 Radiography:
   - renal and bladder sonography
   - voiding cystourethrography (VCUG)
   - spine radiograph – ultrasound <3 months of age; magnetic resonance imaging (MRI) >3 months.

5 Urodynamics:
   - flow rate
   - residual urine (via ultrasound or catheterization)
   - cystometrogram
   - external urethral sphincter electromyography (EMG)
   - static/filling/voiding urethral pressure profile.

Of paramount importance in the work-up of children with neuropathic bladder dysfunction are the history and physical examination. The child's voiding habits prior to any injury and the current pattern of bladder emptying should be delineated. It is imperative to note whether the child voids voluntarily, spontaneously, or only with a Credé maneuver. Does the child have periods of dryness between voiding, or is there constant urinary leakage? Is the incontinence characterized by urgency and an inability to reach the toilet on time? Does the urine flow with a steady or intermittent stream or only dribble out during emptying? Does leakage occur with crying or laughing?

Has the child had a urinary infection? How much urine is produced each day? What is the pattern of bowel emptying? Is there small- or large-volume fecal soiling?

A careful assessment is made of perianal and perineal sensation, anal sphincter tone, and the presence of bulbocavernosus and anocutaneous reflexes. Placing one's finger just at or slightly inside the external anal sphincter and briskly squeezing the glans penis or compressing the clitoris elicits the bulbocavernosus reflex. If the reflex is present, the external anal sphincter should contract. The anocutaneous reflex is elicited by scratching the pigmented skin directly adjacent to the anal opening, which results in a contraction of the perianal muscle. In children with suspected neuropathic bladder dysfunction, complete evaluation of the back, including looking for agenesis of the sacrum, abnormalities of the gluteal cleft, or a cutaneous manifestation of an underlying occult spinal dysraphism, is an important diagnostic aid.[8–10] Examination of the lower extremities, comparing muscle mass and strength of each leg, eliciting deep tendon reflexes, pinpointing sensory losses, and observing the gait, may provide clues to the presence of an occult spinal dysraphism affecting not only the sacral but also the lumbar cord. Left-handedness in a family in which all members are right-handed, learning disabilities at school, poor fine and/or gross motor coordination, and attention deficit disorders all suggest the possibility of a central nervous system (CNS) disorder that might adversely affect lower urinary tract function.

Classification of neuropathic bladder

The classification of neuropathic bladder dysfunction used in this chapter is that which has been adopted by the Urology Section of the American Academy of Pediatrics (AAP) in conjunction with the Urodynamic Society's classification, the International Continence Society (ICS),[11,12a] and, most recently, with the International Children's Continence Society (ICCS).[12b]

Under normal conditions, all portions of the lower urinary tract (detrusor, bladder neck, and external sphincter mechanism) function as a coordinated unit for adequate storage and efficient evacuation of urine. When a neurourologic lesion exists, these components usually fail to act in unison. A classification has been adopted based on dysfunction of a specific area of the vesicourethral unit rather than on a specific etiology:

1 Storage:
   (a) detrusor tone
      - normal
      - increased
         - non-elastic
         - overactive
         - hyperreflexic
         - decreased
   (b) urethral closing mechanism
      - incompetent
         - bladder neck
         - external sphincter
         - non-reciprocal
         - periodic hypoactivity.
2 Evacuation:
   (a) detrusor contraction
      - normoactive
      - underactive
         - areflexic (non-reactive)
         - hypoactive (unsustained)
   (b) urethral closing mechanism
      - non-synchronous
         - bladder neck
         - external sphincter.

Improper storage may be related to an alteration in detrusor function or an inadequate urethral closure mechanism. The bladder may have increased tone secondary to loss of elasticity of the muscle, overactivity from excessive or unopposed sympathetic discharges, or hyperreflexia due to a CNS lesion above the sacral cord, the brainstem, or cerebral cortex that prevents the normal inhibitory centers from influencing the sacral reflex arc. Incontinence may occur with any one of these conditions despite a normal level of resistance in the bladder neck and urethra. Alternatively, incontinence may occur when the bladder neck and external sphincter areas do not provide adequate resistance during filling of the bladder or do not generate a reciprocal increase in outflow resistance as the bladder fills or abdominal pressure is raised. An injury to the spinal cord or nerve roots affecting the sympathetic, parasympathetic, or sacral somatic nervous system may alter both bladder neck and urethral sphincter tone. Periodic relaxation of the external urethral sphincter during filling of the bladder, the result of loss of CNS inhibition, may also lead to urinary incontinence.

Incomplete evacuation of the bladder may be due to a hypoactive or an areflexic detrusor muscle. A CNS lesion affecting the parasympathetic efferents may be responsible. However, non-synchronous relaxation of the bladder neck or external urethral

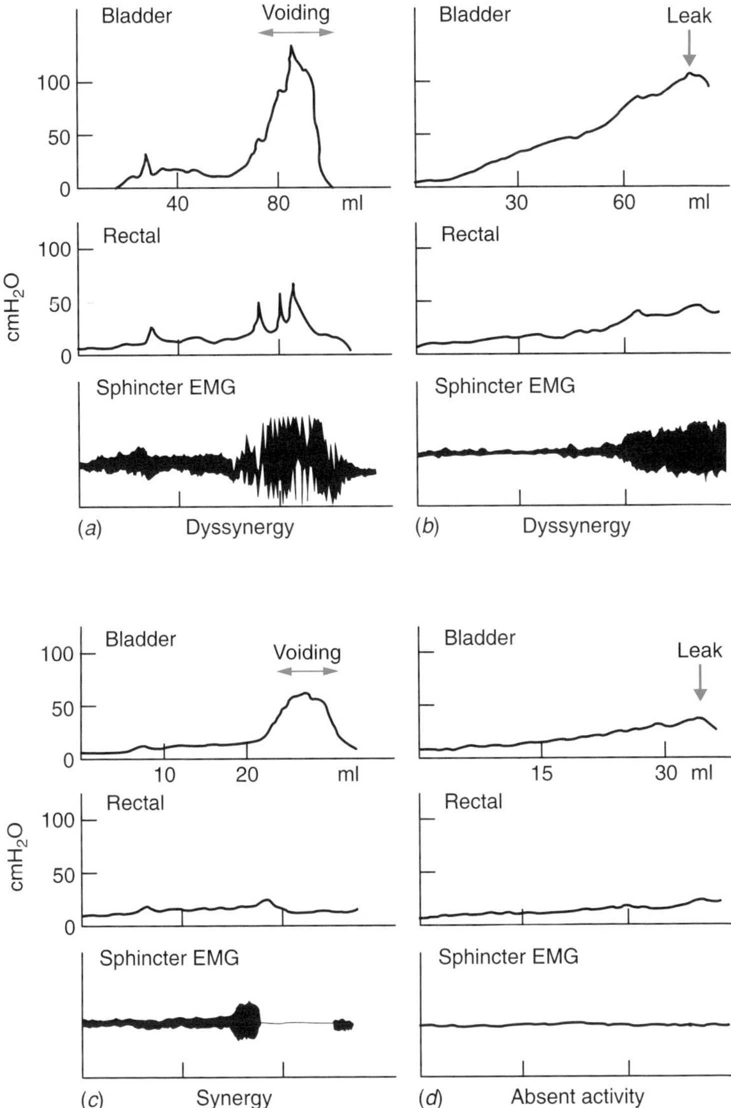

Figure 53.1 (*a–d*) Various patterns of urodynamic findings in newborns with myelodysplasia. Note that a hypertonic detrusor with a non-relaxing sphincter (*b*) is also labeled dyssynergy. (From Bauer.[13])

sphincter area mechanisms (dyssynergia) (Figure 53.1) resulting from a lesion in the CNS above the sacral cord, for example the pontine center or the cerebral cortex, can produce a similar effect. Myogenic failure occurs as the detrusor muscle hypertrophies and then decompensates owing to persistent bladder outflow resistance. Eventually, this mechanism may produce an overflow type of incontinence.

In general, medical management of neuropathic bladder dysfunction is based on the functional impairment produced by the specific neurourologic defect (Table 53.1). Lowering detrusor tone or abolishing uninhibited contractions with anticholinergic medications such as oxybutynin, tolterodine, trospium, glycopyrrolate, hyoscyamine, or propantheline, may enhance inadequate storage capacity. These drugs block cholinergic receptor sites in the detrusor muscle, diminishing its tone and suppressing involuntary contractions of the bladder. Other drugs, for example flavoxate, act directly on the smooth muscle cells and lower detrusor tone without affecting contractility. Failure of drug therapy to increase bladder capacity and lower detrusor tone results in the need for augmentation cystoplasty to enhance bladder storage capability. This procedure is appropriate as long as bladder outflow resistance is normal or increased.

If inadequate urethral resistance is the primary reason for impaired storage of urine, the bladder neck mechanism or the external sphincter area, or both, may be responsible. α-Sympathomimetic agents such as ephedrine sulfate, pseudoephedrine, and phenylpropanolamine stimulate α_1 receptors concentrated in the bladder neck area to enhance the tone of the muscles in this region. No drugs are commercially available that will increase the tone of denervated skeletal muscle in the external sphincter region.

Table 53.1 Drug therapy in neuropathic bladder dysfunction

Type	Minimum dosage	Maximum dosage
Cholinergic		
Bethanechol (Urecholine)	0.7 mg/kg t.i.d.	0.8 mg/kg q.i.d.
Anticholinergic		
Propantheline (Pro-Banthine)	0.5 mg/kg b.i.d.	0.5 mg/kg q.i.d.
Oxybutynin (Ditropan)	0.2 mg/kg b.i.d.	0.2 mg/kg q.i.d.
Glycopyrrolate (Robinul)	0.01 mg/kg b.i.d.	0.03 mg/kg t.i.d.
Hyoscyamine (Levsin)	0.03 mg/kg b.i.d.	0.1 mg/kg q.i.d.
Tolterodine (Detrol)	0.01 mg/kg b.i.d.	0.04 mg/kg b.i.d.
Trospium (Sanctura)	0.1 mg/kg b.i.d.	0.3 mg/kg b.i.d.
Sympathomimetic		
Phenylpropanolamine (alpha) (Ornade)	2.5 mg/kg t.i.d.	2.5 mg/kg b.i.d.
Ephedrine (alpha) (Ephedrine)	0.5 mg/kg b.i.d.	1.0 mg/kg t.i.d.
Pseudoephedrine (alpha) (Sudafed)	0.4 mg/kg b.i.d.	0.9 mg/kg t.i.d.
Sympatholytic		
Prazosin (alpha) (Minipress)	0.05 mg/kg b.i.d.	0.1 mg/kg t.i.d.
Phenoxybenzamine (alpha)	0.3 mg/kg b.i.d.	0.5 mg/kg t.i.d.
Propranolol (beta)	0.25 mg/kg b.i.d.	0.5 mg/kg b.i.d.
Doxazosin (alpha) (Cardura)	0.01 mg/kg q.d.	0.02 mg/kg q.d.
Smooth muscle relaxant		
Flavoxate (Urispas)	3.0 mg/kg b.i.d.	3.0 mg/kg t.i.d.
Dicyclomine (Bentyl)	0.1 mg/kg t.i.d.	0.3 mg/kg t.i.d.
Other		
Imipramine (Tofranil)	0.7 mg/kg b.i.d.	1.2 mg/kg t.i.d.

Incomplete emptying of the bladder may also be due to an areflexic bladder, unsustained detrusor contractions, or uncoordinated activity at the bladder neck or external sphincter area. α-Sympatholytic agents or skeletal muscle relaxants may facilitate emptying. Although conflicting reports have been published regarding the efficacy of bethanechol, it does seem to improve emptying of the bladder in most instances. It should be administered with α-sympatholytic agents because bethanechol also increases urethral resistance at the bladder neck. α-Sympatholytic agents such as phenoxybenzamine or prazosin act primarily in the bladder neck area, whereas diazepam and baclofen diminish skeletal muscle tone at the external sphincter region to lower outlet resistance to voiding.

Most neurologic conditions affecting vesicourethral function in children, including myelomeningocele, lipomeningocele, sacral agenesis, and occult lesions, are called congenital neurospinal dysraphisms:

1 Neuropathic:
  - (a) spinal cord
    - (i) congenital
      - neurospinal dysraphism
      - other anatomic
    - (ii) acquired
      - trauma
      - tumor
      - infection
      - vascular
      - miscellaneous
  - (b) supraspinal cord
    - anatomic/congenital
    - trauma
    - tumor
    - infection
    - vascular
    - degenerative
    - miscellaneous
    - temporary
  - (c) peripheral
    - trauma
    - tumor
    - degenerative
    - Guillain–Barré syndrome.

2 Non-neuropathic:
  - anatomic
  - myopathic
  - psychological
  - endocrinologic
  - toxic.

Occasionally, bladder dysfunction is seen in conjunction with other neurologic lesions. Cerebral palsy is an acquired non-progressive form of dysfunction as a result of a CNS insult occurring in the perinatal period as a consequence of cerebral anoxia from a variety of conditions.

Children without obvious neurologic disease may have a voiding abnormality on a functional or maturational basis. Most children gain urinary control before the age of 5 years. Persistent day and night incontinence without a prolonged period of dryness or the recurrence of nocturnal wetting lasting into puberty are indications for urodynamic evaluation in neurologically normal children. Although an overwhelming number have normal findings, a significant percentage may have a dysfunctional voiding state. The types of abnormality are discussed separately along with individual approaches to therapy.

Neurospinal dysraphisms

Myelodysplasia

The most common etiology of neuropathic bladder dysfunction in children is abnormal spinal column development. Formation of the spinal cord and vertebrae begins around the 18th day of gestation. The canal closes in a caudal direction from the cervical region, and is complete by 35 days. Although the exact mechanism causing a dysraphic state is unknown at present, numerous factors, including genetic influences,[14,15] have been implicated. The incidence has been reported to be 1 in 1000 births in the United States,[16] but there has been a definite decrease in this occurrence.[17] Two explanations are possible for this phenomenon: first, with the advent of prenatal screening, many families are electing to terminate their pregnancies when they have affected fetuses;[18] secondly, the addition of folic acid supplements to the diet of women of childbearing age has reduced the incidence of spina bifida by more than 50%.[19,20] In some cases, despite increased folic acid intake, women may still have a fetus with spina bifida owing to antibodies that develop to folate, which negates its salutatory effect.[21] If spina bifida is already present in one member of a family, there is a 2–5% chance of a second sibling being born with the same condition.[22] The incidence doubles when more than one family member has a neurospinal dysraphism (Table 53.2).

Table 53.2 Familial risk of myelodysplasia in the United States per 1000 live births

Relationship	Incidence
General population	0.7–1.0
Mother with one affected child	30–50
Mother with two affected children	100
Patient with myelodysplasia	40
Mother older than 35 years	30
Sister of mother with affected child	10
Sister of father with affected child	3
Nephew who is affected	2

Adapted from Kroovand et al.[23]

Pathogenesis

Myelodysplasia is an all-inclusive term used to describe the various abnormal conditions of the vertebral column that affect spinal cord function. More specific labels regarding each abnormality include the following:

- a meningocele occurs when just the meninges extend beyond the confines of the vertebral canal without any neural elements contained inside it
- a myelomeningocele implies that neural tissue, either nerve roots and/or portions of the spinal cord, have evaginated with the meningocele
- a lipomyelomeningocele denotes that fatty tissue has developed with the cord structures and both are protruding into the sac.

Myelomeningocele accounts for >90% of all the open spinal dysraphic states.[24] Most spinal defects occur at the level of the lumbar vertebrae, with the sacral, thoracic, and cervical areas being affected in decreasing order of frequency (Table 53.3).[25] An overwhelming number of meningoceles are directed posteriorly, but on rare occasions, the meningocele may protrude anteriorly, particularly in the sacral area. Usually the meningocele is made up of a flimsy covering or transparent membrane, but it may be open and leaking cerebrospinal fluid (CSF). For this reason,

Table 53.3 Spinal level of myelomeningocele

Location	Incidence (%)
Cervical–high thoracic	2
Low thoracic	5
Lumbar	26
Lumbosacral	47
Sacral	20

Adapted from Kroovand et al.[23]

urgent repair after birth is necessary, with sterile precautions being followed in the interval to closure. In 85% of affected children an associated Arnold–Chiari malformation is present; in such cases the cerebellar tonsils have herniated down through the foramen magnum, obstructing the fourth ventricle, and thus preventing the CSF from entering the subarachnoid space surrounding the brain and spinal cord.

The neurologic lesion produced by this condition can be quite variable. It depends on what neural elements, if any, have protruded with the meningocele sac. The bony vertebral level often gives little or no clue as to the exact neurologic level or deficits that are produced. The height of the bony level and the highest extent of the neurologic lesion may vary from one to three vertebrae in one direction or another.[25] There may be differences in function from one side of the body to the other at the same neurologic level, and from one neurologic level to the next, as a result of asymmetry of affected neural elements. In addition, 20% of affected children have a vertebral bony or intraspinal abnormality occurring more cephalad from the vertebral defect and meningocele, which can affect functional changes in those portions of the cord. Children with thoracic and upper lumbar meningoceles often have complete reconstitution of their spine in the sacral area and these individuals will frequently have intact sacral reflex arc function involving the sacral spinal roots. In fact, it is more likely for children with upper thoracic or cervical lesions to have just a meningocele and no myelocele, with no demonstrable loss of function. Finally, the differential growth rates between the vertebral bodies and the elongating spinal cord add a factor of dynamicism in the developing fetus that further complicates the picture.[26] Superimposed on all this is the Arnold–Chiari malformation, which may have profound effects on the brainstem and pontine center areas involved in the control over lower urinary tract function.

Thus, the neurologic lesion produced by this condition influences lower urinary tract function in a variety of ways and cannot be predicted just by looking at the spinal abnormality or the neurologic function of the lower extremities. This wide spectrum of dysfunction is evident when looking at babies with sacral level lesions.[27] Even careful assessment of the sacral area may not provide sufficient information to make a concrete inference. Therefore, urodynamic evaluation in the neonatal period is now performed at most pediatric centers in the United States and worldwide. This is because urodynamics not only provides a clear picture of the function of the sacral spinal cord and lower urinary tract but also has predictive value regarding babies at risk for future urinary tract deterioration and progressive neurologic change.[6,7,27–30]

Newborn assessment

Ideally, it would be best to perform urodynamic testing immediately after the baby is born, but the risk of spinal infection and the urgency for closure has not made this a viable option at this time. In a 1990 study, preoperative testing showed that fewer than 5% of children experience a change in their neurologic status as a result of the spinal canal closure.[31] Therefore, renal ultrasonography and a measurement of residual urine are performed as early as possible after birth, either before or immediately after the spinal defect is closed, with urodynamic studies delayed until it is safe to transport children to the urodynamic suite and place them on on their backs or sides for the test. For infants who cannot empty their bladder following a spontaneous void, intermittent catheterization is begun, even before urodynamic studies are conducted. The normal bladder capacity in the newborn period is between 10 and 15 ml; thus, an acceptable residue of urine is <5 ml. Other tests that should be performed in the neonatal period include a urine analysis and culture, and a determination of the serum creatinine level.[32]

Once the spinal closure has healed sufficiently, renal scintigraphy is performed to assess upper urinary tract function and drainage. VCUG is conducted if there is any element of hydronephrosis and/or the urodynamic study demonstrates risk factors for upper urinary tract deterioration. Thus, urodynamic studies fulfill several objectives:[6,7,29,33]

- They provide baseline information about the radiologic appearance of the upper and lower urinary tract, as well as the condition of the sacral spinal cord and the CNS.
- The studies can then be compared with later assessments, so that early signs of deteriorating urinary tract drainage and function, or of progressive neurologic denervation, can be detected.
- They help to identify babies at risk for urinary tract deterioration as a result of detrusor hypertonicity or outflow obstruction from detrusor–sphincter dyssynergy, which then allows prophylactic measures to be initiated before the changes actually take place.
- They help the physician to counsel parents with regard to their child's future bladder and sexual function.

Findings

Ten to 15 percent of newborns have an abnormal radiographic appearance to their urinary tract when first evaluated;[34] 3% have hydroureteronephrosis secondary to spinal shock, probably from the closure procedure,[35] whereas 10% have abnormalities that developed in utero as a result of abnormal lower urinary tract function in the form of outlet obstruction.

Urodynamic studies in the newborn period have shown that 57% of infants with myelomeningocele have bladder contractions. This is especially true in children with upper lumbar or thoracic lesions who have sparing of the sacral spinal cord, 83% of whom have detrusor contractions.[36] Forty-three percent have an areflexic bladder, and compliance during bladder filling is either good (25%) or poor (18%) in this subgroup.[7] EMG assessment of the external urethral sphincter demonstrates an intact sacral reflex arc with no evidence of lower motor neuron denervation in 47% of newborns, whereas partial denervation is seen in 24% and complete loss of sacral cord function is noted in 29%.[37]

Combining bladder contractility and external sphincter activity results in three categories of lower urinary tract dynamics: synergic; dyssynergic, with and without detrusor hypertonicity; and complete denervation (see Figure 53.1).[7,29] Synergy is characterized by complete silencing of the sphincter during a detrusor contraction or when capacity is reached at the end of filling. Voiding pressures are usually within the normal range. Dyssynergy occurs when the external sphincter fails to decrease, or actually increases its activity during a detrusor contraction or a sustained increase in intravesical pressure, as the bladder is filled to capacity.[38] Frequently, a poorly compliant bladder with high intravesical pressure is seen in conjunction with a dyssynergic sphincter, resulting in a bladder that empties only at high intravesical pressures.[28,29] Complete denervation is noted when no bioelectric potentials are detectable in the region of the external sphincter at any time during the micturition cycle or in response to a Credé maneuver or sacral reflex stimulation.

Categorizing lower urinary tract function in this way is extremely useful because it defines which children are at risk for urinary tract changes, who should be treated prophylactically, who needs close surveillance, and who can be followed at greater intervals without fear of deterioration. On initial assessment or subsequent studies, 71% of newborns with dyssynergic voiding had urinary tract deterioration within the first 3 years of life, whereas only 17% of synergic voiders and 23% with a completely denervated sphincter developed similar changes (Figure 53.2). The infants in the synergic group whose upper urinary tract deteriorated did so only after they converted to a dyssynergic pattern. Among the infants with complete denervation, the only babies who showed hydronephrosis were those who had elevated levels of urethral resistance, presumably due to fibrosis of the skeletal muscle component of the external sphincter. Thus, it appears that outlet obstruction is a major contributor to the development of urinary tract deterioration in these children (Figure 53.3). Bladder tonicity plays an important but somewhat less critical role in this regard,[6] although detrusor compliance seems to be worse in children with high levels of outlet resistance.[39] This combination of parameters (poor compliance and high outlet resistance) is very provocative for the development of hydroureteronephrosis,[40,41] whereas detrusor–sphincter dyssynergia is a significant factor in the onset of vesicoureteral reflux (VUR)[42] (see Figure 53.3). First Bloom and associates[43] and then Park and associates[44] noted an improvement in compliance when outlet resistance was lowered following gentle urethral dilation in these children; however, the reasons for this are unclear and the long-term effect of this maneuver on ultimate continence and upper urinary tract function remains uncertain. Another form of therapy advocated for high-risk children has been botulinum A toxin injected into the detrusor muscle to paralyze bladder activity and improve compliance. Despite an

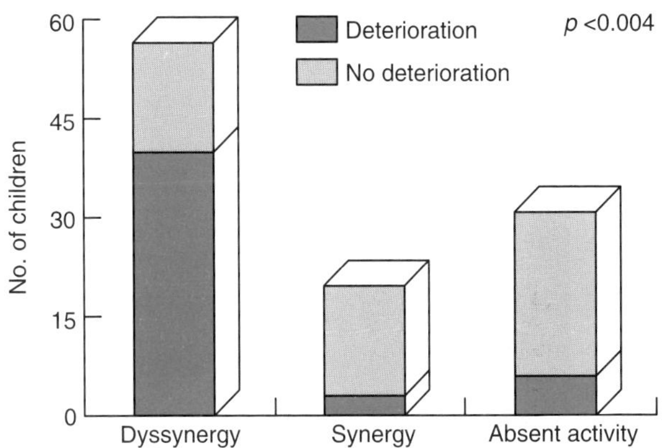

Figure 53.2 Urinary tract deterioration is related to outflow obstruction and most often associated with dyssynergy. Children with synergy converted to dyssynergy and patients with complete bladder denervation developed fibrosis with a fixed high-outlet resistance in the external sphincter, before any changes occurred in the urinary tract. (From Bauer.[13])

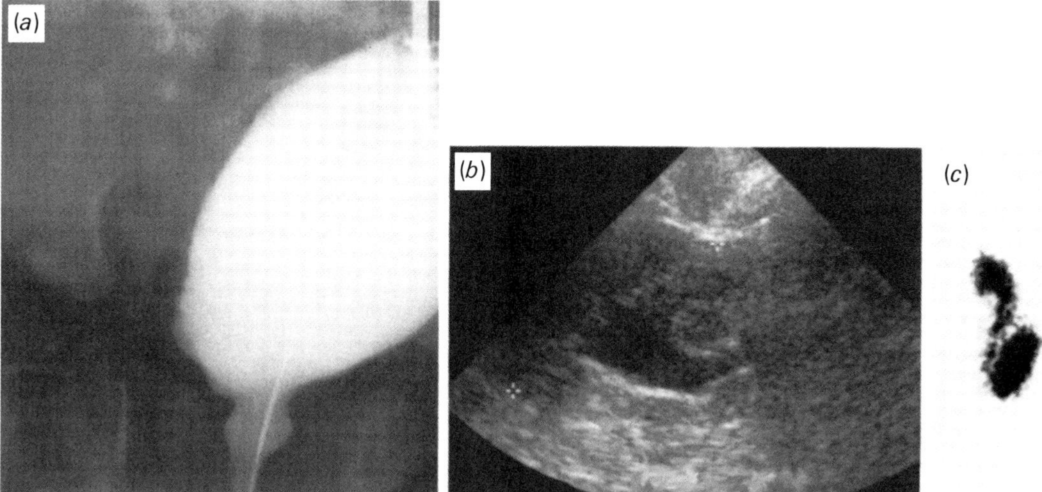

Figure 53.3 (*a*) Voiding cystourethrography in a newborn girl with dyssynergy and elevated voiding pressures demonstrated no reflux and a smooth-walled bladder. Her initial renal echogram was normal. She was started on clean intermittent catheterization and oxybutynin (Ditropan) but did not respond. Within 1 year, she had right hydronephrosis (*b*) and severe reflux on a radionuclide cytogram (*c*).

early excellent response, the effects are short-lived and repeated injections are necessary.[45]

Recommendations

Because expectant treatment has revealed that infants with outlet obstruction in the form of detrusor–sphincter dyssynergy or denervation fibrosis are at considerable risk for urinary tract deterioration, the idea of prophylactically treating the children has emerged as an important alternative to expectant therapy. When CIC is begun in the newborn period, it becomes easy for parents to master, even in uncircumcised boys, and for children to accept as they grow older.[46] Complications of meatitis, epididymitis, or urethral injury are rarely encountered, and symptomatic urinary infection occurs in fewer than 30%,[47] although asymptomatic bacteriuria can be seen in almost 70%.[48]

CIC alone or in combination with anticholinergic agents, when detrusor filling pressures are >40 cmH_2O and voiding pressures reach levels >80–100 cmH_2O, has resulted in only an 8–10% incidence of urinary tract deterioration (Figure 53.4).[47,49,50] This represents a significant drop in the occurrence of detrimental changes compared with the group of children followed expectantly.[6,7,29] Oxybutynin hydrochloride is administered in a dose of 1.0 mg per year of age, every 12 hours, in order to help lower detrusor filling pressure. In neonates or children younger than 1 year of age, the dose is lowered to below 1.0 mg in relation to the child's age at the time and increased proportionately as the child approaches 1 year. No side effects were seen when oxybutynin was administered according to this schedule.[46,47] When a hyperreflexic or hypertonic bladder fails to respond to these measures, augmentation cystoplasty may be required. However, the need for this operative modality in children managed proactively has been substantially reduced to 17%, as compared with a 41% incidence in children followed expectantly[30,51] (see Figure 53.4). Furthermore, the use of vesicostomy drainage has been almost completely eliminated since this approach has been adopted.

Neurologic findings and recommendations

The neurourologic lesion in myelodysplasia is a dynamic disease process with changes taking place throughout childhood,[52–54] especially in early infancy,[37] and then at puberty,[55] when the linear growth rate accelerates again. When a change is noted on neurologic, orthopedic, or urodynamic assessment, radiologic investigation of the CNS often reveals: (1) tethering of the spinal cord; (2) a syrinx or hydromyelia of the cord; (3) increased intracranial pressure due to a shunt malfunction; or (4) partial herniation of the brainstem and cerebellum. Children with completely intact or only partially denervated sacral cord function are particularly vulnerable to progressive changes. MRI reveals anatomic details of the spinal column and CNS, but it is not a functional study. Therefore, when used alone, it cannot provide

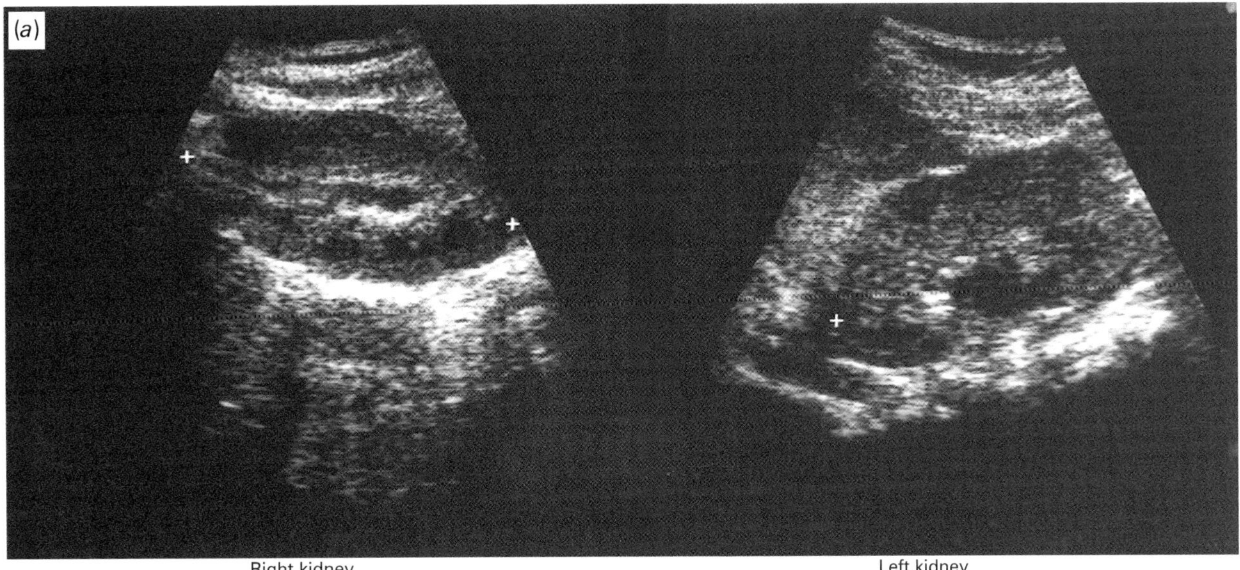

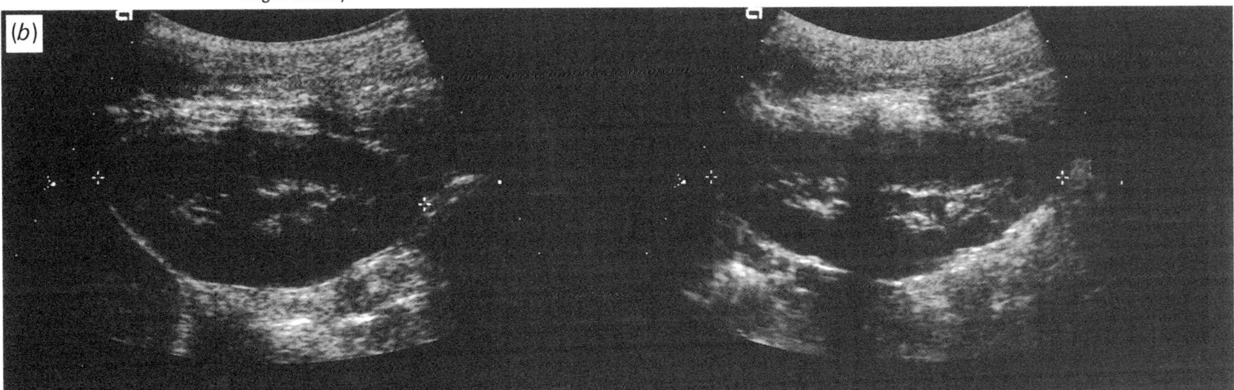

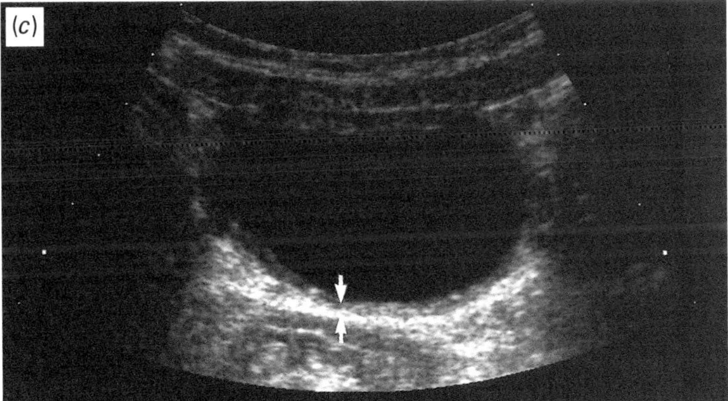

Figure 53.4 Another newborn boy with detrusor–sphincter dyssynergia was successfully treated with clean intermittent catheterization and oxybutynin. Over a 14-year period, his kidneys have remained normal by renal ultrasound (*a*, *b*) and his bladder wall has not increased its thickness (*c*).

exact information with regard to a changing neurologic lesion.

Sequential urodynamic testing on a yearly basis, beginning in the newborn period and continuing until 5 years of age, provides the means for carefully following these children to detect signs of change, thus offering the hope that early detection and neurosurgical intervention may help to arrest or even reverse a progressive pathologic process. Changes occurring in a group of newborns followed in this manner involved both the sacral reflex arc and the pontine–sacral reflex interaction[37,56] (Figure 53.5). Most children who change tend to do so in the first 3 years of life (Figure 53.6). Twenty-two of 28 children who exhibited a worsening in their neurologic picture underwent a second neurosurgical procedure: 50% had a beneficial effect from the surgery, with 11 of these 22 showing improvement in urethral sphincter function.[56]

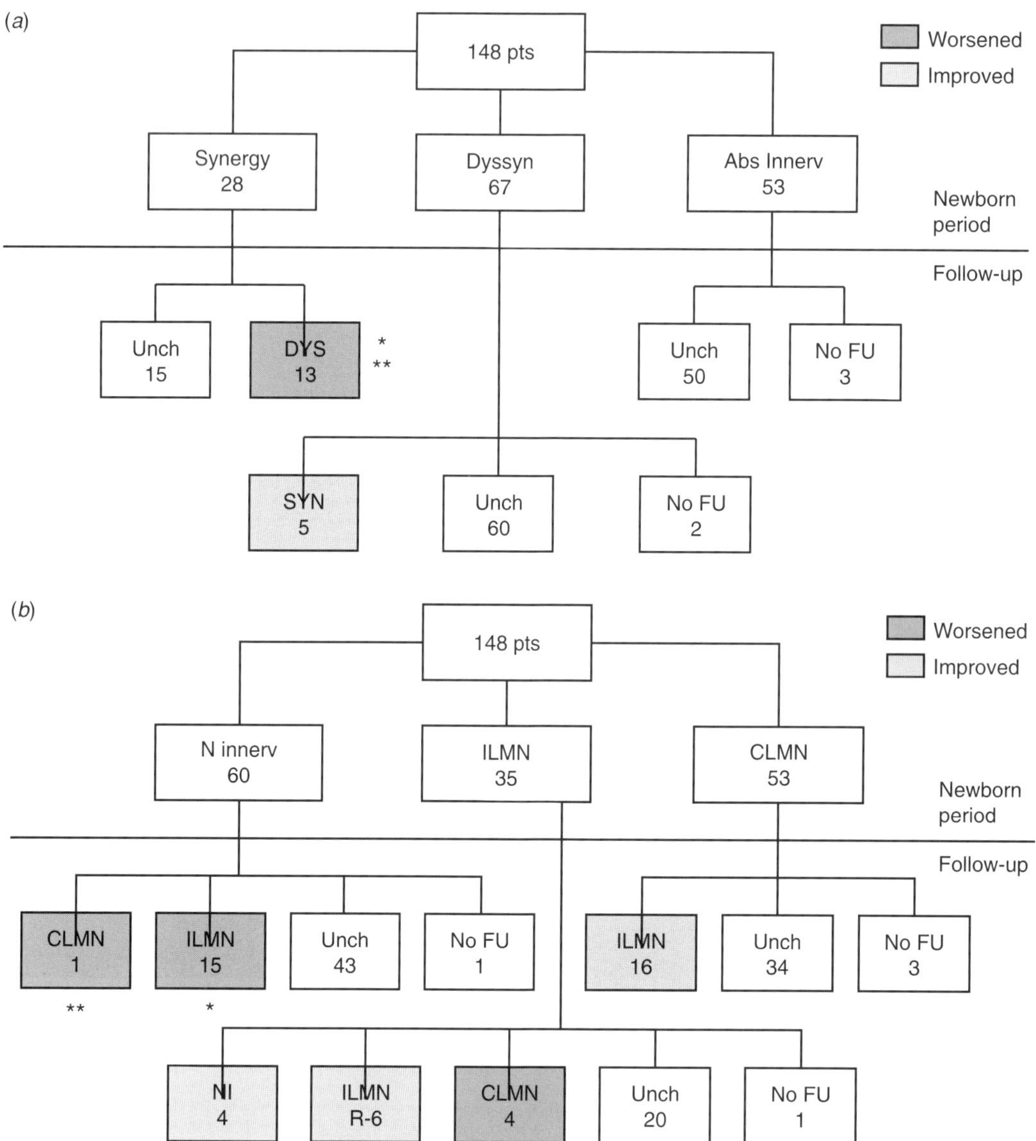

Figure 53.5 (*a*) Pontine–sacral reflux arc changes that occurred in a group of children with myelodysplasia followed with sequential urodynamic studies between the newborn period and 3 or more years of age. Dyssyn = dyssynergy; Abs Innerv = absence of innervation; Unch = unchanged; DYS = dyssynergy; FU = follow-up; Syn = synergy; * = one patient who changed from normal innervation to partial and then complete denervation; ** = four patients who changed from normal innervation to partial denervation. (*b*) Sacral reflex arc pathway changes that occurred in the same group of children. N innerv = normal innervation; ILMN = incomplete lower motor neuron; CLMN = complete lower motor neuron; Unch = unchanged; FU = follow-up; N = normal; * = four of 15 patients who changed from synergy to dyssynergy; ** = one patient who changed from synergy to dyssynergy.

As a result of these developments, all babies with myelodysplasia should be observed according to the guidelines set forth in Table 53.4. It is not enough to look at just the radiographic appearance of the urinary tract; critical scrutiny of the functional status of the lower urinary tract is important as well. In addition to the reasons cited above, it may be necessary to repeat a urodynamic study when the upper urinary tract dilates secondary to impaired drainage from a hypertonic detrusor or urinary incontinence occurs after a prolonged period of dryness on intermittent catheterization and medical therapy.

Management of reflux

VUR occurs in 3–5% of newborns with myelodysplasia, usually in association with detrusor hypertonicity and/or dyssynergia. It is rare to find reflux in

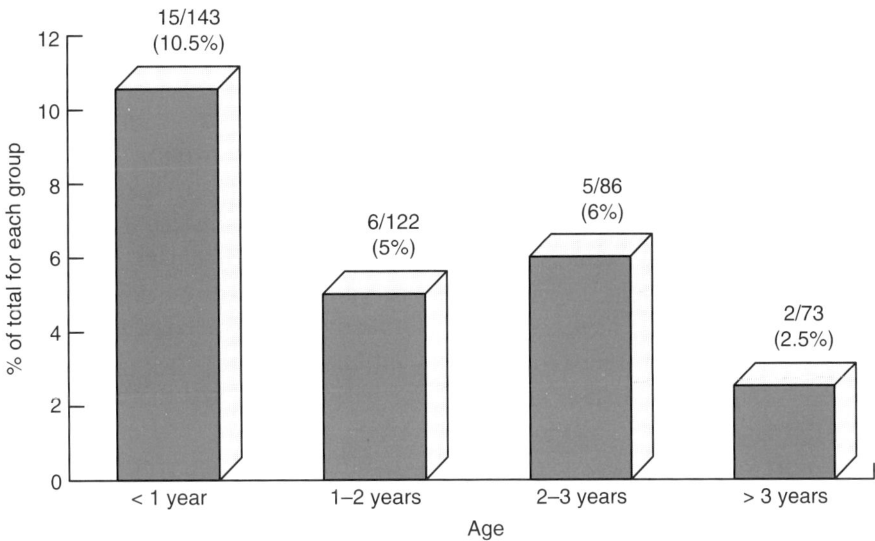

Figure 53.6 Propensity for deterioration in external urethral sphincter innervation is greatest in the first year of life, with a decreasing incidence noted subsequently. (From Bauer.[13])

Table 53.4 Surveillance in infants with myelodysplasia[a]

Sphincter activity	Recommended tests	Frequency
Intact – synergic	Postvoiding residual	Every 4 months
	IVP or renal echo	Every 12 months
	UDS	Every 12 months
Intact – dyssynergic[b]	IVP or renal echo	Every 12 months
	UDS	Every 12 months
	VCUG or RNC[c]	Every 12 months
Partial denervation	Postvoiding residual	Every 4 months
	IVP or renal echo	Every 12 months
	UDS[d]	Every 12 months
	VCUG or RNC[c]	Every 12 months
Complete denervation	Postvoiding residual	Every 6 months
	Renal echo	Every 12 months

[a] Until the age of 5 years.
[b] Patients on intermittent catheterization and anticholinergic agents.
[c] If detrusor hypertonicity or reflux already present.
[d] Depending on degree of denervation.
IVP = intravenous pyelography; echo = sonography; UDS = urodynamic study; VCUG = voiding cystourethrography; RNC = radionuclide cystography.

any neonate with a spinal cord lesion without dyssynergy or poor compliance.[49,57] If left untreated, the incidence of reflux in these at-risk infants increases with time until 30–40% are afflicted by 5 years of age,[57] with even higher levels noted in older children.[42]

In children with mild to moderate grades of reflux (I–III), who void spontaneously or who have complete lesions with little or no outlet resistance and empty their bladder completely, management consists of antibiotic prophylaxis to prevent recurrent infection. When these children have high-grade reflux (grade IV or V), intermittent catheterization is begun to ensure complete emptying. Children who cannot empty their bladders spontaneously, regardless of the grade of reflux, are catheterized intermittently to ensure complete emptying. Children with detrusor hypertonicity, with or without hydroureteronephrosis, are also treated with oxybutynin to lower intravesical pressure and ensure adequate upper urinary tract decompression. When managed in this manner, reflux resolves in 30–55% and renal function does not become impaired.[46,57–61] Although bacteriuria can be seen in as many as 56% of children on intermittent catheterization, generally it is not harmful except in the presence of high-grade reflux because symptomatic urinary infection and renal scarring rarely occur with lesser grades of reflux.[58,62]

Credé voiding is to be avoided in children with reflux and a reactive external sphincter. Under these conditions, the Credé maneuver results in a reflex response of the external sphincter that increases urethral resistance and raises the pressure needed to expel urine from the bladder[63] (Figure 53.7). This has the effect of aggravating the degree of reflux and increasing upper urinary tract dilatation. Vesicostomy drainage[8,64] is reserved for (1) those infants who have such severe reflux that intermittent catheterization and anticholinergic medication fail to improve upper urinary tract drainage; or (2) those children whose parents cannot adapt to the catheterization program.

The indications for antireflux surgery are not very different from those for children with normal bladder function and include recurrent symptomatic urinary infection while on adequate antibiotic therapy and appropriate catheterization techniques, persistent hydroureteronephrosis despite effective emptying of the bladder and lowering of intravesical pressure, severe reflux with an anatomic abnormality at the ureterovesical junction, and reflux persisting into puberty. In addition, children with any grade of reflux who are being considered for implantation of an artificial urinary sphincter or any other procedure designed to increase bladder outlet resistance should have the reflux corrected at the time of or prior to the anti-incontinence surgery.

Jeffs et al[65] noted that antireflux surgery could be very successful in children with neuropathic bladder dysfunction as long as it is combined with measures to ensure complete bladder emptying. Since the advent of intermittent catheterization, success rates for antireflux surgery have approached 95%.[58,66–68] Unilateral reflux does not warrant bilateral reimplantation, because the incidence of contralateral reflux postoperatively is insignificant.[67] The endoscopic injection of Deflux (dextranomer microspheres in sodium hyaluronan solution) has altered the management of reflux in children with myelomeningocele but

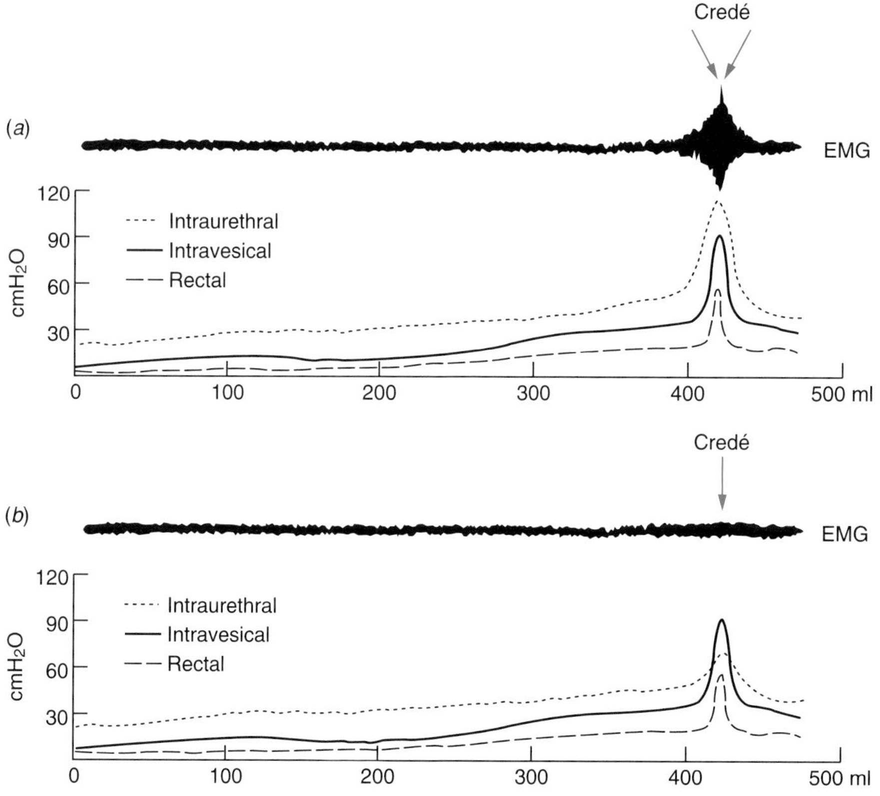

Figure 53.7 (*a*) When the external sphincter is reactive, a Credé maneuver produces a reflex increase in electromyographic (EMG) activity of the sphincter and a concomitant rise in urethral resistance, resulting in high voiding pressure. (*b*) A child whose sphincter is denervated and non-reactive will not have a corresponding rise in EMG activity, urethral resistance, or voiding pressure. A Credé maneuver here will not be detrimental. (From Bauer.[13])

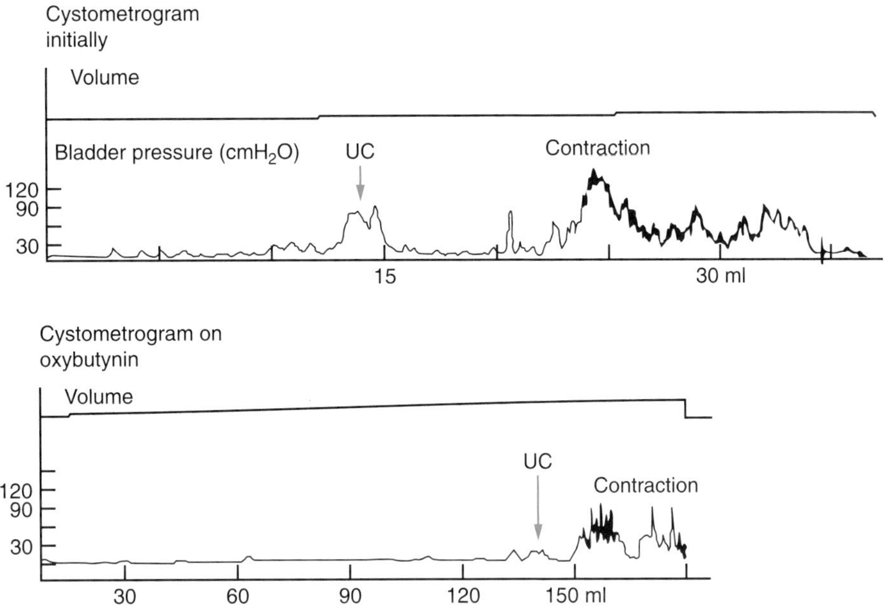

Figure 53.8 Oxybutynin is a potent anticholinergic agent that dramatically delays detrusor contractions and lowers contraction pressure, as demonstrated on these two graphs from a 6-month-old girl with myelodysplasia. UC = uninhibited contraction. (From Bauer.[13])

long-term salutary effects are yet to be appreciated.[69,70]

Continence

Urinary and fecal continence is becoming an increasingly important issue to deal with at an early age as parents try to mainstream their handicapped children. Initial attempts at achieving urinary continence include CIC and drug therapy designed to maintain low intravesical pressure and a reasonable level of urethral resistance (Figures 53.8 and 53.9). Although this approach can be conducted on a trial-and-error basis, it is more efficient to have exact treatment protocols based on specific urodynamic findings. As a result, urodynamic testing is performed if initial attempts with CIC and oxybutynin fail to achieve continence. Without urodynamic studies, it is hard to know whether (1) a single drug is effective, (2) the drug dosage should be increased, (3) a second drug should be added to the regimen, or (4) alternative methods of treatment, i.e. augmentation cystoplasty, should be contemplated.

If urodynamic testing reveals that urethral resistance is inadequate to maintain continence because there is either a failure of the sphincter to react to increases in abdominal pressure or a drop in resistance with bladder filling, then α-sympathomimetic agents are added to the regimen (see Table 53.1). Endoscopic treatment using various bulking agents has

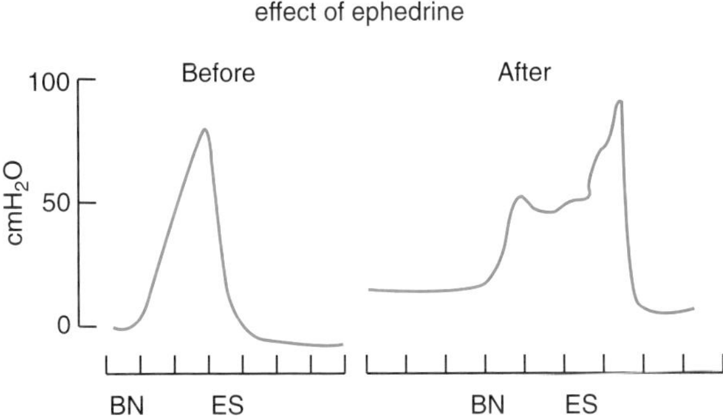

Figure 53.9 α-Sympathomimetic agents potentially have their greatest effect in the bladder neck region where the highest concentration of α-receptor sites exist. They can raise outlet resistance and improve continence in many individuals. (From Bauer.[13]) BN = bladder neck; ES = external sphincter function.

been employed to increase bladder outlet resistance. A positive response has been seen most notably with an areflexic good compliant bladder, but so far a truly long-lasting effect has not been demonstrated.[71–73]

Fecal continence has become a very important social issue for these children as they reach their teenage years.[74] In addition to dietary maneuvers, intravesical bladder stimulation has helped with fecal continence,[75] but the most impressive results have come from the Malone antegrade continence enema or MACE procedure. A continent catheterizable conduit is created from the cecum to the anterior abdominal wall using the appendix or a narrowed reconfigured small segment of bowel. The cecal end of the conduit is implanted in such a manner as to prevent leakage. An enema solution consisting of either GoLYTELY, saline, or tap water is instilled nightly or every other night, cleansing the distal bowel within a short time, and resulting in fecal continence for up to 2–3 days at a time. Older children readily become independent in managing their bowel function, which leads to improved self-esteem and sociability.[76]

Sexuality

Sexuality in this population has become an increasingly important issue to deal with as more and more individuals have reached adulthood and want either to marry or to have meaningful long-term relationships.[77] Few studies are available, however, that look critically at sexual function in these patients.

In one study, researchers interviewed a group of affected teenagers and reported that at least 28% of them had one or more sexual encounters, and almost all had a desire to marry and ultimately bear children.[77] In a more recent study,[78] 57 men were questioned regarding their sexual history: 41 (72%) had erections and 27 of them (66%) had ejaculations. Twenty men said they had had sexual intercourse but only 11 attempted to father children, of whom eight were successful. Overall, 12 men (21%) were married. Another study revealed that 70% of myelodysplastic women were able to become pregnant and have an uneventful pregnancy and delivery, although urinary incontinence in the latter stages of gestation and cesarean section were common.[79] In the same study, 17% of males claimed that they were able to father children. It is more likely for males to have problems with erectile and ejaculatory function because of the frequent neurologic involvement of the sacral spinal cord, whereas reproductive function in the female, which is under hormonal control, is not affected. However, the level of the neurologic lesion is not predictive of ultimate sexual function in men.[78]

As important as knowing what the precise sexual function is in an individual, sexuality or the ability to interact with the opposite sex in a meaningful and lasting way is just as important. Sexual identity, education, and social mores are issues that have been taken out of the realm of secrecy and are now openly discussed and taught to handicapped people.[80–82] Boys reach puberty at an age similar to that for normal males, whereas breast development and menarche tend to start as much as 2 years earlier than usual in myelodysplastic females. The etiology of this early hormonal surge is uncertain, but it may be related to pituitary function changes in girls secondary to their hydrocephalus.[83] The degree of sexuality attained by most is inversely proportional to the level of neurologic function.

Lipomeningocele and other spinal dysraphisms

Diagnosis

A group of congenital defects that affects the formation of the spinal column but does not result in an open vertebral canal has been labeled occult spinal dysraphisms,[84] and includes:

- lipomeningocele
- intradural lipoma
- diastematomyelia or split cord syndrome
- tight filum terminale
- dermoid cyst/sinus
- aberrant nerve roots
- anterior sacral meningocele (when occurring in conjunction with sacral agenesis = Currarino syndrome)
- cauda equina tumor.

These lesions may exist with no obvious outward signs. But 90% of the children manifest a cutaneous abnormality overlying the lower spine.[85] This may vary from a small dimple or skin tag to a tuft of hair, a dermal vascular malformation, or a very noticeable subcutaneous lipoma (Figure 53.10). In addition, on careful inspection of the legs, one may note a high arched foot or alterations in the configuration of the toes, with hammer or claw digits. Other signs include a discrepancy in muscle size and strength between the legs with weakness at the ankle, and/or a gait abnormality, especially in older children, as a result of shortness of one leg.[86–88] Absent perineal sensation and back pain are not uncommon symptoms in older children or young adults.[87,89,90] Lower urinary tract function is abnormal in 40% of affected individuals.[91]

The child may experience difficulty with urinary control (especially during the pubertal growth spurt), urinary retention, recurrent urinary infection, and/or fecal soiling after an initial period of dryness.

Findings

When these children are evaluated in the newborn or early infancy period, the majority have a perfectly normal neurologic examination. Urodynamic testing,

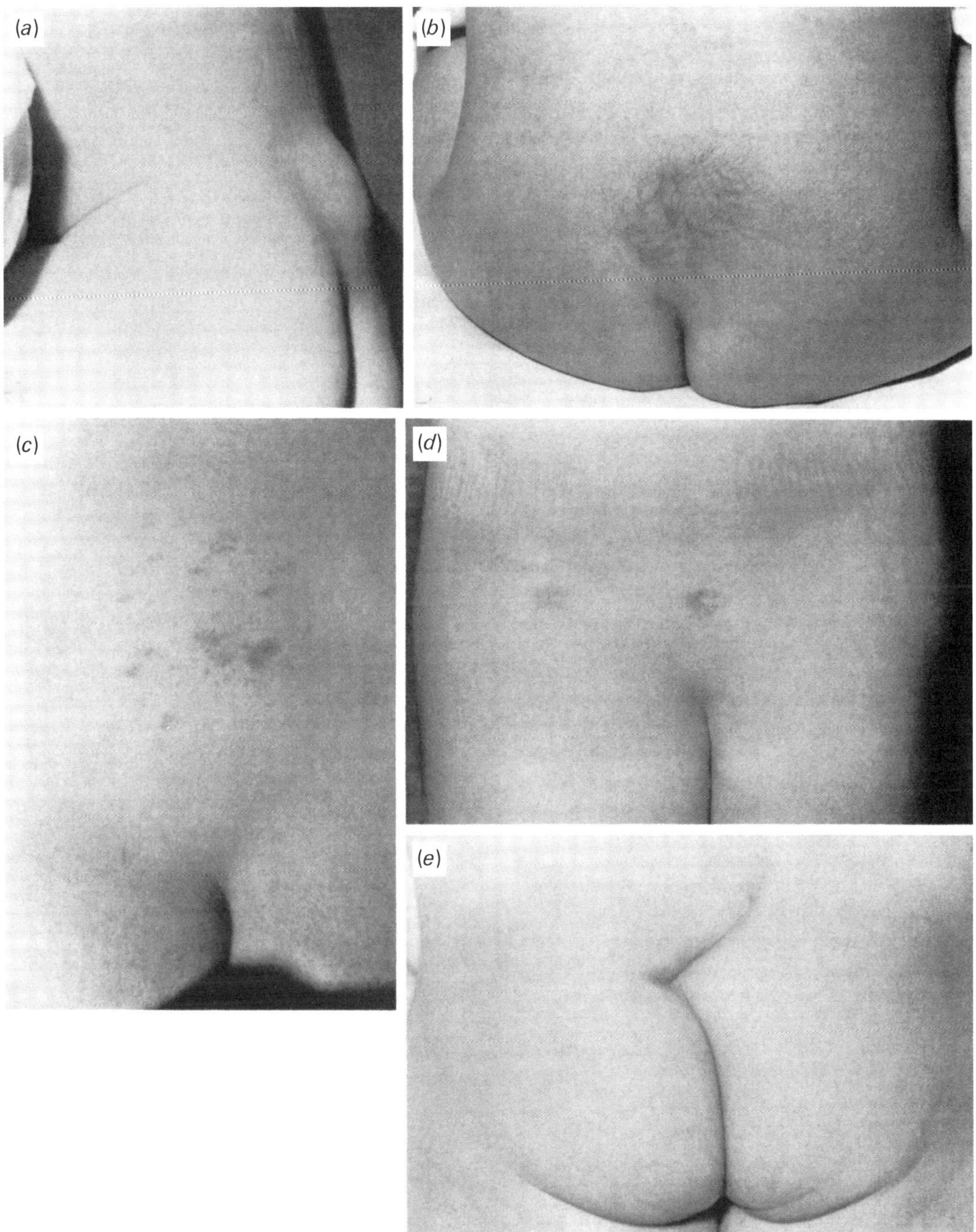

Figure 53.10 Cutaneous lesions occur in 90% of children with various occult dysraphic states. These lesions may vary from a small lipomeningocele (*a*) to a hair patch (*b*), a dermal vascular malformation (*c*), a dimple (*d*), or an abnormal gluteal cleft (*e*).

however, will reveal abnormal lower urinary tract function in about one-third of the babies younger than the age of 18 months[10,92] (Figure 53.11). These studies may provide the only evidence for a neurologic injury involving the lower spinal cord.[92–94] When present, the most likely abnormality is an upper motor neuron lesion characterized by detrusor hyperreflexia and/or hyperactive sacral reflexes, with mild forms of detrusor–sphincter dyssynergy being noted less often. Lower motor neuron signs with denervation potentials in the sphincter, or detrusor areflexia, occur in only 10% of very young children.

In contrast, practically all individuals in the group >3 years of age who have not been operated upon or have been belatedly diagnosed as having an occult dysraphism will have either an upper motor neuron and/or lower motor neuron lesion on urodynamic testing (92%) (see Figure 53.11), or neurologic signs

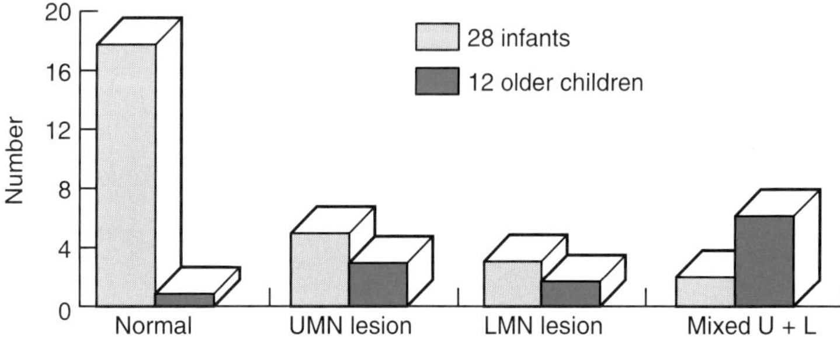

Figure 53.11 Most newborns with a covered spinal dysraphism have normal lower urinary tract function, whereas older children tend to have both upper and lower motor neuron lesions. UMN = upper motor neuron; LMN = lower motor neuron; U + L = upper and lower motor neuron.

of lower extremity dysfunction.[89,92,94–96] There does not seem to be preponderance for one type of lesion over the other (upper versus lower motor neuron); each occurs with equal frequency, and often the child manifests signs of both.[95,97]

Pathogenesis

The reason for this difference in neurologic findings may be related to (1) compression on the cauda equina or sacral nerve roots by an expanding lipoma or lipomeningocele,[98] or (2) tension on the cord from tethering secondary to differential growth rates between the bony and neural elements.[86] The overt stretching that invariably occurs when there is forcible flexion and/or extension of the spinal cord leads to changes in oxidation/reduction of cytochrome oxidase, most notably in the lumbosacral spinal neurons.[99] Under normal circumstances, the conus medullaris ends just below the L-2 vertebra at birth and recedes upwards to T-12 by adulthood.[100] When the cord does not 'rise' secondary to one of these lesions, ischemic injury may ensue.[99,101] Correction of the lesion in infancy has resulted in not only stabilization but also improvement in the neurologic picture in some instances (Figure 53.12). Sixty percent of the babies with abnormal urodynamic findings preoperatively reverted to normal postoperatively, with improvement noted in 30%, whereas 10% worsened with time. In the older child, there is a less dramatic change following surgery, with only 27% becoming normal, 27% improving, 27% stabilizing, but 19% worsening with time[92] (see Figure 53.12). The response to surgical untethering seems to be age related with infants being more likely to improve than older children.[94] Older individuals with hyperreflexia tend to improve, whereas those with areflexic bladders do not.[95,97,102] Finally, fewer than 5% of the children operated on in early childhood developed secondary tethering when observed for several years, suggesting that early surgery has both a beneficial and sustaining effect with these conditions.

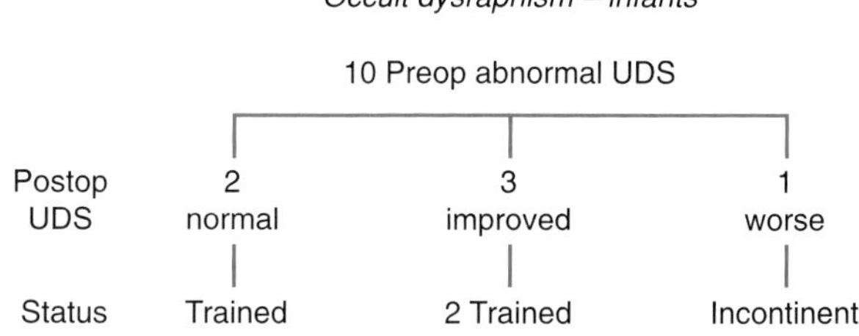

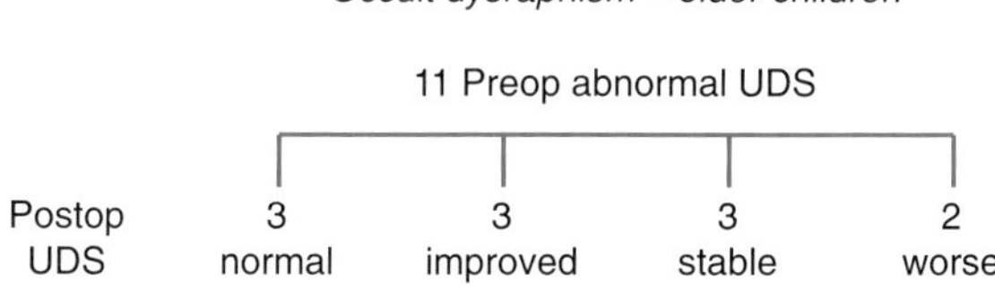

Figure 53.12 Potential for recoverable function is greatest in infants [6/10 (60%)] and less in older children [3/11 (27%)]. The risk of damage to neural tissue at the time of exploration to those with normal function is small [2/19 (11%), not shown]. UDS = urodynamic study.

As a result of these findings, it is apparent that urodynamic testing may be the only way to document that an occult spinal dysraphism is affecting lower spinal cord function.[92,103] Some investigators have shown that posterior tibial somatosensory evoked potentials are an even more sensitive indicator of tethering and should be an integral part of the urodynamic evaluation.[104] The implication of this recommendation is that early detection and intervention are both associated with a reversibility to the lesion that is lost in the older child.[98,101,105,106] and a degree of protection from subsequent tethering, which seems to be a frequent occurrence when the lesion is not dealt with expeditiously in infancy.[107]

Recommendations

Both MRI[108] and urodynamic testing should be conducted in everyone who has a questionable skin or bony abnormality of the lower spine.[109–112] It is the most reliable way to detect a neurologic deficit involving the lumbosacral spinal cord initially, following surgical correction and as a means of predicting and identifying subsequent tethering, which can occur in 10–20% of children.[112]

If the child is younger than 4–6 months of age, ultrasonography may be useful to image the spinal canal before the vertebral bones have had a chance to ossify.[113,114] At this age there is good correlation between the ultrasound and MRI findings, but the latter gives much better definition of the lesion affecting the spinal cord.[115] Thus, ultrasound provides a good screening test, but MRI is the definitive study.

In the past, removing only the superficial skin lesions without dissecting further into the spinal canal to remove or repair the entire abnormality usually treated these conditions. Today, most neurosurgeons advocate laminectomy and removal of the intraspinal process as completely as possible without injuring the nerve roots or cord as soon as feasible after the diagnosis is made. They recommend this in order to release the tethering and to prevent further injury that might ensue with subsequent growth.[88,90,93–95,106]

Sacral agenesis

Sacral agenesis has been defined as absence of part or all of two or more lower vertebral bodies. Although the etiology of this condition is still uncertain, a number of factors have been implicated. Teratogenic factors may play a role in that insulin-dependent mothers have a 1% chance of giving birth to a child with this disorder. In addition, 16% of children with sacral agenesis have a diabetic mother,[116,117] although it may only have been gestational, insulin-dependent diabetes. Sacral agenesis has been reproduced in chicks when exposed as embryos to insulin.[118,119] Maternal insulin–antibody complexes have been noted to cross the placenta, and their concentration in the fetal circulation is directly correlated with macrosomia.[120] It is possible that a similar cause-and-effect phenomenon is occurring in sacral agenesis. Maternal drug exposure, i.e. minoxidil, has been reported to cause sacral agenesis.[121]

In familial cases of sacral agenesis associated with the Currarino syndrome (presacral mass, sacral agenesis, and anorectal malformation), deletions in chromosome 7 (7q) resulting in *HLXB9* genetic mutations have been found.[14] A mutation in *HLXB9*, a homeodomain gene of a 403 amino acid protein which appears to be responsible for neural plate infolding has been identified in 20 of 21 patients with familial and in 2 of 7 sporadic cases of Currarino syndrome.[122,123] Heterozygote carriers within these families have also been identified.[124] Thus, sacral agenesis may represent one point on a spectrum of abnormalities that encompasses sacral meningoceles and anorectal malformations.[125]

Diagnosis

The diagnosis is often delayed until failed attempts at toilet training bring the child to the attention of a physician. Sensation, including perianal dermatomes, is usually intact, and lower extremity function is normal.[126–128] Sacral vertebral bony ossification begins at 15 weeks, so it is possible to detect the abnormality after 18 weeks of gestation by prenatal ultrasonography and then confirm by fetal MRI.[129] Because these children have normal sensation and little or no orthopedic deformity involving the lower extremities (although high arched feet and/or claw or hammer toes may be present), the underlying lesion is often overlooked. In fact, 20% of children escape detection until the age of 3 or 4 years, when parents begin to question their ability to train their child.[117] The only clue, requiring a high index of suspicion, is flattened buttocks and a low short gluteal cleft[130] (Figure 53.13). Palpation of the coccyx will detect the absent vertebrae.[119] The diagnosis is most easily

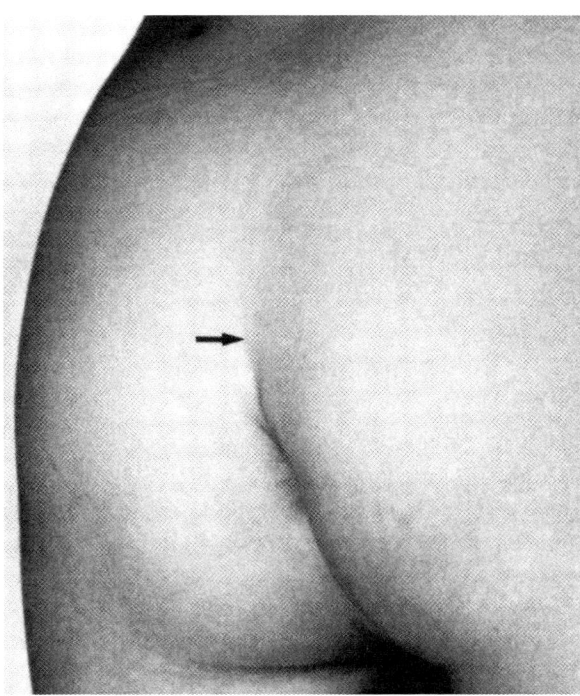

Figure 53.13 Characteristically, the gluteal crease is short and seen only inferiorly (below arrow) as a result of the flattened buttocks in sacral agenesis.

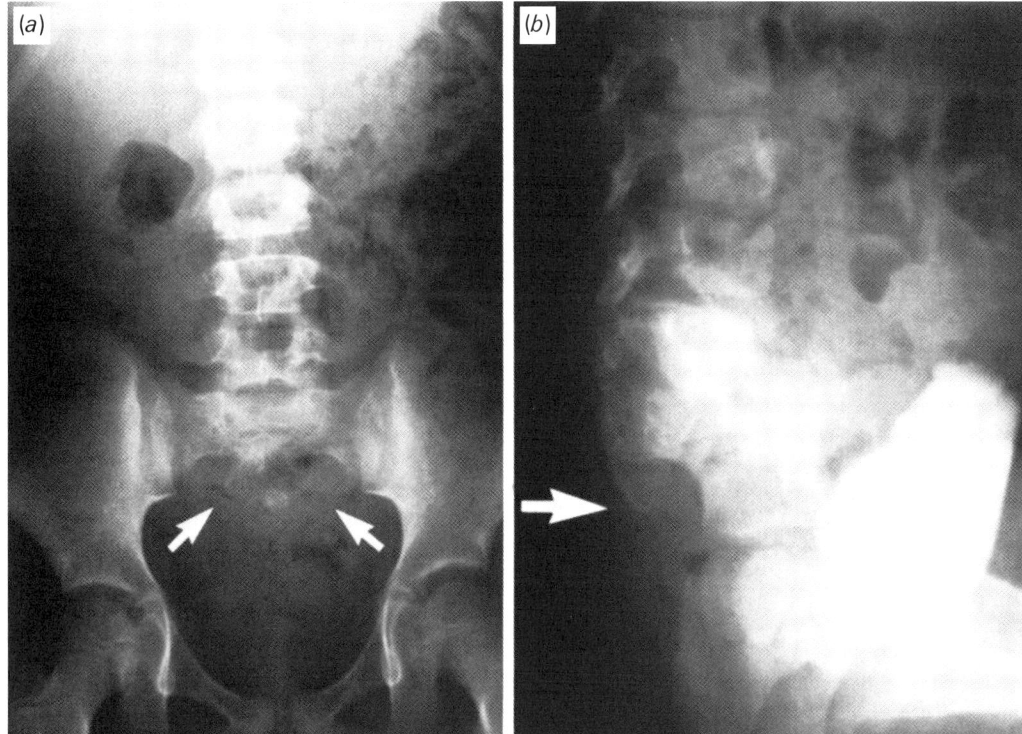

Figure 53.14 The diagnosis is easily confirmed on an anteroposterior (*a*) or lateral (*b*) film of the spine (the latter is performed if bowel gas obscures the sacral area) (arrows).

confirmed with a lateral film of the lower spine, because this area is often obscured by the overlying gas pattern on an anteroposterior projection[117,119] (Figure 53.14). MRI has been used to visualize the spinal cord in these cases, and a sharp cut-off of the conus opposite the T-12 vertebra seems to be a consistent finding[131] (Figure 53.15).

Urodynamic findings

When urodynamic studies are undertaken, almost an equal number of individuals will manifest an upper or lower motor neuron lesion (35% vs 40%, respectively), whereas 25% have no signs of denervation at all.[117] The upper motor neuron lesion is characterized by detrusor hyperreflexia, exaggerated sacral reflexes, absence of voluntary control over sphincter function, detrusor–sphincter dyssynergy, and no electromyographic evidence of denervation potentials in the urethral sphincter.[117,119,126,128] VUR occurs almost exclusively in children with hyperreflexia with or without dyssynergy.[132] A lower motor neuron lesion is noted when detrusor areflexia and partial or complete denervation of the external urethral sphincter with diminished or absent sacral reflexes are seen. The bladder is usually small and smooth-walled, with an open bladder neck a common finding.[132] The number of affected vertebrae does not seem to correlate with the type of motor neuron lesion present (Figure 53.16). The lesion usually appears to be stable and rarely shows signs of progressive denervation.

Recommendations

Management depends on the specific type of neurourologic dysfunction seen on urodynamic testing. Anticholinergic agents should be given to those children with upper motor neuron findings of uninhibited contractions, whereas intermittent catheterization and α-sympathomimetic medication may need to be initiated in individuals with lower motor neuron deficits who can neither empty their bladder nor stay dry between catheterizations. When anticholinergic medication is ineffective in controlling the hyperactive detrusor, augmentation cystoplasty may be required to attain an adequate organ for urinary storage. Failure of α-sympathomimetic agents may require either endoscopic injection of bulking agents or even artificial urinary sphincter implantation to increase bladder outlet resistance. The bowel manifests a similar picture of dysfunction and needs as much characterization and treatment as the lower urinary tract. Anorectal manometry has identified abnormalities in the internal anal sphincter and in vol-

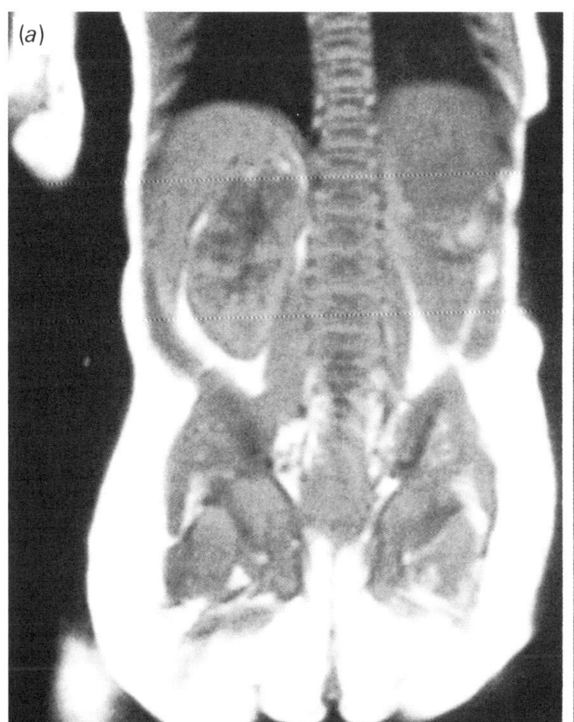

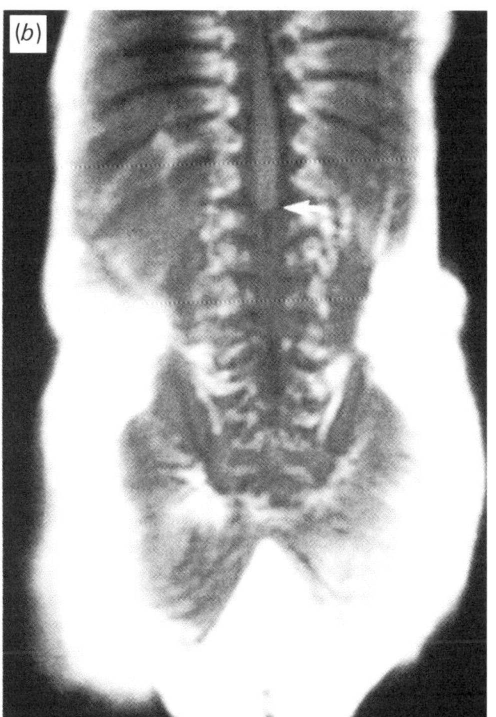

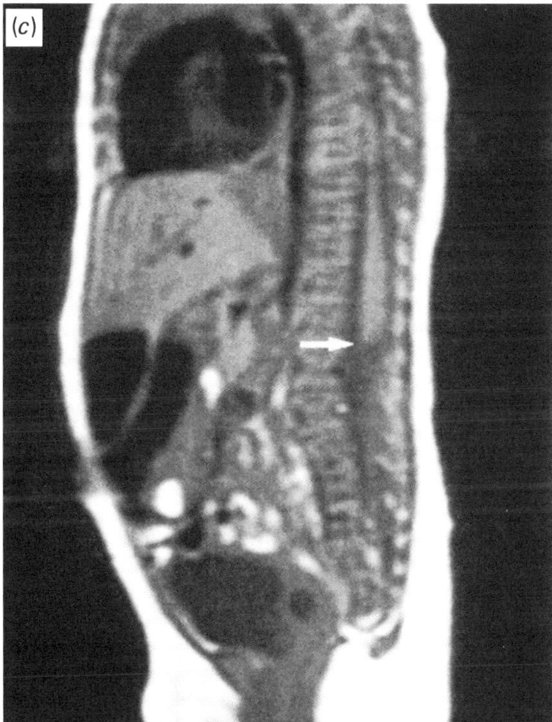

Figure 53.15 Coronal (*a*, left and right) and sagittal (*b*) magnetic resonance images in a 6-month-old girl with sacral agenesis at S-1 reveal a squared lower limit of the cord adjacent to T-12 (arrow). Note a solitary right kidney (*a*, left).

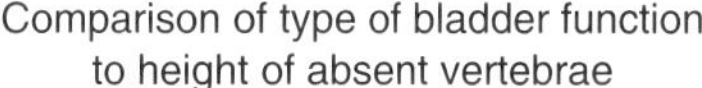

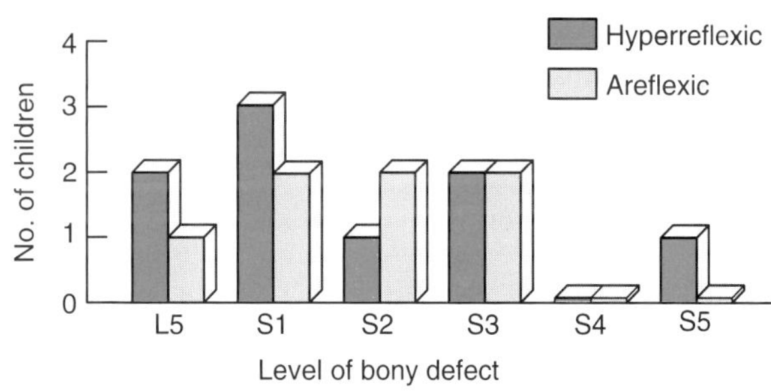

Figure 53.16 Bladder contractility is unrelated to the number of absent vertebrae. (From Bauer.[13])

untary anal sphincter squeeze pressure, leading to weakness of the muscle and concomitant fecal incontinence.[133] It is important to identify these individuals as early as possible so that they can be rendered continent and out of diapers at an appropriate age, thus avoiding the social stigmata of fecal and/or urinary incontinence.

Associated conditions

Imperforate anus

Imperforate anus is a condition that can occur alone or as part of a constellation of anomalies that has been called the VATER or VACTERL syndrome.[134] This mnemonic stands for all of the organs that possibly can be affected (V = vertebral, A = anal, C = cardiac, TE = tracheo-esophageal fistula, R = renal, L = limb). This may be part of a spectrum of hindgut abnormalities that includes sacral agenesis and even a presacral mass or meningocele recently labeled as Currarino syndrome,[123] which has genetic implications.[14] Urinary incontinence is not common unless the spinal cord is involved or the pelvic floor muscles and/or nerves are injured during the imperforate anus repair.[135] A plain film of the abdomen and an ultrasonic image of the spine and kidneys are obtained in the neonatal period in all children regardless of the

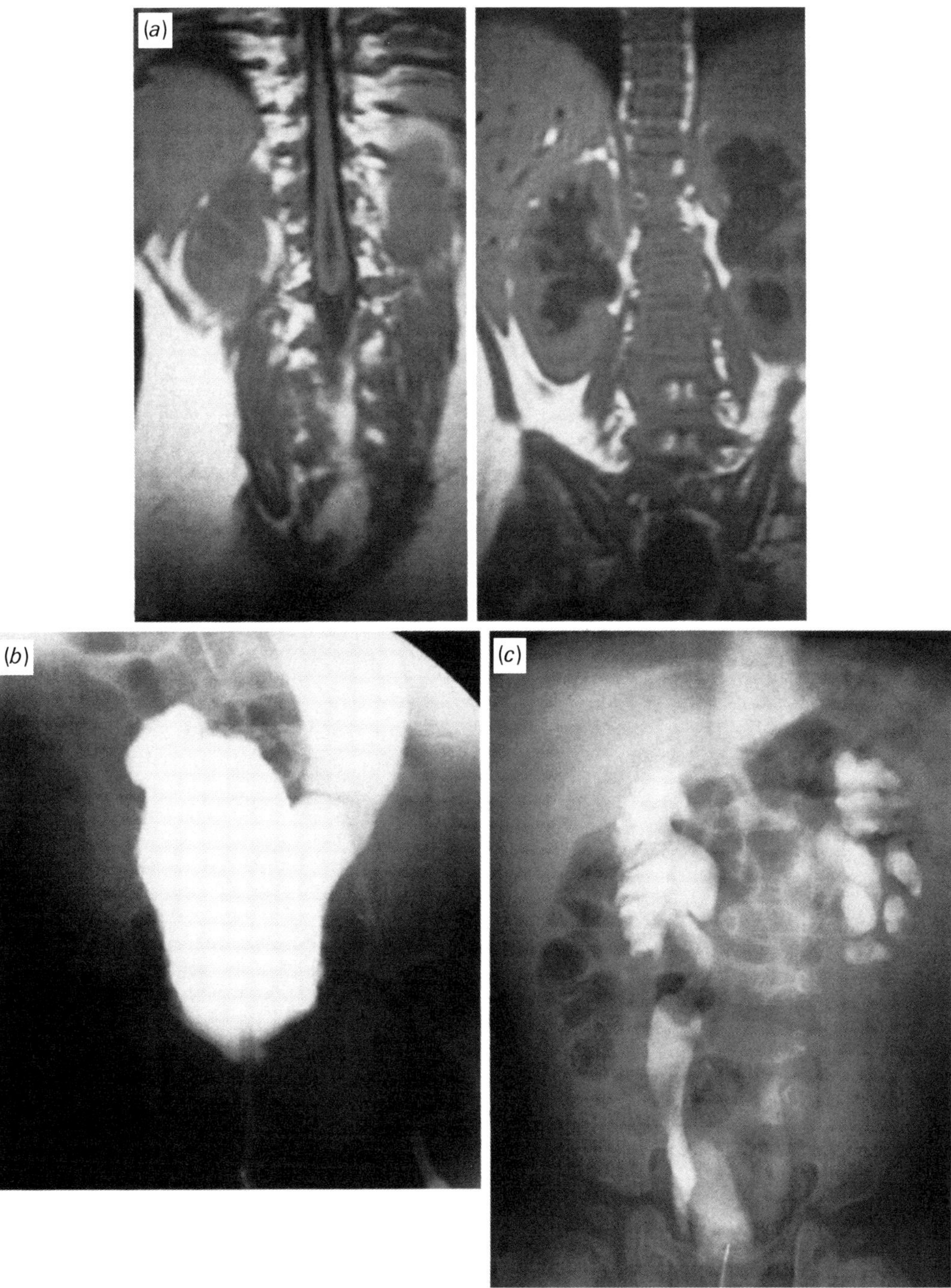

Figure 53.17 (*a*, right and left) This 1-year-old girl with an imperforate anus and bony vertebral abnormalities has bilateral hydronephrosis and a tethered cord on this magnetic resonance imaging scan. (*b*) Her voiding cystourogram reveals significant trabeculation and reflux on the left, whereas her excretory urogram (*c*) demonstrates bilateral hydronephrosis secondary to the reflux on the left and a ureterovesical junction obstruction on the right. Her urodynamic study manifested detrusor hypertonicity and dyssynergy.

level of the rectal atresia, once the child has either stabilized or has had a colostomy performed.[136–138] Vertebral bony anomalies often signify an underlying spinal cord abnormality. Because the vertebral segments have not fully calcified at this time, ultrasonography can readily image the spinal cord. Any hint of an abnormality on these studies or the presence of a lower midline skin lesion overlying the spine warrants an MRI to delineate any pathologic intraspinal process[139] (Figure 53.17). If radiographic images demonstrate an abnormality, urodynamic studies are conducted soon thereafter. Urodynamic studies are also indicated before repair in the child with a high imperforate anus who has undergone an initial colostomy. Abnormal findings may provide a reason to explore and treat any intraspinal abnormality in order to improve the child's chances of becoming continent of both feces and urine. In addition, they furnish a baseline for comparison, especially if incontinence should become a problem in the future, particularly in those children needing extensive surgery for their imperforate anus.

EMG studies of the perianal musculature at this time help to define the optimal location for the future anus. Before the Peña operation, which uses a posterior midline approach, was developed to correct a high imperforate anus, rectal incontinence was thought to be due to an injury involving the pelvic nerves that innervate the levator ani muscles.[140–142] Because the dissection is confined to the midline area, this procedure has reduced the chance of traumatizing the nerve fibers that course laterally and around the bony pelvis from the spine to the urethral and rectal sphincter muscles. Despite careful dissection techniques, 37% of patients still have long-term problems with fecal incontinence.[143] Urodynamic and perianal EMG studies are repeated after the imperforate anus repair, if fecal and/or urinary continence has not been achieved by a reasonable age or if urinary incontinence develops secondarily.

Thirty to 70 percent of these children have a spinal abnormality even though they may not have any other associated anomalies.[144,145] The incidence of neurovesical dysfunction is related to the presence (64%) or absence (31.5%) of a sacral bony defect. Similarly, the level of the anal atresia determines the incidence of bladder dysfunction, with supralevator atresia having a higher risk (70%) than infralevator (35%) lesions.[138] Boemers et al[146] found impaired lower urinary tract function in 24% of 90 children; all but one had a sacral bony abnormality, suggesting an even closer association of dysfunction with abnormal bony spinal development. This abnormality may range from tethering of the spinal cord secondary to an intraspinal dysraphism, which produces an upper motor neuron type of dysfunction involving the bladder and external urethral sphincter, to an atrophic abnormality of the conus medullaris, which leads to a partial or complete lower motor neuron lesion involving the lower urinary tract.[147] In these circumstances, urinary and fecal incontinence might be the child's only complaints. Because lower extremity function may be totally normal, an examination of the legs alone can be misleading.[145] In one review, 20% of children with neuropathic bladder dysfunction and imperforate anus had a normal bony spine, suggesting that postnatal spinal ultrasonography should be performed in all newborns with imperforate anus.[148]

Central nervous system insults

Cerebral palsy

Etiology

Cerebral palsy is a non-progressive injury to the brain in the perinatal period that produces a neuromuscular disability or a specific symptom complex of cerebral dysfunction. Its incidence is approximately 1.5 per 1000 births but may be increasing as more smaller and younger premature infants are surviving in intensive care units. It is usually due to a perinatal infection or period of anoxia (or hypoxia) that affects the CNS.[149,150] It most commonly appears in babies who were premature, but it may be seen following a seizure, infection, or intracranial hemorrhage in the neonatal period.

Diagnosis

Affected children have delayed gross motor development, abnormal fine motor performance, altered muscle tone, abnormal stress gait, and exaggerated deep tendon reflexes. These findings can vary substantially from being very obvious to exquisitely subtle with no discernible lesion present unless a careful neurologic examination is performed. Among the more overtly affected individuals, spastic diplegia is the most common of the five types of dysfunction that characterize this disease, accounting for nearly two-thirds of the cases.

Findings

Most children with cerebral palsy develop total urinary control. Incontinence is a feature in some, but

Table 53.5 Lower urinary tract function in cerebral palsy[a]

Type of dysfunction	No. (%)
Upper motor neuron lesion	49 (86)
Mixed upper and lower motor neuron lesion	5 (9)
Incomplete lower motor neuron lesion	1 (2)
No urodynamic lesion	2 (3.5)

[a] The study comprised 57 children.

the exact incidence has never been truly determined.[151,152] In a recent survey of questionnaires sent to over 600 families with an affected child aged 4–18 years, 23.5% had persistent urinary incontinence.[153] When urinary continence was achieved, its development was delayed when compared with normal children of similar age. With further analysis of the data, 80% of children with spastic diplegia, 54% with tetraplegia, and 38% with low intellectual capacity attained continence. The presence of incontinence was related in part to the extent of the physical impairment because the physical handicap prevents the individuals from reaching the toilet before they have an episode of wetting. If the children are intellectually handicapped they either do not recognize the need to void or relate this fact to caregivers early enough to be toileted.[153] Some children have such a severe degree of mental retardation that they are not trainable, but the majority have sufficient intelligence to learn basic societal protocol with patient and persistent handling. Continence is achievable, albeit at a later than expected age, with diurnal continence being attained first and nocturnal continence occurring within the subsequent year.[153] Therefore, urodynamic evaluation is reserved for children who appear trainable and do not seem to be hampered too much by their physical impairment, but who have not achieved continence by later childhood or early puberty.

One review of urodynamic studies, performed in 57 children with cerebral palsy (Table 53.5),[152] revealed that 49 (86%) of the children presented with the expected picture of a partial upper motor neuron lesion type of dysfunction, with exaggerated sacral reflexes, detrusor hyperreflexia, and/or detrusor–sphincter dyssynergia (Figure 53.18), even though they manifested voluntary control over voiding. Six of the 57 (11%), however, had evidence of both upper and lower motor neuron denervation with detrusor areflexia and/or abnormal motor unit potentials on sphincter EMG assessment (Table 53.6). When their

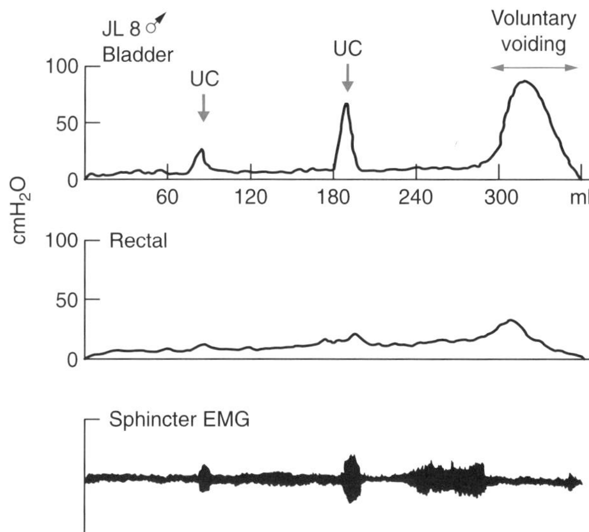

Figure 53.18 An 8-year-old boy with spastic diplegia has a typical partial upper motor neuron lesion-type bladder with uninhibited contractions (UCs) associated with increased sphincter activity but normal voiding dynamics at capacity. Wetting is due to these contractions when unaccompanied by the heightened sphincter activity. EMG = electromyography. (From Bauer.[13])

records were analyzed on a retrospective basis, most of the children who exhibited these latter findings had experienced an episode of cyanosis in the perinatal period (Table 53.7). Thus, a lower motor neuron lesion may be seen in addition to the expected upper motor neuron dysfunction.

In a more recent review of 29 children with cerebral palsy undergoing urodynamic studies,[154] including 23 who had incontinence and/or urinary infection and six who were asymptomatic, urodynamic studies demonstrated poor compliance in 21 of the 23 symp-

Table 53.6 Urodynamic findings in cerebral palsy[a]

Finding	Number
Upper motor neuron	
Uninhibited contractions	35
Detrusor–sphincter dyssynergy	7
Hyperactive sacral reflexes	6
No voluntary control	3
Small-capacity bladder	2
Hypertonia	2
Lower motor neuron	
Excessive polyphasia	5
Increased amplitude and increased duration potentials	4

[a] The study comprised 57 children; some children exhibited more than one finding.

Table 53.7 Perinatal risk factors in cerebral palsy

Factor	UMN	LMN
Prematurity	10	1
Respiratory distress/arrest/apnea	9	2
Neonatal seizures	5	
Infection	5	
Traumatic birth	5	
Congenital hydrocephalus	3	
Placenta previa/abruption	2	2
Hypoglycemia with or without seizures	2	
Intracranial hemorrhage	2	
Cyanosis at birth	1	3
No specific factor noted	15	

UMN = upper motor neuron lesion; LMN = lower motor neuron lesion.

tomatic and two of the six asymptomatic children. In the same study, uninhibited contractions were found in all symptomatic and five of six asymptomatic children, and high leak point pressure in 16 of 23 and four of six symptomatic and asymptomatic children, respectively. VCUG revealed bladder trabeculation in 58% and VUR in 9% of symptomatic, and trabeculation in 50% but no reflux in asymptomatic children. In a meta-analysis of all published reports of urodynamic findings in children with cerebral palsy, detrusor overactivity was seen in 80%, dyssynergy between the bladder and sphincter in 5%, and normal function in only 12%.[152,154–156] From these reports it is apparent that urodynamic studies can be very revealing in all children, whether or not they have urinary symptoms,[154] but are especially useful if frequent toileting or initial anticholinergic treatment fails to improve incontinence, the child develops urinary infection, or renal ultrasonography reveals hydronephrosis.

Recommendations

Treatment usually centers around abolishing the uninhibited contractions with anticholinergic medication, but residual urine volume must be monitored closely to ensure complete evacuation with each void. Intermittent catheterization may be required for those who cannot empty their bladders. Selective dorsal sacral rhizotomy has helped with spasticity and incontinence, with only <5% developing incontinence if careful mapping of dorsal sacral nerve roots is identified.[157,158]

Traumatic injuries to the spine

Despite the exposure and potential for a traumatic spinal cord injury, this condition is rarely encountered in children; the incidence in Sweden is 2.6 cases per million children per year.[159] When an injury does occur, it is most likely to happen as a result of a motor vehicle accident (24–52%), a gunshot wound, or a diving incident.[159–162] Infants are more prone to an injury from a motor vehicle accident (71%), toddlers and children secondary to a fall (48% and 34%, respectively), and adolescents due to a sport-related event (29%).[161] It has also occurred iatrogenically following surgery to correct scoliosis, kyphosis, or other intraspinal problems as well as congenital aortic arch anomalies or patent ductus arteriosus.[160,163] Newborns are particularly prone to hyperextension injuries during a high forceps delivery.[164,165] The lower urinary tract dysfunction that ensues is not likely to be an isolated event but, rather, is usually associated with loss of sensation and paralysis of the lower limbs. Radiologic investigation of the spine may not reveal any bony abnormality, even though momentary subluxation of osseous structures due to the high elasticity of vertebral ligaments can result in a neurologic injury.[166] This has been labeled spinal cord injury without radiologic abnormality or SCIWORA, and can account for up to 38% of spinal cord injuries in children.[162] Myelography and computed tomography (CT) will show swelling of the cord below the level of the lesion, central disk herniation, spinal stenosis, or contusion.[164,165,167] Often, what appears initially as a permanent lesion turns out instead to be a transient phenomenon. Although sensation and motor function in the lower extremities may be restored relatively soon, the dysfunction involving the bladder and rectum may persist for a considerable period.

If urinary retention occurs immediately following the injury, an indwelling Foley catheter is passed into the bladder and left in place for as short a period of time as possible, until intermittent catheterization can be started safely on a regular basis.[168,169] When the child starts voiding again, the timing of catheterization can be such that it is used as a means of measuring the residual urine volume after a spontaneous void. Residual urine volumes of 25 ml or less are considered safe enough to allow for a reduction in the frequency and even cessation of the catheterization program.[169] If there is no improvement in urinary tract function after 4–6 weeks, urodynamic studies are conducted to determine whether or not this condition is the result of spinal shock or actual nerve root or spinal cord injury. Detrusor areflexia is not uncommon under these circumstances.[170] EMG recording of the sphincter often reveals normal motor units without fibrillation potentials, but absent sacral reflexes and a non-relaxing sphincter with bladder filling, a sign that transient spinal shock has occurred.[170] The outcome from this condition is guarded but good, inasmuch as most cases resolve completely as edema of the cord in response to the injury subsides, leaving no permanent damage.[170,171]

Most permanent traumatic injuries involve either the upper thoracic or cervical spinal cord, but some affect the cauda equina region. The sacral cord injury most likely produces a lower motor neuron deficit of the striated sphincter that usually leads to low-pressure bladder emptying with little risk of upper urinary tract deterioration. However, it probably necessitates medical and/or surgical therapy to achieve continence. On the other hand, upper spinal cord injuries produce an upper motor neuron-type lesion with detrusor hyperreflexia and detrusor–sphincter dyssynergia. The potential danger from this outflow obstruction is obvious.[172] Substantial residual urine volumes, detrusor hypertonicity, high voiding pressure, high-pressure reflux, urinary infections, and their sequelae are the leading cause of long-term morbidity and mortality in spinal cord-injured patients. Urodynamic studies will identify those patients at risk.[169] Even if the child is continent and voiding to completion or requires intermittent catheterization to empty, it is imperative to measure detrusor compliance, the presence of hyperreflexia, and actual voiding pressures (if appropriate) to determine the potential risk for hydroureteronephrosis and/or reflux.[173] Early identification and proper management may prevent the signs and effects of bladder outlet obstruction before they become apparent on X-ray examination of the urinary tract.[174–176]

Functional voiding disorders

Urinary incontinence is defined by the ICCS as the uncontrolled leakage of urine; it can be continuous or intermittent, occurring during the daytime or nighttime. Continuous incontinence means leakage of urine all the time and denotes the probability of an ectopic ureter. It is abnormal at any age because even infants have a degree of cortical control over bladder emptying, void in reasonably spaced intervals, and stay dry between voidings. Daytime or diurnal incontinence may be on an urgent or sudden basis, associated with stress activity such as coughing or running, or occur just after voiding (only in girls, resulting from the vaginal trapping of urine during voiding that drips out afterwards). Nocturnal incontinence or enuresis means the leakage of urine while asleep at an age when urinary control is expected. It is difficult, however, to say when this should occur. Studies of large groups of children have provided some guidelines for expectations, but there are no absolute milestones for the individual child.[177,178] Girls tend to become trained before boys, and daytime continence is achieved before nighttime control. It is rare to achieve control before 18 months of age.[179] Thereafter, urinary control is gained by approximately 20% of children for each year of life up to 4.5 years, with a smaller percentage of the population attaining complete continence every year after that. By the age of 10, about 5% of children still have some nocturnal wetting, but this diminishes to 2% after puberty.[180] Recently, evidence has come to light that there may be a genetic basis for the development of urinary control.[181–183]

The evaluation of the incontinent child begins with a comprehensive history. The history includes details of any family history of enuresis, the mother's pregnancy, including the presence of maternal insulin-dependent diabetes mellitus, stage of gestation at the time of delivery, Apgar scores at birth, or difficulties occurring peri- or early postnatally, and developmental milestones such as school performance. History of fine and gross motor incoordination, previous continence, social setting and sibling interaction, parental expectations, and characterization of the wetting episodes are also important. If there is a suspicion of an ectopic ureter in a girl (normal voiding, but constant dampness), then renal and bladder ultrasonography is performed. Boys who have a question of bladder outflow obstruction (urgency or urge incontinence with enuresis beyond the age of 5 years) are evaluated by voiding cystography. One group of clinicians has developed a comprehensive questionnaire that accurately identifies and quantifies children with abnormal voiding patterns and has been used successfully in determining responses to therapy.[184] The indications for performing urodynamic studies are as follows: any suspicion of a neurologic condition, diurnal incontinence with no associated pathology, fecal and urinary incontinence at any age, persistent voiding difficulties long after a urinary infection has been treated, recurrent urinary infection despite continuous antibiotics, and bladder trabeculation and/or 'sphincter spasm' on VCUG (Figure 53.19).

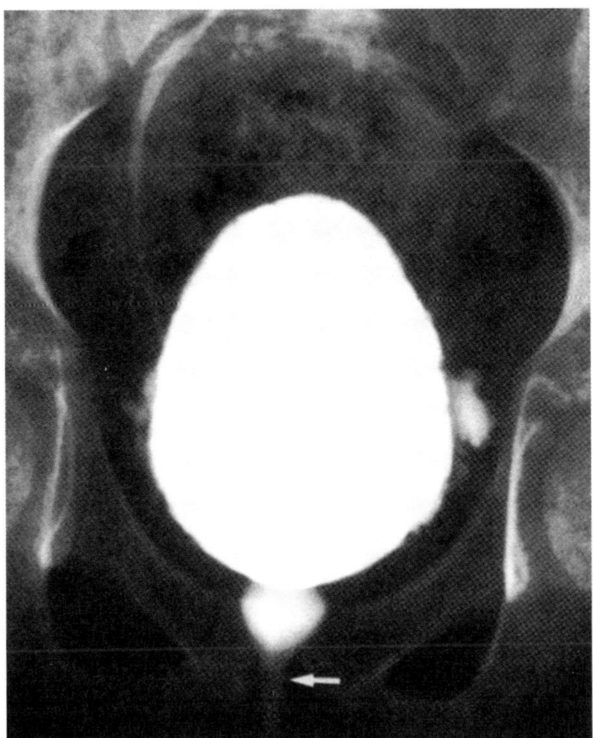

Figure 53.19 This 10-year-old girl with recurrent urinary tract infections has spasm of the sphincter during voiding, with narrowing in the distal urethra, demonstrated on this voiding cystourethrogram (arrow). Note grade II/V right-sided reflux.

When urodynamic studies are performed on a group of children who have these findings without an obvious systemic neurologic disorder, a spectrum of voiding pattern abnormalities emerges:[185]

- small-capacity bladder
- detrusor overactivity
- infrequent voider–lazy bladder syndrome
- psychological non-neuropathic bladder (Hinman syndrome).

Classification and a detailed description of these disorders help one to understand and treat each condition specifically.

Small-capacity hypertonic bladder

Children with recurrent urinary infection without an anatomic abnormality may have symptoms of voiding dysfunction, including frequency, urgency, urge incontinence, staccato or intermittent voiding, nocturia and/or enuresis, and dysuria, long after the infection has cleared. Sometimes, persistence of these symptoms with their associated abnormal voiding dynamics can lead to repeated infections.[186]

An inflammatory reaction in the bladder wall may produce an irritability that affects the sensory threshold and increases the need to void sooner than anticipated. If the detrusor muscle is affected as well, the increased irritability may lead to overactivity of the muscle and eventually to poor compliance.[155] When children attempt to hold back urination because it is either painful or inappropriate to void, they may actually tighten or only partially or intermittently relax the external sphincter muscle during voiding. This retention may result in a functional outflow obstruction that disrupts the laminar flow pattern that normally exists[186–188] (Figure 53.20). This stop-and-start (staccato) voiding (Figure 53.21) is a prominent pattern of dysfunction in girls leading to recurrent infection[189] because bacteria can be carried back up into the bladder from the meatus as a result of the 'milk-back' phenomenon occurring within the urethra when urination is interrupted in this manner.[190] Theoretically, if unrecognized or left untreated in young girls, this may become the forerunner of interstitial cystitis seen in many adult females and may even be the precursor of prostatitis in males.

Radiologic investigation often reveals a normal upper urinary tract, but the bladder may be small and have varying degrees of trabeculation on excretory urography or a thickened wall on ultrasonography.[185,191] During the voiding phase of cystourethrography, the posterior urethra may show signs of intermittent dilatation at its upper end, with a uniform narrowing occurring toward the external

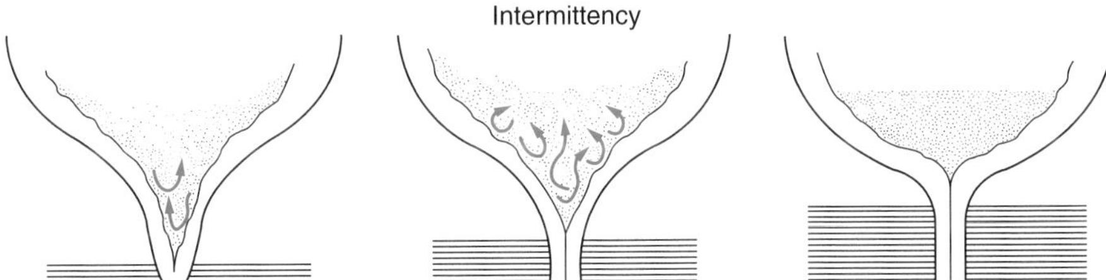

Figure 53.20 Non-laminar flow secondary to periodic tightening and relaxation of the external sphincter leads to eddy current and the 'milk-back' phenomenon, which can carry bacteria colonized at the urethral meatus up into the bladder and cause infection of the residual urine.

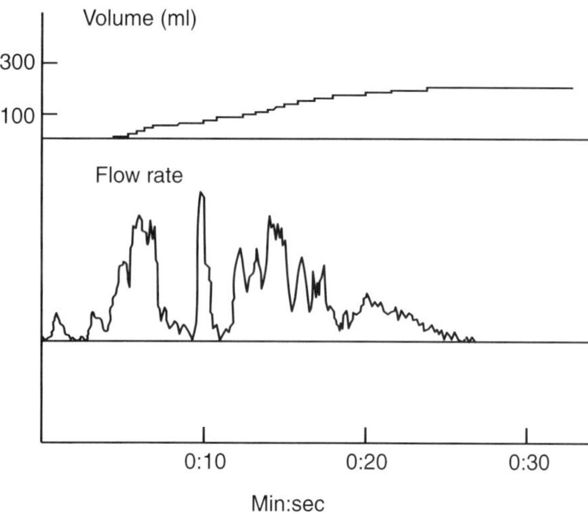

Figure 53.21 Staccato voiding is seen in this 8-year-old girl with recurrent infection.

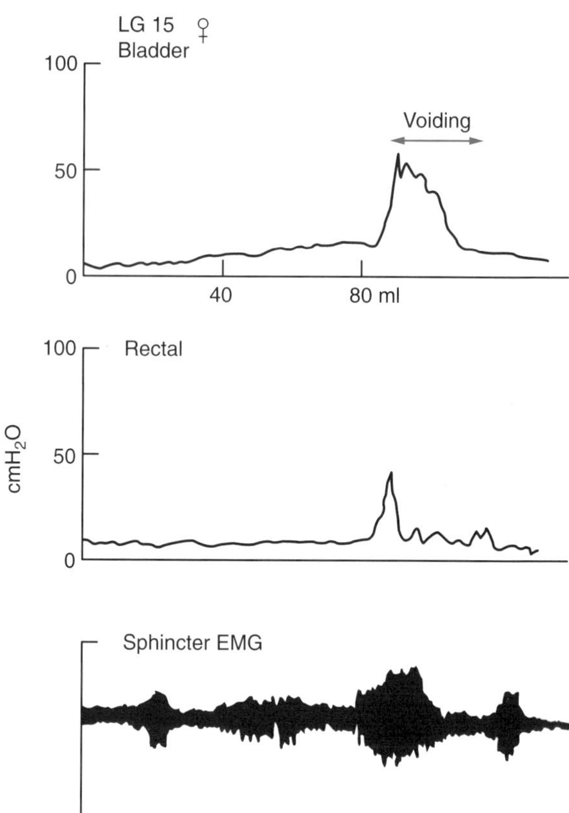

Figure 53.22 This urodynamic picture in a teenage female with recurrent infections reveals a small-capacity bladder and a hypertonic sphincter that relaxes only partially during voiding. EMG = electromyography.

sphincter region. In girls, this 'spinning-top' deformity has raised the question of an obstructed meatus[187,188] (see Figure 53.19), whereas in boys, it has often been mistaken for posterior urethral valves. This appearance is due to failure of complete relaxation of the external sphincter and persistence of a relative obstruction at the distal end of the posterior urethra in an attempt by the child to suppress voiding[192] and has no correlations with meatal size.

Urodynamic studies demonstrate a bladder of small capacity (when adjusted for age) and elevated detrusor pressure during filling[185,188] (Figure 53.22). At capacity, the child has an uncontrolled urge to void that may not be suppressed despite tightly contracting the external sphincter. The bladder contraction is usually sustained, with pressures reaching higher than normal values. Emptying may not always be complete despite these high pressures. The baseline sphincter EMG activity is normal at rest, but there may be complex repetitive discharges (pseudomyotonia)[193] or periodic relaxation of the muscle during filling, contributing to the sense of urgency or actual incontinent episodes. During a voluntary void, the sphincter may relax intermittently or even completely at first, but then contract in response to discomfort, preventing complete emptying[186,194] (see Figure 53.22).

Treatment is based on trying to eliminate the recurrent infections, minimize any possible environmental influences that predispose the individual to infection, and improve the child's voiding pattern and bathroom habits. Girls should learn to take showers instead of baths, or at least to bathe alone without other siblings, wipe from front to back, try to completely relax when they void so that a steady stream is produced, and take the time to empty completely each time they urinate.[186] Biofeedback training to teach these children to relax the sphincter when they void has been used with success.[195–198] In addition to antibiotics, antispasmodic/anticholinergic agents are administered for periods ranging from 6 to 9 months.

Detrusor overactivity

Children with long-standing symptoms of daytime frequency, urgency, or sudden incontinence and squatting, in addition to nocturia and/or enuresis, may have detrusor overactivity. Vincent's curtsy, a characteristic posturing by these children in an attempt to prevent voiding, is a commonly described behavior pattern.[199,200] One or more of the child's parents or siblings often have a history of delayed control over micturition. These affected family members may compensate for their own abnormality by displaying continued daytime frequency or nocturia, or both. Although the child's physical examination may be normal, hyperactive deep tendon reflexes in the lower and/or upper extremities, tight heel cords, ankle clonus, posturing with a stress gait, or difficulty with tandem walking, and mirror movements (similar motion in the contralateral hand when the individual is asked rapidly to pronate and supinate one hand) may be evident. Left-handedness, left-footedness, or left-eyedness in a family in which all other members are right-handed may signify crossed dominance from a previously unrecognized perinatal insult. Attention deficit disorders, poor writing ability and/or incoordination, and learning difficulties are more commonly encountered in these children as well.[201,202] Carefully questioning parents about perinatal events or reviewing birth history records may uncover such an insult that has affected the CNS system and caused these findings. The DVSS or dysfunctional voiding symptom score devised by the group in Toronto has been successfully used in identifying and treating children with subtle effects of such insults.[184]

X-ray evaluation usually reveals no abnormality other than a mildly trabeculated or thick-walled bladder. Urodynamic studies demonstrate premature contractions of the bladder during filling, which the child may or may not sense and/or abolish by increasing the activity of the external urethral sphincter[185,194] (see Figure 53.18). Alternatively, periodic relaxation of the sphincter, the initial phase of an uninhibited contraction, that leads to a sense of urgency or to an episode of leaking, may be the only clue to an overactive bladder (Figure 53.23). During filling, capacity may be reached sooner than expected, at which time

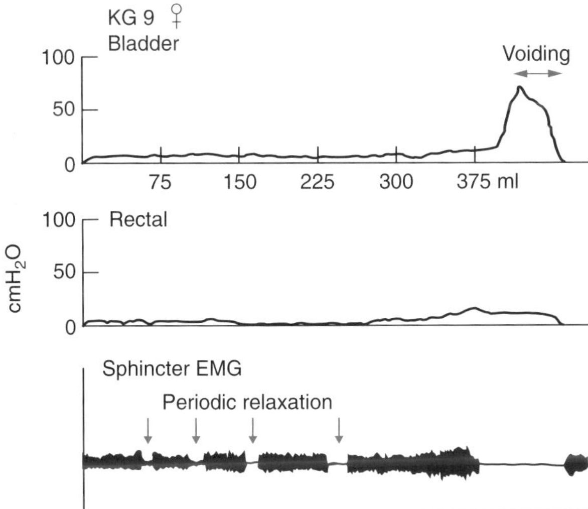

Figure 53.23 Some children only manifest periodic relaxation of the sphincter without a rise in detrusor pressure as an early phase of a hyperreflexic bladder producing urgency and incontinence. EMG = electromyography.

a normal detrusor contraction occurs with a sustained relaxation of the sphincter, resulting in complete emptying. Some children will not be able to suppress this contraction even though the bladder has not been filled to its intended capacity. Sometimes, detrusor overactivity may only be elicited following a cough or strain, or when the child assumes a change in posture.[200] The overactivity is thought to be responsible for the symptoms.[203]

These findings may be the result of a cerebral insult, however mild, in the neonatal (or even prenatal) period, but they are linked more commonly to delayed maturation of the reticulospinal pathways and the inhibitory centers in the midbrain and cerebral cortex. Thus, total control over vesicourethral function may be lacking.[179,180,204] Several investigators have found a similar urodynamic picture in a significant number of adults with nocturnal enuresis and/or daytime symptoms.[205] Parents who exhibit the same behavior pattern as their children may have a genetically determined delayed rate of CNS maturation.[182]

On occasion, children with profound constipation develop detrusor overactivity that leads to urinary incontinence.[206] The etiology of this condition is unclear, but treatment of the bowel distention has resulted in a dramatic improvement in the bladder dysfunction.[207]

Sometimes, repeated urinary infection may produce an identical urodynamic picture. Detrusor overactivity occurs as a result of the inflammatory response in the bladder wall that irritates the receptors located in the submucosa and/or detrusor muscle layers.[208] Therefore, these children should be screened for infection. It has been postulated that an overactive detrusor may lead to inappropriate voiding. The child realizes what is happening, and tightens the sphincter to reverse this process, which shuts the distal urethra first and the bladder neck second, causing the 'milk-back' phenomenon and the potential for urinary infection, as presented in the previous discussion, to occur.[190,208]

Anticholinergic medications alone or in combination have been used successfully to manage this condition.[200] Oxybutynin has been highly successful with tolterodine somewhat less so, primarily due to underdosing, but the latter is better tolerated than the former and constipation is less of an issue.[209,210] Recently, biofeedback training using computer technology has been employed successfully in achieving continence and in reducing the need for medication in children refractory to anticholinergic medication.[196–198,211] If infection is present, it should be eradicated and antibacterial prophylaxis should be employed.[155,185,212–214]

The infrequent voider–lazy bladder syndrome

Most children urinate four or five times per day, and defecate daily or at least every other day. Some children, primarily girls, may void only twice a day, once in the morning (either at home or after they are in school), and again at night.[215] It is not uncommon to find children who do not void at all while in school. These children exhibited normal voiding patterns as infants, but after toilet training, they learned to withhold micturition for extended periods. As a result, a few develop a fear of strange bathrooms or mimic their mother's pattern of infrequent urination and defecation.[185] Others have experienced an aversive event or had an infection associated with dysuria around the time of training, which led to the infrequent pattern of micturition. Some children are excessively neat or have a fetish for cleanliness that causes them to avoid bathrooms. Often, they only void enough to relieve the pressure to urinate and do not empty their bladder completely. The decrepit conditions in many school bathrooms predispose children, mainly girls, to limit the number of times that they use these facilities during the school day; consequently, they become infrequent voiders all of the time.

The infrequent voiding and incomplete emptying produce an ever-increasing bladder capacity and a diminished stimulus to urinate.[190] The chronically distended bladder is at risk for urinary infection and/or overflow or stress incontinence. Sometimes, these signs are the first manifestations of the abnormal voiding pattern. When the child is carefully questioned, the aberrant micturition is easily detected. More often, the problem is diagnosed following VCUG or radionuclide cystography performed for an assessment of urinary tract infection. A larger than normal capacity (for age) and/or a high residual urine volume on initial catheterization is noted. When the child is questioned about voiding habits, this infrequent pattern of elimination is detected[190] (Figure 53.24). The cystogram, however, usually reveals a smooth-walled bladder without reflux.

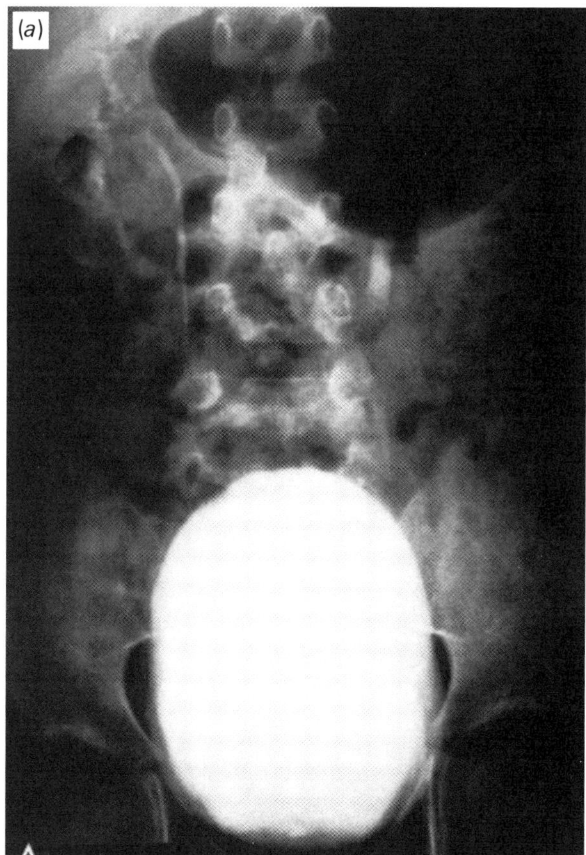

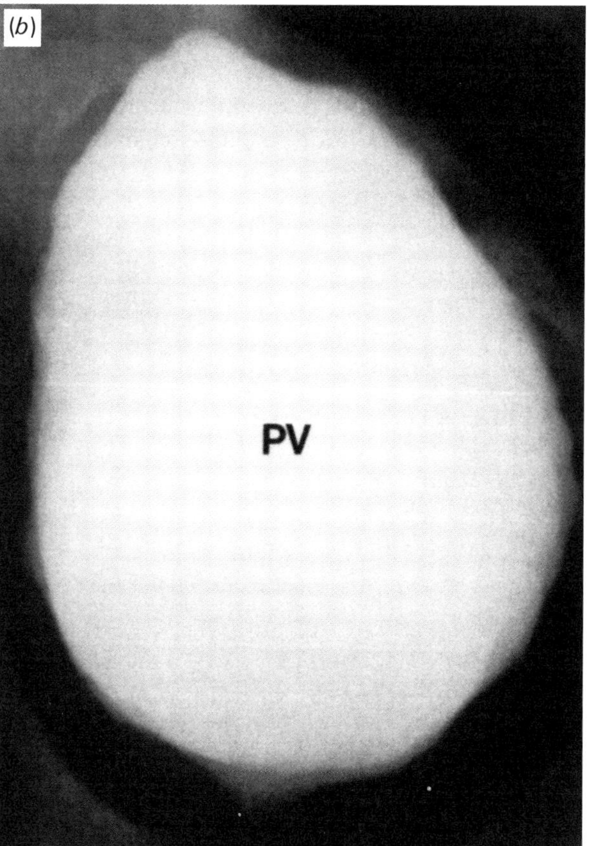

Figure 53.24 (*a*) Excretory urogram in a girl who urinates infrequently, demonstrates a large-capacity bladder with a normal upper urinary tract. (*b*) Her postvoiding (PV) residual is quite large.

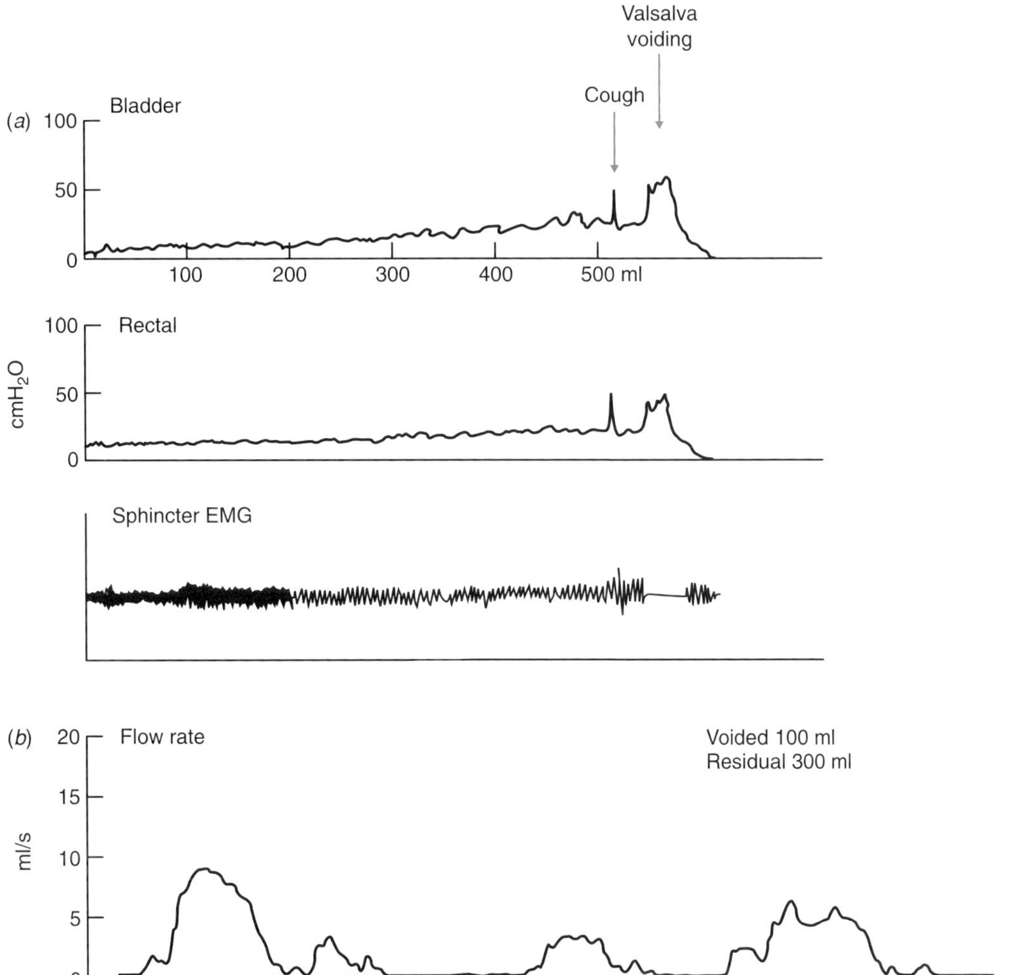

Figure 53.25 (*a*) Urodynamic evaluation reveals a very large-capacity, low-pressure bladder. The girl empties entirely by straining after relaxing the sphincter with no apparent detrusor contraction. EMG = electromyography. (*b*) Her intermittent urinary flow rate is characteristic of this effort to empty and leads to a considerable volume of residual urine.

Urodynamic studies demonstrate a very large-capacity, highly compliant bladder with either normal, unsustained, or absent detrusor contractions[185] (Figure 53.25a). Straining to void is a common form of emptying. Sphincter EMG reveals normal motor unit potentials at rest and normal responses to various sacral reflexes, bladder filling, and attempts at emptying. The urinary flow rate may be intermittent, with sudden peaks coinciding with straining, or it may be normal but short lived, secondary to an unsustained detrusor contraction.[190] Unless strongly encouraged, the child will not completely empty the bladder during voiding[185] (Figure 53.25b). This picture is consistent with myogenic failure from chronic distention.[216]

Changing the child's voiding habits is the first approach to therapy.[217] Keeping to a rigid schedule of toileting and encouraging children to empty each time they void are mandatory.[195] Behavioral therapy techniques to encourage compliance are helpful. Rarely, intermittent catheterization may be necessary to allow the detrusor muscle to regain its contractility and ability to empty.[218] Antibiotics are needed when urinary infection is present and are continued until the voiding pattern improves.

Psychological non-neuropathic bladder (Hinman syndrome)

Hinman[219] described an apparent 'syndrome' of voiding dysfunction that mimics neuropathic bladder disease but may be a learned disorder. At first, this syndrome was believed to be caused by an isolated neurologic lesion,[220–222] but now it is felt to be an acquired abnormality.[185,219,223,224] It is produced by an active contraction of the sphincter during voiding, creating a degree of outflow obstruction. Some investigators think that this phenomenon may be the result of persistence of the transitional phase of gaining control in which the child learns to prevent voiding by voluntarily contracting the external urethral sphincter.[194,223] Others believe that this pattern results from the child's normal response to uninhibited contractions.[203] This behavior becomes habitual because the child has difficulty in distinguishing between involuntary and voluntary voiding; as a consequence, the inappropriate sphincter activity occurs all the time.[185] Jayanthi et al[225] reported similar findings in a group of younger children, newborn to 30 months of age and Bauer et al[226] noted these same findings in five newborns and children under 1 year of age. All were managed by either vesicostomy, urinary diversion, or intermittent catheterization, with spontaneous improvement after vesicostomy closure or urinary undiversion in some.

In general, the children have urgency, urge and/or stress incontinence, infrequent voluntary voiding, intermittent urination associated with straining, recurrent urinary infection, and irregular bowel movements, with fecal soiling in between.[185] Most striking is the similarity in the pattern of family dynamics that is disclosed on carefully observing and questioning.[224] The Hinman syndrome has been applied to many children with any degree of voiding dysfunction, but it should only be diagnosed as such when many of the following conditions are present:

1 Clinical features:
   - day and night wetting
   - encopresis/constipation/impaction
   - recurrent urinary tract infections
   - parental characteristics
     - domineering/exacting
     - divorce
     - alcoholism
     - punishments (mental and physical) inflicted for wetting
   - previous surgery
     - ureteral reimplantation
     - bladder neck plasty
     - diversion.

2 Radiologic features:
   - hydronephrosis, with or without pyelonephritis
   - reflux: III/V in degree
   - large-capacity, trabeculated bladder
   - large residual urine volume
   - posterior urethra sometimes dilated with narrowing at external sphincter
   - heavily loaded colon.

3 Urodynamic features:
   - elevated detrusor filling and voiding pressures
   - ineffective detrusor contractions
   - high resting sphincter EMG
   - unsustained sphincter relaxation during voiding
   - large residual volume.

4 Treatment (individualized):
   - bladder retraining
     - behavioral modification
     - double voiding
     - biofeedback techniques for sphincter relaxation
     - intermittent catheterization
   - drugs
     - oxybutynin
     - tolterodine
     - trospium
     - glycopyrrolate
     - flavoxate
     - bethanechol
     - prazosin
     - diazepam
     - α blockers
   - bowel reregulation program
     - stool softeners
     - bulking agents
     - laxatives, enemas.

The parents, especially the father, tend to be domineering, exacting, unyielding, and intolerant of weakness or failure. Divorce and alcoholism are common threads that only exacerbate the situation. Wetting is perceived as immature, defiant, and/or purposeful behavior that the parents feel must be counteracted with stern reprimands. The children are often punished, both mentally and physically, for their ineptness. Confusion, depression, and withdrawal for fear of wetting with its added punitive response become the children's prevalent attitudes because they do not know how to, nor can they prevent this provocative behavior. They try to withhold urination and defecation further by keeping the sphincter muscle tight, aggravating the situation. Thus, wetting becomes more commonplace, and abdominal pain from chronic constipation is likely.

X-ray evaluation reveals profound changes within the urinary tract. Hydroureteronephrosis with or without pyelonephritic scarring from recurrent infection occurs in two-thirds of the children[185] (Figure

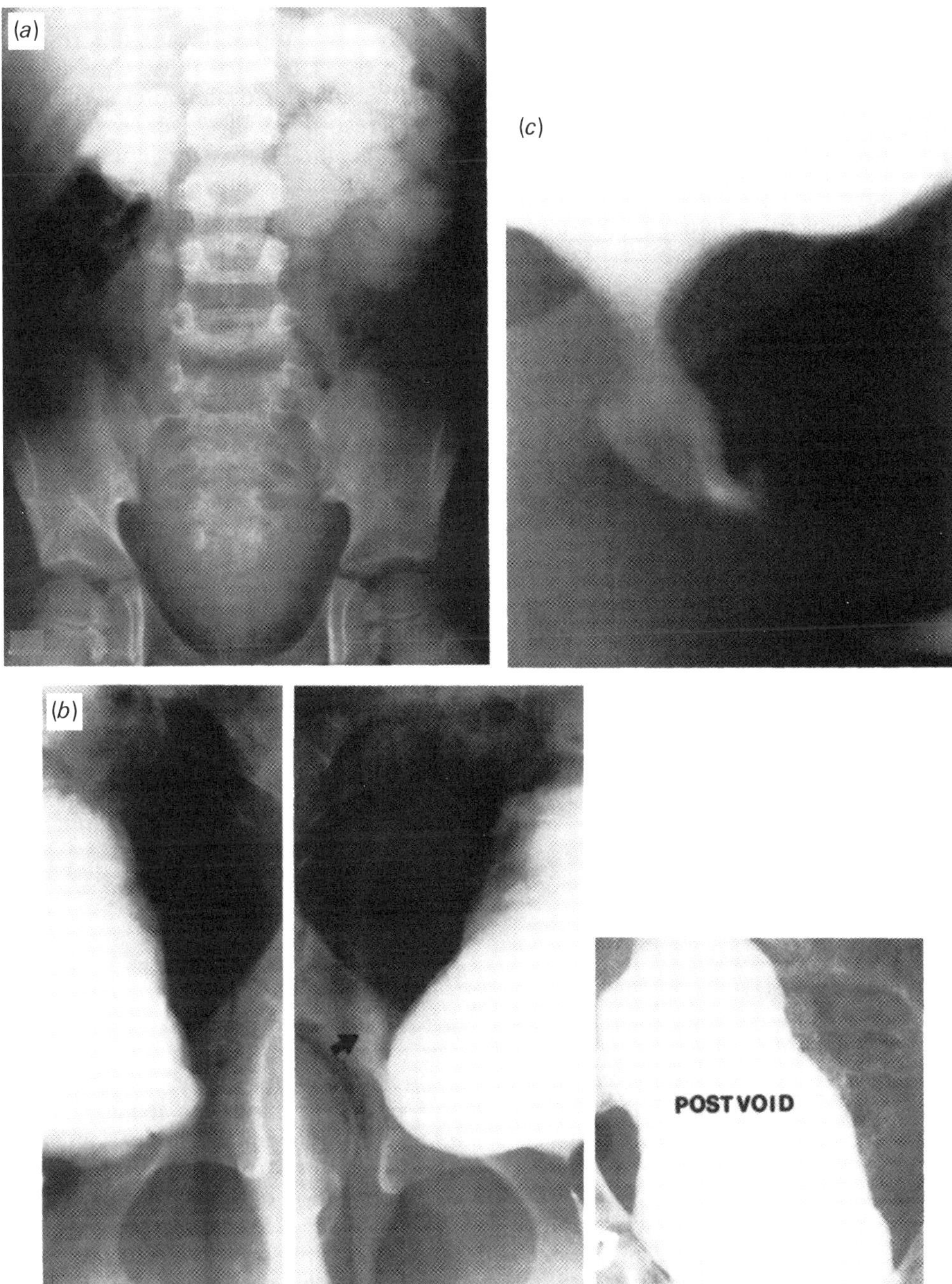

Figure 53.26 (*a*) Excretory urogram in a 14-year-old male with daytime and night-time incontinence and encopresis. Note the impression of a faintly opacified distended bladder. (*b*) His voiding cystourethrogram reveals trabeculation, mild right vesicoureteral reflux (arrow), and a large postvoiding residual urine volume. (*c*) A film during voiding demonstrates intermittent relaxation of the external sphincter area.

53.26). Fifty percent have severe VUR. Nearly every child has a grossly trabeculated, large-capacity bladder with a considerable postvoiding residual urine volume (see Figure 53.26b). Voiding films show either persistent or intermittent narrowing in the region of the external sphincter in almost half of the children (see Figure 53.26c). Finally, the scout film from the excretory urogram displays considerable fecal material in the colon, consistent with chronic constipation and a normal vertebral column.

Urodynamic studies demonstrate a large-capacity bladder with poor compliance, an overactive detrusor, and either high-pressure or ineffective detrusor contractions during voiding[185,214] (Figure 53.27a). Sometimes, Valsalva voiding is needed to empty the bladder. The urinary flow rate is often intermittent as

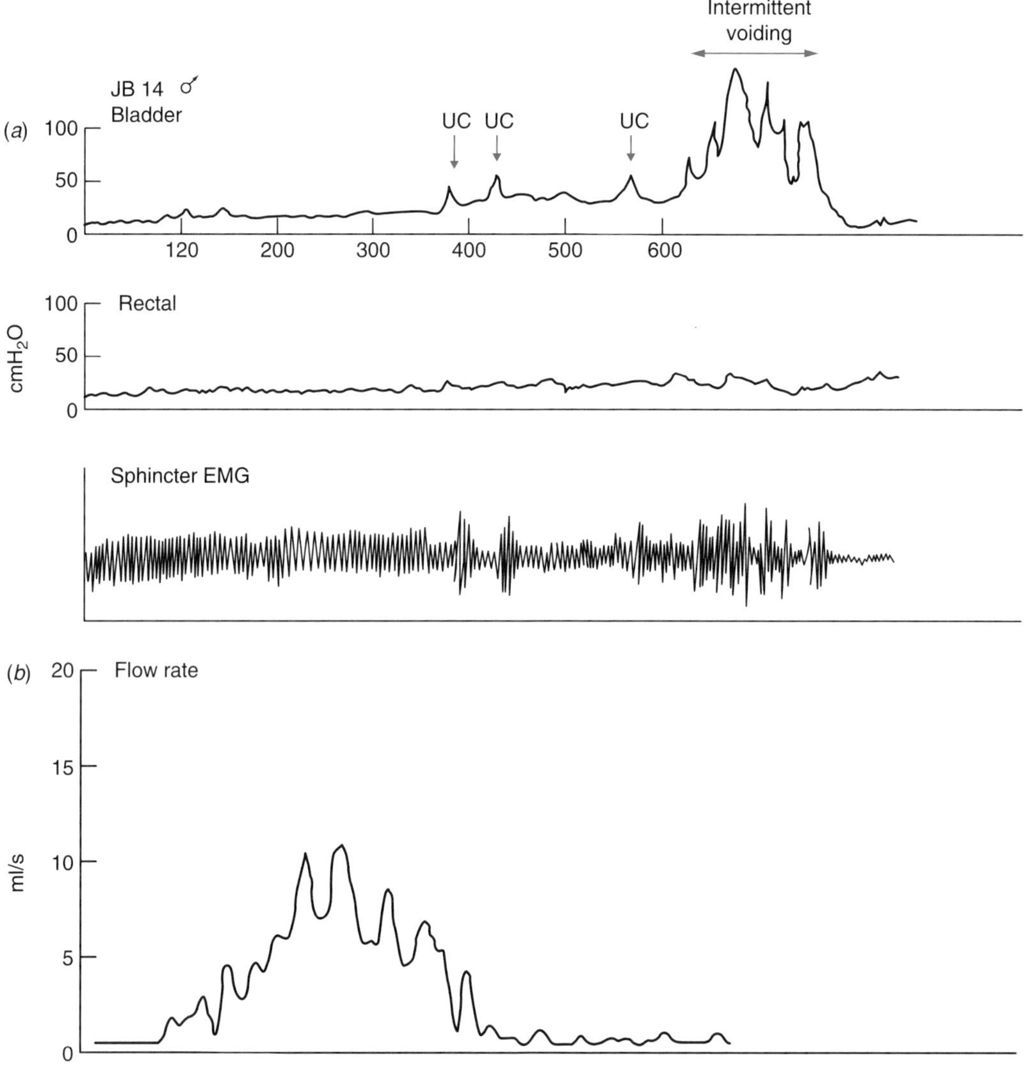

Figure 53.27 (*a*) Uninhibited detrusor contractions (UC) and increases in external urethral sphincter electromyography (EMG) activity are noted as the bladder is filled. During voluntary voiding, very high bladder pressures (>100 cmH_2O) are generated owing to increased activity and then intermittent relaxation of the external sphincter. (*b*) The urinary flow rate reflects the voiding pattern seen on urodynamic evaluation.

a result of the failure of the external sphincter to relax completely throughout voiding (Figure 53.27b). The bethanechol supersensitivity test may be positive; in the past, this response led to the belief that these children had neuropathic bladder dysfunction.[221] EMG recordings, however, reveal normal external urethral sphincter innervation and exclude the possibility of a sacral spinal cord lesion. The sphincter fails to relax completely and may actually tighten episodically once voiding commences;[194] this finding, along with the premature contractions, suggests an upper motor neuron lesion, but usually, no other signs are present to confirm this urodynamic hypothesis. MRI has failed to reveal any intraspinal process as a cause for the voiding dysfunction in these children.[227]

The dyssynergy created by the incoordination between the bladder and sphincter muscles leads to high voiding pressures initially and, later, to ineffective detrusor contractions.[194] Depending on which point of the spectrum one is at, a low or intermittent flow rate and either a minimal or significant postvoiding residual urine volume is noted.

Before this 'syndrome' was recognized and the pathophysiology elucidated, many children underwent multiple operations to improve bladder emptying and correct VUR. Failure of these procedures to succeed led to urinary diversion in a number of instances. Some of these individuals were eventually able to be undiverted at an older age after they outgrew the conditions that caused their dysfunction in the first place.[228] Today, an entirely different approach is taken. Treatment is focused on improving the child's ability to empty the bladder and bowel and alleviating the psychosocial pressures that contribute to the aggravation of the voiding dysfunction.[195,227] A frequent emptying schedule accompanied by biofeedback techniques to relax the sphincter during voiding,[196,198] anticholinergic drugs to abolish detrusor overactivity, and improved bowel emptying regimens are instituted.[185] Despite these measures, intermittent catheterization may be needed in children who fail to respond and in those individuals who require immediate decompression of their upper urinary tract.[218,229] In some cases, the outflow obstruction may have produced severe renal damage and even chronic kidney failure, which must be managed accordingly.

Psychotherapy is an integral part of the rehabilitative process to re-educate both the child and the parents in appropriate voiding habits. Punishments are stopped and a reward system is initiated in order to improve the child's self-image and confidence.[195] This comprehensive urotherapy approach provides the best means for rehabilitating the child's lower urinary tract and for preserving and maintaining renal health.[230]

References

1. Lapides J, Diokno AC, Silber SJ, Lowe BS. Clean intermittent self-catheterization in the treatment of urinary tract disease. J Urol 1972; 107:458.
2. Gierup J, Ericsson NO. Micturition studies in infants and children: intravesical pressure, urinary flow and urethral resistance in boys with intravesical obstruction. Scand J Urol Nephrol 1970; 4:217.
3. Blaivas JG, Labib KB, Bauer SB, Retik AB. Changing concepts in the urodynamic evaluation of children. J Urol 1977; 117:777.
4. Blaivas JG. A critical appraisal of specific diagnostic techniques. In: Krane RJ, Siroky MB, eds. Clinical Neurourology. Boston: Little, Brown & Co, 1979: 69.
5. Smith ED. Urinary prognosis in spina bifida. J Urol 1972; 108:115.
6. McGuire EJ, Woodside JR, Borden TA, Weiss RM. The prognostic value of urodynamic testing in myelodysplastic patients. J Urol 1981; 126:205.
7. Bauer SB, Hallet M, Khoshbin S et al. The predictive value of urodynamic evaluation in the newborn with myelodysplasia. JAMA 1984; 152:650.
8. Mandell J, Bauer SB, Colodny AH, Retik AB. Cutaneous vesicostomy in infancy. J Urol 1981; 126:92.
9. Bauer SB. Urodynamics in children: indication and methods. In: Barrett DM, Wein AJ, eds. Controversies in Neuro-urology. New York: Churchill Livingstone, 1983: 193.
10. Satar N, Bauer SB, Scott RM et al. Late effects of early surgery on lipoma and lipomeningocele in children less than one year old. J Urol 1997; 157:1434.
11. Abrams P, Cardozo L, Fall M et al. The standardisation of terminology in lower urinary tract function. Neurourol Urodyn 2002; 21:167.

12a. Abrams P, Cardozo L, Fall M et al; Standardisation Sub-Committee of the International Continence Society. The standardisation of terminology in lower urinary tract function: report from the standardisation sub-committee of the International Continence Society. Urology 2003; 61:37.

12b. Nevéus T, von Gontard A, Hoebeke P, et al. The standardization of terminology of lower urinary tract function in children and adolescents: report from the standardization committee of the International Children's Continence Society. J Urol 2006; 176:314–24.

13. Bauer SB. Early evaluation and management of children with spina bifida. In: King LR, ed. Urologic Surgery in Neonates and Young Infants. Philadelphia: WB Saunders, 1988: 252.
14. Ross AJ, Ruiz-Perez V, Wang Y et al. A homeobox gene, HLXB9, is the major locus for dominantly inherited sacral agenesis. Nature Genet 1998; 20:358.
15. Catala M. Genetic control of caudal development. Clin Genet 2002; 61:89.
16. Stein SC, Feldman JG, Freidlander M et al. Is myelomeningocele a disappearing disease? Pediatrics 1982; 69:511.
17. Laurence KM. A declining incidence of neural tube defects in U.K. Z Kinderchir 44(Suppl 1):51.
18. Palomaki GE, Williams JR, Haddow JE. Prenatal screening for open neural-tube defects in Maine (Letter). N Engl J Med 1999; 340:1049.
19. MRC Vitamin Study Group. Prevention of neural tube defects: results of the Medical Research Council Vitamin Study. Lancet 1991; 338:131.
20. AAP Committee on Genetics. Folic acid for the prevention of neural tube defects. Pediatrics 1999; 104:325.
21. Rothenberg SP, da Costa MP, Sequeira JM et al. Autoantibodies against folate receptors in women with a pregnancy complicated by a neural-tube defect. N Engl J Med 2004; 350:134.
22. Scarff TB, Fronczak S. Myelomeningocele: a review and update. Rehabil Lit 1981; 42:143.
23. Kroovand RL, Walsh PC, Gittes RF. Myelomeningocele. In: Walsh PC et al, eds. Campbell's Urology, 5th edn. Philadelphia: WB Saunders, 1986: 2193.
24. Stark GD. Spina Bifida: Problems and Management. Oxford: Blackwell Scientific, 1977.
25. Bauer SB, Labib KB, Dieppa RA et al. Urodynamic evaluation in a boy with myelodysplasia and incontinence. Urology 1977; 10:354.
26. Pontari MA, Keating M, Kelly M et al. Retained sacral function in children with high level myelodysplasia. J Urol 1995; 154:775.
27. Dator DP, Hatchett L, Dyro FM et al. Urodynamic dysfunction in walking myelodysplastic children. J Urol 1992; 148:362.
28. Van Gool JD, Kuijten RH, Donckerwolcke RA, Kramer PP. Detrusor–sphincter dyssynergia in children with

myelomeningocele: a prospective study. Z Kinderchir 1982; 37:148.
29. Sidi AA, Dykstra DD, Gonzalez R. The value of urodynamic testing in the management of neonates with myelodysplasia: a prospective study. J Urol 1986; 135:90.
30. Kaefer M, Pabby A, Kelly M et al. Improved bladder function after prophylactic treatment of high risk neurogenic bladder in newborns with myelodysplasia. J Urol 1999; 162:1068.
31. Kroovand RL, Bell W, Hart LJ, Benfeld KY. The effect of back closure on detrusor function in neonates with myelodysplasia. J Urol 1990; 144:423.
32. Bauer SB. Evaluation and management of the newborn with myelomeningocele. In: Gonzales ET, Roth DVR, eds. Common Problems in Urology. St Louis: Mosby Year Book, 1991: 169.
33. Bauer SB. Myelodysplasia: newborn evaluation and management. In: McLaurin RL, ed. Spina Bifida: A Multidisciplinary Approach. New York: Praeger, 1984: 262.
34. Bauer SB. The management of spina bifida from birth onwards. In: Whitaker RH, Woodard JR, eds. Paediatric Urology. London: Butterworths, 1985: 87.
35. Chiaramonte RM, Horowitz EM, Kaplan GA et al. Implications of hydronephrosis in newborns with myelodysplasia. J Urol 1986; 136:427.
36. Keating MA, Bauer SB, Krarup C et al. Sacral sparing in children with myelodysplasia. Presented at the annual meeting of the American Urological Association, Anaheim, May 18, 1987.
37. Spindel MR, Bauer SB, Dyro FM et al. The changing neuro-urologic lesion in myelodysplasia. JAMA 1987; 258:1630.
38. Blaivas JG, Sinka HP, Zayed AH et al. Detrusor–sphincter dyssynergia: a detailed electromyographic study. J Urol 1986; 125:545.
39. Ghoniem GM, Bloom DA, McGuire EJ, Stewart KL. Bladder compliance in meningocele children. J Urol 1989; 141:1404.
40. McLorie GA, Perez-Morero R, Csima AL, Churchill BM. Determinants of hydronephrosis and renal injury in patients with myelomeningocele. J Urol 1986; 140:1289.
41. Steinhardt GF, Goodgold HM, Samuels LD. The effect of intravesical pressure on glomerular filtration rates in patients with myelomeningocele. J Urol 1986; 140:1293.
42. Seki N, Akazawa K, Senoh K et al. An analysis of risk factors for upper urinary tract deterioration in patients with myelodysplasia. Br J Urol 1999; 84:679.
43. Bloom DA, Knechtel JM, McGuire EJ. Urethral dilation improves bladder compliance in children with myelomeningocele and high leak point pressures. J Urol 1990; 144:430.
44. Park JM, McGuire EJ, Koo HP et al. External urethral sphincter dilation for the management of high risk myelomeningocele: 15 year experience. J Urol 2001; 165:2383.
45. Schulte-Baukloh H, Michael T, Sturzebecher B, Knispel HH. Botulinum-A toxin detrusor injection as a novel approach in the treatment of bladder spasticity in children with neurogenic bladder. Eur Urol 2003; 44:139.
46. Joseph DB, Bauer SB, Colodny AH et al. Clean intermittent catheterization in infants with neurogenic bladder. Pediatrics 1989; 84:78.
47. Kasabian NG, Bauer SB, Dyro FM et al. The prophylactic value of clean intermittent catheterization and anticholinergic medication in newborns and infants with myelodysplasia at risk of developing urinary tract deterioration. Am J Dis Child 1992; 146:840.
48. Schlager TA, Clark M, Anderson S. Effect of a single-use sterile catheter for each void on the frequency of bacteriuria in children with neurogenic bladder on intermittent catheterization for bladder emptying. Pediatrics 2001; 108:E71.
49. Geraniotis E, Koff SA, Enrile B. Prophylactic use of clean intermittent catheterization in treatment of infants and young children with myelomeningocele and neurogenic bladder dysfunction. J Urol 1988; 139:85.
50. Edelstein RA, Bauer SB, Kelly MD et al. Long-term urologic response of neonates with myelodysplasia treated proactively with intermittent catheterization and anticholinergic therapy. J Urol 1995; 150:1500.
51. Wu H-Y, Baskin LS, Kogan BA. Neurogenic bladder dysfunction due to myelomeningocele: neonatal versus childhood treatment. J Urol 1997; 157:2295.
52. Epstein F. Meningocele: pitfalls in early and late management. Clin Neurosurg 1982; 30:366.
53. Reigel DH. Tethered spinal cord. Concepts Pediatr Neurosurg 1983; 4:142.
54. Venes JL, Stevens SA. Surgical pathology in tethered cord secondary to meningomyelocele repair. Concepts Pediatr Neurosurg 1983; 4:165.
55. Begeer JH, Meihuizen de Regt MJ, HogenEsch I et al. Progressive neurological deficit in children with spina bifida aperta. Z Kinderchir 1986; 41(Suppl 1):13.
56. Lais A, Kasabian NG, Dyro FM et al. Neurosurgical implications of continuous neuro-urological surveillance of children with myelodysplasia. J Urol 1993; 150:1879.
57. Bauer SB. Vesico-ureteral reflux in children with neurogenic bladder dysfunction. In: Johnston EH, ed. International Perspectives in Urology, Vol. 10. Baltimore: Williams & Wilkins, 1984: 159.
58. Kass EJ, Koff SA, Lapides J. Fate of vesicoureteral reflux in children with neuropathic bladders managed by intermittent catheterization. J Urol 1981; 125:63.
59. Flood HD, Ritchey ML, Bloom DA et al. Outcome of reflux in children with myelodysplasia managed by bladder pressure monitoring. J Urol 1994; 152:1574.
60. Agarwal SK, McLorie GA, Grewal D et al. Urodynamic correlates of resolution of reflux meningomyelocele patients. J Urol 1997; 158:580.
61. Hopps CV, Kropp KA. Preservation of renal function in children with myelomeningocele managed with basic newborn evaluation and close followup. J Urol 2003; 169:305.
62. Cohen RA, Rushton HG, Belman AB et al. Renal scarring and vesicoureteral reflux in children with myelodysplasia. J Urol 1990; 144:541.
63. Barbalias GA, Klauber GT, Blaivas JG. Critical evaluation of the Credé maneuver: a urodynamic study of 207 patients. J Urol 1983; 130:720.
64. Duckett JW. Cutaneous vesicostomy in childhood. Urol Clin North Am 1974; 1:485.

65. Jeffs RD, Jones P, Schillinger JF. Surgical correction of vesico-ureteral reflux in children with neurogenic bladder. J Urol 1976; 115:449.
66. Woodard JR, Anderson AM, Parrott TS. Ureteral reimplantation in myelodysplastic children. J Urol 1981; 126:387.
67. Bauer SB, Colodny AH, Retik AB. The management of vesico-ureteral reflux in children with myelodysplasia. J Urol 1984; 128:102.
68. Kaplan WE, Firlit CF. Management of reflux in myelodysplastic children. J Urol 1983; 129:1195.
69. Elder JS, Diaz M, Caldamone AA et al. Endoscopic therapy for vesicoureteral reflux: a meta-analysis. Presented at the annual meeting of the American Academy of Pediatrics, Section on Urology, San Francisco, Abstract #53, October 10, 2004.
70. Schlussel R. Cystoscopic correction of reflux. Curr Urol Rep 2004; 5:127.
71. Caione P, Capozza N. Endoscopic treatment of urinary incontinence in pediatric patients: 2-year experience with dextranomer/hyaluronic acid copolymer. J Urol 2002; 168:1868.
72. Guys JM, Fakhro A, Louis-Borrione C et al. Endoscopic treatment of urinary incontinence: long-term evaluation of the results. J Urol 2001; 165:2389.
73. Silveri M, Capitanucci ML, Mosiello G, Broggi G, De Gennaro M. Endoscopic treament for urinary incontinence in children with a congenital neuropathic bladder. Br J Urol 1998; 82:694.
74. Krogh K, Lie HR, Bilenberg N, Laurberg S. Bowel function in Danish children with myelomeningocele. APMIS Suppl 2003; 109:81.
75. Han SW, Kim MJ, Kim JH et al. Intravesical electrical stimulation improves neurogenic bowel dysfunction in children with spina bifida. J Urol 2004; 171:2648.
76. Aksnes G, Diseth TH, Helseth A et al. Appendicostomy for antegrade enema: effects on somatic and psychosocial functioning in children with myelomeningocele. Pediatrics 2002; 109:484.
77. Cromer BA, Enrile B, McCoy K et al. Knowledge, attitudes and behavior related to sexuality in adolescents with chronic disability. Dev Med Child Neurol 1990; 32:602.
78. Decter RM, Furness PD, Nguyen TA et al. Reproductive understanding, sexual functioning and testosterone levels in men with spina bifida. J Urol 1997; 157:1466.
79. Cass AS, Bloom BA, Luxenberg M. Sexual function in adults with myelomeningocele. J Urol 1986; 136:425.
80. Woodhouse CJR. Sexual function in boys born with exstrophy, myelomeningocele and micropenis. Urology 1998; 52:3.
81. Joyner BD, McLorie GA, Khoury AE. Sexuality and reproductive issues in children with myelomeningocele. Eur J Pediatr Surg 1998; 8:29.
82. Palmer JS, Kaplan WE, Firlit CF. Sexuality of the spina bifida male and female: anonymous questionnaire. Presented at, Section on Urology, annual meeting of American Academy of Pediatrics, Washington, DC, October 9, 1999 (Abstract No. 13).
83. Hayden P. Adolescents with meningomyelocele. Pediatr Rev 1985; 6:245.
84. James CM, Lassman LP. Spinal Dysraphism: Spina Bifida Occulta. New York: Appleton-Century-Crofts, 1972.
85. Anderson FM. Occult spinal dysraphism: a series of 73 cases. Pediatrics 1975; 55:826.
86. Dubrowitz V, Lorber J, Zachary RB. Lipoma of the cauda equina. Arch Dis Child 1965; 40:207.
87. Weissert M, Gysler R, Sorensen N. The clinical problem of the tethered cord syndrome – a report of 3 personal cases. Z Kinderchir 1989; 44:275.
88. Jindal A, Mahapatra AK. Spinal lipomatous malformations. Indian J Pediatr 2000; 67:342.
89. Yip CM, Leach GE, Rosenfeld DS et al. Delayed diagnosis of voiding dysfunction: occult spinal dysraphism. J Urol 1985; 124:694.
90. Linder M, Rosenstein J, Sklar FH. Functional improvement after spinal surgery for the dysraphic malformations. Neurosurgery 1982; 11:622.
91. Mandell J, Bauer SB, Hallett M et al. Occult spinal dysraphism: a rare but detectable cause of voiding dysfunction. Urol Clin North Am 1980; 7:349.
92. Keating MA, Rink RC, Bauer SB et al. Neuro-urologic implications of changing approach in management of occult spinal lesions. J Urol 1988; 140:1299.
93. Foster LS, Kogan BA, Cogan PH, Edwards MS. Bladder function in patients with lipomyelomeningocele. J Urol 1990; 143:984.
94. Nogueira M, Greenfield SP, Wan J et al. Tethered cord in children: a clinical classification with urodynamic correlation. J Urol 2004; 172:1677.
95. Kondo A, Kato K, Kanai S, Sakakibara T. Bladder dysfunction secondary to tethered cord syndrome in adults: is it curable? J Urol 1986; 135:313.
96. Satar N, Bauer SB, Shefner J et al. Effects of delayed diagnosis and treatment in patients with occult spinal dysraphism. J Urol 1995; 154:754.
97. Hellstrom WJ, Edwards MS, Kogan BA. Urologic aspects of the tethered cord syndrome. J Urol 1986; 135:317.
98. Yamada S, Knierim D, Yonekura M et al. Tethered cord syndrome. J Am Paraplegia Soc 1983; 6(Suppl 3):58.
99. Yamada S, Won DJ, Yamada SM. Pathophysiology of tethered cord syndrome: correlation with symptomatology. Neurosurg Focus 2004; 16:E6.
100. Barson AJ. The vertebral level of termination of the spinal cord during normal and abnormal development. J Anat 1970; 106:489.
101. Yamada S, Zincke DE, Sanders D. Pathophysiology of 'tethered cord syndrome.' J Neurosurg 1981; 54:494.
102. Flanigan RF, Russell DP, Walsh JW. Urologic aspects of tethered cord. Urology 1989; 33:80.
103. Khoury AE, Hendrick EB, McLorie GA et al. Occult spinal dysraphism: clinical and urodynamic outcome after division of the filum terminale. J Urol 1990; 144:426.
104. Roy MW, Gilmore R, Walsh JW. Evaluation of children and young adults with tethered spinal cord syndrome: utility of spinal and scalp recorded somatosensory evoked potentials. Surg Neurol 1986; 26:241.
105. Tami S, Yamada S, Knighton RS. Extensibility of the lumbar and sacral cord. Pathophysiology of the tethered cord in cats. J Neurosurg 1987; 66:116.
106. Kaplan WE, McLone DG, Richards I. The urologic man-

ifestations of the tethered spinal cord. J Urol 1988; 140:1285.
107. Seeds JW, Jones FD. Lipomyelomeningocele: prenatal diagnosis and management. Obstet Gynecol 1986; 67(Suppl):34.
108. Tracey PT, Hanigan WC. Spinal dysraphism: use of magnetic resonance imaging in evaluation. Clin Pediatr 1990; 29:228.
109. Packer RJ, Zimmerman RA, Sutton LN et al. Magnetic resonance imaging of spinal cord diseases of childhood. Pediatrics 1986; 78:251.
110. Campobasso P, Galiani E, Verzerio A et al. A rare cause of occult neuropathic bladder in children: the tethered cord syndrome. Pediatr Med Chir 1988; 10:641.
111. Hall WA, Albright AL, Brunberg JA. Diagnosis of tethered cord by magnetic resonance imaging. Surg Neurol 1988; 30(Suppl 1):60.
112. Meyrat BJ, Tercier S, Lutz N et al. Introduction of a urodynamic score to detect pre- and postoperative neurological deficits in children with a primary tethered cord. Childs Nervous System 2003; 19:716.
113. Raghavendra BN, Epstein FJ, Pinto RS et al. The tethered spinal cord: diagnosis by high-resolution real-time ultrasound. Radiology 1983; 149:123.
114. Scheible W, James HE, Leopold GR, Hilton SW. Occult spinal dysraphism in infants: screening with high-resolution real-time ultrasound. Radiology 1983; 146:743.
115. Hughes JA, De Bruyn R, Patel K, Thompson D. Evaluation of spinal ultrasound in spinal dysraphism. Clin Radiol 2003; 58:227.
116. Passarge E, Lenz K. Syndrome of caudal regression in infants of diabetic mothers: observations of further cases. Pediatrics 1966; 37:672.
117. Guzman L, Bauer SB, Hallett M et al. The evaluation and management of children with sacral agenesis. Urology 1983; 23:506.
118. Landauer W. Rumplessness of chicken embryos produced by the injection of insulin and other chemicals. J Exp Zool 1945; 98:65.
119. White RI, Klauber GT. Sacral agenesis: analysis of twenty-two cases. Urology 1976; 8:521.
120. Menon RK, Cohen RM, Sperling MA et al. Transplacental passage of insulin in pregnant women with insulin-dependent diabetes mellitus. N Engl J Med 1990; 323:309.
121. Rojansky N, Fasouliotis SJ, Ariel I, Nadjari M. Extreme caudal agenesis. Possible drug related etiology? J Reprod Med 2002; 47:241.
122. Kochling J, Karbasiyan M, Reis A. Spectrum of mutations and genotype–phenotype analysis in Currarino syndrome. Eur J Hum Genet 2001; 9:599.
123. Hagan DM, Ross AJ, Strachan T et al. Mutation analysis and embryonic expression of the HLXB9 Currarino syndrome gene. Am J Hum Genet 2000; 66:1504.
124. Lynch SA, Wang Y, Strachan T et al. Autosomal dominant sacral agenesis: Currarino syndrome. J Med Genet 2000; 37:561.
125. Bernbeck B, Schurfeld-Furstenberg K, Ketteler K, Kemperdick H, Schroten H. Unilateral pulmonary atresia with total sacral agenesis and other congenital defects. Clin Dysmorphol 2004; 13:47.
126. Koff SA, DeRidder PA. Patterns of neurogenic bladder dysfunction in sacral agenesis. J Urol 1977; 118:87.
127. Jakobson H, Holm-Bentzen M, Hald T. Neurogenic bladder dysfunction in sacral agenesis and dysgenesis. Neurourol Urodynam 1985; 4:99.
128. Capitanucci ML, Silveri M, Nappo S et al. [Total agenesis of the sacrum and neurogenic bladder dysfunction]. Pediatr Med Chir 1997; 19:113. [in Italian]
129. De Biasio P, Ginocchio G, Aicardi G et al. Ossification timing of sacral vertebrae by ultrasound in the mid-second trimester of pregnancy. Prenat Diagn 2003; 23:1056.
130. Bauer SB. Urodynamics in children. In: Ashcraft KW, ed. Pediatric Urology. Orlando, Florida: Grune & Stratton, 1990: 49.
131. Diel J, Ortiz O, Losada RA et al. The sacrum: pathologic spectrum, multimodality imaging, and subspecialty approach. Radiographics 2001; 21:83.
132. Wilmshurst JM, Kelly R, Borzyskowski M. Presentation and outcome of sacral agenesis: 20 years' experience. Dev Med Child Neurol 1999; 41:806.
133. Morera C, Nurko S. Rectal manometry in sacral agenesis. J Pediatr Gastroenterol Nutr 2003; 37:47.
134. Barry JE, Auldist AW. The Vater association: one end of a spectrum of anomalies. Am J Dis Child 1974; 128:769.
135. Hulthen de Medina V, Mellstam L, Amark P et al. Neurovesical dysfunction in children after surgery for high or intermediate anorectal malformations. Acta Pediatr 2004; 93:43.
136. Tunnell WP, Austin JC, Barnes TP, Reynolds A. Neuroradiologic evaluation of sacral abnormalities in imperforate anus complex. J Pediatr Surg 1987; 22:58.
137. Karrer FM, Flannery AM, Nelson MD Jr et al. Anal rectal malformations: evaluation of associated spinal dysraphic syndromes. J Pediatr Surg 1988; 23:45.
138. Emir H, Soylet Y. Neurovesical dysfunction in patients with anorectal malformations Eur J Pediatr Surg 1998; 8:95.
139. Barnes PD, Lester PD, Yamanashi WS, Prince JR. MRI in infants and children with spinal dysraphism. AJR Am J Roentgenol 1986; 147:339.
140. Williams DI, Grant J. Urologic complications of imperforate anus. Br J Urol 1969; 41:660.
141. Parrott T, Woodard J. Importance of cystourethrography in neonates with imperforate anus. Urology 1979; 13:607.
142. Peña A. Posterior sagittal approach for the correction of anal rectal malformations. Adv Surg 1986; 19:69.
143. Peña A, Hong A. Advances in the management of anorectal malformations. Am J Surg 2000; 180:370.
144. Uehling DT, Gilbert E, Chesney R. Urologic implications of the VATER syndrome. J Urol 1983; 129:352.
145. Carson JA, Barnes PD, Tunell WP et al. Imperforate anus: the neurologic implication of sacral abnormalities. J Pediatr Surg 1984; 19:838.
146. Boemers TM, de Jong TP, van Gool JD et al. Urologic problems in anorectal malformations. Part 2: functional urologic sequelae. J Pediatr Surg 1996; 31:634.
147. Greenfield SP, Fera M. Urodynamic evaluation of the imperforate anus patient: a prospective study. J Urol 1991; 146:539.
148. Sheldon C, Cormier M, Crone K, Wacksman J. Occult

neurovesical dysfunction in children with imperforate anus and its variants. J Pediatr Surg 1991; 26:49.
149. Nelson KB, Ellenberg JH. Antecedents of cerebral palsy. N Engl J Med 1986; 315:81.
150. Naeye RL, Peters EC, Bartholomew M, Landis R. Origins of cerebral palsy. Am J Dis Child 1989; 143:1154.
151. McNeal DM, Hawtrey CE, Wolraich ML, Mapel JR. Symptomatic neurogenic bladder in a cerebral-palsied population. Dev Med Child Neurol 1983; 25:612.
152. Decter RM, Bauer SB, Khoshbin S et al. Urodynamic assessment of children with cerebral palsy. J Urol 1987; 138:1110.
153. Roijen LE, Postema K, Limbeek VJ et al. Development of bladder control in children and adolescents with cerebral palsy. Dev Med Child Neurol 2001; 43:103.
154. Bross S, Pomer S, Doderlein L et al. [Urodynamic findings in patients with infantile cerebral palsy]. Aktuelle Urologie 2004; 35:54. [in German]
155. Mayo ME, Burns MW. Urodynamic studies in children who wet. Br J Urol 1990; 65:641.
156. Reid CJD, Borzyskowski M. Lower urinary tract dysfunction in cerebral palsy. Arch Dis Child 1993; 68:739.
157. Liu M, Hu TZ, Wei FK. A review on the treatment of spastic cerebral palsy with selective posterior rhizotomy. Chinese J Repar Reconstr Surg 1999; 13:183.
158. Huang JC, Deletis V, Vodusek DB, Abbott R. Preservation of pudendal afferents in sacral rhizotomies. Neurosurgy 1997; 41:411.
159. Augutis M, Levi R. Pediatric spinal cord injury in Sweden: incidence, etiology and outcome. Spinal Cord 2003; 41:328.
160. Cass AS, Luxenberg M, Johnson CF, Gleich P. Management of the neurogenic bladder in 413 children. J Urol 1984; 132:521.
161. Cirak B, Ziegfeld S, Knight VM et al. Spinal cord injuries in children. J Pediatr Surg 2004; 39:607.
162. Brown RL, Brunn MA, Garcia VF. Cervical spine injuries in children: a review of 103 patients treated consecutively at a level 1 pediatric trauma center. J Pediatr Surg 2001; 36:1107.
163. Batista JE, Bauer SB, Shefner JM et al. Urodynamic findings in children with spinal cord ischemia. J Urol 1995; 154:1183.
164. Adams C, Babyn PS, Logan WJ. Spinal cord birth injury: value of computed tomographic myelography. Pediatr Neurol 1988; 4:109.
165. Lanska MJ, Roessmann U, Wiznitzer M. Magnetic resonance imaging in cervical cord birth injury. Pediatrics 1990; 85:760.
166. Pollack IF, Pang D, Sclabassi R. Recurrent spinal cord injury without radiographic abnormalities in children. J Neurosurg 1988; 69:177.
167. Hendey GW, Wolfson AB, Mower WR et al. Spinal cord injury without radiographic abnormality: results of the National Emergency X-Radiography Utilization Study in blunt cervical trauma. J Trauma 2002; 53:1.
168. Guttmann L, Frankel H. The value of intermittent catheterization in the early management of traumatic paraplegia and tetraplegia. Paraplegia 1966; 4:63.
169. Barkin M, Dolfin D, Herschorn S et al. The urologic care of the spinal cord injury patient. J Urol 1983; 129:335.
170. Iwatsubo E, Iwakawa A, Koga H. Functional recovery of the bladder in patients with spinal cord injury – prognosticating programs of an aseptic intermittent catheterization. Acta Urol Jpn 1985; 31:775.
171. Fanciullacci F, Zanollo A, Sandri S, Catanzaro F. The neuropathic bladder in children with spinal cord injury. Paraplegia 1988; 26:83.
172. Donnelly J, Hackler RH, Bunts RC. Present urologic status of the World War II paraplegic: 25-year follow-up comparison with status of the 20-year Korean War paraplegic and 5-year Vietnam paraplegic. J Urol 1972; 108:558.
173. Pannek J, Diederichs W, Botel U. Urodynamically controlled management of spinal cord injury in children. Neurourol Urodyn 1997; 16:285.
174. Pearman JW. Urologic follow-up of 99 spinal cord injury patients initially managed by intermittent catheterization. Br J Urol 1976; 48:297.
175. Ogawa T, Yoshida T, Fujinaga T. Bladder deformity in traumatic spinal cord injury patients. Acta Urol Jpn 1988; 34:1173.
176. Watanabe T, Rivas DA, Chancellor MB. Urodynamics of spinal cord injury. Urol Clin North Am 1996; 23:459.
177. Bellman N. Encopresis. Acta Paediatr Scand 1966; 70(Suppl 1):1.
178. Fergusson DM, Hons BA, Horwood LJ, Shannon FT. Factors related to the age of attainment of nocturnal bladder control: an eight year longitudinal study. Pediatrics 1986; 78:884.
179. Yeats WK. Bladder function in normal micturition. In: Kolvin I, MacKeith RL, Meadow SR, eds. Bladder Control and Enuresis. Philadelphia: JB Lippincott, 1973; 28.
180. MacKeith RL, Meadow SR, Turner RK. How children become dry. In: Kolvin I, MacKeith RL, Meadow SR, eds. Bladder Control and Enuresis. Philadelphia: JB Lippincott, 1973: 3.
181. Von Gontard A, Eiberg H, Hollmann E et al. Molecular genetics of nocturnal enuresis: linkage to a locus on chromosome 22. Scand J Urol Nephrol 1999; 202(Suppl):76.
182. Butler RJ, Galsworthy MJ, Rijsdijk F, Plomin R. Genetic and gender influences on nocturnal bladder control – a study of 2900 3-year-old twin pairs. Scand J Urol Nephrol 2001; 35:177.
183. Von Gontard A, Schaumberg H, Hollmann E et al. The genetics of enuresis: a review. J Urol 2001; 166:2438.
184. Farhat W, McLorie GA, O'Reilly S, Khoury A, Bagli DJ. Reliability of the pediatric dysfunctional voiding symptom score in monitoring response to behavioral modification. Can J Urol 2001; 8:1401.
185. Bauer SB, Retik AB, Colodny AH et al. The unstable bladder of childhood. Urol Clin North Am 1980; 7:321.
186. Hansson S, Hjalmas K, Jodal U, Sixt R. Lower urinary tract dysfunction in girls with untreated asymptomatic or covert bacteriuria. J Urol 1990; 143:333.
187. Tanagho EA, Miller EA, Lyon RP. Spastic striated external sphincter and urinary tract infection in girls. Br J Urol 1971; 43:69.
188. Van Gool JD, Tanagho EA. External sphincter activity and recurrent urinary tract infection in girls. Urology 1977; 10:348.
189. Borer JG, Butler A, Zurakowski D et al. Predominant

urodynamic patterns in girls with recurrent urinary tract infection. Presented at the American Urological Meeting, Dallas, Texas, May 3, 1999. Abstract No. 622.

190. Webster GD, Koefoot RB, Sihelnik S. Urodynamic abnormalities in neurologically normal children with micturition dysfunction. J Urol 1984; 132:74.
191. Lebowitz RL, Mandell J. Urinary tract infection in children: putting radiology in its place. Radiology 1987; 165:1.
192. Saxton HM, Borzyskowski M, Mundy AR, Vivian GC. Spinning top deformity: not a normal variant. Radiology 1988; 168:147.
193. Dyro FM, Bauer SB, Hallett M, Khoshbin S. Complex repetitive discharges in the external urethral sphincter in a pediatric population. Neurourol Urodynam 1983; 2:39.
194. Rudy DC, Woodside JR. Non-neurogenic neurogenic bladder: the relationship between intravesical pressure and the external sphincter EMG. Neurourol Urodyn 1991; 10:169.
195. Masek BJ. Behavioral management of voiding dysfunction in neurologically normal children. Dialog Pediatr Urol 1985; 8:7.
196. McKenna PH, Herndon CDA, Connery S et al. Pelvic floor muscle retraining for pediatric voiding dysfunction using interactive computer games. J Urol 1999; 162:1056.
197. Yamanishi T, Yasuda, K. Murayama N et al. Biofeedback training for detrusor overactivity in children. J Urol 2000; 164:1686.
198. Herndon CD, Decambre M, McKenna PH. Interactive computer games for treatment of pelvic floor dysfunction. J Urol 2001; 166:1893.
199. Vincent SA. Postural control of urinary incontinence. The curtsy sign. Lancet 1966; ii:631.
200. Kondo A, Kobayashi M, Otani T et al. Children with unstable bladder: clinical and urodynamic observation. J Urol 1983; 129:88.
201. Crimmins CR, Rathbun SR, Husmann DA. Management of urinary incontinence and nocturnal enuresis in attention-deficit hyperactivity disorder. J Urol 2003; 17:1347.
202. Duel BP, Steinberg-Epstein R, Hill M, Lerner M. A survey of voiding dysfunction in children with attention deficit-hyperactivity disorder. J Urol 2003; 17:1521.
203. McGuire EJ, Savastano JA. Urodynamic studies in enuresis and non-neurogenic bladder. J Urol 1984; 132:299.
204. Mueller SR. Development of urinary control in children. JAMA 1960; 172:1256.
205. Torrens MJ, Collins CD. The urodynamic assessment of adult enuresis. Br J Urol 1975; 47:433.
206. O'Regan S, Yazbeck S, Schick E. Constipation, unstable bladder, urinary tract infection syndrome. Clin Nephrol 1985; 5:154.
207. O'Regan S, Yazbeck S, Hamburger B, Schick E. Constipation: a commonly unrecognized cause of enuresis. Am J Dis Child 1986; 140:260.
208. Koff SA, Murtagh DS. The uninhibited bladder in children: effect of treatment on recurrence of urinary infection and vesicoureteral reflux resolution. J Urol 1983; 130:1158.
209. Persson de Geeter C. [Overactive bladder syndrome in children]. Urologe A 2004; 43:807. [in German]
210. Nijman RJ, Borgstein NG, Ellsworth P, Djurhuus JC. Tolterodine treatment for children with symptoms of urinary urge incontinence suggestive of detrusor overactivity: results from 2 randomized, placebo controlled trials. J Urol 2005; 173:1334.
211. Schulman SL, Von Zuben PC, Plachter N, Kodman-Jones C. Biofeedback methodology: does it matter how we teach children how to relax the pelvic floor during voiding? J Urol 2001; 166:2423.
212. Buttarazzi PJ. Oxybutynin chloride (Ditropan) in enuresis. J Urol 1977; 118:46.
213. Firlit CF, Smey P, King LR. Micturition: urodynamic flow studies in children. J Urol 1978; 119:250.
214. Kass EJ, Diokno AC, Montealegre A. Enuresis: principles of management and results of treatment. J Urol 1979; 121:794.
215. DeLuca FG, Swenson O, Fisher JH, Loutfi AH. The dysfunctional 'lazy' bladder syndrome in children. Arch Dis Child 1962; 37:117.
216. Koefoot RB, Webster GD, Anderson EE, Glenn JF. The primary megacystis syndrome. J Urol 1981; 125:232.
217. De Paepe H, Renson C, Van Laecke E et al. Pelvic-floor therapy and toilet training in young children with dysfunctional voiding and obstipation. BJU Int 2000; 85:889.
218. Pohl HG, Bauer SB, Borer JG et al. The outcome of voiding dysfunction managed with clean intermittent catheterization in neurologically and anatomically normal children. Br J Urol 2002; 89:923.
219. Hinman F. Urinary tract damage in children who wet. Pediatrics 1974; 54:142.
220. Johnston JH, Farkas A. Congenital neuropathic bladder: practicalities and possibilities of conservational management. Urology 1975; 5:719.
221. Williams DI, Hirst G, Doyle D. The occult neuropathic bladder. J Pediatr Surg 1975; 9:35.
222. Mix LW. Occult neuropathic bladder. Urology 1977; 10:1.
223. Allen TD. The non-neurogenic bladder. J Urol 1977; 117:232.
224. Allen TD, Bright TC. Urodynamic patterns in children with dysfunctional voiding problems. J Urol 1978; 119:247.
225. Jayanthi VR, Khoury AE, McLorie CA et al. The non-neurogenic neurogenic bladder of early infancy. J Urol 1997; 158:1281.
226. Bauer SB, Dyro FM, Krarup C et al. Unrecognized neuropathic bladder of infancy. J Urol 1989; 142:589.
227. Hinman F. Non-neurogenic bladder (the Hinman syndrome) fifteen years later. J Urol 1986; 136:769.
228. Yang CC, Mayo ME. Morbidity of dysfunctional voiding syndrome. Urology 1997; 49:445.
229. Snyder H McC, Caldamone AA, Wein AJ, Duckett JW Jr. The Hinman syndrome – alternatives for treatment. Presented at the annual meeting of the American Urological Association, Kansas City, May 16, 1982.
230. Homsy Y, Hellstrom A-L, Hoebeke P, Gray M, McKenna P. Panel Discussion: Urotherapy center organization and management. Annual meeting of American Academy of Pediatrics, Section on Urology, Boston, October 10, 2002.

Diurnal and nocturnal enuresis

54

Mark Horowitz and Rosalia Misseri

Diurnal enuresis

In the infant, a simple reflex controls bladder function without input from the supraspinal centers. A full bladder elicits a detrusor contraction via a signal that is sent along afferent pathways to the spinal cord, which then triggers the appropriate motor response and simultaneous relaxation of the external sphincter muscles. In the absence of an anatomic obstruction, this allows for low-pressure bladder emptying without resistance to flow. The adult pattern of urinary control evolves over time and continence is first achieved by voluntary constriction of the external striated sphincter and later by supraspinal inhibition of the voiding reflex. The adult pattern of voiding is characterized by the absence of bladder contractions during bladder filling and relaxation of the external sphincter just before and throughout bladder emptying. Bladder capacity increases over time to permit the bladder to function as an adequately sized reservoir. In the first 2 years of life, one can predict the bladder's capacity by multiplying the patient's weight in kilograms by 8 to estimate the capacity in milliliters. After 2 years of age, bladder capacity can be accurately estimated and expressed by the formula:

bladder capacity (in ounces) = age (in years) + 2.[1] Multiplying this value by 30 gives the amount in milliliters.

Most children achieve day and night control by 4 years of age. The sequence of development of bowel and bladder control is:

- nocturnal bowel control
- daytime bowel control
- daytime urinary control
- nocturnal urinary control.

There are numerous causes for incontinence including neurological, anatomic and functional, but in children incontinence is most often secondary to problems at the level of the bladder, bladder neck and external striated sphincter, or any combination.

Incontinence may be either diurnal, nocturnal, or both. Patients with daytime incontinence often begin having symptoms 3–6 months after achieving urinary control. Children who are not yet able to inhibit the voiding reflex, stay dry by voluntarily contracting their external sphincter during uninhibited bladder contractions. In many children, persistence of this learned behavior leads to voiding dysfunction. This dyssynergia between the bladder and external sphincter results in high bladder pressures, during filling and emptying. These patients often void in stacatto or fractionated voiding patterns. Instability of the bladder, increased bladder wall thickness, high postvoid residual volumes (PVR), and recurrent infections are often the sequelae of this discordance between the bladder and sphincter. There is a strong association between dysfunctional voiding and urinary tract infections (UTIs), as well as vesicoureteral reflux. More severe forms of this disorder were described as the non-neurogenic neurogenic bladder or the Hinman syndrome.[2] Clinical features that originally characterized the Hinman syndrome included wetting during the day as well as at night with fecal retention and soiling, UTI, radiologic abnormalities of the bladder and/or kidneys, no demonstrable neurologic disease or bladder outlet obstruction and improvement after re-education and suggestive therapy. In addition to features seen in the Hinman syndrome, the Ochoa syndrome is associated with an unusual inversion of facial expression with smiling and a hereditary transmission. In both the Hinman syndrome and Ochoa syndrome upper tract damage may occur.

Urinary frequency and small voided volumes are most often secondary to bladder instability that is either primary, or secondary to the bladder sphincter dysynergia. Patients with primary instability (sometimes referred to as the urge syndrome) have bladder overactivity without any voiding phase problems. Primary instability is commonly seen after a viral or bacterial infection somewhere other than the bladder where the bladder becomes a secondary target. These children experience the urge to void several times an hour and the symptoms resolve spontaneously.

Giggle incontinence (enuresis risoria) is the involuntary loss of urine induced by laughter. The urine is normal and the upper tracts are not affected. Chandra et al reported on a large cohort of children with giggle incontinence, of which 95% had concomitant dysfunctional voiding symptoms.[3] They concluded that detrusor instability contributes to the wetting. Therapy therefore should include timed voiding, anticholinergic therapy, and a bowel program. They reported an 89% remission rate within 10 weeks. Some have reported success with the use of methylphenidate (Ritalin) for the treatment of giggle incontinence.

Enuresis is only one of many symptoms seen in the complex of voiding dysfunction. Others include urinary frequency, urgency, urge associated incontinence, and other lower urinary tract symptoms (LUTS). Additionally, many patients with voiding dysfunction exhibit signs and symptoms of bowel dysfunction. The term dysfunctional elimination syndrome has been used to describe patients with bladder and bowel dysfunction.

Daytime urinary incontinence is a major source of concern for families and has potential to disrupt everyday life at home and school. Approximately 20% of children 4–6 years of age wet their pants, 3% wetting twice or more weekly.[4] As children get older the incidence of enuresis declines but society is less tolerant of the wetting. Pediatric urologists are second in line to treat children with this problem, often after treatment failure by the primary caregiver. Identifying the etiology of the symptoms helps to formulate a specific solution to improve the situation. It is important to remain minimally invasive and offer a treatment plan that is within reach of both the patient and the family, with minimal side effects.

Constipation and enuresis

Until proven otherwise, all patients with lower urinary tract disorders have constipation. Constipation is defined by the hard nature of the stool, the pain associated with its passage, or the failure to pass three stools per week.[5] Voluntary withholding of feces, most of the time caused by fear of painful defecation, is the most common cause of constipation. Encopresis or fecal soiling occurs when loose stool leaks per rectum after passing retained harder stool. Because of the close proximity of the bladder to the rectum, impacted stool in the rectum causes instability, which impedes bladder filling. Patients void smaller amounts with greater frequency. The frequency of bowel movements and consistency of the stool must be included in the history. Parents often know the voiding pattern of their children and the number of urinary and fecal accidents but have little knowledge of their children's frequency of bowel movements. Failure to diagnose and treat constipation often hinders the success of therapy for voiding dysfunction.

Loening-Baucke et al correlated resolution of voiding dysfunction symptoms with treatment of constipation.[6] Successful treatment of constipation leads to resolution of daytime incontinence in 89%, nighttime incontinence in 63% and UTI in 100% of patients. Recommendations included reconditioning the child's bowel movements with timed attempts to defecate, teaching proper toilet sitting positions, and modification of dietary habits. Initial therapy adds more fiber to the diet in the form of high-fiber foods, fiber additives, or laxatives that make bowel movements soft and easy to pass. The use of enemas, fecal disimpaction, and a variety of oral agents such as MiraLax (polyethylene glycol 3350), mineral oil, milk of magnesia, and sorbitol are often necessary for success.

Clinicians use a variety of regimens for the initial clean-out, where the goal is evacuation of retained stool;

1. Mineral oil alone (15–30 ml/kg/day up to 8 ounces once or twice daily for 3 days).
2. Hypertonic enemas and/or suppositories daily for 2–3 days.
3. Polyethylene glycol 3350 (MiraLax) orally, up to 1.5 g/kg/day to a maximum of 100 g for 3 days.
4. An enema each day for 2 days, followed by milk of magnesia 1 ml/kg/dose twice daily for 3 days.

Following the initial clean-out, a maintenance program helps keep the patient defecating on a regular basis. Stool softeners used for a prolonged period include:

- milk of magnesia (1–4 ml/kg/daily)
- mineral oil (2–6 ml/kg/daily)
- sorbitol or lactulose (0.7–3 mg/kg/daily)
- polyethylene glycol 3350 (0.27–1.42 mg/kg/daily).

Work-up

The history is the most important component in the evaluation of a patient with incontinence. A thorough, systematic approach is critical in defining the cause and directing the treatment. The astute clinician can eliminate most anatomic and neurogenic causes of incontinence through a careful history and physical. The following is a list of questions routinely asked of patients or families of children with daytime incontinence.

- How long has the wetting been a problem? We are more inclined to proceed with a full evaluation in a child who has been having accidents for several months than in one who has just recently become symptomatic. Acute onset of bladder instability often resolves spontaneously shortly after the onset of symptoms and does not require intervention.
- How significant is the wetting? Does the child soak through clothing or simply have damp underwear? Many parents are only concerned when soaking is severe enough to require a change of clothes, and consider dampness as either normal or inconsequential. Once children are mature enough to change their own clothes, parents may be less aware of the wetting problem. Dampness is often secondary to patients pulling up their garments before completing the voiding process. These children simply need coaching to encourage them to spend a extra few moments to empty their bladders before getting dressed. We instruct boys to shake their penis after voiding to prevent urine dripping into their underwear. Girls are encouraged to spread their legs and to pause an extra moment to allow for emptying of urine that pools in the vagina.
- How frequently does the child void? Some parents complain that their children go to the bathroom too often. On further questioning, these children state that they can sit through a movie or participate in a sporting event without going to the bathroom. A voiding diary for several days eliminates some of the confusion encountered when the parent's perception of the symptoms conflicts with that of the child. Together, the parent and child record the frequency of voiding, stooling, and hydration. It is sometimes easier for parent and child to record this data over a three-day weekend than during the week when the child is at school. The normal frequency of voiding in a child is 4–7 times per day or about every 2–3 hours. We define increased frequency as voiding more than 8 times per day or more frequently than every 1.5 hours. Infrequent voiding also contributes to recurrent bladder infections and lower urinary tract symptoms seen in children. Many children void only 2–3 times a day and often do not void upon awakening. The treatment for these children is simply a timed voiding schedule.
- Where is the child most symptomatic? Some children are fine at school where they void at least 2–3 times but experience urgency and accidents once they get home because they ignore the need to void while involved in other activities (watching television, playing with friends, playing computer games). Others wet at school because the teachers prevent the use of the bathroom. Some children are afraid to use public restrooms (lack of privacy, poor sanitary conditions, violence in the bathrooms). These children usually come home from school wet, but are able to stay dry at home where they have unlimited access to the bathroom.
- Has the child had associated UTIs? If so, we try to discern whether the child's symptoms followed or preceded an infection. In some cases, the voiding pattern (high PVR volumes and/or high-pressure voiding with turbulent flow) precipitates the infection. High PVR volumes correlate with the number of UTIs.[7] In others, inflammation following the infection results in abnormal voiding with wetting. Deciding who needs a voiding cystourethrogram (VCUG) to rule out vesicoureteral reflux is critical. Our approach has been to obtain a VCUG in all children with a febrile UTI and in all children with one or more infections while still in diapers. If we suspect the infection to be more consistent with cystitis secondary to high residual volumes, i.e. a 5-year-old girl with no history of prior infection who has symptoms consistent with voiding dysfunction and developed some dysuria with a resultant positive culture, a VCUG will not be obtained. This child is studied with a non-invasive flow/electromyelogram (EMG), and therapy is initiated to improve bladder emptying.
- Are the accidents habitual or situational? Stress at home or in the school may cause daytime accidents. In the social history it is important to elicit events such as the death of a friend or relative, parental separation or divorce, recent move to a new neighborhood, etc.
- Is the urinary flow pattern a continuous good urinary stream, or is it choppy and slow? Is there a straining pattern? Does the child feel completely empty after voiding? The clinician must suspect

anatomic conditions such as posterior urethral valves (PUV), meatal stenosis, and stricture disease when the stream is delayed or reduced. In the absence of anatomic conditions, detrusor sphincter dysynergia and primary bladder neck obstruction are the main culprits.

- How much fluid does the child consume over a 24-hour period? Both dehydration and overhydration may result in abnormal patterns and occasional wetting. Some children minimize fluid intake in an attempt to reduce the frequency with which they void.
- Other than incontinence, are there other LUTS? Many children complain of urinary urgency and others wet themselves without a warning or urge. In an attempt to stay dry, many girls either squat or sit on the heel of one foot (Vincent's curtsy) or cross their legs. This squatting behavior is a unique learned response to a sudden detrusor contraction and is an attempt to prevent or minimize urine loss. Boys sometimes grip their penis to stay dry.
- What is the appearance of the urine? Does it have a discrete smell? Dark yellow, strong-smelling urine indicates a relatively dehydrated state or the presence of infection. Children are encouraged to drink more or void with greater frequency. Any infection should be treated with the appropriate antibiotic. Cranberry and cherry juice (or tablets) may help to prevent infection. We suspect bacterial cystitis when symptoms include dysuria, cloudy, foul-smelling urine, and blood or mucus is visible in the urine.

A reliable symptom scoring system should provide accurate, objective, and scientific data that allow us to objectively assess treatment and follow-up of these patients.

We find that the dysfunctional voiding scoring system questionnaire (DVSSQ) is a helpful tool used for diagnosing and monitoring treatment of children with voiding dysfunction. Doubrava et al performed uroflow with pelvic floor electromyography (EMG) and PVR measurements on 51 patients with normal DVSSQ scores for gender.[8] The DVSSQ was able to predict a normal bell-shaped uroflow curve in 73% of patients; however, it correlated poorly with EMG patterns and PVR volumes. Of patients with normal DVSSQ, 65% had abnormal EMG patterns and there was poor correlation between uroflow curves and EMG patterns as well as between uroflow patterns and PVR values.

The dysfunctional voiding symptom score

Over the last month:

1. I have had wet clothes or wet underwear during the day.
2. I wet the bed at night.
3. When I wet myself, my underwear is soaked.
4. I do not have a bowel movement every day.
5. I have to push for my bowel movements to come out.
6. I go to the bathroom only once or twice a day.
7. I can hold onto my pee by crossing my legs, squatting, or doing the 'pee dance'.
8. When I have to pee, I cannot wait.
9. I have to push to pee.
10. When I pee it hurts.

Questions for parents to answer: Has your child experienced any of the following in the past year: new baby, new home, new school, school problems, abuse (sexual/physical), divorce/death, special events (birthday), accident, injury, any other stressful event?

Questionnaires are a practical method for measuring the magnitude of incontinence, and many exist for evaluating and following children with incontinence. Most take just a few moments to complete and augment the evaluation of children with daytime wetting. Use of a questionnaire helps prevent omission of parts of the voiding history. Sureshkumar et al developed a daytime urinary incontinence questionnaire using parent-reported data and demonstrated that it is reproducible.[9] The questionnaire was used in a prevalence survey of Australian primary school children to determine the magnitude of incontinence in those starting school. Farhat et al evaluates the performance of another instrument to quantify or grade the severity of abnormal voiding behaviors in children.[10] In this system, 10 voiding dysfunction parameters were used to assign a score of 0–3, according to prevalence; i.e. scores ranged from 0 to 30. These questionnaires and others help to identify patients with dysfunctional voiding and further direct their investigative studies and treatment.

Examination

Special attention to the evaluation of the abdomen, genitalia, and back is imperative in the evaluation of children with incontinence. Inspection of the lower back for evidence of skin discoloration, dimples, hair patches, subcutaneous lipomas, or spine defects may indicate the presence of an underlying spinal dysraphism. Asymmetry of the buttocks or motor tone of the buttocks may also indicate the presence of neurologic disease. An absent or asymmetrical gluteal cleft suggests sacral agenesis. The neurologic examination includes careful attention to the lower extremities, including strength, sensation, reflexes, and assessment of gait. If a neurologic cause is suspected, strong consideration must be given to obtaining a magnetic resonance imaging (MRI) scan of the lumbosacral spine or requesting a full neurologic consultation. Patients with abnormalities such as tethered cord or lipomas often require neurosurgical intervention. Many patients with spina bifida occulta and a normal spinal cord will experience resolution of their enuresis with conservative management. Ritchey et al compared outcomes for enuretic children with spina bifida occulta to enuretic children with normal spine X-rays.[11] The majority of patients in both groups had resolution of the enuresis with conservative management and only a small percentage of children with spina bifida occulta required neurosurgical intervention.

Examination of the external genitalia may reveal the source of the problem. Boys with significant meatal stenosis may present with LUTS: mainly a decreased, often deflected stream, urinary hesitancy, and incontinence. Observation of the urinary stream and uroflowmetry may help assess the severity of meatal stenosis. Girls with labial fusion may present with LUTS, including dysuria, dribbling, and incontinence. Examination of the vaginal introitus may reveal a ureterocele or an ectopic ureter. Girls with continuous incontinence between normal voids may have an ectopic ureter. Rashes on the genital area or inner thighs may indicate constant exposure of the skin to urine and suggest constant drainage that may be due to an ectopic ureter. Girls with vaginal voiding often present with labiovulvar erythema and/or leukorrhea that may cause burning and itching. Chronic urine irritation leads to urea burns secondary to the action of skin bacteria on the urine.

When examining the child, it is important to inspect the child's undergarments. Some parents believe their child is always wet, and yet when the child is examined, their clothing is dry. When asked to explain this inconsistency, the parents often state that the child knew he or she was going to the doctor and voided several times that day. This is proof to both the child and parents that by going to the bathroom of regular intervals he or she can stay dry. Fecal stains suggest the presence of constipation or encopresis.

A urinalysis is obtained in all patients looking for infection, proteinuria, or glycosuria and if positive, a specimen is sent for culture and sensitivity. Catherized urines greatly improve the specifity of the culture and eliminate treatment for and further investigation of a UTI.

Uroflowmetry, because of its non-invasive nature, is the perfect instrument for revealing voiding disorders in pediatric patients.[12] We have the children void when they have a 'normal' desire to go. We measure peak flow rate, average flow rate, amount voided, and assess the shape of the curve. Voided amounts affect the peak and average flow rates. Patients with significant instability void very small amounts and this can underestimate their true flow rates.

Simultaneous measurement of uroflow rates and pelvic floor EMG tracings (flow/EMG) have been incorporated into the initial assessment of almost every patient we evaluate for daytime incontinence and bladder–kidney infections. The normal, coordinated flow curve is even and bell-shaped in the absence of pelvic floor activity (Figure 54.1). In contrast, a void with simultaneous pelvic floor contraction results in a ragged curve shape, the so-called staccato, interrupted, or irregular curve.[13] EMG studies typically show increased activity during voiding, instead of the expected relaxation (Figure 54.2). Non-invasive flow/EMGs can be performed regularly to monitor the child's response to therapy.

A bladder ultrasound is obtained to document PVR volumes and record bladder wall thickness and/or distal ureteral dilatation. When hydronephrosis is seen on prevoid images, resolution, improvement, or no change in the hydronephrosis is documented after the child voids. The upper tracts are usually normal in patients with voiding dysfunction and a renal sonogram is a quick, non-invasive, inexpensive screening tool to rule out other genitourinary anatomic anomalies.

Cystography is utilized to detect reflux in a child with a UTI. In addition to assessing grade and laterality, cystography provides information about bladder configuration, PVR volumes and urethral anatomy. Causes of bladder outlet obstruction such as PUV, urethral stricture and detrusor–sphincter dyssynergia, are clearly seen. Bladder instability can be detected when at least one of three well-defined radiologic signs are detected: bladder wall irregularity, elongation of bladder shape, and filling of the posterior urethra. The chances of identifying these signs are greatest if fluoroscopy captures images when unstable contractions occur. Opening of the bladder neck with variable degrees of filling of the posterior urethra is due to detrusor contraction, opening of the bladder

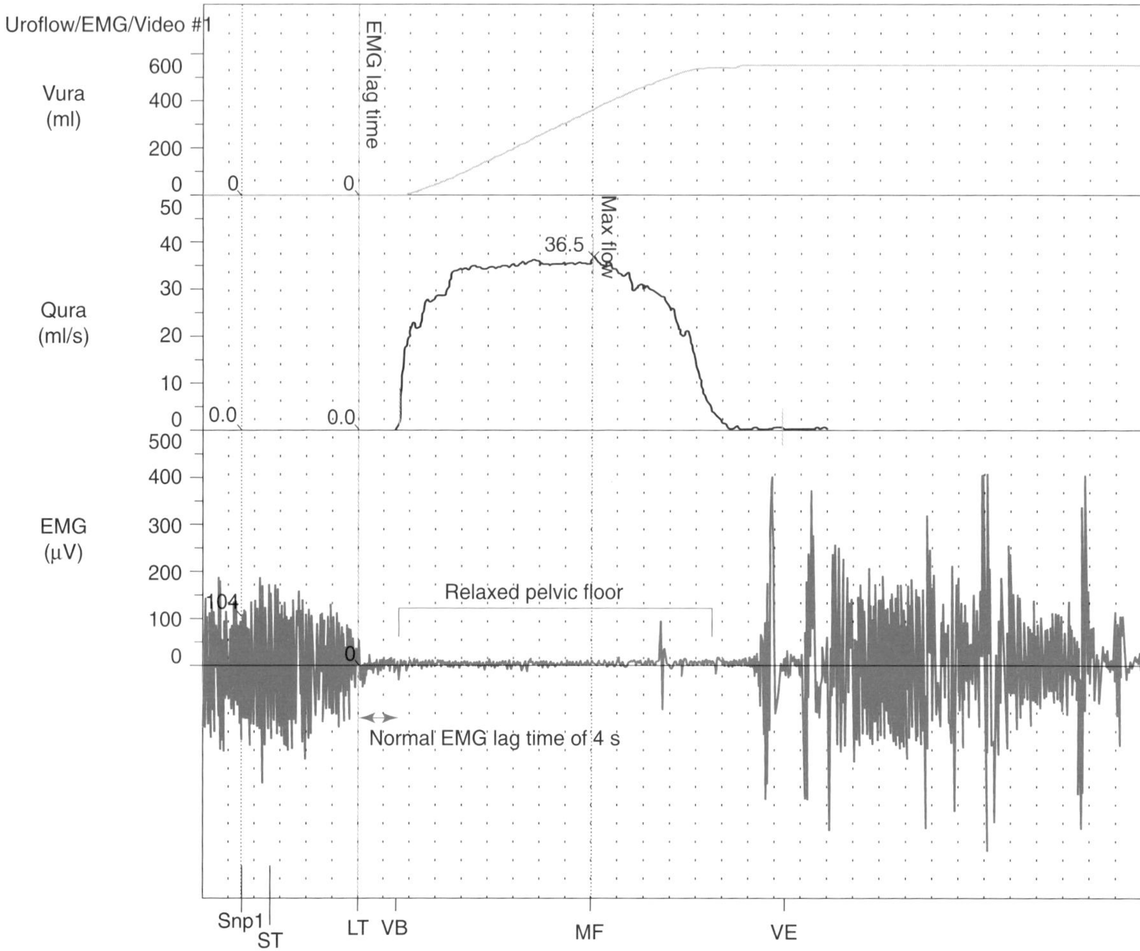

Figure 54.1 Normal voiding pattern. Electromyography (EMG) lag time of 4 seconds. Complete relaxation of pelvic floor muscles with voiding. Normal bell-shaped uroflow curve. Vura = volume of voided urine, Qura = urine flow, ST = start/stop, LT = lag time, VB = voiding begins, MF = maximum flow, VE = voiding ends.

neck, and simultaneous contraction of the external sphincter. Passerini-Glazel et al considered this process a typical and constant sign of bladder instability.[14]

Combs et al reported on the utility of pelvic floor EMG lag time in identifying children with detrusor instability.[15] Pelvic floor EMG lag time is the time interval between pelvic floor relaxation on pelvic floor EMG and the start of flow. Pelvic floor relaxation occurs 1–4 s prior to the start of a voluntary detrusor contraction and the start of flow. Urine flow that occurs instantaneously with or before relaxation of the pelvic floor indicates instability (Figure 54.3). Urodynamics confirms the presence of instability in all patients with a lag time that approaches zero or is in the negative range.

Kakizaki et al measured the internal diameter of the external urethral sphincter on VCUG in children with and without suspected voiding dysfunction to evaluate its diagnostic accuracy as a predictor of detrusor–sphincter incoordination.[16] A diameter <3 mm had satisfactory sensitivity and specificity for detecting detrusor–sphincter incoordination.

We have substituted video-urodynamics (VUDS) for the voiding cystourethrogram (VCUG) in patients being evaluated for febrile UTIs and associated LUTS and in patients not responding to conventional therapy. The advantages of VUDS are its ability to assess detrusor pressures during filling and emptying, monitor EMG activity of the pelvic floor and limit radiation exposure. Monitoring bladder pressure allows us to limit the use of fluoroscopy. We obtain images at the start of the study, two–three times during filling (usually at 25%, 50%, and 75% of expected capacity for age), and when unstable bladder activity on cystometry is seen. We then image during voiding and obtain a single image after completion of voiding to document PVR. In the presence of reflux, a 5 minute delayed KUB is obtained to document drainage of the upper tract.

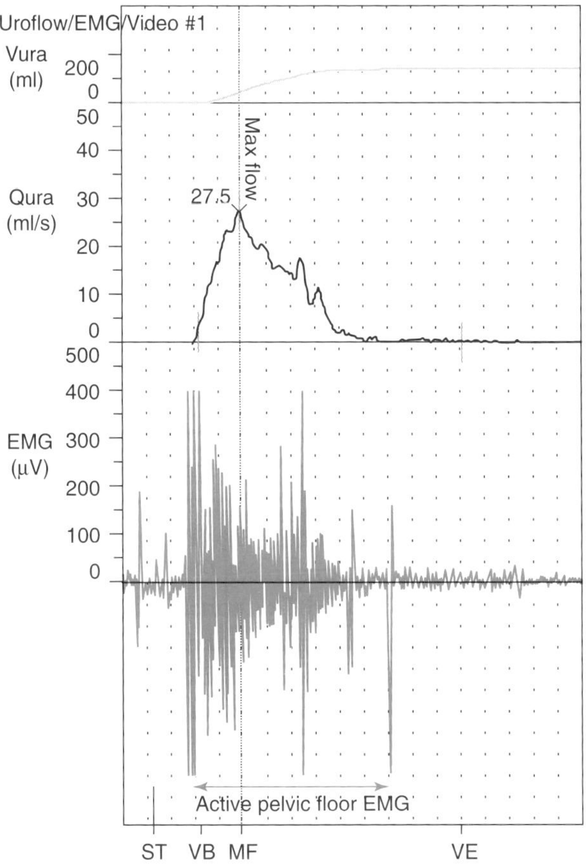

Figure 54.2 Type 1 dysfunctional voiding pattern. Persistent activity (non-relaxation) of pelvic floor muscles during voiding with a staccato uroflow curve.

Primary bladder neck dysfunction (PBND), PUV, urethral stricture and meatal stenosis are considered in boys with poor uroflow rates despite a relaxed pelvic floor. VUDS is obtained in these children to further define their problem.

Children with symptoms of bladder neck dysfunction exhibit narrowing at the bladder neck in addition to high voiding pressures and low flow rates with an obstructive pattern. Some children are able to maintain high enough voiding pressures to achieve normal flow rates. Studies typically show detrusor instability and high voiding pressures. In patients with a long history of LUTS, we may see impaired compliance and/or inefficient detrusor contractions. Urinary flow is often intermittent and there is often a prolonged opening time, which we define as the time between the start of a contraction and the start of urine flow. Pelvic floor EMG lag time correlates with the opening time seen on VUDS.[17] Prolonged pelvic floor EMG lag time associated with abnormal uroflowmetry is highly suggestive of PBND (Figure 54.4). There may be a disparity between peak pressure and peak flow.

Treatment options

The first step is to ask the child to void on a timed schedule. We instruct children to void every 2–3 hours during the day even if they do not have the urge. A multiple alarm watch is a helpful novelty to remind a child to go to the bathroom. We send a letter to school requesting permission for the child to use the bathroom every 3 hours. Timed voiding requires a great deal of cooperation from parents, teachers, and children. In addition to timed voiding, the child must spend at least 30 s to 1 minute voiding, and must relax to ensure efficient emptying. Rewards (stickers, gold stars, etc.) are given each time the child performs satisfactorily. We urge girls to pull their pants/skirts down to their ankles and sit with their legs apart. Commercial and domestic toilets are designed for adults, not for children. It is difficult for a child to void with a relaxed pelvic floor when sitting on a toilet that they are nervous about falling through. Vaginal voiding causes postvoid dribbling because the urine that enters the lower vagina leaks into the underwear when they stand up. Toilet seat adaptors and footstools should be available at both home and school. We instruct girls to sit backwards on the toilet (straddling the toilet seat) to help relax the pelvic floor muscles.

Patients with LUTS sometimes require drug therapy in addition to timed voiding. Patients with severe frequency and/or urgency often report little change with timed voiding alone. Anticholinergics act by blocking the muscarinic receptors on the detrusor muscle, which are stimulated by acetylcholine released from activated cholinergic (parasympathetic) nerves. Anticholinergic medications act mainly during bladder filling by decreasing urge and increasing bladder capacity. In the dose range needed for beneficial effect in the overactive bladder, there is little evidence for a significant reduction of the voiding contraction during bladder emptying.[18] Ditropan (oxybutynin) is a potent anticholinergic agent with strong independent smooth muscle antispasmodic activity at a site distal to the cholinergic receptor. In young children who cannot swallow pills, we initiate treatment with oxybutynin suspension 2–3 times/day. Children who can swallow pills are treated with the extended-release oxybutynin (Ditropan XL) once a day. Patients on oxybutynin experience a decrease in the frequency and intensity of uninhibited bladder contractions.

with documented poor emptying as a result of various etiologies, including both neurogenic and non-neurogenic causes. With the use of an α_1-ANRB, bladder symptoms and/or emptying improved in 82% of patients and was well tolerated by most. Because of this success, they looked at a larger group of 55 patients with voiding dysfunction and poor bladder emptying.[24] There was an 88% reduction in the pretreatment PVR volume, with only 3 patients showing no change in PVR. There was improvement in diurnal continence in 83% of patients and urgency in 70%. They concluded that selective α_1-ANRB therapy might be used as either replacement for, or in addition to, biofeedback in patients with significant PVR volumes. At this time, α blockers have yet to be Food and Drug Administration (FDA) approved and are used off label.

Yucel et al compared the efficacy of biofeedback and α_1-ANRB therapy in children with PVR who had symptoms of incontinence, urgency, and UTIs.[25] There was no statistical difference between the two arms ($p > 0.05$) when looking at post-treatment reduction in PVR as the endpoint. Combined treatment of biofeedback and α_1-ANRB helped 83% of the children with refractory high PVR treated with either biofeedback or α-blocker therapy alone. Children with PBND respond well to α_1-ANRB. Donohoe et al used α_1-ANRB to treat 26 patients with PBND.[26] With α_1-ANRB, average and maximum flow rates improved from 5.5 to 12.6 ml/s and from 10.3 to 19.7 ml/s, respectively. PVR volumes decreased from 98.9 to 8.9 ml ($p < 0.001$). No patient experienced any major adverse side effects.

Diet can have a profound effect on voiding patterns, and dietary changes can alleviate symptoms associated with bladder dysfunction. Avoiding the '4 C's' (caffeine, chocolate, carbonated beverages, and citrus beverages) is an integral part of therapy, as they are known to cause urgency, frequency, and/or incontinence.

Clean intermittent catheterization (CIC) is a last option in a subset of patients that do not respond to standard treatment modalities. Alpert et al reported their experience with 20 patients requiring CIC.[27] CIC was an easy technique for 80% of the children to learn in a single visit and master in a short period. If necessary, CIC is used as a temporary measure until the patients learn to void correctly. If all these modalities fail, surgical intervention may be necessary. Augmentation cystoplasty with CIC provides a large-capacity, low-pressure, compliant bladder that allows for preservation of renal function and urinary continence. However, this is a long haul for a problem with no neurologic or anatomic etiology.

There are numerous approaches for the treatment of urinary incontinence in children. The aggressiveness of evaluation and intervention usually depend on the age of the patient, the chronicity of the problem, and other associated issues such as recurrent infections. A systematic review of randomized controlled trials led to the conclusion that there is a lack of proof for optimal treatment of pediatric incontinence.[28] Historically, antimuscarinic drugs have been the first line of treatment for urinary urgency, frequency, and urge-associated incontinence. Although they are associated with side effects that limit their use in some children, these drugs have undisputed effectiveness for the small numbers of children with overactive bladder that fail urotherapy. Children tolerate these medications better with the newer extended formulations. We sometimes use them in combination with other treatment modalities, including α_1-ANRBs, antibiotics, and bladder and bowel retraining. Newer, once daily, M_3 selective receptor antagonist agents are now available for the treatment of overactive bladder: with greater affinity for the M_3 receptors than the M_1 and M_2 receptors, there is less theoretical risk of central nervous system and cardiac side effects. The use of botulinum types A and B toxin injections into the detrusor muscle has been studied extensively for the treatment of incontinence from neurogenic causes. These treatments are safe, minimally invasive, and can be injected repeatedly, but to date have had no role in the treatment of non-neurogenic voiding disorders.

Summary

Voiding dysfunction is a common childhood problem. Use of a checklist for both the history and physical examination is highly recommended. Patience, diligence, and consistency are critical in the evaluation of these patients. Most children will respond to simple measures such as timed voiding and relaxation techniques to facilitate bladder emptying. In a select population of patients in whom single-modality therapy fails, we advise multiple-modality therapy, including timed voiding, biofeedback, and medications. In our experience, we treat almost all children successfully with combination therapy, frequently with no medication. The objective improvements we aim for are a decrease in PVR volumes, increased uroflow rates, and normalization of EMG patterns. Effective treatment also helps control the secondary complications of reflux, UTIs, and, in extreme cases, urinary tract deterioration.

Nocturnal enuresis

One of the most common urologic complaints in children is nocturnal enuresis (NE). Most children achieve night-time continence by 5 years old. The significance of NE is dependent upon the patient's age, the parents' and child's expectations, and the child's social situation.

Our understanding of the pathophysiology of NE has progressed greatly in recent years and we now know the disorder to be heterogeneous and genetically complex in nature. Abnormalities in nocturnal urine production, bladder reservoir function, arousability, molecular genetics, or a combination of these may be responsible for night-time wetting. This new understanding of NE has had enormous impact on both the diagnosis and treatment of the disorder. Nevertheless, we have much to learn and many controversies remain.

Definitions

In accordance with the International Children's Continence Society recommendations, we use the term primary nocturnal enuresis (PNE) to describe bedwetting in a child who has never had a dry period of >6 months. A child with secondary nocturnal enuresis is one that wets the bed but had previously been dry for at least 6 months prior.[29] Monosymptomatic nocturnal enuresis (MNE) describes bedwetting in children with no daytime urinary symptoms to suggest an underlying voiding dysfunction. Non-monosymptomatic or polysymptomatic nocturnal enuresis is used to describe nocturnal enuresis associated with bladder overactivity.[30]

Epidemiology

The overall prevalence of NE declines with age. By the age of 4 years, 20–25% of children frequently wet the bed. This decreases to 5–10% by the age of 7.[31–34] Fourteen percent of children between the ages of 5 and 9 years and 16% between 10 and 19 years will stop wetting the bed annually.[35] In this longitudinal cohort study, the authors followed 92% of 1129 children born in 1 year for 6 years, with PNE remission rates of approximately 15% per year.[35]

Although spontaneous cure occurs throughout childhood and adolescence, the problem may persist in 0.5–3% of the adult population.[36–39]

Although PNE is more common in young boys, by adolescence the incidence in males is equivalent to that in females.[40] The prevalence of NE is similar throughout the world.

Psychological impact

PNE may have a profound psychological and social impact on children and their families: enuresis may affect a child's normal activities and development; this, in turn, may affect the child's family.[41–43] There is some controversy regarding how enuresis affects self-esteem. A recent review concluded that there is no evidence that bedwetting leads to lower self-esteem.[43] Conversely, some studies have shown that children with NE have worse self-esteem and significantly more behavioral and psychological problems such as anxiety, depression, aggressiveness, and attention-deficit disorder when compared with normal age-matched non-enuretic patients.[41–43] After a successful cure, abnormal behavioral and psychological problems improve in some studies, possibly indicating that the problems are a result of the NE and not vice versa.[42,44,45] Surely, attaining dryness will not negatively impact a child's self-esteem. The child's age itself may change his/her attitude towards enuresis. Butler reported that younger children focus on the immediate consequences of enuresis, whereas older children are more likely to be affected by the social and emotional aspects of the condition.[46] Interestingly, comorbid psychiatric disorders are present in up to 75% of secondary nocturnal enuretics.[41,47] At least 46% of parents have some concern about NE, whereas 17% worry a great deal.[34,48]

In a study by Haque et al 1981, the mean anticipated age of dryness according to parents was 3.18 years. When asked for possible causes for their child's NE, parents believed that emotional problems (35.5%), heavy sleeping (38.2%), physical problems (21.4%), familial problems (28.9%), and small bladders (10.7%) may be responsible for their child's wetness.[49]

NE may also lead to punishment. Some mothers believe that their child is wetting on purpose and choose not to treat their children and may even punish them.[48] The reported rates of punishment in the 1980s were 37% in the UK and 35.8% in the United States.

Etiology

Family studies have repeatedly demonstrated high rates of relatives affected by enuresis. The risk for a child to be enuretic is 40% if one parent and 70% if both parents had been enuretic.[50] Early studies reported that 32% of fathers and 23.9% of mothers of children with enuresis were enuretic as children.[51]

Based on twin studies, the most common mode of transmission is autosomal dominant with high (90%)

Arginine vasopressin (AVP or ADH) is a polypeptide produced in the hypothalamus and released from the pituitary gland. Its release is caused by hyperosmolality or a low effective circulating blood volume. The polypeptide's effect is on V_2 receptors of the collecting ducts and distal tubules to enhance water reabsorption.[115] It also is a potent vasopressor, through independent actions on V_1 receptors.

Desmopressin is an analog of vasopressin. Unlike ADH, this analog has increased antidiuretic activity without vasopressor activity. The half-life is 1.5–3.5 hours. Desmopressin is commercially available in an oral and intranasal formula. The usual dose is 0.2–0.6 mg orally or 10–40 μg intranasally at bedtime with immediate clinical effects. Fluid intake should be limited when the drug is used. A simple suggestion is to avoid drinking for 2 hours before bedtime and to limit fluid intake to 8 ounces after evening meal.

Desmopressin is regarded safe for use in children. In most cases, children tolerate the medication well, with few adverse reactions reported in short- or long-term use.[107,108] Klauber reported no serious adverse reactions in 516 cases.[116] In another study, only 6 of 242 children (2.5%) withdrew, as a result of very mild adverse events, during long-term intranasal treatment. All monitored clinical and laboratory parameters remained within normal limits in this study.[107]

The risk of water intoxication should be discussed with parents prior to initiating DDAVP therapy and, consequently, fluid intake during evening meal and before bedtime should be limited. In this case, hyponatremia results from a large amount of fluid intake while taking the drug.[117]

Although children with nocturnal polyuria and low nocturnal urine osmolality should respond best to DDAVP treatment, some studies have not found any differences in urine output, osmolality, or vasopressin secretion in responders and non-responders.[118,119]

Before labeling a child as a non-responder, it is important to know whether the child received the medication correctly. In children that do not respond to treatment with DDAVP, nocturnal hypercalciuria and hypernatriuria should be suspected.[67,90]

Predictors of good response to desmopressin therapy include larger bladder capacities,[75] older children,[120,121] fewer wet nights at presentation,[120,122] and normal functional bladder capacity.[119,121] Other predictors include primary as opposed to secondary NE,[123] only one wet episode during the night, enuresis that occurs during the first 2 hours of sleep,[119] a family history of NE,[124,125] and initial good response to the smallest dose of desmopressin used in the study (20 μg intranasal).[126]

Several controlled studies have demonstrated the effectiveness of desmopressin in the treatment of nocturnal enuresis,[56,127–129] regardless of the route of administration. Positive response (defined as >50% reduction of wet nights) was reported in 60–70% of patients.[58,64,107] A review of randomized trials comparing desmopressin with placebo found that desmopressin was better in 13 of the 14 studies.[64] Based on the Cochrane report by Glazener and Evans, patients treated with DDAVP were 4.6 times more likely to achieve 14 consecutive dry nights compared with placebo.[130] With a more selected population of children with primary NE, Caione et al found a 79% success rate after the administration of desmopressin.[131]

When DDAVP treatment is successful, we stop the drug for 1 week every 3 months to evaluate whether the problem persists. The annual cure rate in children treated with DDAVP is approximately 30%.[107] Permanent cure may increase to 74.5% by gradually discontinuing the drug and positively reinforcing dry nights over a 10-week period.[132]

Unfortunately, relapse after the cessation of treatment is common, and long-term treatment may yield a better response. Of 399 enuretic children recruited in the Swedish Enuresis Trial (SWEET),[107] 61% responded to desmopressin treatment initially, and of those responders, 61% were dry after 1 year of treatment. However, using an intent-to-treat analysis, only 19% of patients remained dry after the cessation of therapy.[107]

Desmopressin may be helpful in children that have failed alarm therapy or in families where motivation to use the alarm is lacking. In the short term, desmopressin produces more rapid improvement than alarm therapy. As children that do poorly with the alarm may do well with DDAVP, the converse may also be true.

Oxybutynin

The antimuscarinic agent oxybutynin is often used as part of combination therapy in enuretic children with a small bladder capacity, daytime incontinence, or detrusor overactivity. Oxybutynin should not be the first recommended therapy for a child with MNE. Yeung et al found that ≥ 30% of enuretic children refractory to therapy had detrusor overactivity at night.[77] When using oxybutynin, we recommend bladder training, since in unselected populations of children with NE, oxybutynin has not been effective in randomized controlled studies.[133] Watanabe et al[134] reported a 67% success rate with oxybutynin in a group of children with bladder instability as a cause of their NE. Kass et al[135] reported a 90% success rate. The drug may also be considered in children with day- and night-time incontinence and for DDAVP non-responders. The efficacy may improve when combined with desmopressin.[136,137]

Tricyclic antidepressants

Tricyclic antidepressants such as imipramine were extensively used in the treatment of enuresis in the 1970s and 1980s. Imipramine has fallen out of favor for several reasons, including cardiotoxic side effects, risk of death with overdose, and its psychopharmacologic properties. The mechanism of action for this drug in the treatment of NE is unclear, although it may act by reducing detrusor activity and increasing bladder capacity secondary to anticholinergic and smooth muscle relaxant effects.

Additionally, it may enhance arousal and suppress rapid eye movement (REM) sleep or decrease urine production by a stimulating vasopressin release.[138,139]

Because of the lower efficacy and more dangerous side-effect profile of this drug compared with desmopressin (only 17% of children who were dry during treatment with imipramine remained dry 6 months after cessation of medication and alarm therapy), we only use it when all other management has failed.

Other therapies

Combination therapy

Some children with NE may have more than one cause for their condition. The most common combined cause of NE is lack of AVP with poor arousability. In these children, combined therapy may be more successful than a single therapy alone.

Studies using combined desmopressin and the enuresis alarm on unselected groups of children have been published. In study by Bradbury, 71 children were randomized to alarm plus desmopressin (40 μg) or alarm monotherapy for 6 weeks.[140] The combined therapy was more effective than the alarm alone, particularly where the child had severe NE and behavioral problems. Sukhai et al,[141] with a crossover design, randomized children into two treatment groups: i.e. alarm + desmopressin or alarm + placebo. The results suggested that alarm + desmopressin was better ($p = 0.05$) than alarm + placebo in treating NE. In a double-blind placebo-controlled study, Leebeek-Groenewegen et al,[142] examined 93 children with MNE. Children were treated with alarm + desmopressin or alarm + placebo for 9 weeks. Based on the results of this study, it was concluded that desmopressin does not result in higher cure rates and that combined treatment is not justified in all enuretic children at the outset of treatment.

For children with enuresis associated with bladder overactivity, a combination of bladder training coupled with anticholinergic therapy yields success rates of 67–100%.[78,135,137] Combination therapy with oxybutynin and desmopressin has also been found to be effective in this subgroup of patients.[131]

Behavioral therapies

Houts suggested that the addition of selected behavioral procedures produces better outcomes than alarm monotherapy.[143] Houts names four main behavioral procedures. These include arousal training, which reinforces waking and toileting in response to the alarm's trigger, and normalized voiding, which encourages children to increase their fluid intake and time their voiding during the daytime in an attempt to increase cognitive control over voiding. One other procedure, dry-bed training uses the enuresis alarm, and encourages the children to take responsibility for removing wet sheets and re-making the bed, and two waking schedules, to ease arousability from sleep.[144] However, Bollard and Nettelbeck[145] found that the enuresis alarm accounted for most of the success achieved through dry-bed training.

Alternative therapies

Numerous studies using traditional Chinese acupuncture and laser acupuncture for the treatment of NE have been published.[146,147] In a prospective randomized study comparing laser acupuncture with desmopressin in patients with nocturnal polyuria, laser acupuncture was found to be as efficacious as desmopressin.[147]

Treatment for non-responders

Absorptive nocturnal hypercalciuria may be responsible for NE in some children that remain non-responders despite therapy with DDAVP and anticholinergics. Pace et al demonstrated that some enuretic patients with hypercalciuria who failed to respond to DDAVP became desmopressin responders once they were treated with a low-calcium diet.[148]

Abnormalities in aquaporin 2 (AQP2) urinary excretion have been recently reported as another possible cause of nocturnal enuresis.[67] Urinary AQP2 and hypercalciuria levels correlated with the severity of enuresis in children. Valenti et al further strengthened the association between AQP2 and hypercalciuria in a recent study.[149] Enuresis resolved in 80% of patients after 6 months of combined treatment with desmopressin and a low-calcium diet. Arginine vasopressin levels returned to normal, hypercalciuria resolved, and day/night AQP2 ratios returned to near normal levels. Based on these recent reports, Hjalmas and colleagues suggest that:[107]

> it may become mandatory to study the CaU/CrU ratio to determine if the enuretic patient is hypercalciuric or not, as a first step to a correct therapeutic strategy for nocturnal enuresis.

Conclusion

Despite advances in our understanding of NE, the condition remains complex. The key to success involves a motivated patient and family.

References

1. Koff SA. Estimating bladder capacity in children. Urology 1983; 21:248.
2. Hinman F, Baumann FW. Vesical and ureteral damage from voiding dysfunction in boys without neurologic or obstructive disease. J Urol 1973; 109:727–32.
3. Chandra M, Saharia R, Shi Q, Hill V. Giggle incontinence in children: a manifestation of detrusor instability. J Urol 2002; 168(5):2184.
4. Sureshkumar P, Craig JC, Roy LP, Knight JF. Daytime urinary incontinence in primary school children: a population-based survey. J Pediatr 2000; 137:814–18.
5. Abi-Hanna A, Lake AM. Constipation and encopresis in childhood. Pediatric Rev 1998; 19(1):23–30.
6. Loening-Baucke V. Urinary incontinence and urinary tract infection and their resolution with treatment of chronic constipation of childhood. Pediatrics 1997; 100:228–32.
7. Shaikh N, Abedin S, Wise B et al. Can ultrasonography or urowflowmetry predict which children with voiding dysfunction will develop recurrent urinary tract infections? Presented at the American Academy of Pediatrics Annual Meeting, Section on Urology, San Francisco, 2004.
8. Doubrava RG, Bartkowski DP. Ability of the dysfunctional voiding scoring system questionaire to predict uroflowometry and external urinary sphincter electromyography patterns in normal children. Presented at the Society for Pediatric Urology annual meeting, San Francisco, 2004.
9. Sureshkumar P, Craig JC, Roy LP, Knight J. A reproducible pediatric daytime urinary incontinence questionnaire. J Urol 2001; 165:569–73.
10. Farhat W, Bagli DJ, Capolichio G et al. The dysfunctional voiding scoring system: quantitative standardization of dysfunctional voiding symptoms in children. J Urol 2000; 164:1011.
11. Ritchey ML, Sinha A, DiPietro MA et al. Significance of spina bifida occulta in children with diurnal enuresis. J Urol 1994; 15:815–18.
12. Griffiths DJ, Scholtmeijer RJ. Place of the free flow curve in the urodynamic investigation of children. Br J Urol 1984; 56:474–7.
13. Norgaard JP, van Gool JD, Hjalmas K, Djurhuus JC, Hellstrom AL. Standardization and definitions in lower tract dysfunction in children. International Children's Continence Society. Br J Urol 1998; 81:1–16.
14. Passerini-Glazel G, Cisternino A, Camuffo MC. Videourodynamic studies of minor voiding dysfunctions in children: an overview of 13 years' experience. Scand J Urol Nephrol Suppl 1992; 141:70–84.
15. Combs AJ, Misseri R, Horowitz M, Glassberg KI. Pelvic floor EMG lag time and it's utility in diagnosing children with detrusor instability. Presented at the American Academy of Pediatrics Annual Meeting, San Francisco, 2004.
16. Kakizaki H, Moriya K, Ameda K et al. Diameter of the external urethral sphincter as a predictor of detrusor sphincter incoordination in children: comparative study of voiding cystourethrography. J Urol 2003; 169:655–8.
17. Combs AJ, Grafstein N, Horowitz M, Glassberg KI. Primary bladder neck dysfunction in children and adolescents I: pelvic floor electromyography lag time – a new noninvasive method to screen for and monitor therapeutic response. J Urol 2005; 173:207–10, discussion 210–11.
18. Anderson KE. Antimuscarinics for treatment of overactive bladder. Lancet Neurol 2004; 3:46.
19. Wiener JS, Scales MT, Hampton J et al. Long-term efficacy of simple behavioral therapy for daytime wetting in children. J Urol 2000; 164:786–90.
20. Nelson JD, Cooper CS, Boyt MA, Hawtrey CE, Austin JC. Improved uroflow parameters and post-void residual following biofeedback therapy in pediatric patients with dysfunctional voiding does not correspond to outcome. J Urol 2004; 172:1653–6, discussion 1656.
21. Herndon CD, DeCambre M, McKenna PH. Interactive computer games for treatment of pelvic floor dysfunction. J Urol 2001; 166(5):1893.
22. De Gennaro M, Capitanucci ML, Mastracci P et al. Percutaneous tibial nerve neuomodulation is well tolerated in children and effective for treating refractory vesical dysfunction. J Urol 2004; 171:1911–13.
23. Austin PF, Homsy YL, Masel JL et al. α-Adrenergic blockade in children with neuropathic and nonneuropathic voiding dysfunction. J Urol 1999; 163:1064–7.
24. Cain MP, Wu SD, Austin PF, Herndon CD, Rink RC. Alpha blocker therapy for children with dysfunctional voiding and urinary retention. J Urol 2003; 170:1514–15, discussion 1516–17.
25. Yucel S, Akkaya E, Guntekin E et al. Can alpha blocker therapy be an alternative therapy to biofeedback in dysfunctional voiding and urinary retention: a prospective study. Presented at the American Academy of Pediatrics annual meeting, Section on Urology, San Francisco, 2004.

26. Donohoe JM, Combs AJ, Glassbergh KI. Primary bladder neck dysfunction in children and adolescents II: results of treatment with alpha-adrenergic antagonists. J Urol 2005; 173:212–16.
27. Alpert SA, Cheng EY, Zebold KF, Kaplan WE. Clean intermittent catheterization in sensate children: patient's experience and health related quality of life. Presented at the American Academy of Pediatrics annual meeting, Section on Urology, San Francisco, 2004.
28. Sureshkumar P, Bower W, Craig JC, Knight JF. Treatment of daytime urinary incontinence in children: a systematic review of randomized controlled trials. J Urol 2003; 170:196–200, discussion 200.
29. van Gool JD, Bloom DA, Butler RJ et al. Conservative management in children. In: Abrams P, Khoury S, Wein A, eds. 1st International Consultation on Incontinence, Monaco, June 28 to July 1, 1998. Plymouth, United Kingdom: Health Publication, 1999: 495.
30. van Gool JD, Nieuwenhuis E, ten Doeschate IOM, Messer TP, de Jong TPVM. Subtypes of monosymptomatic nocturnal enuresis. Scand J Urol Nephrol Suppl 1999; 202:8–11.
31. Hellstrom AL, Hansson E, Hansson S et al. Micturition habits and incontinence in 7-year-old Swedish school entrants. Eur J Pediatr 1990; 149:434–7.
32. Fergusson DM, Hons BA, Horwood LJ, Shannon FT. Factors related to the age of attainment of nocturnal enuresis. Behav Psychother 1986; 78:884–90.
33. de Jonge GA. Epidemiology of enuresis: a survey of the literature. In: Kovin I, MacKeith RC, Meadows SR, eds. Bladder Control and Enuresis. London: Heinemann, 1973: 39–46.
34. Foxman B, Valdez RB, Brook RH. Childhood enuresis: prevalence, perceived impact, and prescribed treatments. Pediatrics 1986; 77:482–7.
35. Forsythe WI, Redmond A. Enuresis and spontaneous cure rate: study of 1129 patients. Arch Dis Child 1974; 49:259–63.
36. Tietjen DN, Husmann DA. Nocturnal enuresis: a guide to evaluation and treatment. Mayo Clin Proc 1996; 71:857–62.
37. van Son MJ, Mulder G, van Londen A. The effectiveness of dry bed training for nocturnal enuresis in adults. Behav Res Ther 1990; 28:347–9.
38. Cushing FC Jr, Baller WR. The problem of nocturnal enuresis in adults: special reference to managers and managerial aspirants. J Psychol 1975; 89:203–13.
39. Hirasing RA, van Leerdam FJ, Bolk-Bennink L, Janknegt RA. Enuresis nocturna in adults. Scand J Urol Nephrol 1997; 31(6):533–6.
40. Moore KH, Richmond DH, Parys BT. Sex distribution of adult idiopathic detrusor instability in relation to childhood bedwetting. Br J Urol 1991; 68:479–82.
41. von Gontard A, Pluck J, Berner W, Lehmkuhl G. Clinical behavioral problems in day and night wetting children. Pediatr Nephrol 1999; 13:662–7.
42. Hagglof B, Andren O, Bergstrom E et al. Self-esteem before and after treatment in children with nocturnal enuresis and urinary incontinence. Scand J Urol Nephrol 1997; 183:79–82.
43. Redsell SA, Collier J. Bedwetting, behavior and self-esteem: a review of the literature. Child Care Health Dev 2000; 27:149–62.
44. Hagglof B, Andren O, Bergstrom E et al. Self-esteem in children with nocturnal enuresis and urinary incontinence: improvement of self-esteem after treatment. Eur Urol 1998; 33(Suppl. 3):16–19.
45. Longstaffe S, Moffat M, Whalen J. Behavioral and self-esteem changes after six months of enuresis treatment: a randomized, controlled trial. Pediatrics 2000; 105:935–40.
46. Butler RJ. Impact of nocturnal enuresis on children and young people. Scand J Urol Nephrol 2001; 35:169–76.
47. von Gontard A. Annotation: day and night wetting in children – a paediatric and child psychiatric perspective. J Child Psychol Psychiatry 1998; 39:439–51.
48. Butler RJ, Brewin CR, Forsythe WI. Maternal attributions and tolerance for nocturnal enuresis. Behav Res Ther 1986; 24(3):307–12.
49. Haque M, Ellerstein NS, Gundy JH et al. Parental perceptions of enuresis. A collaborative study. Am J Dis Child 1981; 135(9):809–11.
50. Bakwin H. Enuresis in twins. Am J Dis Child 1971; 121(3):222–5.
51. Frary G. Enuresis. A genetic study. Am J Dis Child 1935; 49:557.
52. Hublin C, Kaprio J, Partinen M, Koskenvuo M. Nocturnal enuresis in a nationwide twin cohort. Sleep 1998; 21:579–85.
53. Arnell H, Hjalmas K, Jagervall M et al. The genetics of primary nocturnal enuresis: inheritance and suggestion of a second major gene on chromosome 12q. J Med Genet 1997; 34(5):360–5.
54. Eiberg H. Total genome scan analysis in a single extended family for primary nocturnal enuresis. Evidence for a new locus (ENUR3) for primary nocturnal enuresis on chromosome 22q11. Eur J Urol 1998; 33(Suppl 3):34–6.
55. von Gontard A, Eiberg H, Hollmann E, Rittig S, Lehmkuhl G. Molecular genetics of nocturnal enuresis: clinical and genetic heterogeneity. Acta Paediatr 1998; 87:571–8.
56. Rittig S, Knudsen UB, Norgaard JP, Pedersen EB, Djurhuus JC. Abnormal diurnal rhythm of plasma vasopressin and urinary output in patients with enuresis. Am J Physiol 1989; 256:F664–71.
57. Rittig S, Knudsen UB, Sorensen S et al. Long-term double-blind crossover study of desmopressin intranasal spray in the management of nocturnal enuresis. In: Meadow SR, ed. Desmopressin in Nocturnal Enuresis. UK: Horus Medical Publications, 1989: 43–55.
58. Norgaard JP, Pedersen EB, Djurhuus JC. Diurnal antidiuretic hormone levels in enuretics. J Urol 1985; 134:1029–31.
59. Devitt H, Holland P, Butler RJ et al. Plasma vasopressin and response to treatment in primary nocturnal enuresis. Arch Dis Child 1999; 80:448–51.
60. Butler RJ, Holland P. The three systems: a conceptual way of understanding nocturnal enuresis. Scand J Urol Nephrol 2000; 34:270–7.
61. Norgaard JP, Rittig S, Djurhuus JC. Nocturnal enuresis: an approach to treatment based on pathogenesis. J Pediatr 1989; 114:705–10.

62. Hansen MN, Rittig S, Siggaard C et al. Intra-individual variability in nighttime urine production and functional bladder capacity estimated by home recordings in patients with nocturnal enuresis. J Urol 2001; 166:2452–5.
63. Oredsson AF, Jorgensen TM. Changes in nocturnal bladder capacity during treatment with the bell and pad for monosymptomatic nocturnal enuresis. J Urol 1998; 160:166–9.
64. Moffatt MEK, Harlos S, Kirshen AJ, Burd L. Desmopressin acetate and nocturnal enuresis: How much do we know? Pediatrics 1993; 92:420–5.
65. Natochin YV, Kuznetsova AA. Nocturnal enuresis: correction of renal function by desmopressin and diclofenac. Pediatr Nephrol 2000; 14:42–7.
66. Radetti G, Paganini C, Rigon F et al. Urinary aquaporin-2 excretion in nocturnal enuresis. Eur J Endocrinol 2001; 145:435–8.
67. Valenti G, Laera A, Pace G et al. Urinary aquaporin 2 and calciuria correlate with the severity of enuresis in children. J Am Soc Nephrol 2000; 11:1873–81.
68. Cinar U, Vural C, Cakir B et al. Nocturnal enuresis and upper airway obstruction. Int J Pediatr Otorhinolaryngol 2001; 59:115–18.
69. Lackgren G, Hjalmas K, van Gool J et al. Nocturnal enuresis: a suggestion for a European treatment strategy. Acta Paediatr 1999; 88:679–90.
70. Rittig S, Matthiesen TB, Pedersen EB, Djurhuus JC. Sodium regulating hormones in enuresis. Scand J Urol Nephrol Suppl 1999; 202:45–6.
71. Neveus T, Tuvemo T, Lackgren G, Stenberg A. Bladder capacity and renal concentrating ability in enuresis: pathogenic implications. J Urol 2001; 165:2022–5.
72. Wolfish NM, Pivik RT, Busby KA. Elevated sleep arousal thresholds in enuretic boys: clinical implications. Acta Paediatr 1997; 86(4):381–4.
73. Von Gontard A, Schmelzer D, Seifen S, Pukrop R. Central nervous system involvement in nocturnal enuresis: evidence of general neuromotor delay and specific brainstem dysfunction. J Urol 2001; 166:2448–51.
74. Rushton HG, Belman AB, Zaontz MR et al. The influence of small functional bladder capacity and other predictors on the response to desmopressin in the management of monosymptomatic nocturnal enuresis. J Urol 1996; 156 (Suppl 2):651–5.
75. Eller DA, Austin PF, Tanguay S, Homsy YL. Daytime functional bladder capacity as a predictor of response to desmopressin in monosymptomatic nocturnal enuresis. Eur Urol 1998; 33(Suppl 3):25–9.
76. Yeung CK, Chiu HN, Sit FKY. Bladder dysfunction in children with refractory monosymptomatic primary nocturnal enuresis. J Urol 1999; 162:1049–55.
77. Yeung CK, Sit FKY, To LKC et al. Reduction in nocturnal functional bladder capacity is a common factor in the pathogenesis of refractory nocturnal enuresis. BJU Int 2002; 90:302–7.
78. Watanabe H, Kawauchi A, Kitamori T, Azuma Y. Treatment system for nocturnal enuresis according to an original classification system. Eur Urol 1994; 25:43–50.
79. Torrens MJ, Collins CD. The urodynamic assessment of adults enuresis. Br J Urol 1975; 47:433–40.
80. Sakamoto K, Blaivas JG. Adult onset nocturnal enuresis. J Urol 2001; 165:1914–17.
81. Hjalmas K, Arnold T, Bower W et al. Nocturnal enuresis: an international evidence based management strategy. J Urol 2004; 171(6 Pt 2):2545–61.
82. Bower WF, Moore KH, Adams RD, Shepherd RB. Frequency volume chart data from incontinent children. Br J Urol 1997; 80:658–62.
83. Neveus T, Lackgren G, Tuvemo T et al. Enuresis – background and treatment. Scand J Urol Nephrol Suppl 2000; 206:1–44.
84. Koff SA, Wagner TT, Jayanthi VR. The relationship among dysfunctional elimination syndromes, primary vesicoureteral reflux and urinary tract infections in children. J Urol 1998; 160:1019–22.
85. Hoebeke P, Van Laeke E, Raes A, Van Gool JD, Vande Walle J. Anomalies of external urethral meatus in girls with non-neurogenic bladder sphincter dysfunction. BJU Int 1999; 83:294–8.
86. Forbes FC. Children with enuresis. Nowadays, a strong suspicion of sexual abuse would prompt full investigation. BMJ 1998; 316(7133):777.
87. Klevan JL, De Jong AR. Urinary tract symptoms and urinary tract infection following sexual abuse. Am J Dis Child 1990; 144(2):242–4.
88. Butler RJ, Strenberg A. Treatment of childhood nocturnal enuresis: an examination of clinically relevant principles. BJU Int 2001; 88:563–71.
89. Longstaffe S, Moffat M, Whalen J. Behavioral and self-concept changes after six months of enuresis treatment: a randomized, controlled trial. Pediatrics 2000; 105: 935–40.
90. Aceto G, Penza R, Coccioli MS et al. Enuresis subtypes based on nocturnal hypercalciuria: a multicentric study. J Urol 2003; 170:1670–3.
91. Glazener CM, Evans JH. Simple behavioural and physical interventions for nocturnal enuresis in children. Cochrane Database Syst Rev 2002; 2:CD003637.
92. Loening-Baucke V. Urinary incontinence and urinary tract infection and their resolution with treatment of chronic constipation of childhood. Pediatrics 1997; 100:228–32.
93. Mellon MW, McGrath ML. Empirically supported treatments in pediatric psychology: nocturnal enuresis. J Pediatr Psychol 2000; 25:193–214.
94. Kruse S, Hellstrom AL, Hjalmas K. Daytime bladder dysfunction in therapy-resistant nocturnal enuresis. A pilot study in urotherapy. Scand J Urol Nephrol 1999; 33:49–52.
95. Robson LM, Leung AK. Urotherapy recommendations for bedwetting. J Natl Med Assoc 2002; 94:577–80.
96. Evans JHC. Evidence based management of nocturnal enuresis. BMJ 2001; 323:1167–9.
97. Butler RJ, Robinson JC. Alarm treatment for childhood nocturnal enuresis, an investigation of within-treatment variables. Scand J Urol Nephrol 2002; 36:268–72.
98. Forsythe WI, Butler RJ. Fifty years of enuretic alarms. Arch Dis Child 1989; 64:879–85.
99. Johnson SB. Enuresis. In: Daitzman RD, ed. Clinical Behaviour Therapy and Behaviour Modification. London: Garland STPM Press, 1980: 81–142.

100. Butler RJ, Forsythe WI, Robertson J. The body worn alarm in the treatment of nocturnal enuresis. Br J Clin Pract 1990; 44:237–41.
101. Glazener CM, Evans JH. Alarm interventions for nocturnal enuresis in children Cochrane Database Syst Rev 2003; 3:CD002117.
102. Butler RJ, Brewin CR, Forsythe WI. Maternal attributions and tolerance for nocturnal enuresis. Behav Res Ther 1986; 24:307–12.
103. Morgan RT, Young GC. Parental attitudes and the conditioning treatment of childhood enuresis. Behav Res Ther 1975; 13:197–9.
104. Butler RJ. Establishment of working definitions in nocturnal enuresis. Arch Dis Child 1991; 66(2):267–71.
105. Moffatt ME. Nocturnal enuresis: a review of the efficacy of treatments and practical advice for clinicians. J Dev Behav Pediatr 1997; 18:49–56.
106. Houts AC, Berman JS, Abramson H. Effectiveness of psychological and pharmacological treatments for nocturnal enuresis. J Consult Clin Psychol 1994; 62(4):737–45.
107. Hjalmas K, Hanson E, Hellstrom AL, Kruse S, Sillen U. Long-term treatment with desmopressin in children with primary monosymptomatic nocturnal enuresis: an open multicentre study. Swedish Enuresis Trial (SWEET) Group. Br J Urol 1998; 82:704–9.
108. Lackgren G, Lilja B, Neveus T, Stenberg A. Desmopressin in the treatment of severe nocturnal enuresis in adolescents – a 7-year follow-up study. Br J Urol 1998; 81(Suppl 3):17–23.
109. Wagner WG, Johnson JT. Childhood nocturnal enuresis: the prediction of premature withdrawal from behavioral conditioning. J Abnorm Child Psychol 1988; 16:687–92.
110. Geffken G, Johnson SB, Walker D. Behavioral interventions for childhood nocturnal enuresis: the differential effect of bladder capacity on treatment progress and outcome. Health Psychol 1986; 5:261–72.
111. Devlin JB, O'Cathain C. Predicting treatment outcome in nocturnal enuresis. Arch Dis Child 1990; 65:1158–61.
112. Young GC, Morgan RTT. Reasons for appointment failure among enuretic patients. Comm Med 1972; 129:23–5.
113. Neveus T, Lackgren G, Tuvemo T et al. Enuresis – background and treatment. Scand J Urol Nephrol Suppl 2000; 206:1–44.
114. Hansen AF, Jorgensen TM. A possible explanation of wet and dry nights in enuretic children. Br J Urol 1997; 80:809–11.
115. Kamsteeg EJ, Deen PM, van Os CH. Defective processing and trafficking of water channels in nephrogenic diabetes insipidus. Exp Nephrol 2000; 8:326–31.
116. Klauber GT. Clinical efficacy and safety of desmopressin in the treatment of nocturnal enuresis. J Pediatr 1989; 114:719–22.
117. Robson WL, Norgaard JP, Leung AK. Hyponatremia in patients with nocturnal enuresis treated with DDAVP. Eur J Pediatr 1996; 155(11):959–62.
118. Hunsballe JM, Hansen TK, Rittig S, Pedersen EB, Djurhuus JC. The efficacy of DDAVP is related to the circadian rhythm of urine output in patients with persisting nocturnal enuresis. Clin Endocrinol (Oxf) 1998; 49:793–801.
119. Neveus T, Lackgren G, Tuvemo T, Stenberg A. Osmoregulation and desmopressin pharmacokinetics in enuretic children. Pediatrics 1999; 103:65–70.
120. Post EM, Richman RA, Blackett PR, Duncan KP, Miller K. Desmopressin response of enuretic children. Effects of age and frequency of enuresis. Am J Dis Child 1983; 137:962–3.
121. Rushton HG, Belman AB, Skoog S, Zaontz MR, Sihelnik S. Predictors of response to desmopressin in children and adolescents with monosymptomatic nocturnal enuresis. Scand J Urol Nephrol 1995; 173:109–10.
122. Butler R, Holland P, Devitt H et al. The effectiveness of desmopressin in the treatment of childhood nocturnal enuresis: predicting response using pretreatment variables. Br J Urol 1998; 81(Suppl 3):29–36.
123. Moffatt ME, Harlos S, Kirshen AJ, Burd L. Desmopressin acetate and nocturnal enuresis: how much do we know? Pediatrics 1993; 92:420–5.
124. Hogg RJ. Genetic factors as predictors for desmopressin treatment success. Scand J Urol Nephrol 1997; 183:37–9.
125. Chiozza ML, Plebani M, Scaccianoce C, Biraghi M, Zacchello G. Evaluation of antidiuretic hormone before and after long-term treatment with desmopressin in a group of enuretic children. Br J Urol 1998; 81(Suppl 3): 53–5.
126. Kruse S, Hellstrom AL, Hanson E, Hjalmas K. Treatment of primary monosymptomatic nocturnal enuresis with desmopressin: predictive factors. BJU Int 2001; 88:572–6.
127. Fjellestad-Paulsen A, Wille S, Harris AS. Comparison of intranasal and oral desmopressin for nocturnal enuresis. Arch Dis Child 1987; 62:674–717.
128. Wille S. Comparison of desmopressin and enuresis alarm for nocturnal enuresis. Arch Dis Child 1986; 61:30–3.
129. Janknegt RA, Zweers HM, Delaere KP et al. Oral desmopressin as a new treatment modality for primary nocturnal enuresis in adolescents and adults: a double-blind, randomized, multicenter study. The Dutch Enuresis Study Group. J Urol 1997; 157:513–17.
130. Glazener CM, Evans JH. Desmopressin for nocturnal enuresis in children. Cochrane Database Syst Rev 2002; 2:CD002217.
131. Caione P, Arena F, Biraghi M et al. Nocturnal enuresis and daytime wetting: a multicentric trial with oxybutynin and desmopressin. Eur Urol 1997; 31:459–63.
132. Butler RJ, Holland P, Robinson J. Examination of the structured withdrawal program to prevent relapse of nocturnal enuresis. J Urol 2001; 166:2463–6.
133. Lovering JS, Tallett SE, McKendry JB. Oxybutynin efficacy in the treatment of primary enuresis. Pediatrics 1988; 82:104–6.
134. Watanabe H, Kawauchi A. Nocturnal enuresis: social aspects and treatment perspectives in Japan. Scand J Urol Nephrol Suppl 1994; 163:29–38.
135. Kass EJ, Diokno AC, Montealegre A. Enuresis: principles of management and result of treatment. J Urol 1979; 121:794–6.
136. Neveus T. Oxybutynin, desmopressin and enuresis. J Urol 2001; 166:2459–62.
137. Kosar A, Arikan N, Dincel C. Effectiveness of oxybutynin

hydrochloride in the treatment of enuresis nocturna. Scand J Urol Nephrol 1999; 33:115–18.
138. Kales A, Kales JD, Jacobson A, Humphrey FJ 2nd, Soldatos CR. Effects of imipramine on enuretic frequency and sleep stages. Pediatrics 1977; 60(4):431–6.
139. Tomasi PA, Siracusano S, Monni AM, Mela G, Delitala G. Decreased nocturnal urinary antidiuretic hormone excretion in enuresis is increased by imipramine. BJU Int 2001; 88:932–7.
140. Bradbury M. Combination therapy for nocturnal enuresis with desmopressin and alarm device. Scand J Urol Nephrol Suppl 1997; 183:61–3.
141. Sukhai RN, Mol J, Harris AS. Combined therapy of enuresis alarm and desmopressin in the treatment of nocturnal enuresis. Eur J Pediatr 1989; 148:465–7.
142. Leebeek-Groenewegen A, Blom J, Sukhai R, Van Der Heijden B. Efficacy of desmopressin combined with alarm therapy for monosymptomatic nocturnal enuresis. J Urol 2001; 166(6):2456–8.
143. Houts AC. Behavioural treatment for enuresis. Scand J Urol Nephrol Suppl 1995; 173:83–8.
144. Azrin NH, Sneed TJ, Foxx RM. Dry-bed training: rapid elimination of childhood enuresis. Behav Res Ther 1974; 12:147–56.
145. Bollard J, Nettelbeck T. A comparison of dry-bed training and standard urine-alarm conditioning treatment of childhood bedwetting. Behav Res Ther 1981; 19:215–26.
146. Björkström G, Hellstrom AL, Andersson S. Electro-acupuncture in the treatment of children with monosymptomatic nocturnal enuresis. Scand J Urol Nephrol 2000; 34:21–6.
147. Radmayr C, Schlager B, Studen M, Bartsch G. Prospective randomized trial using laser acupuncture versus desmopressin in the treatment of nocturnal enuresis. Eur Urol 2001; 40:201–5.
148. Pace G, Aceto G, Cormio L et al. Nocturnal enuresis can be caused by absorptive hypercalciuria. Scand J Urol Nephrol 1999; 33:111–14.
149. Valenti G, Laera A, Gouraud S et al. Low-calcium diet in hypercalciuric enuretic children restores AQP2. Am J Physiol Renal Physiol 2002; 283:F895–903.

Operations for the weak bladder outlet

55

Anthony J Casale

Introduction

Surgery to correct urinary incontinence began in 1852 with a procedure to divert the ureters into the sigmoid colon of a boy with exstrophy.[1] Our understanding of the physiology and cause of urinary incontinence has grown slowly over the past century and more has been learned in the past 25 years than in prior medical history. Early surgeons did not have the necessary technology to define the physiology of the bladder neck but they were keen observers of anatomy. As early as 1906 the German surgeon Trendelenburg had suggested to divide the symphysis pubis to gain access for surgical narrowing of the bladder outlet in epispadias patients with the goal of improving urinary control.[2] Hugh Hampton Young was the first American urologist to identify the abnormal anatomy of the bladder neck as the cause of the patient's urinary incontinence and devise surgery to correct it in 1908. In 1919, Young presented his original procedure to provide continence in patients with bladder outlet incompetence.[3]

By examining these patients with early cystoscopes and at the time of open surgery, Young noted that the bladder neck and proximal urethra was enlarged and funnel shaped. The remainder of the bladder appeared healthy. He surmised that if he could restore the bladder neck and proximal urethra to a more normal appearance, then function would improve. He excised a wedge of mucosa from the posterior urethra and bladder below the trigone and narrowed the muscle with a single layer of sutures.

Since Young's bold procedure, surgery for the weak bladder outlet has progressed from the goal of re-creating normal anatomy to that of constructing continence mechanisms that bear no resemblance to the normal bladder outlet. Other developments in urinary tract reconstruction, such as intermittent catheterization, bladder augmentation, and continent catheterizable stomas, have made new procedures to repair the weak bladder outlet possible and offer solutions to problems that early surgeons saw as incurable.

After decades of becoming bolder in our approach to the bladder neck, the last few years have seen a realization of the limitations of reconstructive surgery to the bladder outlet and a turn to less aggressive and disruptive bladder surgery. Better understanding of the physiology of the bladder and stresses on the bladder outlet has led to a more selective approach to increasing bladder outlet resistance. Increased awareness of long-term negative consequences of altered anatomy and physiology have led surgeons to aspire to alter the bladder outlet anatomy only enough to achieve the desired result of socially acceptable continence.

Indications and evaluation

Urinary incontinence may be the result of bladder outlet inadequacy in conditions such as epispadias, exstrophy, cloacal exstrophy, traumatic injuries of the urethra and bladder neck, urogenital sinus, bilateral ectopic ureters, and neurologic conditions. Indications for bladder outlet surgery in these conditions include evidence that weakness of the outlet is a cause of incontinence and the failure of maximal medical therapy to correct the problem.

The bladder outlet includes the bladder neck and proximal urethra: together, they may be considered as a unit and normally function as a sphincter in both boys and girls. There is no identifiable anatomic sphincter but a mixture of smooth and striated muscle, intracellular matrix, and mucosal factors that combine to make up a functional sphincter.[4] Compression of the urethral lumen and the resultant outlet resistance depends on several factors. Among the components that make up the normal sphincter mechanism are smooth and striated muscle tone and contractions, elastic properties of the urethra, mechanical forces transmitted from the abdomen, and structural support of the posterior urethral wall and bladder neck against which the urethra is compressed with increased abdominal pressure. The conditions that cause incontinence in children often present inadequacies in several if not all of these components.

In health, the bladder neck provides a variable resistance to the flow of urine through the urethra. The resistance is stable when the bladder pressure is low and increases as the pressure rises with bladder filling. It also increases reflexively with increased bladder pressure due to coughing or Valsalva's maneuver, and it decreases dramatically when the patient begins to void. For the bladder neck to maintain continence it must be able to generate pressure within the lumen that is greater than the pressure within the bladder at all times except during voiding.

There are several methods to evaluate the competency of the bladder outlet. Just as Young noted, the cystoscopic appearance of the bladder neck reflects its function. When viewing from the proximal urethra, the posterior lip of the bladder neck should be elevated above the level of the urethra and the base of the bladder. The bladder neck should close easily when fluid flow through the cystoscope is stopped. Although these observations are helpful, they are by no means completely reliable in predicting continence.

The bladder outlet may also be evaluated by imaging with a radiographic cystogram. A competent bladder outlet appears closed as the bladder is filled and contrast should not leak into the urethra. The incompetent bladder outlet may remain open and funnel shaped during the filling process or may open with Valsalva's maneuver or suprapubic pressure[5] (Figure 55.1). Lateral views of the cystogram may reveal the lack of adequate elevation and suspension of the posterior bladder outlet.

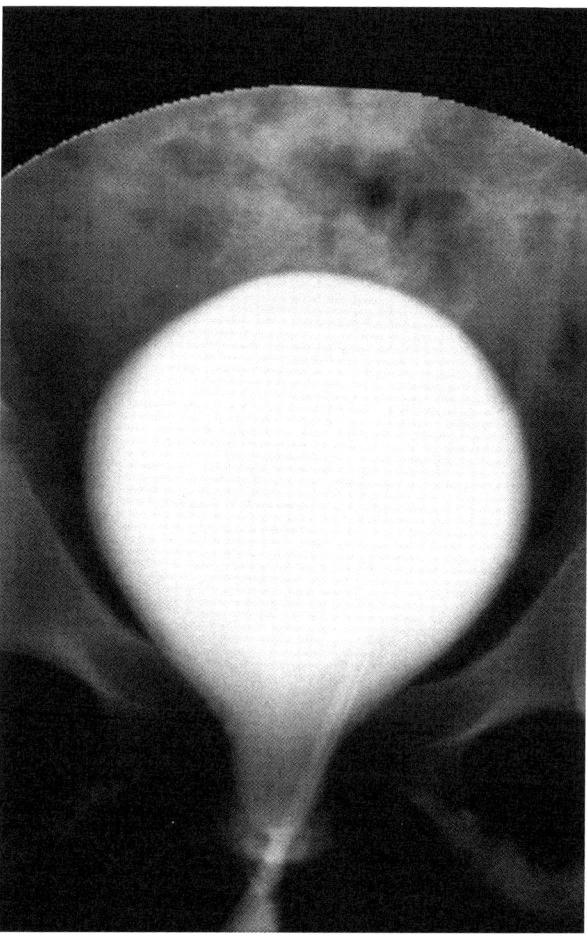

Figure 55.1 Voiding cystourethrogram of a patient with an open bladder neck during filling with contrast. The bladder neck is funneled during the entire study.

Urodynamic studies of the bladder are important in determining causes of incontinence. Bladder leak point pressure and sphincter electromyography (EMG) are commonly used to measure bladder neck function. Leak point pressure is simply the pressure within the bladder at which fluid begins to leak through the bladder outlet into the urethra. Sphincter EMG is the measurement of electrical activity of the striated muscle of the sphincter. The sphincter EMG is most helpful in evaluating coordination of the detrusor and sphincter and may be of some benefit to document neural innervation of the sphincter in incontinent children. It is seldom helpful in children who are candidates for bladder outlet surgery.

On the other hand, bladder leak point pressure is the most reliable objective study in incontinent children due to bladder outlet dysfunction. Low leak point pressures indicate incompetence of the bladder outlet and may cause incontinence independent of detrusor function. McGuire et al defined the importance of leak point pressure in children with myelodysplasia and neuropathic bladder when they found that high leak point pressures >40 cmH_2O resulted in upper tract deterioration due to reflux and hydronephrosis.[6] Children with pressures <40 cmH_2O were protected from such changes but were prone to leak urine easily owing to weak bladder outlet. They also found that the radiographic appearance of an open bladder neck did not correlate well with measured leak point pressures.

McGuire found that children with myelomeningocele have fixed bladder outlet resistance that is located distal to the bladder neck and does not vary with filling or leaking. When these children were treated with intermittent catheterization and anticholinergic medications, patients with closed bladder necks on cystogram were uniformly continent whereas only 60% of those with an open bladder neck became continent. This finding was independent of leak point pressure, indicating its limits in predicting continence in all patients.

Leak point pressure should be measured with a small urethral catheter (5 or 7 Fr). The water should be infused with a pump rather than by gravity. The technique should be standardized for each measurement, since Decter and Harpster have demonstrated that measured values of leak point pressures in children vary with catheter size and with rate and method of infusion.[7] Patients should be encouraged to cough and sit or stand if possible to measure leak point pressures in a dynamic, more normal, setting. The volume at which leaking occurs is important because it reflects the functional capacity of the bladder and prognosis for continence.

Other urodynamic measurements are critical in diagnosing the cause of incontinence. Bladder pressures and volumes indicate storage capacity of the bladder and must be adequate for continence. Compliance may be considered the inverse of stiffness and is a helpful indicator of bladder adaptability. Poorly compliant bladders tend to produce higher pressures with lower volumes of urine, making patients more prone to upper tract deterioration and incontinence.[8] Detrusor measurements in children with completely incompetent bladder necks may be performed by inflating the balloon of a Foley catheter at the bladder neck and pulling it down to occlude the bladder outlet.[9] It is fruitless to consider treatment of bladder outlet incompetence unless the bladder itself has adequate volume and pressure characteristics for the storage of urine.

When evaluating incontinent children as candidates for bladder outlet surgery, a voiding/catheterizing diary can yield invaluable and practical information. Unlike radiographic and urodynamic examinations, these diaries represent the level of incontinence during normal activity. Some parameters, such as functional storage capacity of the bladder, may be quite different from values that hospital tests may imply. We have patients measure voided/catheterized amounts of urine obtained, the times that the bladder is emptied, when incontinence occurs, the degree of incontinence, and activities associated with leaking. This information, along with urodynamic data, examination by cystogram, and cystoscopy, may be needed to define the cause or causes of incontinence.

If incontinence is due to incompetence of the bladder outlet, the physician has two basic treatments available, medical and surgical. Medical treatment must always be exhausted completely before considering surgery. This is important not only because some patients will become dry with medical management alone but also because medical regimens requiring family and patient participation may demonstrate that the family is committed and willing to comply with similar catheterization and medicine schedules that necessarily accompany most surgical procedures to create continence. If the family can give medication and catheterize the child prior to surgery, it is likely that they will do so after bladder outlet surgery.

Medical therapy

Children found to have inadequate bladder outlet resistance may be treated with various non-surgical modalities. Some therapy helpful in incontinent adults has no role in children. Pelvic floor exercises, biofeedback, and electric stimulation of the bladder outlet have not been helpful in children with incontinence who suffer from anatomic and neuropathic conditions.

There are medications that have been effectively used to stimulate muscles of the weak bladder outlet. They include α-sympathomimetic agents such as ephedrine and ephedrine-like compounds that stimulate the large number of α-adrenergic receptor sites found in the proximal urethra and bladder neck and cause smooth muscle contraction.[10] These compounds produce troublesome side effects in some patients such as hypertension, anxiety, and palpitations. Results have not been reliable in this group of children because most have severe anatomic and neurologic defects at the bladder outlet. We have had little success with medical stimulation of the bladder outlet to improve continence.

Other non-surgical therapies include clean intermittent catheterization (CIC) to completely empty the bladder on a prearranged schedule. Intermittent catheterization remains the single most important contribution to the treatment of incontinence in children. In children with neuropathic bladder, intermittent catheterization alone will provide continence in 19–24%.[11,12] The addition of anticholinergic medications, which lower bladder pressures and inhibit detrusor contractions, to CIC programs raised the continence rates to 68–89%.[13,14] It is important to recognize that various authors have defined continence differently in the past. Whereas most patients gain some social or daytime continence with medical therapy, complete dryness is possible in less than one-third. Even if bladder outlet function is marginal, continence may be improved by maximizing other aspects, such as bladder storage capacity, with medication and emptying the bladder regularly with catheterization.

Procedures to increase bladder outlet resistance

Once the bladder outlet has been identified as a cause of incontinence and medical therapy has been exhausted without acceptable improvement, the next options are surgical procedures to enhance bladder outlet resistance. This may be done by three basic surgical methods: procedures to change the suspension, support, or angle of the bladder outlet; procedures to compress the lumen of bladder outlet with either an external compression device or by injection of material under the mucosa; and procedures to reconfigure the bladder outlet into a more efficient continence valve.

Procedures to suspend the bladder outlet

For the past century inadequate support or insufficient elevation of the bladder neck and proximal urethra has been identified as a cause of urinary incontinence.[15] Inadequate suspension contributes to incontinence by making the bladder outlet too mobile, allowing it to descend into the pelvis. Normal suspension of the posterior bladder outlet is necessary to provide resistance from below to counter increased abdominal pressures from above and thus compress the lumen. Suspension of the bladder outlet may be accomplished in several ways, including procedures that fasten the existing periurethral fascia to the anterior pelvic wall and procedures that reinforce the posterior bladder outlet with a sling made of fascia or some other external material.

In 1949, Marshall, Marchetti, and Krantz (MMK) introduced a procedure to improve stress incontinence by surgically elevating and suspending the bladder neck and proximal urethra.[16] The procedure is based on sewing the anterior vaginal fascia just lateral to the urethra and bladder neck to the cartilaginous portion of the symphysis pubis (Figure 55.2). These

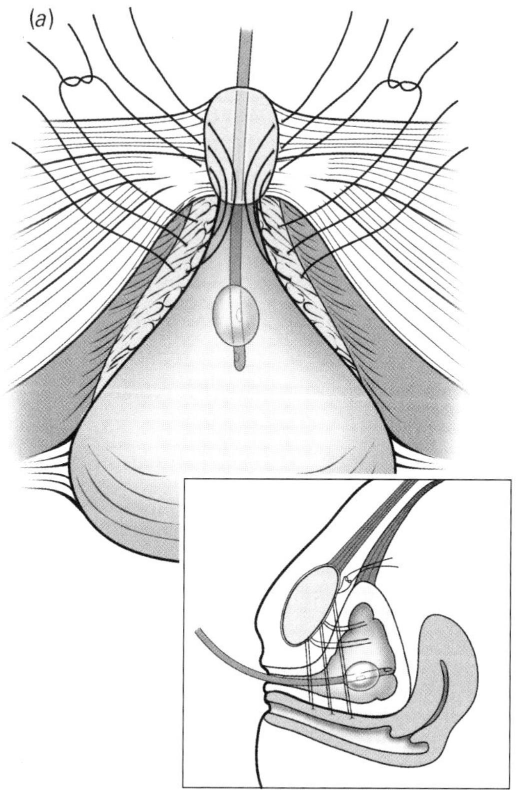

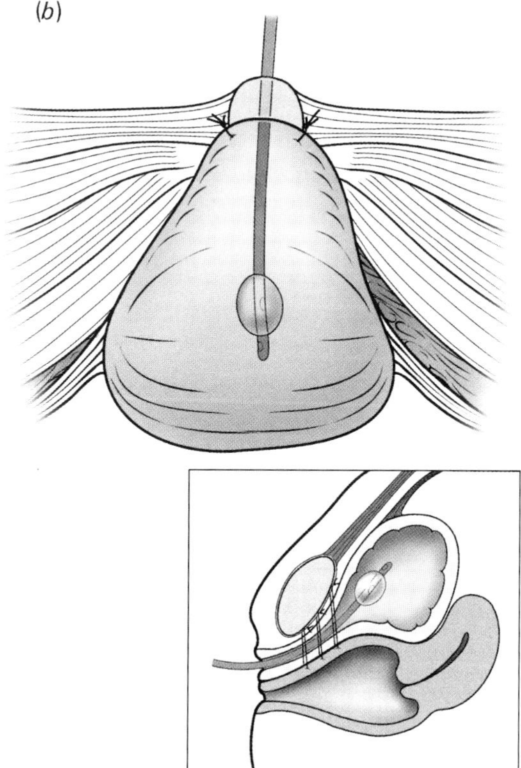

Figure 55.2 The Marshall–Marchetti–Krantz procedure elevates and suspends the bladder outlet, including the proximal urethra, by sewing the anterior vaginal fascia to the underside of the symphysis pubis. These are permanent sutures and re-create the posterior angle of the bladder neck. The concept of bladder neck suspension is still a cornerstone in incontinence surgery. (*a*) Placement of sutures between the anterior vaginal fascia and underside of the pubis. (*b*) Suspension and elevation of the bladder outlet.

sutures suspend and support the bladder outlet and recreate its posterior angle. The MMK procedure was for many years the gold standard of incontinence surgery and the concept is still critical in correcting these problems. Burch's procedure to suspend the bladder outlet from Cooper's ligament was another form of suspension that gained wide acceptance.[17] Both suspension surgeries produce cure rates in patients with pure stress incontinence of >90%.[18] Today, suture suspension of the bladder outlet in children is utilized usually as an adjunct procedure with other incontinence surgery and helps to produce continence in up to 88% of patients.[19,20]

Pereya (1959), Stamey (1973), and Raz (1981) developed procedures that were also designed to elevate and suspend the weak bladder outlet.[21–23] They supported and elevated the bladder neck using sutures from the perivesical and periurethral fascia to the rectus abdominal fascia. These procedures were clear advances because they could be done through small incisions using long needles to place the suspension sutures (Figure 55.3). The surgeons could confirm correct suture placement at the time of the procedure with the cystoscope and the patients suffered minimal discomfort.

McGuire improved on a concept introduced in 1911 by Goebell of suspending the bladder outlet with a sling of fascia or muscle.[24] McGuire developed a method of passing an isolated strip of rectus fascia beneath the bladder neck and reattaching it to the anterior abdominal wall at the insertion of the rectus fascia and the pubis[25] (Figure 55.4). Slings may improve continence by compressing the urethra, elevating the bladder outlet into the abdomen, or by providing a stable point against which the urethra is compressed during increases in abdominal pressure.

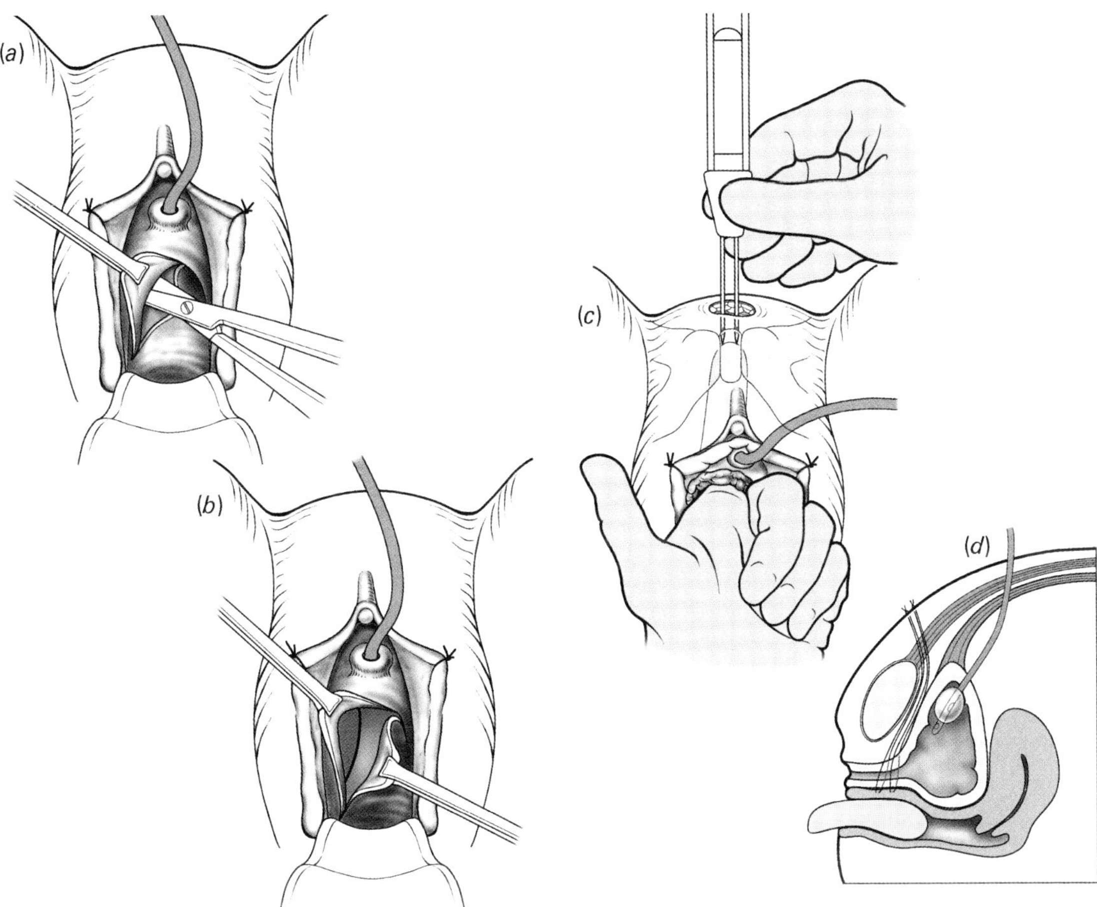

Figure 55.3 The Raz sling suspension uses long needles to pass permanent sutures from the anterior rectus fascia to suspend the bladder outlet from the anterior abdominal wall. The sutures support and elevate the bladder outlet and re-create the normal position and anatomy of the posterior bladder neck. They are dependent on the strength of the fascia surrounding the bladder neck and posterior urethra. (*a* and *b*) Exposure of the anterior vaginal fascia on either side of the bladder outlet. (*c*) Passing a needle from the anterior abdominal fascia to the vaginal incision in order to place sutures. (*d*) Suture suspension of the bladder outlet.

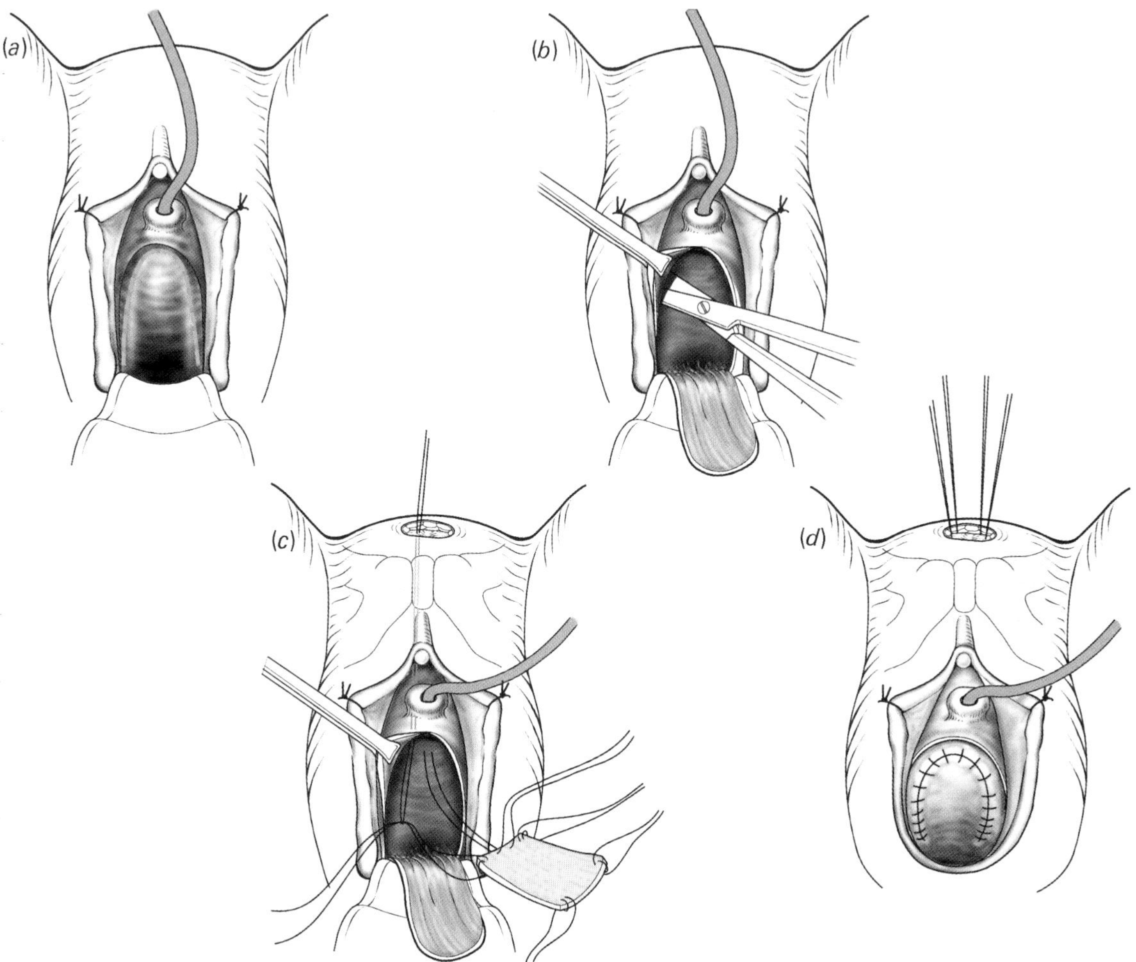

Figure 55.4 McGuire developed a suspension procedure that uses long sutures from the anterior abdominal wall to support a short strip of fascia. This fascia is passed posterior to the bladder outlet and supports and elevates the bladder outlet. This procedure provides more uniform support to the posterior bladder neck and does not rely on the native fascia around the bladder neck and urethra. (*a*) Vaginal incision to expose anterior vaginal fascia. (*b*) Dissection on either side of the bladder outlet. (*c*) Placement of the sling. (*d*) Sutures that elevate and suspend the bladder outlet.

This fascial sling and its variations have proven valuable for children with bladder outlet incompetence.[26] The use of fascia under the bladder neck is more reliable in these children than sutures alone, which must rely on the strength of the native fascia adjacent to the bladder neck and proximal urethra to hold the suspension sutures.

At the time of open surgery, the most popular form of sling suspension involves a long strip of rectus fascia that is passed around the bladder outlet and sewn to the anterior abdominal wall fascia on each side. This suspension depends completely upon the fascia to support the bladder outlet and is done entirely through a lower abdominal incision (Figure 55.5).

Slings may also be placed transvaginally in girls, just as is done in adults with good results.[27] This procedure would seem to be limited somewhat by the age of the child and size of the introitus. It is a useful approach in adolescent girls who are not undergoing simultaneous bladder reconstruction.

Bladder neck suspension, usually in the form of a rectus fascia sling, has been most helpful in girls with myelomeningocele on intermittent catheterization.[28] The female urethra is more easily manipulated in this way and results have been good in this population, with continence rates of 78–90%.[29–31] The success rate in males in our hands has been considerably less than in females when suspension is used alone, although some authors report good experiences.[32–34] The combination of slings with other bladder neck surgery, such as narrowing the outlet, has been successful for some surgeons.[35] In

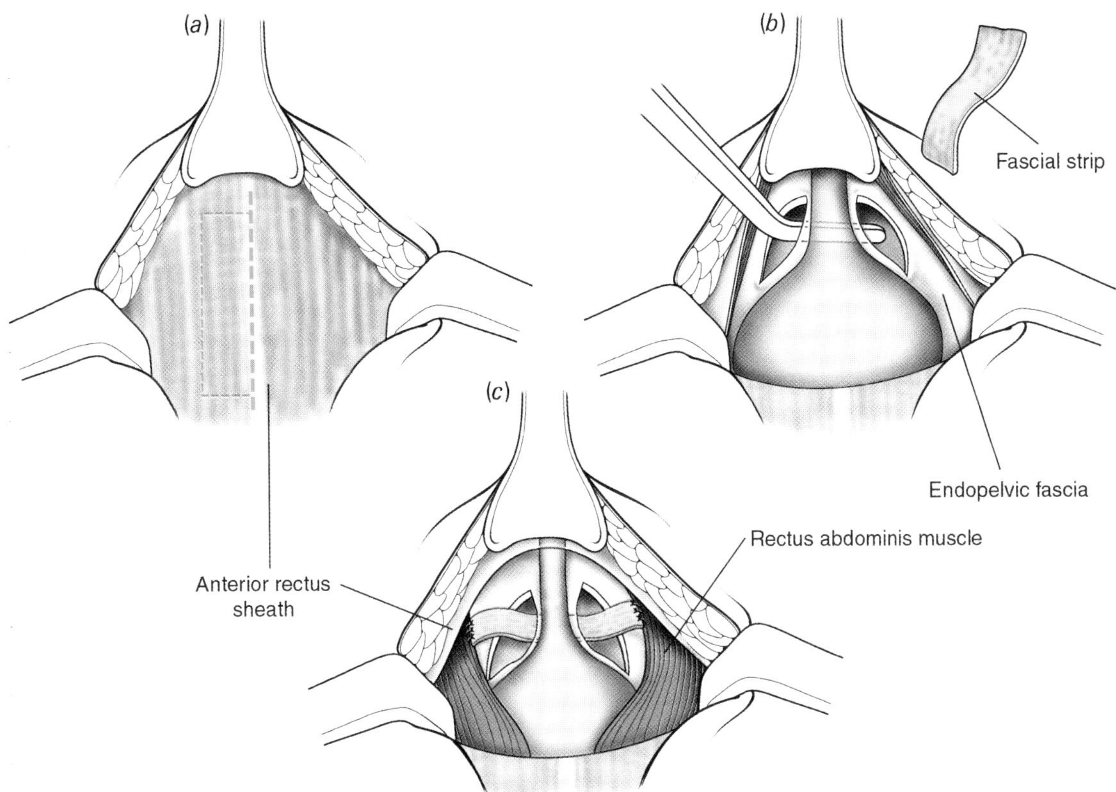

Figure 55.5 Fascial slings may be harvested from the anterior rectus fascia at the time of open surgery and used to suspend the bladder outlet from the anterior abdominal wall. (*a*) A single strip of fascia can be taken from the lateral aspect of a midline incision and (*b*) passed behind the bladder outlet. (*c*) Each end of the sling can then be sewn to the anterior rectus fascia on each side to elevate and support the bladder neck and urethra.

the author's experience the one group of patients who most often fail sling suspension are males who subject their bladder outlet to very high pressures that result from physical activity such as ambulation and play.

Fascial sling suspension of the bladder outlet is not without complications. Decter has reported erosion of the sling into the bladder and late degeneration of detrusor compliance after sling placement.[36] Often patients have difficulty catheterizing through the urethra after sling placement owing to the altered angle of the urethra. We have also witnessed the sling break during physical activity, acutely returning the child to a state of incontinence. There has been concern about the effects of slings on erectile function in males with spina bifida, but this function appears to be preserved in over 90% in one series of 14 patients.[37] Like many other procedures to improve bladder outlet resistance, augmentation cystoplasty has often been required to provide a large low-pressure reservoir for optimal continence.

Slings made of exogenous material have been introduced at various times and include true synthetic and processed biologic material such as porcine small intestinal submucosa. The early-generation pure synthetics such as silicone rubber and Gore-Tex have a high risk of erosion into the urinary tract and are not in common use today.[38] A new generation of material is available, including synthetic polypropylene mesh tape. This material has been useful in adult stress incontinence and has a much lower risk of erosion than prior synthetic materials.[39,40] The use of newer synthetic mesh slings has yet to be documented in children but its use in full-grown adolescents would seem to be promising.

The processed porcine biomaterial, small intestinal submucosa, has been in use for some time and has similar efficacy for producing continence. It offers an off-the-shelf replacement for rectus fascia, thus shortening surgical time and simplifying abdominal wall closure at the time of reconstruction.[41]

Procedures to compress the weak bladder outlet

Surgery to compress the bladder neck externally can take one of two forms: variable or fixed. Since the normal bladder neck offers variable outlet resistance, this form is the most desirable, so that the resistance can be relaxed to allow voiding or easy catheterization. The artificial urinary sphincter developed by Scott in 1972 has been valuable in the management of incontinence for many years.[42]

Artificial urinary sphincter

The artificial urinary sphincter is a hydraulic device that is composed of three parts: an inflatable cuff that surrounds and compresses the bladder neck or bulbous urethra; a pressure-generating balloon; and a pump control module (Figure 55.6). The artificial sphincter gives the patient the ability to deflate the cuff and reduce the compression of the bladder neck at will. The pump is placed in the scrotum or labia and the entire device is contained within the body. Continence rates are close to 90% after placement of the device.[43–45]

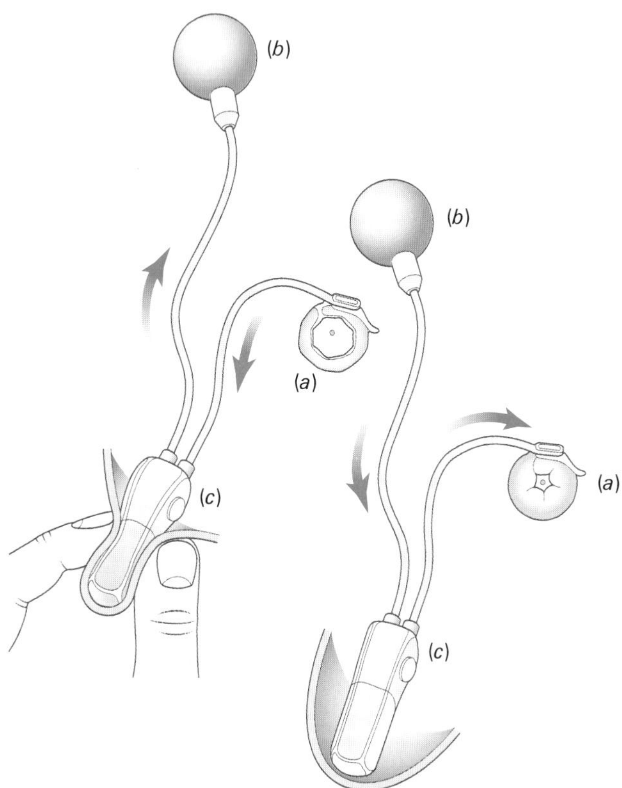

Figure 55.6 The artificial urinary sphincter is a mechanical device composed of three components: (*a*) an inflatable cuff, (*b*) a pressure-regulating reservoirballoon, and (*c*) a control pump. It functions by using hydraulic pressure to inflate the cuff, which compresses the urethra and provides continence. By squeezing the pump (implanted in the scrotum or labia), the patient can manually deflate the cuff and allow voiding or catheterization through the urethra. The pressure in the balloon then restores pressure throughout the system and reinflates the cuff in 3 minutes.

The bladder neck is the preferred site of placement in children (Figure 55.7). The usual minimal age for placement of artificial sphincters is 6 years for boys and 8 or 9 years for girls.[46] The pressure exerted on the urethra is regulated by the balloon/reservoir and most children need 61–70 cmH_2O pressure to safely control the bladder outlet. The device is not activated immediately, as cuff pressure immediately after surgery may cause erosion of the cuff into the bladder. The sphincter may be activated after 6–8 weeks with less risk of erosion.[47]

Initially, there were concerns that performing intermittent catheterization through the implanted sphincter could cause damage to the tissue compressed by the cuff and lead to erosion. Sphincters were only placed in patients who could void, but as many as 50% of children cannot void efficiently after sphincter placement, making catheterization necessary.[48] Barrett and Furlow reported a series of children with neuropathic bladders who could not void after artificial sphincter surgery and found that intermittent catheterization could be performed safely if the cuff was deflated to pass the catheter.[49,50] Continence was good and no patients suffered erosion due to catheterization. It appears that the ability to void may deteriorate with time, particularly in boys with neurogenic bladder. Gonzalez et al reported that 74% of patients followed for a mean of 8 years after sphincter placement required intermittent catheterization.[44] Upsizing the sphincter cuff size in adolescent boys who suffer delayed voiding failure after sphincter placement has not been successful in restoring the ability to void.[51]

Historically, there has been a higher rate of reoperation with artificial sphincters than with bladder outlet reconfiguration.[52] This rate appears to be improving with better technique and newer devices. Kryger et al reported an average of 0.03 revisions per year with the newest model and 70% of children who had sphincters placed since 1987 have not required revision.[53] The long-term (7–10 years) survival of the artificial sphincter in children in two large series is approximately 80%, with most being lost to the complications of device infection and erosion.[45,54] Eventually, all devices will wear out and fail, requiring replacement, but if complications can be avoided the mean survival of the new devices in children is over 12 years.[43] The newest model (AS 800), with a narrow backing cuff, was developed in 1988. It had a

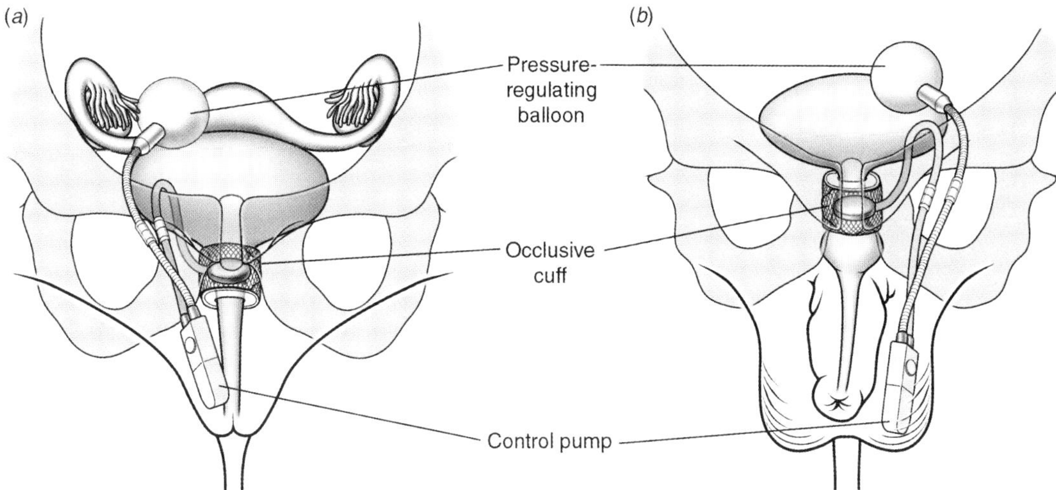

Figure 55.7 (*a*) Artificial urinary sphincter components in a female with the pump implanted in the labia. (*b*) Artificial urinary sphincter components in a male with the pump implanted in the scrotum. Both examples show the cuff implanted around the bladder neck.

mechanical failure rate of 7.6%, a non-mechanical failure rate of 9%, and a sphincter survival rate of 92% in 184 adult patients with a mean follow-up of 40.8 months.[55]

Roth and others reported an important complication of artificial sphincter placement in 1986 when they discovered that some patients suffered late deterioration of the upper urinary tracts.[56–58] This deterioration was due to two factors: a failure to void efficiently in some patients and the new development of detrusor hypertonicity in others. Deterioration of detrusor function after sphincter placement occurs in as many as 20% of patients and there is currently no reliable method to predict which patients will undergo these changes or the timetable for risk.[54,59] Because of this threat it is necessary to follow patients with artificial sphincters with upper tract imaging and urodynamics, as needed indefinitely after placement of the sphincter.

Augmentation cystoplasty, as either a simultaneous or later procedure with artificial sphincter placement, is necessary in approximately 30% of children.[44,60] Augmentation increases storage volume and decreases storage pressures of the bladder due to poor compliance or hypercontractatility of the detrusor. Augmentation may be performed at the same time as sphincter placement but has been associated with an increased risk of device infection if colon and small bowel are used for the augmentation.[61] Apparently, augmentation with stomach does not present an increased risk of infection in simultaneous sphincter placement.[62]

Patient selection for artificial urinary sphincter is important. Although there has been an increased risk of erosion with girls who had prior bladder neck surgery, Bosco et al have demonstrated that the risk to girls and boys is similar if they have not had prior bladder surgery.[63] The condition of the bladder outlet that will be compressed with the cuff is critical, and prior bladder neck surgery or excessive scarring increases the risk of erosion and infection.[64] Castera et al have reported that prior bladder neck surgery also impacts the continence rate after sphincter placement, resulting in only 37.5% continence in this group.[65]

The artificial urinary sphincter is the only method of producing variable bladder outlet resistance and thereby allowing volitional voiding. Its main indication today is in children who have the ability to void prior to surgery and the potential to do so after placement of the device. Use of the artificial sphincter in patients who require augmentation and intermittent catheterization offers little advantage over other methods to increase bladder outlet resistance.

Bladder outlet wraps

There have been a few attempts to compress the bladder neck with a fixed resistance and these have usually been in conjunction with bladder neck reconstruction surgery. Silicone rubber sheaths have been placed around the narrowed bladder neck, but in early series over 60% eroded into the lumen and required removal.[66] Quimby et al presented a large series of 94 patients treated with silicone sheaths used in conjunction with a Young–Dees–Leadbetter (YDL) bladder neck reconstruction. The authors continued to

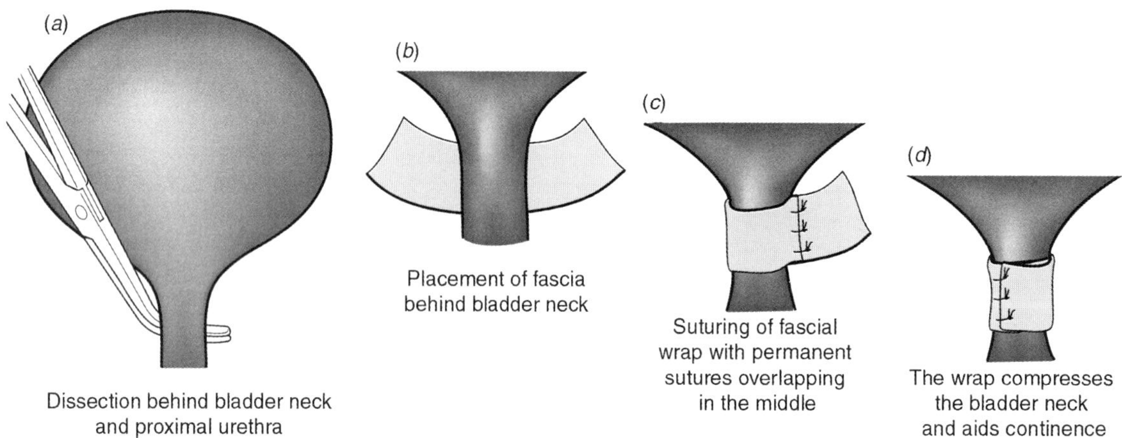

Figure 55.8 Walker described a fascial wrap of the bladder outlet in incontinent children. A strip of rectus fascia was harvested and wrapped around the bladder outlet and sewn together with permanent sutures. This provides consistent compression of the open bladder outlet and constant outlet resistance. Some patients with wide bladder outlets required bladder neck narrowing.

modify their technique until the erosion rated dropped to 7% in 35 patients. This improvement was attributed to using omentum to wrap the sheath and using a single-layer short silicone wrap. Satisfactory continence in this group was achieved in 72% of patients with this method[67] (Figure 55.8). Two other groups have reported synthetic constrictors or cuffs. de O Vilar et al reported a new device called a constrictor that compresses the bladder neck. It produced continence in all of the 42 patients in whom it was used; however, it had to be removed in 4 patients because of erosión or infection.[68] Kohn et al presented a series of children treated with a purse-string cuff around the bladder neck made of polytetrafluoroethylene (PTFE) tubing surrounding woven polyester tape:[69] 75% of patients were dry after surgery, but 30% of the devices had to be removed because of complications.

Walker et al described a procedure to wrap and compress the bladder neck circumferentially with rectus fascia with good results.[70] Some of their patients also needed bladder neck narrowing at the same time. Unlike silicone rubber, there were no erosions of the fascia, and post-surgery urodynamics showed that 70% of patients could not be made to leak at any pressure. Long-term follow-up of these patients indicates that the facial wrap and bladder dynamics are stable.[71] Bugg and Joseph presented a rectal fascia cinch that wraps around the bladder neck and is anchored to the pubis.[72] This procedure produced 60% continence. A myofascial flap made from rectus muscle can be used as a vascularized wrap and has been wrapped around the bladder neck and anchored to the pubic bone. This method has produced 75% continence in limited numbers.[73] Finally, a flap of bladder detrusor has been harvested and used to wrap around the bladder neck to compress the bladder neck.[74] Of course, any increase in fixed resistance at the bladder neck almost always precludes voiding and requires that the patient rely on CIC.

Injection therapy of the bladder outlet

Several substances have been injected under the mucosa of the bladder neck in order to increase intraluminal pressure generated by the weak bladder outlet and provide continence. The first substance used in significant numbers of patients was PTFE paste or Polytef.[75] Politanto et al popularized its use in adults and eventually applied the concept to children.[76,77] They reported 86% success rates in patients who were incontinent from bladder neck surgery and 50% in patients with neuropathic bladder. Injection therapy was relatively easy to perform and required no incision, so it could be done on an outpatient basis. Unfortunately, particles of Polytef were found to migrate to other organs in animal studies and particles were found in pulmonary granulomas in a human after periurethral injection.[78,79] Safety concerns have caused its abandonment in the United States. A newer form of silicone, polydimethylsiloxane or Macroplastique, has been used in Europe with continence achieved in 34% of patients.[80] It is not currently available in the United States. Other agents have been used, including autologous fat and collagen. Gonzalez de Garibay et al reported periurethral injection of fat

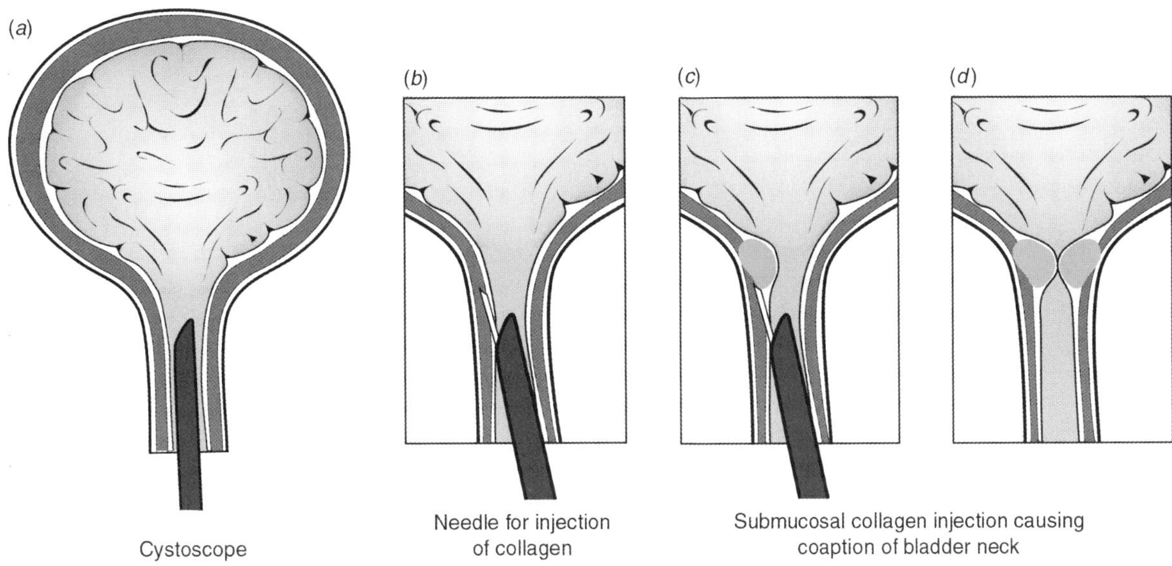

Figure 55.9 Injection of the bladder neck with various materials such as Polytef paste and collagen solutions has been used with more success in adults than in children. The needle is passed through a cystoscope and the material is injected submucosally either from the urethra or from a suprapubic approach. The material provides passive pressure to help to occlude the bladder outlet.

obtained from liposuction of the abdominal wall in 1989.[81] Initial success in treating incontinence was never as good as with Polytef, and the effects diminished with time because the fat did not survive due to poor neovascularity.[82] Eventually 80–90% of the injected fat was absorbed by the local tissue.

Gluteraldehyde cross-linked collagen has been one of the most common agents used to increase bladder outlet resistance. It has been used in the same manner as Polytef paste and is injected beneath the mucosa using a needle passed through a cystoscope (Figure 55.9). The success in treating children with incontinence has been inconsistent, with around 50–88% of patients considered to have a good result and 20–63% becoming dry.[83,84] Bomalaski et al reported a large series of collagen injections in children in 1996.[85] They reported a 22% cure rate of incontinence in 40 children, with improvement in another 54%. Of those patients with a mean follow-up of 4.5 years, the cure or improvement rate remained stable over time. Other clinicians have noted the biologic degradation of collagen and expressed concern about long-term durability.[86] Kassouf et al demonstrated poor results with collagen injections, in children with neuropathic bladder dysfunction. Only 20% of their patients improved after injection, and all of these eventually deteriorated within 2 months after treatment.[87]

The limited success and potential degradation should be explained to the patient and family. Also, 2.5% of patients are allergic to the collagen from dietary exposure and an additional 0.9% may develop late hypersensitivity.[88] Preoperative skin testing is necessary to establish that the patient does not have antibodies to the collagen and is less likely to react to the injection.

The newest agent to be used for injection of the bladder neck for incontinence is Deflux (dextranomer/hyaluronic acid copolymer). We have injected Deflux into the bladder neck of 16 children with bladder outlet incompetence. Of the 12 with neuropathic bladder, 25% were dry and an additional 33% improved after injection therapy, with a mean follow-up of only 9 months. None of the patients with other causes of incontinence achieved continence, whereas 33% showed improvement. No patients who performed intermittent catheterization through their urethra improved.[89]

With the widespread use of catheterizable urinary stomas in children with neuropathic incontinence, antegrade bladder neck injection of bulking agents through the catheterization channel has merit. The visualization of the bladder outlet from above is superior to the visualization from the urethra.

These mixed findings have limited injection therapy in most pediatric urologist's hands to incontinent patients who have had failed bladder neck reconstruction surgery. Up to 50% of these patients may become dry with injection therapy but some require

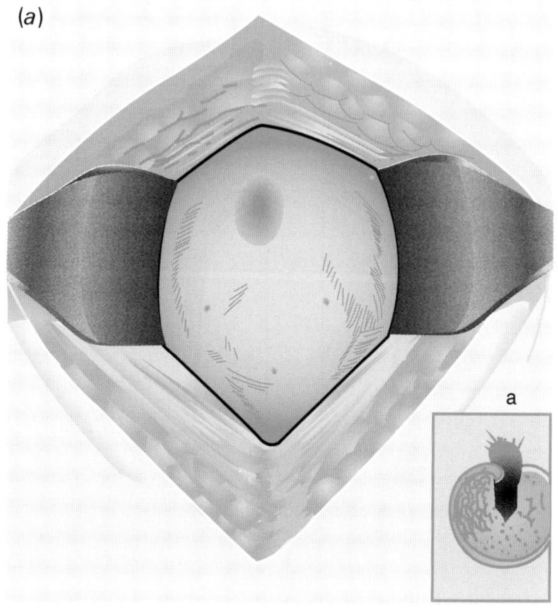

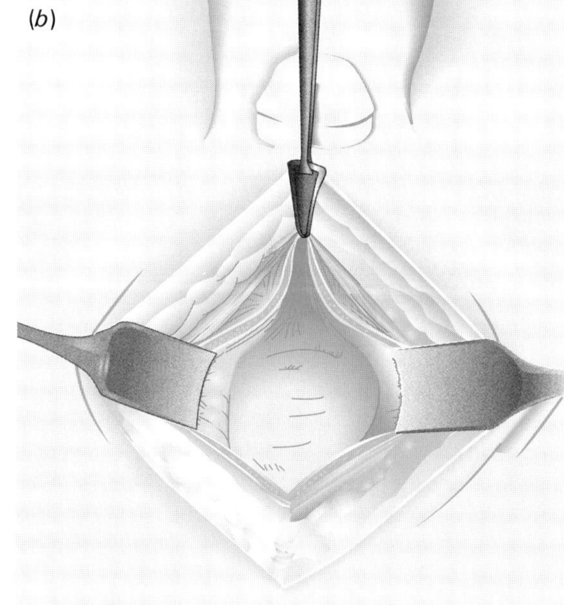

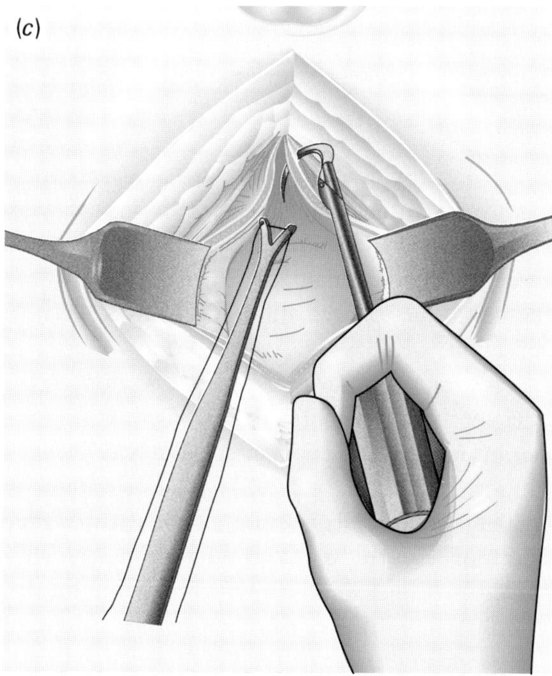

Figure 55.10 Young's original bladder neck repair was essentially an excision and narrowing of the outlet. He excised a full-thickness strip of mucosa and muscle from the bladder neck and proximal urethra and closed it with a single row of sutures to create a more normal-appearing bladder neck when viewed from within the bladder. This, in essence, lengthened the urethra and placed the bladder neck higher in the pelvis. (*a*) The open bladder outlet viewed from above. Inset shows Young's view of epispadias with incontinence. (*b*) Excision of the strip of mucosa and muscle. (*c*) Narrowing of the bladder outlet using Young's instrument to pass suture.

multiple injections.[90] This is a simple and safe outpatient procedure, but the results may degrade with time and its effects diminish.

Surgical reconfiguration of the bladder outlet

Young–Dees–Leadbetter procedure

In 1922 Hugh Young presented a refined procedure to reconfigure the inadequate bladder outlet in epispadiac patients who were incontinent due to bladder outlet incontinence.[91] Young had altered his approach from narrowing the posterior bladder outlet to narrowing the anterior urethral and bladder neck. He excised a full-thickness strip of tissue from the 'funnel-like neck' of the bladder and reapproximated the sides with a single row of chromic catgut sutures to create a more normal appearance (Figure 55.10). Ureterosigmoidostomy diversion was the accepted surgical treatment of incontinence due to epispadias and exstrophy prior to Young's procedure.[92] Young was obviously pleased with the results of his proce-

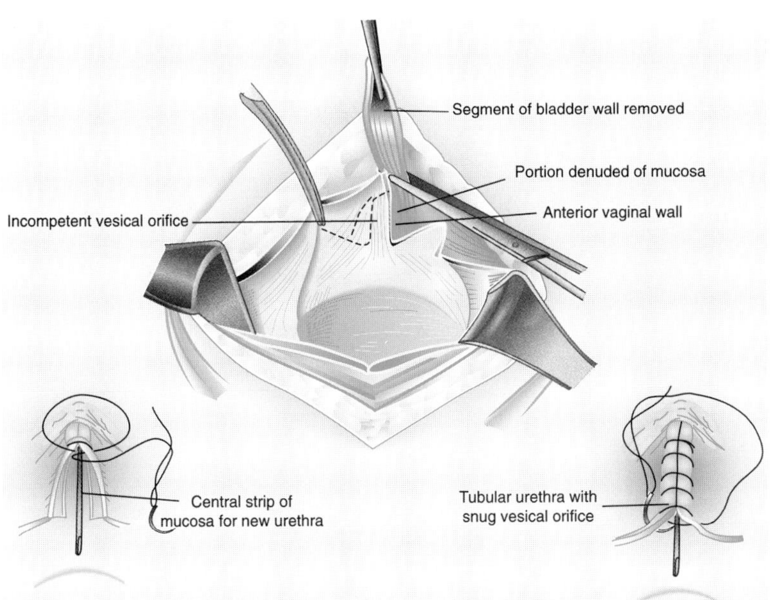

Figure 55.11 Dee's revision of Young's procedure extended the posterior urethral flap into the bladder and allowed a longer neourethra. He removed the mucosa from the muscle on the lateral aspect of this flap and, after closing the central flap of mucosa into a tube, he closed the muscle over the mucosa in a second layer. This provided additional muscle around the neourethra.

dure and reported, 'No fistula, no stricture, perfect urinary control, sexual powers normal'. For over 25 years after Young first presented his method to reconfigure the bladder neck for epispadias, his procedure remained the best surgical treatment for urinary incontinence due to a weak bladder outlet.

In 1949, John Dees improved upon Young's procedure by extending the posterior urethral flap into the bladder and removing the mucosa from the muscle on the lateral aspect of this flap. This posterior strip of urethra and bladder was then closed in two layers, mucosa and muscle, to form a neourethra[93] (Figure 55.11). Whereas Young had been content to narrow the proximal urethra and bladder neck, Dees changed the position of the bladder neck itself. He created a long neourethra from tissue that normally would have been the posterior bladder wall. The result was to move the bladder outlet higher into the pelvis and provide a longer, more muscular, urethra.

In 1964, Guy Leadbetter advanced this concept further by extending the posterior bladder flap even higher into the bladder.[94] This was made possible by moving the ureters from their normal location to a more cranial position further from the urethra and original bladder neck. The position of the ureters had been the limiting factor when Dees created his neourethra and moved the bladder neck above its natural location. Leadbetter moved the ureters out of the way by mobilizing them and reimplanting them transversely across the posterior bladder wall well above the trigone.

By extending the neourethra higher in the bladder, Leadbetter was also presented with a wider strip of bladder to use for his neourethra. A narrow strip of mucosa was left in the central portion of the neourethra. This was tubularized, the entire mucosa lateral to the strip was excised, and the two flaps of muscle lateral to the neourethra were then wrapped over the mucosa in an overlapping fashion, providing additional muscular support to the neourethra and bladder neck (Figure 55.12). With few changes today, the Young–Dees–Leadbetter bladder neck repair remains the gold standard of bladder neck reconstruction. Continence has been obtained in 78% of patients with neuropathic bladders and in 80% of exstrophy patients.[95–97] It must be noted that augmentation cystoplasty was necessary to obtain this degree of continence in 90% of the neuropathic bladder children in our series and in 50% of the exstrophy–epispadias patients in the Mayo Clinic series.

Disadvantages of the YDL bladder neck reconstruction include loss of significant bladder capacity that results from the reallocation of bladder wall tissue to the urethral continence mechanism. The neourethra may be tortuous and difficult to catheterize.

Variations of the Young–Dees–Leadbetter procedure

Of the many variations to the YDL, that of Mollard is closest to the original.[98] He creates a 7 cm long urethral strip that is wide enough to close over a 10 Fr catheter and removes the mucosa from the triangular muscle flaps lateral to the strip. He then incises one of the periurethral muscular flaps vertically parallel to the strip and rotates it horizontally across the midline

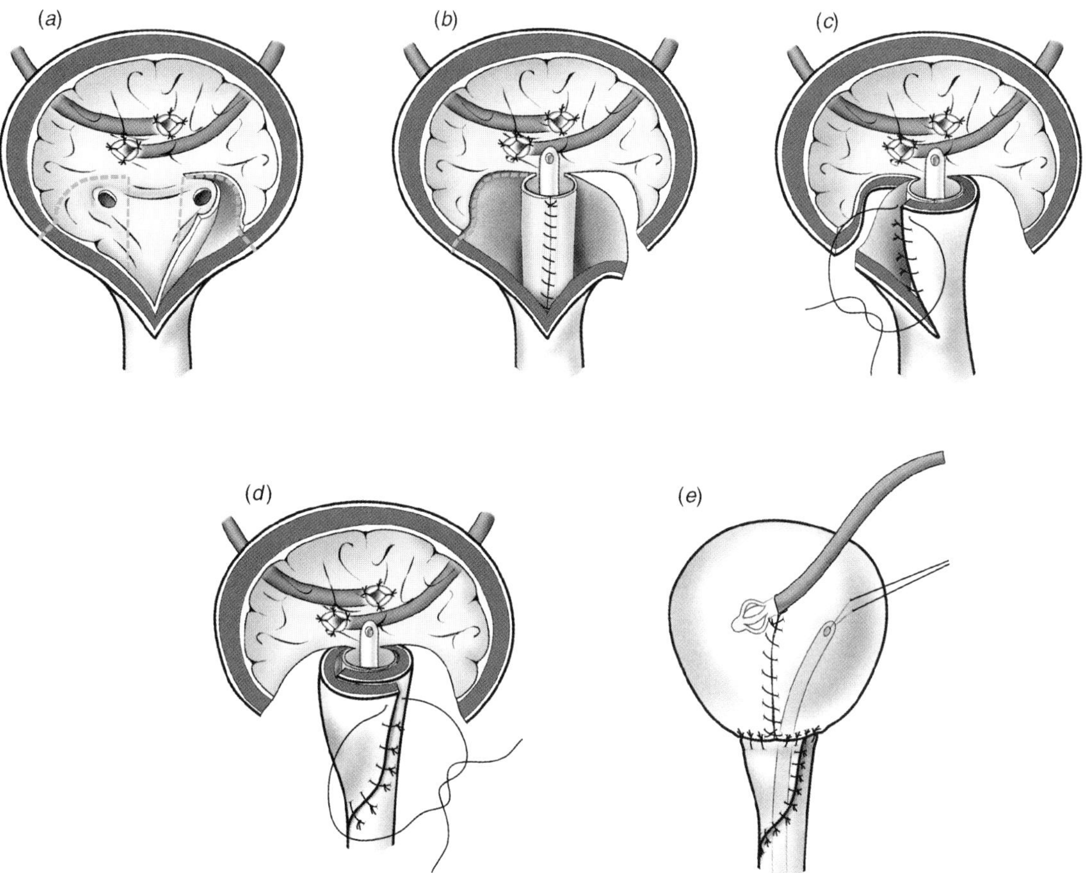

Figure 55.12 Leadbetter further improved upon the Young–Dees bladder neck repair by moving the ureters to a new location higher along the posterior bladder wall and away from the urethra. This maneuver allowed the posterior bladder strip to be even longer and produce a long neourethra and a much higher bladder neck. (*a* and *b*) Leadbetter removed the mucosa from the triangular flaps of bladder muscle on each side of the mucosal strip that was to be used for the neourethra. (*c*) After rolling the strip into a tube for the neourethra, he closed the lateral muscle flaps over the neourethra in layers to provide even more muscle at the bladder outlet. (*d*) Muscle is rotated over the neourethra in an overlapping fashion. (*e*) Dependable bladder drainage is necessary.

in order to develop an anterior bladder neck angle (Figure 55.13). Mollard's procedure has been applied mostly to exstrophy patients, and he has achieved a 70% continence rate.

Koff's variation on the YDL also differs from the original in its use of the periurethral muscle flaps.[99] Koff's initial incision is on the lateral aspect of the bladder neck, rather than the midline, and this produces a single long muscle flap on one side of the bladder. After he moves the ureters cephalad, Koff then strips the mucosa from the long muscle flap, leaving a midline strip of urethra and bladder to tubularize for the neourethra. The long muscle flap is then wrapped around the neourethra, producing what he has termed 'the cinch' (Figure 55.14). Koff has achieved 80% continence rates in mostly exstrophy patients. All of the patients have had significant difficulties voiding. Forty percent of the children required bladder augmentation and intermittent catheterization. Bladder capacity is lost to a similar degree as in the YDL procedure.

Mitchell returned to Young's original concept of a narrowed neourethra without added muscular support.[100] He noted that overlapping bladder muscle flaps used to create more outlet resistance made the bladder smaller by reducing the bladder itself. Mitchell's procedure is the only bladder neck repair that does not decrease bladder capacity as the anterior bladder and urethral flap is incorporated into the bladder (Figure 55.15). He mobilized a triangular full-thickness flap of anterior urethra and bladder neck and then narrowed the bladder outlet. The flap was then rotated cephalad and integrated into the bladder. Continence was achieved in 64% of patients who all voided, and were a mixed group of children including neuropathic bladders and exstrophy.

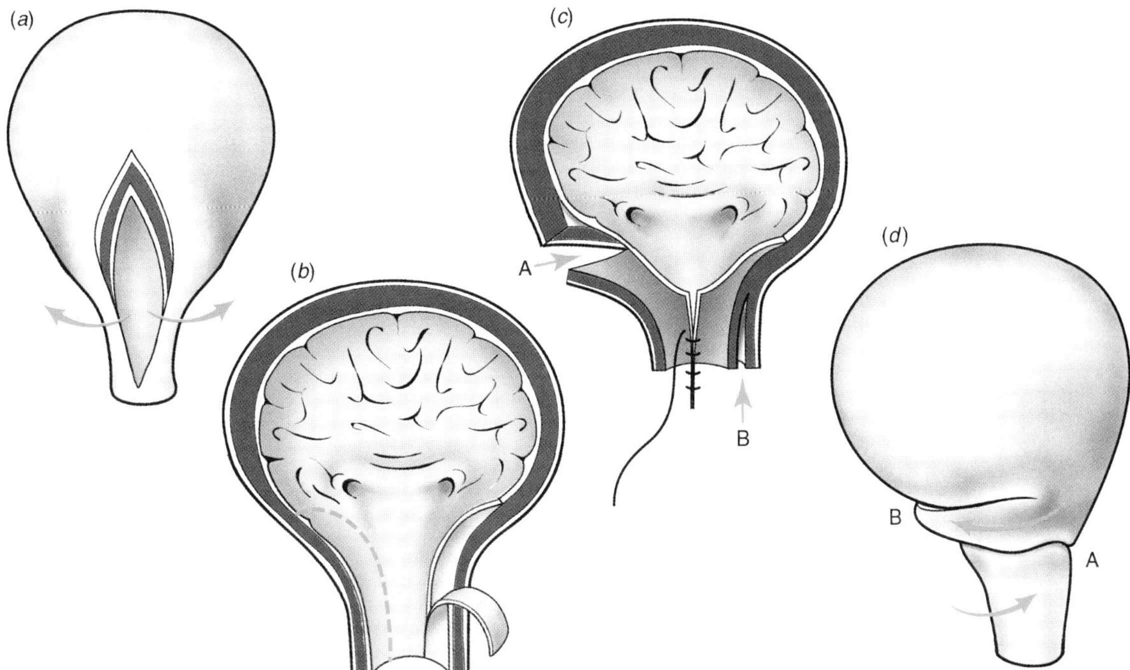

Figure 55.13 Mollard's variation of the Young–Dees–Leadbetter procedure is similar in the construction of the neourethra from a long posterior strip of urethra and bladder. It differs in that one of the two triangular flaps is incised vertically and parallel to the neourethra. This flap is then rotated horizontally across the midline to create an angle of the anterior bladder neck. (*a*) The bladder is opened in the midline. (*b*) The mucosa lateral to the central urethal strip is excised. (*c*) The two lateral muscle flaps are incised, one vertically and one horizontally. (*d*) Flap (A) is wrapped around the neourethra like the YDL operation, while flap (*b*) is rotated horizontally across the repair to create an anterior bladder neck.

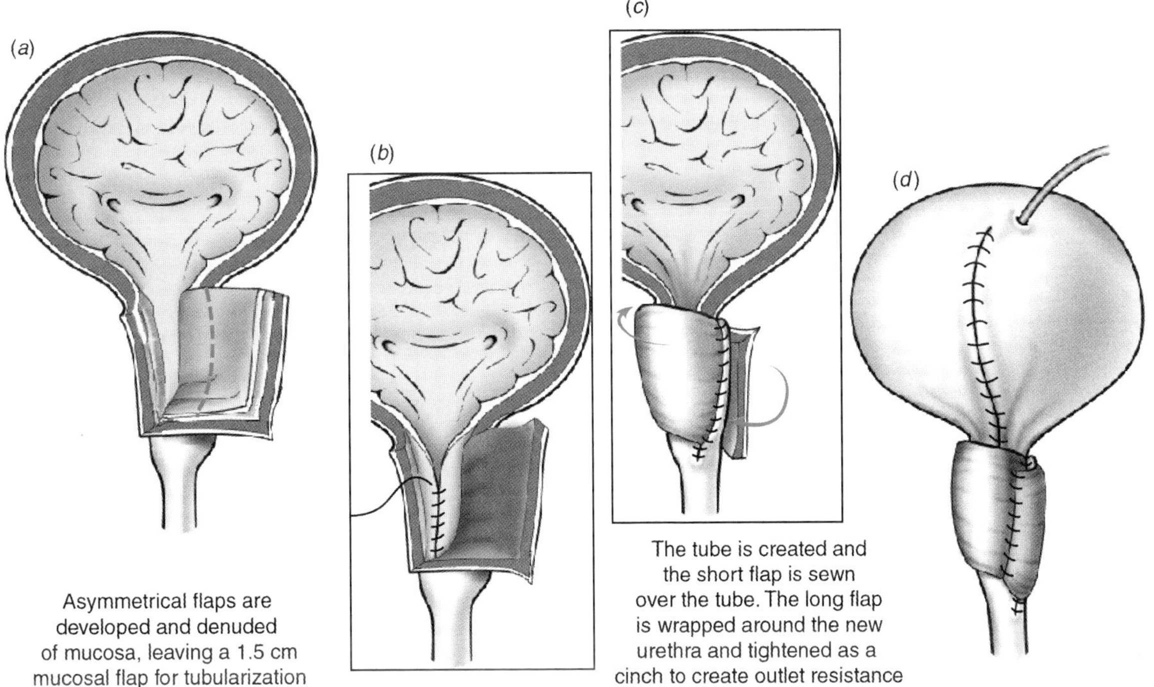

Figure 55.14 Koff's variation of the Young–Dees–Leadbetter procedure also creates the neourethra from a posterior flap of urethra and bladder and covers it with a flap of demucosalized muscle. The construction of this flap is different to other repairs that rely on two flaps. Koff makes a lateral incision of the bladder neck instead of opening the midline. This creates a single long flap on one side of the neourethra. The flap is then wrapped around the neourethra and sewn to itself with permanent sutures. It acts as a constant compression of the bladder outlet. (*a*) The bladder outlet is opened on one side. (*b*) A midline mucosal strip is tubularized and the mucosa is dissected from the remaining muscle flap. (*c* and *d*) The muscle flap is then rotated around the bladder outlet.

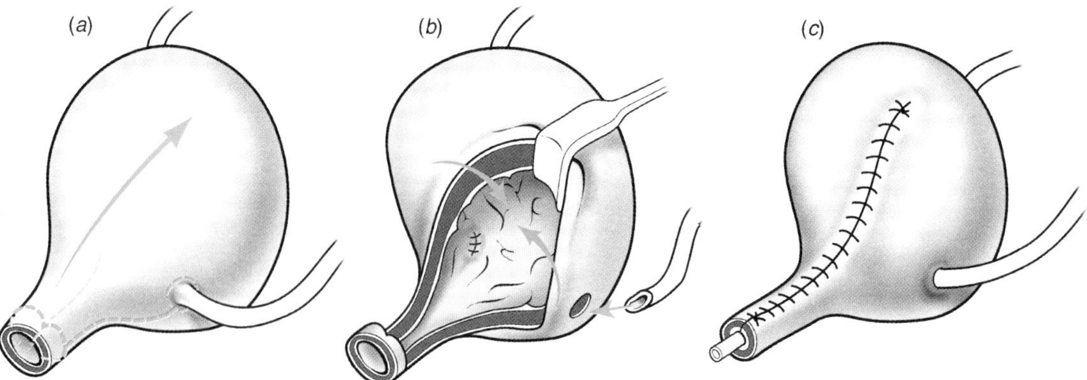

Figure 55.15 Mitchell returned to Young's original concept of a narrowed bladder neck that is not reinforced with additional muscle layers. His repair mobilizes a triangular flap of anterior bladder and urethra based on the bladder-side blood supply and then rotates the flap into the bladder. It is the only repair that does not decrease bladder volume. (*a*) An incision is made across the anterior urethra, extending up along the posterior lateral wall of the bladder outlet on each side. (*b*) The flap of bladder and urethra is rotated back into the bladder. (*c*) The incision is closed in the midline.

Some other variations of the YDL procedure have been developed, including Koyle's Thiersch–Duplay type-tubularization of the posterior bladder wall.[101] This procedure isolates and rolls a strip of mucosa into a tube in situ and then closes muscle and mucosa over the tube by rolling in the lateral tissue (Figure 55.16). He calls this the reverse Kropp or pPork repair, and has achieved 82% continence in neuropathic bladder patients. There may be problems with catheterization per urethra, and therefore all of his patients had an alternative access for bladder catheterization.

Arap et al presented the most radical variation of the YDL posterior-tube bladder neck repair for use in the most severe cases of exstrophy with tiny bladder plates.[102] Their procedure is performed in two stages: the first stage is creation of a colon conduit with antirefluxing uretero-colonic anastomosis; the second procedure creates a tube in the same manner as the YDL procedure but uses the entire bladder except for the dome, which is left open as a wide funnel (Figure 55.17).

The previously created colon conduit is then reconfigured as a reservoir and attached to the funneled

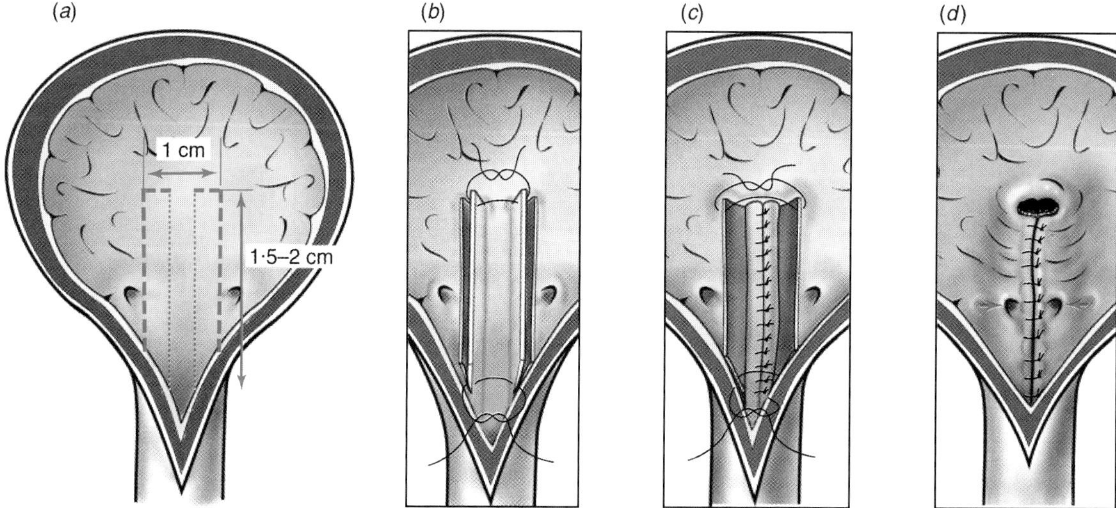

Figure 55.16 Koyle presented a bladder neck reconfiguration that isolates a strip of posterior mucosa in the posterior midline of the bladder. This strip is then rolled into a tube, creating a neourethra. Finally, the neourethra is covered with flaps of muscle and mucosa that have been mobilized lateral to the neourethra. (*a*) A mucosal flap is outlined. (*b*) The flap is then tubularized. (*c*) A second layer of muscle is closed. (*d*) Lateral mucosa is closed over the tube.

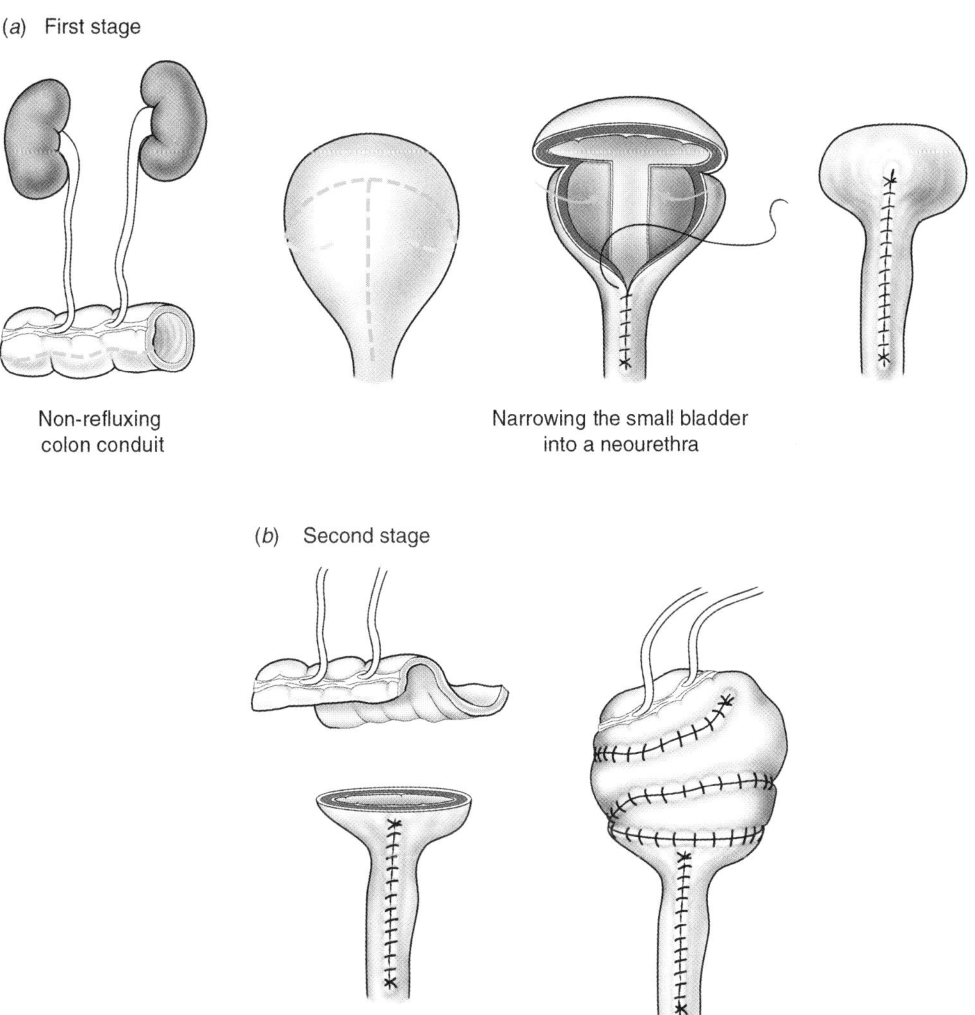

Figure 55.17 Arap's staged bladder reconstruction is the most radical reconfiguration of the bladder outlet. In the first stage the ureters are transplanted from the bladder plate to a non-refluxing anastomosis into a colon conduit. The second procedure creates a neourethra from the entire bladder except for the dome, which is left open as a wide funnel. The colon conduit is then reconfigured as a reservoir and sewn to the funneled bladder.

bladder plate. Arap reported a 75% continence rate with patients voiding frequently. Intermittent catheterization has provided continence and allowed a long dry interval in our limited experience with the Arap procedure.

Tanagho bladder neck repair

In 1968, Tanagho was studying function and anatomy of bladder muscle when he noticed 'a condensation of circle fibers above the internal meatus'.[103] He then designed the first anterior bladder tube repair for incontinence and perfected it in dogs.[104] Three years later he presented his experience in patients, including postprostatectomy adults.[105]

Tanagho intended to capture the muscle fibers of the anterior bladder and incorporate them into the bladder neck. He created a bladder-based flap from the anterior bladder just proximal to the urethra and rolled it into a tube for the neourethra (Figure 55.18). He then divided the urethra from the original bladder neck and anastomosed the neourethra to the native urethra end to end. The effect of this maneuver was to lengthen the urethra and to create a new, more cephalad bladder neck.

Tanagho achieved a 72% continence rate and patients voided well. He compared his long-term results in 50 patients to the YDL procedure performed in 25 patients and found a 70% success with the Tanagho anterior bladder tube compared with

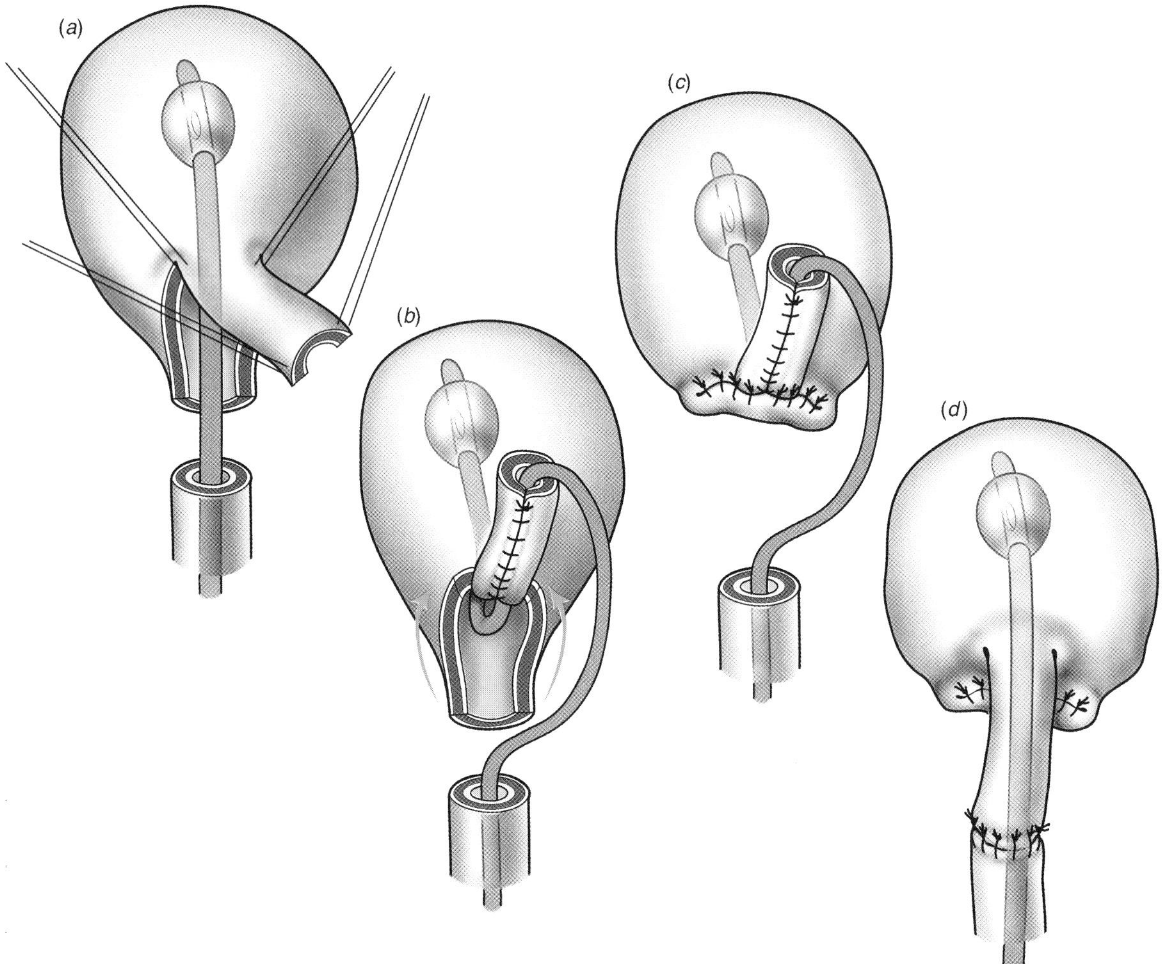

Figure 55.18 Tanagho's procedure created a neourethra from a strip of the anterior bladder neck and bladder. This allowed the creation of an angle at the posterior bladder neck. It required complete separation of the bladder from the urethra and a reanastomosis of the neourethra to the native urethra. (*a*) The bladder outlet is divided from the urethra and an anterior bladder-based tube is formed. (*b*) The flap is tubularized. (*c*) The posterior bladder is closed. (*d*) The tube is sewn to the urethra.

52% with the YDL posterior tube.[106] One advantage of Tanagho's bladder-based anterior flap was its applicability to short urethras, as demonstrated by Diamond and Ransley in urogenital sinus patients.[107] This application remains as the most likely use of the Tanagho repair in children today. Disadvantages include the necessity to divide the bladder from the urethra, possibly resulting in difficult catheterization, and loss of bladder volume.

Kropp bladder neck repair

In 1972, Jack Lapides made a contribution that changed forever our attitude and approach toward incontinence surgery.[108] His introduction of CIC controlled infection, decreased bladder pressure, and made many patients continent without further surgery.[109] CIC made voiding an option rather than a requirement, and changed the goals and results of incontinence surgery.

Kropp was the first surgeon to develop a new bladder neck reconstruction designed to take full advantage of CIC.[110] The goals of the surgery had changed. Dryness was foremost and voiding was no longer a consideration. CIC had been used in patients with other forms of bladder neck reconstruction before this, but they were all procedures that allowed the patient to void, at least in theory. The Kropp procedure was the first to preclude voiding.

The Kropp procedure uses a full-thickness flap of anterior bladder muscle. This flap is based on the urethra, unlike Tanagho's flap, which is based on the bladder. The full-thickness bladder flap is isolated from the bladder and rolled into a tube of the same

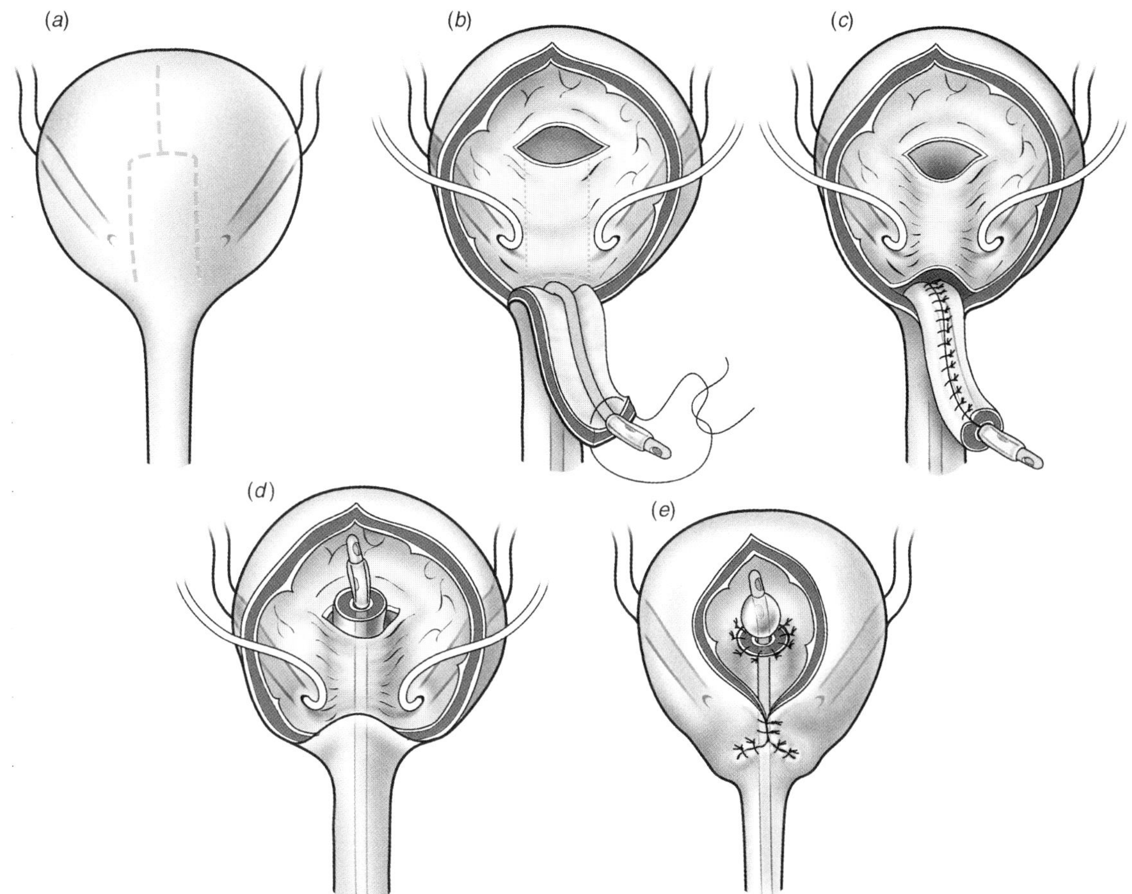

Figure 55.19 Kropp also creates a neourethra from a flap of anterior bladder neck and bladder but, unlike Tanagho, Kropp's flap is based on the urethra. The flap is tubularized and then placed in a submucosal tunnel created along the midline of the posterior bladder wall. (*a*) An anterior urethral-based flap is mobilized. (*b* and *c*) The flap is tubularized. A submucosal tunnel is made in the posterior bladder wall. (*d* and *e*) The tube is placed in the tunnel.

diameter as the urethra. The tube is then reimplanted in a submucosal tunnel in the midline of the posterior bladder wall between the ureters (Figure 55.19).

Advantages of Kropp's reconstruction included a very high continence rate of 80–94%.[111,112] Kropp's strict definition of continence has been complete dryness or rare leakage. The reoperation rate was high in the original series but most secondary procedures involved the storage function of the bladder and only 20% of patients required additional surgery to the bladder outlet. To facilitate storage and to compensate from bladder volume lost in construction of the tube, Kropp now suggests that all patients undergo a simultaneous bladder augmentation. There have been problems catheterizing through the repair but the improvement of leaving lateral attachments at the bladder neck intact and not completely separating the neourethra from the bladder has minimized this difficulty.

In 1997, Snodgrass reported a series of 22 children treated with the modified Kropp procedure described by Belman and Kaplan.[112,113] Snodgrass created a urethral-based flap of anterior bladder wall and rolled it into a tube. He did not divide the bladder neck from the remainder of the bladder. The posterior bladder mucosa is then incised in the midline to create a trough and the tube is laid in this trough with the mucosa closed over the tube (Figure 55.20) No attempt is made to tunnel the tube. He reported a 91% continence rate, defined as dry intervals of 3 hours. Snodgrass notes that these patients are socially continent and will have slight leakage when catheterization is delayed. Bladder augmentation was performed in 91% of his patients at the same time as bladder outlet surgery. Just as in the original Kropp procedure, voiding is impossible.

Pippi Salle bladder neck repair

Pippi Salle developed a bladder outlet repair for incontinence by creating a neourethra composed of both

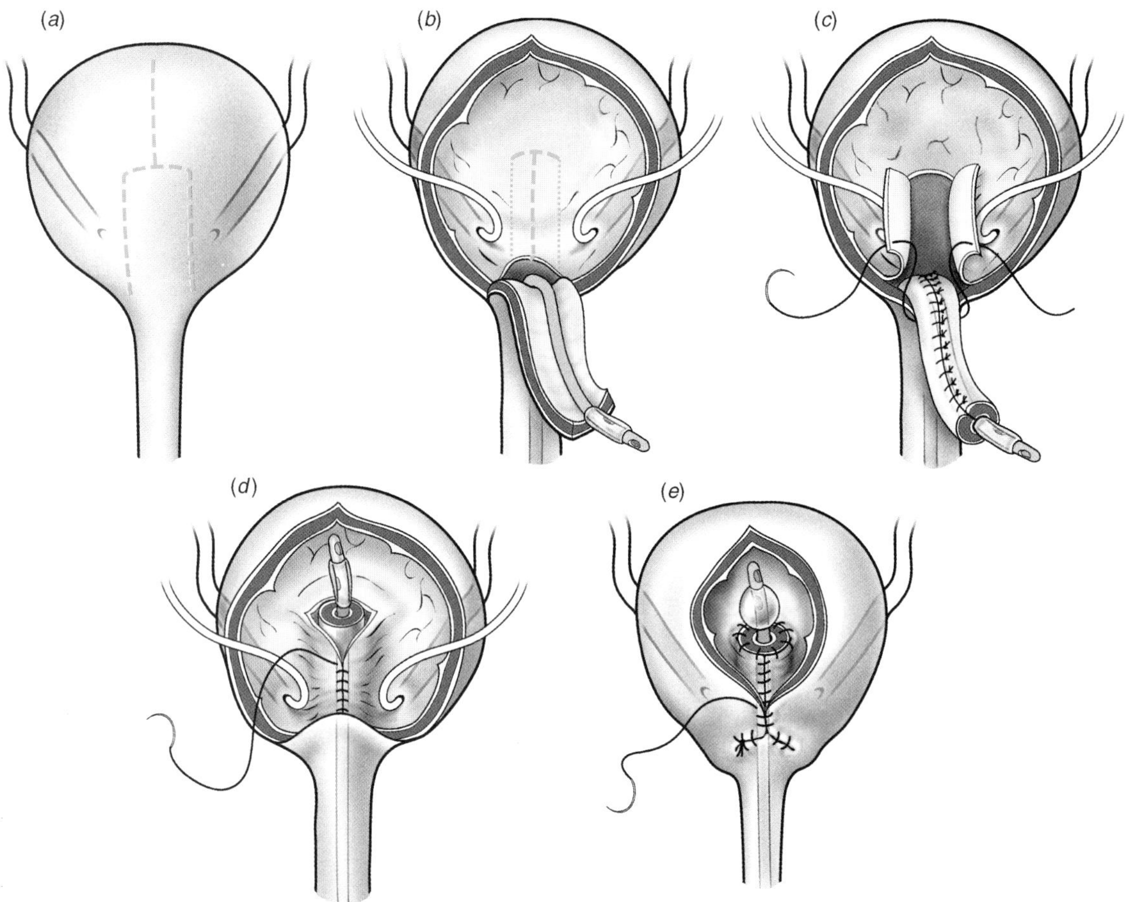

Figure 55.20 The Snodgrass variation of the Kropp procedure lays the Kropp tube in a trough instead of a tunnel. Construction of the tube is identical to Kropp. Creation of the trough shown in figures b, c and d is the only different maneuver.

anterior and posterior bladder flaps.[114] This flap valve continence mechanism produces the only neourethra made of two separate flaps. Both anterior and posterior strips of bladder are isolated and the anterior flap is completely mobilized as a flap based on the urethra. The posterior flap is outlined with two parallel mucosal incisions and the posterior bladder muscle is left intact. The anterior bladder flap is then flipped down to oppose the posterior flap at the level of the posterior bladder wall. The two flaps are sewn together, creating a neourethra, which extends above the level of the ureters (Figure 55.21). Mucosa on either side of the strip of posterior bladder wall is mobilized and the muscle from the anterior strip is sewn to the muscle of the posterior bladder. The complete-thickness bladder tube is then covered with the previously mobilized bladder mucosa just lateral to the tube.

The Pippi Salle repair produces continence rates of 80%, and this repair is easy to catheterize primarily because the posterior wall remains intact.[115] Bladder volume is decreased by the use of bladder wall to create the continence mechanism. This repair also requires the patient to catheterize, as voiding is impossible. McLorie and Khoury have warned about the potential danger of damaging the blood supply while isolating the long thin anterior bladder flap.[116]

Bladder neck closure

The ultimate bladder neck reconfiguration is complete closure of the bladder outlet. Today, after years of experience, we feel that most but not all bladder necks can be made continent. Those, that cannot be repaired can be closed. The concept of bladder neck closure was made a viable option in 1980 when Paul Mitrofanoff constructed the continent appendicovesicostomy and combined it with bladder neck closure in patients with neurogenic bladder[117] (Figure 55.22). Duckett and Snyder presented variations of bladder neck closure and continent stomas and Van Savage et al presented a series of 46 children with closure of bladder neck.[118,119]

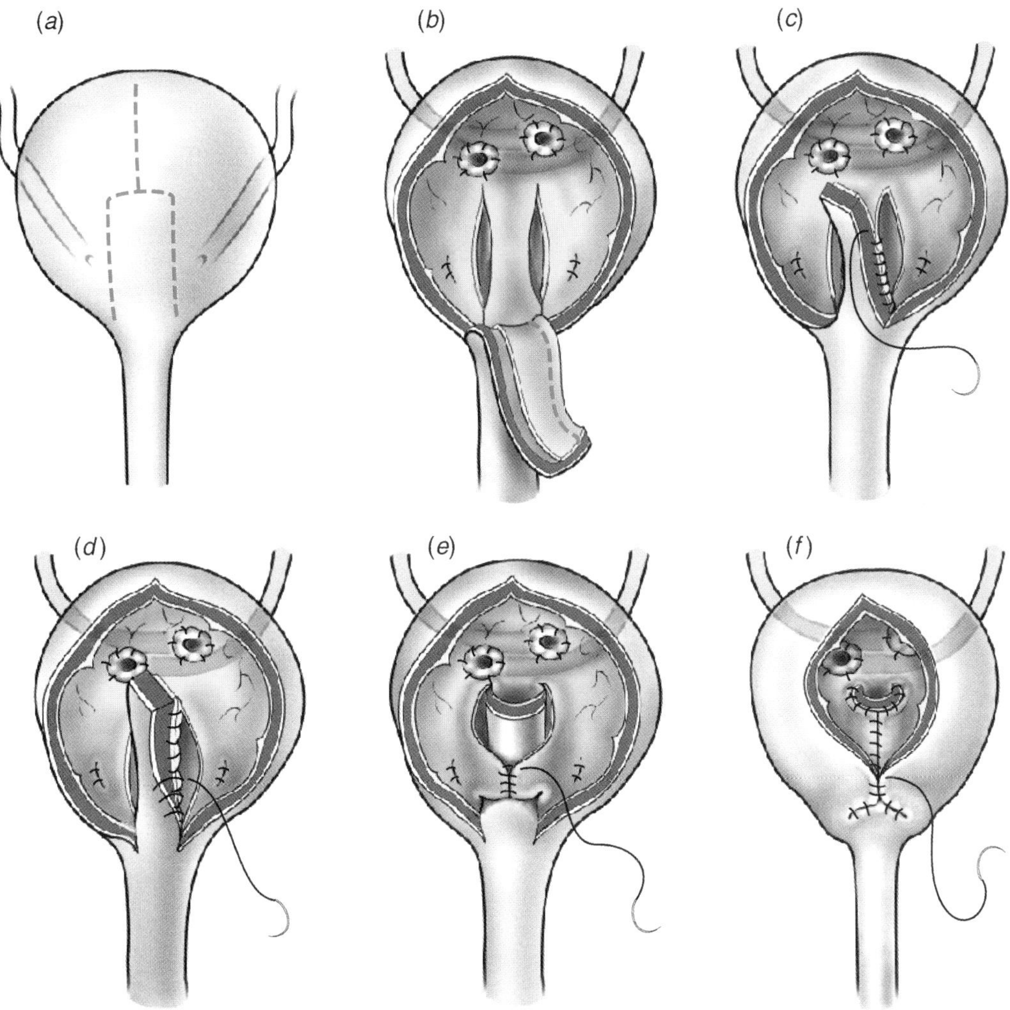

Figure 55.21 Pippi Salle creates a neourethra from an anterior and a posterior strip of bladder neck and bladder. The two are sewn together but only the anterior flap is mobilized completely. The posterior flap is isolated but not mobilized from the posterior bladder wall. The neourethra is then covered with mucosa and some muscle which is mobilized on each side. (*a*) An anterior bladder flap is mobilized. (*b*) A posterior bladder mucosal flap is mobilized. (*c*) The mucosa of the anterior and posterior flaps are sewn together. (*d*) The muscle of the flaps is sewn together. (*e* and *f*) The bladder mucosa in closed over the neourethra.

In general, bladder neck closure is a procedure of last resort and is utilized after other more flexible options in bladder neck reconstruction have been exhausted.[120,121] The indications for bladder neck closure are intractable urinary incontinence resistant to maximal medical management and reasonable surgical management. Patients usually have failed previous incontinence surgery or suffer from a primary condition that projects failure. The obvious advantage is complete urethral continence in as many as 96% of patients. Eighty-nine percent have stable upper urinary tracts and no bladder capacity is lost in the creation of a continence mechanism.[122] Disadvantages include a complete lifelong reliance on an extra-anatomic method of bladder emptying and no pressure pop-off valve. Bladder neck closure does have complications, with one series reporting initial results of 20% with stomal incontinence and 40% with urethral fistulas and persistent urethral leakage.[123] With surgical revision, 85% became completely continent. In reviewing multiple reports, 65% of patients with closed bladder necks require additional surgery for complications such as fistulas, stones, augmentation, ruptures, and other revisions.

The Mitrofanoff principle

Mitrofanoff's contribution, now termed the Mitrofanoff principle, has had a profound effect on incontinence surgery in children. His development of

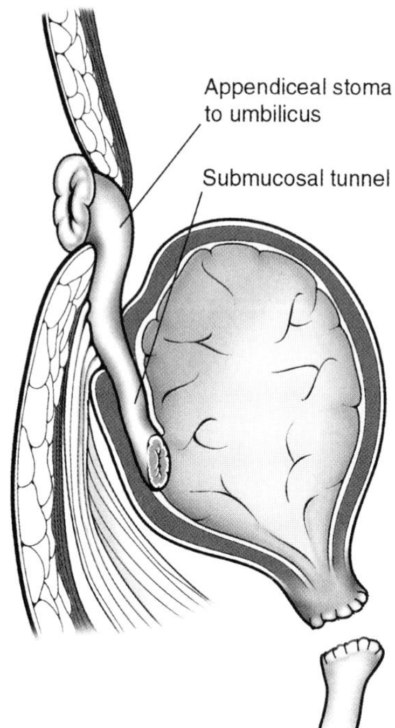

Figure 55.22 Mitrofanoff used a continent catheterizable stoma to empty the bladder. By implanting the appendix into the bladder in a continent manner, he allowed efficient bladder emptying without relying on the urethra. This allowed him to close the bladder neck surgically, leaving the appendix as the only access with which to empty the bladder.

alternative continent bladder access through a continent stoma has relieved the necessity for the patient to either void efficiently or to catheterize through the reconstructed bladder neck. There have been other alternatives to Mitrofanoff's original use of appendix for extra-anatomic access to the bladder. Other options for continent bladder access include ureter, fallopian tube, bladder tubes, and tubularized bowel.[124–126] With the recent interest in the Malone antegrade continence enema (MACE) for patients with neuropathic bowel and bladder, the appendix has been used more often as access to the colon.[127] Tubularized ileum and Yang/Monti tubes have been the most dependable and flexible method of bladder access for these patients[128] (Figure 55.23). We have developed a longer ileal tube for patients with a greater distance between the bladder and skin[129] (Figure 55.24). Today, an easily accessible, continent, catheterizable access for emptying the bladder is available for almost all patients.

We believe that catheterizable abdominal stomas promote continence by avoiding manipulation of the reconstructed bladder neck. In some cases they encourage patient compliance with intermittent catheterization because catheterizing through an abdominal stoma is easier and less time consuming than urethral catheterization for many patients. Regular catheterization keeps

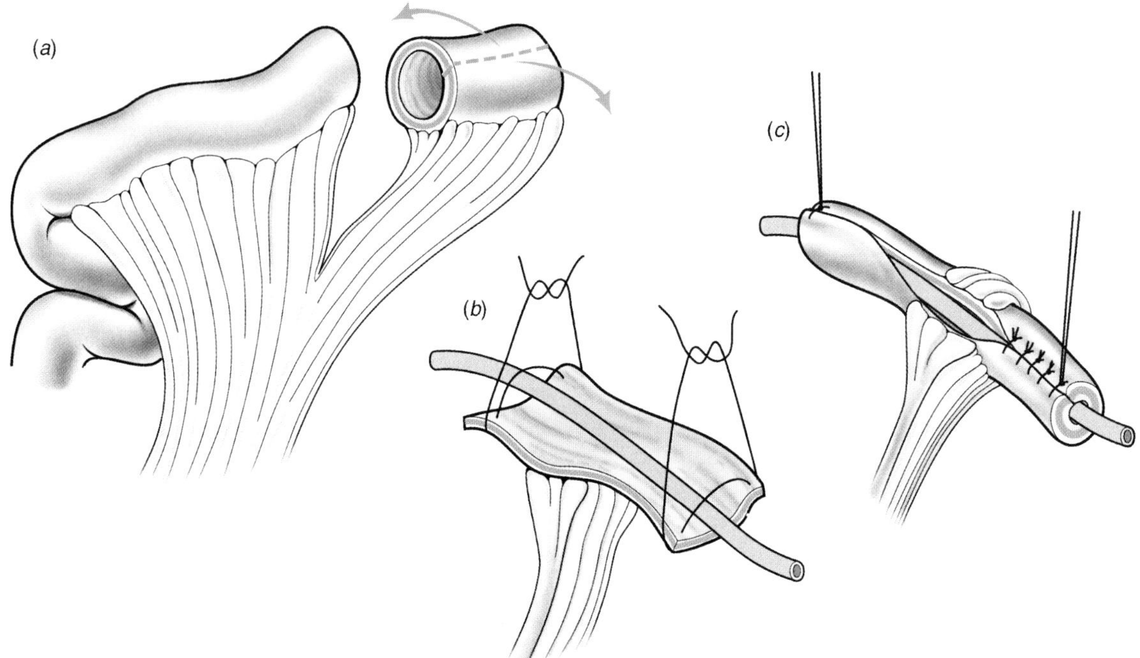

Figure 55.23 Monti popularized a concept originally described by Yang, who created a catheterizable tube from small bowel. (*a*) A 3–4 cm section of bowel is isolated on its mesentery and split on the antimesenteric border. (*b*) It is then closed along the transverse axis, 90° from the original. (*c*) This doubles the length of tube produced from a piece of bowel. The tube may then be implanted into the bladder for continent catheterizable access.

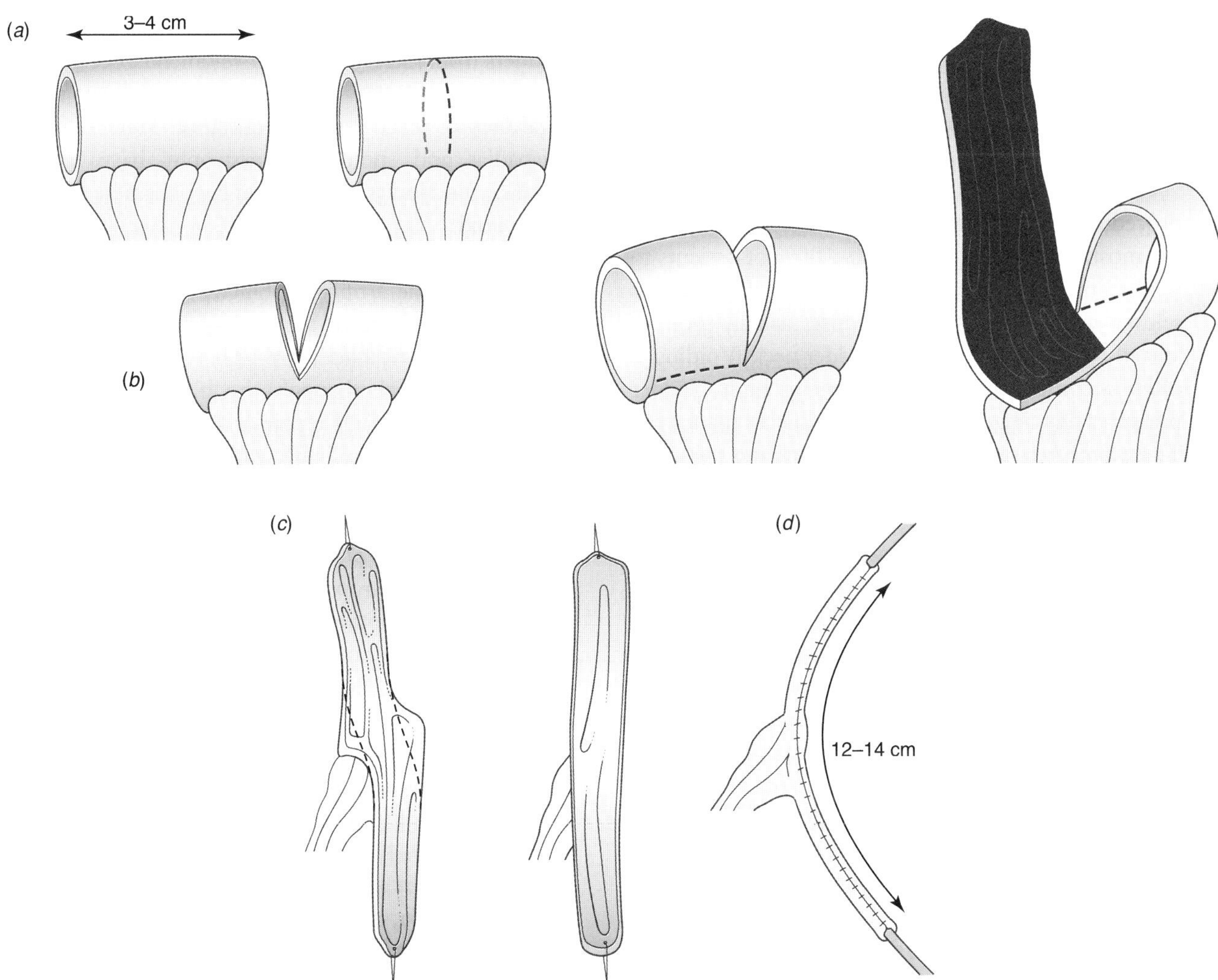

Figure 55.24 Casale presented a variation of the reconfigured ileal tube. (*a*) A 3–4 cm section of ileum is partially split into two rings, leaving the bowel over the mesentery intact. (*b*) The two rings are then split on opposite sides, allowing the bowel to be unfolded into a much longer flap. (*c*) Corners of bowel along the mesentery are trimmed off to make the strip uniform in width before it is tubularized. (*d*) The longer tube allows more flexibility in placement of the anastomosis, mesentery, and stoma.

bladder pressures low and minimizes stress on reconstruction done at the bladder neck. Stomas allow the surgeon to be more aggressive in creating resistance at the bladder outlet because the urethra will not be needed as the primary access for catheterization. The combination of continent stomas and augmentation has allowed patients who have suffered multiple failed continence surgeries to be salvaged with good results.[130]

Indicators for success

The definition of continence has changed over the years and is open to interpretation by each surgeon. 'Social continence' was felt to be adequate in the past and if a child used several continence pads per day but was free of diapers most pediatric urologists considered their treatment successful. Our tolerance of wetness has been modified over the years; perhaps in response to the change in public policy in the 1970s to mainstream the education of children with disabilities. In more modern reviews, surgeons have been more specific in defining successful continence. Dryness, without the odor of urine, has become the expected goal. This evolution of the definition of success makes comparing results from different eras and series difficult.

The effectiveness of procedures to treat the weak bladder outlet cannot be judged easily. Ultimate success is of course based on continence, but also

alone will improve continence in this patient population even if the bladder outlet is weak.[134] In our experience, augmentation alone has not provided reliable continence even in patients with reasonable bladder outlet resistance. For this reason, we believe that in most cases of reconstruction for incontinence, the surgeon should maximize both bladder outlet resistance and the storage capacity of the bladder.

In preparing the revised edition of this chapter, I was struck by the change in emphasis in surgical treatment of severe anatomic or neuropathic incontinence. New work in this field is directed toward less-aggressive surgical intervention such as slings, wraps, and injection therapy. There have been few advances in the area of major bladder outlet reconstruction in the past 8 years and, if anything, this surgery has become less radical as in the modifications of the YDL procedure.

Procedures to improve resistance at the incompetent bladder outlet have been advanced greatly by the development of associated procedures such as bladder augmentation over the past 25 years. Two singular contributions in this field came from Lapides, with his concept of CIC, and Mitrofanoff, whose novel idea to create a continent catheterizable stoma allowed a non-urethral method of bladder emptying. Finally, the predictors of success in bladder outlet reconstruction remain unchanged despite any new advances. They are sufficient resistance at the bladder outlet, a low-pressure reservoir of adequate size, and a reliable means to empty the bladder efficiently.

References

1. Simon J. Ectropia vesicae (absence of the anterior walls of the bladder and pubic abdominal parietes); operation for directing the orifices of the ureters into the rectum; temporary success; subsequent death; autopsy. Lancet 1852; 2:568.
2. Trendedenburg F. The treatment of ectopia vesicae. Ann Surg 1906; 44:281–9.
3. Young H. An operation for the cure of incontinence of urine. Surg Gynecol Obstet 1919; 28:84–90.
4. Blaivas J, Romanzi L, Heritz D. Urinary incontinence: pathophysiology, evaluation, treatment overview, and nonsurgical management. In: Walsh P, Retik A, Vaughn E, Wein A, eds. Campbell's Urology, Vol 7. Philadelphia: WB Saunders, 1998: 1007–36.
5. Gonzalez R, Sidi A. Preoperative prediction of continence after enterocystoplasty or undiversion in children with neurogenic bladder. J Urol 1985; 134:705–7.
6. McGuire E, Woodside J, Borden T, Weis R. Prognostic value of urodynamic testing in myelodysplastic patients. J Urol 1981; 126:205–9.
7. Decter R, Harpster L. Pitfalls in determination of leak point pressure. J Urol 1992; 148:588–91.
8. Ghoniem G, Bloom D, McGuire E, Stewart K. Bladder compliance in meningomyelocele children. J Urol 1989; 141:1404–6.
9. Woodside J, McGuire E. Technique for detection of detrusor hypertonia in the presence of urethral sphincteric incompetence. J Urol 1982; 127:740–3.
10. Andersson K. Pharmacology of lower urinary tract smooth muscles and penile erectile tissues. Pharmacol Rev 1993; 45:253–308.
11. Purcell M, Gregory J. Intermittent catheterization: evaluation of complete dryness and independence in children with myelomeningocele. J Urol 1984; 132:518–20.
12. Hilwa N, Perlmutter A. The role of adjunctive drug therapy for intermittent catheterization and self-catheterization in children with vesical dysfunction. J Urol 1978; 119:551–4.
13. Wang S, McGuire E, Bloom D. A bladder pressure management system for myelodysplasia – clinical outcome. J Urol 1988; 140:1499–502.
14. Mulcahy J, James H, McRoberts J. Oxybutynin chloride combined with intermittent clean catheterization in the treatment of myelomeningocele patients. J Urol 1977; 118:95–6.
15. Blaivas J. Pubovaginal slings. In: Kursh ED, McGuire EJ, eds. Female Urology. Philadelphia: JB Lippincott, 1994: 235.
16. Marshall V, Marchetti A, Krantz K. Correction of stress incontinence by simple vesicourethral suspension. Surg Gynecol Obstet 1949; 88:509–18.
17. Burch J. Urethrovaginal fixation to Cooper's ligament for correction of stress incontinence, cystocele, and prolapse. Am J Obstet Gynecol 1961; 81:281–90.
18. Webster G, Khoury J. Retropubic suspension surgery for female sphincteric incontinence. In: Walsh P, Retik A, Vaughn E, Wein A, eds. Campbell's Urology, Vol 7. Philadelphia: WB Saunders, 1998: 1095–102.
19. Freedman E, Singh G, Donnell S, Rickwood A, Thomas D. Combined bladder neck suspension and augmentation cystoplasty for neuropathic incontinence in female patients. Br J Urol 1994; 73:621–4.
20. Raz S, Ehrlich E, Zeidman E, Alarcon A, McLaughlin S. Surgical treatment of the incontinent female patient with myelomeningocele. J Urol 1988; 139:524–7.
21. Stamey T. Endoscopic suspension of the vesical neck for urinary incontinence. Surg Gynecol Obstet 1973; 136:547–54.
22. Pereya A, Ledherz T. Combined urethrovesical suspension and vaginal urethroplasty for correction of urinary stress incontinence. Obstet Gynecol 1967; 30:537–46.
23. Raz S. Modified bladder neck suspension for female stress incontinence. Urology 1981; 17:82–5.
24. Goebell R. Zur operativen beseritigung der angerborenen incontinentia vesical. Ztsch Gynak 1911; 2:187.
25. McGuire E, Lytton B. Pubovaginal sling for stress incontinence. J Urol 1978; 119:82–4.
26. McGuire E, Wang C, Usitalo H, Savastano J. Modified pubovaginal sling in girls with myelodysplasia. J Urol 1986; 135:94–6.
27. Dik P, Klijn A, van Gool J, de Jong T. Transvaginal sling suspension of bladder neck in female patients with neuro-

genic sphincter incontinence. J Urol 2003; 170:580–1, discussion 581–2.
28. Woodside J, Borden T. Pubovaginal sling procedure for the management of urinary incontinence in a myelodysplastic girl. J Urol 1982; 127:744–6.
29. Bauer S, Peters C, Colodny A, Mandell J, Retik A. The use of rectus fascia to manage urinary incontinence. J Urol 1989; 142:516–19.
30. Gormley E, Bloom D, McGuire E, Ritchey M. Pubovaginal slings for the management of urinary incontinence in female adolescents. J Urol 1994; 152:822–5.
31. Elder J. Periurethral and puboprostatic sling repair for incontinence in patients with myelodysplasia. J Urol 1990; 144:434–7.
32. Ludlow J, Keating M, Wahle G et al. Fascial slings in children – the gender gap. J Urol 1995; 153:279A (Abstract 201).
33. Raz S, McGuire E, Ehrilch R et al. Fascial sling to correct male neurogenic sphincter incompetence: the McGuire/Raz approach. J Urol 1988; 139:528–31.
34. Kakizaki H, Shibata T, Shinno Y et al. Fascial sling for the management of urinary incontinence due to sphincter incompetence. J Urol 1995; 153:644–7.
35. Herschorn S, Randomski S. Fascial slings and bladder neck tapering in the treatment of male urologic incontinence. J Urol 1992; 147:1073–5.
36. Decter R. Use of the fascial sling for neurogenic incontinence: lessons learned. J Urol 1993; 150:683–6.
37. Van Gool D, De Jong T. Urinary continence and erectile function after bladder neck sling suspension in male patients with spinal dysraphism. Br J Urol Int 1999; 83:971.
38. Godbole P, MacKinnon A. Expanded PTFE bladder neck slings for incontinence in children: the long-term outcome. Br J Urol Int 2004; 93:139–41.
39. Volkmer B, Nesslauer T, Rinnab L et al. Surgical intervention for complications of tension-free vaginal tape procedure. J Urol 2003; 169:570–4.
40. Cetinel B, Demirkesen O, Kural A, Onal B, Alan C. Polypropylene mesh tape for male sphincteric incontinence. Scand J Urol Nephrol 2004; 38:396–400.
41. Colvert J 3rd, Kropp B, Cheng E et al. The use of small intestinal submucosa as an off-the-shelf urethral sling material for pediatric urinary incontinence. J Urol 2002; 168:1872–5, discussion 1875–6.
42. Scott F, Bradley W, Timm G. Treatment of urinary incontinence by an implantable prosthetic urinary sphincter. J Urol 1974; 112:75–80.
43. Levisque P, Bauer S, Atala A et al. Ten year experience with the artificial urinary sphincter in children. J Urol 1996; 156:625–8.
44. Gonzalez R, Merino F, Vaughn M. Long term results of the artificial urinary sphincter in male patients with neurogenic bladder. J Urol 1995; 154:769–70.
45. Herndon C, Rink R, Shaw M et al. The Indiana experience with artificial urinary sphincters in children and young adults. J Urol 2003; 169:650–4, discussion 654.
46. Barrett D, Licht M. Implantation of the artificial genitourinary sphincter in men and women. In: Walsh P, Retik A, Vaughn E, Wein A, eds. Campbell's Urology, Vol 7. Philadelphia: WB Saunders, 1998: 1121–34.
47. Barrett D, Furlow W. Implantation of a new semi-automatic artificial genitourinary sphincter. Experience with patients utilizing a new concept of primary and secondary activation. Prog Clin Biol Res 1981; 78:375–86.
48. Gonzalez, R, Koleilat, N, Austin C, Sidi A. The artificial sphincter AS800 in congenital urinary incontinence. J Urol 1989; 142:512–15.
49. Barrett D, Furlow W. Incontinence, intermittent self-catheterization and the artificial genitourinary sphincter. J Urol 1984: 132:268–9.
50. Barrett D, Furlow W. The management of severe urinary incontinence in patients with myelodysplasia by implantation of the AS 791/792 urinary sphincter device. J Urol 1982; 128:484–6.
51. Kaefer M, McLaughlin K, Rink R, Adams M, Keating M. Upsizing of the artificial urinary sphincter cuff to facilitate spontaneous voiding. Urology 1997; 50:106–9.
52. Sidi A, Reinberg Y, Gonzalez R. Comparison of artificial sphincter implantation and bladder neck reconstruction in patients with neurogenic urinary incontinence. J Urol 1987; 138:1120–2.
53. Kryger J, Spencer Barthold J, Fleming P, Gonzalez R. The outcome of artificial sphincter placement after a mean 15-year follow-up in a paediatric population. BJU Int 1999; 83:1026–31.
54. Hafez A, McLorie G, Bagli D, Khoury A. A single-center long-term outcome analysis of artificial urinary sphincter placement in children. BJU Int 2002; 89:82–5.
55. Elliott D, Barrett D. Mayo Clinic long-term analysis of the functional durability of the AMS 800 artificial urinary sphincter: A review of 323 cases. J Urol 1998; 159: 1206–8.
56. Roth D, Vyas P, Kroovand R, Perlmutter A. Urinary tract deterioration associated with the artificial urinary sphincter. J Urol 1986; 135:528–30.
57. Kronner K, Rink R, Simmons G et al. Artificial urinary sphincter in the treatment of urinary incontinence: preoperative urodynamics do not predict the need for future bladder augmentation. J Urol 1998; 160:1093–5.
58. Bauer S, Reda E, Colodny A, Retik A. Detrusor instability: a delayed complication in association with the artificial sphincter. J Urol 1986; 135:1212–15.
59. Light K, Pietro T. Alteration in detrusor behavior and the effect on renal function following insertion of the artificial urinary sphincter. J Urol 1986; 136:632–5.
60. Barrett D, Parulkar B, Kramer S. Experience with AS 800 artificial sphincter in pediatric and young adult patients. Urology 1993; 42:431–6.
61. Light J, Lapin S, Vohra S. Combined use of bowel and the artificial urinary sphincter in reconstruction of the lower urinary tract: infectious complications. J Urol 1995; 153:331–3.
62. Miller E, Mayo M, Kwan D, Mitchel M. Simultaneous augmentation cystoplasty and artificial urinary sphincter placement: infection rates and voiding mechanisms. J Urol 1998; 160:750–3.
63. Bosco P, Bauer S, Colodny A, Mandell J, Retik A. The long-term results of artificial sphincters in children. J Urol 1991; 146:396–9.
64. Holmes N, Kogan B, Baskin L. Placement of artificial urinary sphincter in children and simultaneous gastrocystoplasty. J Urol 2001; 165:2366–8.

65. Castera R, Podesta M, Ruarte A Herrera M, Medel R. 10-Year experience with artificial urinary sphincter in children and adolescents. J Urol 2001; 165:2373–6.
66. Kropp B, Rink R, Adams M, Keating M, Mitchell M. Bladder outlet reconstruction: fate of the silicone sheath. J Urol 1993; 150:703–4.
67. Quimby G, Diamond D, Mor Y, Zaidi Z, Ransley P. Bladder neck reconstruction: long-term followup of reconstruction with omentum and silicone sheath. J Urol 1996; 156:629–32.
68. de O Vilar F, Araujo I, Lima S. Periurethral constrictor in pediatric urology: long-term followup. J Urol 2004; 171:2626–8.
69. Kohn I, Balsara R, Rabinovitch H. Placement of a bladder neck purse-string cuff for the management of incontinence in children with myelodysplasia. Urology 1998; 51:1027–30.
70. Walker R, Flack C, Hawkins-Lee B et al. Rectus fascial wrap: early results of modification of the rectus fascial sling. J Urol 1995; 154:771–4.
71. Walker R, Erhard M, Starling J. Long-term evaluation of rectus fascial wrap in patients with spina bifida. J Urol 2000; 144:485–6.
72. Bugg C Jr, Joseph D. Bladder neck cinch for pediatric neurogenic outlet deficiency. J Urol 2003; 170:1501–3, discussion 1503–4.
73. Kolligian M, Palmer L, Cheng E, Firlit C. Myofascial wrap to treat intractable urinary incontinence in children. Urology 1998; 52:1122–7.
74. Kurzrock E, Lowe P, Hardy B. Bladder wall pedicle wraparound sling for neurogenic urinary incontinence in children. J Urol 1996; 155:305–8.
75. Berg S. Polytef augmentation urethroplasty. Arch Surg 1973; 107:379–81.
76. Politano V, Small M, Harper J, Lynn C. Periurethral Teflon injection for urinary incontinence. J Urol 1974; 111:180–3.
77. Vorstman, B, Lockhard J, Kaufman M, Politano V. Polytetrafluoroethylene injection for urinary incontinence in children. J Urol 1985; 133:248–50.
78. Malizia A Jr, Reiman H, Meyers R et al. Migration and granulomatous reaction after periurethral injection of polytef (Teflon). JAMA 1984; 251:3277–81.
79. Mittleman R, Marraccini J. Pulmonary Teflon granulomas following periurethral Teflon injection for urinary incontinence. Arch Pathol Lab Med 1983; 107:611–12.
80. Guys J, Fakhro A, Louis-Borrione C, Prost J, Hauter A. Endoscopic treatment of urinary incontinence: long-term evaluation of the results. J Urol 2001; 165:2389–91.
81. Gonzalez de Garibay A, Jimeno C, York M, Gomez P, Borruell S. Endoscopic autotransplantation of fat tissue in the treatment of urinary incontinence in the female. J Urol 1989; 95:363–6.
82. Bartynski J, Marion M, Wang T. Histopathologic evaluation of adipose autografts in a rabbit ear model. Otolaryngology 1990; 102:314–21.
83. Perez L, Smith E, Parrott T et al. Submucosal bladder neck injection of bovine dermal collagen for stress urinary incontinence in the pediatric population. J Urol 1996; 156:633–6.
84. Wan J, McGuire E, Bloom D, Ritchey M. The treatment of urinary incontinence in children using glutaraldehyde cross-linked collagen. J Urol 1992; 148:127–30.
85. Bomalaski M, Bloom D, McGuire E, Panzl A. Glutaraldehyde cross-linked collagen in the treatment of urinary incontinence in children. J Urol 1996; 155:699–702.
86. Gorton E, Stanton S, Monga A et al. Periurethral collagen injection: a long-term follow-up study. BJU Int 1999; 84:966–71.
87. Kassouf W, Capolicchio G, Berardinucci G, Corcos J. J Urol 2001; 165:1666–8.
88. Strothers L, Goldenberg S. Delayed hypersensitivity and systemic arthralgia following transurethral collagen injection for stress urinary incontinence. J Urol 1998; 159:1507–9.
89. Misseri R, Casale A, Cain M, Rink R. Alternate uses of Deflux, the efficacy of bladder neck injection for urinary incontinence. Abstract presented at the American Academy of Pediatrics, Section on Urology, San Francisco, October 2004.
90. Ben-Chaim J, Jeffs R, Peppas D, Gearhart JL. Submucosal bladder neck injections of glutaraldehyde cross-linked bovine collagen for the treatment of urinary incontinence in patients with the exstrophy/epispadias complex. J Urol 1995; 154:862–4.
91. Young H. An operation for the cure of incontinence associated with epispadias. J Urol 1922; 7:1–32.
92. Culp O. Treatment of epispadias with and without urinary incontinence: experience with 46 patients. J Urol 1973; 100:120–5.
93. Dees J. Congenital epispadias with incontinence. J Urol 1949; 62:513–22.
94. Leadbetter G Jr. Surgical correction of total urinary incontinence. J Urol 1964; 91:261–4.
95. Gearhart J, Jeffs R. Management of the exstrophy–epispadias complex and urachal anomalies. In: Walsh P, Retik A, Vaughn E, Wein A, eds. Campbell's Urology, Vol 6. Philadelphia: WB Saunders, 1992: 1772.
96. Donnahoo K, Rink R, Cain M, Casale A. The use of the Young–Dees–Leadbetter bladder neck repair in patients with neurogenic incontinence. J Urol 1999; 161:1946–9.
97. McMahon D, Cain M, Husmann D, Kramer S. Vesical neck reconstruction in patients with the exstrophy–epispadias complex. J Urol 1996; 155:1411–13.
98. Mollard P. Bladder reconstruction in exstrophy. J Urol 1980; 124:525–9.
99. Koff S. A technique for bladder neck reconstruction in exstrophy: the cinch. J Urol 1990; 144:546–9.
100. Jones J, Mitchell M, Rink R. Improved results using a modification of the Young–Dees–Leadbetter bladder neck repair. Br J Urol 1993; 71:555–61.
101. Koyle M. Flap valve techniques in bladder neck reconstruction. Dialog Pediatr Urol 1998; 21:6.
102. Arap S, Martins Giron A, Menezes de Goes G. Initial results of the complete reconstruction of bladder exstrophy. Urol Clin North Am 1980; 7:477–88.
103. Tanagho E, Smith D. Mechanism of urinary continence. I. Embryologic, anatomic and pathologic considerations. J Urol 1968; 100:640–6.
104. Tanagho E, Smith D, Meyers F, Fisher R. Mechanism of urinary continence. II. Technique for surgical correction of incontinence. J Urol 1969; 101:305–13.

105. Tanagho E, Smith D. Clinical evaluation of a surgical technique for the correction of complete urinary incontinence. J Urol 1972; 107:402–11.
106. Tanagho E. Bladder neck reconstruction for total urinary incontinence: 10 years of experience. J Urol 1981; 125:321–4.
107. Diamond D, Ransley P. Use of the anterior detrusor tube in managing urogenital sinus anomalies. J Urol 1987; 138:1057–9.
108. Lapides J, Diokno A, Silber S, Lowe B. Clean, intermittent catheterization in the treatment of urinary tract disease. J Urol 1972; 107:458–61.
109. Charney E, Kalichman M, Snyder H. Multiple benefits of clean intermittent catheterization for children with myelomeningocele. Z Kinderchir 1982; 37:145.
110. Kropp K, Angwafo F. Urethral lengthening and reimplantation for neurogenic incontinence in children. J Urol 1986; 135:533–6.
111. Nill T, Peller P, Kropp K. Management of urinary incontinence by bladder tube urethral lengthening and submucosal reimplantation. J Urol 1990; 144:559–63.
112. Belman A, Kaplan G. Experience with the Kropp anti-incontinence procedure. J Urol 1989; 141:1160–2.
113. Snodgrass W. A simplified Kropp procedure for incontinence. J Urol 1997; 158:1049–52.
114. Salle J, De Fraga J, Amarante A et al. Urethral lengthening with anterior bladder wall flap for urinary incontinence: a new approach. J Urol 1994; 152:803–4.
115. Rink R, Adams M, Keating M. The flip-flap technique to lengthen the urethra (Salle procedure) for treatment of neurogenic urinary incontinence. J Urol 1994; 152:799–802.
116. McLorie G, Khoury A. Anterior bladder wall flap (Sallee procedure). Dialog Pediatr Urol 1998; 21:5.
117. Mitrofanoff P. Cystostomie continente trans-appendiculaire dans le traitement des vesses neurologiques. Chir Pediatr 1980; 21:297–305.
118. Duckett J, Snyder H. Continent urinary diversion: variations on the Mitrofanoff principle. J Urol 1986; 136:58–62.
119. Van Savage J, Khoury A, McLorie G, Churchill B. Outcome analysis of Mitrofanoff principle applications using appendix and ureter to umbilical and lower quadrant stomal sites. J Urol 1996; 156:1794–7.
120. Gearhart J, Peppas D, Jeffs R. The application of continent urinary stomas to bladder augmentation or replacement in the failed exstrophy reconstruction. Br J Urol 1995; 75:87–90.
121. Hensle T, Kirsch A, Kennedy W, Reiley E. Bladder neck closure in association with continent urinary diversion. J Urol 1995; 154:883–5.
122. Jayanthi V, Churchill B, McLorie G, Khoury A. Concomitant bladder neck closure and Mitrofanoff diversion for the management of intractable urinary incontinence. J Urol 1995; 154:886–8.
123. Nguyen H, Baskin L. The outcome of bladder neck closure in children with severe urinary incontinence. J Urol 2003; 169:1114–16, discussion 1116.
124. Casale A. Continent vesicostomy: a new method utilizing only bladder tissue (Abstract 72). Presented at the 60th annual meeting of the American Academy of Pediatrics, New Orleans, 1991.
125. Yang W. Yang needle tunneling technique in creating antireflux and continent mechanisms. J Urol 1993; 150:830–4.
126. Monti P, Lara R, Dutra M, De Carvalho J. New techniques for construction of efferent conduits based on the Mitrofanoff principle. Urology 1997; 49:112–15.
127. Malone P, Ransley P, Kiely E. Preliminary report: the antegrade continence enema. Lancet 1990; 336:1217–18.
128. Cain M, Casale A, Rink R. Initial experience utilizing a catheterizable ileovesicostomy (Monti procedure) in children. Urology 1998; 52:870–3.
129. Casale A. A long continent ileovesicostomy made of a single piece of bowel. J Urol 1999; 162:1743–5.
130. Gearhart J, Canning D, Jeffs R. Failed bladder neck reconstruction: options for management. J Urol 1991; 146:1082–4.
131. Kaefer M, Andler R, Bauer S et al. Urodynamic findings in children with isolated epispadias. J Urol 1999; 162:1172–5.
132. Diamond D, Bauer S, Dinlecn C et al. Normal urodynamics in patients with bladder exstrophy: are they achievable? J Urol 1999; 162:841–5.
133. Grady R, Carr M, Mitchell M. Complete primary closure of bladder exstrophy. Epispadias and bladder exstrophy repair. Urol Clin North Am 1999; 26; 95–109.
134. Cher M, Allen T. Continence in the myelodysplastic patient following enterocystoplasty. J Urol 1993; 149:1103–6.

Bladder augmentation: current and future techniques

56

Bradley P Kropp and Earl Y Cheng

Introduction

The surgical management of the child with a neuropathic bladder can be a formidable task, but major advances in surgical technique have been made in recent decades. The ability to augment the capacity of the bladder with a piece of reconfigured bowel in conjunction with clean intermittent catheterization (CIC) has dramatically altered our ability to form a compliant urinary reservoir that protects the integrity of the upper urinary tract and promotes urinary continence. Conventional enterocystoplasty uses detubularized segments of small or large bowel. Despite the functional success of intestinocystoplasty, clinical experience has demonstrated that numerous complications can result from the incorporation of small and large bowel and their associated heterotopic epithelium into the urinary tract. To avoid some of these deleterious side effects of the use of bowel for bladder augmentation, several procedures have now been developed to augment the bladder without the use of bowel, including gastrocystoplasty, autoaugmentation, seromuscular enterocystoplasty, and ureterocystoplasty. In addition, recent advances in tissue engineering techniques have increased the possibility of regenerating new bladder tissue that is clinically useful for augmentation purposes. This chapter reviews the relevant surgical anatomy and physiology, advantages and disadvantages, surgical technique, and clinical results of conventional enterocystoplasty and each of the alternative procedures that avoid the use of bowel. These are summarized in Table 56.1. Since the care of the child with a neuropathic bladder can be complex and requires individualization that is dependent on the desires of the patient and family, familiarity with each of these procedures is extremely important for the pediatric urologist when considering augmentation cystoplasty.

Indications and preoperative assessment

Enterocystoplasty is performed when there is a need to enlarge and/or decrease the storage pressure in the native bladder. This can result from a host of conditions, including spina bifida, spinal cord trauma, posterior urethral valves (PUV), dysfunctional voiding, radiation, and infectious or other chronic inflammatory processes. Enterocystoplasty is intended to relieve high-pressure and low-capacity characteristics. There are two major indications for enterocystoplasty. The first is the presence or risk of upper tract deterioration secondary to a poorly compliant bladder. The second indication is when the bladder is a causative factor in urinary incontinence. All patients who are being considered for enterocystoplasty should be thoroughly studied with preoperative urodynamics and initially treated by medical alternatives such as anticholinergic medications and/or intermittent catheterization. It is extremely important that patients understand that, in most instances, enterocystoplasty will not result in normal voiding and a lifelong commitment to intermittent catheterization will be required.[1]

Lapides' landmark studies in the early 1970s, demonstrating that intermittent catheterization can be performed safely and effectively in children,[2,3] have had the single greatest impact on the ability to perform enterocystoplasties in children. If a patient is not dedicated to performing lifelong intermittent catheterization, then a non-continent form of urinary diversion should be chosen instead of enterocystoplasty.

The goals of enterocystoplasty are to change the native bladder environment by reducing storage pressure and increasing volume. A thorough preoperative evaluation will help to determine which type of augmentation is most appropriate and beneficial for each

Bowel function

A thorough evaluation of bowel function, including a history of constipation or diarrhea, must be carried out prior to enterocystoplasty. Postoperative bowel dysfunction can occur in up to 50% of patients who have undergone enterocystoplasty.[14] In addition, King[15] found that removal of the ileocecal segment in children with spina bifida causes severe diarrhea in approximately 10% of patients. However, in a more recent series of 63 patients who underwent ileal cecal cystoplasty, bowel complication was found to be only 3%.[16] Nevertheless, before undertaking any type of urinary reconstruction that involves the use of a bowel segment, discussion with the patient and family should include potential gastrointestinal complications. The type of augmentation should be chosen with these potential complications in mind.

Ability to catheterize

Since most patients who undergo enterocystoplasty will not be able to void completely without lifelong intermittent catheterization, one should consider the formation of a catheterizable stoma at the time of the augmentation. This is especially important in patients who are sensate or are in wheelchairs. Clinical experience has shown that when both the native urethra and a catheterizable stoma are present, the majority of patients will choose to use the catheterizable stoma. In addition, assessment of the physical and mental capacities of the patient and family must be undertaken to make sure that they will be able to perform intermittent catheterization on a regular schedule.

Families want to believe that their child will become continent after enterocystoplasty and that the kidneys will be protected. However, the amount of time and effort that will be required is often not appreciated preoperatively. Therefore, all must understand the risks and benefits of enterocystoplasty prior to surgery and the lifelong commitment to a rigorous schedule of intermittent catheterization. Since there are many potential problems associated with failure to catheterize, including spontaneous bladder rupture and death, urinary reconstruction should be deferred until the patient has the physical and mental maturity needed to care for him or herself.

Intestinocystoplasty

Small bowel

Currently, ileum is the most commonly used bowel segment for enterocystoplasty. The abundant supply of small bowel, easy workability, mobility, reliable blood supply, and compliance of the reconfigured ileum have led most reconstructive surgeons to choose ileum over other bowel segments. Although the jejunum can be used for urinary reconstruction, the high incidence of metabolic complications (hyponatremic, hypochloremic, and hyperkalemic acidosis) associated with use of this segment make it less desirable and thus it is rarely used. The major contraindications to the use of ileum are a history of short gut syndrome, inflammatory bowel disease, pelvic and/or abdominal radiation, and significant renal insufficiency. Under these conditions, alternative segments such as stomach are more appropriate.

Anatomy and physiology

The proximal two-fifths of the small bowel proper is jejunum and the distal three-fifths is ileum. The coils of mid-ileum usually lie in the pelvis, whereas the terminal 30 cm of ileum, the most commonly used portion for enterocystoplasty, usually rises out of the pelvis to lie in close relationship to the cecum and the ascending colon.

The mesentery of the small bowel attaches to the posterior abdominal wall. The 'root' of the small bowel mesentery runs obliquely across the abdomen. As the root of the mesentery runs obliquely from left to right, it crosses, in order, the abdominal aorta, the vertebral column, and the third portion of the duodenum. The mid-portion of the small bowel has the longest mesentery, whereas the segments of the small bowel closest to the cecum and the duodenojejunal flexure have the shortest. Therefore, in patients in whom the mesentery is short, a segment of ileum 30 cm or more above the ileocecal valve will be the most mobile and will reach the furthest into the pelvis.

The arterial supply to the entire small bowel is derived from the superior mesenteric artery (Figure 56.1). There are usually 12–16 branches of the superior mesenteric artery running to the jejunum and ileum and entering the small bowel at its mesenteric border. The ileocolic artery is the most distal segment of this vessel. It is found in the right lower abdominal quadrant, where it gives off branches that supply the terminal ileum, the cecum and appendix, and the proximal ascending colon. Venous drainage of the small bowel occurs through multiple mesenteric channels that coalesce to form the superior mesenteric vein. It is this abundant and redundant blood supply that makes the use of different segments of ileum viable for urinary reconstruction.

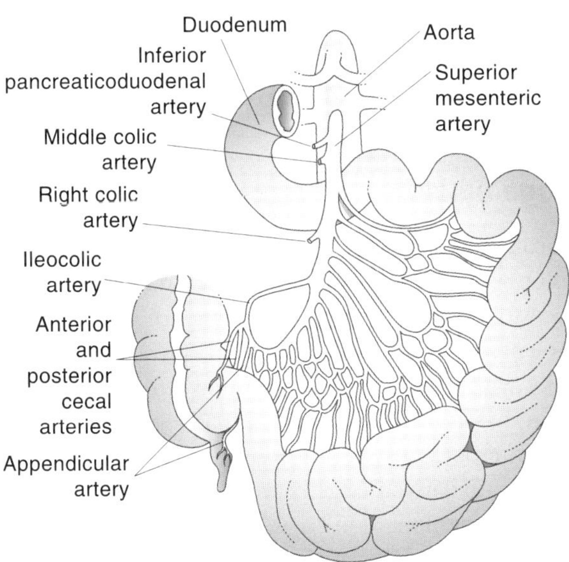

Figure 56.1 Arterial blood supply to the small intestine. The portion of the ileum with the longest mesentery that is commonly used for intestinocystoplasty is around 20–30 cm proximal to the ileocecal valve. (Adapted from Lindner,[17] with permission.)

The small intestine is innervated from the autonomic plexuses grouped around the 'take-off' of the superior mesenteric artery from the aorta. These plexuses include preganglionic parasympathetic nerves from the vagus as well as postganglionic sympathetic fibers from the celiac plexus. The submucosa of the small intestine contains the nerve plexus of Meissner. Between the longitudinal and circular muscle of the small bowel is the intramuscular myenteric (Auerbach's) plexus, consisting of non-myelinated nerve fiber plus numerous ganglion cells.

The bowel wall is made up of an outer serosal coat, two layers of muscle (outer longitudinal smooth muscle and inner circular smooth muscle), a submucosal layer, and a mucous membrane composed of a single layer of columnar epithelial cells. Since the muscle and epithelial layers are relatively thin, the plane between these layers is difficult to establish surgically; therefore, tunneling procedures for ureters and catheterizable stomas may be quite difficult in small bowel.

The physiology of the small and large intestine involves an intricate balance of water and electrolyte shifts. The major mechanisms of intestinal transport of water and electrolytes are illustrated in Figure 56.2. Water and electrolyte movement varies throughout the length of the bowel. These changes can be accounted for by both structural and functional differences between the small and large bowel. The

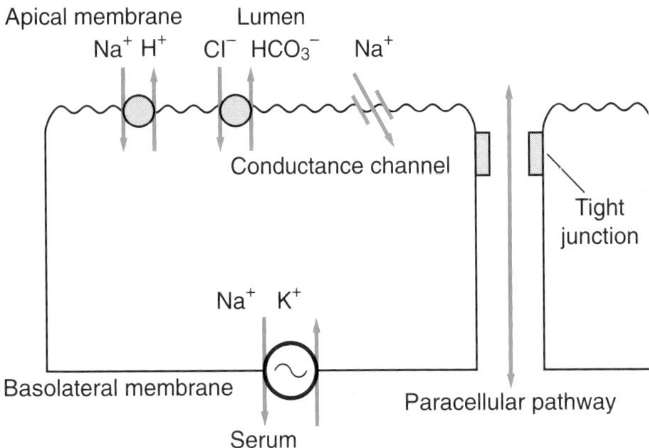

Figure 56.2 Intestinal transport mechanisms. Sodium absorption in both the small and large bowel is transcellular and occurs via a Na^+–H^+ exchanger on the apical membrane and a Na^+–K^+ pump on the basolateral membrane. The colon has an additional pathway of entry for Na^+ via conductance channels, which allows for non-coupled sodium absorption. Chloride and bicarbonate transport is coupled, which is pertinent in the development of metabolic acidosis following intestinocystoplasty. Water and electrolyte movement also occurs via paracellular pathways associated with tight junctions between the cells. Paracellular movement occurs more in the ileum than in the colon owing to leakier tight junctions. (Adapted from Lindner,[17] with permission.)

major structural difference between the small and large bowel involves the 'tight' junctions that join the epithelial cells (see Figure 56.2). These tight junctions have characteristic permeabilities and ionic conductance that form the basis for paracellular ion and water movement.[18] Because such junctions are tightest in the colon and more permeable or leaky in the proximal small bowel, paracellular movement may account for a significant portion of water and electrolyte transport in the small bowel, and not play as an important role in the colon.

Although paracellular movement accounts for some of the bidirectional water and electrolyte transport, most of these shifts are thought to occur via transcellular mechanisms that occur through the intestinal absorptive cell. A characteristic example of the intestinal absorptive mechanism is the Na^+/K^+-ATPase enzyme, which is located on the basolateral membrane. This pump maintains low intracellular sodium concentrations and thus creates an electrochemical gradient for sodium absorption as well as passive transport of other electrolytes and water.

Sodium entry in the small bowel is accomplished by way of a Na^+–H^+ countertransport system in the apical membrane. In addition, a significant portion of the sodium entry into the colon also occurs via electrogenic Na^+ conductance channels that allow for non-coupled sodium absorption. The presence of this channel in the colon probably accounts for its ability to transport Na^+ and water against large gradients.

Chloride is absorbed throughout the entire small and large bowel. Bicarbonate is absorbed in large quantities in the jejunum but secreted in the ileum and colon. Chloride absorption in exchange for HCO_3^- secretion plays a large role in the transport of these electrolytes in the ileum and colon. Na^+–H^+ exchange and Cl^-–HCO_3^- exchange occur together. The net result is the electroneutral absorption of Na^+ and Cl^-.

Metabolic acidosis may develop whenever urine is in contact with ileal or colonic mucosa. The mechanism by which this hyperchloremic metabolic acidosis occurs is thought to be directly related to ammonium (NH_4^+) reabsorption that can occur along the entire small and large bowel. It is likely that the inhibitory effect of ammonium on Na^+–H^+ exchange allows ionized ammonium transport where it substitutes for sodium in the Na^+–H^+ exchanger.[19] The result of this ammonium absorption is increased Cl^- absorption in order to maintain electrical neutrality. This leads to hyperchloremia and eventual metabolic acidosis. Although the exact physiologic mechanisms of electrolyte transport continue to be defined, it must be remembered that the major function of the intestine, regarding this transport, does not change when intestine is used for urinary reconstruction. Continued fluid and electrolyte fluxes account for the majority of the physiologic problems associated with the use of intestine in the urinary tract.

Advantages and disadvantages

Ileum is the most commonly used bowel segment for bladder augmentation. The advantages realized with use of ileum are (1) large quantity available; (2) ease in handling and reconfiguration; (3) predictable and abundant blood supply; (4) most compliant segment of bowel; (5) moderate mucus production compared with colon; (6) less severe metabolic complications than colon or stomach; and (7) fewer gastrointestinal complications than cecum.

The disadvantages in using ileum include (1) occasional short mesentery that cannot reach the pelvis; (2) possible development of diarrhea and vitamin B_{12} deficiency when the most distal ileum is used; (3) difficulty with creation of submucosal tunnels; and (4) metabolic acidosis; as well as (5) bowel obstruction; (6) stone formation; (7) mucus production; (8) urinary tract infections (UTIs); and (9) tumor formation, all of which are risks with large bowel segments as well.

Large bowel

Through the early 1980s, the cecum and sigmoid colon were more commonly used than ileum for enterocystoplasty. However, because of the shorter mesenteries, increased mucus production, and difficulty with configuration associated with large bowel, ileum has come to be the preferred segment of bowel for enterocystoplasty for most surgeons. Nevertheless, detubularized large bowel is still used for simple bladder augmentation in select patients, and in the hands of some surgeons, sigmoid colon may be the preferred segment.

Anatomy and physiology

Anatomically, the large bowel can be divided into five sections: (1) the cecum and vermiform appendix; (2) the ascending colon and the hepatic flexure; (3) the transverse colon and mesocolon; (4) the splenic flexure and descending colon; and (5) the sigmoid colon.

The colon is 1.4–1.7 m in length. Its diameter is greatest on the right side and gradually decreases as it approaches the sigmoid colon. The diameter of the sigmoid colon is often no wider than a loop of terminal ileum. The large bowel is made up of five distinct layers: serosa, muscularis externa, submucosa, muscularis mucosa, and mucosa. The outer serosal coat is a component of the peritoneum and normally completely covers the cecum, the appendix, and the transverse and sigmoid colon segments. The muscularis externa of the large bowel is composed of a complete inner circular and incomplete outer longitudinal layer of smooth muscle. The submucosa is composed of areolar tissue and lies between the muscularis externa and the muscularis mucosa. This layer contains the blood and lymphatic vessels supplying the bowel and is also the most important layer when developing an anastomotic site. The thin muscularis mucosa is made up of circular and longitudinal smooth muscle. The mucosa is composed of a layer of simple columnar epithelium containing goblet cells and is smooth and devoid of villi.

The muscle layers of the colon are notably different from those of the stomach, small intestine, and rectum. Longitudinal smooth muscle covers the large bowel incompletely. The longitudinal fibers are arranged in three narrow but distinct bands called teniae coli. The teniae of the cecum and ascending colon have a constant position relative to the bowel circumference. One band lies on the ventral surface of the colon, whereas the other two lie medial and lateral to the ventral band. The teniae of the transverse colon are less constant in position. Near the rectosigmoid junction the teniae become quite indistinct. The unique anatomy of the teniae facilitates reimplantation of ureters, appendix, and catheterizable stomas to create a reliable flap-valve continence mechanism. The deep circular muscular coat of the colon wall is visible between the longitudinal muscle fibers of the teniae. Contractions of the colon produce a pouching or sacculations of the bowel between the teniae. These pouchings, or haustra, are randomly distributed and are easily noted on gross examination and visible on X-ray studies.

Cecum and vermiform appendix

The cecum measures approximately 6 cm in length and lies caudal to the entrance of the ileum into the colon. It is the thinnest portion of the colon. The cecum is normally mobile. In over 90% of individuals it is completely covered with peritoneum and possesses no mesentery. In some patients, such as children with spina bifida and ventroperitoneal shunts, the cecum can become fused with the posterior abdominal wall. This in turn causes foreshortening of the peritoneal attachments, resulting in the cecum becoming more superiorly located in the right colic gutter.[20]

The terminal 14 cm of ileum, the cecum, appendix, and the ascending colon are supplied by the ileocolic artery, which is the terminal segment of the superior mesenteric artery. The ileocolic artery ends just proximal to the ileocecal junction and then divides into four major branches. The most superior branch, the colic artery, passes to the ascending colon, anastomosing with the descending branches of the right colic artery initiating the right colic portion of the marginal artery of Drummond or mesenteric arcade (Figure 56.3.).

The three bands of teniae coli originate at the base of the appendix. The appendix varies in length from

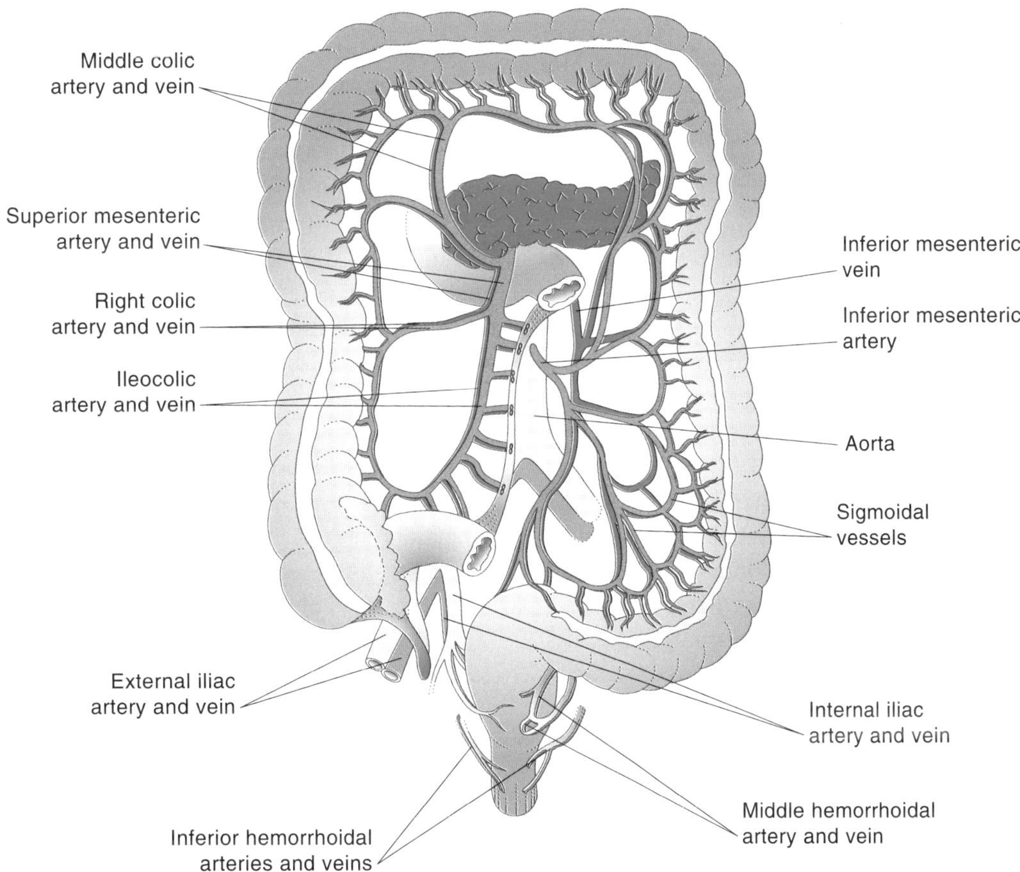

Figure 56.3 Arterial blood supply to the large bowel. Preservation of the marginal artery is extremely important when isolating portions of colon for intestinocystoplasty. (Adapted from Lindner,[17] with permission.)

2 to 20 cm, with an average of 9 cm. In the majority of patients, the appendix is held in position by the posterior inferior ileocecal fold. In about 5% of patients, the mesentery of the appendix runs directly from the posterior peritoneum in the region of the ileocecal junction onto the midportion of the appendix, at which point it is usually joined by the appendicular artery, a branch of the ileocolic artery. The appendicular artery arises either as a branch of the posterior cecal artery or directly from the main ileocolic trunk. It may also arise from the ileal branch of the ileocolic artery. Regardless of its site of origin, the appendicular artery will usually pass dorsal to the most distal segment of the terminal ileum before it enters the mesoappendix.

Ascending colon and transverse colon

The ascending colon occupies most of the right side of the abdominal cavity and extends from the cecum to the hepatic flexure. The blood supply to the ascending colon comes from the colic branches of the ileocolic artery, the right colic artery, and the right branches of the middle colic artery. The right colic artery is the most variable vessel in the colon and is absent in 5–7% of people. The transverse colon receives blood from the left colic artery; however, the major supplier is the middle colic artery, which is a more direct branch of the superior mesenteric artery.

Sigmoid colon

The sigmoid colon frequently has an S-shape, and is divided into a fixed superior and a mobile inferior portion. The fixed portion of the sigmoid colon begins at the level of the iliac crest. The mobile portion of the sigmoid colon begins at the medial border of the left psoas major muscle and ends where it joins the rectum. The length, location of loops, degree of redundancy, relationship to other structures, and mobility of the sigmoid colon are markedly variable. It is very common in the spina bifida population to encounter sigmoid colon so enlarged and redundant that the mobile portion crosses the midline and lies anterior to the cecum.

The inferior mesenteric artery is the major vessel to the left transverse colon, the splenic flexure, the left colon, the sigmoid colon, and the rectum. The left colic artery is the first branch of the inferior mesenteric artery and runs in the direction of the superior half of the descending colon. The ascending branch of the left colic artery runs superiorly and parallel with the left colon, contributing to the marginal artery of Drummond. The descending branch of the left colic artery supplies the fixed segment of the sigmoid. The sigmoid arteries, which are second branches of the inferior mesenteric, supply the lower portion of the descending colon, the sigmoid colon, and a small segment of the upper rectum.

Advantages and disadvantages

The ileocecal segment and cecum have been used extensively in reconstructive urology. One major advantage of these segments is utilization of the portion of bowel that has the largest diameter, which results in a capacious and compliant reservoir that often fits the bladder base neatly. It has a well-defined blood supply that is reliable. The modified ileocecal valve can also be used as an antireflux or continence mechanism.

The major disadvantage in using the ileocecal segment is related to the loss of the ileocecal valve in the intestine. Patients with neurologic disorders or short gut may have an increased incidence of diarrhea and difficulty with fecal continence following removal of this segment from the intestinal tract. In addition, it is not available in the cloacal exstrophy population who have little or no hindgut. The ileocecal segment also reabsorbs urinary wastes, which may result in hyperchloremic acidosis. Finally, cecum usually produces more mucus than the ileum, which can lead to increased infections and stone formation.

The major advantage in using sigmoid colon is the redundancy that is present, especially in the spina bifida population. The mobile portion of the sigmoid is so redundant in such children that it often lies in the right lower quadrant. It can be easily opened and reconfigured into a U-shape to increase compliance. The thicker muscle can be used to create an antireflux ureteral anastomosis as well as for placement of a tunneled continent catheterizable stoma such as the appendix.

The major disadvantage in using the sigmoid colon is the reduced ability to create a large-capacity, compliant reservoir. The diameter of the sigmoid may be only as large as the ileum. In this circumstance, a segment of colon at least 20–28 cm is required to create an adequately sized reservoir. This amount of sigmoid colon can occasionally be difficult to obtain in the non-spina bifida population. Mucus production from the sigmoid is increased compared with small bowel. This may increase the potential for the development of UTI and bladder stones. In the Indiana series the highest spontaneous perforation rate occurred among those with sigmoid cystoplasties.[21] However, this has not been observed in other large series. Finally, hyperchloremic acidosis is more common when the sigmoid colon is used, compared with other bowel segments. Frequently, patients will need lifelong alkalizing agents, but this is also true after cecocystoplasty or ileocystoplasty.[22]

Surgical technique

The goals of bladder augmentation are to provide a large-capacity, low-pressure urinary reservoir. Hinman[23] and Koff,[24] in particular, have documented the importance of detubularization and reconfiguration of the small and large bowel to facilitate maximum gains in capacity and compliance. Detubularization of bowel segments prevents synchronous contractions of the circular muscle of the gut. Since the radius of the reservoir is directly related to the volume, a greater radius in the augmented bladder translates into a larger low-pressure reservoir. The diameter of the reconfigured bowel segment increases with the number of folds that are incorporated during the reconfiguration (Figure 56.4).

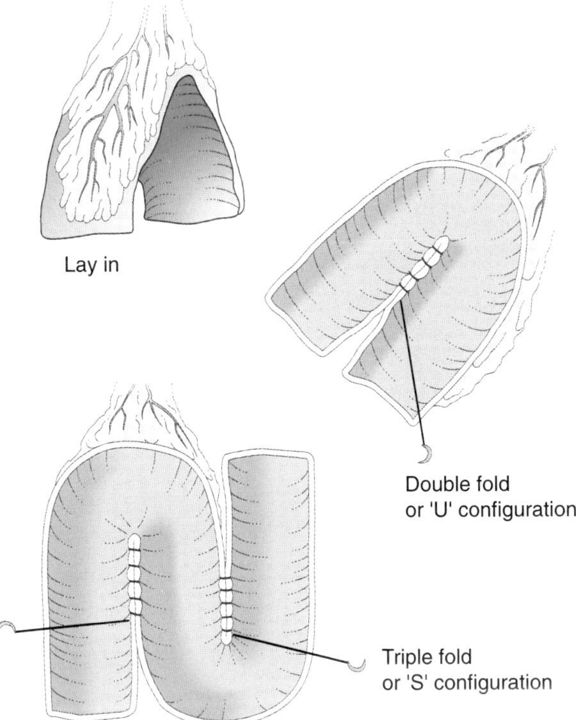

Figure 56.4 The detubularized ileum can be reconfigured in numerous ways. Each additional fold increases the potential radius of the augmented bladder. (Adapted from Rink and Adams,[25] with permission of WB Saunders.)

Regardless of the bowel segment used for augmentation, detubularization and reconfiguration should always be employed.

Ileocystoplasty

Enterocystoplasty is very reliable in lowering storage pressures and expanding the capacity of the non-compliant bladder. Ureteral reimplantations and procedures to increase outlet resistance can safely be undertaken at the same time. However, not every augmentation is completely successful. This may be related to the bladder having a great tendency to reform itself, turning the augmentation into a diverticulum with a relatively small opening. To prevent this, the bladder should be bivalved ('clamshelled') from the bladder neck ventrally to the trigone posteriorly. Alternatively, when the bladder is small and thick walled, the 'star' modification can be performed[26] (Figure 56.5). The star procedure involves opening the bladder in the sagittal plane. A second incision is then made in the coronal plane. If ureteral reimplantation or bladder neck reconstruction is being performed, the second incision is not made until after these procedures are completed. The authors will also occasionally employ an upside-down U-shaped or a Boari flap modification for the initial bladder opening when a catheterizable stoma is being positioned at the umbilicus. In severely diseased bladders from tuberculosis, schistosomiasis, interstitial cystitis, and rarely bladder exstrophy, supratrigonal bladder excision is

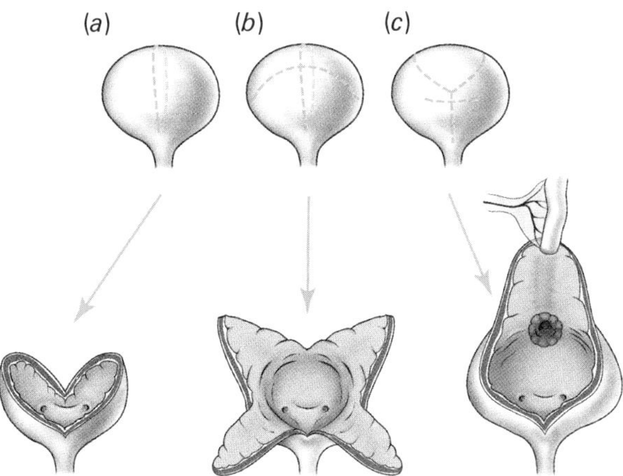

Figure 56.5 The native bladder can be opened in several ways: (*a*) bivalved in a 'clam'-like fashion with full extension of the incision into the bladder neck to prevent an hourglass deformation of the augmented bladder; (*b*) the 'star' modification; (*c*) a 'U' incision to create a flap of bladder that can be used for tunneling when creating a continent catheterizable stoma to the umbilicus.

sometimes necessary, as in neuropathic bladders when the walls are very thick. Whatever type of bladder opening is used, the goal is the same: to provide a wide bladder plate to which the bowel segment can be sewn, thus preventing a narrow anastomosis or hourglass deformity that might result in the augmentation becoming a diverticulum.

When using ileum for enterocystoplasty, the segment chosen should be at least 15 cm proximal to the ileocecal valve to prevent vitamin B_{12} malabsorption, diarrhea due to malabsorption of bile salts, and potential injury to the blood supply to the cecum. Guidelines on the length of ileum required to obtain the appropriate size and shape of the augmentation vary.[24,27] Most commonly, an ileal segment between 20 and 35 cm in length is used. However, a slightly longer segment may be required in an older child or an individual with a severely diseased and contracted bladder.

Prior to harvesting the ileal segment, it is important to ensure the mesentery reaches well down into the pelvis. Extensive mobilization of the mesentery is sometimes required if it is foreshortened. This is most common in the spina bifida population, often secondary to spinal abnormalities and the intraperitoneal adhesions that occur from the ventriculoperitoneal shunt. Once the appropriate bowel segment has been selected, the bowel is divided between straight clamps. The authors prefer to perform a single-layer hand-sewn ileoileostomy. A two-layer hand-sewn or a stapled anastomosis can also be used. Closure of the mesenteric window with interrupted permanent

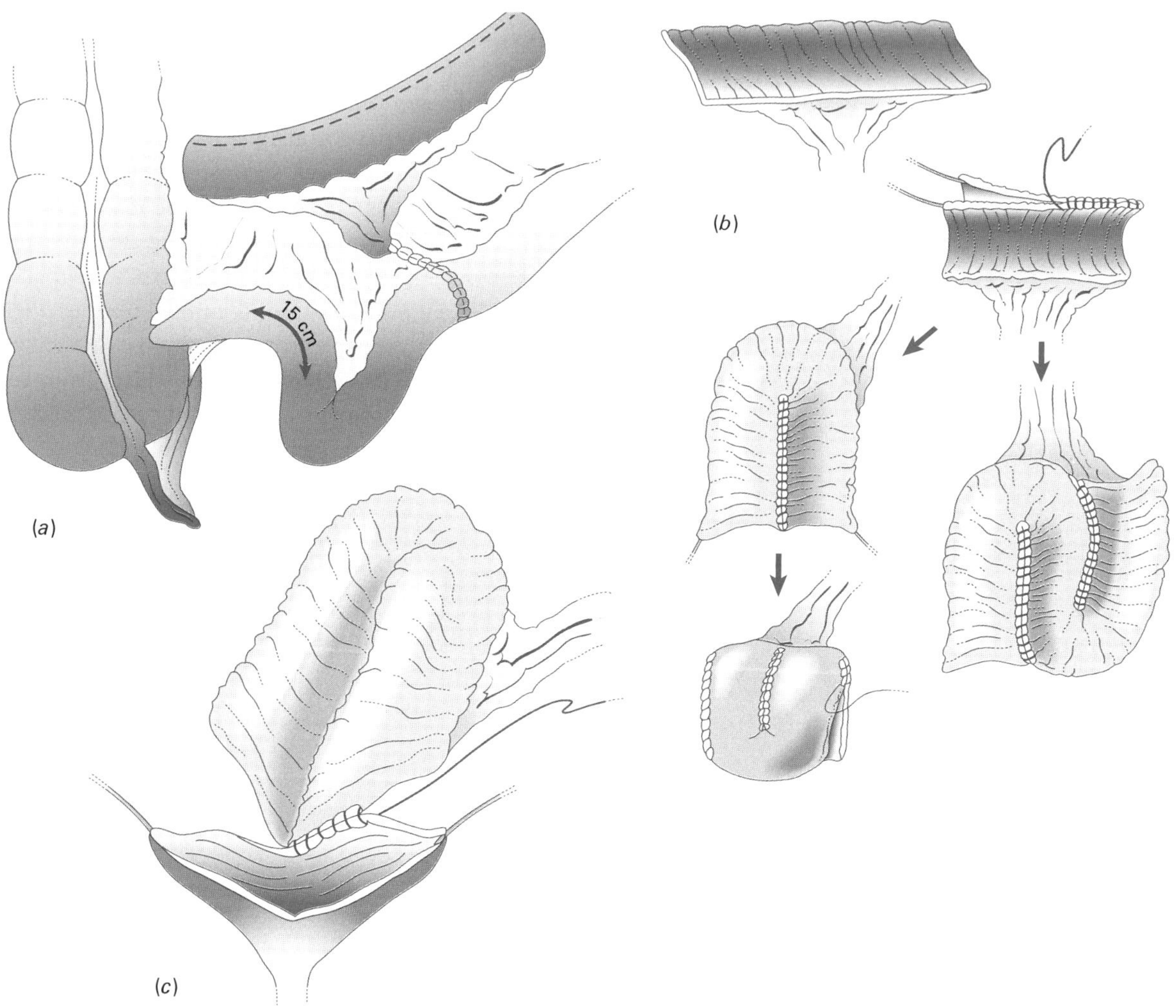

Figure 56.6 Ileocystoplasty. (*a*) A dependent portion of the ileum that is 20–30 cm long and a minimum of 15 cm proximal to the ileocecal valve is isolated and detubularized. Bowel continuity is reestablished with an end-to-end ileoileostomy. (*b*) Depending on the size of the ileal segment, it can be reconfigured and folded in several ways, including the U, S, and W (not illustrated) configurations. In addition, the edges of the reconfigured bowel can be sewn together to create a cup patch. (*c*) The anastomosis of the reconfigured bowel to the native bladder begins in the posterior apex of the opened bladder. (Adapted from Rink and Adams,[25] with permission of WB Saunders.)

sutures then completes the anastomosis. The isolated ileal segment is detubularized along its antimesenteric border after thorough intraluminal irrigation with normal saline. The ileal segment is then reconfigured into a U, S, or W (Figure 56.6).

After opening the native bladder as described above, the reconfigured bowel segment is anastomosed to the bladder with a full-thickness absorbable suture beginning at the posterior apex of the opened native bladder. Once the posterior aspect of the running, locking anastomosis has been completed, a second running, locking suture beginning at the bladder neck apex is begun and carried along the lateral aspect to meet the previous suture. Before final closure of the anastomosis, a suprapubic tube is brought out through the native bladder wall. After completion of the augmentation, the bladder is inflated and a watertight anastomosis confirmed by irrigation. A Penrose or closed suction drain is usually left in place along the posterior and anterior aspects of the bladder. The bowel is then examined to confirm its integrity and the abdomen is closed in an anatomic fashion using heavy, running, absorbable sutures.

Ileocecocystoplasty and cecocystoplasty

The ileocecal segment and cecum have frequently been used for augmentation cystoplasty. The cecum alone is rarely used. Simple detubularization and reconfiguration can be performed. The terminal ileum can be detubularized and incorporated into the cecal segment to increase total volume (Figure 56.7). Continuity of the bowel is re-established with an end-to-side ileocolostomy. The reconfigured ileocecal segment is then anastomosed to the bivalved bladder with a single or double layer of running, locking, absorbable suture. Alternatively, the terminal ileum can be used for ureteral replacement when the ureters are short or the ileum can be tapered and used as a continent catheterizable stoma.

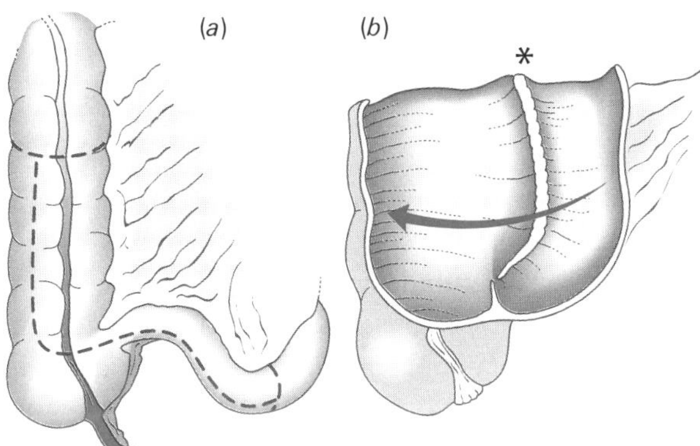

Figure 56.7 Ileocecocystoplasty: the ileum and cecum are isolated as a single unit (*a*) and reconfigured to form a 'cup' for augmentation (*b*). * = suture line between ileum and cecum. (Adapted from Rink and Adams,[25] with permission of WB Saunders.)

Sigmoid cystoplasty

The sigmoid colon easily reaches the bladder and can be used for augmentation cystoplasty. It is especially valuable when reimplantation of ureters or a catheterizable stoma is not possible in the native bladder because the sigmoid musculature can easily be separated from the muscosa, facilitating tunneling. Twenty cm of sigmoid is usually sufficient to achieve an adequate capacity after the segment is reconfigured. It is important to detubularize the sigmoid in order to prevent high-pressure coordinated contractions. Several techniques of sigmoid reconfiguration have been described (Figure 56.8). The authors prefer the U or S configuration because of simplicity and the possibility of significant contractile activity that may result from the method described by Mitchell[28] (see Figure 56.8c). When the sigmoid segment has been isolated, colon continuity is re-established with a single-layer, hand-sewn, end-to-end colocolostomy. The reconfigured sigmoid segment is then anastomosed to the native bladder in a similar fashion as described for ileum.

Postoperative care

Following enterocystoplasty, parenteral antibiotics are continued for 48 hours unless the intraoperative urine culture is positive. Then, a full 7 days of culture-sensitive coverage is used. A nasogastric tube is left in place until bowel function returns. Urinary drainage is maintained through the suprapubic tube and a secondary catheter through either the native urethra or the appendicovesicostomy (when performed). Diligent observation is needed during the immediate postoperative period to ensure that obstruction of the catheters does not occur secondary to blood clots or mucus. Daily bladder irrigations are important to decrease mucus build-up in the bladder, which can lead to infection, stone formation, and inefficient emptying. Bladder irrigations can begin immediately after surgery with 30 ml three times a day. This is increased to 60 ml twice a day after discharge. Both the suprapubic tube and secondary catheter are left to gravity drainage for 2–3 weeks. The suprapubic tube is then plugged and the patient begins intermittent catheterization. Before this, a cystogram can be performed to

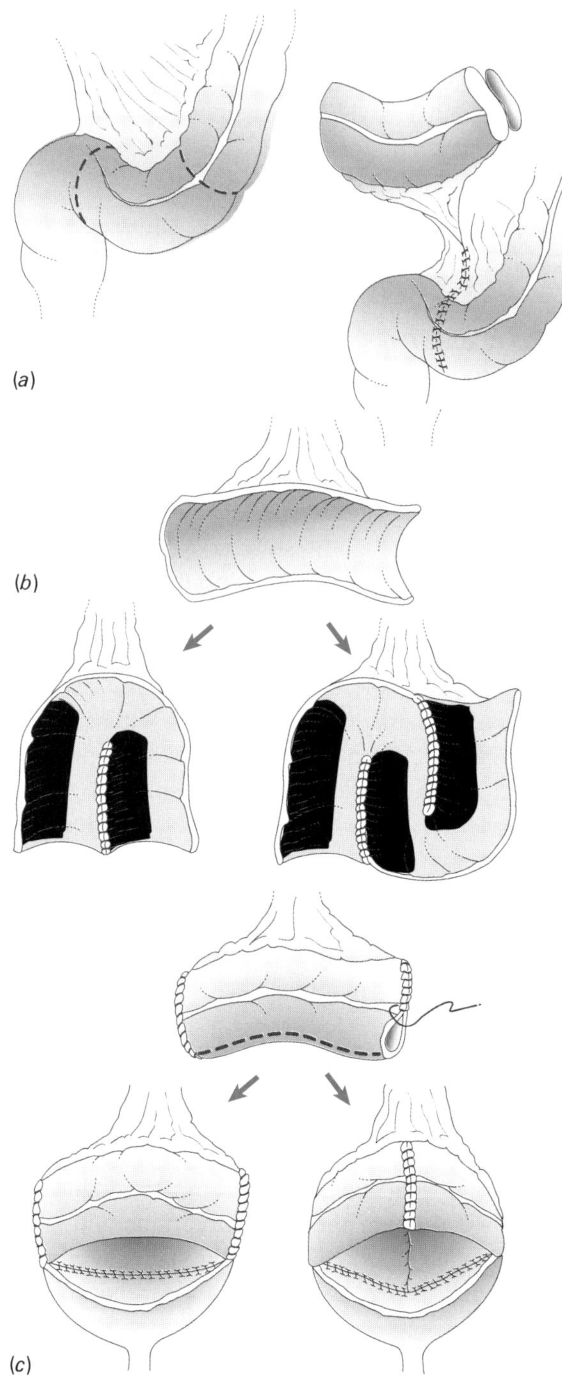

Figure 56.8 Sigmoid cystoplasty. (*a*) A portion of sigmoid colon is isolated. (*b*) The sigmoid can then be reconfigured in a similar fashion as is performed for ileocystoplasty with detubularization and folding back on itself. (*c*) Alternatively, the colonic segment can be closed at both ends, opened along the antimesenteric border, and then anastomosed to the bladder. This latter method is less optimal, owing to the persistence of high intraluminal pressures following augmentation. (Adapted from Rink and Adams,[25] with permission of WB Saunders.)

ensure adequate healing and the absence of extravasation; however, it is not absolutely necessary. Adequate emptying of the bladder with catheterization can be confirmed by checking residual urine via the indwelling suprapubic tube. Once the patient demonstrates proficiency at performing intermittent catheterization, the suprapubic tube is removed. Daily irrigations to clear the bladder of mucus are then recommended. Patients are told to catheterize every 2–3 hours during the daytime and once at night for the next few weeks. The time interval between catheterizations is gradually lengthened, depending on the compliance of the augmented bladder and the gradually increasing storage volumes. In general, adequate stretching of the augmented bladder occurs within 6 months so that most patients need only catheterize approximately four to six times during the day to stay dry and maintain safe filling pressures. If a patient is going to attempt spontaneous voiding, one should wait until at least 3 months after surgery and then follow postvoid residuals to ensure adequate emptying. Radiographic imaging of the augmented bladder and the upper urinary tract is performed approximately 3 months postoperatively.

Results of ileocystoplasty and colocystoplasty

Bladder capacity and compliance

The most common preoperative urodynamic finding in the pediatric patient with a neuropathic bladder in need of bladder augmentation is a small-capacity, poorly compliant bladder with or without evidence of hyperreflexia and bladder instability. Both small and large bowel segments, when detubularized and reconfigured, have been found to provide adequately compliant tissue for enterocystoplasty that ameliorates or eliminates these adverse characteristics.[29] Flood et al[30] reported on 22 augmentation cystoplasties performed over a period of 8 years. Mean age at surgery was 37 years, with a range of 2–82 years. The major indication for augmentation cystoplasty was reduced bladder compliance. A detubularized ileal augmentation was performed in 67% of the patients, 30% had a detubularized ileocecocystoplasty, and the remainder had detubularized sigmoid augmentation. Mean follow-up was 37 months. Bladder capacities increased from a preoperative mean of 108 ml to 438 ml postoperatively. Excellent or improved results by all parameters were achieved in 95% of these patients.[30] Kilic et al[31] reported on 30 children who underwent intestinocystoplasty. Sigmoid was used in 11 cases, ileum in six, and ileocecum in two. Postoperative evaluations revealed a mean postoperative capacity of 237 ml in the colonic group, 240 ml in the ileal group, and 250 ml in the ileocecal group. Mean compliance was 20.6 ml/cmH_2O in the colonic group, 21.6 ml/cmH_2O in the ileal group, and 25.5 ml/cmH_2O in the ileocecal group. They concluded that ileal, ileocecal, and colonic augmentations all provided high-volume reservoirs of similar compliance. More recently, Quek and Ginsberg reported long-term results on 26 patients with neurogenic voiding dysfunction who underwent enterocystoplasty. Mean follow-up in these patients was 8.0 years. Ninety-six percent of the patients had near or complete resolution of urinary incontinence. Mean total bladder capacity increased from 201 ml to 615 ml. They concluded that bladder augmentation provides durable clinical and urodynamic improvement for patients with neurogenic bladder dysfunction.[32]

It is apparent that all segments of intestine, when appropriately reconfigured, can adequately increase the capacity of the native bladder. However, enterocystoplasty does not guarantee that the bladder will be free of hyperreflexia. Robertson et al[33] reported the persistence of hyperreflexia in 23% of patients after enterocystoplasty and documented regular phasic contractions in 77% of the augmented bladders despite bowel detubularization. It should be mentioned that in a majority of the patients in this series an ileocecal segment was used. Recently, Pope et al[34] reported on 19 of 323 patients who had undergone primary enterocystoplasty but required a secondary augmentation owing to the persistence of high pressures. Twelve of the 19 patients had had colocystoplasties (14% of the total colocystoplasties), four had gastrocystoplasties (10% of the total gastrocystoplasties), and two had undergone ileocystoplasty. Cecum was used in one (1%). It is apparent in this large series that colocystoplasties are more likely to allow high storage pressures to persist. However, it must be noted that not all of the colocystoplasties were completely detubularized but instead reconfigured after the ends were closed with the colon opened along the antimesenteric border. Given this, it is difficult in this series to compare colon to ileum that was reconfigured into an S or W shape. Nevertheless, these studies emphasize the importance of careful functional and urodynamic follow-up in patients after enterocystoplasty, since some will require anticholinergics or secondary augmentation due to failure of the original procedure to improve bladder capacity and compliance adequately.

In summary, it appears that both small and large bowel, when detubularized, can be used for cystoplasty to provide a compliant and large-capacity reservoir. However, the large bowel may retain increased contractile activity despite detubularization.[21,29] It appears that detubularized ileum has less energetic phasic contractions than colon and therefore has potentially less risk for persistent high storage pressures.[34] Given these advantages of ileum over colon, it is the authors' preference to use ileum whenever possible when performing simple enterocystoplasty.

Metabolic issues

Electrolytes

The major function of intact small and large bowel is to absorb food, fluid, and electrolytes. When urine is stored in the bowel for prolonged periods, there is increased absorption of urinary solutes, which increases the risk of metabolic derangement. Koch and McDougal[35] hypothesized that ammonium reabsorption plays a key role in the development of hyperchloremic metabolic acidosis in patients following intestinocystoplasty. In support of this hypothesis, Stampfer and McDougal[19] demonstrated in a rat model that ammonium inhibits the sodium/hydrogen exchanger, resulting in ionized ammonium transport where it substitutes for sodium in the exchanger. This then leads to the increased absorption of chloride to maintain electrolyte neutrality, resulting in the development of hyperchloremic metabolic acidosis. In patients with normal renal function, serum electrolytes are usually unaffected by enterocystoplasty.[36–38] However, in patients with impaired renal function, metabolic acidosis can be profound. Careful preoperative evaluation and judicious use of bowel is recommended in patients with chronic renal insufficiency.[39] A gastric segment or cutaneous diversion may be safer. Owing to the electrolyte problems that can often develop in patients with significant renal insufficiency, the authors recommend gastrocystoplasty rather than conventional enterocystoplasty in this patient population.

Bone growth

Impaired bone growth and demineralization are major concerns related to prolonged acidosis. Demineralization occurs secondary to the increased excretion of titratable acid (bony buffers). These concerns have received a large amount of attention in the last decade. Hochstetler et al[40] demonstrated in a rat model that animals with ileocystoplasty, when given an acid challenge, developed bone demineralization and decreased bone growth that can be corrected with bicarbonate therapy. Current basic science literature demonstrated that enterocystoplasty in rats neither impairs skeletal growth nor bone quantity, but leads to significant loss of bone mass when combined with resection of the ileocaecal segment.[41] This same group has also reported histomorphometrically that bone loss occurs after enterocystoplasty in the rat model.[42]

The more recent clinical literature has not clarified the true incidence or effect on bone growth. Mundy and Nurse[43] reported an average of 20% reduction in growth potential in three of six children who had colocystoplasties. However, no decrease in growth potential was noted in 10 children who had ileocystoplasties. They concluded that bone growth impairment after colocystoplasty was more likely than after ileocystoplasty. Two other reports demonstrated no impairment of bone growth or demineralization in children and adults after urinary reconstruction with various bowel segments.[38,44] However, two series have demonstrated variable degrees of reduction in bone mineral density in children with enterocystoplasties.[45,46] Finally, four other series have not demonstrated any effects on bone growth.[47–50] Interestingly, two of these reports are in bladder exstrophy patients; both of them report growth retardation in this population with or without augmentation.[47,48] In a large study that compared linear growth in bladder exstrophy patients with and without augmentation, using pre- and postaugmentation growth velocities, a statistically significant decrease in linear growth after intestinal bladder augmentation was demonstrated.[51] Further longitudinal studies will be required to clarify this issue. Therefore, until such studies are available, close observation for the development of acidosis and the treatment of any electrolyte abnormalities following intestinocystoplasty with bicarbonate therapy is recommended.

Bowel dysfunction

Bowel dysfunction is known to occur occasionally after enterocystoplasty. Diarrhea can develop after resection of large segments of ileum, removal of the ileocecal valve, and extensive colonic resections. The incidence of bowel dysfunction following enterocystoplasty in all patients, including adults, has been reported to be between 10 and 54%.[14,52,53] In the spina bifida population, the incidence is approximately 20%. Since the overall incidence of bowel problems in children with spina bifida is further increased when the ileocecal valve is removed, one should try to avoid the use of ileocecal segments for augmentation in this patient population. Osmotic diarrhea has been theorized to occur after removal of the ileocecal valve, which results in a decreased transit time within the intestine.[54] It should be noted that these original data were not supported in a recent report by Husmann and Cain[16] in which only 3% of their 63 ileal cecal cystoplasty patients had worsening of their bowel function. Despite this encouraging recent report, the authors feel that careful preoperative screening of patients with spina bifida with regard to their bowel habits is extremely important.

The diarrhea that develops postoperatively can be osmotic or secretory in nature. Secretory diarrhea is thought to occur because of decreased resorption of bile salts and subsequent fat malabsorption, resulting in steatorrhea. Barrington et al[55] reported on 14 patients who developed bowel difficulties after enterocystoplasty. They showed a direct correlation in many of these patients between their diarrhea and interruption of the enterohepatic circulation of bile acids. They also found that these patients can be identified by using bowel frequency charts and can be treated with anion-exchange resins.

Vitamin B_{12} deficiency

Concerns regarding the development of vitamin B_{12} deficiency following small bowel resection or the use of small bowel for urinary reconstruction are well documented. The distal ileum is the major site of vitamin B_{12} absorption. It has previously been reported that up to 35% of patients will develop vitamin B_{12} deficiency following the construction of a Kock pouch, which uses about 80 cm of small bowel.[56] Despite theoretical and legitimate concerns about the development of vitamin B_{12} deficiency in children following ileocystoplasty, it has yet to be reported in the literature. Stein et al[44] reported on 51 children who had undergone such reconstructions, but no significant drop in vitamin B_{12} levels was noted following surgery. From the available published data, it appears that the use of shorter segments of ileum, about 35 cm, as used for the Camey type 1 enterocystoplasty and conventional ileocystoplasty in children, does not place the patient at significant risk for vitamin B_{12} deficiency, even in the long term.[37]

Despite the lack of evidence of any vitamin B_{12} deficiencies developing in children undergoing enterocystoplasty, the authors recommend harvesting small bowel segments that are at least 15 cm away from the ileocecal valve. The vitamin B_{12} receptor sites are clustered in the most terminal portion of the ileum. If large amounts of small bowel are required for reconstruction of the bladder, periodic vitamin B_{12} levels should be obtained postoperatively. Alternatively, a vitamin B_{12} injection can be given prophylactically 3 years after enterocystoplasty. There is no evidence that the use of sigmoid colon for augmentation places patients at risk for vitamin B_{12} deficiency.

Mucus production and stone formation

Mucus production and bladder stone formation are both complications related to the use of the gastrointestinal tract for urinary reconstruction. All segments of bowel produce mucus. However, mucus production from the ileum is less than from the colon.[25] This has been confirmed clinically by several authors.[21,57] Mucus in the urinary tract is associated with an increased risk of infection.[58] Mucus production also increases during an acute infection, resulting in poor bladder emptying, especially when small catheters are used to drain the bladder.[27] Clinically, mucus production appears to decrease over time following ileocystoplasty. This is probably because of villus atrophy that occurs in the ileum. Colonic epithelium does not appear to undergo this type of change. Significant mucus production in colonic augmentations continues throughout the life of the patient.

The risk of stone formation after enterocystoplasty ranges between 7 and 52%.[59–64] The usual stone composition reported is magnesium ammonium phosphate (struvite), although several other stone compositions have been reported. Since the majority of stones are struvite in origin, it appears that chronic bacteriuria with urease-producing organisms may have a contributory role. However, it is also clear that the presence of mucus has an important role in the development of bladder stones following intestinocystoplasty. Mucus may serve as a biofilm that can harbor bacteria and promote further growth in a protected environment. Khoury et al[65] have also demonstrated that the mucus from stone formers has increased levels of calcium, phosphate, and magnesium, and an increase in the calcium to phosphate ratio, compared with non-stone formers. This increased calcium to phosphate ratio may be clinically important in predicting which patients are at risk for stone formation. Given these findings, it appears that mucus has strong lithogenic properties and is a nidus for stone formation. Daily irrigation of the augmented bladder to prevent excess mucus build-up can be an effective measure to reduce the risk of stone formation in the augmented bladder. Hensle et al[66] recently reported that an irrigation protocol consisting of saline twice a week (240 ml) and gentamicin sulfate solution once a week (240–480 mg of gentamicin/L of saline, at 120–240 ml per irrigation, depending on patient age and reservoir size) significantly reduced the number of reservoir calculi from 43% to 7%. However, Brough et al[61] did not observe a decreased incidence of stone formation when they instituted a regular bladder washout program in children following intestinocystoplasty.

Palmer et al[60] identified an additional risk factor for the development of bladder stones in the augmented bladder. They noted the presence of hypocitraturia in some of their stone-forming patients. Treatment with oral potassium citrate returned urinary citrate levels to within normal values and no recurrent calculi were then seen. Woodhouse and Robertson[67] have also reported that a metabolic screen in their augmented patients demonstrated that 80% of patients have risk factors for at least three different types of stones. All of the patients were found to have an increase in urinary pH and hypocitraturia.

Bladder calculi in the augmented bladder are amenable to both open surgery and endoscopic management.[59,60,63,68,69] Neither procedure appears to have a clear advantage at this time. An open procedure is usually simpler when the stones are large, although new energy sources for the endoscopic treatment of stones, such as the holmium laser, may enhance the ability to manage bladder stones non-invasively. Miller and Park[70] have also described a method of using a laparoscopic entrapment sac percutaneously to control the loss of multiple fragments. This method has been used by the authors and has been highly successful. Treatment of bladder calculi needs to be individualized. Factors that should influence the surgical approach include number and size of calculi, previous bladder outlet procedure, availability of endoscopic equipment, availability of energy sources, and the surgeon's experience with endoscopic techniques.

Infections

Bacteriuria following enterocystoplasty is the rule, since these patients are being intermittently catheterized. If the bladder is not emptied completely, symptomatic UTI may result. It is not known whether one type of bowel segment is at greater risk for the development of UTIs than another. Hirst[71] reported the presence of bacteriuria in 50% of sigmoid augmentations, whereas only 25% of ileocystoplasties had bacteriuria at any one time. In a series of 231 augmentation patients, Rink et al[21] reported a symptomatic UTI rate of 22.7% following ileocystoplasty, 17.3% following sigmoid cystoplasty, 12% following cecocystoplasty, and 8% following gastrocystoplasty. They reported an overall 14% incidence of febrile UTIs with no statistical difference in the incidence between the various bowel segments. It appears that all augmented bladders are at risk for infection.

Tumors

Many fear that there may be an increased risk of malignancy in bladders after enterocystoplasty, as is the case after conventional ureterosigmoidostomy. Adenocarcinoma is the predominant tumor that develops after ureterosigmoidostomy, found most frequently at the site of the ureteral orifice. The latency period for tumor formation in the ureterosigmoidostomy patients ranges between 3 and 53 years, with a mean of 26 years. It is estimated that there is a 7000-fold increased risk of developing adenocarcinoma following ureterosigmoidostomy. It is with great trepidation that we enter the new millennium with hundreds of children having received enterocystoplasties without knowing whether there is an increased risk for the development of cancer. Filmer and Spencer[72] reported on 14 patients with tumor formation in the augmented bladder: nine of these patients had ileocystoplasty and colon was used in five. The exact etiology and pathogenesis of these tumors are unknown but they seem analogous to cancers occurring after uterosigmoidostomy. Nurse and Mundy[73] studied 34 patients who had undergone augmentation cystoplasty or colonic substitution cystoplasty. A high incidence of histologic abnormalities in the intestinal segment was reported to occur along the anastomotic suture line and in the remaining bladder. Such abnormalities were directly correlated with heavy mixed bacterial growth in the urine and high levels of urinary *N*-nitrosamines. Woodhams et al[74] have reported that there are no diurnal or long-term variations in urinary *N*-nitrosamine levels. They also found that levels were consistently higher in patients with inflamed or infected cystoplasties, those using intermittent self-catheterization, and those not taking antibiotic prophylaxis. Shokeir et al[75] and Ali-El-Dein et al[76] demonstrated that all bowel segments exposed to urine, regardless of their position (bladder or ureteral substitution), are at risk for malignant changes, and that urine cytologies may be a useful diagnostic tool in this setting. Barrington et al[77] reported on four patients who developed tumors in augmented bladders. All of the tumors were adenocarcinomas and were located on the bladder side of the anastomosis. It was concluded that these tumors were derived from the native urothelium. It was also demonstrated that transitional epithelium could undergo intestinal mucosal-like changes throughout the exposed native urothelium, including the renal pelvis, which was observed in one patient who had vesicoureteral reflux (VUR). Soergel et al[78] reported from the Indiana Augmentation database of 483 cases, three new cases of transitional cell carcinoma (TCC). Mean time from augmentation to TCC was 19 years. None of these patients had any additional risk factors. Thus, it is felt that development of bladder cancer is a real issue and that all patients should undergo endoscopic surveillance beginning 10 years after initial surgery.

Barrington et al[79] showed that there are elevated levels of transforming growth factor-β (TGF-β) in the enterocystoplasty population. It is believed that TGF-β increases cellular proliferation and/or phagocytic activity, producing nitrosamines and oxygen free radicals. It has been demonstrated that urinary TGF-β levels can be decreased with the administration of pentosan polysulfate sodium.[80] Therefore, if further research demonstrates elevated TGF-β as a risk factor, potential treatment options would be available. Barrington et al[81] have also demonstrated a decreased serum level of selenium, a free oxygen radical scavenger, in the neuropathic bladder population. These may be possible reasons for augmented bladders being at increased risk for tumor formation.

The issue of potential malignancy in augmented bladders cannot be overlooked or ignored. This is a potentially disastrous complication for children in whom one hopes to provide a surgically reconstructed bladder that will last for life. Future research is needed to determine the true risk of tumor formation, which children are at greatest risk, and whether premalignant changes can be detected endoscopically or with urine markers or cytology. Although the incidence of tumor formation following enterocystoplasty is unknown, lifelong follow-up and yearly cystoscopic evaluation and urine cytologies from the augmented bladder should be considered beginning no later than 6–10 years after the augmentation.[82] All malignant tumors reported have occurred after this time lapse.[72]

Perforation

Many complications can occur following enterocystoplasty. However, no complication is more potentially devastating or life threatening than unsuspected spontaneous bladder perforation. Although the exact incidence of perforation is not known, nearly every large series of enterocystoplasties includes at least one patient.[25,83–89] Amongst these reports, seven deaths have been directly attributed to such perforation.[90] Most of these deaths were due, at least in part, to delay in diagnosis. Therefore, a high index of suspicion is needed in any patient with a history of enterocystoplasty who presents with abdominal and/or shoulder pain.

It is not known whether one type of bowel is particularly prone to perforation after cystoplasty. Rink[28] reported a higher incidence of spontaneous perforations in sigmoid cystoplasties. They initially felt that the sigmoid colon was inherently at greater risk for perforation, but they now feel that this higher incidence may be more directly related to their initial technique of sigmoid detubularization. Others have reported that the highest incidence of perforation occurred when ileum was used.[89] DeFoor et al believe that gastrocystoplasty may be at a lower risk for perforation.[91] However, it appears that no segment of bowel, tubularized or detubularized, is immune from this complication.

The etiology of bladder perforation is unknown. Initially, perforations were thought either to be linked to traumatic catheterization or as a consequence of failure to catheterize on a timely basis.[83,87] However, perforation has been reported in patients who do not perform intermittent catheterization.[85] Another contributing factor in bladder perforation may be vascular compromise in the bowel wall. Crane et al[92] reported that specimens from perforated bladders demonstrated histologic evidence of bowel wall ischemia. Also supporting the theory of bowel wall ischemia is an arterial perfusion study in a canine augmentation model, where a decrease in blood flow to the bowel wall was seen when the reservoir was overdistended and intravesical pressures were increased.[93] The perfusion change was most striking at the antimesenteric border in the detubularized bowel. In addition to overdistention, high pressures due to bladder hyperreflexia may lead to an increased risk of perforation. Bauer et al[89] noted the presence of postoperative hyperreflexia in 40% of their patients who suffered a spontaneous perforation.

Some authors have suggested that a low urethral resistance is protective against both the high pressures associated with bladder hyperreflexia and failure to empty the reservoir on a timely basis.[88] However, Jayanthi et al[94] reported on 28 patients who underwent complete bladder neck ligation in conjunction with enterocystoplasty with a catheterizable stoma. In this series the one bladder perforation that occurred was associated with blunt trauma and was not spontaneous in origin. Therefore, achieving total urinary continence surgically without a pop-off valve mechanism does not in itself increase the risk for spontaneous rupture.

There does not appear to be one single etiology or risk factor that makes some individuals more prone to bladder perforation than others. Multiple factors are probably involved. Repetitive overdistention secondary to poor compliance, bladder hyperreflexia, and chronic infection all appear to place the augmented bladder at increased risk for spontaneous perforation.

The diagnosis of bladder perforation can be difficult at times, and a high index of suspicion is required to make the diagnosis quickly. Most pediatric patients who undergo enterocystoplasty are neurologically impaired. Lower abdominal sensation is diminished. Therefore, the clinical presentation may be non-specific. Nausea, vomiting, fever, oliguria, and possibly referred pain to the shoulder secondary to diaphragmatic irritation may be presenting complaints.[95]

On physical examination the abdomen is distended, with pain and irritation above the level of anesthesia. It may be difficult to distinguish pyelonephritis from a spontaneous bladder perforation. Thus, a standard or computed tomographic (CT) cystogram is recommended in any patient with an augmented bladder who presents with the above symptoms. Although the diagnostic role of a cystogram has been questioned in the past,[86,87] it is the most specific diagnostic radiographic test.[85,89] Braverman and Lebowitz[96] have recommended fluoroscopy during the filling phase to make sure that the bladder is completely distended in order to diagnosis the perforation accurately. Residual contrast in the abdomen after the bladder has been drained establishes the diagnosis. Alternatively, an abdominal CT scan can be diagnostic and is helpful in demonstrating the extent of the extravasation.

When spontaneous perforation of the augmented bladder is suspected clinically and/or confirmed radiographically, immediate treatment is required. Catheter drainage, fluid resuscitation, and broad-spectrum antibiotics should be started immediately. In a stable patient, non-operative management with catheter drainage, antibiotics, and serial physical evaluations may be all that is needed.[97] This non-operative approach should be used only in selected patients in whom a small rupture is suspected. In the majority of patients, immediate exploration and closure of the bladder leak is safer. Intra-abdominal lavage, and irrigation and placement of intra-abdominal drains should then be done. Finally, all patients with an augmented bladder must be educated on the potentially lethal complications associated with delay in diagnosis of a spontaneous perforation. They should be instructed to inform a treating physician that they have an augmented bladder, and are at some risk for bladder perforation.

Surgical alternatives to intestinocystoplasty

As discussed above, bladder augmentation with small and large bowel segments may result in electrolyte abnormalities, UTIs, mucus production, stones, and tumor formation. Most long-term complications are attributable to the presence of intestinal mucosa in a urinary tract reservoir for urine storage. In an effort to avoid the unwanted effects of enterocystoplasty, several other surgical procedures have been developed: these include gastrocystoplasty, ureterocystoplasty, autoaugmentation, and seromuscular enterocystoplasty.

Gastrocystoplasty

Gastric tissue was first reported to be applied to the urinary tract in 1956 when Sinaiko described the use of a stomach segment for urinary diversion.[98] Leong and Ong[99,100] subsequently reported the successful use of stomach for augmentation of the bladder in both dogs and humans. More recently, Mitchell and colleagues have modified Leong's original techniques for gastrocystoplasty and popularized its use in pediatric patients.[101,102] Since then, experience from multiple institutions over the past two decades indicates that the use of stomach is feasible and effective in augmenting the neuropathic bladder. However, widespread use of stomach tissue as an alternative to intestine has been limited by the findings that the hematuria–dysuria syndrome (HDS) can be problematic in many patients (especially those that are sensate) and that, in the long term, gastrocystoplasty does not appear to result in a reservoir that is as capacious and compliant as that which is achieved with conventional intestinocystoplasty. Nevertheless, the use of stomach tissue can be very advantageous and appropriate in some patients. For example, in patients with renal insufficiency and metabolic acidosis, gastrocystoplasty helps to buffer the adverse effects of the acidosis because of its ability to secrete acid into the urine. Thus, in select patients, the use of stomach for augmentation is a viable and appropriate alternative to the use of intestine.

Anatomy and physiology

Anatomically, the stomach can be divided into five parts: the lesser curvature, greater curvature, fundus, body, and antrum. The layers of the gastric wall include the outer serosal coat, a muscular coat, the submucosal layer, and the epithelium. The muscular coat consists of smooth muscle fibers oriented in a longitudinal, circular, and an oblique fashion. The epithelium of the gastric mucosa consists of a single layer of tall columnar epithelial cells and smaller acid-secreting cells. Loose areolar tissue in the submucosa lies between the mucosal and muscular layers. This loosely arranged layer allows technically simple separation of the mucosa from underlying muscle, permitting implantation of ureters in an antireflux fashion and tunneling of continent catheterizable stomas.

The entire arterial supply of the stomach is based on branches of the celiac artery, including the gastric, splenic, and hepatic arteries (Figure 56.9). The right and left gastroepiploic arteries supply the greater curvature and are pertinent for use in gastrocystoplasty. The gastroepiploic arteries arise from the right gastric and splenic arteries, respectively. They usually do not anastomose directly but are connected through small arterial branches.

The main physiologic function of the stomach is to digest food mechanically and chemically. Given this, the muscle of the stomach functionally contracts in a manner that is different from the rest of the intestinal tract in that it acts to churn its contents as opposed to moving the bolus of food along a peristaltic wave. This unique pattern of contractility may be the cause of the phasic contractions that are seen in the augmented bladder following gastrocystoplasty.

The stomach chemically digests food through the secretion of acid. The exact mechanisms responsible for the control of acid secretion from the stomach are still not completely understood. Current evidence suggests that parietal cells, which are mainly located in the body of the stomach, secrete acid in response to

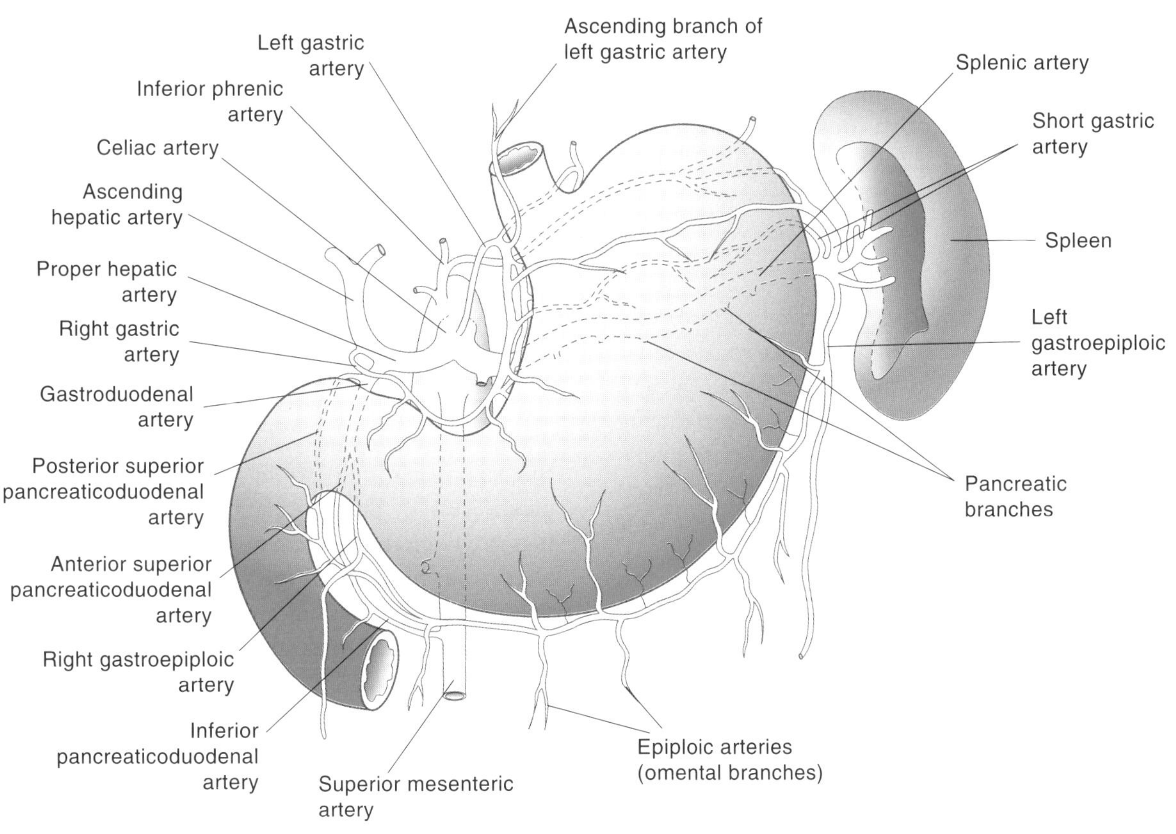

Figure 56.9 Arterial blood supply to the stomach. (Adapted from Lindner,[17] with permission.)

gastrin that is released from G cells located in the antral mucosa. G cells, in turn, are stimulated to release gastrin by direct contact of the mucosa with food, antral distention, and vagal stimulation. Acid secretion can also be stimulated by acetycholine and histamine. The latter is important in that acid secretion from gastric segments following gastrocystoplasty can be inhibited with H_2 receptor blockers.

In addition to the stomach's ability to secrete chloride, other metabolic properties of importance include its barrier function to ammonium and chloride reabsorption. The combination of hydrogen ion and chloride secretion predisposes patients to the development of hypochloremic, hypokalemic, and metabolic alkalosis following gastrocystoplasty. However, this secretion of acid is beneficial in patients who have chronic acidosis associated with renal insufficiency.

Advantages and disadvantages

Surgically, the stomach is relatively thick and easy to work with. Use of stomach for bladder augmentation has clear advantages in patients with renal insufficiency owing to its ability to secrete acid. This allows for buffering of systemic acidosis and reduces the need for bicarbonate supplementation. The resultant acid urine also appears to decrease the incidence of bacteriuria. In comparison to other intestinal segments, there is decreased mucus production and stone formation. The inherent musculature of the gastric segment may offer an additional advantage over small and large bowel by increasing the possibility for spontaneous voiding. This may result in more efficient emptying, less residual urine, and decreased need for intermittent catheterization.[103,104] Lastly, gastrocystoplasty can potentially be accomplished laparoscopically, which offers significant advantages in more rapid patient recovery following surgery.[105]

The main disadvantage of gastrocystoplasty that currently limits its widespread use in children with neuropathic bladders is the high incidence of HDS. This is most troublesome in patients who have a sensate urethra and perineum. Given this, caution should be exercised in selecting patients who are sensate and are at risk for incontinence (i.e. bladder exstrophy) when other enteric segments are available. This also applies when considering gastrocystoplasty in a patient with end-stage renal disease in need of transplantation, since ulcer formation and perforation of defunctionalized bladders have been reported.[106]

Postoperative studies suggest that gastrocystoplasty results in a less compliant and capacious reservoir than that usually achieved with conventional enterocystoplasty. Gastrocystoplasty may therefore be less useful in patients with a very small, non-compliant bladder plate.[31,107]

Surgical technique

The original gastrocystoplasty, as described by Leong and Ong,[99,100] used the antrum of the stomach. Since incorporation of antral tissue may increase cyclical secretion of acid because of antral distention during bladder filling, more recent forms of gastrocystoplasty[102,108] favor utilization of a wedge taken from the greater curvature of the stomach that incorporates more body and less antrum (Figure 56.10). Depending on the individual vascular supply, this wedge of tissue may be based on either the right or left gastroepiploic artery. There is usually a vascular window between these arteries that defines which artery is dominant. Since the right gastroepiploic artery is longer and dominant in the majority of cases, this is more commonly used. A 10–15 cm length of stomach along the greater curvature is chosen, with special care being taken to minimize inclusion of antral tissue. Branches of the gastroepiploic artery that are not directly supplying the wedge to be harvested are ligated. The wedge of stomach is isolated with the use of bowel clamps or an automatic stapler. The authors prefer the latter. The apex of the gastric wedge should be at least 1 cm below the lesser curvature to prevent injury to the vagus nerve and the right gastric vessels. Before isolation of the gastric wedge, it is advisable to ligate branches of the right gastric artery near the apex of the wedge, since failure to do this can result in significant blood loss.[109] A flap of greater omentum must also be mobilized along with the gastric wedge. The stomach is then closed in two layers. Alternatively, Raz et al[110] have described a technique using an automatic stapler to harvest a gastric segment along the greater curvature of the stomach without opening the stomach.

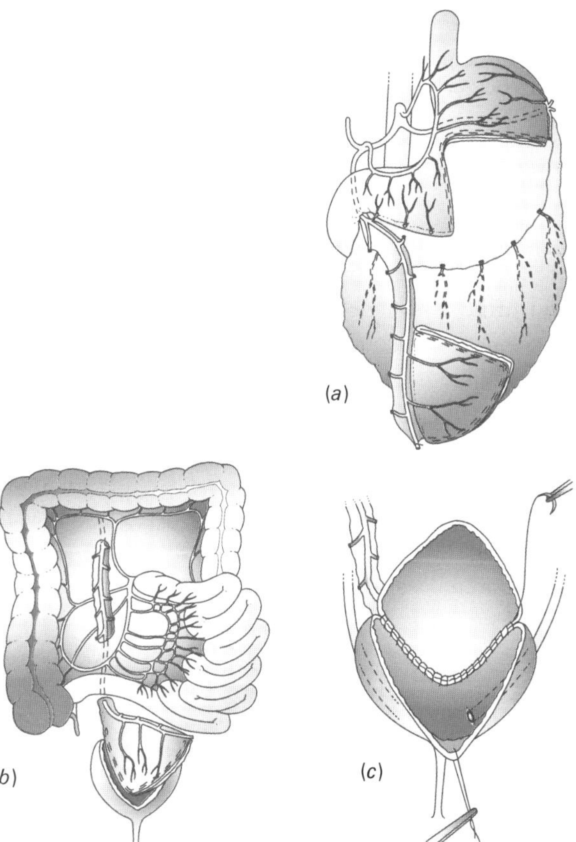

Figure 56.10 Gastrocystoplasty. (*a*) A wedge of stomach is isolated along the greater curvature of the stomach with its blood supply based on either the right or left gastroepiploic artery. (*b*) The flap is brought through the mesenteries of the small and large bowel or retroperitonealized following complete mobilization of the small and large bowel. (*c*) The flap is then anastomosed to the bivalved bladder.

Once the gastric segment is isolated, it is retroperitonealized by bringing it through the mesenteries of the transverse colon and small bowel. Special care should be taken to close these defects in the mesentery to prevent internal intestinal herniation. Alternatively, the right colon and duodenum can be mobilized up to the root of the small bowel mesentery, which allows placement of the gastric segment and its trailing vascular supply entirely in the retroperitoneal space. After the segment has been relocated inferiorly into the pelvis, it is rotated 90° to straighten the mesentery and vessels. The staples are then removed and the posterior tip of the stomach is sutured to the posterior aspect of the bivalved bladder using a running, interlocking 3–0 polyglactin suture.

Postoperatively, the augmented bladder should be adequately drained with a suprapubic tube and urethral catheter. A nasogastric suction tube is maintained for 3–5 days postoperatively. Following removal of the nasogastric tube and resumption of oral intake, the patient should be encouraged to eat small, frequent meals for the first few weeks to months.

Results

The urodynamic results of gastrocystoplasty are somewhat variable. Some authors report that it is useful in increasing capacity and compliance, similar to large and small bowel.[111] In studies that have analyzed both preoperative and postoperative urodynamics, gastrocystoplasty has been shown to increase bladder capacity by approximately 150–200%.[112–114] However, it should be noted that there is a wide range of results reported with regard to increased bladder capacity following gastrocystoplasty.[31,108,111,113–115] In a recent series comparing the urodynamic findings and clinical outcomes following augmentation with stomach versus intestine, it was shown that both stomach and intestine are efficacious in improving compliance, but that the use of ileum and colon results in a higher volume reservoir. Intestinal segments appear to expand more readily following augmentation than does stomach.[31] Some of the differences in the literature regarding improvements in capacity and compliance following gastrocystoplasty may be in part explained by the variable amounts of stomach that have been harvested in individual patients. However, less volume expansion seems inherent to gastric segments when compared with ileum and colon.

A unique postoperative urodynamic finding after gastrocystoplasty is the presence of low-amplitude, rhythmic contractions during bladder filling. These contractions are usually <30 cmH_2O.[102,115] However, contractions >30 cmH_2O have been noted to be present in 10% of patients.[113–115]

Taken together, experience with gastrocystoplasty demonstrates that it is clearly an effective procedure in providing improvements in bladder compliance and capacity. However, in comparison to ileum and colon, stomach often results in a reservoir that is less capacious and perhaps less compliant.

HDS is unique to gastrocystoplasty. It is defined as the presence of pain in the bladder, suprapubic, or genital area, coffee-brown or bright-red hematuria in the absence of infection, skin irritation or excoriation, and painful urination or pain with catheterization. HDS occurs in up to one-third of patients and is the major factor that has limited the more widespread use of gastrocystoplasty in children requiring enterocystoplasty. In the largest series to date with long-term follow-up, Plaire et al[116] reported that 24% of patients following gastrocystoplasty had some element of this syndrome. Other retrospective series have reported the incidence of HDS to be as low as 2% and as high as 50%.[22,111,117] The disparity in these numbers probably relates to the variable makeup of the patient populations in each study. Also, longer-term follow-up may result in an increased incidence of complications.[118] In all studies evaluating HDS following gastrocystoplasty, a uniform finding is that HDS is much more prevalent in patients who have a sensate urethra and perineum, whereas it is less common in patients who are insensate, as in patients with a neuropathic bladder secondary to spina bifida or spinal cord injury. Despite the relatively high incidence of HDS following gastrocystoplasty, most patients respond well to either H_2 receptor blockers or hydrogen ion pump blockers such as omeprazole.[119] In some patients, alkaline irrigation of the bladder can also be used effectively.[120] A small percentage of patients may be refractory to all forms of conservative medical management, necessitating conversion to a different form of augmentation or diversion.[121]

The etiology of HDS is not entirely clear. Bogaert et al[122] demonstrated that the gastric mucosa in the augmented bladder is stimulated in the same way as the native stomach. With this in mind, some authors have proposed that hypergastrinemia may be a causative or major contributing factor in patients with HDS. The association of hypergastrinemia and HDS has been demonstrated in several patients.[114,119,123–125] Despite this association, there has never been a direct correlation between this syndrome and aciduria and/or hypergastrinemia.[111,117]

Another potential complication associated with the use of stomach is peptic ulcer disease of the gastric patch with subsequent perforation.[106] It has been postulated that *Helicobacter pylori* infection may be an important etiologic factor in patients who develop ulcerative changes in the gastric portion of the augmented bladder.[126] Although patients are at significant risk for the development of HDS following gastrocystoplasty and other related complications associated with acid secretion by the stomach segment, it is rarely necessary to remove the gastric patch. Medical management of these problems is usually successful.

The beneficial effects of gastrocystoplasty in patients with reduced renal function and systemic acidosis are well documented.[102,103] However, the metabolic losses of acids and chloride may be overabundant, resulting in significant hypochloremic, hypokalemic, and metabolic alkalosis in some. This metabolic imbalance has been severe enough to warrant hospitalization in up to 7% of patients with gastrocystoplasty.[111,112] The mechanisms responsible for the development of a severe form of hypochloremic, hypokalemic alkalosis have not been precisely or sequentially elucidated. Significant risk factors appear to be recent viral illness associated with vomiting and other gastrointestinal losses, urinary concentrating defect,[102] renal insufficiency,[127] and the absence of acidosis prior to gastrocystoplasty.

As is the case with HDS, the development of hypergastrinemia following gastrocystoplasty has been postulated, although not definitively proven, to play a significant etiologic role in the development of metabolic alkalosis.[119,123,125] Clinical management of patients with hypochloremic, hypokalemic alkalosis includes aggressive intravenous rehydration with normal saline, replenishment of sodium and chloride, and use of H_2 receptor blockers. Once again, it is unusual to have an electrolyte abnormality that is so severe and unresponsive to medical therapy that removal of the gastric segment becomes necessary.

In comparison to conventional enterocystoplasty with small and large bowel, the incidence of bacteriuria, mucus production, and the development of bladder stones are significantly less following gastrocystoplasty.[62,102,115,128,129] The combination of decreased mucus, acidic urine, and the potential for spontaneous voiding (thus eliminating the need for intermittent catheterization) may be responsible for this decreased incidence.

Composite gastrocystoplasty and intestinocystoplasty (gastrointestinal composite)

As seen in the previous discussion regarding intestinocystoplasty and gastrocystoplasty, use of single enteric segments for augmentation has unique individual advantages and disadvantages. Since some of the metabolic effects of gastrocystoplasty are directly opposite to those of intestinocystoplasty, it has been proposed that some of these metabolic effects could buffer each other if both enteric segments are placed in combination. This concept was first introduced by Lockhart et al.[130] Ideally, the advantages of each segment could be retained and maximized with concomitant reduction of many of the undesired side effects: i.e. the stomach could still be retained for reimplantation of catheterizable tubes and ureters, whereas incorporation of a piece of ileum could reduce the side effects of increased acid secretion in the bladder (HDS) and enhance the urodynamic effects that are achieved with the use of stomach alone. Over the last decade, several reports have now demonstrated that gastrointestinal composite augmentation is feasible and advantageous in select patients.[131–134] The composite augment can either be constructed primarily or as a secondary procedure following a previous augmentation with a single piece of stomach or bowel. The size of each individual gastrointestinal segment can be varied depending on the individual metabolic and urodynamic needs of each patient. Austin et al[133,134] have demonstrated that the beneficial reduction in acid load in patients with renal insufficiency can still be maintained with the gastrointestinal composite augmentation, while the buffering effects of the incorporated intestine helps to reduce the incidence of HDS. In addition, the incidence of bacteriuria and stone formation is lower in composite reservoirs than intestinocystoplasty alone, presumably in part due to the lessened mucus production from the gastric segment. Although technically demanding, gastrointestinal composite augmentation appears to be a viable and improved form of augmentation in select patients with short bowel syndrome, metabolic acidosis, and renal insufficiency.

Autoaugmentation

Autoaugmentation, also known as vesicomyotomy and vesicomyectomy, was introduced by Cartwright and Snow.[135,136] This is a novel approach to bladder augmentation that aims to enlarge bladder capacity and improve bladder compliance without using a patch graft or opening the bladder. In essence, this procedure creates a large bladder diverticulum by removal of the bladder muscle from the dome. The most important advantage of this procedure is the avoidance of intestinal epithelium with its associated complications. The native urothelium is preserved. The major drawback of autoaugmentation is that experience has failed to identify the most appropriate patients for this procedure. Mixed results have been obtained clinically with regard to postoperative symptomatic and urodynamic improvement in the autoaugmented bladder. Evaluation of the available data indicates that there is no direct correlation between preoperative urodynamic findings and success. It works well in some patients while it fails in others. Nevertheless, it appears that this procedure is best suited for patients with reduced compliance in combination with a near-normal preoperative bladder capacity.[137–139]

Despite the problems in predicting surgical success preoperatively, it seems reasonable to consider autoaugmentation as an option in some patients in whom bladder augmentation is needed and there is a desire to avoid the use of bowel. However, patients need to be aware of the relatively high failure rate of autoaugmentation in comparison to conventional enterocystoplasty. Patients that should be excluded from consideration for autoaugmentation include those with failed bladder exstrophy repair, those who have had multiple previous bladder operations, and patients with very small bladder capacities. Autoaugmentation in these children is more difficult technically and results in general have been poor.[137,139]

Anatomy and physiology

Autoaugmentation preserves the native bladder urothelium. The metabolic and physiologic properties of this urothelium following autoaugmentation are not well studied, although available data suggest that no significant changes occur. Following autoaugmentation, the mucosal herniation has been shown in both experimental animals and humans to have evidence of collagen deposition, neovascularity, variable inflammatory changes, and occasional muscle fibers.[139–141] No significant metaplastic or dysplastic changes in the native urothelium have been reported.

Advantages and disadvantages

The primary advantage of autoaugmentation over conventional enterocystoplasty is preservation of the patient's native urothelium in the augmented segment. This avoids the complications associated with enterocystoplasty related to the presence of heterotopic epithelium in contact with the urine noted previously. Technically, autoaugmentation can be an extraperitoneal procedure performed through a Pfannenstiel incision, avoiding the complications of transperitoneal bowel surgery. Although autoaugmentation is usually performed without a formal cystotomy, other bladder procedures such as ureteral reimplantation and appendicovesicostomy can be carried out (intravesically or extravesically) at the same time. Lastly, it is important to note that autoaugmentation does not preclude further augmentation procedures if unsuccessful.

The main disadvantage of autoaugmentation is the inability to predict which patients will do well with this technique. An additional concern is the theoretical risk of bladder rupture that has been demonstrated in animal studies.[142,143] Although perforation of the autoaugmented bladder has been reported in only one patient to date,[144] the overall increased risk of bladder rupture compared with other types of bladder augmentation has yet to be defined.

Surgical technique

Patients should receive a full bowel preparation preoperatively and be counseled on the possible need to perform an alternative type of augmentation if intraoperative findings dictate that autoaugmentation is not technically feasible. Specifics regarding the technique of autoaugmentation have been well described by Snow and Cartwright.[139] The procedure is usually performed through a Pfannenstiel incision and is done extraperitoneally. Once the bladder is mobilized, the peritoneal covering is entirely detached. Snow and Cartwright advocate the performance of intraoperative urodynamics, both before and after the autoaugmentation. Although not definitive, intraoperative urodynamics can be useful in making an assessment of potential success. It also assists in establishing the maximum volume following autoaugmentation to which the bladder can be safely distended during the immediate postoperative period.

Once the initial intraoperative urodynamic study is completed, the bladder is filled and a needle-tipped electrocautery device is used to divide the detrusor

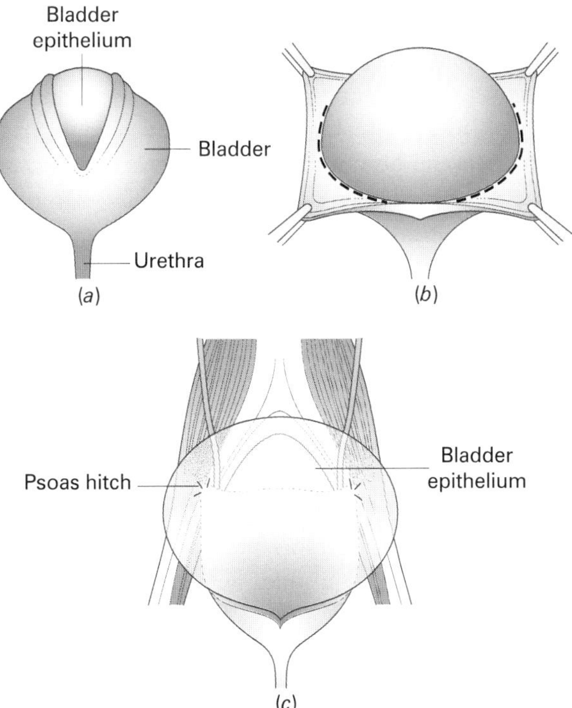

Figure 56.11 Autoaugmentation. (*a*) The detrusor muscle is incised in the midline and a plane is established between the muscle and the underlying mucosa. (*b*) This plane is further developed and a large mouth diverticulum is created. (*c*) The remaining detrusor muscle is fixed posteriorly to prevent its coaptation. (Adapted from Cartwright and Snow,[135] with permission.)

musculature from the underlying epithelium (Figure 56.11). This is usually started ventrally in a vertical fashion. The plane between the underlying epithelium and the overlying muscle is then identified and further developed using both blunt and sharp dissection. Special care is taken to avoid tears in the urothelium, since this can be difficult to repair in some cases and urinary extravasation postoperatively is associated with inflammation. Inability to distend the bladder postoperatively may result in contraction. When perforation does occur, it should be repaired with fine, absorbable suture. Removal of overlying muscle fibers continues until the detrusor musculature is removed from at least one-half of the bladder. Optimally, as much musculature is removed as possible. At this juncture, intraoperative urodynamics is repeated once again. If there is minimal to no improvement in bladder capacity and/or compliance, autoaugmentation should be abandoned and conventional enterocystoplasty undertaken following excision of the redundant bladder epithelium.

After autoaugmentation is completed, either one can excise the detached detrusor musculature or the remaining lateral bladder muscle can be attached to the psoas muscles. However, neither of these steps has been found to be essential for success.[139,145] Postoperatively, a urethral catheter and Penrose drain are left in place. Suprapubic tubes are avoided, as the bladder should be watertight. Experience has shown that bladder distention during initial healing is important for surgical success. This can be accomplished either by intermittent distention of the bladder to the capacity that was determined appropriate intraoperatively or by maintaining catheter drainage with constant bladder distention at an intravesical pressure of 20–40 cmH_2O. The catheter can generally be removed in 1–2 weeks. It is recommended that a cystogram be performed before catheter removal to exclude urinary extravasation.

Recently, several authors have demonstrated that technically successful bladder autoaugmentation can be accomplished laparoscopically.[146–149] Although a laparoscopic approach is feasible, further experience is necessary to determine whether this approach is clinically successful and cost-effective.

Results

The efficacy of autoaugmentation in improving bladder capacity and compliance has been varied. Cartwright and Snow[137] have reported follow-up of greater than 1 year in 30 patients, 19 of whom had a neuropathic bladder secondary to spina bifida. All patients had preoperative urodynamic evidence of reduced bladder compliance and detrusor hyperreflexia. Whereas clinical success has been dramatic in some patients, the overall results have been less impressive. One-third of the patients had a significant increase in bladder capacity, an additional one-third were unchanged, while one-third had loss of capacity. Evaluation of bladder compliance revealed that 60% had an improvement in compliance by >50% compared with preoperative measurements, 20% had a 20–50% improvement, and the remainder did not change significantly. Following autoaugmentation, the majority of patients remained on intermittent catheterization, although 20% demonstrated the ability to void spontaneously. Seven of these 30 patients have required secondary enterocystoplasty.

Snow and Cartwright have re-evaluated preoperative parameters in these patients in an effort to identify specific factors that would help to prognosticate eventual outcome following autoaugmentation. Unfortunately, they were unable to identify any such factors. However, certain generalizations can be made from this analysis. Autoaugmentation appears to be poorly suited to patients with a history of bladder exstrophy or multiple prior bladder operations, since in these patients it is difficult to develop a plane between the bladder muscle and mucosa. Results have also been relatively poor in these groups. The ideal candidate is the patient with a near-normal bladder capacity but reduced compliance.

Since the original publications describing the autoaugmentation technique, several other centers have reported their experiences with autoaugmentation in children. Stothers et al[150] performed autoaugmentations in 12 pediatric patients. They observed a mean increase in bladder capacity of 40% and a mean decrease in leak point pressure of 33%. Skobejko-Wlodarska et al[151] have reported on the use of autoaugmentation in 21 children with spina bifida and found a modest increase in bladder capacity in two-thirds of patients and significant improvements in bladder compliance in another two-thirds. Two recent series with long-term follow-up in children with myelomeningocele have demonstrated less favorable results.[152,153] Both studies demonstrated that a majority of patients were considered surgical failures due to a lack of clinical and/or urodynamic improvement and a high incidence of patients requiring subsequent enterocystoplasty.

The experience with autoaugmentation in the adult population appears to be more predictable and consistently favorable than the results described thus far in children. Stohrer et al[154,155] reported on 50 adult patients from their spinal cord injury center. In patients with neuropathic hyperreflexive bladders that were refractory to medical therapy, bladder autoaugmentation was found to increase mean bladder capacity from 121 to 406 ml with concomitant improvements in bladder compliance. McGuire and colleagues[156] recently compared the efficacy of enterocystoplasty to autoaugmentation in adults. They reported on over 60 patients undergoing either autoaugmentation or conventional enterocystoplasty. There were no significant differences in postoperative urodynamic parameters between enterocystoplasty and autoaugmentation in patients with refractory detrusor instability, interstitial cystitis, radiation cystitis, and other forms of neuropathic bladder. An important finding was that enterocystoplasty was uniformly superior to autoaugmentation in patients with a history of myelodysplasia. The overall improvement in the results of autoaugmentation in adults may be related to differences in the bladder disease processes and patient population. Autoaugmentation is mostly performed in children with a neuropathic bladder from congenital causes, whereas in adults the neuropathic bladder is usually an acquired condition. It may be that autoaugmentation is more successful in adults because surgery is undertaken earlier in the disease process prior to irreversible histologic and functional changes in the bladder wall.

Seromuscular enterocystoplasty

Seromuscular enterocystoplasty involves the use of a demucosalized flap of colon, stomach, or ileum. The removal of the gastrointestinal mucosa results in a denuded seromuscular flap that can either (1) be used alone as an augmentation flap that is subsequently re-epithelialized with native urothelium from the native bladder or (2) used in conjunction with autoaugmentation in which the seromuscular flap is placed over the exposed bladder mucosa of an autoaugmented bladder. The use of a demucosalized segment of bowel for bladder augmentation was first described by Shoemaker in 1955.[157,158] He was able to show that seromuscular bowel flaps, when placed into the bladder wall with the denuded side either inward or reversed, such that the serosa faced the lumen of the bladder, were re-epithelialized by urothelium. Unfortunately, subsequent long-term studies in small and large animals have consistently demonstrated that seromuscular bowel segments alone scar and contract.[159–162] Histologic evaluation suggests that the scarring is due to the trauma associated with the demucosalization process and/or a prolonged inflammatory response in the denuded bowel before the re-epithelialization of the seromuscular flap from the native bladder urothelium occurs.

The intention of seromuscular enterocystoplasty is to combine the advantages of conventional enterocystoplasty while preserving the native urothelium of the bladder. This procedure ideally results in a muscle-backed augmentation flap that is lined with urothelium. Contraction of the seromuscular flap is hopefully avoided by either rapid regrowth of native urothelium over the demucosalized surface or adherence of the native urothelium to the demucosalized gastrointestinal segment (when combined with autoaugmentation). Numerous animal studies have demonstrated that seromuscular enterocystoplasty with or without autoaugmentation can successfully augment the bladder, with elimination of the complications related to retained intestinal epithelium.[163–167] However, clinical experience thus far has been mixed and varied. Early experience with this procedure suggested that the success may be limited by the same factors that give rise to inconsistent results with autoaugmentation. More recent modifications of the technique, including improved methods for demucosalization and constant distention of the seromuscular flap during the initial postoperative period, have demonstrated that more reliable results are possible. Further experience with long-term follow-up is needed to better determine the factors that are important in predicting success and whether this type of augmentation remains stable without future fibrosis, loss of compliance, and/or metaplastic changes. Nevertheless, seromuscular enterocystoplasty represents an intriguing advancement in bladder augmentation techniques whose appropriateness for routine use in children is currently being defined.

Anatomy and physiology

Seromuscular enterocystoplasty has been accomplished with stomach, ileum, and colon. The metabolic consequences of seromuscular enterocystoplasty are presumed to be minimal, since the native urothelium is kept intact. This assumption is supported in part by animal studies.[166] Histology from these studies reveals that the urothelium covering the seromuscular flap appears normal.[167,168] Whether or not late metaplastic changes will occur in the bladder urothelium when it is placed in direct contact with a seromuscular segment of

seromuscular flap from the outside using an intraluminal Foley balloon during this important dissection, routine postoperative distention of the bladder, and diversion of the urine for 2–3 weeks. Jednak et al[179] have also reported favorable results in 32 patients: all were done in conjunction with autoaugmentation; mean follow-up was 1.6 years; and a near twofold increase in bladder capacity was noted with a 12.5% reaugmentation rate. A more recent report from the same group has also demonstrated the ability to combine seromuscular enterocystoplasty with placement of an artificial sphincter with no increase in the complication rate.

Recurrent or persistent intestinal mucosa has been found in several patients after seromuscular enterocystoplasty.[171,179] Whether this partial intestinal regrowth is progressive or clinically relevant remains to be determined. As mentioned above, it has been suggested and supported by animal studies that removal of the submucosa may prevent re-epithelialization of the seromuscular flap with islands of native enteric mucosa.[171]

Ureterocystoplasty

The use of ureteral tissue for bladder augmentation was first described in 1992.[180,181] Since then, its use in children has become more popular.[182–184] For many reasons native ureter is the best tissue available for augmentation cystoplasty. It is autologous, lined with urothelium, backed by muscle, distensible, and compliant. However, few patients in need of bladder augmentation have widely dilated ureters available for such use. Patients who are candidates for ureterocystoplasty should have either a non-functional renal unit that can be removed, making the ureter and renal pelvis available, or a functional renal unit that is associated with a massively dilated, tortuous, and elongated ureter.[182,185] The lower ureter can then be used for augmentation while kidney drainage is re-established either by reimplantation of the straightened upper ureter into the bladder or by transureteroureterostomy.

One of the challenges that one faces in selecting the appropriate patient for ureterocystoplasty is determination of whether the ureter that is to be used is going to be adequate for successful augmentation. Recent clinical experience and long-term urodynamic follow-up suggests that the detubularized and reconstructed ureter following ureterocystoplasty remains compliant, but that the overall compliance, distensibility, and volume may not increase significantly as compared with the dilated intact ureter in its preoperative state. Thus, postoperative urodynamic studies in a patient with a refluxing ureter that was used for ureterocystoplasty may not show a significant increase in volume and compliance of the augmented bladder compared with preoperative studies (when the ureter was refluxing and intact).[186] However, if the ureter that is to be used is not refluxing, then improvement in urodynamics following ureterocystoplasty would be expected and may be directly related to the degree of ureteral dilatation that is present preoperatively. Given this, preoperative urodynamic studies can be very valuable in select patients in predicting success or failure following ureterocystoplasty, especially in the setting of refluxing ureter.

Ureterocystoplasty can also be appropriate in patients with end-stage renal failure on dialysis who are awaiting transplantation and are in need of augmentation owing to bladder dysfunction. As is the case with conventional intestinocystoplasty, the augmented bladder following ureterocystoplasty and subsequent transplantation has been shown to function adequately.[187]

Anatomy and physiology

Preservation of the ureteral blood supply is paramount when performing ureterocystoplasty. The normal ureter receives its blood supply from branches of numerous vessels including the aorta and renal, gonadal, and common iliac arteries (Figure 56.13). The upper ureter receives its blood supply medially, whereas the lower ureter receives it posterolaterally. There are extensive anastomosing plexuses in the adventitia of the ureter that are important to preserve if viability of the ureter is to be maintained. Careful attention to these vessels allows for long segments of ureter to be mobilized without vascular compromise. Ureteral urothelium is contiguous with the urothelium from the bladder and has similar physiologic characteristics. Peristalsis of the ureter depends on autonomic innervation and input from intrinsic pacemaker sites in the minor calices of the renal collecting system.[188] Although the ureter is detubularized and its inherent innervation is disrupted with ureterocystoplasty, it appears that the ureteral tissue still maintains some ability to contract.

Advantages and disadvantages

There are several advantages in using the ureter for augmentation. As is the case with autoaugmentation, the major advantage of ureterocystoplasty is that the

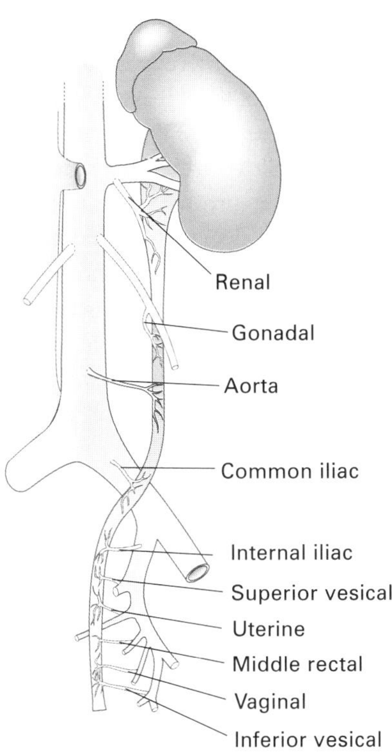

Figure 56.13 Arterial blood supply to the ureter. (Adapted from Lindner,[17] with permission.)

native urothelium is preserved, thereby avoiding the specific potential problems associated with the use of bowel. Unlike some cases following autoaugmention, the full-thickness opened ureter does not tend to shrink with time, unless the vascular supply is compromised. In patients with end-stage renal disease, the procedure can be performed extraperitoneally, thus preserving the peritoneum for future peritoneal dialysis. Alternatively, it can also be performed with laparoscopic assistance for the nephrectomy and upper ureter mobilization.[20,189,190] When needed, concomitant procedures in the bladder may also be performed. It seems likely that the risk of tumor formation will be avoided, and perforation of the augmented bladder may be less probable. However, long-term follow-up will be needed to confirm these possibilities.[182] Finally, there is increased potential for spontaneous voiding postoperatively, especially in patients who are able to empty their bladders adequately preoperatively.

The main disadvantage of ureterocystoplasty is that it is only applicable in a minority of patients. More recently, the use of ureterocystoplasty has been expanded in an attempt to take advantage of this valuable tissue and make it available to more surgical candidates. Its use has been reported in patients with a duplex system in which either the upper or lower pole is non-functioning.[191] In patients with a duplex system and a dilated ureter in conjunction with a functioning renal segment, drainage of that segment can be accomplished with an ipsilateral pyeloureterostomy or a ureteropyelostomy with preservation of the distal portion of the ureter for augmentation. Ahmed et al[192] also described the tandem use of bilateral megaureters for ureterocystoplasty.

Efforts are being made to produce dilated ureters to make ureterocystoplasty available to more patients. Lailas et al[193] have demonstrated in a rabbit model that a temporary cutaneous ureterostomy can be used to perform hydrostatic distention of the ureter with subsequent successful ureterocystoplasty. Others have reported that placement of a tissue expander in pig ureters adequately dilates the ureter.[194,195]

Surgical technique

Patients undergoing ureterocystoplasty should have a full bowel preparation and sterilization preoperatively in case the ureter is not suitable for augmentation. The procedure can be performed either through a midline incision with transperitoneal approach to the urinary tract or via two incisions such as is used for nephroureterectomy.[196] The latter approach is extraperitoneal. This may be advantageous in patients with severe renal insufficiency who may subsequently require peritoneal dialysis. A nephrectomy is performed initially, preserving the renal pelvis. The upper portion of the ureter and renal pelvis are then mobilized (Figure 56.14). Efforts should be made to preserve as much renal pelvis as possible since this increases the surface area of the augmentation. One should include any available periureteral tissue to protect the network of vessels within the ureteral adventitia. Although the blood supply from the lower ureter (which is derived posterolaterally) can maintain the viability of the upper ureter via this adventitial network, efforts should also be made to preserve collaterals from the gonadal vessels and the main renal vessels. These vessels supply the renal pelvis and upper ureter directly and their preservation helps to ensure adequate vascular supply to the upper portion of the ureter. As Churchill et al[197] have noted, preservation of the upper ureteral blood supply is most important when previous reconstructive surgery has compromised the collaterals involving the distal ureter.

Following mobilization of the renal pelvis and ureter, the ureter is detubularized and reconfigured to form a patch. The bladder is then opened. The bladder incision extends from the ipsilateral ureteral

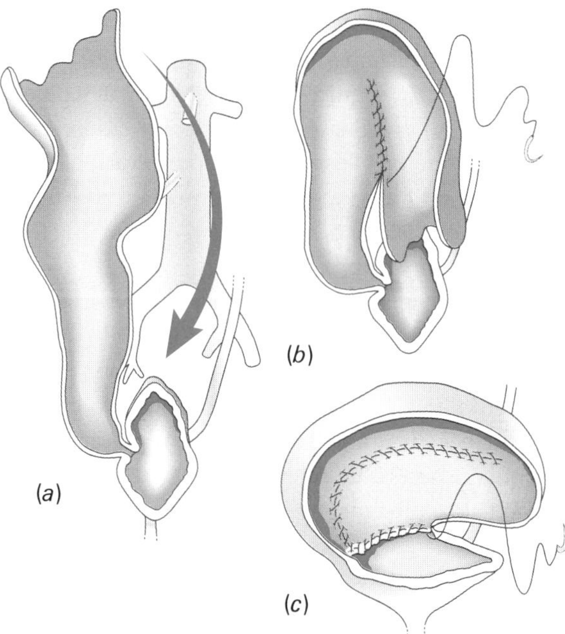

Figure 56.14 Ureterocystoplasty. A standard nephrectomy is performed with preservation of the renal pelvis. (*a*) The proximal ureter is mobilized, with preservation of the medial blood supply. (*b*) The ureter is then detubularized, with the incision for detubularization connecting with the off-center cystostomy. (*c*) The ureter is folded on itself and anastomosed to the opened bladder.

orifice to the contralateral ventral quadrant of the bladder. The incision is carried through the ipsilateral ureteral orifice so that it unroofs the intravesical ureter and meets the detubularization incision in the ureter. This allows the bladder to be opened sufficiently for ureterocystoplasty without much risk of an hourglass deformity. Alternatively, to preserve vascularity, the incision can stop short of the orifice, maintaining the normal configuration of the distal ureter for a few centimeters.[181] Once the bladder is adequately opened, the reconfigured ureteral segment is sutured to the defect in the bladder, creating a wide anastomosis. Prior to closure, a suprapubic tube is placed through the native bladder, and left indwelling for 2–3 weeks. Postoperative care is essentially the same as for routine enterocystoplasty, except that daily irrigation for mucus is not required.

Results

Since its original description in 1992, wide experience has been gained with ureterocystoplasty. Early reports demonstrating its efficacy have led to increased enthusiasm for this technique and a desire to use ureter instead of intestinal segments whenever adequate ureteral tissue is available. Churchill et al[182] initially reported on 16 patients: there was a 218% increase in bladder capacity, a 284% increase in pressure-specific bladder capacity, and a 227% increase in bladder compliance. In a follow-up to this study, Landau et al[198] compared the urodynamic results between patients treated with ileocystoplasty and those with ureterocystoplasty. They reported no significant differences in the postoperative mean increase in bladder capacity and pressure-specific bladder volume. Both procedures produced in excellent functional results. Hitchcock et al[199] described similar excellent short-term results in eight patients.

Subsequent reports have also demonstrated that ureterocystoplasty can be an effective augmentation procedure, but have further clarified which patients are most appropriate for the procedure and what amount of ureter is needed for success. Pascual et al[200] described 22 patients in which only the distal ureter of a single ureter was utilized for augmentation. Whereas increases in capacity and improvement in compliance were noted, only 50% of the patients reached the expected age capacity of the bladder and the overall results were less successful than other reported previous series in which the entire ureter was utilized. In the largest series to date, Hussman et al[186] reported on 64 patients from multiple institutions. In 40 of the patients, augmentation was performed with a complete single or double collecting system. In 9/40 patients, reflux was not present and postoperative success directly correlated with a preoperative ureteral diameter of >1.5 cm. In the remaining 31 patients, reflux was present preoperatively. In these refluxing patients, if the system on preoperative urodynamics demonstrated only mild non-compliance (>20 ml/cmH_2O), ureterocystoplasty improved compliance onefold and was adequate. However, if the system preoperatively demonstrated poor compliance, ureterocystoplasty did not adequately improve capacity and compliance, resulting in 81% of patients having either undergone or being considered for reaugmentation.

Collectively, these results suggest that the ideal patient for ureterocystoplasty is one with a massively dilated ureter in which most (or all) of the ureter can be used for augmentation purposes. If reflux is present preoperatively, then preoperative urodynamics can be predictive of future success. If a poorly compliant system is present in the setting of a dilated refluxing ureter, then failure and the need for reaugmentation are likely. Novel techniques to make ureterocystoplasty more readily available for patients that do not have massive dilation of the ureter are currently being investigated.

Tissue-engineered bladder

The complications associated with using various portions of the gastrointestinal tract for genitourinary reconstruction in both adults and children, described in this chapter, have stimulated the development of tissue-engineering techniques for bladder reconstruction. Current research efforts are focused on the development of biodegradable materials that are well characterized with predictable behavior. Although attempts at bladder reconstruction via bladder regeneration are not new,[201] the major obstacle has been the lack of a biomaterial, either permanent or biodegradable, that will function as a suitable scaffold to allow the process of regeneration to occur either naturally or with the addition of cultured cells. The ideal graft material is one that would be replaced by the host tissue, provide a low-pressure reservoir, and serve as a scaffold for regeneration of the bladder wall with normal functional characteristics. If a suitable graft material were developed, the need for autogenous tissue and the associated complications of intestinal segments could be eliminated. Currently, two types of tissue-engineering technology have been shown to induce bladder regeneration in preliminary studies: 'unseeded' and 'seeded' technologies.

Unseeded technology

The first technique currently being investigated for bladder regeneration is unseeded technology. This involves the use of tissue matrix grafts that are biodegradable, acellular, collagen based, autologous, or xenogenic.[202–204] This technology involves placement of the graft into the wall of the host bladder. The body then provides the needed environment for subsequent cell growth and tissue generation. This represents an unseeded bladder regenerating process.

Thus far, the major obstacle to unseeded tissue-engineering technology has been the inability to develop an optimal biomaterial that will act as a suitable scaffold for the 'natural' process of regeneration. Synthetic non-biodegradable materials such as silicone, rubber, polytetrafluoroethylene, and polypropylene have been tried without success because of host–foreign body reactions.[205–209] As a consequence of these failures with non-biodegradable materials, synthetic biodegradable materials were developed. It is anticipated that these grafts will allow the host bladder adequate time for regeneration but dissolve before the onset of foreign body reactions. These materials have been used experimentally and have shown less graft encrustation and fewer infectious complications than non-biodegradable materials. However, graft shrinkage still limits the potential clinical utility of these materials.[210] Non-synthetic biodegradable materials such as placenta, amnion, and pericardium have been investigated and have shown a clear ability to host bladder regeneration.[211–214] However, despite initial encouraging laboratory results, none of these materials has been found to be suitable for clinical use. The reasons for this are not entirely clear. It can only be speculated from the available literature that long-term experimental results with these biodegradable materials did not replicate the initial results and, therefore, clinical trials were not undertaken.

Recently, new types of biodegradable material have been developed that have shown tremendous potential for the induction of bladder regeneration with unseeded tissue-engineering technology. These materials are acellular extracellular matrix (ECM) grafts that are derived from various organs. The graft is made acellular by a mechanical process that lyses the cells and/or by detergent and enzymatic extraction. These types of ECM grafts have been derived from full-thickness bladder and stomach and the submucosal layer of small intestine.[202,215,216]

The most thoroughly studied collagen-based ECM graft for bladder augmentation and urinary reconstruction using unseeded technology is small intestinal submucosa (SIS).[217] SIS is a xenogenic membrane derived from pig small intestine in which the mucosa is mechanically removed from the inner surface and the serosa and muscularis are mechanically removed from the outer surface. This results in a thin, translucent membrane (0.1 mm wall thickness) composed mainly of the submucosal layer of the intestinal wall. Production of SIS is reminiscent of the manufacture of sausage casing. This unique material has been shown to function well as an arterial or venous graft, with rapid replacement by native tissues and evidence of tissue-specific regeneration.[218–220]

SIS grafts have been shown to promote full-thickness bladder regeneration in both rat and canine animal models.[221] The regenerated bladder tissue is composed of all three layers of the normal bladder wall (urothelium, smooth muscle, and serosa). In addition, the regenerated segment is contractile, compliant, and functionally innervated. Urodynamic studies in a long-term canine augmentation model have demonstrated that the

SIS augmented bladder maintains normal bladder capacity and compliance for at least 15 months postoperatively.[222] In-vitro muscle strip studies on the regenerated portions of the bladders also demonstrate contractility and compliance that is similar to normal bladder.[223]

SIS has been shown to be non-immunogenic, with over 1000 cross-species transplants and direct challenge testing elucidating no response.[224–226] In addition, SIS is unique from other biomaterials that have been studied thus far in that it contains a combination of active intrinsic growth factors, cytokines, structural proteins, glycoproteins, and proteoglycans that may assist in cell migration, cell-to-cell interaction, and cell growth and differentiation during the regenerative process.[227–229] These inherent elements within SIS may prove to be vital to the regenerative process. It has been recently published that different segments of SIS may have different regenerative potentials for the bladder. Kropp et al[230] have been able to show more reliable bladder regeneration when utilizing distal ileum from a 3-year-old sow as compared with the proximal jejunal segment from the same age sow.[231] The reasons for this variable regeneration are not yet clear and are under investigation.

Acellular ECM grafts similar to SIS have also been shown to induce bladder regeneration. Preliminary work by Sutherland et al[203] and Piechota et al[232] demonstrated successful morphologic and functional regeneration of the rat urinary bladder with homologous bladder acellular matrix grafts (BAMG). Reddy et al[216] also reported on partial bladder substitution with porcine bladder acellular matrix allografts (BAMA) in a porcine model. They demonstrated that the regenerated urothelium with BAMA was multilayered and that there was also histologic evidence of organized smooth muscle regeneration and neoangiogenesis at 30 days.

The above experience with SIS and other similar ECM-derived biomaterials clearly demonstrates that bladder regeneration using unseeded tissue-engineering technology is feasible without the complications of graft shrinkage, encrustation, and infection. These observations have significant clinical ramifications. The ability to augment the bladder without the use of bowel or other native host tissue would eliminate many of the complications of conventional enterocystoplasty and would simplify the technical aspects of this operation. Further research into the individual composition of the various biomaterials,[233,234] the cell-to-cell interactions, and the growth factors[203,235–237] that are involved in the bladder regenerative process will be required before clinical use of these grafts. Advances in this type of mechanistic research will bring us closer to having an off-the-shelf, acellular, clinically available product for bladder augmentation.

Seeded technology

The second type of tissue-engineering technology, the seeded technique, involves the use of biodegradable materials that act as cell-delivery vehicles for cultured cells from the patient. This technique has been applied to the urinary bladder. Initially, this process is begun by harvesting native bladder tissue for the establishment and expansion of primary cultures of both bladder smooth muscle and epithelial cells. Cilento et al[238] demonstrated that it is possible to expand a bladder epithelial cell culture from a single biopsy specimen such that the cultured cells could cover a surface area of over 400 m^2 within 8 weeks. Once the cells are grown, they are seeded on a biodegradable membrane in vitro and then transplanted back into the host for continuation of the regenerative process. Atala et al[239] demonstrated the successful use of non-woven polyglycolic acid polymer sheets that allow the seeded growth of rabbit and human bladder epithelium and smooth muscle cells. Further work demonstrated that these cell–polymer constructs could then be implanted into athymic mice, with the subsequent formation of organized layers of bladder epithelial and smooth muscle cells. Yoo et al[240] and Oberpenning et al[241] reported on the feasibility of dog bladder augmentation using allogenic bladder submucosa or polyglycolic acid polymers seeded with urothelial and smooth muscle cells. Organized bladder histology was noted in the regenerated bladder tissue. More importantly, the regenerated bladder tissue was found to increase bladder capacity and was urodynamically compliant.

Recently, many other materials have been shown to support the growth of bladder cells, both in vitro and in vivo.[242,243] In addition to research looking at different types of biomaterials to support cell growth, both biologic and synthetic new approaches to deliver cells back to the host are being explored. These include the development of a capsule around the bladder and the use of de-epithelialized bowel segments.[244–247] The importance of new or pre-existing vasculature to provide a conduit for nutrients to the regenerating tissue is evident. This has initiated new research efforts to create a vascularized matrix[248] and other novel methods to induce neovascularization in the regenerating tissue. Further advancements in biomaterial development, methods of cell attachment, and angiogenesis will be areas of intense future research aimed at improving the type of tissue regeneration that results from seeded technology.

It is clear that bladder regeneration is possible using both unseeded and seeded tissue-engineering technologies. Further advances in current techniques will eventually revolutionize urologic reconstructive surgery as we know it today. Additional work is needed before clinical application of these techniques. One of the concerns that has been expressed is that all of the animal studies performed thus far have been in animals with a normal bladder. It is not known whether normal bladder regeneration can be achieved with either unseeded or seeded technology in an animal or a patient with a neuropathic bladder. Lin et al[249] recently demonstrated that cultured cells from the neuropathic bladder retain functional differences in vitro. Ongoing work is aimed at determining whether these functional differences are retained in vivo when these cells are utilized in a seeded fashion to regenerate bladder tissue. This must be understood before tissue-engineering technologies can be applied clinically. Additional information is needed to understand the differences between the unseeded and seeded approaches and the resultant regenerated bladder, such that the best aspects of each technology may be used to achieve a superior result. It is hoped that future chapters on bladder augmentation will discuss the use of intestinal segments as an historical footnote, and the major focus will be on the indications and methods for various types of tissue-engineering technologies.

References

1. Gleason DM, Gittes RF, Bottaccini MR, Byrne JC. Energy balance of voiding after cecal cystoplasty. J Urol 1972; 108:259–64.
2. Lapides J, Diokno AC, Silber SJ, Lowe BS. Clean, intermittent self-catheterization in the treatment of urinary tract disease. J Urol 1972; 107:458–61.
3. Lapides J, Diokno AC, Gould FR, Lowe BS. Further observations on self-catheterization. J Urol 1976; 116:169–71.
4. Nasrallah PF, Aliabadi HA. Bladder augmentation in patients with neurogenic bladder and vesicoureteral reflux. J Urol 1991; 146:563–6.
5. Lopez PP, Martinez UMJ, Lobato RR et al. Should we treat vesicoureteral reflux in patients who simultaneously undergo bladder augmentation for neuropathic bladder? J Urol 2001; 165:2259–61.
6. Simforoosh N, Tabibi A, Basiri A et al. Is ureteral reimplantation necessary during augmentation cystoplasty in patients with neurogenic bladder and vesicoureteral reflux? J Urol 2002; 168:1439–41.
7. Soylet Y, Emir H, Yesildag E et al. Quo vadis? Ureteric reimplantation or ignoring reflux during augmentation cystoplasty. BJU Int 2004; 94:379–80.
8. de Badiola FI, Castro-Diaz D, Hart-Austin C, Gonzalez R. Influence of preoperative bladder capacity and compliance on the outcome of artificial sphincter implantation in patients with neurogenic sphincter incompetence. J Urol 1992; 148:1493–5.
9. Kronner KM, Rink RC, Simmons G et al. Artificial urinary sphincter in the treatment of urinary incontinence: preoperative urodynamics do not predict the need for future bladder augmentation. J Urol 1998; 160:1093–5, discussion 1103.
10. Firlit CF. Use of defunctionalized bladders in pediatric renal transplantation. J Urol 1976; 116:634–7.
11. MacGregor P, Novick AC, Cunningham R et al. Renal transplantation in end stage renal disease patients with existing urinary diversion. J Urol 1986; 135:686–8.
12. Serrano DP, Flechner SM, Modlin CS et al. Transplantation into the long-term defunctionalized bladder. J Urol 1996; 156:885–8.
13. de Badiola FI, Denes ED, Ruiz E et al. New application of the gastrostomy button for clinical and urodynamic evaluation before vesicostomy closure. J Urol 1996; 156:618–20.
14. N'Dow J, Leung HY, Marshall C, Neal DE. Bowel dysfunction after bladder reconstruction. J Urol 1998; 159:1470–4, discussion 1474–5.
15. King L Protection of the upper tracts in children. In: King LR, Stone AR, Webster GD, eds. Bladder Reconstruction and Continent Urinary Diversion. Chicago, IL: Year Book Medical Publishers, 1987: 127.
16. Husmann OA, Cain MP. Fecal and urinary continence after ileal cecal cystoplasty for the neurogenic bladder J Urol 2001; 165:922–5.
17. Lindner H. Clinical Anatomy. Norwalk, CT: Appleton and Lange, 1989.
18. Powell DW. Intestinal water and electrolyte transport. In: Johnson LR, ed. Physiology of the Gastrointestinal Tract, 2nd edn. New York: Raven Press, 1987: 1267.
19. Stampfer DS, McDougal WS. Inhibition of the sodium/hydrogen antiport by ammonium ion. J Urol 1997; 157:362–5.
20. Hedican SP, Schulam PG, Docimo SG. Laparoscopic assisted reconstructive surgery. J Urol 1999; 161: 267–70.
21. Rink RC, Hollensbe D, Adams MC. Complications of bladder augmentation in children and comparison of gastrointestinal segments. AUA Update Ser 1995; 14:122–7.
22. Di Benedetto V, Monfort G. Stomach versus sigmoid colon in children undergoing major reconstruction of the lower urinary tract. Pediatr Surg Int 1997; 12:393–6.
23. Hinman F Jr. Selection of intestinal segments for bladder substitution: physical and physiological characteristics. J Urol 1988; 139:519–23.
24. Koff SA. Guidelines to determine the size and shape of

intestinal segments used for reconstruction. J Urol 1988; 140:1150–1.
25. Rink RC, Adams MC. Augmentation cystoplasty. In: Walsh PC, Retik AB, Vaughan ED, Wein AJ, eds. Campbell's Urology, 7th edn. Philadelphia: WB Saunders, 1998: 3167–89.
26. Keating MA, Ludlow JK, Rich MA. Enterocystoplasty: the star modification. J Urol 1996; 155:1723–5.
27. Rink R, Mitchell M. Role of enterocystoplasty in reconstructing the neurogenic bladder. In: Gonzales E, Roth D, eds. Common Problems in Pediatric Urology. St. Louis: Mosby Year Book, 1990: 192–204.
28. Rink RC. Bladder augmentation. Options, outcomes, future. Urol Clin North Am 1999; 26:111–23, viii–ix.
29. Goldwasser B, Barrett DM, Webster GD, Kramer SA. Cystometric properties of ileum and right colon after bladder augmentation, substitution or replacement. J Urol 1987; 138:1007–8.
30. Flood HD, Malhotra SJ, O'Connell HE et al. Long-term results and complications using augmentation cystoplasty in reconstructive urology. Neurourol Urodyn 1995; 14:297–309.
31. Kilic N, Celayir S, Elicevik M et al. Bladder augmentation: urodynamic findings and clinical outcome in different augmentation techniques. Eur J Pediatr Surg 1999; 9:29–32.
32. Quek ML, Ginsberg DA. Long-term urodynamics followup of bladder augmentation for neurogenic bladder. J Urol 2003; 169:195–8.
33. Robertson AS, Davies JB, Webb RJ, Neal DE. Bladder augmentation and replacement. Urodynamic and clinical review of 25 patients. Br J Urol 1991; 68:590–7.
34. Pope JC, Keating MA, Casale AJ, Rink RC. Augmenting the augmented bladder: treatment of the contractile bowel segment. J Urol 1988; 160:854–7.
35. Koch MO, McDougal WS. The pathophysiology of hyperchloremic metabolic acidosis after urinary diversion through intestinal segments. Surgery 1985; 98:561–70.
36. Mitchell ME, Piser JA. Intestinocystoplasty and total bladder replacement in children and young adults: followup in 129 cases. J Urol 1987; 138:579–84.
37. Salomon L, Lugagne PM, Herve JM et al. No evidence of metabolic disorders 10 to 22 years after Camey type I ileal enterocystoplasty. J Urol 1997; 157:2104–6.
38. Kockum CC, Helin I, Malmberg L, Malmfors G. Pediatric urinary tract reconstruction using intestine. Scand J Urol Nephrol 1999; 33:53–6.
39. Stampfer DS, McDougal WS, McGovern FJ. The use of in bowel urology. Metabolic and nutritional complications. Urol Clin North Am 1997; 24:715–22.
40. Hochstetler JA, Flanigan MJ, Kreder KJ. Impaired bone growth after ileal augmentation cystoplasty. J Urol 1997; 157:1873–9.
41. Gerharz EW, Gasser JA, Mosekilde L et al. Skeletal growth and long-term bone turnover after enterocystoplasty in a chronic rat model. BJU Int 2003; 9293:306–13.
42. Gerharz EW, Mosekilde L, Thomsen JS et al. The effect of enterocystoplasty on bone strength assessed at four different skeletal sites in a rat model. Bone 2003; 33(4):549–56.
43. Mundy AR, Nurse DE. Calcium balance, growth and skeletal mineralisation in patients with cystoplasties. Br J Urol 1992; 69:257–9.
44. Stein R, Lotz J, Andreas J et al. Long-term metabolic effects in patients with urinary diversion. World J Urol 1998; 16:292–7.
45. Haafez AT, McLorie G, Laudenberg B et al. Long-term evaluation of metabolic profile and bone mineral density after ileocystoplasty in children. J Urol 2003; 170:1639–41.
46. Abes M, Sarihan H, Madenci E. Evaluation of bone mineral density with dual x-ray absorptiometry for osteoporosis in children with bladder augmentation. J Pediatr Surg 2003; 38:230–2.
47. Canturk F, Tander B, Tander B et al. Bladder exstrophy: effects on bone age, bone mineral density, growth, and metabolism. Bone 2005; 36:69–73.
48. Feng AH, Kaar S, Elder JS. Influence of enterocystoplasty on linear growth in children with exstrophy. J Urol 2002; 167:2552–5.
49. Mingin G, Nguyen HT, Mathias RS et al. Growth and metabolic consequences of bladder augmentation in children with myelomeningocele and bladder exstrophy. Pediatrics 2002; 110:1193–8.
50. Mingin G, Maroni P, Gerharz EW et al. Linear growth after enterocystoplasty in children and adolescents: a review. World J Urol 2004; 22:196–9.
51. Gros DA, Dodson JL, Lopatin U et al. Decreased linear growth associated with intestinal bladder augmentation in children with bladder exstrophy. J Urol 2000; 164:917–20.
52. Singh G, Thomas DG. Bowel problems after enterocystoplasty. Br J Urol 1997; 79:328–32.
53. Herschorn S, Hewitt RJ. Patient perspective of long-term outcome of augmentation cystoplasty for neurogenic bladder. Urology 1998; 52:672–8.
54. King LR, Webster GD, Bertram RA. Experiences with bladder reconstruction in children. J Urol 1987; 138:1002–6.
55. Barrington JW, Fern-Davies H, Adams RJ et al. Bile acid dysfunction after clam enterocystoplasty. Br J Urol 1995; 76:169–71.
56. Akerlund S, Delin K, Kock NG et al. Renal function and upper urinary tract configuration following urinary diversion to a continent ileal reservoir (Kock pouch): a prospective 5 to 11-year followup after reservoir construction. J Urol 1989; 142:964–8.
57. Hendren WH, Hendren RB. Bladder augmentation: experience with 129 children and young adults. J Urol 1990; 144:445–53, discussion 460.
58. Bruce AW, Reid G, Chan RC, Costerton JW. Bacterial adherence in the human ileal conduit: a morphological and bacteriological study. J Urol 1984; 132:184–8.
59. Blyth B, Ewalt DH, Duckett JW, Snyder HM 3rd. Lithogenic properties of enterocystoplasty. J Urol 1992; 148:575–7, discussion 578–9.
60. Palmer LS, Franco I, Kogan SJ et al. Urolithiasis in children following augmentation cystoplasty. J Urol 1993; 150:726–9.
61. Brough RJ, O'Flynn KJ, Fishwick J, Gough DC. Bladder washout and stone formation in paediatric enterocystoplasty. Eur Urol 1998; 33:500–2.

62. Kaefer M, Hendren WH, Bauer SB et al. Reservoir calculi: a comparison of reservoirs constructed from stomach and other enteric segments. J Urol 1998; 160:2187–90.
63. Kronner KM, Casale AJ, Cain MP et al. Bladder calculi in the pediatric augmented bladder. J Urol 1998; 160:1096–8, discussion 1103.
64. Defoor W, Minvich E, Reddy P et al. Bladder calculi after augmentation cystoplasty: risk factors and prevention strategies. J Urol 2004; 172:1964–6.
65. Khoury AE, Salomon M, Doche R et al. Stone formation after augmentation cystoplasty: the role of intestinal mucus. J Urol 1997; 158:1133–7.
66. Hensle TW, Bingham J, Lam J et al. Preventing reservoir calculi after augmentation cystoplasty and continent urinary diversion: the influence of an irrigation protocol. BJU Int 2004; 93:585–7.
67. Woodhouse CR, Robertson WG. Urolithiasis in enterocystoplasties. World J Urol 2004; 22:215–21.
68. Palmer LS, Franco I, Reda EF et al. Endoscopic management of bladder calculi following augmentation cystoplasty. Urology 1994; 44:902–4.
69. Docimo SG, Orth CR, Schulam PG. Percutaneous cystolithotomy after augmentation cystoplasty: comparison with open procedures. Tech Urol 1998; 4:43–5.
70. Miller EC, Park JM. Percutaneous cystolithotomy using a laparoscopic entrapment sac. Urology 2003; 62:333–6.
71. Hirst G. Ileal and colonic cystoplasties. In: Rowland RB, ed. Problems in Urology. Hagerstown: JB Lippincott, 1991: 223.
72. Filmer RB, Spencer JR. Malignancies in bladder augmentations and intestinal conduits. J Urol 1990; 143:671–8.
73. Nurse DE, Mundy AR. Assessment of the malignant potential of cystoplasty. Br J Urol 1989; 64:489–92.
74. Woodhams SD, Greenwell TJ, Smalley T et al. Factors causing variation in urinary N-nitrosamine levels in enterocystoplasties. BJU Int 2001; 88:187–91.
75. Shokeir AA, Shamaa M, el-Mekresh MM, el-Baz M, Ghoneim MA. Late malignancy in bowel segments exposed to urine without fecal stream. Urology 1995; 46:657–61.
76. Ali-El-Dein B, El-Tabey N, Abdel-Latif M, Abdel-Rahim M, El-Bahnasawy MS. Late uro-ileal cancer after incorporation of ileum into the urinary tract. J Urol 2002; 167:84–8.
77. Barrington JW, Fulford S, Griffiths D, Stephenson TP. Tumors in bladder remnant after augmentation enterocystoplasty. J Urol 1997; 157:482–5, discussion 485–6.
78. Soergel TM, Cain MP, Misseri R et al. Transitional cell carcinoma of the bladder following augmentation cystoplasty for the neuropathic bladder. J Urol 2004; 172:1649–51.
79. Barrington JW, Fraylin L, Fish R et al. Elevated levels of basic fibroblast growth factor in the urine of clam enterocystoplasty patients. J Urol 1996; 155:468–70.
80. Barrington JW, Fulford S, Fraylin L. Reduction of urinary basic fibroblast growth factor using pentosan polysulphate sodium. Br J Urol 1996; 78:54–6.
81. Barrington JW, Jones A, James D. Antioxidant deficiency following clam enterocystoplasty. Br J Urol 1997; 80:238–42.
82. Vajda P, Kaiser L, Magyarlaki T et al. Histological findings after colocystoplasty and gastrocystoplasty. J Urol 2002; 168:698–701.
83. Elder JS, Snyder HM, Hulbert WC, Duckett JW. Perforation of the augmented bladder in patients undergoing clean intermittent catheterization. J Urol 1988; 140:1159–62.
84. Glass RB, Rushton HG. Delayed spontaneous rupture of augmented bladder in children: diagnosis with sonography and CT. AJR Am J Roentgenol 1992; 158:833–5.
85. Rosen MA, Light JK. Spontaneous bladder rupture following augmentation enterocystoplasty. J Urol 1991; 146:1232–4.
86. Sheiner JR, Kaplan GW. Spontaneous bladder rupture following enterocystoplasty. J Urol 1988; 140:1157–8.
87. Rushton HG, Woodard JR, Parrott TS et al. Delayed bladder rupture after augmentation enterocystoplasty. J Urol 1988; 140:344–6.
88. Anderson PA, Rickwood AM. Detrusor hyper-reflexia as a factor in spontaneous perforation of augmentation cystoplasty for neuropathic bladder. Br J Urol 1991; 67:210–12.
89. Bauer SB, Hendren WH, Kozakewich H et al. Perforation of the augmented bladder. J Urol 1992; 148:699–703.
90. Couillard DR, Vapnek JM, Rentzepis MJ, Stone AR. Fatal perforation of augmentation cystoplasty in an adult. Urology 1993; 42:585–8.
91. Defoor W, Tackett L, Minevich E, Wacksman J, Sheldon C. Risk factors for spontaneous bladder perforation after augmentation cystoplasty. Urology 2003; 62:737–41.
92. Crane JM, Scherz HS, Billman GF, Kaplan GW. Ischemic necrosis: a hypothesis to explain the pathogenesis of spontaneously ruptured enterocystoplasty. J Urol 1991; 146:141–4.
93. Essig KA, Sheldon CA, Brandt MT et al. Elevated intravesical pressure causes arterial hypoperfusion in canine colocystoplasty: a fluorometric assessment. J Urol 1991; 146:551–3.
94. Jayanthi VR, Churchill BM, McLorie GA, Khoury AE. Concomitant bladder neck closure and Mitrofanoff diversion for the management of intractable urinary incontinence. J Urol 1995; 154:886–8.
95. Fontaine E, Leaver R, Woodhouse CR. Diagnosis of perforated enterocystoplasty. J R Soc Med 2003; 96:393–4.
96. Braverman RM, Lebowitz RL. Perforation of the augmented urinary bladder in nine children and adolescents: importance of cystography. AJR Am J Roentgenol 1991; 157:1059–63.
97. Slaton JW, Kropp KA. Conservative management of suspected bladder rupture after augmentation enterocystoplasty. J Urol 1994; 152:713–15.
98. Sinaiko ES. Artificial bladder from segment of stomach and study effect of urine on gastric secretion. Surg Gynecol Obstet 1956; 102:433–8.
99. Leong CH, Ong GB. Gastrocystoplasty in dogs. Aust N Z J Surg 1972; 41:272–9.
100. Leong CH, Ong GB. Proceedings: gastrocystoplasty. Br J Urol 1975; 47:236.
101. Piser JA, Mitchell ME, Kulb TB et al. Gastrocystoplasty and colocystoplasty in canines: the metabolic conse-

quences of acute saline and acid loading. J Urol 1987; 138:1009–13.
102. Adams MC, Mitchell ME, Rink RC. Gastrocystoplasty: an alternative solution to the problem of urological reconstruction in the severely compromised patient. J Urol 1988; 140:1152–6.
103. Sheldon CA, Gilbert A, Wacksman J, Lewis AG. Gastrocystoplasty: technical and metabolic characteristics of the most versatile childhood bladder augmentation modality. J Pediatr Surg 1995; 30:283–7, discussion 287–8.
104. Kajbafzadeh AM, Quinn FM, Duffy PG, Ransley PG. Augmentation cystoplasty in boys with posterior urethral valves. J Urol 1995; 154:874–7.
105. Docimo SG, Moore RG, Adams J, Kavoussi LR. Laparoscopic bladder augmentation using stomach. Urology 1995; 46:565–9.
106. Reinberg Y, Manivel JC, Froemming C, Gonzalez R. Perforation of the gastric segment of an augmented bladder secondary to peptic ulcer disease. J Urol 1992; 148:369–71.
107. El-Ghoneimi A, Muller C, Guys JM et al. Functional outcome and specific complications of gastrocystoplasty for failed bladder exstrophy closure. J Urol 1998; 160:1186–9.
108. Dewan PA, Chacko J, Ashwood P. Gastrocystoplasty: technical and metabolic characteristics of the most versatile childhood bladder augmentation modality (Letter; Comment). J Pediatr Surg 1995; 30:1531–2.
109. Rink RC. Gastrocystoplasty. In: Hinman FJ, ed. Atlas of Pediatric Urologic Surgery. Philadelphia: WB Saunders, 1994: 472–3.
110. Raz S, Ehrlich RM, Babiarz JW, Payne CK. Gastrocystoplasty without opening the stomach. J Urol 1993; 150:713–15.
111. Kurzrock EA, Baskin LS, Kogan BA. Gastrocystoplasty: is there a consensus? World J Urol 1998; 16:242–50.
112. Kurzrock EA, Baskin LS, Kogan BA. Gastrocystoplasty: long-term followup. J Urol 1998; 160:2182–6.
113. Atala A, Bauer SB, Hendren WH, Retik AB. The effect of gastric augmentation on bladder function. J Urol 1993; 149:1099–102.
114. Gosalbez R Jr, Woodard JR, Broecker BH et al. The use of stomach in pediatric urinary reconstruction. J Urol 1993; 150:438–40.
115. Bogaert GA, Mevorach RA, Kogan BA. Urodynamic and clinical follow-up of 28 children after gastrocystoplasty. Br J Urol 1994; 74:469–75.
116. Chadwick Plaire J, Snodgrass WT, Grady RW, Mitchell ME. Long-term followup of the hematuria–dysuria syndrome. J Urol 2000; 164:921–3.
117. Nguyen DH, Bain MA, Salmonson KL. The syndrome of dysuria and hematuria in pediatric urinary reconstruction with stomach. J Urol 1993; 150:707–9.
118. Mingin GC, Stock JA, Hanna MK. Gastrocystoplasty: long-term complications in 22 patients. J Urol 1999; 162:1122–5.
119. Kinahan TJ, Khoury AE, McLorie GA, Churchill BM. Omeprazole in post-gastrocystoplasty metabolic alkalosis and aciduria. J Urol 1992; 47:435–7.
120. Mitchell ME. Gastrocystoplasty. In: Hinman FJ, ed. Atlas of Pediatric Urologic Surgery. Philadelphia: WB Saunders, 1994:473.
121. Leonard MP, Dharamsi N, Williot PE. Outcome of gastrocystoplasty in tertiary pediatric urology practice. J Urol 2000; 164:947–50.
122. Bogaert GA, Mevorach RA, Kim J, Kogan BA. The physiology of gastrocystoplasty: once a stomach, always a stomach. J Urol 1995; 153:1977–80.
123. Gosalbez R Jr, Woodard JR, Broecker BH, Warshaw B. Metabolic complications of the use of stomach for urinary reconstruction. J Urol 1993; 150:710–12.
124. Ortiz V, Goldenberg S. Hypergastrinemia following gastrocystoplasty in rats. Urol Res 1995; 23:361–3.
125. Plawker MW, Rabinowitz SS, Etwaru DJ, Glassberg KI. Hypergastrinemia, dysuria–hematuria and metabolic alkalosis: complications associated with gastrocystoplasty. J Urol 1995; 154:546–9.
126. Celayir S, Goksel S, Unal T, Buyukunal SN. *Helicobacter pylori* infection in a child with gastric augmentation. J Pediatr Surg 1997; 32:1757–8.
127. McDougal WS. Metabolic complications of urinary intestinal diversion. J Urol 1992; 147:1199–208.
128. Lewis AG, Gardner B, Gilbert A et al. Relative microbial resistance of gastric, ileal and cecal bladder augmentation in the rat. J Urol 1995; 154:1895–9.
129. Palmer LS, Palmer JS, Firlit BM, Firlit CF. Recurrent urolithiasis after augmentation gastrocystoplasty. J Urol 1998; 159:1331–2.
130. Lockhart JL, Davies R, Cox C et al. The gastroileoileal pouch: an alternative continent urinary reservoir for patients with short bowel, acidosis and/or extensive pelvic radiation. J Urol 1993; 150:46–50.
131. McLaughlin KP, Rink RC, Adams MC, Keating MA. Stomach in combination with other intestinal segments in pediatric lower urinary tract reconstruction. J Urol 1995; 154:1162–8.
132. Austin PF, DeLeary G, Homsy YL, Persky L, Lockhart JL. Long-term metabolic advantages of a gastrointestinal composite urinary reservoir. J Urol 1997; 158:1704–7, discussion 1707–8.
133. Austin PF, Rink RC, Lockhart JL. The gastrointestinal composite urinary reservoir in patients with myelomeningocele and exstrophy: long-term metabolic followup. J Urol 1999; 162:1126–8.
134. Austin PF, Lockhart JL, Bissada NK et al. Multi-institutional experience with the gastrointestinal composite reservoir. J Urol 2001; 165:2018–21.
135. Cartwright PC, Snow BW. Bladder autoaugmentation: partial detrusor excision to augment the bladder without use of bowel. J Urol 1989; 142:1050–3.
136. Cartwright PC, Snow BW. Bladder autoaugmentation: early clinical experience. J Urol 1989; 142:505–8, discussion 520–1.
137. Cartwright PC, Snow BW. Autoaugmentation cystoplasty. In: Dewan PA, Mitchell ME, eds. Bladder Augmentation. London: Edward Arnold, 1999: 83–92.
138. Duel BP, Gonzalez R, Barthold JS. Alternative techniques for augmentation cystoplasty. J Urol 1998; 59:998–1005.
139. Snow BW, Cartwright PC. Bladder autoaugmentation. Urol Clin North Am 1996; 23:323–31.
140. Dewan PA, Stefanek W, Lorenz C, Byard RW. Autoaug-

mentation omentocystoplasty in a sheep model. Urology 1994; 43:888–91.
141. Dewan PA, Owen AJ, Stefanek W et al. Late follow up of autoaugmentation omentocystoplasty in a sheep model. Aust N Z J Surg 1995; 65:596–9.
142. Rivas DA, Chancellor MB, Huang B et al. Comparison of bladder rupture pressure after intestinal bladder augmentation (ileocystoplasty) and myomyotomy (autoaugmentation). Urology 1996; 48:40–6.
143. Chancellor MB, Rivas DA, Bourgeois IM. Laplace's law and the risks and prevention of bladder rupture after enterocystoplasty and bladder autoaugmentation. Neurourol Urodyn 1996; 15:223–33.
144. Ahmed S, Sripathi V, Sen S. Perforation of an autoaugmented bladder. Aust N Z J Surg 1998; 68:617–19.
145. Johnson HW, Nigro MK, Stothers L. Laboratory variables of bladder autoaugmentation in an animal model. Urology 1994; 44:260–3.
146. Ehrlich RM, Gershman A. Laparoscopic seromyotomy (auto-augmentation) for non-neurogenic neurogenic bladder in a child: initial case report. Urology 1993; 42:175–8.
147. Braren V, Bishop MR. Laparoscopic bladder autoaugmentation in children. Urol Clin North Am 1998; 25:533–40.
148. Britanisky RG, Poppas DP, Shichman SN, Mininberg DT, Sora RE. Laparoscopic laser-assisted bladder autoaugmentation. Urology 1995; 46:31–5.
149. McDougall EM, Clayman RV, Figenshau RS, Pearle MS. Laparoscopic retropubic auto-augmentation of the bladder. J Urol 1995; 153:123–6.
150. Stothers L, Johnson H, Arnold W et al. Bladder autoaugmentation by vesicomyotomy in the pediatric neurogenic bladder. Urology 1994; 44:110–13.
151. Skobejko-Wlodarska L, Strulak K, Nachulewicz P, Szymkiewicz C. Bladder autoaugmentation in myelodysplastic children. Br J Urol 1998; 81(Suppl 3):114–16.
152. MacNeily AE, Afshar K, Coleman GU, Johnson HW. Autoaugmentation by detrusor myotomy: its lack of effectiveness in the management of congenital neuropathic bladder. J Urol 2003; 170:1643–6, discussion 1646.
153. Marte A, Di Meglio D, Cotrufo AM et al. A long-term follow-up of autoaugmentation in myelodysplastic children. BJU Int 2002; 89:928–31.
154. Stohrer M, Kramer A, Goepel M et al. Bladder auto-augmentation – an alternative for enterocystoplasty: preliminary results. Neurourol Urodyn 1995; 14:11–23.
155. Stohrer M, Kramer G, Goepel M et al. Bladder autoaugmentation in adult patients with neurogenic voiding dysfunction. Spinal Cord 1997; 35:456–62.
156. Leng WW, Blalock HJ, Fredriksson WH et al. Enterocystoplasty or detrusor myectomy? Comparison of indications and outcomes for bladder augmentation. J Urol 1999; 161:758–63.
157. Shoemaker WC. Reversed seromuscular grafts in urinary tract reconstruction. J Urol 1955; 74:453–75.
158. Shoemaker WC, Marucci HD. The experimental use of seromuscular grafts in bladder reconstruction: preliminary report. J Urol 1955; 73:314–21.
159. Cheng E, Rento R, Grayhack JT et al. Reversed seromuscular flaps in the urinary tract in dogs. J Urol 1994; 152:2252–7.
160. Oesch I. Neourothelium in bladder augmentation. An experimental study in rats. Eur Urol 1988; 14:328–9.
161. Salle JL, Fraga JC, Lucib A et al. Seromuscular enterocystoplasty in dogs. J Urol 1990; 144:454–6, discussion 460.
162. de Badiola F, Manivel JC, Gonzalez R. Seromuscular enterocystoplasty in rats. J Urol 1991; 146:559–62.
163. Close CE, Anderson PD, Edwards GA, Mitchell ME, Dewan PA. Autoaugmentation gastrocystoplasty: further studies of the sheep model. BJU Int 2004; 94:658–62.
164. Kibar Y, Tahmaz L, Onguru O, Dayanc M. Prevention of colonic mucosal regrowth after seromuscular enterocystoplasty. J Urol 2001; 165:2059–62.
165. Vastyan AM, Pinter AB, Farkas AP et al. Seromuscular gastrocystoplasty in dogs. Urol Int 2003; 71:215–18.
166. Denes ED, Vates TS, Freedman AL, Gonzalez R. Seromuscular colocystoplasty lined with urothelium protects dogs from acidosis during ammonium chloride loading. J Urol 1997; 158:1075–80.
167. Dewan PA, Lorenz C, Stefanek W, Byard RW. Urothelial lined colocystoplasty in a sheep model. Eur Urol 1994; 26:240–6.
168. Buson H, Manivel JC, Dayanc M et al. Seromuscular colocystoplasty lined with urothelium: experimental study. Urology 1994; 44:743–8.
169. Di Sandro MJ, Li Y, Baskin LS et al. Mesenchymal–epithelial interactions in bladder smooth muscle development: epithelial specificity. J Urol 1998; 160:1040–6, discussion 1079.
170. Baskin LS, Hayward SW, Sutherland RA et al. Mesenchymal–epithelial interactions in the bladder. World J Urol 1996; 14:301–9.
171. Dewan PA, Close CE, Byard RW et al. Enteric mucosal regrowth after bladder augmentation using demucosalized gut segments. J Urol 1997; 158:1141–6.
172. Gonzalez R, Jednak R, Franc-Guimond J, Schimke CM. Treating neuropathic incontinence in children with seromuscular colocystoplasty and an artificial urinary sphincter. BJU Int 2002; 90:909–11.
173. Carr MC, Docimo SG, Mitchell ME. Bladder augmentation with urothelial preservation. J Urol 1999; 162:1133–6, discussion 1137.
174. de Badiola F, Ruiz E, Puigdevall J et al. Sigmoid cystoplasty with argon beam without mucosa. J Urol 2001; 165:2253–5.
175. Lima SV, Araujo LA, Vilar FO, Kummer CL, Lima EC. Nonsecretory sigmoid cystoplasty: experimental and clinical results. J Urol 1995; 153:1651–4.
176. Lima SV, Araujo LA, Vilar FO. Nonsecretory intestinocystoplasty: a 10-year experience. J Urol 2004; 171:2636–9; discussion 2639–40.
177. Dewan PA, Stefanek W. Autoaugmentation gastrocystoplasty: early clinical results. Br J Urol 1994; 74:460–4.
178. Gonzalez R, Buson H, Reid C, Reinberg Y. Seromuscular colocystoplasty lined with urothelium: experience with 16 patients. Urology 1995; 45:124–9.
179. Jednak R, Schimke CM, Barroso U Jr, Barthold JS, Gonzalez R. Further experience with seromuscular colocystoplasty lined with urothelium. J Urol 2000; 164:2045–9.

180. Mitchell ME, Rink RC, Adams MC. Augmentation cystoplasty implantation of artificial urinary sphincter in men and women and reconstruction of the dysfunctional urinary tract. In: Walsh PC, Retik AB, Stamey TA, Vaughn ED, eds. Campbell's Urology, 6th ed. Philadelphia: WB Saunders, 1992:2654–716.
181. Wolf JS Jr, Turzan CW. Augmentation ureterocystoplasty. J Urol 1993; 149:1095–8.
182. Churchill BM, Aliabadi H, Landau EH et al. Ureteral bladder augmentation. J Urol 1993; 150:716–20.
183. Bellinger MF. Ureterocystoplasty: a unique method for vesical augmentation in children. J Urol 1993; 149: 811–13.
184. Bellinger MF. Ureterocystoplasty update. World J Urol 1998; 16:251–4.
185. Gosalbez R Jr, Kim CO Jr. Ureterocystoplasty with preservation of ipsilateral renal function. J Pediatr Surg 1996; 31:970–5.
186. Husmann DA, Snodgrass WT, Koyle MA et al. Ureterocystoplasty: indications for a successful augmentation. J Urol 2004; 171:376–80.
187. Nahas WC, Lucon M, Mazzucchi E et al. Clinical and urodynamic evaluation after ureterocystoplasty and kidney transplantation. J Urol 2004; 171:1428–31.
188. Kabalin JN. Surgical anatomy of the retroperitoneum, kidneys, and ureters. In: Walsh PC, Retik AB, Vaughn ED, Wein AG, eds. Campbell's Urology, 7th edn. Philadelphia: WB Saunders, 1998: 49–89.
189. Chung SY, Meldrum K, Docimo SG. Laparoscopic assisted reconstructive surgery: a 7-year experience. J Urol 2004; 171:372–5.
190. Cilento BG Jr, Diamond DA, Yeung CK et al. Laparoscopically assisted ureterocystoplasty. BJU Int 2003; 91:525–7.
191. Ben-Chaim J, Partin AW, Jeffs RD. Ureteral bladder augmentation using the lower pole ureter of a duplicated system. Urology 1996; 47:135–7.
192. Ahmed S, Neel KF, Sen S. Tandem ureterocystoplasty. Aust N Z J Surg 1998; 68:203–5.
193. Lailas NG, Cilento B, Atala A. Progressive ureteral dilation for subsequent ureterocystoplasty. J Urol 1996; 156:1151–3.
194. Ikeguchi EF, Stifelman MD, Hensle TW. Ureteral tissue expansion for bladder augmentation. J Urol 1998; 159:1665–8.
195. Stifelman MD, Ikeguchi EF, Hensle TW. Ureteral tissue expansion for bladder augmentation: a long-term prospective controlled trial in a porcine model. J Urol 1998; 160:1826–9.
196. Reinberg Y, Allen RC Jr, Vaughn M, McKenna PH. Nephrectomy combined with lower abdominal extraperitoneal ureteral bladder augmentation in the treatment of children with the vesicoureteral reflux dysplasia syndrome. J Urol 1995; 153:177–9.
197. Churchill BM, Jayanthi VR, Landau EH et al. Ureterocystoplasty: importance of the proximal blood supply. J Urol 1995; 154:197–8.
198. Landau EH, Jayanthi VR, Khoury AE et al. Bladder augmentation: ureterocystoplasty versus ileocystoplasty. J Urol 1994; 152:716–19.
199. Hitchcock RJ, Duffy PG, Malone PS. Ureterocystoplasty: the 'bladder' augmentation of choice. Br J Urol 1994; 73:575–9.
200. Pascual LA, Sentagne LM, Vega-Perugorria JM et al. Single distal ureter for ureterocystoplasty: a safe first choice tissue for bladder augmentation. J Urol 2001; 165:2256–8.
201. Tizzoni G, Poggi A. Die Wiederherstellung der Harnblase: experimentelle Untersuchungen. Centralbl Chir 1888; 15:921.
202. Kropp BP, Eppley BL, Prevel CD et al. Experimental assessment of small intestinal submucosa as a bladder wall substitute. Urology 1995; 46:396–400.
203. Sutherland RS, Baskin LS, Hayward SW, Cunha GR. Regeneration of bladder urothelium, smooth muscle, blood vessels and nerves into an acellular tissue matrix. J Urol 1996; 156:571–7.
204. Piechota HJ, Dahms SE, Nunes LS. In vitro functional properties of the rat bladder regenerated by the bladder acellular matrix graft. J Urol 1998; 159:1717–24.
205. Bohne AW, Osborn RW, Hettle PJ. Regeneration of the urinary bladder in the dog, following total cystectomy. Surg Gynecol Obstet 1955; 100:259–64.
206. Bohne AW, Urwiller KL. Experience with urinary bladder regeneration. J Urol 1957; 77:725–32.
207. Kudish HG. The use of polyvinyl sponge for experimental cystoplasty. J Urol 1957; 78:232.
208. Swinney J, Tomlinson BE, Walder DN. Urinary tract substitution. Br J Urol 1961; 33:414–27.
209. Ashkar L, Heller E. The silastic bladder patch. J Urol 1967; 98:679–83.
210. Agishi T, Nakazono M, Kiraly RJ et al. Biodegradable material for bladder reconstruction. J Biomed Mater Res 1975; 9:119–31.
211. Scott R, Mohammed R, Gorham SD et al. The evolution of a biodegradable membrane for use in urological surgery. A summary of 109 in vivo experiments. Br J Urol 1988; 62:26–31.
212. Kambic H, Kay R, Chen JF et al. Biodegradable pericardial implants for bladder augmentation: a 2.5-year study in dogs. J Urol 1992; 148:539–43.
213. Gorham S, McCafferty I, Baraza R, Scott R. Preliminary development of a collagen membrane for use in urological surgery. Urol Res 1984; 12:295–9.
214. Fishman IJ, Flores FN, Scott B et al. Use of fresh placental membranes for bladder reconstruction. J Urol 1987; 138:1291.
215. Probst M, Dahiya R, Carrier S, Tanagho EA. Reproduction of functional smooth muscle tissue and partial bladder replacement. Br J Urol 1997; 79:505–15.
216. Reddy PP, Barrieras DJ, Wilson G. Regeneration of functional bladder substitutes using large segmented acellular matrix allografts in a porcine model. J Urol 2000; 164:936–41.
217. Kropp BP. Small-intestinal submucosa for bladder augmentation: a review of preclinical studies. World J Urol 1998; 16:262–7.
218. Badylak SF, Lantz GC, Coffey A, Geddes LA. Small intestinal submucosa as a large diameter vascular graft in the dog. J Surg Res 1989; 47:74–80.
219. Lantz GC, Badylak SF, Coffey AC et al. Small intestinal submucosa as a small-diameter arterial graft in the dog. J Invest Surg 1990; 3:217–27.

220. Lantz GC, Badylak SF, Coffey AC et al. Small intestinal submucosa as a superior vena cava graft in the dog. J Surg Res 1992; 53:175–81.
221. Kropp BP, Badylak S, Thor KB. Regenerative bladder augmentation: a review of the initial preclinical studies with porcine small intestinal submucosa. Adv Exp Med Biol 1985; 385:229–35.
222. Kropp BP, Rippy MK, Badylak SF et al. Regenerative urinary bladder augmentation using small intestinal submucosa: urodynamic and histopathologic assessment in long-term canine bladder augmentations. J Urol 1996; 155:2098–104.
223. Kropp BP, Sawyer BD, Shannon HE et al. Characterization of small intestinal submucosa regenerated canine detrusor: assessment of reinnervation, in vitro compliance and contractility. J Urol 1986; 156:599–607.
224. Badylak SF. The immunogenic response of SIS (pers comm), 1994.
225. Metzger DW, Moyad TF, McPherson T, Badylak SF. Cytokine and antibody responses to xenogeneic SIS transplants. In: First SIS Symposium, Orlando, Florida, 1996.
226. Badylak SF. Xenogeneic extracellular matrix as a scaffold for tissue reconstruction. Transpl Immunol 2004; 12:367–77.
227. Badylak SF. Speculation (with a little evidence) for the roles of cell proliferation, differentiation, neovascularization, and environmental stressors in SIS-induced remodeling. In: First SIS Symposium, Orlando, Florida, 1996.
228. Voytik-Harbin SL, Brightman AO, Kraine MR et al. Identification of extractable growth factors from small intestinal submucosa. J Cell Biochem 1997; 67:478–91.
229. Hodde JP, Badylak SF, Brightman AO, Voytik-Harbin SL. Glycosaminoglycan content of small intestinal submucosa: a bioscaffold for tissue replacement. Tissue Eng 1996; 2:209–17.
230. Kropp BP, Cheng EY, Lin HK et al. Reliable and reproducible bladder regeneration using unseeded distal small intestinal submucosa. J Urol 2004; 172:1710–13.
231. Raghavan D, Kropp BP, Lin HK et al. Physical characteristics of small intestinal submucosa scaffolds are location-dependent. J Biomed Mater Res A 2005; 73:90–6.
232. Piechota HJ, Dahms SE, Probst M et al. Functional rat bladder regeneration through xenotransplantation of the bladder acellular matrix graft. Br J Urol 1998; 81:548–59.
233. Thapa A, Miller DC, Webster TJ, Haberstroh KM. Nano-structured polymers enhance bladder smooth muscle cell function. Biomaterials 2003; 24:2915–26.
234. Hutmacher DW. Scaffold design and fabrication technologies for engineering tissues – state of the art and future perspectives. J Biomater Sci Polym Ed 2001; 12:107–24.
235. Pope JC, Davis MM, Smith ER Jr et al. The ontogeny of canine small intestinal submucosa regenerated bladder. J Urol 1997; 158:1105–10.
236. Master VA, Wei G, Liu W et al. Urothelium facilitates the recruitment and trans-differentiation of fibroblasts into smooth muscle in acellular matrix. J Urol 2003; 170:1628–32.
237. Kanematsu A, Yamamoto S, Noguchi T et al. Bladder regeneration by bladder acellular matrix combined with sustained release of exogenous growth factor. J Urol 2003; 170:1633–8.
238. Cilento BG, Freeman MR, Schneck FX et al. Phenotypic and cytogenetic characterization of human bladder urothelia expanded in vitro. J Urol 1994; 152:665–70.
239. Atala A, Vacanti JP, Peters CA et al. Formation of urothelial structures in vivo from dissociated cells attached to biodegradable polymer scaffolds in vitro. J Urol 1992; 148:658–62.
240. Yoo JJ, Meng J, Oberpenning F, Atala A. Bladder augmentation using allogenic bladder submucosa seeded with cells. Urology 1998; 51:221–5.
241. Oberpenning F, Meng J, Yoo JJ, Atala A. De novo reconstitution of a functional mammalian urinary bladder by tissue engineering. Nat Biotechnol 1999; 17:149–55.
242. Zhang YY, Kropp BP, Lin HK et al. Bladder regeneration with cell-seeded small intestinal submucosa. Tissue Eng 2004; 10:181–7.
243. Pariente JL, Kim BS, Atala A. In vitro biocompatibility evaluation of naturally derived and synthetic biomaterials using normal human bladder smooth muscle cells. J Urol 2002; 167:1867–71.
244. Schoeller T, Neumeister MW, Huemer GM et al. Capsule induction technique in a rat model for bladder wall replacement: an overview. Biomaterial 2004; 25: 1663–73.
245. Walker BR, Gardner MP, Gatti HM et al. Bladder augmentation in dogs using the tissue capsule formed around a perivesical tissue expander. J Urol 2002; 168:1534–6.
246. Fraser M, Thomas DF, Pitt E et al A surgical model of composite cystoplasty with cultured urothelial cells: a controlled study of gross outcome and urothelial phenotype. BJU Int 2004; 93:609–16.
247. Aktug T, Ozdemir T, Agartan C et al. Experimentally prefabricated bladder. J Urol 2001; 165:2055–8.
248. Schultheiss D, Gabouev AI, Cebotari S et al. Biological vascularized matrix for bladder tissue engineering: matrix preparation, reseeding technique and short-term implantation in a porcine model. J Urol 2005; 173:276–80.
249. Lin HK, Cowan R, Moore P et al. Characterization of neuropathic bladder smooth muscle cells in culture. J Urol 2004; 171:1348–52.

Urinary diversion

57

Mark P Cain, Peter D Metcalfe, and Richard C Rink

Introduction

The past 30 years have seen unprecedented advances in lower urinary reconstruction in children. The majority of congenital urologic abnormalities can now be addressed by primary reconstruction with the exception of urinary and fecal continence. These procedures can be performed even in small infants. Thus, the need for permanent conduit diversion with the storage receptacle outside the body as a bag has dwindled, and is now used primarily in children who can never live an independent lifestyle. In children where permanent urinary diversion is required, it is nearly always with a continent urinary reservoir that is then emptied by intermittent catheterization. This chapter will focus primarily on continent urinary reservoirs (CURs).

Some urologic problems are still encountered where severe urinary obstruction in the neonate may prevent definitive reconstruction. In this patient population temporary diversion may be necessary. Intubated diversions are generally reserved for patients requiring a short duration (weeks to a few months) of urinary drainage. These may be especially useful in the setting of an unstable or a small premature child that requires relief of obstruction, or when renal function cannot be adequately assessed without first alleviating the obstruction. These non-continent urinary diversions will be briefly discussed.

Temporary urinary diversion

Temporary intubated diversions

Urethral catheter

The most frequently used intubated urinary diversion is the urethral catheter. The most common pediatric urologic condition managed initially with a urethral catheter in the neonate is posterior urethral valves (PUV). A 5 or 8 Fr feeding tube is usually placed to drain the bladder temporarily prior to endoscopic valve fulguration. In males with dilatation of the posterior urethra, the catheter will occasionally coil in the prostatic urethra and incompletely drain the bladder. In this scenario, a small lacrimal duct probe can be used as a catheter guide. It is sometimes helpful to place a finger in the rectum to elevate and straighten the prostatic urethra during catheter placement. Whenever the catheter is difficult to pass, it is appropriate to obtain an abdominal radiograph, after injecting a small amount of contrast through the catheter, to ensure its proper position in the bladder. In the older child who requires bladder drainage, a 6 or 8 Fr balloon (Foley) catheter is a reasonable alternative. Intermittent catheterization is another option for children with urinary retention and has proven to be safe in even the neonate.

Complications of urethral catheters in children are usually related to improper placement or prolonged use, and include urethral injury, urethritis or meatitis, urinary tract infection (UTI), urethral stricture, and bladder stones. Care must be taken when using a feeding tube as a catheter in the small infant/neonate to avoid coiling the catheter in the bladder, which can result in a knot in the tube that will often require a cystotomy to remove.

Percutaneous suprapubic cystotomy

In rare circumstances when a urethral catheter is contraindicated or cannot be placed, a suprapubic cystotomy tube can provide short- or long-term bladder drainage. Percutaneous cystotomy is very useful in the infant or child with urethral trauma or following a reconstructive procedure for epispadias or complex hypospadias in the older child. Kits are available that allow catheter placement either simultaneously with the trocar (Stamey percutaneous suprapubic catheter set; Cook Urological, Spencer, Indiana, USA) or through it (Cystocath suprapubic drainage system; Dow Corning, Midland, Michigan, USA). A full bladder is an absolute prerequisite to percutaneous catheter placement and can be confirmed sonographically if needed. If necessary, the bladder can be filled with a small urethral catheter or by placing a small percutaneous angiocatheter or spinal needle into the bladder for localization, and filling the bladder until it is easily palpable. When attempting to place a suprapubic tube in the awake child, conscious sedation and infiltration of the skin and fascia with 1% lidocaine can be used to prevent anxiety and pain. It is helpful to establish the distance from the skin to the bladder lumen with a small needle to prevent injury to structures posterior to the bladder. The trocar is passed with gentle pressure until urine is obtained and the catheter is passed 1–2 cm beyond the trocar. Alternatively, the percutaneous cystotomy tube and obturator needle are passed together into the bladder until urine is obtained, then the catheter is advanced over the obturator. A recently described technique using the light from a flexible cystoscope to help localize the position of the bladder dome may allow percutaneous tube cystotomy in the more difficult cases.[1] In children with a history of prior reconstruction bladder surgery, it is often safest to use the site of a prior suprapubic tract that is fixed to the posterior abdominal fascia to place a suprapubic tube. The catheter is fixed to the skin with permanent suture. These tubes are designed for temporary bladder drainage, and long-term use has been associated with bladder wall thickening and contracture, UTI, bladder stones, and upper urinary tract dilatation.[2,3]

Surgically placed cystotomy

Because of the relative ease and safety of percutaneous cystotomy tube placement, open suprapubic tube placement is rarely used except in the context of a more extensive reconstructive procedure, or for placement of a large-bore drainage tube following urethral or bladder trauma. Another indication for the open technique is in a patient that has had prior extensive pelvic procedures which may have resulted in bowel adhesions to the anterior dome of the bladder.

With the patient in the supine position, the prevesical space is exposed using either a low transverse abdominal incision or a low vertical midline incision for those that may later undergo a transabdominal reconstructive procedure. After mobilizing the bladder dome, stay sutures are placed and a small cystotomy is made. The catheter is first brought through a small skin incision and then through the rectus fascia and muscle. After the tube has been placed in the bladder, it is pulled to the dome of the bladder, and secured with a purse-string suture at the bladder. Bladder muscle adjacent to the tube is secured to the posterior fascial wall with absorbable suture, and the suprapubic tube is sutured to the skin.

Ureteral stents

Ureteral stents are frequently used for temporary upper tract drainage following reconstruction, trauma, or stone surgery in children. There are two general options available: either an entirely internal stent or an external ureteral stent with one end brought out through the skin or via the urethra. External stents have traditionally been used more frequently in children following open surgery, as they do not require an anesthetic for removal and do not carry the same risk of proximal migration found with internal stents. Problems that can be associated with JJ stents in children[4] include:

- obstruction
- encrustation/stone formation
- infection
- proximal migration
- stent fragmentation
- discomfort/bladder spasms
- requirement of anesthesia for removal of stent
- hematuria.

Internal JJ stents can be placed either at the time of open surgery, endoscopically, or by means of an antegrade approach through a percutaneous nephrostomy tract. Endoscopic placement of internal stents is usually done fluoroscopically over a wire in the small patient because of the smaller size of the working port of pediatric cystoscopes that will not permit passage of the stent under direct vision.

Percutaneous nephrostomy

Improvements in the expertise and availability of pediatric interventional radiologists has led to percutaneous nephrostomy tube drainage almost completely replacing the need for open nephrostomy tube placement in children. Indications for nephrostomy tube drainage in children include obstruction, renal/ureteral calculi, pyonephrosis, fungal bezoar, or for a diagnostic Whitaker test. Although general anesthesia will often be required in the young or uncooperative child, the procedure can frequently be performed with sedation only,[5] and has been performed with just local anesthesia in small neonates in the intensive care unit.[6] The technique most commonly used is the Seldinger technique. A small needle is placed into the renal pelvis with radiographic guidance. A small guidewire is then passed into the renal pelvis and the tract is dilated until a nephrostomy tube can be easily advanced. Several types of nephrostomy tubes are commercially available, most of which rely on a 'pigtail' curl to maintain their position within the renal pelvis. It is critical that broad-spectrum intravenous antibiotics be initiated before tube placement, especially in the child with obstruction and infection to prevent urosepsis. Complications directly related to the procedure are rare[7,8] and include:

- hemorrhage
- urosepsis
- arteriovenous fistula/pseudoaneurysms
- urinary extravasation
- pneumothorax
- bowel injury
- air embolism.

Percutaneous nephrostomy tube placement and irrigation with antifungal agents comprise the first-line therapy for neonates with obstructing fungal bezoars.[9–12] In addition to draining the obstruction and providing access for intermittent irrigation of the obstructed collecting system, the fungal ball can be fragmented with the guidewire at the time of tube placement, which will lead to more rapid clearance of the fungal debris.

Open nephrostomy tube

Open nephrostomy tube placement is rarely necessary, and only utilized when nephrostomy is technically not possible, or carries an unacceptable risk. High-risk conditions include low platelet count, a solitary kidney, abnormal renal position following a complicated reconstruction of the renal pelvis, and exploration for renal trauma when significant injury to the ureter or pelvis has occurred. The kidney is exposed through a flank incision and mobilized until the renal pelvis is identified. Stay sutures are placed, and the renal pelvis is opened. A clamp is placed into an inferior calyx. A small nephrotomy is made and the Malecot catheter is advanced into the renal pelvis, as shown in Figure 57.1. The catheter is secured to the renal capsule with a purse-string chromic suture. The nephrostomy tube is brought out through a stab incision in the skin and secured. A small Penrose drain is left in the renal fossa. Some newer catheters come preassembled as either simple nephrostomy catheters or nephrostents, often with an attached trocar that can be advanced in a retrograde fashion out of the selected calyx.

Temporary non-intubated diversion

Cutaneous vesicostomy

Cutaneous vesicostomy continues to be the most widely used and simplest method for temporary bladder drainage. Most commonly it is used for patients

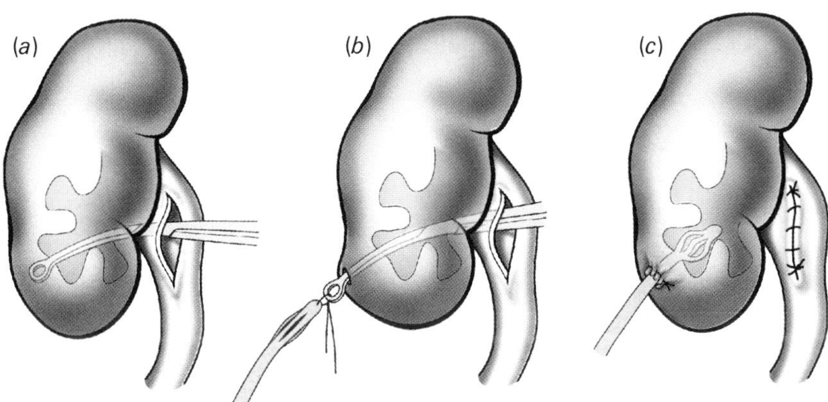

Figure 57.1 Technique for open nephrostomy. A small Randall forcep or right angle clamp is passed through an inferior calyx via a small pyelotomy incision. The renal capsule is incised with electrocautery and the catheter is advanced into the calyx. The catheter is secured to the renal capsule with absorbable suture. The pyelotomy is closed with either running or interrupted, absorbable suture.

with a neuropathic bladder or PUV, in situations where clean intermittent catheterization (CIC) is not possible. In multiple series temporary diversion with vesicostomy has resulted in significant improvement in urinary tract dilatation, stabilization of renal function, and decrease in the frequency and severity of febrile UTIs.[3,13–15] The introduction of CIC in early infancy has limited the role of vesicostomy in some centers, and has provided equivalent long-term results.[16] One concern regarding temporary cutaneous vesicostomy is potential impairment in bladder function due to inadequate cycling of the detrusor during the period of diversion.[17] Jayanthi et al reported on a large group of patients who underwent cutaneous vesicostomy and eventual bladder closure. They found no significant alteration in eventual bladder capacity or function.[18] These findings were also supported in a series of patients with PUV managed with either valve ablation or urinary tract diversion, with no evidence of bladder dysfunction based on urodynamics findings in those who had diversion with vesicostomy.[19]

Two basic techniques have been described for cutaneous vesicostomy in children. The procedure described by Lapides involves creation of extensive skin flaps to allow a tension-free anastomosis of the bladder to the skin, and a very wide stoma that is less prone to stenosis.[20] This procedure was initially intended as a semi-permanent form of vesicostomy in the adult patient, where the bladder position is deeper in the bony pelvis. Because of the complexity of both creating and taking down the Lapides vesicostomy, there is limited application for the majority of pediatric patients. The more popular technique for vesicostomy in children was described by Blocksom and modified by Duckett, as outlined in Figure 57.2.[3,21] Key technical points are adequate mobilization of the bladder dome for a tension-free anastomosis to the fascia and skin, use of the dome of the bladder to create the stoma, and creating an adequate caliber stoma (at least 22 Fr) that is flush with the skin.[3,22]

Common problems following vesicostomy are listed in Table 57.1. The majority of complications that lead to stomal revision are secondary either to technical errors of stomal placement inferior to the dome of the bladder, inadequate stomal diameter, or primary bladder pathology that results in an extremely thick-walled bladder that does not allow for straightforward creation of an adequate-caliber stoma.

Bladder prolapse through the vesicostomy stoma is usually due to placement of the stoma too inferior, allowing the posterior bladder wall to evert through the stoma. Acute prolapse can usually be managed with manual decompression and bladder drainage with a catheter through the vesicostomy until the edema subsides. On rare occasions, the prolapsed bladder will incarcerate due to vascular congestion. This requires emergency reduction under anesthesia. Revision of the vesicostomy by moving the stoma to a more superior position in the dome of the bladder will prevent recurrence.

Table 57.1 Complications of cutaneous vesicostomy

Complication	Frequency (%)
Stomal prolapse	9–17
Stomal stenosis	3–12
Peristomal dermatitis	3–14
Stone formation	3–7
Parastomal hernia	3–4

From Skoog.[22]

Stomal stenosis will often present with either UTI or hydronephrosis. Stenosis is thought to occur secondary to excess tension on the skin anastomosis or too small of a fascial opening, and is more frequent in patients with very thick-walled bladder or patients with prune belly syndrome.[3,22] Simple revision with creation of a wider-caliber stoma or use of a small V-shaped skin flap to disrupt the circumferential stomal scar tissue will usually correct the problem and prevent recurrence.

Cutaneous ureterostomy

The indications and need for temporary and permanent urinary diversion with cutaneous ureterostomy or pyelostomy have been significantly reduced over the past several decades. Advances in percutaneous and endoscopic techniques and the ability to perform these procedures even in the smallest neonates or infants have contributed to the trend away from cutaneous upper tract diversion. In addition, we have a better understanding of the pathophysiology and natural history of the dilated ureter in childhood, which has led to observation with radiographic surveillance instead of early surgical intervention in many circumstances. There are still clear indications for ureterostomy to decompress massively dilated upper tracts, for example in the neonate or infant who is not a candidate for reconstruction because of size or acute UTI, or when there is a question of recoverable function in the involved kidney. In this latter instance, an interval of diversion may help one to decide between reconstruction and nephrectomy.[23]

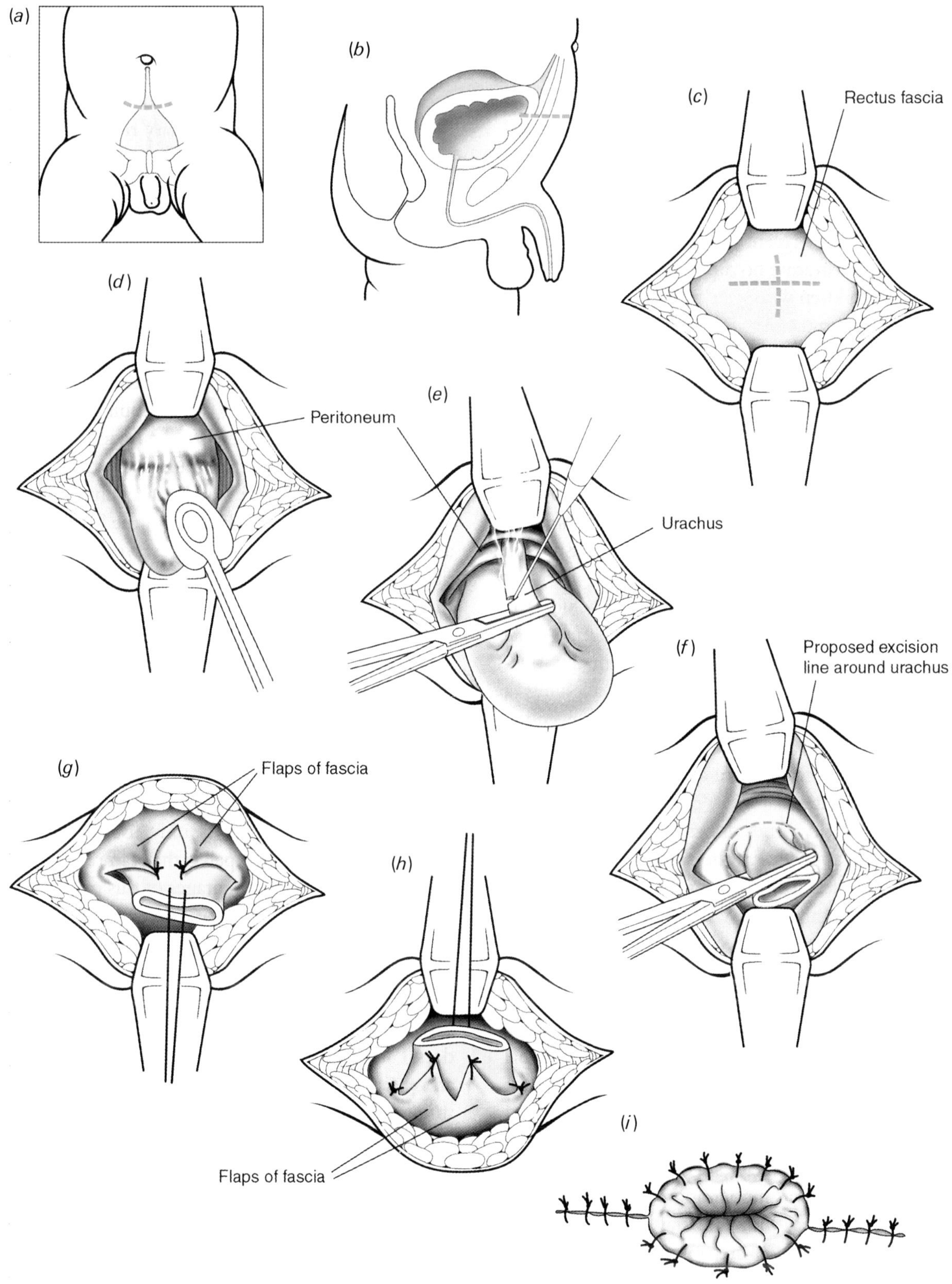

Figure 57.2 Technical points for Blocksom vesicostomy. (*a* and *b*) A small transverse skin incision is made midway between the pubis and umbilicus. (*c*) The rectus fascia is opened vertically and horizontally and the muscle is retracted laterally. (*d*) Stay sutures are placed in the bladder and the peritoneum is bluntly mobilized superiorly, exposing the bladder dome. (*e*) The urachus is identified and divided. The urachal segment is mobilized until it reaches the skin without tension. (*f*) The urachus is excised, ensuring an adequate caliber opening into the bladder (22–24 Fr). (*g*) The detrusor is circumferentially secured to the rectus fascia. (*h*) The lateral edges of the fascia are closed, allowing easy passage of a 22–24 Fr sound. (*i*) The bladder mucosa and detrusor are secured to the skin, and the lateral skin edges are closed in layers.

Figure 57.16 Caption opposite

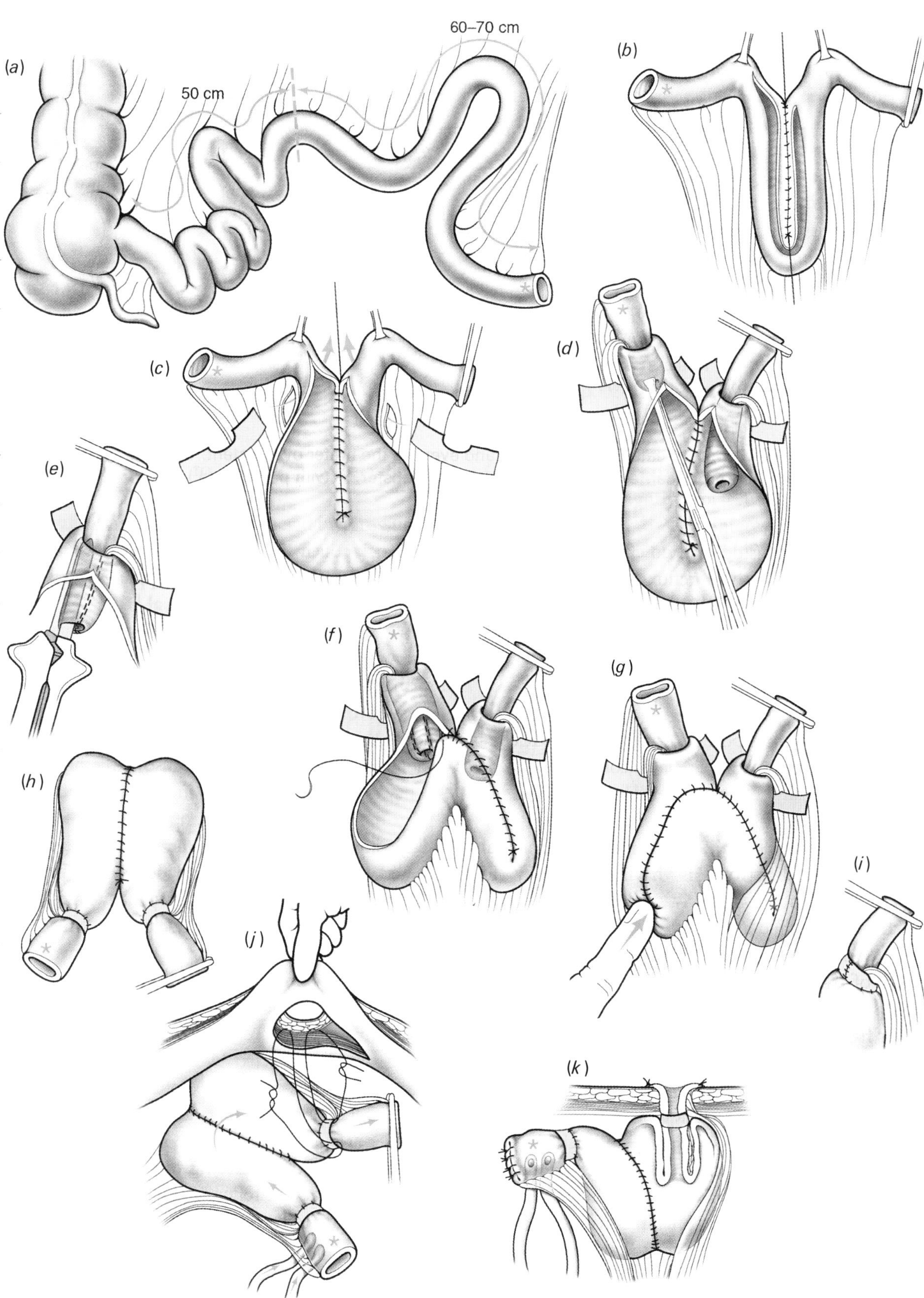

Figure 57.16 Kock pouch (continent ileal reservoir). (*a*) Bowel segment measuring 60–70 cm is isolated approximately 50 cm from the ileocecal valve and positioned as the letter U with the terminal end directed toward the head of the patient and the bottom of the U toward the left side of the patient. (*b*) The legs of the U are united at the antimesenteric border with continuous 3–0 polyglycolic acid sutures. (*c*) The intestine is divided adjacent to the suture line and the incision is continued for 3 cm on the afferent limb. The mucous membrane is sutured with continuous 3–0 polyglycolic acid sutures. Openings are made in the mesentery supplying the future base of the nipple valves. (*d*) Intussusception of the afferent and efferent segments into the future reservoir. (*e*) The nipple valves are secured with staples. (*f*) The reservoir is closed with two continuous inverting 3–0 polyglycolic acid sutures. (*g–h*) The reservoir is brought into its final position by pushing the corners of the reservoir downwards between mesenteric leaves. (*i*) A fascia of Marlex mesh encircles the base of the nipple valve, and the ends are approximated with three or four non-absorbable sutures. The reservoir wall is sutured to the cylinder with 3–0 polyglycolic acid sutures. (*j*) The cylinder at the efferent segment is attached to the opening and anterior rectus sheath with non-absorbable sutures. (*k*) The completed continent ileal reservoir.

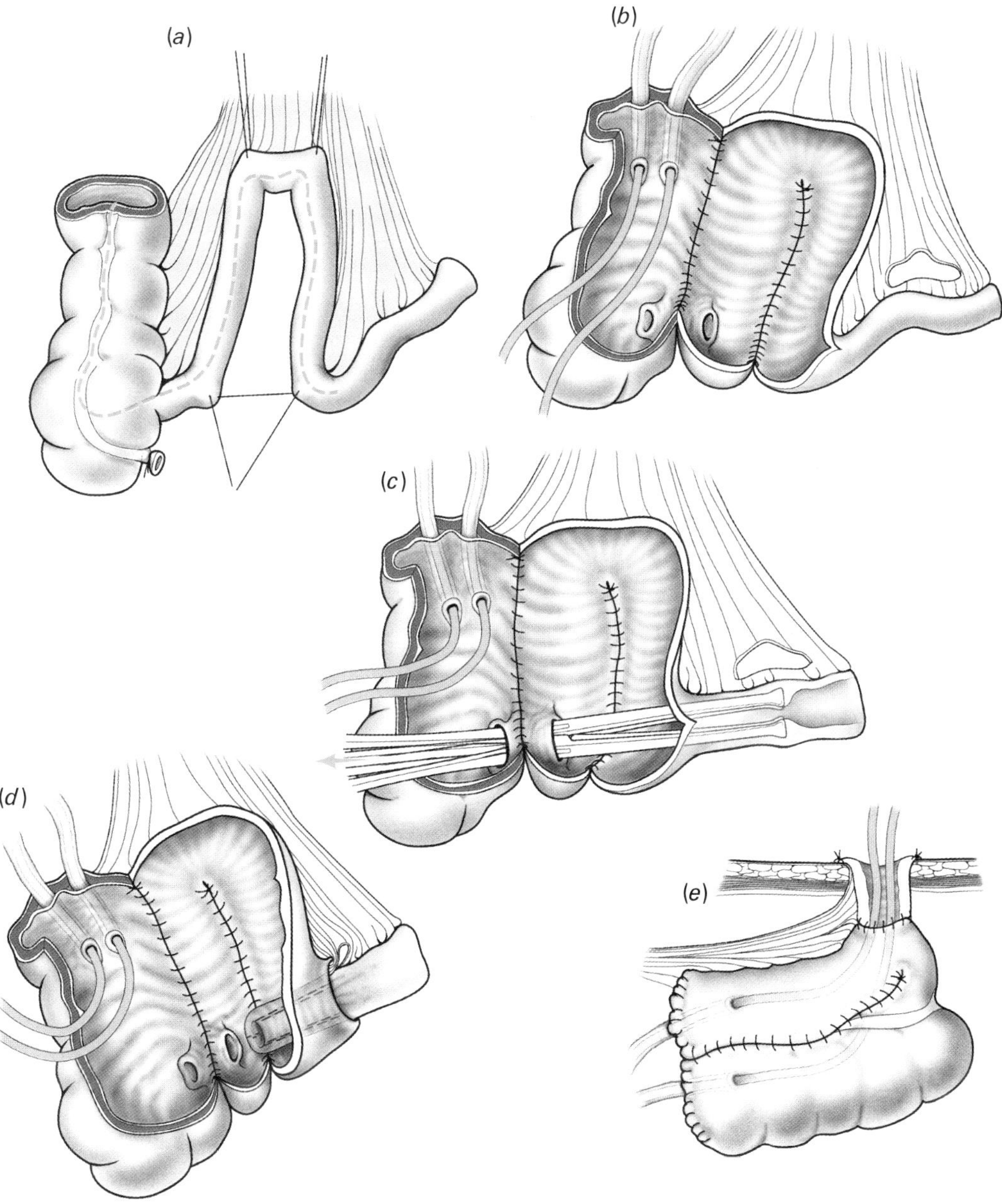

Figure 57.17 The Mainz pouch utilizes intussuscepted ileum pulled through the ileocecal valve (*c*) as the continence mechanism.

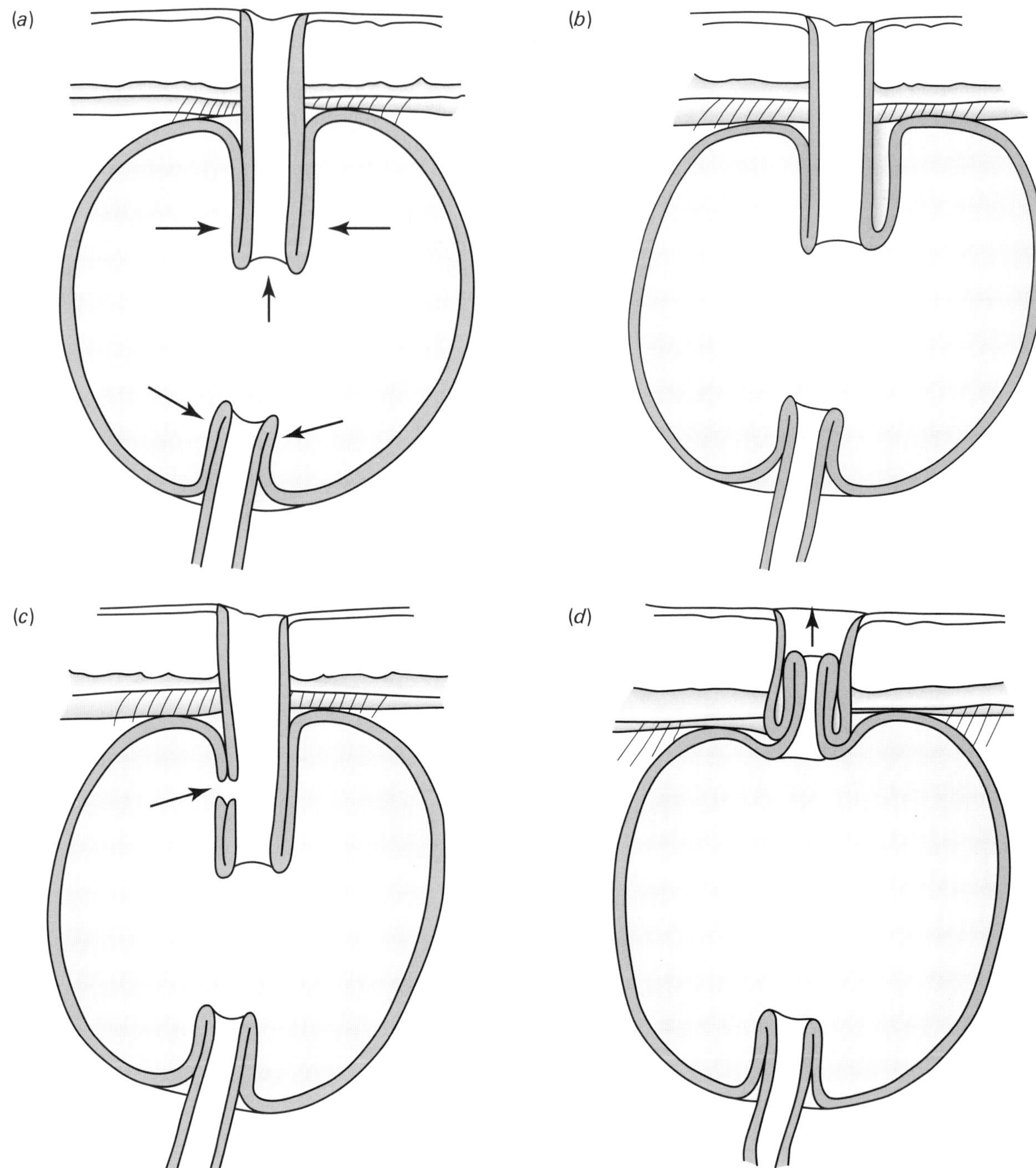

Figure 57.18 Nipple valves. (*a*) Hydrostatic forces exerted on the nipple to provide continence. (*b*) Breakdown of nipple, yielding incontinence. (*c*) Fistula of nipple, yielding incontinence. (*d*) Prolapse of nipple, resulting in inability to catheterize.

patients, with the vast majority involving the efferent nipple.[63] The large amount of ileum required (78 cm), the complexity of the procedure, and the requirement for two nipples with stapling and collar fixation, have deterred its widespread use in children, but it does provide the least contractile and most compliant reservoir, with pouch capacities ultimately over 700 ml.[67] Hanna and Bloiso achieved success in a small series in children, but modified the nipple to avoid the use of staples and Marlex.[157] Benson and Olsson noted that nipple failure occurs in approximately 15% in the best of hands, with the three most common complications of the nipple being pinhole fistulae at the base of the nipple, nipple valve prolapse, and shortening of the nipple length.[67] Because of this high complication rate, they no longer recommend its routine use.[151]

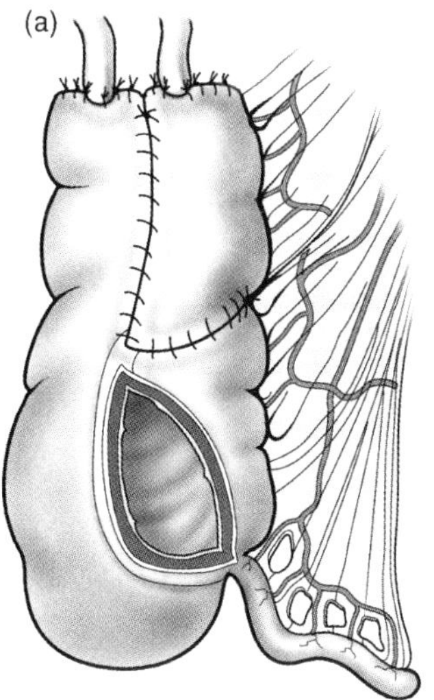

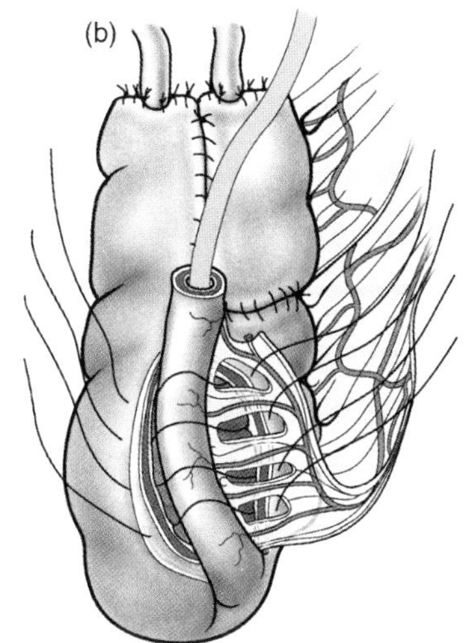

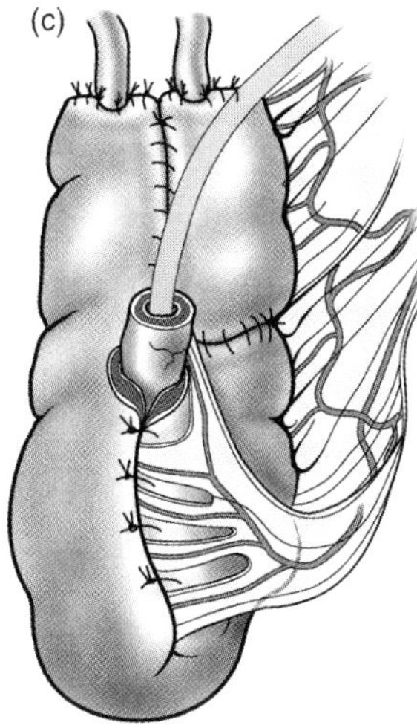

Figure 57.19 Mainz pouch with appendix. (*a*) The cecum has been patched with ileum. A seromuscular incision is made in the tenia. (*b*) Mesenteric windows are made in the mesoappendix. (*c*) The appendix is placed in the submucosal tunnel and the cecum is closed over it, avoiding the appendiceal vasculature.

The ileocecal valve is commonly used as a continence mechanism with the cecum acting as the reservoir. However, in its native form it is functionally adequate in only 25% of the population.[158,159] Rendelmen et al found that at 25 cmH_2O, the valve is incompetent in 25%.[159] This incompetence increases such that only 7% are continent at 50 cmH_2O pressure.[159] Reinforcement to achieve continence was achieved by Zinman and Libertino by wrapping the cecum around the ileum.[160] Intussusception of the ileocecal valve as a nipple to enhance its continence is the basis for the pouch described by Mansson et al.[154] The Mainz pouch (mixed augmentation with ileum and cecum) uses tunneled ureteral implants to prevent ureteral reflux and an unusual nipple valve for continence with the reservoir created by combining the cecum and ileum (see Figure 57.17). The ileum is intussuscepted to create a nipple, which is then pulled through the ileocecal valve and secured by stapling. Continence rates have been greater than 95% and reservoir capacities greater than 600 ml in 179 patients, 41 of whom were children.[161–163] Again, owing to nipple complications and the difficulty in constructing them, the Mainz group no longer uses the nipple but instead an in-situ appendix, which is imbricated in the cecum, as the continence mechanism (Figure 57.19). Stein et al reported 374 patients undergoing a Mainz pouch in which 116 had the appendix as the continence mechanism with 6.7% having early complications and 25% late complications.[164] All of the incontinence occurred with use of the nipple valves, while none of the appendiceal efferent stomas were incontinent. Gerharz et al[165] compared the two continence mechanisms in the Mainz pouch (96 appendiceal stomas, 106 ileal nipples) and noted that 17% of the appendiceal stomas required 23 reinterventions with all but two being for stenosis. Nipple valves required a second operation in 12.3%, but the revisions were much simpler in the appendiceal group and this has become their preferred method. If the appendix is not available, a Lampel tube of cecum (Figure 57.20a) or submuscular tube (Figure 57.20b) is now used.[166] The Mainz group also looked at vitamin A, B, B_2, B_6, D, and E and folic acid levels, as well as bone density, after these diversions, and all were within normal limits.[167] Vitamin B_{12} levels and bone density were normal in the 51 children, but dropped significantly in adults. They recommend checking vitamin B_{12} levels after 4 years.[167]

The appendix has also been used by others to create an intussuscepted nipple as a continence mechanism for a right colon pouch.[168–170] There is only minimal intussusception in the Bissada technique,[169] but Issa et al reinforced this with a mesh wrap similar to the ileal nipple in the Kock pouch.[168] Tillem et al reinforce the appendix only if leakage is demonstrated after filling the cecum to 60 cmH_2O.[170]

An interesting nipple valve was developed by Benchekroun[171,172] and modified by Guzman et al.[173] The ileum is inverted into itself to create an 'inkwell' system whereby urine enters between the walls and compresses the inner layer for continence (Figure 57.21). Benchekroun et al reported 136 patients with

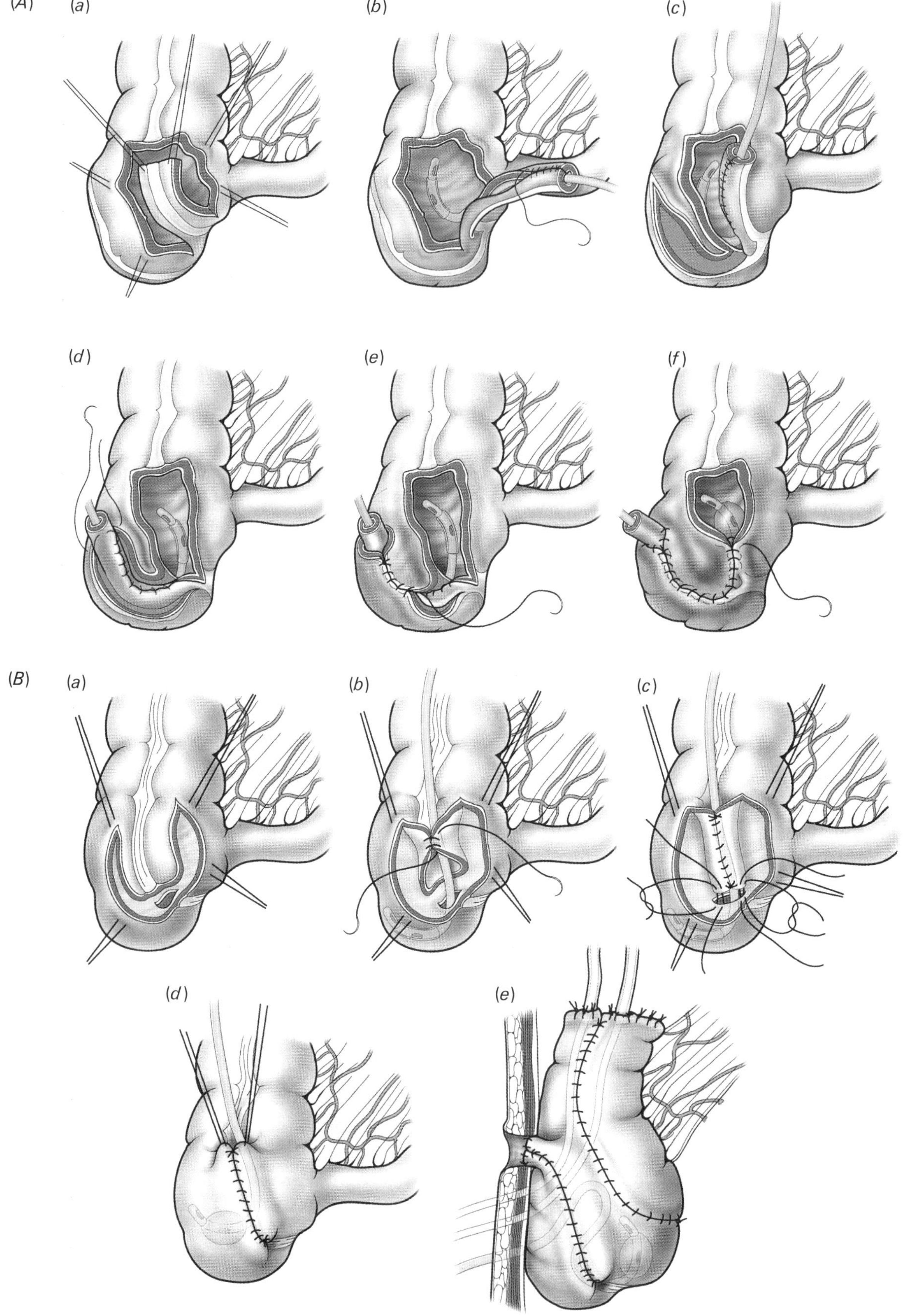

Figure 57.20 (*A*) Lampel tube. (*a–c*) A full-thickness bowel flap is elevated and tubularized over an 18 Fr catheter. (*d–f*) It is then placed in a submucosal subtineal tunnel and the bowel wall is closed. (*B*) Lampel seromuscular tube. (*a* and *b*) The elevated seromuscular layer is tubularized over an 18 Fr catheter and (*c*) anastomosed at its base to the mucosal opening. (*d*) The bowel wall is closed over the tube and (*e*) brought to the umbilicus as a catheterizable stoma. (Reproduced from Lampel et al,[166] with permission.)

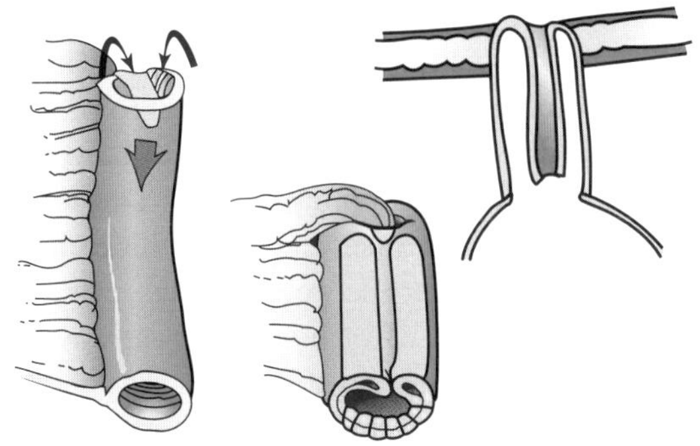

Figure 57.21 The Benchekroun ileo-nipple.

75% continence after the initial operation.[171] Another 17.6% achieved continence after revision. The results with this technique by the Johns Hopkins group were not nearly as good and, after initially recommending this procedure, they have now abandoned it, as stomal stenosis in children and destabilization are problems.[174,175] This hydraulic nipple valve, while ingenious, has not gained wide acceptance.

Plication techniques have been widely accepted as reliable continence mechanisms and have been popularized by the Indiana group in what has become known as the Indiana pouch. This pouch is based on a modification of Gilcrest and Merrick's cecoileal reservoir. It has undergone several modifications since the initial report in 1985.[176] In this procedure the cecum is detubularized and used as the reservoir. Reflux prevention is obtained by tunneling the ureters into the tenia or by the Le Duc technique.[177] The continence mechanism is based on plication of the ileum to the level of the ileocecal valve. The native ileocecal valve is reinforced by Lembert sutures (Figure 57.22). A very similar technique has been used by Lockhart et al in the Florida pouch.[178] The advantage of this procedure is its ease of construction, using techniques familiar to all urologists. Carroll and Presti compared plicated vs stapled ileal segments and noted that mean contraction pressures were higher in the stapled group (63 ± 27 cmH_2O at 41 ± 21 cmH_2O).[179] They have previously shown the contractions in the ileal segment always precede or are concomitant with cecal reservoir contractions.[180] Mean reservoir volumes were 675 ml, with mean reservoir contractions being 24 cmH_2O and mean plicated ileal pressures 40 cmH_2O in the reservoir. As would be expected from these data, continence rates have been quite good. Rowland reviewed several series and noted that one of 17 patients (6%) required repair of the efferent limb for leakage.[181]

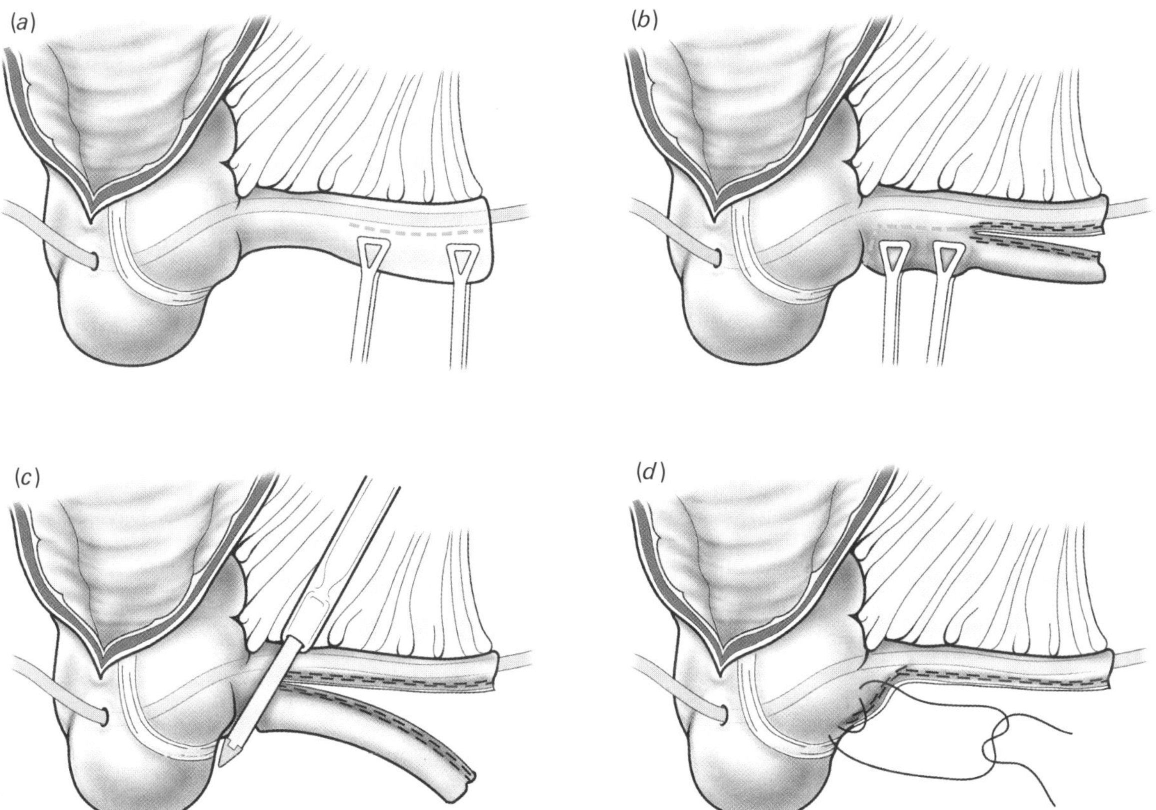

Figure 57.22 Continence is achieved by plicating the ileum to the level of the ileocecal valve. The ileocecal valve is reinforced (*d*).

However, Canning, reported that leakage occurs more readily with this mechanism than with nipples.[182] Ring and Hensle achieved a 95% continence rate in 29 children undergoing the Indiana pouch.[183] In Rowland's most recent report, five of the last 81 patients had incontinence secondary to high reservoir pressures;[184] however, the cecal reservoir with ileum may correct this.

Koff et al reported a technique to provide hydraulic compression to the efferent ileal limb of the Indiana pouch.[185] A segment of ileum is used to wrap around the efferent limb and is anastomosed to the cecal pouch. While this would increase resistance further, it adds complexity to an otherwise easily performed procedure that already has a high continence rate. Koff's approach has not gained widespread use.

Without question, the most commonly used continence mechanism in children is based on the flap-valve principle as introduced by Mitrofanoff.[186] Mitrofanoff reported the use of the appendix to tunnel into the neuropathic bladder (similar to a ureteral reimplantation to prevent reflux) to provide a continent catheterizable stoma into the native bladder. The procedure was popularized by Duckett and Snyder,[187,188] who extended the use of this technique to create a continent ileocecal pouch, the Penn pouch[189] (Figure 57.23). Since these early reports, many authors from around the world have reported their experience using not only appendix but also ureter, tapered ileal, colonic or gastric tubes, fallopian tubes, and vas deferens.[190–199] The continence mechanism is based on placing a supple tube in a submucosal tunnel with a 5:1 ratio of length to tube diameter. Firm muscle backing of the tube prevents reflux (Figure 57.24). It was initially thought that the tube itself must also be muscular, but bladder urothelium, colonic mucosa, and preputial skin alone have all been used successfully.[200–202]

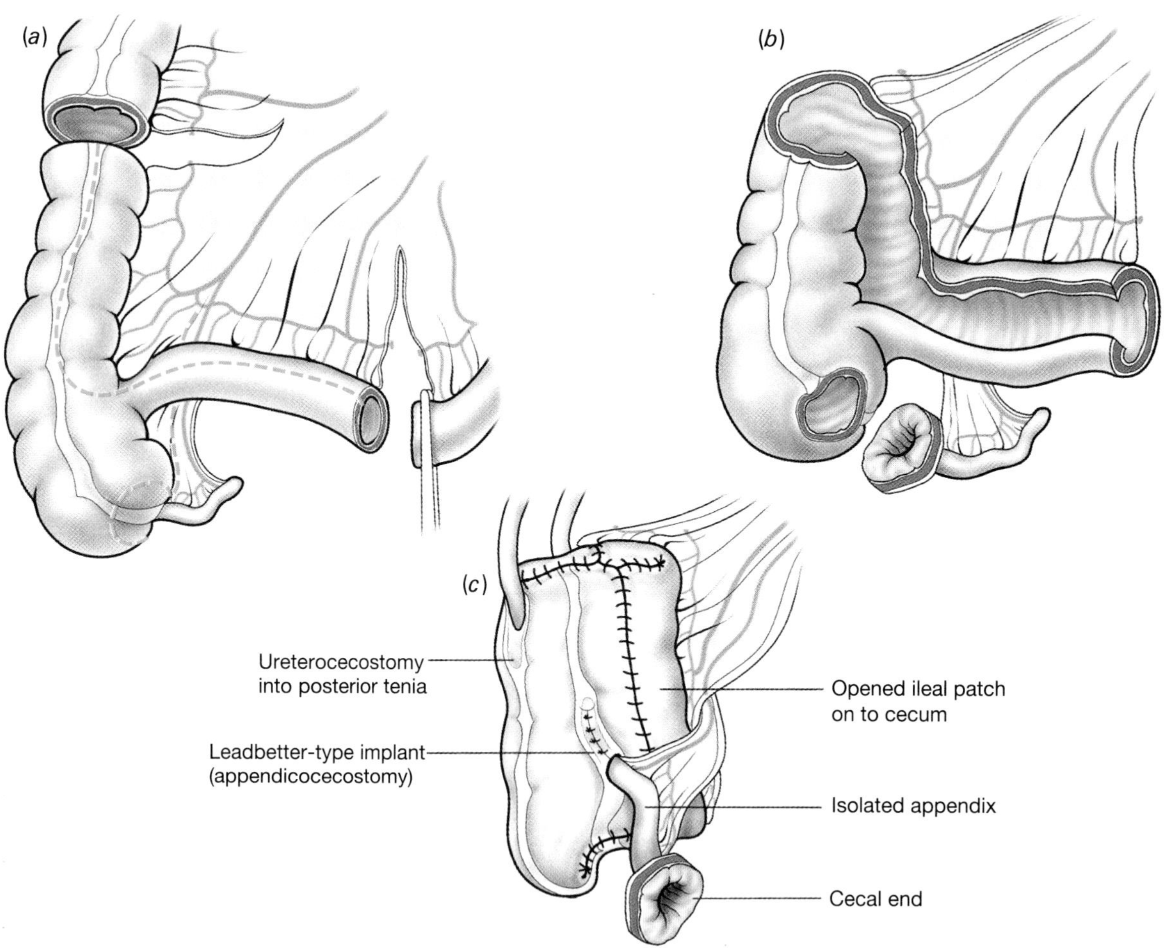

Figure 57.23 The Penn pouch. (*a*) The ileocecal segment is isolated and incised on its antimesenteric border; the ureters are implanted into the colonic segment. (*b*) The appendix is isolated in its mesentery. (*c*) The ileocecal segments are joined and the appendix is implanted into the cecum; the cecal end is brought to the skin as a catheterizable stoma.

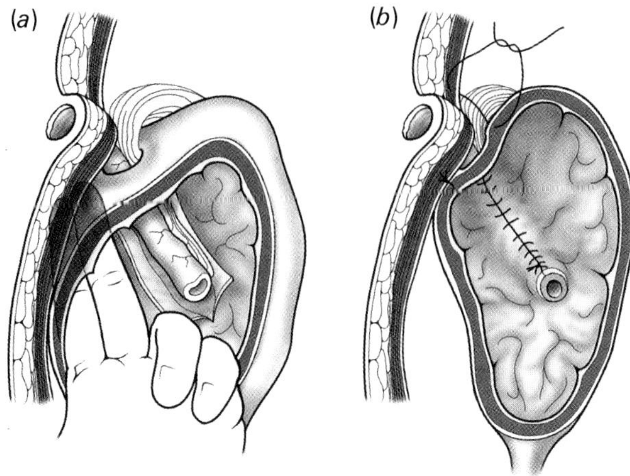

Figure 57.24 Appendicovesicostomy is performed by tunneling the appendix submucosally into the bladder. (Reprinted from Keating et al,[194] with permission.)

This is a relatively simple procedure using techniques familiar to pediatric urologists. It is also particularly useful in children who, as noted previously, often are not candidates for use of the ileocecal valve or long segments of ileum. Kaefer and Retik reviewed several series and found that continence rates ranged from 86 to 96%.[196] The most common complication reported is stomal stenosis. Khoury et al noted stomal stenosis in 5–57% of patients and described a technique of placing the stoma at the umbilicus.[203] The Mainz group concluded that the stomal stenosis is slightly higher when placed at the umbilicus. A high risk for stenosis has also been seen when using the appendix compared with tapered ileum.[204,205] The Great Ormond Street group has reported a decrease in the incidence of stomal stenosis using a VQZ skin-flap technique[206] (see Figure 58.3). Using the concealed umbilical stoma technique, the Pittsburgh group has seen a stomal revision rate of 7% at nearly 3 years mean follow-up.[207] At a minimum, a skin flap should be placed into the spatulated tube. In the authors' last 100 patients in whom the Mitrofanoff principle has been applied, there is a 99% continence rate. Stomal stenosis has occurred in 12% (5/57 appendix, 1/22 ileum, and 6/21 bladder).[208] In the Boston experience, five of 50 patients leaked at the stomal level, five had stomal stenosis, and one an appendiceal stricture.[196]

Since the introduction of the MACE procedure (Malone antegrade colonic enema), which used the appendix brought to the skin for irrigation of the cecum, it has become necessary to find other tissue to form a catheterizable urinary stoma. The Yang–Monti technique,[209,210] which uses only 2 cm of reconfigured ileum to form a tube, has been a great advance, and the technique has been used successfully[211] (Figure 57.25). Tunneling of these tubes into colon or stomach is easily accomplished but is difficult in ileum. A seromuscular trough for implantation has been described[194] and Plaire et al[212] have described a serosal reimplant similar to the Abol-Enein and Ghoneim ureteral reimplant (see Figure 57.14). It is now clear that the Mitrofanoff principle is a major advance and that virtually any supple tube placed in a tunnel that has adequate muscular backing will successfully provide continence.

Complete gastric reservoirs have been popularized by Mitchell's group,[143] and they have recently described three techniques to provide continence[213] (Figures 57.26 and 57.27). Two of these are based on the Mitrofanoff principle and one on a nipple valve.

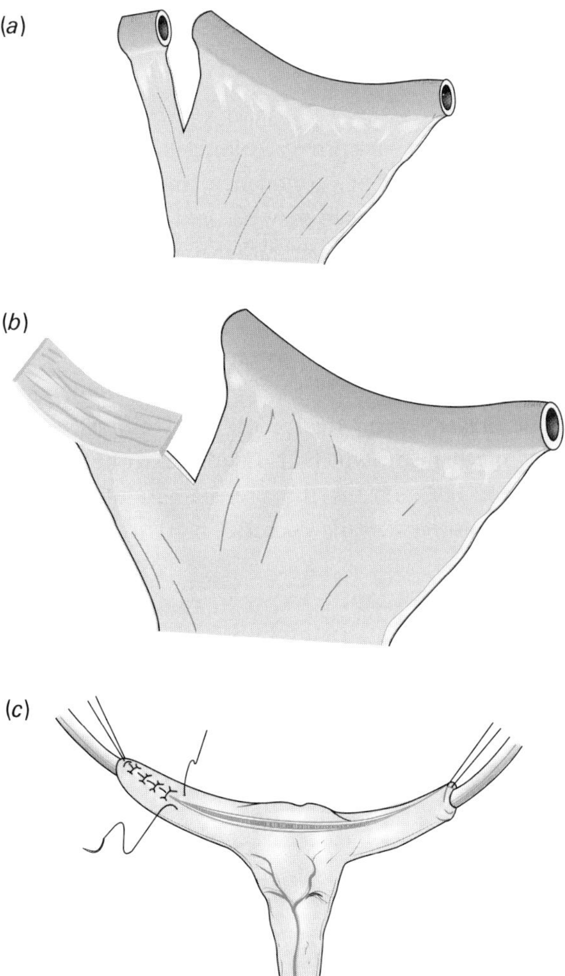

Figure 57.25 Yang–Monti. (*a*) A 2 cm segment of small bowel is isolated on its mesentery. (*b*) It is opened on its antimesenteric border. (*c*) The segment is retubularized by closing it in a longitudinal fashion (see also Figures 55.23 and 55.24).

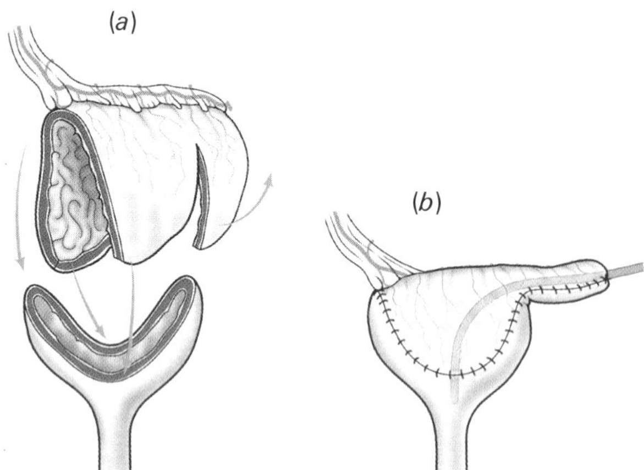

Figure 57.26 Gastric continence mechanisms. (*a*) A gastric wedge is harvested from the greater curvature of the stomach with an anterior strip mobilized for tubularization. (*b*) The anterior strip is tubularized with two sutured layers over a 12 Fr catheter. The proximal end is formed into a nipple for the continence mechanism. (Reproduced from Close and Mitchell,[213] with permission.)

Stomach is very receptive at tunneled reimplants for either antireflux or continence mechanisms. To reduce acidity, stomach may be used in combination with ileum as the reservoir, rather than using stomach alone.[142,143] Applying a Yang–Monti ileal tube tunneled into the stomach as the continence mechanism prevents the peristomal irritation sometimes seen with gastric tubes.[198,213]

The only reservoir that provides a volitional continence mechanism, which also happens to be the first continent reservoir, is the ureterosigmoidostomy.[52] Since its introduction, over 60 modifications have been proposed. Because of the problems with upper tract deterioration, occasional incontinence, acidosis, and the risk for adenocarcinoma, it has been largely abandoned. However, the opportunity to control continence without CIC continues to make it very attractive. It cannot be used in spinal dysraphism, as a neurologically intact anal sphincter is required. In children it has been used almost exclusively in the exstrophy population when continence cannot be achieved with bladder neck surgery. It has been suggested that oatmeal enemas be given preoperatively to check anal continence.[214] Classically, ureterosigmoidostomy has been done by simply tunneling the ureters into the rectum. However, the risk of cancer at the anastomotic site and night-time incontinence led surgeons to pursue other efforts to provide more of a reservoir effect and avoid direct contact of the ureters with the stool. Development of neoplasms seems to require urine to be in contact with stool and bowel mucosa.[215,216] Of 94 children with ureterosigmoidostomy followed at the Children's Hospital of Boston, seven developed adenocarcinoma of the colon, four of whom died.[217] Rink and Retik proposed that an ileocecal conduit be initially constructed and the conduit later anastomosed to the intact sigmoid by end-to-end colocolostomy.[217] Kock et al described a 'valved-rectum' with the colon intussuscepted at the rectosigmoid junction to prevent reflux of rectal contents and an ileal patch anastomosed to the anterior rectal wall.[218] This allowed the rectal capacity to increase from 200 to 700 ml with maximal pressures of only 24 cmH_2O and minimal metabolic disturbances.[218]

A hemi-Kock pouch anastomosed to the rectum has also been described,[218] but the complexity of cre-

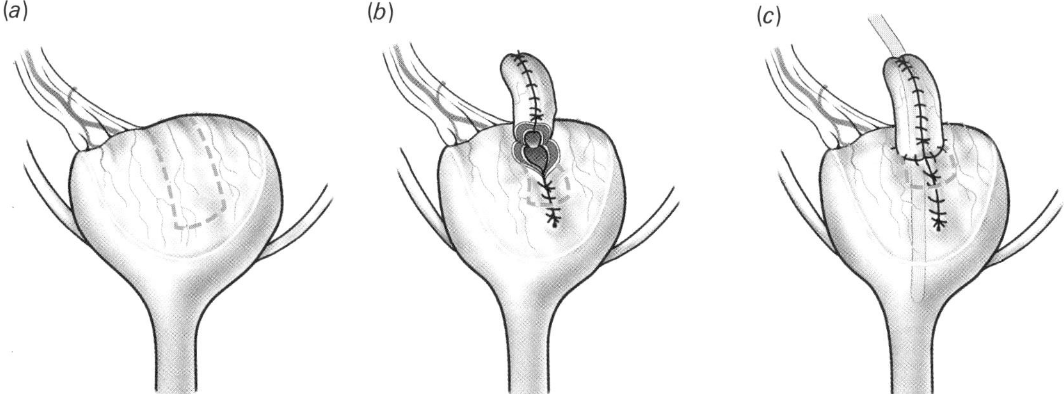

Figure 57.27 Gastroileal pouch with a Monti tube. (*a*) The flap to be tubularized is indicated on existing gastrocystoplasty. (*b*) The flap is raised and tubularized, and the bladder defect is closed. (*c*) Creation of a continent nipple valve by intussusception of gastric tissue as a cuff around the base of the gastric tube. (Reproduced from Close and Michell,[213] with permission.)

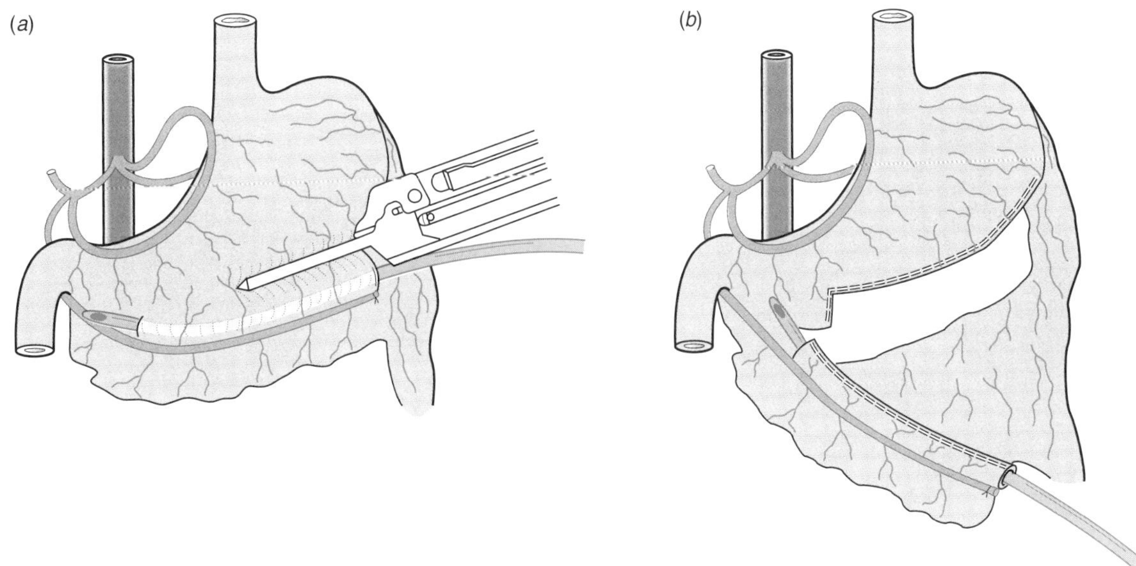

Figure 57.28 (*a*) An isolated gastric tube is harvested with a GIA-90 stapler over a 12 Fr catheter. (*b*) The mobilized isolated gastric tube is ready for placement into an augmented bladder or reservoir.

ating the colonic nipple in these two procedures makes them less attractive. The sigma rectum (Mainz pouch II) has been proposed from the group from Mainz as a means of lowering the very high pressures in the intact rectosigmoid colon without the need for nipples or augmentation[219] (Figures 57.28 and 57.29). Continence was achieved in 40 of 47 patients, with voiding five times per day, and extracolonic pressures remained low. The results in 34 patients of the Mainz II were reported by Gerharz et al.[220] All were continent during the day. One had night-time soiling and had creation of an ileal conduit due to recurrent septicemia. One ureteral obstruction led to a nephrectomy and two had mild hyperchloremic acidosis. Although lower pressures with the new procedures should reduce the risk for upper tract changes, the risk for adenocarcinoma still weighs heavily when contemplating any type of ureterocolonic diversion.

Postoperative care

In the early postoperative interval ureteral drainage is provided by stents, which are left indwelling for at least 1 week. Antibiotics are given until all tubes are removed. H_2 blockers are given temporarily if stomach is used. A large-bore silastic tube drains the reservoir for 3 weeks. The reservoirs are irrigated three times a day for the first 3 weeks and then slowly decreased to daily, for the rest of the patient's life. A pouch-o-gram is obtained before removal of the stents. The indwelling reservoir drainage tube is maintained until the patient and family demonstrate that they can easily catheterize the stoma and empty the reservoir. Demonstration of complete emptying is mandatory to prevent long-term problems of infection, stone formation, incontinence, and perforation, and to maintain stable renal function.

Renal and pouch sonography, abdominal radiographs, and serum creatinine and electrolytes are all obtained 3 months postoperatively, repeated at 6-month intervals, twice, and yearly thereafter. Vitamin B_{12} levels should be checked in the long term and somatic growth monitored. Endoscopic evaluation of the pouch should be carried out annually, starting 5–10 years postoperatively.

Summary

Tremendous advances have been made in lower urinary tract reconstruction in children. The entire urinary tract can now be completely replaced. Bladders can be constructed that are continent, ureters can be replaced with antireflux mechanisms easily achieved, and kidneys can be transplanted. Direct cutaneous diversion is generally only used as a temporary means to provide drainage. Non-continent diversion is only used in children who are incapable of independent care. It is ideal to maintain the native urinary tract intact, and reconstructive efforts should be directed to achieve this. If this cannot be achieved, a CUR should be provided. The limits of reconstruction are based

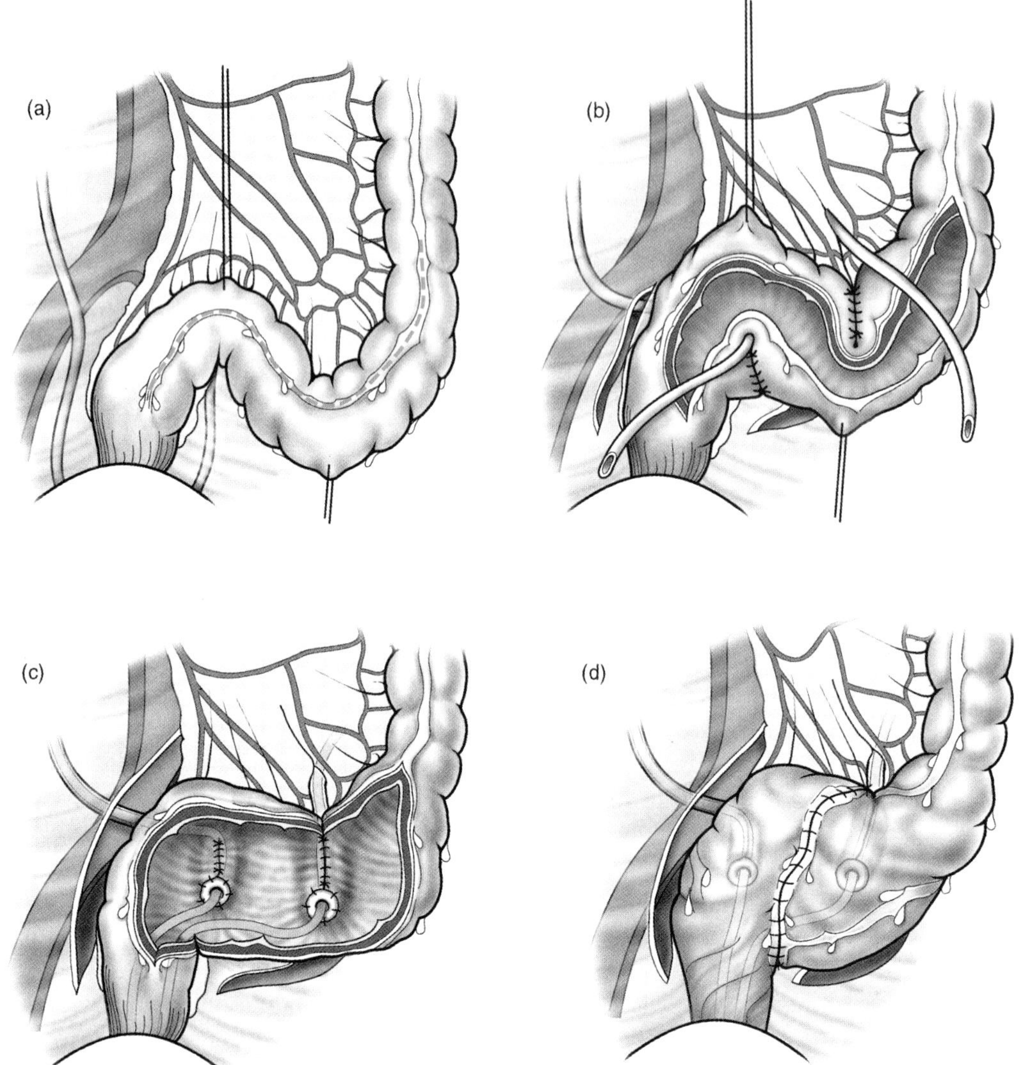

Figure 57.29 The Mainz pouch II (sigma rectum) has been presented as a means of reconstructing a low-pressure ureterosigmoidostomy.

only on the surgeon's imagination and skills. As long as the principles of CUR construction outlined in this chapter are met, a successful surgical result can almost always be achieved. True success, however, will always require the cooperation of a well-motivated child and equally motivated parents. Furthermore, this type of major reconstruction necessitates that the surgeon be surrounded by dedicated personnel who function as a team for the betterment of the health of these children.

References

1. Alagiri M, Seidmon EJ. Percutaneous endoscopic cystostomy for bladder localization and exact placement of a suprapubic tube. J Urol 1998; 159(3):963–4.
2. Belman A. Temporary diversion. In: Kelalis PP, King LR, Belman AB, eds. Clinical Pediatric Urology. Philadelphia: WB Saunders, 1985: 582.
3. Ducket J, Ziylan O. Uses and abuses of vesicostomy. AUA Update Ser 1995; 14:130–5.
4. Slaton JW, Kropp KA. Proximal ureteral stent migration: an avoidable complication? J Urol 1996; 155(1):58–61.
5. Stanley P, Diament MJ. Pediatric percutaneous nephrostomy: experience with 50 patients. J Urol 1986; 135(6):1223–6.
6. Morelli G, Felipetto R, Biver P, Bottone U, Minervini R. Use of new nephrostomy catheter for treatment of renal neonatal candidiasis. Eur Urol 1997; 32(4):485–6.
7. Farrell TA, Hicks ME. A review of radiologically guided percutaneous nephrostomies in 303 patients. J Vasc Interv Radiol 1997; 8(5):769–74.
8. Papanicolaou N. Urinary tract imaging and interventions: basic principles. In: Walsh PC, Retik AB, Vaughan ED, Wein AG, eds. Campbell's Urology, 7th edn. Philadelphia: WB Saunders, 1998: 170–260.

9. Bell DA, Rose SC, Starr NK, Jaffe RB, Miller FJ Jr. Percutaneous nephrostomy for nonoperative management of fungal urinary tract infections. J Vasc Interv Radiol 1993; 4(2):311–15.
10. Bartone FF, Hurwitz RS, Rojas EL, Steinberg E, Franceschini, R. The role of percutaneous nephrostomy in the management of obstructing candidiasis of the urinary tract in infants. J Urol 1988; 140(2):338–41.
11. Bartone PT, Adler AB, Vaitkus MA. Dimensions of psychological stress in peacekeeping operations. Mil Med 1998; 163(9):587–93.
12. Ducret A, Bartone N, Haynes PA, Blanchard A, Aebersold R. A simplified gradient solvent delivery system for capillary liquid chromatography–electrospray ionization mass spectrometry. Anal Biochem 1998; 265(1):129–38.
13. Noe HN, Jerkins GR. Cutaneous vesicostomy experience in infants and children. J Urol 1985; 134(2):301–3.
14. Krahn CG, Johnson HW. Cutaneous vesicostomy in the young child: indications and results. Urology 1993; 41(6):558–63.
15. Hutton KA, Thomas DF. Selective use of cutaneous vesicostomy in prenatally detected and clinically presenting uropathies. Eur Urol 1998; 33(4):405–11.
16. Edelstein RA, Bauer SB, Kelly MD et al. The long-term urological response of neonates with myelodysplasia treated proactively with intermittent catheterization and anticholinergic therapy. J Urol 1995; 154(4):1500–4.
17. Close CE, Carr MC, Burns MW, Mitchell ME. Lower urinary tract changes after early valve ablation in neonates and infants: is early diversion warranted? J Urol 1997; 157(3):984–8.
18. Jayanthi VR, McLorie GA, Khoury AE, Churchill BM. The effect of temporary cutaneous diversion on ultimate bladder function. J Urol 1995; 154(2 Pt 2):889–92.
19. Kim YH, Horowitz M, Combs A et al. Comparative urodynamic findings after primary valve ablation, vesicostomy or proximal diversion. J Urol 1996; 156(2 Pt 2):673–6.
20. Lapides J, Ajemian EP, Lichtwardt JR. Cutaneous vesicostomy. J Urol 1960; 84:609–14.
21. Blocksom BH Jr. Bladder pouch for prolonged tubeless cystostomy. J Urol 1957; 78(4):398–401.
22. Skoog S. Pediatric vesical diversion. In: Graham SD, ed. Glenn's Urologic Surgery. Philadelphia: Lippincott-Raven, 1998: 822–8.
23. Cendron M. Discussion: temporary cutaneous urinary diversion in children. Dialog Pediatr Urol 1995; 18:1–8.
24. Krueger RP, Ash JM, Silver MM et al. Primary hydronephrosis. Assessment of diuretic renography, pelvis perfusion pressure, operative findings, and renal and ureteral histology. Urol Clin North Am 1980; 7(2):231–42.
25. Joyner B, Khoury A. The role of urinary diversion in childhood: temporary, continent, or otherwise. Gonzalez ET, Bauer S, eds. Pediatric Urology Practice. Baltimore: Lippincott, Williams & Williams, 1999: 687–704.
26. Reinberg Y, de Castano I, Gonzalez R. Influence of initial therapy on progression of renal failure and body growth in children with posterior urethral valves. J Urol 1992; 148(2 Pt 2):532–3.
27. Smith GH, Canning DA, Schulman SL, Snyder HM 3rd, Duckett JW. The long-term outcome of posterior urethral valves treated with primary valve ablation and observation. J Urol 1996; 155(5):1730–4.
28. Tietjen DN, Gloor JM, Husmann DA. Proximal urinary diversion in the management of posterior urethral valves: is it necessary? J Urol 1997; 158(3 Pt 2):1008–10.
29. Sober I. Pelvioureterostomy-en-Y. J Urol 1972; 107(3):473–5.
30. Rink RC, Keating MA. Cutaneous ureterostomy. Fowler J, ed. Urologic Surgery. Boston: Little, Brown, and Co, 1992: 315–20.
31. Pfeffer P, Caldamone A. Management of the dilated ureter in children. Fowler J, ed. Urologic Surgery. Boston, Little, Brown, and Co, 1992: 221–7.
32. Shapiro SR, Lebowitz R, Colodny AH. Fate of 90 children with ileal conduit urinary diversion a decade later: analysis of complications, pyelography, renal function and bacteriology. J Urol 1975; 114(2):289–95.
33. Husmann DA, McLorie GA, Churchill BM. Nonrefluxing colonic conduits: a long-term life-table analysis. J Urol 1989; 142(5):1201–3.
34. Koch MO, McDougal WS, Hall MC et al. Long-term metabolic effects of urinary diversion: a comparison of myelomeningocele patients managed by clean intermittent catheterization and urinary diversion. J Urol 1992; 147(5):1343–7.
35. Pitts WR Jr, Muecke EC. A 20-year experience with ileal conduits: the fate of the kidneys. J Urol 1979; 122(2):154–7.
36. Elder DD, Moisey CU, Rees RW. A long-term follow-up of the colonic conduit operation in children. Br J Urol 1979; 51(6):462–5.
37. Schwarz GR, Jeffs RD. Ileal conduit urinary diversion in children: computer analysis of follow up from 2 to 16 years. J Urol 1975; 114(2):285–8.
38. Grune M, Taylor R. Aspects of urinary diversion: the current role of conduits. AUA Update Ser 1996; 15:166–71.
39. McDougal WS. Use of intestinal segments and urinary diversions. In: Walsh PC, Retik AB, Vaughan ED, Wein AJ, eds. Campbell's Urology, 7th edn. Philadelphia: WB Saunders, 1998: 3121–61.
40. DeFoor W, Minevich E, McEnery P et al. Lower urinary tract reconstruction is safe and effective in children with end stage renal disease. J Urol 2003; 170(4 Pt 2):1497–500, discussion 1500.
41. Sheldon CA, Gonzalez R, Burns MW et al. Renal transplantation into the dysfunctional bladder: the role of adjunctive bladder reconstruction. J Urol 1994; 152(3):972–5.
42. Rink R, McLaughlin K. Indications for enterocystoplasty and choice of bowel segment. Prob Urol 1994; 8:389–403.
43. Regan JB, Barrett DM. Stented versus nonstented ureteroileal anastomoses: is there a difference with regard to leak and stricture? J Urol 1985; 134(6):1101–13.
44. Levy J, Van Arsdalen K. Ureteral and ureteroenteral strictures. AUA Update Ser 1994; 13:230–5.
45. Razvi H, Martin T, Sosa R, Vaughan E. Endourologic management of complications of urinary intestinal diversion. AUA Update Ser 1996; 15:174–9.
46. Fitzgerald J, Malone MJ, Gaertner RA, Zinman LN.

Stomal construction, complications, and reconstruction. Urol Clin North Am 1997; 24(4):729–33.
47. Webster GD. Conduit urinary diversion. In: Webster GD, Goldwasser B, eds. Urinary Diversion. Oxford: Isis Medical Media, 1995: 318–29.
48. Filmer RB, Spencer JR. Malignancies in bladder augmentations and intestinal conduits. J Urol 1990; 143(4): 671–8.
49. Bricker E. Bladder substitution after pelvic exonteration. Surg Clin North Am 1950; 30:1511–21.
50. Wallace DM. Ureteroileostomy. Br J Urol 1970; 42(5): 529–34.
51. Williams O, Vereb M, Libertino JA. Incontinent urinary diversion. Urol Clin North Am 1997; 24:735–44.
52. Simon J. Ectropia vesicae (absence of the anterior abdominal walls of the bladder and pubic abdominal parietes); operation for directing the orifices of the ureters into the rectum; temporary success; subsequent death, autopsy. Lancet 1852; ii:568.
53. Gilcrest R, Merricks J, Hamlin H, Rieger I. Construction of a substitute bladder and urethra. Surg Gynecol Obstet 1950; 90:752–60.
54. Harper JG, Berman MH, Hertzberg AD, Lerman F, Brendler H. Observations on the use of the cecum as a substitute urinary bladder. J Urol 1954; 71(5):600–2.
55. Wells CA. The use of the intestine in urology, omitting ureterocolic anastomosis. Br J Urol 1956; 28(4):335–50, discussion 406–16.
56. Sullivan H, Gilchrist RK, Merricks JW. Ileocecal substitute bladder. Long-term follow up. J Urol 1973; 109(1): 43–5.
57. Merricks J. A continent substitute bladder and urethra. In: King LR, Stone AR, Webster GD, eds. Bladder Reconstruction and Continent Urinary Diversion. Chicago: Yearbook Medical Publishers, 1987: 179–203.
58. Lapides J, Diokno AC, Siber SJ, Lowe BS. Clean, intermittent self-catheterization in the treatment of urinary tract disease. J Urol 1972; 107(3):458–61.
59. Blaivas JG, Labib KL, Bauer SB, Retik AB. Changing concepts in the urodynamic evaluation of children. J Urol 1997; 117(6):778–81.
60. Hendren WH. A new approach to infants with severe obstructive uropathy: early complete reconstruction. J Pediatr Surg 1970; 5(2):184–99.
61. Hendren WH. Reconstruction of previously diverted urinary tracts in children. J Pediatr Surg 1973; 8(2):135–50.
62. Kock NG, Nilson AE, Nilsson LO, Norlen LJ, Philipson BM. Urinary diversion via a continent ileal reservoir: clinical results in 12 patients. J Urol 1982; 128(3):469–75.
63. Skinner DG, Lieskovsky G, Boyd S. Continent urinary diversion. J Urol 1989; 141(6):1323–7.
64. Skinner DG, Boyd SD, Lieskovsky G. Clinical experience with the Kock continent ileal reservoir for urinary diversion. J Urol 1984; 132(6):1101–17.
65. Skinner DG, Lieskovsky G, Boyd SD. Continuing experience with the continent ileal reservoir (Kock pouch) as an alternative to cutaneous urinary diversion: an update after 250 cases. J Urol 1987; 137(6): 1140–5.
66. McLaughlin KP, Rink RC, Adams MC, Keating MA. Stomach in combination with other intestinal segments in pediatric lower urinary tract reconstruction. J Urol 1995; 154(3):1162–8.
67. Benson M, Olsson C. Continent urinary diversion. In: Walsh PC, Retik AB, Vaughan FD, Wein AJ, eds. Campbell's Urology, 7th edn. Philadelphia: WB Saunders, 1998: 3190–245.
68. Ferris D, Odel H. Electrolyte abnormality of the blood after ureterosigmoidostomy. JAMA 1950; 142:634–40.
69. Koch MO, McDougal WS. The pathophysiology of hyperchloremic metabolic acidosis after urinary diversion through intestinal segments. Surgery 1985; 98(3):561–70.
70. Demos MP. Radioactive electrolyte absorption studies of small bowel; comparison of different segments for use in urinary diversion. J Urol 1962; 88:638–43.
71. Mitchell ME, Piser JA. Intestinocystoplasty and total bladder replacement in children and young adults: follow up in 129 cases. J Urol 1987; 138(3):579–84.
72. Rink R, Hollensbe D, Adams M. Complications of augmentation in children and comparison of gastrointestinal segments. AUA Update Ser 1995; 14:122–8.
73. Allen T, Peters P, Sagalowsky A. The Camey procedure, preliminary results in patients. World J Urol 1985; 3:167.
74. McDougal WS. Bladder reconstruction following cystectomy by uretero-ileo-colourethrostomy. J Urol 1986; 135(4):698–701.
75. Asken M. Urinary cecal reservoir. In: King LR, Stone AR, Webster GD, eds. Bladder Reconstruction and Urinary Diversion. Chicago: Yearbook Medical Publishers, 1987: 288–251.
76. Thuroff J, Alken P, Hohenfellner K. The MAINZ pouch (mixed augmentation with ileum 'n' zecum) for bladder augmentation and continent diversion. Chicago: Yearbook Medical Publishers, 1987: 252.
77. Boyd SD, Schiff WM, Skinner DG et al. Prospective study of metabolic abnormalities in patient with continent Kock pouch urinary diversion. Urology 1989; 33(2):85–8.
78. Nurse DE, Mundy AR. Metabolic complications of cystoplasty. Br J Urol 1989; 63(2):165–70.
79. Hall MC, Koch MO, McDougal WS. Metabolic consequences of urinary diversion through intestinal segments. Urol Clin North Am 1991; 18(4):725–35.
80. Gros DA, Dodson JL, Lopatin UA et al. Decreased linear growth associated with intestinal bladder augmentation in children with bladder exstrophy. J Urol 2000; 164(3 Pt 2):917–20.
81. Wagstaff KE, Woodhouse CR, Duffy PG, Ransley PG. Delayed linear growth in children with enterocystoplasties. Br J Urol 1992; 69(3):314–17.
82. Feng AH, Kaar S, Elder JS. Influence of enterocystoplasty on linear growth in children with exstrophy. J Urol 2002; 167(6):2552–5; discussion 2555.
83. Mingin GC, Nguyen HT, Mathias RS et al. Growth and metabolic consequences of bladder augmentation in children with myelomeningocele and bladder exstrophy. Pediatrics 2002; 110(6):1193–8.
84. Mingin G, Maroni P, Gerharz EW, Woodhouse CR, Baskin LS. Linear growth after enterocystoplasty in children and adolescents: a review. World J Urol 2004; 22(3):196–9.
85. Rink R, Mitchell M. Role of enterocystoplasty in recon-

structing the neurogenic bladder. In: Gonzalez ET, Roth D, eds. Common Problems in Pediatric Urology. St. Louis: Mosby Year Book, 1990: 192–204.
86. Rink RC. Bladder augmentation: options, outcomes, future. Urol Clin North Am 1999; 26(1):111–23, viii–ix.
87. Rink R, Adams M. Augmentation cystoplasty. In: Walsh P, Retik A, Vaughan E, Wein A, eds. Campbell's Urology, 7th edn. Philadelphia: WB Saunders, 1998: 3167–89.
88. Hensle TW, Ring KS. Urinary tract reconstruction in children. Urol Clin North Am 1991; 18(4):701–15.
89. Horowitz M, Kuhr CS, Mitchell ME. The Mitrofanoff catheterizable channel: patient acceptance. J Urol 1995; 153(3 Pt 1):771–2.
90. Fowler JE Jr. Continent urinary reservoirs. Surg Ann 1988; 20:201–25.
91. Camey M, Richard F, Botto H. Ileal replacement of bladder. In: King LS, Stone AB, Webster GD, eds. Bladder Reconstruction and Continent Urinary Diversion. St. Louis, Mosby Yearbook, 1991: 389–410.
92. Kock NG. Intra-abdominal 'reservoir' in patients with permanent ileostomy. Preliminary observations on a procedure resulting in fecal 'continence' in five ileostomy patients. Arch Surg 1969; 99(2):223–31.
93. Light JK, Engelmann UH. Reconstruction of the lower urinary tract: observations on bowel dynamics and the artificial urinary sphincter. J Urol 1985; 133(4):594–7.
94. Pope J, Albers P, Rink R et al. Spontaneous rupture of the augmented bladder: from silence to chaos. European Society of Pediatric Urology, Istanbul, Turkey, 1999.
95. McGuire EJ, Woodside JR, Borden TA, Weiss RM. Prognostic value of urodynamic testing in myelodysplastic patients. J Urol 1981; 126(2):205–9.
96. Haberstroh KM, Kaefer M, Bizios R. Inhibition of pressure induced bladder smooth muscle cell hyperplasia using CRM197. J Urol 2000; 164(4):1329–33.
97. Haberstroh KM, Kaefer M, Retik AB, Freeman MR, Bizios R. The effects of sustained hydrostatic pressure on select bladder smooth muscle cell functions. J Urol 1999; 162(6):2114–18.
98. Backhaus BO, Kaefer M, Haberstroh KM et al. Alterations in the molecular determinants of bladder compliance at hydrostatic pressures less than 40 cm. H_2O. J Urol 2002; 168(6):2600–4.
99. Hinman F Jr. Selection of intestinal segments for bladder substitution: physical and physiological characteristics. J Urol 1988; 139(3):519–23.
100. Koff SA. Guidelines to determine the size and shape of intestinal segments used for reconstruction. J Urol 1988; 140(5 Pt 2):1150–1.
101. Lytton B, Green DF. Urodynamic studies in patients undergoing bladder replacement surgery. J Urol 1989; 141(6):1394–7.
102. Sidi AA, Reinberg Y, Gonzalez R. Influence of intestinal segment and configuration on the outcome of augmentation enterocystoplasty. J Urol 1986; 136(6):1201–4.
103. Goldwasser B, Webster GD. Augmentation and substitution enterocystoplasty. J Urol 1986; 135(2):215–24.
104. Berglund B, Kock NG. Volume capacity and pressure characteristics of various types of intestinal reservoirs. World J Surg 1987; 11(6):798–803.
105. Pope JC, Keating MA, Casale AJ, Rink RC. Augmenting the augmented bladder: treatment of the contractile bowel segment. J Urol 1998; 160(3 Pt 1):854–7.
106. Rink R. Choice of materials for bladder augmentation. Curr Opin Urol 1995; 9:300–5.
107. Kulb T, Rink R, Mitchell M. Gastrocystoplasty in azotemic canines. American Urological Association, North Central Section, Palm Springs, Florida, 1986.
108. Rowland R. Intestine for bladder augmentation and substitution. In: King LR, Stone AR, Webster GD, eds. Bladder Reconstruction and Continent Urinary Diversion. St. Louis, Mosby Yearbook, 1996: 12–28.
109. Sheldon C, Snyder HI. Principles of urinary tract reconstruction. In: Gillenwater JY, Graghack JT, Howards SS, Duckett JW, eds. Adult and Pediatric Urology. St. Louis, Mosby, 1996.
110. Akerlund S. Urinary diversion via the continent ileal reservoir. Functional characteristics and long-term outcome. Scand J Urol Nephrol Suppl 1989; 121:1–36.
111. Canning DA, Perman JA, Jeffs RD, Gearhart JP. Nutritional consequences of bowel segments in the lower urinary tract. J Urol 1989; 142(2 Pt 2):509–11, discussion 20–1.
112. Steiner MS, Morton RA. Nutritional and gastrointestinal complications of the use of bowel segments in the lower urinary tract. Urol Clin North Am 1991; 18(4):743–54.
113. Roth S, Semjonow A, Waldner M, Hertle L. Risk of bowel dysfunction with diarrhea after continent urinary diversion with ileal and ileocecal segments. J Urol 1995; 154(5):1696–9.
114. Baker L, Gearhart J. Continent urinary diversion. Prog Pediatr Urol 1998; 1:67–9.
115. King L. Protection of the upper tracts in children. In: King LR, Stone AR, Webster GD, eds. Bladder Reconstruction and Continent Urinary Diversion. Chicago: Year Book Medical, 1987: 127.
116. Gonzalez R, Cabral B. Rectal continence after enterocystoplasty. Dialog Pediatr Urol 1987; 10:3–4.
117. Hirst G. Ileal and colonic cystoplasties. Prob Urol 1991; 5:223.
118. Shekarriz B, Upadhyay J, Demirbilek S, Barthold JS, Gonzalez R. Surgical complications of bladder augmentation: comparison between various enterocystoplasties in 133 patients. Urology 2000; 55(1):123–8.
119. Bauer SB, Hendren WH, Kozakewich H et al. Perforation of the augmented bladder. J Urol 1992; 148(2 Pt 2):699–703.
120. Mitchell ME. Use of bowel in undiversion. Urol Clin North Am 1986; 13(2):349–59.
121. Adams MC, Mitchell ME, Rink RC. Gastrocystoplasty: an alternative solution to the problem of urological reconstruction in the severely compromised patient. J Urol 1988; 140(5 Pt 2):1152–6.
122. Adams M, Birhle R, Rink R. The use of stomach in urologic reconstruction. AUA Update Ser 1995; 27:218–33.
123. Kaefer M, Hendren WH, Bauer SB et al. Reservoir calculi: a comparison of reservoirs constructed from stomach and other enteric segments. J Urol 1998; 160(6 Pt 1):2187–90.
124. DeFoor W, Minevich E, Reddy P et al. Bladder calculi after augmentation cystoplasty: risk factors and prevention strategies. J Urol 2004; 172(5 Pt 1):1964–6.

125. Kronner KM, Casale AJ, Cain MP et al. Bladder calculi in the pediatric augmented bladder. J Urol 1998; 160(3 Pt 2):1096–8, discussion 1103.
126. Piser JA, Mitchell ME, Kulb TB et al. Gastrocystoplasty and colocystoplasty in canines: the metabolic consequences of acute saline and acid loading. J Urol 1987; 138(4 Pt 2):1009–13.
127. Kennedy HA, Adams MC, Mitchell ME et al. Chronic renal failure and bladder augmentation: stomach versus sigmoid colon in the canine model. J Urol 1988; 140(5 Pt 2):1138–40.
128. Ganeson G, Mitchell M, Adams M, Rink R. Use of stomach for the reconstruction of the lower urinary tract in patients with compromised renal function. American Association of Pediatrics, New Orleans, Louisiana, 1991.
129. Castro-Diaz D, Froemming C, Manivel JC et al. The influence of urinary diversion on experimental gastrocystoplasty. J Urol 1992; 148(2 Pt 2):571–4.
130. Reinberg Y, Manivel JC, Froemming C, Gonzalez R. Perforation of the gastric segment of an augmented bladder secondary to peptic ulcer disease. J Urol 1992; 148(2 Pt 1):369–71.
131. Atala A, Bauer SB, Hendren WH, Retik AB. The effect of gastric augmentation on bladder function. J Urol 1993; 149(5):1099–102.
132. Leonard MP, Dharamsi N, Williot PE. Outcome of gastrocystoplasty in tertiary pediatric urology practice. J Urol 2000; 164(3 Pt 2):947–50.
133. Nguyen DH, Bain MA, Salmonson KL et al. The syndrome of dysuria and hematuria in pediatric urinary reconstruction with stomach. J Urol 1993; 150(2 Pt 2):707–9.
134. Ngan JH, Lau JL, Lim ST et al. Long-term results of antral gastrocystoplasty. J Urol 1993; 149(4):731–4.
135. Sheldon CA, Gilbert A, Wacksman J, Lewis AG. Gastrocystoplasty: technical and metabolic characteristics of the most versatile childhood bladder augmentation modality. J Pediatr Surg 1995; 30(2):283–7, discussion 287–8.
136. Kinahan TJ, Khoury AE, McLorie GA, Churchill BM. Omeprazole in post-gastrocystoplasty metabolic alkalosis and aciduria. J Urol 1992; 147(2):435–7.
137. Dykes EH, Ransley PG. Gastrocystoplasty in children. Br J Urol 1992; 69(1):91–5.
138. DeFoor W, Minevich E, Reeves D et al. Gastrocystoplasty: long-term followup. J Urol 2003; 170(4 Pt 2):1647–9, discussion 1649–50.
139. Gosalbez R Jr, Woodard JR, Broecker BH, Parrott TS, Massad C. The use of stomach in pediatric urinary reconstruction. J Urol 1993; 150(2 Pt 1):438–40.
140. Rink R, Adams M. Augmentation cystoplasty. In: Marshall F, ed. Textbook of Operative Urology. Philadelphia: WB Saunders, 1996: 914–26.
141. Lockhart JL, Davies R, Cox C et al. The gastroileoileal pouch: an alternative continent urinary reservoir for patients with short bowel, acidosis and/or extensive pelvic radiation. J Urol 1993; 150(1):46–50.
142. Austin PF, DeLeary G, Homsy YL, Persky L, Lockhart JL. Long-term metabolic advantages of a gastrointestinal composite urinary reservoir. J Urol 1997; 158 (5):1704–7; discussion 1707–8.
143. Austin PF, Rink RC, Lockhart JL. The gastrointestinal composite urinary reservoir in patients with myelomeningocele and exstrophy: long-term metabolic followup. J Urol 1999; 162(3 Pt 2):1126–8.
144. Walker R. Antireflux mechanisms into continent urinary diversion. AUA Update Ser 1994; 13:294–9.
145. Coffey R. Physiologic implantation of the severed ureter or common bile duct into the intestine. JAMA 1911; 56:397–403.
146. Le Duc A, Camey M, Teillac P. An original antireflux ureteroileal implantation technique: long-term followup. J Urol 1987; 137(6):1156–8.
147. Abol-Enein H, Ghoneim MA. A novel uretero-ileal reimplantation technique: the serous lined extramural tunnel. A preliminary report. J Urol 1994; 151(5):1193–7.
148. Stone AR, MacDermott JP. The split-cuff ureteral nipple reimplantation technique: reliable reflux prevention from bowel segments. J Urol 1989; 142(3):707–9.
149. Warwick RT, Ashken MH. The functional results of partial, subtotal and total cystoplasty with special reference to ureterocaecocystoplasty, selective sphincterotomy and cystocystoplasty. Br J Urol 1967; 39(1):3–12.
150. Lockhart JL, Pow-Sang JM, Persky L, Sanford E, Helal M. Results, complications and surgical indications of the Florida pouch. Surg Gynecol Obstet 1991; 173(4):289–96.
151. Benson M, Olsson C. Continent urinary diversion. Urol Clin North Am 1999; 26:125–47.
152. Sagalowsky A. Mechanisms of continence in continent urinary diversions. AUA Update Ser 1992; 11:34–9.
153. Austin PF, Lockhart JL. Continence mechanisms in urinary reconstruction. AUA Update Ser 1998; 29:226–31.
154. Mansson W, Davidsson T, Colleen S. The detubularized right colonic segment as urinary reservoir: evolution of technique for continent diversion. J Urol 1990; 144(6):1359–61.
155. Hendren WH. Reoperative ureteral reimplantation: management of the difficult case. J Pediatr Surg 1980; 15(6):770–86.
156. Kock NG. Construction of a continent ileostomy. Schweiz Med Wochenschr 1971; 101(20):729–34.
157. Hanna MK, Bloiso G. Continent diversion in children: modification of Kock pouch. J Urol 1987; 137(6): 1206–8.
158. Cohen S, Harris LD, Levitan R. Manometric characteristics of the human ileocecal junctional zone. Gastroenterology 1968; 54(1):72–5.
159. Rendelman D, Anthony J, Davis CJ. Reflux pressure studies on the ileocecal valve of dogs and humans. Surgery 1958; 44:640–3.
160. Zinman L, Libertino JA. Ileocecal conduit for temporary and permanent urinary diversion. J Urol 1975; 113(3):317–23.
161. Thuroff JW, Alken P, Engelmann U et al. The Mainz pouch (mixed augmentation ileum 'n zecum) for bladder augmentation and continent urinary diversion. Eur Urol 1985; 11(3):152–60.
162. Thuroff JW, Alken P, Riedmiller H, Jacobi GH, Hohenfellner R. 100 cases of Mainz pouch: continuing experience and evolution. J Urol 1998; 140(2):283–8.
163. Hohenfellner R, Riedmiller H, Thuroff JW. Commentary: the MAINZ pouch. In: Whitehead ED, ed. Current Operative Urology. Philadelphia: JP Lippincott, 1990: 168.

164. Stein R, Matani Y, Doi Y. Continent urinary diversion using the MAINZ pouch I technique – ten years later. J Urol 1995; 153:251.
165. Gerharz EW, Kohl U, Weingartner K et al. Complications related to different continence mechanisms in ileocecal reservoirs. J Urol 1997; 158(5):1709–13.
166. Lampel A, Hohenfellner M, Schultz-Lampel D, Thuroff JW. In situ tunneled bowel flap tubes: 2 new techniques of a continent outlet for Mainz pouch cutaneous diversion. J Urol 1995; 153(2):308–15.
167. Stein R, Lotz J, Andreas J et al. Long-term metabolic effects in patients with urinary diversion. World J Urol 1998; 16(4):292–7.
168. Issa MM, Oesterling JE, Canning DA, Jeffs RD. A new technique of using the in situ appendix as a catheterizable stoma in continent urinary reservoirs. J Urol 1989; 141(6):1385–7.
169. Bissada NK. New continent ileocolonic urinary reservoir: Charleston pouch with minimally altered in situ appendix stoma. Urology 1993; 41(6):524–6.
170. Tillem SM, Kessler OJ, Hanna MK. Long-term results of lower urinary tract reconstruction with the ceco-appendiceal unit. J Urol 1997; 157(4):1429–33.
171. Benchekroun A, Essakalli N, Faik M et al. Continent urostomy with hydraulic ileal valve in 136 patients: 13 years of experience. J Urol 1989; 142(1):46–51.
172. Benchekroun A. Continent caecal bladder. Br J Urol 1982; 54(5):505–6.
173. Guzman JM, Montes de Oca L, Gonzalez R, Ercole CJ. Modified Benchekroun technique for continent ileal stoma. J Urol 1989; 142(6):1431–3.
174. Leonard MP, Gearhart JP, Jeffs RD. Continent urinary reservoirs in pediatric urological practice. J Urol 1990; 144(2 Pt 1):330–3.
175. Sanda M, Jeffs R, Gearhart JP. Evaluation of outcomes with the ileal hydraulic continent diversion: reevaluation of the Bechkroun catheterizable stoma. World J Urol 1988; 14:108–11.
176. Rowland R, Mitchell ME, Birhle R. The cecoileal continent reservoir. World J Urol 1985; 3:(185).
177. Rink RC, Birhle R. Continent urinary diversion in children and the Indiana pouch. Probl Urol 1990; 4:663–75.
178. Lockhart JL, Pow-Sang JM, Persky L et al. A continent colonic urinary reservoir: the Florida pouch. J Urol 1990; 144(4):864–7.
179. Carroll PR, Presti JC Jr. Comparison of plicated and stapled continent ileocecal stoma. Urology 1992; 40(2):107–9.
180. Carroll PR, Presti JC Jr, McAninch JW, Tanagho EA. Functional characteristics of the continent ileocecal urinary reservoir: mechanisms of urinary continence. J Urol 1989; 142(4):1032–6.
181. Rowland R. Present experience with the Indiana pouch. World J Urol 1995; 14:92–8.
182. Canning D. Continent urinary diversion. In: King LR, ed. Urologic Surgery in Infants and Children. Philadelphia: WB Saunders, 1998: 139–61.
183. Ring K, Hensle T. Urinary diversion. In: Kelalis P, King LE, Belman AB, eds. Clinical Pediatric Urology, 3rd edn. Philadelphia: WB Saunders, 1992.
184. Rowland R. Present experience with the Indiana pouch. World J Urol 1996; 14:92–8.
185. Koff SA, Cirulli C, Wise HA. Clinical and urodynamic features of a new intestinal urinary sphincter for continent urinary diversion. J Urol 1989; 142(2 Pt 1):293–6.
186. Mitrofanoff P. [Trans-appendicular continent cystostomy in the management of the neurogenic bladder]. Chir Pediatr 1980; 21(4):297–305.
187. Duckett JW, Snyder HM 3rd. Use of the Mitrofanoff principle in urinary reconstruction. Urol Clin North Am 1986; 13(2):271–4.
188. Duckett JW, Snyder HM 3rd. The Mitrofanoff principle in continent urinary reservoirs. Semin Urol 1987; 5:55–62.
189. Duckett JW, Snyder HM 3rd. Continent urinary diversion: variations on the Mitrofanoff principle. J Urol 1986; 136(1):58–62.
190. Monfort G, Guys JM, Morrison Lacombe G. Appendicovesicostomy: an alternative urinary diversion in the child. Eur Urol 1984; 10(6):361–3.
191. Bihrle R, Klee LW, Adams MC, Foster RS. Early clinical experience with the transverse colon–gastric tube continent urinary reservoir. J Urol 1991; 146(3):751–3.
192. Cendron M, Gearhart JP. The Mitrofanoff principle. Technique and application in continent urinary diversion. Urol Clin North Am 1991; 18(4):615–21.
193. Dykes EH, Duffy PG, Ransley PG. The use of the Mitrofanoff principle in achieving clean intermittent catheterisation and urinary continence in children. J Pediatr Surg 1991; 26(5):535–8.
194. Keating MA, Rink RC, Adams MC. Appendicovesicostomy: a useful adjunct to continent reconstruction of the bladder. J Urol 1993; 149(5):1091–4.
195. Woodhouse CR, Malone PR, Cumming J, Reilly TM. The Mitrofanoff principle for continent urinary diversion. Br J Urol 1989; 63(1):53–7.
196. Kaefer M, Retik A. The Mitrofanoff principle in continent urinary reconstruction. Urol Clin North Am 1997; 24:795–811.
197. Suzer O, Vates TS, Freedman AL, Smith CA, Gonzalez R. Results of the Mitrofanoff procedure in urinary tract reconstruction in children. Br J Urol 1997; 79(2):279–82.
198. Bihrle R, Klee LW, Adams MC, Steidle CP, Foster RS. Transverse colon–gastric tube composite reservoir. Urology 1991; 37(1):36–40.
199. Sumfest JM, Burns MW, Mitchell ME. The Mitrofanoff principle in urinary reconstruction. J Urol 1993; 150(6):1875–7, discussion 1877–8.
200. Perovic S. Continent urinary diversion using preputial penile or clitoral skin flap. J Urol 1996; 155(4):1402–6.
201. Casale A, Rink R. Continent vesicostomy. Dialog Pediatr Urol 1999; 22:5–6.
202. Sen S, Ahmed S. Construction of continent catheterizable urinary conduit from an isolated segment of colon. Aust N Z J Surg 1998; 68(5):367–8.
203. Khoury AE, Van Savage JG, McLorie GA, Churchill BM. Minimizing stomal stenosis in appendicovesicostomy using the modified umbilical stoma. J Urol 1996; 155(6):2050–1.
204. Kaefer M, Rink R, Cain M, Casale A. Stomal stenosis: is ileum the ideal substrate for efferent limb construction? American Association of Pediatrics, Washington, DC, October 1999.

compliance to the washout regimen was a major contributory factor to failure in 9 patients in the early Southampton and Colorado experience. Detailed preoperative counseling and continued intensive postoperative support, ideally provided by a nurse practitioner, are essential to ensure adequate and continued motivation, without which the MACE is doomed to failure. It is an advantage to introduce the potential patient to a child and family with a functioning MACE prior to the surgical procedure.

In summary, the ideal patient for a MACE should be over 5 years of age, have a diagnosis of neuropathic bowel, an anorectal malformation or Hirschsprung's disease, be well motivated with a dedicated family, and have tried and failed all conservative measures first.

Operative technique

An aggressive preoperative bowel preparation is essential to facilitate the initial postoperative enema. A cleanout from below is often necessary, especially in the patient where constipation is the primary problem. Broad-spectrum prophylactic antibiotics that cover bowel bacteria are always administered perioperatively. In most instances, since coincidental urinary tract reconstruction is performed, a lower midline or Pfannenstiel incision is selected, depending upon the patient's body habitus, prior surgical scars, and preference. In the patient in whom a MACE only is indicated, without a urinary operation, a laparoscopic approach or an appendectomy incision can be employed.

It has been reported that it is not necessary to construct an antireflux mechanism, and some surgeons simply pull the appendix out to an abdominal stomal site. This may be done using a laparoscopic approach.[17] Both authors have attempted not using an antireflux mechanism on a number of occasions and, in some cases, the stoma was incontinent of flatus and/or stool, but in the majority the stoma was continent. It is recommended that an antireflux mechanism is constructed in open surgery, but this may be omitted to reduce technical difficulty if a laparoscopic approach is used. It is no longer necessary to disconnect the appendix from the cecum and reimplant it as one would for a continent appendicovesicostomy, as initially had been proposed by Malone. Rather, the in-situ appendix can be folded over with the cecal wall wrapped around it to produce the antireflux mechanism. This is an adaptation of the technique originally described for the Mainz pouch urinary reservoir.[12] This procedure is performed in slightly different ways by the two authors. Koyle simply wraps the cecal wall around the folded appendix using permanent sutures, similar to the technique for a Nissen fundoplication, On the other hand, Malone continues to produce a submucosal tunnel along one of the tenia and inlays the appendix into this, finally closing the seromuscular layer over it with absorbable sutures (Figure 58.1). Both authors recommend catching the serosa of the appendix wall with covering sutures in order to prevent it from pulling out of the tunnel. The mesentery of the appendix is fenestrated to prevent the wrap from compromising the blood supply to the appendix. Currently both these techniques are performing satisfactorily without significant long-term leakage. Once the antireflux mechanism has been constructed, the cecum or colon is sutured to the posterior aspect of the anterior abdominal wall to ensure that the conduit is not lying free in the peritoneal cavity, as this can lead to kinking and difficulties with catheterization. The technique needs to be modified if simultaneous MACE and appendicovesicostomy procedures are being performed. If the appendix is long enough and the vascular anatomy is suitable, it is possible to split the appendix, and both authors have done this successfully.

If the appendix is not suitable to split, or if it is absent, another technique must be instituted. The tubularized cecal or colonic flap[18] is no longer recommended because of the unacceptably high complication rates associated with this technique.[3] There are two options to using the appendix that are worthy of serious consideration. The first is the Monti procedure.[19] This is an ingenious technique where a segment of ileum is harvested on its pedicle and transversely detubularized on its antimesenteric border (see Chapter 55). The rectangular patch is tubularized along its longitudinal axis to create a catheterizable conduit of approximately 7 cm in length. The internal valvulae coniventes run in the longitudinal direction of the conduit, thus facilitating easy catheterization. Both ends of the conduit are free of mesentery and this makes the creation of the antireflux mechanism easy. When a Monti conduit is used, the Mitrofanoff flap valve principle is followed and a submucosal tunnel is created along one of the tenia, which is wrapped around it. This is similar to the original description of the MACE.[13] If the patient is obese, it is possible to use two segments of ileum or colon and produce a 14 cm conduit ('The Full Monti'), which is long enough for virtually all

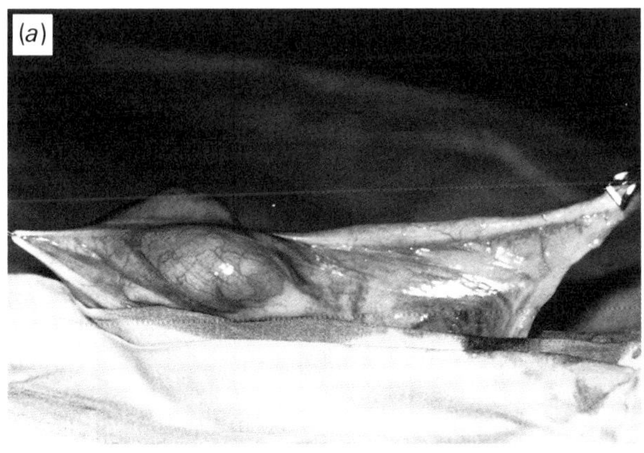

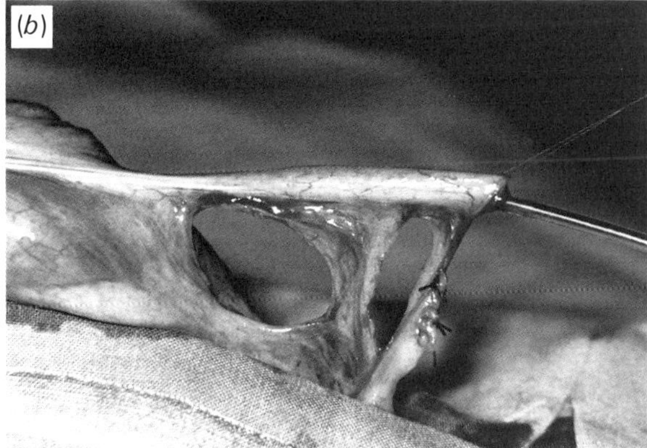

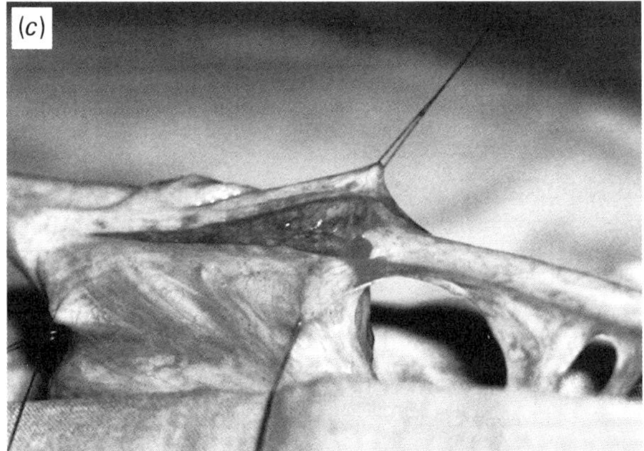

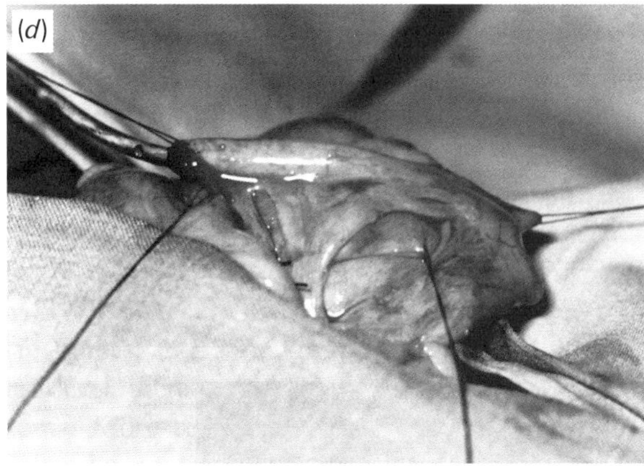

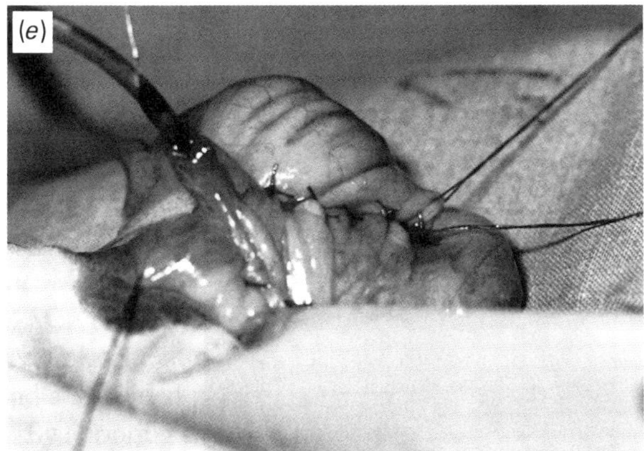

Figure 58.1 In-situ formation of the MACE: (*a*) the in-situ appendix attached to the cecum; (*b*) the fenestrated appendix mesentery; (*c*) the submucosal tunnel along one of the tenia; (*d*) the appendix folded into the tunnel; (e) the completed tunnel (note the short length of appendix).

patients. This is the procedure of choice when the appendix is not available.[20]

The other technique worthy of consideration is the use of a cecostomy tube and cecal button. Shandling et al[21] described a technique for the percutaneous placement of a cecal tube that could be changed at a later date to a low-profile cecal button (similar to a gastrostomy button), which is then used to administer the enema. A number of patients in both the Colorado and Southampton series manage their MACEs using a button, with results no different from those obtained using an appendiceal MACE (Figure 58.2). The indications for the button were:

- sloughing of cecal tubes formed when the appendix was absent,
- refusal by children/caretakers to catheterize their stomas, and thus the buttons are being used semipermanently in these cases,
- patients who developed stomal stenosis on at least one occasion and the families have preferred the non-operative button option to that of repair under anesthesia.

Our greatest worry has been erosion or skin problems as the abdominal wall girth increases with age; hence, a close follow-up is mandatory The tubes are

22. Chait PG, Shandling B, Richards HF. The cecostomy button. J Pediatr Surg 1997; 32:849–51.
23. Fonkalsrud EW, Dunn JC, Kawaguchi AE. Simplified technique for antegrade continence enemas for fecal retention and incontinence. J Am Coll Surg 1998; 187:457–60.
24. Mouriquand P, Mure PY, Feyaerts A et al. The left Monti-Malone. BJU Int 2000; 85(suppl):65.
25. Liloku RB, Mure PY, Braga L et al. The left Monti-Malone procedure: preliminary results in seven cases. J Pediatr Surg 2002; 37:228–31.
26. Churchill BM, De Ugarte DA, Atkinson JB. Left-colon antegrade continence enema (LACE) procedure for fecal incontinence. J Pediatr Surg 2003; 38:1778–80.
27. Roberts JP, Moon S, Malone PS. Treatment of neuropathic urinary and faecal incontinence with synchronous bladder reconstruction and the antegrade continence enema procedure. Br J Urol 1995; 75:386–9.
28. Malone PSJ, Curry JI, Osborne A. The antegrade continence enema procedure why, when and how? World J Urol 1999; 16:274–8.
29. McAndrew HF, Malone PS. Continent catheterizable conduits which stoma, which conduit and which reservoir? BJU Int 2002; 89:86–9.
30. Barqawi A, deValdenebro M, Furness PD 3rd, Koyle MA. Lessons learned from stomal complications in children with cutaneous catheterizable continent stomas. BJU Int 2004; 94:1344–47.
31. Hunter MF, Ashton MR, Roberts JP et al. Hyperphosphataemia following enemas in childhood: prevention and treatment. Arch Dis Child 1993; 68:233–34.
32. Shankar KR, Losty PD, Kenny SE et al. Functional results following the antegrade continence enema procedure. Br J Surg 1998; 85:980–2.
33. Aksnes G, Diseth TH, Helseth A et al. Appendicostomy for antegrade enema: effects on somatic and psychosocial functioning in children with myelomeningocele. Pediatrics 2002; 109:484–9.
34. Kajbafzadeh AM, Chubak N. Simultaneous Malone antegrade continent enema and Mitrofanoff principle using the divided appendix: report of a new technique for prevention of stoma complications. J Urol 2001; 165:2404–9.

Minimally invasive approaches to lower urinary tract reconstruction

59

Christina Kim and Steven G Docimo

Introduction

In the past 30 years, minimally invasive surgery in pediatric urology has evolved from simple diagnostic procedures to a method for performing complex reconstructive surgery. The goals of laparoscopy are to maintain the principles of open procedures while minimizing morbidity for the patient. This chapter discusses the indications, techniques, and outcomes for minimally invasive lower urinary tract reconstruction.

Principles of bladder reconstruction

Pediatric bladder reconstruction is commonly indicated for patients with neurogenic or non-neurogenic voiding dysfunction associated with high pressures or low volume. In order to protect the upper tracts from damage, and to enhance or enable urinary continence, surgery is sometimes necessary to enlarge the bladder and lower the filling pressures. In addition, surgery is sometimes necessary to enhance outlet resistance and provide for methods of emptying.

Bladder enlargement may be achieved with or without the use of bowel segments. If a bowel segment is needed, it is detubularized and reconfigured to minimize internal contractions and maximize volume.[1,2] When the circular muscle fibers are divided in a longitudinal fashion, the source for the strongest generation of contractions is stopped.[3] Theoretically, detubularization doubles the volume of the original segment. Although studies have shown the detubularized segments ultimately retain some internal contractions, detubularization is the best method available to decrease its frequency and strength.[4]

Emptying the bladder regularly will reduce the risk of infections and protect renal function. Emptying may be through voiding or may require intermittent catheterization. Catheterization may be achieved through the native urethra or a constructed Mitrofanoff or Monti continent stoma.[5] If bladder outlet resistance is low, this can be treated with bladder neck reconstruction, insertion of an artificial sphincter, placement of a periurethral sling, or bladder neck closure.

Benefits of laparoscopic reconstruction

By creating a continent system, bladder reconstruction allows the patient more independence and better quality of life. Traditionally, the only way to access appendix, small bowel, stomach, colon, as well as other pelvic organs was by making a long midline incision.[6,7] Laparoscopic assistance allows the same access and manipulation through 5 mm ports and a lower midline or Pfannenstiel incision.

The number of visible scars has been shown to inversely correlate with pediatric patients' level of happiness and satisfaction.[8] In addition, scars associated with reconstructive surgery have been associated with lower self-esteem and poor body image.[9] It is reasonable to consider that these associations and outcomes are even greater in the pediatric and adolescent populations. Not only surgical scars but also the appearance of stomas can have an impact. The development of a concealed umbilical stoma is a major step towards improving body image,[10] as well as decreasing the likelihood of stomal stenosis.[11]

Laparoscopy is associated with decreased morbidity and improved cosmesis. The outcomes in pediatrics have mirrored the outcomes in adults. The use of laparoscopy has been associated with lower narcotic requirements, shorter hospital stays, and quicker return to normal activities. In addition, and perhaps

The biggest concerns with a purely laparoscopic approach are the technical challenges of bowel manipulation, irrigation, and anastomosis. This can be intricate and time consuming. In addition to time, reconstructive urologists are concerned about the technical ability to match the outcomes of open procedures. The goal of laparoscopic-assisted surgery is to combine the morbidity and cosmetic benefits of laparoscopy with the technical precision of open reconstruction.[29]

By using laparoscopy, the required bowel segments can be isolated and mobilized quickly with small access ports. Once the bowel segment is freed, ureter or stomach harvested, and omentum mobilized, the more precise aspects of the surgery can be performed through a small lower abdominal incision. If a bladder augmentation is planned without any bladder neck reconstruction, ureteral reimplantation, or continent stoma, this can often be done simply with a lower abdominal incision and no laparoscopy is required.

The biggest benefit of laparoscopy is the ability to quickly mobilize the necessary bowel segments without the upper aspect of a large abdominal incision. Many of the pediatric patients requiring bladder reconstruction have an underlying neurologic disorder such as myelomeningocele. These patients often have an abnormally rotated cecum and appendix with position in the right upper quadrant.[30] Although challenging to reach through a lower abdominal incision, the high cecum can easily be reached with laparoscopy. In addition, patients with spina bifida may have severe lordosis, which can inhibit the mobilization of the cecum.[31] In addition, laparoscopy can easily allow lysis of adhesions that may have developed because of prior surgeries or long-term ventriculoperitoneal shunts. The presence of a shunt is not a contraindication to laparoscopic surgery.[15]

Once the needed segments are harvested, a lower midline or Pfannenstiel incision is used to mobilize the bladder and bladder neck and to assemble the anastomosis. The lower abdominal incision may incorporate one of the lower abdominal ports as well (Figure 59.10).

The technique allows similar dissection to the open technique, with smaller incisions and lower morbidity.[10,32]

Using laparoscopic assistance to create an appendicovesicostomy was first described in 1993.[32] Since that time, there have been other reports of successful laparoscopic bladder reconstructions with creation of continent stomas.[29,31,33,34] The only large reported series is from Docimo and colleagues.[33]

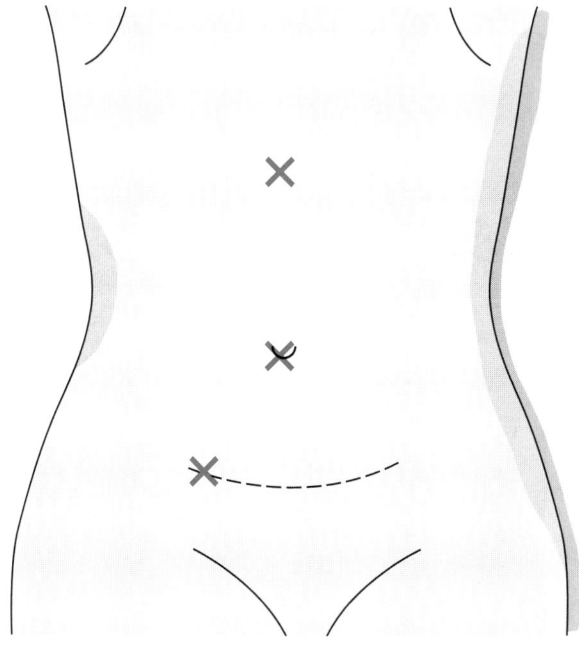

Figure 59.10 After harvesting the necessary bowel segments, the lower working port can be incorporated into a Pfannenstiel incision. (Reproduced from Hedican et al,[29] with permission.)

Technique

Preoperatively, the patient undergoes a mechanical and antibiotic bowel preparation. Intraoperatively, the patient is positioned in low lithotomy to perform a cystoscopy. If there is no active cystitis, the patient is repositioned supine. If a concominant nephrectomy or ureterocystoplasty is anticipated, the patient may be positioned in a modified flank position. The patient is padded with foam and gel pads to protect any pressure points. In addition, the patient is secured to the table to allow repositioning with steep Trendelenburg and lateral rotation as needed.

Intravenous antibiotics are given to cover Gram-positive and Gram-negative bacteria. After induction of general anesthesia, a nasogastric tube is placed. If possible, an epidural catheter is also placed.

The first step is to obtain peritoneal access. If a concealed umbilical stoma is anticipated, a U-shaped flap is created on the lower umbilicus.[11] For the purposes of achieving a straight stoma, the fascia inferior to the umbilicus is opened and the peritoneum entered under direct vision. A radially dilating trocar sleeve is inserted into the peritoneum, and dilated using the trocar insert. This should be 10 or 12 mm in size to allow easy passage of the stomal segment without creating too large a defect, which would risk parastomal herniation.

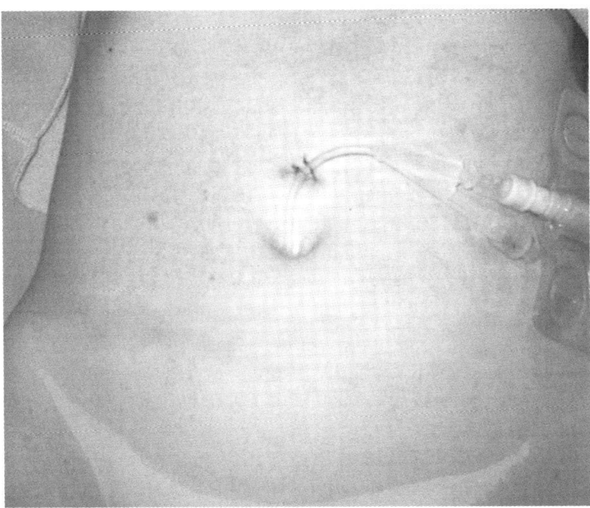

Figure 59.11 After incorporating the lower port into a Pfannenstiel incision, the visible scars are minimized. Here the umbilical port site was used for the continent stoma and the lower port healed within the Pfannenstiel scar. (Reproduced from Chung et al,[33] with permission.)

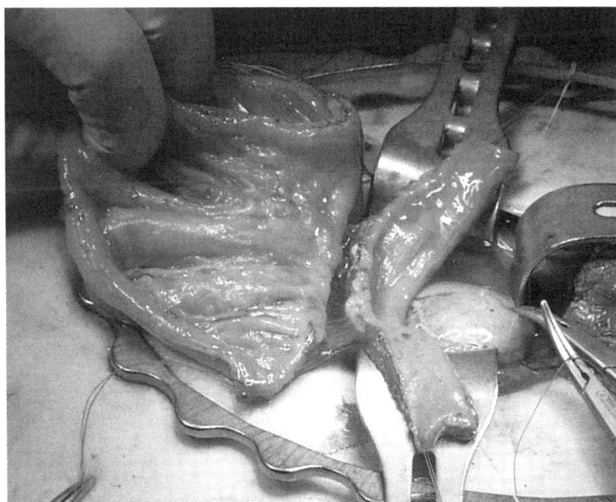

Figure 59.12 The majority of bowel manipulation can be done through a lower midline or Pfannenstiel incision. (Reproduced from Chung et al,[33] with permission.)

Placement of the working ports depends on the type of repair planned and the bowel segments needed. Most commonly, two working ports are used. A 3 or 5 mm epigastric port is placed between the umbilicus and the xyphoid. An additional port in the lower abdomen can be of variable size because it will be incorporated into the abdominal incision (Figure 59.11). If an additional stoma is created (i.e. ACE), another U-shaped incision is made in the right lower quadrant and a 10 mm port placed at this site.

Laparoscopy is for bowel manipulation, lysis of adhesions, performing nephrectomies, harvesting ureter, and harvesting omentum.

If appendix is needed, the right colon is mobilized until the appendix can reach the lower abdominal incision. Through the open incision, the appendix can be divided from the cecum. An alternative is to isolate and divide the appendix using an Endo-GIA stapler. If this approach is chosen, care must be taken to avoid disruption of the mesoappendix (Figure 59.12). If laparoscopic examination reveals an appendix in the deep pelvis, easily accessed through a Pfannenstiel incision, further laparoscopic dissection is not necessary.

After the laparoscopic portion of the procedure is completed, a 4–5 cm Pfannenstiel incision is made. This can incorporate the lower working port (see Figure 59.12). To minimize bowel manipulation, the peritoneum is left intact and any bladder work is completed first. This may include bladder neck division or reconstruction, ureteral reimplantation, and cystolitholapaxy. The next step is opening the bladder, implanting the continent stomal segment, and creating the anastomosis to the augment. All stomas are matured to the skin and any redundancy is addressed to allow easy catheterization. The bladder stoma is spatulated dorsally and then secured to the U-shaped flap. This helps conceal the stoma and reduce the chance of stenosis. The entry site of the stoma to the bladder is secured to the anterior abdominal wall to decrease the likelihood of eventual tortuosity and difficulty with catheterization.

Postoperatively, most patients are left with a nasogastric tube, suprapubic tube, and a 10 Fr stomal catheter. Drains are rarely used. The stomal catheter is secured to the skin with the balloon deflated to avoid excess tension on the continence mechanism.

Results

Laparoscopic-assisted bladder reconstruction allows patients to resume a normal diet faster and leave the hospital earlier. These outcomes exist without an increase in operative time or perioperative complications.[29,35]

The only large series of minimally invasive bladder reconstruction is the Pittsburgh series reported by the Docimo group in 2004. This series consisted of 31 patients with a mean age of 14 years: 29 of 31 patients had at least one stoma created; 10 patients had both a Mitrofanoff and an ACE stoma created;

19 patients had additional procedures performed (e.g. fascial sling, bladder neck reconstruction, revision of epispadias, ureteral reimplantation, and revision of orchidopexy).

Mean hospital stay was 6 days. Mean follow-up was 32 months. Of all stomas, 94.9% were continent of either urine or stool and easy to catheterize. Improved compliance and capacity were maintained at last follow-up. There were no late bowel obstructions or other sequelae of problematic adhesion formation. Stomal stenosis occurred in 5.1% of patients, 7.7% required stomal revision secondary to incontinence or difficulty with catheterization, and minor procedures were required in 25.6% of stomas.

Complications occurred in five patients, including ileus, partial small bowel obstruction, delayed bladder perforation, deep vein thrombosis, and wound infection.[33]

Conclusions

Minimally invasive bladder reconstruction has become our standard approach. The outcomes match or exceed those of open operations with recovery and cosmetic benefits. Long-term benefits of decreased intra-abdominal adhesions will be hard to measure, but may be the most important reason to continue to pursue these techniques. Further advances may allow purely laparoscopic techniques to achieve a more prominent role, but complex reconstruction will probably remain too time consuming for the near future. The ability of reconstructive surgeons to achieve consistent results depends on the precision of reconstructive techniques. Perhaps robotics and other advances will eventually allow performance of even complex operations with equivalent outcomes. For now, laparoscopic-assisted reconstruction is the only minimally invasive technique with well-documented outcomes, and should be considered the state of the art. One thing that is certain: in this era, there is no need for a large abdominal incision in the majority of children who require bladder reconstruction.

References

1. Koff SA. Guidelines to determine the size and shape of intestinal segments used for reconstruction. J Urol 1988; 140(5 Pt 2):1150–1.
2. Hinman F Jr. Selection of intestinal segments for bladder substitution: physical and physiological characteristics. J Urol 1988; 139(3):519–23.
3. Hensle TW, Ring KS. Urinary tract reconstruction in children. Urol Clin North Am 1991; 18(4):701–15.
4. Pope JC 4th, Keating MA, Casale AJ, Rink RC. Augmenting the augmented bladder: treatment of the contractile bowel segment. J Urol 1998; 160(3 Pt 1):854–7.
5. Mitrofanoff P. [Trans-appendicular continent cystostomy in the management of the neurogenic bladder]. Chir Pediatr 1980; 21:297–305. [French]
6. Aksnes G, Diseth TH, Helseth A et al. Appendicostomy for antegrade enema: effects on somatic and psychosocial functioning in children with myelomeningocele. Pediatrics 2002; 109(3):484–9.
7. Horowitz M, Kuhr CS, Mitchell ME. The Mitrofanoff catheterizable channel: patient acceptance. J Urol 1995; 153(3 Pt 1):771–2.
8. Abdullah A, Blakeney P, Hunt R et al. Visible scars and self-esteem in pediatric patients with burns. J Burn Care Rehabil 1994; 15(2):164–8.
9. Sarwer DB, Whitaker LA, Pertschuk MJ, Wadden TA. Body image concerns of reconstructive surgery patients: an underrecognized problem. Ann Plast Surg 1998; 40(4):403–7.
10. Ben-Chaim J, Rodriguez R, Docimo SG. Concealed umbilical stoma: description of a modified technique. J Urol 1995; 154(3):1169–70.
11. Glassman DT, Docimo SG. Concealed umbilical stoma: long-term evaluation of stomal stenosis. J Urol 2001; 166(3):1028–30.
12. Garrard CL, Clements RH, Nanney L, Davidson JM, Richards WO. Adhesion formation is reduced after laparoscopic surgery. Surg Endosc 1999; 13(1):10–13.
13. Docimo SG, Moore RG, Adams J, Kavoussi LR. Laparoscopic orchiopexy for the high palpable undescended testis: preliminary experience. J Urol 1995; 154(4):1513–15.
14. Pattaras JG, Moore RG, Landman J et al. Incidence of postoperative adhesion formation after transperitoneal genitourinary laparoscopic surgery. Urology 2002; 59(1):37–41.
15. Jackman SV, Weingart JD, Kinsman SL, Docimo SG. Laparoscopic surgery in patients with ventriculoperitoneal shunts: safety and monitoring. J Urol 2000; 164(4):1352–4.
16. Griffiths DM, Malone PS. The Malone antegrade continence enema. J Pediatr Surg 1995; 30(1):68–71.
17. Cartwright PC, Snow BW. Bladder autoaugmentation: early clinical experience. J Urol 1989; 142(2 Pt 2):505–8, discussion 20–1.
18. Ehrlich RM, Gershman A. Laparoscopic seromyotomy (auto-augmentation) for non-neurogenic neurogenic bladder in a child: initial case report. Urology 1993; 42(2):175–8.
19. Braren V, Bishop MR. Laparoscopic bladder autoaugmentation in children. Urol Clin North Am 1998; 25(3):533–40.
20. Diamond DA, Price HM, McDougall EM, Bloom DA. Retroperitoneal laparoscopic nephrectomy in children. J Urol 1995; 153(6):1966–8.
21. Britanisky RG, Poppas DP, Shichman SN, Mininberg DT, Sosa RE. Laparoscopic laser-assisted bladder autoaugmentation. Urology 1995; 46(1):31–5.

22. Poppas DP, Uzzo RG, Britanisky RG, Mininberg DT. Laparoscopic laser assisted auto-augmentation of the pediatric neurogenic bladder: early experience with urodynamic followup. J Urol 1996; 155(3):1057–60.
23. Mikulicz J. Zur Operation der angeborenen Blasenspalte. Zentralbl Chir 1899; 26:641.
24. Docimo SG, Moore RG, Adams J, Kavoussi LR. Laparoscopic bladder augmentation using stomach. Urology 1995; 46(4):565–9.
25. Meng MV, Anwar HP, Elliott SP, Stoller ML. Pure laparoscopic enterocystoplasty. J Urol 2002; 167(3): 1386.
26. Elliott SP, Meng MV, Anwar HP, Stoller ML. Complete laparoscopic ileal cystoplasty. Urology 2002; 59(6): 939–43.
27. Rackley RR, Abdelmalak JB. Laparoscopic augmentation cystoplasty. Surgical technique. Urol Clin North Am 2001; 28(3):663–70.
28. Gill IS, Rackley RR, Meraney AM, Marcello PW, Sung GT. Laparoscopic enterocystoplasty. Urology 2000; 55(2):178–81.
29. Hedican SP, Schulam PG, Docimo SG. Laparoscopic assisted reconstructive surgery. J Urol 1999; 161(1): 267–70.
30. Brown SF. Congenital malformations associated with myelomeningocele. J Iowa Med Soc 1975; 65:101–4.
31. Seifman BD, Wolf JS Jr. Use of bowel in laparoscopic urology. Urol Clin North Am 2001; 28(1):159–65.
32. Jordan GH, Winslow BH. Laparoscopically assisted continent catheterizable cutaneous appendicovesicostomy. J Endourol 1993; 7:517–20.
33. Chung SY, Meldrum K, Docimo SG. Laparoscopic assisted reconstructive surgery: a 7-year experience. J Urol 2004; 171(1):372–5.
34. Strand WR, McDougall EM, Leach FS, Allen TD, Pearle MS. Laparoscopic creation of a catheterizable cutaneous ureterovesicostomy. Urology 1997; 49(2):272–5.
35. Cadeddu JA, Docimo SG. Laparoscopic-assisted continent stoma procedures: our new standard. Urology 1999; 54(5):909–12.

syndrome. Whereas Wilms' tumor is the most common malignancy associated with BWS, in the first 7 years of life RMS, adrenocortical carcinoma and hepatoblastoma may be seen.

Li–Fraumeni syndrome is associated with a known *p53* mutation with autosomal dominant transmission. These patients are predisposed to multiple tumors, which often retain a normal *p53* allele, suggesting an alternate additional tumorgenic mechanism is involved in *p53* inactivation. Malkin et al evaluated two patients with multiple tumors in the presence of Li-Fraumeni syndrome who had a heterozygous germline *p53* mutation and found that they both were heterozygous for *p53* mutation, and tumors that they developed, which maintained *p53* heterozygosity, were noted on immunostaining to contain the DNA tumor virus SV40. The authors postulate that *p53* inactivation by viral proteins may contribute to tumor formation in these genetically susceptible patients.[13–15] Some concern has been raised for an increased risk of breast cancer in the mothers of children with soft tissue sarcomas; however, this has not been demonstrated by the International Rhabdomyosarcoma Study Groups (IRSG).[1]

Environmental factors associated with RMS include ionizing radiation and alklyating agents. The increased risk of secondary malignancies in those patients with neurofibromatosis and Li–Fraumeni syndromes after treatment with alkylating agents and radiation therapy for RMS draws a link between the likely dual causation of malignancy by genetics and environment. It is therefore desirable to limit the use of alkylating agents and radiotherapy in these particular populations.[1]

Molecular and cellular biology

Somatically acquired genetic changes underlie all forms of cancer; however, until recently, the genetic characteristics of RMS were largely unknown. With improved cytogenetic techniques, it is now clear that the chromosomes of this tumor contain both numerical and structural abnormalities.[16–18] Recent advances in the molecular and cell biology of RMS have helped in understanding the pathogenesis of this tumor and will aid in its diagnosis, staging, and management.

RMS appears to develop from a derangement in the final steps of myogenic differentiation. Genes of the *MyoD* family are crucial in the early differentiation of skeletal muscle precursors.[19,20] These genes express DNA-binding proteins that facilitate the production of myogenic proteins such as desmin, creatine kinase, and myosin. *MyoD* expression is higher in rhabdomyosarcoma cells. Activation of p38 MAP kinase, which is required for muscle differentiation, is absent in RMS cells.[21] Failing to differentiate completely, the rhabdomyosarcoma cells continue to produce forms of actin seen only transiently in normal-developing skeletal muscle cells.[22] *MyoD1*, a recently described myogenic regulatory protein, maps on chromosome 11p15.4 and is expressed during skeletal muscle development. Steroid receptor coactivator SRC-2 is necessary for skeletal muscle differentiation. RMS cell lines have demonstrated aberrant transcription factor SRC localization and expression.[23]

Myogenin is a myogenic regulatory protein whose expression determines differentiation of primitive mesenchymal cells into skeletal muscle. It is regulated by pathways involving p38, calcium–calmodulin-dependent protein kinase (CaMK), or calcineurin, and its expression may be down-regulated with terminal differentiation. The activation of myogenin by CaMK and calcineurin pathways fails in RMS cell lines.[24] Myf5 is an additional transcription factor which is useful in differentiating RMS from other sarcomas.[1]

MAGE, *BAGE*, and *GAGE* are active genes expressed in RMS which encode tumor-associated antigens and may have therapeutic potential in tumor immunotherapy.[25] The MDM2 protein binds p53 (tumor suppressor) and deactivates it. It may be seen frequently in RMS but not ERMS, and its splice variants are present in up to 82% of RMS tumors.[26–28] MDM2 increased resistance to vincristine, etoposide and doxorubicin, but not cisplatin in RMS cell lines.[29]

ARMS may be distinguished from ERMS and other tumors on the basis of structural abnormalities. Cytogenetic analysis of ARMS tumors revealed a translocation involving chromosomes 2 and 13, t(2;13)(q35;q14) in 70–80% of cases (Figure 60.1).[30–33] There have also been several reports of a

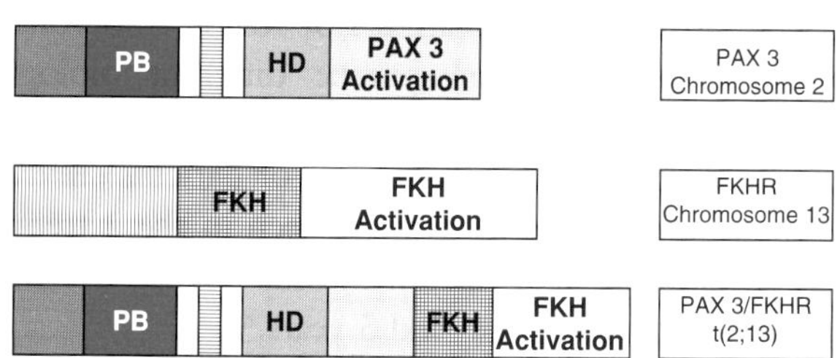

Figure 60.1 Structure of PAX3 on chromosome 2, the fork head in rhabdomyosarcoma (FKHR) on chromosome 13, and the fusion product PAX–FKHR of the t(2;13) in alveolar rhabdomyosarcoma. PB = paired box; HD = homeodomain.

t(1;13)(p36;q14) variant translocation,[32,34,35] and single reports of cases with other related alterations.[32,35,36] The t(2;13) and t(1;13) translocations have not been associated with any other tumor and appear to be specific markers for ARMS.

In a series of mapping experiments, the chromosome 2 locus disrupted by the t(2;13) was found to be *PAX3*, and translocation breakpoints were localized to the final intron of the *PAX3* gene.[37] This gene is a member of the paired box family and encodes a transcription factor with an *N*-terminal DNA-binding domain containing paired box and homeobox motifs. Its presumed function is that of transcriptional regulation strictly during embryogenesis, important in the development of mesenchymal precursors.[38] Northern analysis of ARMS tumors with 5′ PAX3 probes demonstrated a 7.2 kb transcript that is the product of the rearranged *PAX3* gene located on the derivative chromosome 13[der(13)].[37,39–41] Cloning of the corresponding cDNA revealed a fusion of exons 5′ to the t(2;13) breakpoint with a novel sequence from the 13q14 chromosomal region. A full length cDNA of the wild-type chromosome 13 gene was cloned and found to be a novel widely expressed member of the fork head transcription factor family.[42,43] This family is characterized by a conserved DNA-binding motif termed the 'fork head' domain. Based on homology to this family, the chromosome 13 gene was named FKHR for 'fork head in rhabdomyosarcoma'.[42] These combined findings indicate that the t(2;13) results in a chimeric transcript composed of 5′ PAX3 and 3′ FKHR exons (see Figure 60.1). The PAX3–FKHR fusion in ARMS is characterized by a rearrangement of chromosome 2 and 13, t(2;13)(q35;q14), in which the *PAX3* gene within band 2q35 is fused with the *FKHR* gene within band 13q14. Both of the PAX3 DNA-binding regions (the paired box and the homeodomain) are retained in the fusion gene, whereas the carboxyl-terminal sequences are replaced by the bisected fork head DNA-binding sequences of FKHR.[5,44] In PAX7–FKHR fusions, a chromosome 1 locus encoding PAX7,[43] another member of the paired box family, is rearranged and fused to FKHR in the t(1;13) conscript, consisting of 5′ PAX7 and 3′ FKHR regions, which is very similar structurally to the 5′PAX3– 3′FKHR transcript formed by the t(2;13) translocation.[45,46]

Assays of expression during embryogenesis demonstrate that PAX3 and PAX7 are expressed with specific temporal and spatial patterns in early skeletal muscle progenitors, the presumed origin of ARMS, and in the developing nervous system.[47,48] PAX3–FHKR fusion proteins have been identified to interfere with normal embryonic development prior to transformation.[49] Several putative target genes for PAX3 and PAX3–FHKR have been identified, including *Itm2A*, *Fath*, *FLT1*, *TGFA*, *BVES*, *EN2*, and *GLUT4*, which all may be involved with PAX3 regulation during embryogenesis and tumorigenesis.[50,51] In ARMS, studies indicate that the alteration of the *PAX3* gene by the t(2;13) results in a gain of function. These studies are consistent with the hypothesis that the t(2;13) activates the oncogenic potential of PAX3, by dysregulating or exaggerating its normal function in the myogenic lineage. Studies indicate that the PAX3–FKHR and PAX7–FKHR proteins affect the cellular activities of growth, differentiation, and apoptosis, and enhance cellular proliferation and invasion, with the potential to exert oncogenic effects through multiple pathways.[33,52,53]

PAX–FKHR fusions result in potent transcriptional activators.[54] FHKR may be overexpressed due to increased transcription on the PAX3–FKHR fusion protein and with in-vivo amplification of PAX7–FKHR. As opposed to FKHR, these fusion proteins are resistant to regulation by AKT, altering function and increasing expression.[33] The PAX7 *N*-terminus has repressor function which inhibits transactivation by its *C*-terminus and is only partially effective at inhibiting the C-terminus of PAX7–FKHR. This is similar to the mechanism for gain of function with PAX3–FKHR.[54] PAX3–FKHR is capable of inducing myogenin and MyoD. It is also associated with up-regulation of *Six1*, *Slug*, and *Igfbp5*, which are all genes associated with muscle development and noted to be up-regulated in ARMS.[54]

The matrix metalloproteinases (MMPs) are a family of enzymes that degrade extracellular matrix and are important in neoplastic cell invasion and metastasis. It has been shown that ARMS strongly expresses MMP-1, -2, and -9 compared with ERMS. These seem to contribute to the more aggressive nature of alveolar rhabdomyoblastic cells.[55]

PAX3–FHKR has become a potential target for ARMS therapy. Repression of *PAX3* target genes, using PAX3–KRAB fusion proteins in ARMS cell lines, has resulted in tumor repression in mice, and the engineered repressor approach targeting the genes deregulated by PAX3–FHKR may be useful to identify target genes critical for ARMS tumorigenesis.[56,57] Insulin-like growth factor-1 (IGF-1) has an important role in muscle development and in the etiology of ARMS. PAX3–FHKR has been shown to transactivate the IGF-1 receptor gene (*IGF-1R*) promoter in sarcoma cell lines with a higher potency than PAX3.[58]

Sorenson et al determined the PAX3–FKHR/PAX7–FKHR fusion status in 171 patients enrolled in IRS IV with reverse transcription polymerase chain reaction (RT-PCR). PAX3–FKHR and PAX7–FHKR were detected in 55% and 22% of the 78 patients with alveolar histology, respectively, and none with other than ARMS. Fusion status was a prognosticator for metastatic but not local disease between the two transcripts, with an estimated overall 4-year survival rate of 75% for PAX7–FKHR vs 8% for PAX3–FKHR. Failure, death, and bone marrow involvement were all significantly increased on multivariate analysis in patients with metastatic disease harboring PAX3–FKHR compared with PAX7–FKHR.[59] This corroborated results by Anderson et al, who had previously evaluated 91 RMS tumors with unequivocal evidence of the presence or absence of PAX3/PAX7–FKHR fusion transcripts: 37 had PAX3–FHKR, 8 had PAX7–FHKR, and 46 had neither. The authors found a statistically significant association between PAX3–FKHR and higher-stage disease and its absence and lower-stage disease (p = 0.06 when grouping stages 1 and 2 and stages 3 and 4). PAX7–FKHR transcript numbers were too small to reach statistical significance, but stage results were similar to the group without a translocation. PAX3–FHKR was in statistically significantly older children (p = 0.001, median 9 years old) than the other two groups (3 and 4 years for PAX7–FHKR and no translocation, respectively), whereas translocation status was not associated with disease site. Among 66 patients with non-metastatic disease, overall and event-free survival were significantly worse in the PAX3–FKHR group.[60] Collins et al found that, compared with PAX7–FKHR, PAX3–FKHR RMS demonstrated greater cell cycle dysregulation, related to both increased cell proliferation and apoptosis, and concluded that this contributes to the poorer prognosis in the PAX3–FHKR group.[61]

Evaluation of 23 ARMS tumors lacking PAX3–FHKR or PAX7–FHKR fusions identified seven cases with low expression, atypical presentation of standard fusions, or variant fusions with other genes, suggesting a genetic heterogeneity in this subset of RMS tumors.[30]

ERMS has not been associated with consistent chromosomal alterations. Ten percent of ERMS demonstrate EWS–ETS fusion anomalies that are sometimes seen simultaneously with PAX–FKHR fusions.[1] EWS/ETS is a chimeric protein identified in most Ewing's sarcoma. These are characterized by specific chromosomal translocations wherein the EWS (Ewing's sarcoma) gene on chromosome 22 is fused to one of the five members of the ETS gene family. The ETS family of transcriptional factors is so named because the first gene was uncovered in E26 avian retrovirus. Molecular genetic analyses have revealed frequent allelic loss on chromosome 11.[62] Loss of heterozygosity (LOH) at chromosome 11 is also seen in Wilms' tumor and hepatoblastoma. This genetic feature is not found in ARMS.[18] The smallest region of consistent allelic loss in ERMS cases has been localized to chromosomal region 11p15.5.[63] The deletion may be detected by cytogenic or loss of heterozygosity analysis.[38] Alterations in this chromosome region are also noted in BWS and Wilms' tumor.[64] Whereas ERMS over ARMS is more commonly associated with BWS, there is a report of three cases in the literature where ARMS without PAX–FHKR fusion was associated with BWS, with two of the cases having an 11p15 defect, suggesting that chromosome 11 alterations may play a role in this particular subset of ARMS as well as ERMS.[65]

Usually, the presence of a consistent region of allelic loss suggests the presence of a tumor suppressor gene that is inactivated in the associated malignancy. Studies have confirmed the presence of a tumor suppressor gene locus in the region previously demonstrated to show allelic loss in ERMS.[66,67] Comparing allelic loss pattern in ERMS tumors to allelic status of the patients' parents has revealed that ERMS tumors preferentially maintain the paternally inherited allele and lose the maternal allele.[17,18] The presence of the paternal allele suggests imprinting, the process by which individual genes from one parent are preferentially expressed over genes from the other. Even in close proximity to the genome, two genes can be oppositely imprinted, as is the case with the insulin-like growth factor-2 gene (*IGF-2*) vs *H19* and *CDKN1C* genes, which all map to chromosome 11p15.5. The *H19* gene product is an RNA molecule that is widely expressed during fetal development in association with cell differentiation but is apparently not translated into a protein product.[68] It controls the *IGF-2* gene, and is deactivated in several pediatric tumors, including Wilms' tumor and ERMS.[69] The *CDKN1C* gene is expressed during development in several tissues, including skeletal muscle, and encodes a cyclin-dependent kinase inhibitor that negatively regulates cell cycle progression by binding to and inhibiting the activity of several G1 cyclin/cyclin-dependent kinase complexes.[70] *H19* and *CDKN1C* are preferentially expressed from the maternally inherited allele and *IGF-2* is imprinted in the opposite direction, so that the paternally inherited alleles are expressed preferentially.[68] Recently, another gene, *GOK*, has been identified at chromosome 11p15.5. *GOK* may act as a tumor-suppressor gene in RMS and rhabdoid tumors. It has been shown that *GOK* is not expressed in many RMS cell lines, which contrasts with high expression of *GOK* in skeletal muscle.[71] Therefore, down-regulation of *GOK* expression may also play a role in the pathogenesis of RMS. *STIM-1* is another gene which maps to 11p15.5 and is a candidate growth suppressor gene with the features of a regulatory cell surface phosphoprotein. In RMS cell lines, *STIM-1* overexpression has resulted in growth arrest.[72,73] Results of these allelic loss studies suggest that ERMS tumorigenesis frequently involves inactivation of an imprinted tumor suppressor by allelic loss of the maternal active allele and retention of the paternally inactive allele.

In a small study of RMS, CD44, a membrane glycoprotein involved in cell–substrate and cell–cell interactions, was identified in 11/20 favorable and 1/7 unfavorable histology RMS ($p = 0.07$). Of the 12 patients with CD44+ve tumors, 11 were alive and in first remission, significantly less than 5/15 patients with CD44–ve tumors ($p = 0.001$). In this small study, CD44 expression in RMS correlated directly with prognosis.[74]

The combined data indicate that RMS tumorigenesis involves a variety of genetic alterations within a chromosomal region encompassing several genes. Some alterations serve to increase the number of active *IGF-2* alleles, thereby overexpressing this fetal growth factor, whereas other alterations serve to mutate or inactivate expression of growth-suppressive loci such as *H19*, *CDKN1C*, *GOK*, and *STIM-1*.

Although the *PAX3/PAX7–FKHR* gene fusions and allelic loss at chromosome 11p15.5 are the consistent, and possible defining, genetic alterations in ARMS and ERMS, other alterations have also been detected. These alterations include both mutations that activate proto-oncogenes and mutations that inactivate tumor suppressor genes. These additional genetic changes indicate that ARMS and ERMS arise and evolve by a multistep process.

Studies of genomic amplification have shown differences between ARMS and ERMS. Using chromosome scanning techniques of comparative genomic hybridization, there are frequent examples of whole chromosome gains in ERMS involving chromosomes 2, 7, 8, 11, 12, 13, 17, 18, 19, and 20.[75,76] Examination of ARMS tumors reveals few examples of chromosomal gains but evidence of amplification in almost every sample tested.[76] In contrast, in a study of 23 ARMS and 22 ERMS cases, gains and losses of chromosomal regions were found to be equally distributed between ARMS and ERMS with the exception of 7/7 q and 11/11 q gains, which were chiefly seen in ERMS. Additionally, amplifications were identified in 26% of ARMS and 23% of ERMS, with nearly all of the ERMS subset demonstrating anaplastic features.[75] In 50% of ARMS, amplification of chromosomal region 12q13–15 was detected; this region contains numerous growth-related genes, including *MDM2*, *CDK4*, and *GLI*.[77–79] Also, *MYCN* gene amplification has been found in 10 of 40 ARMS cases and in no ERMS cases.[40,80–82] This particular amplification may prognosticate a poor outcome. Among 15 ARMS patients, lack of *MYCN* amplification was associated with 66% survival compared with 11% ($p < 0.05$) for those who had it.[74] The locus for IGF-IR, 15q25–26, has been shown to be one of the amplicons that may be present in these cell lines.[75]

Another group of proto-oncogenes that are genetically altered in RMS are members of the *Ras* gene family. Mutations of members of this family (*K-ras*, *N-ras*, and *H-ras*) have been detected in some ERMS tumors, whereas none were detected in ARMS tumors.[83–85] Of the tumor suppressor genes, alterations of the *p53* gene have been most extensively studied in RMS. Using immunohistochemical assays of *p53* expression that screen for tumors in which missense mutations increase the p53 protein half-life, p53 staining was detected in approximately 70% of RMS tumors.[86,87] Diller et al corroborated previous findings that *p53* germline mutations are seen with increased frequency in sporadic cases of RMS and that these alterations are almost uniquely seen in children <3 years of age.[88] The combined results of these studies indicate that germline and acquired *p53* mutations contribute to the development of both ERMS and ARMS.

Other known tumor suppressor loci have also been investigated in RMS. A genome-wide screen of 32 RMS cases revealed several regions of allelic loss in addition to the expected 11p15 region.[89] In at least 25% of cases the regions showing allelic loss were 6p, 11q, 14q, 16q, and 18p. The overall frequency of allelic loss was lower in ARMS tumors than in ERMS tumors, again supporting the view that different molecular mechanisms are involved in the development of these two RMS subtypes. The *DCC* gene, initially identified as a tumor suppressor gene in colorectal cancer, is noted to have a mutation in 6/10 RMS cell lines.[90]

IGF-2 is overexpressed in RMS cell lines and inhibited by IGF-binding protein 6 (IGFBP6), which is associated with myoblast quiescence. IGFBP6 expression is low in RMS cell lines, and studies have demonstrated that it induced a decrease in growth and increase in apoptosis in RMS cell lines that were partially reversed with the IGF-2.[91] Several growth factors in addition to IGF have been identified to play a role in RMS tumor biology. Transforming growth factor-β (TGF-β) is an inhibitor of myogenic differentiation and an autocrine product in RMS cell lines. Inhibiting the activation of latent TGF-β in these cell lines has induced growth arrest and myogenic differentiation, whereas its elimination induces arrest, but not differentiation, indicating that there is a critical concentration required for myogenesis and this concentration is much higher in human primary muscle cells than in RMS cell lines.[92] Both high- and low-affinity receptors for nerve growth factor (NGF) have been identified in RMS cell lines. NGF has been associated with decreased apoptosis without altering differentiation in these lines.[93]

In conclusion, molecular genetic studies of RMS support the premise that ARMS and ERMS represent distinct entities. These tumors are associated with specific molecular alterations, namely PAX3/PAX7–FKHR gene fusions in ARMS and 11p15.5 allelic loss in ERMS. The gene fusions in ARMS represent gain-of-function oncogenic mutations that generate potent transcriptional activators of target genes with PAX3/PAX7 binding sites. On the other hand, the 11p15 allelic loss in ERMS acts on an imprinted region to inactivate expression of putative tumor suppressor loci. Genomic hybridization techniques may be utilized to identify genomic gains and losses in ERMS. In addition, secondary genetic alterations of other genes occur in both ARMS and ERMS, indicating that these tumors arise in a multistep process. Both the primary and secondary events affect gene products that function in signal transduction and gene expression regulatory pathways, altering numerous key pathways in the cell to ultimately generate the phenotypic changes of growth autonomy, abnormal differentiation, and motility.[94] Molecular techniques identifying these changes will be useful in differentiating ERMS and ARMS from each other and other soft tissue sarcomas as well as detecting occult bone marrow and peripheral blood metastasis, and evaluating surgical margins, both at initial resection and with second-look procedures.

Pathology

The significant difference in survival between embryonal RMS and alveolar RMS makes it imperative for the pathologist to accurately diagnose variants of RMS so that the biologic course of the disease can be predicted and appropriate therapy initiated.

In 1995, a consensus classification of RMS was published[8] that was based on a review of a large number of tumors from IRS II by 16 international pathologists from eight pathology groups. This produced a classification that was both reproducible and could predict outcome by univariate analysis. A multivariate analysis of this new International Classification of Rhabdomyosarcoma (ICR) indicated that a survival model that included the ICR along with known prognostic factors of primary site, clinical group, and tumor size was significantly better at predicting survival than a model with only the known prognostic factors.[8] The ICR classification is shown in Table 60.1, along with the IRSG addition (anaplastic variant). The data presented in this table are from ICR-related publications and IRSG publications on specific RMS subtypes.[7,8,95–97]

Table 60.1 International classification of rhabdomysarcoma

Diagnosis	Histology	Incidence (%)	5-year survival (%)	Prognosis
Embryonal, botryoid	Favorable	6	95	Superior
Embryonal, spindle cell	Favorable	3	88	Superior
Embryonal, not otherwise specified (NOS)	Favorable	49	66	Intermediate
Alveolar, NOS, or solid variant	Unfavorable	31	53	Poor
Anaplasia, diffuse	Unfavorable	2	45	Poor
Undifferentiated sarcoma	Unfavorable	3	44	Poor

Total incidence is only 94%: remaining 6% are sarcomas (NOS category) that had insufficient or inadequate tissue to make a more specific diagnosis.

Embryonal rhabdomyosarcoma

These tumors have variable amounts of spindle and primitive round cells, which may be either tightly packed or loosely dispersed in a myxoid background. The rhabdomyoblast, the more mature embryonal component, is characterized by bright eosinophilic cytoplasm and may appear in a variety of unusual shapes, termed 'tadpole', 'racquet', or 'strap' cells.[8,98] Cross-striations are seen in 50–60% of cases. Embryonal RMS represents the most common genitourinary RMS variant. These tumors rarely metastasize and respond well to current therapy. On fine needle aspiration (FNA), the embryonal subtype is suggested in specimens with large tissue fragments containing abundant eosinophilic material and small, tightly packed cells with oval nuclei.[99] ERMS stains positively for myoglobin, desmin, and vimentin. Classic ERMS with a polypoid growth pattern was associated with a more favorable prognosis than a diffuse intramural (endophytic) growth pattern in 65 cases of bladder and vaginal RMS (92% vs 68% 10-year survival, $p = 0.02$).[95]

Botryoid embryonal rhabdomyosarcoma

The ICR criterion for diagnosis of botryoid embryonal RMS requires demonstration of a cambium (condensed layer of rhabdomyoblasts) tumor layer underlying an intact epithelium in at least one microscopic field (Figure 60.2). This microscopic criterion supersedes any gross demonstration of a 'grape-like' tumor mass. An extensive degree of rhabdomyoblastic differentiation can be evident both in the cambium layer and elsewhere in the tumor. The importance of diagnosing this subtype is evident given its superior prognosis, with a 95% 5-year survival. There remains debate as to whether BRMS is a distinct entity or a variant of ERMS, and biologic studies have not demonstrated a molecular distinction.[100]

Spindle cell embryonal rhabdomyosarcoma

The spindle cell variant of RMS also enjoys a superior prognosis, with an 88% 5-year survival rate. It has only been recognized in the literature since 1993.[101] This neoplasm has a fascicular, spindled 'leiomyomatous' growth pattern that can show a marked degree of rhabdomyoblastic differentiation. Some tumors show marked collagen deposition. This variant almost exclusively occurs in the paratesticular region, although it can rarely occur at other body sites. These tumors are immunopositive for titin, a marker for terminal differentiation.[102]

Alveolar (solid) rhabdomyosarcoma

A review comparing IRSG pathologic diagnosis with institutional diagnosis performed between 1984 and 1997 showed concordance in only 63% of cases. The high level of discordant diagnosis (37%) reflects the need for better recognition of the solid alveolar variant of this RMS subtype. The classic cleft-like spaces lined by rhabdomyoblasts (Figure 60.3) that are traditionally described[7,8] for alveolar RMS may merge with spaces filled with tumor cells that sit on thin fibrovascular septae. This latter solid variant is rarely present without the classic finding of cleft-like spaces and can be recognized with adequate tumor sampling. The key criterion is to recognize palisading of tumor cells

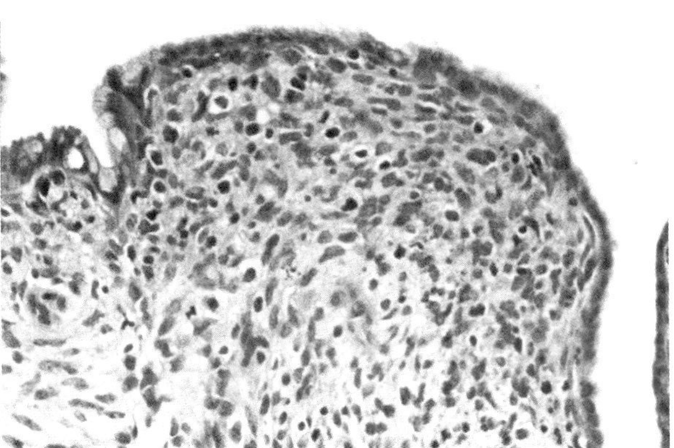

Figure 60.2 Botryoid embryonal rhabdomyosarcoma demonstrating the cambium (condensed layer of rhabdomyoblasts) tumor layer underlying an intact epithelium.

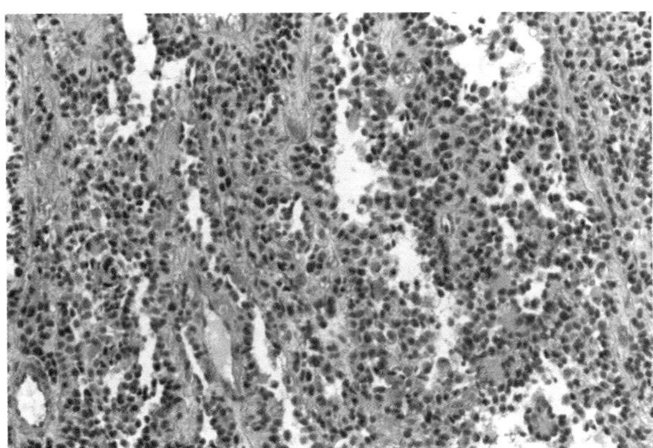

Figure 60.3 Alveolar rhabdomyosarcoma showing palisading of tumor cells with a coarse chromatin pattern about fibrovascular cores.

about fibrovascular cores. The tumor cells have a coarse chromatin pattern to their nuclei, with less-evident myogenesis than in embryonal RMS.[8] FNA biopsies of ARMS demonstrate predominantly two architectural patterns: either completely dissociated cells or many chance formations of cells. However this is non-specific, and any RMS diagnosis on FNA requires immunohistochemical confirmation.[99]

The prognosis for both the classic and solid variants is the same. Both carry a poor prognosis, with only a 53% 5-year survival rate. Improved concordance of review and institutional diagnosis is crucial for this malignancy, as they receive intensified therapy on current IRSG protocols.

Anaplastic rhabdomyosarcoma

This variant also has a high rate of discordance(62%).[7] Using the IRS I–III material, anaplastic RMS was defined using the following criteria:

- large, lobate hyperchromatic nuclei of at least three times the size of neighboring nuclei
- atypical multipolar mitotic figures.[7,96]

It is also defined further by its distribution as focal (group I), consisting of single or few anaplastic cells, or diffuse (group II), where anaplastic cells aggregate in clusters or form a continuous sheet.[7,96] The occurrence of anaplasia is independent of both RMS tumor site and histopathologic subtype, although it occurs preferentially in embryonal RMS. The overall incidence of anaplasia in IRS I–III was 3%, and it will be assessed as a new diagnostic feature of RMS in IRS V therapeutic trials.[7]

Undifferentiated sarcoma

This category, which also has a high rate of discordance (62%),[7] is included in the ICR classification only because its response to therapy is similar to that of RMS.[8]

These tumors are mainly composed of sheets of medium-packed cells with no discernible architectural structure except for delicate fibrovascular septae or a vague spindled-storiform pattern. Necrosis and inflammation are not prominent, cellularity is high with high mitotic activity [>10 mitoses per 10 high-power field(hpf)], and the nuclei are predominantly oval with prominent chromocenters and indistinct cytoplasm.[7,97] The tumors stain only with vimentin antisera (77%), if at all.

This entity is rare (3% of cases) and, like ARMS, occurs more often in males (62%), in patients ≥ 5 years old (65%), and is more common in the extremities (53%).[97] Five-year survival with localized disease is 72%, but with disseminated disease is only 44%.[7] Early identification of this histologic subtype, enabling prompt, intensified therapy, is an important component of the IRS V studies.

Ectomesenchymoma

A rare malignant neoplasm, consisting of RMS with a neural component, ectomesenchymoma (EM) is probably underdiagnosed and has a similar outcome to the RMS component of the tumors. Boue et al, in their report of 15 cases, noted that there were previously only 21 other cases reported in the literature. They noted that, of their 15 cases, only two had an originating institutional diagnosis of EM, with 12 diagnosed as RMS, and one diagnosed as undifferentiated sarcoma. Five of these cases were of external genital origin and six were pelvic/abdominal.[103]

Other diagnostic studies

Ancillary studies performed on histopathologic tissues are useful in confirming the diagnosis and in providing prognostic information on the course of the malignancy. A comprehensive study using commercially available and experimental antibodies was undertaken in the IRS IV study, which included 100 cases of RMS representing all subtypes.[7] The incidence of immunopositivity for the various antisera is summarized in Table 60.2. Around 20% of RMS cases required the use of immunohistochemistry to establish the final diagnosis.[7]

Table 60.2 Incidence of immunopositivity for antisera in rhabdomyosarcoma diagnostic studies

Antibody	Percentage
Polyclonal desmin	99
Monoclonal desmin	62
Muscle-specific actin	94
α-Smooth muscle actin	4
Myoglobin	78
Wide-spectrum keratin	7
Epithelial membrane antigen	2
S-100 protein	19
Neuron-specific enolase	6
Leukocyte common antigen	0
MIC-2	14
p53	16

Immunostaining

Myogenin is specific for rhabdomyoblastic differentiation and may help in the differentiation of small round cell tumors. It is strongly expressed in ARMS nuclei but demonstrates little or no staining in ERMS, where it has a variable staining pattern and intensity. The extent of myogenin staining in RMS is much greater than in non-RMS tumors, making it a useful marker.[104–107] In contrast to other studies, Cessna et al did note some rare non-RMS (7/107) focal nuclear reactivity to myogenin.[105] Pseudosarcomatous myofibroblastic tumors (PMTs) of the urogenital tract are rare benign tumors which may be mistaken for RMS. Myogenin is expressed in RMS but not PMTs and may be useful in differentiating these distinct clinical entities.[108]

MyoD1 expression is a distinguishing characteristic of RMS. It is now possible, through RT-PCR assay to evaluate expression of *MyoD1* mRNA. This has been found to be highly sensitive and specific in detecting minimal residual disease, as well as bone marrow and peripheral blood stem cell involvement, regardless of histologic subtype.[109] This is in contrast to a report by Gattenloehner et al, who described that *MyoD1* mRNA could be amplified from many other tissues and childhood tumors ex vivo.[110] Cessna et al reported that while all RMS stained for *MyoD1*, there was diagnostic difficulty on paraffin-embedded specimens studied due to cytoplasmic and non-specific background staining of non-myoid tissues.[105]

Polyclonal antidesmin (P-DES) antibody was positive in all but one rhabdomyosarcoma (99%). Monoclonal antidesmin (M-DES) antibody was negative in many of the same tumors (38%). Antimuscle-specific actin (MSA) antibody was positive in 94% of the RMS. Antimyoglobin (MYO) antibody was positive in 78% and was negative mostly in the less differentiated tumors. Anti-α smooth muscle actin (SMA) antibody reacted positively only in a minority (4%) of embryonal RMS.[7]

The current approach at the IRSG Pathology Center in cases where the diagnosis of RMS is in question is to screen the case with immunostaining for three antibodies: P-DES, MSA, and MIC-2; the latter helps to rule out the diagnosis of an extraosseous Ewing's sarcoma or primitive neuroectodermal tumor.[111] Around 14% of RMS stain positive to MIC-2 antisera, but this is only a weak granular intracytoplasmic immunopositivity, whereas Ewing's sarcoma and primitive neuroectodermal tumors show discreet plasma membrane staining.[111] Antibodies to the various myogenic transcription factors (MyoD1, etc.) are not tested because of their noted negativity with paraffin sections.[112]

Monoclonal antibody to p53 protein was also studied in pediatric RMS.[113] Positive immunostaining is seen in only 16% of RMS specimens.[7,114] On the other hand, immunopositivity at the grade 3–4 level (6% of RMS) was significantly associated with occurrence of any anaplasia in alveolar RMS and diffuse anaplasia in embryonal RMS, independent of fusion gene status.[115] The potential linkage of p53 abnormalities with anaplasia in RMS will be further studied in the IRS V study.

Molecular studies

Tobar et al analyzed RMS samples from nine patients (two ERMS, four ARMS, three undifferentiated sarcoma) with RT-PCR to identify the PAX3–FKHR transcript (Table 60.3). As expected, all patients diagnosed with ARMS demonstrated the chimeric transcript. However, positivity in one patient diagnosed with ERMS (with LOH at 11p15.5) and two diagnosed with undifferentiated sarcoma prompted histologic review. In the ERMS patient and one of the undifferentiated sarcoma patients, areas consistent with ARMS were identified on histologic review and patients were reclassified as ARMS, whereas the second undifferentiated sarcoma patient's diagnosis was substantiated.[38] RT-PCR for PAX3–FKHR and PAX7–FKHR on tumor tissue, bone marrow, and body fluids obtained at initial presentation and relapse in 13 ARMS patients was found to be sensitive and specific in identifying residual disease and micrometastases. Rate of detection of micrometastases in this study of three pediatric sarcomas using RT-PCR was 95% compared with 70% for morphologic methods. In three of the ARMS patients, micrometastases were

Table 60.3 Rhabdomyosarcoma immunodifferentiation

ERMS	ARMS	Poorly differentiated RMS
Myoglobin	Desmin in solid variant	*MyoD1* gene
Desmin	Vimentin	
Vimentin	Actin	
11p15.5 deletion	HHF35	
	α-1-actin	
	t(2;13)(q35;q14)	

From Tobar et al.[38]

identified with RT-PCR alone and no patient diagnosed with localized disease was found to have micrometastases on RT-PCR evaluation of bone marrow. The significance of molecularly detectable disease is unclear.[116]

In IRS V the emphasis will be on the incidence of t(1;13) and t(2;13) and their fusion genes in RMS.[7] RT-PCR methodology will be employed in detecting fusion genes in frozen and archived tissue.[117] The t(1;13) (PAX7) translocation may predict a different clinical phenotype and longer event-free survival and predilection for younger patients and extremity tumors than the t(2;13) (PAX3) translocation.[7,38]

As determined by flow cytometry, approximately two-thirds of alveolar tumors have near-tetraploid DNA content. The remaining cases are usually diploid.[118] Interestingly, near-tetraploidy is almost never observed in embryonal RMS.[5] LoH for closely linked foci of chromosome 11p5.5 is seen in embryonal RMS.

Post-treatment pathologic studies

The most difficult assessment by pathologists is the prognostic significance of residual rhabdomyoblasts in post-therapeutic RMS tissue specimens. Studies support the concept that post-therapeutic cytodifferentiation occurs more frequently in botryoid or embryonal RMS.[119–121] In botryoid RMS, cytodifferentiation and decreased proliferation activity were associated with favorable outcome. Unchanged or increased post-therapeutic proliferation activity suggested aggressive biologic potential in embryonal or alveolar RMS.

Smith et al reported on the post-treatment cytodifferentiation and clinical outcome from 19/31 IRS IV cases which were adequate for evaluation. None of the 10 cases with extensive cytodifferentiation (two BRMS, eight ERMS) failed, whereas among the five cases with moderate cytodifferentiation, only the two ARMS patients failed, and all four patients (one ERMS, three ARMS) with mild or no cytodifferentiation failed. The authors concluded that post-treatment cytodifferentiation is more common in both ERMS and BRMS than in ARMS, and postulated that this difference is due to different mechanisms of cellular response to therapy. They also noted that sparse persistent tumor cells in ARMS/BRMS did not appear to affect outcome.[121] Myoglobin is specific for terminally differentiated myocytes, and as such is a useful marker for differentiated tissue in organs such as bladder and prostate, which normally do not contain skeletal muscle. As the expression of myogenin and MyoD is down-regulated with terminal differentiation, they are less helpful to identify differentiated cells.[100] In another study, sequential evaluation of six patients with pelvic (four bladder/prostate, two vulvovaginal) RMS who had persistent well-differentiated rhabdomyoblasts without mitotic activity during and after the completion of therapy demonstrated rhabdomyoblast persistence, but decrease in number with time. All six patients were alive, with no evidence of disease from 37 to 233 months after the completion of therapy. The authors conclude that, while the biologic nature of these cells is not known, their presence is not an indication for further therapy.[122]

These phenomena will be further studied in IRS V.

Staging of rhabdomyosarcoma

Both the surgically based clinical grouping system employed in IRS I, II, and III, and the site-based TNM staging system have been used.[123–125]

Table 60.4 Clinical group staging system for rhabdomyosarcoma

Clinical	Group	Extent of disease
I	A	Localized tumor, confined to site of origin, completely resected
I	B	Localized tumor, infiltrating beyond site of origin, completely resected
II	A	Localized tumor, gross total resection, microscopic residual disease
II	B	Locally extensive tumor (spread to regional lymph nodes), completely resected
II	C	Locally extensive tumor (spread to regional lymph nodes), gross total resection, but microscopic residual disease
III	A	Localized or locally extensive tumor, gross residual disease after biopsy only
III	B	Localized or locally extensive tumor, gross residual disease after major resection (>50% debulking)
IV		Any size primary tumor, with or without regional lymph node involvement, with distant metastases, without respect to surgical approach to primary tumor

Table 60.5 Clinical grouping system for rhabdomyosarcoma

Clinical Group	Extent of disease
I	*Localized, completely resected* A Confined to site of origin B Infiltration beyond site of origin
II	*Micro residual or regional spread* A Localized with micro positive margins, grossly resected B Regional disease with complete resection, most distal node negative C Regional disease resected with micro residual or most distal resected nodes involved
III	*Gross residual* A Biopsy only B Gross/major primary resection (>50%)
IV	*Distant metastasis at diagnosis* (lung, liver, BM, bone, brain, distant muscle or + cytology CSF, pleural fluid, peritoneal fluid)

BM = bone marrow; CSF = cerebrospinal fluid.

The clinical grouping system (CGS) (Tables 60.4 and 60.5) is a surgicopathologic staging system based on whether surgical resection has been accomplished, with modifiers related to clinical and pathologic findings.[123,124]

The CGS is used to plan radiation therapy and relies on the pathologic findings determining if the tumor is confined to the primary site, with or without local invasion, and if the surgical resection is complete with tumor-free margins.

The TNM staging system (Table 60.6) takes into account tumor location, size, clinical lymph node involvement, and the presence or absence of metastases. It is used to plan therapy and is highly predictive of outcome.[123–125]

Per IRS V protocol, representative portions of the tumor should be submitted for light microscopy or fixed for electron microscopy, placed in tissue culture medium for potential chromosome studies, and frozen and stored for molecular studies.[7] When a tumor is resected, evaluation of the margins is mandatory. Recording the three-dimensional tumor size is of utmost importance as it influences staging and outcome. The distance of the tumor from the nearest resection margins is also important for staging. The pathologist has an important role in the proper staging/grouping of RMS as well as its proper histopathologic classification. Also, rapid pathology review is important for patients diagnosed with ARMS or undifferentiated sarcoma who receive additional cytotoxic therapy and radiation based on the IRS V therapeutic trials.[126] Figure 60.4 outlines the treatment algorithm for IRS V low-risk genitourinary sarcoma at diagnosis.

Presentation: bladder/prostate

- Urinary tract obstruction, hematuria, abdominal mass.
- Typically >5 cm and invasive at presentation.

Table 60.6 TNM staging of childhood genitourinary rhabdomyosarcoma

Stage	Sites	T invasiveness	T size	Regional nodes	Metastases
I	Genitourinary (non-bladder/prostate)	T1 or T2	a or b	N0, N1 or NX	M0
II	Bladder/prostate	T1 or T2	a	N0 or NX	M0
III	Bladder/prostate	T1 or T2	a	N1	M0
		T1 or T2	b	N0, N1 or NX	M0
IV	All	T1 or T2	a or b	N0 or N1	M1

T tumor: T1 = confined to anatomic site of origin; T2 = extension.
Size: a = <5 cm in diameter; b = >5 cm in diameter.
Regional nodes: N0 = not clinically involved; N1 = clinically involved; NX = clinical status unknown.
Metastases: M0 = no distant metastasis; M1 = distant metastasis present.

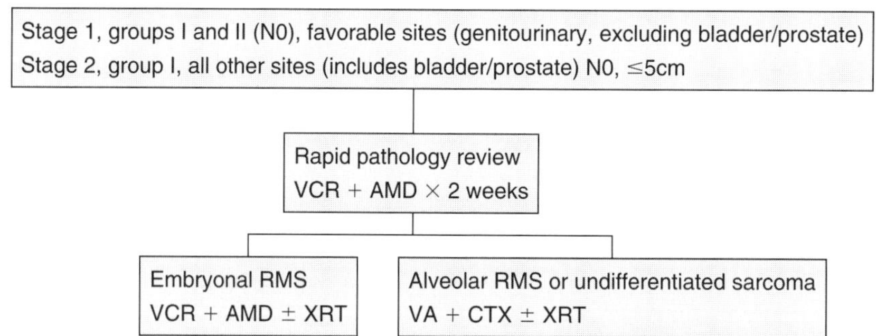

Figure 60.4 Treatment algorithm for low-risk genitourinary sarcoma in IRS V. RMS = rhabdomyosarcoma; VCR = vincristine; AMD = actinomycin D, CTX = cytoxan; XRT = radiotherapy.

A rare neonatal RMS presentation has been described, with several cases reported in the literature. It presents in the neonatal period, frequently of alveolar subtype associated with multiple cutaneous metastases, lacking characteristic RMS translocations, and has been fatal with current therapy.[21,127] In general, cutaneous metastasis of non-hematopoietic neoplasms is rare; however on review of this entity, RMS was noted to be the most common pediatric neoplasm to metastasize to the skin.[128]

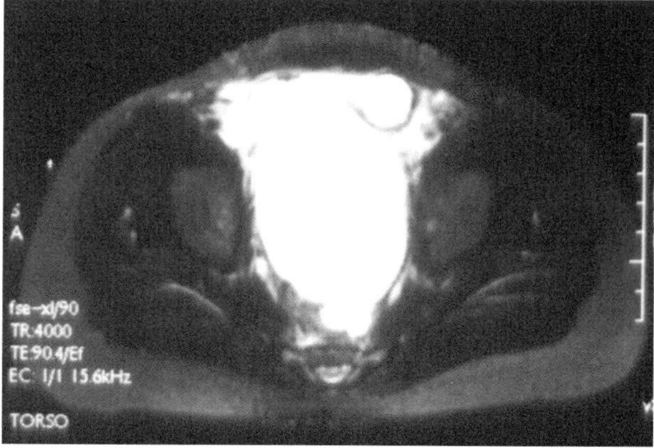

Figure 60.5 Magnetic resonance imaging scan finding in a 4-year-old male with embryonal group III rhabdomyosarcoma. On T2-weighted images the extent of the tumor is well visualized.

Diagnostic evaluation

Imaging

The first diagnostic procedure performed in patients who present with an abdominal or pelvic mass and/or symptoms of urinary obstruction is to perform a pelvic and renal ultrasound. This will usually show a solid tumor, which may be hyperechoic or hypoechoic, and will also evaluate the status of the bladder, the postvoid residual, and the upper tracts. Bladder BRMS may appear as a polypoid intraluminal mass resembling a cluster of grapes, which is characteristic but not pathognomonic of this entity.[129]

The remainder of the radiographic evaluation is to determine the extent of the local and regional disease as well as to identify metastatic foci. Magnetic resonance imaging (MRI) is replacing computed tomography (CT) as the examination of choice for accurate presurgical assessment of the extent and volume of disease. An accurate pretreatment tumor volume is necessary to plan later for adequate radiation treatment, if necessary. The extent of the tumor around the bladder and prostate can be determined by MRI T2-weighted images, with sagittal views demonstrating urethral tumor extent[130] (Figures 60.5–60.8). RMS has intermediate signal intensity on T1-

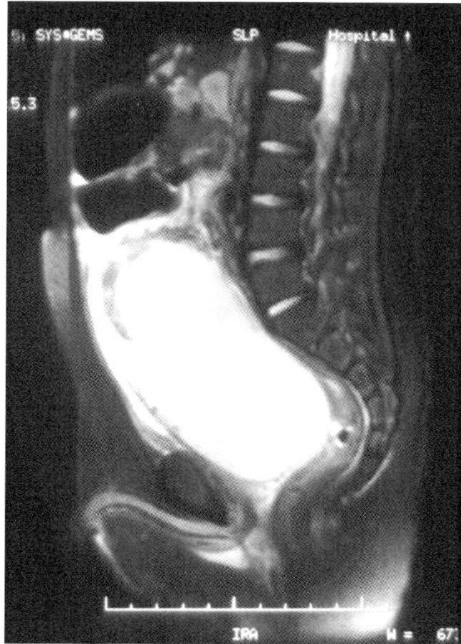

Figure 60.6 Magnetic resonance imaging scan in a 4-year-old child with embryonal group III rhabdomyosarcoma. In this sagittal view, the extent of the tumor into the membranous urethra is well delineated.

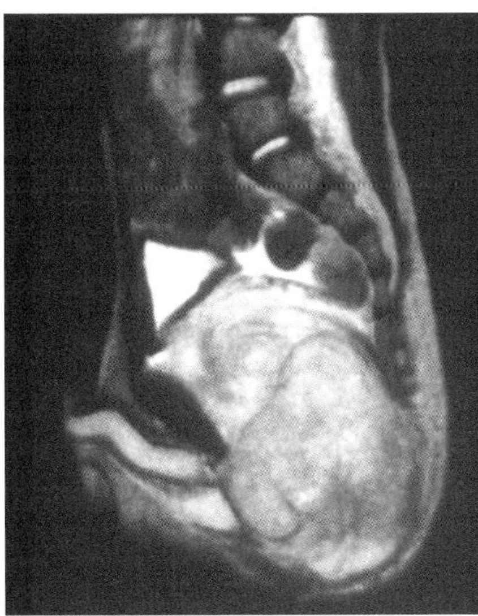

Figure 60.7 Magnetic resonance imaging scan in a 6-year-old child with embryonal group III rhabdomysarcoma. This sagittal view on T2-weighted image shows the extent of the tumor distally in the membranous urethra.

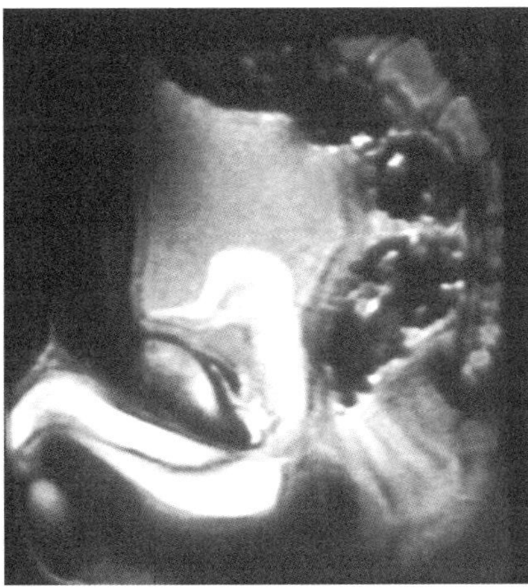

Figure 60.8 Magnetic resonance imaging scan in a 5-year-old child with embryonal group III rhabdomyosarcoma after 16 weeks chemotherapy. The tumor is visualized extending into the bladder and its extent into the urethra is also well seen.

weighted images and intermediate to high signal intensity on T2-weighted images with significant enhancement with gadolinium diethylenetriamine penta-acetic acid (Gd DTPA). ARMS demonstrates a lobular appearance on post-contrast images. Although these characteristics are non-specific and indistinguishable from other soft tissue sarcomas, MRI is useful for staging and therapeutic response assessment in RMS.[129]

Metastases occur most commonly to the lungs, bone, and lymph nodes followed by bone marrow and liver. Prostatic primaries are more likely than bladder primaries to metastasize to the lungs or bone marrow.[129] Metastatic assessment may be achieved by a CT scan of the chest, an MRI or CT of the abdomen and pelvis, bone marrow aspiration, and, if indicated, a bone scan. A CT scan may identify inguinal or retroperitoneal nodes as well as pulmonary metastases. The absence of ascites does not exclude peritoneal involvement.[131] Bone metastases in RMS are identified on imaging as ill-defined lytic lesions.[129]

In a retrospective review of 301 consecutive patients from the UK Children's Cancer Study Group, only one asymptomatic patient had evidence of metastasis on bone scan in the absence of other identifiable metastatic disease. Based on these findings, McHugh et al suggest that a routine bone scan may not be justified in patients without symptoms attributable to bone metastases (back or limb pain, limp, or hypercalcemia) or other demonstrable metastatic disease, but may be reserved for older patients or those with high-risk RMS, bone pain, alveolar histology, or poor prognostic sites outside of the head and neck.[132] These findings and recommendations were further supported by Jager et al in their study of 109 soft tissue sarcoma patients.[133] Bone marrow aspirate and biopsy are mandatory for IRS protocols, and bone marrow involvement at diagnosis is a poor prognosticator, with $<10\%$ survival. Any bone medullary defects noted on MRI require biopsy, even in the presence of a normal bone scan.[1] Routine CT or MRI of the head to evaluate for metastatic RMS of extracranial origin, required for the IRS IV protocol, is now recommended only for clinically symptomatic patients or those with paraspinal tumors.[134]

Biopsy

Tissue diagnosis of RMS is confirmed by biopsy. Specimens can be obtained either cystoscopically or with a needle biopsy. During endoscopic biopsy, it is preferable to utilize a cold-cup biopsy forceps or cold knife to avoid coagulation-induced histologic artifacts. An ultrasound-guided needle biopsy through the perineum or the extraperitroneal suprapubic route may also be used. Vaginal tumors are diagnosed and biopsied endoscopically; the extent of distortion and/or infiltration of the bladder by the tumor can also be assessed by cystoscopy. Uterine tumors can be biopsied either at the time of vaginoscopy or by performing a cervical dilatation and curettage.

Confer with the pathologist to ensure that ample tissue is obtained in order to identify the histologic subgroups of RMS and allow adequate grading to direct therapy. Needle biopsies that are performed to establish the diagnosis of RMS must include a sufficient number of cores.

Brahmi et al effectively differentiated RMS from other malignant round blue cell tumors, including Ewing's sarcoma, neuroblastoma, non-Hodgkin's lymphoma, peripheral neuroectodermal tumor, and Wilms' tumor, but not from retinoblastoma on FNA, using nuclear image morphometry.[135]

Suprapubic catheter drainage should not be used in children with RMS who present in urinary retention, to avoid the risk of tumor spread along the suprapubic track. A urethral Foley catheter can usually be used, and can be removed after chemotherapy reduces the tumor and the child is able to void.

Treatment

The outcome of children with RMS has improved dramatically over the past 30 years. Despite more frequently presenting with larger, invasive tumors and positive lymph nodes, children of ethnic minorities have enjoyed similar 5-year failure-free survivals as white children on IRS protocols in the period 1984–1997.[136] In the 1960s when therapy was local in the form of surgery and irradiation, only around one-third of all patients survived.[137] The subgroup of patients with tumors in selected primary sites such as the bladder or the orbit was treated with radical surgery, with 70% survival.[138,139] During the 1960s combined chemotherapy was initiated, with vincristine, dactinomycin, and cyclophosphamide (VAC) yielding promising results.[140,141] These early encouraging results, combined with the heterogeneity and rarity of RMS, prompted implementation in 1972 of the first national cooperative trial.

The IRS committee has reported the results of four consecutive trials, encompassing 3680 patients: IRS I (1972–1978, n = 686), IRS II (1978–1984, n = 999), IRS III (1984–1991, n = 1062),[6,9,10] and IRS IV (1991–1997, n = 883).[142] The results of the fifth consecutive trial IRS V have not been published yet. The estimated 5-year overall survival rates steadily and significantly increased in each of the first three trials: 55% in IRS I, 63% in IRS II, and 71% in IRS III, whereas the fourth trial only showed benefit over prior studies in specific subgroups of intermediate-risk ERMS, with an overall 3-year survival of 86%.[142]

In IRS I, treatment assignment was based on the postsurgical extent of disease, with no stratification for specific risk subgroups. The IRS II study recognized the prognostic significance of certain risk factors (clinical group, site, and histology), and stratified patients accordingly. Patients with primary tumors in 'special pelvic' sites (bladder, prostate, vagina, and uterus) received VAC chemotherapy. The IRS III further stratified patients into nine distinct risk subgroups according to extent of disease, primary tumor site, and histology. IRS IV evaluated new upfront window chemotherapy regimens and the effectiveness of hyperfractionated radiation therapy compared with conventional radiation.[142] IRS V, now also named the Soft Tissue Sarcoma (STS) studies of the Children's Oncology Group, has three primary protocols that are based on the risk of disease recurrence with the overall aims of reducing cyclophosphamide and radiation in low-risk groups, evaluating new regimens for unfavorable disease, and applying molecular studies for occult metastasis. The low-risk protocol will target localized embryonal and botryoid histology patients and will evaluate the efficacy of treating node-negative, favorable-site (GU non-bladder/prostate) clinical group I or II, and unfavorable-site clinical group I $\leq$ 5 cm with vincristine and actinomycin D, reserving the three-drug VAC regimen for favorable sites with gross residual or positive nodes and unfavorable sites with tumor >5 cm, microscopic residual, or positive nodes. It is also evaluating the efficacy of reduced radiation doses in microscopic residual low-risk disease. The intermediate-risk protocol will compare VAC to VAC alternating with vincristine, topotecan, and cyclophosphamide as the chemotherapeutic regimen in conjunction with radiotherapy and surgery for localized ARMS stages 1–3, ERMS stage 2 or 3 with gross residual, or patients <10 years old with stage 4 ERMS. The high-risk protocol is a phase II trial of irinotecan followed by VAC and radiation, with responders receiving additional irinotecan for stage 4 patients with ARMS as well as patients >10 years of age with ERMS.

Clinical group I

This group consists of children whose tumors were completely resected and who were expected to have an excellent prognosis.[6] In the IRS I trial it was concluded that the 5-year overall and disease-free survival did not change with the addition of radiotherapy to VAC chemotherapy. Therefore, radiotherapy was omitted in children with clinical group I tumors.[9] In this subset of patients, the IRS II study showed that vincristine and dactinomycin chemotherapy (VA) was equivalent to VAC chemotherapy. The IRS III study showed that the 5-year progression-free survival (PFS) and survival for those treated with VA for 1 year was similar to VAC for 2 years or VA for 2 years.[6] IRS IV treatment protocols, with an increased cyclophosphamide/ifosfamide intensity over IRS III, demonstrated improved 3-year failure-free survival (FFS) in group I and II unfavorable site ERMS from 71% to 86%.[143] Thus, patients with completely resected embryonal histology tumors at favorable sites (GU non-bladder prostate) can be treated safely and effectively with two drugs (VA) for 1 year. Those with bladder/prostate group I should receive cyclophosphamide, potentially at an intensified dose, and those with alveolar or undifferentiated histology should receive radiotherapy in addition to VAC.[143]

Clinical group II

Children in this category usually received postoperative radiotherapy at various time points during treatment, resulting in a local control rate of 90%.[6,9,10] Based on findings of IRS I and IRS II studies, VA with radiotherapy remains the therapeutic standard for children with clinical group II disease who present with a favorable histology tumor in a favorable site. IRS III compared VA + adriamycin and radiotherapy to VA only + radiotherapy. Even though there seemed to be an advantage to adding adriamycin, this was not statistically significant.[6] The Cooperative Soft Tissue Sarcoma Study Group (CWS) reviewed the benefits of radiotherapy for group II patients over four trials in the period 1981–1998. In this study of 203 group II patients, 110 received radiotherapy and 93 did not. Local control rates were 83% with and 65% without radiotherapy ($p < 0.004$), whereas the difference in overall survival was not statistically significant (84% vs 77%). In these studies the distribution of patients with unfavorable histology or sites was significantly higher in the groups that received radiotherapy than in those that did not, and despite this difference, the trends were for better outcome in the groups that received radiotherapy. This group was not able to identify a subset of group II patients in whom radiotherapy may be spared.[144] In IRS IV, which evaluated higher-dose cyclophosphamide as well as ifosfamide and etoposide, the intensified cyclophosphamide therapy from IRS III to IRS IV provided similar survival for patients with local or regional tumors in all IRS IV treatment groups, with a lower overall toxic death rate in IRS IV (1%). However, IRS IV was associated with improved overall survival and FFS than IRS III for the subgroup of patients with intermediate-risk (stage II/III, group 1/2) embryonal RMS (93% vs 76% 3-year FFS).[142]

As part of the Italian Cooperative Study RMS-88, 25 patients with microscopic residual RMS after primary excision were reviewed. Microscopic residuals were difficult to manage because of the lack of a measurable target. Primary re-excision with chemotherapy was the treatment of choice for children <3 years old who could not receive radiation. It was not effective for tumors >5 cm where adequate radiotherapy and chemotherapy were found to be effective.[145]

Clinical group III

This is the largest group of patients enrolled in IRS I, II, and III.[9,10,146] In IRS I, all group III patients were randomized to receive either VAC chemotherapy and radiation, or VAC with doxorubicin (VADRC–VAC) and radiation. Addition of doxorubicin failed to improve the 5-year overall survival.[9] In IRS II, patients were randomized to receive intensified VAC or VADRCV–VA therapy. Prognosis was not different between those two regimens, but the intensified treatments were superior in inducing complete responses and prolonged survival compared with IRS-I.[10] In IRS III, patients were randomized to receive either pulsed VAC or VADRC–VAC–cisplatin or VADRC–VAC–cisplatin–VP16 and radiotherapy. At 5 years, the overall survival rate was the same for all three regimens.[6] Several patients among these study arms received alternate induction chemotherapy with one of three drug pairs (doxorubicin–dacarbazine, dactinomycin–VP16, or dactinomycin–dacarbazine) and second-look surgery.[6,146] Outcome of these children was improved compared with that of patients who were treated in IRS II. In IRS IV, regimens including ifosfamide and etoposide and higher cyclophosphamide doses than in IRS III resulted in similar outcomes for group III patients among the IRS IV treatment groups and between IRS III and IRS IV. The standard remains VAC and radiation therapy for these patients.[142] However, whereas unfavorable-site group III patients demonstrated no improvement in survival on IRS IV compared with IRS III, the subset of group III or resectable node-positive ERMS with a GU non-bladder/prostate primary improved from 72% to 92% 3-year FFS.[143]

Clinical group IV

With the exception of a subset of intermediate-risk patients (<10 years old, embryonal), the 5-year survival for patients with metastatic disease continues to be poor, in spite of intensified therapy and new drug combinations. The combined-agent regimens in the first three IRS studies led to 5-year overall survival and PFS rates of below 30%.[6,9,10]

In a pilot study for IRS IV, doxorubicin and ifosfamide were used in an upfront window prior to VAC for metastatic RMS, resulting in an ultimate complete response rate of 53% and one-third survival, similar to prior regimens. Factors in this study contributing to a better prognosis included age <10 years old, embryonal histology, a GU primary, lack of nodal disease, and absence of bone or bone marrow metastasis.[147] IRS IV evaluated the effectiveness of an upfront window of ifosfamide and etoposide (IE) compared with vincristine and melphalan (VM) for metastatic presentations. This initial therapy was followed by VAC, surgery, and radiotherapy and then a repeat of VM or IE in initial responders. Whereas initial response in both groups was high, overall survival was better in the IE group, with 3-year FFS and overall survival of 33 and 55% in the IE group compared with 19 and 27% for the VM group, respectively.[148] Retrospective multivariate analysis of 137 group IV patients enrolled in IRS IV identified the presence of two or fewer metastatic sites as a predictor of survival. The subgroup with embryonal histology and two or fewer metastatic sites demonstrated a 3-year FFS of 40% and overall survival of 47%, compared with 25% and 39% for all patients studied. The authors suggest that this subgroup, whose survival approaches that of selected patients with nonmetastatic disease, might not be appropriate candidates for consideration in highly toxic or unproven antitumor investigational regimens.[149]

Topotecan in an upfront window prior to VAC and continued for responders, in 48 patients with metastatic RMS, resulted in a 46% overall response rate with an acceptable toxicity profile; in particular, efficacy was greater against ARMS than ERMS (65% vs 28% response, $p = 0.08$).[150]

IRS V is investigating new drugs such as irinotecan and topotecan.[126] It is also exploring the role of surgery after induction chemotherapy (12 weeks for most group III patients) as a strategy to reduce local failure risk. The decision for resection is determined by chemotherapy response, and whether form and function can be preserved. If such surgery is performed, postoperative radiotherapy is required, with doses determined by resection margin status: gross residual 50.4 Gy; microscopic residual 41.4 Gy; and clear margins 36 Gy.[151]

The European Collaborative Studies MMT4–89 and MMT4–91 failed to demonstrate a statistically significant improvement in 3-year event-free survival comparing consolidative megatherapy (high-dose chemotherapy and stem cell rescue) and standard chemotherapy (30% vs 19% of 53 and 44 patients) in the treatment of metastatic disease.[152] The lack of benefit of this modality was further verified by Weigel et al, who completed a meta-analysis of 389 metastatic RMS patients treated with high-dose chemotherapy and stem cell rescue; this treatment conferred no survival advantage for stage IV patients compared with IRS II and III.[153]

A novel treatment strategy for these patients includes immunotherapy. Research at the National Cancer Institute has demonstrated that blocking the IGF-1 receptor using the antibody α-IR-3 can inhibit RMS cell proliferation.[154]

Special pelvic tumors

Early on in the IRS studies, it became apparent that certain pelvic tumors (bladder, prostate, vagina, and uterus) responded better to therapy than other sites. The 5-year overall survival rate in this group of patients was 74%. However, this outcome was achieved at the expense of numerous bladder extirpations for patients with GU tumors, and only 23% of the patients had functional bladders 3 years after therapy.[155] In IRS II, the treatment strategy changed to primary chemotherapy with 4 months of VAC followed by delayed radiation and/or surgery. This treatment approach failed to improve the bladder salvage rate, with a 3-year bladder retention rate of only 25% and a survival rate similar to IRS I.[156,157] In IRS III, patients in clinical group III received an either intensified VADRC–VAC regimen + cisplatin to induce a complete response. Second-look surgery was recommended at 20 weeks. Alternate induction therapy with dactinomycin alone or dactinomycin and VP16 was initiated if tumor remained. The 3-year bladder preservation rate (60%), 5-year PFS estimate (74 ± 5%) and overall survival (83 ± 4) were strikingly superior to those of IRS I and IRS II.[6,9,10]

The extent of surgical intervention in RMS of the bladder, vagina, and prostate remains controversial. In a series of 15 patients with tumors confined to one of these three organs, Fisch et al have shown that, after chemotherapy, radical operative intervention with multiple biopsies at the resection margins permits complete tumor resection with excellent long-term results.[158] This radical operative approach is in contrast to the IRS protocol. The main advantage of this treatment protocol is that radiotherapy – which is often used in conjunction with organ-sparing surgery, and can be associated with severe complications, including radiation-induced cystitis and impaired growth of the pelvic bone – is avoided.[3] Fichtner and Hohenfellner reported a 10% rate of radiation-induced cystitis when radiation was used alone and 30% when it was used in conjunction with chemotherapy.[159]

Bladder/prostate

Prior to multiagent chemotherapy, bladder/prostate RMS was treated with radical cystectomy or pelvic exenteration. Encouraging results with primary chemotherapy have prompted a paradigm shift toward organ preservation when possible without negatively impacting long-term survival.

Heyn et al reviewed the outcome of 28 patients with group III bladder RMS. All received 20 weeks of multiagent chemotherapy and 4 weeks of radiotherapy. Of these, 13 underwent cystectomy. Cystectomy specimens demonstrated diminished tumor cells with varying degrees of maturation. They concluded that primary bladder RMS is very responsive to chemotherapy and radiotherapy, and that these tumors show further maturation following treatment, thus allowing preservation of larger proportions of bladders with residual disease.[119] Similarly, Lobe et al examined the role of conservative surgery in localized prostatic RMS and have shown a high cure rate with relatively good bladder salvage rate without aggressive early surgery.[160]

Arndt et al reported the results from the IRS IV study. They reviewed the records of 88 patients with non-metastatic bladder/prostate RMS. Tumors commonly arose in the bladder (70%) and had favorable histology (80% embryonal or botryoid). Of these tumors, 69% were >5 cm in diameter, 84% were group III, and 56% were invasive T2 tumors. The survival rate at 6 years was 82%, and event-free survival at 6 years was 77%. Of all the patients entered in the study, 40% (36/88) survived event free, with apparently normal functioning bladders. The authors state that more precise long-term evaluation of bladder and sexual function will be required using such tools as urodynamic studies and validated patient surveys.[161]

In an outcome analysis of 13 patients with lower urinary tract RMS at the Hospital for Sick Children in Toronto, the authors proposed a strategy of induction chemotherapy followed by surgical excision and reconstruction without radiotherapy, which provided a high cure rate without the late sequelae of pelvic radiotherapy.[162] The survival rate in this small group of patients was 80%. They suggested reserving radiotherapy for residual and metastatic disease and for patients with unresectable disease and those with microscopic disease. Their approach included performing re-excision should microscopic disease be found in the final pathology report.

Arndt et al reviewed bladder function retention with a bladder preservation approach in patients with non-metastatic bladder or prostate RMS enrolled in IRS IV.[161] Of 90 patients, 88 had sufficient information for review, with most tumors in the bladder, large, favorable histology, unresectable, and invasive. All received alkylating-based chemotherapy, and 74 received radiation. As one of the goals of the protocol was organ preservation, initial radical resection was not recommended. Patients underwent initial biopsy with initial complete resection only if organ preservation was possible, with extirpation reserved for biopsy-proven residual after completion of therapy, or progression of disease and early treatment failure after chemotherapy and radiotherapy, Overall and event-free survival rates at a median follow-up of 6.1 years were 82% and 77%, respectively. Events included three second malignancies, one toxic death, and 18 relapses (14 (78%) deaths with relapse). Bladder preservation without relapse was achieved in 55 patients, 40% of whom had normal bladder function defined as lack of incontinence, dribbling, hydronephrosis, or enuresis after age 10 years at a median follow-up of 9 years. The authors advocated conservative delayed surgery in this group of patients and recognized the need for continued long-term evaluation of bladder function in these patients as radiation treatment may have late effects.

Female genital tract

From 1972 to 1996, with the advent of effective chemotherapeutic regimens, the rate of surgical tumor resection for vaginal/uterine RMS decreased from 100% to 13%. Management with chemotherapy and restrictive surgery has demonstrated excellent long-term survival and frequent uterine preservation. Arndt et al reviewed the 151 patients with RMS of the female genital tract out of the 4272 enrolled in IRS I–IV with RMS. Overall 5-year survival was 82%. Chemotherapy was primarily VAC based. Local control was surgery alone in 42%, surgery and radiotherapy in 19%, biopsy and radiotherapy in 12%, and biopsy without radiotherapy in 21% (no local therapy). Many patients with primary vaginal tumors received delayed radiotherapy or had it omitted with excellent outcome. Hysterectomy rates decreased from 48% in IRS I–II to 22% in IRS III–IV, with an increase in radiotherapy from 23% in IRS II to 45% in IRS IV. There was no significant difference in survival over the course of the four trials for patients with localized embryonal/botryoid tumors. Prognostic factors included improved prognosis for age 1–9 years, embryonal histology, N0 disease, non-invasive tumors, and the use of IRS III or IV treatment protocols. Patients outside of the 1–9 year age range particularly benefited from the intensified treatment of IRS III or IV (5-year survival 67% IRS I–II vs 90% IRS III–IV); 43% of deaths of patients with group I–III tumors were from toxicity. Unlike RMS at other sites, in this subgroup of patients, 67% of those who developed recurrent disease were salvaged with multimodal treatment, including chemotherapy, surgery, and radiotherapy if not previously received. The authors recommend continued use of primary chemotherapy of VA for group I or II embryonal RMS and VAC for group III disease, with individualized local treatment plans based on tumor site and histology. Non-embryonal female genital tract RMS should receive intensified chemotherapy, as they are of intermediate recurrence risk. Delayed radiotherapy is recommended for selected patients, such as those with positive margins after chemotherapy and local surgery, those with vulvar embryonal group II or III tumors, and all those with embryonal lesions who are lymph node positive.[163]

Unfavorable histology clinical groups I and II tumors

The poor outcome for children with clinical group I alveolar tumors was recognized in IRS I.[9] All these children therefore received intensive VAC chemotherapy in IRS II. This treatment modification increased the 3-year disease-free survival rate from 43% to 69%.[10] In IRS III, therapy was further intensified with the use of a VADRC–VAC–cisplatin-containing regimen. The 5-year PFS (71 ± 6%) and overall survival (80 ± 6) rates were significantly improved over those for comparable patients treated on IRS II protocols.[6]

Despite using an intensified chemotherapy regimen in IRS III compared with the first two studies, patients with unfavorable histology (alveolar or undifferentiated) who did not receive radiotherapy fared worse than those who received radiotherapy in this study or historically. Pooled data from IRS I, II, and III on all undifferentiated and alveolar RMS demonstrated that radiotherapy was associated with improved FFS (73 vs 44%, 10 years; $p = 0.03$), with fewer local, regional, and distant relapses.[54] In a review of IRS I, II, and III group 1 patients, Wolden et al identified that tumors >5 cm and alveolar histology were associated with poorer FFS. GU primary site conferred both an overall survival and FFS advantage for embryonal RMS but not for alveolar RMS or undifferentiated sarcoma.[164] IRS IV found no improved survival in alveolar histology compared with IRS III.[142]

Local therapy: results of multi-institutional trials

Although RMS is a chemosensitive tumor, drugs alone cannot cure most children who have this disease. Surgical resection alone or in combination with irradiation is necessary for local control of the tumor, which is essential as nearly half of those children who die of this tumor fail at the primary site.

Radiotherapy

Radiotherapy has been used to eradicate residual microscopic or macroscopic tumor cells following surgery or chemotherapy. In response to the results of several trials, radiotherapy doses now vary according to the patient age, tumor site, and amount of residual tumor.[165]

Intensified chemotherapy and second-look surgery have decreased the use of radiotherapy and extensive primary surgery for patients with vaginal and vulvar RMS.[166] In addition, the use of early radiotherapy, aggressive chemotherapy, and second-look surgery has dramatically decreased the use of radical surgery to treat children with genitourinary RMS.[6,166]

Currently, microscopic residual disease is treated with 40 Gy of radiation to the tumor bed and a 2 cm margin. In IRS IV, radiotherapy of completely resected tumors with unfavorable features (large size, unfavorable site, nodal involvement) was mandated, with gross residual disease requiring higher doses of 45–55 Gy, depending on the site and size of the tumor.[5,44]

Further, to increase local control and decrease the acute and late adverse effects of radiotherapy, IRS IV evaluated hyperfractionated radiotherapy in patients with unresectable or metastatic disease. A total of 559 patients with group III RMS were enrolled, of which

490 were eligible for randomization. Of these 239 were randomized to hyperfractionated radiation therapy and 251 to conventionally fractionated radiotherapy. There was no statistical difference in overall survival or FFS between the two radiation treatment methods, and no difference between the two treatment groups when analyzed for age, gender, tumor size, invasiveness, nodal status, histology, or primary site. The recommendation from the analysis is that the standard of care for group III RMS remains chemotherapy and conventionally fractionated radiation therapy.[149]

Surgery

Surgical approaches to the treatment of RMS have also been influenced by the multi-institutional studies. Nodal involvement is very common among patients with GU tumors; therefore, nodal sampling should be considered at the time of initial staging.[124,167] If performed within 35 days of the primary procedure, surgical re-excision may benefit patients with microscopic positive residual tumor; however, such re-excision may be difficult with the lack of a measurable target.[145,162,168]

Summary

IRS III trials in patients with group III special pelvic primary tumors (bladder, prostate, vagina, and uterus) clearly demonstrated that these patients benefited from the more complex therapy. Addition of doxorubicin (ADR) and cisplatin (CDDP), with or without second-look surgery, or dactinomycin (AMD) + VP16 to VAC improved outcome as compared with the results with VAC with or without second-look surgery in IRS II (83% vs 72% 5-year survival rate). Of the 90 patients who achieved complete response (CR), 29% (26/90) were rendered tumor free by second-look surgery. They also concluded that the introduction of radiotherapy in patients with tumors in the bladder neck/trigone or prostate may have had a favorable impact on outcome. Finally, there was a more than doubling of the bladder salvage rate, which was attributed to the more intensive therapy used in IRS III.

Figure 60.4 summarizes the protocol for low-risk genitourinary RMS in the present IRS trial.

Chemotherapeutic agents

Doxorubicin

IRS I, II, and III randomized group III and IV tumor patients to VAC with or without doxorubicin with similar radiotherapy. No benefit to doxorubicin was detected.

Cisplatin and etoposide

IRS III evaluated VAC vs VAC–doxorubicin + cisplatin vs VAC–doxorubicin–cisplatin + etoposide, with all patients receiving radiotherapy. There was no benefit of any of the additional agents over VAC alone.

Ifosfamide

Severe acute renal tubular toxicity was noted for ifosfamide when combined with carboplatin in children with sarcomas compared with ifosfamide alone or with cisplatin, whereas combination use with cisplatin was associated with delayed renal tubular toxicity.[169] Skinner et al identified risk factors associated with nephrotoxicity from ifosfamide in 148 young sarcoma patients. Reduction of risk for nephrotoxicity was noted with doses <84 g/m,[2] whereas doses >119 g/m^2 were associated with a very high risk of severe toxicity.[170]

Melphalan

Melphalan is active in previously untreated RMS and was combined with vincristine in IRS IV in comparison with ifosfamide–etoposide and ifosfamide–doxorubicin (DOX) for metastatic disease in an upfront window. Despite high response rates, the melphalan group required more dose reduction of cyclophosphamide and had higher rates of secondary malignancy and inferior overall survival.[126,148]

Topotecan

Chastagner et al reported that topotecan potentiates the radiation response of two different human RMS tumors xenografted into nude mice. Five days of concomitant topotecan and radiotherapy had a synergistic therapeutic effect, with the efficiency of the combined regimen resulting in similar effect at a radiation dose of 20 Gy to the 40 Gy of radiation alone.[171] Topotecan administered to 40 patients with stage 4 RMS resulted in a 45% complete and partial response rate.[126] Fifteen patients with recurrent or refractory RMS were treated with a combination of topotecan and cyclophosphamide, with 10 achieving a partial or complete response.[172]

Investigational

Differentiation therapy is a novel approach for cancer treatment in which the principle is to transform malignant cells into mature cells and decrease side effects of classical chemotherapy such as drug resistance and cytotoxicity. This technique has shown in-vitro effectiveness using GR-891 and QF-3602, 5-fluorouracil acyclonucleoside derivatives, against RMS cell lines, by inducing terminal myogenic differentiation with no cytotoxicity, increased adhesion capability, and no induction of *MDR1*, a gene that induces multidrug resistance.[173,174]

Antiangiogenesis therapy is a novel treatment approach of great research interest. The angiogenesis stimulators, vascular endothelial growth factor (VEGF), basic fibroblast growth factor (bFGF), and interleukin-8 (IL-8), have all been identified as products of ERMS, and effective antiangiogenic therapies may require multiple drugs to target several angiogenic factors.[175] Landuyt et al induced tumor necrosis in subcutaneous RMS in rats using the angiogenesis inhibitor TNP-470, with both tumor volume and drug dose affecting treatment outcome and therapy found to be potentially useful in treating progressive tumor growth and large tumors.[176] Antibodies to VEGF have been shown to decrease growth of RMS cell lines; however, there is up-regulation of host VEGF in response to hypoxia, indicating a need to completely block VEGF for maximum tumor inhibition.[177] VEGF and VEGF receptor 2 (fetal liver kinase 1 (Flk-1)) play a role in tumor angiogenesis. Dc101, an anti-Flk-1 antibody, in conjunction with doxorubicin demonstrated greater antitumor activity in RMS cell lines xenografted in immunodeficient mice than doxorubicin alone.[178]

An alternative method of targeting tumor-specific vascularization is antivascular therapy, which would target inadequate and ill-structured tumor vasculature. Combretastatin A4 phosphate is an antivascular drug that when administered systemically to rats induced growth delay in solid RMS with a greater effectiveness with larger tumor volume.[179] As opposed to small or medium tumors, large tumors had a better response with the addition of radiotherapy to combretastatin A4 phosphate. The addition of the antiangiogenesis drug TNP-470 demonstrated no added therapeutic effect.[180]

Late effects of therapy

Because of the improved long-term survival and the use of intensified chemotherapeutic regimens, several serious and potentially life-threatening therapy-related complications have emerged. In IRS IV pilot studies, the incorporation of ifosfamide into front-line therapeutic protocols for children with unresectable tumors was associated with a 14% incidence of renal toxicity. Factors that contributed to that toxicity included high doses of ifosfamide (>72 g/m^2), age younger than 3 years, and pre-existing renal abnormalities such as hydronephrosis.[181,182] Toxicities for the final IRS IV trial included >90% myelosuppression, 55% severe infections, and only 2% severe renal toxicity. Toxic deaths were highest in the VAC regimen in patients with pre-existing renal abnormalities (3/56), with rates for other regimens <1% (neutropenia with septicemia = 6, metabolic = 1, and other = 1).[142]

Of the 109 patients with bladder and prostate tumors who were treated in IRS I and II, 29% developed post-therapy hematuria, 29% showed evidence of delayed pubertal development, and 10% had growth retardation.[183]

The occurrence of second malignant neoplasms is one of the most devastating sequelae of successful contemporary therapy. Of the 1770 patients enrolled in IRS I and II, 22 developed second malignant neoplasms (10-year cumulative incidence rate of 1.7%). The most common malignancies were bone sarcomas ($n = 11$) and acute non-lymphoblastic leukemia ($n = 5$). The median time to development of these neoplasms was 7 and 4 years, respectively.[184] In the IRS III trial, acute myeloid leukemia occurred in 5 of the 1062 patients enrolled. All of the patients received the alkylating agent cyclophosphamide, and four received etoposide. The median time to development of acute myeloid leukemia was 39 months; median follow-up was 3.7 years.[185] IRS IV had 10 second malignancies in the initial report (myelodysplastic syndrome/acute myeloid leukemia = 4, acute lymphoid leukemia = 1, lymphoblastic lymphoma = 1, osteogenic sarcoma = 1, leiomyosarcoma = 1, undifferentiated sarcoma = 1, and primitive neuroectodermal tumor = 1), for a 3-year cumulative risk in locoregional disease on IRS IV of 2%.[142] A large review of secondary malignancies in long-term survivors of childhood RMS was performed by Scaradavou et al.[186] They reported on 130 patients, with a median follow-up of 9 years. Seven patients (5.4%) developed secondary malignancies, including three with acute non-lymphoblastic leukemia and four with solid tumors. This study identified an increased risk of secondary neoplasms in patients receiving the chemotherapeutic agents carmustine and doxorubicin. They did not find radiotherapy to be a significant risk factor in contrast to the findings from the Late Effect Study Group, which reported an increased incidence of secondary neoplasms within prior radiation fields. Additionally, there are case reports in the literature of other secondary malignancies after RMS treatment, including adenocarcinoma of the colon associated with radiation colitis 13 years after treatment for bladder RMS, bladder transitional cell carcinoma 8 years after cyclophosphamide for ERMS, and Hodgkin's disease after childhood RMS therapy.[187]

Residual disease

Residual disease after treatment is a risk factor for local recurrence. Differentiation of residual tumor from fibrosis can be very difficult on CT and MRI. Positron emission tomography (PET) scanning with fluorodeoxyglucose (FDG), which has been found to have a high uptake in many different tumors, may help with this differentiation in the future. These techniques may also be useful in screening for metastatic disease.[132]

Recurrence

Review of IRS I–III for group 1 patients found 86/439 patients relapsed, with median follow-up of 12.9 years for IRS I, 9.1 years for IRS II, and 4.6 years for IRS III. Relapses in these patients occurred within 1 year in 48% and 3 years in 93% of patients, while two patients relapsed as late as 10 years after diagnosis.[164] In IRS III, the estimated 5-year cumulative incidence of local failure was 19%, regional nodal was 2%, and distant recurrence was 11%. Lymph node involvement at diagnosis was the single factor most predictive of increased total local failure risk (5-year cumulative incidence of 32%), compared with children with negative nodes or unknown node status (16%). The 5-year FFS and overall survival rates were 70% and 78%, respectively.[151]

IRS IV had a 3-year estimated cumulative incidence of local, regional, and distant failures of 10%, 4%, and 7%, respectively.[142] Retrospective analysis of survival for 605 patients after relapse in IRS III and IV revealed that 5-year survival depended significantly on histology (64% of botryoid, 26% of embryonal, and 5% of alveolar). Within the embryonal group, stage and group at presentation affected probability of relapse survival (52% stage 1/group I; 12% stage 4/group IV), but the type of relapse was only influential in initial stage 1/group 1 disease, with local relapse survival 72% and distant 30%. Relapse in alveolar RMS was associated with better survival after an initial group 1 tumor compared with other initial presentations despite location of recurrence (40% vs 3%).[188]

From the IRS trials III, IV, pilot and IV, the 10-year late event (disease recurrence, second malignant neoplasm, or death from other causes) rate was estimated at 9%. The estimated cumulative incidence of the specific subtypes of failures at 5 and 10 years were 2.4% and 2.7% for recurrence, 1.9% and 2.4% for second malignant neoplasms, and 0.8% and 3.5% for death as a first event, respectively. Patients with both advanced disease (group III/IV) and large primary tumors at diagnosis (>5 cm) were at the highest risk for late events. The probability of a late event in that high-risk group of patients was 19%.[189] Relapse in ARMS continues to have a dismal clinical outcome, prompting ongoing evaluation of novel therapies. Dagher et al evaluated the effectiveness and toxicity of a peptide pulsed vaccination targeting the breakpoint region of fusion proteins administered concomitantly with continuous IL-2 infusion. Treatment did not alter the poor outcome for all 16 translocation positive Ewing sarcoma and ARMS patients who continued to have progressive disease after immunization. All patients in this trial were significantly immunocompromised and had large bulky tumors.[190]

Conclusion

The advances in understanding the biologic and genetic features of RMS, as well as the development and scheduling of new drugs, have improved the survival of these children. However, several challenges still remain. These include the refinement of risk-directed therapy based on the understanding of newly recognized biologic and clinical features. The use of newly developed hematopoietic growth factors will allow dose intensification, which may offer improvement in children with metastatic or recurrent disease. Finally, genetic abnormalities such as translocation (PAX3–FKHR and PAX7–FKHR) in alveolar tumors may provide molecular targets for future therapies.

Other pelvic tumors

Transitional cell carcinomas

Bladder tumors rarely occur in the first two decades of life and are commonly of mesodermal origin. These are low-grade transitional cell carcinomas that seldom recur.[191–197] Some of these tumors occur secondary to cyclophosphamide therapy.[146,198–201] In more than 90% the lesions are solitary. Pathologically, 80% of these tumors are grade I or papilloma, 20% are grade I–II tumors, and only 3% are invasive through the lamina propria. The recurrence rate is low (2–5%).

Presenting symptoms include gross hematuria in 80% of the patients, irritative voiding symptoms or recurrent urinary tract infections in 15%, and microscopic hematuria in 8% of patients.[202]

The initial diagnosis can be made by ultrasound, which in some series was found to be 100% sensitive. Intravenous pyelography and CT scans may not be able to detect small tumors. Cytologic evaluation is of limited value, as most of these tumors are low-grade transitional cell carcinoma.[191,202]

Cystoscopy allows definitive diagnosis, staging, and treatment of these tumors. Its role in surveillance remains ill defined, particularly because it requires general anesthesia and because the risk of recurrence is low.

Nephrogenic adenoma of the bladder

This rare, benign lesion of the bladder occurs as an epithelial response to infection or trauma. It presents as a papillary lesion resembling a low-grade, low-stage transitional cell carcinoma.[203–206] There is a significant predominance of girls to boys (5:1). The medical history in all cases is remarkable for previous bladder surgery or inflammation. This benign lesion is believed to represent urothelial transformation in response to trauma or inflammation.[203]

Most children present with unspecific symptoms of gross hematuria, dysuria, and bladder instability. Final diagnosis is established after cystoscopy and histopathologic review of a tumor biopsy specimen. Tumor recurrence develops in 80% of the children, with a latency period of 4 years. Therapy consists of transurethral resection, long-term antibiotic therapy, and periodic cystoscopy.[203–206]

Leiomyosarcoma

These tumors are rare in the pediatric age group and account for <2% of all soft tissue sarcomas; their diagnostic features and biologic behavior appear similar to those in adults. The most important features in assessing malignant potential are tumor size and mitotic counts. Local excision usually provides adequate therapy.[207–210]

Urachal adenocarcinoma

This very rare tumor accounts for only 0.17–0.34% of all bladder neoplasms. It usually occurs in adults, but there are several reported cases in children. This mucin-producing or colloid adenocarcinoma arises from the juxtavesical segment of the urachus and invades the bladder. The presenting symptoms are hematuria and bladder irritative symptoms. The primary treatment is surgical resection. The prognosis is poor because its location predisposes to extensive local spread before detection and diagnosis.[211,212]

Adenocarcinoma of the extrophied bladder

This tumor occurs more frequently in adults than in children. It occurs in patients who have not had bladder reconstruction and is rarely found in a reconstructed bladder.[213–223]

Pathologically, the epithelial lining of the bladder is replaced with colonic epithelium. The histochemistry comprises cells containing colon-specific mucin and carcinoembryonic antigen. In many of these tumors dysplasia of the colonic epithelium is found, with an area of colonic exophytic adenocarcinoma.

Mesonephric adenocarcinoma of the female genital tract

This rare and highly malignant tumor can occur at any age. Approximately 30% of such tumors occur in children. Evidence that these tumors originate from the mesonephric (wolffian) rests includes their tubular structure and their occurrence along the tract of the mesonephric duct or its remnants (vagina, cervix, uterus, and salpinx). The clinical, gross pathologic, and radiographic presentations of vaginal mesonephric carcinomas may be indistinguishable from those of ERMS. The presenting symptoms are vaginal bleeding or a vaginal mass. Radiographic features are similar to RMS and include grape-like clusters of tumor nodules within the vagina. Treatment includes radical excision, radiotherapy, or both.[224–226]

Clear cell adenocarcinoma of the vagina or cervix

Maternal diethylstilbestrol (DES) prior to 18 weeks' gestation has been strongly implicated in the etiology of this tumor. The age of the DES-exposed patients has varied from 7 to 34 years old, with the highest frequency from 14 to 22 years old. The risk among the exposed is in the order of 1 in 1000.[227–229]

The rarity of this tumor among exposed women suggests that DES is not a complete carcinogen but that some other factors are also involved in the pathogenesis of clear cell adenocarcinoma of the vagina and cervix.[229–236]

Cavernous hemangiomas of the bladder

This hamartoma is a rare benign tumor of the bladder that usually presents with macroscopic hematuria. In about 30% of cases, the bladder tumor is associated with angiomatous lesions in other parts of the body. The diagnosis may be suspected on ultrasound examination but it is generally made at cystoscopy.[237–240] Blood-pool scintigraphy using technetium 99m (^{99m}TC) human serum albumin combined with DTPA usually reveals an area of increased activity in the bladder.[241] Biopsy and transurethral resection must be avoided because of the risk of hemorrhage. Laser treatment of hemangiomas has been reported and should be the initial management.[241] Should laser coagulation fail, partial cystectomy appears to be the most effective method of treatment.[239,242]

References

1. Ruymann FB, Grovas AC. Progress in the diagnosis and treatment of rhabdomyosarcoma and related soft tissue sarcomas. Cancer Invest 2000; 18(3):223–41.
2. Julian JC, Merguerian PA, Shortliffe LM. Pediatric genitourinary tumors. Curr Opin Oncol 1995; 7(3):265–74.
3. Agarwal SK, Prowse OA, Merguerian PA. Pediatric genitourinary tumors. Curr Opin Oncol 1997; 9(3):307–12.
4. Angell SK, Pruthi RS, Merguerian PA. Pediatric genitourinary tumors. Curr Opin Oncol 1996; 8(3):240–6.
5. Pappo AS, Shapiro DN. Rhabdomyosarcoma: biology and therapy. Cancer Treat Res 1997; 92:309–39.
6. Crist W, Gehan EA, Ragab AH et al. The Third Intergroup Rhabdomyosarcoma Study. J Clin Oncol 1995; 13(3):610–30.
7. Qualman SJ, Coffin CM, Newton WA et al. Intergroup Rhabdomyosarcoma Study: update for pathologists. Pediatr Dev Pathol 1998; 1(6):550–61.
8. Newton WA Jr, Gehan EA, Webber BL et al. Classification of rhabdomyosarcomas and related sarcomas. Pathologic aspects and proposal for a new classification – an Intergroup Rhabdomyosarcoma Study. Cancer 1995; 76(6):1073–85.
9. Maurer HM, Beltangady M, Gehan EA et al. The Intergroup Rhabdomyosarcoma Study-I. A final report. Cancer 1988; 61(2):209–20.
10. Maurer HM, Gehan EA, Beltangady M et al. The Intergroup Rhabdomyosarcoma Study-II. Cancer 1993; 71(5):1904–22.
11. Sung L, Anderson JR, Arndt C et al. Neurofibromatosis in children with rhabdomyosarcoma: a report from the Intergroup Rhabdomyosarcoma study IV. J Pediatr 2004; 144(5):666–8.
12. Gripp KW, Scott CI Jr, Nicholson L et al. Five additional Costello syndrome patients with rhabdomyosarcoma: proposal for a tumor screening protocol. Am J Med Genet 2002; 108(1):80–7.
13. Malkin D, Chilton-MacNeill S, Meister LA et al. Tissue-specific expression of SV40 in tumors associated with the Li–Fraumeni syndrome. Oncogene 2001; 20(33): 4441–9.
14. Malkin D. p53 and the Li–Fraumeni syndrome. Biochim Biophys Acta 1994; 1198(2–3):197–213.
15. Malkin D. p53 and the Li–Fraumeni syndrome. Cancer Genet Cytogenet 1993; 66(2):83–92.
16. Pappo AS, Crist WM, Kuttesch J et al. Tumor-cell DNA content predicts outcome in children and adolescents with clinical group III embryonal rhabdomyosarcoma. The Intergroup Rhabdomyosarcoma Study Committee of the Children's Cancer Group and the Pediatric Oncology Group. J Clin Oncol 1993; 11(10):1901–5.
17. Scrable H, Cavenee W, Ghavimi F et al. A model for embryonal rhabdomyosarcoma tumorigenesis that involves genome imprinting. Proc Natl Acad Sci USA 1989; 86(19):7480–4.
18. Scrable H, Witte D, Shimada H et al. Molecular differential pathology of rhabdomyosarcoma. Genes Chromosomes Cancer 1989; 1(1):23–35.
19. Parham DM. The molecular biology of childhood rhabdomyosarcoma. Semin Diagn Pathol 1994; 11(1):39–46.
20. Parham DM, Dias P, Bertorini T et al. Immunohistochemical analysis of the distribution of MyoD1 in muscle biopsies of primary myopathies and neurogenic atrophy. Acta Neuropathol (Berl) 1994; 87(6):605–11.
21. Puri PL, Wu Z, Zhang P et al. Induction of terminal differentiation by constitutive activation of p38 MAP kinase in human rhabdomyosarcoma cells. Genes Dev 2000; 14(5):574–84.
22. Schurch W, Bochaton-Piallat ML, Geinoz A et al. All histological types of primary human rhabdomyosarcoma express alpha-cardiac and not alpha-skeletal actin messenger RNA. Am J Pathol 1994; 144(4):836–46.
23. Chen SL, Wang SC, Hosking B, Muscat GE. Subcellular localization of the steroid receptor coactivators (SRCs) and MEF2 in muscle and rhabdomyosarcoma cells. Mol Endocrinol 2001; 15(5):783–96.
24. Xu Q, Yu L, Liu L, Cheung CF et al. p38 Mitogen-activated protein kinase-, calcium-calmodulin-dependent protein kinase-, and calcineurin-mediated signaling pathways transcriptionally regulate myogenin expression. Mol Biol Cell 2002; 13(6):1940–52.
25. Dalerba P, Frascella E, Macino B et al. MAGE, BAGE and GAGE gene expression in human rhabdomyosarcomas. Int J Cancer 2001; 93(1):85–90.
26. Bartel F, Taylor AC, Taubert H, Harris LC. Novel mdm2 splice variants identified in pediatric rhabdomyosarcoma tumors and cell lines. Oncol Res 2000; 12(11–12): 451–7.
27. Taylor AC, Shu L, Danks MK et al. P53 mutation and MDM2 amplification frequency in pediatric rhabdomyosarcoma tumors and cell lines. Med Pediatr Oncol 2000; 35(2):96–103.
28. Xia SJ, Pressey JG, Barr FG. Molecular pathogenesis of rhabdomyosarcoma. Cancer Biol Ther 2002; 1(2):97–104.
29. Cocker HA, Hobbs SM, Tiffin N et al. High levels of the MDM2 oncogene in paediatric rhabdomyosarcoma cell lines may confer multidrug resistance. Br J Cancer 2001; 85(11):1746–52.

155. Hays DM. Bladder/prostate rhabdomyosarcoma: results of the multi-institutional trials of the Intergroup Rhabdomyosarcoma Study. Semin Surg Oncol 1993; 9:520–3.
156. Raney RB Jr, Crist W, Hays D et al. Soft tissue sarcoma of the perineal region in childhood. A report from the Intergroup Rhabdomyosarcoma Studies I and II, 1972 through 1984. Cancer 1990; 65:2787–92.
157. Raney RB Jr, Gehan EA, Hays DM et al. Primary chemotherapy with or without radiation therapy and/or surgery for children with localized sarcoma of the bladder, prostate, vagina, uterus, and cervix. A comparison of the results in Intergroup Rhabdomyosarcoma Studies I and II. Cancer 1990; 66:2072–81.
158. Fisch M, Burger R, Barthels U, Gutjahr P, Hohenfellner R. Surgery in rhabdomyosarcoma of the bladder, prostate and vagina. World J Urol 1995; 13(4):213–18.
159. Fichtner J, Hohenfellner R. Damage to the urinary tract secondary to irradiation. World J Urol 1995; 13(4): 240–2.
160. Lobe TE, Wiener E, Andrassy RJ et al. The argument for conservative, delayed surgery in the management of prostatic rhabdomyosarcoma. J Pediatr Surg 1996; 31(8):1084–7.
161. Arndt C, Rodeberg D, Breitfeld PP et al. Does bladder preservation (as a surgical principle) lead to retaining bladder function in bladder/prostate rhabdomyosarcoma? Results from intergroup rhabdomyosarcoma study iv. J Urol 2004; 171(6 Pt 1):2396–403.
162. Merguerian PA, Agarwal S, Greenberg M et al. Outcome analysis of rhabdomyosarcoma of the lower urinary tract. J Urol 1998; 160(3 Pt 2):1191–4, discussion 1216.
163. Arndt CA, Donaldson SS, Anderson JR et al. What constitutes optimal therapy for patients with rhabdomyosarcoma of the female genital tract? Cancer 2001; 91(12):2454–68.
164. Wolden SL, Anderson JR, Crist WM et al. Indications for radiotherapy and chemotherapy after complete resection in rhabdomyosarcoma: a report from the Intergroup Rhabdomyosarcoma Studies I to III. J Clin Oncol 1999; 17(11):3468–75.
165. Pappo AS, Bowman LC, Furman WL et al. A phase II trial of high-dose methotrexate in previously untreated children and adolescents with high-risk unresectable or metastatic rhabdomyosarcoma. J Pediatr Hematol Oncol 1997; 19(5):438–42.
166. Andrassy RJ, Hays DM, Raney RB et al. Conservative surgical management of vaginal and vulvar pediatric rhabdomyosarcoma: a report from the Intergroup Rhabdomyosarcoma Study III. J Pediatr Surg 1995; 30(7):1034–6, discussion 1036–7.
167. Lawrence W Jr, Hays DM, Heyn R et al. Lymphatic metastases with childhood rhabdomyosarcoma. A report from the Intergroup Rhabdomyosarcoma Study. Cancer 1987; 60(4):910–15.
168. Hays DM, Lawrence W Jr, Wharam M et al. Primary reexcision for patients with 'microscopic residual' tumor following initial excision of sarcomas of trunk and extremity sites. J Pediatr Surg 1989; 24(1):5–10.
169. Marina NM, Poquette CA, Cain AM et al. Comparative renal tubular toxicity of chemotherapy regimens including ifosfamide in patients with newly diagnosed sarcomas. J Pediatr Hematol Oncol 2000; 22(2):112–18.
170. Skinner R, Cotterill SJ, Stevens MC. Risk factors for nephrotoxicity after ifosfamide treatment in children: a UKCCSG Late Effects Group study. United Kingdom Children's Cancer Study Group. Br J Cancer 2000; 82(10):1636–45.
171. Chastagner P, Merlin JL, Marchal C et al. In vivo potentiation of radiation response by topotecan in human rhabdomyosarcoma xenografted into nude mice. Clin Cancer Res 2000; 6(8):3327–33.
172. Saylors RL 3rd, Stine KC, Sullivan J et al. Cyclophosphamide plus topotecan in children with recurrent or refractory solid tumors: a Pediatric Oncology Group phase II study. J Clin Oncol 2001; 19(15):3463–9.
173. Marchal JA, Prados J, Melguizo C et al. GR-891: a novel 5-fluorouracil acyclonucleoside prodrug for differentiation therapy in rhabdomyosarcoma cells. Br J Cancer 1999; 79(5–6):807–13.
174. Marchal JA, Melguizo C, Prados J et al. Modulation of myogenic differentiation in a human rhabdomyosarcoma cell line by a new derivative of 5-fluorouracil (QF-3602). Jpn J Cancer Res 2000; 91(9):934–40.
175. Pavlakovic H, Havers W, Schweigerer L. Multiple angiogenesis stimulators in a single malignancy: implications for anti-angiogenic tumour therapy. Angiogenesis 2001; 4(4):259–62.
176. Landuyt W, Theys J, Nuyts S et al. Effect of TNP-470 (AGM-1470) on the growth of rat rhabdomyosarcoma tumors of different sizes. Cancer Invest 2001; 19(1):35–40.
177. Gerber HP, Kowalski J, Sherman D, Eberhard DA, Ferrara N. Complete inhibition of rhabdomyosarcoma xenograft growth and neovascularization requires blockade of both tumor and host vascular endothelial growth factor. Cancer Res 2000; 60(22):6253–8.
178. Zhang L, Yu D, Hicklin DJ et al. Combined anti-fetal liver kinase 1 monoclonal antibody and continuous low-dose doxorubicin inhibits angiogenesis and growth of human soft tissue sarcoma xenografts by induction of endothelial cell apoptosis. Cancer Res 2002; 62(7): 2034–42.
179. Landuyt W, Verdoes O, Darius DO et al. Vascular targeting of solid tumours: a major 'inverse' volume-response relationship following combretastatin A-4 phosphate treatment of rat rhabdomyosarcomas. Eur J Cancer 2000; 36(14):1833–43.
180. Landuyt W, Ahmed B, Nuyts S et al. In vivo antitumor effect of vascular targeting combined with either ionizing radiation or anti-angiogenesis treatment. Int J Radiat Oncol Biol Phys 2001; 49(2):443–50.
181. Heyn R, Raney RB Jr, Hays DM et al. Late effects of therapy in patients with paratesticular rhabdomyosarcoma. Intergroup Rhabdomyosarcoma Study Committee. J Clin Oncol 1992; 10(4):614–23.
182. Ashraf MS, Brady J, Breatnach F, Deasy PF, O'Meara A. Ifosfamide nephrotoxicity in paediatric cancer patients. Eur J Pediatr 1994; 153(2):90–4.
183. Raney B Jr, Heyn R, Hays DM et al. Sequelae of treatment in 109 patients followed for 5 to 15 years after diagnosis of sarcoma of the bladder and prostate. A report

from the Intergroup Rhabdomyosarcoma Study Committee. Cancer 1993; 71(7):2387–94.
184. Heyn R, Haeberlen V, Newton WA et al. Second malignant neoplasms in children treated for rhabdomyosarcoma. Intergroup Rhabdomyosarcoma Study Committee. J Clin Oncol 1993; 11(2):262–70.
185. Heyn R, Khan F, Ensign LG et al. Acute myeloid leukemia in patients treated for rhabdomyosarcoma with cyclophosphamide and low-dose etoposide on Intergroup Rhabdomyosarcoma Study III: an interim report. Med Pediatr Oncol 1994; 23(2):99–106.
186. Scaradavou A, Heller G, Sklar CA, Ren L, Ghavimi F. Second malignant neoplasms in long-term survivors of childhood rhabdomyosarcoma. Cancer 1995; 76(10): 1860–7.
187. Park SS, Kim BK, Kim CJ et al. Colorectal adenocarcinoma as a second malignant neoplasm following rhabdomyosarcoma of the urinary bladder: a case report. J Korean Med Sci 2000; 15(4):475–7.
188. Pappo AS, Anderson JR, Crist WM et al. Survival after relapse in children and adolescents with rhabdomyosarcoma: A report from the Intergroup Rhabdomyosarcoma Study Group. J Clin Oncol 1999; 17(11):3487–93.
189. Sung L, Anderson JR, Donaldson SS et al. Late events occurring five years or more after successful therapy for childhood rhabdomyosarcoma: a report from the Soft Tissue Sarcoma Committee of the Children's Oncology Group. Eur J Cancer 2004; 40(12):1878–85.
190. Dagher R, Long LM, Read EJ et al. Pilot trial of tumor-specific peptide vaccination and continuous infusion interleukin-2 in patients with recurrent Ewing sarcoma and alveolar rhabdomyosarcoma: an inter-institute NIH study. Med Pediatr Oncol 2002; 38(3):158–64.
191. Serrano-Durba A, Dominguez-Hinarejos C, Reig-Ruiz C, Fernandez-Cordoba M, Garcia-Ibarra F. Transitional cell carcinoma of the bladder in children. Scand J Urol Nephrol 1999; 33(1):73–6.
192. Keetch DW, Manley CB, Catalona WJ. Transitional cell carcinoma of bladder in children and adolescents. Urology 1993; 42(4):447–9.
193. Yanase M, Tsukamoto T, Kumamoto Y et al. Transitional cell carcinoma of the bladder or renal pelvis in children. Eur Urol 1991; 19(4):312–14.
194. Quillin SP, McAlister WH. Transitional cell carcinoma of the bladder in children: radiologic appearance and differential diagnosis. Urol Radiol 1991; 13(2):107–9.
195. Khasidy LR, Khashu B, Mallett EC, Kaplan GW, Brock WA. Transitional cell carcinoma of bladder in children. Urology 1990; 35(2):142–4.
196. Madgar I, Nativ O, Hanani Y, Jonas P. Transitional cell carcinoma of the bladder in children under ten years of age. A case report. Eur Urol 1988; 14(3):216–17.
197. Benson RC Jr, Tomera KM, Kelalis PP. Transitional cell carcinoma of the bladder in children and adolescents. J Urol 1983; 130(1):54–5.
198. Durkee C, Benson R Jr. Bladder cancer following administration of cyclophosphamide. Urology 1980; 16(2):145–8.
199. Cox PJ. Cyclophosphamide cystitis and bladder cancer. A hypothesis. Eur J Cancer 1979; 15(8):1071–2.
200. Fairchild WV, Spence CR, Solomon HD, Gangai MP. The incidence of bladder cancer after cyclophosphamide therapy. J Urol 1979; 122(2):163–4.
201. Pearson RM, Soloway MS. Does cyclophosphamide induce bladder cancer? Urology 1978; 11(5):437–47.
202. Hoenig DM, McRae S, Chen SC et al. Transitional cell carcinoma of the bladder in the pediatric patient. J Urol 1996; 156(1):203–5.
203. Heidenreich A, Zirbes TK, Wolter S, Engelmann UH. Nephrogenic adenoma: a rare bladder tumor in children. Eur Urol 1999; 36(4):348–53.
204. Azumi M, Tokumitsu M, Saga Y et al. [Nephrogenic adenoma of the bladder in children]. Nippon Hinyokika Gakkai Zasshi 2002; 93(3):495–8. [in Japanese]
205. de Jong EA, Scholtmeijer RJ. Nephrogenic adenoma of the bladder in children. Eur Urol 1984; 10(3):187–90.
206. Nold SR, Terry WJ, Cerniglia FR et al. Nephrogenic adenoma of the bladder in children. J Urol 1989; 142(6):1545–7.
207. Borzi PA, Frank JD. Bladder leiomyosarcoma in a child: a 6 year follow-up. Br J Urol 1994; 73(2):219–20.
208. Lack EE. Leiomyosarcomas in childhood: a clinical and pathologic study of 10 cases. Pediatr Pathol 1986; 6(2–3):181–97.
209. Laurenti C, De Dominicis C, Dal Forno S, Bologna G. Leiomyosarcoma of the bladder in a girl. Eur Urol 1982; 8(3):185–7.
210. Weitzner S. Leiomyosarcoma of urinary bladder in children. Urology 1978; 12(4):450–2.
211. Sheldon CA, Clayman RV, Gonzalez R, Williams RD, Fraley EE. Malignant urachal lesions. J Urol 1984; 131(1):1–8.
212. Rankin LF, Allen GD, Yuppa FR, Pirozzi MJ, Hajjar JR. Carcinoma of the urachus in an adolescent: a case report. J Urol 1993; 150(5 Pt 1):1472–3.
213. de Riese W, Warmbold H. Adenocarcinoma in extrophy of the bladder. A case report and review of the literature. Int Urol Nephrol 1986; 18(2):159–62.
214. Allen LE. Adult exstrophy of the bladder with adenocarcinoma. J Indiana State Med Assoc 1977; 70(8): 639–41.
215. Beare JB, Tormey AR Jr, Wattenberg CA. Exstrophy of the urinary bladder complicated by adenocarcinoma. J Urol 1956; 76(5):583–94.
216. Beynon J, Zwink R, Chow W, Sturdy DE. The late presentation of adenocarcinoma in bladder exstrophy. Br J Surg 1985; 72(12):989.
217. Davillas N, Thanos A, Liakatas J, Davillas E. Bladder exstrophy complicated by adenocarcinoma. Br J Urol 1991; 68(1):107.
218. Goyanna R, Emmett JL, McDonald DJ. Exstrophy of the bladder complicated by adenocarcinoma. J Urol 1951; 65(3):391–400.
219. Jakobsen BE, Olesen S. Bladder exstrophy complicated by adenocarcinoma. Dan Med Bull 1968; 15(8):253–6.
220. Kandzari SJ, Majid A, Orteza AM, Milam DF. Exstrophy of urinary bladder complicated by adenocarcinoma. Urology 1974; 3(4):496–8.
221. McIntosh IJ, Worley G Jr. Adenocarcinoma arising in exstrophy of the bladder: report of two cases and review of the literature. J Urol 1955; 73(5):820–9.
222. Nielsen K, Nielsen KK. Adenocarcinoma in exstrophy of

the bladder – the last case in Scandinavia? A case report and review of literature. J Urol 1983; 130(6):1180–2.
223. Paulhac P, Maisonnette F, Bourg S, Dumas JP, Colombeau P. Adenocarcinoma in the exstrophic bladder. Urology 1999; 54(4):744.
224. Droegemueller W, Makowski EL, Taylor ES. Vaginal mesonephric adenocarcinoma in two prepubertal children. Am J Dis Child 1970; 119(2):168–70.
225. Shaaban MM. Primary adenocarcinoma of the vagina of mesonephric pattern. Report of a case and review of literature. Aust N Z J Obstet Gynaecol 1970; 10(1):55–8.
226. Nix HG, Wright HL. Mesonephric adenocarcinoma of the vagina. Am J Obstet Gynecol 1967; 99(7):893–9.
227. Senekjian EK, Frey K, Herbst AL. Pelvic exenteration in clear cell adenocarcinoma of the vagina and cervix. Gynecol Oncol 1989; 34(3):413–16.
228. Melnick S, Cole P, Anderson D, Herbst A. Rates and risks of diethylstilbestrol-related clear-cell adenocarcinoma of the vagina and cervix. An update. N Engl J Med 1987; 316(9):514–16.
229. Herbst AL, Cole P, Colton T, Robboy SJ, Scully RE. Age-incidence and risk of diethylstilbestrol-related clear cell adenocarcinoma of the vagina and cervix. Am J Obstet Gynecol 1977; 128(1):43–50.
230. Herbst AL. DES-associated clear cell adenocarcinoma of the vagina and cervix. Obstet Gynecol Surv 1979; 34(11):844.
231. Herbst AL, Anderson D. Clear cell adenocarcinoma of the vagina and cervix secondary to intrauterine exposure to diethylstilbestrol. Semin Surg Oncol 1990; 6(6):343–6.
232. Herbst AL, Cole P, Norusis MJ, Welch WR, Scully RE. Epidemiologic aspects and factors related to survival in 384 Registry cases of clear cell adenocarcinoma of the vagina and cervix. Am J Obstet Gynecol 1979; 135(7):876–86.
233. Herbst AL, Norusis MJ, Rosenow PJ, Welch WR, Scully RE. An analysis of 346 cases of clear cell adenocarcinoma of the vagina and cervix with emphasis on recurrence and survival. Gynecol Oncol 1979; 7(2):111–22.
234. Herbst AL, Robboy SJ, Scully RE, Poskanzer DC. Clear-cell adenocarcinoma of the vagina and cervix in girls: analysis of 170 registry cases. Am J Obstet Gynecol 1974; 119(5):713–24.
235. Herbst AL, Scully RE, Robboy SJ. The significance of adenosis and clear-cell adenocarcinoma of the genital tract in young females. J Reprod Med 1975; 15(1):5–11.
236. Hanselaar A, van Loosbroek M, Schuurbiers O et al. Clear cell adenocarcinoma of the vagina and cervix. An update of the central Netherlands registry showing twin age incidence peaks. Cancer 1997; 79(11):2229–36.
237. Fuqua F, Alexander JC, King KB, Ware EW Jr. Cavernous hemangioma of the bladder in a child: a case report. J Urol 1955; 74(1):82–4.
238. Fuqua J, Alexander JC, King KB, Ware EW Jr. Cavernous hemangioma of the bladder in a child: a case report. Trans South Cent Sect Am Urol Assoc 1954; 49:140–3.
239. Ikeda T, Shimamoto K, Tanji N et al. Cavernous hemangioma of the urinary bladder in an 8-year-old child. Int J Urol 2004; 11(6):429–31.
240. Kogan MG, Koenigsberg M, Laor E, Bennett B. US case of the day. Cavernous hemangioma of the bladder. Radiographics 1996; 16(2):443–7.
241. Ishikawa K, Saitoh M, Chida S. Detection of bladder hemangioma in a child by blood-pool scintigraphy. Pediatr Radiol 2003; 33(6):433–5.
242. Legraverend JM, Canarelli JP, Boudailliez B et al. [Cavernous hemangioma of the bladder in children. Apropos of a case]. Ann Urol (Paris) 1986; 20(4):265–6. [in French]

Exstrophy and epispadias

61

Linda A Baker and Richard W Grady

Introduction

The exstrophic diseases, referred to collectively as the exstrophy–epispadias complex,[1] are considered a spectrum of embryologic malformations related by certain principal anatomic features. This complex includes:

- Epispadias – the urethra is a partial or complete open plate on the dorsal surface of the phallus.
- Classic bladder exstrophy – the bladder is an open plate on the low abdominal wall and the urethra is epispadic.
- Cloacal exstrophy – the bladder and the ileocecal junction of the bowel are an open plate on the low abdominal wall associated with other malformations.
- Exstrophy variants – partial manifestations are seen of the above malformations.

Formal historical descriptions of exstrophy date back to at least 1597 with Sherk Von Grafenberg's description of this congenital defect; possible depictions of exstrophy also exist on Assyrian tablets from 2000 BC. Chaussier first coined the term 'exstrophie' to describe this defect in 1780 following detailed descriptions of it by Mowat in 1748. Because exstrophy can be a non-lethal defect, its natural history is known and has been well described. Since the 19th century, various efforts to manage exstrophy have been described. Because exstrophic conditions are rare, these approaches were empiric and often unsuccessful. Until the 20th century, no effective surgical remedy was available to consistently ameliorate the morbidity associated with bladder exstrophy.

As we enter a second century of surgical care of the child affected by bladder exstrophy, epispadias, or cloacal exstrophy, a review of this history is a triumphant story for pediatric urology and pediatric surgery alike. These birth defects represent some of the most complex that pediatric urologists manage Although great strides in management have been made, many challenges still exist.

Anatomic pathology

Bladder exstrophy

Brock and O'Neill described exstrophy as 'if one blade of a pair of scissors were passed through the urethra of a normal person; the other blade were used to cut through the skin, abdominal wall, anterior wall of the bladder and urethra, and the symphysis pubis; and the cut edges were then folded laterally as if the pages of a book were being opened.'[2] (Figure 61.1)

Anatomic features of exstrophy include the presence of a layer of urothelium on the anterior abdominal wall representing the bladder and urethra. At birth, the urothelium is usually normal in appearance. However, ectopic bowel mucosa or polypoid lesions consistent with cystitis cystica and/or glandularis may be present. If left untreated and without meticulous protection after birth, the exposed urothelium will undergo squamous metaplasia in response to acute and chronic inflammation. Other inflammatory changes such as cystitis cystica and/or glandularis will also be seen.[3] When left chronically exposed to the environment, the areas of squamous metaplasia often undergo malignant degeneration to adenocarcinoma or squamous cell carcinoma.[4,5]

Associated anomalies

Classic exstrophy and epispadias have a relatively low incidence of associated anomalies. In contrast, patients with cloacal exstrophy have associated anomalies more often than not.[6,7] These anomalies can

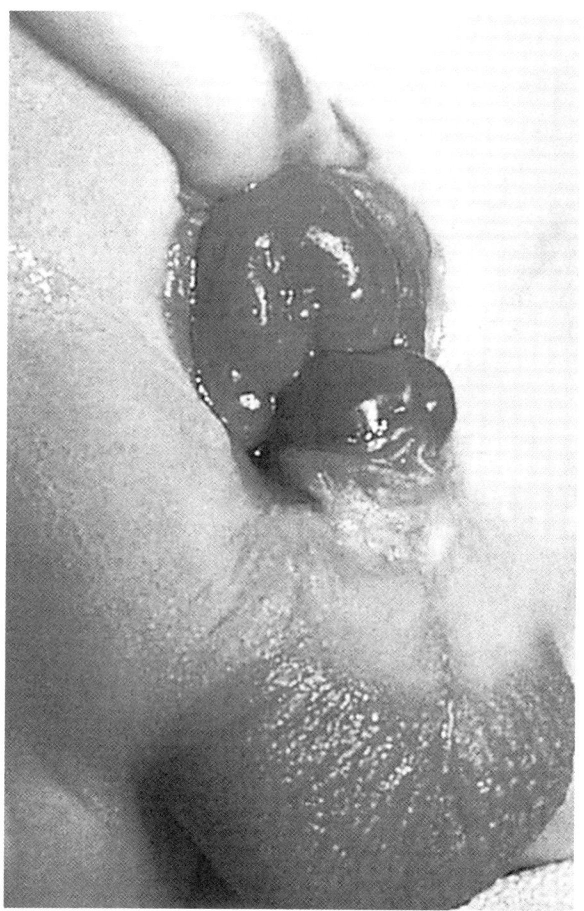

Figure 61.1 Newborn boy with classic bladder exstrophy. Note evidence of anterior placement of the bladder and epispadic urethra.

affect the upper urinary tract, intestines, skeletal system, and neurologic system.

Kidneys and upper urinary tract

Renal anomalies can occur with bladder exstrophy but they are not characteristic. Associated renal abnormalities include cystic dysplasia, ureteropelvic junction (UPJ) obstruction, pelvic kidney, megaureter, renal hypoplasia, and horseshoe kidney.[8] In contrast, vesicoureteral reflux (VUR) occurs almost universally after exstrophy closure owing to the lateral placement of the ureters on the bladder plate in association with the lateral and inferior approach of the ureters into the bladder.

Genitalia

In males the penis is broad and shortened because the corpora cavernosa are splayed laterally, attached to the separated pubic bones. The penis is deflected dorsally and may have true intrinsic dorsal chordee

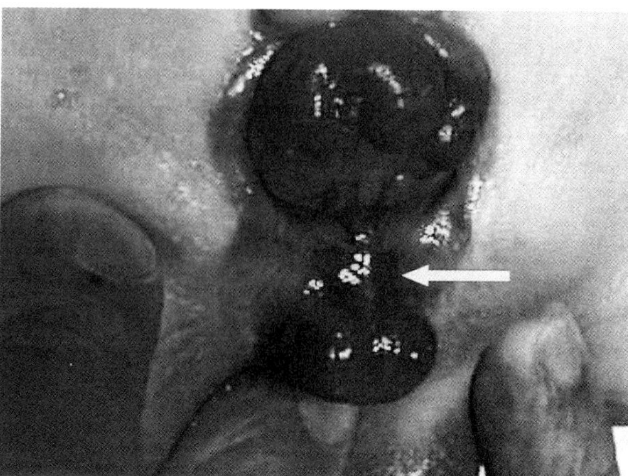

Figure 61.2 Newborn boy with classic bladder exstrophy. The phallus is pulled downward. The white arrow indicates the posterior urethra and location of verumontanum.

(Figure 61.2). Because of the varying degree of diastasis associated with exstrophy, the penis appears variably foreshortened. Further, magnetic resonance imaging (MRI) evaluation of the penile length of adult male exstrophy and epispadias patients reveals that the total corporeal length is significantly shorter than in a control population. This corporeal shortening apparently results from a foreshortened anterior segment (distal to the pelvic attachment); the posterior corporeal segment is unaffected in exstrophy patients (Figure 61.3).[9] It seems that in most cases, the length of the penis and the size of the exstrophic bladder plate are inversely related.

The short urethral plate also creates the appearance of the glans penis lying in close approximation to the prostatic utricle. The ejaculatory ducts empty at the prostatic utricle exposed on the urethral plate. The vas and ejaculatory ducts are probably unaffected in classic exstrophy unless iatrogenically damaged.[10] Innervation to the penis is also preserved. The cavernosal nerves are located on the lateral aspects of the corporeal bodies. In the normal situation, these nerves can be found on the dorsal aspect of the penis after they traverse the posterolateral aspects of the prostate and the membranous urethra.[11] The prostate is also incompletely formed in exstrophy.[12,13] The scrotum is usually not affected, although most exstrophy patients have an increased distance between the base of the penile shaft and the scrotum and a broadening of the scrotum dependent on the degree of diastasis. The testes may be undescended. Because of the underlying bladder neck anomalies, exstrophic males may have impaired fertility. A particular problem is retrograde

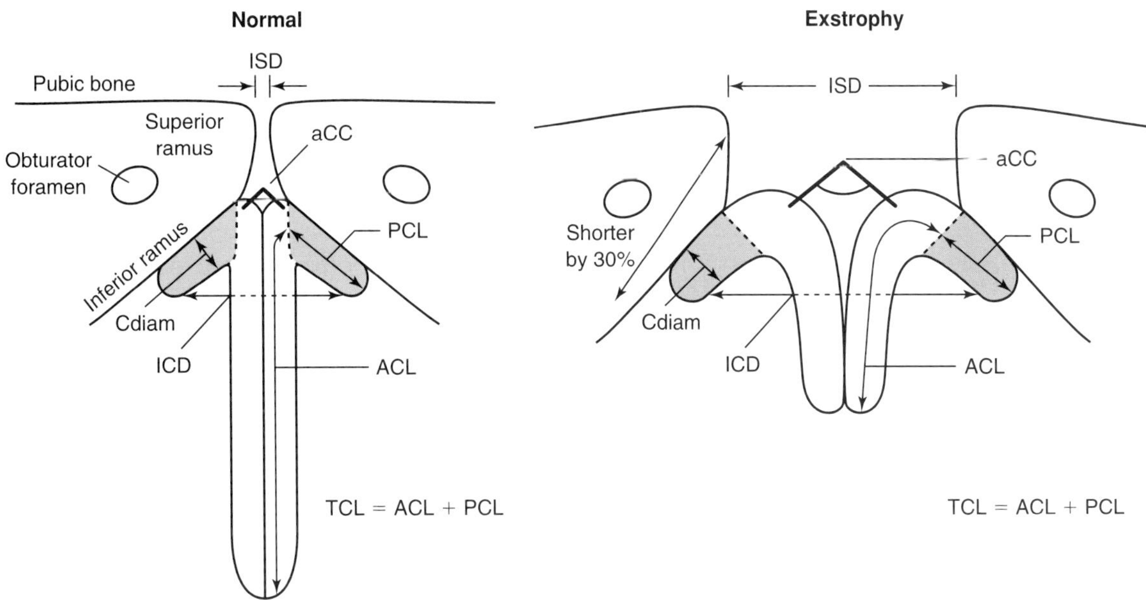

Figure 61.3 Penile and pelvic measurements in normal men and patients with exstrophy. ISD, intersymphyseal distance; aCC, corpora cavernosa subtended angle; Cdiam, corpus cavernosum diameter; PCL, posterior corporeal length; ICD, intercorporeal distance; ACL, anterior corporeal length; TCL, total corporeal length.[9]

ejaculation if the bladder neck cannot close completely following bladder reconstruction.[14–16]

In the female with bladder exstrophy or female epispadias (Figure 61.4), the mons pubis is absent. In association with a bifid clitoris, the anterior labia are laterally displaced although they fuse in the midline posteriorly. The vagina and introitus are also displaced anteriorly from their usual position. The vaginal opening may be stenotic in these patients but we have not found this to be a characteristic feature. Stenosis can result from improper primary closure. Internal female genital structures (uterus, cervix, fallopian tubes, and ovaries) are unaffected in classic exstrophy. Uterine prolapse as a result of deficient pelvic floor support can occur in the older exstrophy patient and poses particular problems with pregnancy.[17] Early primary bladder reconstruction with pelvic closure may decrease this risk. Uterine suspension procedures such as sacrocolpopexy can be employed in these situations as well.

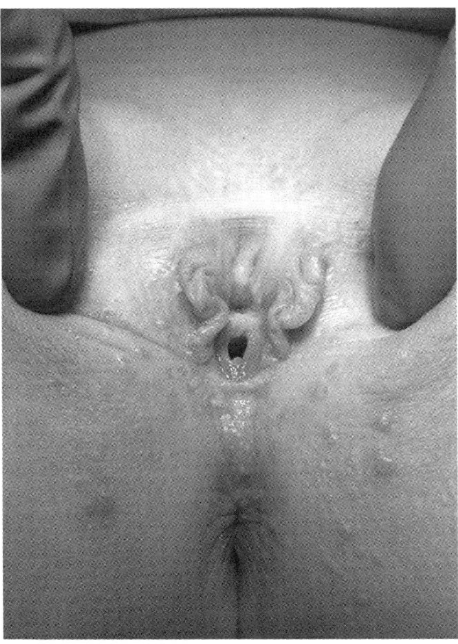

Figure 61.4 Female epispadias in a 5-year-old. Chronic perineal skin changes are due to lifelong frank urinary incontinence. Note the depressed mons pubis, bifid clitoris, outwardly rotated labia minora, and open gaping urethral meatus just above the vaginal introitus.

Anorectal and intestinal abnormalities

The anus is often located anteriorly in the exstrophy complex. Surgical procedures involving these patients should preserve the anal sphincter mechanism. However, a few exstrophic patients will have insufficient anal continence due to the underlying abnormalities of the pelvic floor support structures including the levator ani and puborectalis muscles. Anal sphincter weakness impacts not only fecal continence but also limits the use of ureterosigmoidostomy and its variants; i.e. rectal bladder, ileocecal ureterosigmoidostomy, etc. In untreated patients rectal prolapse can also occur owing to insufficient pelvic floor support.

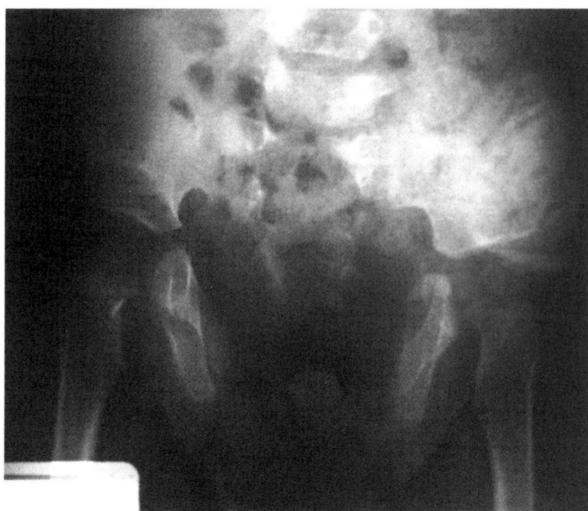

Figure 61.5 Plain abdominal radiograph demonstrating pubic diastasis in a patient with bladder exstrophy.

This is usually definitively treated with formal exstrophy repair that corrects the lack of anterior pelvic support. In the interim, most rectal prolapse is intermittent and reducible.[1]

Skeletal abnormalities

Diastasis of the pubic symphysis occurs as part of the exstrophy complex (Figure 61.5). This results from outward rotation of the innominate bones along both sacroiliac joints. Outward rotation of the pubic rami at the iliac and ischial junctions is also seen. Sponseller et al have quantified the differences in the pelvic anatomy of patients with exstrophy, noting (1) a 12° external rotation of the innominate bones on the sagittal axis, (2) retroversion of the acetabula, (3) increased distance between the triradiate cartilage, (4) 18° external rotation and shortening (by 30%) of the anterior segment of the iliac bone, and (5) external rotation of the posterior segment of ileum (Figure 61.6).[18] These pelvic bone abnormalities contribute to splaying of the penis noted with exstrophy and epispadias and cause the penis to appear foreshortened. Gait abnormalities in these children arise as a consequence of these bone abnormalities. Many of these children learn to ambulate with a wide waddling gait. This gait abnormality resolves as the children grow. Orthopedic procedures to reapproximate the pubis symphysis do not appear to offer any long-term benefits to these patients from an orthopedic viewpoint. Osteotomies to reapproximate the pubis symphysis do, however, increase the chance of successful primary bladder closure in selected patients and may have a significant role in securing continence and support of the pelvic diaphragm.[19,20]

Fascial abnormalities

Fascial abnormalities include the rectus fascial defect associated with the exposed bladder. Inferiorly, the pelvic floor support structures are also compromised. At the inferior portion of the fascial defect, these patients possess an anteriorly located intersymphyseal ligament or band representing the attenuated urogenital diaphragm. The rectus muscles diverge laterally with the widened pubis symphysis. This abdominal defect is most severe in cloacal exstrophy.

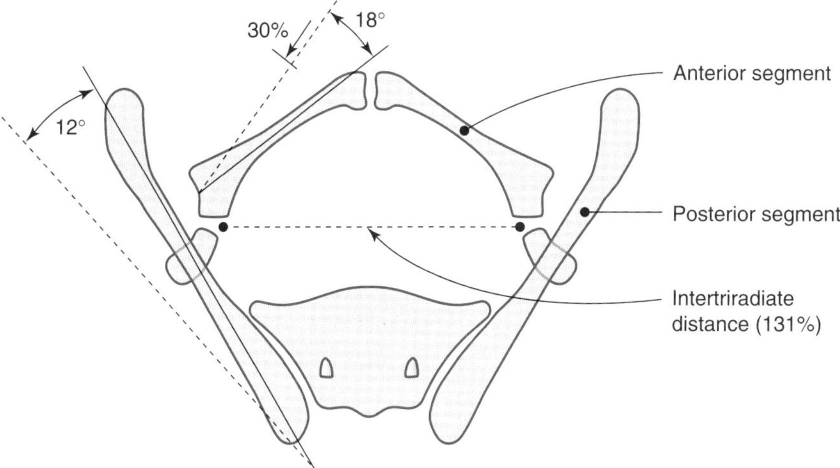

Figure 61.6 The anatomy of the normal bony pelvis is seen in transverse view. Superimposed are the deviations observed in the pelvis of classic bladder exstrophy patients. In the posterior segment, each half is externally rotated 12°. The acetabulae are retroverted, yielding an increased intertriradiate distance. In the anterior segment, each half is externally rotated 18° and is on average 30% shorter.[18]

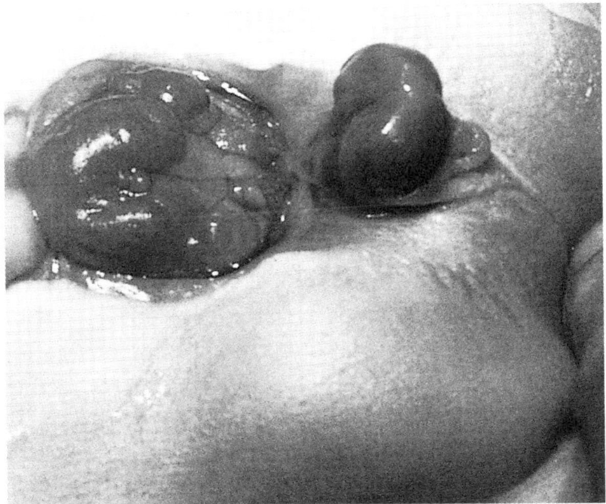

Figure 61.7 Evidence of an inguinal hernia in this newborn male with bladder exstrophy, as demonstrated by the inguinal bulge.

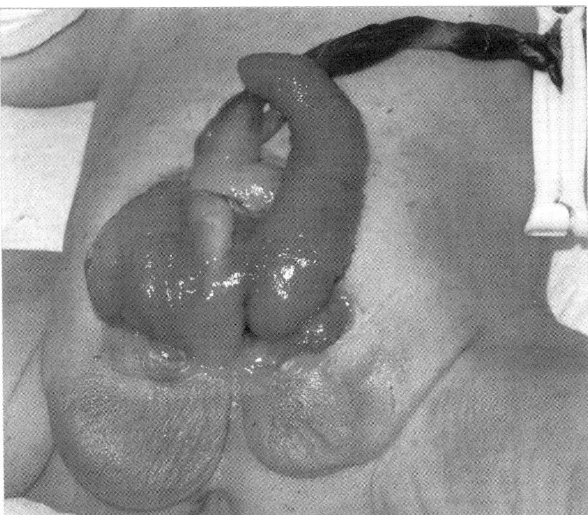

Figure 61.8 Newborn male with cloacal exstrophy. The omphalocele is small. The terminal ileum is intussusepted and is the long 'trunk' to the patient's left. Each hemipenis is small, the left being smaller than the right.

Inguinal hernias are commonly associated with exstrophy in both male and female patients[21,22] (Figure 61.7). The majority of these hernias occur indirectly. They probably occur as a consequence of the enlarged internal and external inguinal rings noted in these patients in conjunction with compromised fascial support and lack of obliquity of the inguinal canal.[23] In a review of patients from Toronto Sick Children's Hospital, 56% of classic male exstrophy patients and 15% of classic female exstrophy patients developed inguinal hernias over a 10-year period. The authors recommended these hernias be repaired at the time of primary bladder closure to prevent incarcerated hernias, which could affect up to 50% of these patients in the first 2 years of life.[24] Reinforcement of the transversalis and internal oblique fascia during hernia repair decreases the incidence of later direct inguinal hernias. Umbilical hernias also uniformly occur with exstrophy and are repaired at the time of the primary repair.

An omphalocele can also be found in association with classic bladder exstrophy, although this is rare.[25]

Neurologic system

Spinal cord abnormalities are the exception rather than the rule in bladder exstrophy. Occult spina bifida and even myelomeningocele can be seen in combination with bladder exstrophy, but this is a rare occurrence.[26]

Cloacal exstrophy

The bladder plate associated with cloacal exstrophy is divided in half by the hindgut plate; the hindgut plate represents the deformation in the development of the colon that occurs with cloacal exstrophy. Ileum enters and intussuscepts into the middle of the hindgut, creating the 'trunk of an elephant's face' appearance with appendiceal appendages located laterally to give the impression of 'tusks on the face of the elephant'[27] (Figure 61.8).

With cloacal exstrophy, the bladder neck (internal urethral sphincter) and external urethral sphincter are not fully developed owing to the failed development of the bladder and urethral remnant located on the anterior and dorsal surfaces of the body wall and penis, respectively. However, because the innervation to these structures is usually intact, anatomic closure theoretically offers the possibility of achieving urinary continence.[17,28,29] The urethral plate is characteristically short as well.

Associated anomalies

Kidneys and upper urinary tract

Renal anomalies are much more common with cloacal exstrophy. They include anomalies of location such as pelvic kidneys or crossed fused ectopia. Horseshoe kidneys, renal agenesis, and UPJ obstruction may also occur.[17]

Genitalia

In cloacal exstrophy the penis is often separated into two hemiphalluses owing to the wide pubic diastasis (see Figure 61.8). This can make subsequent reconstructive efforts technically more challenging if a male phenotype is preserved. Cryptorchidism is the rule with cloacal exstrophy.

For girls, in addition to the genital pathology described above with bladder exstrophy, uterus didelphys and other fusion anomalies of the müllerian duct structures are seen in up to two-thirds of cloacal exstrophy patients. Vaginal agenesis occurs in one-third of girls with cloacal exstrophy.

Anorectal and intestinal abnormalities

Associated intestinal abnormalities specific to cloacal exstrophy include imperforate anus, foreshortening of the midgut, bowel duplication, malrotation, intestinal atresia, and Meckel's diverticulum.[17] These are in addition to the exstrophy of hindgut, ileal intussusception, and exposed appendices that are considered part of the primary pathology of cloacal exstrophy.

Skeletal abnormalities

In addition to the features seen with bladder exstrophy, patients with cloacal exstrophy can have other skeletal abnormalities. Skeletal anomalies are seen in as many as 50% of patients with cloacal exstrophy. Anomalies include congenital hip dislocation, talipes equinovarus, and a variety of limb deficiencies.[18]

Fascial abnormalities

The fascial anomalies associated with cloacal exstrophy include those described above for bladder exstrophy. Further, omphaloceles often occur in association with cloacal exstrophy.[30,31] These can be closed during the initial bladder closure if they are small. If the omphalocele is large, it may require closure as a primary procedure with the reapproximated bladder halves acting as a silo to decompress intra-abdominal pressure. Alternatively, omphaloceles may be treated with antiseptic paint to promote skin overgrowth. Our preference is to proceed with a staged surgical omphalocele correction, with primary reconstruction of the bladder at a later date if the infant is a surgical candidate. In our experience, intra-abdominal pressure following omphalocele closure determines whether we may proceed with primary bladder closure at the same time as the omphalocele repair or whether these operations must be staged. Aggressive one-stage closure of a cloacal exstrophy can lead to organ ischemia from increased intra-abdominal pressure. Rupture of an omphalocele clearly requires immediate attention in these patients and would take precedence over other considerations. Fortunately, this occurs rarely.

Neurologic abnormalities

Neurologic involvement of the lower spinal cord in the cloacal exstrophy population is reported to occur in 50–100% of patients.[31–33] Most patients have lumbar or sacral cord involvement, but thoracic-level myelodysplasia has been reported.[31] Management of cloacal exstrophy in these situations must be coordinated with neurosurgical plans to close the neural tube defect.

Epispadias

Epispadias can be considered the least severe form of exstrophy. It does not involve the body of the bladder. However, the urethra is represented as a plate of tissue located dorsally on the penis (Figure 61.9). The genital anomalies described above are noted with epispadias. These include lateral splaying of the penis and dorsal chordee in boys. In affected girls, the clitoris is bifid, the perineal body is broadened, and the vagina is anterior to its orthotopic or typical position (see Figure 61.4). Widening of the pubic diastasis occurs as well. Importantly, the bladder neck is also frequently involved – it is often wide and incompetent. This directly affects the continence mechanism of these children and impacts the ability to achieve urinary continence. In boys with epispadias, primary continence is possible if the epispadias is located distally and the bladder neck is normally formed. In girls, however, continence is invariably affected to some degree because of the associated urethral and bladder

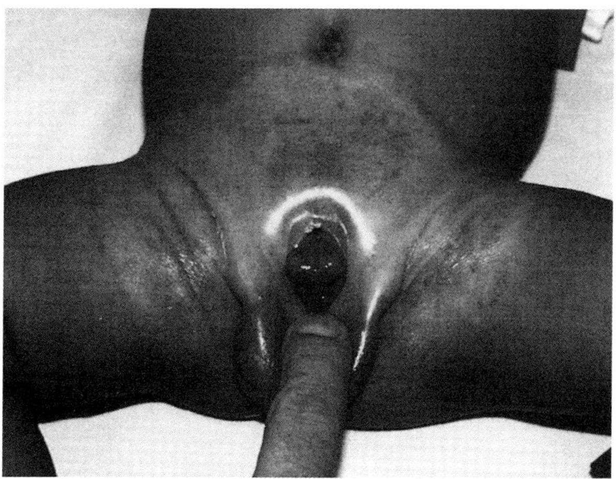

Figure 61.9 Penopubic epispadias in a 3-month-old male. Skin demarcation is due to chronic urine contact dermatitis in this patient.

neck ectasia. Because the features of epispadias are shared with bladder exstrophy, clinicians consider these anomalies as part of a spectrum of the exstrophy–epispadias complex.

Exstrophy variants

In the exstrophy–epispadias complex, variations in bladder plate size and compliance are commonplace but no system to quantify these differences is currently in use. Phallic size and degree of phallic separation also vary from patient to patient. However, despite these variations the underlying features of this disease are consistent for classic forms of the exstrophy complex.

Variants from these findings have also been recognized. Patients with atypical physical findings are referred to as exstrophy variant patients. These patients have some but not all of the typical features of bladder or cloacal exstrophy as well as other features not typically associated with bladder exstrophy. These include covered exstrophy and superior vesical fissure. Patients with exstrophy variants may have anatomically normal genitalia despite their bladder and colon anomalies.

Bladder exstrophy variants include patients whose anatomic features resemble classic exstrophy in regard to the fascial and/or symphyseal defects but who do not have any significant anomaly associated with the urinary tract. These patients are considered to have pseudoexstrophy.[34,35] If these patients also have an isolated ectopic bowel segment in association with these findings they are referred to as covered exstrophy variants.[36] Patients with superior vesical fissure also have the muscular and skeletal defects associated with bladder exstrophy, but only the upper portion of the bladder is affected, so that the urethra is intact and the genitalia are less significantly affected than with classic exstrophy.[37] Duplicate exstrophy may occur. Patients with this variation have a superior vesical fissure associated with normal fascial abdominal wall development, so that components of the bladder remain ectopic such as urothelial elements. These patients can have genital anomalies consistent with classic exstrophy as well, but this association is variable.[38–41]

Cloacal exstrophy variants also exist. These patients possess some of the features of cloacal exstophy such as an exposed hindgut plate and bladder plate but may not have the typical genital involvement.[42–44] Hypospadias has been described in association with cloacal exstrophy as well as normal genitalia in both male and female patients. Some have been reported with intact anal innervation, permitting a Peña procedure.[45] These patients may also have other atypical features such as accessory appendages or limb malformation. These findings, in association with prenatal ultrasound examinations that document twin gestations early in some pregnancies, suggest that aborted conjoined twinning may be the underlying cause of cloacal exstrophy variation in some case[46–48] (Figure 61.10).

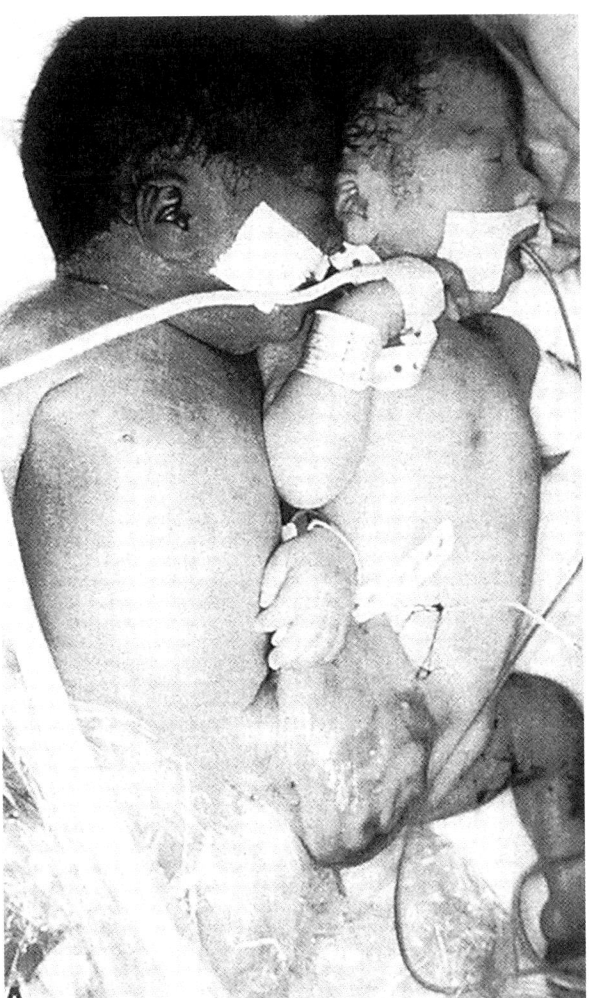

Figure 61.10 Conjoined twins connected by a membranous omphalocele sac containing a shared segment of distal ileum, cecum, and colon draining to a common exstrophic cloaca; an example of an exstrophy variant.

Embryology

Normal bladder development

Normal bladder development results in an organ that functions to store and evacuate urine. This process, known as bladder cycling, requires the bladder to store urine at low intravesical pressures during filling while maintaining continence at the level of the bladder neck. Subsequent evacuation of urine from the bladder requires a coordinated contraction of the detrusor in conjunction with relaxation of the bladder outlet. Both normal storage and emptying require intact innervation of the bladder, sphincter mechanisms, and urethra.[49]

During embryogenesis, components of the urinary system such as the ureteral buds first appear during the 4th week of gestation. At this time the bladder has not completely formed from the anterior urogenital sinus. Before the bladder is completely formed, mesenchyme grows inward toward the midline between the bilaminar (ectoderm and endoderm) layers of the cloacal membrane. This mesenchyme later differentiates into the abdominal wall musculature and fascia. Subsequent to this, the urorectal septum separates the bladder from rectum by growing downward between them. Abnormalities in the appearance, timing, and function of the cloacal membrane are implicated in the creation of exstrophy. In this fashion, the urinary bladder arises during the 8th week of fetal development when the ventral portion of the urogenital sinus begins to expand.[49] With bladder filling, the mesenchymal tissue surrounding this structure differentiates into smooth muscle, which will eventually become the detrusor muscle. Ingrowth of neuronal tissue into this smooth muscle to form motor units is critical to the development of a functional bladder.[50] Embryogenesis of the pelvic floor is also important in normal fetal bladder development and function; the pelvic floor acts as a dynamic support for the bladder, which aids in both continence and volitional voiding.[51]

Theories of pathogenesis of exstrophy

Improvements in our understanding of embryogenesis have led to some insight into the cause of exstrophy. In the premodern era, trauma to the unborn child or ulceration of the abdominal wall and bladder between the 2nd and 3rd months of life was felt to be the underlying cause of exstrophy. Current theories implicate an error in embryogenesis rather than an event of arrested development, since the developing human embryo does not normally pass through a stage that corresponds to exstrophy.[52] Animal models suggest that exstrophy results from pathophysiologic events involving the cloacal membrane. This membrane serves to separate the coelomic cavity from the amniotic space in early development. The cloacal membrane can first be identified during development at 2–3 weeks of gestation. By the 4th week of development, it forms the ventral wall of the urogenital sinus, with the unfused primordia of the genital tubercles sitting cephalad and lateral to it. With further development, the primordia grow and fuse in the midline, and mesoderm grows toward the midline, creating an infraumbilical abdominal wall. Simultaneous to this process, the urorectal septum develops medially and caudally to separate the cloaca into the urogenital sinus and rectum.[49]

In 1962, Marshall proposed that exstrophy was caused by persistence of this cloacal membrane during fetal development based on autopsy studies of fetuses with bladder exstrophy done earlier in the century.[53] Persistence of the membrane would create a wedge effect that would keep the medially encroaching mesoderm from fusing in the midline.[52] To further study this hypothesis, Muecke subsequently created an animal model of cloacal exstrophy using the developing chick embryo. By placing a plastic graft in the region of the tail bud, he created cloacal exstrophy in these animals and concluded that exstrophy was due to persistence of the cloacal membrane, as Marshall had originally postulated.[52]

Other experimental models implicate the cloacal membrane in the pathophysiology of exstrophy as well. Thomalla and co-workers developed a model of cloacal exstrophy in the developing chick embryo by using a CO_2 laser to create an early dehiscence in the tail bud caudal to the omphalomesenteric vessels. Their results suggest that exstrophy may be caused by failure of the mesodermal ingrowth between the ectoderm and endoderm of the cloacal membrane, which later ruptures to produce exstrophy. They hypothesize that such an event could be caused by early hypoxemic infarction in the region of the tail bud, with subsequent cellular loss of the mesoderm, and herniation of the developing bladder or cloaca.[54] This type of ischemic injury has been implicated as the cause of gastroschisis and could explain the spectrum of exstrophy–epispadias complex.[55]

Other proposed theories for exstrophy include caudal displacement of the paired primordia of the genital tubercles. Exstrophy occurs by this mechanism when the primordia of the genital tubercles fuse caudal to their usual location relative to where the urorectal fold divides the cloaca into the urogenital sinus and rectum.[56] This theory readily explains the spectrum of variation seen in the exstrophy–epispadias complex. However, it fails to explain the higher incidence of exstrophy compared with epispadias; one would anticipate a higher incidence of epispadias if caudal displacement were the underlying cause of exstrophy–epispadias because it would represent the most minimal example of this phenomenon.[2]

In 2005, a new maldevelopment theory was put forth for cloacal exstrophy based on a suramin-exposed chick model.[57] When these chick embryos were examined at 1 or 2 days after pericardial injection of suramin, ~8% were noted to have a midline infraumbilical opening into the cloaca and allantois, abnormal leg bud abduction, hypoplastic tail and allantois, broad infraumbilical pelvic region, and large aneurysmal dilation of the paired dorsal aortae at the level of the leg buds. The aortic dilation is transient, resolving on the 2nd and 3rd days after drug exposure, but leaving maldevelopment. These authors implicate the aneurysmal paired dorsal aorta as the primary defects leading to cloacal exstrophy in this animal model.

The chick model to study bladder exstrophy has inherent limitations. Chicks normally possess a cloaca, which precludes the creation of a bladder exstrophy vs a cloacal exstrophy. Other animal models to study bladder exstrophy have been difficult to create. Slaughenhoupt and colleagues created an exstrophy model using fetal sheep. A significant increase in the ratio of collagen-to-smooth muscle was noted in exstrophic vs normal control bladders ($p < 0.05$). There was no significant difference in the ratios of types I and III collagen in the two groups of sheep bladders. These histologic changes are similar in part to changes seen in human bladder exstrophy tissue.[58,59] The underlying cause of human exstrophy remains in question.

Incidence and genetics

Bladder exstrophy occurs at a rate of 1 in 10 000 live births to 1 in 50 000 live births.[60,61] This anomaly has long been recognized to occur more commonly in males than females, with a ratio of 3–6:1 reported in the literature.[62,63] Cloacal exstrophy occurs even more rarely, with an incidence of 1 in 200 000 to 1 in 400 000 live births,[64] but is higher in stillborns, at 1 in 10 000 to 1 in 50 000.[65]

Genetic factors involved in exstrophy remain incompletely defined. Because of the associated physical anomalies with this condition, patients with bladder exstrophy often have to overcome significant obstacles to reproduce. Men may need to resort to assisted reproductive techniques (such as intracytoplasmic sperm injection[66]) because their seminal emissions drain from their ejaculatory ducts located at the base of their bladder plate, if at all. Further, sexual intercourse due to the accompanying deformity of the phallus can be difficult for some of these patients, although the majority have the capacity for satisfactory sexual relations. In the 1800s the prevailing thought declared males with bladder exstrophy as completely impotent because of the associated deformities of the penis.[67] Women with exstrophy were (and still are) prone to uterine prolapse and miscarriage. In the mid-19th century, few reported cases of women with bladder exstrophy successfully conceiving are documented. Difficulty with conception and pregnancy are still a problem today despite in vitro fertilization and careful obstetric care.[68,69]

These issues combined may explain, in part, why familial patterns of inheritance of exstrophy–epispadias complex are noted infrequently. To date, 37 familial cases of bladder exstrophy have been reported.[70] Five cases of an affected parent–child pair have been reported.[70–72] Another 18 cases with bladder exstrophy have been reported in twin pairs.[70] In 1984, a survey of pediatric urologists and surgeons reported nine cases related to 2500 index cases of bladder exstrophy; this same series also reported on cases of twins, and noted discordance in both fraternal as well as identical twinships.[71] In a study population of greater than 6 million births with 208 reported cases of exstrophy, no case had a family history for this anomaly.[73] Current recommendations on counseling about risk of recurrence in a sibling of a patient with exstrophy cite an estimate of about 1%[74] and a 1:70 chance of transmission to the progeny of an affected parent.[72] A Florida population-based study found multiple births had a 46% increased risk of birth defects, with bladder exstrophy being the fifth highest adjusted relative risk.[75]

A genetic basis is further supported by several reports of karyotypic anomalies. Of 39 cases karyotyped at Johns Hopkins, two patients with exstrophy–epispadias complex had anomalies, including 47XYY and a balanced translocation 46XY,t(8;9)(p11.2;q13).[74] A candidate gene on 9q13, contactin associated protein-like 3 (CNTNAP3), was evaluated, but a causal relationship could not be proven in bladder exstrophy.[76] A recent report of cloacal exstrophy with a de-novo unbalanced translocation yielding monosomy from 9q34.1-qter[77] may indicate this as a potential genetic locus. Given the multi-organ maldevelopment in cloacal exstrophy, it is not surprising that aneuploidies such as 47XXX,[78] 45XO/46XX, or 47XX,+21 have been found.[79,80] Based on these findings, the exstrophy–epispadias complex appears to be multifactorial, with a strong genetic predisposition for susceptibility. Collaborative efforts are underway to further investigate the causes of exstrophy–epispadias complex. If environmental factors play a role, they have not yet been identified.

Antenatal diagnosis

Prenatal detection of bladder exstrophy is possible. Ultrasonography can reliably detect exstrophy before the 20th week of gestation[81–89] (Figure 61.11). Absence of bladder filling in the presence of normal kidneys and in association with a low-set umbilical cord suggests the diagnosis. Sonographic examination may also reveal a semisolid mass protruding from the abdominal wall in association with the findings above.[90,91] Gearhart and co-workers reviewed the antenatal ultrasonographic studies of 25 women who delivered live infants with exstrophy and found:

- an absent bladder in 71% of the studies
- a lower abdominal protrusion in 47% of the studies
- an anteriorly displaced scrotum with a small phallus in 57% of the male fetuses
- a low-set umbilical cord in 29% of the studies
- an abnormal iliac crest widening in 18%.[85]

Amniotic fluid levels are normal since urine production is normal for these fetuses. Prenatal diagnosis is valuable in the management of bladder exstrophy because it allows optimal perinatal management of these infants at a center equipped to treat this unusual anomaly. Unfortunately, many affected fetuses are not detected antenatally.[92]

Antenatal diagnosis also allows the parents the opportunity to discuss termination of the pregnancy. It is our opinion that such a discussion should include a pediatric urologist experienced in the treatment of bladder exstrophy. The overall prognosis of these children is excellent if they are treated at medical centers with physicians experienced in the treatment of this disorder. Unfortunately, because of the rarity of bladder exstrophy, healthcare providers who lack insight and knowledge of this disorder often counsel prospective parents of these patients. For example, in one article, the authors state '... the point of termination (of

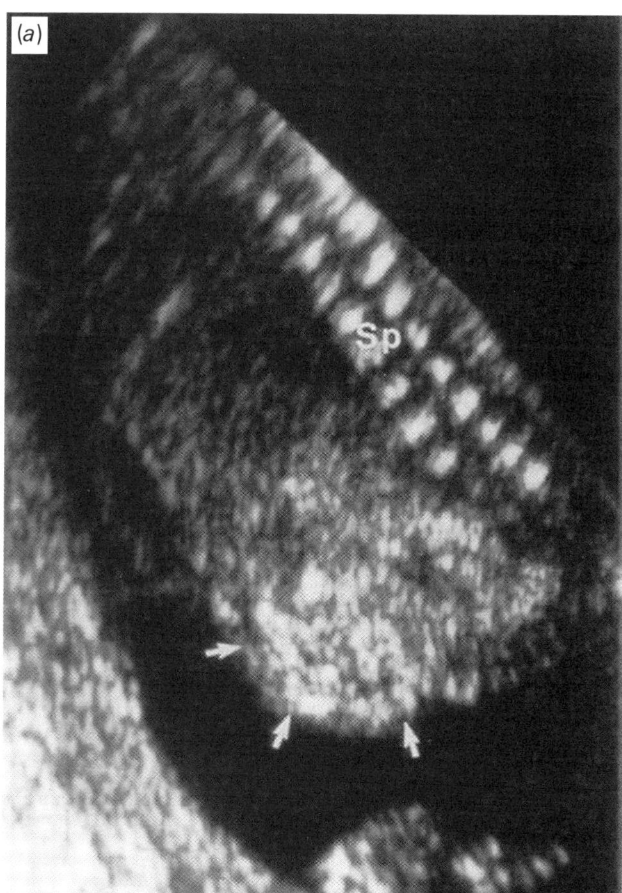

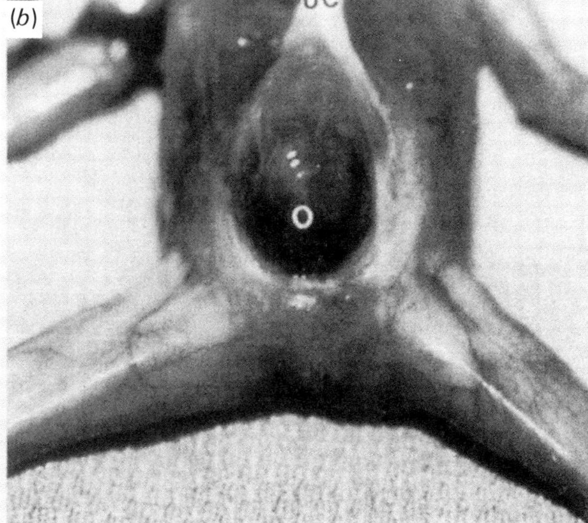

Figure 61.11 (*a*) Antenatal sonogram of a fetus with exstrophy. (*b*) Photograph of a fetus with confirmed exstrophy at autopsy. (Adapted from Mirk et al,[89] with permission.) Sp = spine; O = omphalocele.

the pregnancy) may be underlined by the poor long term results in boys, who mostly end up with severe sexual dysfunction.'[72] Such recommendations are based on an outdated understanding of bladder exstrophy. We believe that recommending abortion for exstrophy would be akin to recommending therapeutic termination in a child diagnosed antenatally with a cleft lip/palate or ventricular septal defect. Unfortunately, the counseling of these families by healthcare providers who are unaware of the true prognosis of patients with bladder exstrophy has led to an increase in the abortion rate of these fetuses, who have a treatable condition with a satisfactory long-term outcome and life expectancy when appropriately managed.[84]

Treatment philosophies

Goals of reconstruction of exstrophy–epispadias

In the treatment of exstrophy, objectives for reconstruction can be placed broadly in the following categories:

Principal objectives:

- urinary continence
- volitional voiding
- low-pressure urine storage
- preservation of kidney function
- functionally and cosmetically acceptable external genitalia.

Secondary objectives:

- avoid urinary tract infections (UTIs)
- reduce risk of urinary calculi
- minimize the risk for malignancy associated with the urinary tract
- integrity of the abdominal wall fascia
- integrity of the pelvic floor.

Successful achievement of these goals remains challenging. Numerous operations have been devised for the treatment of bladder exstrophy, testing the ingenuity of the physicians and the resilience of the patients themselves. The objectives have expanded since the first operations were proposed and attempted in the 1800s. These objectives address the primary pathology and problems associated with exstrophy and its management. These problems include:

Primary pathophysiology (untreated):

- urinary incontinence
- UTI/renal scarring
- urinary calculi
- bladder malignancy
- pelvic floor prolapse
- inguinal herniation
- inadequate phallus and ejaculatory dysfunction in males, with subsequent sexual, social, and psychological sequelae.

Potential complications (associated with management of exstrophy):

- malignancy (related to the use of intestine in bladder reconstruction)
- UTI
- urinary tract obstruction
- inadequate bladder emptying
- urinary incontinence
- uterine prolapse
- severe penile shortening with dorsal chordee
- ejaculatory dysfunction
- urinary calculi
- renal scarring
- abdominal wall hernia
- epididymo-orchitis.

Natural history of exstrophy

Bladder exstrophy–epispadias complex is not a lethal anomaly; reports exist of untreated patients with classic bladder exstrophy living into their eighth decade.[5] Far from debilitated, these children are often quite intelligent, with many achieving postgraduate education degrees. In contrast, until recently, patients born with cloacal exstrophy died shortly after birth from electrolyte abnormalities and malnutrition. Because bladder exstrophy is a serious anomaly, the morbidity these patients experienced was often severe and included the problems noted above. Patients left untreated covered the exposed bladder with a variety of undergarments, including linament-soaked rags, cotton, and wool bolsters, etc. The surrounding skin around the exstrophic bladder was often inflamed and broken down from urine contact dermatitis and secondary infection. These patients were often social pariahs because of the odor and hygiene problems. Up to the 20th century, many considered bladder exstrophy irreparable, as evidenced by these comments by Gross in 1876:[67]

> Exstrophy of the bladder, unless the patient is willing to assume the (often mortal) risk of an autoplastic operation, is utterly irremediable; all

that can be done is to palliate the patient's suffering by attention to cleanliness, and by the use of a closely-fitting flexible gutta-percha shield, furnished with a gum-elastic bottle for receiving urine... When this cannot be obtained, the part must be kept constantly covered with a thick, soft compress, renewed as often as it becomes wet and disagreeable. The skin around may be protected, if necessary, with pomatum, simple cerate, or zinc treatment.

Early attempts at surgical reconstruction

The morbidity of exstrophy led surgeons to begin empiric approaches to the operative correction of this anomaly. Surgeons in the 19th century attempted urinary reconstructive or diversion procedures to treat these patients. Initial efforts were directed at partial reconstruction of the abdominal wall to allow the application of a urinary receptacle to collect urine. The first successful record of this form of repair is attributed to Dr Pancoast in 1859. He used skin flaps from the abdominal wall:

> In the treatment of exstrophy of the bladder the principal objects aimed at are either to establish a channel for the conveyance of the urine to the rectum or perineum, or to cover its exposed and sensitive mucus membrane with flaps of skin, thereby protecting it from contact of the clothing, and preventing excoriation of the surrounding parts, as well as facilitating the adjustment of an apparatus for receiving the urine.[67]
>
> A flap is taken from one side of the abdomen or groin, dissected up, and turned over like the leaf of a book so that the epidermis comes into contact with the mucous membrane. A second flap is then taken from the groin on the opposite side and its raw surface applied to the raw surface of the former flap ... thus a thick bridge is formed over the cleft.[93]

Dr John Wood and Maury also described variations on the use of skin flaps to reconstruct the abdominal wall.[67,94] Wood used a full-thickness skin graft from the abdominal wall followed by a lateral, pyriform flap from each groin held in place with hare-lip pins, wire sutures, and broad straps of adhesive plaster which were removed 6–8 days after surgery (Figure 61.12). In contrast, Maury created perineal and scrotal skin flaps to repair bladder exstrophy. These procedures represented early attempts at anatomic closure but did not address the functional reconstruction of these bladders – namely to achieve satisfactory storage and emptying of urine. Van Buren and Keyes aptly stated the common sentiment of the time:

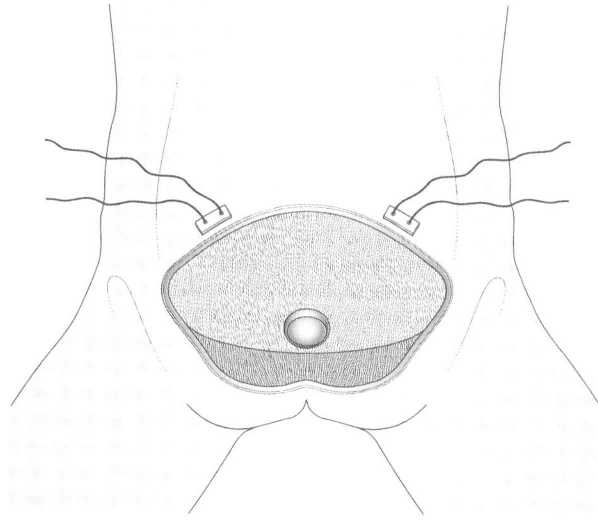

Figure 61.12 Early operation for bladder exstrophy, as proposed by Maury in the mid-19th century.

> The most that can be promised by operative interference is to leave behind a fistula, more or less large, over which a urinal must be constantly worn. The patient's virility is not returned to him, nor is his condition very materially bettered. A less dangerous and equally efficacious mode of treatment seems to be to adapt a suitable urinal to the parts as they are left by Nature, such a one as shall shield them from injury, and keep the patient dry and clean.[95]

Others, such as Simon, approached the surgical treatment by attempting urinary diversion in these patients through the creation of a ureteral sigmoid fistula. Results were poor; one patient died of peritonitis in the immediate postoperative period and the other died of renal failure secondary to chronic pyelonephritis.[67]

These early efforts suffered from lack of understanding of the physiology of the urinary tract and bladder and subsequently how these operations would affect urine storage and emptying, kidney function, electrolyte homeostasis, the propensity for UTI or calculus formation, fertility, and sexual function. Complications from these operations as noted above were often life threatening. The fact that patients were willing to assume the risk of surgical death demonstrates the impact this anomaly had on their lives.

The modern era – operative procedures in the management of exstrophy

A host of operations for exstrophy have been proposed and attempted, which may be broadly characterized into two approaches:

- in the first approach, operations are designed to remove the exstrophic bladder and replace it with a form of urinary diversion.
- in the second approach, the operations are anatomically oriented and designed to reconstruct the bladder either in multiple stages or in a single stage.

Surgeon preference, patient anatomy, previous surgical procedures, availability of tertiary care facilities, and access to medical care all play a role in which operative procedure is chosen for a particular patient. Even in the 21st century, no standard of care exists for this patient population. However, because of the complexity of care involved and the rarity of this congenital defect, specialists with an interest in the exstrophy–epispadias complex usually manage these patients most effectively.[96]

Perioperative care of the patient with exstrophy

Preoperative care

With rapid referrals and, in some cases, prenatal diagnoses, neonates with bladder exstrophy should be evaluated for surgical reconstruction promptly. To prevent trauma to the exposed bladder plate after delivery, the umbilical cord should be ligated with silk suture rather than a plastic or metal clamp. An ideal protective covering for the exstrophic bladder is a hydrated gel dressing such as Vigilon, if available. If a hydrated dressing is unavailable, covering the exposed bladder with plastic wrap (Saran Wrap), especially for transportation, is an acceptable alternative. These protect the bladder plate effectively and allow handling of the infant with minimal risk of trauma to the bladder. In some circumstances, Vigilon has been used for over 2 months with minimal inflammation of the bladder noted at the time of repair. The dressing should be replaced daily and the bladder irrigated with normal saline with each diaper change. Others advocate the use of a humidified air incubator with no dressing at all to minimize bladder trauma.[24] Often, the keratinized skin around the bladder plate becomes inflamed from the chronic urine exposure; barrier creams (zinc oxide) help prevent this.

Some exstrophic bladders are extremely small, acontractile, and non-distensibile.[97] Although bladder cycling is known to stimulate bladder growth, in some cases an early attempt at closure will only result in upper tract deterioration. Although this is a subjective decision, delay of closure may give more time for bladder plate growth. Two reports have also indicated that exstrophy closure in the premature infant should be discouraged owing to higher complication rates.[98,99]

Routine use of intravenous antibiotic therapy in the pre- and postoperative period decreases the chance for bacterial infection; however, candidal infection may supersede. A baseline sonogram should be obtained to assess the kidneys preoperatively for later comparisons. A preoperative KUB (kidney, ureter, and bladder) X-ray can delineate the extent of pubic symphysis diastasis. A spinal sonographic examination should also be obtained if sacral dimpling or other signs of spina bifida occulta are noted on physical examination in the child under the age of 6 months. After this age, MRI will be necessary to image the spinal cord. Orthopedic consultation is advisable to plan osteotomies if needed and neurosurgical consultation is required for children with spinal anomalies.

Operative considerations

Most children with epispadias and bladder exstrophy have no additional anesthetic risk factors, but cloacal exstrophy patients often have comorbidities. Cloacal exstrophy patients with short gut will probably require long-term central venous access at the time of surgery. Exstrophy closure is performed using general inhalation anesthesia, avoiding nitrous oxide to minimize bowel and peritoneal distention and maximize surgical exposure. The use of a nasogastric tube to minimize abdominal distention is controversial.[100,101] Regional anesthesia can be achieved by a one-time caudal block to reduce the inhaled anaesthetic requirement during the operation or, in the older child, via a continuous infusion epidural.

General comments on osteotomies

Trendelenberg first recognized the importance of osteotomies in exstrophy closure at the start of the 20th century. Osteotomies optimize pubic symphysis apposition, diminish tension on the closure, and optimize anatomic placement of the bladder, bladder neck, and urethra in the pelvis. They also improve the

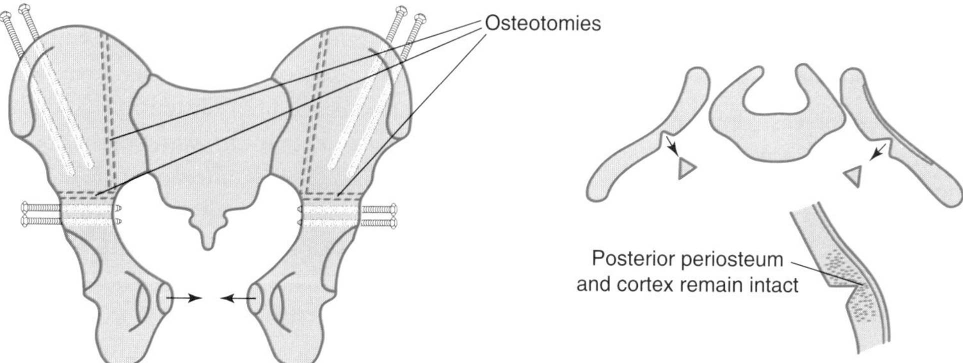

Figure 61.13 Osteotomy sites for combined vertical iliac and transverse innominate osteotomies showing the placement of intrafragmentary pins.[103]

reapproximation of the corporeal and clitoral bodies. Finally, osteotomies may decrease the chance for later uterine prolapse because the anterior closure brings the pelvic diaphragm into a more normal anatomic position to offer more support.

The need for osteotomy is best determined under general anesthesia. Candidates for osteotomy include infants more than 72 hours old, newborns with a wide pubic diastasis, newborns with cloacal exstrophy, and patients who have had a previously failed closure. Osteotomies are usually performed at the same setting as bladder closure to help secure the closure.

Osteotomies may be performed by an anterior or posterior approach or a combination of approaches. Posterior iliac osteotomies are performed with the patient in a prone position, after which the patient is then repositioned for the bladder closure. However, increased blood loss and occasional malunion of the ileum has caused this approach to fall out of favor. Anterior iliac osteotomies offer the advantage of a single position and sterile field preparation (see Figures 61.37 and 61.38). Anterior diagonal iliac osteotomies have been preferred by the Seattle group. Compared with posterior iliac osteotomies, an anterior approach has also been shown to result in less blood loss and better apposition and mobility of the pubic rami. The group at Johns Hopkins uses bilateral combined anterior innominate and vertical iliac osteotomies (Figure 61.13) because of superior initial and long-term results compared with anterior iliac osteotomies alone.[102,103] Both osteotomies may be performed through the same anterior skin incision on each side, and with minimal blood loss, and 4% complication rate[102,104] (Figure 61.14). McKenna et al have also described the use of a diagonal mid-iliac osteotomy performed through the same incision as

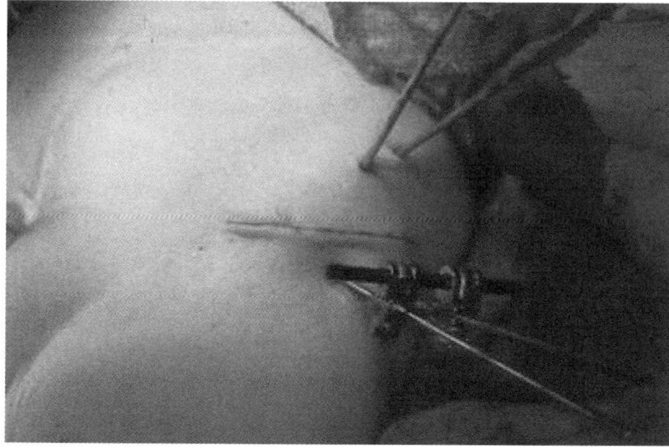

Figure 61.14 Single postoperative incision for combined vertical iliac and transverse innominate osteotomies with interfragmentary pins. (Photo courtesy of John Gearhart MD.)

the exstrophy closure.[105] Division of the superior pubic ramus has also been described; it is not as effective as the other methods described but may be used in the newborn period.[106,107]

Postoperative considerations

Several methods have been used to maintain pelvic ring closure and prevent external hip rotation following bladder closure without osteotomies. Although most agree that mummy wrapping is unreliable and should not be used,[101] high-volume exstrophy centers debate over the best method. The two most commonly employed methods in the newborn period are modified Bryant's traction for 4 weeks[1] (Figure 61.15) and spica casting for 3 weeks[100] (Figure 61.16). If osteotomies are performed, they are secured with interfragmentary pins and external fixation with light Buck's traction for 2–4 weeks (Figure 61.15). Some fit the newborn with a 'sled' to be used when the child

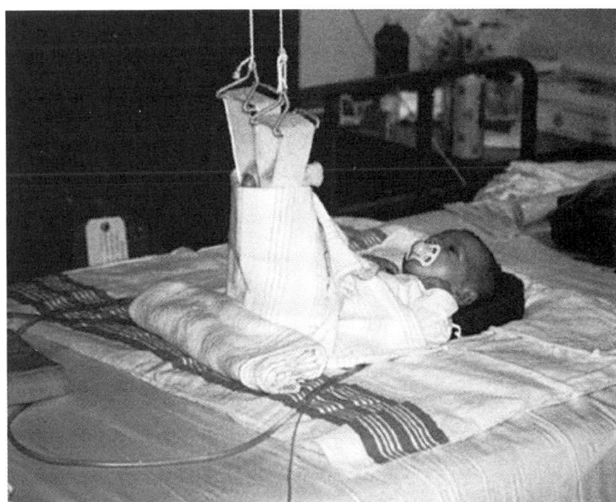

Figure 61.15 Patient seen in Bryant's traction after exstrophy closure without osteotomies. (Photo courtesy of John Gearhart.)

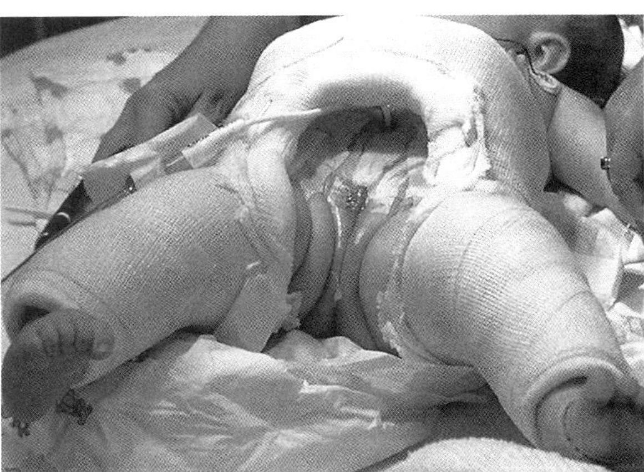

Figure 61.16 Use of a spica cast following complete primary repair for exstrophy to reduce tension on the closure by preventing hip abduction in the postoperative period.

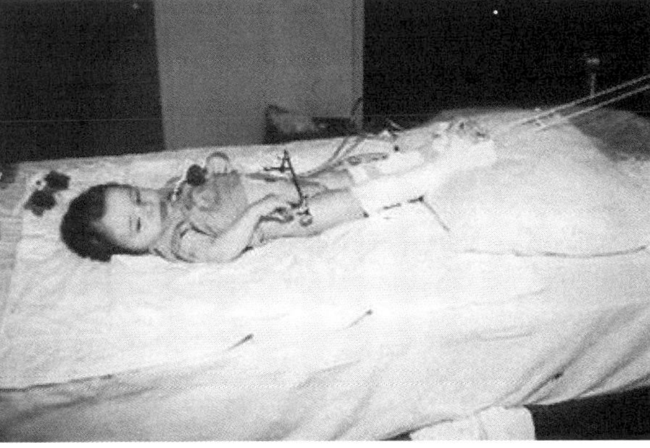

Figure 61.17 Patient seen with an external fixator and in modified Buck's traction. (Photo courtesy of John Gearhart.)

is out of traction for feeding and bathing in these situations. Traction does make performing daily activities and routine care difficult, but spica casting can permit more mobility of the infant pelvis.

Low-dose antibiotic prophylaxis should be prescribed, since VUR is nearly universal. This is continued until VUR is corrected or resolves spontaneously.

Postoperative factors recognized to increase the success of the initial reconstruction[108] include:

- use of osteotomies (in selected cases) or newborn closure (<24–48 hours)
- postoperative immobilization
- use of postoperative antibiotics
- ureteral stenting catheters
- adequate postoperative pain management
- avoidance of abdominal distention
- adequate nutritional support
- secure fixation of urinary drainage catheters.

Exstrophy closure: anatomic reconstruction

The first efforts at anatomic reconstruction of the exstrophic bladder are usually attributed to Trendelenberg.[109] In 1881, he described an exstrophy closure that emphasized the importance of pubic reapproximation in front of the reconstructed bladder to achieve continence and prevent dehiscence. This effort ultimately proved unsuccessful. Because of discouraging results such as this, bladder reconstruction in exstrophy was largely abandoned and replaced by urinary diversion, most notably ureterosigmoidostomy, in the early part of the 20th century.

Not all attempts at bladder reconstruction for exstrophy were abandoned. Various surgeons reported occasional successful attempts at bladder reconstruction during this time. However, these results were uncommon and difficult to reproduce. For example, Young reported the first successful primary bladder closure in 1942. He achieved urinary continence after reconstruction in a young girl.[110] Primary reconstructive efforts by others remained inconsistent and largely unsuccessful during this period. Since Young's successful report in 1942, other investigators have intermittently achieved a satisfactory result with a one-stage reconstructive effort to repair the exstrophied bladder. Ansell reported on a one-stage closure in 1971 with a successful outcome in a newborn female.[111] Ansell was also one of the early advocates for primary closure of bladder exstrophy in the newborn period, and reported 28 cases closed in this fashion.[112] Montagnani described a one-stage functional bladder reconstruction in two female babies aged 8 and 13 months. His bladder reconstruction procedure included innominate osteotomy, bladder closure, an antireflux procedure, and narrowing of the bladder outlet followed by pubic reapproximation. Continence was achieved in one of the two patients. The second patient required further bladder neck reconstruction (BNR) to achieve continence.[113] Fuchs et al also achieved urinary continence in 8 of 15 patients who were also repaired in a single-stage effort.[114] However, several large series of patients who underwent single-stage reconstruction in the 1960s and 1970s reported continence rates of only 10–30%.[115–120] Renal damage was as high as 90% in these series, generally because of bladder outlet obstruction.[115]

Because of these complications and the low rate of urinary continence, reconstructive surgical efforts were subsequently directed toward planned staged bladder reconstruction, an approach pioneered and advocated by Jeffs, Chisholm, and Ansell in the 1970s and further refined by Gearhart and others as the modern staged repair of exstrophy (MSRE).[19,112,121,122] Recent advances in single-stage reconstruction for neonatal and older exstrophy have been advocated by Fuchs et al,[114] Kelly,[123] and others; as such, the complete primary repair for exstrophy (CPRE) by Mitchell has gained favor.[114,123,124]

All approaches aim to reconstruct and achieve anatomic and functional normalcy with minimal surgical morbidity. In the subsequent section, the two currently favored surgical techniques, the CPRE and the MSRE, are detailed. In reality, closure of the female with bladder exstrophy is not significantly different in the CPRE and MSRE methods; the end result is closure of the bladder, urethra, and abdominal wall. In contrast, closure of the male with bladder exstrophy is quite different in the CPRE and MSRE. The CPRE closes and repositions the bladder and entire urethra at one stage. In contrast, the MSRE closes and repositions the bladder and posterior urethra at the first stage, with the remainder of the urethra closed at a later stage.

Complete primary repair for exstrophy

In the late 1980s, an anatomic approach to exstrophy repair that combined simultaneous bladder closure, bladder neck remodeling, and epispadias repair was initiated by Mitchell.[124] This operation evolved out of a technique developed for the treatment of epispadias – the complete penile disassembly technique.[125]

Complete primary reconstruction of the exstrophied bladder is best done in the newborn period. Primary reconstruction in the newborn period is technically easier than when done in an older child. It also offers theoretical advantages, as it may maximize the opportunity for 'normal' bladder development and the potential for urinary continence. The bony pelvis remains pliable in the newborn period, so that osteotomies may be avoided in some cases – usually if closure can be performed within the first 72 hours of life.

Clinical experience with patients with posterior urethral valves (PUV) suggests that early restoration of non-obstructive emptying and filling of the bladder allows the bladder to regain some or all of its normal physiologic and developmental potential.[126] This, in turn, implies that the bladder progresses through developmental milestones that occur in the first few months of life and which may be irreversibly lost if missed. Precedence for this form of organ development is noted in the brain with the acquisition of language and visual perception. Finally, early primary bladder reconstruction creates a more normal-appearing baby that fosters improved bonding between the parents and infant.

In the complete primary repair or Mitchell technique,[124] the bladder, bladder neck, and urethra are moved posteriorly within the pelvis. This movement positions the proximal urethra within the pelvic diaphragm in an anatomically more normal position to maximize the effect of the pelvic muscles and support structures in the achievement of urinary continence. Posterior movement of the bladder neck and urethra also facilitates reapproximation of the pubic symphysis, which in turn helps prevent anterior migration of the urethra and bladder neck and provides a more anatomically normal muscular pelvic diaphragm.

Total penile disassembly reduces anterior tension on the urethra because it is separated from its attachments to the underlying corporeal bodies. These attachments otherwise pull the urethral plate anteriorly, preventing posterior placement of the proximal urethra and bladder neck in the pelvis. Tension reduction theoretically decreases the risk of bladder dehiscence and also temporarily reduces the dorsal tension on the corporeal bodies that may contribute to dorsal chordee in males. Combining the epispadias repair with primary closure allows for the most important aspect of primary closure – division of the intersym-

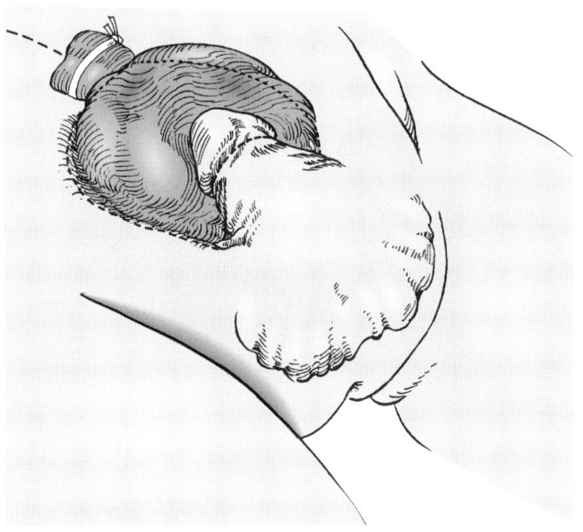

Figure 61.18 Initial lines of dissection for male complete primary exstrophy repair technique – ventral perspective.

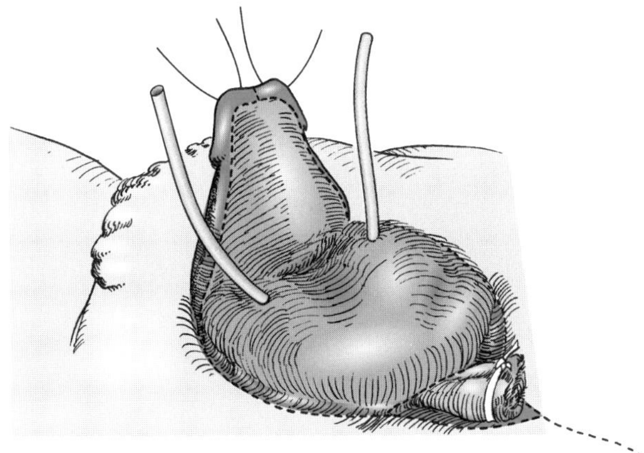

Figure 61.19 Initial lines of dissection for male complete primary exstrophy repair – dorsal perspective. Lines at the bladder neck indicate approximate tailoring that may be needed to exclude dysplastic tissue in this area.

physeal ligament or band located posterior to the urethra in these patients. Advocates of CPRE feel that division of this ligament and deep dissection is optimized when the urethra is separated from the corpora cavernosa.

Neonatal closure employing this technique optimizes the chance for early bladder cycling and consequent normal bladder development. It may also obviate the need for a multistaged repair of the exstrophied bladder, including further BNR, bladder augmentation, and penile reconstructive surgery.

Male CPRE technique

The surgical technique of CPRE and the Mitchell complete penile disassembly technique for epispadias follow the same principles and thus are discussed simultaneously. After standard preparation of the surgical field, 3.5 Fr umbilical artery catheters are placed into both ureters and secured with 5.0 chromic sutures. A marking pen outlines the planned lines of dissection (Figures 61.18 and 61.19). Initial dissection begins superiorly and proceeds inferiorly to separate the bladder plate from the adjacent skin and fascia using fine-tip electrocautery (Colorado tip). The umbilical cord usually needs to be mobilized on its vessels in a cephalad direction such that the resulting umbilicus will be at the level of a line drawn between the two iliac crests. The relocated umbilicus will also be the cutaneous site for bringing out the suprapubic tube. The dissection in classic exstrophy patients is extraperitoneally.

To aid in dissection, traction sutures are placed into each hemiglans of the penis. These sutures are placed at the beginning of the operation and are initially oriented transversely in the hemiglans. The sutures will rotate to a parallel vertical orientation as the corporeal bodies rotate medially following dissection of the corporeal bodies and the urethral wedge (urethral plate + underlying corpora spongiosa) from each other.

To begin the penile dissection, a circumcising incision is made along the ventral aspect of the penis. This should precede dissection of the urethral wedge from the corporeal bodies because it is easier to identify Buck's fascia ventrally. The initial plane of dissection is developed just above Buck's fascia. Buck's fascia stops at the corpora spongiosum during the dissection. So, as the dissection progresses medially, the plane shifts subtly from above Buck's fascia to just above the tunica albuginea. Dorsally, methylene blue or brilliant green helps differentiate urothelium from squamous epithelium. Injection of the surrounding tissues with 0.25% lidocaine and 1:200 000 U/ml epinephrine also improves hemostasis, which assists the dissection. The margins of the dorsal urethra are usually obvious. The surgeon must take care not to narrow the urethral wedge as this will be tubularized later. Urethral wedge dissection is carried proximally to the bladder neck. Careful lateral dissection of the penile shaft skin and dartos fascia from the corporeal bodies is paramount; the lateral dissection of the penis is always superficial to Buck's fascia because the neurovascular bundles are located laterally in the epispadic penis. Medially, under the urethral wedge, the

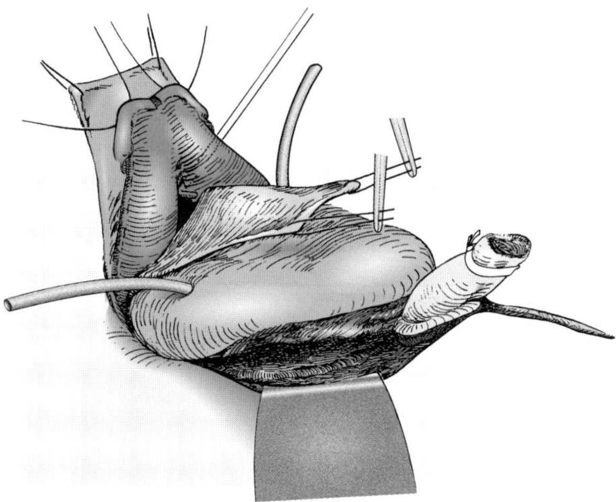

Figure 61.20 Disassembly of the urethral wedge (urethral plate with underlying corpora spongiosa) from corporeal bodies. The plane of dissection should remain on the corporeal bodies to allow the corpora spongiosa to remain with the urethra.

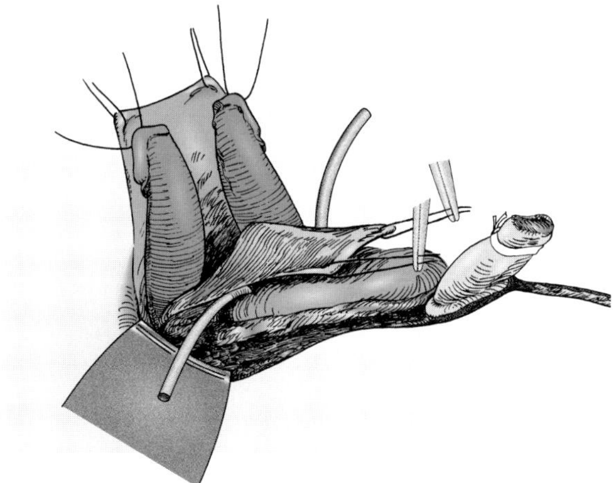

Figure 61.21 Distal separation of the corporeal bodies and urethral wedge. This maneuver may not always be required. Complete separation allows maximal exposure to the pelvis and optimizes the dissection and posterior positioning of the bladder, bladder neck, and urethra in the pelvis.

dissection plane is on the tunica albuginea of the corpora cavernosa.

The penis is surgically disassembled into three components – the right and left corporeal bodies, with their respective hemiglans, and the urethral wedge (urothelium with underlying corpora spongiosa).[125] This is done primarily to provide exposure to the intersymphyseal band and to allow adequate proximal dissection. It is easiest to initiate the dissection proximally and ventrally, on the underside of the corpora cavernosa (Figure 61.20). The plane of dissection should be carried out at the level of the tunica albuginea on the corpora. After a plane is established between the urethral wedge and the corporeal bodies, this dissection is carried distally to separate the three components from each other (Figure 61.21). This maximizes the degree of freedom for the best repair. The corporeal bodies may be completely separated from each other, since they exist on a separate blood supply. It is important to keep the underlying corpora spongiosa with the urethral plate; the blood supply to the urethral plate is based on this corporeal tissue, which should appear wedge-shaped after its dissection from the adjacent corpora cavernosa. The urethral–corporal spongiosal component will later be tubularized and placed ventral to the corporeal bodies. Paraexstrophy skin flaps should not be used for urethral lengthening, because this maneuver may devascularize the distal urethra. Because the bladder and urethra are moved posteriorly into the pelvis as a unit, division of the urethral wedge should never be necessary. However, in some cases, a male patient will be left with a hypospadias that will require later surgical reconstruction (short distal urethra).

Proximal dissection of the urethral wedge from the corporeal cavernosa bodies facilitates exposure of the intersymphyseal ligament, which must be incised. The dissection may be carried into the pelvis following the planes along the medial aspects of the corporeal bodies (Figure 61.22). Deep incision of the intersymphyseal ligaments posterior and lateral to each side of the urethral wedge is absolutely necessary to allow the bladder to achieve a posterior position in the pelvis

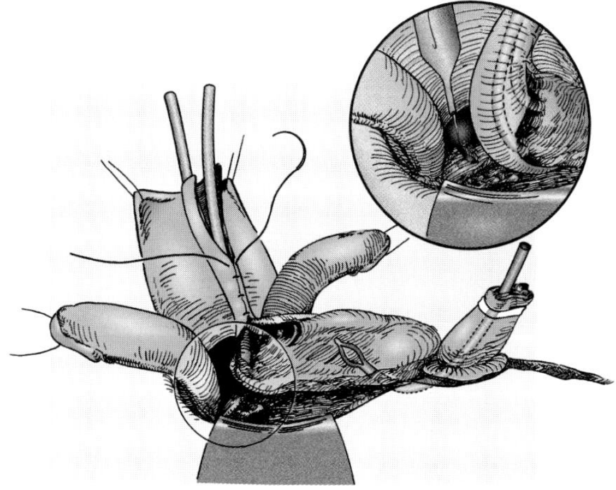

Figure 61.22 Division of the intersymphyseal band (condensation of anterior pelvic fascia) and deep pelvic dissection. The inset demonstrates division of the intersymphyseal band. Division of this band allows posterior placement of the bladder without tension.

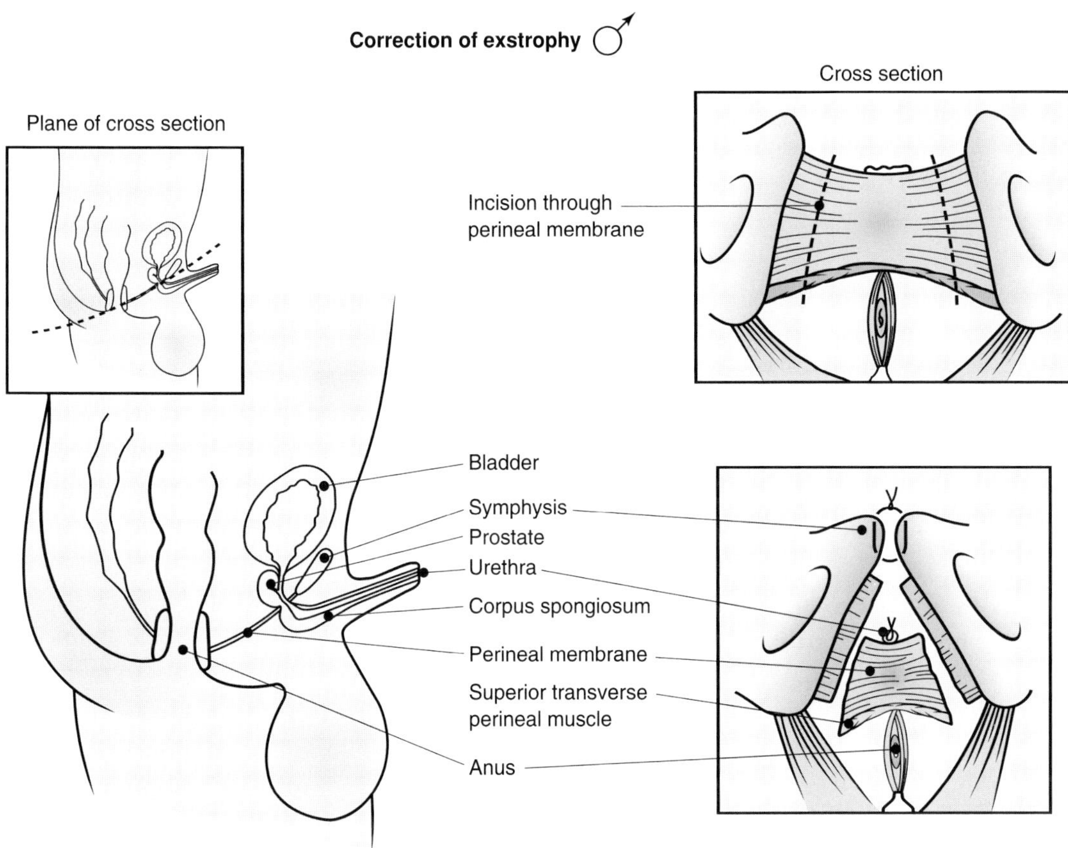

Figure 61.23 This cross section represents an idealized positioning of the urethra and bladder neck in the pelvis.

(Figure 61.23). This dissection should be carried until the pelvic floor musculature becomes visible (i.e. the intersymphyseal ligament is completely incised). Computed tomography (CT) of the pelvis demonstrates that these ligaments lie posterior to the bladder neck and urethra. Failure to adequately dissect the bladder and urethral wedge from surrounding structures will create anterior tension along the urethral plate and prevent posterior movement of the bladder in the pelvis.

Once the bladder and urethral wedge are adequately dissected from the surrounding tissues, the majority of the procedure is done and the closure is straightforward and anatomic. The importance of recognizing the proper location of the bladder neck is key: in boys, proximal to the verumontanum; in girls, just distal to the trigone. Prior to reapproximating the bladder, a suprapubic tube is placed and brought out through the umbilicus. The primary closure of the bladder is achieved using a three-layer closure with monofilament absorbable suture (i.e. Monocryl and Vicryl). The urethra is tubularized using a two-layer running closure with monofilament and Vicryl suture as well (Figure 61.24). The tubularized urethra is then placed ventral to the corpora in an anatomically normal position.

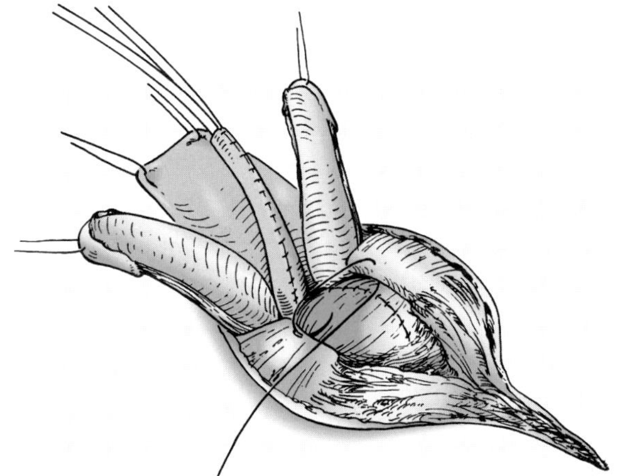

Figure 61.24 The bladder and urethra are closed in two layers using absorbable suture. The ureteral catheters are brought out throught the urethral closure. The suprapubic tube may be brought out through the umbilicus.

Then the pubic symphysis is reapproximated using 0–0 polydiaxonone interrupted figure-of-eight

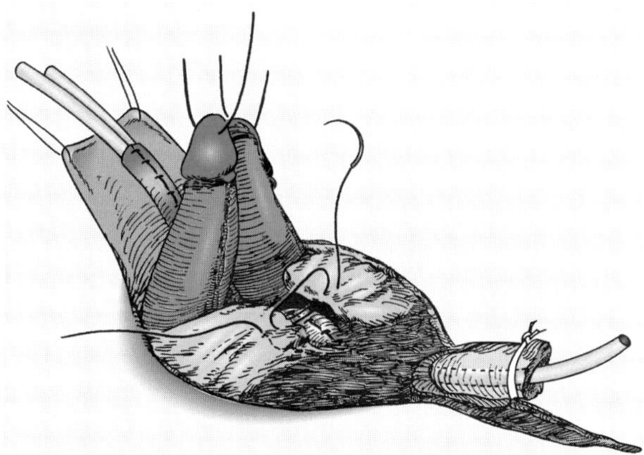

Figure 61.25 Reapproximation of pubis symphysis using absorbable suture. Note medial rotation of glans that occurs after dissection.

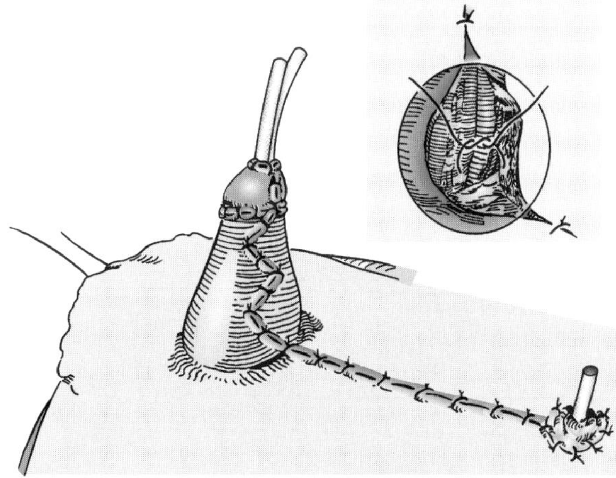

Figure 61.26 Skin reapproximation can be challenging. Tacking sutures placed between the dermal tissue and the corporeal bodies can assist in anchoring the penile shaft skin to the base of the penis. Z-plasty incisions can also be useful to approximate the shaft skin ventrally.

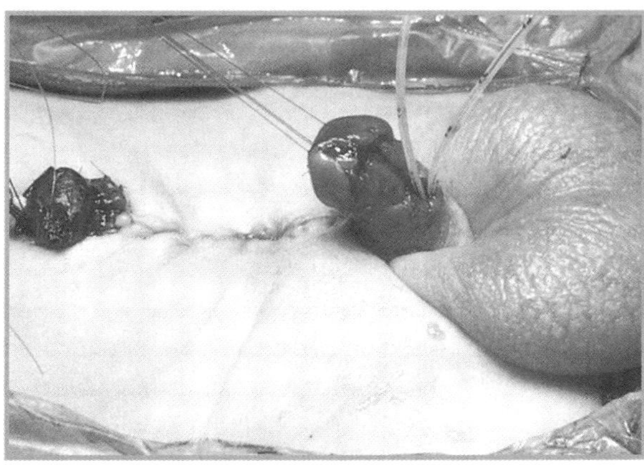

Figure 61.27 Hypospadias occurs in this situation because the urethra is too short after the bladder has been positioned posteriorly in the pelvis.

sutures. Knots are anterior to prevent suture erosion into the bladder neck (Figure 61.25). Rectus fascia is reapproximated using a running 2–0 polydiaxonone suture. Penile shaft skin is reconfigured using either a primary dorsal closure or reversed Byars flaps if needed to provide dorsal skin coverage. Skin covering the abdominal wall is reapproximated using a two-layer running closure of absorbable monofilament suture.

The corporeal bodies will tend to rotate medially with closure when the lateral margins of Buck's fascia of each corpora cavernosa are approximated. This rotation will assist in correcting the dorsal deflection and can be readily appreciated by observing the vertical lie of the previously horizontally placed glans traction sutures. Occasionally, significant discrepancies in the dorsal and ventral lengths of the corpora will require dermal graft insertion. However, this is rarely needed in the newborn closure. The corpora are reapproximated with fine interrupted suture along their dorsal aspect.

The urethra can then be brought up to each hemiglans ventrally to create an orthotopic meatus (Figure 61.26). The glans is reconfigured using interrupted mattress sutures of polydiaxonone suture (i.e. PDS) followed by horizontal mattress sutures of 7–0 monofilament suture (i.e. Maxon) to reapproximate the glans epithelium. The neourethra is matured with 7–0 braided polyglactin suture (i.e. Vicryl) similar to a standard hypospadias repair. In some cases, the glans tissue is reduced to create a conical-appearing glans. In roughly half of cases, the urethra lacks enough length to reach the glans. In this situation, the urethra may be matured along the ventral aspect of the penis to create a hypospadias (Figure 61.27). This can be corrected at a later date as a second-stage procedure and options for hypospadias repair are detailed in other chapters. The redundant shaft skin is maintained ventrally in these patients to assist in later penile reconstructive procedures.

Female CPRE technique

The principles and timing of repair are analogous for boys and girls (Figure 61.28). To perform this technique, the lines of initial dissection are depicted in Figure 61.29. In an effort to clearly define the bladder neck, the bladder neck dissection is tailored. The bladder neck, urethra, and vagina are mobilized as a unit.

Figure 61.32 P
place a suprap
drainage. The
the umbilicus.
brought out th
gravity drainag

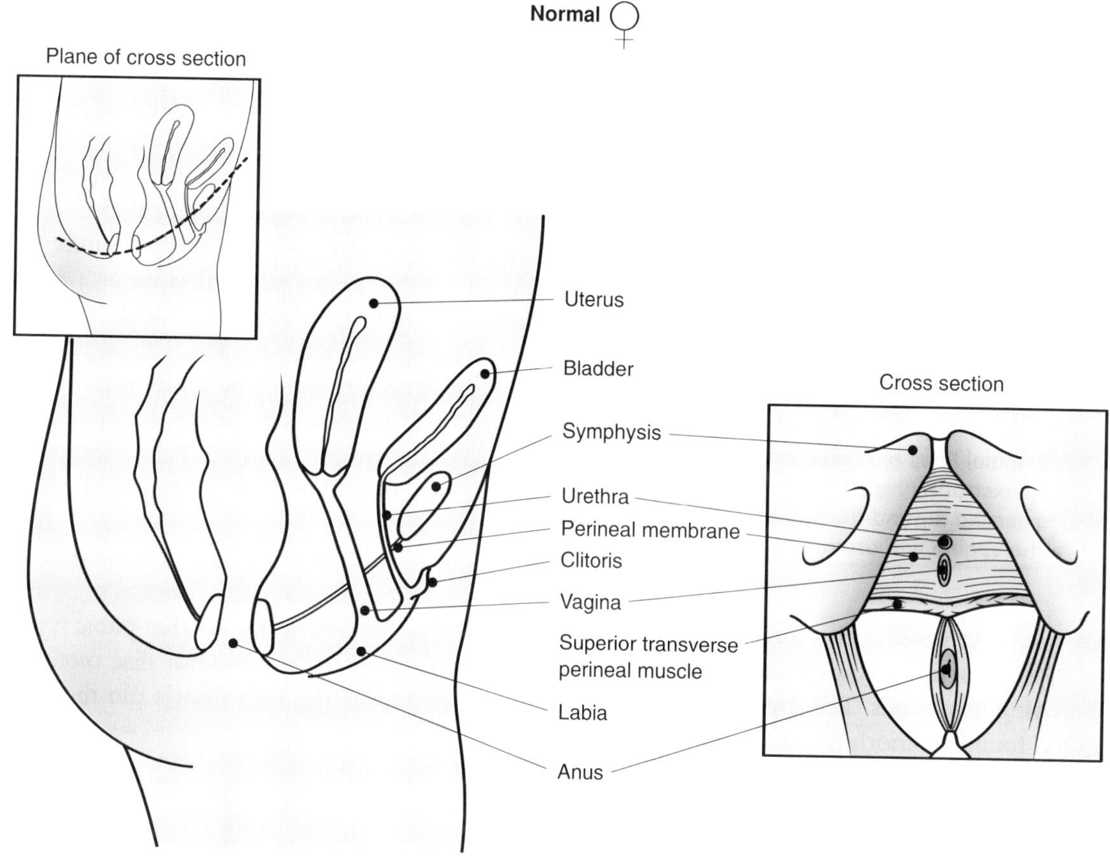

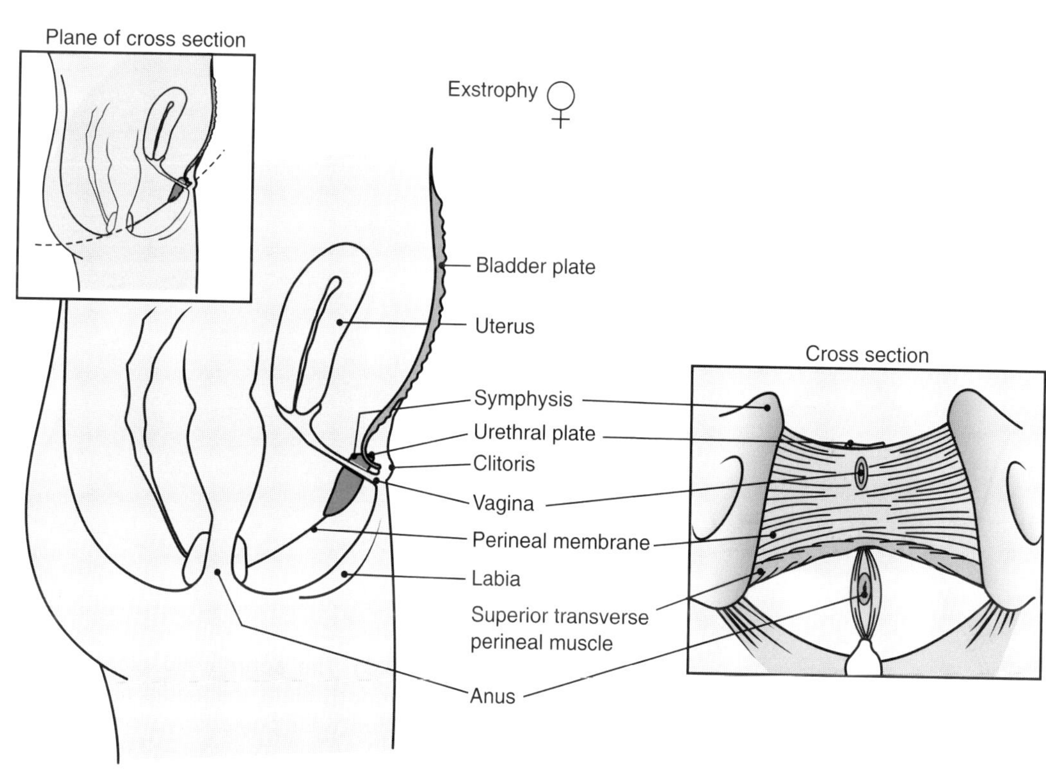

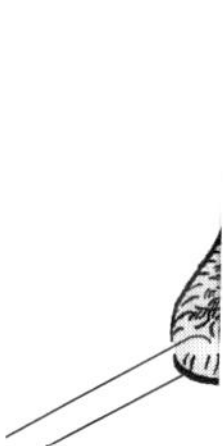

Figure 61.33
should be p
quate dissect

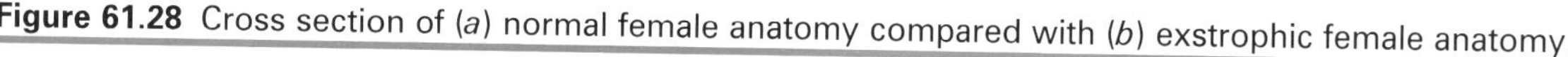

Figure 61.28 Cross section of (*a*) normal female anatomy compared with (*b*) exstrophic female anatomy.

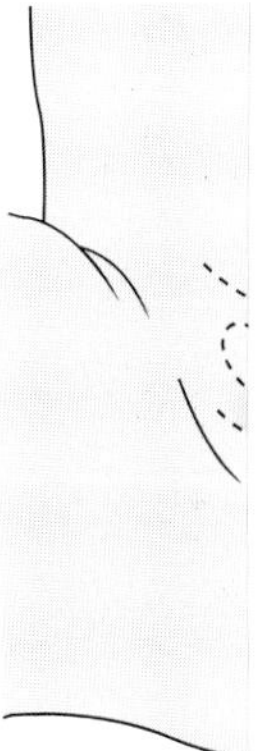

Modifications of the CPRE technique

In an effort to improve the results of the CPRE technique, several authors have reported modifications. Caione and colleagues described the use of an electrical muscle stimulator during deep pelvic dissection to preserve and reconfigure the periurethral muscle complex. Long-term results of this patient series have not yet been reported but preliminary results are promising.[127]

El-Sherbiny and Hafez have described a modification of the penile disassembly technique preserving the connection between the distal urethral wedge and the corporeal bodies to decrease the incidence of hypospadias.[128] Proposed by Emir and colleagues, one solution for intraoperatively anticipated hypospadias is to generate parameatal-based inner preputial skin flaps which do not require anastomosis to the urethral plate.[129]

Outcomes of CPRE

The longest series reporting outcomes of CPRE is from Children's Hospital & Regional Medical Center in Seattle, Washington, spanning 13 years: of 29 patients, 17 are >5 years of age and have 76% continence (defined as a dry interval >2 hours and spontaneous voiding without catheterization); only 3% (1 of 29) required augmentation, which compared favorably with 27% of 77 staged exstrophy closures at this institution requiring augmentation, although admittedly the latter group has been followed longer. However, this report does not mention the number of patients requiring BNR to achieve this continence rate. In 2003, preliminary outcomes from the Seattle group were presented in abstract form. In this series, bladder neck modification was performed in 72% of females and 86% of males prior to achieving continence; overall, 86% of children achieved daytime continence with volitional voiding. The majority of these bladder neck modifications were perfomed at the same time as ureteral reimplantation procedures and were performed using a Mitchell bladder neck technique.[130] A 14% complication rate and 16% moderate or severe hydronephrosis rate was also noted. Of note, in the majority of these patients the hydronephrosis remains a transient phenomenon that the authors believe represents a reaction to bladder cycling.[130] One other report from the Boston group provides an 8-year follow-up of CPRE outcomes. Borer and colleagues noted that 5 of 8 patients (63%) ≥ 4 years old had grossly inadequate bladder outlet resistance and either had or would require BNR. This same group also reported on urodynamic findings between patients who had undergone exstrophy repair using a complete primary repair technique compared with a modern stage repair technique. They found that patients undergoing a complete primary repair universally had better bladder stability and bladder compliance than those who had been repaired with a staged technique. Bladder capacity was equivalent between the two groups. Interestingly, patients repaired with a complete repair technique also had normal electromyelography (EMG) results during this study.[98]

After CPRE, hypospadias rates have ranged from 50 to 82%.[98,124,131] Borer and colleagues have decreased this rate by using interrupted urethral sutures instead of running sutures.[98] Reconstruction of the hypospadic defect can be challenging[98,132] owing to paucity of skin. Hafez and El-Sherbiny have found tubularized penile flap urethroplasty to be superior to Thiersch–Duplay urethroplasty.[132] Bladder neck fistula have been observed in as many as 41% of CPRE repairs,[133] 78% of which required fistulectomy. Partial or complete hemiglans and corporeal loss have been reported by several authors,[133,134] which is probably the most feared complication. However, this complication may not be unique to CPRE, and can be seen in any bladder exstrophy closure method.[135] Borer and colleagues reported 75% of 16 males and 29% of seven females undergoing newborn CPRE required blood transfusion.

Some surgeons have criticized the staged approach as requiring a greater number of surgical procedures than the CPRE.[135] Given the 'relative newness' of the CPRE technique, long-term studies will further delineate the number of patients who require hypospadias reconstruction and BNR to achieve urinary continence. As the male children progress through puberty, phallic growth, presence of chordee, erectile function, and ejaculatory function will be outcomes to closely monitor. Given exstrophy is a complex birth defect to reconstruct, no matter which method is chosen, complications will occur,[134,136] most of which require further surgical interventions.[98]

Complete penile disassembly for the treatment of isolated male epispadias

Mitchell performed his first complete penile disassembly or Mitchell technique for epispadias repair in 1989. Mitchell and Bagli first reported their results in 1996.[125] Complete penile disassembly offers several advantages over the modified Cantwell–Ransley tech-

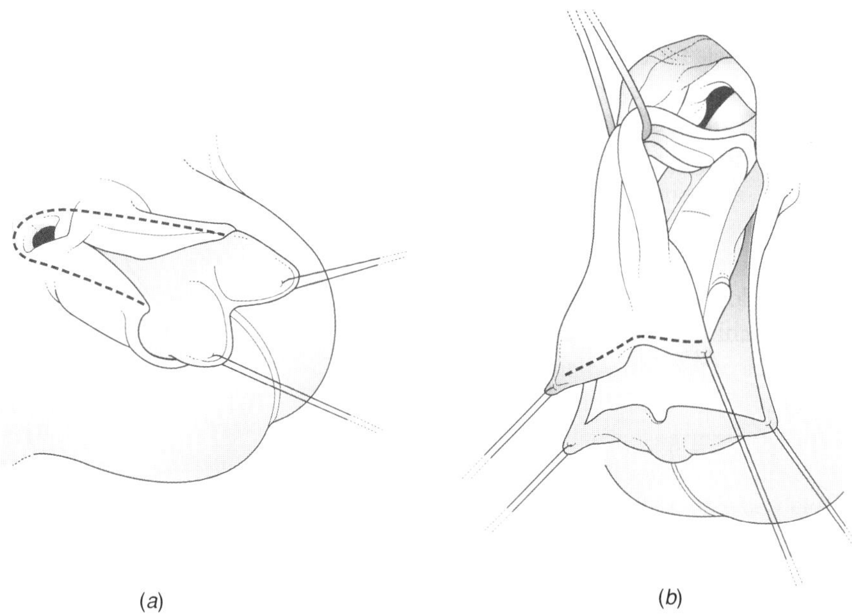

Figure 61.36 Complete penile disassembly technique. (*a*) Lines of initial dissection circumscribing the urethral plate and bladder neck. (*b*) Careful dissection of the urethra from the underlying corporeal bodies. Dotted line indicates the site of distal incision to free the urethra entirely from the glans. (Adapted from Mitchell and Bagli,[125] with permission.)

nique. The planes of dissection extend anatomically to the bladder neck. This facilitates its use with BNR. Complete mobilization of the urethral wedge from the corporeal bodies by disassembly also creates a more normal appearance of the penis by allowing ventral placement of the urethra (Figures 61.36–61.38). A detailed description of the surgical technique is included in the section on complete primary repair of

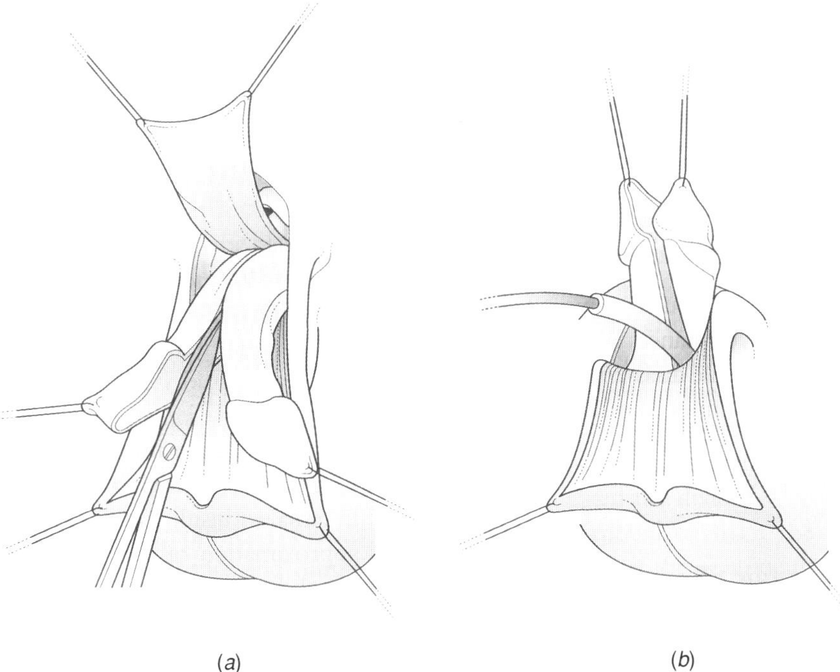

Figure 61.37 Complete penile disassembly technique. (*a*) Corporeal bodies and two hemiglans are separated by a longitudinal midline incision. (*b*) The urethra is tubularized and brought to the ventrum. The corpora are reapproximated dorsally. They will rotate medially when adequately dissected from each other. (Adapted from Mitchell and Bagli,[125] with permission.)

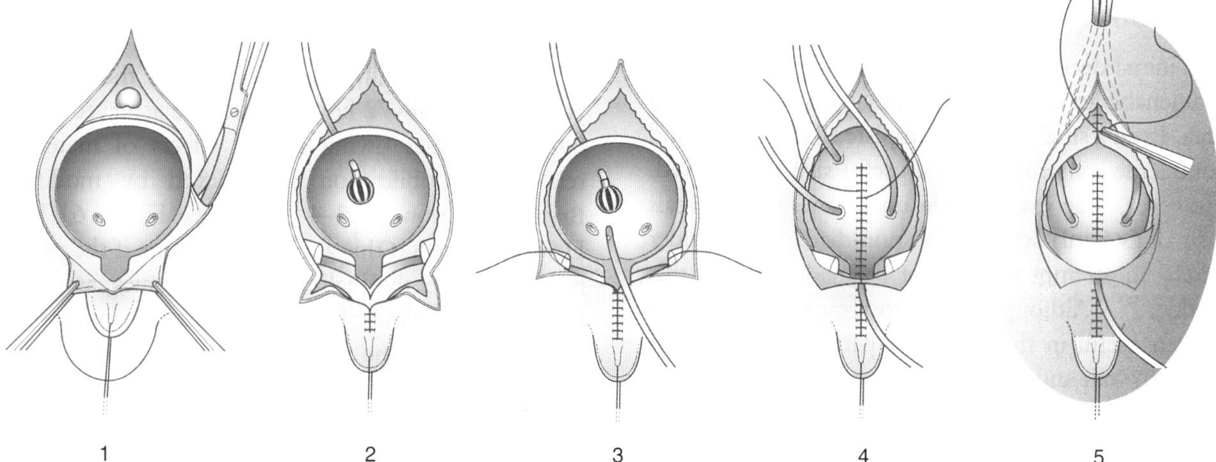

Figure 61.39 Primary bladder closure. These diagrams demonstrate the sequence of initial bladder closure in a staged repair for bladder exstrophy in the male patient. From left to right: (1) completion of dissection around the bladder and urethral plate; (2) placement of a suprapubic drainage tube after corporeal reapproximation; (3) tubularization of the urethral plate over the catheter; (4) following two-layer closure of the bladder and urethral plate, the bladder is reduced in the pelvis and fixed with sutures; (5) drainage tubes are brought out superiorly and the fascia, subcutaneous tissue, and skin are reapproximated. (Adapted from Brock and O'Neill,[2] with permission.)

posterior urethra–bladder neck. The urogenital diaphragm fibers and the intersymphyseal band must be completely taken down from the pubic subperiosteum bilaterally to the pelvic floor, or the posterior urethra and bladder will not be recessed within the deep pelvis.

At this point the posterior urethra must be assessed. If the urethral groove is adequate in length, no transverse incision is made to transect the urethral plate. If the child has severe chordee and a short urethra that inhibits attempts at penile lengthening, an incision of the urethral plate may be necessary. Management of this is best assessed after extensive mobilization of the bladder and prostatic plate from the rectus fascia, the pubic bones, and the inferior ramus of the pubis. Once radical division of the urogenital diaphragm fibers from the posterior urethra–bladder neck area is accomplished, the prostatic urethra can be displaced posteriorly into the pelvis. In some cases, division of the anterior attachments of the crura and the suspensory tissue of the penis is needed and displays the gap to be bridged between the prostatic plate and the penile plate. This lack of urethral plate length can be managed by dividing the prostatic plate distal to the verumontanum in a V-shaped fashion. After corporeal mobilization and midline reapproximation, the penile urethral plate is fashioned from a lateral rotational flap generated after a single lateral incision into the paraexstrophy skin; therefore, less tissue redundancy and dissection are necessary. Whereas this has been reconstructed after the manner of Johnston[152] or Duckett,[153] paraexstrophy skin flaps should be used with great caution. The authors have noted a 40% complication rate associated with their use and significant comorbidity.[154]

The corporeal bodies are not sewn together at this time, since this will be achieved after the urethra has been transposed beneath the corpora at the time of epispadias closure. Once the dissection appears complete, a sound on the posterior urethra can be compressed and the pelvis manually approximated to roughly assess completeness of mobilization of the posterior urethra and urogenital diaphragm.

After a silicone Malecot suprapubic tube has been placed, the umbilicus is excised and the bladder is closed in the midline in multiple layers with a running 3–0 Vicryl suture. The posterior urethra is also closed onto the base of the penis, sizing it to accept a 12–14 Fr sound. The intersymphyseal stitch is then placed but initially is not tied. A No. 2 nylon suture is recommended. It is key to perform a horizontal mattress closure, planning for the knot to be placed on the anterior surface of the pubis. This technique prevents the suture or knot from eroding into the urethra or bladder neck. Once the suture is in but not tied, three surgical personnel are needed to reapproximate the pubis symphysis. One individual applies pressure over each greater trochanter to push the pubic rami to the midline. A second individual depresses the posterior urethra and bladder neck. The third individual ties the nylon suture. If the rectus fascia is strong, a second No. 2 nylon suture is placed just above the symphysis. The abdominal wall, subcutaneous tissues, and skin are then closed in multiple layers. A V-shaped flap of skin is fashioned in the midline for the neoumbilicus at the level of the iliac crests. The neoumbilicus is used as the site to bring the three urinary drainage catheters out to the skin. Inguinal hernias, seen in up to 82% of males, may be surgically repaired at the time of initial exstrophy closure.[21] This can be done through separate incisions or via the midline exstrophy closure incision.

Female MSRE bladder and posterior urethral closure technique

In stage 1 of the MSRE of the female child, the surgical techniques of bladder, pelvic ring, and abdominal wall closure are identical to those described for the male. However, the closure of the female differs from the male closure in that the female urethra is completely reconstructed at stage 1.[1,151] The urethral plate mucosal incision is 2 cm wide, traversing from the distal trigone to the vaginal orifice in the female. Paraexstrophy skin flaps are unnecessary in female exstrophy closures.[155] The medial aspect of each hemiclitoris is de-epithelialized to permit approximation of the two glans clitori and reconstruction of the mons. The bladder and female urethra are closed in a two-layer Vicryl closure and the pubic bones, abdominal wall, subcutaneous tissue, and skin are closed as outlined in the male. The monsplasty and genitoplasty are then performed.

Postoperative care of stage 1 MSRE

In male and female cases of initial closure, a suprapubic tube and ureteral stents are placed via the neoumbilicus, since intubation of the urethra is discouraged. Additional factors that are important to the success of the initial closure include pelvic immobilization and fixation, adequate pain control, prevention of abdominal distention, and postoperative antibiotics.[149,156] The ureteral stents are maintained for 2–3 weeks. Adequate urethral caliber and minimal postvoid residuals are assured prior to removal of the suprapubic tube at 4 weeks. The status of the upper tracts is documented by ultrasound prior to discharge and is followed by ultrasound at 3 months and every 6 months to 1 year. The successfully closed child is continued on prophylactic antibiotics, for essentially all have VUR. Increasing hydronephrosis, worsening VUR, retained urine in the bladder, and recurrent UTIs should prompt further evaluation for suture erosion or outlet obstruction. Between the ages of 1 and 3 years old, yearly cystograms under anesthesia are performed to assess the degree of reflux and, more importantly, to assess the growth of the bladder. By this age, it is hoped that the capacity will achieve 60–85 ml.

MSRE stage 2: epispadias repair

Since the initial description by Jeffs of the staged reconstructive approach to exstrophy, the timing of the epispadias repair has changed. Originally, Jeffs advocated epispadias repair as the last stage of reconstruction. However, he later recognized that earlier epispadias repair increased the success of later continence procedures by stimulating bladder growth and increasing bladder capacity.[141] In the MSRE, epispadias repair (stage 2) is now typically performed at 12–18 months of age via the modified Cantwell–Ransley technique (Figure 61.40). Epispadias repair can prove challenging. The goals of epispadias repair include a straight penis and urethra, easy urethral catheterization, normal erectile function, and a cosmetically satisfactory phallus. These goals allow the patient to stand while voiding and to have intromission during intercourse.

Preoperative considerations

In preparation for this repair, the following questions must be addressed:

1 Would preoperative stimulation of penile growth with testosterone benefit the repair?
2 Is penile straightening and lengthening required at this time?
3 Is the current posterior urethral meatus ideal, i.e. without and/or not prone to stricture?

Prior to performing the epispadias repair, several surgeons use topical or intramuscular testosterone to increase the size of the phallus and the phallic skin.[139,157,158] Intramuscular testosterone enanthate in oil (2 mg/kg) can be administered at 5 and 2 weeks prior to epispadias closure. The decision as to the need for penile lengthening can then be made after the response to testosterone has been observed. Penile lengthening can be achieved almost always at this time by division of all remnants of the suspensory ligament and scar tissue as well as further release of the crura from the inferior pubic rami. It is surprising how much of this tissue is intact at the onset of the epispadias repair. In some situations, further urethral

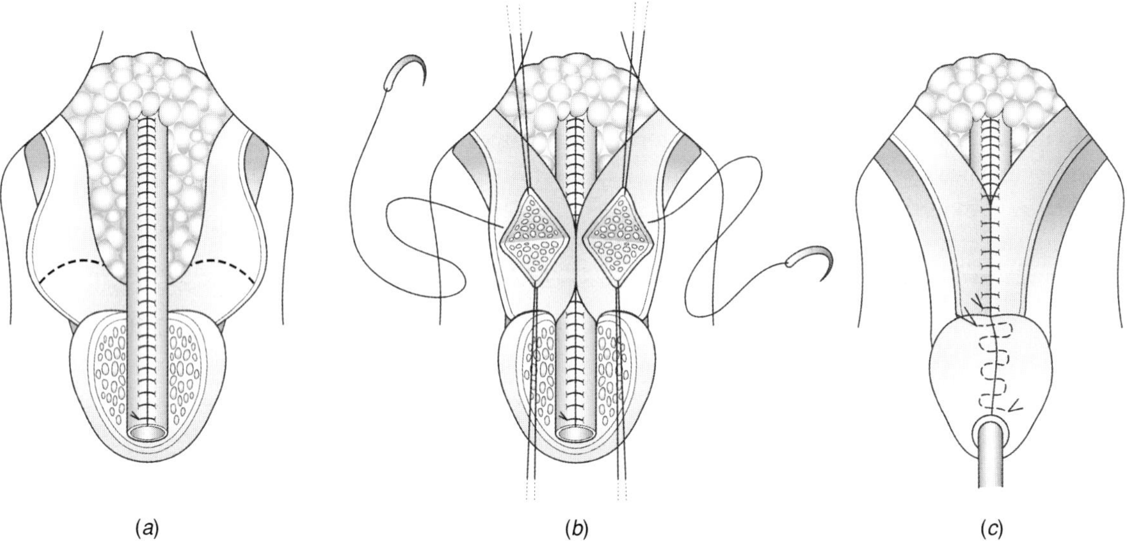

Figure 61.40 The steps for the Cantwell–Ransley repair for epispadias. (*a*) The tubularized urethral plate is placed in a dorsal groove incision in the glans penis. The dotted lines indicate the site of incision for the cavernosa – cavernosotomies; (*b*) approximation of the corpora cavernosa and performance of cavernosal anastomosis; (*c*) glans closure over urethra and skin closure. (Adapted from Brock and O'Neill,[2] with permission.)

lengthening may require free skin grafts, buccal mucosal grafts, ureteral grafts, or pedicle skin flaps. These same maneuvers can be used to repair the scarred or stenosed posterior urethra.

The modified Cantwell–Ransley technique

Cantwell first described mobilization of the urethra and moving it ventrally for epispadias repair.[159] Ransley and Woppin subsequently modified this technique and reported on their results in 1988.[160] To begin this procedure, a stay suture is placed into the glans penis (see Figure 61.40). A reverse MAGPI (meatal advancement-glanuloplasty) or IPGAM procedure at the distal urethral plate allows advancement of the urethral meatus onto the glans. Following this, skin incisions are made on the lateral edges of the urethral plate and around the epispadic meatus. This plate is dissected from the corporeal bodies up to the level of the glans distally and to the prostatic urethra proximally. Glandular wings should be developed distally as well. The corporeal bodies are then separated from each other. This allows them to be rotated medially. The urethra is then tubularized over a 6 or 8 Fr urethral catheter, using running 6–0 absorbable suture. The corporeal bodies are rotated over the urethra and reapproximated using 5–0 absorbable suture in an interrupted fashion.

Cavernocavernosotomies may be performed prior to reapproximating the corporeal bodies to help correct persistent chordee. These are performed at the point of maximal angulation. The neurovascular bundles may require mobilization to avoid injuring them if cavernosotomies are performed. The glans wings are then closed over the urethra using interrupted 5–0 absorbable suture. Penile shaft skin can be trimmed and tailored to cover the penis using interrupted 5–0 or 6–0 absorbable sutures. Z-plasties at the level of the pubis may decrease the chance of a dorsal retractile scar at the base of the penis. Postoperative care includes bladder antispasmodics, broad-spectrum antibiotics, and removal of the urethral catheter at 2 weeks.

Outcomes of this technique have revealed urethrocutaneous fistula rates ranging from 5.5 to 42%. In Lottmann and colleagues' series of 40 patients, a successful anatomic and functional result was seen in 90% of the patients at a mean follow-up period of 3 years. These authors also reported complications requiring further procedures in 45%. Complications were more common in those patients who underwent this procedure as part of an exstrophy closure vs isolated epispadias.[161] A recent review of the 10-year Johns Hopkins experience with the modified Cantwell–Ransley procedure[162] found 79 patients with classic bladder exstrophy and 14 with complete epispadias; 23% developed early urethrocutaneous fistulae, with a 19% fistula rate at 3 months postoperatively; 7.5% developed urethral stricture proximally and 83% had a straight urethra by cystoscopy or catheterization; 93.5% had a horizontal or downward-angled penis when standing. Long-term experience with 93 patients with the modified Cantwell–Ransley repair finds a conical glans, a straight penis, and urethra below the corporeal bodies with an acceptable complication rate.[162]

MSRE stage 1+ 2: combined exstrophy and epispadias closures

In the event of a significantly delayed primary closure or an initial bladder closure failure, a simultaneous closure of the exstrophy bladder and the epispadias can be performed. The advantages to this approach include one less anesthetic exposure and increasing outlet resistance to stimulate bladder growth. Again, in this scenario, the combined horizontal innominate and the posterior vertical osteotomies are necessary for a secure bladder, abdominal wall, and posterior urethral closure and can allow transposition of the urethra to beneath the corpora with some dissection. This combined approach of simultaneous exstrophy and epispadias closures has been performed in 38 patients at Johns Hopkins Hospital with comparable results (i.e. fistula rate, BNR rate, augmentation rate, and continence rate) to age-matched patients who underwent the classic staged approach after failed initial closure.[143]

Bladder neck reconstruction

Preoperative assessment

In incontinent children after CPRE or MSRE, a continence procedure is indicated when (1) the urethra is stricture-free and capable of catheterization if necessary, (2) under anesthesia, the bladder capacity has achieved a minimum volume of 60–85 ml, and (3) the child is mature enough to participate in the postoperative voiding program.[163] This is typically around age 4–5 years. Following a careful history and physical examination, cystourethroscopy and gravity cystogram under anesthesia is performed for all patients before proceeding to open BNR. Cystoscopy and gravity cystogram provide information regarding bladder capacity and the status of any previous repairs, including correction of epispadias. Advocates of staged reconstruction emphasize the importance of achieving adequate bladder capacity prior to performing BNR. A bladder capacity of <60 ml under anesthesia or during urodynamic evaluation decreases the success of BNR.[103,135] BNR requires adequate bladder capacity because some volume is lost during construction of the bladder neck. Factors that increase the potential for the bladder to achieve adequate capacity prior to BNR include:

- avoidance of UTIs
- complete bladder emptying with institution of clean intermittent catheterization if bladder emptying is incomplete.
- epispadias repair
- avoidance of bladder prolapse.[24]

Preoperative urodynamic evaluation should be considered because it allows detection of detrusor hyperactivity or atony as well as assessment of functional bladder capacity and leak point pressures. However, the urethra of these patients may be difficult to catheterize. In these situations, a urodynamic catheter can be placed suprapubically at the time of the cystourethroscopic examination to be used later that day for the urodynamic evaluation.

Ureteroneocystostomy may be required at the time of BNR to correct VUR and to move the ureters from the lower bladder where BNR will occur. The Cohen technique is often employed. However, others have described a cephalotrigonal technique that is particularly applicable to exstrophy patients because of the angle of ureteral entry into the bladder.[164] The Marshall–Marchetti–Krantz bladder neck suspension or a bladder neck wrap using rectus muscle or fascia or gracilis may be combined with BNR as well. It is also necessary to reassess whether osteotomy might stabilize the intersymphyseal bar and improve continence at the time of BNR.

The following section describes the most commonly employed BNR techniques, including the modified Young–Dees–Leadbetter (Figures 61.41 and 61.42) and the Mitchell repairs (Figure 61.43).

MSRE stage 3: modified Young–Dees–Leadbetter bladder neck reconstruction

The modified Young–Dees–Leadbetter (YDL) bladder neck plasty[165] and the transtrigonal/cephalotrigonal bilateral ureteral reimplantation[164] are the surgical techniques employed in the MSRE stage 3. As evidenced by the name, the combined thoughts of several surgeons spanning over an 82-year period has led to the modern YDL BNR.[163] To perform a modified YDL procedure (see Figures 61.41 and 61.42),[165] the bladder neck is extensively dissected and a vertical cystotomy is made. Occasionally, a portion of the inter-

Approximately 20–30% of patients with posterior urethral valves go on to develop ESRD. Studies suggest that if by 1 year old the serum creatinine level has reached a nadir value of ≤0.8, ESRD will be avoided.[82] Although such renal insufficiency is present in the neonatal period, there is usually enough GFR to support growth and development. The pediatric urologist and nephrologist must work together to closely follow boys whose creatinine level approaches these values. On occasion, these boys suffer from tubular acidosis, and require bicarbonate replenishment. For those with more advanced renal insufficiency, growth hormone may be required. As the renal failure advances, calcium metabolism and bone development must be closely monitored. Long before the time for transplantation approaches, the urology and nephrology team must begin to address the function of the lower urinary tract, and its ability to safely sustain an allograft with low storage pressures.

Most series report a substantial delay in the acquisition of daytime and night-time continence for all patients with posterior urethral valves.[82,96] For patients with less severe posterior urethral valves, the bladder and renal function combined allow for continence, usually around 6–7 years old. However, persistent urinary incontinence is an ominous sign in patients with a diagnosis of posterior urethral valves.[99] Given the pathophysiology of upper and lower urinary tract obstruction outlined at the beginning of this chapter, this incontinence is more readily understood. Because of the bladder wall fibrosis and poor storage capabilities, an increasing volume of urine is stored at higher pressures within the upper urinary tract. The severe polyuria that these patients exhibit due to distal tubular injury in utero worsens this problem. Ironically, the boy himself may also unwittingly aggravate the condition in his desire to be dry. As he struggles to achieve dryness by suppressing the desire to void, and retain urine, he contributes to upper tract dilatation and increasing storage pressures. For many boys, a regimen of timed voiding is effective. In others with upper tract dilatation, double voiding will safely result in dryness. Instructing the boy to void in the ultrasound suite, with pre- and postvoid views of the kidneys, ureters, and bladder provides a powerful teaching tool for the boy who would benefit from double voiding and his family.

It has become clear in recent years that, for many of these patients, overnight catheter drainage[100,101] and CIC will provide continence, lower storage pressures, and preserve renal function. For all these reasons, a critical time to follow a boy with posterior urethral valves closely is around the time he begins to express an interest in potty training. This is even truer for boys with borderline renal function.

Videourodynamics

For the posterior urethral valve patient who has persistent urinary incontinence, or is approaching ESRD, videourodynamics offers an invaluable tool to optimize the chances for achieving dryness[92,102] and

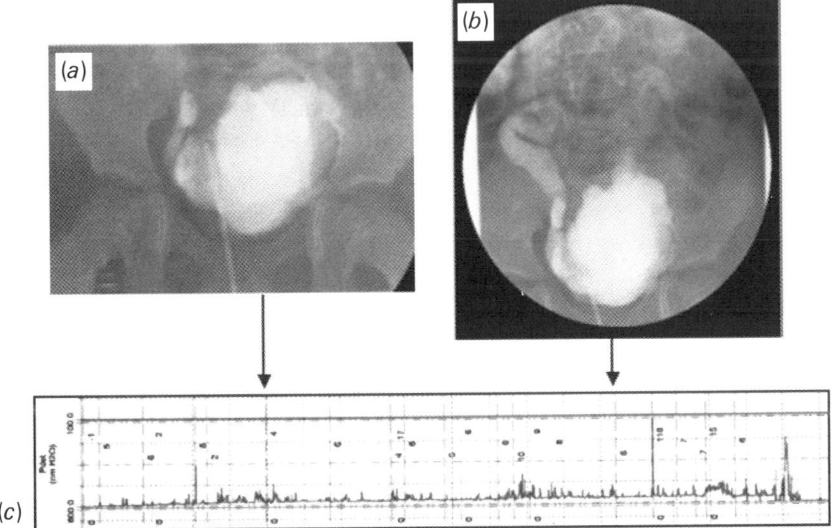

Figure 63.14 This videourodynamics study demonstrates the benefit of the fluoroscopic examination (*a*, *b*). At first glance, it appears to be a very compliant cystometrogram (*c*); however close examination reveals that compliance is augmented by the reflux into the upper tracts (*b*).

for successful transplantation. Before ordering videourodynamics, it is essential to have the patient and family complete a thorough diary, which includes not only the urinary output but also the fluid intake. This helps to determine the average urinary volume produced on an hourly basis by day and night, and what voiding frequency will be required. In contrast to conventional urodynamics, a videourodynamics study will help to determine what part of the storage capacity is provided by the bladder, and compare that with is contributed by the ureters, renal pelvis, and calices.

We have demonstrated this concept with the study shown in Figure 63.14. This study, if done conventionally, would suggest that the boy has a very compliant bladder. In fact, when the video images are considered, it is clear that the bladder has poor compliance and there is high-grade reflux early in filling. The high-grade reflux into his native kidneys augmented this boy's storage capacity and masked poor bladder compliance. Despite attempts at double and triple voiding, his diurnal urinary incontinence persisted in part due to his polyuria. He resisted our attempts to teach him urethral CIC, which is typical in this population of patients with a sensate perineum and a dilated posterior urethra (see Figure 63.9). Based on this study, we recommended an appendicovesicostomy to allow intermittent catheterization every 2–3 hours by day, and overnight catheter drainage. As long as this boy was compliant with his daytime catheterization schedule, he remained dry. Following transplantation he is continent due in large part to the improved concentrating ability of his allograft. In this case, the videourodynamic study altered this boy's care in two ways: first, the study made it clear that native nephroureterectomy would compromise his ability to achieve safe storage pressures; secondly, the large residual urine measured by the study reflected storage in his upper tracts that would not respond to double-voiding regimens. Given these findings, clean catheterization via an appendicovesicostomy offered him the optimal management for achieving dryness in the short term, while preparing for the inevitable renal transplant that followed.

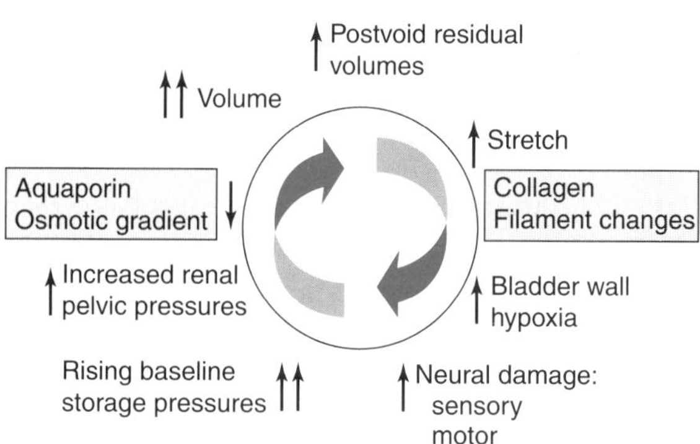

Figure 63.15 The integration of upper and lower urinary tract dysfunction in boys with posterior urethral valves. The cycle of gradual increasing postvoid residual volumes leads to increased resting prevoid pressures, which in turn leads to increasing renal medullary pressures. The resulting loss of concentrating ability results in increasing diuresis, which aggravates the cycle by subjecting the bladder to increasing stretch.

Postobstructive diuresis

Boys with a history of posterior urethral valves often have persistent dilation of the upper urinary tract that worsens as they begin to toilet train. For some boys, the imposition of daytime dryness achieved by delaying voiding and conscious use of the external sphincter places additional burden on the upper tracts. This worsens during sleep. What produces a reward for the child in terms of dry sheets in the morning and clean underwear at the end of the day may contribute to worsening of renal function. For some boys this leads to a cycle (Figure 63.15) in which increasing bladder storage pressures result in higher renal pelvic pressures. This in turn aggravates renal medullary concentrating ability, which is already compromised,[38] and thus results in additional diuresis.

Clinical and experimental evidence supports these concepts. In a videourodynamic assessment of partial bladder outlet obstruction, decompensated rabbit bladders had good compliance, defined as $\Delta V/\Delta P$. They also required much larger volumes (with a higher prevoid baseline pressure) to initiate their voids, which were small and associated with high residuals. Within this group, the postvoid residual urine recorded exceeded the infused volume.[103] This led us to consider these cystometrograms on an individual basis, and to classify them according to their baseline pressure before voiding. For the subset of obstructed bladders (30%) in which the baseline pressure >10 cmH_2O, the postvoid residual urine exceeded the infused volume by an average of 30 ml (Figure 63.16). How could the residual volume exceed the infused volume by nearly 40%? In performing these experiments, we emptied the bladder under fluoroscopic control before initiating slow-fill cystometry at 1–2 ml/min. During the filling period, the diuresis from the upper tracts was pronounced in those bladders with an elevated baseline pressure

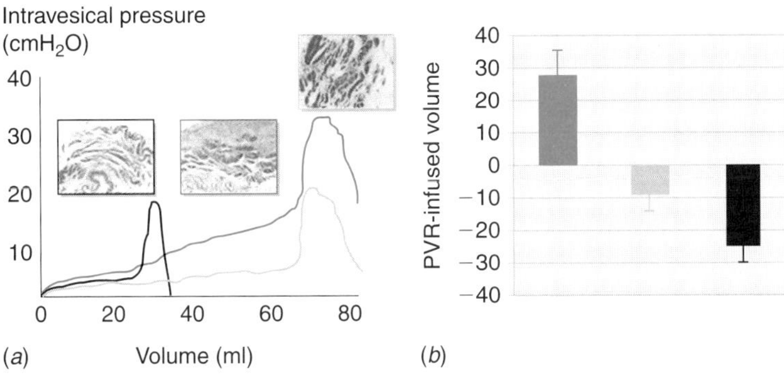

Figure 63.16 Experimental work demonstrates the relationship between a non-compliant bladder and postobstructive diuresis. (*a*) Following partial bladder outlet obstruction in rabbits, we performed videourodynamics free of any sedation 24 hours after placement of bladder and peritoneal catheters. For the sham control (——) we recorded a normal slow-fill CMG terminating in a voluntary void to completion. For decompensated bladders, we observed two populations of curves. In one group of bladders, compliance was preserved if expressed as $\Delta P/\Delta V$; however, the resting pressure just before voiding was higher (——). However for a second group of decompensated bladders, a non-compliant pattern was observed with a much higher resting pressure before void (——). In each instance, we recorded an accurate postvoid residual with fluoroscopic confirmation. Note the increased deposition of extracellular matrix elements in the two decompensated bladders. (*b*) If one subtracts the infused volume from the postvoid residual, and exceeds zero, this is evidence of a diuresis that occurs during bladder filling. We observed the presence of a postobstructive diuresis only in those non-compliant decompensated bladders whose resting pressure before voiding exceeded 10 cmH_2O. (Adapted from Stein,[104] with permission.)

before voiding. Although the majority of these bladders demonstrated 'good compliance', these rabbits were spending most of their time at the far right of their cystometry curves, and thus subjecting their upper tracts to the same higher baseline pressure. This postobstructive diuresis was also observed in 30% of the rabbits following reversal of outlet obstruction in a subsequent group of experiments.[104]

We have observed similar findings in boys with posterior urethral valves. During a videourodynamic study of a boy with urinary incontinence following valve ablation, we noted that despite having initiated the study by aspirating all urine from the system, the postvoid residual urine exceeded the volume infused. We also observed this phenomenon in another boy with posterior urethral valves in whom we had created a unilateral end-cutaneous ureterostomy. We recorded this boy's ureterostomy output and correlated it with the catheterization status of the bladder. When this boy slept without an indwelling catheter, we recorded larger volumes of urine from the ureterostomy. In contrast, when sleeping with an indwelling catheter, the overnight volumes recorded from the ureterostomy dropped by almost 40%. This finding supports our conclusion[100] and that of others[101,105,106] who feel that overnight catheter drainage can eliminate a substantial volume and hence pressure burden on the upper tract (Figure 63.17). Taken over a period of time, and with recovery of some concentrating ability, the total 24-hour urine volumes often drop, offering both the benefits of improved daytime continence and optimizing renal function.

Pretransplant evaluation

Even today, despite antenatal diagnosis, the incidence of ESRD for patients with posterior urethral valves remains at about 20%. The pediatric urologist caring for these boys must continue to remain actively involved with the nephrology transplant team. Boys undergoing transplantation with a poorly functioning bladder have higher complication rates and graft loss than those in whom lower urinary tract function has been optimized.[107,108] We recommend videourodynamic assessment for any boy in whom transplantation is imminent. This allows us to calculate the safe bladder storage pressures and to assess whether CIC is required. Videourodynamic studies may also reveal that high-grade reflux into the native ureters provides additional compliance to the system (see Figure 63.14). For this reason, we rarely recommend nephrectomy. The principal indications for pretransplant native nephrectomy are the presence of severe polyuria or hypertension that is difficult to control. We have rarely witnessed new urinary tract infection into the native kidney following transplantation if infection was not common before the transplant. If

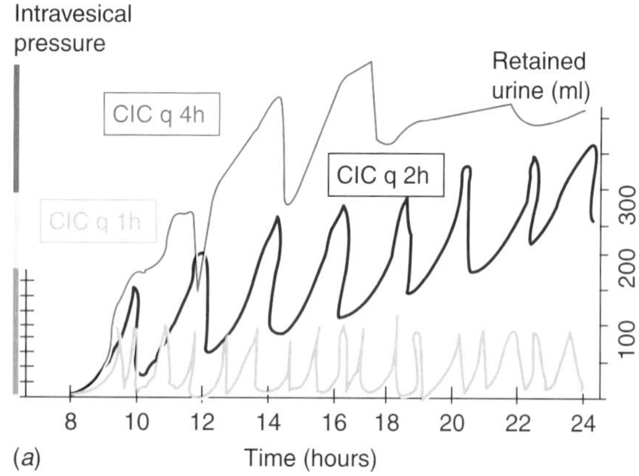

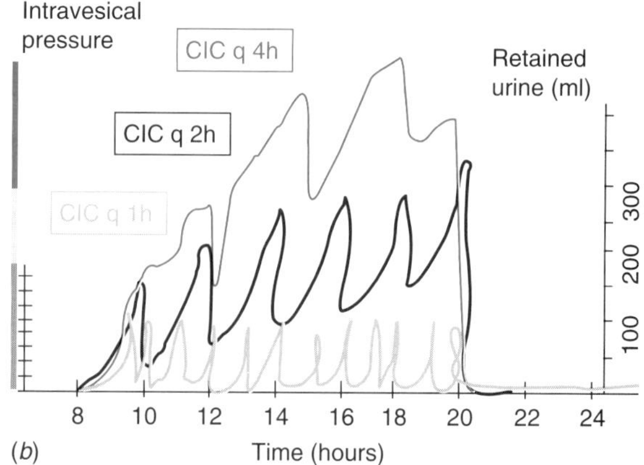

Figure 63.17 The concepts of (*a*) a safe pressure storage zone and (*b*) the role of overnight catheter drainage. As is shown in both (*a*) and (*b*), maintaining a safe storage pressure (mid-blue on the left) for a patient with this severe polyuria is possible only with a regimen of clean intermittent catheterization (CIC) at 1-hour intervals. As the intervals move to CIC at 2-hour intervals, the daytime hours drift upwards from the mid-blue to the pale-blue pressure zones. However, at 4-hour CIC intervals, the dark blue zone of high intravesical pressures is reached during the waking hours, and prolonged exposures to high dark blue zone pressures are maintained during the overnight hours. However, with overnight catheter drainage (*b*), the hours of exposure at high pressure at night are minimized. An additional benefit with this particular patient was that renal-concentrating ability improved and the total volume produced in 24 hours dropped, making daytime dryness easier to attain and at lower intravesical pressures.

nephrectomy is indicated, we preserve the ureters for catheterization, augmentation, or for anastomosis to the transplanted kidney should problems arise within the transplanted ureter.

If videourodynamics reveals that the bladder capacity must be expanded to provide safe storage pressures, ureteral augmentation is an option.[109] Very rarely, augmentation using a bowel segment may be necessary. In the past, dogma required that total bladder reconstruction, including augmentation if required, must occur before transplant. Our experience has been different. We have been pleased with the results of transplantation to the vesicostomy in the unusual cases where low bladder volume and poor compliance resulted in lower tract diversion. Under these conditions the transplant team should not hesitate to reimplant the transplant ureter into a diverted bladder that is draining via a vesicostomy.[110] With this approach, we have successfully postponed reconstruction with the associated CIC to an age-appropriate date, and in some cases, with the addition of overnight catheterization, we have avoided the need for augmentation altogether.

References

1. Young HH, Frontz WA, Baldwin JC. Congenital obstruction of the posterior urethra. J Urol 1919; 3:289.
2. Imaji R, Moon DA, Dewan PA. Congenital posterior urethral membrane: variable morphological expression. J Urol 2001; 165:1240.
3. Imaji R, Dewan PA. The clinical and radiological findings in boys with endoscopically severe congenital posterior urethral obstruction. BJU Int 2001; 88:263.
4. Stephens FD, Smith ED, Hutson JM. Congenital intrinsic lesions of the posterior urethra. In: Stephens FD, Smith ED, Hutson JM, eds. Congenital Anomalies of the Kidney, Urinary, and Genital Tracts, 2nd edn. London: Martin Dunitz, 2002: 91–106.
5. Krishnan A, de Souza A, Konijeti R et al. The anatomy and embryology of posterior urethral valves. J Urol 2006; 175:1214–20.
6. Sullivan MP, Yalla SV. Detrusor contractility and compliance characteristics in adult male patients with obstructive and nonobstructive voiding dysfunction. J Urol 1996; 155:1995.
7. Gonzalez R, Reinberg Y, Burke B et al. Early bladder outlet obstruction in fetal lambs induces renal dysplasia and the prune-belly syndrome. J Pediatr Surg 1990; 25:342.
8. Kirsch AJ, Macarak EJ, Chaqour B et al. Molecular response of the bladder to obstruction. Adv Exp Med Biol 2003; 539:195.
9. Bogaert GA, Mevorach RA, Kogan BA. Renal hemodynamic and functional effects of 10 days' partial urinary obstruction in the fetal lamb. J Urol 1994; 152:220.
10. Thiruchelvam N, Wu C, David A et al. Neurotransmission and viscoelasticity in the ovine fetal bladder after in utero bladder outflow obstruction. Am J Physiol Regul Integr Comp Physiol 2003; 284:R1296.
11. Levin RM, Macarak E, Howard P et al. The response of fetal sheep bladder tissue to partial outlet obstruction. J Urol 2001; 166:1156.
12. Rohrmann D, Monson FC, Damaser MS et al. Partial

bladder outlet obstruction in the fetal rabbit. J Urol 1997; 158:1071.

13. Rohrmann D, Zderic SA, Duckett JW Jr et al. Compliance of the obstructed fetal rabbit bladder. Neurourol Urodyn 1997; 16:179.
14. Workman SJ, Kogan BA. Fetal bladder histology in posterior urethral valves and the prune belly syndrome. J Urol 1990; 144:337.
15. Holmes N, Harrison MR, Baskin LS. Fetal surgery for posterior urethral valves: long-term postnatal outcomes. Pediatrics 2001; 108:E7.
16. Park JM, Yang T, Arend LJ et al. Cyclooxygenase-2 is expressed in bladder during fetal development and stimulated by outlet obstruction. Am J Physiol 1997; 273:F538.
17. Park JM, Yang T, Arend LJ et al. Obstruction stimulates COX-2 expression in bladder smooth muscle cells via increased mechanical stretch. Am J Physiol 1999; 276:F129.
18. Capolicchio G, Aitken KJ, Gu JX, Reddy P, Bagli DJ. Extracellular matrix gene responses in a novel ex vivo model of bladder stretch injury. J Urol 2001; 165:2235.
19. Adam RM, Eaton SH, Estrada C et al. Mechanical stretch is a highly selective regulator of gene expression in human bladder smooth muscle cells. Physiol Genomics 2004; 20:36.
20. Greenland JE, Brading AF. The effect of bladder outflow obstruction on detrusor blood flow changes during the voiding cycle in conscious pigs. J Urol 2001; 165:245.
21. Azadzoi KM, Pontari M, Vlachiotis J, Siroky MB. Canine bladder blood flow and oxygenation: changes induced by filling, contraction and outlet obstruction. J Urol 1996; 155:1459.
22. Ghafar MA, Anastasiadis AG, Olsson LE et al. Hypoxia and an angiogenic response in the partially obstructed rat bladder. Lab Invest 2002; 82:903.
23. Azadzoi KM, Tarcan T, Siroky MB, Krane RJ. Atherosclerosis-induced chronic ischemia causes bladder fibrosis and non-compliance in the rabbit. J Urol 1999; 161:1626.
24. Levin RM, Agartan CA, Leggett RE. Effect of partial outlet obstruction on nitrotyrosine content and distribution within the rabbit bladder. Mol Cell Biochem 2005; 276:143.
25. Hutcheson JC, Stein R, Chacko S et al. Murine in vitro whole bladder model: a method for assessing phenotypic responses to pharmacologic stimuli and hypoxia. Neurourol Urodyn 2004; 23:349.
26. Zhang EY, Stein R, Chang S et al. Smooth muscle hypertrophy following partial bladder outlet obstruction is associated with overexpression of non-muscle caldesmon. Am J Pathol 2004; 164:601.
27. Coplen DE, Howard PS, Duckett JW et al. Cultured bladder cells and their response to mechanical strain. Adv Exp Med Biol 1995; 385:207.
28. Coplen DE, Macarak EJ, Howard PS. Matrix synthesis by bladder smooth muscle cells is modulated by stretch frequency. In Vitro Cell Dev Biol Anim 2003; 39:157.
29. Peters CA, Freeman MR, Fernandez CA et al. Dysregulated proteolytic balance as the basis of excess extracellular matrix in fibrotic disease. Am J Physiol 1997; 272:R1960.
30. Sillen U, Hjalmas K, Aili M et al. Pronounced detrusor hypercontractility in infants with gross bilateral reflux. J Urol 1992; 148:598.
31. Angell SK, Pruthi RS, Shortliffe LD. The urodynamic relationship of renal pelvic and bladder pressures, and urinary flow rate in rats with congenital vesicoureteral reflux. J Urol 1998; 160:150.
32. Norregaard R, Jensen BL, Li C et al. COX–2 inhibition prevents downregulation of key renal water and sodium transport proteins in response to bilateral ureteral obstruction. Am J Physiol Renal Physiol 2005; 289: F322.
33. Li C, Wang W, Kwon TH et al. Downregulation of AQP1, –2, and –3 after ureteral obstruction is associated with a long-term urine-concentrating defect. Am J Physiol Renal Physiol 2001; 281:F163.
34. Nguyen HT, Hsieh MH, Gaborro A et al. JNK/SAPK and p38 SAPK–2 mediate mechanical stretch-induced apoptosis via caspase–3 and –9 in NRK–52E renal epithelial cells. Nephron Exp Nephrol 2005; 102:e49.
35. Sweeney P, Young LS, Fitzpatrick JM. An autoradiographic study of regional blood flow distribution in the rat kidney during ureteric obstruction – the role of vasoactive compounds. BJU Int 2001; 88:268.
36. Hwang SJ, Haas M, Harris HW Jr et al. Transport defects of rabbit medullary thick ascending limb cells in obstructive nephropathy. J Clin Invest 1993; 91:21.
37. Li C, Klein JD, Wang W et al. Altered expression of urea transporters in response to ureteral obstruction. Am J Physiol Renal Physiol 2004; 286:F1154.
38. Dinneen MD, Duffy PG, Barratt TM et al. Persistent polyuria after posterior urethral valves. Br J Urol 1995; 75:236.
39. Gobet R, Bleakley J, Cisek L et al. Fetal partial urethral obstruction causes renal fibrosis and is associated with proteolytic imbalance. J Urol 1999; 162:854.
40. Furness PD 3rd, Maizels M, Han SW et al. Elevated bladder urine concentration of transforming growth factor-beta1 correlates with upper urinary tract obstruction in children. J Urol 1999; 162:1033.
41. MacRae Dell K, Hoffman BB, Leonard MB, Ziyadeh FN, Schulman SL. Increased urinary transforming growth factor-beta(1) excretion in children with posterior urethral valves. Urology 2000; 56:311.
42. Gagliardini E, Benigni A. Role of anti-TGF-beta antibodies in the treatment of renal injury. Cytokine Growth Factor Rev 2005; 17:89.
43. Yu L, Border WA, Anderson I et al. Combining TGF-beta inhibition and angiotensin II blockade results in enhanced antifibrotic effect. Kidney Int 2004; 66:1774.
44. Harrison MR, Golbus MS, Filly RA et al. Fetal surgery for congenital hydronephrosis. N Engl J Med 1982; 306:591–3.
45. Ichikawa I, Kuwayama F, Pope JC 4th, Stephens FD, Miyazaki Y. Paradigm shift from classic anatomic theories to contemporary cell biological views of CAKUT. Kidney Int 2002; 61:889.
46. Peruzzi L, Lombardo F, Amore A et al. Low renin–angiotensin system activity gene polymorphism and dysplasia associated with posterior urethral valves. J Urol 2005; 174:713.

47. Bajpai M, Pratap A, Tripathi M, Bal CS. Posterior urethral valves: preliminary observations on the significance of plasma renin activity as a prognostic marker. J Urol 2005; 173:592.
48. Abbott JF, Levine D, Wapner R. Posterior urethral valves: inaccuracy of prenatal diagnosis. Fetal Diagn Ther 1998; 13:179.
49. Cassart M, Massez A, Metens T et al. Complementary role of MRI after sonography in assessing bilateral urinary tract anomalies in the fetus. AJR Am J Roentgenol 2004; 182:689.
50. Poutamo J, Vanninen R, Partanen K et al. Diagnosing fetal urinary tract abnormalities: benefits of MRI compared to ultrasonography. Acta Obstet Gynecol Scand 2000; 79:65.
51. Zaretsky M, Ramus R, McIntire D et al. MRI calculation of lung volumes to predict outcome in fetuses with genitourinary abnormalities. AJR Am J Roentgenol 2005; 185:1328.
52. Harrison MR, Ross N, Noall R et al. Correction of congenital hydronephrosis in utero. I. The model: fetal urethral obstruction produces hydronephrosis and pulmonary hypoplasia in fetal lambs. J Pediatr Surg 1983; 18:247.
53. Glick PL, Harrison MR, Adzick NS, Noall RA, Villa RL. Correction of congenital hydronephrosis in utero IV: in utero decompression prevents renal dysplasia. J Pediatr Surg 1984; 19:649.
54. Harrison MR. The University of California at San Francisco Fetal Treatment Center: a personal perspective. Fetal Diagn Ther 2004; 19:513.
55. Adzick NS, Harrison MR, Glick PL, Villa RL, Finkbeiner W. Experimental pulmonary hypoplasia and oligohydramnios: relative contributions of lung fluid and fetal breathing movements. J Pediatr Surg 1984; 19:658.
56. Nakayama DK, Glick PL, Harrison MR, Villa RL, Noall R. Experimental pulmonary hypoplasia due to oligohydramnios and its reversal by relieving thoracic compression. J Pediatr Surg 1983; 18:347.
57. Agre P, Kozono D. Aquaporin water channels: molecular mechanisms for human diseases. FEBS Lett 2003; 555:72.
58. Glick PL, Harrison MR, Golbus MS et al. Management of the fetus with congenital hydronephrosis II: prognostic criteria and selection for treatment. J Pediatr Surg 1985; 20:376.
59. Freedman AL, Bukowski TP, Smith CA et al. Use of urinary beta-2-microglobulin to predict severe renal damage in fetal obstructive uropathy. Fetal Diagn Ther 1997; 12:1.
60. Freedman AL, Johnson MP, Gonzalez R. Fetal therapy for obstructive uropathy: past, present and future? Pediatr Nephrol 2000; 14:167.
61. Biard JM, Johnson MP, Carr MC et al. Long-term outcomes in children treated by prenatal vesicoamniotic shunting for lower urinary tract obstruction. Obstet Gynecol 2005; 106:503.
62. Freedman AL, Johnson MP, Smith CA et al. Long-term outcome in children after antenatal intervention for obstructive uropathies. Lancet 1999; 354:374.
63. Elder JS. Antenatal surgical intervention for urinary obstruction: a critical analysis. In: Smith AD, ed. Smith's Textbook of Endourology, 1st edn, Vol 2. St Louis: Quality Medical Publishing, 1996: 1464.
64. Chevalier RL. Biomarkers of congenital obstructive nephropathy: past, present and future. J Urol 2004; 172:852.
65. Nakayama DK, Harrison MR, de Lorimier AA. Prognosis of posterior urethral valves presenting at birth. J Pediatr Surg 1986; 21:43.
66. Cameron D, Lupton BA, Farquharson D et al. Amnioinfusions in renal agenesis. Obstet Gynecol 1994; 83:872.
67. Tabsh KM, Theroux NL. Obstructive fetal hydronephrosis managed by amnioinfusions and bladder aspirations. Obstet Gynecol 1997; 90:679.
68. Coplen DE, Hare JY, Zderic SA et al. 10-year experience with prenatal intervention for hydronephrosis. J Urol 1996; 156:1142.
69. Hutton KA, Thomas DF, Davies BW. Prenatally detected posterior urethral valves: qualitative assessment of second trimester scans and prediction of outcome. J Urol 1997; 158:1022.
70. Cromie WJ, Lee K, Honde K et al. Implications of prenatal ultrasound screening in the incidence of major genitourinary malformations. J Urol 2001; 165:1677–80.
71. Schober JM, Dulabon LM, Woodhouse CR. Outcome of valve ablation in late-presenting posterior urethral valves. BJU Int 2004; 94:616.
72. Bomalaski MD, Anema JG, Coplen DE et al. Delayed presentation of posterior urethral valves: a not so benign condition. J Urol 1999; 162:2130.
73. Dinneen MD, Dhillon HK, Ward HC et al. Antenatal diagnosis of posterior urethral valves. Br J Urol 1993; 72:364.
74. Moslehi J, Herndon CD, McKenna PH. Posterior urethral valves presented at birth despite normal prenatal ultrasound scans. Urology 2001; 57:1178.
75. Hoover DL, Duckett JW Jr. Posterior urethral valves, unilateral reflux and renal dysplasia: a syndrome. J Urol 1982; 128:994.
76. Rittenberg MH, Hulbert WC, Snyder HM 3rd et al. Protective factors in posterior urethral valves. J Urol 1988; 140:993.
77. Kaefer M, Keating MA, Adams MC et al. Posterior urethral valves, pressure pop-offs and bladder function. J Urol 1995; 154:708.
78. Hulbert WC, Rosenberg HK, Cartwright PC et al. The predictive value of ultrasonography in evaluation of infants with posterior urethral valves. J Urol 1992; 148:122.
79. Kaefer M, Peters CA, Retik AB et al. Increased renal echogenicity: a sonographic sign for differentiating between obstructive and nonobstructive etiologies of in utero bladder distension. J Urol 1997; 158:1026.
80. Cuckow PM, Dinneen MD, Risdon RA et al. Long-term renal function in the posterior urethral valves, unilateral reflux and renal dysplasia syndrome. J Urol 1997; 158:1004.
81. Zderic SA. Endoscopic approach to anterior and posterior urethral valves. In: Smith AD, ed. Smith's Textbook of Endourology, 1st edn, Vol 2. St Louis: Quality Medical Publishing, 1996: 1323.

82. Smith GH, Canning DA, Schulman SL et al. The long-term outcome of posterior urethral valves treated with primary valve ablation and observation. J Urol 1996; 155:1730.
83. Kim YH, Horowitz M, Combs A et al. Comparative urodynamic findings after primary valve ablation, vesicostomy or proximal diversion. J Urol 1996; 156:673.
84. Krueger RP, Hardy BE, Churchill BM. Growth in boys and posterior urethral valves. Primary valve resection vs upper tract diversion. Urol Clin North Am 1980; 7:265.
85. Close CE, Carr MC, Burns MW et al. Lower urinary tract changes after early valve ablation in neonates and infants: is early diversion warranted? J Urol 1997; 157:984.
86. Duckett JW. Are 'valve bladders' congenital or iatrogenic? Br J Urol 1997; 79:271.
87. Podesta M, Ruarte AC, Gargiulo C et al. Bladder function associated with posterior urethral valves after primary valve ablation or proximal urinary diversion in children and adolescents. J Urol 2002; 168:1830: discussion 1835.
88. Podesta ML, Ruarte A, Herrera M, Medel R, Castera R. Bladder functional outcome after delayed vesicostomy closure and antireflux surgery in young infants with 'primary' vesico-ureteric reflux. BJU Int 2001; 87:473.
89. Wiswell TE, Geschke DW. Risks from circumcision during the first month of life compared with those for uncircumcised boys. Pediatrics 1989; 83:1011.
90. Wiswell TE, John K. Lattimer Lecture. Prepuce presence portends prevalence of potentially perilous periurethral pathogens. J Urol 1992; 148:739.
91. Noe HN, Spivey OS Jr, Jerkins GR. Use of ureter of non-functioning renal unit in pediatric urinary reconstruction. Urology 1984; 23:144.
92. Kim YH, Horowitz M, Combs AJ et al. Management of posterior urethral valves on the basis of urodynamic findings. J Urol 1997; 158:1011.
93. Kim YH, Horowitz M, Combs AJ, Nitti VW, Glassberg KI. The management of unilateral poorly functioning kidneys in patients with posterior urethral valves. J Urol 1997; 158:1001.
94. Coleman JW, McGovern JH. Ureterovesical reimplantation in children. Surgical results in 491 children. Urology 1978; 12:514.
95. Puri P, Kumar R. Endoscopic correction of vesicoureteral reflux secondary to posterior urethral valves. J Urol 1996; 156:680.
96. Nguyen HT, Peters CA. The long-term complications of posterior urethral valves. BJU Int 1999; 83(Suppl 3):23.
97. Misseri R, Combs AJ, Horowitz M, Donohue JM, Glassberg KI. Myogenic failure in posterior urethral valve disease: real or imagined? J Urol 2002; 168:1844, discussion 1848.
98. Gibbons MD, Horan JJ, Dejter SW Jr, Keszler M. Extracorporeal membrane oxygenation: an adjunct in the management of the neonate with severe respiratory distress and congenital urinary tract anomalies. J Urol 1993; 150:434.
99. Parkhouse HF, Barratt TM, Dillon MJ et al. Long-term outcome of boys with posterior urethral valves. Br J Urol 1988; 62:59.
100. Nguyen MT, Pavlock CL, Zderic SA, Carr MC, Canning DA. Overnight catheter drainage in children with poorly compliant bladders improves post-obstructive diuresis and urinary incontinence. J Urol 2005; 174:1633.
101. Koff SA, Mutabagani KH, Jayanthi VR. The valve bladder syndrome: pathophysiology and treatment with nocturnal bladder emptying. J Urol 2002; 167:291.
102. Peters CA, Bolkier M, Bauer SB et al. The urodynamic consequences of posterior urethral valves. J Urol 1990; 144:122.
103. Stein R, Gong C, Hutcheson J et al. The fate of urinary bladder smooth muscle after outlet obstruction – a role for the sarcoplasmic reticulum. Adv Exp Med Biol 2003; 539:773.
104. Stein R, Hutcheson JC, Krasnopolsky L et al. The decompensated detrusor V: molecular correlates of bladder function after reversal of experimental outlet obstruction. J Urol 2001; 166:651.
105. Koff SA, Gigax MR, Jayanthi VR. Nocturnal bladder emptying: a simple technique for reversing urinary tract deterioration in children with neurogenic bladder. J Urol 2005; 174:1629.
106. Montane B, Abitbol C, Seeherunvong W et al. Beneficial effects of continuous overnight catheter drainage in children with polyuric renal failure. BJU Int 2003; 92:447.
107. Sheldon CA, Gonzalez R, Burns MW et al. Renal transplantation into the dysfunctional bladder: the role of adjunctive bladder reconstruction. J Urol 1994; 152:972.
108. Mendizabal S, Estornell F, Zamora I et al. Renal transplantation in children with severe bladder dysfunction. J Urol 2005; 173:226.
109. Nahas WC, Lucon M, Mazzucchi E et al. Clinical and urodynamic evaluation after ureterocystoplasty and kidney transplantation. J Urol 2004; 171:1428.
110. Rigamonti W, Capizzi A, Zacchello G et al. Kidney transplantation into bladder augmentation or urinary diversion: long-term results. Transplantation 2005; 80:1435.

Prune belly syndrome

64

R Guy Hudson and Steven J Skoog

Introduction

Prune belly syndrome is classically defined by three abnormalities: deficiency of the abdominal wall musculature, bilateral cryptorchidism, and a dilated, dysmorphic urinary tract (Figure 64.1). The scope of involvement of the genitourinary system, combined with the visible appearance of the abdominal wall, sets the stage for the intense interest that surrounds this developmental anomaly.

A rich history surrounds the recognition of the essential components of the prune belly syndrome (Table 64.1). In 1839, Frolich noted the abdominal wall 'tumidity'.[1] Parker, in 1895, recognized the essential element of the syndrome to include a large flaccid abdominal wall with absent musculature, undescended testes, and a hypertrophied bladder and dilated renal collecting system without urethral obstruction.[2] William Osler is credited with giving the syndrome its name 'prune belly' in 1901. Prune belly syndrome is, at present, the most widely accepted appellation.[3] Other popular synonyms – Eagle–Barrett syndrome, urethral obstruction malformation complex, the triad syndrome, abdominal muscle deficiency syndrome, and mesenchymal dysplasia syndrome – reflect the etiologic biases of the respective authors.[4–7]

Prune belly syndrome is not confined to the male gender. Females constitute about 3–5% of recorded cases.[8] The strict criterion of cryptorchidism would effectively eliminate the syndrome in female patients, but the descriptive term 'prune belly' is applicable. Omphalocele and bladder outlet obstructive lesions are often seen in female patients with prune belly syndrome.[9] In a review by Reinberg et al, 40% of female patients had anorectal anomalies and the perinatal mortality was 40%.[10] The term 'pseudoprune' has been suggested to define females and males who do not have the complete triad of prune belly syndrome.[3] Hence, males with a lax abdominal wall but without undescended testes or without a dilated urinary tract and all affected females are considered pseudoprunes. The principles of management in females are essentially the same as in the male patient. The underlying uropathy and clinical course in patients with pseudoprune belly syndrome are unpredictable and in one series 63% went on to renal failure.[11]

The incidence of prune belly syndrome is 1 in 29 000 to 1 in 40 000 live births.[12,13] An increased incidence has been reported in Nigeria[14] as well as in Saskatchewan, Canada.[7] In a population-based study from New York State the live birth prevalence was 3.2 per 100 000. Twins, blacks, and children born to younger mothers appear to be at higher risk.[15] Maternal

Table 64.1 History of prune belly syndrome

Year	Author	Discovery
1839	Frolich	Described abdominal wall abnormality
1895	Parker	Recognized all three components of the syndrome
1901	Osler	Coined the name prune belly syndrome
1903	Strumme	Proposed obstructive hypothesis of prune belly syndrome
1961	Nunn and Stephens	Proposed theory of mesodermal arrest as an etiology of prune belly syndrome

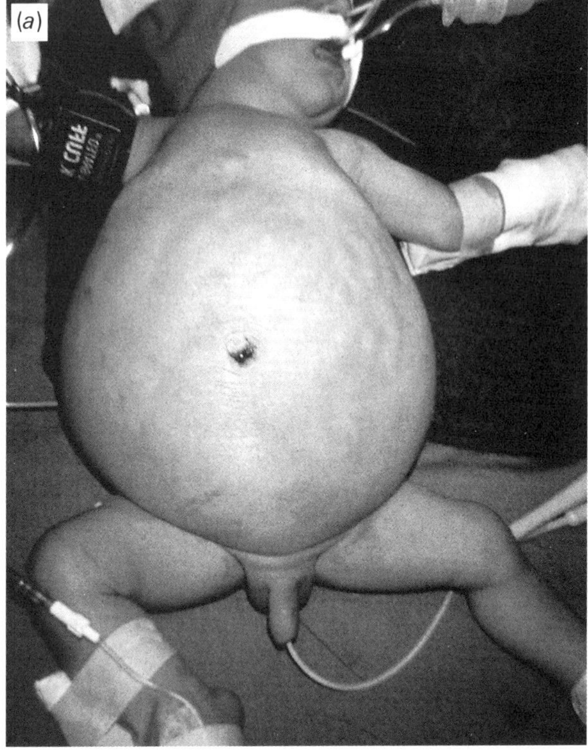

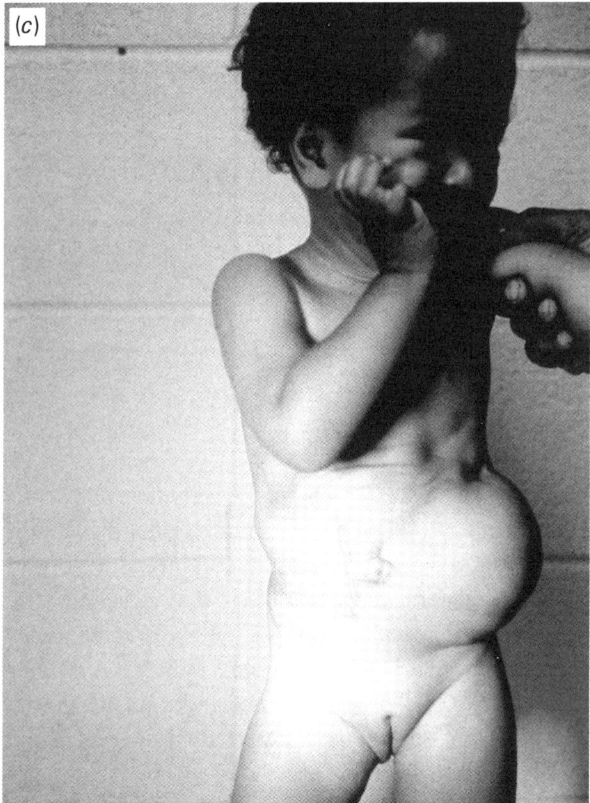

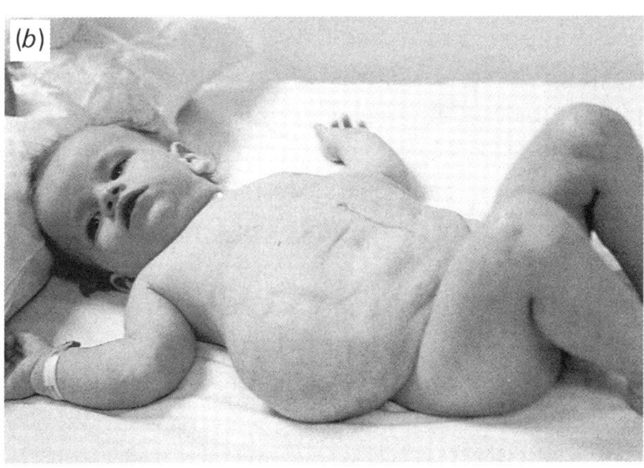

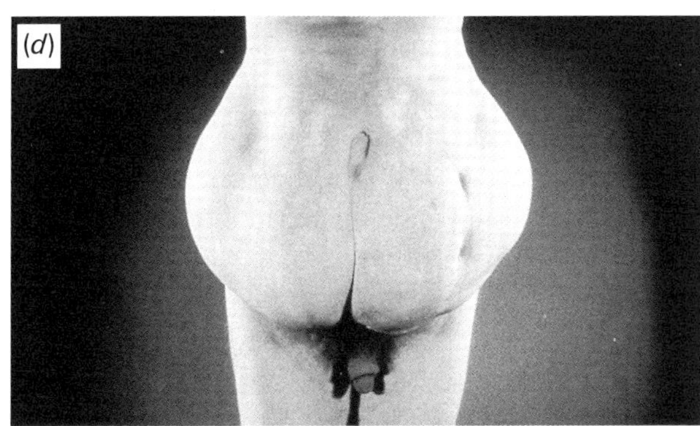

Figure 64.1 (*a*) A newborn with prune belly syndrome, urinary ascites, and pulmonary hypoplasia. Outline of the bowel is visible through the abdominal wall. (*b*) A 6-month old infant with prune belly syndrome before comprehensive reconstruction. (*c*) A 4-year-old female with hemiprune belly. (*d*) An adult with prune belly syndrome exhibiting 'pot belly' configuration.

cocaine abuse during pregnancy has been associated with prune belly syndrome.[16]

Unfortunately, patients with prune belly syndrome can have many associated conditions that have a significant clinical impact. These can include pulmonary hypoplasia, renal dysplasia/insufficiency, cardiac anomalies, lower extremity musculoskeletal malformations, imperforate anus, and intestinal malrotation/malfixation. These conditions impart a significant morbidity in prune belly patients and often influence urologic management.

One major area of controversy in the management of prune belly syndrome is the role of surgical reconstruction. Early series stressed the importance of relief of obstruction and stasis by high ureterostomies or catheter drainage. Indwelling catheter drainage often met with infectious complications, with an additional 30% mortality reported in the first 2 years of life.[17,18] Later reports of successful, early urinary reconstruction demonstrated both improved urinary drainage and radiologic configuration of the urinary tract. Long-term follow-up demonstrated stabilization of renal function.[6,19–22]

Prevention of urinary infection and preservation of renal function may also be achieved with 'watchful waiting.'[23–26] With the development of improved prophylactic antibiotic therapy and utilization of advanced urodynamic equipment, the need for extensive tailoring of the urinary tract has been questioned. In fact, Woodhouse et al reported a normal serum creatinine in 27 patients with prune belly syndrome who had limited surgical intervention over a 29-year period.[27] However, mindful of psychological and fertility considerations, current practice dictates an early surgical role in correction of the abdominal wall defect and the cryptorchid testes.[28–31]

A further improvement in the treatment of prune belly syndrome has been the application of dialysis and renal transplantation. Transplantation offers hope to patients with poor renal function due to initial renal dysplasia or progressive chronic renal insufficiency, despite appropriate urologic intervention.

This chapter reviews proposed etiologies of the syndrome and associated malformations, and illustrates the spectrum of management of these patients.

Theories of etiology and embryogenesis

Inheritance

A variety of genetic inheritance patterns have been suggested in prune belly syndrome. The majority of cases are sporadic and have a normal karyotype.[13,32] Prune belly syndrome has been reported in male siblings, cousins, and twins.[14,33–36] However, the majority of affected twin pairs are discordant for prune belly syndrome, which speaks against a purely genetic etiology. Ives noted 11 pairs of twins discordant for the syndrome: six were monozygous and five were of unknown zygosity. Of the 250 cases of prune belly syndrome reviewed, 11 cases or 4% occurred in twins, compared with the 1.25% incidence of twinning in the general population. Unequal division of mesoderm cells, occurring at the primitive streak formation, may explain the discordant monozygotic twinning phenomena.[7]

Williams was one of the first to suggest that prune belly syndrome was due to a sex-linked recessive trait. This would explain the male predominance of the syndrome, its occurrence in male siblings, in concordant twins, and in association with Turner's syndrome.[23,37] The presence of prune belly syndrome in three females with documented 46,XX karyotype speaks strongly against this pattern of inheritance.[38]

Autosomal dominant and autosomal recessive inheritance have also been reported.[14] Male predominance, lack of consanguinity, and lack of extensive pedigrees in new cases due to associated infertility, make any association with single gene inheritance uncertain at this time.[13] Riccardi and Grum suggested a two-step autosomal dominant mutation with sex-limited expression that partially mimics X-linkage. This genetic inheritance pattern would explain male predominance, as well as the small number of affected family members.[35]

Specific chromosomal abnormalities are rare. Trisomy 18 and trisomy 21 have been demonstrated in prune belly syndrome.[39–42] Trisomy 18 is also associated with other genitourinary abnormalities, including renal dysplasia and hypoplasia, horseshoe kidney, duplication anomalies, and persistent nodular renal blastema.[43] A cause-and-effect relationship is only speculative. A careful analysis of incidence and birth rates suggests that these are independent events, occurring together by chance alone.[44]

An association with Turners' syndrome suggests that the gene responsible for the syndrome may be located on the X chromosome and is recessively transmitted. However, it probably represents the occurrence of the prune belly phenotype in the female as a result of other causes of abdominal distention, such as impaired lymphatic development with chylous ascites.[4,14,37] Although mosaicism for a monosome of chromosome number 16 in two male siblings with prune belly syndrome has been documented, its importance etiologically cannot be determined.[45] An extracentric chromosomal fragment was reported in association with prune belly syndrome. However, the same aberration was present in two phenotypically normal male family members.[46]

Prune belly syndrome has been reported in association with other syndromes, chromosomal aberrations, and conditions. Perlman syndrome, Beckwith–Wiedemann syndrome, VACTERL association, Pfeiffer syndrome type 3, and megacystis–microcolon–intestinal hypoperistalsis syndrome have all been described in patients with prune belly syndrome, suggesting the possibility of a common pathogenesis.[47–50]

Fetal development

Three major theories have been proposed to explain the clinical features of the prune belly syndrome. As with most theories, none completely explains the entire constellation of findings in the syndrome, and all are marred by conjecture and speculation.

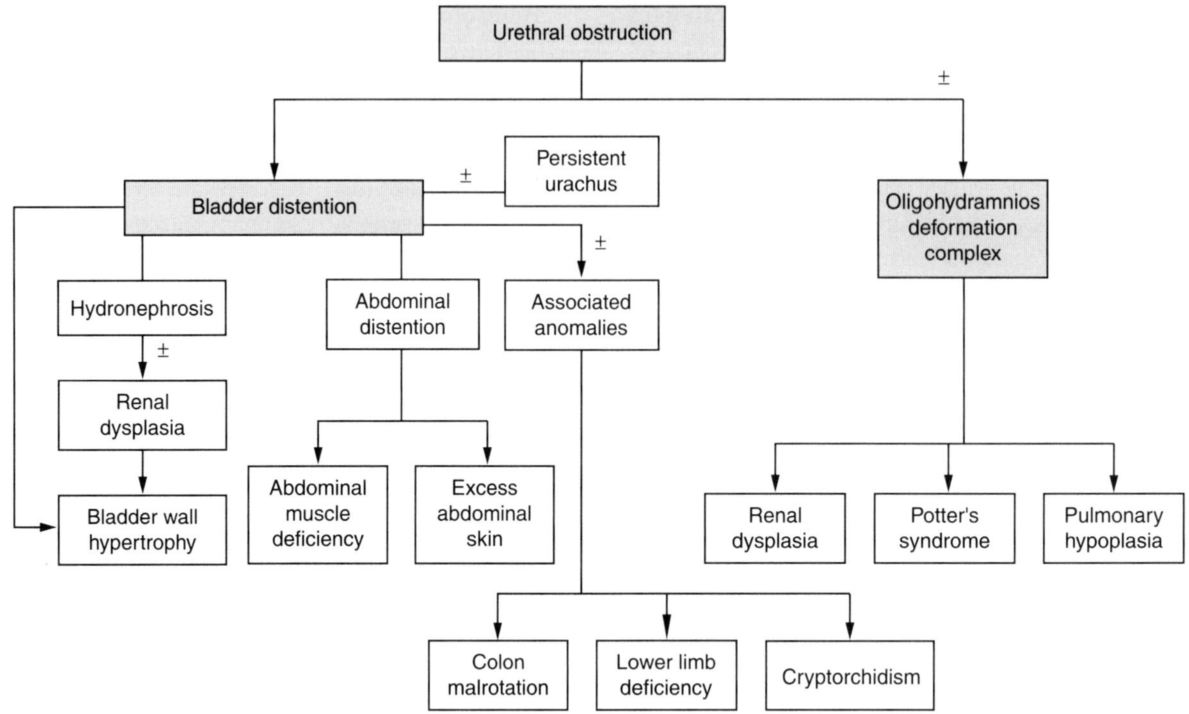

Figure 64.2 Urethral obstruction, whether anatomic or functional, is a proposed etiology of prune belly syndrome and its associated anomalies.

Fetal outlet obstruction

In 1903, Strumme proposed that prune belly syndrome was the final expression of an obstructive urologic lesion producing significant back pressure at a critical time during development. The dilatation of the urinary tract and secondary pressure atrophy of the abdominal wall produced the clinical features common to prune belly syndrome (Figure 64.2).[51] Subsequent clinical reviews reflected this belief and called attention to the need to alleviate the obstructing lesions commonly found in the posterior urethra.[18,52–54] Improved methods of radiographic diagnosis of obstruction with the voiding cystourethrogram (VCUG), postmortem anatomic en-bloc dissections, and the application of urodynamic studies cast doubt on the anatomic presence of obstruction.[5,23,24,55] More recent clinical reports have found evidence of an obstructing lesion in 10–20% of patients, contrasted with up to 80% in earlier series.[26,52] It has been proposed that those infants with the most severe manifestations of the syndrome have the 'lethal variant' (an anatomic obstructing lesion), leading to pulmonary hypoplasia, renal dysplasia, and death.[53] This distinction is particularly important when studying the theories of pathogenesis, as most articles that indicate obstruction as the primary cause are based on autopsy information.[54,56–59]

The source of the obstruction may be true areas of stenosis, atresia, valves, or pinpoint diaphragms at the junction of the posterior and membranous urethra. Recent theories have suggested a 'functional obstruction' present in utero, secondary to prostatic hypoplasia, as the specific etiology of the syndrome. This 'obstruction' is thought to be the result of conformational changes in the prostatic urethra during voiding, creating a valve-like mechanism.[57,60] Another etiology suggested in prune belly syndrome is a transient obstruction at the junction of the glandular and penile urethra. This was based on evidence of anterior urethral dilatation in patients with prune belly syndrome measured on radiographs from a VCUG. Comparisons were made with children with urinary tract infections and children with posterior urethral valves.[61] This theory is supported by the high incidence of megalourethra seen with prune belly syndrome.[62,63]

The obstructive theory contends that the abdominal wall findings are secondary to the pressure effects of the distended bladder on the developing myotomes of the abdominal wall. The muscles directly over the bladder – transversus abdominis, obliques, and lower rectus – are most severely affected, supporting this theory. However, histologic studies and electron microscopy of the abdominal wall do not demonstrate a pattern of atrophy, but one of developmental arrest.[64–66] In addition, the absence histologically of any aponeurotic layer of the affected muscles opposes an atrophic cause.[66]

Evidence from prenatal ultrasound in patients with prune belly syndrome and other disease processes associated with the prune belly phenotype suggest that the abdominal wall laxity is due to abdominal distention. A transient ascitic distention explains patients with the syndrome who lack evidence of urethral obstruction.[4,67–70] Urinary ascites has been demonstrated in utero in patients with prune belly syndrome. The urine is theorized to leak into the abdomen via the distended urinary tract and spontaneously reabsorbs at the end of gestation, which explains its clinical absence at birth.[67,68,71–73] Other causes of in-utero abdominal wall distention and the prune belly phenotype include non-immune ascites, intestinal duplication, posterior urethral valves, amniotic band syndrome, visceromegaly, polycystic kidneys, impaired lymphatic drainage in Turner's syndrome, giant liver cyst, and cystic adenomatoid malformation of the lung.[4,69,74–76]

The 'urethral obstruction malformation complex' is applied to the theory of fetal outlet obstruction as the etiology of prune belly syndrome. The timing and severity of the obstructive phenomena is critical. Distension of the urinary tract at 13–15 weeks of gestation could produce the degenerative changes in the abdominal wall and urinary tract, preventing gut rotation and prostatic development.[77] This broader application of Strumme's original hypothesis fails to explain (1) the lack of hypertrophy and hyperplasia present in the obstructed urinary tract, (2) the replacement of smooth and skeletal muscle by fibrous and collagenous tissue, (3) normal or low intravesical pressures assessed urodynamically, (4) absent obstruction but presence of renal dysgenesis in the majority of patients, (5) other causes of in-utero outlet obstruction not associated with abdominal wall laxity, and (6) the excessively high incidence of cryptorchid testes. All these factors are common in prune belly syndrome and cannot be completely explained on the basis of obstruction alone.[5,23,55,78,79]

Theory of mesodermal arrest

This theory suggests that the etiology of prune belly syndrome is an embryologic aberration of mesenchymal development (Figure 64.3).[5] Urinary tract obstruction occurs in some patients as a consequence of the primary defect and may increase the pathologic severity.[77] Stephens and Gupta have proposed that the genitourinary tract, the testes, and the abdominal wall would be vulnerable to a mesodermal defect occurring between the 6th and 10th weeks of gestation.[80] A noxious insult occurring when the lateral plate mesoderm has already extended to the midline, with failure of myoblast differentiation and migration ventrally and caudally, would explain the abdominal wall findings.[56] At the same time, the urinary tract is developing from the visceral layer of the lateral plate mesoderm. The same insult would impair differentiation of the mesoderm that forms the smooth muscle of the urinary tract, resulting in the characteristic dilatation and dysmorphic features common to the

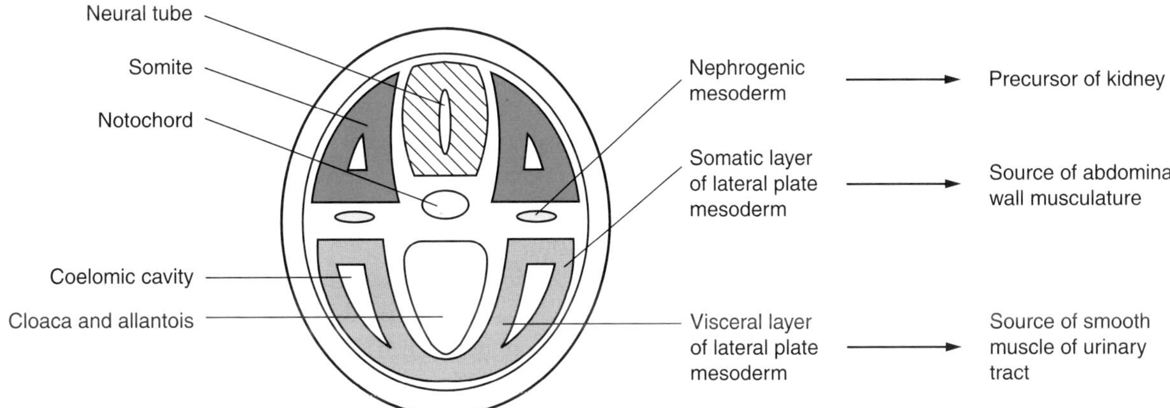

Figure 64.3 Cross section of a fetus at 6–10 weeks of gestation. An embryologic insult to both layers of the lateral plate mesoderm and the nephrogenic mesoderm could explain the majority of findings seen in the prune belly syndrome.

syndrome. The kidneys are concurrently differentiating from the para-axial mesoderm. A defect in induction by the ureteral bud or an abnormality in the metanephric blastema, with or without subsequent urinary tract obstruction, would account for the renal dysplasia commonly associated with prune belly syndrome.[12,56,80]

Some authors have suggested that this insult must occur early in the 3rd week of embryogenesis, at the primitive streak stage of development. At the division of the embryonic disk, an unequal distribution of mesoderm could explain the discordant occurrence in monozygotic twins.[7] This localized defect in mesodermal development would also explain the abnormalities seen in the prostate, urethra, and in testicular descent. According to this theory, the prostatic hypoplasia with poor glandular development, and abnormalities in the mesenchyme of the testicular gubernaculum, result in unresponsiveness of these tissues to hormonal stimulation.[56,81–83] This unresponsiveness of the gubernaculum to hormonal stimulation, the diminished intra-abdominal pressure, and potential mechanical obstruction by an enlarged bladder, all contribute to the maldescent of the testes in the prune belly syndrome.

The mesodermal arrest theory is further supported by histologic findings in the abdominal wall, the urinary tract, and the male genital tract. The abundance of fibrous tissue, collagen, and connective tissue, in association with sparse smooth muscle throughout the urinary tract, indicates an inherent problem with mesodermal differentiation. Bladder outlet obstruction, as seen in posterior urethral valves, results in hypertrophy and hyperplasia in the urinary tract, with normally developed seminal ducts, seminal vesicles, and prostate glands proximal to the obstruction. These features are noticeably absent in the prune belly syndrome.[5,55,65,80,81,84] The absence of anatomic obstruction in the majority of patients and the demonstration of urodynamically unobstructed urinary tracts support this theory. This theory also provides an adequate explanation for the high association with megalourethra.[5,63,85]

Nevertheless, the mesodermal arrest theory does not explain the male predominance of the syndrome. It also fails to explain the myriad associated anomalies and the presence of the abdominal wall abnormalities with a normal urinary tract. In addition, obstructive urethral lesions, whether anatomic or functional, are sometimes associated with the syndrome. The development of an animal model, created by urethral ligation, has been reported with all the features of the syndrome.[57,60,86]

The yolk sac theory

Stephens proposed an additional theory to explain the features of the prune belly syndrome. It is based on an error in embryogenesis of the yolk sac and allantois. Inherent in this theory is the contention that the bladder and prostatic urethra are derived, to a greater degree than customarily accepted, from the allantois. If an abnormally large amount of the yolk sac is retained inside the embryo, due to overgrowth of the lateral folds of the discoid embryo, it could affect the development of the abdominal wall, resulting in the prune belly phenotype. A critical aspect of this theory is the overdevelopment of the allantoic diverticulum. This structure grows out from the yolk sac contiguous with the body stalk. If it becomes excessively large due to the oversized intra-abdominal yolk sac, it would become incorporated into the urinary tract as the redundant enlarged urachus, bladder, and prostatic urethra which characterizes the syndrome.[66,80] Unfortunately, this theory does not explain the errors in development of the upper urinary tract or male genital tract.

Spectrum of disease

Prune belly syndrome represents a spectrum of disease severity. Classification systems based on this clinical spectrum have been formulated by numerous authors and all take into consideration initial and subsequent renal function.[31,54,87,88] The classifications have similar, clinically distinctive parameters to segregate the patients prognostically. The clinical classification of prune belly syndrome provides a framework for a more rational approach to overall management, which is determined on an individual basis.[12] Based on Woodard's classification, three major categories can be broadly defined (Table 64.2).

Category I patients exhibit the most severe form of the prune belly syndrome, with pulmonary hypoplasia and severe renal dysplasia. Most patients in this category do not survive beyond the first few days of life. The stillborn births are often associated with oligohydramnios and the classic features of Potter's syndrome are observed.[89,90] In this subset of patients with severe renal dysplasia, high urinary diversion, when performed, is generally to no avail.[6] Initial normal serum creatinine progressively rises in spite of urinary diversion. These patients may also have complete urethral obstruction or atresia, which is the 'lethal variant' of the syndrome unless associated with a patent urachus.[53]

Table 64.2 Spectrum of prune belly syndrome

Category classification	Distinguishing characteristics
I	Oligohydramnios, pulmonary hypoplasia or pneumothorax. May have urethral obstruction or patent urachus and clubfoot
II	Typical external features. Uropathy of the full-blown syndrome but no immediate problem with survival. May have mild or unilateral renal dysplasia. May or may not develop urosepsis or gradual azotemia
III	External features may be mild or incomplete. Uropathy less severe. Stable renal function

The next group, category II, includes those infants who do not have pulmonary hypoplasia but have significant involvement of the urinary tract. This can include mild to severe renal dysplasia with potential azotemia and failure to thrive. The clinical course is one of either stabilization of renal function or progressive azotemia. Surgical intervention to tailor the urinary tract, in order to provide unimpeded drainage and decrease stasis, has been successfully performed. The impact of surgical intervention on long-term renal function remains a source of continued controversy.[17,21,91]

Category III patients with prune belly syndrome are associated with the external abdominal features and undescended testes but neither pulmonary nor renal function is severely impaired. They constitute the majority of patients with prune belly syndrome.[30,88] Although these infants may have severe dilatation of the urinary tract, they have stable renal function and usually do not require reconstructive urologic surgery.[31]

Clinical features

Genitourinary manifestations

Kidneys

Renal dysplasia and hydronephrosis are the common characteristics of the upper urinary tract in prune belly syndrome. Both grossly and radiographically, cystic dilatation of the calices and renal pelvis is present. Infundibular narrowing without obstruction and occasional ureteropelvic junction obstruction may be evident.[21] Wide variations may exist in individual renal unit appearance, function, location, and rotation (Figure 64.4).[56]

Prognosis is directly related to renal function and the degree of renal dysplasia. Stephens proposed pathogenic mechanisms to explain the development of renal dysplasia. These include (1) defects of the ureteric bud or its branches, (2) qualitative or quantitative deficiencies of the nephrogenic mesenchyme, and (3) vascular ischemic insults with resultant ureteric obstruction and renal cystic dysplasia. He suggested that the renal dysplasia of the prune belly syndrome is due to a combination of a ureteric bud and metanephric defect.[66]

The most severe degree of renal dysplasia is recognized from autopsy studies and associated with both Potter's type II and IV renal cystic changes.[56,78] These patients have associated distal outlet obstruction (urethral atresia) with a non-patent urachus, and they are usually stillborn. The kidneys are small, with disorganized histologic features consistent with dysplasia, and are most likely injured at the stage of ampullary development prior to significant nephron formation.[54]

In contrast, some patients have hydronephrosis but adequate renal function (Figure 64.5). The degree of hydronephrosis may not correlate with the ureteral dilatation or the abdominal wall deficiency. The renal parenchyma is often well preserved despite a grossly abnormal drainage system. Urinary infection rather than obstruction represents the greatest threat to the renal parenchyma. The dilatation is attributed to the mesenchymal defect and deficient smooth muscle, not to obstruction. Consequently, some resolution in the degree of dilatation can occur spontaneously in follow-up.

Ureters

The ureters are elongated, tortuous, and dilated, representing the radiographic hallmark of the syndrome (Figure 64.6).[92] The lower one-third of the ureter is more profoundly affected than the proximal portion and occupies the flared-out flanks of the abdomen. Although fluoroscopic studies demonstrate ineffective peristalsis over its entire length, true obstructive lesions of the ureter are the exception. However, pleat-like valves at the ureterovesical junction (UVJ) have been documented in two cases.[93]

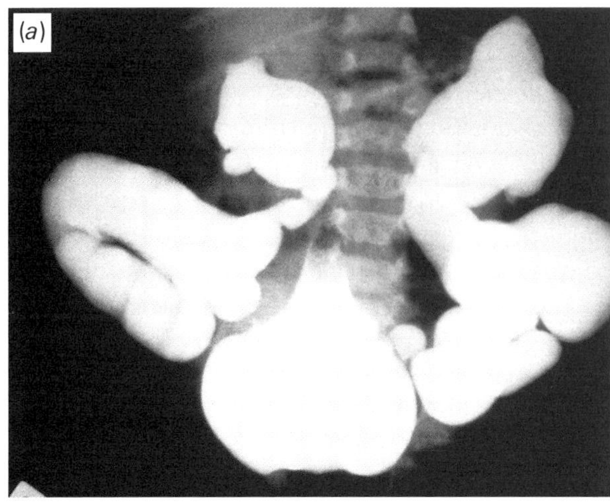

Figure 64.4 (*a*) Retrograde cystogram demonstrates the dilated, tortuous, refluxing ureters; enlarged, floppy, renal pelvis; and distended bladder, with urachal remnant. (*b*) Retrograde cystogram demonstrates vesicoureteral reflux into a dilated, dysmorphic ureter. Renal pelvis indicative of pseudoureteropelvic junction obstruction. (*c*) Same patient as (*b*) with entire left ureter and renal pelvis visualization.

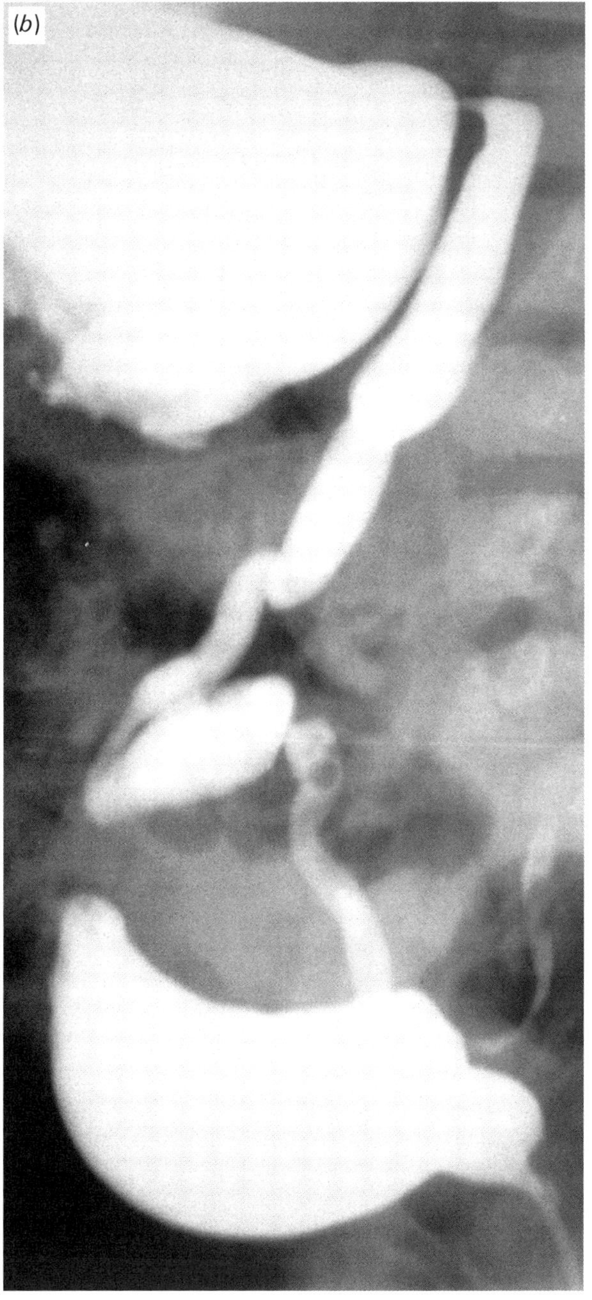

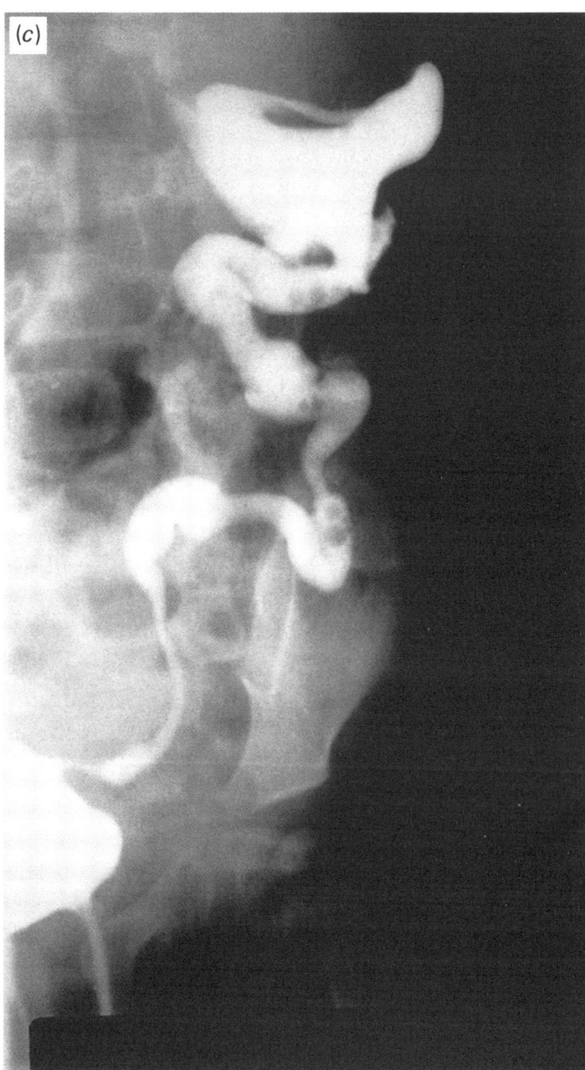

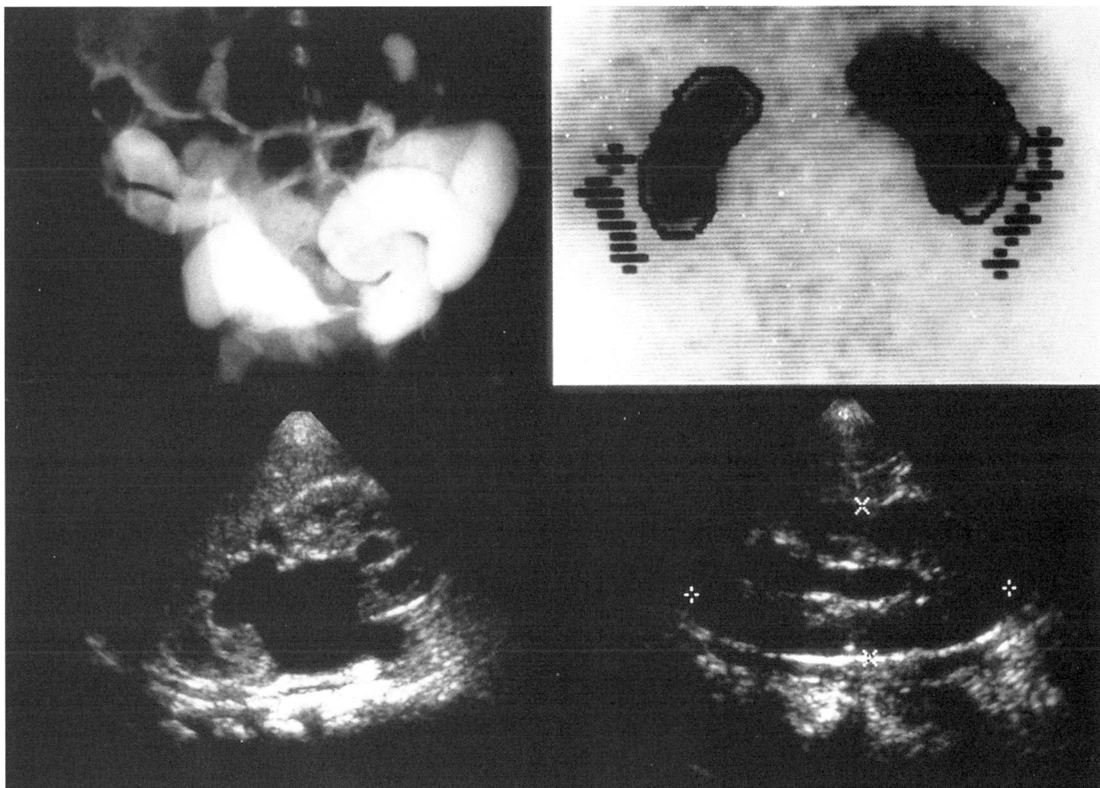

Figure 64.5 Intravenous pyelogram, DMSA renal scan, and renal sonogram of a 1-year-old child with prune belly syndrome. Despite gross dilatation and dysmorphic features of the renal pelvis and ureters, the renal scan and renal function were remarkably normal. The renal sonogram demonstrates evidence of hydronephrosis with preserved renal parenchyma.

Vesicoureteral reflux is seen in up to 85% of patients. The conventional system of grading reflux is difficult to apply, due to the dysmorphic features of the ureter, renal pelvis, and calices.[29]

Histologic examination of the ureter demonstrates a profound alteration in the content and architecture of the ureteral wall. The hypertrophy and hyperplasia of the smooth muscle cells seen in dilated ureters due to obstruction or vesicoureteral reflux are absent in the prune belly syndrome. A diffuse increase in the connective tissue with replacement of the smooth muscle is present. The ratio of collagen to smooth muscle, especially in refluxing ureters, is markedly elevated.[94] There is no differentiation into longitudinal and circular muscle layers. The patchy distribution of smooth muscle is present in both the dilated and narrowed ureteral segments. The upper ureter has more smooth muscle cells than the lower portion.[5,79] A marked decrease in the number of nerve plexuses, with degeneration of non-myelinated Schwann fibers, has been reported. This may contribute to the poor ureteral peristalsis even after corrective surgery.[95] Ultrastructural examination of the smooth muscle cells of the ureter reveals a decrease in the number of thick and thin myofilaments, which contributes to poor muscle cell performance.[79,96] The histologic and pathologic features are important to remember during genitourinary reconstructive efforts. Because the upper ureter is potentially the best, its future should not be risked by using it for temporary cutaneous diversion. The dilatation and ineffective peristalsis of the ureters result in urinary stasis and a heightened risk of infection.

Bladder

The bladder is thick walled and grossly enlarged, but trabeculations are usually absent (Figure 64.7). The normal bladder contour is deviated by a pseudodiverticulum, consisting of the urachal remnant and giving the bladder an hourglass configuration. A patent urachus may be present, especially in association with

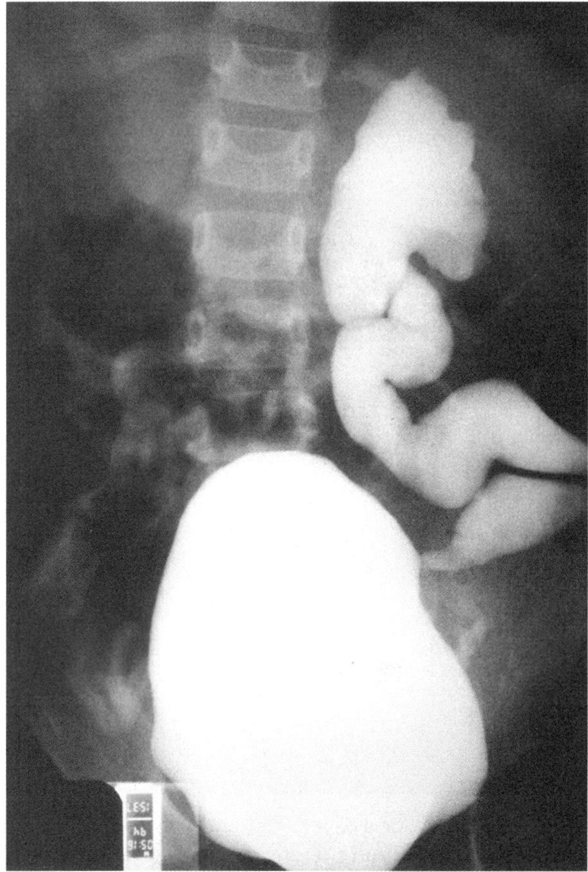

Figure 64.6 Voiding cystourethrogram of a 1-year-old child with prune belly syndrome exhibiting the classic elongated, tortuous, and dilated ureter representing one of the radiographic hallmarks of the syndrome. The large, distended bladder is thick walled. (Courtesy of George W Kaplan MD.)

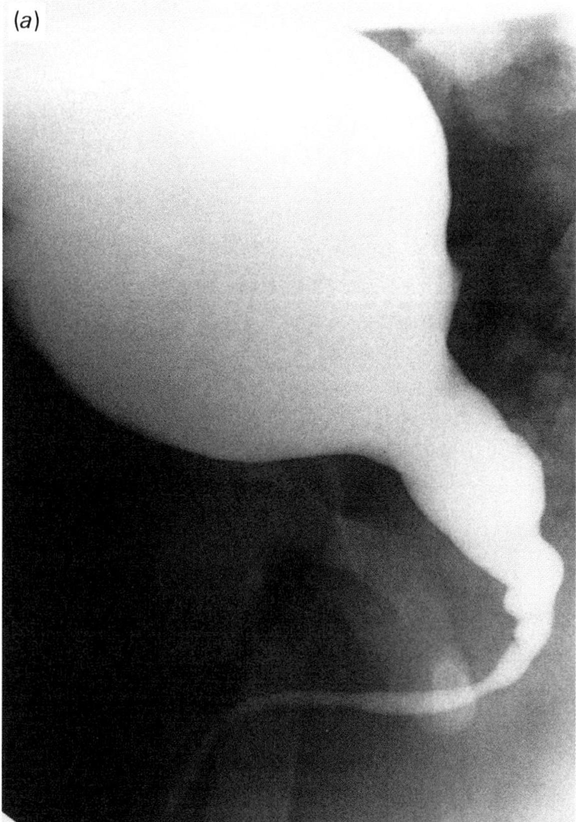

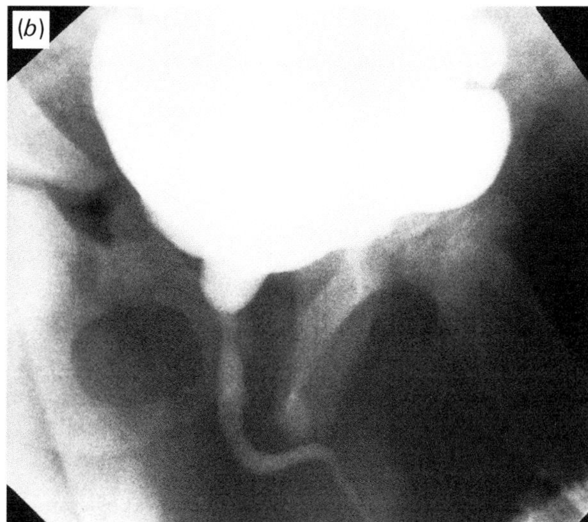

Figure 64.7 (*a* and *b*) The voiding cystourethrograms detail the grossly enlarged, but non-trabeculated bladder. The bladder neck is widely patent, with dilatation of the posterior urethra. No valves or stenosis is present.

urethral atresia or microurethra. The trigone is splayed and the ureteric orifices are located laterally, which explains the common association with vesicoureteral reflux.[66] The bladder neck is characteristically quite wide at its junction with the prostatic urethra.

Histologic evaluation of the bladder demonstrates an alteration in the ratio of connective tissue to smooth muscle. The extent of involvement is less than the ureter, and smooth muscle hypertrophy can be present.[56,97] The increased bladder thickness is largely due to fibrocytes and collagen. The anatomic innervation of the bladder is normal. No abnormality in the distribution of ganglion cells is present.[5,24]

The bladder in prune belly syndrome has efficient low-pressure storage and good compliance. However, its ability to empty is compromised by vesicoureteral reflux and poor contractility.

Urodynamic assessment of the bladder has demonstrated normal balanced voiding in some patients regardless of the gross anatomic and radiologic features.[5] Three distinct patterns of voiding have been observed: normal, prolonged voiding with a low peak, and an intermittent pattern. The voiding pattern did not correlate with residual urine volume.[98]

Maximum urinary flow rates and voiding pressures can be within normal limits for age. The filling phase of the cystometrogram is shifted to the right, with a markedly delayed first sensation to void. Bladder instability with uninhibited contractions is infrequent and usually not the explanation for urinary incontinence.[23,85,98] In those patients with unbalanced voiding manifested by urinary incontinence, an increase in residual urine with a decreased flow rate may be noted. Changes in voiding efficiency are not unusual and mandate the need for regular urodynamic assessment. Surgical intervention or intermittent self-catheterization may be necessary.

Prostate and posterior urethra

The radiographic appearance of the prostatic urethra is quite distinctive. The bladder neck is open and the posterior urethra is dilated, elongated, and tapered at the membranous urethra (Figures 64.7 and 64.8). The anterior wall of the prostate is shorter than the posterior wall. It frequently has a localized sacculation, which represents a utricular diverticulum. Reflux into the vas deferens may be present and the verumontanum is small or absent. True obstructive lesions at the junction of the prostate and membranous urethra have been described in 20% of infants, usually those with the worst prognosis. These obstructions have been described as stenosis, true valves, atresia, diaphragms, and diverticula.[52,54,56,99] A kinking of the prostatic urethra during voiding, as a result of asymmetry of its anterior and posterior walls, has been suggested as a functional obstruction in prune belly syndrome. Stephens assigned a type IV valve classification to these lesions.[57,66]

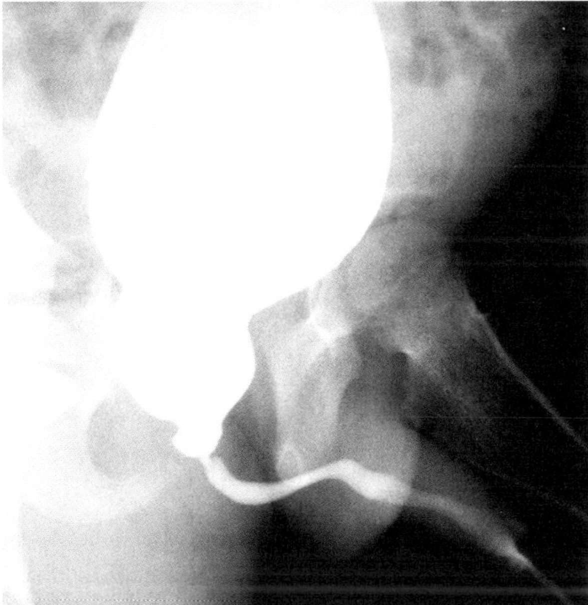

Figure 64.8 Voiding cystourethrogram of a 1-year-old child demonstrating the classic radiographic appearance of the posterior urethra in prune belly syndrome. The open bladder neck and dilated prostatic/posterior urethra is evident. No urethral obstruction is present. (Courtesy of George W Kaplan MD.)

Lack of development of the epithelial portion of the prostate is a constant component of the syndrome. When compared with normal children and children with posterior urethral valves, patients with prune belly syndrome have either absent or sparsely distributed prostatic epithelial glands.[5,80,81] The prostatic hypoplasia results from an inability of the urogenital mesenchyme to induce epithelial differentiation.[81] Prostatic hypoplasia is one of the etiologies of infertility in this syndrome.[100]

Accessory male sexual organs

As with the other mesenchyme-derived genitourinary organs in the prune belly syndrome, abnormalities of the epididymis, seminal vesicles, and vas deferens have been noted. Autopsy findings have noted lack of continuity between the ductuli efferentes and rete testis. The body of the epididymis is frequently detached from the testis, a common finding with abdominal undescended testes. The vas deferens is abnormally thickened and may drain ectopically.[101] The seminal vesicles may be dilated with diverticular formation but usually are atretic or absent, which may be a diagnostic feature of prune belly syndrome.[80] All of these findings have significance in regards to the known infertility associated with prune belly syndrome.[66]

Anterior urethra

The recognized abnormalities of the anterior urethra in prune belly syndrome range from urethral atresia to fusiform megalourethra (Figure 64.9). Surviving patients with urethral atresia or microurethra have a patent urachus. It has been suggested that the microurethra is normally formed but unused and can be progressively dilated to a functional caliber.[102]

Bulbous urethral dilatation was evident in 68% of patients with prune belly syndrome.[63] Two of these patients had a fusiform megalourethra. Comparative measurements of anterior urethral diameters in patients with prune belly syndrome with normal patients have confirmed a dilated anterior urethra in prune belly syndrome patients (Figure 64.10).[103] A

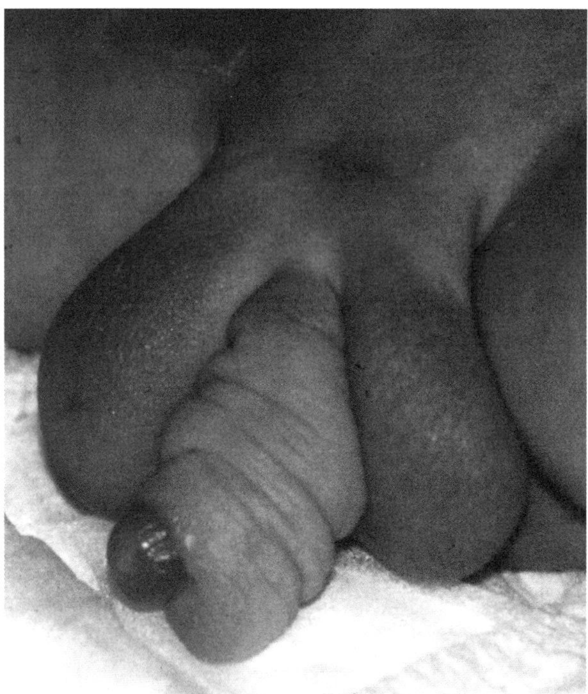

Figure 64.9 A newborn with prune belly syndrome with evidence of megalourethra and penoscrotal transposition. (Courtesy of George W Kaplan MD.)

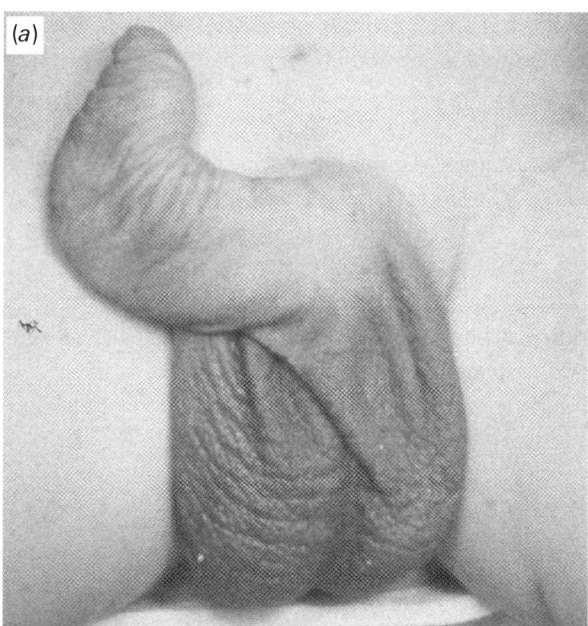

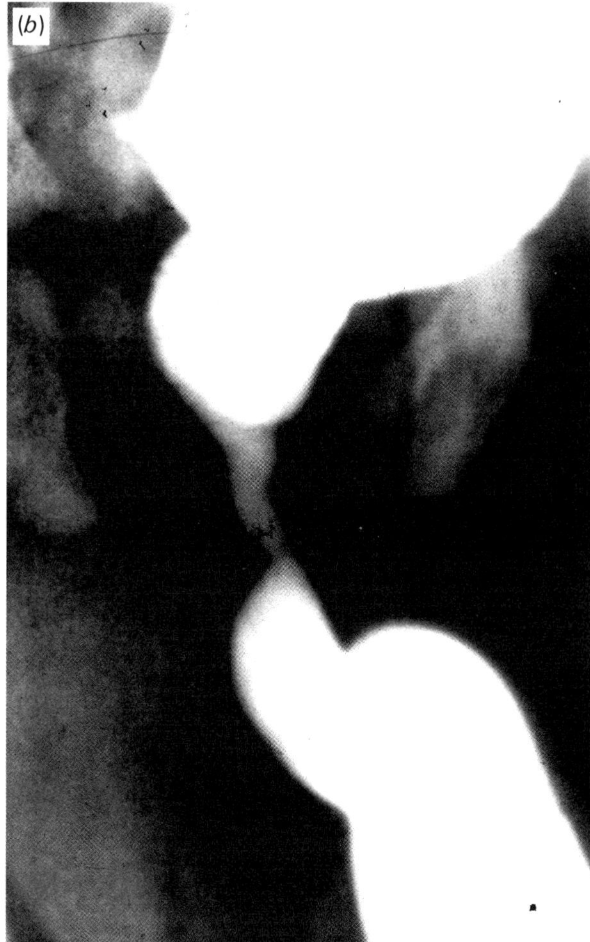

Figure 64.10 (*a*) A newborn with prune belly syndrome and megalourethra. (*b*) The voiding cystourethrogram in this patient demonstrates a large dilated bladder, open bladder neck, dilated posterior urethra, and wide, patent megalourethra. (Courtesy of George W Kaplan MD.)

transient obstruction during fetal development at the junction of the glandular and penile urethra may explain this common radiographic finding, as well as the known association of prune belly syndrome with megalourethra.[62]

Both types of megalourethra – scaphoid and fusiform – are associated with prune belly syndrome. The fusiform megalourethra, accompanied by deficient corpora cavernosa, is a more severe defect frequently associated with renal dysplasia and lethal anomalies. Scaphoid megalourethra is characterized as a deficiency of the corpus spongiosum with normal glans and fossa navicularis. In a series of 26 patients with this anomaly, 10 had prune belly syndrome.[104] It has been suggested that the mesenchymal developmental arrest that accounts for the major features of the syndrome could also explain the urethral malformations.[63]

Testis

Bilateral cryptorchidism is an essential component of the prune belly syndrome. In the majority of patients the testes are intra-abdominal, overlying the ectatic ureters at the pelvic inlet. The epididymal abnormalities associated with abdominal undescended testis are present.[1] The intra-abdominal position of the testes predisposes these patients to increased risk of malignant degeneration of 30–50 times that of a normally descended testes.[105] At least three documented cases of testis tumor in prune belly syndrome have been reported, one of which was retroperitoneal.[3,106,107] The gubernaculum is normally attached proximally to the tail of the epididymis, travels via the inguinal canal, and attaches distally at the pubic tubercle.[66] No histologic abnormality has been noted, and the nerve supply of the gubernaculum is intact.[108]

Comparative, quantitative analysis of spermatogonia in fetuses with prune belly syndrome has demonstrated a significantly decreased number of spermatogonia and marked Leydig cell hyperplasia. These changes are evident before expected testicular descent, implying intrinsically abnormal testes.[109] Absent spermatogenesis due to prolonged intra-abdominal location has been histologically documented.[110] Azoospermia was present in adults when a semen sample was obtained.[111] Early orchidopexy is advocated for these patients to optimize potential spermatogenesis, to improve evaluation for possible malignancy, and to promote better psychological health.[29,112] With assisted reproductive techniques, specifically intracytoplasmic sperm injection (ICSI), paternity in prune belly patients is possible.[113]

The etiology of testicular maldescent in prune belly syndrome is multifactorial. Mechanical obstruction by the enlarged bladder is contributory, as the incidence of cryptorchidism is increased in other diseases associated with an enlarged bladder, such as posterior urethral valves.[114] The mechanical effects of the intramuscular pressure of the abdominal muscles pushing the testis toward the scrotum are obviously deficient in the prune belly syndrome. In addition, given the mesenchymal abnormalities of the syndrome, the ability of the gubernaculum to respond hormonally to guide the testes to the scrotum may be impaired.[82]

Sexual function and fertility

Woodhouse and Snyder studied sexual function in nine adult patients with prune belly syndrome. All had normal libido, with normal erections and orgasms. Seven had retrograde ejaculation. All patients studied to date have been azoospermic.[28,111] These patients all had orchidopexy performed late in childhood. Earlier orchidopexy may improve spermatogenesis, as germ cells have been demonstrated in these patients.[112]

There is no report of a patient with prune belly syndrome becoming a father naturally. However, the first reported case of paternity in a prune belly patient involved the use of ICSI and produced twins.[113] Patients with prune belly syndrome have multiple factors, other than spermatogenesis, that contribute to infertility. An open bladder neck and poorly developed prostate result in retrograde ejaculation. Associated abnormalities of the prostatic epithelium and seminal vesicles affect the amount and content of the seminal fluid. Vas deferens obstruction and epididymal abnormalities associated with maldescent affect sperm delivery and maturation.

Extragenitourinary manifestations

Abdominal wall

The wrinkled, floppy abdominal wall that characterizes the syndrome results from a deficiency of the underlying musculature. The functionally impaired abdominal wall can result in significant morbidity. These infants are unable to sit up directly from the supine position, and this delays the onset of walking.[3] The lack of mechanical assistance from the abdominal wall contributes to the noted difficulties with respiratory infections and to chronic constipation.[115] In addition, the long-term psychosocial effects of poor body image have been addressed.[30,31]

Autopsy studies have shown that the muscles most severely affected are those ventrally and laterally located. The epaxial and hypaxial trunk muscles develop normally. The order of severity of involvement from most to least involved is: transversus abdominis, rectus abdominus below the umbilicus, internal oblique, external oblique, and rectus abdominis above the umbilicus (Figure 64.11).[2,18] There is cephalic displacement of the umbilicus due to unopposed contraction of the upper rectus abdominis muscle. The diminished muscle mass, if severe, allows one to observe spontaneous contraction of the underlying bowel and easily palpate the abdominal organs and kidneys. Because the muscular deficiency may not be symmetric, a more dominant flank bulge on one side of the abdomen is often present and coincides with the dilated distal ureter (Figure 64.12).

Electromyographic studies of the abdominal wall have confirmed the anatomic findings. The lower midline musculature demonstrates the least amount of electrical activity. Recruitment of voluntary motor units is greatest in the upper lateral musculature.[116]

Autopsy studies of the abdominal wall have demonstrated normal segmental nerve distribution and normal blood supply.[56,66] The distribution of muscle fibers is haphazard. In more severe cases, the

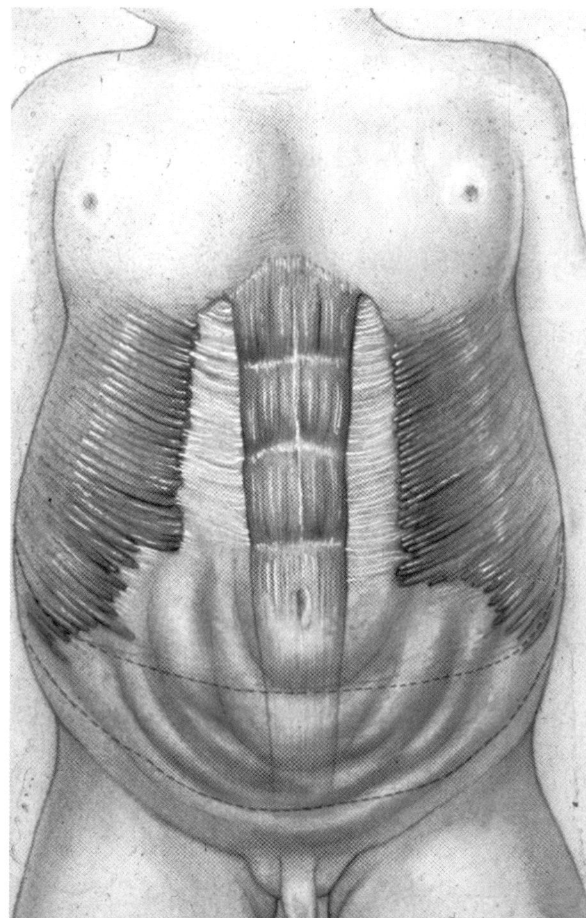

Figure 64.11 The abdominal wall deficiencies in prune belly syndrome. The epaxial and hypaxial trunk muscles develop normally. The order of severity of involvement from most to least involved is: transversus abdominis, rectus abdominis below the umbilicus, internal oblique, external oblique, and rectus abdominis above the umbilicus. (Reproduced from Randolph,[116] with permission.)

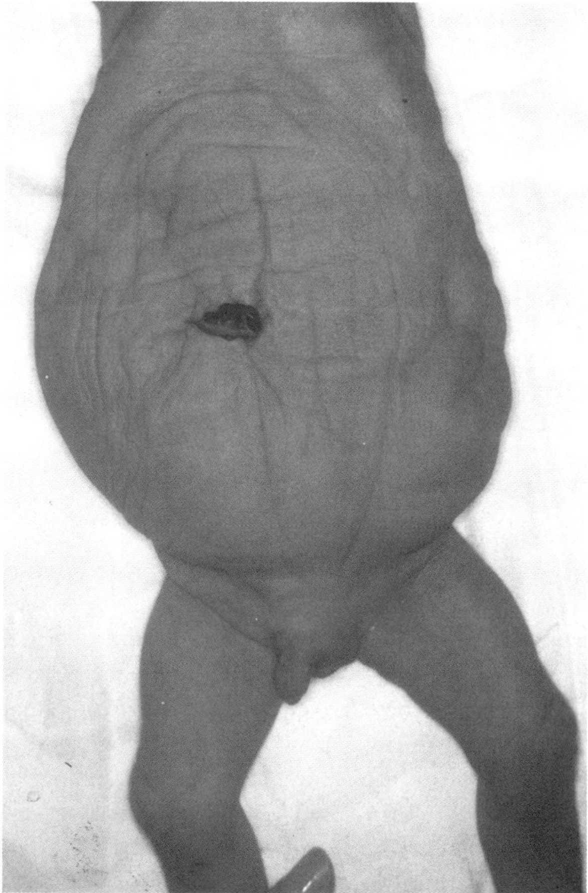

Figure 64.12 A newborn with prune belly syndrome. The classic abdominal deficiency exists, with a dilated, tortuous, and easily palpable left ureter exhibited along the left flank. (Courtesy of George W Kaplan MD.)

entire thickness of the abdominal wall consists of skin, connective tissue, superficial fascia, and peritoneum (Figure 64.13). In the infant there is no aponeurotic layer that might represent atrophied muscle.[23] Fortunately, the poorly developed abdominal wall heals well after incision despite the muscular layer deficiencies.

Microscopic examination demonstrates fatty infiltration interdigitated with muscle fibers. These fibers have been characterized as hypoplastic, atrophic, and hypertrophic, which adds further confusion to an apparent etiology.[65,117] Others have found the muscle cells to be clear and normal in appearance and at times associated with myotubular embryonic cells similar to that seen in the fetus of about 10 weeks' gestation.[64,66] Ultrastructural abnormalities demonstrated by electron microscopy include loss of coherence and orientation of the Z-bands, mitochondrial disruption, and clumping of glycogen granules. These changes are non-specific, but are consistent with hypoplastic histologic changes.[65]

Associated anomalies

Abnormalities of other organ systems result in long-term morbidity for as many as 75% of patients with prune belly syndrome (Table 64.3).[115] Growth was impaired in 32% of surviving patients in one large series and was poorly correlated with renal function. This impairment was most manifest in the first year of life, with subsequent stabilization but incomplete catch-up growth.[115] Developmental delay has also been documented in selected patients.

The non-urologic associated anomalies in patients with prune belly syndrome are a major source of morbidity and mortality. Care of these patients requires close cooperation with all caregivers. The urologic

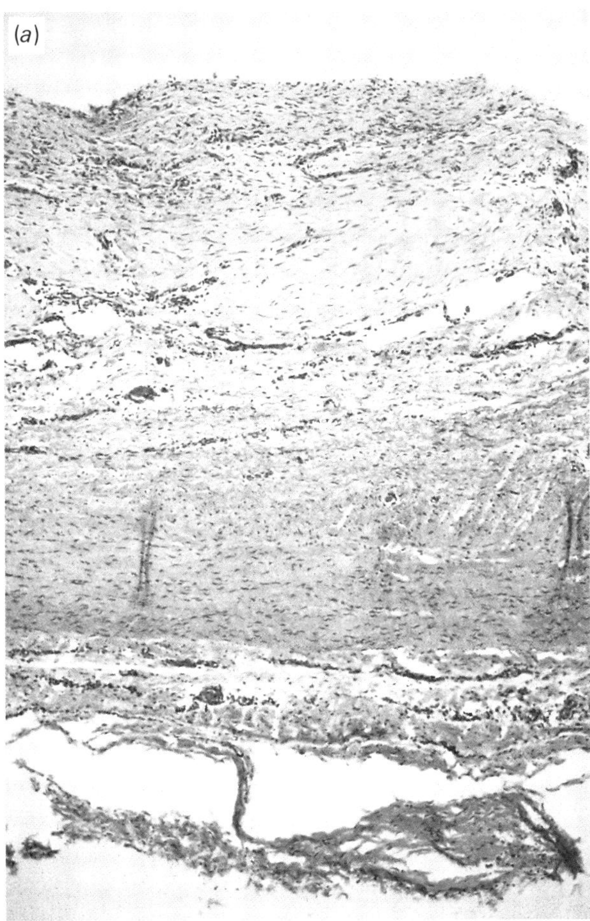

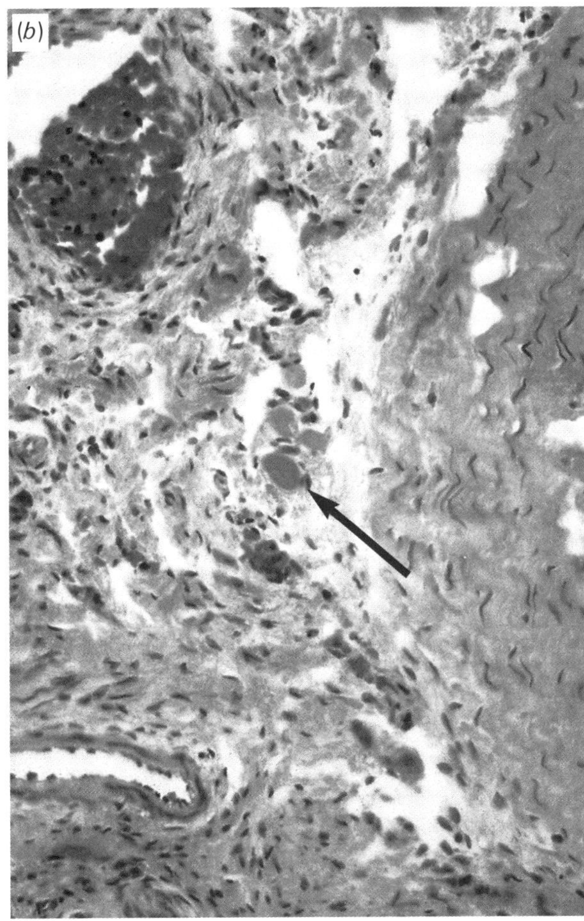

Figure 64.13 (*a*) A cross section of the abdominal wall of an infant with prune belly syndrome. Note the scant and haphazard arrangement of muscle fibers. (*b*) A high-power view of abdominal wall composed largely of collagen and fibrous tissue. The arrow points to scant skeletal muscle fibers.

manifestations of prune belly syndrome rarely require emergent treatment.

Orthopedic

Orthopedic-related problems in prune belly syndrome are present in 45–63% of cases.[118] In most series, musculoskeletal anomalies predominate, with congenital dislocation of the hips the most frequent finding. This requires early treatment and may be resistant to conventional therapy.[118] Lateral dimples of the elbows and knees are the mildest manifestation of the compression effect of intrauterine oligohydramnios (Figure 64.14). More severe deformities, attributed to oligohydramnios and intrauterine compression, are recognized usually at autopsy as lower limb deficiencies and arthrogryposis.[4,119] Talipes equinovarus, polydactyly, syndactyly, and torticollis have been reported.[24,56] Pectus carinatum and pectus excavatum deformities are frequently present. Scoliosis is the most common spinal deformity. In one instance, scoliosis was associated with thoracic segmental insensibility.[120] As prognosis improves in these patients, orthopedic interventions will play a greater role in management.

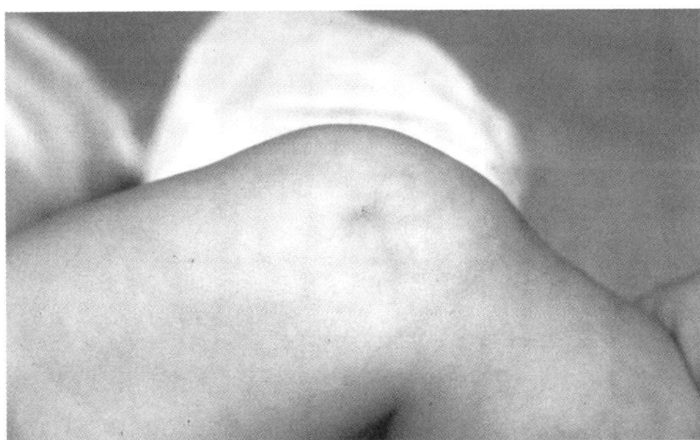

Figure 64.14 Lateral dimple of the knee in this infant with prune belly syndrome is a mild manifestation of the compression effect of intrauterine oligohydramnios.

Table 64.3 Extragenitourinary abnormalities in prune belly syndrome

Organ system	Frequency (%)	Manifestations
Pulmonary	55	Pulmonary hypoplasia Pneumothorax Pneumomediastinum Lobar atelectasis Pneumonia Chronic bronchitis
Orthopedic	45–63	Congenital dislocation of hips Chest wall deformity: Pectus excavatum Pectus carinatum Scoliosis Genu valgum Talipes equinovarus Severe leg maldevelopment: Arthrogryposis
Gastro-intestinal	30	Malrotation Intestinal atresia Intestinal stenosis Volvulus Anorectal agenesis Imperforate anus Omphalocele Gastroschisis Hepatobiliary anomalies Acquired megacolon
Cardiac	10	Patent ductus arteriosus Atrial septal defect Ventricular septal defect Tetrology of Fallot

Gastrointestinal

Gastrointestinal anomalies are present in over 30% of autopsied patients with prune belly syndrome. These anomalies are commonly recognized in the postnatal period. The majority of anomalies such as malrotation, atresia, stenosis, and volvulus are due to persistence of the embryonic wide mesentery, with absent fixation to the posterior abdominal wall.[121] This same suspension abnormality allows the spleen to wander freely in the abdominal cavity and acute splenic torsion has been reported on two occasions.[122] It has been recommended that all patients with prune belly syndrome have radiographic assessment of their alimentary tract.[121] Anorectal agenesis, imperforate anus, omphalocele, and gastroschisis have been reported in association with prune belly syndrome.[121,123–125] Chronic constipation is a frequent problem with these children, and is attributed to a decrease in abdominal wall pressure aiding evacuation. Acquired megacolon can result. Chronic constipation requires continuous attention with dietary and cathartic intervention.[12,115]

Cardiac

Cardiac anomalies have been reported in up to 10% of patients with prune belly syndrome. Patent ductus arteriosus, atrial and ventricular septal defects, and tetralogy of Fallot occur with increased frequency in prune belly syndrome.[126,127] The severity of the cardiac involvement will dictate initial care of the infant, as the urologic anomalies rarely demand immediate treatment.

Pulmonary

Pulmonary and respiratory difficulties pervade the lives of these patients from birth to adulthood. Severe pulmonary hypoplasia, with associated oligohydramnios and renal dysplasia, is incompatible with life. Initial prognosis depends upon pulmonary development. A review of most series demonstrates that approximately 20% of newborns will die in the perinatal period as a consequence of pulmonary complications.[21,28,29] Of those that survive the newborn period, clinically significant pulmonary problems were noted in 55% of patients.[115] Pneumothorax and pneumomediastinum may be present at birth, with or without pulmonary hypoplasia, and an early chest X-ray is advised. Chest wall deformities and abdominal muscle deficiency impair mechanical ventilation, which results in a ventilatory limitation and a high incidence of lobar atelectasis and pneumonia.[128,129] Chronic bronchitis and the development of respiratory insufficiency following upper respiratory infections or anesthetics are well recognized, and appropriate pulmonary support must be provided.[115,128]

Patient evaluation

Prenatal

Prenatal diagnosis of prune belly syndrome has been made as early as 11 weeks of gestation on ultrasound.[130] With improved ultrasonic capability and surveillance protocols, the ability to diagnose major genitourinary abnormalities in the early gestational period is increased.[131] However, definite distinction from other causes of hydronephrosis, such as posterior urethral valves, can be difficult. Previous ultrasonic diagnostic accuracy varies from 30 to 85%.[132]

The development of vesicoamniotic shunt procedures makes possible in-utero treatment of patients with obstructive uropathy.[133–135] Specific criteria for in-utero intervention include normal karyotype, severe oligohydramnios, and predicted good renal function.[133,136] The timing for intervention is critical, as renal dysplasia is more pronounced with increasing gestational age. Although several reports of vesicoamniotic shunt procedures for fetal obstructive uropathy exist, reviews have failed to document a beneficial effect of fetal intervention on subsequent renal function or pulmonary development.[132,137]

Hence, prenatal intervention to relieve potential obstruction in a fetus is difficult to justify. As the majority of patients with prune belly syndrome have no demonstrable evidence of obstruction, and renal function does not correlate with the amount of dilatation present in the urinary tract, the risks and benefits of in-utero intervention must be carefully weighed.[138–140]

Newborn

The appearance of the abdominal wall leaves little doubt as to the diagnosis in the newborn. Given the wide range of disease severity, a multisystem evaluation to rule out significant cardiac, pulmonary, or other associated malformations must take place in the neonatal period.[141] An immediate chest X-ray is necessary to exclude associated pneumothorax and pneumomediastinum. The presence of severe pulmonary hypoplasia with progressive inability to oxygenate the infant immediately affects prognosis. This is usually associated with the antenatal demonstration of oligohydramnios, which indicates impaired renal function.[90]

Initial creatinine measurements reflect maternal renal function and repetitive sampling is necessary. If after 48–72 hours the serum creatinine is >1.0 mg/dl in the term infant or 1.5 mg/dl in the preterm infant, a degree of renal insufficiency is present. A progressive rise in serum creatinine over the first few weeks of life portends a poor prognosis. If initial nadir creatinine is <0.7 mg/dl, then subsequent renal failure is unlikely.[142] Urine is sent for baseline culture and antibiotic prophylaxis is initiated. Measurement of serum and urinary electrolytes at birth can be helpful in assessing sodium conservation, implying adequate renal function.[143] In the premature and full-term infant, the glomerular filtration rate (GFR) is initially low, then rapidly increases.[144] This must be remembered in relation to the administration of intravenous contrast agents, which may rapidly elevate plasma osmolality, causing intraventricular hemorrhage as well as further impairment of renal function.[145]

Diagnostic evaluation

A thorough urologic evaluation proceeds after stabilization of the patient's comorbidities. Physical examination and ultrasonography of the urinary tract are initially required. Renal sonograms provide information on cortical thickness, presence of cystic changes, and renal size. Sonographic examinations before and after voiding give a clue to the presence of vesicoureteral reflux and postvoid residual urine. Serial serum electrolyte determinations, urinalysis, and urine culture are essential.

Radiologic assessment in the newborn is tempered by the known risks of intravenous contrast and the introduction of infection with retrograde studies. Initially, a VCUG is performed in those infants with abnormal renal function to insure that a true anatomic, urethral obstruction is not present. This 'lethal variant' and the potential confusion with posterior urethral valves 'masquerading' as prune belly syndrome must be differentiated, as treatment changes dramatically.[53,146,147] In addition, the VCUG demonstrates vesicoureteral reflux in up to 85% of patients and assesses bladder emptying. All infants are treated with antibiotics prior to VCUG to decrease the risk of infection. In general, the radiologic assessment of the urinary tract is tailored by the management philosophy of the individual urologic surgeon. Contrast studies requiring risky instrumentation are avoided in those infants with good renal function.

After initial evaluation, a technetium 99m (^{99m}Tc) diethylene triaminepenta-acetic acid (DTPA) renal scan and a mercaptoacetyltriglycine (MAG3) renal scan can provide both functional and anatomic information. Blood flow, differential renal function, and drainage in response to furosemide (Lasix) can be assessed and compared with subsequent studies (Figure 64.15). The limitations of diuresis renography in demonstrating obstruction in patients with prune belly syndrome have been noted. A Whitaker test is occasionally necessary as the definitive study to

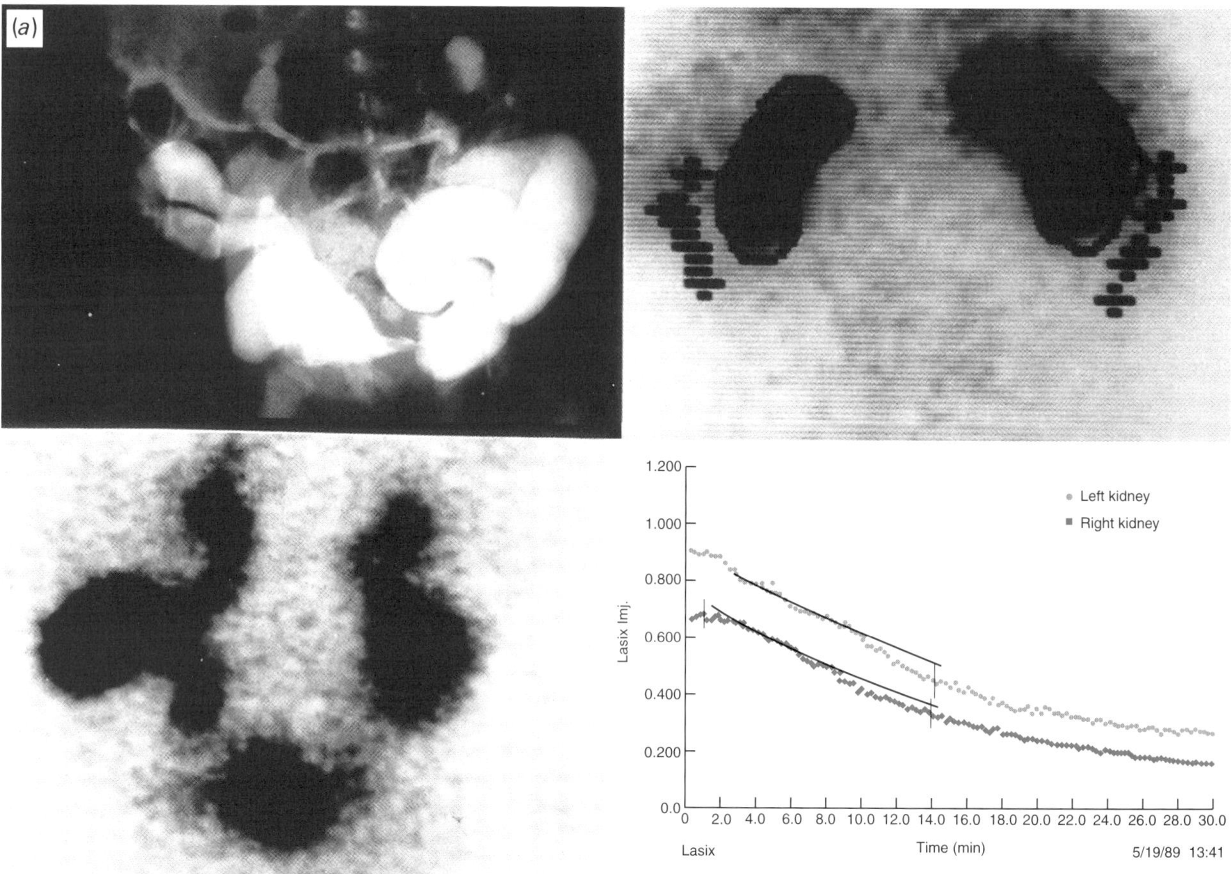

Figure 64.15 (*a*) Intravenous pyelogram and Lasix (furosemide) renal scan in a child with prune belly syndrome (top). Note the anatomic definition of the renal scan (bottom) and adequate drainage of the upper collecting system (graph). Renal function was normal.

demonstrate significant obstruction.[92] A dimercapto-succinic (DMSA) acid renal scan is performed rather than an intravenous pyelogram (IVP) to evaluate renal size, tubular mass, and differential function. Longitudinal studies are invaluable to assess renal growth and scarring, as these patients require long-term follow-up.[148]

Patient management

The overall goals of initial management are to preserve renal function and prevent infection. The attainment of these goals is possible via a variety of therapeutic approaches, which range from watchful waiting to immediate surgical reconstruction of the urinary tract.[17,22,27]

Early surgical intervention in the neonate is avoided, unless a rising creatinine or infection intervenes, requiring early vesicostomy. Unless salvaged by extraordinary means (extracorporeal membrane oxygenation with or without dialysis), patients with category I disease associated with prenatal oligohydramnios and postnatal pulmonary hypoplasia usually die in the immediate postnatal period due to pulmonary complications. In those few infants surviving the pulmonary insult, high urinary diversion by cutaneous pyelostomy has been attempted to provide optimal urinary drainage.[91] Unfortunately, recovery of renal function is not usually possible as a result of severe underlying renal dysplasia.

Patients with category II involvement are serially monitored for infection and a decrease in renal function. These infants and children are placed on long-term prophylactic antibiotics. With documentation of infection, failure of adequate renal growth, or decreasing renal function, aggressive reconstruction of the urinary tract is pursued. To allow pulmonary maturation, surgical reconstruction is usually delayed until the infant is 3 months of age or more. Our approach involves a surgical remodeling to eliminate urinary stasis and vesicoureteral reflux, and promote optimal

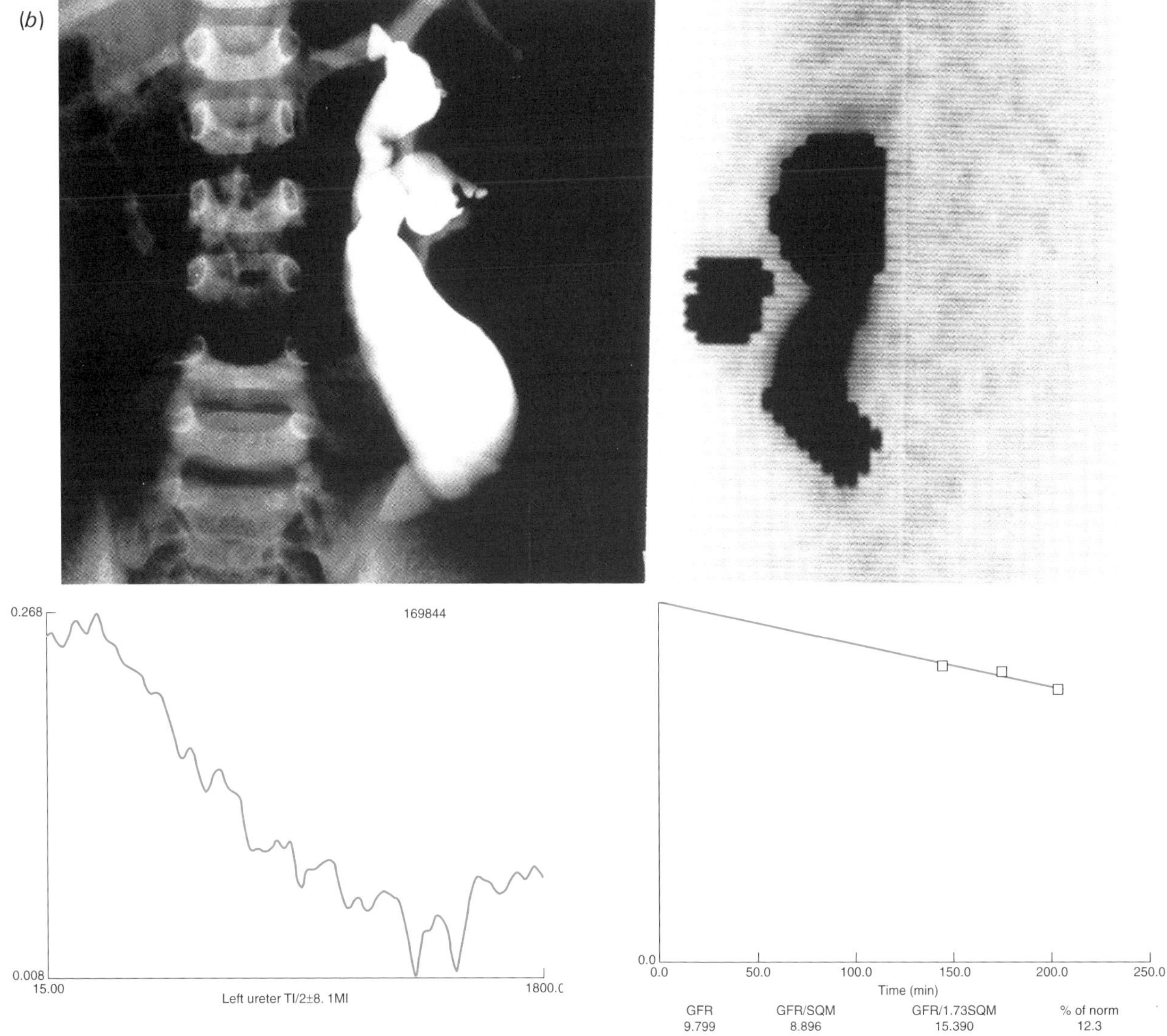

Figure 64.15 (*b*) Cystogram and Lasix renal scan with glomerular filtration rate (GFR) in a patient with poor renal function. The scan demonstrates adequate drainage, but a solitary kidney functions poorly (GFR = 15.3 ml/min/ 1.73 m^2).

urinary drainage (Figures 64.16 and 64.17).[22] If renal insufficiency is severe or infection is initially present, a period of urinary diversion by means of cutaneous vesicostomy is recommended.[149] Cutaneous ureterostomies probably add little to improve drainage. In addition, the upper ureter is anatomically and histologically the most normal and should be preserved if later tailored reconstruction is elected.[79,96] Combining urinary tract reconstruction, orchidopexy, and abdominoplasty at or prior to 1 year of age is our preferred approach. This optimizes the potential for improved urinary drainage, as well as addressing the issues of subsequent fertility and psychological well-being.[29]

Patients with category III prune belly syndrome demonstrate good renal function, despite gross dilatation of the upper and lower urinary tract and constitute the majority of patients. Serial assessment of renal function by selective imaging techniques is performed. Surgical intervention to reconstruct the urinary tract is not usually necessary. Antibiotic prophylaxis is recommended. Development of urinary infections or decrease in renal function mandates urodynamic assessment of the urinary tract. The demonstration of significant residual urine with unbalanced voiding warrants surgical intervention to promote emptying.[85,88] Upper tract stasis should be evaluated and a Whitaker test performed, if necessary, to rule out obstruction.[150] The results of these specific tests will help determine the type of surgical intervention. These patients benefit from early orchidopexy and

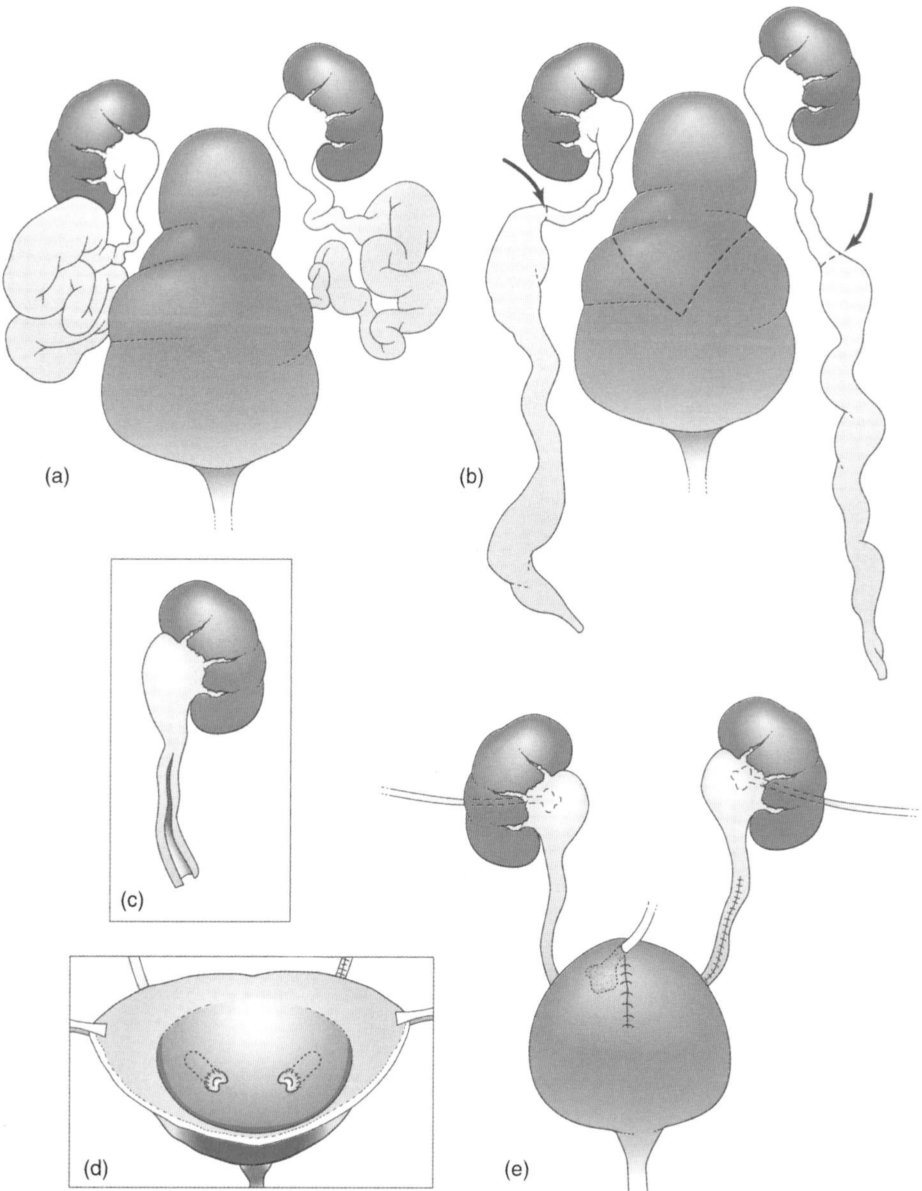

Figure 64.16 *(a–e)* Surgical technique used for extensive reconstruction of prune belly uropathy. The operation is performed transperitoneally. No attempt is made to straighten the lower ureter, inasmuch as only the upper portion of the ureter is needed for reimplantation. The ureter may require tapering. The dome of the bladder is excised (*b*; dotted line) in most patients. Ureteral stents (not shown) are used; nephrostomy tubes are rarely required.

abdominoplasty, as correction of the abdominal wall may improve defecation and voiding efficiency.[151]

Anesthetic considerations

The patient with prune belly syndrome presents unique problems to the anesthesiologist. Several reports have commented on respiratory difficulties due to the abnormal mechanics of pulmonary ventilation. The deficient abdominal musculature weakens the ability to cough effectively and predisposes these patients to postoperative atelectasis and infection.[152] In one case, prolonged, postoperative ventilation was necessary to effectively clear secretions and adequately oxygenate the patient.[153] In a review of 36 patients with prune belly syndrome, postoperative respiratory infection developed following eight of 133 anesthetics, all of which resolved with antibiotics and physiotherapy.[154] There were no intraoperative respiratory difficulties. Three deaths occurred in the postoperative period, one of which was partially due to pneumonia, as a result of ineffective cough.

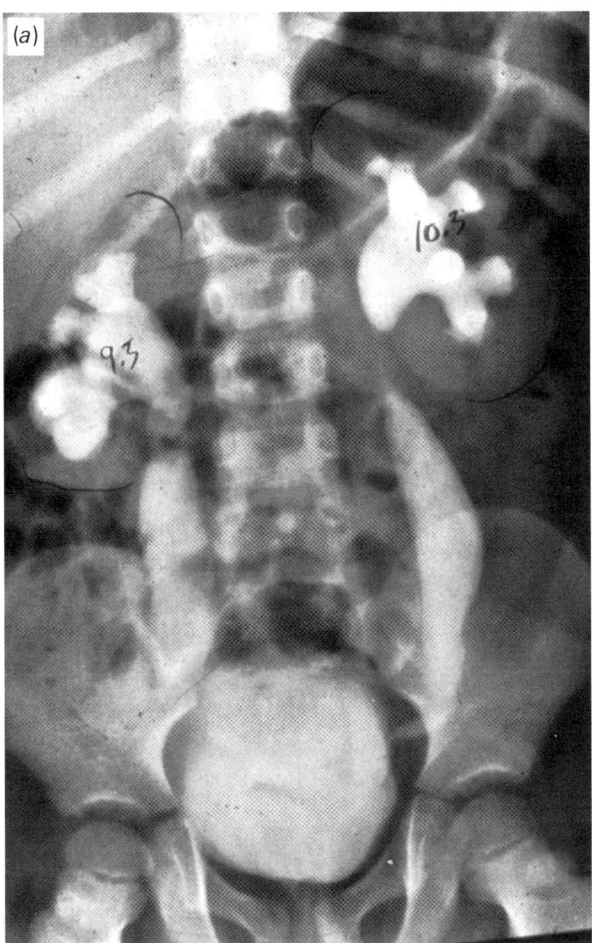

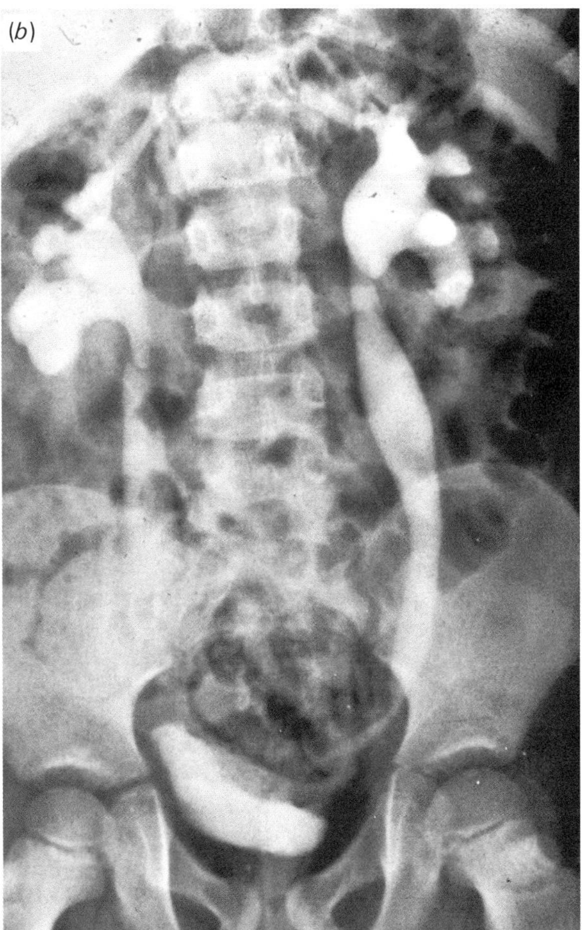

Figure 64.17 (*a* and *b*) Intravenous pyelogram (two views) obtained postoperatively in a child with prune belly syndrome after a single, comprehensive surgical reconstruction.

All patients with prune belly syndrome require careful preoperative pulmonary assessment. An antecedent history of recurrent respiratory infections warrants aggressive physiotherapy, postural drainage, and intermittent positive pressure breathing treatments. Specific antibiotic therapy should be given.[153] Judicious use of postoperative analgesics, which may produce respiratory depression, is advised.

Operative interventions in prune belly syndrome

Vesicourethral dysfunction

Internal urethrotomy

In rare cases, an internal urethrotomy is indicated in patients with an anatomic urethral obstruction. At the junction of the prostatic and membranous urethra, a 'type 4' valve may be present. This redundancy partially obstructs the membranous urethra. A transurethral incision at the 12 o'clock position has been advised to improve voiding and decrease residual urine.[155]

Urodynamic assessment, including pressure–flow studies, in patients with prune belly syndrome may prove valuable.[5,23,85] The demonstration of residual urine with infection indicates the need for further testing. If a low flow rate is associated with significant residual urine and normal voiding pressure, then intervention to lower urethral resistance is warranted.[85] Endoscopic urethrotomy by hot or cold knife, to decrease outlet resistance, was successful in 10 of 11 cases in improving emptying.[156] Most authors that advocate minimal surgical intervention stress the need to closely monitor patients in follow-up. Assessment of lower urinary tract dynamics, routine urinary flow rates, and the amount of residual urine are monitored with follow-up. Internal urethrotomy is a potential first step to balanced voiding, but clean intermittent catheterization should be considered if the urodynamic criteria of outlet obstruction are not present.[27,85,156,157]

Vesicostomy

When the patient's condition is complicated by urinary infection or deteriorating renal function in the perinatal period, a cutaneous vesicostomy is the drainage procedure of choice.[3,158] This provides a vent that decompresses the entire urinary tract. The vesicostomy is performed through a small transverse incision midway between the umbilicus and the pubic symphysis. The rectus fascia is incised and a small amount of it and the skin removed. The dome of the bladder is mobilized and brought to the skin. The wall of the bladder is sewn to the fascia and matured to the skin. A generous stoma is advocated to prevent stomal stenosis.[92] A urachal diverticulum can be excised, if present. The vesicostomy can serve as an initial temporary drainage procedure prior to more extensive reconstruction.[159] A potential disadvantage is ineffective drainage of the redundant, tortuous, upper ureters or an associated ureteropelvic junction obstruction. These are unlikely, as true supravesical obstruction is rarely a component of prune belly syndrome.

Reduction cystoplasty

Reduction cystoplasty has been suggested in order to reduce volume and improve emptying.[97] Bladder volumes in excess of 3 L have been recorded in children with prune belly syndrome.[85] Concomitant removal of a dilated urachal diverticulum, which contributes to inefficient voiding, is performed. According to the law of LaPlace, a spherical shape of the bladder should allow maximal intravesical pressure with each detrusor contraction. A variety of techniques to reduce bladder volume and produce a more efficient spherical shape have been proposed.[32,97,160] A vest-over-pants closure of the bladder wall after removal of bladder epithelial strips or simple resection and watertight closure have been performed in the majority of cases.

Reduction cystoplasty has clinically resulted in fewer hospitalizations for urinary infections and initially improved voiding. However, the long-term bladder capacity and voiding efficiency were not improved.[161] Comparison of urodynamic voiding parameters between reconstructed voiding patients and non-reconstructed voiding patients did not show significant differences. Consequently, some authors do not recommend reduction cystoplasty in light of the effective and safe application of clean intermittent catheterization, except for the removal of a urachal pseudodiverticulum.[92,157]

Anterior urethra

Prune belly syndrome is associated with microurethra and megalourethra. Utilization of the unused 'micro' anterior urethra is advocated. Successful progressive soft dilatation of the urethra with normal voiding has been reported.[102] If the anterior urethra is not usable, urethroplasty techniques combining skin flaps and grafts are necessary to bridge the anterior urethral defect. Megalourethra can be repaired by application of hypospadias operative techniques.

Upper urinary tract

Vesicoureteral dysfunction

Vesicoureteral dysfunction is manifested most commonly as vesicoureteral reflux, occurring in up to 85% of patients. Ureteral valves and ureterovesical junction obstruction have been described.[93] Both conditions potentially contribute to urinary stasis and increased risk of infection. The indications for surgical correction of obstructing lesions should be based on the demonstration of decreasing renal function, infection, or a positive Whitaker test.

Surgery to repair vesicoureteral reflux has been contested because of the poor peristaltic activity of the ureters and their dissipation of voiding pressure due to increased capacity.[3] Observation of prune belly patients who remain infection free on prophylactic antibiotics has confirmed preservation of renal function.[26,88] When urinary infection becomes problematic, correction of reflux and reduction of urinary stasis become necessary. Formal tapering and reimplantation, as well as ureteral imbrication, have been used as part of the comprehensive approach to management.[29] We found no difference in the complication rate with either procedure, and 9 of 13 patients had successful elimination of their reflux. Ureteral imbrication may produce fewer problems with stenosis.[3] However, the imbricated ureter is very bulky and requires a long, wide subepithelial tunnel for reimplantation.

Temporary diversion of the upper tract by pyelostomy or ureterostomy is rarely necessary. Vesicostomy is preferred, but in those neonates with unresponsive urosepsis, high diversion to optimize drainage may be required.

Comprehensive reconstruction

Comprehensive recontruction in the prune belly patient involves reduction cystoplasty, resection of the

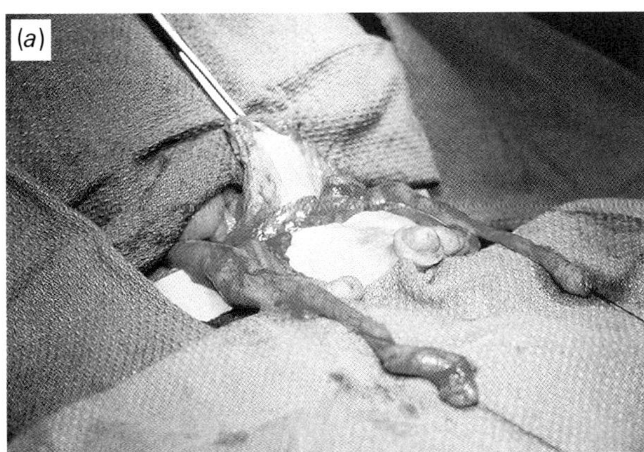

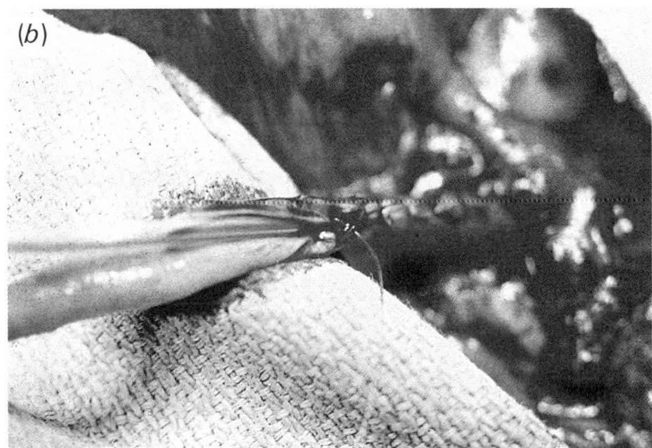

Figure 64.18 (*a*) Both ureters have been mobilized prior to reimplantation and tapering. (*b*) The ureter is closed in two layers with a running, locking suture.

distal ureter, and bilateral ureteral tapered reimplantation (see Figure 64.16). Reconstruction may be combined with the performance of the abdominoplasty and bilateral orchidopexy, usually prior to 2 years of age.[22,30] This aggressive approach was utilized in 15 patients in our series. Serial measurements of creatinine up to 13 years later documented preservation of renal function.[29] Vesicoureteral reflux was corrected in 9 of 13 patients and improved in three patients. Because of the known urinary stasis that occurs in these children, all are maintained on antibiotic prophylaxis. Therefore, our ability to decrease urinary infection cannot be totally attributed to the surgical result.

Complete surgical reconstruction, as reported by Denes et al, involved abdominoplasty, urinary tract reconstruction, and orchiopexy in a select group of 32 patients. A morbidity rate of 18.7% and a reoperation rate of 15.6% was reported. Thirty of 32 patients demonstrated stable or improved renal function at a mean follow-up of 5 years.[162]

Our proposed surgical approach is similar to that proposed by Woodward (see Figure 64.16). A wide lower abdominal incision is made that extends from the tip of the 12th rib, along the anterior superior iliac spine to the pubis and then curves upward to the opposite 12th rib.[116] This tends to spare the segmental nerve and vascular supply of the abdominal wall left for reconstruction. In addition, at the time of excision of the redundant abdominal wall, that portion with the most muscle fibers is preserved. The exposure of the urinary tract provided with this incision is exceptional and plays a role in our decision to reconstruct the urinary tract.

The posterior peritoneum is incised along the length of the ureters. The spermatic vessels are mobilized distally, care being taken not to compromise the peritoneal attachments of the vas deferens if a Fowler–Stephens orchidopexy is required. The bladder is opened in the midline with cautery. The laterally placed ureteral orifices are recognized and each ureter is mobilized. The extreme length of the mobilized ureters allows for resection of its distal third, usually the most abnormal portion. Formal tapering or imbrication is performed (Figure 64.18).[163,164] The ureters are then reimplanted, using a transtrigonal or Politano–Leadbetter technique. Stenting of the operated ureters is performed and these are brought out through the bladder and separate abdominal incisions.

Prior to reduction cystoplasty, the testes are mobilized with a wide apron of posterior peritoneum (Figure 64.19). If the reconstruction is performed prior to 2 years of age, a standard orchidopexy with intact spermatic vessels can be performed in 80% of cases.[21,29] Otherwise, a delayed or formal Fowler–Stephens orchidopexy will be necessary.[165]

The bladder is reduced in size by resection of the urachal remnant and the huge bladder dome. A strip of bladder epithelium can be removed from one of the lateral walls and closed by the vest-over-pants technique. The bladder is drained with a Malecot catheter. The previously mobilized testes are brought up through the distal abdominal wall at the pubic tubercle. A dartos pouch is created in the scrotum and each testis is secured in the pouch with permanent sutures.

The redundant abdominal wall is then held taut and marked in the midline and laterally at the costovertebral angles to outline the tissue to be excised (Figure 64.20).[116] Avoidance of removal of excessive amounts of abdominal wall is critical. The second line of incision parallels the previous incision. A large

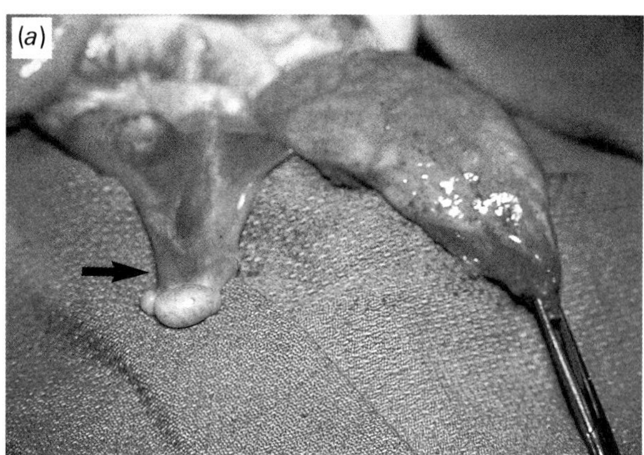

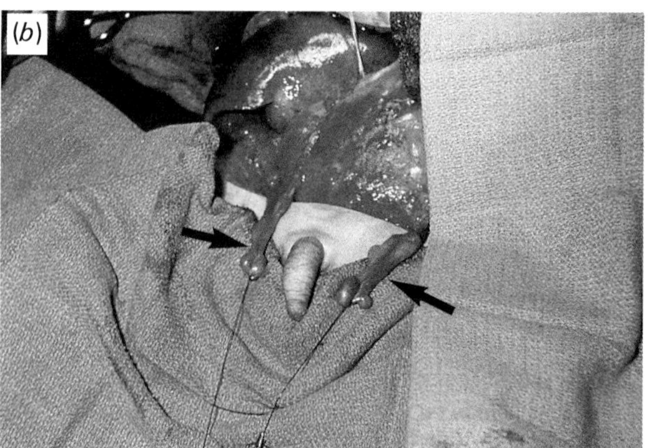

Figure 64.19 (*a*) The widely mobilized peritoneum with intact spermatic vessels (arrows) ensures good blood supply to the testis. (*b*) Achieving adequate length to secure the testes in the scrotum is usually not difficult in the child less than 2 years of age.

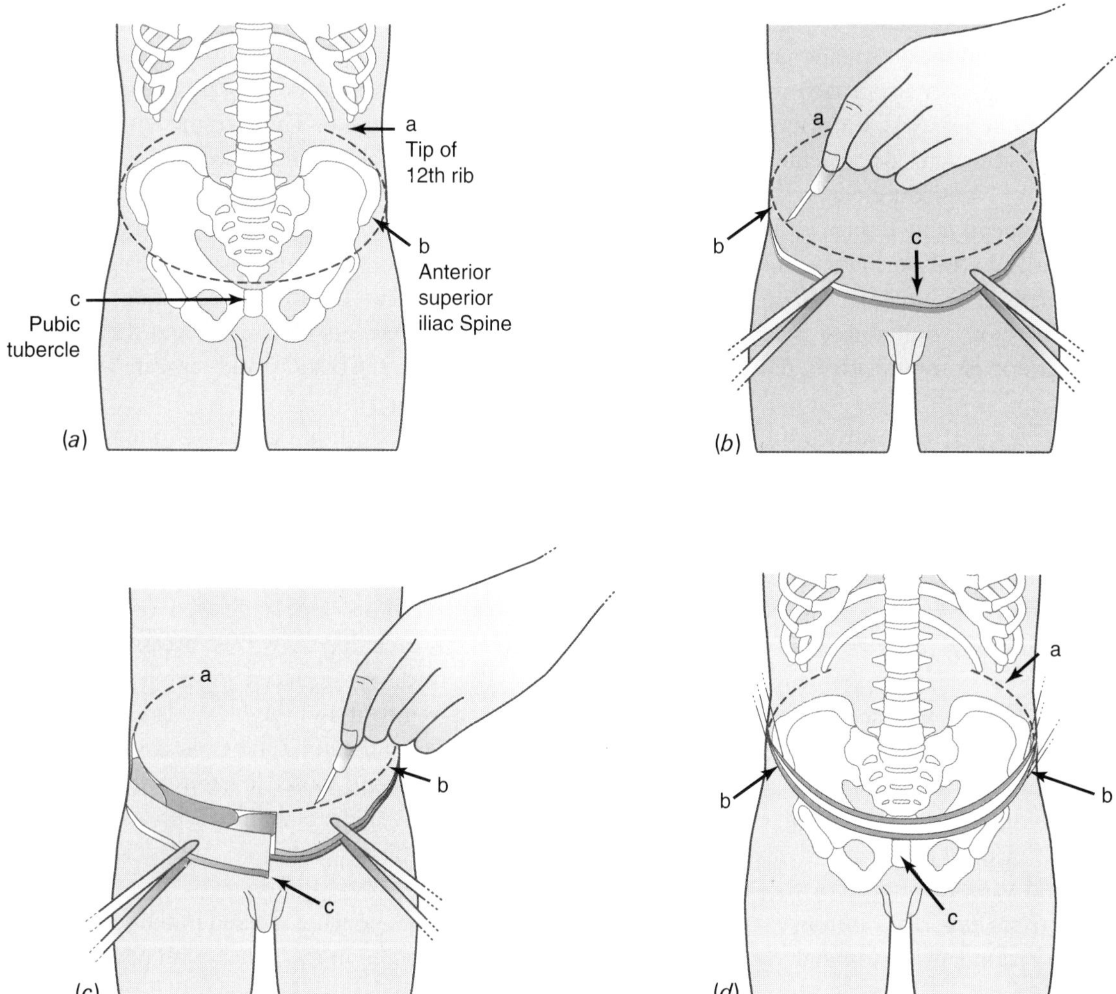

Figure 64.20 Technique of Randolph abdominoplasty. (*a*) A curvilinear incision extends from the tip of the 12th rib, along the anterior superior iliac spine to the pubic tubercle and onto the opposite 12th rib. (*b*) A parallel incision is made, avoiding removal of too much abdominal wall. (*c*) Rhomboid-like pieces of abdominal wall are removed. (*d*) Critical non-absorbable sutures are placed at the anterior iliac spines and pubic tubercle. These are placed through full thickness of the abdominal wall including the periosteum.

wedge of full-thickness abdominal wall is removed. The closure of the abdominal wall is commenced by placement of key sutures of 0 or 1–0 non-absorbable sutures at the anterior iliac spines and at each pubic tubercle. These sutures should include the periosteum of the bone and a full thickness of the proximal opposing tissue edge. The tension created occasionally allows for removal of additional lateral redundant abdominal wall. Each section between the key sutures is closed with interrupted sutures apposing the full thickness of the abdominal tissue. The subcutaneous tissue is closed to prevent dead space and the skin is approximated with a subcuticular absorbable suture.

All patients undergo preoperative enemas to clear the colon, and require good bowel decompression postoperatively. Postoperative abdominal distention must be avoided and a rectal tube placed during surgery is often valuable.

Cryptorchidism

The early correction of the cryptorchid intra-abdominal testes by a transabdominal approach is recommended to optimize spermatogenesis, facilitate examination for testicular malignancy, and improve testicular salvage. If orchidopexy is performed in the first year of life, a standard technique with preservation of the spermatic vessels can usually be performed. Orchidopexy in older children frequently requires division of the spermatic vessels, with results based on a one- or two-stage Fowler–Stevens technique.[166–168] To avoid atrophy, a broad, peritoneal pedicle mobilized with the long-looping vas, combined with early ligation of the spermatic vessels above the point of confluence of the vas and spermatic artery, is recommended.[169] Utilizing this two-stage approach, an 80–83% success rate for intra-abdominal testes has been attained.[166,167] Overall, successful orchidopexy can be expected in the majority of patients. Open and laparoscopic techniques have been described with similar results.[165,170,171] Orchiopexy can be performed at the time of comprehensive reconstruction with a high success rate.[16,21,22,29]

Microvascular testicular autotransplantation has been utilized in patients with prune belly syndrome. The spermatic vessels are anastomosed to the inferior epigastric vessels, with microsurgical vascular techniques.[172] This has normally been performed in older patients as a last salvage effort.[159] Prior to 1999, all boys with prune belly syndrome were considered infertile. However, with recent advances in male factor infertility and assisted reproductive techniques, the first assisted conception of a man with prune belly syndrome was reported.[113] Consequently, an early orchiopexy to preserve spermatogonia and testicular function in these patients is warranted.

Abdominal wall reconstruction

Abdominal wall reconstruction has a significant role in the treatment of patients with prune belly syndrome. Abdominoplasty had previously been performed to improve body image, self-esteem, and psychological well-being.[30,31] Recent studies suggest that the improved abdominal contour, with repositioning of the most functional musculature, improves voiding efficiency.[120,151] The decrease in residual urine has obvious benefit in the prevention of urinary infection. In addition, abdominoplasty was subjectively felt to improve defecation and sensation of bladder fullness.

The surgical approaches to performance of the abdominoplasty are based on preservation of the lateral and upper parts of the abdominal wall, the sites of most normal musculature. Our experience has been quite positive with the cosmetic and functional results provided by the abdominoplasty as described by Randolph et al.[116] This technique excises the most abnormal segment of redundant abdominal wall, provides excellent exposure for urinary reconstruction and orchidopexy, and preserves segmental motor nerves to the retained abdominal musculature. In 16 patients where this technique was utilized, nine had an excellent cosmetic improvement in abdominal contour, and in seven a slight protuberance remained. There were no serious complications related to the abdominoplasty procedure (Figures 64.20 and 64.21).[29] The major criticisms of this technique are that it does not improve abdominal wall thickness, and lateral bulging is not completely eliminated. However, this technique has been favored by a number of surgeons.[3,92]

The surgical approach to abdominal wall reconstruction, utilizing a midline incision with extensive subcutaneous dissection and a pants-over-vest closure has been described (Figures 64.22 and 64.23).[173,174] This technique preserves the umbilicus, uses the full thickness of abdominal wall, and provides narrowing at the waist. Excellent cosmetic results with a high degree of patient satisfaction have been reported with both the Ehrlich and Monfort techniques (Figure 64.24).[31,173–175] An adaptation utilizing an extraperitoneal plication of the abdominal wall through a midline incision decreases the extent of facial dissection,

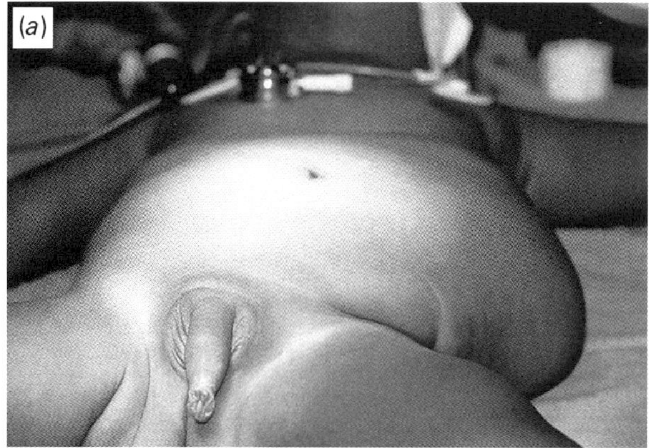

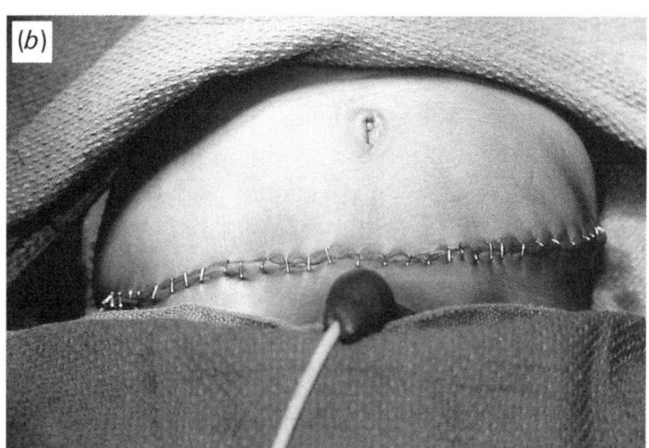

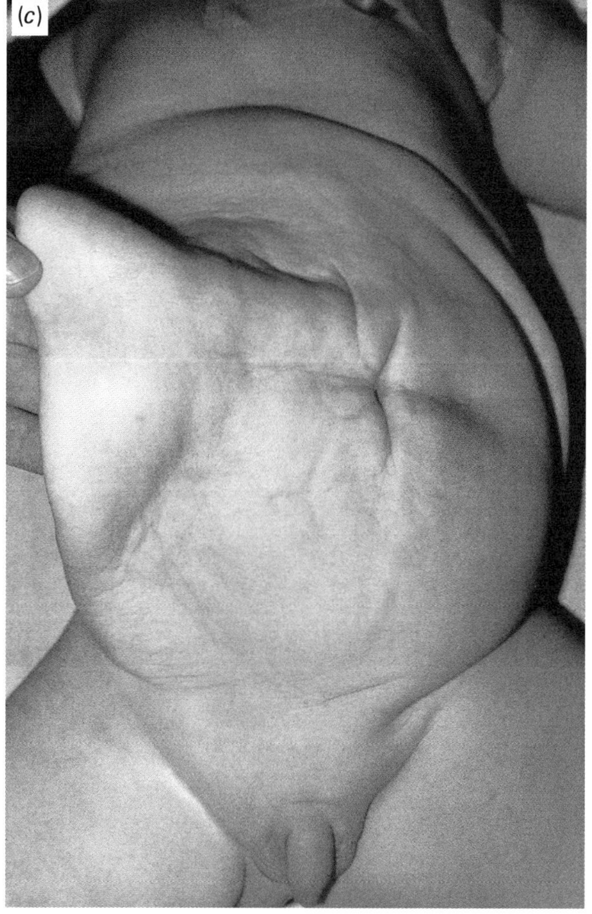

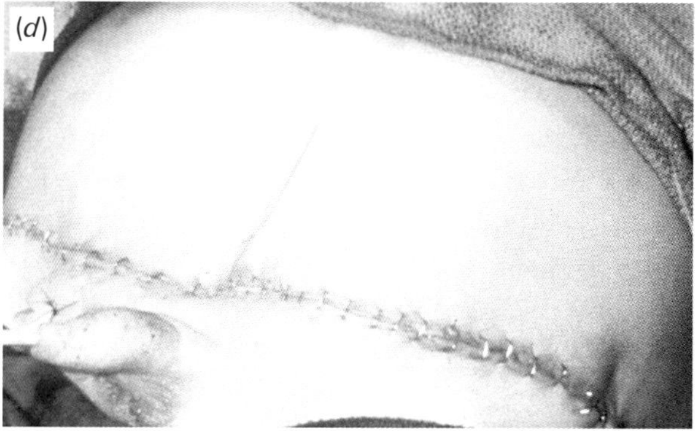

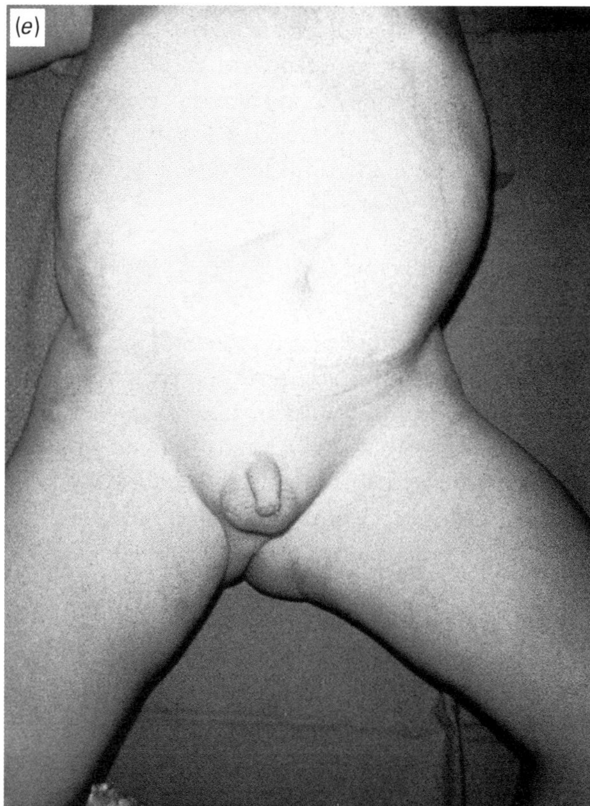

Figure 64.21 (*a,b*) Preoperative and immediate postoperative results of Randolph abdominoplasty. (*c–e*) Preoperative, postoperative, and 18 months following Randolph abdominoplasty in a 9-month-old-child.

avoids entering the peritoneal cavity and, decreases postoperative recovery time.[176] This simplification seems most appropriate for patients not requiring other concomitant surgical procedures. A modification of the Monfort abdominoplasty includes a neoumbilical modification to provide a normal anatomic placement of the umbilicus.[177]

Other treatment possibilities include abdominal binders and elasticized corsets (Figure 64.25). These aids do not address the psychological implications of

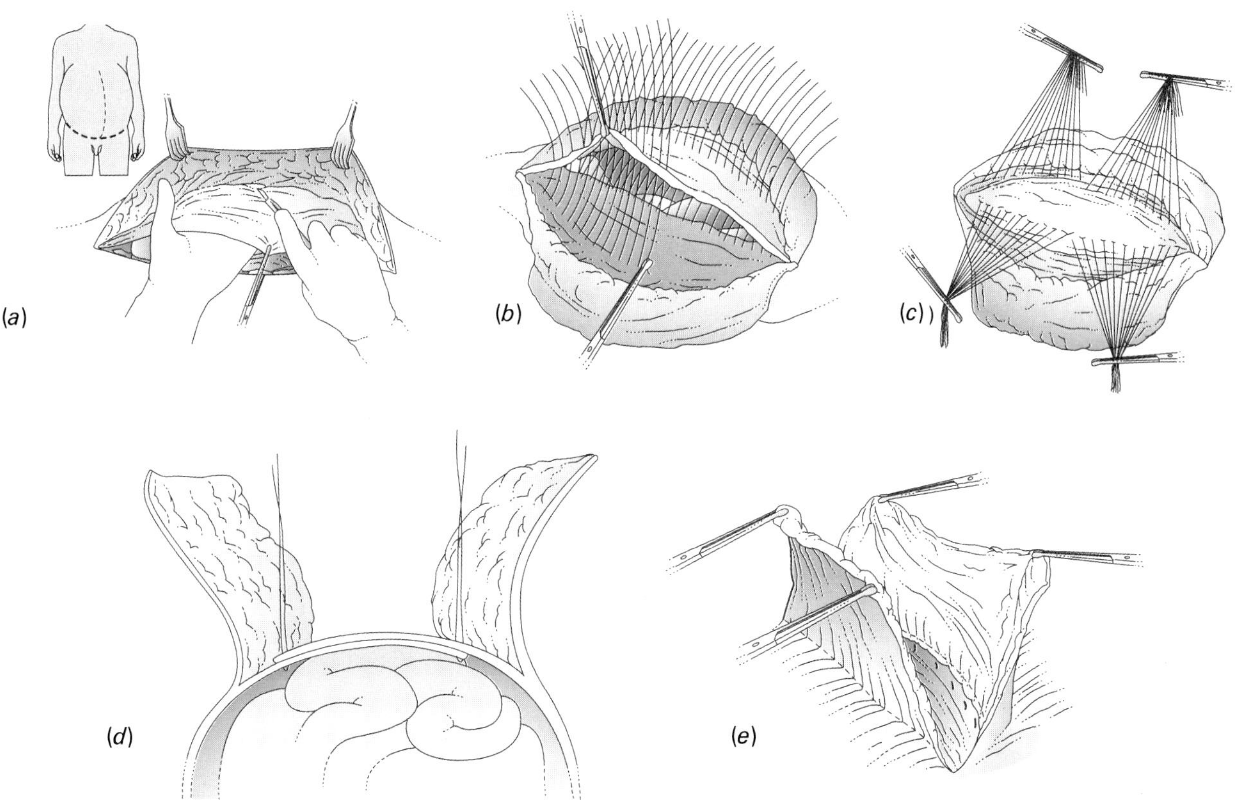

Figure 64.22 Ehrlich abdominoplasty. (*a*) Sharp dissection separates the skin and subcutaneous tissue from the musculofascial layer. (*b–d*) A 'vest-over-pants' closure of the musculofascial layers. The umbilicus can be saved on a separate pedicle. (*e*) The excess abdominal skin is removed. (Reproduced from Ehrlich et al,[173] with permission from Williams & Wilkins.)

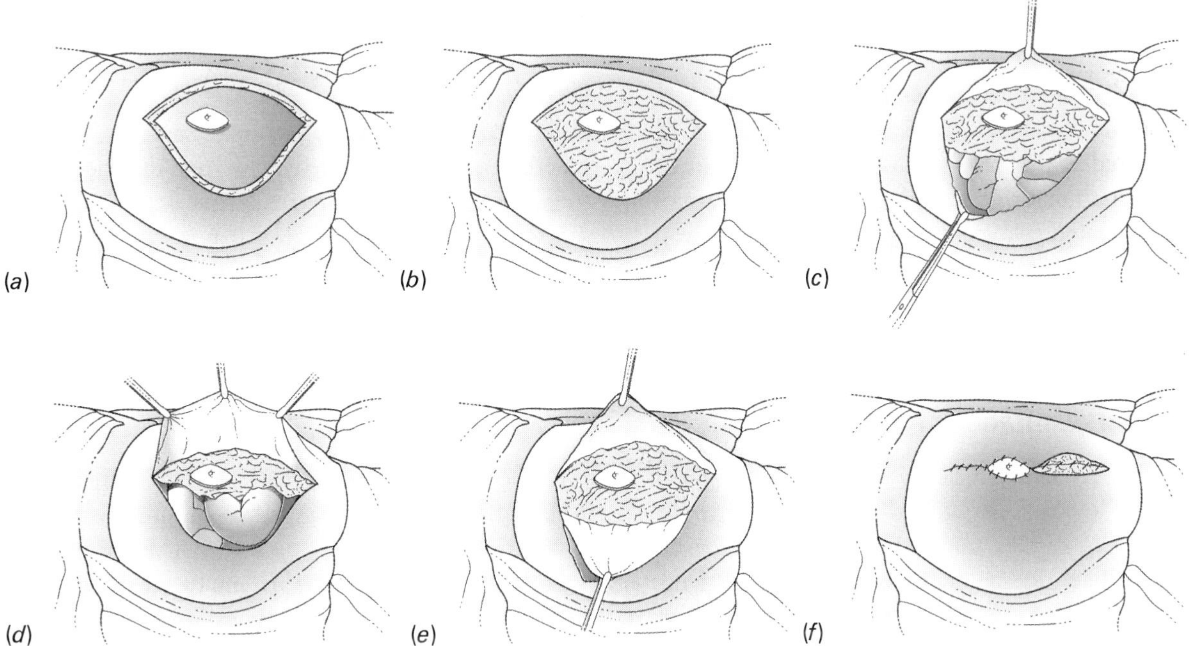

Figure 64.23 Monfort abdominoplasty. (*a*) An almond-shaped incision is made on the abdomen from the xyphoid to the pubic symphysis. (*b*) The full thickness of skin is removed, sparing the umbilicus. (*c*) The peritoneum is opened lateral to the musculofascial layer. Intra-abdominal surgery can be easily performed through these incisions. (*d*) The parietal peritoneum is incised at a level to achieve a normal-appearing waistline. (*e*) The edges of the musculofascial plate are sewn to the peritoneal incisions. (*f*) The lateral skin flaps are trimmed and sutured together in the midline. (From Monfort et al,[174] with permission from Williams & Wilkins.)

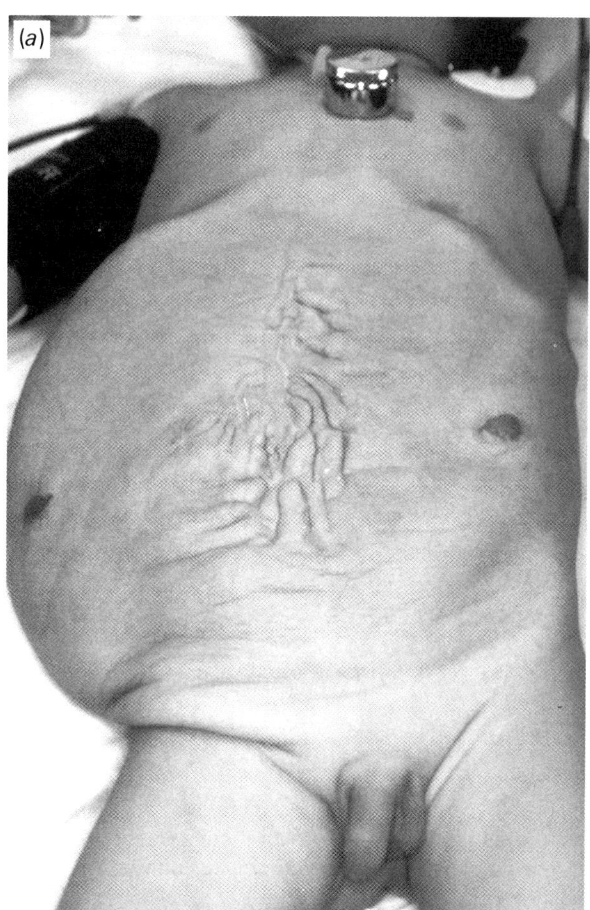
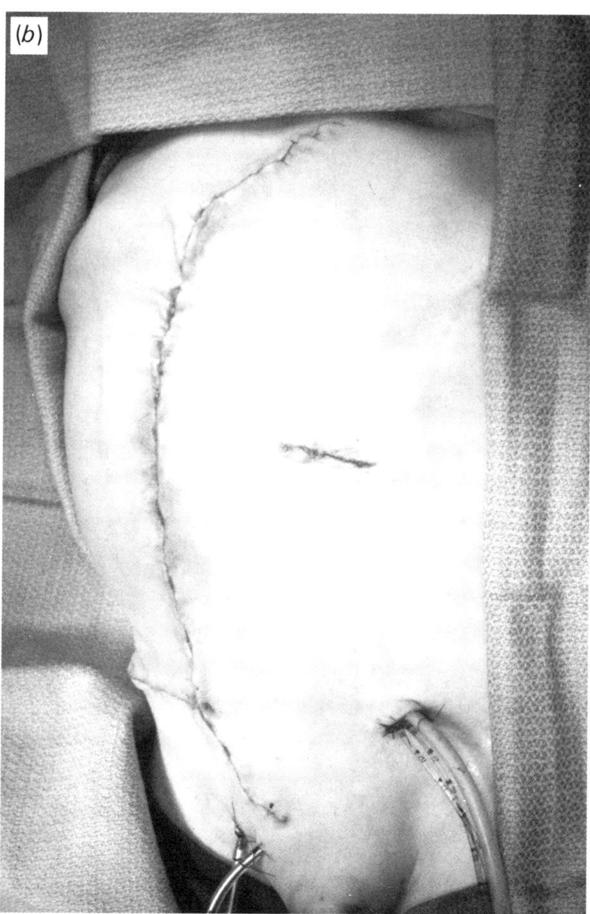

Figure 64.24 (*a*) Preoperative depiction of a 2-year-old child with bilateral cutaneous loop ureterostomies prior to comprehensive surgical reconstruction. (*b*) Same child after comprehensive reconstruction of the urinary tract and Monfort abdominoplasty. (Courtesy of George W Kaplan MD.)

the abdominal disfigurement, which have generally been ignored in the past.[173] The importance of body image during the formative years of childhood cannot be overestimated. The abdominoplasty provides these males with freedom from abdominal binders, a more natural waisted physique, ability to wear normal pants, and participate in sports.[29]

Renal transplantation

Progressive renal insufficiency resulting from renal dysplasia, reflux nephropathy, and recurrent pyelonephritis can be successfully treated by renal transplantation. Renal transplantation in patients with prune belly syndrome was first reported in 1976.[178] The age at transplantation has ranged from 8 months to 21 years of age.[179,180] Both cadaver and living-related donor kidneys have been successfully transplanted. In a retrospective review of eight patients with prune belly syndrome who underwent transplantation, there was no statistically significant difference in patient deaths, graft survival, or graft function when compared with age-matched controls.[180] A more recent retrospective analysis of graft survival at 10 years of 47% was not statistically significantly different from age-matched controlled patients.[181] The success of renal transplantation was in part attributed to the low-pressure urine storage provided by the bladder in prune belly syndrome.[182]

Prior to transplantation, bilateral nephroureterectomies were performed in all reported cases. Radiographic and urodynamic assessment of the lower urinary tract is recommended to insure absence of obstruction and balanced voiding.[183] The use of clean intermittent catheterization to empty the decompensated bladder is not a contraindication to renal transplantation.[180,184] All patients should be kept on antibiotic prophylaxis. An unusual complication of transplantation in prune belly syndrome is allograft torsion.[185] The torsion, with resultant graft loss, is a result of lack of abdominal wall tone. Nephropexy has been recommended to avoid this disastrous complication.

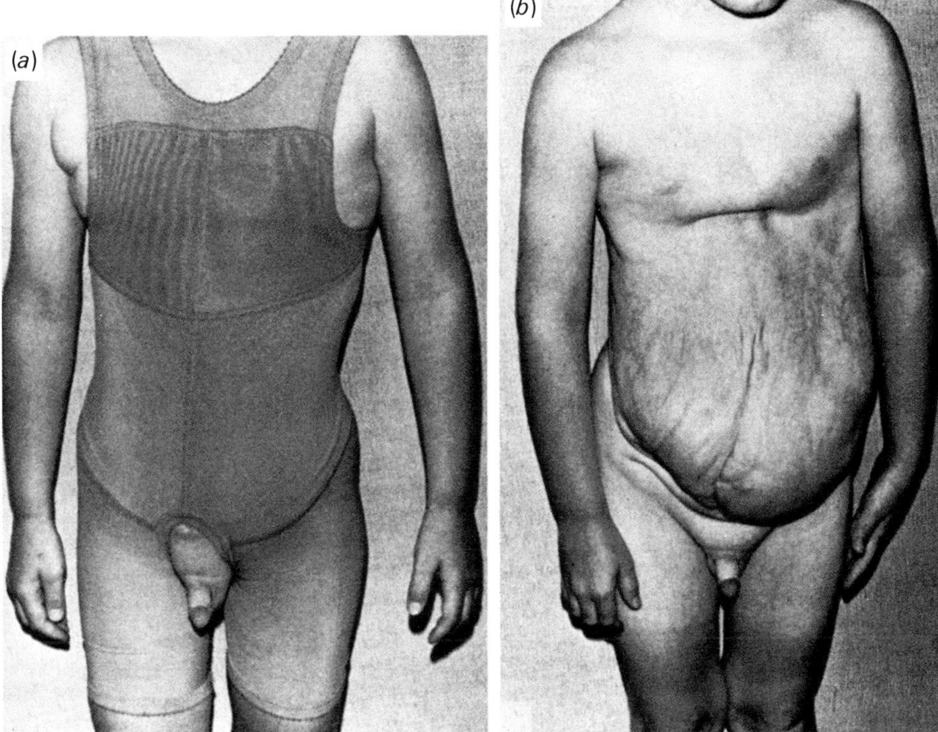

Figure 64.25 A 4-year-old boy with prune belly syndrome, (*a*) with and (*b*) without his elasticized corset.

Conclusions

The treatment of prune belly syndrome has become refined as a result of significant improvements in antibiotic therapy, diagnostic capabilities, urodynamic assessment of the urinary tract, and our understanding of the natural history of the disease. Given the wide spectrum of disease, each patient requires individualized management. When infection and stasis compromise renal growth or function, aggressive surgical intervention to promote drainage is advised. Because of the changing urodynamic condition of the lower urinary tract and its effects on renal function and urinary infection, all patients with prune belly syndrome require careful lifelong urologic surveillance.

References

1. Frolich F. Der Mangel der Muskeln, insbesondere der Seitenbauch muskeln. Dissertation. Wurzburg: C.A. Zurn, 1839.
2. Parker RW. Case of an infant in whom some of the abdominal muscles were absent. Trans Clin Soc Lond 1895; 28:201–3.
3. Duckett JW. Prune belly syndrome. In: Welsh KJ, Randolph JG, Ravich MM, O'Neill JA, Rowe MI, eds. Pediatric Surgery. Chicago: Year Book Medical Publishers, 1986: 1193–203.
4. Pagon RA, Smith DW, Shepard TH. Urethral obstruction malformation complex: a cause of abdominal muscle deficiency and the 'prune belly.' J Pediatr 1979; 94:900–6.
5. Nunn IN, Stephens FD. The triad syndrome: a composite anomaly of the abdominal wall, urinary system and testes. J Urol 1961; 86:782–94.
6. Welsh K, Kearney GP. Abdominal musculature deficiency syndrome: prune belly. J Urol 1974; 111:693–7.
7. Ives EJ. The abdominal muscle deficiency triad syndrome – experience with ten cases. Birth Defects 1974; 10:127–35.
8. Rabinowitz R, Schillinger JF. Prune belly syndrome in the female subject. J Urol 1977; 115:454–6.
9. Guvenc M, Guvenc H, Aygun AD et al. Prune-belly syndrome associated with omphalocele in a female newborn. J Pediatr Surg 1995; 30(6):896–7.
10. Reinberg Y, Shapiro E, Manivel JC. Prune belly syndrome in females: a triad of abdominal musculature deficiency and anomalies of the urinary and genital systems. J Pediatr 1991; 118:395–8.
11. Bellah RD, States LJ, Duckett JW. Pseudoprune belly syndrome: imaging, findings and outcome. AJR Am J Roentgenol 1996; 167:1389–93.
12. Greskovich FJ, Nyberg LM. The prune belly syndrome: a review of its etiology, defects, treatment and prognosis. J Urol 1988; 140:707–12.
13. Garlinger P, Ott J. Prune belly syndrome: possible genetic implications. Birth Defects 1974; 10:173–80.
14. Adeyokunnu AA, Familuse JB. Prune belly syndrome in

two siblings and a first cousin: possible genetic implications. Am J Dis Child 1982; 136:23–5.
15. Druschel CM. A descriptive study of prune belly in New York State 1983 to 1989. Arch Pediatr Adolesc Med 1995; 149:70–6.
16. Greenfield SP, Rutigliano E, Steinhardt G et al. Genitourinary tract malformations and maternal cocaine abuse. Urology 1991; 37:455–9.
17. Waldbaum RS, Marshall VS. The prune belly syndrome: a diagnostic therapeutic plan. J Urol 1970; 103:668–74.
18. Eagle JF, Barrett GS. Congenital deficiency of abdominal musculature with associated genitourinary abnormalities. A syndrome: a report of 9 cases. Pediatrics 1950; 6:721–36.
19. Jeffs RD, Comisarow RH, Hanna MK. The early assessment for individualized treatment in the prune belly syndrome. Birth Defects 1977; 13:97–9.
20. Rabinowitz R, Barkin M. Urinary tract reconstruction in the prune belly syndrome. Urology 1978; 12:333–5.
21. Woodard JR, Parrott TS. Reconstruction of the urinary tract in prune belly uropathy. J Urol 1978; 119:824–8.
22. Randolph JG, Cavett C, Eng G. Surgical correction and rehabilitation for children with 'prune belly syndrome.' Ann Surg 1981; 193: 757–62.
23. Williams DI, Burkholder GV. The prune belly syndrome. J Urol 1967; 98:244–9.
24. Burke EC, Shin MH, Kelalis PP. Prune belly syndrome: clinical findings and survival. Am J Dis Child 1969; 117:668–71.
25. Duckett JW Jr. The prune belly syndrome. In: Kelalis PP, King LR, Belman AB, eds. Clinical Pediatric Urology. Philadelphia: WB Saunders, 1976: 615–35.
26. Tank ES, McCoy GB. Limited surgical intervention in the prune belly syndrome. J Pediatr Surg 1983; 18:688–91.
27. Woodhouse CRJ, Kellett MJ, Williams DI. Minimal surgical interference in the prune belly syndrome. Br J Urol 1979; 51:475–80.
28. Burbidge KA, Amodio J, Berdon WE et al. Prune belly syndrome: 35 years of experience. J Urol 1987; 137:86–90.
29. Fallat ME, Skoog SJ, Belman AT et al. The prune belly syndrome: a comprehensive approach to management. J Urol 1989; 142:802–5.
30. Woodard JR. Editorial: lessons learned in 3 decades of managing the prune belly syndrome. J Urol 1998; 159:1680.
31. Woodard JR, Smith EA. Prune belly syndrome. In: Walsh PC, Retik AB, Vaughan ED Jr, Wein AJ, eds. Campbell's Urology. Philadelphia: WB Saunders, 1998: 1917–38.
32. Woodard JR, Trulock TS. Prune belly syndrome. In: Walsh PC, Retik AB, Vaughan ED Jr, Wein AJ, eds. Campbell's Urology. Philadelphia: WB Saunders, 1996: 2159–67.
33. Sladezyk VE. Das gehaufte familiare Duftreten des angeborenen Bauchmuskel-wanddefektes. Zbl Chir 1967; 92:426–8.
34. Petersen DS, Fish L, Cass AS. Twins with congenital deficiency of abdominal musculature. J Urol 1972; 107:670–2.
35. Riccardi VM, Grum CM. The prune belly syndrome: heterogeneity and superficial X-linkage mimicry. J Med Genet 1977; 14:266–70.
36. Balaji KC, Patil A, Townes PL et al. Concordant prune belly syndrome in monozygotic twins. Urology 2000; 55(6):949.
37. Lubinsky M, Doyle K, Trunca C. The association of prune belly with Turner's syndrome. Am J Dis Child 1980; 134:1171–2.
38. Rabinowitz R, Shillinger JR. Prune belly syndrome in the female subject. J Urol 1977; 115:454–6.
39. Hoagland MH, Frank KA, Hutchins GM. Prune belly syndrome with prostatic hypoplasia, bladder wall rupture, and massive ascites in a fetus with trisomy 18. Arch Path Lab Med 1988; 112:1126–8.
40. Curry CJR, Jensen K, Holland J et al. The Potter sequence: a clinical analysis of 80 cases. Am J Med Genet 1984; 19:679–702.
41. Amacker EA, Grass FS, Hickey DE et al. An association of prune belly anomaly with trisomy 21. Am J Med Genet 1986; 23:919–23.
42. Al Harbi NN. Prune-belly anomalies in a girl with Down syndrome. Pediatr Nephrol 2003; 18(11):1191–2.
43. Moerman P, Fryns KP, Godderis PI. Spectrum of clinical and autopsy findings in trisomy 18 syndrome. J Genet Hum 1982; 30:17–38.
44. Baird PA, Sadovnick AD. Letter to the editor: prune belly anomaly in Down syndrome. Am J Med Genet 1987; 26:747–8.
45. Harley LM, Chen Y, Rattner WH. Prune belly syndrome. J Urol 1972; 108:174–6.
46. Halbrecht I, Komulus L, Shabtai F. Prune belly syndrome with chromosomal fragment. Am J Dis Child 1972; 123:518.
47. Fahmy J, Kaminsky CK, Parisi MT. Perlman syndrome: a case report emphasizing its similarity to and distinction from Beckwith–Wiedemann and prune-belly syndrome. Pediatr Radiol 1998; 28(3):179–82.
48. Shah D, Sharma S, Faridi MM, Mishra K. VACTERL association with Prune-Belly syndrome. Indian Pediatr 2004; 41(8):845–7.
49. Levin TL, Soghier L, Blitman NM, Vega-Rich C, Nafday S. Megacystis–microcolon–intestinal hypoperistalsis and prune belly: overlapping syndromes. Pediatr Radiol 2004; 34(12):995–8.
50. Silengo M, Barberis L, Ferrero GB, Sorasio L, Valenzise M. A possible relationship between Beckwith–Wiedemann syndrome and prune belly syndrome. Clin Dysmorphol 2002; 11(4):293–4.
51. Strumme EG. Über die symmetrischen krongenitalen Bauchmuskeldefekte unt über die Kombination derselben mit anderen Bildungsanomalien des Rumpfres. Mitt Grenzigeb Med Chir 1903; 11:548–51.
52. Lattimer JK. Congenital deficiency of the abdominal musculature and associated genitourinary anomalies: a report of 22 cases. J Urol 1958; 79:343–52.
53. Rogers LW, Ostrow PT. The prune belly syndrome: report of 20 cases and description of a lethal variant. J Pediatr 1973; 83:786–83.
54. Berdon WE, Baker DH, Wigger HJ et al. The radiologic and pathologic spectrum of prune belly syndrome. Radiol Clin North Am 1977; 15:83–92.

55. Straub E, Spranger J. Etiology and pathogenesis of the prune belly syndrome. Kidney Int 1981; 20:695–9.
56. Wigger JH, Blanc WA. The prune belly syndrome. Pathol Ann 1977; 12:17–39.
57. Hoagland MH, Hutchins GM. Obstructive lesions of the lower urinary tract in the prune belly syndrome. Arch Pathol Lab Med 1987; 111:154–6.
58. Volmar KE, Nguyen TC, Holcroft CJ, Blakemore KJ, Hutchins GM. Phimosis as a cause of the prune belly syndrome: comparison to a more common pattern of proximal penile urethra obstruction. Virchows Arch 2003; 442:169–72.
59. Volmar KE, Fritsch MK, Perlman EJ, Hutchins GM. Patterns of congenital lower urinary tract obstructive uropathy: relation to abnormal prostate and bladder development and the prune belly syndrome. Pediatric Dev Pathol 2001; 4:467–72.
60. Moerman P, Fryns JP, Goddeeris P et al. Pathogenesis of the prune-belly syndrome: a functional urethral obstruction caused by prostatic hypoplasia. Pediatrics 1984; 73:470–5.
61. Beasley SW, Henay F, Hutson JM. The anterior urethra provides clues to the aetiology of prune belly syndrome. Pediatr Surg Int 1988; 3:169.
62. Sellers BB, McNeal R, Smith RV et al. Congenital megalourethra associated with prune belly syndrome. J Urol 1796; 116:814–15.
63. Kroovand RL, Al-Ansari RM, Perlmutter AD. Urethral and genital malformations in prune belly syndrome. J Urol 1982; 127:94–6.
64. O'Kell RT. Embryonic abdominal musculature associated with anomalies of the genitourinary and gastrointestinal system. Am J Obstet Gynecol 1969; 105:1283–4.
65. Mininberg DT, Montoya F, Okada K et al. Subcellular muscle studies in the prune belly syndrome. J Urol 1974; 109:524–6.
66. Stephens FD. Triad (prune belly) syndrome. In: Stephens FD, ed. Congenital Malformations of the Urinary Tract. New York: Praeger, 1983:485–511.
67. Monie IW, Monie BJ. Prune belly and fetal ascites. Teratology 1979; 19:111–17.
68. Smythe AR. Ultrasonic detection of fetal ascites and bladder dilatation with resulting prune belly. J Pediatr 1981; 98:978–80.
69. Nakayama DK, Harrison MR, Chinn DH et al. Pathogenesis of prune belly. Am J Dis Child 1984; 138:834–6.
70. Cazorla E, Ruiz F, Abad A et al. Prune belly syndrome: early antenatal diagnosis. Eur J Obstet Gynecol Reprod Biol 1997; 72:31–3.
71. Symonds DA, Driscoll SG. Massive fetal ascites, urethral atresia and cytomegalic inclusion disease. Am J Dis Child 1974; 127:895–7.
72. Golbus MS, Harrison MR, Filly RA et al. In utero treatment of urinary tract obstruction. Am J Obstet Gynecol 1982; 142:383–8.
73. Fitzsimmons RB, Keohane C, Galvin J. Prune belly syndrome with ultrasound demonstration of reduced megacystis in utero. Br J Radiol 1985; 58:374–6.
74. Kuruvilla AC, Kesler KR, Williams JW et al. Congenital cystic adenomatoid malformation of the lungs associated with prune belly syndrome. J Pediatr Surg 1987; 22:370–1.
75. Chen CP, Liu FF, Jan SW et al. First report of distal obstructive uropathy and prune belly syndrome in an infant with amniotic band syndrome. Am J Perinatol 1997; 14:31–3.
76. Yamamoto H, Sera Y, Ikeda S. Giant liver cyst in a fetus with prune belly syndrome. Pediatr Surg Int 1994; 9:417.
77. Wheatley JM, Stephens FD, Hutson JM. Prune-belly syndrome: ongoing controversies regarding pathogenesis and management. Semin Pediatr Surg 1996; 5:95–106.
78. Osathanondh V, Potter EL. Pathogenesis of polycystic kidneys. Arch Pathol 1964; 77:510–12.
79. Palmer JM, Tesluck H. Ureteral pathology in the prune belly syndrome. J Urol 1974; 111:701–7.
80. Stephens FD, Gupta D. Pathogenesis of the prune belly syndrome. J Urol 1994; 152:2328–31.
81. Deklerk DP, Scott WW. Prostatic maldevelopment in the prune belly syndrome: a defect in prostatic stromal–epithelial interaction. J Urol 1978; 120:341–4.
82. Elder JS, Isaacs JT, Walsh PC. Androgenic sensitivity of the gubernaculum testis: evidence for hormonal/mechanical interactions in testicular descent. J Urol 1982; 127:170–6.
83. Fallon B, Welton M, Hawtrey C. Congenital anomalies associated with cryptorchidism. J Urol 1982; 127:91–3.
84. Cussen LJ. The morphology of congenital dilatation of the ureter: intrinsic ureteral lesions. Aust N Z J Surg 1971; 41:185–94.
85. Snyder HM, Harrison NW, Whitfield HN et al. Urodynamics in the prune belly syndrome. Br J Urol 1976; 48:663–70.
86. Gonzalez R, Reinberg Y, Burke B et al. Early bladder outlet obstruction in fetal lambs induces renal dysplasia and the prune belly syndrome. J Pediatr Surg 1990; 25: 342–5.
87. Welsh K, Kearney GP. Abdominal musculature deficiency syndrome: prune belly. J Urol 1974; 111:693–7.
88. Woodhouse CRJ, Ransley PG, Williams DI. Prune belly syndrome – report of 47 cases. Arch Dis Child 1982; 57:856–9.
89. Potter EL. Abnormal development of the kidney. In: Potter EL, ed. Normal and Abnormal Development of the Kidney. Chicago: Year Book Medical Publishers, 1972: 154–220.
90. Perlman M, Levin M. Fetal pulmonary hypoplasia, anuria, and oligohydramnios: clinicopathologic observations and review of the literature. Am J Obstet Gynecol 1974; 118:1119–22.
91. Randolph JG. Total surgical reconstruction for patients with abdominal muscular deficiency ('prune belly') syndrome. J Pediatr Surg 1977; 12:1033–43.
92. Snow BS, Duckett JW. Prune belly syndrome. In: Gillenwater JY, Grayhack JT, Howards SS, Duckett JW, eds. Adult and Pediatric Urology. Chicago: Year Book Medical Publishers, 1987: 1709–25.
93. Maizels M, Stephens FD. Valves of the ureter as a cause of primary obstruction of the ureter: anatomic, embryologic and clinical aspects. J Urol 1980; 123:742–7.
94. Gearhart JP, Lee BR, Partin AW et al. The quantitative histological evaluation of the dilated ureter of childhood. II: Ectopia, posterior urethral valves and the prune belly syndrome. J Urol 1995; 153:172–6.

95. Ehrlich RM, Brown WJ. Ultrastructural anatomic observations of the ureter in prune belly syndrome. Birth Defects 1977; 13:101–3.
96. Hanna MK, Jeffs RD, Sturgess JM et al. Ureteral structure and ultrastructure. Part III. The congenitally dilated ureter (megaureter). J Urol 1977; 117:24–7.
97. Perlmutter AD. Reduction cystoplasty in prune belly syndrome. J Urol 1976; 116:356–62.
98. Kinahan TJ, Churchill BM, McLorie GA et al. The efficiency of bladder emptying in prune belly syndrome. J Urol 1992; 148:600–3.
99. Bourne CW, Cerny JC. Congenital absence of abdominal muscles: report of six cases. J Urol 1967; 98:252–5.
100. Hinman F. Alternatives to orchiectomy. J Urol 1980; 123:548–51.
101. Cabral B, Majidi A, Gonzales R. Ectopic vasa deferentia in an infant with the prune belly syndrome. J Urol (Paris) 1988; 94:223–6.
102. Passerini-Glazel G, Araguna F, Chiozza L et al. The P.A.D.U.A. (progressive augmentation by dilating the urethral anterior) procedure for the treatment of severe urethral hypoplasia. J Urol 1988;140:1247–9.
103. Hutson JM, Beasley SW. Aetiology of the prune belly syndrome. Aust Paediatr J 1987; 23:309–10.
104. Shrom SH, Cromie WJ, Duckett JW. Megalourethra. Urology 1981; 17:152–6.
105. Batata MS, Chu FCH, Hilaris BI et al. Testicular cancer in cryptorchids. Cancer 1982; 49:1023–32.
106. Woodhouse CRJ, Ransley PG. Teratoma of the testis in the prune belly syndrome. Br J Urol 1983; 55:580–1.
107. Sayre R, Stephens R, Chonko AM. Prune belly syndrome and retroperitoneal germ cell tumor. Am J Med 1986; 81:895–7.
108. Tayakkanontak K. The gubernaculum and its nerve supply. Aust N Z J Surg 1963; 33:61–3.
109. Orvis BR, Bottles K, Kogan BA. Testicular histology in fetuses with prune belly syndrome and posterior urethral valves. J Urol 1988; 139:335–7.
110. Uehling DT, Zadina SP, Gilbert E. Testicular histology in triad syndrome. Urology 1984; 23:364–6.
111. Woodhouse CRJ, Snyder HM III. Testicular and sexual function in adults with prune belly syndrome. J Urol 1985; 133:607–9.
112. Woodard JR, Parrott TS. Orchidopexy in the prune belly syndrome. Br J Urol 1978; 50:348–51.
113. Kolettis PN, Ross JH, Kay R, Thomas AJ Jr. Sperm retrieval and intracystoplasmic sperm injection in patients with prune-belly syndrome. Fertil Steril 1999; 72(5):948–9.
114. Krueger RP, Hardy BE, Churchill BM. Cryptorchidism in boys with posterior urethral valves. J Urol 1980; 124:101–2.
115. Geary DF, MacLusky IB, Churchill BM et al. A broader spectrum of abnormalities in the prune belly syndrome. J Urol 1986; 135:324–6.
116. Randolph JG, Cavett C, Eng G. Abdominal wall reconstruction in the prune belly syndrome. J Pediatr Surg 1981; 16:960–4.
117. Afifi AK, Rebeiz JM, Adonia SJ et al. The myopathy of prune belly syndrome. J Neurol Sci 1972; 15:153–65.
118. Brinker MR, Palutsis RS, Sarwark JF. The orthopedic manifestations of prune belly (Eagle–Barrett) syndrome. J Bone Joint Surg Am 1995; 77:251–7.
119. Carey JC, Eggert L, Curry CJR. Lower limb deficiency and the urethral obstruction sequence. Birth Defects 1982; 18:19–28.
120. Joller R, Scheier H. Complete thoracic segmental insensibility accompanying prune belly syndrome with scoliosis. Spine 1986; 11:496–8.
121. Wright JR, Barth RF, Neff JC et al. Gastrointestinal malformations associated with prune belly syndrome: three cases and a review of the literature. Pediatr Pathol 1986; 5:421–8.
122. Teramoto R, Opas LM, Andrassy R. Splenic torsion with prune belly syndrome. J Pediatr 1981; 98:91–2.
123. Short KL, Groff DB, Cook L. The concomitant presence of gastroschisis and prune belly syndrome in a twin. J Pediatr Surg 1985; 20:186–7.
124. Walker J, Prokurat AI, Irving IM. Prune belly syndrome associated with exomphalos and anorectal agenesis. J Pediatr Surg 1987; 22:215–17.
125. Salihu HM, Tchuinguem G, Aliyu MH, Kouam L. Prune belly syndrome and associated malformations. West Indian Med J 2003; 52(4):281–4.
126. Adebonojo FO. Dysplasia of the abdominal musculature with multiple congenital anomalies: prune belly or triad syndrome. J Nat Med Assoc 1973; 65:327–9.
127. Welsh KJ. Abdominal musculature deficiency syndrome. In: Ravich MM, Welch KJ, Benson CD, Aberdeen E, Randolph JG, eds. Pediatric Surgery, 3rd edn. Chicago: Year Book Medical Publishers, 1979: 1220–32.
128. Alford BA, Peoples WM, Resnick JS et al. Pulmonary complications associated with the prune-belly syndrome. Radiology 1978; 129:401–7.
129. Ewig JM, Grissom NT, Wohl ME. The effect of the absence of abdominal muscles on pulmonary function and exercise. Am J Respir Crit Care Med 1996; 153:1314–21.
130. Yamamoto H, Nishikawa S, Hayashi T, Sagae S, Kudo R. Antenatal diagnosis of prune belly syndrome at 11 weeks of gestation. J Obstet Gynaecol Res 2001; 27(1):37–40.
131. Cromie WJ. Implications of antenatal ultrasound screening in the incidence of major genitourinary malformations. Semin Pediatr Surg 2001; 10(4):204–11.
132. Elder JS. Intrauterine intervention for obstructive uropathy. Kidney 1990; 22:19–24.
133. Leeners BL, Sauer I, Schefels J, Cotarelo CL, Funk A. Prune-belly syndrome: therapeutic options including in utero placement of a vesicoamniotic shunt. J Clin Ultrasound 2000; 28(9):500–7.
134. Makino Y, Kobayashi H, Kyono K, Oshima K, Kawarabayashi T. Clinical results of fetal obstructive uropathy treated by vesicoamniotic shunting. Urology 2000; 55(1):118–22.
135. Kaplan BS. In utero intervention in prune-belly syndrome. Pediatr Nephrol 1999; 13(2):138.
136. Johnson MP, Bukowski TP, Reitleman C. In utero surgical treatment of fetal obstructive uropathy: a new comprehensive approach to identify appropriate candidates for vesicoamniotic shunt therapy. Am J Obstet Gynecol 1994; 170:1770–6, discussion 1776–9.
137. Kramer SA. Current status of fetal intervention for hydronephrosis. J Urol 1983; 130: 641–6.

138. Gadziala NA, Kavade CY, Doherty FJ et al. Intrauterine decompression of megalocystis during the second trimester of pregnancy. Am J Obstet Gynecol 1982; 144:355–6.
139. Prescia G, Cruz JM, Weeks D. Prenatal diagnosis of prune belly syndrome by means of raised maternal alphafetoprotein level. J Genet Hum 1982; 30:271–3.
140. Golbus MS, Harrison MR, Filly RA et al. In utero treatment of urinary tract obstruction. Am J Obstet Gynecol 1982; 142:383–8.
141. Alford BA, Peoples WM, Resnick JS et al. Pulmonary complications associated with the prune-belly syndrome. Radiology 1978; 129: 401–7.
142. Noh PH, Cooper CS, Zderic SA et al. Prognostic factors in patients with prune belly syndrome. J Urol 1999; 162:1399–401.
143. Appleman Z, Golbus MS. The management of fetal urinary tract obstruction. Clin Obstet Gynecol 1986; 29:483–6.
144. Arant BS Jr. Development patterns of renal functional maturation compared in the human neonate. J Pediatr 1978; 92:705–12.
145. Chevalier RL. Perinatal renal development and physiology. AUA Update Ser 1989; 8:58–60.
146. Aaronson IA. Posterior urethral valve masquerading as the prune belly syndrome. Br J Urol 1983; 55:508–12.
147. Krueger RP. Posterior urethral valves masquerading as prune belly syndrome. Urology 1981; 18:182–4.
148. Rushton HG, Majd M, Chandra R, Yim D. Evaluation of 99m technetium dimercaptosuccinic acid renal scans in experimental acute pyelonephritis in piglets. J Urol 1988; 140:1169–74.
149. Duckett JW Jr. Cutaneous vesicostomy in childhood. Urol Clin North Am 1974; 1:485–92.
150. Whitaker RH. Methods of assessing obstruction in dilated ureters. Br J Urol 1973; 45:15–22.
151. Smith CA, Smith EA, Parrott TS et al. Voiding function in patients with the prune belly syndrome after Monfort abdominoplasty. J Urol 1998; 159:1675–9.
152. Hannington-Kiff JG. Prune belly syndrome and general anesthesia. Br J Anaesth 1970; 42:649–52.
153. Karamanian A, Kravath R, Nagashima H et al. Anesthetic management of prune belly syndrome: a case report. Br J Anaesth 1974; 46:897–9.
154. Henderson AM, Vallis CJ, Sumner E. Anesthesia in the prune belly syndrome: a review of 36 cases. Anesthesia 1987;42:54–60.
155. King LR. Idiopathic dilatation of the posterior urethra in boys without bladder outlet obstruction. J Urol 1969; 102:783–7.
156. Cukier J. Resection of the urethra with the prune belly syndrome. Birth Defects 1977; 13:95–6.
157. Kinahan TJ, Churchill BM, McLorie GA et al. The efficiency of bladder emptying in the prune belly syndrome. J Urol 1992; 148:600–3.
158. Duckett JW Jr, Knutrud O, Hohenfellner R et al. Prune belly syndrome. Dialog Pediatr Urol 1980; 3:1–7.
159. Woodard JR. Prune-belly syndrome. In: Kelalis PP, King LR, Belman AB, eds. Clinical Pediatric Urology. Philadelphia: WB Saunders, 1985: 805–24.
160. Binard JE, Zoedler D. Treatment of hypotonic decompensated urinary bladder. Int Surg 1968; 50:502–7.
161. Bukowski TP, Perlmutter AD. Reduction cystoplasty in the prune belly syndrome: a long-term follow-up. J Urol 1994; 152:2113–16.
162. Denes FT, Arap MA, Giron AM, Silva FA, Arap S. Comprehensive surgical treatment of prune belly syndrome: 17 years' experience with 32 patients. Urology 2004; 64(4):789–93, discussion 793–4.
163. Hendren WH. Functional restoration of decompensated ureters in children. Am J Surg 1970; 119:477–82.
164. Ehrlich RM. The ureteral folding technique for megaureter surgery. J Urol 1985; 134:668–70.
165. Ransley PG, Vordermark JS, Caldamone AA, Bellinger MF. Preliminary ligation of the gonadal vessels prior to orchidopexy for the intra-abdominal testicle: a staged Fowler–Stephens procedure. World J Urol 1984; 2:266–9.
166. Patil AA, Duffy PG, Woodhouse CRJ, Ransley PG. Long-term outcome of Fowler–Stephens orchiopexy in boys with prune-belly syndrome. J Urol 2004; 171:1666–9.
167. Gibbons DM, Cromie WJ, Duckett JW. Management of the abdominal undescended testicle. J Urol 1979; 122:76–9.
168. Docimo SG. The results of surgical therapy for cryptorchidism: a literature review and analysis. J Urol 1995; 154:1148–52.
169. Fowler R, Stephens FD. The role of testicular vascular anatomy in the salvage of high undescended testes. Aust NZ J Surg 1959; 29:92–6.
170. Bloom DA. Two step orchiopexy with pelviscopic clip ligation of the spermatic vessels. J Urol 1991; 145: 1030–3.
171. Yu TJ, Lai MK, Chen WF et al. Two stage orchiopexy with laparoscopic clip ligation of the spermatic vessels in prune belly syndrome. J Pediatr Surg 1995; 30:870–2.
172. Wacksman J, Dinner M, Staffon RA. Technique of testicular autotransplantation using a microvascular anastomosis. Surg Obstet Gynecol 1980; 150:399–401.
173. Ehrlich RM, Lesavoy MA, Fine RN. Total abdominal wall reconstruction in the prune belly syndrome. J Urol 1986; 136:282–5.
174. Monfort G, Guys JM, Bocciardi A et al. A novel technique for reconstruction of the abdominal wall in prune belly syndrome. J Urol 1991; 146:639–40.
175. Parrott TS, Woodard JRR. The Monfort operation for the abdominal wall reconstruction in the prune belly syndrome. J Urol 1992; 148:688–90.
176. Furness PD III, Cheng EY, Franco I et al. The prune belly syndrome: a new and simplified technique for abdominal wall reconstruction. J Urol 1998; 160: 1195–7.
177. Bukowski TP, Smith CA. Monfort abdominoplasty with neoumbilical modification. J Urol 2000; 164:1711–13.
178. Shenasky JH, Whelchel JD. Renal transplantation in prune belly syndrome. J Urol 1976; 115:112–13.
179. Dreikorn K, Palmtag H, Rohl L. Prune belly syndrome: treatment of terminal renal failure by hemodialysis and renal transplantation. Eur Urol 1978; 3:245–7.
180. Reinberg Y, Manivel JC, Fryd P et al. The outcome of renal transplantation in children with the prune belly syndrome. J Urol 1989; 142:1541–2.

181. Fontaine E, Salomon L, Gaganadoux MF et al. Long term results of renal transplantation in children with the prune belly syndrome. J Urol 1997; 158:892–4.
182. Gonzales R. Editorial: renal transplantation into abnormal bladders. J Urol 1997; 158:895.
183. Messing EM, Dibbell DG, Belzer FO. Bilateral rectus femoris pedicle flaps for detrusor augmentation in the prune belly syndrome. J Urol 1985;134:1202–4.
184. Kogan SJ, Weiss R, Hanna M et al. Successful renal transplantation into a patient with neurogenic bladder managed by clean intermittent catheterization. J Urol 1986; 135:563–5.
185. Marvin RG, Halff GA, Elshihabi I. Renal allograft torsion associated with prune belly syndrome. Pediatr Nephrol 1995; 9:81–2.

SECTION VI

Urethra, External Genitalia, and Retroperitoneum

Basic science of the genitalia

65

Laurence S Baskin

Introduction

Genital anomalies are the most common birth defects with the exception of cardiac malformations. Hypospadias is defined as an arrest in normal development of the urethra, foreskin, and ventral aspect of the penis; it is the most common genital anomaly, occurring in approximately 1:250 newborns or roughly 1 out of 125 live male births.[1] Hypospadias results in a wide range of abnormalities, with the urethral opening located anywhere along the shaft of the penis, within the scrotum or even in the perineum (Figure 65.1a–c). Hypospadias is also associated with ventral penile curvature (chordee). Left uncorrected, patients with severe hypospadias may need to sit down to void and tend to shun intimate relationships because of fears related to abnormal sexuality. Babies born with severe hypospadias and penile curvature may have 'ambiguous genitalia' in the newborn period, making an immediate and accurate sex assignment difficult.

Epispadias is a urethral defect on the dorsal aspect of the penis (Figure 65.1d). Epispadias is associated with a short penis, dorsal penile curvature, and, in the most severe forms, bladder exstrophy. Females (as

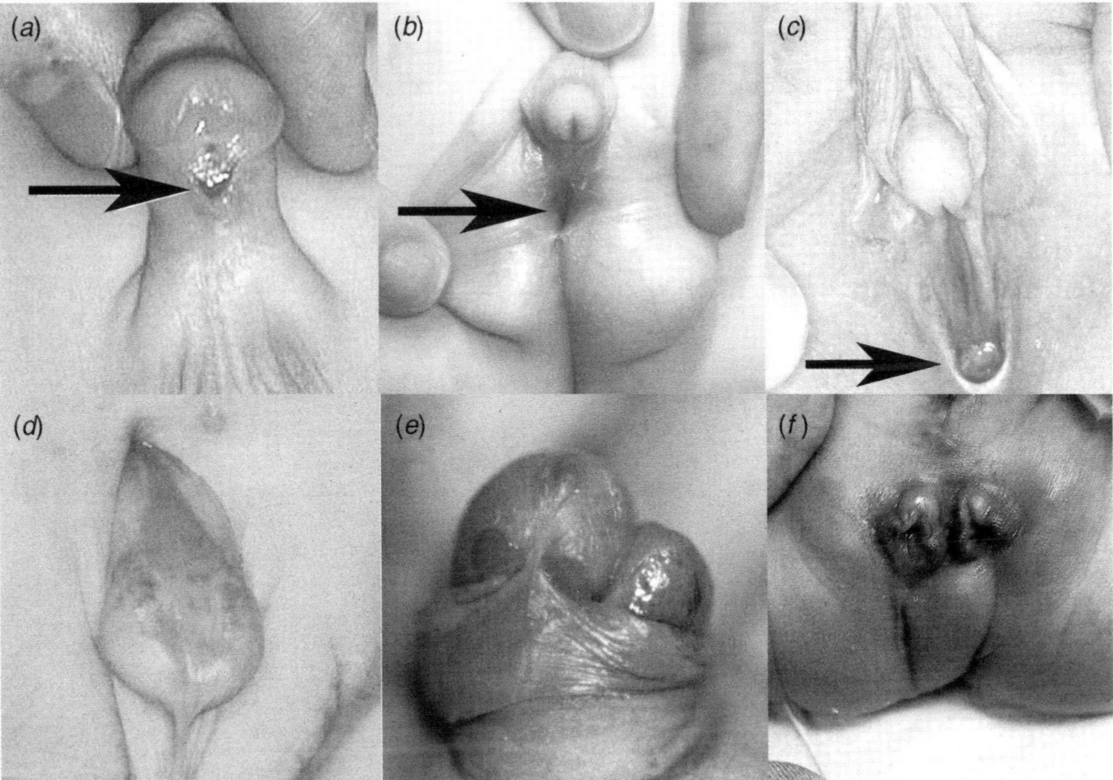

Figure 65.1 Genital abnormalities: (*a*) distal hypospadias; (*b*) scrotal hypospadias; (*c*) perineal hypospadias secondary to type II 5α-reductase deficiency; (*d*) epispadias; (*e*) penile duplication anomaly; (*f*) Complete duplication of the female external genitalia.

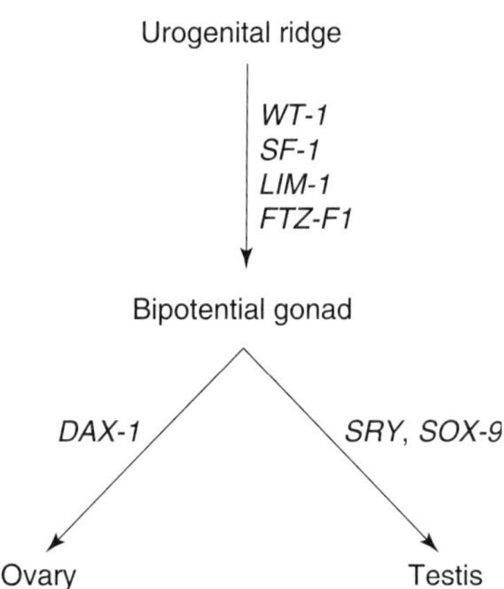

Figure 65.2 Sex-determining genes involved in testes and ovarian development.

well as males) can also suffer from these genital anomalies, and others such as genital duplication or malformations, but these problems are extremely rare (Figure 65.1e,f). To understand abnormal development of the external genitalia requires a concise knowledge of normal genital development.

Normal sexual differentiation

Chromosomal sex

The genetic material necessary for the development of the male phenotype is normally located on the short arm of the Y chromosome. The critical gene or sex-determining region on the Y chromosome is known as the *SRY* region.[2] The gene products of the *SRY* genetic cascade will subsequently direct the development of the testis by interacting with multiple other genes such as *SOX-9*. Genetic information that is necessary for male and female development beyond gonadal differentiation is located on the X chromosome and on the autosomes.

Gonadal differentiation

The gonads develop from the urogenital ridges (Figure 65.2), which are formed during the 4th week of gestation by the proliferation of the coelomic epithelium and condensation of the underlying mesenchyme along the mesonephros. The germ cells located in the endoderm of the yolk sac migrate to the genital ridges. At the early stage of development the gonad is bipotential, capable of forming into either a testis or ovary. During the 6th to 7th week of gestation, at least four different genes – Wilms' tumor suppressor gene (*WT-1*), Fushi–Tarza factor-1 (*FTZ-F1*) steroidogenic factor-1 (*SF-1*), and *LIM-1* – induce the development of the testis. The primordial germ cells differentiate into the Sertoli cells and associated Leydig cells, which aggregate into spermatogenic cords. Loose mesenchymal tissue condenses into a thick layer, the tunica albuginea, that surrounds the testis and separates it from the coelomic epithelium,

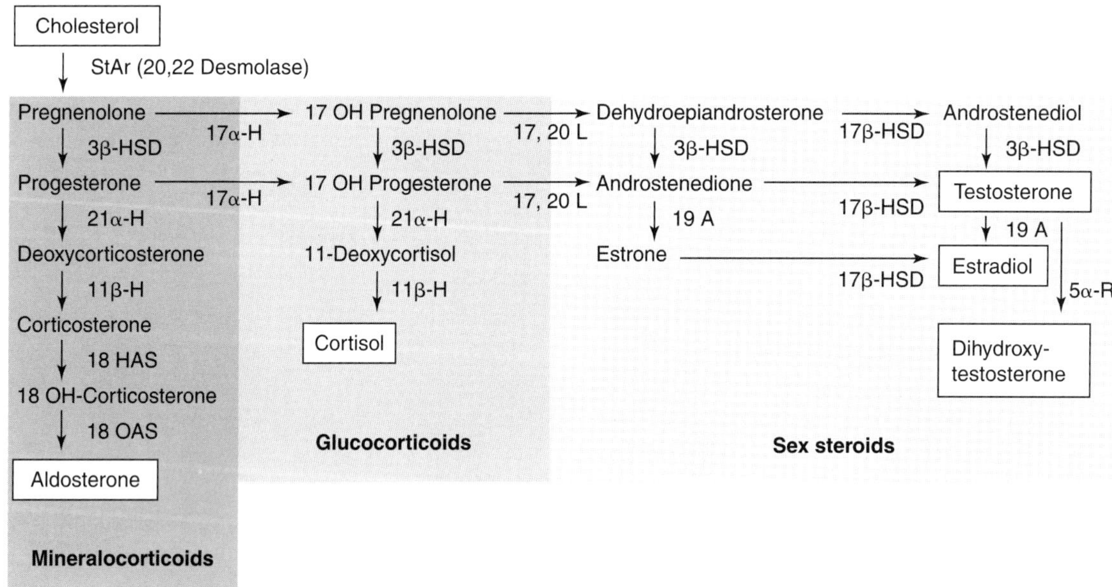

Figure 65.3 Pathway of steroid hormone biosynthesis and possible enzyme deficiencies: 3β-HSD = 3β-hydroxysteroid dehydrogenase; 17α-H = 17α-hydroxylase; 21α-H = 21α-hydroxylase; 11β-H = 11β-hydroxylase; 17, 20 L = 17, 20-lyase; 17β-HSD = 17β-hydroxysteroid dehydrogenase; 18 HAS = 18-hydroxyaldosterone synthetase; 18 OAS = 18 oxidase-aldosterone synthetase, 5α-R = 5α-reductase; 19 A = 19-aromatase.

thereby preventing further migration of mesonephric cells into the testis.

Classic teaching is that the female phenotype is the default developmental pathway in the absence of the *SRY* cascade. It is now known that at least one gene – dosage sensitive sex reversal (*DAX-1*) – is essential for ovarian development. *DAX-1* is located on the short arm of the X chromosome. The gene products of SRY and *DAX-1* compete to stimulate the steroidogenic acute regulatory protein (StAR). The StAR protein is the first step in steroidogenesis, facilitating the conversion of cholesterol to pregnenolone (Figure 65.3). In the normal XY male, *SRY* overwhelms the one functional *DAX-1* gene, stimulating testicular development and subsequent testosterone production. In the normal XX female, two *DAX-1* genes are present without the competitive SRY, down-regulating StAR and hence inhibiting testicular development, which results in ovarian development. In the fetal ovaries, the germ cells differentiate and are arrested in the last phase of meiotic prophase, forming the oocytes. The cells in the genital ridges develop into granulosa cells, which surround the oocytes and complete the formation of the ovaries.

Hormones

At 3.5 weeks' gestation, the wolffian system appears as two longitudinal ducts connecting cranially to the mesonephros and caudually draining into the urogenital sinus (Figure 65.4). At approximately the 6th week of gestation, the müllerian duct develops as an evagination in the coelomic epithelium just lateral to the wolffian duct.

During the 8th–9th week of gestation Sertoli cells of the fetal testis secrete a glycoprotein, müllerian-inhibiting substance (MIS) or anti-müllerian hormone. This protein induces the regression of the müllerian ducts through the dissolution of the basement membrane and condensation of mesenchymal cells around the müllerian duct. Because MIS acts locally, müllerian duct regression occurs only on the ipsilateral side of the fetal testis, producing this hormone. MIS also induces the formation of seminiferous tubules and further differentiation of the testis. At the 9th or 10th week of gestation, the Leydig cells appear in the testis and begin to synthesize testosterone. This hormone transforms the wolffian duct into the male genital tract, which is completed by the end of the 11th week of gestation.

Beginning in the 9th week of gestation, testosterone also induces the development of the external genitalia (Figure 65.5) from the genital tubercle, urogenital sinus, and genital swellings. At the molecular level, testosterone is converted to 5α-dihydrotestosterone (DHT) by the microsomal enzyme, type 2 5α-reductase, which is responsible for complete differentiation of the penis with a male-type urethra and glans. Testosterone dissociates from its carrier proteins in the plasma and enters cells via passive diffusion. Once in the cell, testosterone binds to the androgen receptor (AR) and induces changes in conformation, protecting it from degradation by proteolytic enzymes. This conformational change is also required for AR dimerization, DNA binding, and transcriptional activation, which are all necessary for testosterone to be expressed. Androgen binding also displaces heat shock proteins, possibly relieving constraints on receptor dimerization or DNA binding. After entering the nucleus, the AR complex then binds androgen response element DNA regulatory sequences within the androgen responsive genes and

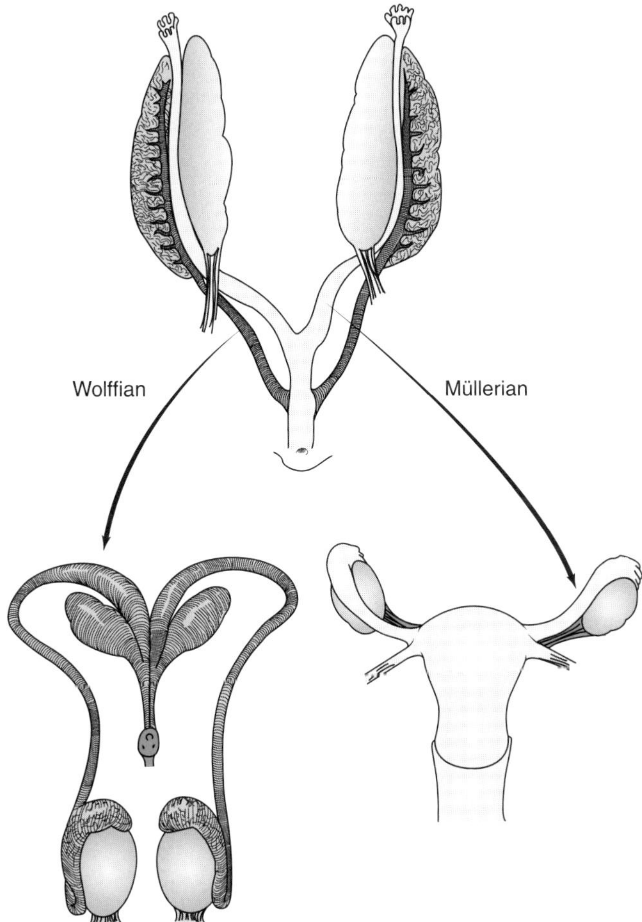

Figure 65.4 Schematic of male (wolffian) and female (müllerian) internal and external genital development from a common origin.

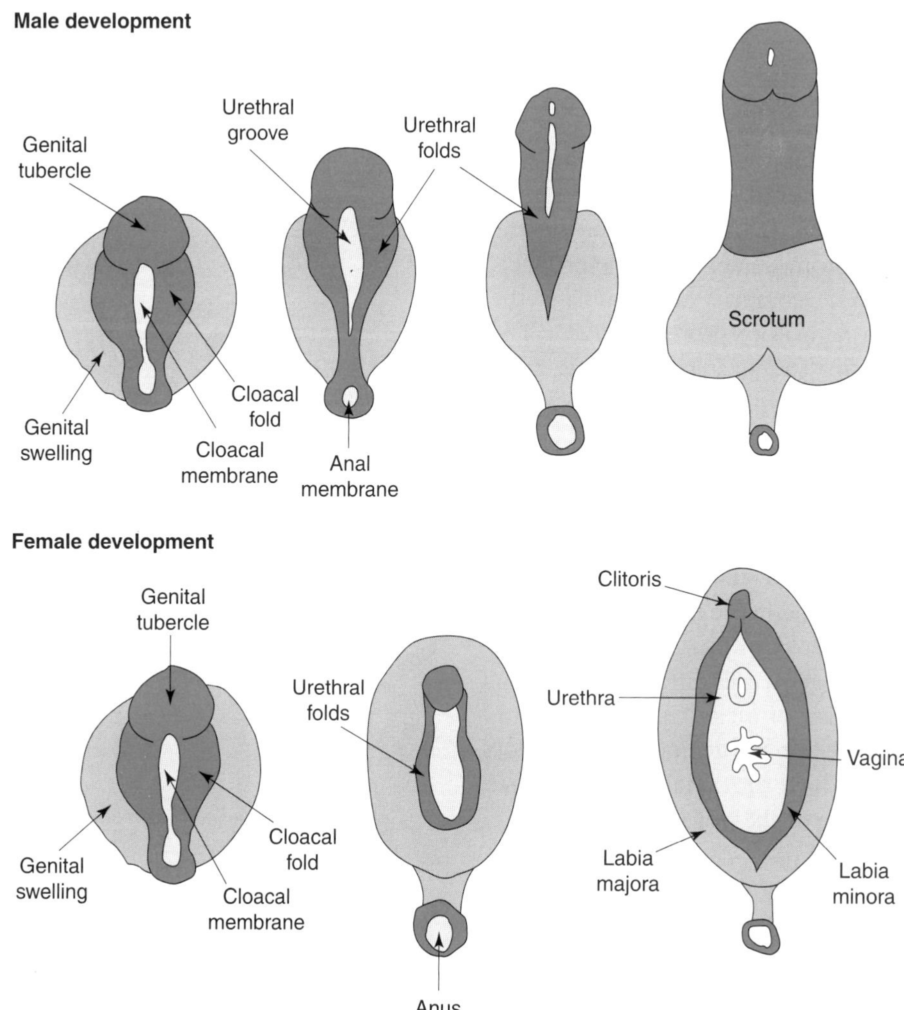

Figure 65.5 Differentiation of the male and female external genitalia from the indifferent stage to full differentiation (8–16 weeks).

activates them. DHT also binds the AR, with greater androgenic activity than testosterone, in part because of its slow dissociation rate from the AR.

DHT then binds to nuclear receptors, forming a complex that regulates the transformation of these tissues into the glans penis, penile and cavernous urethra, Cowper's glands, prostate, and scrotum. At the 28th–37th week of gestation, testicular descent into the scrotum begins. Although its mechanism is not completely understood, it is clearly an androgen-dependent-process.

The female internal genitalia develop from the müllerian ducts. Without the hormones produced by the testis, the wolffian ducts regress at the 9th week of gestation. At the same time, the müllerian ducts begin to differentiate; the cranial portions form the fallopian tubes, while the caudal portions fuse to form the uterus, cervix, and the upper portion of the vagina. Concurrently, the external genitalia, defined as the lower portion of the vagina, the vestibule, Bartholin's and Skene's glands, the clitoris, and labia minora and majora, develop from the urogenital sinus and genital tubercles. Like the testis, the ovary undergoes a partial transabdominal descent. However, transinguinal descent of the ovary does not occur, leaving the ovaries just below the rim of the true pelvis. The role of estrogen in the differentiation of the female phenotype is unclear.

Embryology: development of the male external urogenital system

Formation of the external male genitalia is a complex developmental process involving genetic programming, cell differentiation, hormonal signaling,

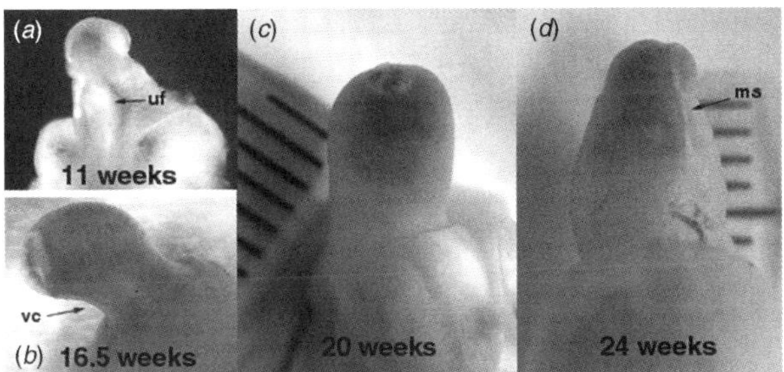

Figure 65.6 Male human fetal external genitalia during gestation. (*a*) At 11 weeks' gestation, note the urethra is open and the urethral fold (uf) and groove are prominent in the transillumination view of the phallus. (*b*) At 16.5 weeks' gestation, note the normal ventral curvature (vc) is shown and the foreskin, which is almost completely formed. (*c*) At 20 weeks' gestation, penile and urethral development looks complete, with the prepuce covering glans and the penile curvature resolving. (*d*) At 24 weeks, the prepuce covers the whole glans; note the midline seam (ms). Note the progression of natural curvature to a straight phallus during development.

enzyme activity, and tissue remodeling.[3] By the end of the 1st month of gestation, the hindgut and future urogenital system reach the ventral surface of the embryo at the cloacal membrane.[4] The cloacal membrane divides the urorectal septum into a posterior, or anal half, and an anterior half, the urogenital membrane. Three protuberances appear around the latter. The most cephalad is the genital tubercle. The other two, the genital swellings, flank the urogenital membrane on each side. Up to this point, the male and female genitalia are indistinguishable. Under the influence of testosterone in response to a surge of luteinizing hormone from the pituitary, masculinization of the external genitalia takes place (see Figure 65.5). One of the first signs of masculinization is an increase in the distance between the anus and the genital structures, followed by elongation of the phallus, formation of the penile urethra from the urethral groove, and development of the prepuce.[5,6]

At 8 weeks' gestation the external genitalia remain in the indifferent stage (see Figure 65.5). The urethral groove on the ventral surface of the phallus is between the paired urethral folds (Figure 65.6). The penile urethra forms as a result of fusion of the medial edges of the endodermal urethral folds. The ectodermal edges of the urethral groove fuse to form the median raphe. By 12 weeks the coronal sulcus separates the glans from the shaft of the penis. The urethral folds have completely fused in the midline on the ventrum of the penile shaft. During the 16th week of gestation the glandular urethra appears. The mechanism of the glandular urethral formation remains controversial. Evidence suggests two possible explanations: endodermal cellular differentiation or primary intrusion of the ectodermal tissue from the glans (Figure 65.7).

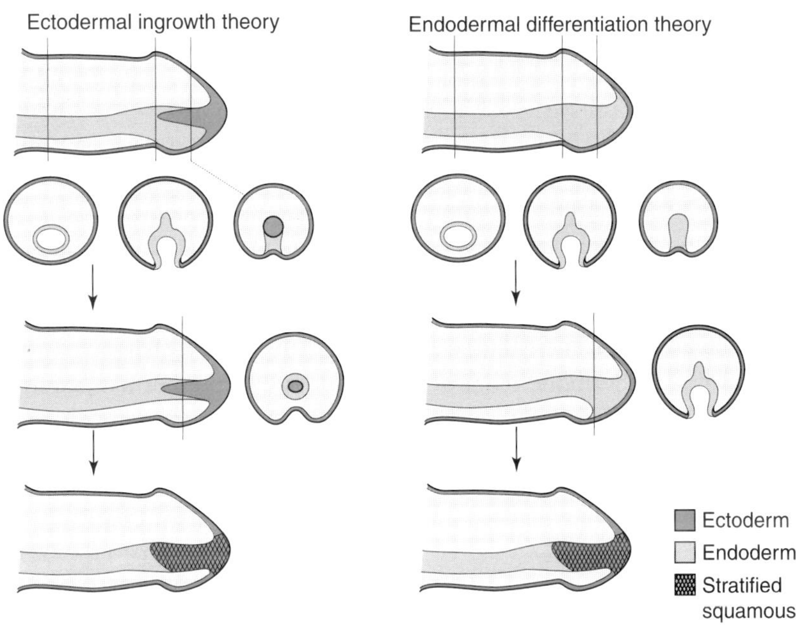

Figure 65.7 Theories of human penile urethral development. The ectodermal ingrowth theory, as described in most textbooks of embryology, postulates that the glandular urethra is formed by ingrowth of epidermis. More recent data support the formation of the entire urethra via endodermal differentiation alone.

Anatomic and immunohistochemical studies advocate the new theory of endodermal differentiation, which shows that epithelium of the entire urethra is of urogenital sinus origin.[7] The entire male urethra, including the glandular urethra, is formed by dorsal growth of the urethral plate into the genital tubercle and ventral growth and fusion of the urethral folds. Under proper mesenchymal induction, urothelium has the ability to differentiate into a stratified squamous phenotype with characteristic keratin staining, thereby explaining the cell type of the glans penis.[8] There is no evidence of an ectodermal ingrowth, as was historically proposed (old theory).[9]

The future prepuce is forming at the same time as the urethra and is dependent on normal urethral development. At about 8 weeks' gestation, low preputial folds appear on both sides of the penile shaft, which join dorsally to form a flat ridge at the proximal edge of the corona. The ridge does not entirely encircle the glans because it is blocked on the ventrum by incomplete development of the glandular urethra. Thus, the preputial fold is transported distally by active growth of the mesenchyme between it and the glandular lamella. The process continues until the preputial fold (foreskin) covers all of the glans (see Figure 65.6). The fusion is usually present at birth, but subsequent desquamation of the epithelial fusion allows the prepuce to retract. If the genital folds fail to fuse, the preputial tissues do not form ventrally; consequently, in hypospadias, preputial tissue is absent on the ventrum and is excessive dorsally.

Genital malformations

Unfortunately, to date there is no sound understanding of the etiology of genital anomalies and specifically hypospadias (which is the most common defect) that can inform primary prevention efforts and improve therapeutics. However, much is known about the genetics of hypospadias, hormone requirements for normal development, and environmental toxins, and a possible explanation for the increasing incidence of hypospadias that has already been noted.

Genetic impairment

Uncertainty about the etiology of hypospadias is in part a reflection of the complicated and incompletely understood molecular and cellular basis for normal phallus and urethral development.[10] It is well established that the urethral folds fuse during the formation of the penile urethra in the 7th–12th week after ovulation.[3] Fusion of the folds eventually leads to a fully formed penis, a process that is dependent on the synthesis of testosterone by the fetal testis. Adequate virilization of the urogenital sinus and external genitalia during embryogenesis is also dependent on the conversion of testosterone to DHT by 5α-reductase.

Increasingly, researchers are examining the role of cellular signals other than testosterone and DHT in the morphogenesis of the phallus and the etiology of hypospadias. Normal embryogenesis of the urogenital system depends on epithelial–mesenchymal interactions, and it has been hypothesized that aberrant signaling between epithelium and mesenchyme could lead to hypospadias.[8] For example, prostate development requires 'testosterone-dependent Sonic hedgehog (Shh) expression in the epithelium of the urogenital sinus'.[11] In the mouse null for Shh not only is penile development inhibited but also there is a cloacal defect.[12,13] Mice null for fibroblast growth factor 10 have a proximal urethra opening and a flattened glans consistent with the hypospadias defect.[12] It is likely that researchers may find similar genetic, signaling molecules involved in epithelial–mesenchymal interactions in the phallus that play a role in its development.

Another area of investigation with respect to the etiology of hypospadias is the expression and regulation of homeobox (*Hox*) genes. These genes are transcriptional regulators that play an essential role in directing embryonic development. Genes of the *Hox A* and *Hox D* clusters are expressed in regionalized domains along the axis of the urogenital tract. Transgenic mice with loss of function of single *Hox A* or *Hox D* genes exhibit homeotic transformations and impaired morphogenesis of the urogenital tract.[14–17] Human males with hand–foot–genital (HFG) syndrome, an autosomal dominant disorder characterized by a mutation in *HOXA13*, exhibit hypospadias of variable severity, suggesting that *HOXA13* may be important in the normal patterning of the penis.[18–20] Furthermore, recent research has shown that the embryonic expression of certain *Hox* genes is regulated by hormonal factors.[21] Estrogen and the synthetic estrogen diethylstilbestrol (DES), for example, inhibit *HOXA9*, *HOXA10*, *HOXA11*, and *HOXA13* genes in mice. Thus, in addition to defects in *Hox* genes, it is possible that improper regulation or expression of hormonal factors during embryogenesis could disrupt normal expression of *Hox* genes and lead to reproductive tract anomalies.

Hormone receptor impairment

Studies examining the androgen receptor have yielded even less insight into the etiology of hypospadias. In fact, a number of studies have concluded that defects in the AR or mutations in the AR coding sequence are rare in patients with hypospadias.[22,23] In addition, Bentvelsen et al measured AR expression in the foreskins of boys with hypospadias and age-matched controls and found no significant difference in mean AR content.[24]

Enzyme impairment

Despite the central role that testosterone plays, attempts to ascribe all hypospadias to an underlying genetic defect in this pathway have only rarely been successful. Holmes et al determined the incidence of defects in three major enzymes in the biosynthetic pathway of testosterone: 3β-hydroxysteroid dehydrogenase, 17α-hydroxylase, and 17,20 lyase (see Figure 65.3). Morning fasting serum samples of pregnenolone, progesterone, 11-deoxycorticosterone, 17-hydroxypregnenolone, 17-hydroxyprogesterone, 11-deoxycortisol, cortisol, dehydroepiandrosterone (DHEA), androstenedione, androstenediol, testosterone, and DHT were obtained.[25] No significant differences in the androgen precursors and metabolites were found between the controls and the individuals with hypospadias. The response to adrenocorticotropic hormone (ACTH) was variable, without a significant difference between the patients with different degrees of hypospadias and/or published controls. These data indicate that enzymatic defects in the steroidogenic steps from cholesterol to DHT are not a frequent etiology of hypospadias.

Environmental factors and endocrine disruptors

In the past, environmental factors were generally ruled out as causes for hypospadias.[26,27] More recently, multicausality models include environmental contaminants to determine the risk of developing a given phenotype. For example, familial clustering of hypospadias among first-degree relatives has been perceived as under the influence of a strong genetic and heritable component, but there have been many exceptions where genetics were ruled out. More recently, it has been suggested that environmental influences should be considered as well, taking into consideration that families share similar exposure: especially in those cases where the effects are the most profound, genetic predisposition exacerbated by environmental exposure should be considered.[28,29]

Attempts to determine risk factors for hypospadias have yielded a number of maternal and paternal risk factors. Among traditional studies of maternal risk factors for congenital anomalies, maternal age and primiparity are significantly associated with hypospadias, although some studies have contested the maternal age effect.[26] Paternal risk factors associated with hypospadias include abnormalities of the father's scrotum or testes[30] and low spermatozoa motility and abnormal sperm morphology.[28] It has been suggested that the recent increase in hypospadias reflects the improvement in fertility treatment, contributing to more subfertile men fathering children. As the authors state, this 'relaxed-selection hypothesis, which states that there is a redistribution in the number of children born to fertile and infertile (subfertile) couples, may account for the increasing number of other defects and cancers of male genitalia observed today and the fall in sperm counts'.[28]

In addition to parental risk factors, there is strong consensus in the literature that boys with hypospadias have lower birth weight.[31] Fredell et al examined hypospadias in discordant monozygotic twins and found that the twin with hypospadias weighed 78% of the twin without hypospadias. The birth weight difference was still significant when compared with birth weight difference between healthy monozygotic twins. Another study found that boys with hypospadias have a lower placental weight than control boys.[27] A 1995 meta-analysis of first-trimester exposure to progestins and oral contraceptives did not indicate an increased risk of hypospadias.[32] Exposure to DES was excluded in this study. However, a number of studies do list gestational exposure to progestins as a causal agent. Another recent study links a maternal vegetarian diet during pregnancy with an increase in the incidence of hypospadias.[33] This study looked at 51 boys with hypospadias from a group of 7928 boys born to mothers taking part in the Avon Longitudinal Study of Pregnancy and Childhood (ALSPAC). The authors hypothesize that vegetarians have a greater exposure to phytoestrogens than omnivores. The phytoestrogens may come in the form of soy, which is high in isoflavones, or be related to endocrine disrupters in pesticides and fertilizers.[34]

Whereas these risk factors do not reveal direct information about the etiology of hypospadias, they provide additional information that may reveal a common developmental pathway and can inform future research. For example, there is growing evidence that androgens play a central role in the lower birth weight of girls than boys.[35] They are also crucial to the development of the male reproductive tract; thus, perhaps exposure to an agent that compromises the weight-gaining advantage of an androgen during gestation could play a role in the development of hypospadias and lowered birth weight.

Increasing rates of hypospadias have paralleled reports of other untoward endpoints related to male reproductive health, including increases in testicular cancer,[36] increasing incidence of cryptorchidism, and decreasing semen and sperm quality.[37] In another study, 8% of patients diagnosed with undescended testes (n = 252) had urogenital anomalies and over 50% of those had hypospadias.[38] The increasing incidence over the past 50 years of multiple endpoints, co-occurring with increasing production and use of synthetic chemicals, has raised concerns that environmental factors may play a role in the etiology of these problems.[29,39] It is now well documented, from wildlife studies and accompanying laboratory data, that a number of synthetic and natural chemicals commonly found in the environment can mimic or antagonize hormones or otherwise interfere with the development and function of the endocrine and reproductive systems.[40,41] Pregnant mice subjected to in-utero exposure to both estrogen and prednisone have been shown to develop hypospadias.[42] Whether endocrine disruptors are having an impact on human male reproductive health and on hypospadias in particular is difficult to determine.[43] Regardless, public health agencies worldwide are increasingly concerned about endocrine disruption and it remains an active area of research.[44–46]

Conclusion

Great strides have been made in understanding the molecular mechanism of genital formation. Understanding normal development is necessary to elucidate the etiology of abnormalities such as hypospadias. Recent work suggests that environmental exposure to endocrine disruptors may account for the increase in incidence of hypospadias cases. Prevention by reducing exposure may be the best strategy to reverse the increasing incidence of hypospadias.

References

1. Paulozzi L, Erickson D, Jackson R. Hypospadias trends in two US surveillance systems. Pediatrics 1997; 100:831–834.
2. Grumbach MM, Conte FA, Hughes IA. Disorders of sex differentiation. In: Reed Larsen P, Kronenberg H, Melmed S, Polonsky K, eds. Williams, Textbook of Endocrinology, 10th edn. Amsterdam: Elsevier, 2003: 842–1002.
3. Baskin LS. Hypospadias and urethral development. J Urol 2000; 163:951–6.
4. Cunha G, Baskin L. Development of the penile urethra. In: Baskin LS, ed. Hypospadias and Genital Development. Philadelphia: Kluwer Academic/Plenum, 2004:87–100.
5. Jirasek J, Raboch J, Uher J. The relationship between the development of gonads and external genitals in human fetuses. Am J Obstet Gynecol 1968; 101:830–3.
6. Hinman FJ. Penis and male urethra. In: Hinman FJ, ed. Atlas of UroSurgical Anatomy. Philadelphia: WB Saunders, 1993:418–70.
7. Kurzrock EA, Baskin LS, Cunha GR. Ontogeny of the male urethra: theory of endodermal differentiation. Differentation 1999; 64:115–22.
8. Kurzrock EA, Baskin LS, Li Y, Cunha GR. Epithelial–mesenchymal interactions in development of the mouse fetal genital tubercle. Cells Tissues Organs 1999; 164:1015–20.
9. Glenister T. The origin and fate of the urethral plate in man. J Anat 1954; 288:413–18.
10. Wilson JD, George FW, Griffin JE. The hormonal control of sexual development. Science 1981; 211:1278–84.
11. Podlasek CA, Barnett DH, Clemens JQ, Bak PM, Bushman W. Prostate development requires Sonic hedgehog expressed by the urogenital sinus epithelium. Dev Biol 1999; 209:28–39.
12. Yucel S, Liu W, Cordero D, Donjacour A, Cunha G, Baskin L. Anatomical studies of the fibroblast growth factor-10 mutant, sonic hedgehog mutant, and androgen receptor mutant mouse genital tubercle. In: Baskin L, ed. Hypospadias and Genital Development. Philadelphia: Kluwer Academic/Plenum, 2004:123–45.
13. Baskin L, Liu W, Bastacky J, Yucel S. Anatomical studies of the mouse genital tubercle. In: Baskin LS, ed. Hypospadias and Genital Development. Philadelphia: Kluwer Academic/Plenum, 2004:103–20.
14. Dolle P, Izpisua-Belmonte JC, Brown JM, Tickle C, Duboule D. HOX-4 genes and the morphogenesis of mammalian genitalia. Genes Dev 1991; 5:1767–7.
15. Benson GV, Lim H, Paria BC et al. Mechanisms of reduced fertility in Hoxa-10 mutant mice: uterine homeosis and loss of maternal Hoxa-10 expression. Development 1996; 122:2687–96.
16. Hsieh-Li HM, Witte DP, Weinstein M et al. Hoxa 11 structure, extensive antisense transcription, and function in male and female fertility. Development 1995; 121:1373–85.
17. Podlasek CA, Duboule D, Bushman W. Male accessory sex organ morphogenesis is altered by loss of function of Hoxd-13. Dev Dyn 1997; 208:454–65.
18. Mortlock DP, Innis JW. Mutation of HOXA13 in hand-foot-genital syndrome [see comments]. Nat Genet 1997; 15:179–80.
19. Donnenfeld AE, Schrager DS, Corson SL. Update on a family with hand-foot-genital syndrome: hypospadias and

urinary tract abnormalities in two boys from the fourth generation. Am J Med Genet 1992; 44:482–4.

20. Fryns JP, Vogels A, Decock P, van den Berghe H. The hand-foot-genital syndrome: on the variable expression in affected males. Clin Genet 1993; 43:232–4.
21. Ma L, Benson GV, Lim H, Dey SK, Maas RL. Abdominal B (AbdB) Hoxa genes: regulation in adult uterus by estrogen and progesterone and repression in müllerian duct by the synthetic estrogen diethylstilbestrol (DES). Dev Biol 1998; 197:141–54.
22. McPhaul MJ, Marcelli M, Zoppi S, Griffin JE, Wilson JD. Genetic basis of endocrine disease. 4. The spectrum of mutations in the androgen receptor gene that causes androgen resistance. J Clin Endocrinol Metab 1993; 76:17–23.
23. Hiort O, Klauber G, Cendron M et al. Molecular characterization of the androgen receptor gene in boys with hypospadias. Eur J Pediatr 1994; 153:317–21.
24. Bentvelsen FM, Brinkmann AO, van der Linden JE, Schroder FH, Nijman JM. Decreased immunoreactive androgen receptor levels are not the cause of isolated hypospadias. Br J Urol 1995; 76:384–8.
25. Holmes NM, Miller WL, Baskin LS. Lack of defects in androgen production in children with hypospadias. J Clin Endocrinol Metab 2004; 89:2811–16.
26. Harris EL. Genetic epidemiology of hypospadias. Epidemiol Rev 1990; 12:29–40.
27. Stoll C, Alembik Y, Roth MP, Dott B. Genetic and environmental factors in hypospadias. J Med Genet 1990; 27:559–63.
28. Fritz G, Czeizel AE. Abnormal sperm morphology and function in the fathers of hypospadiacs. J Reprod Fertil 1996; 106:63–6.
29. Baskin LS, Himes K, Colborn T. Hypospadias and endocrine disruption: is there a connection? Environ Health Perspect 2001; 109:1175–83.
30. Sweet R, Schrott H, Kurland R, Culp O. Study of the incidence of hypospadias in Rochester, Minnesota 1940–1970, and a case-control comparison of possible etiologic factors. Mayo Clin Proc 1974; 49:52–8.
31. Fredell L, Lichtenstein P, Pedersen NL, Svensson J, Nordenskjold A. Hypospadias is related to birth weight in discordant monozygotic twins. J Urol 1998; 160:2197–9.
32. Raman-Wilms L, Tseng AL, Wighardt S, Einarson TR, Koren G. Fetal genital effects of first-trimester sex hormone exposure: a meta-analysis. Obstet Gynecol 1995; 85:141–9.
33. North K, Golding J. A maternal vegetarian diet in pregnancy is associated with hypospadias. The ALSPAC Study Team. Avon Longitudinal Study of Pregnancy and Childhood. BJU Int 2000; 85:107–13.
34. Price K, Fenwick G. Naturally occurring oestrogens in foods – a review. Food Addit Contam 1985; 2:73–106.
35. de Zegher F, Francois I, Boehmer AL et al. Androgens and fetal growth. Horm Res 1998; 50:243–4.
36. Bergstrom R, Adami HO, Mohner M et al. Increase in testicular cancer incidence in six European countries: a birth cohort phenomenon. J Natl Cancer Inst 1996; 88:727–33.
37. Carlsen E, Giwercman A, Keiding N, Skakkebaek NE. Declining semen quality and increasing incidence of testicular cancer: is there a common cause? Environ Health Perspect 1995; 103(Suppl 7):137–9.
38. Cheng W, Mya GH, Saing H. Associated anomalies in patients with undescended testes. J Trop Pediatr 1996; 42:204–6.
39. Toppari J, Larsen JC, Christiansen P et al. Male reproductive health and environmental xenoestrogens [see comments]. Environ Health Perspect 1996; 104(Suppl 4):741–803.
40. Rolland R, Gilbertson M, Colborn T. Environmentally induced alternations in development: a focus on wildlife. Environ Health Perspect 1995; 103(Suppl 4): 90–105.
41. Colborn T, Short P, Gilbertson M. Health effects of contemporary-use pesticides: the wildlife/human connection. Toxicol Ind Health 1999; 15:240–75.
42. Kim KS, Torres CR, Yucel S et al. Induction of hypospadias in a murine model by maternal exposure to synthetic estrogens. Environ Res 2004; 94(3):267–75.
43. Skakkebaek NE, Rajpert-De Meyts E, Jorgensen N et al. Germ cell cancer and disorders of spermatogenesis: an environmental connection? APMIS 1998; 106:3–11, discussion 12.
44. Jensen K. European Parliament's Committee on the Environment, Public Health and Consumer Protection. Report on Endocrine Disrupting Chemicals, Rapporteur, 1998.
45. Groshart C, Okkerman P, Folkers G. Report to the European Commission: identification of endocrine disruptors, first draft interim report. Delft, The Netherlands: BKH Consulting Engineers, 1999.
46. EPA. Endocrine Disruptor Screening and Testing Advisory Committee (EDSTAC). Final Report: United States Environmental Protection Agency, 1998.

Basic science of the testis

66

Julia Spencer Barthold

Introduction

Development of the mammalian gonad is an active process in both sexes that requires precise timing and coordination of diverse signaling mechanisms.[1] Although the details are not completely understood, understanding of this process has surged in recent years with routine availability of transgenic mouse models and sophisticated techniques for studying gene expression. Failure of the normal program due to delayed and/or insufficient expression of gene products may cause profound, long-term deficiencies in testicular function. It has been known for more than a decade that the sex-determining region on the Y chromosome (*SRY*) is the switch that triggers testis determination.[2] Subsequent work has identified many additional genes that participate in gonadal, testicular and/or ovarian development, the complex mechanisms involved, and the importance of cell–cell interactions in the development of cell types.[3,4] Although some species differences are apparent, knowledge of the basic mechanisms of development will aid in understanding the etiology and pathology of testicular and sexual differentiation disorders in children, such as intersex and other disorders of testicular development and descent.

Gonadal determination

Formation of the indifferent gonadal ridge anterior to the mesonephros begins at 33 days postovulation in human fetuses.[5] Germ cell migration from the extraembryonic ectoderm to the gonadal ridge is completed by about 5 weeks' gestation.[6] Expression of two genes required for gonadal determination, *WT1* (Wilms' tumor 1) and *SF1* (steroidogenic factor 1), is present by day 32 in both male and female gonads.[5] *WT1* is a transcription factor required for normal development of the urogenital ridge and for germ cell development. Homozygous deletion of *Wt1* in mice causes failure of gonadal and renal development, whereas selective deletions affecting production of specific isoforms leads to development of ovaries or dysgenic (hypoplastic, poorly differentiated, or 'dysgenetic') testes in XY fetuses[7] (Table 66.1). Therefore, *Wt1* function is critical for stabilization of the gonad but also for testis determination via expression of *SRY* and other downstream testis-determining genes. In man, *WT1* gene mutations are found in the Denys–Drash syndrome, Frazier syndrome, and WAGR syndrome (a syndrome of Wilms' tumor, aniridia, genital anomalies, and mental retardation), associated with a similar spectrum of gonadal disorders ranging from cryptorchidism and dysgenic testes without genital ambiguity to gonadal dysgenesis (streak gonads with sex reversal).[8]

Sf1, another transcription factor with similarly global effects on maintenance of the gonadal primordium, is also required for development of the adrenal, hypothalamus, and pituitary.[9] *Sf1* interacts with other key transcription factors and regulates transcription of other important genes involved in development and regulation of the reproductive tracts (Figure 66.1), including *Sry*, *Sox9* (SRY-type high-mobility group (HMG) box 9), *DAX1* (dosage-sensitive sex reversal/adrenal hypoplasia congenita critical region on chromosome X), *AMH* (anti-müllerian hormone), and *INSL3* (insulin-like 3), whose functions are discussed in more detail below. Deletion of the murine *Sf1* gene produces gonadal and adrenal agenesis in both XX and XY fetuses as well as gonadotropin deficiency.[9] In man, mutations of *SF1* cause XY gonadal dysgenesis, but are not associated with failure of adrenal or ovarian development.[10]

Homozygous deletion of patterning genes with more generalized functions during embryogenesis, including several homeodomain proteins that function as transcriptional regulators such as Emx2 (empty spiracles homolog 2),[11] Pbx1 (pre-B-cell leukemia transcription factor 1),[12] the LIM (lin-11/Islet-1/mec-3) homeobox proteins Lhx1[13] and Lhx9[14] and M33[15] (polycomb-like protein/chromobox homolog 2,

Table 66.1 Genetic regulation of gonadal development

Gene	Function	Transgenetic mouse gonadal development		Clinical gonadal phenotype
		Male	*Female*	
Gonadal determination				
Wt1	Transcription factor; regulator of urogenital ridge and early germ cell development	Gonadal/renal agenesis in complete knockout +KTS isoform knockout: ovaries –KTS isoform knockout: gonadal dysgenesis		Cryptorchidism, dysgenic testis, or gonadal dysgenesis
Sf1	Transcription factor; regulator of gonadal ridge and adrenal development	Gonadal and adrenal agenesis		Gonadal dysgenesis, primary adrenal failure
Emx2	Homeodomain transcription factor	Agenesis of kidneys, gonads, and reproductive tract		No gonadal pathology reported
Pbx1	Transcription factor	Agenesis of kidneys, gonads, and reproductive tract		NA
Lhx1	Homeodomain transcription factor	Gonadal/renal agenesis		NA
Lhx9	Homeodomain transcription factor; regulation of *SF1*	Gonadal agenesis		NA
M33/Cbx2	Regulation of homeotic genes	Ovaries, ovotestes or gonadal dysgenesis	Small ovaries or ovarian agenesis	NA
Pod1 (capsulin/ epicardin/ *Tcf21*)	Basic helix–loop–helix transcription factor; antagonizes *SF1*	Up-regulation of steroidogenic cells; disorganization of gonad; increased apoptosis; female phenotype in XY fetuses		NA
Igf1r/Ir/Irr	Insulin receptor tyrosine kinase signaling; cell proliferation	Ovaries in triple homozygotes Ovotestes or testes in double homozygotes	Small ovaries	NA
Gonadal development				
Sry	Transcriptional regulator; initiates testis determination	Gonadal dysgenesis	Gain of function: testis	Pure or partial gonadal dysgenesis (15–20% of cases studied)
Sox9	Transcription factor; *Sry* target; necessary and sufficient for testis determination	Ovary, gonadal dysgenesis or dysgenic testis	Gain of function: testis	Dysplastic ovary; ovotestis or dysgenic testis
Sox8	Transcription factor; functions cooperatively with *Sox9*	*Sox8/Sox9* double knockout more severe than *Sox9* alone	NA	NA
Gata4/Fog2	Transcription factor and cofactor; mediate male and female gonadal development	Gonadal dysgenesis; dysgenic testis	Abnormal ovaries	NA
Fgf9	Fibroblast growth factor receptor (FGFR2) signaling; Sertoli cell proliferation	Ovary; gonadal dysgenesis or dysgenic testis	Normal ovaries	NA

Table 66.1 *continued*

Gene	Function	Transgenetic mouse gonadal development		
		Male	*Female*	*Clinical gonadal phenotype*
Pdgfrα	Growth factor receptor; mesonephric cell migration and Leydig cell differentiation	Disorganization of testis cords; no Leydig cells	Normal ovaries	NA
Arx	Homeobox gene; Leydig cell development	Inhibition of Leydig cell differentiation	NA	Dysgenic testes
Dhh	Desert hedgehog; signaling through Patched receptor; Leydig cell development	Dysgenic testis or hypospermatogenesis; loss of Leydig cells	Normal ovaries	Gonadal dysgenesis
Dmrt1/ *Dmrt2*	Transcription factors; contain phylogenetically conserved sex differentiation domains	Overproliferation of immature Sertoli cells; loss of post-meiotic germ cells	Normal ovaries	9p monosomy associated with gonadal dysgenesis, ovotestis, dysgenic or cryptorchid testis
Dax1	Orphan nuclear receptor; dose-dependent anti- and pro-testis functions	Progressive loss of spermatogenesis Gain of function: ovotestes	Normal ovaries	Loss of spermatogenesis Gain of function: XY gonadal dysgenesis
Wnt4	Signaling through Frizzled receptor; required for testis and ovary development	Dysgenic testes Gain of function: disordered vasculature and reduced steroidogenesis	Androgen synthesis with masculinization Gain of function: normal ovaries	Müllerian dysgenesis and virilization in XX Gain of function: cryptorchidism, dysgenic testis or gonadal dysgenesis
Amh	Growth factor; member of transforming growth factor-β family; müllerian duct regression in males	Leydig cell hyperplasia; loss of spermatogenesis Gain of function: inhibition of Leydig cell differentiation	Normal ovaries Gain of function: ovarian degeneration, Sertoli cell and tubule development	Persistent müllerian duct syndrome with testicular dysgenesis and infertility

Known genes regulating gonadal determination and testicular development are based on murine knockout studies and reported human mutations. Transgenic mouse gonadal phenotype describes the effects of homozygous deletion, unless indicated otherwise. Clinical gonadal phenotype refers to loss of function mutations in males, unless otherwise indicated. NA, not available; Wtl, Wilms' tumor 1; *Sf1*, steroidogenic factor 1; *Emx2*, empty spiracles homolog 2; *Pbx1*, pre-B-cell leukemia transcription factor 1; *Lhx1*, LIM homeobox 1; *Lhx9*, LIM homeobox 9; *M33/Cbx2*, M33 polycomb-like protein/chromobox homolog 2; *Tcf21*, transcription factor 21; *Igf1r*, insulin growth factor 1 receptor; *Ir*, insulin receptor; *Irr*, insulin-related receptor; *Sry*, sex-determining region Y chromosome; *Sox8/9*, SRY-box containing genes 8 and 9; *Gata4*, GATA transcription factor 4; *Fog2*, Friend of *Gata2*; *Fgf9*, fibroblast growth factor 9; *Pdgfrα*, platelet-derived growth factor receptor α; *Arx*, aristaless related homeobox gene; *Dhh*, desert hedgehog; *Dmrt*, doublesex and mab-3 related transcription factor; *Dax1*, dosage-sensitive sex reversal/adrenal hypoplasia congenita X chromosome; *Wnt4*, wingless-type MMTV integration site family, member 4; *Amh*, anti-müllerian hormone. See text for references.

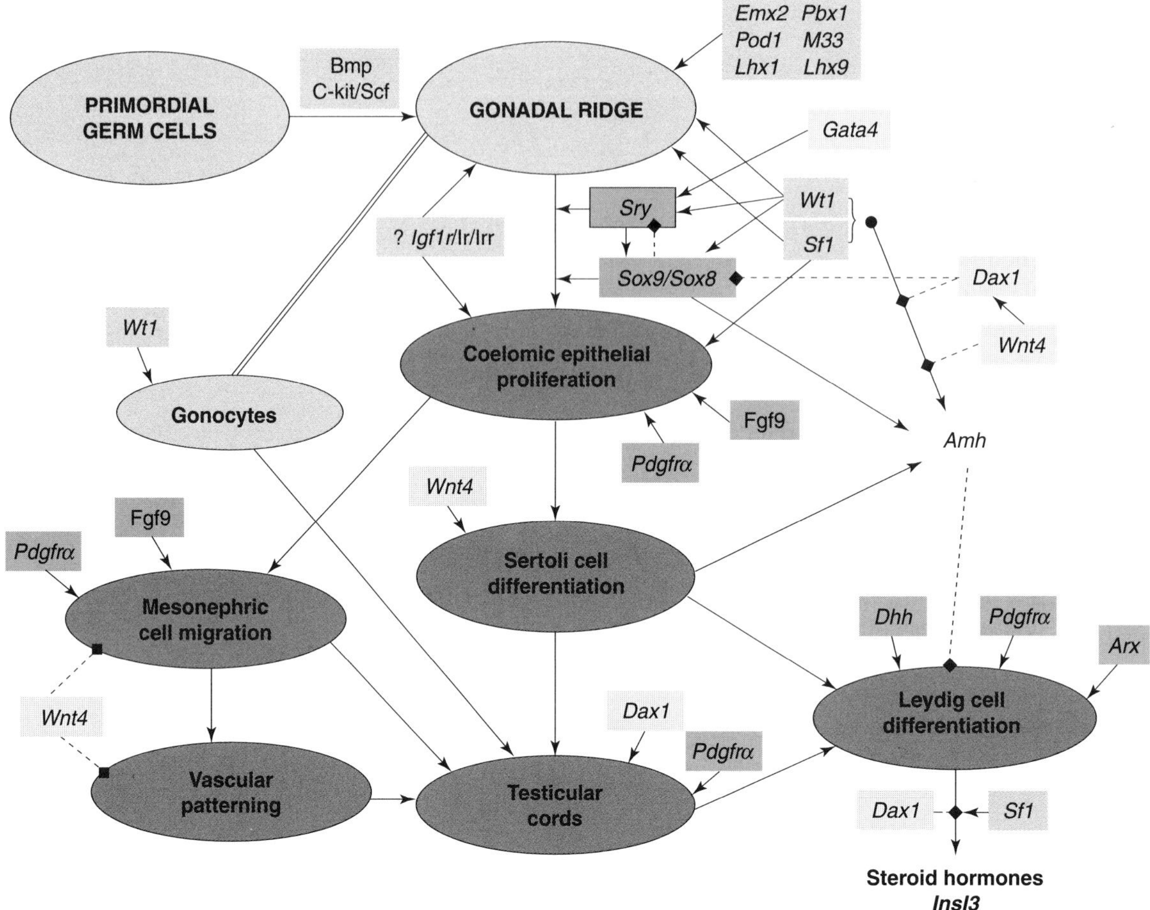

Figure 66.1 Key events and regulatory mechanisms of gonadal and testicular determination based on studies in mice. Solid arrows denote pathways that are directly or indirectly activated by specific events or signals, whereas inhibitory processes are specified by dashed lines. Structure/genes active prior to sex determination (light gray), testis-specific development (dark gray), genes regulating testis development (dark blue), and genes that have roles in both testis and ovarian development (light blue) are noted as such. Bmp, bone morphogenetic proteins; SCF, stem cell factor; *Emx2*, empty spiracles homolog 2; *Pbx1*, pre-B-cell leukemia transcription factor 1; *Pod1*, capsulin/epicardin/*Tcf21*; M33, M33 polycomb-like protein/chromobox homolog 2; *Lhx*, *LIM* homeobox; *Wt1*, Wilms' tumor 1; *Sf1*, steroidogenic factor 1; *Sry*, sex-determining region Y chromosome; *Sox8/9*, *SRY*-box containing gene 8/9; *Gata4*, *GATA* transcription factor 4; *Igf1r*, insulin growth factor 1 receptor; *Ir*, insulin receptor; *Irr*, insulin-related receptor; Fgf9, fibroblast growth factor 9; *Dax1*, dosage-sensitive sex reversal/adrenal hypoplasia congenita X chromosome; *Wnt4*, wingless-type MMTV integration site family, member 4; *Pdgfrα*, platelet-derived growth factor receptor α; *Amh*, anti-müllerian hormone; *Dhh*, desert hedgehog; *Arx*, aristaless related homeobox gene; *Insl3*, insulin-like 3. For further details, see Table 66.1 and text.

CBX2), is associated with severe dysmorphogenesis or absence of gonads (see Table 66.1). Affected fetuses are not viable due to other severe anomalies, including renal agenesis in some cases. The exact function of these proteins in stabilization and development of the gonadal ridge is not known but probably involves a role in cell proliferation.[1] Similarly, defective cell proliferation may be the cause of failed gonadal determination in mice lacking insulin-like receptor signaling following deletion of the insulin growth factor receptor 1 (*Igf1r*), insulin receptor (*Ir*), and insulin-related receptor (*Irr*).[1,16] *Pod1* (capsulin/epicardin/*Tcf21*), a basic helix–loop–helix transcription factor, functions as a repressor of *SF1* in the genital ridge. *Pod1* knockouts of both sexes have gonads that show failed development with aberrant up-regulation of steroidogenic cells and increased apoptosis.[17]

Testis determination

The first definitive step in testis determination is expression of *SRY* by pre-Sertoli cells followed by their subsequent differentiation.[1,2] Sertoli cells then direct differentiation of other cell types and induce mitotic arrest of germ cells. Testicular organogenesis involves a complex interplay of many genes, some of which influence development of both gonadal types (see Figure 66.1). Careful studies of gonadal architecture, concomitant gene expression, and transgenic phenotypes indicate that precision in the timing and degree of gene expression is crucial. Functional redundancy of critical pathways is also evident.

SRY is expressed in the human XY gonad at 41 days' gestation.[5] Although downstream signaling pathways have not been precisely delineated, it is known that murine *Sry* rapidly induces expression of the related HMG-box gene *Sox9*,[18] which is also expressed concurrently with *SRY* in the human fetal testis.[5] Both genes are essential and sufficient for initiating the testis development pathway in indifferent XY and XX gonads.[19] In both mice and human fetuses, *Sox9* expression is closely linked to that of *Sry*; however, humans appear to be more susceptible than mice to changes in dosage of both genes. Another important SRY-like gene, *Sox8*, has been shown to function cooperatively with *Sox9* in regulation of downstream signaling, and gonad-specific targeted deletion of *Sox8* and *Sox9* produces a more severe phenotype than knockout of *Sox 9* alone.[19,20] Despite its key role in testis development, mutations of *SRY* are found in only 15–20% of individuals with XY gonadal dysgenesis. *SOX9* mutations in humans are associated with the campomelic dysplasia in addition to gonadal dysgenesis[2] and a possible role for *SOX8* in clinical XY gonadal dysgenesis has not been reported. Therefore, other genetic and/or environmental factors must influence the process of testicular determination. Some candidate genes have been identified, as discussed below, but additional uncharacterized autosomal loci may also modulate function of these critical genes and produce the phenotype of XY gonadal dysgenesis.[21]

The earliest indication of testis determination is proliferation of the coelomic epithelium adjacent to the primordial gonad[1] (see Figure 66.1). In the fetal mouse, proliferating cells migrate into the gonad, stimulated by *Fgf9* (fibroblast growth factor 9) and *Pdgfrα* (platelet-derived growth factor) signaling, and differentiate into Sertoli and other gonadal cell lineages. *Pdgfrα* is also required for later formation of testis cords and Leydig cell differentiation. Homozygous deletion of either gene produces partial or complete failure of testis development or, in *Fgf9* knockout mice, development of ovaries.[22,23] Two other genes required during the early phases of testicular determination are the transcription factor *Gata4* (GATA-binding protein 4) and *Wnt4* (wingless-type MMTV integration site family, member 4). *Gata4* directly or indirectly enhances SRY function via interaction with its cofactor, Friend of GATA (*Fog2*) and enhances Sertoli cell proliferation and differentiation; functional knockouts have gonadal dysgenesis or dysgenic testes.[24] *Gata4* also influences ovarian development by a mechanism that remains poorly defined. Similarly, *Wnt4* is required for Sertoli cell differentiation, but has other functions that promote ovarian differentiation (see below).[25] In man, *GATA4* expression in Leydig, Sertoli, and germ cells is already present in the fetal testis at 12 weeks' gestation, the earliest time point studied, and peaks 6 weeks later.[26] Expression is reduced in testes of males with androgen receptor defects, suggesting hormonal control, but is normal in testes of cryptorchid boys.

Differentiation of adequate numbers of Sertoli cells is critical for downstream events in testicular differentiation. *Fgf9* and *Pdgfrα* signaling stimulates mesonephric cells to migrate into the developing gonad, a process that is sexually dimorphic and necessary for formation of the testicular cords and the testis-specific vasculature.[1,22,23] These processes are blocked in ovaries by Wnt4 and in testes of XY fetuses exposed to increased Wnt4 dosage.[27,28] Sertoli cells surround gonocytes already present within the gonad to form testicular cords, with subsequent inhibition of germ cell mitosis. Germ cells located in an ectopic extratubular position either fail to survive or inappropriately enter meiosis. Testicular cord formation also requires *Dax1*, an orphan nuclear receptor that maps to the Xp21 duplication region associated with clinical XY sex reversal and therefore previously considered an ovarian determination or antitestis gene.[29] Transgenic mouse studies confirm that *Dax1* overexpression may lead to ovotestis formation in XY fetuses.[30] However, loss of *Dax1* function in mice is associated with spermatogenic failure in testes, but normal ovaries, data that support a role for this gene in development of the testis but not the ovary.[31] *Dax1* also inhibits expression of *Sf1* and genes involved in hormone production by Leydig and Sertoli cells.[32] In humans, *DAX1* is expressed in the indifferent fetal gonad and transcription persists at low levels in both sexes throughout the period of sexual differentiation.[5] Clinically, *DAX1* mutations are associated with hypogonadotropic hypogonadism, but an intrinsic abnormality in germ cell differentiation is also present, which precludes spermatogenic response to gonadotropin therapy.[33]

DMRT1 and *DMRT2* (*doublesex* and *mab-3* related transcription factors 1 and 2) are genes located within the 9p deletion critical region associated with clinical XY gonadal dysgenesis and sex reversal. They are therefore candidate genes for testis determination downstream of *SRY*.[34] Although specific mutations have not yet been identified in these genes, they contain highly conserved DNA-binding domains that are also present in the sex-determining genes *doublesex* (*Drosophila*) and *mab-3* (*C. elegans*). In mice with homozygous deletion of *Dmrt1* alone, testes form but Sertoli cell maturation and postmeiotic spermatogenesis are abnormal.[35] It is not clear if both genes are needed for testis determination or if there are species-specific differences in DMRT function.

Proper differentiation of the testicular cords and vasculature is also necessary for establishment of the interstitial cell compartment.[1] Desert hedgehog (*Dhh*),[36] a *Drosophila* homolog in the hedgehog signaling pathway, *Pdgfrα*[22] and the homeobox gene *Arx*[37] are required for Leydig cell development. However, human mutations in the *DHH*[38] and *ARX*[37] genes are associated with more generalized failure of testicular development (see Table 66.1). *Dhh* and *Pdgfrα* function via paracrine mechanisms, as they are expressed in Sertoli and interstitial cells, respectively. These data indicate that interaction between the various testicular cell types is essential for normal development and function of the testis.

Anti-müllerian hormone (AMH, or müllerian-inhibiting substance) is a sensitive indicator of the function of Sertoli cells at the time of their differentiation and in postnatal life.[1,39,40] Moreover, secretion of AMH is regulated by many genes important in the testis determination pathway and is inhibited by Wnt4 and Dax1 in the ovary. Like Wnt4 and Dax1, Amh has been shown to have variable effects in murine testis and ovary that are dose-related. Males

Table 66.2 Genetic regulation of testicular descent

Gene	*Function*	*Transgenic mouse phenotype*	*Clinical phenotype*
Insl3	Insulin-like growth factor; stimulates development of the mesenchymal gubernaculum	Perirenal testes	Mutations rare in isolated cryptorchidism
Great/Lgr8	Receptor for insl3, present in gubernacular cells	Perirenal testes	Mutations rare in isolated cryptorchidism
Desrt/ARID5B	AT-rich interaction domain DNA-binding protein	Inguinal testes	NA
HoxA10/HoxA11	Homeobox genes involved in embryo patterning	Perirenal, abdominal, or inguinal testes; epididymal and vasal anomalies	Mutations rare in isolated cryptorchidism
Tgfβ$_2$	Transforming growth factor signaling	Failure of abdominal descent in male fetus	NA
Ar	Androgen receptor signaling	Spontaneous genetic mutation; testes at internal ring	Pelvic, abdominal, inguinal, or labial testes
Aromatase	Conversion of testosterone to estradiol	Overexpression: cryptorchidism	One case of inguinal cryptorchidism
Gata1	Transcription factor	No gonadal phenotype; expressed in Sertoli cells	Familial dyserythropoietic anemia; one report of associated inguinal cryptorchism in brothers

Candidate genes regulating testicular descent are based on transgenic mouse studies and human mutations associated with cryptorchidism. Transgenic mouse phenotype describes the effects of homozygous deletion, unless specified otherwise. Clinical phenotype refers to loss of function mutations. NA, not available; *Insl3*, insulin-like 3; *Great/Lgr8*, G-coupled protein receptor affecting testicular descent/leucine-rich repeat-containing G-protein coupled receptor 8; *Desrt/ARID5B*, developmentally and sexually retarded with transient immune abnormalities/AT-rich interaction domain 5B; *HoxA10/A11*, homeobox A10/A11; *TGFβ$_2$*, transforming growth factor β_2; *Ar*, androgen receptor; *Gata1*, GATA transcription factor 1. See text for references.

with deletion of *Amh* have impaired testicular development, characterized by reduced spermatogenesis and Leydig cell hyperplasia, in addition to persistence of müllerian ducts. Although not well studied, lack of AMH in humans may also adversely affect testicular development, given that males with persistent müllerian duct syndrome are prone to infertility and testicular tumors.[41] Transgenic overexpression of Amh in mice causes inhibition of Leydig cell differentiation in testes and sex reversal in ovaries.[39]

Mechanisms of testicular descent

The human fetal testis is located adjacent to the internal inguinal ring at the end of the first trimester.[42] During the second trimester, a dramatic increase in size of the gubernaculum testis occurs, which allows dilation of the inguinal canal and migration of the processus vaginalis.[43] Finally, starting at 24 weeks' gestation, testes begin a rapid traversal through the inguinal canal. The anatomic and biochemical changes involved in development of the gubernaculum have been studied extensively in rodent and pig fetuses,[44] but the signaling pathways involved remain poorly understood. It is known that gubernacular function depends upon testicular hormones and/or factors that induce its growth, proliferation, and subsequent migration, with the testis, into the scrotum.

Genetic diseases typically associated with gonadal dysgenesis, such as *WT1* mutations,[8] *WNT4* (gain of function) mutations,[28] and 9p monosomy[45] may also present with isolated cryptorchidism. Similarly, mutations of the androgen receptor (AR) may be associated with impaired testicular descent, but phenotypes are variable.[46] Many loci are linked to syndromes associated with cryptorchidism.[47] However, until recently, there were no gene candidates for non-syndromic cryptorchidism. One promising candidate has been identified as INSL3 (insulin-like 3),[48] a hormone in the relaxin family that is probably the non-androgenic testicular factor that is the primary stimulus to gubernacular growth.[49] INSL3 binds to a specific receptor, *Rxfp2* (also known as G-protein coupled receptor affecting testicular descent, or GREAT) that is present in the gubernaculum.[50] Homozygous deletion of *Insl3* or *Rxfp2* in mice is associated with perirenal testes and failure of prenatal development of the gubernaculum. Although *INSL3* and *RXFP2* appear to be ideal candidates for human non-syndromic cryptorchidism, a mutation in one of these genes is present in less than 5% of cases (Table 66.2).[51] It is likely that variants in multiple genes, and possibly environmental exposures,[52] contribute to failure of testis descent.

Some progress in identifying mechanisms of testicular descent has been made by screening fetal mouse gubernacula for expression of cytoplasmic and receptor tyrosine kinases and members of the insulin receptor family.[53] These data indicate that many genes, including *Pdgfrα*, *Igf1r*, *Ir*, and members of the *Eph* and *Egfr* (epidermal growth factor receptor) signaling pathways are expressed in the gubernaculum during development. Characterization of the relative importance and roles of these signals awaits further studies. Additional potential members of signaling pathways involved in testicular descent have been identified from transgenic mouse models and clinical studies. These include the transcription factors *HoxA10*,[54] *HoxA11*[55] (homeobox genes), *Gata1*[56] (GATA binding protein 1), and *Desrt/Arid5B*[58] (developmentally and sexually retarded with transient immune abnormalities/AT-rich interaction domain 5B), and *Tgfβ*$_2$[57] (transforming growth factor β_2) (see Table 66.2). Transgenic deletion of *HoxA10* or *HoxA11* is associated with cryptorchidism and anomalies of wolffian duct derivatives, but mutations of the human homologs of these genes are uncommon in boys with cryptorchidism[59,60] (unpublished observations). A *GATA1* mutation was reported in a family with hematologic abnormalities and cryptorchidism, but it is not clear if failure of testicular descent was a consequence of the mutation. *AR* variants that reduce but do not eliminate function, such as increased GGN repeats, may increase the risk for cryptorchidism.[61] Similarly, experimental up-regulation of the aromatase gene[62] is associated with increased estrogen production and cryptorchidism but a reported loss of function mutation in this same gene produced inguinal cryptorchidism in an affected man.[63] As with testis determination, experimental and clinical data do not necessarily correlate, and so far the factors contributing to failure of testicular descent in human fetuses remain unknown in most cases.

Calcitonin gene-related peptide (CGRP) is expressed in the muscular portion of the rat gubernaculum and in the sensory nucleus of the genitofemoral nerve.[64] A role for CGRP in migration of the rat gubernaculum is supported by data showing differential expression of this signaling molecule in rats with cryptorchidism. However, no studies have examined the effect of loss of function of the *CGRP* gene on testicular descent. It remains unclear whether changes in expression of *CGRP* is a cause or effect of failure of descent in rats, or if its role in cremaster muscle function is applicable to the etiology of human cryptorchidism.[65] Preliminary analysis of the *CGRP* gene has failed to show mutations associated with clinical cryptorchidism.[66]

Early testicular development

Survival and proliferation of primordial germ cells is dependent on bone morphogenetic proteins (BMPs), signaling via the C-kit receptor tyrosine kinase and its ligand, stem cell factor (SCF), and other signaling molecules.[67] In human fetuses, these cells become localized within the testicular cords by the 8th week of gestation.[6] By the second trimester, three distinct subpopulations of germ cells – gonocytes, prespermatogonia, and intermediate spermatogonia – are distinguishable within the tubules based on immunohistochemical characteristics. Along with differentiation, apoptosis (programmed cell death) is an ongoing process throughout gestation in human germ cells as well as in Sertoli and Leydig cells and has an important role in establishing a normal population of cells in the testis.[68]

In mice, migration of undifferentiated germ cells to the tubule periphery and association with Sertoli cells via adhesion molecules occurs in the 1st week of life.[69] The process of migration is not well characterized but requires Sertoli cell signaling, thyroid hormone, and perhaps other hormones and/or testicular factors. Germ cell survival within tubules in neonatal mice is also mediated by C-kit and SCF. Maturation to spermatogonial stem cells is a process that is critical for long-term maintenance of adequate spermatogenesis.[70] Failure of maturation leads to excess apoptosis or persistence of undifferentiated cells that may predispose to future malignant transformation. Direct evidence for regulation of this process in newborn boys by specific factors is lacking. However, failure of germ cell maturation has been identified as a negative prognostic factor in human cryptorchidism.[71]

Maturation of Sertoli and Leydig cells is also essential for spermatogenesis. Active proliferation of Sertoli cells occurs in the perinatal and peripubertal periods and support of sufficient numbers of germ cells depends on subsequent maturation of these cells.[72] Mature Sertoli cells can be identified by expression of Wt1, GATA1, $p27^{Kip1}$ (a cyclin-dependent kinase inhibitor) and AR, whereas persistent expression of AMH, aromatase, NCAM (neural cell adhesion molecule), and cytokeratin-18 is associated with Sertoli cell immaturity. Similarly, the Leydig cell population is composed of distinct fetal and adult types.[73] Adult Leydig cells differentiate from interstitial mesenchymal precursors during the postnatal period through a series of maturational steps. This process is regulated by gonadotropins, androgens, AMH, thyroid hormone, and growth factors. Failed maturation of Sertoli and/or Leydig cells may be the underlying cause of testicular dysfunction, also called 'testicular dysgenesis syndrome', which is observed in cases of cryptorchidism, testicular cancer, and/or hypospermatogenesis.[72]

Conclusions

Normal testicular development and descent requires multiple signaling pathways, many of which have not been elucidated. Failure or reduced expression of only one of these signals may produce a wide spectrum of phenotypic abnormalities that is indistinguishable from other causes. As development is normally associated with phases of proliferation, differentiation, and apoptosis, alterations in any of these programs may ultimately reduce testicular hormone secretion and/or spermatogenesis. Moreover, primary defects in development of one testicular cell type may affect patterning and long-term function of the entire organ. In the future, genetic analysis of boys with abnormalities of testicular development and descent may define more precisely the severity and prognosis of disease among individuals with similar phenotypes, and improve our therapeutic approach to these cases.

Key points

- Establishment of the mammalian gonad is an active process that involves expression of multiple urogenital patterning genes and migration of primordial germ cells.
- Testis determination, triggered by *Sry*, requires coelomic epithelial migration for establishment of Sertoli cells, formation of testicular cords, vascular patterning, establishment of interstitial cells within the gonad, and both differentiation and apoptosis of all cell types.
- Many genes, some of which have dual roles in promoting or inhibiting testis-specific events, regulate testis development.
- The ligand/receptor pair INSL3/Great is critical for testicular descent.
- Postnatal spermatogonial differentiation is critical for establishing spermatogenesis.

References

1. Brennan J, Capel B. One tissue, two fates: molecular genetic events that underlie testis versus ovary development. Nat Rev Genet 2004; 5:509–21.
2. Harley VR, Clarkson MJ, Argentaro A. The molecular action and regulation of the testis-determining factors, SRY (sex-determining region on the Y chromosome) and SOX9 [SRY-related high-mobility group (HMG) box 9]. Endocr Rev 2003; 24:466–87.
3. Park SY, Jameson JL. Minireview: transcriptional regulation of gonadal development and differentiation. Endocrinology 2005; 146:1035–42.
4. Ross AJ, Capel B. Signaling at the crossroads of gonad development. Trends Endocrinol Metab 2005; 16:19–25.
5. Hanley NA, Hagan DM, Clement-Jones M et al. SRY, SOX9, and DAX1 expression patterns during human sex determination and gonadal development. Mech Dev 2000; 91:403–7.
6. Gaskell TL, Esnal A, Robinson LLL, Anderson RA, Saunders PTK. Immunohistochemical profiling of germ cells within the human fetal testis: identification of three subpopulations. Biol Reprod 2004; 71:2012–21.
7. Natoli TA, Alberta JA, Bortvin A et al. Wt1 functions in the development of germ cells in addition to somatic cell lineages of the testis. Dev Biol 2004; 268:429–40.
8. Lim HN, Hughes IA, Hawkins JR. Clinical and molecular evidence for the role of androgens and WT1 in testis descent. Mol Cell Endocrinol 2001; 185:43–50.
9. Parker KL. The roles of steroidogenic factor 1 in endocrine development and function. Mol Cell Endocrinol 1998; 145:15–20.
10. Ozisik G, Achermann JC, Jameson JL. The role of SF1 in adrenal and reproductive function: insight from naturally occurring mutations in humans. Mol Genet Metab 2002; 76:85–91.
11. Miyamoto N, Yoshida M, Kuratani S, Matsuo I, Alzawa S. Defects of urogenital development in mice lacking Emx2. Development 1997; 124:1653–64.
12. Schnabel CA, Selleri L, Cleary ML. Pbx1 is essential for adrenal development and urogenital differentiation. Genesis 2003; 37:123–30.
13. Shawlot W, Behringer RR. Requirement for Lim1 in head-organizer function. Nature 1995; 374:425–30.
14. Birk OS, Caslano DE, Wassif CA et al. The LIM homeobox gene Lhx9 is essential for mouse gonad development. Nature 2000; 403:909–13.
15. Katoh-Fukui Y, Tsuchiya R, Shiroishi T et al. Male-to-female sex reversal in M33 mutant mice. Nature 1998; 393:688–92.
16. Nef S, Verma-Kuvari S, Merenmies J et al. Testis determination requires insulin receptor family function in mice. Nature 2003; 426:291–5.
17. Cui S, Ross A, Stallings N et al. Disrupted gonadogenesis and male-to-female sex reversal in Pod1 knockout mice. Development 2004; 131:4095–105.
18. Sekido R, Bar I, Narvaez V, Penny G, Lovell-Badge R. SOX9 is up-regulated by the transient expression of SRY specifically in Sertoli cell precursors. Dev Biol 2004; 274:271–9.
19. Chaboissier M-C, Kobayashi A, Vidal VIP et al. Functional analysis of Sox8 and Sox9 during sex determination in the mouse. Development 2004; 131:1891–901.
20. Schepers G, Wilson M, Wilhelm D, Koopman P. SOX8 is expressed during testis differentiation in mice and synergizes with SF1 to activate the AMH promoter in vitro. J Biol Chem 2003; 278:28101–8.
21. Eicher EM, Washburn LL, Schork NJ et al. Sex-determining genes on mouse autosomes identified by linkage analysis of C57BL/6J-Y^{POS} sex reversal. Nat Genet 1996; 14:206–9.
22. Covin JS, Green RP, Schmahl J, Capel B, Ornitz DM. Male-to-female sex reversal in mice lacking fibroblast growth factor 9. Cell 2001; 104:875–89.
23. Brennan J, Tilmann C, Capel B. Pdgfr-α mediates testis cord organization and fetal Leydig cell development in the XY gonad. Genes Dev 2003; 17:800–10.
24. Tevosian SG, Albrecht KH, Crispino JD et al. Gonadal differentiation, sex determination and normal Sry expression in mice require direct interaction between transcription partners GATA4 and FOG2. Development 2002; 129:4627–34.
25. Jeays-Ward K, Dandonneau M, Swain A. Wnt4 is required for proper male as well as female sexual development. Dev Biol 2004; 276:431–40.
26. Ketola I, Pentikainen V, Vaskivuo T et al. Expression of transcription factor GATA-4 during human testicular development and disease. J Clin Endocrinol Metab 2000; 85:3925–31.
27. Jordan BK, Shen JH-C, Olaso R, Ingraham HA, Vilain E. Wnt4 overexpression disrupts normal testicular vasculature and inhibits testosterone synthesis by repressing steroidogenic factor1/β-catenin synergy. PNAS 2003; 100:10866–71.
28. Jordan BK, Mohammed M, Ching ST et al. Up-regulation of WNT-4 signaling and dosage-sensitive sex reversal in humans. Am J Hum Genet 2001; 68:1102–9.
29. Ludbrook LM, Harley VR. Sex determination: a 'window' of DAX1 activity. Trends Endocrinol Metab 2004; 15:116–21.
30. Swain A, Narvaez V, Burgoyne P, Camerino G, Lovell-Badge R. Dax1 antagonizes Sry action in mammalian sex determination. Nature 1998; 391:761–7.
31. Meeks JJ, Crawford SE, Russell TA et al. Dax1 regulates testis cord organization during gonadal differentiation. Development 2003; 130:1029–36.
32. Lalli E, Sassone-Corsi P. DAX-1, an unusual orphan receptor at the crossroads of steroidogenic function and sexual differentiation. Mol Endocrinol 2003; 17:1445–53.
33. Seminara SB, Achermann JC, Genel M, Jameson JL, Crowley Jr WF. X-linked adrenal hypoplasia congenita: a mutation in DAX1 expands the phenotypic spectrum in males and females. J Clin Endocrinol Metab 1999; 84:4501–9.
34. Ounap K, Uibo O, Zordania R et al. Three patients with 9p deletions including DMRT1 and DMRT2: a girl with XY complement, bilateral ovotestes, and extreme growth retardation, and two XX females with normal pubertal development. Am J Med Genet 2004; 130A:415–23.

35. Raymond CS, Murphy MW, O'Sullivan MG, Bardwell VJ, Zarkower D. Dmrt1, a gene related to worm and fly sexual regulators, is required for mammalian testis differentiation. Gene Dev 2000; 14:2587–95.
36. Clark AM, Garland KK, Russell LD. Desert hedgehog (DHH) gene is required in the mouse testis for formation of adult-type Leydig cells and normal development of the peritubular cells and seminiferous tubules. Biol Reprod 2000; 63:1825–38.
37. Kitamura K, Yanazawa M, Sugiyama N et al. Mutation of ARX causes abnormal development of forebrain and testes in mice and X-linked lissencephaly with abnormal genitalia in humans. Nat Genet 2002; 32:359–69.
38. Canto P, Söderlund D, Reyes E, Méndez JP. Mutations in the Desert hedgehog (DHH) gene in patients with 46,XY complete pure gonadal dysgenesis. J Clin Endocrinol Metab 2004; 89:4480–3.
39. Josso N, Racine C, di Clemente N, Rey R, Xavier F. The role of anti-Müllerian hormone in gonadal development. Mol Cell Endocrinol 1998; 145:3–7.
40. Lee MM, Misra M, Donahoe PK, MacLaughlin DT. MIS/AMH in the assessment of cryptorchidism and intersex conditions. Mol Cell Endocrinol 2003; 211:91–8.
41. Martin EL, Bennett AH, Cromie WJ. Persistent Müllerian duct syndrome with transverse testicular ectopia and spermatogenesis. J Urol 1992; 147:1615–17.
42. Arey LB. Developmental Anatomy. Philadelphia: WB Saunders, 1974: 315–41.
43. Heyns CF. The gubernaculum during testicular descent in the human fetus. J Anat 1987; 153:93–112.
44. Wensing CJ. The embryology of testicular descent. Horm Res 1988; 30:144–52.
45. Muroya K, Okuyama T, Goishi K et al. Sex-determining gene(s) on distal 9p: clinical and molecular studies in six cases. J Clin Endocrinol Metab 2000; 85:3094–100.
46. Barthold JS, Kumasi-Rivers K, Upadhyay J, Shekarriz B, Imperato-McGinley J. Testicular position in androgen insensitivity syndrome: implications for the role of androgens in testicular descent. J Urol 2000; 164:497–501.
47. Klonisch T, Fowler PA, Hombach-Klonisch S. Molecular and genetic regulation of testis descent and external genitalia development. Dev Biol 2004; 270:1–18.
48. Zimmerman S, Steding G, Emmen JMA et al. Targeted disruption of the Insl3 gene causes bilateral cryptorchidism. Mol Endocrinol 1999; 13:681–91.
49. Fentener van Vlissingen JM, van Zoelen EJ, Ursem PJ, Wensing CJ. In vitro model of the first phase of testicular descent: identification of a low molecular weight factor from fetal testis involved in proliferation of gubernaculum testis cells and distinct from specified polypeptide growth factors and fetal gonadal hormones. Endocrinology 1988; 123:2868–77.
50. Overbeek PA, Gorlov IP, Sutherland RW et al. A transgenic insertion causing cryptorchidism in mice. Genesis 2001; 30:26–35.
51. Foresta C, Ferlin A. Role of INSL3 and LGR8 in cryptorchidism and testicular function. Reprod Biomed Online 2004; 9:294–8.
52. Sharpe RM, Irvine DS. How strong is the evidence of a link between environmental chemicals and adverse effects on human reproductive health? BMJ 2004; 328:447–51.
53. Verma-Kurvari S, Parada LF. Identification of tyrosine kinases expressed in the male mouse gubernaculum during development. Dev Dyn 2004; 230:660–5.
54. Satokata I, Benson G, Maas R. Sexually dimorphic sterility phenotypes in Hoxa10-deficient mice. Nature 1995; 374:460–3.
55. Hsieh-Li HM, Witte DP, Weinstein M et al. Hoxa-11 structure, extensive antisense transcription, and function in male and female fertility. Development 1995; 121:1373–85.
56. Nichols KE, Crispino JD, Punex M et al. Familial dyserythropoietic anaemia and thrombocytopenia due to an inherited mutation in GATA1. Nat Genet 2000; 24:266–70.
57. Lahoud MH, Ristevski S, Venter DJ et al. Gene targeting of Desrt, a novel ARID class DNA-binding protein, causes growth retardation and abnormal development of reproductive organs. Genome Res 2001; 11:1327–34.
58. Sanford LP, Ormsby I, Gittenberger-de Groot AC et al. TGFβ2 knockout mice have multiple developmental defects that are nonoverlapping with other TGFβ phenotypes. Development 1997; 124:2659–70.
59. Kolon TF, Wiener JS, Lewitton M et al. Analysis of homeobox gene HOXA10 mutations in cryptorchidism. J Urol 1999; 161:275–80.
60. Bertini V, Bertelloni S, Valetto A et al. Homeobox HOXA10 gene analysis in cryptorchidism. J Pediatr Endocrinol Metab 2004; 17:41–5.
61. Aschim EL, Nordenskjöld A, Giwercman A et al. Linkage between cryptorchidism, hypospadias and GGN repeat length in the androgen receptor gene. J Clin Endocrinol Metab 2004; 89:5105–9.
62. Li X, Makela S, Streng T, Santti R, Poutanen M. Phenotype characteristics of transgenic male mice expressing human aromatase under ubiquitin C promoter. J Steroid Biochem Mol Biol 2003; 86:469–76.
63. Maffei L, Murata Y, Rochira V et al. Dysmetabolic syndrome in a man with a novel mutation of the aromatase gene: effects of testosterone, alendronate, and estradiol treatment. J Clin Endocrinol Metab 2004; 89:61–70.
64. Hrabovszky Z, Farmer PJ, Hutson JM. Undescended testis is accompanied by calcitonin gene related peptide accumulation within the sensory nucleus of the genitofemoral nerve in trans-scrotal rats. J Urol 2001; 165:1015–18.
65. Husmann DA. Cryptorchidism – problems extrapolating experimental animal data to the clinical undescended testicle. J Urol 1998; 159:1029–30.
66. Zuccarello D, Morini E, Douzgou S et al. Preliminary data suggest that mutations in the CgRP pathway are not involved in human sporadic cryptorchidism. J Endocrinol Invest 2004; 27:761–4.
67. Zhao GQ, Garbers DL. Male germ cell specification and differentiation. Dev Cell 2002; 2:537–47.
68. Helal MA, Mehmet H, Thomas NS et al. Ontogeny of human fetal testicular apoptosis during first, second, and third trimesters of pregnancy. J Clin Endocrinol Metab 2002; 87:1189–93.
69. Orth JM, Jester WF, Li LH, Laslett AL. Gonocyte–Sertoli cell interactions during development of the neonatal rodent testis. Curr Top Dev Biol 2000; 50:103–24.

70. Ryu BY, Orwig KE, Kubota H, Avarbock MR, Brinster RL. Phenotypic and functional characteristics of spermatogonial stem cells in rats. Dev Biol 2004; 274:158–70.
71. Hadziselimovic F, Herzog B. The importance of both an early orchidopexy and germ cell maturation for fertility. Lancet 2001; 358:1156–7.
72. Sharpe RM, McKinnell C, Kivlin C, Fisher JS. Proliferation and functional maturation of Sertoli cells, and their relevance to disorders of testis function in adulthood. Reproduction 2003; 125:769–84.
73. Mendis-Handagama SML, Ariyaratne HB. Differentiation of the adult Leydig cell population in the postnatal testis. Biol Reprod 2001; 65:660–71.

Gonads, genital ducts, and genitalia

67

Steven E Lerman, Irene M McAleer, and George W Kaplan

Formation of the gonads begins during the first 3 weeks. Approximately 30–50 germ cells become recognizable among the endodermal cells of the caudal portion of the yolk sac near the allantoic stalk. These begin to migrate by ameboid motion towards the genital ridge.

The hindgut begins to develop during this same time frame. Its development was described in Chapter 49. To briefly recapitulate, the hindgut which is endoderm, sends a blind extension caudally which meets the ectoderm of the body wall at the cloacal membrane. The cloacal membrane initially extends from the tail bud to the body stalk, but as the mesoderm grows the extent of the cloacal membrane becomes smaller.

The gonads continue to develop during the 4th week but remain in an indifferent stage. At this time it is impossible to determine the sex of an embryo by examination. The ventromedial surface of the urogenital ridge begins to thicken and bulge into the coelom as a separate genital ridge, which lies medial and parallel to the mesonephric ridge.

The germ cells, which have been migrating dorsally in the wall of the yolk sac and gut, reach the gonadal ridge by the middle of the 5th week (Figure 67.1). It is during this time that the genital tubercle appears on

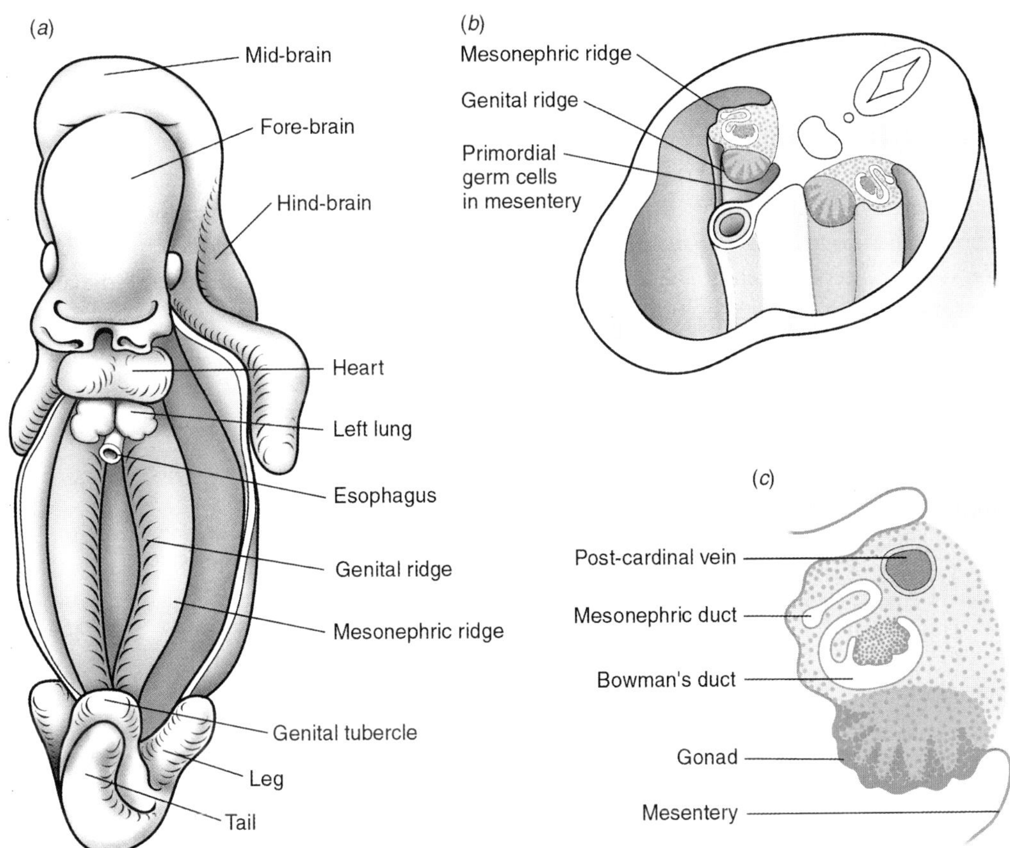

Figure 67.1 Urogenital ridge in the human: (*a*) 9 mm ventral view; (*b*) 7 mm transverse view; and (*c*) 10 mm transverse view. (Reproduced from Arey,[1] with permission.)

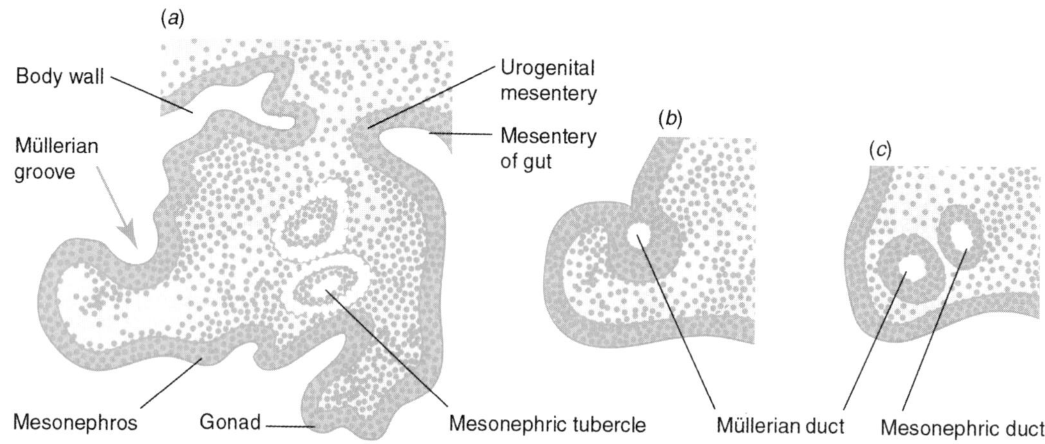

Figure 67.2 Origin of the human müllerian duct at the 12 mm stage: (*a*) through the open groove; (*b*) slightly lower level, showing closure; and (*c*) still lower, showing a tube. (Reproduced from Arey,[1] with permission.)

the ventral midline between the umbilical cord and the tailbud. The tubercle has a thin urogenital groove caudally, the floor of which is the cloacal membrane and the sides are the urogenital folds. At the same time the cloaca is divided into an anterior urogenital sinus and a posterior rectum by the urorectal septum.

During the 6th week an indifferent gonad is recognizable in both sexes and consists of superficial germinal epithelium and an internal blastema derived from ingrowth of coelomic epithelium. The blastema forms into primary or medullary sex cords, and the germ cells and mesenchyme come to lie between these cords. The urogenital ridge is attached broadly near the root of the mesentery. In both sexes a groove appears in the urogenital ridge, located laterally on the mesonephros near the cephalic end. The cranial end of this groove remains open while caudally it begins to close into a tube (the müllerian duct) (Figure 67.2). There is progressive caudal growth of the solid, blind end of the müllerian duct, guided by the mesonephros. Near the cloaca the urogenital ridges swing mesiad into the genital cord. The cranial end of the müllerian duct is forced laterally by the enlarging suprarenal glands and kidneys. Hence, each müllerian duct has two bends, a cranial one and a caudal one (Figure 67.3).

During the 7th week in the male the attachment of the gonads to the mesonephros becomes the mesorchium. The medullary sex cords fuse with mesonephric tubules to form ductuli efferentes (Figure 67.4). Some mesonephric tubules cephalad to this area persist as vestigial structures associated with the epididymis and spermatic cord (the appendix epididymis, the superior and inferior vasa aberrantia, and

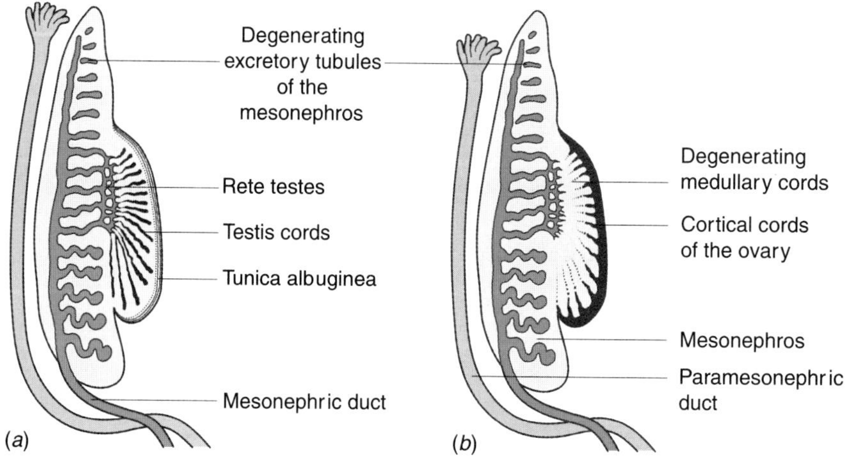

Figure 67.3 Diagram of the genital ducts in the 6th week of development in the male (*a*) and female (*b*). The mesonephric and müllerian ducts are present in both. Note the excretory tubules of the mesonephros and their relationship to the developing gonad in both sexes. (Reproduced from Sadler,[2] with permission.)

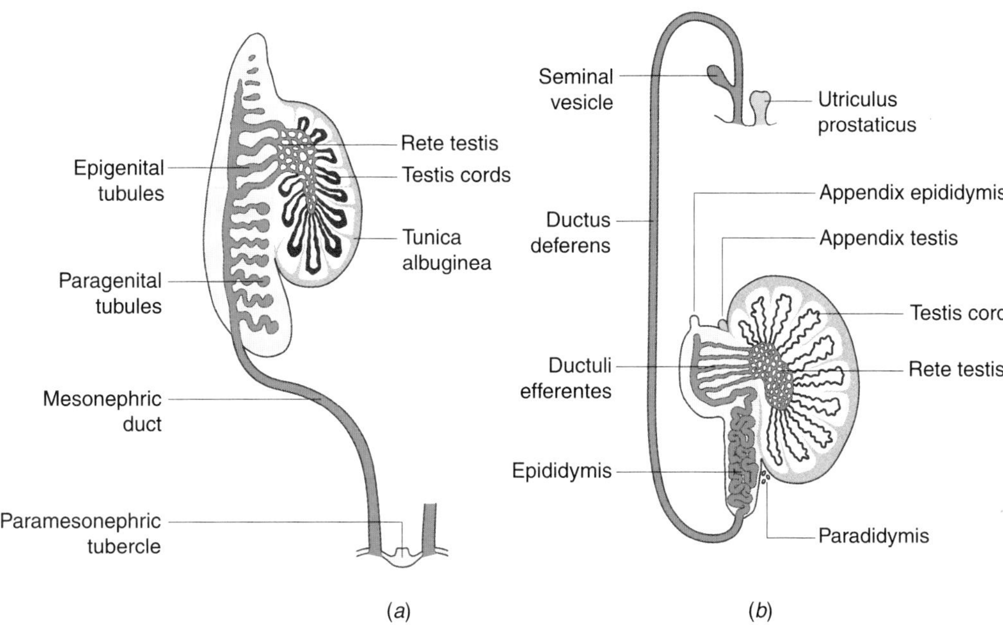

Figure 67.4 (*a*) Diagram of the genital ducts in the male in the 4th month of development. Cranial and caudal (paragenital tubule) segments of the mesonephric system regress. (*b*) Diagram of the genital ducts after descent of the testis. Note the horseshoe-shaped testis cords, rete testis, and efferent ductules entering the ductus deferens. The paradidymis is formed by remnants of the paragenital mesonephric tubules. The müllerian duct has degenerated except for the appendix testis. The prostatic utricle is an outpocketing from the urethra. (Reproduced from Sadler,[2] with permission.)

the paradidymis). The sex cords become separated from the surface epithelium of the gonad by small cells that eventually form the tunica albuginea. The primordial germ cells become incorporated into the testis cords, and these cords become arranged radially, separated by a proliferation of mesenchyme. The cords eventually converge towards the blastemal mass, emerging as the primordia of the rete testis. In the female at this time the round ligament begins to form.

The genital tubercle elongates into a phallus and its tip rounds into the glans (Figure 67.5). Genital swellings appear lateral to the phallic base. The urogenital sinus opens at the base of the phallus by rupture of the cloacal membrane. In the male the corpora cavernosa begin to appear from mesenchymal columns in this area.

The upper five-sixths of the mesonephric ridge has been lost by the 8th week and becomes the diaphragmatic ligament of the mesonephros, which eventually will become the suspensory ligament of the gonad.

In the male, the tunica albuginea has formed a definite encapsulating layer on the gonad, and the gubernaculum begins to form. The phallus elongates, as does the urethral groove and the genital swellings rotate caudad.

In the female, clusters of indifferent cells and primordial germ cells appear. These fall into a dense primary cortex and a looser primary medulla. A mass bulges from the medulla into the mesovarium to form the rete ovarii (Figure 67.6). The suspensory ligament of the ovary is formed from the cephalic end of the genital ridge, while the proper ligament of the ovary is formed from the terminal part of the genital ridge and unites the caudal end of the ovary to the transverse bend of the müllerian duct and eventually to the uterus.

The mesonephros consists of 34 pairs of tubules by the 9th week, but half of them are non-functional. This is the end of the stage of maximal mesonephric development. The cranial eight to 15 pairs project against the rete testis or rete ovarii. The caudal ends of the müllerian ducts have now fused medially and end blindly at Müller's tubercle. The mesonephric ducts are now lateral to the müllerian duct caudally.

Cowper's gland in the male and Bartholin's gland in the female, which are homologues, arise as a pair of solid buds from the endodermal epithelium of the urogenital sinus distal to Müller's tubercle. In the male, they extend backwards, paralleling the urogenital sinus, and penetrate the mesenchyme of the corpus cavernosum urethrae and become glandular. They open into the bulbus urethra. In the female, they open into the vestibule near the hymen.

By the 10th week all of the mesonephric tubules have become discontinuous. The gonads in both sexes lie at the boundary of the pelvis and the abdomen. In

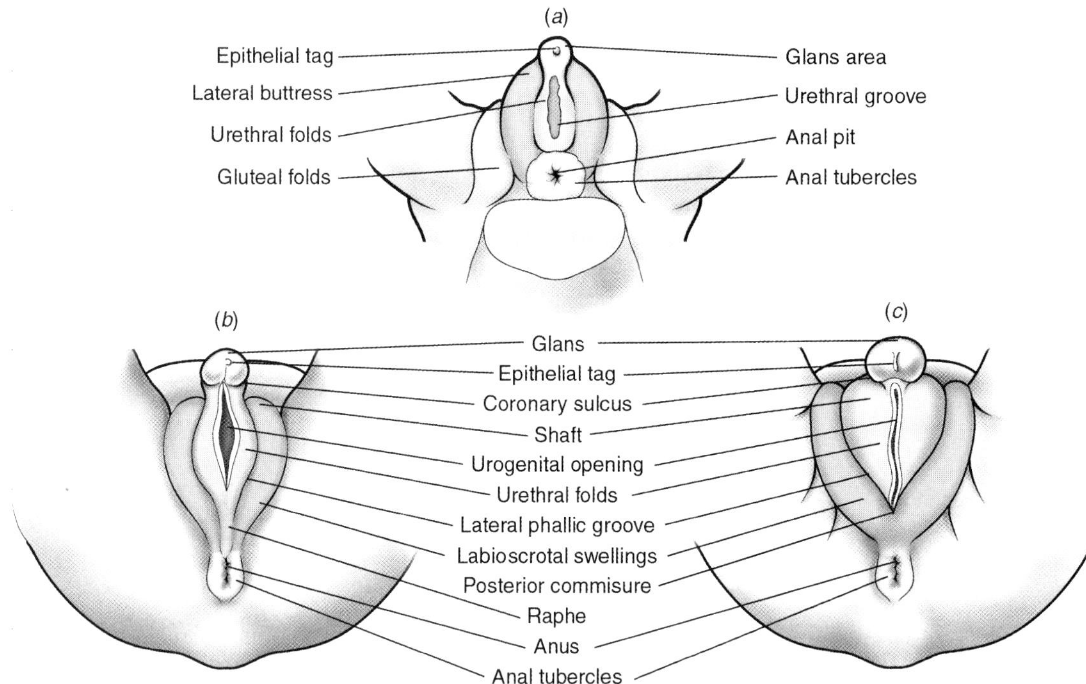

Figure 67.5 Developing external genitalia of the human: (*a*) 7th week; (*b*) male, 10th week; and (*c*) female, 11th week. (Reproduced from Gray and Skandalakis,[3] with permission.)

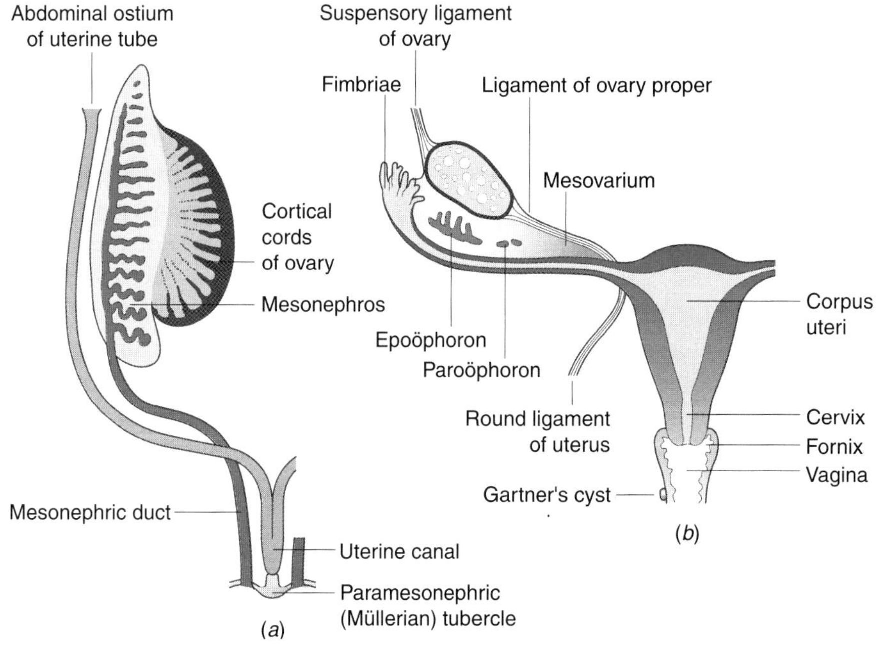

Figure 67.6 (*a*) Drawing of the genital ducts in the female at the end of the 2nd month of development. Note the müllerian tubercle and formation of the uterine canal. (*b*) Drawing of the genital ducts after descent of the ovary. The only parts remaining from the mesonephric system are the epoöphoron, paroöphoron, and Gartner's duct. Note the suspensory ligament of the ovary, ligament of the ovary proper, and round ligament of the uterus. (Reproduced from Sadler,[2] with permission.)

the male, the external genitalia are becoming visible as male structures as a result of secretion of testosterone by the fetal testis. The phallus has become the penis. The edges of the urethral folds begin to fuse progressively from posterior to anterior, forming the urethra and the median raphe. The genital swellings become scrotal swellings, which fuse to form a scrotal septum and raphe.

Table 67.1 Embryologic remnants

Male	Müllerian remnants	Appendix testis Prostatic utricle
Female	Wolffian remnants	Epoöphoron Paraoöphoron Gartner's duct

In the 11th week the prostate arises as multiple outgrowths of endoderm both above and below the mesonephric ducts. These outgrowths arise in five different groups, each of which corresponds to a future prostatic lobe. The buds grow into the surrounding mesenchyme, which in turn provides both connective tissue and smooth muscle. In the female, the homologues of the prostate are the urethral glands, which are drained by Skene's ducts on each side.

Littre's glands bud from the male urethra in the 12th week. In the female, homologues of Littre's glands bud into the vestibule. In the male the processus vaginalis appears as an outpouching at the internal inguinal ring, and the testis lies nearby. The gubernaculum has already formed. The müllerian ducts degenerate owing to the secretion, by Sertoli cells, of müllerian inhibiting factor (MIF). Müllerian remants in the male are the appendix testis from the cranial end and the prostatic utricle from the caudal end of the müllerian duct (Table 67.1).

In the female, the secondary ovarian cortex begins to form in the 12th week by division of cells of the ovarian blastema and by new growth of germinal epithelium. The early ova regress and form the medulla. The ovaries at this time lie at the pelvic brim. The round ligament is complete. Vaginal and uterine musculature appears from the mesenchyme surrounding the müllerian ducts. The distal portions of the müllerian ducts have fused below the caudal bend (Figure 67.7).

In the 13th week, in the male, the seminal vesicles develop as lateral branches off the mesonephric duct. Branching of these seminal vesicles is evident by the 4th month of fetal life, and eventually a muscular coat is gained from the mesenchyme. In the female, the mesonephric ducts begin to regress. Elongation of the fetal pelvis causes a solid epithelial cord to form between the end of the müllerian ducts and the urogenital sinus; this cord will become the upper vagina.

During the 14th week, the penile shaft continues to elongate in the male, and the urethra has fused to the base of glans penis. The penile shaft has a ventral deflection.[4] The prepuce now begins to form as a fold of skin that grows distally. By 5 months of gestational age, preputial formation is complete. The prepuce then fuses to the glans and reseparates from it under the influence of testosterone by the formation of small clefts in the preputial sac. This procedure of separation is incomplete at birth and continues for several years thereafter.

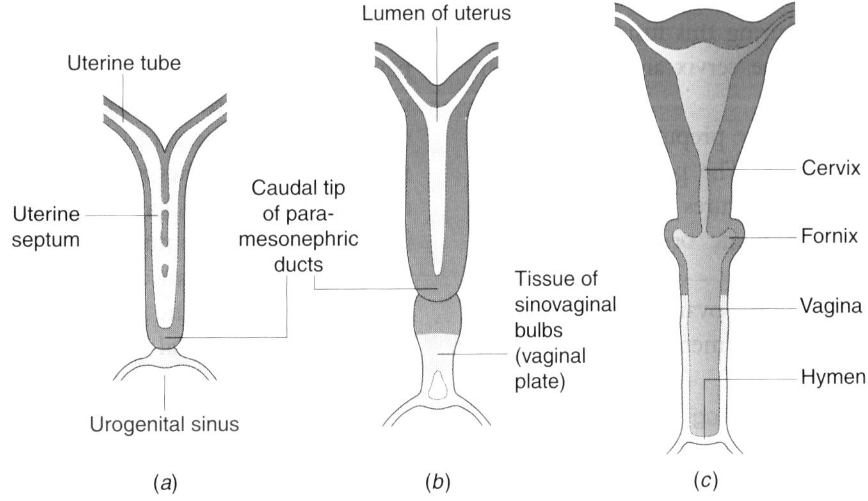

Figure 67.7 Schematic drawing showing formation of the uterus and vagina: (*a*) at 9 weeks, note the disappearance of the uterine septum; (*b*) at the end of the 3rd month, note the tissue of the sinovaginal bulbs; and (*c*) in the newborn, the fornices and the upper portion of the vagina are formed by vacuolization of the müllerian tissue and the lower portion of the vagina is formed by vacuolization of the sinovaginal bulbs. (Reproduced from Sadler,[2] with permission.)

Male pseudohermaphrodite

Complete androgen insensitivity

Patients with CAIS present as young girls either with a hernia or with amenorrhea. CAIS can be due to a spontaneous mutation or can be an X-linked recessive disorder. Since the androgen receptor is defective and the testes make MIS, both the wolffian and müllerian systems involute, and the upper vagina, fallopian tubes, and uterus are usually absent. The vagina is short and blind ending. Serum LH, FSH, and testosterone are all elevated, since testosterone is unable to feedback to the hypothalamus. Patients have a clearly female gender identity, presumably because they also lack androgen receptor in the brain. At puberty, the abundant testosterone is converted to estradiol, leading to normal female breast development, without pubic hair development ('hairless women'). Once the diagnosis is made, gonadectomy is recommended to prevent eventual malignant degeneration of an undescended testis, usually a seminoma[12] (Figure 68.14). If the diagnosis is made prepubertally and gonadectomy is carried out, exogenous estrogen will be required to bring on puberty. An alternative is to leave the gonads in place and remove them after puberty. Since gonadectomy is easier to perform in infancy, assists in making the diagnosis of CAIS, and eliminates the risk of tumor formation, most patients who are diagnosed prepubertally undergo an early gonadectomy. Adult patients all require estrogen supplementation. Patients are not fertile, since no uterine tissue is present. If sexual function is impaired due to the short vagina, a substitution, skin flap, or Frank (dilatation) vaginoplasty can be carried out.[14]

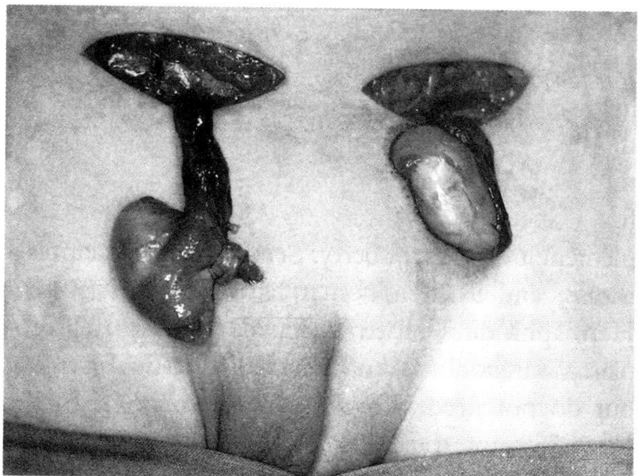

Figure 68.14 Complete androgen insensitivity syndrome: bilateral inguinal explorations revealed apparently normal testes.

Partial androgen insensitivity

Patients with partial loss of androgen receptor activity were previously diagnosed with Reifenstein syndrome, Lub's syndrome, or Gilbert–Dreyfus syndrome, which are now categorized as PAIS. Phenotypically, the genitals range from mildly virilized to fully male. There is no pathognomonic enzyme abnormality that can be used to define PAIS. Depending on the response to testosterone stimulation, patients may be raised as male or female. The response to exogenous testosterone is not impressive.[15]

5α-Reductase deficiency

This disorder is also known as pseudovaginal perineoscrotal hypospadias. 5α-Reductase has two forms: type 1 is found in non-genital tissue and type 2 is found in the genitals. Boys with 5α-reductase type 2 deficiency have low levels of DHT, so they are born with perineal hypospadias, a blind-ending vagina, and testes that are usually palpable. At puberty, a rise in testosterone level leads to phallic enlargement due to peripheral conversion by the normal 5α-reductase type 1. Pubic hair does not develop well, and the prostate does not enlarge.[16,17] The diagnosis is made by a high testosterone: DHT ratio of 50:1, compared with the normal ratio of 5–10:1.[7] Children with this disorder in the Dominican Republic and Papua New Guinea are initially raised as females and then change their gender identity at puberty to male. There are rare reports of fertility in affected men, since most men have low-volume ejaculates. Preoperative testosterone stimulation to lengthen the penis has been used before hypospadias repair. An improved understanding of how gender identity changes during development in patients with 5α-reductase deficiency has resulted in most of these individuals being raised as males.

Persistent müllerian duct syndrome

Also known as hernia uteri inguinalis, this presents as either an undescended testis or an inguinal hernia in a boy. Lack of MIS synthesis or a defective MIS receptor is felt to be the cause. The müllerian structures (fallopian tube, uterus, and upper vagina) are intimately associated with the wolffian structures. There is no risk of malignant degeneration of the müllerian structures since there is no ovarian tissue, so excision is not necessary, and would risk injury to the vas and testis. Orchiopexy is felt to be the optimal surgical management, since some men have had children without assisted reproductive techniques.[18] The testes are at risk for tumor formation, as are other abdominal undescended testes, so if the testis cannot be successfully placed in the scrotum for monitoring, orchiectomy should be considered.

Congenital lipoid adrenal hyperplasia

Previously thought to be due to a defect in 20,22-desmolase activity, this condition is actually due to a protein – known as steroid acute reaction protein (StAR) – controlling the metabolism of 20,22-desmolase. Patients are 46,XY, but appear as phenotypic newborn girls, and present with diarrhea, salt wasting, and shock, similar to patients with salt-wasting CAH. Their adrenals are massively distended with cholesterol, which cannot be further metabolized. They require corticosteroid and mineralocorticoid supplementation, and are usually raised as girls after the testes are removed.[19]

3β-hydroxysteroid dehydrogenase deficiency

This deficiency is discussed above in the section on the female pseudohermaphrodite, and represents the only enzymatic defect to cause genital ambiguity in both males and females.

17β-hydroxylase dehydrogenase (type 3) deficiency

This enzyme is only found in the testis. (17β-Hydroxylase dehydrogenase type 1 is responsible for catalyzing the conversion of estrone to estradiol in the ovary – see Figure 68.6.) Since androstenedione cannot be converted to testosterone and DHT, the external genitalia do not masculinize in 46,XY infants. However, androstenedione is able to keep the wolffian duct from involuting. The perineum is female, with clitoral hypertrophy and a short vaginal pouch. Most patients are Palestinians living in Gaza. The diagnosis is made by an elevated androstenedione/testosterone level. At puberty, increased peripheral (non-testicular) conversion of androstenedione to testosterone results in virilization, and patients change their gender identity from female to male, similar to patients with 5α-reductase deficiency.[20]

17α-Hydroxylase/17,20-lyase deficiency

Females with this disorder have mild clitoral hypertrophy, whereas males have hypospadias. The distinguishing factor is the presence of hypertension, since the pathway is directed toward aldosterone synthesis. Progesterone, deoxycorticosterone, aldosterone, and progesterone/17-hydroxyprogesterone ratio are elevated.[21]

Mixed gonadal dysgenesis

Mixed gonadal dysgenesis is the second most likely diagnosis in a newborn with ambiguous genitalia. Patients have a 45,XO/46,XY karyotype, and present with hypospadias and one palpable gonad (Figure 68.15). Gonadal exploration in the patients with ambiguous genitalia shows a streak gonad and ipsilateral unicornuate uterus, and occasional wolffian structures. The contralateral gonad may be a normal or dysgenetic testis. Müllerian structures can also be found ipsilateral to the testis. Streak gonads and dysgenetic testes are removed, and normal testes are placed into the scrotum (Figures 68.16–68.18).

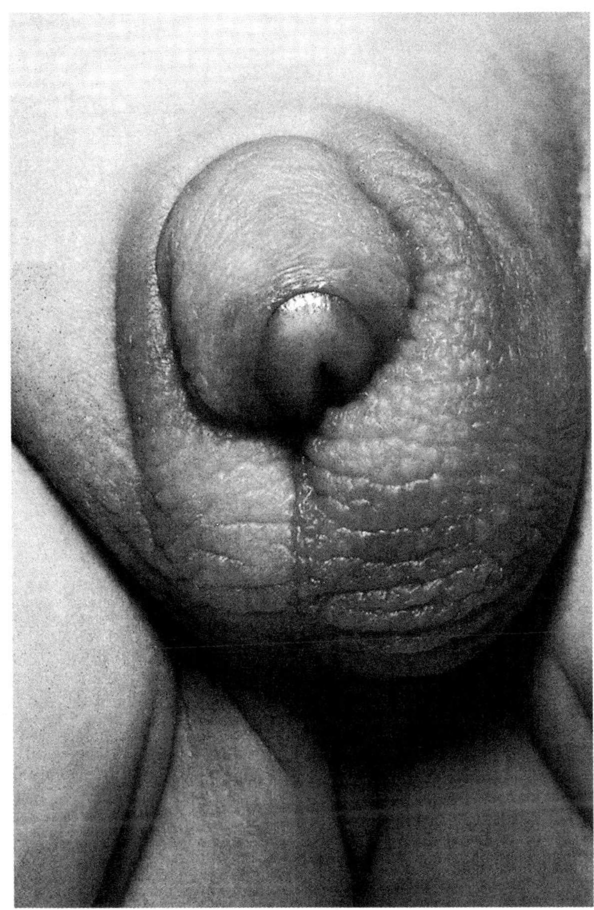

Figure 68.15 Mixed gonadal dysgenesis, showing a flat and empty right hemiscrotum in a boy with hypospadias.

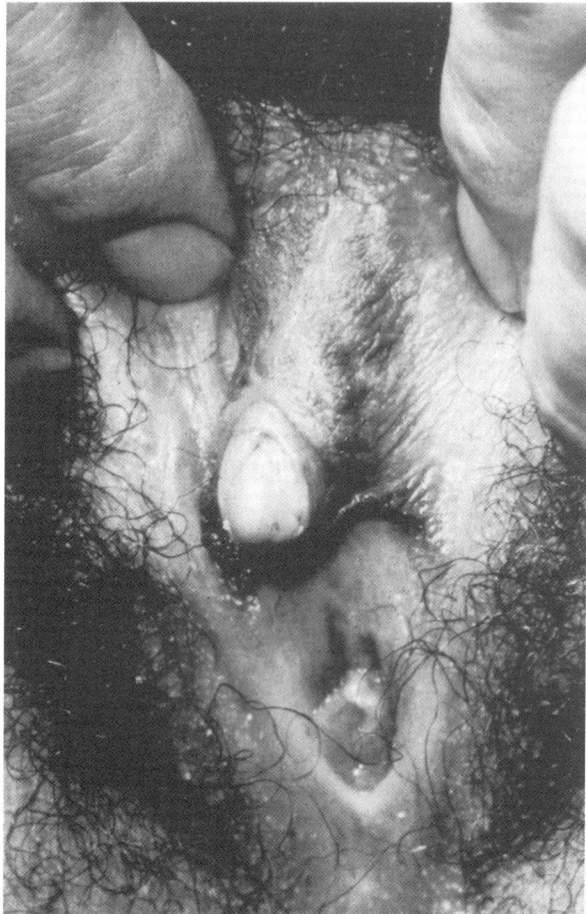

Figure 68.16 Mixed gonadal dysgenesis, postpubertal. Enlarged clitoris. (Reproduced from Snyder,[4] with permission.)

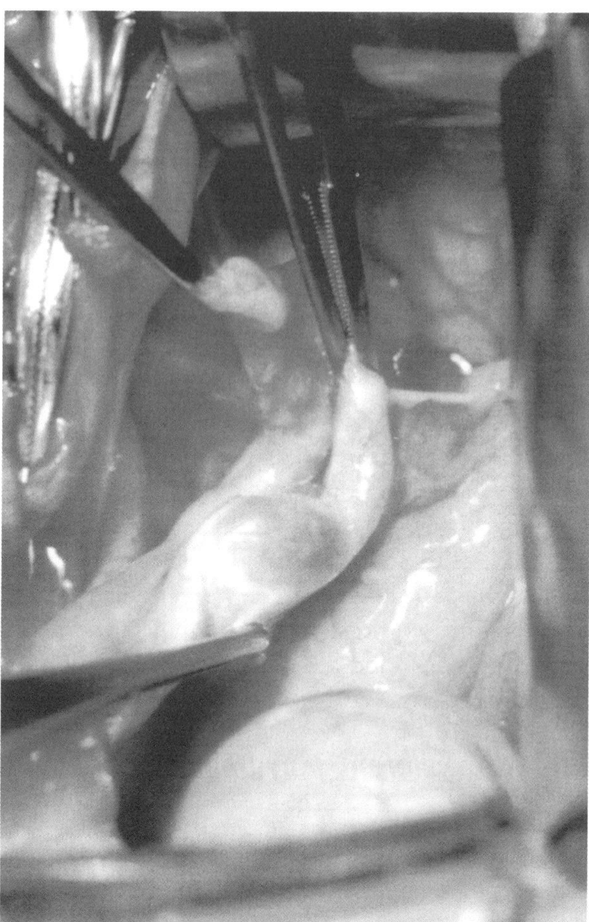

Figure 68.17 Mixed gonadal dysgenesis. Left intra-abdominal testis was removed. (Reproduced from Snyder,[4] with permission.)

Patients are at risk for developing gonadoblastomas, dysgerminomas, and seminomas in the testes. A renal ultrasound is helpful to rule out renal masses if the clinical diagnosis of Denys–Drash syndrome is made (Wilms' tumor, renal failure, ambiguous genitalia.) Testosterone is required after puberty, and patients are usually infertile. If the patient is well virilized, he is usually raised as a male, and the hypospadias is repaired.

Turner's syndrome and pure gonadal dysgenesis

Patients with a 45,XO or 45,XO/46,XY karyotype present with a combination of webbed neck, shield chest, aortic coarctation, horseshoe kidney, and short stature, known as Turner's syndrome. Only 5% have a 45,XO/46,XY karyotype.[22] Both gonads are streaks and are not at risk for tumor unless they are mosaic with 45,XO/46,XY. Because of their characteristic physical findings, these patients are not encountered in the newborn period as intersex patients. Growth hormone and estrogen supplementation are generally required. Patients with gonadal dysgenesis can also have 46,XX and 46,XY karyotypes. Although they are normal phenotypic females without Turner's stigmata and have fallopian tubes and a uterus, the 46,XY patients (Swyer syndrome[23]) are at risk for developing gonadoblastoma, and should have their gonads removed (Figure 68.19).

Gender identity and role: choosing the sex of rearing

The relative importance of environment vs genetics on gender identity has been vigorously debated. The pendulum has swung from believing that gender identity was entirely determined by environment to understanding that both genetics and environment influence ultimate gender identity. In making the

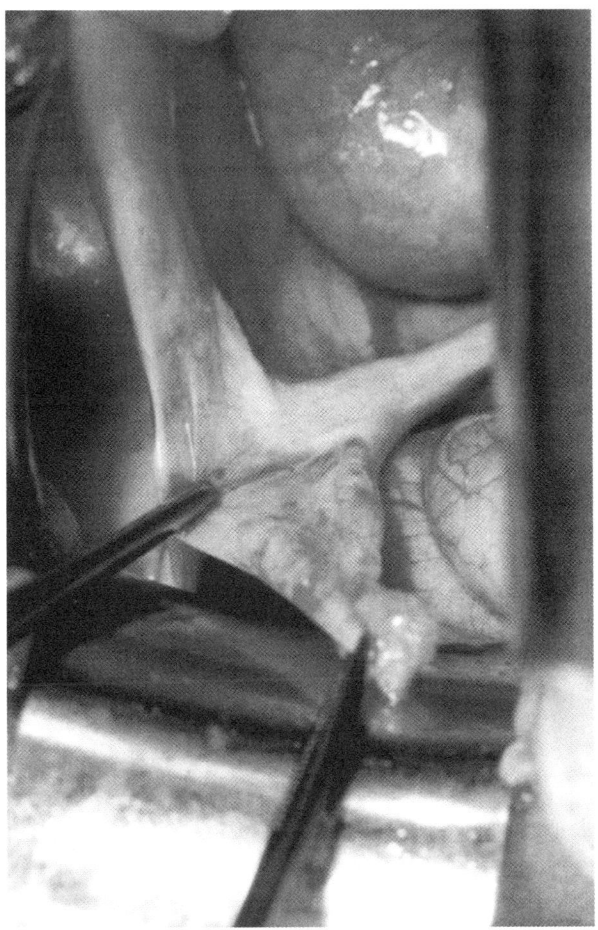

Figure 68.18 Mixed gonadal dysgenesis. Right streak gonad was removed, and cycling with estrogen and progesterone begun. (Reproduced from Snyder,[4] with permission.)

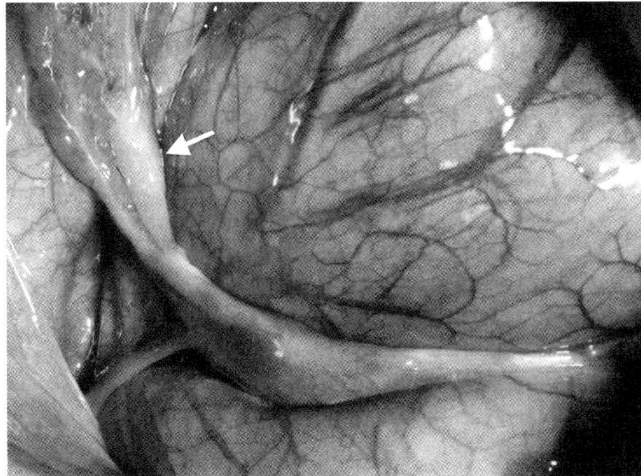

Figure 68.19 XY gonadal dysgenesis: the streak gonad on the left broad ligament (arrow) showed a few testicular elements on microscopy.

decision regarding gender assignment, the following factors should be considered if the 'optimal gender policy' is followed: possible fertility, sexual function, and stable gender identity.[24,25] Whereas fertility is fairly well understood, the data on eventual sexual function are sparse,[26–28] and understanding gender identity long term is even more difficult to predict. Unfortunately, it is difficult to correlate genital virilization with gender identity.

Testosterone undoubtedly 'imprints' the prenatal brain, and the highly publicized cases of gender reassignment have involved genotypic and phenotypic males reassigned as females. Patients choose to identify as male or female (gender identity) and also behave in different ways (gender role) depending on which sex they identify with. Severely virilized CAH patients are more likely to change gender identity later in life, and less significantly affected patients show a more 'tomboyish' gender role than control patients.[29,30] Advocacy groups such as the Intersex Society of North America propose that surgery should be delayed until patients can make the choice for themselves.[31] There is no argument that patients should be assigned a male or female gender at birth. The controversy is over the timing and necessity of genital surgery, which hopefully will become clearer once long-term data on gender identity and gender role are accumulated.[32–34]

Key points

1. Internal genital development depends on the ipsilateral gonad.
2. External genital development depends on the presence of testosterone and DHT.
3. A palpable gonad is usually a testis.
4. Preliminary diagnosis of CAH can usually be made based on physical examination and pelvic ultrasound.
5. There is evidence that testosterone imprints the brain prenatally.

References

1. van Niekerk WA. True hermaphroditism. In: Josso N, ed. The Intersex Child. Basel: Karger, 1981: 80–99.
2. Jost A. Recherches sur la differenciation sexuelle de l'embryon de lapin. Arch d'Anat Microsc Morph Exp 1947; 36:271–2.
3. Jost A. Hormonal factors in the sex differentiation of the mammalian foetus. Phil Trans R Soc Lond B 1970; 259:119–30.

4. Snyder HM. Management of ambiguous genitalia in the neonate. In King LR, ed. Urologic Surgery in Neonates & Young Infants. Philadelphia: WB Saunders, 1988: 346–85.
5. Allen TD. Disorders of sexual differentiation. Urology 1976; 7(4 Suppl):1–32.
6. New MI. Diagnosis and management of congenital adrenal hyperplasia. Annu Rev Med 1998; 49: 311–28.
7. Witchel SF, Lee PA. Ambiguous genitalia. In: Sperling MA, ed. Pediatric Endocrinology. Philadelphia: WB Saunders, 2002: 111–33.
8. Lee P. A perspective on the approach to the intersex child born with genital ambiguity. J Pediatr Endocrinol Metab 2004; 17:133–40.
9. Bongiovanni AM. The adrenogenital syndrome with deficiency of 3 beta-hydroxysteroid dehydrogenase. J Clin Invest 1962; 41:2086–92.
10. Walker AM, Walker J, Adams S et al. True hermaphroditism. J Paediatr Child Health 2000; 36:69–73.
11. Aaronson IA. True hermaphroditism. A review of 41 cases with observations on testicular histology and function. Br J Urol 1985; 57:775–9.
12. Scully RE. Neoplasia associated with anomalous sexual development and abnormal sex chromosomes. In: Josso N, ed. The Intersex Child. Basel: Karger, 1981: 203–17.
13. Krob G, Braun A, Kuhnle U. True hermaphroditism: geographical distribution, clinical findings, chromosomes and gonadal histology. Eur J Pediatr 1994; 153:2–10.
14. Wisniewski AB, Migeon CJ, Meyer-Bahlburg HFL et al. Complete androgen insensitivity syndrome: long-term medical, surgical, and psychosexual outcome. J Clin Endocrinol Metab 2000; 85:2664–9.
15. Gottlieb B, Pinsky P, Beitel LK, Trifiro M. Androgen insensitivity. Am J Med Genet 1999; 87:210–17.
16. Imperato-McGinley J, Peterson R, Stoller R et al. Steroid 5 alpha reductase deficiency in man: an inherited form of male pseudohermaphroditism. Science 1974; 186:1213–15.
17. Walsh PC, Madden JD, Harrod MJ et al. Familial incomplete male pseudohermaphroditism, type 2. Decreased dihydrotestosterone formation in pseudovaginal perineoscrotal hypospadias. N Engl J Med 1974; 291:944–9.
18. Vandersteen DR, Chaumeton AK, Ireland K, Tank ES. Surgical management of persistent müllerian duct syndrome. Urology 1997; 49:941–5.
19. Bose HS, Sugawara T, Strauss JF III et al. The pathophysiology and genetics of congenital lipoid adrenal hyperplasia. International Congenital Lipoid Adrenal Hyperplasia Consortium. N Engl J Med 1996; 335:1970–8.
20. Saez JM, De Peretti E, Morera AM, David M, Bertrand J. Familial male pseudohermaphroditism with gynecomastia due to a testicular 17-ketosteroid reductase defect. I. Studies in vivo. J Clin Endocrinol Metab 1971; 33:604–10.
21. Zachmann M, Vollmin JA, Hamilton W, Prader A. Steroid 17,20-desmolase deficiency: a new cause of male pseudohermaphroditism. Clin Endocrinol (Oxf) 1972; 1:369–85.
22. Kleczkowska A, Dmoch E, Kubien E, Fryns JP, Van den Berghe H. Cytogenetic findings in a consecutive series of 478 patients with Turner syndrome. The Leuven experience 1965–1989. Genet Counsel 1990; 1:227–33.
23. Swyer GI. Male pseudohermaphroditism: a hitherto undescribed form. Br Med J 1955; 2:709–12.
24. Meyer-Bahlburg HFL. Gender assignment in intersexuality. J Psychol Hum Sex 1998; 10:1–21.
25. Meyer-Bahlburg HFL. Gender assignment and reassignment in 46,XY pseudohermaphroditism and related conditions. J Clin Endocrinol Metab 1999; 84:3455–8.
26. Alizai NK, Thomas DFM, Lilford RJ, Batchelor AGG, Johnson N. Feminizing genitoplasty for congenital adrenal hyperplasia: what happens at puberty? J Urol 1999; 161:1588–91.
27. Creighton SM, Minto CL, Steele SJ. Objective cosmetic and anatomical outcomes at adolescence of feminizing surgery for ambiguous genitalia done in childhood. Lancet 2001; 358:124–5.
28. Minto CL, Liao LM, Woodhouse CRJ, Ransley PG, Creighton SM. The effect of clitoral surgery on sexual outcome in individuals who have intersex conditions with ambiguous genitalia: a cross-sectional study. Lancet 2003; 361:1252–7.
29. Zucker KJ, Bradley ST, Oliver G et al. Psychosexual development of women with congenital adrenal hyperplasia. Horm Behav 1996; 30:300–18.
30. Meyer-Bahlburg HF, Dolezal C, Baker SW et al. Prenatal androgenization affects gender-related behavior but not gender identity in 5–12-year old girls with congenital adrenal hyperplasia. Arch Sex Behav 2004; 33:97–104.
31. Intersex Society of North America. www.isna.org
32. Reiner WG. Gender identity and sex assignment: a reappraisal for the 21st century. In: Zderic SA, ed. Pediatric Gender Assignment: A Critical Reappraisal. New York: Kluwer, 2002: 175–97.
33. Meyer-Bahlburg HFL. Gender assignment and reassignment in intersexuality: controversies, data, and guidelines for research. In: Zderic SA, ed. Pediatric Gender Assignment: A Critical Reappraisal. New York: Kluwer, 2002: 199–223.
34. Thomas DFM. Gender assignment: background and current controversies. BJU Int 2004; 93(Suppl 3):47–50.

Anorectal malformation and cloaca 69

Curtis A Sheldon and William R DeFoor Jr

Introduction

The pediatric urologist must be familiar with the management of anorectal malformations (ARMs) and cloacal malformations (CMs). ARMs are commonly associated with surgically relevant urinary tract and vaginal pathology. The pediatric urologist is responsible for the management of these defects. Because these malformations are relatively uncommon, it is vitally important for the reconstructive surgeon to be familiar with the embryology, anatomy, and pathophysiology of each of these. Considerable morbidity ensues if the surgeon fails to manage these defects in a thoughtful, deliberate manner. A multidisciplinary approach to children with complex cloacal malformations is appropriate and involves pediatric general surgeons, pediatric urologists, pediatric anesthesiologists, and pediatric radiologists.

Anorectal malformations occur in approximately 1 in 4000 to 1 in 5000 live births.[1] Cloacal anomalies occur in 1 in 50 000 live births.[2] The incidence of mortality with ARMs has dropped dramatically over time. The morbidity associated with these anomalies is extensive and includes psychosocial developmental disorders, fecal incontinence, urinary incontinence, urinary tract infection (UTI), impaired intercourse, impaired fertility, as well as other abnormalities such as limb anomalies, vertebral anomalies, neurologic deficits, and tracheoesophageal fistulae.

The history of imperforate anus management dates back to the 7th century, where the earliest reports of survival with surgery (rupture of an obstructing anal membrane) may be found. In 1835, Amusset performed a perineal proctoplasty. In the 1850s, various authors reported the use of colostomy, which opened the door for successful management of high ARM. An abdominal–perineal pull-through procedure was undertaken in the 1880s[3,4] and advanced further by Rhoads et al.[5] In 1953, Stevens promoted a direct sacral approach to reconstruction, and in 1967, Kiesewetter combined these approaches into a two-stage sacroabdominoperineal pull-through procedure. Peña and Hendren ushered in the modern era of ARMs as well as cloacal management. They performed their posterior sagittal approach for the treatment of these malformations initially in 1980 and reported the results soon thereafter.[6]

Surgeons recognized the frequent association of urologic abnormalities with ARMs.[7–11] Similar recognition of the high incidence of spinal cord abnormalities, including occult spinal dysraphisms such as tethered cord, lipomas, neurenteric cysts, and diastematomyelia, advanced the management of these patients.[12–15] Patients with ARMs frequently require complex urinary reconstruction, for which unique concerns must be addressed.[16]

The development of the Malone antegrade continence enema or continent cecostomy[17] advanced the management of fecal incontinence and fecal retention in children with neurologic conditions such as myelomeningocele. Surgeons now successfully apply this procedure to enable fecal undiversion in children with ARMs who have previously undergone colostomy for refractory fecal incontinence.[18–19]

Spectrum of abnormalities encountered

We now know that urinary, genital, and anorectal development are intimately interconnected. As early as 1829, Mayer recognized an association between vaginal agenesis and other congenital anomalies.[20] Küster and Rokitansky independently confirmed this observation.[21,22] Hauser and Schreiner[23] emphasized the association of vaginal agenesis with skeletal and renal anomalies. Thus, the final association became known as the Mayer–Rokitansky–Küster–Hauser syndrome. Upper tract anomalies are encountered in

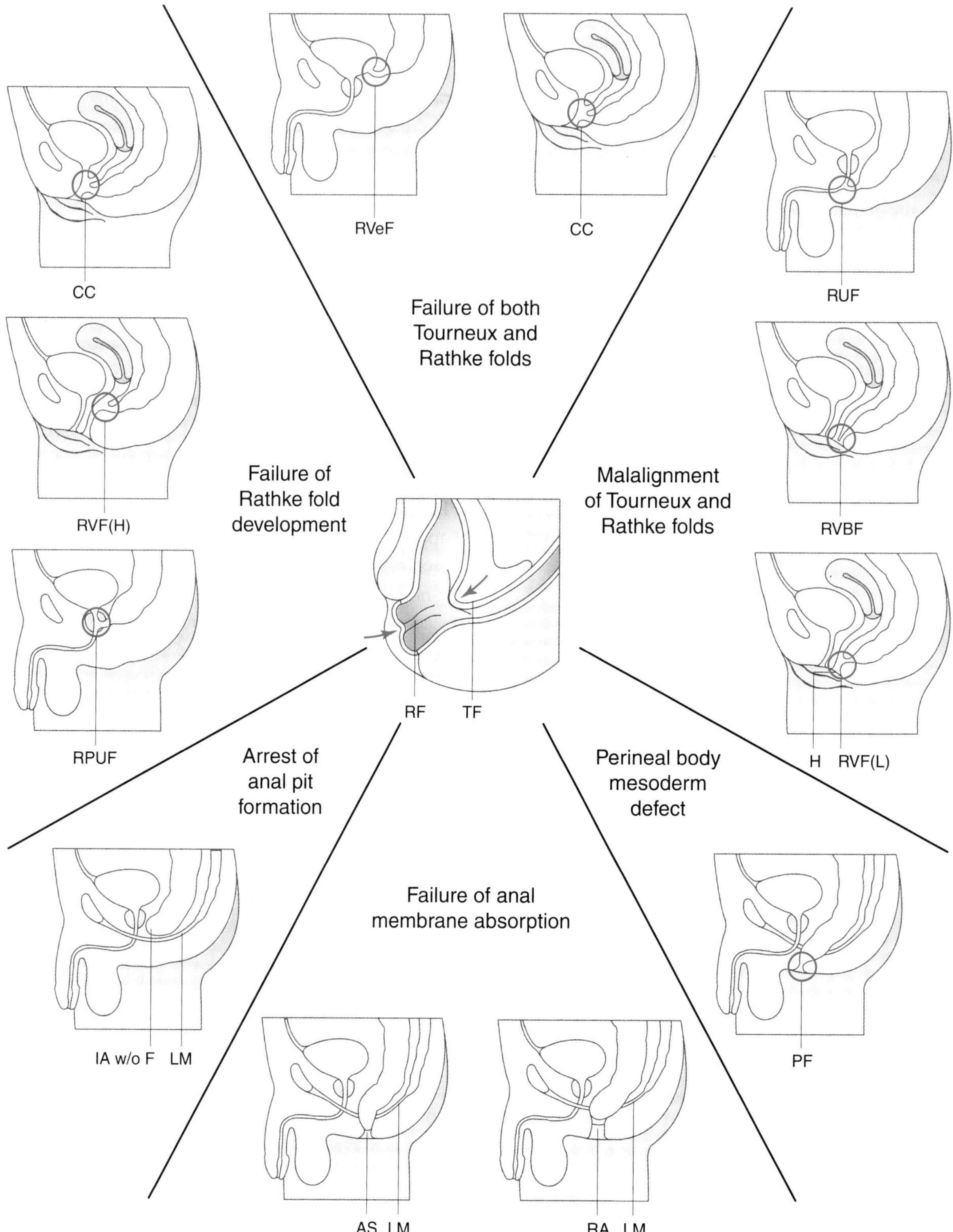

Figure 69.2 Spectrum of anomalies associated with imperforate anus. AS = anal stenosis; CC = common cloaca; IA w/o F = imperforate anus without fistula; RF = Rathke fold; RA = rectal atresia; RPUF = rectoprostatic urethral fistula; RUF = rectourethral fistula; RVF(H) = rectovaginal fistula (high); RVF(L) = rectovaginal fistula (low); RVeF = rectovesical fistula; RVBF = rectovestibular fistula; TF = Tourneux fold; LM = levator muscle; PF = perineal fistula; H = hymen. (Redrawn after Paidas and Peña.[45])

wedge, the medial portion of which (Tourneux fold) is progressively driven caudally toward the cloacal membrane by progressive fusion of the lateral ridges (Rathke folds) which grow inward from the sides of the cloaca. The urorectal septum divides the cloacal membrane into the urogenital membrane and the anal membrane, which subsequently ruptures (see Figure 69.1c,d). Differential growth causes the anal membrane to be displaced caudally and depressed below the surface, forming the anal pit. The pectinate line in the fully developed human represents the level of the anal membrane. Further differential growth separates the urogenital and anal orifices with the formation of the perineal body (see Figure 69.1e).

Paidas and Peña offer an alternative explanation of various ARMs, as outlined in Figure 69.2.[45] In this scheme, failure of the Rathke fold (RF) development results in the rectoprostatic urethral fistula (RPUF) in males, and the high rectovaginal fistula (RVFH) and common cloaca (CC) in females. Similarly, failure of both Rathke and Tourneux fold (TF) development results in the rectovesical fistula in males and common cloaca in females. Malalignment of Tourneux and Rathke folds causes rectourethral fistulae (RUF) in males and rectovestibular (RVBF) and low rectovaginal fistulae (RVFL) in females. A mesodermal defect at the level of the perineal body results in perineal fistulae (PF). Partial or complete failure of anal membrane absorption results in anal stenosis (AS) or rectal atresia (RA), respectively. The arrest of the anal pit formation results in imperforate anus without fistula, while abnormal fusion of the genital folds gives rise to the covered anus.

The developing mesonephric duct induces the formation of the paramesonephric ducts, which arise as coelomic invaginations.[42] The paramesonephric ducts grow caudally to insert into the urogenital sinus. Caudally, they fuse to become the uterus, while cranially the unfused portions become the uterine or fallopian tubes. A sinual tubercle develops at the site of insertion of the solid tip of the paramesonephric duct and the urogenital sinus (see Figure 69.1f–h). This intimate embryologic relationship between the mesonephric and paramesonephric ducts explains the high incidence of upper tract urinary anomalies encountered with anomalous vaginal development.

The vaginal plate occludes the developing vagina (see Figure 69.1i). With differential growth, the vagina elongates and slides caudally down the dorsal surface of the urethra to establish a separate vestibular opening, as the vaginal plate desquamates to create the vaginal lumen. The hymen represents the junction of the sinual tubercle and the urogenital sinus. Failure of the hymen to rupture (imperforate hymen) and failure of vaginal plate canalization (vaginal atresias and vaginal septa) may cause hydrocolpos (obstructive fluid distention of the vagina) or hydrometrocolpos (obstructive fluid distention of both the vagina and uterus). After menarche, vaginal obstruction may result in hematocolpos or hematometrocolpos (obstructive distention with blood). Müllerian (or uterine) aplasia represents absence of the uterus and results from inadequate caudal progression of the developing paramesonephric ducts. Here, the distal most vagina, ovaries, and external genitalia are normal. A unicornuate uterus occurs from developmental failure of one paramesonephric duct, while uterus didelphys (two uteri, two cervices, and two vaginas), uterus duplex bicollis (two uteri, two cervices, and one vagina), and uterus duplex unicollis or bicornuate uterus (two uteri, one cervix, and one vagina) arise from various degrees of failure of paramesonephric duct fusion.

Anomalies of anorectal development: imperforate anus

Imperforate anus exists as a large spectrum of anomalies. For this reason, classification systems are essential. Stephens and Smith[46] presented a classification

Table 69.3 Wingspread classification of anorectal malformations

Female	Male
High	**High**
Anorectal agenesis	Anorectal agenesis
Rectovaginal fistula	Rectoprostatic fistula
No fistula	Rectovesical fistula
Rectal atresia	No fistula
	Rectal atresia
Intermediate	**Intermediate**
Rectovestibular fistula	Rectobulbar fistula
Rectovaginal fistula	Anal agenesis without fistula
Anal agenesis without fistula	
Low	**Low**
Anovestibular fistula	Anocutaneous fistula
Anocutaneous fistula	Anal stenosis
Anal stenosis	Rare malformations
Cloaca	
Rare malformations	

After Stephens and Smith.[46]

Table 69.4 Incidence of anorectal anomalies

Male		Female		Total
High (35%)		High (13%)		High (26%)
Rectourethral fistula	81%	Cloaca	86%	
Rectovesical fistula	10%	Anorectal agenesis without fistula	5%	
Anorectal agenesis without fistula	8%	Rectovaginal fistula	5%	
Rectal atresia	1%	Rectovesical fistula	2%	
		Rectal atresia	2%	
Intermediate (14%)		Intermediate (7%)		Intermediate (11%)
Rectobulbar fistula	56%	Rectovestibular fistula	54%	
Anal agenesis without fistula	38%	Anal agenesis without fistula	21%	
Anorectal stenosis	7%	Rectovaginal fistula	20%	
		Anorectal stenosis	5%	
Low (49%)		Low (72%)		Low (58%)
Anocutaneous fistula	65%	Anovestibular fistula	42%	
Covered anal stenosis	21%	Anocutaneous fistula	30%	
Covered anus	14%	Anovulvar fistula	17%	
		Covered anus	6%	
		Covered anal stenosis	4%	
		Other	1%	
Miscellaneous (2%)		Miscellaneous (8%)		Miscellaneous (5%)

From Endo et al.[47]

for anal rectal malformations, outlined in Table 69.3. This classification is detailed and anatomically precise. A study of 1992 patients with ARMs from Japan[47] demonstrated the incidence of these anomalies (Table 69.4). 'Low' lesions represented 58% of patients; 'high' and 'intermediate' lesions were found in 26% and 11% of patients, respectively. Only 13% of female ARMs were classified as 'high', most of which were CMs. In contrast, 35% of males had 'high' lesions, 81% of whom had rectourethral fistulae. 'Low' lesions occurred in 49% and 72% of males and females, respectively, most of which were anocutaneous or anovestibular fistulae. 'Intermediate' lesions are less common but important because they are managed as high lesions but appear to be low lesions on examination. Brock and Peña[37] promoted a classification system that is useful clinically (Table 69.5), dividing both males and females into those for whom no colostomy is required, for whom colostomy is required, and complex malformations. In both males and females, those patients for whom no colostomy is required represent a rather simple spectrum of ARMs. In contrast, those patients requiring colostomy represent a more diverse population of patients with more difficult anatomic problems.

The management of the patient with imperforate anus is outlined in Figures 69.3 and 69.4. Neonatal evaluation begins with a detailed physical examination followed by a period of observation usually ranging between 18 and 24 hours. This not only enables medical stabilization and exclusion of important associated congenital anomalies but also helps in determining the level of the imperforate anus. Infants who pass meconium through the urethra or into the blad-

Table 69.5 Peña classification of anorectal malformations and fistulae

Female	Male
No colostomy required	No colostomy required
Rectoperineal (cutaneous) fistula	Rectoperineal (cutaneous) fistula
	Anal stenosis
	Anal membrane
Colostomy required	Colostomy required
Vestibular fistula	Rectourethral fistula:
Vaginal fistula	Bulbar
Anorectal agenesis without fistula	Prostatic
Rectal atresia	Rectovesical fistula
Persistent cloaca	Anorectal agenesis without fistula
	Rectal atresia
Complex malformations	Complex malformations

From Brock and Peña.[37]

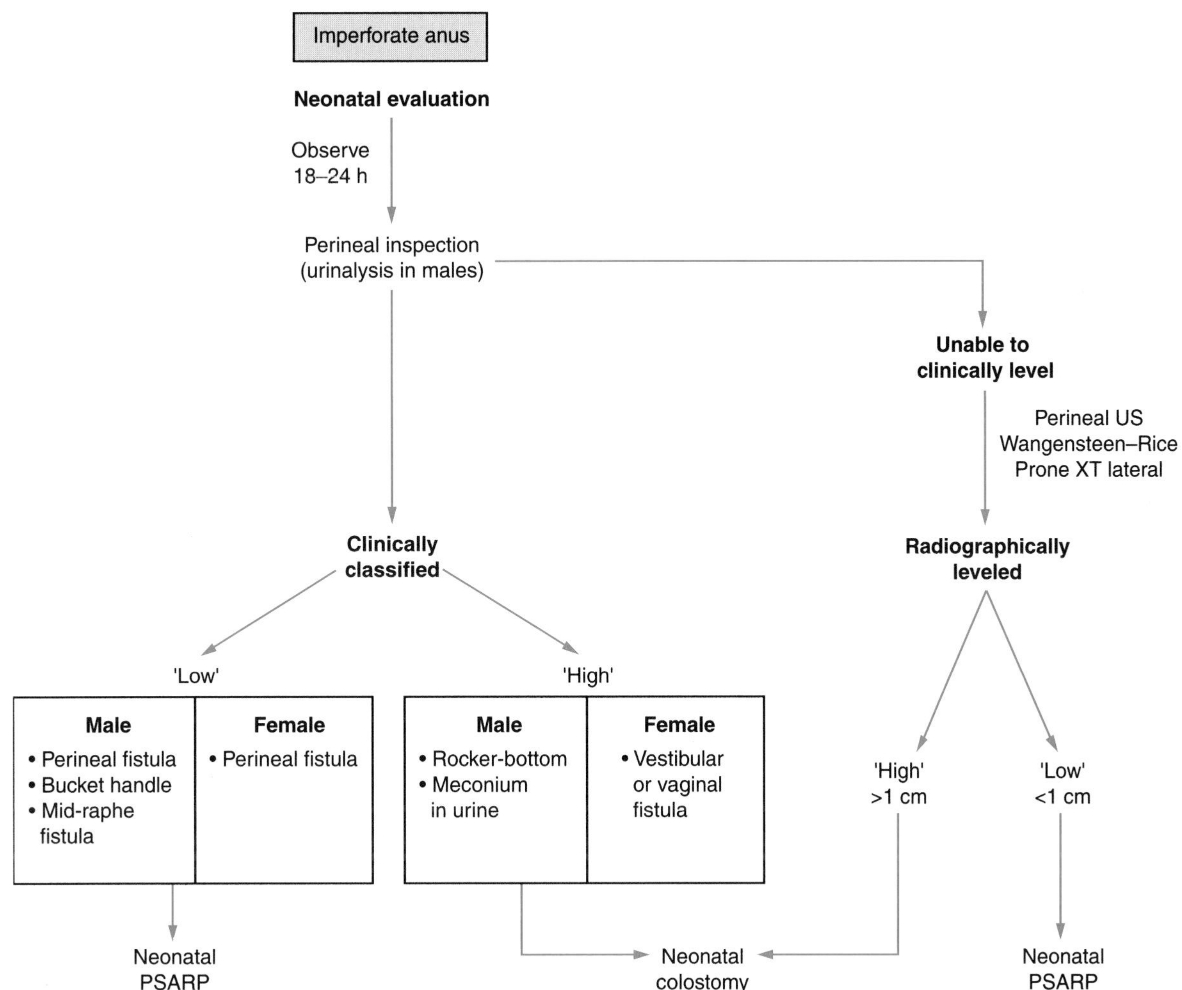

Figure 69.3 Neonatal evaluation and management of patient with imperforate anus. PSARP = posterior sagittal anorectoplasty.

der may be detected by direct inspection or by urinalysis. This indicates a high imperforate anus. In contrast, those patients who pass meconium through a perineal fistula generally have a low imperforate anus. In males, the presence of a 'bucket handle' abnormality or a mid-raphe fistula suggests a low imperforate anus. As noted in Figure 69.3, children with a 'rocker-bottom' anomaly or females with rectovestibular or rectovaginal fistulae usually have a high imperforate anus. Those patients with high lesions require neonatal colostomy, whereas those with a low lesion can be managed with a neonatal posterior sagittal anorectoplasty (PSARP).

Some patients must be clinically classified with radiographic evaluation. In these cases, a perineal ultrasound, a Wangensteen–Rice 'invertogram', or a prone, cross-table, lateral X-ray study is very helpful. Those infants with a radiographically determined distance between the rectal pouch and perineum exceeding 1 cm have high lesions and those with distances less than 1 cm have low lesions. Occasionally, contrast injected into a cutaneous or vestibular lesion may help to distinguish between an intermediate and a low lesion. Recently, magnetic resonance imaging (MRI) has been proposed as a tool for depicting the level of ARM as well as diagnosing associated anomalies of the spinal cord and urogenital system.[48]

As outlined in Figure 69.4, the goals of management in the first few years of life are to protect the upper urinary tracts, ensure low-pressure urinary drainage, normalize anorectal anatomy, and minimize any neurologic deficit that might arise from treatable spinal pathology. We evaluate all patients with an abdominal sonogram to include the kidneys, a contrast voiding cystourethrogram (VCUG), a spinal sonogram, and determination of postvoid residual volume of urine (PVR). Depending on these findings, patients occasionally require intermittent

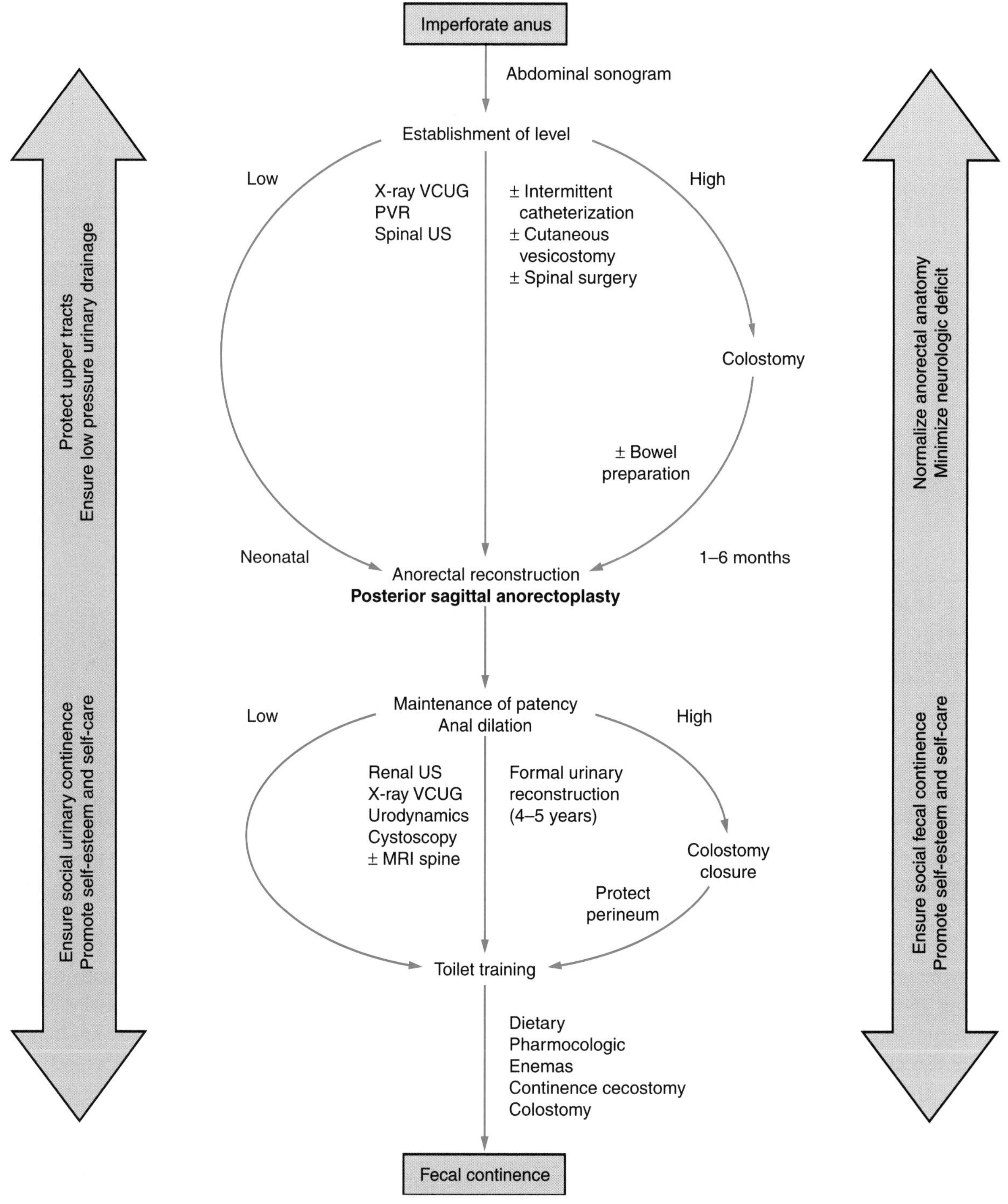

Figure 69.4 Management strategy for imperforate anus (± = possible).

catheterization, cutaneous vesicostomy, or even spinal surgery. Those patients who receive a colostomy will undergo definitive anorectal reconstruction in the form of posterior sagittal anorectoplasty (PSARP), usually between 1 and 6 months of age, but occasionally older, depending on the presence of other congenital anomalies.

The type of colostomy performed is important. Peña[49] recommends a colostomy opened at the junction of the descending colon with the sigmoid, with completely separated stomas. Transverse colostomies are difficult to clean and decompress distally, and loop colostomies are contraindicated owing to the risk of fecal contamination of the urinary tract. Figure 69.5

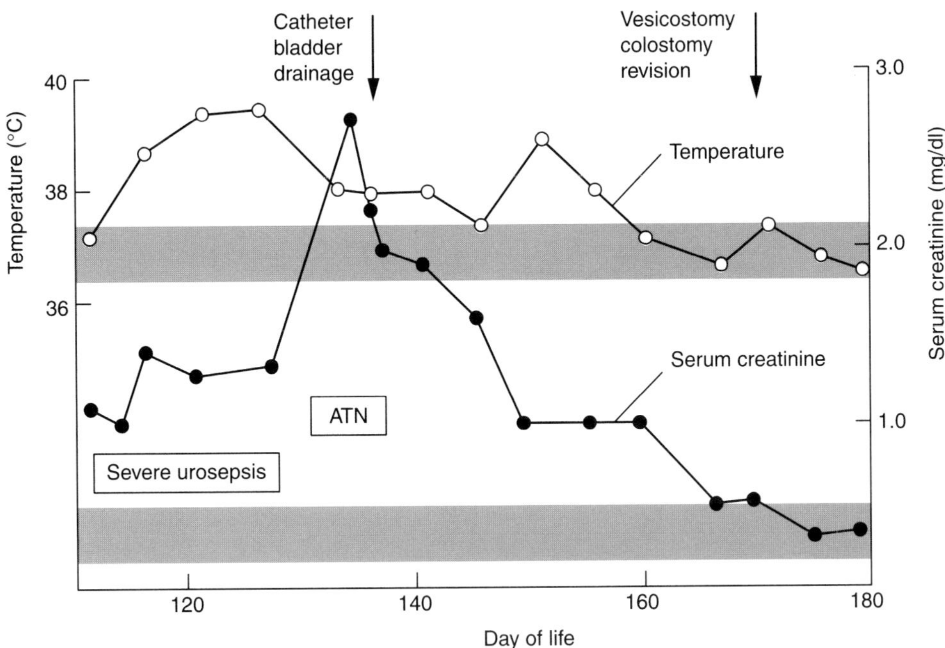

Figure 69.5 This hospital course demonstrates the sequelae of severe urosepsis in a child with imperforate anus in whom chronic urinary retention was unrecognized and a partially diverting colostomy was performed for high imperforate anus. Urosepsis persisted despite antibiotic therapy and resolved only after appropriate drainage had been instituted. (From Sheldon et al.[14])

outlines the course of an infant who received a partially diverting colostomy for high imperforate anus and who had incomplete bladder emptying. This child suffered severe urosepsis, resulting in acute tubular necrosis and significant azotemia that ultimately resolved following creation of a vesicostomy and revision of the colostomy to an end colostomy. Accordingly, patients with rectourinary fistulae, particularly, those with incomplete bladder emptying and/or vesicoureteral reflux (VUR), should be managed with a completely diverting colostomy.

As outlined in Figure 69.4, the goals of management of the preschool and school-aged child with ARMs are to ensure social urinary and fecal continence and to promote self-esteem and self-care. Following PSARP, maintenance of anorectal patency is generally ensured by gentle anal dilation. Children who have previously received a colostomy undergo colostomy closure once healing of the PSARP is complete. These children often develop a severe perineal rash owing to the sudden exposure to feces. We minimize this aggressively by applying antifungal ointment in the early post-colostomy closure period.

Children who fail to attain fecal continence are often managed by dietary or pharmacologic intervention. Occasionally, enemas may be required to achieve continence. Most effective are high cleaning enemas administered at night.[50] Frequently, the child cannot administer the enemas or enemas are not successful. In this case, the creation of a continent cecostomy for an antegrade continence enema has been helpful. This procedure creates a continent, catheterizable channel connecting the cecum and the skin. The appendix is used for this purpose most frequently; however, reconfigured ileum also works successfully. This concept was first developed and presented by Malone et al.[17] We have found this procedure effective in children who have extremely deformed and dysfunctional anal canals,[18] and it has worked even for children who had previously received colostomies for refractory fecal incontinence.

Many children have urinary tract anomalies or fail to attain urinary continence and require urinary reconstruction. They may present to the urologist for the first time after failing toilet training. These children require careful diagnostic evaluation, including renal sonogram, contrast VCUG, urodynamics, and often a cystoscopy before formal urinary reconstruction. Those who have not had previous spinal imaging require an MRI of the spine. Ultrasound evaluation of the spine after age of 6 months is unreliable because of vertebral calcification.

The surgical management of ARMs (PSARP) is illustrated in Figures 69.6 and 69.7.[45] We perform

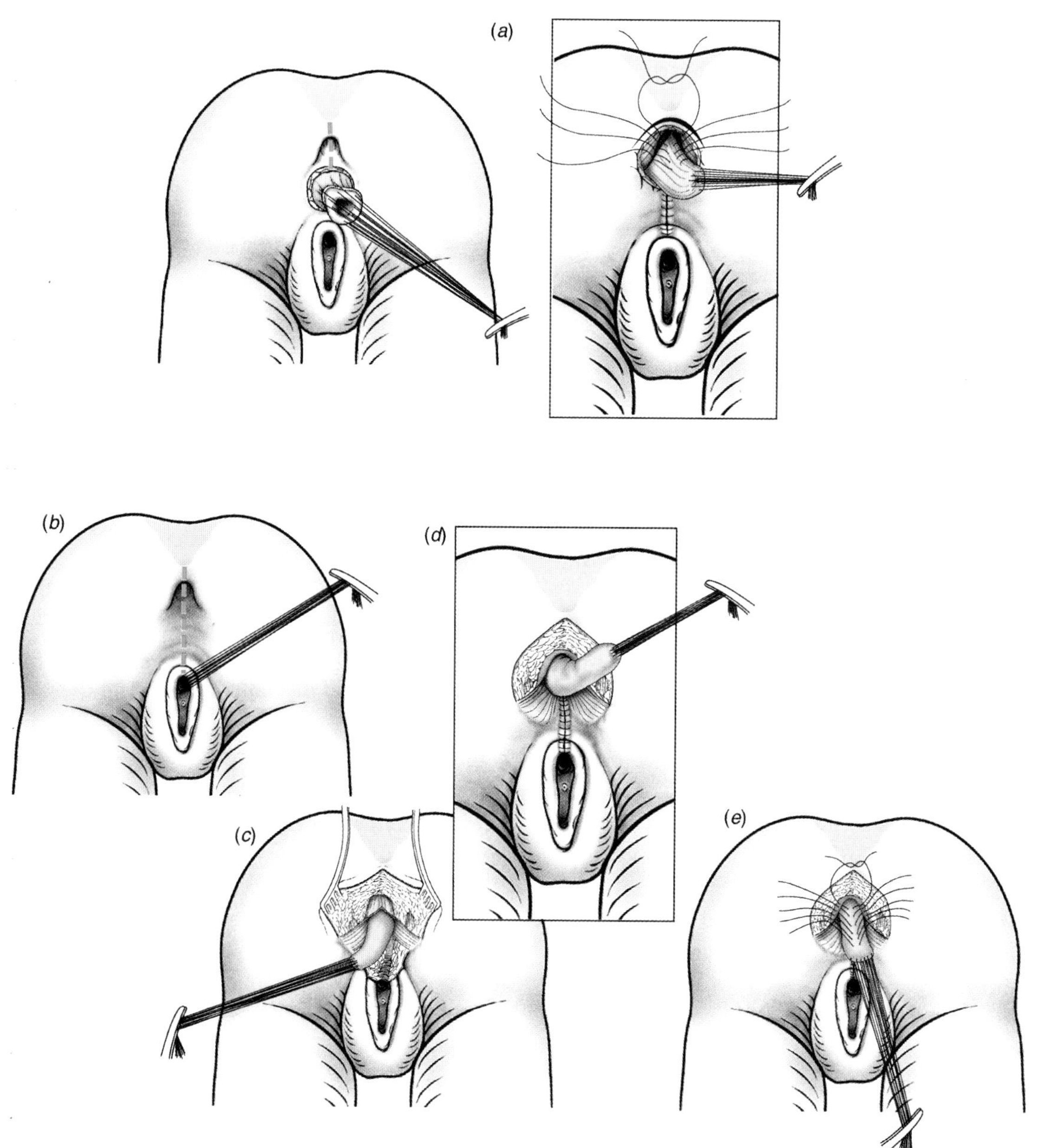

Figure 69.6 Surgical management of anorectal malformations (low lesions). See text. (Redrawn from Paidas and Peña.[45])

these procedures with the patient prone, with the pelvis elevated into a 'jack-knife' position, and with a Foley catheter indwelling. Figure 69.6 shows the approach to low lesions, as illustrated by the anoperineal fistula (see Figure 69.6a) and the anal vestibular fistula (see Figure 69.6b–e). The perineal fistula in both males and females is corrected in the newborn without a diverting colostomy. Electrical stimulation (see Figure 69.7) allows determination of the position of the anal sphincter.

The fistula is mobilized through a circumferential incision. A vertical incision is created in the posterior midline through the external sphincter mechanism, enabling the surgeon to transpose the rectum posterior to the site of the external sphincter mechanism. Similarly, the anovestibular fistula is corrected through a limited posterior sagittal approach. Many surgeons approach this in the newborn period without a protecting colostomy. Others prefer a colostomy, with early subsequent definitive correction of the anorectal malformation. In this case, the fistula is circumscribed (Figure 69.6b) and a vertical midline incision is created, extending through the sphincteric mechanism identified by electrical stimulation.

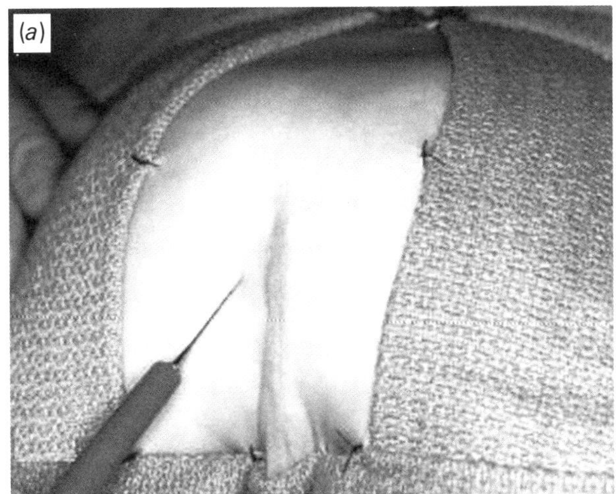

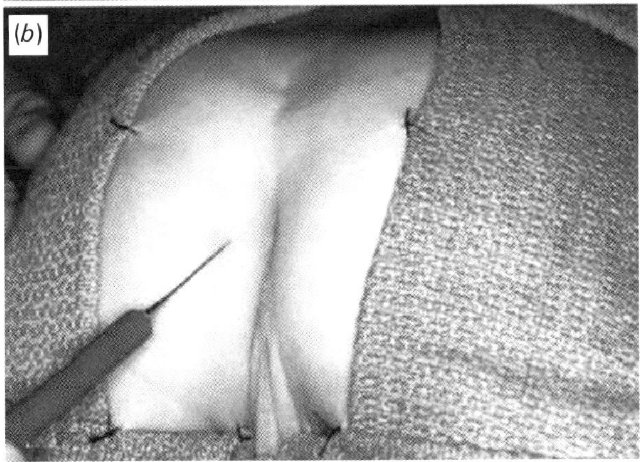

Figure 69.7 Identification of the location of the external striated muscle complex: (*a*) prior to stimulation; (*b*) during stimulation. Dimpling localizes the site of the muscle complex.

The rectum is gently dissected free from the underlying vagina to which it is intimately attached (Figure 69.6c). Once the rectum is sufficiently mobilized to prevent tension, the perineal body is reconstructed in two layers, establishing clear separation between the anus and vagina and the anterior edge of the sphincter muscle is approximated (Figure 69.6d). Posteriorly, the muscle complex is approximated and anchored to the rectum (Figure 69.6e), following which the anocutaneous anastomosis is completed.

Prior to this approach, the only access to these defects was through either the perineum, the abdomen, or a combination of the two. Surgical procedures frequently involved blind maneuvers with the consequent risk of injuring important structures. The rectum was pulled down through a path that was assumed to be the right one.[51]

We manage high lesions with a similar but more extensive approach (Figure 69.8). We illustrate this concept in a boy with a rectourethral fistula who previously had a diverting colostomy. The patient is prone with an indwelling Foley catheter. A midline incision extends from the coccyx (which is divided distally) to a point through and beyond the external sphincter (see Figure 69.8a), identified by electrical stimulation. We divide the sphincteric muscle complex and levator muscle directly in the midline, guided by electrical stimulation to minimize any resultant nerve injury. We open the rectum distally in the midline between traction sutures (see Figure 69.8b), which enables us to identify the rectourethral fistula (see Figure 69.8c,d). We place a series of traction sutures just proximal to the fistula, to help develop a plane between the rectum and the underlying urogenital structures (see Fig 69.8e–g).

Once mobilization is complete, we suture the urethral fistula closed under direct vision with the protection of an indwelling Foley catheter, making urethral injury very unlikely. We construct the perineal body in two layers and approximate the anterior edge of the external muscle complex. We approximate the levator muscle over the rectum (see Figure 69.8h), and then approximate the posterior edge of the external sphincteric muscle complex and anchor it to the rectum to prevent prolapse (see Figure 69.8i). We complete the anocutaneous anastomosis and close the posterior–sagittal incision in layers (see Figure 69.8j–k).

Urologic problems associated with imperforate anus

The incidence of structural anomalies of the urinary tract is 35% (Table 69.6). A 1987 review of 484 patients with imperforate anus detailed several critical

Table 69.6 Structural abnormalities of the genitourinary tract

Series	No.	GU anomaly (%)
Smith[7]	195	60
Santulli et al[8]	1166	26
Belman and King[9]	143	36
Wiener and Kiesewetter[10]	200	28
Hoekstra[52]	150	50
McLorie et al[11]	484	38
Rich et al[53]	244	48
Metts et al[54]	105	41
Total	2687	50

GU = genitourinary.

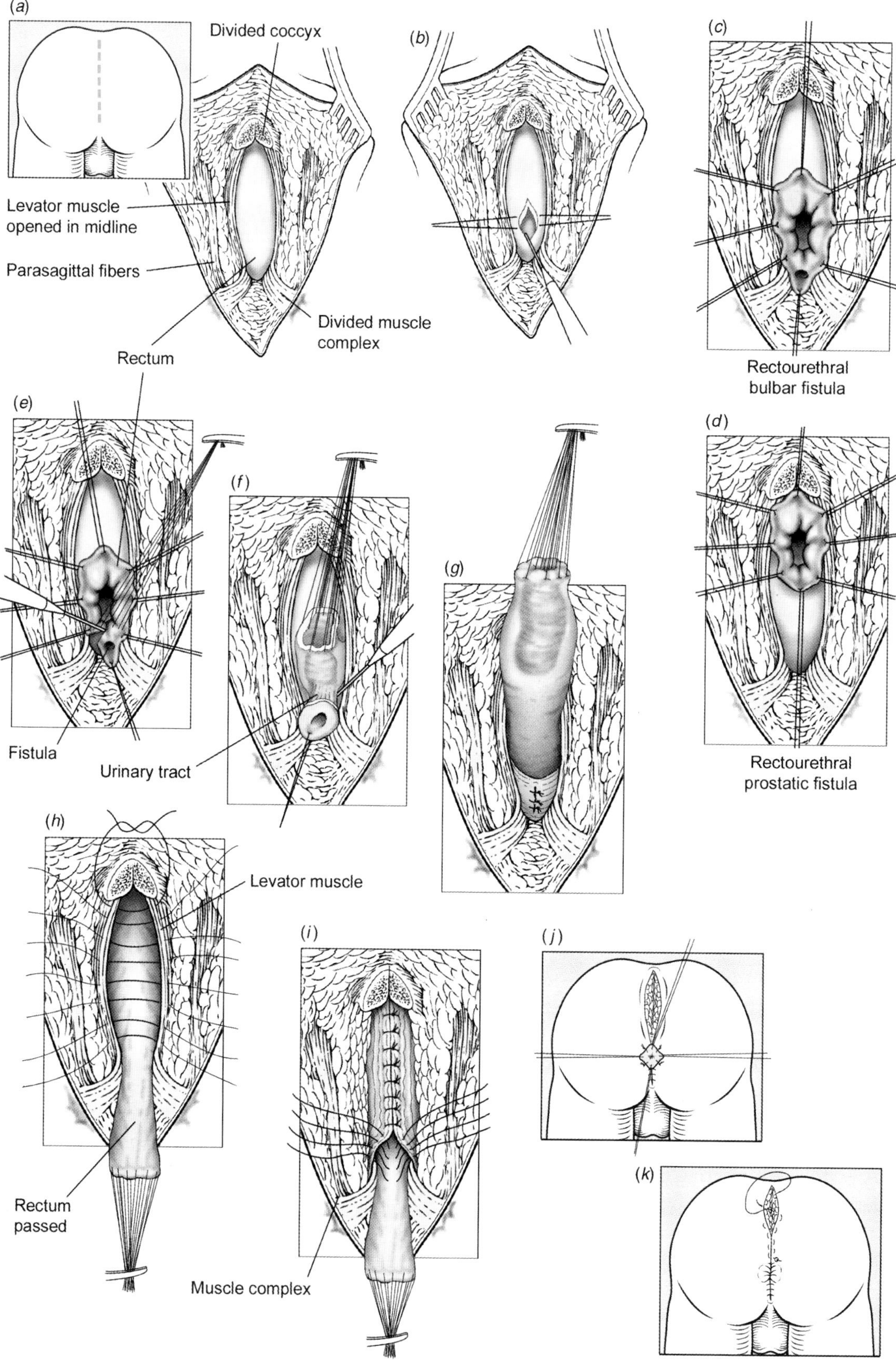

Figure 69.8 Surgical management of anorectal malformations (high lesions). See text. (Redrawn from Paidas and Peña.[45])

Table 69.7 Genitourinary anomalies in patients with imperforate anus

	High			Low			
484 patients	Male	Female	Total	Male	Female	Total	Overall
GU anomalies excluding fistulae	60%	62%	60%	25%	20%	25%	42%
Renal mortality	7.2%	3.8%	6.4%	1.5%	0.8%	1.1%	3.5%

GU = genitourinary.
From McLorie et al.[11]

Table 69.8 Bilateral upper tract urinary abnormalities threatening renal function

Symmetric		Asymmetric	
Pathology	No.	Pathology	No.
Bilateral reflux	22	Reflux/agenesis	14
Bilateral agenesis	16	Reflux/hypoplasia–dysplasia	6
Bilateral UPJ obstruction	5	Reflux/ectopia	3
Hypoplasia–dysplasia	1	Reflux/UPJ obstruction	3
Bilateral duplication		Reflux/primary obstructing megaureter	1
		Dysplasia/UPJ obstruction	1
		Agenesis/hypoplasia–dysplasia	3
		Agenesis/ectopia	1
Total	36 (7%)	Total	32 (7%)

Overall incidence of lesions placing both kidneys at risk = 14%.
True overall incidence of vesicoureteral reflux (patients screened by voiding cystourethrography) = 44/133 (33%).
UPJ = ureteropelvic junction.
From McLorie et al.[11]

relationships between imperforate anus and upper tract urinary anomalies (Tables 69.7 and 69.8). Fistulae connecting the rectum with the urinary tract are frequently encountered abnormalities. Excluding these, structural genitourinary anomalies occurred in 42% of patients. Non-fistula genitourinary anomalies were present in 60% of the patients with high lesions, equally in males and females and in 25% of low lesions (25% for males and 20% for females). Renal mortality occurred in 3.5% of these patients. Death from renal failure occurred in 6.4% of patients with high anorectal abnormalities (7.2% male, 3.8% female). Renal mortality occurred in only 1.1% of patients with low anorectal malformations (1.5% male, 0.8% female). This reflects the high incidence of conditions threatening both kidneys.

Table 69.8 reviews the incidence of bilateral upper tract urinary abnormalities threatening renal function. Symmetric bilateral upper tract urinary abnormalities occurred in 36 patients (7%) and included bilateral reflux, bilateral agenesis, and bilateral hypoplasia–dysplasia. Asymmetric abnormalities occurred in 32 (7%) patients. Most of these had reflux on one side and agenesis, hypoplasia–dysplasia, or obstructive pathology on the other. The overall incidence of lesions threatening both kidneys was 14%.

VUR is important in this population of children, who also frequently develop UTI and voiding dysfunction. The incidence of VUR (i.e. the incidence encountered in patients who received a screening VCUG) was 33%. The presence of a UTI in a child with imperforate anus demands prompt and aggressive evaluation and management. Epididymitis is often overlooked, and may reflect UTI in the presence of dysfunctional voiding, urethral stricture pathology, or may be associated with intermittent catheterization. Epididymitis may also be associated with ectopic ureteral insertion into the genital pathway.

The mean incidence of neurovesical dysfunction is 25% and varies quite widely among reported series (Table 69.9). As expected, high anorectal malformations have the greatest incidence. However, neurovesical dysfunction is frequently present in children with low lesions. Therefore, we screen all patients

Table 69.9 Incidence of neuropathic bladder in anorectal malformation

Series	No.	NVD (%)
Sheldon et al[14]	90	24
Kakizaki et al[55]	21	43
Boemers et al[15]	90	57
Capitanucci et al[56]	14	18
Total	215	25

NVD = neurovesical dysfunction.

with ARM. As previously noted, the recognition of the high incidence of occult spinal dysraphism has had a major impact on the management of these patients.[12–14,57] Such lesions may progress following surgical correction.[57–61] Although the timing of surgical intervention remains controversial, some authors suggest that early surgical intervention results in the best functional neurologic outcome.[62]

Screening ultrasonography has proven useful in the diagnosis of occult spinal dysraphism in infants.[63,64] Older children generally require MRI for diagnosis. The significance of these dysraphic states became apparent in the early 1990s. Table 69.10 outlines an early experience, where dysfunctional voiding occurred in 31% and 5% high and low ARMs, respectively. Structural spinal cord pathology was present in 12% and 4%, respectively. One report[65] suggests that screening by MRI for occult dysraphic myelodysplasia yields an even higher incidence of spinal cord pathology. They encountered dysraphic states in 17% of low ARMs, 34% of high ARMs, 46% of cloacal anomalies, and 100% of patients with cloacal exstrophy. A recent study from Golonka et al[66] reported 27% of those with high lesions and 50% with low lesions had a tethered cord by MRI.

Some surgeons have wondered whether surgical correction of ARMs results in the development of the neuropathic bladder. Ralph et al[67] evaluated 58 patients with imperforate anus who had reached an age of ≥18 years old. Of these, 43 patients had received rectal pull-through procedures while the remainder received cutback procedures. They found evidence for a neuropathic bladder in 32 patients (55%). Ninety-one per cent of these neuropathic bladders were hyper-reflexic in nature. Thirty patients (52%) had spinal deformities, 21 (70%) of which had evidence for neurovesical dysfunction. Only three patients (5%) had hypotonic bladders, normal spinal anatomy, and high ARMs, and were felt likely to have iatrogenic neurovesical dysfunction. Boemers et al[68] evaluated 32 patients with ARMs who underwent PSARP employing urodynamic investigation. In 27 patients, urodynamic investigation was performed both before and after PSARP. No evidence of somatic nerve injury was found in this series. Detrusor failure suggestive of autonomic denervation occurred in three males, two of whom had combined PSARP with transabdominal dissection. The authors concluded that, in the absence of transabdominal dissection and significant retrovesical dissection, PSARP did not affect lower urinary tract function. De Fillipo et al[69] also reported that bladder dysfunction does not appear to follow a properly performed PSARP.

Hyperchloremic metabolic acidosis is another potential problem for these children.[70,71] This condition results from urine passing from the bladder through a rectovesical or rectourethral fistula into the defunctionalized distal limb of colon following initial diverting colostomy. The resultant absorption of urinary constituents by the bowel results in the metabolic abnormality. The occurrence of this complication requires the presence of a urorectal fistula. A long segment of defunctionalized colon (large

Table 69.10 Spinal abnormalities in patients with anorectal malformations

		Dysfunctional voiding		Structural cord lesion[a]	
Type of anorectal malformation	No. of patients	No.	%	No.	%
High	25	8	31	3	12
Low	56	3	5	2	4
Anorectal stenosis	2	1	50	1	50
Cloaca	5	3	60	–	–
Cloacal exstrophy	2	1	50	1	50
Total	90	16	18	7	8

[a] Six tethered cords and one lumbar stenosis.
From Sheldon et al.[14]

absorptive surface) that communicates with the fistula worsens the metabolic imbalance. Distal urinary obstruction, which may be structural (stricture) or functional (neurovesical dysfunction), also worsens this risk. UTI and renal insufficiency may also make this metabolic abnormality more likely. Creation of a low, fully diverting colostomy and ensuring effective bladder drainage helps to avoid hyperchloremic metabolic acidosis. Once established, hyperchloremic metabolic acidosis is treated by the administration of oral alkalinizing agents, intermittent catheterization, vesicostomy, or early anorectal reconstruction with division of the fistula, depending on the clinical setting.

Vaginal problems in patients with imperforate anus

Surgeons often overlook and underestimate the long-term vaginal and reproductive problems that can occur in girls with imperforate anus.[72] Whereas most girls who experience these have cloacal anomalies, these anomalies may occur in girls with imperforate anus alone. Problems may follow scarring from reconstructive vaginal surgery, from primary vaginal anomalies, such as vaginal agenesis, or from the surgical violation of the vagina in the correction of imperforate anus associated with rectovaginal fistula.

Transperitoneal pelvic surgery, needed in many of these children, may result in peritoneal adhesions that may compromise tubal function, impair fertility, and promote ectopic pregnancy. Consequently, it is imperative that the managing physician as well as the patient is aware of the potential of impaired fertility and that the surgeon ensures long-term follow-up. Some children require subsequent introital surgery to facilitate intercourse. We usually defer this surgery until adolescence.

Anomalies of both anorectal and vaginal development: cloaca

> Cloaca is the Latin word for sewer. … A persisting cloaca is normal in birds, reptiles and some fish. However, a persistent cloaca can be disastrous for the human infant if it is not managed properly.[73]

The cloaca is one of the most complex congenital anomalies for which successful restorative surgery is feasible. The approach recognizes that the cloaca represents the combination of an imperforate anus and a urogenital sinus malformation. Accordingly, all the principles already discussed in this chapter are applicable to this complex and highly heterogeneous patient population. Cloacal anatomy is sufficiently diverse to defy meaningful classification. Rather, it is best thought of as a spectrum of abnormalities occurring as a continuum, one gradually blending into the next (Figure 69.9).

From a surgical perspective, the level of insertion of the rectum is generally immaterial, as all patients are managed with an initial diverting colostomy. As with the PSARP for imperforate anus, the rectum is divided from its site of insertion and mobilized to reach the perineum. The configuration of the remaining urogenital sinus, however, has tremendous surgical implications. We manage girls with very short urogenital sinus remnants by total urogenital advancement,[75] with excellent cosmetic and functional outcome. Otherwise, the vagina is dissected away from the urogenital sinus. The urogenital sinus is closed to become the urethra and the vagina is mobilized for exteriorization. A short vagina may require interposition with a tubularized vaginal flap (most appropriate for cloaca with hydrocolpos) or a vaginal switch procedure (most applicable to patients with vaginal and uterine duplication). Occasionally, bowel interposition is necessary.

A rare (and unique) form of cloaca is the posterior cloaca.[74] Here, the cloaca drains through a posterior orifice rather than the usual anterior orifice. This draining orifice may represent a normally positioned anus. The surgical management of these infants is different from that for other cloacal anomalies.

Figure 69.10 outlines the conceptual approach to the management of cloacal malformations. During the first phase of management, the surgeon endeavors to protect the upper urinary tracts, maintain low-pressure urinary drainage, normalize the perineal anatomy, and minimize any neurologic deficit related to spinal cord anomaly. The presence of a cloacal malformation (CM) is an urgent indication for the creation of a colostomy in order to prevent fecal contamination of the urinary tract. The colostomy should be positioned well away from the lower midline abdomen, where a subsequent vesicostomy may be necessary. Contrast cystography, measurement of PVR, and spinal ultrasonography are necessary in all patients. We perform genitoscopy at the time of colostomy in selected patients, particularly those with significant hydrocolpos. Depending on the findings, intermittent catheterization, cutaneous vesicostomy, or spinal surgery may be indicated. Patients with

will not experience a significant change in their social integration. We address these problems concomitantly and in a coordinated fashion, as the treatment of one may have a significant influence on the management of the other. For example, anticholinergic therapy to control uninhibited detrusor contractions may adversely affect anorectal function by causing constipation. Similarly, loss of the ileocecal valve with procedures such as ileocecocystoplasty may exacerbate fecal soilage in patients with ARM by preventing the production of formed stool. Furthermore, sigmoid colocystoplasty in patients with imperforate anus runs the risk of ischemic injury to the anorectum by dividing the descending blood supply.

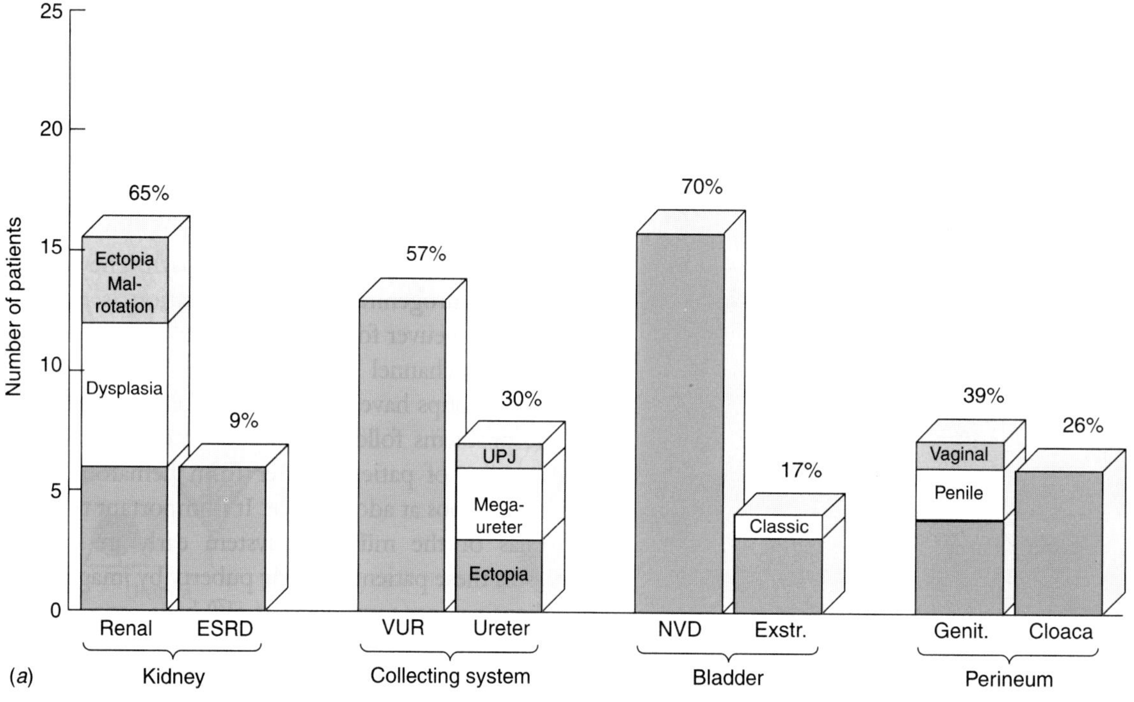

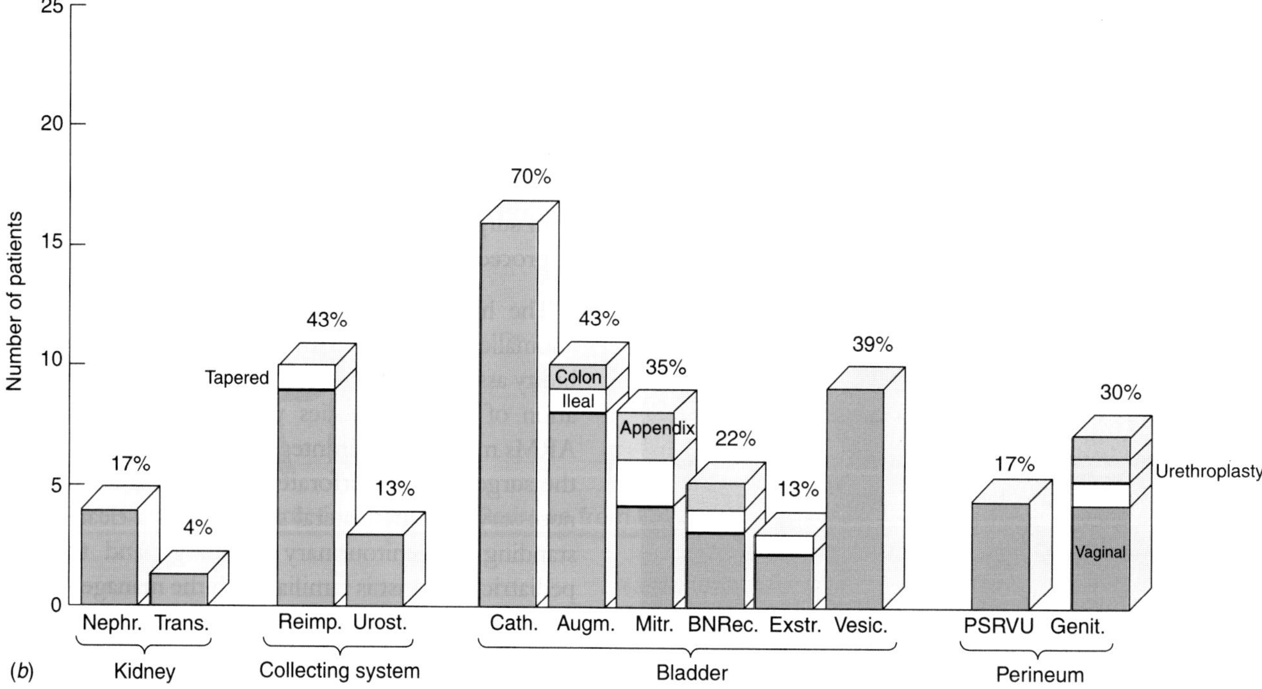

Figure 69.13 (*a*) Genitourinary abnormalities and (*b*) genitourinary surgical procedures in patients with anorectal malformations. NVD = neurovesical dysfunction. (From Sheldon et al.[16])

Incidental appendectomy must be avoided, because the appendix may be needed for either antegrade continence enema or Mitrofanoff neourethral bladder access. Imperforate anus surgery must be performed with an indwelling Foley catheter, because of the risk of inadvertent urethral injury. Inability to pass a catheter at the time of anorectal reconstruction is an indication for a cystoscopic evaluation and guidance in catheter placement. All patients with rectourinary fistulae, but especially those with VUR and/or neurovesical dysfunction, should have a fully diverting colostomy with a short distal colonic limb in order to prevent ongoing fecal urinary contamination. Placement of the colostomy is important. Patients at risk for future vesicostomy (e.g. high-grade VUR, neurovesical dysfunction, and hydrocolpos) should have the colostomy positioned so as not to interfere with a possible subsequent vesicostomy.

Sheldon has previously outlined the implications of genitourinary surgery in patients with ARMs.[16] Figure 69.13a reviews the genitourinary abnormalities encountered in 90 consecutive patients with ARMs managed over a 5-year period. Twenty-three patients had genitourinary anomalies requiring surgical intervention. Of these, 65% had primary renal pathology [9% had end-stage renal disease (ESRD)], 87% had collecting system abnormalities placing the kidneys at risk, 70% had neurovesical dysfunction, and 26% had CMs.

Figure 69.13b shows the genitourinary surgical procedures required for the reconstruction: note that 70% of children requiring urinary reconstruction ultimately required intermittent catheterization. The presence of a rectourethral fistula in the male may impair the ability to perform intermittent catheterization even after the fistula has been divided. Usually, intermittent catheterization can be performed with a coudé catheter. Diverticula, which may result in infection, voiding difficulties, and catheterization problems, may be managed by endoscopic fulguration.[78] Rarely, surgical excision may be required.

More than 40% of these patients required ureteral reimplantation and bladder augmentation. Twenty-two percent required bladder neck reconstruction for incontinence and 35% required a Mitrofanoff neourethra for alternate continent catheterizable bladder access. Nine patients required temporary vesicostomy, three for neonatal urosepsis, four for neurovesical dysfunction and hydronephrosis not responding to intermittent catheterization, one to control hyperchloremic metabolic acidosis, and one to relieve hydrocolpos complicating a CM.

Importantly, none of the 16 patients with neurovesical dysfunction had evidence to support PSARP as a source of bladder denervation. Further, four patients had urethral stricture. At least three of these were congenital. The fourth was suspected to be congenital but this was not proven by preoperative urethrography or endoscopy.

The 18 surgical complications occurring in 14 of these 23 children requiring genitourinary reconstruction are particularly instructive. Nine complications were secondary to surgery performed before referral to the author's institution. Four patients with a cloaca were referred for vaginal reconstruction after previous anorectal pull-through with no effort made to correct the UGSM. Two of these patients subsequently had urogenital sinus surgery using inlay flap techniques, and both of these developed urethrovaginal fistulae. Three patients had ureteral reimplantation before referral, which failed due to the associated neuropathic bladder.

Nine complications occurred following referral. Two children developed delayed small bowel obstruction that necessitated exploratory laparotomy and lysis of adhesions. One child experienced intraoperative vascular collapse from severe latex allergy. One patient developed a lymphocele following transplantation, and one patient developed a mild recurrent urethral stricture following urethroplasty for congenital stricture that urethral dilation addressed. One child developed a urethral calculus that occurred secondary to urethral erosion of a suture placed for approximation of the pubis for cloacal exstrophy reconstruction. Two children developed stenosis of their catheterizable channels corrected by stomal revision. Both had previously undergone incidental appendectomy such that one patient required a ureteral neourethra and the other a tubularized ileal neourethra. One patient reconstructed for a CM developed late vaginal stenosis.

This experience emphasizes several important principles:

1 Most neurovesical dysfunction and urethral strictures encountered in patients with ARMs are not iatrogenic but congenital in origin.
2 VUR is usually bilateral or, if unilateral, occurs in conjunction with a condition that threatens the contralateral kidney. In addition, neurovesical dysfunction often accompanies the VUR.
3 Ureteral reimplantation into a dysfunctional bladder usually fails unless the underlying bladder dysfunction is controlled.

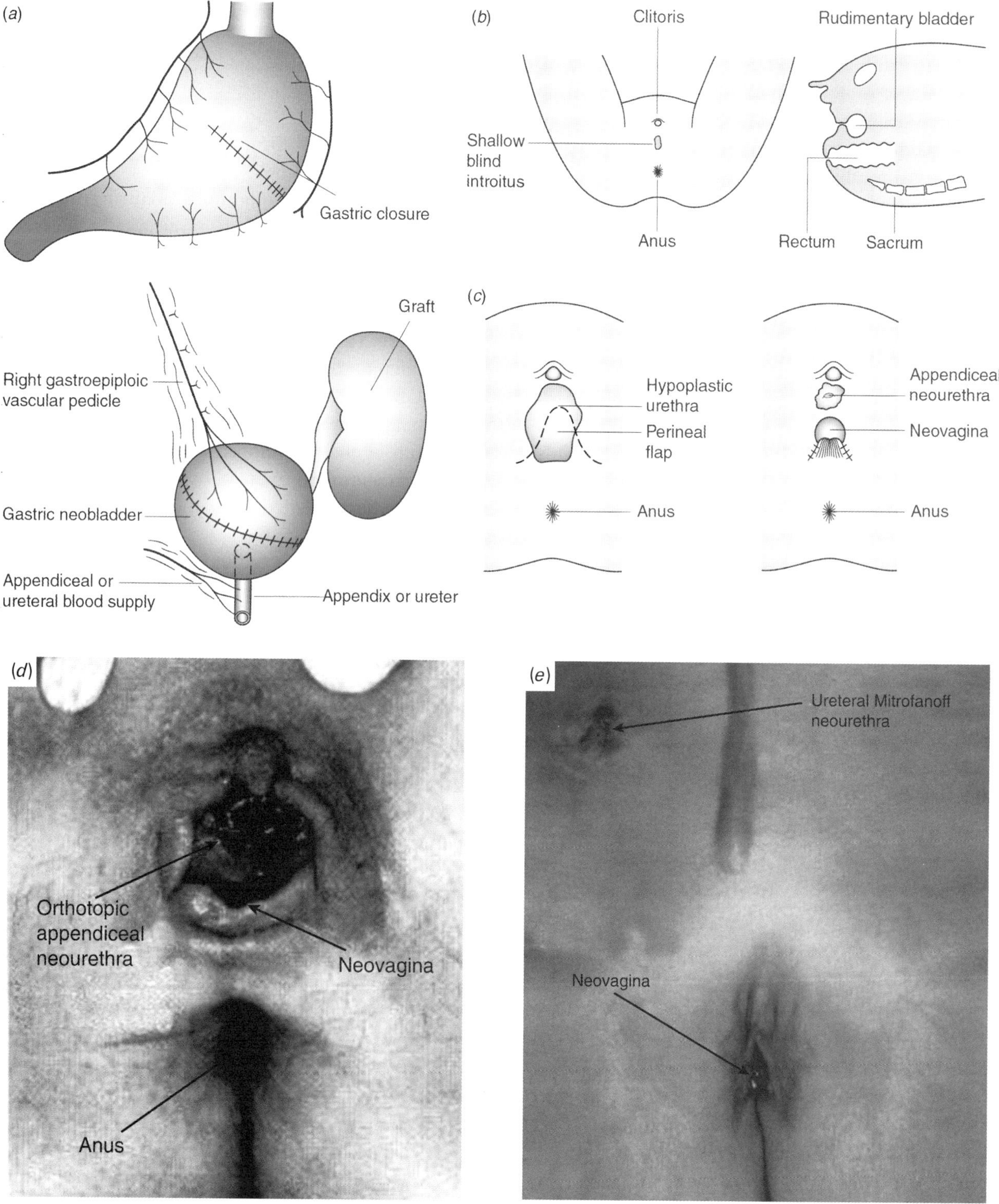

Figure 69.14 Vaginal reconstruction employing a bladder substitution technique: (*a*) total anatomic urinary replacement; (*b*) preoperative anatomy; (*c*) reconstruction employing a perineal inlay flap bladder substitution and an appendiceal neourethra. (From Sheldon et al.[84] and Sheldon and Welch.[85]) (*d*) Appearance of perineum of a child with a urogenital sinus malformation, a tiny hypoplastic bladder, and a rudimentary vaginal remnant employing an inlay flap bladder substitution technique. (From Sheldon et al.[84]) (*e*) Appearance of a child with a urogenital sinus malformation, a tiny hypoplastic bladder, and a rudimentary vaginal remnant reconstructed employing an inlay flap bladder substitution technique. A composite neobladder (stomach and ileum) was constructed along with a ureteral Mitrofanoff neourethra.

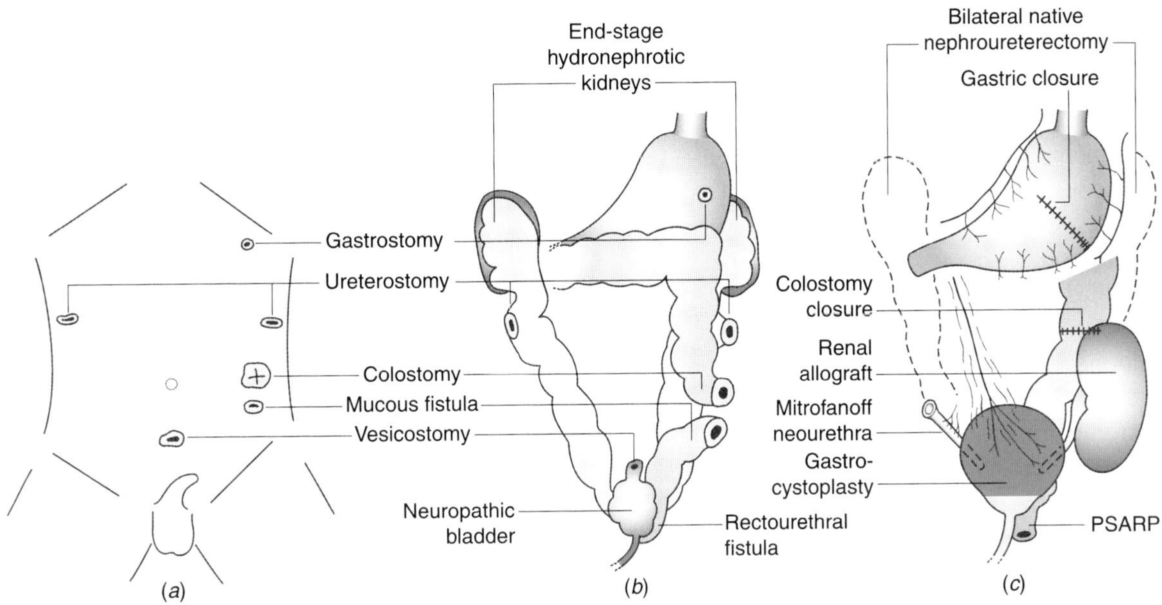

Figure 69.15 Urinary reconstruction and renal transplantation in a patient with the VATER association: (*a*) preoperative appearance; (*b*) preoperative urinary and colonic status; (*c*) postreconstructive status.

4 Prompt and efficient decompression of obstructive hydronephrosis is essential in order to optimize long-term renal function.
5 Patients with ARM have a similar risk for latex allergy as do the myelomeningocele population.
6 The combination of neurovesical dysfunction or urethral stricture and rectourinary fistulae predisposes the patient to critical neonatal illness such as sepsis and hyperchloremic metabolic acidosis.
7 A low, fully diverting colostomy is most protective of the urinary tract.
8 Patients with a cloaca should never have their anorectal and UGSMs corrected separately.

The best results are attained using a single-stage PSARUVP. Those patients who present for correction of a UGSM who have previously undergone an anorectal pull-through procedure are best corrected by reoperative PSARUVP complete with repeat mobilization of the rectum. Both patients managed in this fashion in this series were successfully reconstructed.

Renal transplantation in patients with anorectal malformations

Renal transplantation in the setting of ARMs and CM deserves additional comment. ESRD in this setting may considerably complicate management.[79–81] Peritoneal dialysis is more difficult, or may be impossible in the presence of multiple adhesions from prior transabdominal surgical procedures. Surgeons should make every effort to preserve the peritoneal cavity in the very young, because hemodialysis access is difficult and is associated with long-term complications such as superior vena cava thrombosis.

Renal transplantation in patients with ARMs and UGSMs is extremely challenging, as the majority of these patients with ESRD have major bladder pathology that must be controlled or corrected before transplantation, in order to optimize outcome. In addition, vascular anomalies are relatively common in these children.[82] Successful renal transplantation, however, in the setting of imperforate anus and cloacal anomalies, can be achieved.[79–81,83]

The complex nature of transplant management in these patients is illustrated by the following three cases. The patient in Figure 69.14 presented with a cloacal anomaly with a tiny hypoplastic bladder, a rudimentary vagina, and ectopic ureters draining dysplastic kidneys. She underwent creation of a neovagina using the hypoplastic bladder and then underwent total anatomic urinary replacement with the creation of an appendiceal orthotopic neourethra and an orthotopic gastric neobladder, followed by living related donor transplantation.

The second child was born with cloacal exstrophy and had the cloacal plate removed as an infant. She was managed with an ileostomy and a cutaneous ureterostomy draining a solitary kidney. This kidney was lost over the ensuing years from hydronephrosis and urosepsis. She presented for renal transplantation and underwent creation of an orthotopic neourethra using a segment of ureter and creation of an orthotopic neobladder using a gastric segment. She subsequently underwent renal transplantation. Both of these patients with total anatomic urinary tract replacement continue to have satisfactory renal function and are continent of urine on intermittent catheterization.[85]

The third patient (Figure 69.15) presented after several decompressive procedures at the referring institution. These included a gastrostomy, a colostomy with mucous fistula for imperforate anus, a vesicostomy for neuropathic bladder, and bilateral cutaneous ureterostomies for bilateral hydronephrosis accompanied by profound renal insufficiency. This child presented with ESRD for transplantation. His surgical preparation consisted of posterior sagittal anorectoplasty, followed by takedown of colostomy, gastrocystoplasty, creation of a Mitrofanoff neourethra, and native nephrectomy. He subsequently underwent living related transplantation. He now has excellent renal function and is continent of urine on intermittent catheterization.

Conclusion

The principles outlined in this chapter regarding the management of ARMs and CMs, along with the advancements in the science of perioperative surgical management and transplantation, have enabled even those children born with the most devastating congenital anomalies to be restored to health and a functional social status.

References

1. Trusler GA, Wilkinson RH. Imperforate anus: a review of 147 cases. Can J Surg 1962; 5:269–77.
2. Hendren WH. Further experience in reconstructive surgery for cloacal anomalies. J Pediatr Surg 1982; 17:695–717.
3. McLeod N. A case of imperforate anus, with a suggestion for a new method of treatment. BMJ 1880; ii:657.
4. Hadra R. Demonstration zweier Fälle von Atresie ani vulvalis. Berlin Clin Wochenschr 1885; 22:340.
5. Rhoads JE, Pipes RL, Randall JP. A simultaneous abdominal and perineal approach in operations for imperforate anus with atresia of the rectum and rectosigmoid. Ann Surg 1948; 127:552.
6. Peña A, Devries PA. Posterior sagittal anorectoplasty: important technical considerations and new applications. J Pediatr Surg 1982; 17:796–811.
7. Smith DE. Urinary anomalies and complications in imperforate anus and rectum. J Pediatr Surg 1968; 3:337–49.
8. Santulli TV, Schullinger JN, Kiesewetter WB, Bill AH. Imperforate anus: a survey from the members of the Surgical Section of the American Academy of Pediatrics. J Pediatr Surg 1971; 6:484–7.
9. Belman AB, King L. Urinary tract abnormalities associated with imperforate anus. J Urol 1972; 108:823–4.
10. Wiener ES, Kiesewetter WB. Urologic abnormalities associated with imperforate anus. J Pediatr Surg 1973; 8:151–7.
11. McLorie GA, Sheldon CA, Fleisher M et al. The genitourinary system in patients with imperforate anus. J Pediatr Surg 1987; 22:1100–109.
12. Carson JA, Barnes PD, Tunell WP et al. Imperforate anus: the neurologic implication of sacral abnormalities. J Pediatr Surg 1984; 19:838–42.
13. Karrer FM, Flannery AM, Nelson MD Jr, McLone DG, Raffensperger JG. Anorectal malformations: evaluation of associated spinal dysraphic syndromes. J Pediatr Surg 1988; 23:45–8.
14. Sheldon C, Cormier M, Crone K et al. Occult neurovesical dysfunction in children with imperforate anus and its variants. J Pediatr Surg 1991; 26:49–54.
15. Boemers TM, de Jong TP, van Gool JD et al. Urologic problems in anorectal malformations. Part 2: Functional urologic sequelae. J Pediatr Surg 1996; 31:634–7.
16. Sheldon CA, Gilbert A, Lewis AG et al. Surgical implications of genitourinary tract anomalies in patients with imperforate anus. J Urol 1994; 152:196–9.
17. Malone PS, Ransley PG, Kiely EM. Preliminary report: the antegrade continence enema. Lancet 1990; 336: 1217–18.
18. Sheldon CA, Minevich E, Wacksman J et al. Role of the antegrade continence enema in the management of the most debilitating childhood rectourogenital anomalies. J Urol 1997; 158:1277–9.
19. Malone PSJ, Curry JL. The MACE procedure. Dialog Pediatr Urol 1999; 22:2.
20. Mayer CAJ. Uber verdoppelungen des uterus and ihre arten, nebst bemerkungen uber hasenscarte und wolfsrachen. J Chir Auger 1829; 13:525.
21. Küster H. Uterus bipartitus solidus rudimentarius cum vagina solida. Z Geburtshilfe Perinatol 1910; 67:692.
22. Rokitansky K. Uber die sogenannten verdoppelungen des uterus. Med Jb Ost Staat 1938; 26:39.
23. Hauser GA, Schreiner WE. Das Mayer–Rokitansky–Kuster Syndrome. Schweiz Med Wochenschr 1961; 91:381.
24. Fore SR, Hammond CB, Parker RT. Urologic and genital anomalies in patients with congenital absence of the vagina. Obstet Gynecol 1975; 46:410–16.
25. Griffin JE, Edwards C, Madden JD et al. Congenital absence of the vagina. Ann Intern Med 1976; 85:224–36.
26. Duncan PA, Shapiro LR, Stangel JJ et al. The MURCS association: müllerian duct aplasia, renal aplasia, and cervicothoracic somite dysplasia. J Pediatr 1975; 95:399–402.
27. Say P, Gerald PS. A new polydactyly/imperforate anus/vertebral anomalies syndrome? Lancet 1968; ii:688.

28. Quan L, Smith DW. The VATER association. J Pediatr 1973; 82:104–7.
29. Barry JE, Auldist AW. The Vater association. One end of a spectrum of anomalies. Am J Dis Child 1974; 128: 769–71.
30. Temtamy SA, Miller JD. Extending the scope of the VATER association: definition of the VATER syndrome. J Pediatr 1974; 85:345–9.
31. Wendelken JR, Sethney HT, Halverstadt DB. Urologic abnormalities associated with imperforate anus. Urology 1977; 10:239.
32. Weber TR, Smith W, Grosfeld JL. Surgical experience in infants with the VATER association. J Pediatr Surg 1980; 15:849–54.
33. Uehling DT, Gilbert E, Chesney R. Urologic implications of the VATER association. J Urol 1983; 129: 352–4.
34. Muraji T, Mahour HG. Surgical problems in patients with VATER-associated anomalies. J Pediatr Surg 1984; 19:550–4.
35. Weaver DD, Mapstone CL. The VATER association: analysis of 46 patients. Am J Dis Child 1986; 140:225–9.
36. Beals RK, Rolfe B. Current concepts review – VATER association. J Bone Joint Surg 1989; 71:948–50.
37. Brock WA, Peña A. Cloacal abnormalities and imperforate anus. In: Kelalis PP, King LR, Belman AB, eds. Clinical Pediatric Urology, Vol 2. Philadelphia: WB Saunders, 1992:922.
38. White JJ, Haller JA, Scott JR et al. N-type anorectal malformations. J Pediatr Surg 1978; 13:631–7.
39. Hong AR, Croitoru DP, Nguyen LT et al. Congenital urethral fistula with normal anus: a report of two cases. J Pediatr Surg 1992; 27:1278–80.
40. Raffensberger JG, ed. Swenson's Pediatric Surgery, 5th edn. Norwalk, CT: Appleton & Lange, 1990.
41. Kluth D, Lambrecht W. Current concepts in the embryology of anorectal malformations. Semin Pediatr Surg 1997; 6:180–6.
42. O'Rahilly R, Müller F. Human Embryology and Teratology. New York: Wiley-Liss, 1992:216.
43. Skandalakis JE, Gray SW, eds. Embryology for Surgeons, 2nd edn. Baltimore: Williams & Wilkins, 1994:244.
44. Skandalakis JE, Gray SW, Ricketts R. The colon and rectum. In: Skandalakis JE, Gray S, eds. Embryology for Surgeons, 2nd edn. Baltimore: Williams & Wilkins, 1994:244.
45. Paidas CN, Peña A. Rectum and anus. In: Oldham KT, Colombani PM, Foglia RP, eds. Surgery of Infants and Children: Scientific Principles and Practice. Philadelphia: Lippincott-Raven, 1997:1323–62.
46. Stephens FD, Smith ED. Classification, identification and assessment of surgical treatment of anorectal anomalies. Pediatr Surg Int 1986; 1:200.
47. Endo M, Hayashi A, Ishihara M et al. Analysis of 1,992 patients with anorectal malformations over the past two decades in Japan. J Pediatr Surg 1999; 34:435–41.
48. Nievelstein RA, Vos A, Valk J, Vermeij-Keers C. Magnetic resonance imaging in children with anorectal malformations: embryologic implications. J Pediatr Surg 2002; 37(8):1138–45.
49. Peña A, Migotto-Krieger M, Levitt MA. Colostomy in anorectal malformations: a procedure with serious but preventable complications. J Pediatr Surg 2006; 41(4):748–56.
50. Shandling B, Gilmour RF. The enema continence catheter in spina bifida: successful bowel management. J Pediatr Surg 1987; 22:271–3.
51. Peña A. Atlas of Surgical Management of Anorectal Malformations. New York: Springer, 1990.
52. Hoekstra WJ. Urogenital tract abnormalities associated with congenital anorectal anomalies. J Urol 1983; 130:962–3.
53. Rich MA, Brock WA, Peña A. Spectrum of genitourinary malformations in patients with imperforate anus. Pediatr Surg Int 1988; 3:110.
54. Metts JC, Kotkin L, Kasper S et al. Genital malformations and coexistent urinary tract or spinal anomalies in patients with imperforate anus. J Urol 1997; 158: 1298–300.
55. Kakizaki H, Nonomura K, Asano Y et al. Preexisting neurogenic voiding dysfunction in children with imperforate anus: problems in management. J Urol 1994; 151:1041–4.
56. Capitanucci ML, Rivosecchi M, Silveri M et al. Neurovesical dysfunction due to spinal dysraphism in anorectal anomalies. Eur J Pediatr Surg 1996; 6:159–62.
57. Warf BC, Scott RM, Barnes PD et al. Tethered spinal cord in patients with anorectal and urogenital malformations. Pediatr Neurosurg 1993; 19:25–30.
58. Cumes D. Sacral dysgenesis associated with occult spinal dysraphism causing neurogenic bladder dysfunction. J Urol 1977; 117:127–8.
59. Al-Mefty O, Kandzari S, Fox J. Neurogenic bladder and the tethered spinal cord syndrome. J Urol 1980; 122:112–15.
60. Yoneyama T, Fukui J, Ohtsuka K et al. Urinary tract dysfunctions in tethered spinal cord syndrome: improvement after surgical untethering. J Urol 1985; 133:999–1001.
61. Hellstrom WJ, Edwards MS, Kogan B. Urological aspects of the tethered cord syndrome. J Urol 1985; 135:317–20.
62. Sato S, Shirane R, Yoshimoto T. Evaluation of tethered cord syndrome associated with anorectal malformations. Neurosurgery 1993; 32:1025–7.
63. Raghavendra BN, Epstein FJ, Pinto RS et al. The tethered spinal cord: diagnosis by high-resolution real-time ultrasound. Radiology 1983; 149:123–8.
64. Scheible W, James VE, Leopold GR et al. Occult spinal dysraphism in infants: screening with high-resolution real-time ultrasound. Radiology 1983; 146:743–6.
65. Appignani BA, Jaramillo D, Barnes PD et al. Dysraphic myelodysplasias associated with urogenital and anorectal anomalies: prevalence and types seen with MR imaging. AJR Am J Roentgenol 1994; 163:1199–203.
66. Golonka N, Haga LJ, Keating RP et al. Routine MRI evaluation of low imperforate anus reveals unexpected high incidence of tethered spinal cord. J Pediatr Surg 2002; 37:966–9.
67. Ralph DJ, Woodhouse CR, Ransley PG. The management of the neuropathic bladder in adolescents with imperforate anus. J Urol 1993; 148:366–8.
68. Boemers TML, Bax KM, Rovekamp MH, Van Gool JD.

The effect of posterior sagittal anorectoplasty and its variants on lower urinary tract function in children with anorectal malformations. J Urol 1995; 153:191–3.
69. De Fillipo RE, Shaul DB, Harrison EA, Xie HW, Hardy BE. Neurogenic bladder in infants born with anorectal malformations: comparison with spinal and urologic status. J Pediatr Surg 1999; 34:825–7, discussion 828.
70. Iwai N, Ogita S, Shirasaka S et al. Hyperchloremic acidosis in an infant with imperforate anus and rectourethral fistula. J Pediatr Surg 1978; 13:437–8.
71. Caldamone AA, Emmens RW, Rabinowitz R. Hyperchloremic acidosis and imperforate anus. J Urol 1979; 122:817–18.
72. Fleming SE, Hall R, Gysler M et al. Imperforate anus in females: frequency of genital tract involvement, incidence of associated anomalies, and functional outcome. J Pediatr Surg 1986; 21:146–50.
73. Hendren WH. Management of cloacal malformations. Semin Pediatr Surg 1997; 6:217–27.
74. Peña A, Kessler O. Posterior cloaca: a unique defect. J Pediatr Surg 1998; 33:407–12.
75. Peña A. Total urogenital mobilization: an easier way to repair cloacas. J Pediatr Surg 1997; 32:263–7.
76. Peña A, Levitt MA, Hong A, Midulla P. Surgical management of cloacal malformations: a review of 339 patients. J Pediatr Surg 2004; 39(3):470–9.
77. Warne S, Wilcox DT, Creighton S, Ransley PG. Long-term gynecological outcome of patients with persistent cloaca. J Urol 2003; 170:1493–6.
78. Husmann DA, Allen TD. Endoscopic management of infected enlarged prostatic utricles and remnants of rectourethral fistula tract of high imperforate anus. J Urol 1997; 157:1902–6.
79. Sharma AK, Kashtan CE, Nevins TE. The management of end-stage renal disease in infants with imperforate anus. Pediatr Nephrol 1993; 7:721–4.
80. Sheldon CA, Gonzalez R, Burns MW et al. Renal transplantation into the dysfunctional bladder: the role of adjunctive bladder reconstruction. J Urol 1994; 152:972–5.
81. Sheldon CA. Urinary reconstruction (rather than diversion) for continence in difficult pediatric urologic disorders. Semin Pediatri Surg 1996; 5:8–15.
82. Dykes EH, Oesch I, Ransley PG, Hendren WH. Abnormal aorta and iliac arteries in children with urogenital abnormalities. J Pediatr Surg 1993; 28:696–700.
83. DeFoor W, Minevich E, McEnery P et al. Lower urinary tract reconstruction is safe and effective in children with end stage renal disease. J Urol 2003; 170:1497–500.
84. Sheldon CA, Gilbert A, Lewis AG. Vaginal reconstruction: critical technical principles. J Urol 1994; 152:190–5.
85. Sheldon CA, Welch TR. Total anatomic urinary tract replacement and renal transplantation: a surgical strategy to correct severe genitourinary anomalies. J Pediatr Surg 1998; 33:635–8.

Surgery for intersex disorders and urogenital sinus

70

Mark C Adams and Romano T DeMarco

Introduction

Advances in surgical management have improved both the cosmetic and functional outcomes of patients with urogenital sinus abnormalities and those with varying degrees of intersexuality, at least, when judged by treating surgeons. Descriptions in early textbooks of methods such as clitoridectomy or convenient 'forgetting' of the hypoplastic vagina are now considered archaic because of improved understanding of genital anatomy and function. Better exposure and innovative techniques have produced surgical improvements hardly thought possible half a century ago. While our understanding of these complex problems is better, it is not complete. Much remains to be learned about female genital function, the affects of surgery on genital innervation, and the significant psychological affects of these problems and their reconstruction on the patient.

Genital development and implications for surgery

Normal development in any organ system proceeds through a highly regulated and complex cascade of interactions. Errors in development virtually always occur in a spectrum of severity and can lead to minor, inconsequential aberrancies or profound problems affecting patient survival. Similarly, embryologic errors in the urogenital tract have a wide range of magnitude. Genitourinary embryology is discussed in detail in Chapter 67.

Under the influence of SRY (the sex-determining region of the Y chromosome) the bipotential gonad should differentiate into a testis near the 7th week of gestation. Normal phenotypic expression of male differentiation is then actively controlled by secretion of MIS (müllerian inhibiting substance) by Sertoli cells and testosterone by Leydig cells. MIS causes rapid regression of the paramesonephric (müllerian) ducts between the 8th and 10th weeks. In normal females, the absence of the Y chromosome and SRY protein secretion leads to the formation of ovaries without Sertoli or Leydig cells. The absence of such cell types prevents elaboration of MIS and androgens. Subsequently, the paramesonephric ducts give rise to the fallopian tubes, uterus, and the upper two-thirds of the vagina. The distal third of the vagina is formed from endodermal tissue, the sinovaginal bulb. In simple terms, the female phenotype has been thought of as the passive or default sex, forming in the absence of the Y chromosome. Exceptions to this cascade do exist.[1]

In a sense, normal males have a persistent urogenital sinus with ultimate entry of the wolffian ducts as well as a remnant of the müllerian system at the verumontanum. It would seem, therefore, that the most proximal confluence of a persistent urogenital sinus in a female would be the area of the proximal urethra. Whereas the vast majority of girls with a urogenital sinus anomaly have a confluence at that level or more distally, exceptions do occur. The vagina may be found entering the bladder itself even cephalad to the level of the ureteral orifices. It is not known whether the müllerian duct opening may migrate into the bladder in tandem with the ureteral bud or whether there is simply an abnormal breakdown in communication between these intimate structures.

The normal vagina has two embryologic components. The complex development may contribute to the typical appearance of the vagina in the setting of a urogenital sinus. The distal portion of the vagina is virtually always narrow for a variable length (Figure 70.1). Recognition of that finding is critical in surgical reconstruction. Failure of flaps to reach all the way through the narrow segment and well into the more normal proximal portion may ultimately lead to stenosis. The paramesonephric ducts and entire müllerian

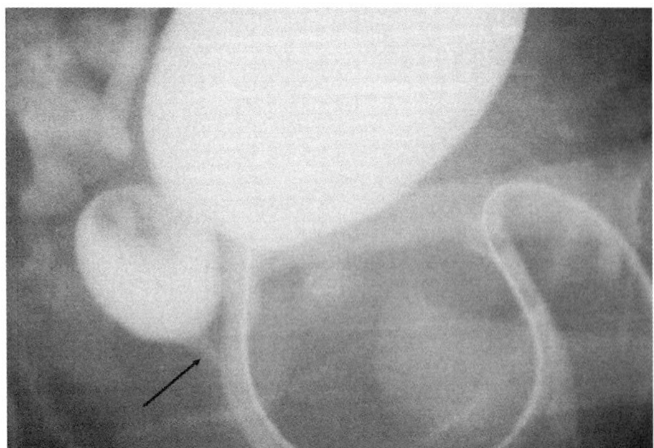

Figure 70.1 Genitogram on a female with a urogenital sinus. No matter the level of confluence, the distal vagina (arrow) is usually narrow.

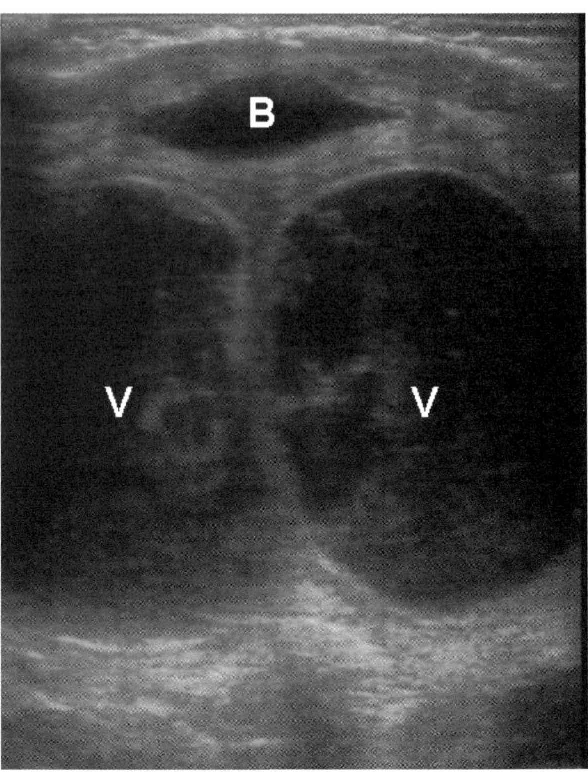

Figure 70.2 Postnatal ultrasound on newborn with urogenital sinus and duplicate vagina (V). Such vaginal distention with urine may be noted on antenatal studies. B = bladder.

system are initially paired structures which should fuse distally in the midline. Errors in fusion do occur,[2] and patients with a persistent urogenital sinus or cloaca may be at increased risk for such problems (Figure 70.2). In the setting of a urogenital sinus, the finding of a vagina to either side of the midline should arouse suspicion that a second vagina, even if obscure or obstructed, may well exist on the other side. Failure to recognize the second vagina at the time of reconstruction may eventually lead to hydrometrocolpos.

Classification scheme

A urogenital sinus abnormality is present when a persistent communication occurs between the genital and urinary tract in the female. Typically, the urethra and vagina are joined and exit to the perineum as a common channel. If there is associated rectal involvement and imperforate anus with a single perineal opening for all three structures, a persistent cloaca or cloacal anomaly exists. A urogenital sinus with an anteriorly displaced rectum may represent the form früste of a persistent cloaca. Such a finding may have implications for rectal function and exposure during surgical reconstruction of the urogenital sinus. Patients with urogenital sinus anomalies commonly have associated abnormalities of the clitoris, labia, and external genitalia. The most common etiology of a persistent urogenital sinus is congenital adrenal hyperplasia (CAH).

The most useful classification schemes for urogenital sinus anomalies relate to the level of the confluence of the urethra and vagina. Hendren made a landmark contribution to genital reconstructive surgery when he divided urogenital anomalies into those with a confluence above or below the female external sphincter and suggested that a different surgical approach was indicated for the two types.[3] In females with extreme virilization related to CAH, the external sphincter may be well developed and quite obvious. In most females, the sphincter mechanism may be indistinct and the level of the pelvic floor a more reliable landmark. The absence of a well-defined external sphincter in such patients has led to subjective classification based on the level of confluence as low, moderate, or high. It is important to recognize that the level of the confluence should be considered relative to the bladder neck and not the external meatus. Virilization of the distal urethra or urogenital sinus may create a confluence that is distant from the meatus yet still relatively low. The critical determinant, therefore, is the distance from the bladder neck to the confluence as it affects reconstructive surgery (Figure 70.3). Rink et al[4] have proposed a more rigid classification scheme based on careful measurements from both directions.

The nature of the urogenital sinus distal to the confluence should also be considered. Hendren described

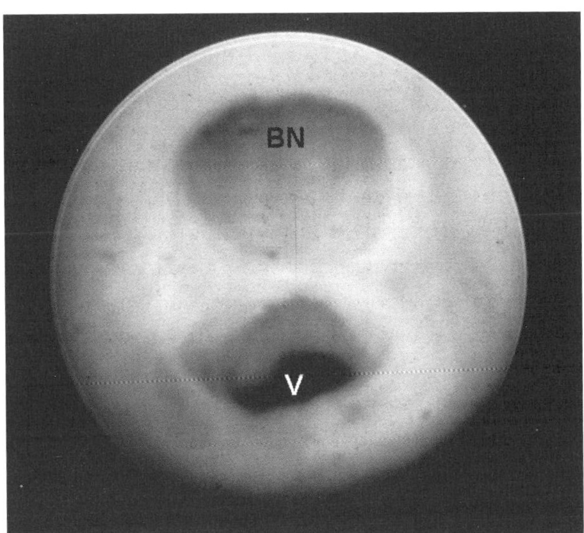

Figure 70.3 Endoscopy. A vaginal opening (V) this close to the bladder neck (BN) represents a high confluence no matter the distance from the external meatus.

the urogenital sinus distal to the confluence as urethra-like or vagina-like based on circumference.[5] This difference has typically been applied in descriptions of a persistent cloaca but may be useful for isolated urogenital sinus anomalies as well. The difference between the two has potential ramifications on surgical reconstruction in terms of the amount of local tissue available for reconstruction of the urethra or vagina.

Evaluation

A thorough evaluation of the newborn with a urogenital sinus should be completed expeditiously. Immediate attention to and stabilization of any fluid or electrolyte imbalance is paramount. Delays in appropriate medical evaluation of those patients with CAH and unrecognized salt wasting carry significant risks. Initial screening studies in such patients include assessment of serum electrolytes, biochemical assays screening for CAH, and evaluation of karyotype using cultured peripheral leukocytes. A multidisciplinary assessment is initiated, including medical professionals from neonatology, endocrinology, child psychiatry, medical genetics, urology, and at times medical ethics. Gender assignment based on karyotype and potential for genitourinary function should be made after discussion within the entire treatment team and the parents. A child should not be named until the appropriate gender assignment is made.

History/physical examination

A careful maternal and family history is mandatory. Maternal use of alcohol or drugs and exposure to androgenic substances as well as a family history of previous neonatal death, infertility, genital ambiguity, abnormal pubertal development or inguinal hernias associated with retained müllerian structures may contribute to proper diagnosis.

Physical examination of the child is important and may provide further clues. The general well being of the child should be assessed. Signs of dehydration and lethargy suggest a diagnosis of CAH. Patients with 11 β-hydroxylase deficiency may be hypertensive. The abdominal examination should note any lower, midline abdominal masses which might represent a distended bladder or vagina. The back should be assessed for any findings associated with an underlying neurologic anomaly. Gonads are palpated to determine location, number, size, and associated structures such as an epididymis and vas deferens. Rectal examination should carefully evaluate the location of the anus, and palpation with the little finger may identify the midline cervical cap or uterine tissue. Careful inspection of the female introitus is required to identify an isolated urogenital sinus if no clitoral or labial abnormalities are present.

Radiographic evaluation

Ultrasound is a valuable adjunct to physical examination in these patients. The newborn period is the optimal time for evaluation because maternal hormones make the ovaries and uterus more prominent.[6] The spinal cord may also be evaluated for cord tethering. Although sometimes helpful, the sensitivity for locating a non-palpable or intra-abdominal gonad with sonography is at best 60%.[7] Hydrocolpos, in this setting usually related to retained urine, and bladder distention are easily seen with sonography. Likewise, the kidneys should be evaluated for hydronephrosis, dysplasia, and agenesis. Additionally, patients with CAH usually have a cerebriform appearance of their adrenal glands that may be helpful in diagnosis.[8]

All patients with a urogenital sinus anomaly should undergo contrast genitography. These studies require interest, skill, and determination on the part of the radiologist. The study may be performed by insertion of the tip of a Foley catheter into the opening of the urogenital sinus. The balloon may then be inflated outside the meatus to prevent spillage of contrast, and retrograde instillation of radiopaque dye used to define the anatomy. In many cases it is then possible to advance a feeding tube into the bladder for formal voiding cystourethrography. Proper studies should define the length of the common sinus and the level of confluence. Pelvic magnetic resonance imaging (MRI) may, at times, add anatomic detail or understanding.

Endoscopic evaluation

Endoscopic evaluation of the anatomy is critical and should be performed on all children with a urogenital sinus. Generally, this is done under the same anesthetic as open reconstruction, particularly for lower or intermediate lesions. If the anatomy is not well understood after radiographic evaluation, particularly in the presence of a high confluence or after failure to identify any vaginal structure on genitography, cystoscopy may be performed alone in order to better understand or delineate the anatomy and better prepare the patient and family for reconstructive surgery.

Further studies

In rare circumstances usually related to the diagnosis of intersex, the definite diagnosis may remain elusive after conventional studies. At times, relatively prolonged hormonal stimulation to evaluate the presence and function of testicular tissue may be indicated. Gonadal biopsy may be necessary for diagnosis. An adequate biopsy requires a full length, deep longitudinal incision into the gonad to ensure adequate tissue sampling. This may be done in an open fashion or laparoscopically. Such a procedure allows for thorough examination of the pelvis and abdomen for müllerian and wolffian structures.

Surgical techniques

Timing

Significant improvements in surgical techniques and outcomes have occurred over the past several decades. Despite these apparent improvements, controversies remain. Intersex advocacy groups, patients, and some medical professionals still question the timing of surgery and whether reconstruction should be performed at all until the patient can contribute to informed consent. Discussions with a multidisciplinary team and parents must address these controversies prior to female genital surgery. Today, most genital reconstructive surgery is performed with respect to genetic sex. Only in very rare situations is gender conversion considered.

Most girls with a urogenital sinus diagnosed as infants have CAH. It is generally accepted that clitoroplasty for those patients is best performed in the first few months of life. Waiting several months allows good stabilization of the patient from an endocrine and metabolic standpoint. Appropriate medical treatment will, at times, produce improvement in the external virilization, but seldom results in complete normalization. Relatively early intervention may carry the benefit of thicker, more vascular skin and easier dissection or manipulation of the clitoris and paravaginal tissue related to maternal estrogen stimulation. There may also be some psychological benefit for the parents from early correction of the virilized external genitalia.

In contrast to timing of clitoral reduction, the optimal age for vaginal reconstruction is more controversial. It is our belief that total genital reconstruction with vaginoplasty should be performed as a single stage with clitoroplasty within the first several months to first year of life. This is particularly true for patients with CAH, most of whom have clitoromegaly and a low to moderate confluence of the urogenital sinus. Potential benefits include improved tissue transfer and reduced scarring secondary to estrogen stimulation, minimization of parental anxiety over the child's condition, and earlier self-acceptance of the child's gender identity and genital anatomy. It must be noted that delayed vaginal construction is recommended by some surgeons.[9] Early vaginal reconstruction may carry an increased risk for an element of vaginal stenosis when evaluated in the adolescent or young adult.[10] Advocates for delayed reconstruction note psychological concerns in older patients with subsequent vaginal stenosis particularly when vaginal dilatation is required. It is not clear that the psychological impact of later, major reconstruction for vaginoplasty will carry a lesser psychological impact on the patient. We favor complete, early repair as we have found the exposure and surgical reconstruction then to be considerably easier than in an older patient and value the increased availability of genital skin from the clitoris for vaginal reconstruction.

Patient preparation

Most children undergoing vaginoplasty for a urogenital sinus anomaly, unless the confluence is extremely low, undergo a full bowel preparation using a polyethylene glycol and electrolyte solution such as GoLYTELY. For young children, this preparation is done as an inpatient with bowel catharsis administered by a nasogastric tube. Adolescent patients may self-administer the bowel preparation orally at home with parental guidance. A series of oral antibiotic doses are often administered as well as perioperative broad-spectrum intravenous antibiotics.

After general anesthesia is administered, the child is usually placed in the dorsal lithotomy position for endoscopy. Even if endoscopy has previously been performed in the newborn period, we generally repeat endoscopy at the time of surgical reconstruction, as the internal genital findings may be much more obvious in an older patient. The rectum and distal colon may be irrigated clear of any residual fecal matter at this time. For higher lesions, a Foley catheter is placed into the bladder, and a second catheter, either a Fogarty or Foley, is placed into the vagina. Cystoscopy aids in confirmation of catheter placement in the appropriate position.

Surgical preparation is dependent on the extent of the planned reconstruction and surgeon preference, as well as on the age of the patient. In all but the lowest of urogenital lesions, we perform a full, lower body prep from the nipple to toes, front and back (Figure 70.4). The catheters are kept sterile and prepped into the surgical field. The feet and lower legs are wrapped, and the patient passed through an aperture in the surgical drape. This preparation allows exposure to the entire lower body in both the prone and supine position. It is simple and safe to move smaller patients between the two positions. It is often helpful to perform the external feminizing genitoplasty with the patient supine, while exposing and repairing the proximal sinus in the prone position. Trying to prep and move a larger teenage patient in a similar fashion may be cumbersome and impractical. If prone positioning is desired for exposure and vaginoplasty in such patients, a modified skydiver position may be used. Positioning and padding must be utilized carefully to avoid injury.

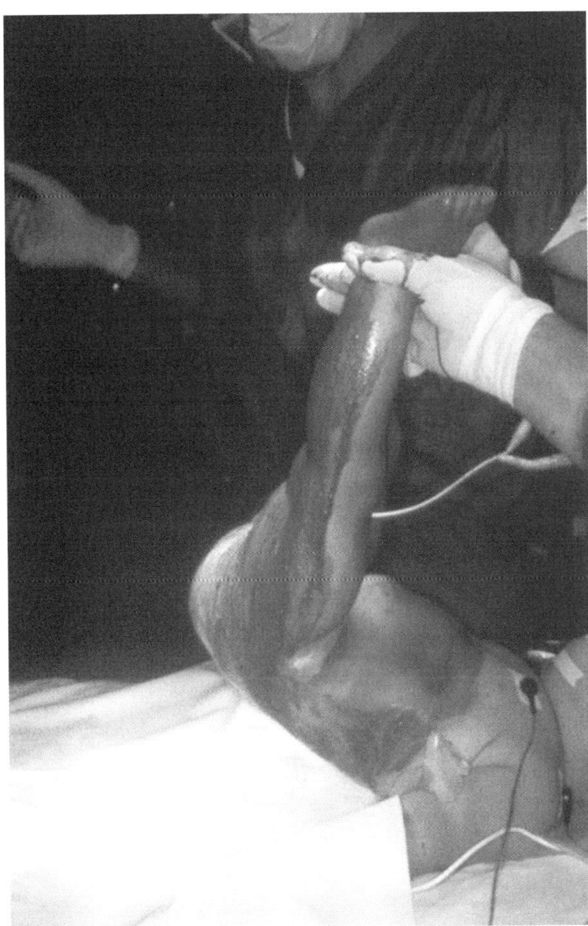

Figure 70.4 Lower body preparation. The preparation allows supine and prone approach. Smaller patients may be easily turned between the two positions.

Feminizing genitoplasty

The surgical management of the child with clitoromegaly has undergone marked evolution from early methods that advocated clitoral amputation.[11,12] Although satisfactory cosmetic results were reported after such procedures,[13] impairment in orgasm and psychosexual development were later noted.[14] The first attempts at sparing the clitoris with modification of the appearance involved clitoral recession or concealment.[15–17] All current techniques have preservation of clitoral sensation and function as their cornerstone. Those repairs are based on Schmid's landmark description of corporeal body excision and neurovascular bundle conservation.[18] Early reports described complete excision of the corpora cavernosa of the phallus, including the tunica, while the neurovascular bundle was preserved only with Buck's fascia.[19] It then became clear that subtunical resection of the corporeal erectile tissue with preservation of the dorsal tunica might protect the glanular nerve and blood supply.[20] Recently Baskin and colleagues have suggested that a more ventral tunical incision may be prudent after carefully demonstrating lateral fanning of the clitoral nerve supply.[21] Other interesting work has helped to define the spatial relationship of the normal clitoris, urethral meatus, vaginal introitus, and other anatomic landmarks,[22] as well as begun to examine which areas of external genital skin may be most involved in genital sensation and orgasm.[23]

Clitoral resection is performed with the child supine with legs spread or in a low lithotomy position. A traction suture is placed in the glans clitoris,

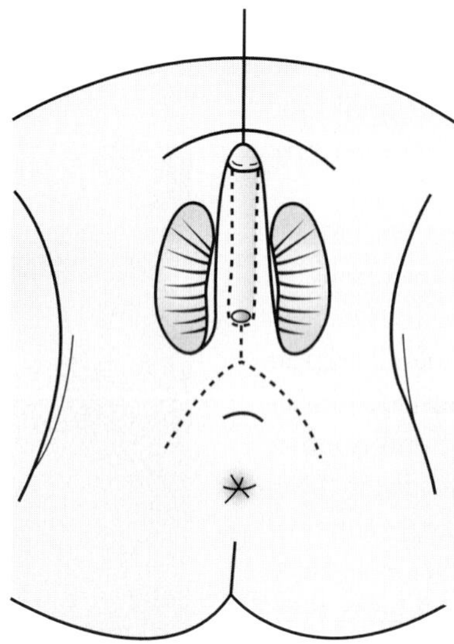

Figure 70.5 Feminizing genitoplasty. The dashed lines mark the initial incisions. (From Rink RC, Adams MC,[26] with permission from Springer Science and Business Media.)

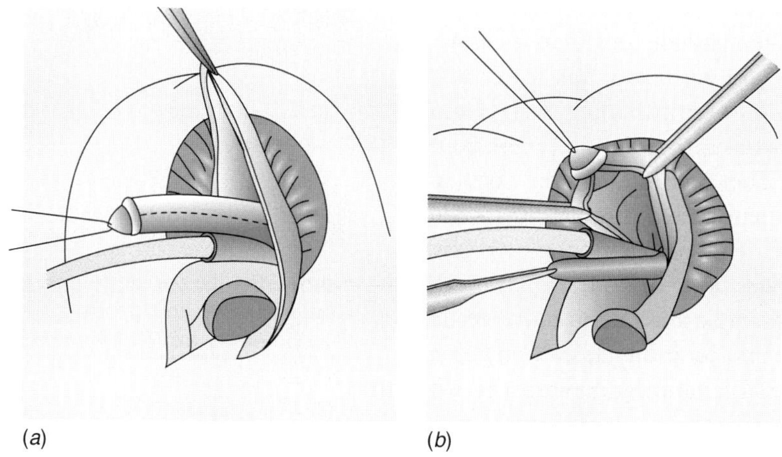

Figure 70.6 Corporeal reduction. (*a*) The urethral plate and spongiosum are mobilized off the ventral corpora. The dashed line shows the ventromedial incision into tunica on either side. (*b*) The erectile tissue is excised with ventral tunica. (Adopted from Rink RC, Kaefer M,[102] with permission from Elsevier.)

and the initial incision is marked and made in a circumcising fashion just off the glans over the dorsum and lateral aspect of the clitoris. Ventrally, the incisions are carried in a parallel fashion from distal to proximal on either side of what would be the urethral plate (Figure 70.5). These incisions are carried proximally to the urethral meatus. The lines of incision and base of the clitoris may be infiltrated with 1:200 000 epinephrine with or without lidocaine for aid in hemostasis. Incisions are carried down to Buck's fascia and the clitoris degloved of phallic skin. The urethra is generally left attached to the glans with consideration of glanular blood supply while the urethral plate with spongiosum is dissected off of the corpora cavernosa to expose the ventral tunica of the cavernosa.

The tunica of the corpora are incised proximally at their bifurcation on the ventromedial side (Figure 70.6). Longitudinal incisions are carried out towards the glans all the way through the tunica to expose the erectile tissue. Erectile tissue is sharply excised from the proximal bifurcation out to the level of the corona along with the ventral tunics. The proximal ends of erectile tissue may be oversewn or suture ligated for hemostasis. Even after treatment with steroids, the glans clitoris may be remarkably enlarged. If so, the

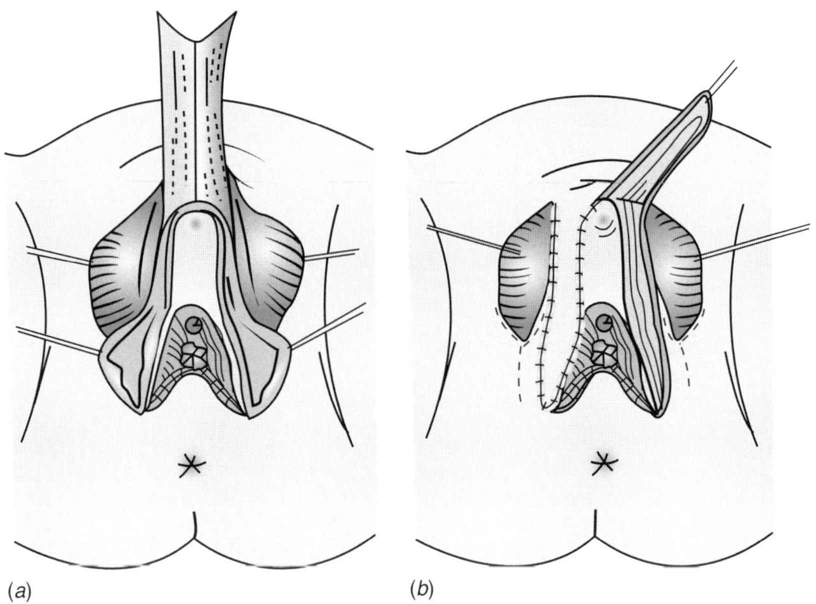

Figure 70.7 Labioplasty. (*a*) Redundant dorsal phallic skin is mobilized and incised in midline. (*b*) The phallic skin is used as labia minora on either side. Y-V plasty is performed on the labia majora. The posterior flap is advanced into the vagina. (Adapted from Rink RC, Adams MC,[26] with permission from Springer Science and Business Media).

glans may be reduced by excising a wedge of glanular tissue on the ventral surface. Baskin et al have shown that ventral excision of the glans is the most appropriate when considering the nerve supply.[21] The reduced glans should be approximated to the base of the corporeal bodies by anchoring sutures. The location of the glans should give consideration to the position of the clitoral hood and symphysis pubis.

Feminizing genitoplasty also involves construction of labia minora from clitoral skin as well as modification of the labia majora (Figure 70.7). The phallic skin is released dorsally and unfurled by mobilizing the inner from outer prepuce. The skin is then usually incised in the dorsal midline. The midline incision is stopped short of the base of the phallus in order to preserve an appropriate hood over the dorsal clitoris. The excess skin is rotated ventrally, trimmed, and approximated to either side of the urethral plate medially as well as the modified labia majora laterally. The flaps, as such, serve as labia minora. Alternatively, the phallic skin may be used for an anterior vaginal flap in more proximal repairs. The labia majora, as the result of virilization, are initially short and rounded. Aggressive incision around the medial, posterior, and lateral aspect of the labia majora on either side allows the labia to be lengthened and narrowed using a Y-V plasty. This plastic reconstruction of the labia is often performed in conjunction with flap vaginoplasty, and modifications in the posteriorly based vaginal flap may allow the labia from either side to swing inwards posteriorly and avoid an overly wide posterior introitus.[24]

Surgical correction of the low confluence

Cutback vaginoplasty

A cutback vaginoplasty is a simple procedure performed in the patient with labial fusion. This technique involves incision of the fused skin posteriorly to the perineum to expose the vaginal orifice. The incised lateral edges are oversewn. Whereas such a procedure is simple and may produce a good result in the appropriate patient, it is only a consideration in patients with a common urogenital sinus on the phallus with confluence of a normal vaginal opening at the level of the perineum. That combination is extraordinarily rare; thus the procedure is very rarely, if ever, indicated.

Flap vaginoplasty

Flap vaginoplasty is best suited for those patients with a low confluence of the urogenital sinus. The perineal skin incision is marked and made as a broad-based, inverted U-flap.[25] The closed end of the flap is created at the posterior lip of the meatus of the urogenital sinus, and the lateral margins should be well inside the ischial rami. The flap may be variable in length, depending on the length of the urogenital sinus; however, the posterior extent should leave a normal-sized

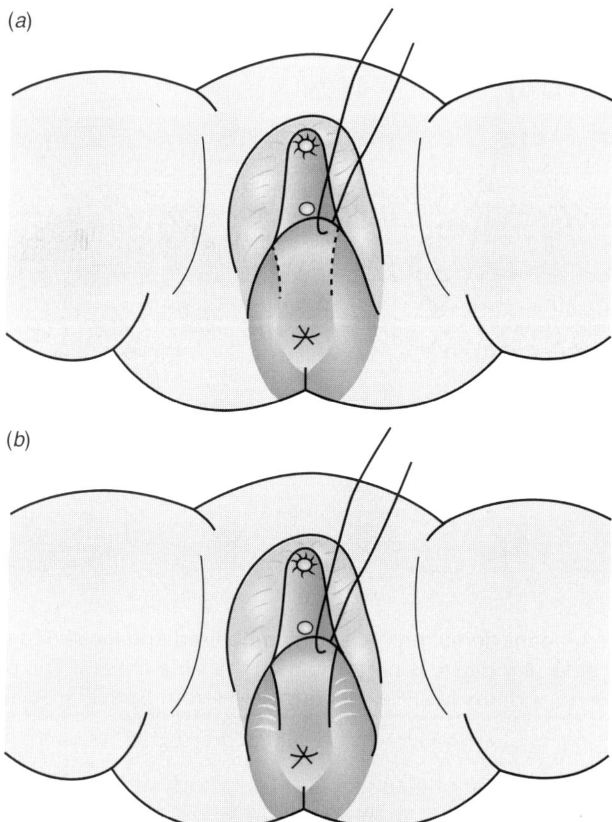

Figure 70.8 Omega flap. Skin elements may be excised carefully at the base of the flap to create a more normal-appearing posterior introitus. Subcutaneous tissue and blood supply should be preserved at the base.

perineal body. Design of the flap should respect considerations of the length versus width so as to ensure a good blood supply. Maintaining a U shape rather than narrow V shape at the tip anteriorly helps to make sure that the end of the flap is not ischemic.[26] The skin flap should be mobilized away from the posterior aspect of the urogenital sinus while maintaining a thick layer of subcutaneous tissue and fat with the flap. This mobilization exposes the urogenital sinus, which is eventually incised in the midline posteriorly. The incision is carried into the vagina and must extend through the distal vagina, which is typically narrow. Failure to place the flap well into the proximal vagina that is normal in circumference may result in stenosis. The flap of perineal skin is advanced into the vagina and secured with interrupted absorbable suture and should reach without tension (see Figure 70.7).

The broad-based flap may create an abnormal appearance to the introitus posteriorly when the labia are spread. Careful trimming of the dermis and epidermis at the base of the flap may allow creation of a rhomboid or omega shape without sacrificing viability of the flap[24] (Figure 70.8). Posterior excision of the skin should not be so extreme as to compromise the vascularity of the flap, and the subcutaneous tissue must be carefully preserved at that level. Modification of the flap allows subsequent use of the labia to provide some posterior closure of the introitus and a more normal appearance.

It should be noted that flap vaginoplasty does not totally correct the urogenital sinus. Without any separation of the vagina from urethra and lengthening or advancement of the urethra itself, the patient is still left with a urogenital sinus. The sinus, however, is much broader distally and may, therefore, not be of any functional or cosmetic significance. Consequently, flap vaginoplasty should not be a viable surgical option for correction of a high-confluence urogenital sinus. One appropriate role for total urogenital mobilization may be to advance the level of confluence towards the perineum in a patient with a moderate-level lesion in order to make conventional flap vaginoplasty an appropriate technique for repair.

Surgical correction of the higher confluence

Pull-through vaginoplasty

This repair, as described by Hendren and Crawford,[3] was a landmark advance in female genital reconstruc-

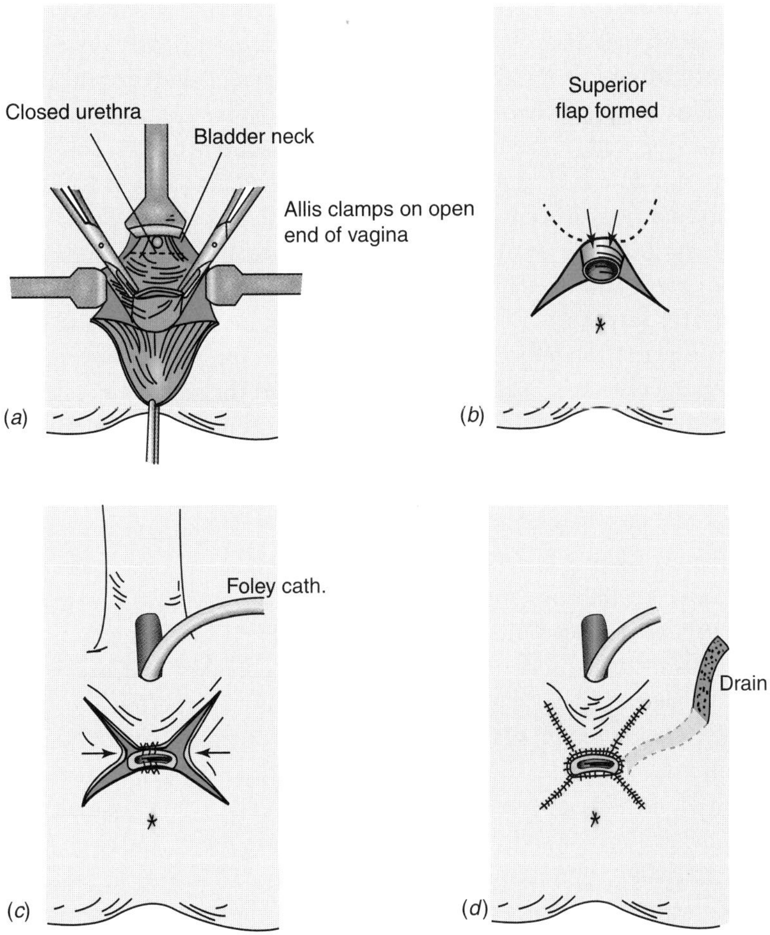

Figure 70.9 Pull-through vaginoplasty. The vagina is mobilized off of the urogenital sinus and advanced to the perineum. The sinus is closed to creat the urethra. (Adapted from Hendren WH, Crawford JD,[3] with permission from Elsevier.)

tive surgery; its basic principles still apply for children with higher lesions. Hendren's initial description includes the use of shallow, opposing U-shaped incisions on the perineum at the spot for placement of the eventual vaginal introitus[3,25] (Figure 70.9). Dissection is then made parallel and slightly posterior to the distal urogenital sinus until the vaginal catheter is encountered. A finger placed in the rectum may help maintain the proper plane of dissection posteriorly. The vagina is divided at its entrance to the sinus and then mobilized extensively. The proximal urogenital sinus at the site of prior confluence is closed, and the urogenital sinus used as a functional urethra. As originally described, the vagina is mobilized extensively in a circumferential fashion. The proper plane of dissection between the proximal urethra and anterior vagina is always quite difficult. For the first several millimeters, there is often virtually no connective tissue between the mucosa of the two structures. Dissection must continue through this difficult area in order to achieve adequate mobilization, and Hendren[3] and others[27] initially promoted mobilization of the vagina to the extent that it could be advanced as is to the perineum. Avoidance of the bladder and urethral sphincter mechanisms is mandatary as one proceeds proximally. In general, it is better to err by dissecting too close to the vagina than on the side of the bladder or urethra. This method is technically challenging, largely as a result of the limited exposure to the critical area of the confluence. Early results produced an isolated and separate vaginal opening that was cosmetically unappealing. Additional problems related to vaginal stenosis have been reported and may be due to tension created by attempts to mobilize a relatively thin vagina all the way to the perineum.[28]

Exposure

Much of the difficulty with pull-through vaginoplasties is related to exposure of the high confluence, and modifications have been described to improve the approach to the critical proximal area. Passerini-Glazel in 1989[28] popularized Monfort's transtrigonal approach in which the vagina is approached from a midline incision in the posterior wall of the bladder. It does provide superb exposure to a very high lesion but is usually not necessary. During dissection from below, simple incision of the posterior wall of the entire urogenital sinus from the meatus to the level of the confluence may improve exposure over that achieved when leaving the distal portion intact. Opening of the entire sinus then necessitates subsequent tubularization of the same structure for use as a urethra and theoretically increases the length over which a urethrovaginal fistula may occur. Most such fistula, however, when they occur, do so at the level of the initial confluence where the exposure and repair are most tenuous. Anything done to improve exposure and the quality of the repair at that level may ultimately be advantageous. This extended incision into the sinus is particularly beneficial when the distal anomaly is vagina-like. Such a lesion requires tapering distally to achieve a more normal urethra.

The persistent cloaca is a more complex lesion than a urogenital sinus because the rectum is also involved. Cloacal anomalies are generally approached and repaired through a posterior sagittal incision extending from the coccyx. Once the rectal fistula has been removed and the more proximal rectum mobilized, the patient is left with a urogenital sinus that is nicely exposed through an incision that is much longer in the sagittal axis. Reports do exist of a posterior sagittal approach to a high urogenital sinus with splitting of the rectum either completely or anteriorly.[29] Such exposure is superb but potentially adds morbidity and is generally not necessary. Rink et al[30] encouraged the use of an anterior sagittal prone approach without division of the rectum. This approach provides excellent exposure during the difficult mobilization of the vagina off of the posterior urethra and bladder neck and does not preclude use of an inverted U-shaped incision as described for flap vaginoplasty. The procedure begins with the child supine, and the initial steps of clitoroplasty, if necessary, are performed. Initial dissection onto the posterior aspect of the more distal sinus is begun in the supine position. The patient, prepped from nipple to toes, front and back, is then turned prone. The dissection, with remarkably better visualization after the change in position alone, is continued between the posterior wall of the urogenital sinus and the rectum in the midline. The intact rectum is displaced superiorly with a malleable retractor, and the urogenital sinus is opened well into the vagina (Figure 70.10). The same malleable retractor can then be placed into the vagina to provide excellent visualization anteriorly. Following aggressive anterior vaginal mobilization, the urogenital sinus is closed in several layers over a urethral catheter, creating a neourethra. Generally, several layers of tissue can then be approximated in the midline to separate the vagina and urethra.

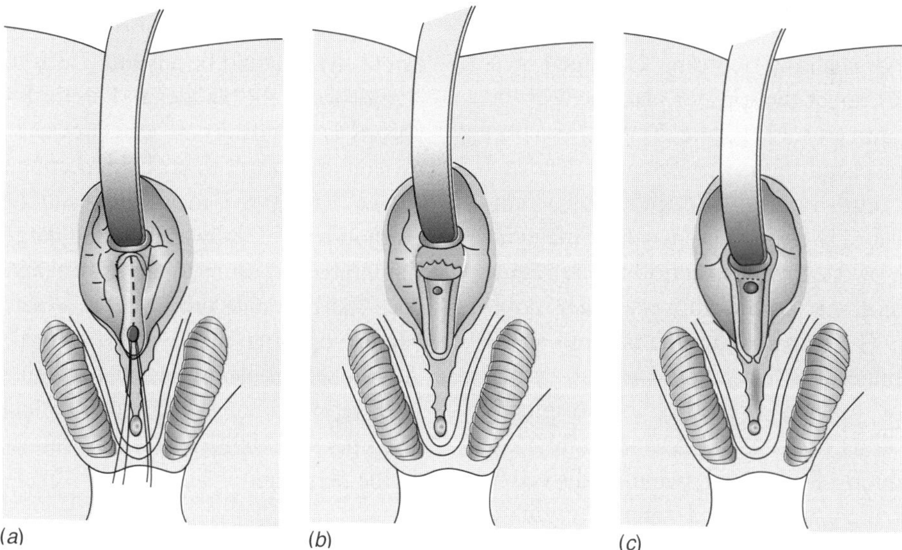

Figure 70.10 Prone exposure to high confluence. (*a*) After creation of a posteriorly based flap, the rectum is retracted to expose the sinus. (*b*) The sinus is opened into the vagina. (*c*) The malleable retractor is placed into the vagina to expose the critical area of dissection (dashed line).

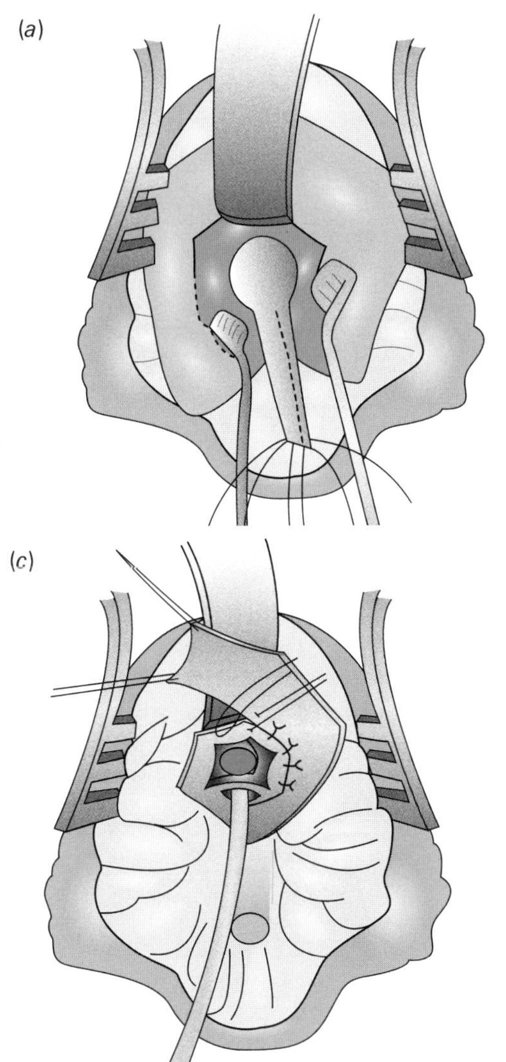

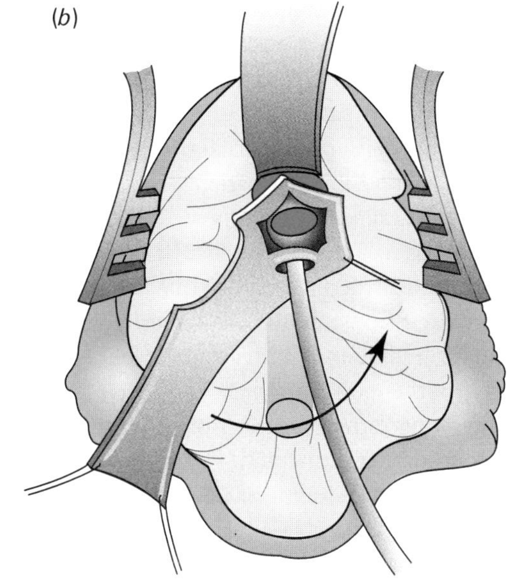

Figure 70.11 Use of distal sinus for vaginoplasty. (*a*) After total urogenital mobilization and exposure of the confluence, a lateral incision in the sinus (dashed line) is planned. (*b*) A healthy flap is created opposite the side of the incision. (*c*) The flap can be utilized in a spiral fashion to create a distal vagina. (b and c reproduced with permission from Indiana University School of Medicine.)

Complex flaps

It is often clear that the short vagina mobilized off of the urethra in a patient with a high-level urogenital sinus may not reach the perineum without tension. The use of flaps to reach the proximal vagina may provide the potential to improve the functional and cosmetic result of pull-through vaginoplasty. Complex flaps of labia majora or buttocks skin from either side may be used to reach the proximal vagina without tension.[31] Such flaps may provide a good result from the standpoint of a functional vagina but can distort the appearance of the introitus. Secondary perineal surgery 6–12 months after initial creation of the flaps may be appropriate to divide the base of such flaps and recreate a more normal appearance of the labia and perineum. Gonzalez[32] used flaps of phallic skin to construct the distal vagina. Passerini-Glazel[28] used the distal urogenital sinus opened anteriorly rather than posteriorly in similar fashion. The sinus was folded back at the proximal end of the anterior incision and combined with phallic skin to tubularize as distal vagina. Such flaps of clitoral skin or distal urogenital sinus may be useful in constructing the anterior vagina in combination with a posteriorly based, U-shaped flap. Rink and Cain[33] have recently described lateral incision into the distal urogenital sinus with spiral construction of a distal vagina that is mucosally lined at the level of the introitus (Figure 70.11).

Total urogenital mobilization

In 1997, Pena described the technique of total urogenital mobilization for repair of urogenital sinus in patients with a cloacal anomaly.[34] Applications for this repair have been expanded to include patients with urogenital sinus abnormalities alone. Such mobilization is generally not necessary for patients with a low confluence, and the best indication for its use may be patients with a mid-level lesion in whom the level of confluence may be converted to a low one suitable for flap vaginoplasty. The role of total urogenital mobilization for patients with a very high lesion remains to be determined. Total urogenital mobilization may be used in such patients to improve exposure at the critical level of confluence. The urethra and vagina can be mobilized towards the perineum, separated, and the structures released back to a proximal position for reconstruction. Total urogenital mobilization for high lesions with advancement of the confluence to the perineum has also been described; however, long-term validation of the results in such patients need be documented. Potential advantages of this technique include improved cosmesis, easier dissection leading to decreased operative time, and less risk of vaginal stenosis or urethrovaginal fistula.[34] There is no question that this operative technique with advancement is potentially easier as it avoids the difficult dissection between the anterior vagina and proximal urethra or bladder neck; an easier operative approach, however, does not necessarily mean a better long-term result for the patient. Rare patients with a urogenital sinus, particularly those related to the persistent cloaca, may suffer from urinary incontinence or poor voiding. Such dysfunction may be related to the anatomic problem, abnormal innervation, or a combination of the two issues. Circumferential dissection of the urogenital sinus to the bladder neck could potentially exacerbate neurologic problems. Even if it does not do so in the short-term, long-term follow-up of girls with high lesions undergoing total urogenital mobilization with advancement distally will be required to determine the risk of stress urinary incontinence.[35,36] Stress incontinence in patients after such a procedure would probably be difficult to treat.

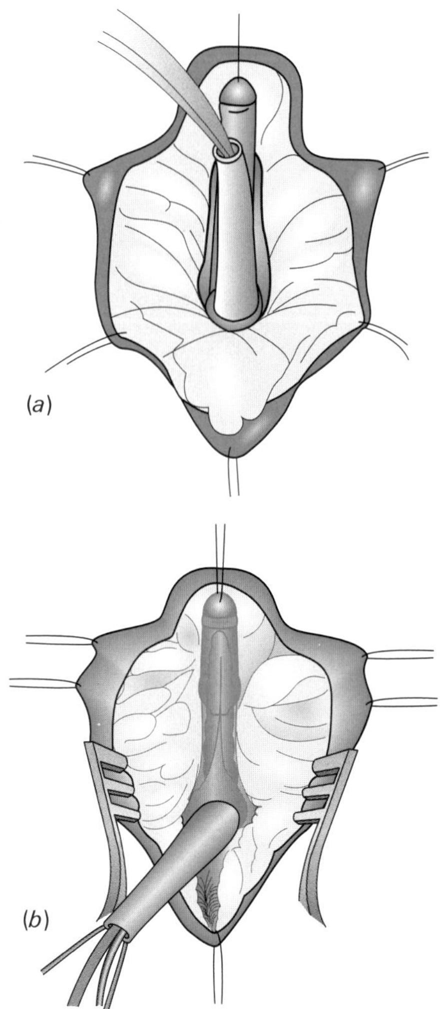

Figure 70.12 Total urogenital mobilization. (*a*) The skin is mobilized and the sinus exposed with a circumferential incision at the meatus. (*b*) The sinus is mobilized from the rectum posteriorly and the corpora anteriorly up to the pubis. (Adapted from Rink RC, Kaefer M,[62] with permission from Elsevier.)

In total urogenital mobilization, the sinus is initially approached from the midline posteriorly, and attachments between the rectum and sinus divided. This exposure may be done from a midline incision or after creation of a posteriorly based flap. The sinus is then circumscribed at the meatus on the clitoris and dissection carried circumferentially from distal to proximal. The distal sinus is carefully mobilized with all spongiosum off of the corpora cavernosa (Figure 70.12). Anteriorly, the ligamentous attachments of the sinus to the pubis are incised, allowing for adequate mobilization to the perineum. It is possible in some cases that anterior dissection may be stopped just short of these attachments.[37] The catheter in the vagina is palpated, identifying the posterior vaginal wall. The vagina is opened posteriorly between stay sutures well through the distal narrow segment. If the vagina reaches the perineum without tension, the sinus can be opened ventrally to create the vestibule. A posteriorly based flap may be useful in some such cases. If the vagina is very high and the urethra very short above the confluence, a decision must be made whether advancement of the intact sinus towards the perineum is appropriate (Figure 70.13). If not, the patient may be turned to the prone position and the vagina separated from the sinus with superb exposure. The distal mobilized sinus may then be incised dorsally or laterally, as previously described,[28,33] and used for vaginoplasty after the more proximal sinus is tubularized as the urethra. The child is usually turned

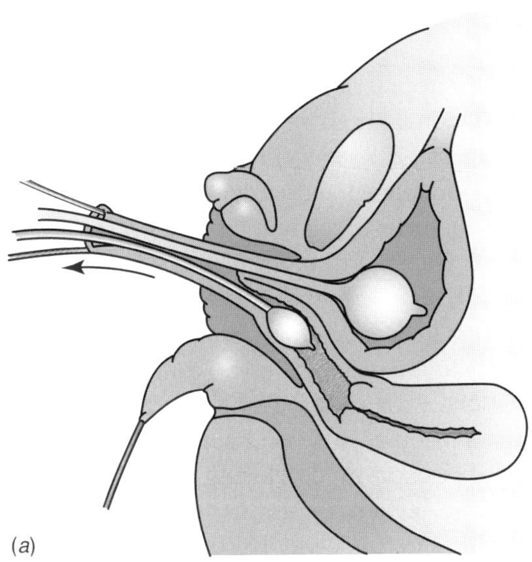

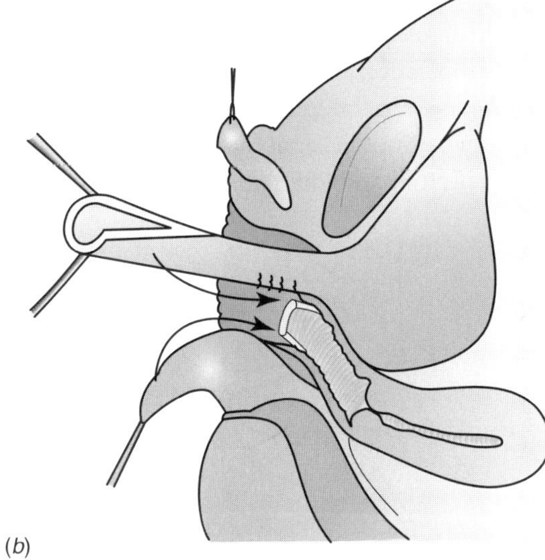

Figure 70.13 Options with total urogenital mobilization. (*a*) After adequate mobilization, the confluence may be advanced to the perineum. (*b*) Alternatively, mobilization allows good exposure for separation of the vagina and urethra. Anterior and posterior flaps may be used for vaginoplasty after releasing the urethra and vagina in a cephalad direction. (Adapted from Rink RC, Kaefer M,[62] with permission from Elsevier.)

back to the supine position to complete the plastic repair of the labia and perineum. Bladder catheter drainage and vaginal packing are usually employed after such complex repairs.

Vaginal replacement

Skin graft

In those patients with absence of the vagina or severe hypoplasia, total vaginal replacement is required. Treatment options have included use of chronic vaginal dilatation,[38] skin grafts,[39,40] rotational flaps,[41] or the use of bowel substitution.[42]

The use of split- or full-thickness skin grafts and rotational flaps remains an option for vaginal replacement. McIndoe described the use of split-thickness skin grafts taken from the thigh and conformed to a cylindrical stent[40] (Figure 70.14). Space is created between the urethra and rectum in which the dermal surface of the skin graft is secured. The vaginal stent is left in place to be removed after a period of 7–10 days. A period of weeks to months of daily vaginal dilatation is usually required to maintain patency and prevent vaginal stenosis. Full-thickness skin grafts have less reliable ingrowth of blood supply but contract less once in place. The full-thickness grafts potentially leave a more obvious cosmetic defect at the donor site. Rotational flaps have been used to create a neovagina. Gracilis myocutaneous flaps,[43] pudendal thigh flaps,[44] labia minora flaps,[45] and flaps raised after tissue expansion have been described.[46] Unfortunately, patients with skin grafts or flaps for vaginal replacement may have problems with lubrication, graft contracture, or dyspareunia, and a need for chronic vaginal dilatation.[47] These difficulties have led to a general acceptance of the superiority of bowel vaginoplasty for replacement, at least among pediatric urologists.

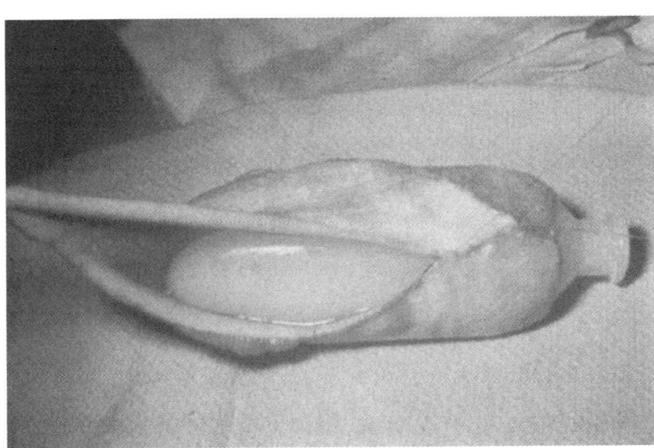

Figure 70.14 McIndoe skin vagina. Split-thickness skin graft is modeled over stent.

Bowel vagina

Advantages of the bowel vaginoplasty include natural lubrication from the intestinal segment, less problems with dyspareunia, and infrequent contracture or stenosis often without any need for routine vaginal dilatation.[42,48,49] The sigmoid colon is generally preferred for vaginoplasty because of its proximity and ease of mobilization. In addition, the bowel segment does not need to be reconfigured. A segment of ileum, if more mobile, may also be useful but may require folding in an older patient.

(a)

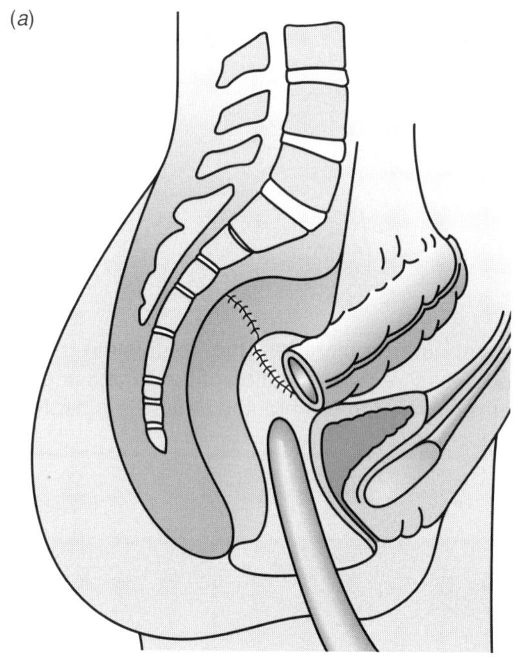

(b)

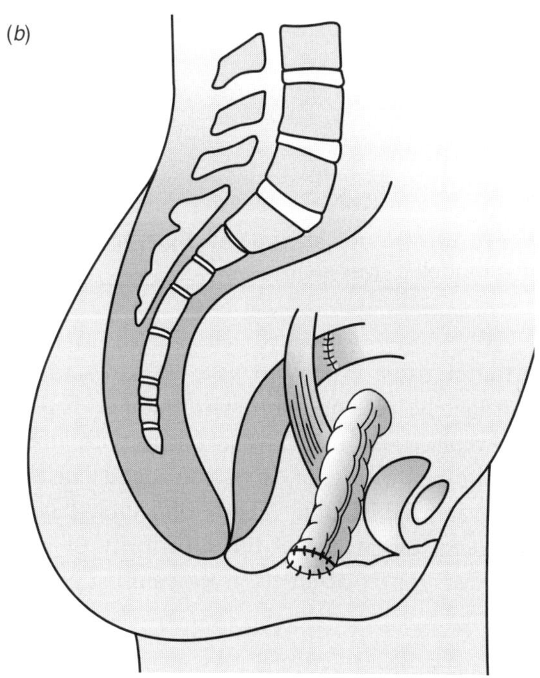

Figure 70.15 Sigmoid vaginal replacement. (*a*) A short segment of colon is isolated and space created from below. (*b*) The bowel vagina is secured in place. (Adapted from Rink RC, Kaefer M,[62] with permission from Elsevier.)

The patient is placed in a modified, low lithotomy position with careful support of the lower extremities to avoid neuropraxia. This position allows for simultaneous abdominal and perineal approach by two surgeons. Through a low Pfannenstiel incision, the sigmoid is identified and evaluated for mobility. An 8–12 cm segment of sigmoid colon is identified and isolated with a window in the mesocolon at either end (Figure 70.15). A short segment is utilized because redundancy in length often results in eventual prolapse at the perineum. Bowel continuity may be reestablished with a stapled or hand-sewn anastomosis. Simultaneously, a second surgeon may perform perineal dissection by developing space between the bladder and rectum to the level of the peritoneal reflection in the cul-de-sac. Palpation of a catheter in the urethra aids in identification of the proper plane. The peritoneum is incised from above and an adequate space created bluntly using a finger initially and then larger dilators. Care must be taken that the space is adequate along the entire length, particularly at the level of the pelvic floor. If an ileal segment is to be used, it is generally opened on its antimesenteric border and folded into a U configuration. Either segment of bowel is checked for viability. Minimal tension at the distal end of the segment reaching to the perineum may not be problematic and may, in fact, help avoid future prolapse. Extreme tension on the mesentery of the bowel segment should be avoided whether using ileum or sigmoid colon. If such tension exists, creation of larger windows in the mesentery may be helpful, although careful identification of mesenteric vessels is critical. Serial transverse myotomies in the isolated sigmoid colon segment may also aid in lengthening of the segment. An inverted U-shaped perineal flap is often used to avoid the appearance of circumferential bowel mucosa at the introitus. The mobilized bowel segment is approximated to the perineal skin, skin flaps, or the remnant of the native vagina with absorbable suture. The neovagina is packed with antibiotic-soaked gauze, which is removed after several days of healing. Irrigation of the bowel segment to avoid accumulation of excess mucus is then begun.

Other procedures

Gonadectomy

A thorough chromosome evaluation is mandatory at the time of initial diagnosis in children with ambiguous genitalia. The presence of all or part of the Y chromosome in patients with disorders of gonadal differentiation places them at increased risk for development of gonadoblastomas and other germ cell tumors.[50,51] Bilateral gonadectomies in such patients are typically performed in the first several years of life; however, no consensus exists in regards to the optimal timing. We have recently noted bilateral gonadoblastomas in a patient with pure gonadal dysgenesis at 6 months of age and prefer early excision. Gonadectomies are also performed in children with severe feminizing male pseudohermaphroditism who have undergone gender conversion. Laparoscopic excision may minimize morbidity and improve the cosmetic result; it also allows for therapeutic visualization of the abdomen, pelvis, and accessory sex organs. Longitudinal biopsy of the gonads may be appropriate in some patients for diagnosis or prior to excision.

Reconstruction for male pseudohermaphroditism

Male pseudohermaphroditism occurs when there is impaired genital differentiation of an XY male with developed testes and may result in a wide range of male and female phenotypes. Treatment of these children must be individualized, and appropriate surgical intervention may include relatively minor hypospadias repair, orchidopexy, or major genital reconstruction including gender conversion. A detailed discussion of the treatment of these patients is found in Chapter 68.

Results of reconstruction

Quality reviews documenting long-term results following feminizing genitoplasty or vaginoplasty in the setting of a urogenital sinus are lacking, particularly any with careful consideration to the initial anatomy or the surgical technique employed. Clitoral nerve conduction studies have identified preservation following clitoral reduction techniques and are encouraging in regards to ultimate clitoral function.[52] Work evaluating orgasm and sexual satisfaction following such reconstruction is rudimentary at best.

More studies have evaluated the vagina after reconstruction in terms of more obvious complications such as vaginal stenosis or urethrovaginal fistula. Studies evaluating the ability of the vagina to accommodate sexual intercourse after such reconstruction have provided sobering results. Jones and colleagues have noted that 30% of patients required surgical revision after initial vaginoplasty in order to achieve satisfactory intercourse,[53] and Azziz et al reported satisfactory coitus in only 62% of patients 20 years following vaginal reconstruction in patients with CAH.[54] Many of those patients, however, had required secondary or tertiary procedures to correct stenosis at the introitus.

Early vaginoplasty may be a factor in the development of vaginal stenosis. Sotiropoulos et al noted that all of their patients operated upon in a prepubertal period required revision of their introitus at a later date.[55] Bailez and colleagues, as well as Azziz et al, noted more revisions among children in whom vaginoplasty was performed prior to 1 year of age.[10,54] These older series included a wide range of patients with variability in the severity of the initial anomaly or even in the surgical techniques that were employed in their repair. It is possible that newer techniques for exposure, tissue handling, and use of flaps for vaginal reconstruction may change the surgical outcomes for the better; however, only long-term follow-up will determine if that is indeed the case. Careful attention must also be paid to defining the severity of vaginal stenosis after reconstruction. Many stenoses may be minor and only result in the necessity for a minor revision usually involving modified Z-plasty at the level of the narrowing. Such secondary procedures are less troublesome than the major rotational flaps that might be required for severe, extensive stenosis. The difference between the two procedures has not always been well indicated in historic series.

The role of routine vaginal dilatation in an attempt to avoid vaginal stenosis remains unclear. Routine dilatation or calibration may help some patients avoid stenosis if done regularly, particularly in patients destined to develop minor stenosis. It is less likely that routine dilatation will avoid problems in patients headed for extensive fibrosis and stenosis. It is quite possible that long-term vaginal dilatation or calibration may cause some psychological trauma for the patient or parent. Proponents of delayed vaginal reconstruction would suggest that the need for dilatation or secondary surgical revision demonstrates the advantages of later reconstruction. It is clear that vaginoplasty, particularly for a patient with a moderate or high confluence urogenital sinus, is a major surgical procedure in an older patient. Such a procedure may likewise have a profound psychological impact on the patient and still carry risk for stenosis or other complications.

Urethrovaginal fistulae can occur following reconstruction of the urogenital sinus but fortunately are much less common than vaginal stenosis. Careful, yet aggressive, separation of the vagina and urethra allows adequate reconstruction of both structures and interposition of layers of tissue in between in order to minimize the risk of fistula. The most likely place to develop such a fistula is the area of the initial confluence. Modern techniques to improve exposure and use more effective flaps for vaginoplasty should lower the risk of fistula formation. Total urogenital mobilization without separation of the proximal urethra from the vagina should carry virtually no risk for the problem.[34]

Controversy

Historically, the decision of gender assignment has been made shortly after birth by the parents in consultation with a multispecialty team. This choice involves many factors and includes genotypic sex and the functional potential of gonadal tissue, reproductive tracts, and the external genitalia. Such a scheme is still utilized in most centers. Sex assignment in infancy has been advocated by many as it allows for early and consistent gender-specific social interactions throughout childhood. Support for this school of thought came from the observations and work of Money and investigators.[56–59] Partially driven by older patients unhappy with their sexual development, some of the lay and medical community have more recently questioned the timing and need for reconstructive surgery. Proponents of waiting and allowing for full participation in such decisions by the patient at a later age have appeared and gained support.[60,61] A few authors have called for a moratorium on genital reconstructive surgery until these concerns can be appropriately addressed.

It is beyond the scope of this chapter to address all of the moral, ethical, and gender identity issues involved with female genital surgery. It is important to note that, while no universal practice policy has gained acceptance, it is incumbent upon the surgeon interested in such problems to be well aware of these issues and discuss them openly with patients and parents. Well-planned, long-term outcome studies are needed to address these problems and should lead to further refinement in the timing and techniques of genital reconstruction.

Conclusions

Significant strides have been made in surgical outcomes of patients with urogenital sinus abnormalities and intersex states. Evaluation of previously employed techniques, improved understanding of genital anatomy, and a greater sensitivity to the complex nature of genital innervation have led to improvements in terms of both cosmesis and, perhaps, function. Although complications, the most common being vaginal stenosis, may still occur following female genital reconstruction, the ultimate expectation for the patient and family should be normal or nearly normal appearing and functioning genitalia. Even when such a result is achieved, the underlying problem and process of reconstruction often have a profound psychological impact on the patient, particularly in terms of sexual identity. It remains to be determined how the best functional endpoint can be achieved for the patient with the least morbidity in that regard.

References

1. Boucekkine C, Toublanc JE, Abbas N et al. Clinical and anatomical spectrum in XX sex reversed patients. Relationship to the presence of Y specific DNA-sequences. Clin Endocrinol (Oxf) 1994; 40:733–42.
2. Golan A, Langer R, Bukovsky I, Caspi E. Congenital anomalies of the müllerian system. Fertil Steril 1989; 51:747–55.
3. Hendren WH, Crawford JD. Adrenogenital syndrome: the anatomy of the anomaly and its repair. J Pediatr Surg 1969; 4:49–58.
4. Rink RC, Adams MC, Misseri R. A new classification for genital ambiguity and urogenital sinus. BJU Int 2005; 95:638–42.
5. Jaramillo D, Lebowitz RL, Hendren WH. The cloacal malformation: radiologic findings and imaging recommendations. Radiology 1990; 177:441–8.
6. Wright NB, Smith C, Rickwood AM, Carty HM. Imaging children with ambiguous genitalia and intersex states. Clin Radiol 1995; 50:823–9.
7. Biswas K, Kapoor A, Karak AK et al. Imaging in intersex disorders. J Pediatr Endocrinol Metab 2004; 17:841–5.
8. Brock JW III, Hernanz-Schulman M, Russel W. Diagnosis of congenital adrenal hyperplasia by ultrasound in the newborn. Presented at the American Academy of Pediatrics, Urology Section Meeting, 1998. [abstract]
9. Alizai NK, Thomas DF, Lilford RJ, Batchelor AG, Johnson N. Feminizing genitoplasty for congenital adrenal hyperplasia: what happens at puberty? J Urol 1999; 161:1588–91.
10. Bailez MM, Gearhart JP, Migeon C, Rock J. Vaginal reconstruction after initial construction of the external genitalia in girls with salt-wasting adrenal hyperplasia. J Urol 1992; 148:680–2.
11. Campbell M. Embryology and anomalies of the urogenital tract. In: Campbell M, ed. Urology, 1st Vol. Philadelphia: WB Saunders, 1954; 227–501.
12. Gross RE, Randolph J, Crigler JF Jr. Clitorectomy for

sexual abnormalities: indications and technique. Surgery 1966; 59:300–8.

13. Allen LE, Hardy BE, Churchill BM. The surgical management of the enlarged clitoris. J Urol 1982; 128:351–4.
14. Lewis VG, Ehrhardt AA, Money J. Genital operations in girls with the adrenogenital syndrome. Obstet Gynecol 1970; 36:11–15.
15. Lattimer JK. Relocation and recession of the enlarged clitoris with preservation of the glans: an alternative to amputation. J Urol 1961; 86:113–16.
16. Kaplan I. A simple technique for shortening the clitoris without amputation. Obstet Gynecol 1967; 29:270–1.
17. Randolph JG, Hung W. Reduction clitoroplasty in females with hypertrophied clitoris. J Pediatr Surg 1970; 5:224–31.
18. Schmid MA. Plastische Korrectur des äussern Genital bei einem männlichen. Scheinzwitter, Langenbecks. Arch Klin Chir 1961; 289:977–82.
19. Spence HM, Allen TD. Genital reconstruction in the female with the adrenogenital syndrome. Br J Urol 1973; 45:126–30.
20. Kogan SJ, Smey P, Levitt SB. Subtunical total reduction clitoroplasty: a safe modification of existing techniques. J Urol 1983; 130:746–8.
21. Baskin LS, Erol A, Li YW et al. Anatomical studies of the human clitoris. J Urol 1999; 162:1015–20.
22. DeCambre M, Gingalewski C, Burke G, Kablik P, McKenna P. Female external genitalia relationships to fixed bony landmarks. Presented at American Academy of Pediatrics, Urology Section Meeting, 2001. [abstract]
23. Schober JM, Meyer-Bahlburg HF, Ransley PG. Self-assessment of genital anatomy, sexual sensitivity and function in women: implications for genitoplasty. BJU Int 2004; 94:589–94.
24. Freitas Filho LG, Carnevale J, Melo CE, Laks M, Calcagno Silva M. A posterior-based omega-shaped flap vaginoplasty in girls with congenital adrenal hyperplasia caused by 21-hydroxylase deficiency. BJU Int 2003; 91:263–7.
25. Hendren WH, Donahoe PK. Correction of congenital abnormalities of the vagina and perineum. J Pediatr Surg 1980; 15:751–63.
26. Rink RC, Adams MC. Feminizing genitoplasty: state of the art. World J Urol 1998; 16:212–18.
27. Raffensperger JG. The cloaca in the newborn. Birth Defects 1988; 24:111–23.
28. Passerini-Glazel G. A new 1-stage procedure for clitorovaginoplasty in severely masculinized female pseudohermaphrodites. J Urol 1989; 142:565–8.
29. Pena A, Filmer B, Bonilla E, Mendez M, Stolar C. Transanorectal approach for the treatment of the urogenital sinus: preliminary report. J Pediatr Surg 1992; 27:681–5.
30. Rink RC, Pope JC, Kropp BP et al. Reconstruction of the high urogenital sinus: early perineal prone approach without division of the rectum. J Urol 1997; 158:1293–7.
31. Dumanian GA, Donahoe PK. Bilateral rotated buttock flaps for vaginal atresia in severely masculinized females with adrenogenital syndrome. Plast Reconstr Surg 1992; 90:487–91.
32. Gonzalez R, Fernandes ET. Single-stage feminization genitoplasty. J Urol 1990; 143:776–8.
33. Rink RC, Cain MP. Further use of the mobilized sinus in total urogenital mobilization procedures. Presented at the American Academy of Pediatrics, Urology Section Meeting, 2002. [abstract].
34. Pena A. Total urogenital mobilization: an easier way to repair cloacas. J Pediatr Surg 1997; 32:263–7.
35. Hamza AF, Elhalaby E, Elshafey I et al. Total urogenital sinus mobilization in complex female urogenital anomalies: long term effects on bladder function. Presented at the American Academy of Pediatrics, General Surgery Section Meeting, 2004. [abstract].
36. Kryger JV, Gonzalez R. Urinary continence is well preserved after total urogenital mobilization. J Urol 2004; 172:2384–6.
37. Rink RC, Baskin L, Schoeber J. Implications of female genital innervation. Presented at the American Academy of Pediatrics, Urology Section Meeting, 2004. [panel discussion]
38. Frank RT. The formation of an artificial vagina without operation. Am J Obstet Gynecol 1938; 35:1053–5.
39. Abbe R. New method of creating a vagina in a case of congenital absence. Med Rec 1898; 54:836–8.
40. McIndoe AH, Banister JB. An operation for the cure of congenital absence of the vagina. J Obstet Gynecol Br Common 1938; 45:490.
41. Frank RT, Geist SH. The formation of an artificial vagina by a new plastic technique. Am J Obstet 1927; 14: 712–18.
42. Baldwin JF. The formation of an artificial vagina by intestinal transplantation. Ann Surg 1904; 40:398–403.
43. McCraw JB, Massey FM, Shanklin KD, Horton CE. Vaginal reconstruction with gracilis myocutaneous flaps. Plast Reconstr Surg 1976; 58:176–83.
44. Joseph VT. Pudendal-thigh flap vaginoplasty in the reconstruction of genital anomalies. J Pediatr Surg 1997; 32:62–5.
45. Flack CE, Barraza MA, Stevens PS. Vaginoplasty: combination therapy using labia minora flaps and lucite dilators – preliminary report. J Urol 1993; 150:654–6.
46. Chudacoff RM, Alexander J, Alvero R, Segars JH. Tissue expansion vaginoplasty for treatment of congenital vaginal agenesis. Obstet Gynecol 1996; 87:865–8.
47. Cali RW, Pratt JH. Congenital absence of the vagina: long-term results of vaginal reconstruction in 175 cases. Am J Obstet Gynecol 1968; 100:752–63.
48. Wesley JR, Coran AG. Intestinal vaginoplasty for congenital absence of the vagina. J Pediatr Surg 1992; 27:885–9.
49. Hensle TW, Reiley EA. Vaginal replacement in children and young adults. J Urol 1998; 159:1035–8.
50. Hall JG, Gilchrist DM. Turner syndrome and its variants. Pediatr Clin North Am 1990; 37:1421–40.
51. Verp MS, Simpson JL. Abnormal sexual differentiation and neoplasia. Cancer Genet Cytogenet 1987; 25:191–218.
52. Gearhart JP, Burnett A, Owen JH. Measurement of pudendal evoked potentials during feminizing genitoplasty: technique and applications. J Urol 1995; 153:486–7.

53. Jones HW Jr, Garcia SC, Klingensmith GJ. Secondary surgical treatment of the masculinized external genitalia of patients with virilizing adrenal hyperplasia. Obstet Gynecol 1976; 48:73–5.
54. Azziz R, Mulaikal RM, Migeon CJ, Jones HW Jr, Rock JA. Congenital adrenal hyperplasia: long-term results following vaginal reconstruction. Fertil Steril 1986; 46:1011–14.
55. Sotiropoulos A, Morishima A, Homsy Y, Lattimer JK. Long-term assessment of genital reconstruction in female pseudohermaphrodites. J Urol 1976; 115:599–601.
56. Money J, Hampson JG, Hampson JL. Sexual incongruities and psychopathology: the evidence of human hermaphroditism. Bull Johns Hopkins Hosp 1956; 98:43–57.
57. Lewis VG, Ehrdardt AA, Money J. Genital operations in girls with the adrenogenital syndrome. Obstet Gynecol 1979; 36:11–15.
58. Money J, Devore H, Norma BP. Gender identity and gender transposition: longitudinal outcome study of 32 male hermaphrodites assigned as girls. J Sex Marital Ther 1986; 12:165–78.
59. Money J, Norman BP. Gender identity and gender transposition: longitudinal outcome study of 24 male hermaphrodites assigned as boys. J Sex Marital Ther 1987; 13:75–92.
60. Diamond M, Sigmundson K. Management of intersexuality: guidelines for dealing with persons with ambiguous genitalia. Arch Pediatr Adolesc Med 1997; 151:1046–50.
61. Diamond M, Sigmundson K. Sex reassignment at birth: long-term review and clinical implications. Arch Pediatr Adolesc Med 1997; 151:298–304.
62. Rink RC, Kaefer M. Surgical management of intersexuality, cloacal malformation, and other malformation of the genitalia in girls. In: Walsh PC, Retik AB, Stamey TA, Darracott Vaughen E. Philadelphia; WB Saunders, 1998.

Hypospadias

71

Warren T Snodgrass, Aseem R Shukla, and Douglas A Canning

Introduction

Hypospadias occurs following abnormal development of the penis. The urethral meatus in hypospadias may be proximal to its normal glanular position anywhere along the penile shaft, scrotum, or perineum. A spectrum of abnormalities including ventral curvature of the penis (chordee), a 'hooded' incomplete prepuce, and abortive corpora spongiosum are commonly associated with hypospadias.

John W Duckett Jr, the former chief of the Division of Urology at the Children's Hospital of Philadelphia (CHOP) and a pioneer in hypospadias repairs, coined the term hypospadiology. Today, hypospadiology encompasses a continuously evolving and expanding discipline. Whereas modern experiments have only recently begun to yield a deeper understanding of the genetic, hormonal, and environmental basis of hypospadias, the quest for a surgical procedure that consistently results in a straight penis with a normally placed glanular meatus has eluded surgeons for over two centuries. Advances in the understanding of the etiology of hypospadias and the current approaches to the correction of hypospadias to provide a cosmetically and functionally satisfactory repair are the focus of this chapter.

Etiology

Hypospadias results from partial or complete failure of urethral folds to form throughout their normal length or a failure of the folds to close distally if they have formed. The extent of the closure determines the position of the urethral orifice.

A unifying etiology for hypospadias remains elusive. Hypospadias probably results from multiple factors. The hypospadiac anatomy appears consistent with incomplete embryologic development as a result of:

- abnormal androgen production by the fetal testis
- limited androgen sensitivity in target tissues of the developing genitalia
- premature cessation of androgenic stimulation due to early atrophy of the Leydig cells of the testes.[1,2]

Endocrine factors

A number of writers have suggested that hypospadias represents a mild form of intersexuality. It could represent one end of a spectrum, the other of which is a completely feminized male.[3] Hypospadias may result from an endocrinopathy in which there is a disruption in the synthetic biopathway of androgens. More than just a focal malformation, hypospadias may be a local manifestation of a systemic endocrinopathy. A qualitative androgen receptor abnormality or defects at a post-receptor level may explain the defect in some boys with hypospadias. For example, the blunted response to human chorionic gonadotropin (hCG) injections seen in many boys with hypospadias may suggest a mutation in the luteinizing hormone (LH) receptor in the testis or perhaps an increase in receptor numbers because of the previous stimulation.[4] In a study of 15 boys under 4 years of age with severe hypospadias, Allen and Griffin diagnosed 11 boys with six distinct endocrine-related abnormalities. The most consistent finding was a subnormal testosterone response to hCG stimulation in seven boys. The authors believe their findings may represent a delay in the maturation of the hypothalamic–pituitary–testicular axis.

Genetic factors

Hypospadias may have a complex genetic background, with gene expression acting in concert with environmental factors. The familial rate of hypospadias is approximately 7%, which reflects a non-familial, sporadic finding in most cases. Recent studies have suggested a role for müllerian inhibiting substance (MIS) in the etiology of hypospadias. There is an inverse relationship between MIS and testosterone, and this may be related to the MIS inhibition of cytochrome P450c17 CYP17, the enzyme that catalyzes the committed step in testosterone synthesis.[5] Indeed, MIS may directly inhibit testosterone production by suppressing the *CYP17* gene.[6] Abnormalities of other genes such as fibroblast growth factor-10 (*FGF-10*) have also been shown to result in hypospadias.[7]

Normal sexual differentiation depends on testosterone and its metabolites as well as functional androgen receptors. Despite a correlation of certain clear defects in the androgen metabolism pathway and hypospadias, as in the 5α-reductase II (5αRII) defect (mutation in *SRD5A2* gene on chromosome 2), such associations have been limited to few cases – underlining the importance of seeking other genetic explanations for this congenital defect.[8]

Environmental factors

The incidence of hypospadias is increasing. One possible explanation is environmental contamination. Insecticides, pharmaceuticals, and plant estrogens contain estrogenic ingredients. Manufacturers of cans used in the canned food industry coat the inside of the cans with plastics known to contain estrogenic substances.[9] These substances are ultimately present in freshwater and seawater in trace amounts that bioaccumulate and concentrate in higher organisms of the food chain. For this reason, predators at the top of the food chain, such as large fish, birds, sea mammals, and humans, accumulate high levels of estrogenic environmental contaminants. Thus, humans and wild animals are constantly exposed to estrogenic compounds that are known to disrupt reproduction – the so-called endocrine disrupters.[7]

Epidemiology

The incidence of hypospadias varies geographically. Prevalence ranges from 0.26 per 1000 births (both male and female births) in Mexico to 2.11 in Hungary and 2.6 per 1000 live births in Scandinavia.[10] A recent study found the rate of hypospadias in a 2-year prospective study to be 38 in 10 000 live births in Netherlands, a number six times higher than previously recorded.[11] Sweet and colleagues reported a much lower incidence in Sweden of 1 in 1250 live male births.[12]

In 1997, two independent surveillance systems in the United States – the nationwide Birth Defects Monitoring Program (BDMP) and the Metropolitan Atlanta Congenital Defects Program (MACDP) – reported a near doubling of the incidence of hypospadias when compared with immediately preceding decades.[13] The incidence of all types of hypospadias increased from 20.2 to 39.7 in 10 000 live male births during the period from 1970–1993; i.e. one in every 250 live male births was a boy with hypospadias (measured by BDMP). MACDP reported a rise in the severe hypospadias rate of between three- and five-fold. These rising trends, however, may simply reflect earlier diagnosis or an increase in reporting to registries of congenital defects. The increased reporting of more proximal than distal hypospadias cases, however, refutes the argument that these findings simply represent more frequent reporting of minor cases.[14]

Recent studies have linked the rising rate of hypospadias in boys born prematurely and small for gestational age, boys with low birth weight, and boys born to mothers over 35 years of age.[15–17] Roberts and Lloyd noted an 8.5-fold increase in hypospadias in one of monozygotic male twins, compared with singleton live male births.[18] This may suggest a discrepancy in the supply of hCG to the fetus where a single placenta is unable to meet the requirements of two developing male fetuses.

Embryology of hypospadias

The genital tubercle appears during the 4th week of gestation as anlagen for development of either the clitoris or penis. Endodermal cells from the cloaca migrate along its ventral midline surface to create the urethral plate, while proliferating mesenchyme on either side establishes the urogenital folds. Subsequent phallic development is dependent upon androgenic stimulation during a critical period from the 9th to 12th weeks. 5αRII in the genital tubercle catalyzes the conversion of testosterone, produced by fetal Leydig cells within the testes, to dihydrotestosterone (DHT). DHT then binds to androgen receptors to initiate a cascade of downstream effects.

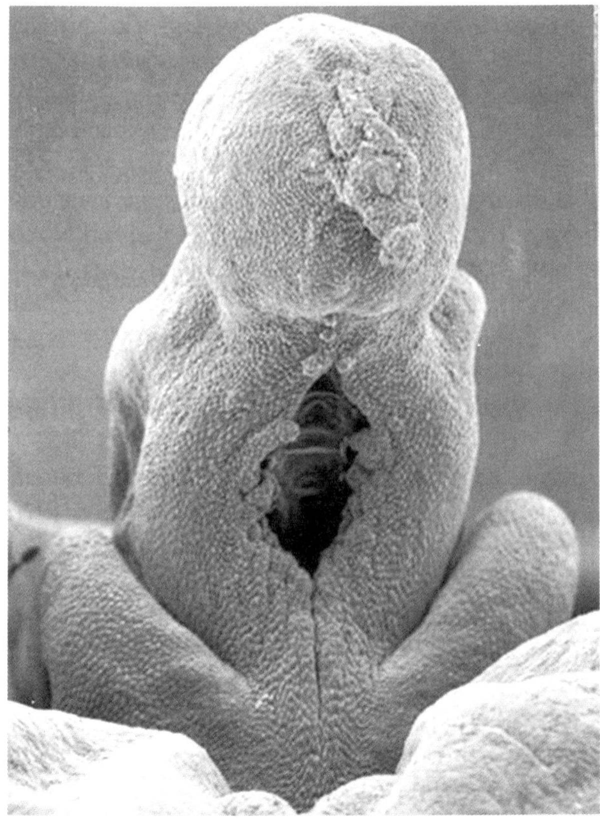

Figure 71.1 Scanning electron micrography demonstrates fusion of the urethral folds proximally while the distal urethral plate remains open before tubularization.

Androgen stimulation causes the genital tubercle to elongate and the urogenital (urethral) folds to migrate toward the midline and fuse, enclosing the urethral groove (Figure 71.1). This process moves proximally to distally creating the pendulous urethra. Some clinicians have disputed the current theories of the formation of the glanular urethra. One theory holds that ectoderm from the glans surface migrates inward to contact the distal urethral plate and establish continuity with the urethra.[19–22] Alternatively, the endodermal plate may continue to canalize distally until surface ectoderm is reached.[23]

Gene knockout studies in mice have further characterized the process of urethral plate tubularization. Concerns that this animal model, with its postnatal formation of an os penis, poorly represent human development were addressed by Baskin et al,[24] who determined that the basic processes of genital tubercle and urethral development were analogous in the two species. Specifically, Baskin's group noted urethral tubularization in mice also extends from proximal to distal, with formation of a urethral seam where the two sides fuse. A proposed mechanism for hypospadias is failure of ventral plate fusion, and *FGF-10*-deficient mice with abnormal seam development have an opened urethra resembling hypospadias[25] (Figure 71.2). Mesenchyme along the midline during seam formation normally expresses this signaling molecule and therefore seems to play an important role in normal urethral development in mice.

In humans, as the plate tubularizes, mesoderm within the urethral folds differentiates into corpus spongiosum, which fuses with the glans distally. Mesoderm also forms the corpora cavernosa. Development of the penis apparently proceeds at different

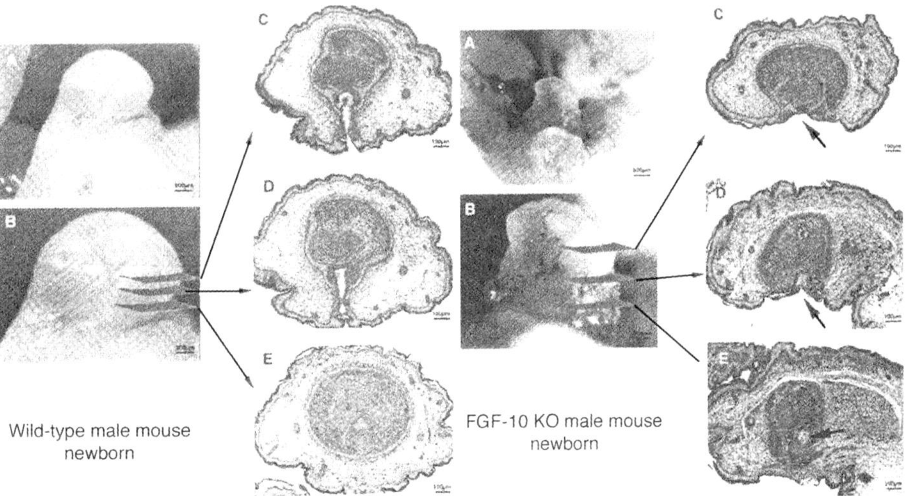

Figure 71.2 Gross and histologic comparison of urethral development in normal wild-type mice versus fibroblast growth factor-10 (*FGF-10*) gene deletion 'null' mice. Normal mouse genital tubercle formation with a distal urethral meatus contrasts with a proximal urethral opening in the knockout model. Histologic sections demonstrate abnormal distal urethral seam formation associated with *FGF-10* deletion.

overlying the penile shaft in proximal hypospadias did not appear suitable for urethroplasty (see Figure 71.14). In two boys, I performed TIP nevertheless, with one wound dehiscence and one contracture of the neourethra resulting in curvature. In this circumstance, there appears to be a paucity of subepithelial tissues and perceived rigidity to the plate. In subsequent patients with this finding, the plate has been excised and a staged urethroplasty performed.[77]

Staged urethroplasty

There are two situations in which the urethral plate cannot be tubularized: most common is penile curvature greater than 30°, which leads to plate transection; less often encountered is an 'unhealthy' incised plate. Options for repair include tubularized preputial flaps or staged urethroplasty, which traditionally has been done using skin flaps from the dorsal prepuce transposed ventrally. However, I now favor use of a buccal graft quilted onto the corpora to create a neourethral plate for tubularization at the second operation. This graft can be placed directly over transverse incisions made into the corpora for straightening. Staged buccal grafts have reliably taken and have not been reported to develop diverticula.

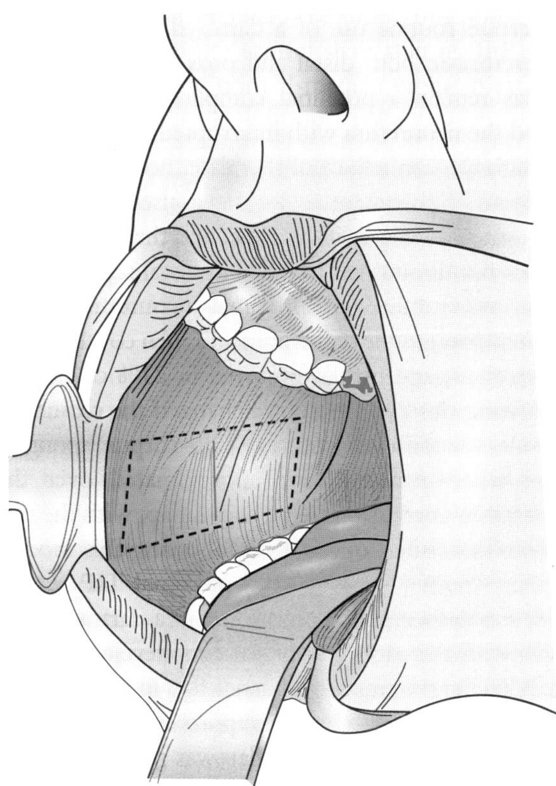

Figure 71.16 Harvesting the buccal mucosa graft for urethroplasty.

Either inner lip or cheek can be used to obtain buccal epithelium, but I prefer to use the thinner lip tissue for grafting in the glans and thicker cheek for the penile shaft. The proposed site is outlined slightly larger than needed and infiltrated with 1:100 000 epinephrine, taking care to identify and avoid injury to the parotid duct near the upper second molar (Figure 71.16). A first-generation cephalosporin is given, along with glycopyrrolate to diminish oral secretions during harvest. Dissection seeks to minimize fat and muscle on the underside of the graft. The donor site is packed until bleeding stops and then coated with fibrin glue for coverage. The cheek or lip wound is not closed. Meanwhile, the graft is further defatted, as shown in Figure 71.17.

We next secure the graft with interrupted polyglactin stitches around the perimeter of the wound and then quilt it into place with additional absorbable sutures 0.5 cm apart down the midline and then to either side between the perimeter and midline stitches. This quilting minimizes the likelihood that hematoma will collect under the graft and prevent revascularization. We leave a 'tie-over' dressing of Vaseline gauze to secure the graft further. We leave this dressing postoperatively with a catheter for urinary diversion for 7–10 days.

In primary repairs, we use the graft to bridge the gap between the proximal urethrostomy and the preserved urethral plate in the glans. We leave the distal aspect of the plate undisturbed until the second stage, or tubularize it at the first stage with the buccal graft interposed between proximal and distal urethros-

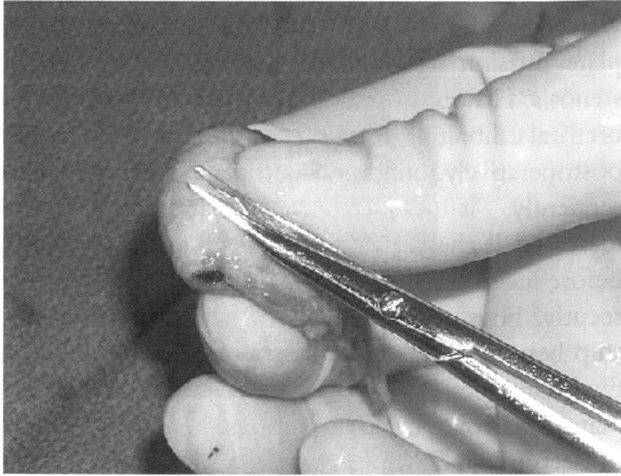

Figure 71.17 Defatting the graft. Although pin boards can be used, the authors find it simpler to defat the graft as shown. Tactile sensation helps determine the depth of excision and avoid inadvertent epithelial holes.

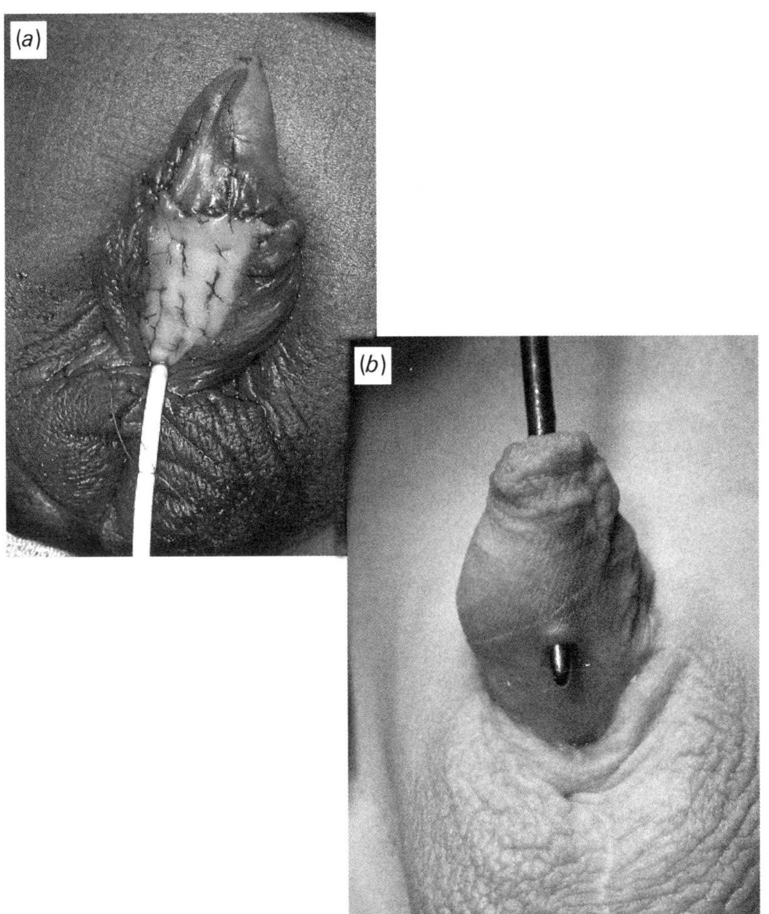

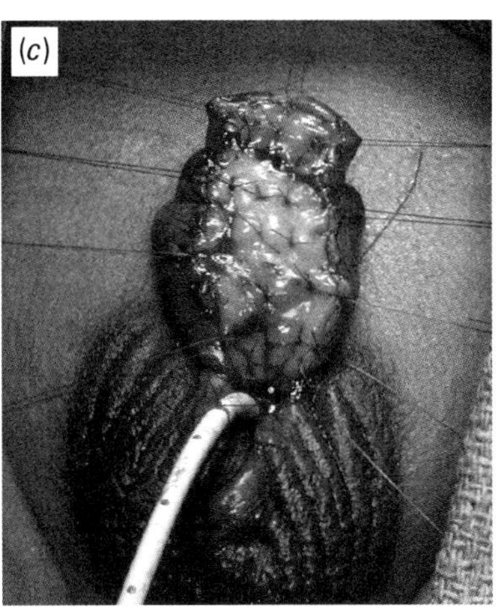

Figure 71.18 Options for buccal grafting in primary hypospadias repair when the urethral plate cannot be used. (*a*) The graft is interposed between the proximal urethrostomy and the distal intact glanular urethral plate. (*b*) The graft from the proximal urethrostomy to the distal tubularized urethral plate. (*c*) The graft from the proximal urethrostomy to the tip of the glans.

tomies. Alternatively, we resect the glanular plate and extend the graft to the tip of the glans (Figure 71.18).

The graft take is visually apparent. The second-stage tubularization of the now-vascularized 'neourethral plate' is done 6 months later using a two-layer closure turning epithelium into the lumen. We cover the neourethra with a dartos flap, or a tunical vaginalis flap if there is not sufficient dartos available. A catheter provides urinary diversion for 7–10 days.

DAC [third author]: The goals of hypospadias repair are to provide a straight penis adequate for sexual function and to move the urethral meatus to the tip of the penis to allow the boy to void with a normal urinary stream.

The glans size, the degree of chordee, the meatal location, and the quality of the foreskin all influence the choice of repair. Surgeons have developed a myriad of hypospadias techniques. My training, the interpretations of the ample body of hypospadias literature, and my clinical experience as tempered by the suggestions of my colleagues have all influenced my choice of procedure for the individual boy. Early in my career, meatal-based urethral flaps and staged repairs were frequent. At the CHOP, which has historically relied on single-stage transverse preputial island flaps and tubes, I began to do more of these and fewer staged repairs.

To avoid the creation of a 'hypospadias cripple', a skilled team with considerable experience must perform the reconstruction. The surgeon should not enter the operating room with an unyielding plan. They should have an abundance of techniques available and a broad fundamental knowledge in the principles required for a successful outcome.

I believe that the reliability of the repair is reduced when the perfusion of the tissue is at risk. I also believe that the repair is jeopardized when tissues are introduced in the repair that are foreign to the urethra.

Since adequate urethral tissue is rarely present in the boy who has had multiple hypospadias repairs, the advantages vs the disadvantages of each technique must be weighed. A preputial flap, for example, introduces well-perfused foreign tissue to the urethra at the expense of a higher risk of diverticulum. On the other hand, the TIP or Snodgrass repair employs local urethral tissue in the reconstruction, which perhaps is less well supplied with blood. To compensate, additional dartos tissue should be moved to cover the repair. Because of the interest in island flaps at our institution, most of our experience with primary repair for hypospadias has been using either an island onlay (the vast majority) or an island tube (less commonly). After our experience broadened with the onlay, we used it even in cases where there was considerable chordee.[95] I am now more cautious with this. In at least one case, after plicating the dorsum of the penis, I have put the penis on compression and therefore shortened it to a degree. For this reason, in boys with considerable chordee and proximal hypospadias, I now rely more on the island tube. I am less resistant to transecting the urethral plate, particularly since having enjoyed improved results with a modification of the island tube.[96] In addition, I have found that what frequently begins as a two-stage repair, in my hands, often results in three stages.[97]

Over time, we have modified both the island onlay and the transverse preputial island flap and now operate on younger children. Studies by some of the best surgeons have shown that adult hypospadias repair is far less successful than repair in younger children.[98] Tissue factors that contribute to near scarless wound healing in the fetus[99] are less likely to be present in the older boy and the adult.

What follows is a description of the major repairs we use at CHOP, in addition to the TIP described above.

Meatal advancement and glanuloplasty

The MAGPI offers reliable cosmesis and long-term success when applied to glanular and selected coronal meatus repairs. Recently, we have used this repair less commonly and will usually opt for a TIP repair in cases where we would have used the MAGPI in the past. Presence of urethral mobility and a rounded glans, along with the absence of significant chordee, should be assessed to ensure an ideal outcome and avoid meatal regression. We assess urethral mobility by distal traction on the meatus with fine forceps.

The MAGPI begins with a circumferential incision 6–8 mm proximal to the corona of the glans and proximal to the meatus (Figure 71.19a). We dissect the penile shaft skin with extreme care ventrally over the corpus spongiosum to avoid urethral injury. A longitudinal incision from the dorsal distal edge of the meatus is carried to the distal glans groove as it transects the transverse bridge of tissue that is often present (Figure 72.19b). We approximate the incised

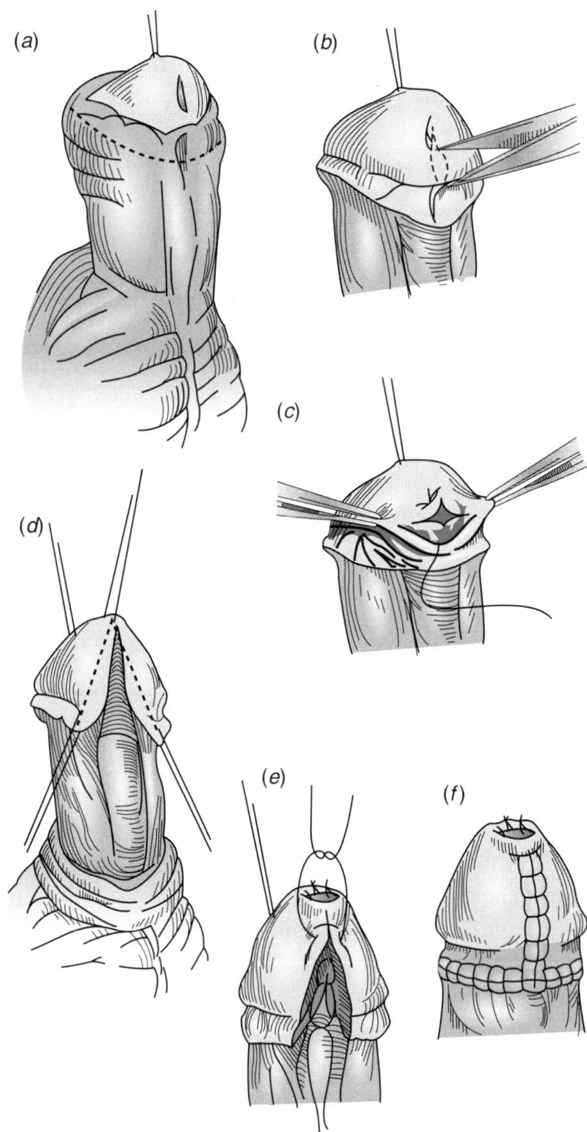

Figure 71.19 Meatoplasty and glanuloplasty repair (MAGPI). (*a*) A circumferential incision 5 cm below the corona. (*b*) The transverse bridge of the tissue distal to the meatus is sharply incised. (*c*) A Heineke–Mikulicz closure opens and advances the meatus. (*d*) The ventral meatal edge is pulled distally and the exposed glans edges are trimmed and approximated. (*e*) Glanuloplasty is performed with subepithelial sutures to leave a rounded, conical glans. (*f*) The dorsal skin is transferred ventrally, excess skin is excised, and no catheter is left in place.

tissue edges in a Heineke–Mikulicz fashion with 7–0 absorbable suture to advance the meatus distally (Figure 72.19c). We pull the medial edge of the ventral meatus distally and the exposed glans edges are trimmed to leave the glans with a cosmetically sound, rounded appearance (Figure 72.19d). The dorsal hooded foreskin is trimmed in the midline to allow adequate ventral skin transfer, and skin is approximated to the glans with absorbable, subcuticular suture to complete the repair (Figures 72.19e,f).

In cases where the urethral meatus is proximal to the corona or if the ventral penile shaft skin is thin, we are less apt to use the TIP repair and tend to use the onlay island flap repair.

Onlay island flap

Numerous alternatives for single-stage neourethral reconstruction for proximal hypospadias, ranging from prepuce-based flaps, the incised plate urethroplasty to free grafts, have been described with varying results.[93,100–102] Whereas surgical innovation has enabled most variants of hypospadias to be repaired with preservation of the urethral plate, proximal hypospadias with severe chordee may still require transection of the urethral plate. From the time Duckett first described the transverse preputial island flap (TPIF) repair in 1980,[65] we have continued to prefer the incorporation of vascularized preputial flaps for these difficult cases.

To ensure hemostasis, we infiltrate a solution of 1:100 000 epinephrine and 1% lidocaine along the marked line. We then incise the skin and deglove the penis to Buck's fascia, beginning the dissection ventrally – from the urethral meatus to the penoscrotal junction – and then dorsally to the penopubic junction. We then incise the urethral meatus proximally until we see normal-appearing vascularized corpora spongiosum and normal bleeding from the native urethra. We then perform an artificial erection with injection of normal saline. If the penis is curved less than 30°, we plicate the dorsum of the penis with a pair of vertical incisions closed horizontally.

Van Hook first introduced the concept of a preputial flap based on a vascular pedicle to repair proximal hypospadias in 1896.[1] Asopa and colleagues developed the effective use of inner preputial skin for a substitution urethroplasty and Duckett furthered this technique by describing a TPIF repair in 1980.[65,103] The island onlay flap evolved from the TPIF as experience demonstrated that repair of the chordee with hypospadias can be accomplished by dissection of the subcutaneous tissue and dorsal midline plication, and that division of the urethral plate is required in only 10% of cases.[52] The concept that spongiosum consists of vascularized tissue and smooth muscle bundles that may be utilized in a hypospadias repair evolved over the 1980s after histologic examination.[104,105] We use the onlay island flap for more than 90% of our patients with subcoronal hypospadias.

The circumferential incision begins dorsally, 6–8 mm proximal to the corona, and extends ventrally just proximal to the meatus (Figure 71.20a). We then

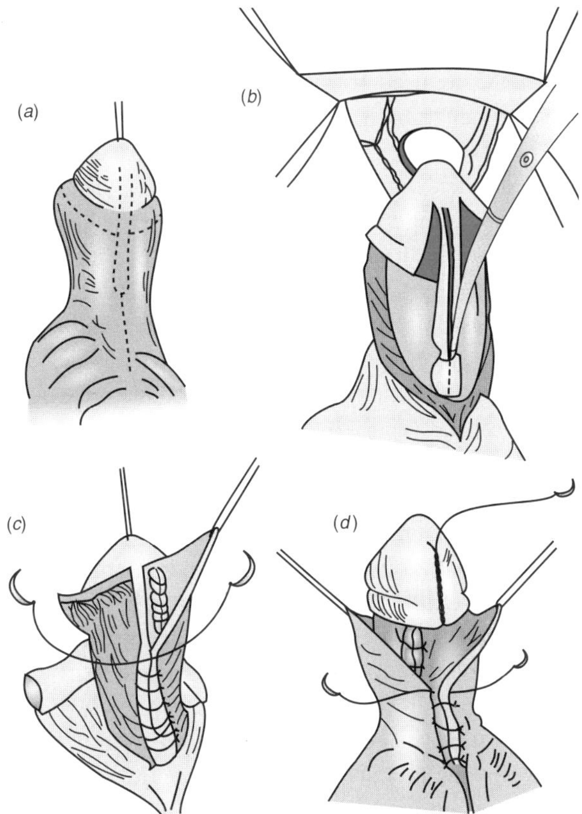

Figure 71.20 Onlay island flap. (*a*) Dashed lines indicate the initial circumcising incision carried along to the ventrum and anteriorly to provide a subcoronal collar. Note the midline incision is carried to the penoscrotal junction to facilitate adequate inspection of spongiosal tissue. (*b*) The penis is degloved and the native urethral meatus is incised back to normal spongiosal tissue. Thin gossamer-like dysplastic urethral tissue is incised until normal, well-vascularized tissue is seen. Stay sutures separate the inner and outer faces of the preputial flap and the onlay flap is mobilized with mesentery intact. A buttonhole in the mesentery allows ventral transposition without increasing torque on the penis. (*c*) The edges of the flap are sutured with subepithelial interrupted sutures. Tailoring of the flap minimizes the risk of diverticulum formation. (*d*) Byars flaps cover the skin-deficient ventrum with subcuticular sutures.

extend the incision further proximally to split ventral shaft skin in the midline to the penoscrotal junction (Figure 71.20b). We make parallel incisions 5 mm wide or narrower along the urethral plate distally to the glans tip at a point where the flat ventral surface of the glans begins to curve around the meatal groove. We take care to keep these incisions superficial to avoid injury to underlying spongiosum. Dissection of the skin should avoid entering a plane into the intrinsic vascularity of the skin to preserve its viability as a preputial flap. As is commonly the case, if dissection of the penile ventrum reveals thinned spongiosal tissue that is nearly transparent, we incise the urethra proximally to what appears to be normal spongiosum. The urethral plate need not be more than 2 mm wide prior to the onlay transfer.

Then we outline the flap on the inner preputial skin surface with interrupted 5–0 polypropylene stay sutures (see Figure 71.20b). We place the sutures to accentuate the fold of tissue between the inner and outer prepuce. The initial incision just beneath the skin at the junction between the inner and outer preputial faces of foreskin sharply divides an 8–10 mm segment of this epithelium. We are careful to harvest the flap following a midline incision on the ventral shaft to the penoscrotal junction, allowing flattening of the shaft skin that facilitates the establishment of the plane between the blood supply to the flap and the blood supply to the penile shaft skin.

The dissection of the vascular pedicle begins at the mid-shaft where we have an easier time separating it from the blood supply to the dorsal penile shaft skin. This approach to the harvest of the flap easily identifies the proper plane and assures preservation of blood supply to the flap. The splitting of ventral shaft skin, completed during the initial circumcising skin incision, releases the base of the dorsal vascular pedicle and allows for wider mobilization of the preputial foreskin for flap isolation. The flap is then rotated ventrally, or more commonly, transferred by creating a window in the vascular mesentery through which the glans is passed, and then tapered proximally and distally (Figure 71.20c). To avoid turbulent voiding that may contribute to fistula formation and diverticulum, we aggressively trim the proximal flap to a wedge shape to provide a consistent caliber of the tube as the neourethra meets the spatulated native urethra. The combined width of the preserved plate and the flap should be about 10 mm and no wider at the anastomosis than at the urethral meatus.

Experience has shown that too wide a neourethra may lead to kinking or diverticulum formation. The appropriately designed flap is then sutured into place using lubricated interrupted 7–0 polyglactic suture at the proximal meatus and then in an interrupted subepithelial fashion along the lateral edges of the plate (see Figure 71.20c). We no longer close the flap over a feeding tube. We prefer to place the tube at the conclusion of the construction of the neourethra. The 8 Fr feeding tube then serves as a spacer to assure an adequately sized glanuloplasty. We complete the glanuloplasty with medial rotation of mobilized glans wings with 6–0 Maxon sutures placed parallel to the cut edge of the glans wing, beginning at the urethral meatus (Figure 71.20d). We place a 6 Fr Kendall urethral stent and the dorsal preputial skin is split in the midline and rotated ventrally to afford adequate circumferential skin coverage.

The transverse preputial island flap

The traditional TPIF creates the neourethra by first tubularizing the dorsal preputial tissue into a neourethra and then transferring the tube to the native urethra proximally and to the glans distally. This repair has been associated with a complication rate of up to 32–42% in some reports.[106–108] In our own experience, we encountered postoperative complications, especially urethral diverticula and meatal stenosis, in a minority of infants when the meatal opening or phallic size was small, or when the chordee was severe.

Recently, we developed a modification of the Duckett transverse island tube that uses one side of the island flap to recreate a urethral plate, with the remainder of the flap tailored and rolled to recreate a neourethra. This modification of Duckett's original procedure has made it easier for us to tailor the urethroplasty to create a more consistent neourethra with less risk for diverticulum and stenosis. We believe that reducing the likelihood of leaving redundant tissue in situ minimizes the risk for diverticulum formation, turbulent voiding, and urethrocutaneous fistula. We perform the TPIF by first placing a glans-holding suture. We next outline a circumcising incision and extend the mark on the midline to the penoscrotal junction. Proximal extension of the ventral incision facilitates subsequent harvesting of the onlay flap by allowing the penile shaft skin to flatten, which results in better visibility of the pedicle of the flap and better separation of the pedicle and the dorsal penile shaft skin. To ensure hemostasis, we infiltrate a solution of 1:100 000 epinephrine and 1% lidocaine along the marked line. We then incise the skin and deglove the

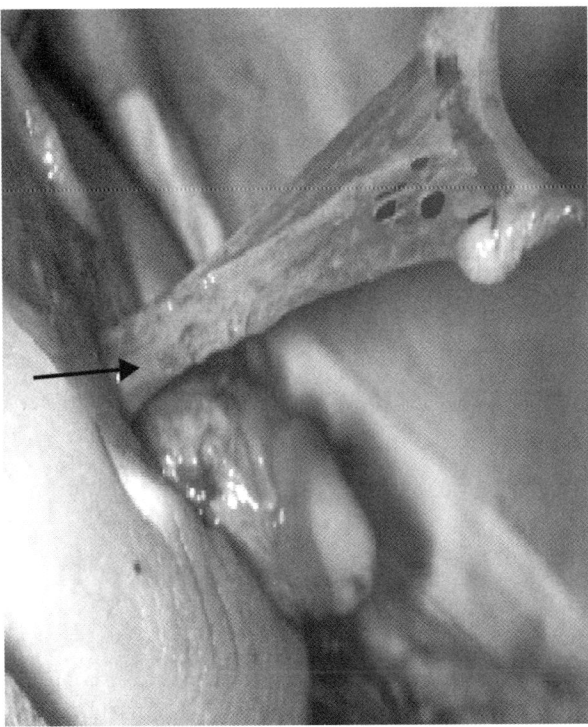

Figure 71.21 An inner preputial skin flap is harvested dorsally. The preputial flap should be harvested beginning at the middle of the penile shaft where the vascular pedicle to the inner prepuce is better defined. The dissection then proceeds proximal to the penopubic junction and distal, completely separating the preputial flap from the distal penile shaft skin. In the past, we rotated the pedicle along one side or the other of the penile shaft. We now create a buttonhole through the vascular pedicle at the penopubic junction, which reduces the extent of the pedicle dissection while minimizing the risk of penile torque after the flap is transferred to the ventrum in preparation for the urethral reconstruction. The arrow indicates the site of the buttonhole for this flap.

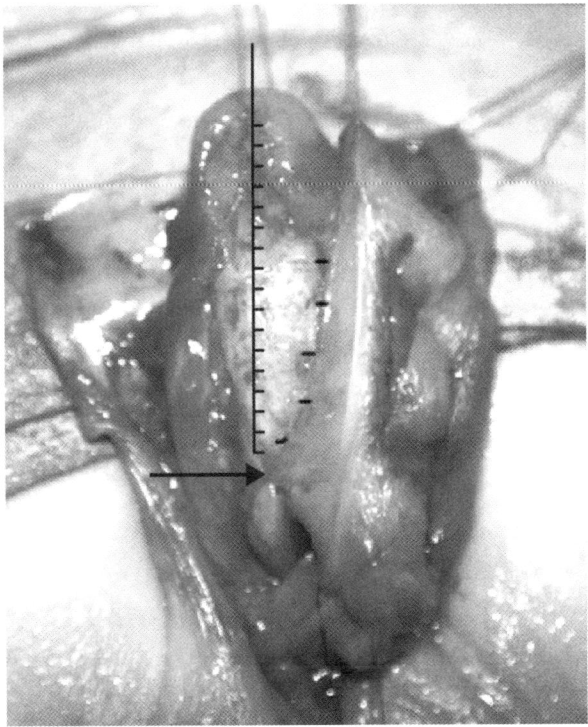

Figure 71.22 The medial margin of the flap is anchored longitudinally to the ventral surface of the corpora cavernosa just to the right or left of the midline using a series of interrupted 7–0 polyglactin sutures. Proposed site of this first suture line is shown by hatched line. These sutures are placed subcuticularly and are not passed through the epithelium of the flap. An arrow indicates the location of the urethral meatus and a vertical solid line represents the proposed plane for placement of a second parallel suture line that completes the tubularization of the neourethra.

penis to Buck's fascia, beginning the dissection ventrally – from the urethral meatus to the penoscrotal junction – and then dorsally to the penopubic junction. We then incise the urethral meatus proximally until we see normal-appearing vascularized corpora spongiosum and normal bleeding from the native urethra. We next perform an artificial erection, and if the chordee is severe, the urethral plate is transected and dissected from the corporeal tissue until the tethering effect of the spongiosum tissue is released. The ventral dissection of the urethral plate sometimes results in a relatively distal urethra displaced to the penoscrotal junction or even to the perineum. We incise the glans deeply in the midline and excess epithelium is trimmed. If required, we make appropriate-length dorsal longitudinal incisions off the midline and close them horizontally to correct chordee. Then we repeat the artificial erection to assure that we have corrected all of the curvature.

When the penis is straight, we harvest the segment of inner prepuce from the redundant dorsal prepuce and buttonhole the mesentery of the flap and transpose the flap to the ventrum (Figure 71.21). We fix the native urethral meatus, which is now in a more proximal location, to the corpora cavernosa with fine absorbable monofilament sutures.

In the past, we constructed the urethra from the island flap by rolling the tissue over a tube and then suturing the proximal end to the native urethral meatus at the penoscrotal junction or at the perineum.[65] We currently modify the construction of the urethra by first anchoring one side of the flap longitudinally to the ventral surface of the corpora cavernosa just to the right or left of the midline using 7–0 polyglactin sutures (Figure 71.22). The anchoring

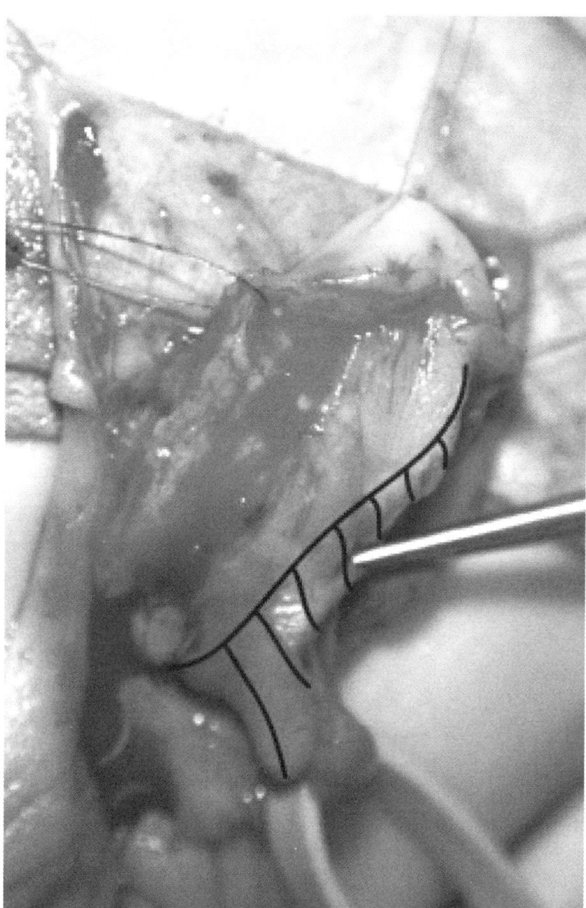

Figure 71.23 The opposite margin of the flap is stretched to accurately tailor the flap to the desired size of the neourethra (marked area indicates portion of flap to be discarded while preserving underlying vascular supply). The narrowed proximal flap is sutured to the spatulated native urethral meatus.

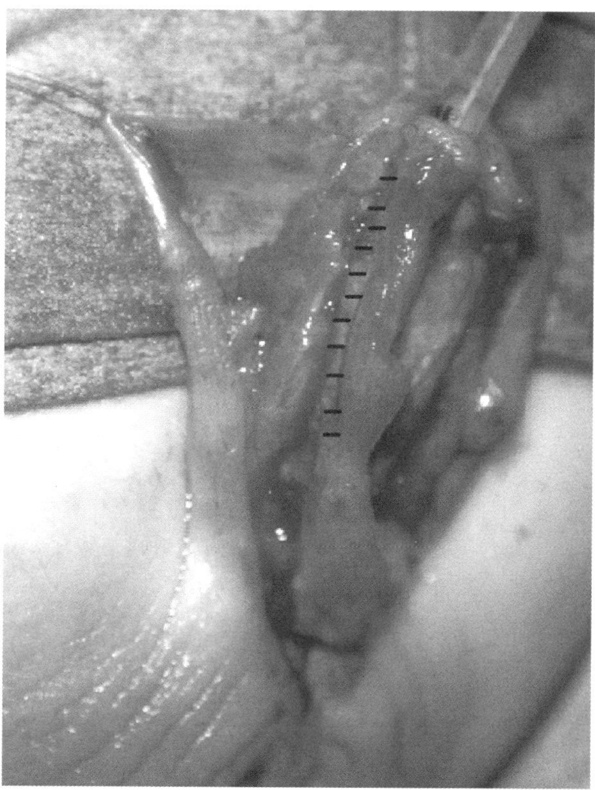

Figure 71.24 The neourethra is constructed over an 8 Fr feeding tube, which is replaced with a 6 Fr urethral stent prior to application of the dressing.

begins at the posterior wall of the native urethra and proceeds distally to the proposed location of the neomeatus in the glans. This maneuver creates a new urethral plate of inner preputial skin, which no longer binds the ventral corpora. The anchored medial edge of the tube allows the opposite end of the flap to flatten, to facilitate the construction of an appropriately sized neourethra (Figure 71.23). The tube must be narrowed substantially at the proximal anastomosis between the new and spatulated native urethra to align the skin edges and to construct a tube of ideal caliber without a diverticulum at the distal extent of the native urethra. For boys reconstructed in the first year, we use an 8 Fr feeding tube as a template to gauge urethral lumen as the closure proceeds.

To construct the neourethra, we place a second interrupted subcuticular suture line adjacent to the first suture line longitudinally along the ventral penile shaft (Figure 71.24). The urethral reconstruction continues proximally to the glans penis. We complete the glanuloplasty over an 8 Fr urethral stent with 6–0 absorbable monofilament horizontal mattress sutures placed parallel to the cut edge of the glans to cover the distal edge of the tube and to provide an accurate appearance. We exchange the 8 Fr stent for a 6 Fr stent that we leave indwelling for 2–2.5 weeks and a dorsal preputial skin is fashioned to provide adequate skin coverage as in all hypospadias repairs (Figure 71.25).

We cover the repair with a dressing that compresses the penis against the lower abdominal wall by placing a thin non-absorbent pad and a folded gauze sponge on top of the penis followed by a bioocclusive dressing. We use trimethoprim–sulfamethoxazole as antimicrobial prophylaxis while the urethral stent remains – usually for 2–2½ weeks.

The ideal surgical correction for penoscrotal or perineoscrotal hypospadias with severe chordee remains elusive. In addition to allowing a single-stage repair with the attendant benefits to the patient, the primary advantage of the modified TPIF over free graft repairs is the incorporation of vascularized preputial flaps.

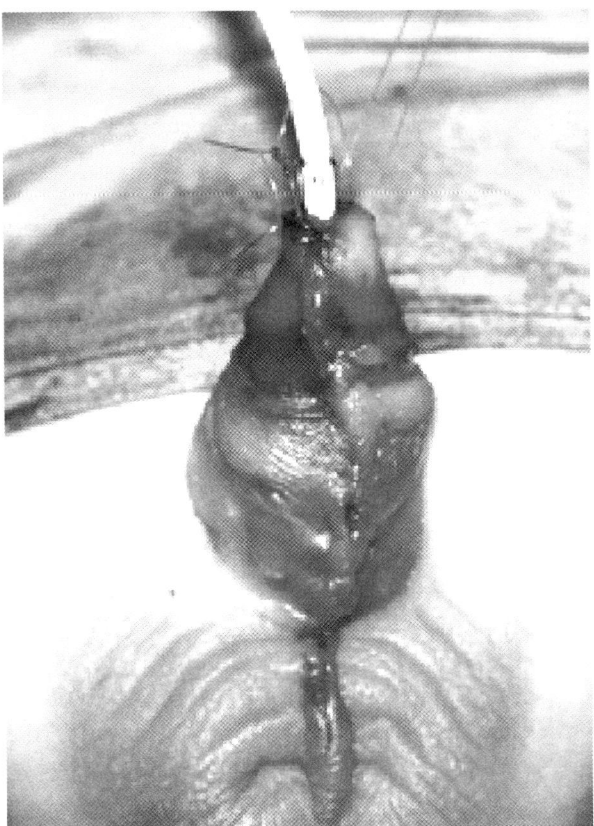

Figure 71.25 The dorsal preputial skin is split in the midline and rotated ventrally to afford adequate circumferential skin coverage with a series of subcuticular sutures.

We recently reported a 20-year review of outcomes utilizing vascularized preputial flaps for severe hypospadias at our institution that confirmed the long-term viability of these flaps.[109] Our preference continues to be to utilize preputial flaps as an island onlay or island tube when the urethral plate is or is not preserved, respectively.[110]

The modified TPIF converts a difficult procedure – the original transverse preputial island tube repair – into a more commonly performed and consistent island onlay repair by recreating a urethral plate with one side of the ventrally transposed inner preputial skin that we anchor to the medial margin of the corpora. By anchoring the medial edge of the flap to the corpora, we can stretch the opposite end of the flap to tailor the neourethra to the size of the native urethra. This minimizes the risk of formation of a urethral diverticulum where the native urethra meets the neourethra, and probably precludes the turbulent voiding that may contribute to formation of urethral diverticula. Furthermore, the adjacent suture lines are dorsal, which may minimize the risk of fistula.

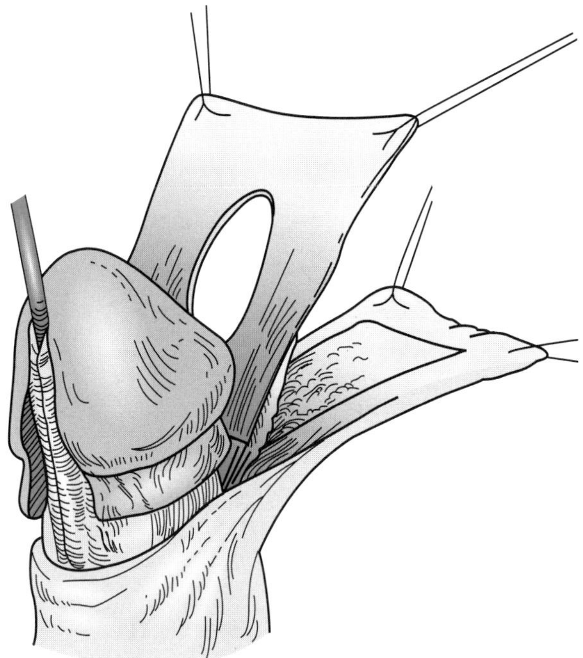

Figure 71.26 Tunica vaginalis flap.

Barrier layers

The most common complication of hypospadias repair is urethrocutaneous fistula. One factor thought to contribute to the development of fistula is overlapping suture lines of the neourethra and overlying shaft skin closure. To prevent fistula, tissue barrier layers are interposed as a preventive measure. In primary repairs, we obtain dartos flaps from the dorsal prepuce and shaft skin and transpose them to the ventrum, either around the side of the penis or via a buttonhole over the glans (Figure 71.26). When we bring these flaps around the penile shaft, proximal dissection extends to the suspensory ligament to avoid penile torsion. We also harvest de-epithelialized dartos flaps from the scrotum. When dartos is not readily available, usually in reoperations, we use tunica vaginalis flaps (Figure 71.27). It is important to dissect these flaps well up the spermatic cord to avoid postoperative traction on the ipsilateral testis, especially during erections.[111]

Skin closures

Hypospadias repair in the United States has traditionally included circumcision to remove the dorsally hooded foreskin, whereas in other countries foreskin reconstruction is preferred so that the penis looks unoperated. However, many ethnic groups in the United States do not prefer routine circumcision.

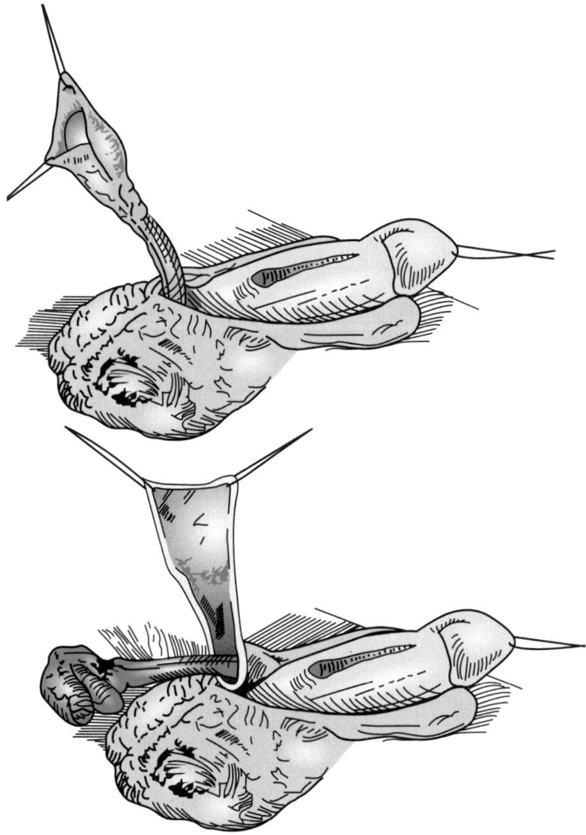

Figure 71.27 Dorsal buccal inlay hypospadias reoperation.

Whenever possible, hypospadiologists should offer families the outcome they desire. If the TIP repair is performed, surgeons can reconstruct the foreskin without increased complications unless there is ventral curvature more than 30° or urethroplasty using preputial skin is anticipated. The main difference between repairs with circumcision is that the initial skin incision does not extend circumferentially, but from the dorsal corners of the hooded prepuce ventrally under the meatus (see Figure 71.12). The ventral shaft is degloved to healthy dartos. After urethroplasty, the prepuce is approximated in three layers, consisting of inner prepuce, middle dartos, and outer skin. The reconstructed foreskin is not manipulated until these suture lines have healed, usually between 6 and 12 weeks. Secondary phimosis is uncommon, and although dorsal dartos is not accessible for a barrier layer, the rate of fistulas has not been increased.[112–114]

Suture tracks have occurred in as many as 40% of patients after hypospadias repair when stitches are placed through the epithelium.[115] These may not be apparent for as long as 1 year postoperatively, as desquamated keratin fills the small tunnel remaining after the sutures dissolve. We advocate use of subepithelial stitches to minimize suture tracks, although they can still occur despite this precaution from the passage of needles through skin appendages.

Two-stage repair

We occasionally encounter challenging cases where severe chordee and a proximal meatus limit the applicability of a one-stage tube repair. In a few cases, injury to the vascular pedicle of the onlay or tube during harvest requires a two-stage repair. Anecdotal and reported experience maintains, in fact, that the two-stage technique offers fewer complications overall and better cosmetic results than the single-stage repair for select cases.[116,117] Our CHOP experience, however, suggests a similar fistula rate following the second stage of a two-stage repair to that following a one-stage island onlay or tube repair.[97]

A two-stage repair often involves a scrotoplasty with an aggressive attempt to relieve penile curvature, including transection and proximal removal of the plate. Either a dermal graft or tunica vaginalis may bridge a gap over an incised Buck's fascia, although this maneuver is very rarely required to bridge any defect in the ventral tunica albuginea surface. Traditionally, the dorsal hooded preputial skin is incised to rotate the resultant flaps ventrally. These flaps are allowed to heal and will be used to create the future urethral plate. Alternatively, an island flap can be sewn into place to be used as a urethral plate later.

The second stage is planned after an interval of about 6 months. At that point, parallel vertical incisions 12–15 mm apart are mapped distally, beginning at the meatus and including the glans. Glans wings are mobilized and the glans may be incised in the midline as with the TIP repair. Incisions are completed and a neourethra is then tubularized to complete the repair using a standard Thiersch–Duplay technique. We cover the repair aggressively with dartos tissue or in some cases with processus vaginalis flaps taken adjacent to the spermatic cord on one side or the other. Rarely, placement of the suture line into the scrotum facilitates healing. The penis is then mobilized from the scrotal flaps in a third stage, usually 3–12 months later.

Grafts

Severe proximal hypospadias and repeat hypospadias repairs may incorporate free grafts to construct a neourethra or augment an existing plate. The versatility of most primary hypospadias repairs using preputial skin or the urethral plate, however, has obviated our use of free grafts for primary hypospadias repairs. At CHOP, we reserve this technique only for reoperations or the rare instances where a paucity of local tissue is evident.[118] Free skin, bladder mucosa, tunica vaginalis, and buccal mucosa have been variously described as appropriate tissue for free graft use.[119–121]

Our experience has been that bladder mucosa is less pliable than buccal mucosa, with the latter being less likely to shrink and requiring a one-to-one ratio for harvest compared with the defect to be repaired. We prefer buccal mucosa also, as thick epithelium, tensile strength, and high levels of type IV collagen favor graft take.[122] We no longer use bladder mucosa and use buccal mucosa exclusively in the rare cases requiring a free graft. Our techniques are similar to those described above. We no longer advocate the use of tubularized buccal mucosal grafts, but prefer staged repairs, as described above.

Metro et al[118] and Hensle et al[98] have reported long-term results for buccal mucosa used as tubularized repairs in complex hypospadias reoperations. Overall complication rates of from 32% to 57% were reported, with graft stricture and meatal stenosis being most common. All complications were evident by 11 months in both groups Buccal mucosa is a viable non-genital tissue alternative for a select subgroup of patients requiring urethral reconstruction, but superior results seem likely if the graft is staged.

Reoperative urethroplasty

Differences in opinion between the authors regarding primary hypospadias repair also influence our recommendations for reoperations.

WTS [first author]: The goal in hypospadias reoperation is the same as in primary surgery, which is a functional penis with a normal cosmetic appearance. I follow the same decision-making process – tubularizing the urethral plate when it is still present and supple, and otherwise creating a neourethral plate for tubularization. As in primary urethroplasty, skin flaps are avoided, especially since their vascularity cannot be assured after prior surgery.[123]

During the past 20 years the trend in primary hypospadias repair has been to conserve the urethral plate for use in urethroplasty. Consequently, in my experience, the plate is most often still present after one or two failed operations. Furthermore, despite prior incision for MAGPI or TIP, the urethral plate may remain grossly supple. We perform cystoscopy before surgery to determine the status of any remnant neourethra or the distal native urethra. Then we outline a Y-shaped incision along the visible junction of the glans to urethral plate, extending 2 mm under the meatus and then continuing in the midline to near the penoscrotal junction. We then incise and tubularize the urethral plate. We mobilize a flip-flap of dartos from the ventrum to cover the neourethra before glansplasty. If a dartos flap is not available, we use tunica vaginalis, since fistulas are more likely without

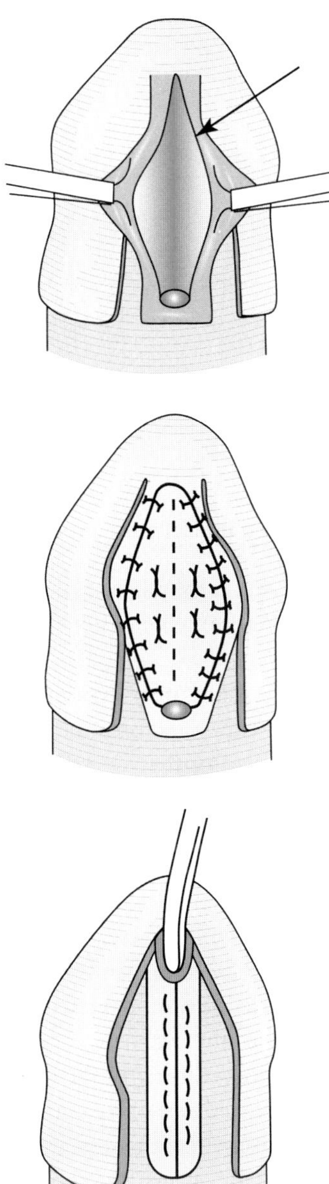

Figure 71.28 Patch grafting regions of focal scar in staged buccal graft urethroplasty. The scarred region is excised and replaced with new buccal graft quilted into place.

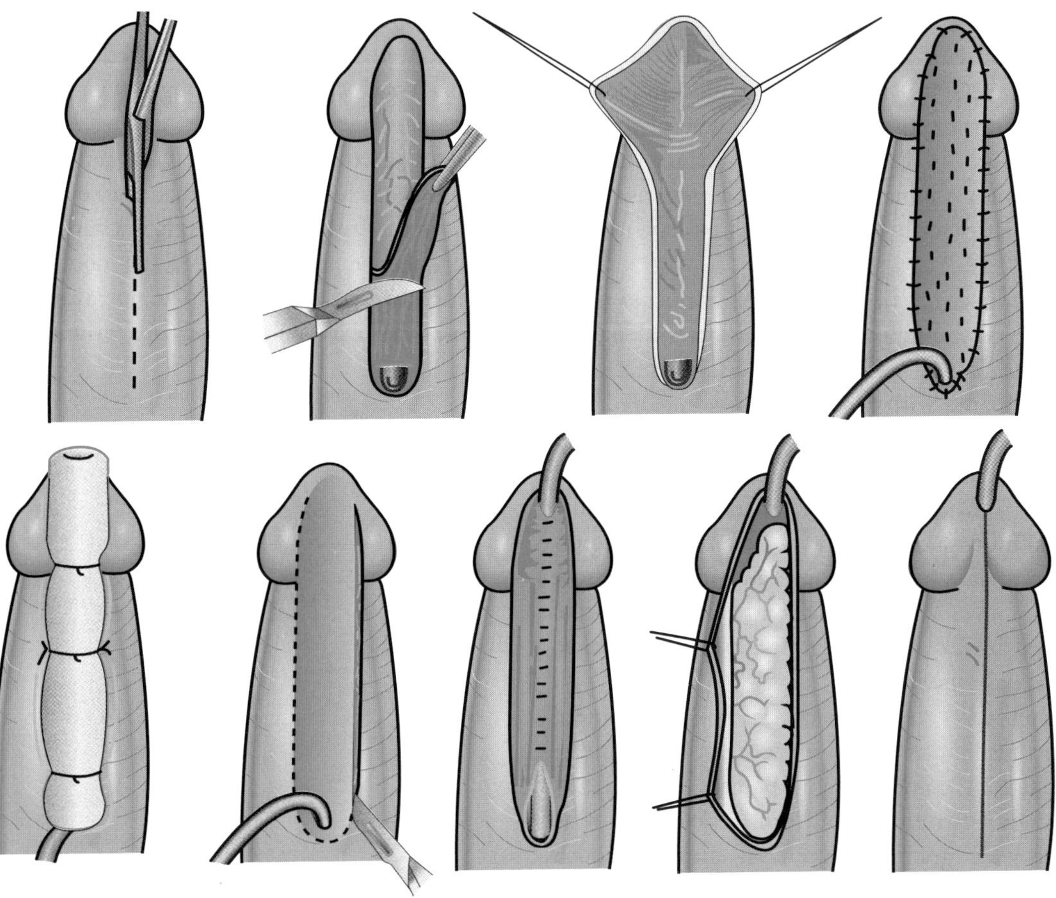

Figure 71.29 Staged buccal graft hypospadias reoperation.

coverage of the urethral reconstruction with a barrier layer.

If the urethral plate was excised previously, a healthy skin strip can sometimes be conserved as a substitute urethral plate. It is incised in the midline, but rather than rely upon spontaneous re-epithelialization, the resultant defect is grafted with buccal mucosa (Figure 71.28). We quilt this buccal inlay graft into place, and then tubularization proceeds for a single-stage repair. Dorsal inlay grafting mimics current trends in adult urethral stricture repair, taking advantage of the reliable take that occurs when a graft is secured dorsally to the corpora.

When there is gross scarring of the urethral plate or residual skin, or any evidence of balanitis xerotica obliterans (BXO), we excise these tissues and replace them with buccal graft for staged urethroplasty (Figure 71.29). In the first operation, we excise unhealthy tissues from prior surgery from the surface of the corpora and between the glans wings, re-establishing a deep glans groove. We create a proximal urethrostomy and we harvest a buccal graft. We use the inner lip to resurface the glans, while cheek covers the penile shaft.

Following the first stage, focal contraction or scar develops in up to 20% of patients. Midline incision and buccal inlay grafting during the planned second-stage urethroplasty can correct partial graft contracture. More extensive contracture or scarring requires a second operation to excise the unhealthy region and regraft (Figure 71.30). Urethroplasty is then performed 6 months later.

At the second stage, margins of the neourethral plate are first infiltrated with 1:100 000 epinephrine. Then the buccal plate is separated from the shaft skin and glans. It is tubularized, turning epithelium into the lumen. I prefer to use a two-layer closure, the first with interrupted and the second with running stitches. We cover the entire neourethra with dartos and/or tunical vaginalis flaps, and then glanuloplasty and shaft skin closures proceed as described above for primary repairs.

A 6 or 8 Fr dripping stent provides urinary diversion in prepubertal boys, but in teens and adults we leave a 10 or 12 Fr stent across the repair with a percutaneous suprapubic tube for urine drainage. We continue diversion for 10 days, and cover with

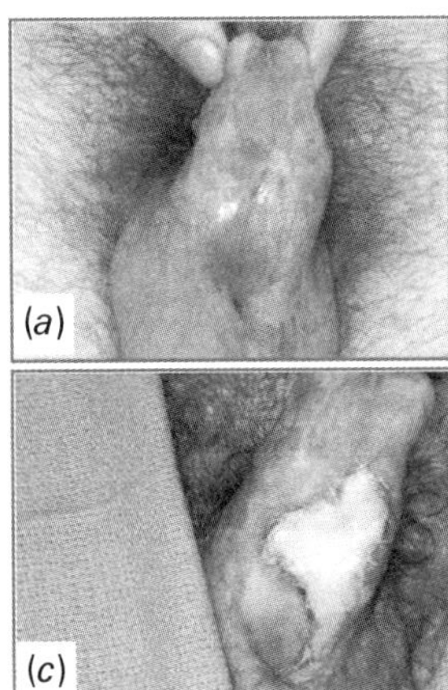

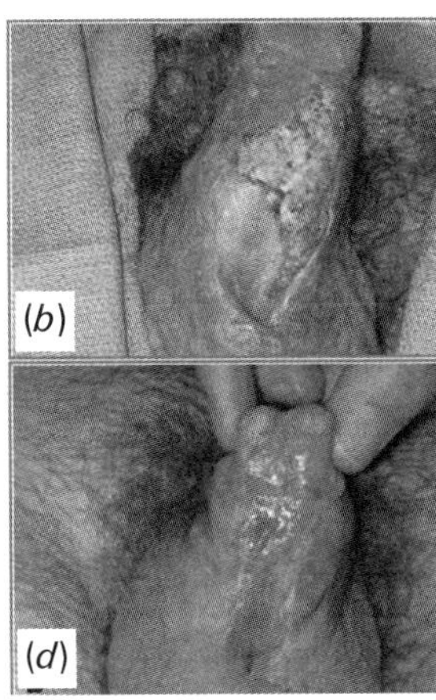

Figure 71.30 (*a*) Scar noted in mid portion of graft. (*b*) Scarred region is excised. (*c*) Scarred region is replaced with new buccal graft quilted into place. (*d*) Patched area now healed, neourethral plate ready to be tubularized.

antimicrobial prophylaxis using trimethoprim–sulfamethoxazole. We have usually prescribed antiandrogens in teens and adults to reduce erections.

Staged buccal graft reoperations result in a vertical slit meatus while preserving penile skin for shaft closure. Consequently, excellent cosmetic outcomes have been achieved despite as many as 15 prior failed operations.[124] Fistulas were noted in only one case in which a tissue barrier layer covered the neourethra, and no strictures or diverticulum occurred.

DAC [third author]: In redo hypospadias repairs, our modification of the flap harvest has led us to feel more confident in harvesting distal penile shaft skin in patients who have already had the foreskin utilized in previous repairs and even in a reharvest of shaft skin following the previous harvest of an island flap in the initial repairs.

Because of the difficulty and high risk of fistula, particularly in the older patient, we prefer to get as much tissue to the ventral penile shaft as possible; hence our commitment to moving tissue, to covering the fistula in most cases with skin taken from the dorsum of the penis on a pedicle flap. If the urethra requires replacement, we separate the flap with half of the flap deployed as the urethral replacement and the other half of the flap used as ventral skin coverage. Successful urethroplasty for a patient that has undergone previous failed hypospadias repairs remains a surgical challenge. These repairs require continued adherence to the surgical principles of urethrocutaneous fistula repair: a sufficient time interval following failed repair; excision of the fistulous tract; closure of the urethral defect with mucosa-inverting sutures; and overlay of the urethral repair with abundantly vascularized tissue.[125] In some cases, however, the absence of preputial skin, paucity of ventral skin, and residual chordee may all contribute to augment the risk of failure following salvage hypospadias surgery.

The split onlay skin (SOS) flap for redo hypospadias repair or fistula

We have attempted to address the dual aims of completing a redo urethroplasty with an onlay island flap using residual penile skin while also rotating adequate skin for ventral penile skin coverage. We place a glans traction suture and mark a circumcising incision line. The line extends ventrally to the midline and then vertically to the penoscrotal junction. The release of this ventral tissue allows the dorsal skin to flatten in an 'open-book' fashion, facilitating proximal dartos mobilization with the island skin flap with minimal risk of damage to the pedicle to the dorsal skin flap. Lidocaine with epinephrine (1:100 000) is infiltrated along the marked line prior to incision. We then deglove the penis by creating a plane of dissection superficial to Buck's fascia and avoiding injury to the preputial skin pedicle (Figure 71.31a).

If the distal urethral coverage is particularly thin, or if a diverticulum is present along with a fistula, we incise the urethra distal to the fistula, from distal to proximal, and the diverticulum is trimmed. If the distal urethra requires reconstruction, we measure the length of the urethral defect to estimate the size of the skin flap that will be required for urethroplasty. We then examine the dorsal penile shaft skin for redundancy, and outline a circumferential flap up to 1 cm wide and longer than the length of the urethral defect. We place interrupted 5–0 polypropylene stay sutures and grasp them so that we accentuate the fold of tissue between the outlined flap skin and the shaft skin. We divide the epithelium with the initial incision and harvest the flap in a plane that preserves the vascular pedicle. The midline incision of the ventral shaft skin completed earlier releases the base of the dorsal vascular mesentery and facilitates flap mobilization.

We then pass the dorsal penile skin flap over the glans through a buttonhole in the mesentery. We divide the flap transversely into superior and inferior segments after ensuring adequate vascularity to both segments (Figure 71.31b,c). We tailor one part of the flap to fit the urethral defect. We suture the urethral segment into place with interrupted 7–0 polyglactin sutures as an island onlay hypospadias repair (Figure 71.31d). After we reconstruct the glans, we place a

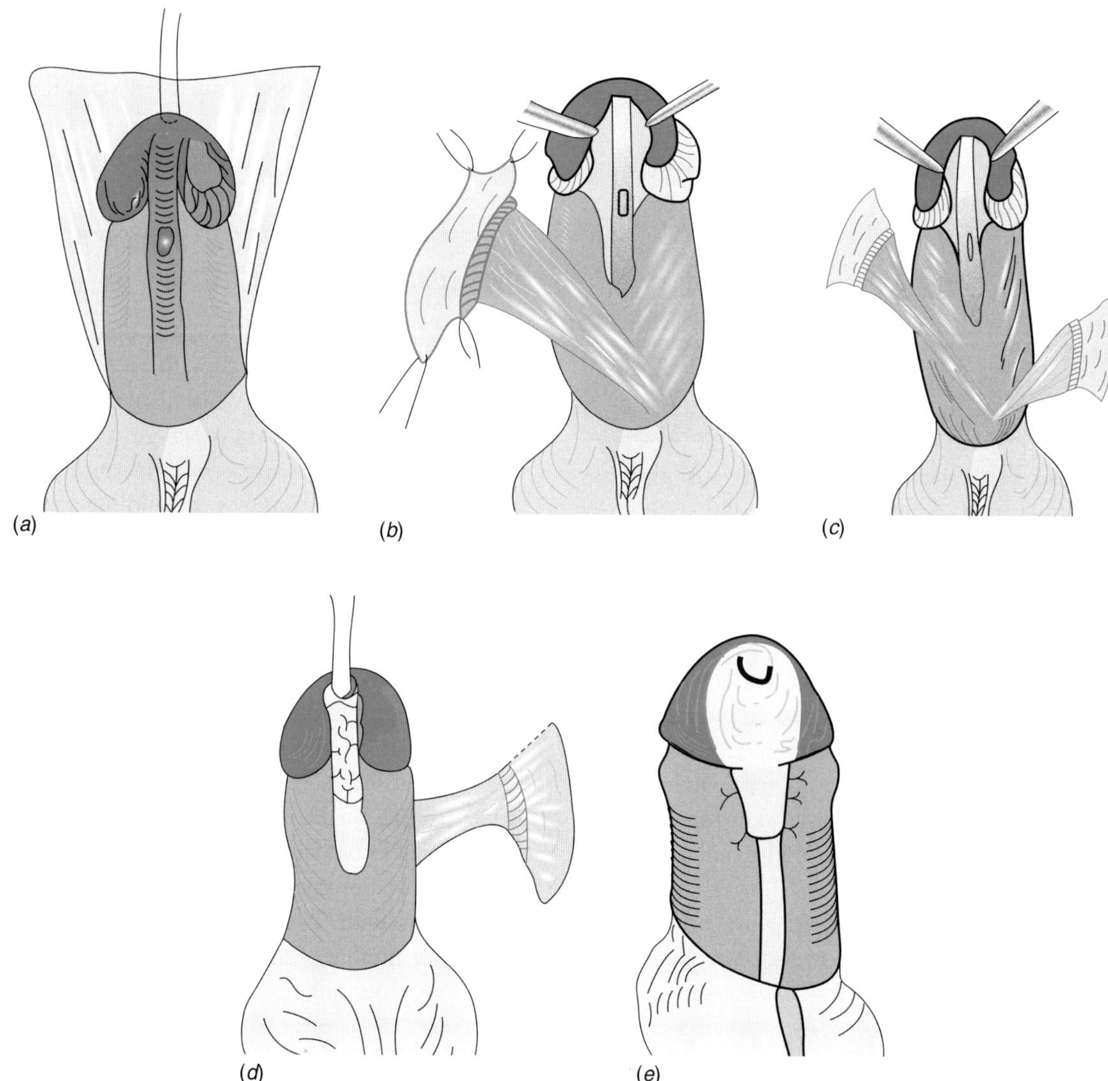

Figure 71.31 The split onlay skin (SOS) hypospadias repair technique. (*a*) The fistula is identified along the ventral surface of the penis following circumferential degloving of the penile skin. (*b*) An approximately 1 cm wide dorsal preputial flap is isolated and harvested, preserving the vascular mesentery. A buttonhole is created in the mesentery and the flap is transposed ventrally. (*c*) The flap is divided transversely into two segments, with the superior segment tailored to correspond to the urethral defect and to be used as an onlay flap. (*d*) The appropriately designed superior segment is sutured into place with interrupted 7–0 polyglactin sutures, as in the standard island onlay hypospadias repair, and a glanuloplasty is completed over a 6 Fr Kendall stent. (*e*) The residual penile skin is reapproximated dorsally and the remaining inferior segment of the rotated flap is used to cover the persistent ventral skin defect.

6 Fr urethral stent and begin the skin closure. A redundant dorsal prepuce is not available in these boys to use to cover the ventral skin defect. Therefore, after reapproximating the dorsal penile shaft skin, we tailor the remaining segment of the dorsal skin flap to provide additional coverage of the ventral penile shaft (Figure 71.31e). A Telfa and gauze dressing that compresses the penis and urethral stent against the lower abdominal wall with Tegaderm ('sandwich dressing') is applied and the patient is discharged with prophylactic antibiotics.

Our preference is to preserve the urethral plate, if possible, and utilize penile skin in repairing the failed hypospadias repair. Our experience has been similar to the reports of Jayanthi et al[123] and Simmons et al[126] that previously relocated penile skin may be successfully rotated as an island onlay flap to repair hypospadias fistula without vascular compromise and with consistently favorable outcomes. We have found that even following multiple previous hypospadias repairs, enough penile shaft skin is usually present dorsally or laterally to transpose ventrally for an island onlay repair.

We have also used acellular dermal matrix (AlloDerm) to augment the flap in cases where the dartos coverage is thin. In complex hypospadias cripples, we have also used this material in conjunction with primary closure or in association with flaps.

Complications of hypospadias repair

Fistulas

Urethrocutaneous fistulas are the most common complication of hypospadias surgery. Several factors have been implicated in their occurrence, including apposing suture lines from neourethral and skin closure, distal obstruction from meatal stenosis or urethral stricture, turbulent urine flow, for example in diverticulum, and locally impaired vascularity. Fistulas are usually apparent within the first few months after surgery, but occasionally develop years later. Some close spontaneously, but most require surgical correction.

Barrier layers to 'waterproof' the neourethra separate overlying suture lines to decrease risk for fistulas. Although helpful, this measure alone is not sufficient, as seen in our report of a 21% incidence of fistulas in proximal repairs despite the use of a dartos barrier flap in every case.[93] In this series no attempt was made to turn epithelium into the lumen of the neourethra and, since making this modification, the fistula rate has diminished by more than 50%.

We have delayed fistula repair for 6 months and longer after hypospadias surgery in older children and adolescents to allow postoperative edema and tissue inflammation to resolve. We perform urethroscopy or sound the urethra to assess the neourethra for obstruction, diverticulum, or unexpected additional fistulas. The surgical field is infiltrated with 1:100 000 epinephrine to minimize bleeding for optimal visualization, and then the fistula opening is circumscribed and the tract dissected to the entrance into the urethra. After excision, we turn back the epithelium of the urethral opening into the lumen, and this closure is then covered with a dartos flap. Fistulas at the coronal margin or on the proximal glans require more extensive repair, opening the distal urethra from the meatus through the fistula. In these cases, we redo the hypospadias with closure of the neourethra, interposition of a dartos flap, and glanuloplasty. Although catheter drainage in not always needed after closure of small fistulas on the penile shaft, we recommend it following reoperative glanuloplasty.

Immediate treatment to seal fistulas was reported in a small series of patients in whom topical corticosteroid was initially applied for 3 days to reduce tissue reaction, and then a catheter was placed and n-butyl cyanoacrylate applied.[127] Durable success, defined as no recurrent fistula at 6 months, was noted in five of eight cases, but the potential role of early therapy will require additional experience.

Small fistulas amenable to simple closure, including coverage with a dartos layer, are successfully repaired in over 90% of cases,[128,129] although larger and multiple fistulas have a higher recurrence rate,[129,130] which may indicate impaired local vascularity. If the neourethra appears otherwise healthy, we would expose the affected area with a more extensive dissection and supplement any available local dartos flap with an additional covering using a tunica vaginalis flap.[131]

Meatal stenosis

Meatal stenosis may result from poor distal vascularity and wound contracture, technical errors in meatoplasty, or less commonly, from BXO. Regardless of urethroplasty technique, the neomeatus should be generously sized and oval, not rounded, allowing for minor postoperative contraction. This precaution applies especially to tubularization procedures where the temptation to suture the neourethra too far distally can lead directly to stenosis. Failure to incise a narrow, flat urethral plate for TIP repair could also result in an inadequate diameter. BXO is not commonly encountered after hypospadias repair in the United States, possibly because of the preference for circumcision, but should be suspected when a typical white scar involves the meatus.

A visually small meatus is not necessarily pathologic, and calibration should be performed to diagnose true stenosis. Meatotomy may be an effective therapy for a limited distal scar, or reoperative glanuloplasty with deep urethral plate incision may be required to increase the distal urethral caliber. BXO occasionally responds to topical corticosteroids, but usually mandates complete excision of the involved tissues with buccal mucosal grafting.[132]

Urethral stricture

We suspect a neourethral stricture when the urinary stream is diminished, although a visibly decreased force of the stream and uroflowmetry in the lower limits of normal can occur despite an adequate urethral diameter determined by urethroscopy and calibration.[88] Circumferential anastomoses are thought to have a greater risk for constriction, but a comparison study of tubularized vs onlay preputial flaps found no significant difference in strictures between the two techniques.[106] Despite initial concerns that the relaxing incision for TIP would create strictures, this complication has only been rarely encountered.[88,92]

Short strictures detected within a few months of surgery can be managed successfully with dilation under anesthesia or optical urethrotomy, with reported success in approximately 50% of cases.[133] However, these interventions are only successful in 16–21% of cases when strictures are detected later.[133,134] Because strictures probably indicate regions of compromised vascularity, we usually recommend open repair incorporating healthy tissues. Following the example of adult stricture repair, it may be preferable to open the diseased area longitudinally to healthy margins and then incise dorsally through the entire stricture, filling the defect with buccal graft. Extensive stricture of the neourethra should prompt consideration for reoperative urethroplasty.

Diverticulum

Diverticulum presents with visible ballooning during voiding and postvoid dribbling. Etiologies include distal obstruction, turbulent flow, and creation of too large a neourethra. Genital skin is elastic to allow erection, and so may balloon proximally from fixed resistance of the non-distensible glanular urethra without anatomic obstruction. Accordingly, Greenfield et al[135] reported a 21% incidence following staged preputial repairs, whereas in a personal series of six patients undergoing staged Byars flap–glanular TIP urethroplasty, diverticulum developed in four cases despite care to avoid making skin flaps wider than 12 mm. A significantly decreased incidence of diverticulum was reported by Weiner et al[106] after onlays rather than tubularized preputial flaps, probably reflecting the use of less genital skin. To our knowledge, diverticula have not been reported after buccal graft urethroplasty, which probably reflects the difference in elasticity of this tissue compared with genital skin.

After excluding distal obstruction, correction involves excision of redundant tissue to restore a normal urethral caliber. Recurrent diverticulum is uncommon.

Dehiscence

Partial or complete dehiscence of the glans has probably been under-reported, or characterized as meatal regression. This wound separation could result from infection, poor vascularity, and/or tension on the repair. In addition, one of us (WTS, unpublished data) has noted that choice of suture material and closure technique for glanuloplasty was related to the incidence of this complication. Among the initial 131 patients undergoing TIP repair, 7–0 chromic mattress sutures were used to approximate glans wings, with a subsequent 5% partial or complete separation. When subepithelial 6–0 polyglactin was substituted in the next 156 cases, the rate of glans dehiscence decreased to 2.5%. Furthermore, since the glanuloplasty technique was changed so that the ventral lip of the meatus was sutured first and not sewn to the underlying neourethra, there has been no dehiscence in a subsequent 75 distal cases.

Recurrent penile curvature

There are very limited data regarding long-term results of currently used techniques for correcting penile curvature. The most important question is whether the straightening achieved in childhood is maintained during puberty, and to date no reports document such outcomes for dorsal plication or the various forms of ventral corporeal grafting.

Baskin and Duckett performed dorsal plication in 182 boys, most during the first year of life, using transverse incisions into the tunica albuginea lateral to the neurovascular bundles. Curvature was diagnosed by artificial erection after shaft skin degloving, and straightening then confirmed after plication by repeat injection. With mean follow-up of 2.7 years, 4% of the boys had recurrent curvature. Only one patient was deemed to have sufficient bending to warrant repeat surgery, and failure in this case was attributed to plication without incision into the tunica albuginea.[136] Nevertheless, Baskin subsequently abandoned this technique for midline plication without tunic incision to minimize potential iatrogenic injury to the sensory nerve complex.[28] In one series[138] of boys undergoing midline plication using one–two stitches of 4–0 or 5–0 polypropylene, 97% of boys with curvature <45° had a straight penis with a median follow-up of 16 months. There were four patients with >45° bending, of which two had persistently severe curvature, leading the authors to recommend other techniques for straightening be used for this extent of curvature.

A survey of pediatric urologists in the United States reported increased reliance on division of the urethral plate and ventral corporeal grafting for curvature >40°.[138] Dermal grafts have most commonly been used to repair the defect created by incising the tunica albuginea of the corpora cavernosa, with straightening achieved in >90% of patients.[79,80] Tunica vaginalis grafts were also reported successful for penile straightening,[81,82] although Caesar and Caldamone[78] noted recurrent curvature in 60% of patients after tunica vaginalis grafting while no patient had bending following dermal repair. Two studies report the use of single-layered small intestinal submucosa (SIS) for corporeal grafting in a total of 24 patients, with straightening confirmed in each by repeat erection during second-stage urethroplasty.[83,84] However, recurrent curvature from graft contracture occurred in two of 12 boys repaired with four-layer SIS.[139]

Contracture of the neourethra can also result in ventral curvature. As mentioned above, this complication occurred in one patient following tubularization of an 'unhealthy' incised urethral plate. Vandersteen and Husmann[140] reported similar contracture of prior tubed graft urethroplasty resulting in curvature in a small series of men evaluated after puberty. Penile tethering in this circumstance requires transection of the neourethra for straightening.

Shaft skin complications

Suture tracks result from epithelialization around suture material before its dissolution. Given the small diameter of sutures currently used for skin closure in hypospadias surgery, it may take as long as 1 year following repair for keratin to fill the sinus and thereby become visually apparent. Consequently, the incidence of this minor complication is unknown and most probably underestimated, but it was reported in 43% of a small series of boys and prompted a recommendation that subepithelial stitches be used.[115] Correction involves unroofing the skin tunnel using sharp pointed scissors.

Secondary phimosis or wound dehiscence can occur after foreskin reconstruction. Most series have noted few such complications,[112–114] although one European center reported 14% dehiscence and increased fistula development.[141] We advise parents not to manipulate the foreskin postoperatively until the surgeon first ascertains sufficient wound healing has occurred 6–12 weeks later to minimize concerns for iatrogenic disruption of the suture line. Although secondary phimosis rarely occurs, when suspected, application of 0.05% betamethasone twice daily to the tip of the prepuce may be advised to ensure it can subsequently be retracted.

Secondary phimosis can also occur following circumcision, usually from a combination of shaft skin swelling and peripenile fat tending to elevate the skin. Steroid creams may resolve the issue, or reoperative circumcision is needed. Sutures tacking skin to the penile shaft dorsally and ventrally may help prevent this complication if there is concern that excess prepubic fat will push the penile shaft skin over the glans.

References

1. Horton CE, Devine CJ, Baran N. Pictoral history of hypospadias repair techniques. In: Horton CE, ed. Plastic and Reconstructive Surgery of the Genital Area. Boston: Little Brown, 1973: 237–48.
2. Devine CJ Jr, Horton CE. Hypospadias repair. J Urol 1977; 118:188.
3. Willis R. Pathology of Tumors. London: Butterworth, 1948.
4. Allen TD, Griffin JE. Endocrine studies in patients with advanced hypospadias. J Urol 1984; 131:310.
5. Austin PF, Siow Y, Fallat ME et al. The relationship between müllerian inhibiting substance and androgens in boys with hypospadias. J Urol 2002; 168:1784.
6. Teixeira J, Maheswaran S, Donahoe P. Müllerian inhibiting substance: an instructive developmental hormone with diagnostic and possible therapeutic applications. Endocr Rev 2001; 22:657.
7. Baskin LS. Hypospadias and urethral development. J Urol 2000; 163:951.
8. Silver RI, Russell DW. 5alpha-reductase type 2 mutations are present in some boys with isolated hypospadias. J Urol 1999; 162:1142.
9. Baskin LS, Erol A, Li YW. Hypospadias and urethral development. J Urol 2000; 163:951.
10. Kallen B. Case control study of hypospadias, based on registry information. Teratology 1988; 38:45.
11. Pierik FH, Burdorf A, Nijman JMR et al. A high hypospadias rate in The Netherlands. Hum Reprod 2002; 17:1112.
12. Sweet RA, Schrott HG, Kurland R et al. Study of the incidence of hypospadias in Rochester, Minnesota, 1940–1970, and a case-control comparison of possible etiologic factors. Mayo Clin Proc 1974; 49:52.
13. Paulozzi LJ, Erickson JD, Jackson RJ. Hypospadias trends in two US surveillance systems. Pediatrics 1997; 100:831.
14. Dolk H. Rise in prevalence of hypospadias. Lancet 1998; 351:770.
15. Gatti JM, Kirsch AJ, Troyer WA et al. Increased incidence of hypospadias in small-for-gestational age infants in a neonatal intensive-care unit. BJU Int 2001; 87:548.
16. Fredell L, Kockum I, Hansson E et al. Heredity of hypospadias and the significance of low birth weight. J Urol 2002; 167:1423.
17. Fisch H, Golden RJ, Libersen GL et al. Maternal age as a risk factor for hypospadias. J Urol 2001; 165:934.
18. Roberts CJ, Lloyd S. Observations on the epidemiology of simple hypospadias. Br Med J 1973; 1:768.
19. Altemus AR, Hutchins GM. Development of the human anterior urethra. J Urol 1991; 146:1085.

20. Glenister TW. The origin and fate of the urethral plate in man. J Anat 1954; 88:413.
21. Rowsell AR, Morgan BD. Hypospadias and the embryogenesis of the penile urethra. Br J Plast Surg 1987; 40:201.
22. Williams DI. The development and abnormalities of the penile urethra. Acta Anat (Basel) 1952; 15:176.
23. Kurzrock EA, Baskin LS, Cunha GR. Ontogeny of the male urethra: theory of endodermal differentiation. Differentiation 1999; 64:115.
24. Baskin LS, Liu W, Bastacky J et al. Anatomic studies of the mouse genital tubercle. In: Baskin LS, ed. Hypospadias and Genital Development. New York: Kluwer Academic/Plenum, 2004: 103.
25. Yucel S, Liu W, Cordero D et al. Anatomical studies of the fibroblast growth factor–10 mutant, Sonic Hedge Hog mutant and androgen receptor mutant mouse genital tubercle. In: Baskin LS, ed. Hypospadias and Genital Development. New York: Kluwer Academic/Plenum, 2004: 123–8.
26. Kaplan GW, Lamm DL. Embryogenesis of chordee. J Urol 1975; 114:769.
27. Hunter RH. Notes on the development of the prepuce. J Anat 1935; 70:68.
28. Baskin LS, Erol A, Li YW et al. Anatomical studies of hypospadias. J Urol 1998; 160:1108.
29. Yang CC, Bradley WE. Innervation of the human glans penis. J Urol 1999; 161:97.
30. Duckett JW, Baskin LS. Hypospadias. In: Gillenwater JY, Grayhack JT, Howards SS, Mitchell ME, eds. Adult and Pediatric Urology, 3rd edn. St. Louis: Mosby, 1996.
31. Duckett JW. Hypospadias. In: Walsh C, Retik AB, Vaughan D, Wein AJ, eds. Campbell's Urology, 7th edn, Vol 2. Philadelphia: WB Saunders, 1998: 2094–6.
32. Aarskog D. Clinical and cytogenetic studies in hypospadias. Acta Paediatr Scand Suppl 1970; 203:1.
33. Rajfer J, Walsh PC. The incidence of intersexuality in patients with hypospadias and cryptorchidism. J Urol 1976; 116:769.
34. Koff SA, Jayanthi VR. Preoperative treatment with human chorionic gonadotropin in infancy decreases the severity of proximal hypospadias and chordee [see comment]. J Urol 1999; 162:1435.
35. American Academy of Pediatrics. Timing of elective surgery on the genitalia of male children with particular reference to the risks, benefits, and psychological effects of surgery and anesthesia. Pediatrics 1996; 97:590.
36. Cote CJ, Zaslavsky A, Downes JJ et al. Postoperative apnea in former preterm infants after inguinal herniorrhaphy. A combined analysis. Anesthesiology 1995; 82:809.
37. Schultz JR, Klykylo WM, Wacksman J. Timing of elective hypospadias repair in children. Pediatrics 1983; 71:342.
38. Liechty KW, Adzick NS, Crombleholme TM. Diminished interleukin 6 (IL–6) production during scarless human fetal wound repair. Cytokine 2000; 12:671.
39. Liechty KW, Crombleholme TM, Cass DL et al. Diminished interleukin–8 (IL–8) production in the fetal wound healing response. J Surg Res 1998; 77:80.
40. Sandberg DE, Meyer-Bahlburg HF, Aranoff GS et al. Boys with hypospadias: a survey of behavioral difficulties. J Pediatr Psychol 1989; 14:491.
41. Gearhart JP, Jeffs RD. The use of parenteral testosterone therapy in genital reconstructive surgery. J Urol 1987; 138:1077.
42. Luo CC, Lin JN, Chiu CH et al. Use of parenteral testosterone prior to hypospadias surgery. Pediatr Surg Int 2003; 19:82.
43. Chalapathi G, Rao KL, Chowdhary SK et al. Testosterone therapy in microphallic hypospadias: topical or parenteral? J Pediatr Surg 2003; 38:221.
44. Koff SA, Jayanthi VR. Preoperative treatment with human chorionic gonadotropin in infancy decreases the severity of proximal hypospadias and chordee. J Urol 1999; 162:1435.
45. Tsur H, Shafir R, Shachar J et al. Microphallic hypospadias: testosterone therapy prior to surgical repair. Br J Plast Surg 1983; 36:398.
46. Hinman F Jr. Atlas of Pediatric Urologic Surgery. Philadelphia: WB Saunders, 1994: 554.
47. Byars LT. A technique for consistently satisfactory repair of hypospadias. Surg Gynecol Obstet 1955; 100:184.
48. Devine CJ Jr, Horton CE. A one stage hypospadias repair. J Urol 1961; 85:166.
49. van Hook W. A new operation for hypospadias. Ann Surg 1896; 23:378.
50. Smith DR, Blackfield HM. A critique on the repair of hypospadias. Surgery 1952; 31:885.
51. Allen TD, Spence HM. The surgical treatment of coronal hypospadias and related problems. Trans Am Assoc Genitourin Surg 1968; 60:78.
52. Gittes RF, McLaughlin AP 3rd. Injection technique to induce penile erection. Urology 1974; 4:473.
53. Baskin LS, Duckett JW, Ueoka K et al. Changing concepts of hypospadias curvature lead to more onlay island flap procedures. J Urol 1994; 151:191.
54. Snodgrass W, Patterson K, Plaire JC et al. Histology of the urethral plate: implications for hypospadias repair. J Urol 2000; 164:988.
55. Nesbit RM. Congenital curvature of the phallus: report of three cases with description of corrective operation. J Urol 1965; 93:230.
56. Thiersch C. Uber die entstehungsweise und operative behandlung der epispadie. Arch Heitkunde 1869; 10:20.
57. Anger T. Hypospadias péno-scrotal, compliqué de caidure de la verge: redressement du pénis et urethra-plastie par inclusion cutanée: guérison. Bull Soc Chir Paris 1875; 179.
58. Backus LH, Defelice CA. Hypospadias – then and now. Plast Reconstr Surg 1960; 25:146.
59. Edmunds A. An operation for hypospadias. Lancet 1913; 1:447.
60. Ombredanne L. Precis Clinique et Operatoie de Chirugie Infantile. Paris: Masson and Cie, 1923: 654.
61. Mathieu P. Traitment en un temps de l'hypospadias balanique ou juxtabalanique. J Chir 1932; 39:481.
62. Horton CE, Devine CJJ. Hypospadias. In: Converse JM, ed. Reconstructive Plastic Surgery, 2nd edn. Philadelphia: WB Saunders, 1977.
63. Duckett JW. MAGPI (meatoplasty and glanuloplasty): a procedure for subcoronal hypospadias. Urol Clin North Am 1981; 8:513.

64. Elder JS, Duckett JW, Snyder HM. Onlay island flap in the repair of mid and distal penile hypospadias without chordee. J Urol 1987; 138:376.
65. Duckett JW Jr. Transverse preputial island flap technique for repair of severe hypospadias. Urol Clin North Am 1980; 7:423.
66. Johanson B, Avellan L. Hypospadias. A review of 299 cases operated 1957–69. Scand J Plast Reconstr Surg 1980; 14:259.
67. Rich MA, Keating MA, Snyder HM et al. Hinging the urethral plate in hypospadias meatoplasty. J Urol 1989; 142:1551.
68. Snodgrass W. Tubularized, incised plate urethroplasty for distal hypospadias. J Urol 1994; 151:464.
69. King LR. Hypospadias – a one-stage repair without skin graft based on a new principle: chordee is sometimes produced by the skin alone. J Urol 1970; 103:660.
70. van Horn AC, Kass EJ. Glanuloplasty and in situ tubularization of the urethral plate: a simple reliable technique for the majority of boys with hypospadias. J Urol 1995; 154:1505.
71. Zaontz MR. The GAP (glans approximation procedure) for glanular/coronal hypospadias. J Urol 1989; 141:359.
72. DiSandro M, Palmer JM. Stricture incidence related to suture material in hypospadias surgery. J Pediatr Surg 1996; 31:881.
73. Cromie WJ, Bellinger MF. Hypospadias dressings and diversions. Urol Clin North Am 1981; 8:545.
74. Van Savage JG, Palanca LG, Slaughenhoupt BL. A prospective randomized trial of dressings versus no dressings for hypospadias repair. J Urol 2000; 164:981.
75. Hakim S, Merguerian PA, Rabinowitz R et al. Outcome analysis of the modified Mathieu hypospadias repair: comparison of stented and unstented repairs. J Urol 1996; 156:836.
76. Montagnino BA, Gonzales ET Jr, Roth DR. Open catheter drainage after urethral surgery. J Urol 1988; 140:1250.
77. Sozubir S, Snodgrass W. A new algorithm for primary hypospadias repair based on tip urethroplasty. J Pediatr Surg 2003; 38:1157.
78. Caesar RE, Caldamone AA. The use of free grafts for correcting penile chordee. J Urol 2000; 164:1691.
79. Kogan SJ, Reda EF, Smey PL et al. Dermal graft correction of extraordinary chordee. J Urol 1983; 130:952.
80. Pope JCI, Kropp BP, McLaughlin KP et al. Penile orthoplasty using dermal grafts in the outpatient setting. Urology 1996; 48:124.
81. Perlmutter AD, Montgomery BT, Steinhardt GF. Tunica vaginalis free graft for the correction of chordee. J Urol 1985; 134:311.
82. Ritchey ML, Ribbeck M. Successful use of tunica vaginalis grafts for treatment of severe penile chordee in children. J Urol 2003; 170:1574.
83. Kropp BP, Cheng EY, Pope JC 4th et al. Use of small intestinal submucosa for corporal body grafting in cases of severe penile curvature. J Urol 2002; 168:1742.
84. Weiser AC, Franco I, Herz DB et al. Single layered small intestinal submucosa in the repair of severe chordee and complicated hypospadias. J Urol 2003; 170:1593.
85. Nguyen MT, Snodgrass WT, Zaontz MR. Effect of urethral plate characteristics on tubularized incised plate urethroplasty. J Urol 2004; 171:1260.
86. Firlit CF. The mucosal collar in hypospadias surgery. J Urol 1987; 137:80.
87. Yerkes EB, Adams MC, Miller DA et al. Y-to-I wrap: use of the distal spongiosum for hypospadias repair. J Urol 2000; 163:1536.
88. Snodgrass W. Does tubularized incised plate hypospadias repair create neourethral strictures? J Urol 1999; 162:1159.
89. Holland AJ, Smith GH. Effect of the depth and width of the urethral plate on tubularized incised plate urethroplasty. J Urol 2000; 164:489.
90. Borer JG, Bauer SB, Peters CA et al. Tubularized incised plate urethroplasty: expanded use in primary and repeat surgery for hypospadias. J Urol 2001; 165:581.
91. Nguyen MT, Snodgrass WT. Tubularized incised plate hypospadias reoperation. J Urol 2004; 171:2404.
92. Lorenzo AJ, Snodgrass WT. Regular dilatation is unnecessary after tubularized incised-plate hypospadias repair. BJU Int 2002; 89:94.
93. Snodgrass WT, Lorenzo A. Tubularized incised-plate urethroplasty for proximal hypospadias. BJU Int 2002; 89:90.
94. Cheng EY, Vemulapalli SN, Kropp BP et al. Snodgrass hypospadias repair with vascularized dartos flap: the perfect repair for virgin cases of hypospadias? J Urol 2002; 168:1723.
95. Hollowell JG, Keating MA, Snyder HM 3rd et al. Preservation of the urethral plate in hypospadias repair: extended applications and further experience with the onlay island flap urethroplasty. J Urol 1990; 143:98.
96. Shukla AR, Patel RP, Canning DA. Hypospadias. Urol Clin North Am 2004; 31:445.
97. Shukla AR, Patel RP, Canning DA. The 2-stage hypospadias repair. Is it a misnomer? J Urol 2004; 172:1714.
98. Hensle TW, Tennenbaum SY, Reiley EA, Pollard J. Hypospadias repair in adults: adventures and misadventures. J Urol 2001; 165:77.
99. Liechty KW, Kim HB, Adzick NS et al. Fetal wound repair results in scar formation in interleukin-10-deficient mice in a syngeneic murine model of scarless fetal wound repair. J Pediatr Surg 2000; 35:866.
100. Powell CR, McAleer I, Alagiri M et al. Comparison of flaps versus grafts in proximal hypospadias surgery. J Urol 2000; 163:1286.
101. Kolon TF, Gonzales ET Jr. The dorsal inlay graft for hypospadias repair. J Urol 2000; 163:1941.
102. Kocvara R, Dvoracek J. Inlay-onlay flap urethroplasty for hypospadias and urethral stricture repair. J Urol 1997; 158:2142.
103. Asopa HS, Elhence IP, Atri SP, Bansal NK. One stage correction of penile hypospadias using a foreskin tube. A preliminary report. Int Surg 1971; 55:435.
104. Avellan L, Knutsson F. Microscopic studies of curvature-causing structures in hypospadias. Scand J Plast Reconstr Surg 1980; 14:249.
105. Snodgrass W, Patterson K, Plaire JC et al. Histology of the urethral plate: implications for hypospadias repair. J Urol 2000; 164:988.
106. Wiener JS, Sutherland RW, Roth DR et al. Comparison

of onlay and tubularized island flaps of inner preputial skin for the repair of proximal hypospadias. J Urol 1997; 158:1172.
107. Dewan PA, Dinneen MD, Winkle D et al. Hypospadias: Duckett pedicle tube urethroplasty. Eur Urol 1991; 20:39.
108. Elbakry A. Complications of the preputial island flap-tube urethroplasty. BJU Int 1999; 84:89.
109. Patel RP, Shukla AR, Snyder HM. The island tube and island onlay hypospadias repairs offer excellent long-term outcomes: a 14 year follow-up. J Urol 2004; 172:1717.
110. Elder JS, Duckett JW, Snyder HM. Onlay island flap in the repair of mid and distal penile hypospadias without chordee. J Urol 1987; 138:376.
111. Pattaras JG, Rushton HG. Penile torque after the use of tunica vaginalis blanket wrap as an aid in hypospadias repair. J Urol 1999; 161:934.
112. Erdenetsetseg G, Dewan PA. Reconstruction of the hypospadiac hooded prepuce. J Urol 2003; 169:1822.
113. Gray J, Boston VE. Glanular reconstruction and preputioplasty repair for distal hypospadias: a unique day-case method to avoid urethral stenting and preserve the prepuce. BJU Int 2003; 91:268.
114. Snodgrass WT, Koyle MA, Baskin LS et al. Foreskin preservation in penile surgery. Presented at the American Urological Association (AUA) Meeting, San Francisco, 2004.
115. Snodgrass W. Suture tracks after hypospadias repair. BJU Int 1999; 84:843.
116. Retik AB, Bauer SB, Mandell J et al. Management of severe hypospadias with a 2-stage repair. J Urol 1994; 152:749.
117. Gershbaum MD, Stock JA, Hanna MK. A case for 2-stage repair of perineoscrotal hypospadias with severe chordee. J Urol 2002; 168:1727.
118. Metro MJ, Wu HY, Snyder HM 3rd et al. Buccal mucosal grafts: lessons learned from an 8-year experience. J Urol 2001; 166:1459.
119. Hendren WH, Keating MA. Use of dermal graft and free urethral graft in penile reconstruction. J Urol 1988; 140:1265.
120. Baskin L, Duckett JW. Mucosal grafts in hypospadias and stricture management. AUA Update Ser 1994; 13:270.
121. Duckett JW, Coplen D, Ewalt D et al. Buccal mucosal urethral replacement. J Urol 1995; 153:1660.
122. Baskin L, Duckett JW. Buccal mucosa grafts in hypospadias surgery. Br J Urol 1995; 76:23.
123. Jayanthi VR, McLorie GA, Khoury AE et al. Can previously relocated penile skin be successfully used for salvage hypospadias repair? J Urol 1994; 152:740.
124. Snodgrass W, Elmore J. Initial experience with staged buccal graft (Bracka) hypospadias reoperations. J Urol 2004; 172:1720.
125. Horton CE, Devine CJ Jr, Graham JK. Fistulas of the penile urethra. Plast Reconstr Surg 1980; 66:407.
126. Simmons GR, Cain MP, Casale AJ et al. Repair of hypospadias complications using the previously utilized urethral plate. Urology 1999; 54:724.
127. Lapointe SP, N-Fekete C, Lortat-Jacob S. Early closure of fistula after hypospadias surgery using N-butyl cyanoacrylate: preliminary results. J Urol 2002; 168:1751.
128. Dennis MA, Walker RD 3rd. The repair of urethral fistulas occurring after hypospadias repair. J Urol 1982; 128:1004.
129. Santangelo K, Rushton HG, Belman AB. Outcome analysis of simple and complex urethrocutaneous fistula closure using a de-epithelialized or full thickness skin advancement flap for coverage. J Urol 2003; 170:1589.
130. Shankar KR, Losty PD, Hopper M et al. Outcome of hypospadias fistula repair. BJU Int 2002; 89:103.
131. Landau EH, Gofrit ON, Meretyk S et al. Outcome analysis of tunica vaginalis flap for the correction of recurrent urethrocutaneous fistula in children. J Urol 2003; 170:1596.
132. Bracka A. A versatile two-stage hypospadias repair. Br J Plast Surg 1995; 48:345.
133. Duel BP, Barthold JS, Gonzalez R. Management of urethral strictures after hypospadias repair. J Urol 1998; 160:170.
134. Scherz HC, Kaplan GW, Packer MG et al. Post-hypospadias repair urethral strictures: a review of 30 cases. J Urol 1988; 140:1253.
135. Greenfield SP, Sadler BT, Wan J. Two-stage repair for severe hypospadias. J Urol 1994; 152:498.
136. Baskin LS, Duckett JW. Dorsal tunica albuginea plication for hypospadias curvature. J Urol 1994; 151:1668.
137. Bar Yosef Y, Binyamini J, Matzkin H et al. Midline dorsal plication technique for penile curvature repair. J Urol 2004; 172:1368.
138. Bologna RA, Noah TA, Nasrallah PF et al. Chordee: varied opinions and treatments as documented in a survey of the American Academy of Pediatrics, Section of Urology. Urology 1999; 53:608.
139. Soergel TM, Cain MP, Kaefer M et al. Complications of small intestinal submucosa for corporal body grafting for proximal hypospadias. J Urol 2003; 170:1577.
140. Vandersteen DR, Husmann DA. Late onset recurrent penile chordee after successful correction at hypospadias repair. J Urol 1998; 160:1131.
141. Klijn AJ, Dik P, de Jong TP. Results of preputial reconstruction in 77 boys with distal hypospadias. J Urol 2001; 165:1255.

Abnormalities of the penis and scrotum

72

Michael F MacDonald, Julie Spencer Barthold, and Evan J Kass

Introduction

Anomalies of the genitalia are common and as a group constitute the most frequent cause of birth defects in males. However, other than cryptorchidism and hypospadias, the majority of congenital malformations of the testis and scrotum are extremely rare and are often associated with anomalies of other organ systems. Fortunately, most of these anomalies are identified at birth and some are occasionally detected in utero.[1] Many other developmental abnormalities affecting the genitalia, such as patency of the processus vaginalis (hernia and/or hydrocele), varicocele, and the bell clapper deformity of testicular suspension, may not be apparent for many years but have the potential for significant long-term morbidity. For most genital defects the etiology remains unknown. Congenital and acquired pediatric abnormalities of male genitalia, excluding intersex disorders, hypospadias, and cryptorchidism, are reviewed here.

Normal development of the penis and scrotum

The external genitalia, including the genital tubercle and labioscrotal swellings, are indistinguishable in the male and female before the 9th week of human gestation.[2] Subsequent development in males proceeds in a proximal to distal fashion. The urethral groove deepens and the urethral folds become distinct and then fuse in the midline. Recent work suggests that creation of the glanular urethra also occurs by fusion of the urethral plate, via the mechanism of epithelial–mesenchymal interaction, and not by the previously suggested ingrowth of surface glanular epithelium.[2–5] The paired labioscrotal swellings attain a more ventral position, either by actual migration or by relative change in position due to lengthening, and are anterior to the genital tubercle by 11 weeks of gestation. Fusion of the urethra up to the coronal sulcus is complete by 12 weeks. Developmental penile curvature is lost and scrotal positioning complete by 13 weeks. Fusion of the urethral folds within the glans proceeds as described for urethral closure in the shaft, and is accompanied by distal growth of the prepuce. By 24 weeks, the meatus is at the glans tip and the prepuce completely covers the glans, to which it is largely adherent.

Penile abnormalities

Prepuce

Normal development

At birth, the normal prepuce is usually unretractable because of physiologic adherence between the glans and inner preputial skin and/or tightness of the preputial ring. Ease of retractability of the prepuce increases with age, with complete retraction possible in at least two-thirds of 11–15-year-old and 95% of 16–17-year-old uncircumcised males.[6–8] Therefore, true phimosis is present in childhood only in cases of secondary fibrosis or balanitis xerotica obliterans of the prepuce, which occur in 0.8–1.5% of uncircumcised boys.[9]

Circumcision

The prevalence of routine neonatal circumcision in the USA has dropped from close to 90% in the mid-1960s to an estimated 64% in 1995.[10,11] Epidemiologic data indicate that there are marked differences in fusion. The use of more complex procedures, such as prepubic liposuction or lipectomy, and closure with Z-plasties or skin flaps not only is rarely indicated but also may cause unnecessary scarring. However, Casale et al[50] reported follow-up from the parents of the patients perspective, at a minimum of 3 years, after the above-mentioned complex surgeries. The parents of infants and toddlers almost uniformly thought that surgical intervention alleviated negative concerns, addressed hygiene issues, and enhanced the appearance of the penis. Surgery was less successful in the adolescent population. Others reported early failure in as many as 35% of cases and long-term results are unknown.[48,51,52]

Micropenis

A penis that measures more than 2 or 2.5 standard deviations below the mean in stretched length for age but is otherwise normally formed is called a micropenis.[53,54] In newborns, a stretched length of <2.0 cm is considered abnormal. Normal development of the urethra and prepuce implies normal first trimester development, with impaired penile growth occurring in the second and third trimesters. Cryptorchidism may also be present. The most common etiology is gonadotropin deficiency with or without panhypopituitarism.[53] Other endocrine causes include growth hormone deficiency, testicular dysgenesis or regression and, rarely, 5α-reductase deficiency[55] or partial androgen insensitivity.[56] Micropenis may be present in gonadal determination disorders, such as Klinefelter's syndrome and XX sex reversal, and in Prader–Willi syndrome, Laurence–Moon–Biedl syndrome, Robinow's syndrome, and other rare syndromes, or it may be idiopathic.[53,54]

Evaluation of patients generally includes karyotype, determination of serum glucose, electrolytes, cortisol, and growth hormone levels, as well as thyroid function tests and pituitary imaging, as indicated.[53,54] Testicular function can be determined by measuring serum luteinizing hormone (LH), follicle-stimulating hormone (FSH), and testosterone before and after human chorionic gonadotropin (hCG) stimulation. The dose of hCG is 500–1500 international units (approx. 3000 IU/m^2) every other day for 5–7 days with serum testosterone measurements before and 24–48 hours after the last dose. Newborns can be evaluated for the normal spontaneous surge in serum gonadotropins and testosterone within the first few weeks of life; absence suggests a central (pituitary or hypothalamic) defect.

After diagnostic studies are complete, androgen stimulation therapy using intramuscular depot testosterone, 25 mg every 3–4 weeks for several months in infants, has been recommended to assess penile growth potential.[54,57] Unfortunately, response to testosterone does not always correlate with adequate penile size in adulthood, and may vary with the etiology of micropenis.[57,58] In this regard, patients with palpable testes[59] and significant response to gonadotropin-releasing hormone (GnRH) and hCG stimulation tests[60] appear more likely to have adequate long-term penile growth, although some do not.[58] Limited data suggest that treatment with dihydrotestosterone cream may be an effective alternative to parenteral testosterone, particularly in peripubertal males and in some patients who have failed testosterone therapy.[61] In patients with isolated growth hormone deficiency, growth hormone replacement appears to be sufficient for adequate penile growth.[62] Concerns that early androgen therapy might itself limit long-term penile growth potential are not supported by observations of males with early androgen excess syndromes.[63]

Until recently, routine gender reassignment was recommended for patients who show no penile growth response to testosterone.[53,54] However, the advisability of routine gender reassignment in genetic males with functioning testes has been questioned in other contexts,[20,32–35] and the long-term results of reassignment for micropenis are not known. Adequate sexual functioning and clear male gender identity in adulthood have been reported in some patients raised as males with persistent small penile size in adulthood,[64] but not in others.[58] Additional long-term follow-up data are critically needed to facilitate clinical decision making in these patients. Therefore, gender reassignment should be performed with caution and should be accompanied by expert ongoing patient and family counseling, including a discussion of the risks and benefits of penile reconstruction (see Chapter 71).

Priapism

Priapism is defined as a prolonged, frequently painful penile erection not sustained by sexual activity. The most common pediatric cause is homozygous sickle cell (SS) disease, but other possible etiologies include other hemoglobinopathies, leukemia, local malignancy, viral infections, pelvic infections or appendicitis, trauma, diabetes, amyloidosis, and Fabry's disease.[65,66] Low-flow priapism (ischemic) is usually present in affected boys with sickle cell disease, whereas a high-flow state (non-ischemic) is typically present in trauma-induced priapism, but may rarely also be present in sicklers.[67,68] The incidence of priapism in males with sickle cell disease is 2–35%.[69–75] Stuttering episodes usually lasting less than 24 hours are common in both pediatric and adult patients. Initial episodes may occur in early childhood.

Priapism can be characterized by the site and degree of blood flow or stasis in the erectile tissues. Tumescence is usually limited to the corpora cavernosa but in some cases may also involve the corpus spongiosum, a situation termed tricorporeal priapism.[72] Spongiosal involvement, described in postpubertal individuals, is characterized by a firm, tender, engorged glans. Voiding difficulty may occur in some patients. Studies used to characterize degree of blood flow include analysis of aspirated penile blood, technetium 99m (^{99m}Tc) penile flow studies, and color Doppler ultrasonography. Low-flow priapism is characterized by acidosis, hypercarbia, and hypoxemia on penile blood gas analysis. The usefulness and reliability of penile nuclear scans and Doppler studies in children remain unclear. Miller et al[73] reported that nuclear scans did not predict outcome in a series of pediatric patients with sickle cell-associated priapism.

In the past, the initial treatment of patients with priapism due to sickle cell disease was hydration, analgesia, and transfusion to achieve a target hemoglobin S concentration of 30% or less.[69,70,73,76] However, in 2003 the Erectile Dysfunction Guideline Update Panel on the management of priapism[77] recommended that intracavernosal treatment should be administered concurrently with the above treatment if the priapism lasts longer than 4 hours. Intracavernosal therapy includes aspiration with irrigation and/or intracavernosal injection of a sympathomimetic drug. Prepubertal boys appear to respond more commonly to medical therapy than older patients.[71] Exchange transfusion has been associated with acute neurologic events characterized by reversible or irreversible cerebral ischemia, termed the ASPEN syndrome (association of sickle cell disease, priapism, exchange transfusion, and neurologic events).[78] Morbidity from this complication may be reduced by gradual or partial exchange transfusion, recognition of prodromal headache, and close monitoring.

With a total lack of response to medical and intracavernosal therapies, the next step should be surgical intervention.[69,73,75,77,79,80] The older view that surgical intervention in prepubertal patients with sickle cell priapism is unnecessary, if not contraindicated,[76] appears unjustified based on documented erectile dysfunction in boys following prolonged episodes of priapism.[79,81] For low-flow priapism, distal shunts (e.g. Winter, Ebbehoj and Al-Ghorab procedures) should be attempted prior to proximal shunts (e.g. Quackels and Grayhack procedures), because the distal shunts have fewer complications and are easier to perform.[77,80] These usually produce detumescence. Available long-term follow-up data suggest that potency is more commonly preserved in prepubertal patients, after episodes of shorter duration, and when successful intervention occurs early.[79,82,83]

For the patient with high-flow priapism, diagnosed by history, corporeal aspiration, and blood gas analysis, the Erectile Dysfunction Guideline Update Panel on the management of priapism[77] recommends observation, along with ice packs and site-specific compression, as the initial management. High-flow priapism is not associated with ischemia and will often resolve without treatment. Selective arterial embolization of the ruptured artery is the next step if observation fails or treatment is requested by the patient and/or family.[77,80]

A variety of other treatments have been suggested for patients with sickle cell disease and priapism; however, data are anecdotal or limited. α-Adrenergic agents such as etilefrine[84,85] have been given orally or intracavernosally with some success. Detumescence with hydroxyurea has been reported[86] but not confirmed in a large series. Other options include treatment with sildenafil,[87] GnRH analogues,[88] or antiandrogens,[89] but the latter two are not recommended in patients who have not achieved full sexual maturation and adult stature.[77]

Persistent, apparently painless penile erection has also been observed in newborns.[90] This condition resolves spontaneously in 2–6 days with no adverse sequelae. Associated, possibly contributing factors include polycythemia and birth trauma, although many reported cases are idiopathic.

Scrotal abnormalities

Two main types of scrotal pathology occur in the pediatric population: the commonly observed acute swelling of a normal scrotum (discussed under Inguinoscrotal disease) and the rare abnormalities of scrotal development.

Defects of number or position

Scrotal agenesis

Complete absence of the scrotum is an extremely rare anomaly, with only three reported cases in the

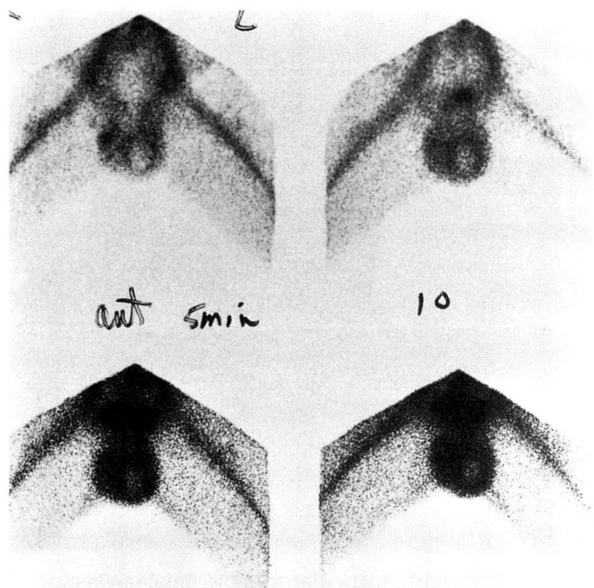

Figure 72.13 Late testicular torsion: nuclear testicular scan showing a 'halo' sign, or increased flow around the avascular left testis.

these conditions may mimic the findings of torsion. In addition, it is of critical importance to localize the exact position of the testis; otherwise, no reliable test is possible. In addition, most centers do not have personnel experienced in the performance or interpretation of nuclear medicine scrotal scans.

Color Doppler sonography has become the most popular diagnostic modality to evaluate a child with an acute scrotum because it is non-invasive and has a diagnostic accuracy at least equal to that of nuclear scanning. It can semiquantitatively characterize blood flow, distinguish intratesticular and scrotal wall flow, and can also be used to assess other pathologic conditions involving the scrotum (Figures 72.14–72.16).[196–198] Proper technique is essential. When color Doppler examinations are not performed correctly, false-positive or false-negative studies may occur. Certain caveats are important to remember. It may not be possible to demonstrate a Doppler signal in the small testes of very young boys. Just seeing color dots does not mean that flow is present; one must see a wave form within the substance of the testis. Reduced flow in a painful testis relative to the normal testis may indicate torsion, and exploration is indicated.

Spermatic cord torsion

The suggested protocol for the evaluation of a child with an acute scrotum (Figure 72.17) states that when the history and physical examination strongly suggest that testicular torsion is present and the duration of the pain is less than 12 hours, urgent surgical intervention is indicated.[199] Imaging studies may delay treatment and thereby jeopardize testicular survival. When pain has been present for more than 12 hours or the diagnosis is unclear, color Doppler ultrasound examination can be helpful in making clinical

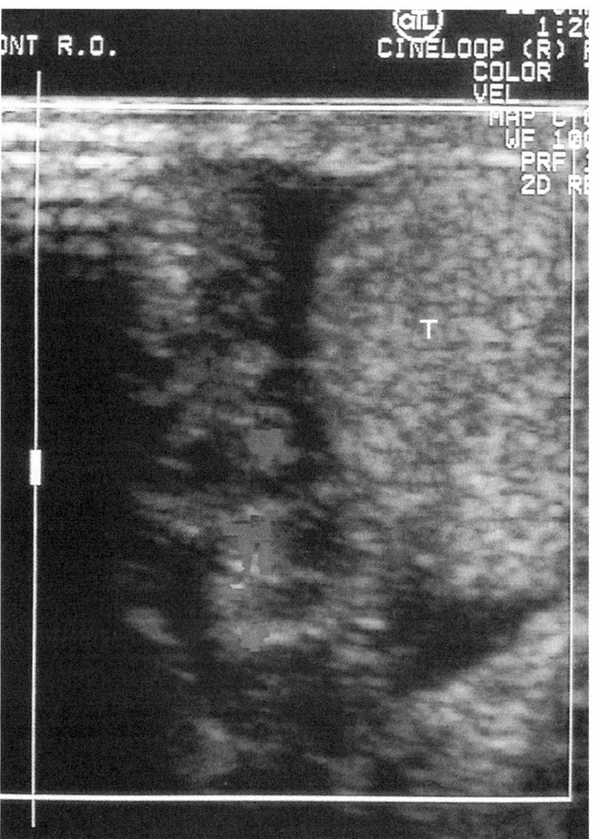

Figure 72.14 Testicular torsion: color Doppler ultrasound showing lack of flow in the testis (T).

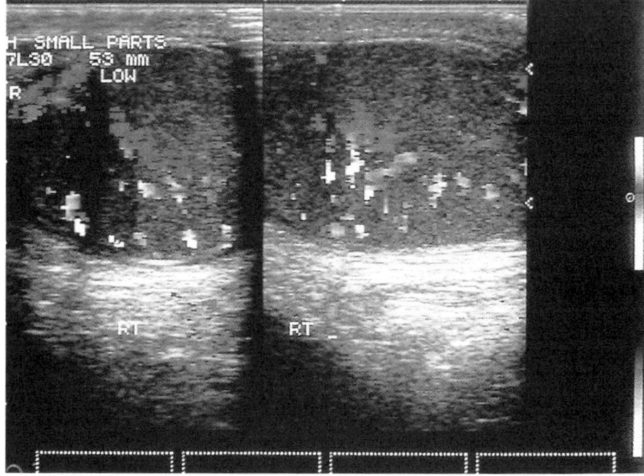

Figure 72.15 Orchitis: color Doppler ultrasound showing increased flow to the right testis.

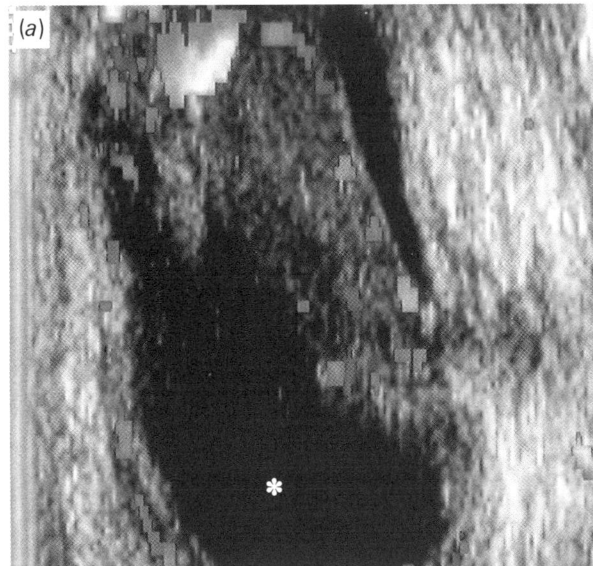

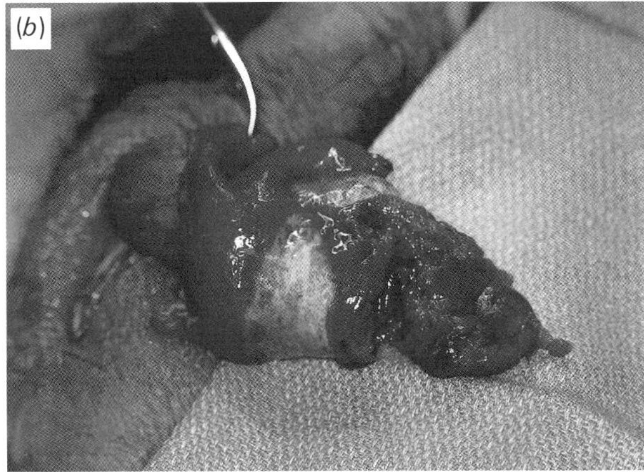

Figure 72.16 Testicular trauma: (*a*) color Doppler ultrasound showing discontinuity of testis and anechoic area at site of hematoma (asterisk); (*b*) intraoperative photograph showing disrupted testis with hematoma.

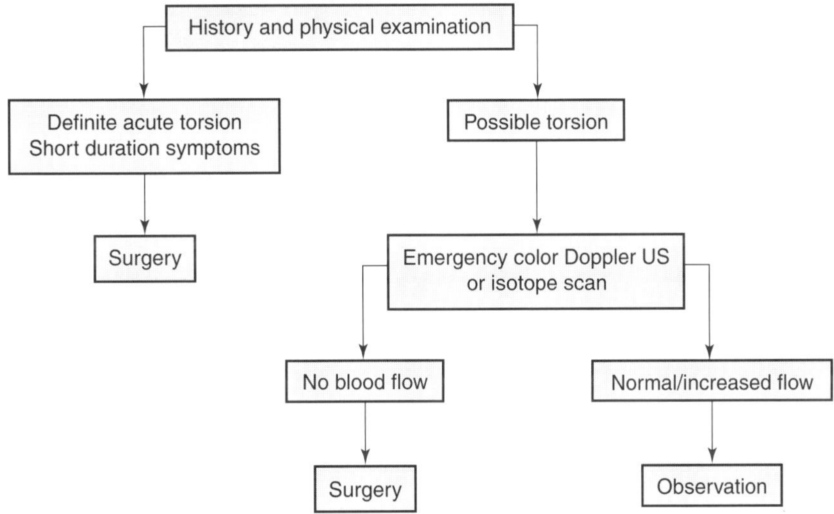

Figure 72.17 Algorithm for evaluation and treatment of patients with acute scrotal pain. (US = ultrasonography.)

decisions. It is important to remember that most patients with an acute scrotum do not have testicular torsion.

The 'bell clapper' deformity is the underlying cause of testicular torsion in older children. In this deformity, the testicle lacks a normal attachment to the tunica vaginalis and therefore hangs freely. As a result, the spermatic cord can twist within the tunica vaginalis (intravaginal torsion).

Surgery is performed to correct torsion in the affected testis and to anchor the other testis to prevent future torsion. Surgical exploration can usually be accomplished through a single, small, midline incision in the scrotal raphe. Testes that are unequivocally necrotic should be removed. Viable testes should be fixed to the scrotal wall with multiple non-absorbable sutures.

Testicular torsion can also occur perinatally before the entire testis complex has fused to the scrotum. In this type of torsion the testis, spermatic cord, and tunica vaginalis twist en bloc (extravaginal torsion) (Figure 72.18). Clinically, extravaginal torsion generally appears as a hard asymptomatic intrascrotal swelling in the newborn. Erythema or a bluish discoloration of the scrotum is also frequently seen and may be confused with a hydrocele.

The management of perinatal torsion remains controversial. Some surgeons advocate a non-operative approach because of the poor potential for testicular salvage. Others argue that leaving a neonatal testis in place may have adverse effects on the contralateral testis and note that cases of bilateral neonatal torsion have been reported.[200] Also controversial is the question as

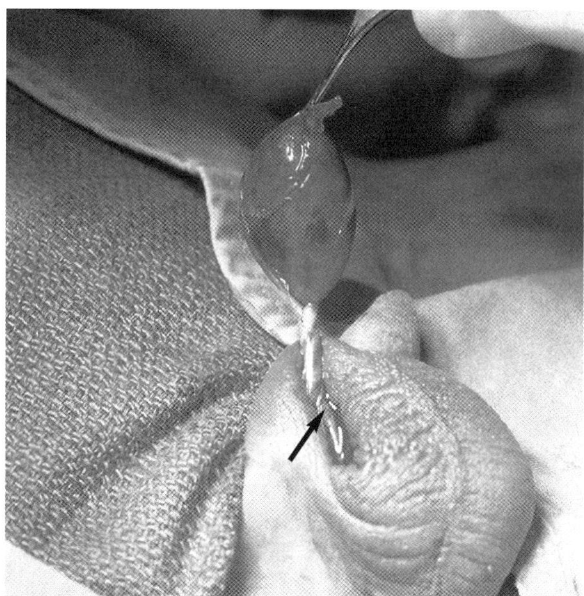

Figure 72.18 Extravaginal torsion (twisted cord – arrow).

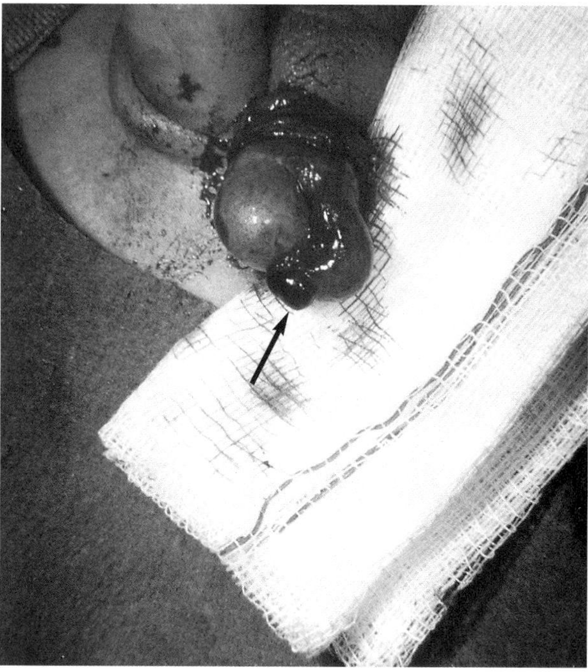

Figure 72.19 Torsion of appendix testis (arrow). Note accompanying enlargement and hyperemia of the epididymis.

to whether or not the remaining solitary testis should be fixed in place, although risk of torsion of that testis is no greater than for the general (adult) population.

Torsion of an appendix of the testis or epididymis

The appendix testis, a müllerian duct remnant located at the superior pole of the testicle, is the most common appendage to undergo torsion (Figure 72.19). The epididymal appendix, located on the head of the epididymis, is a wolffian duct remnant and may also become twisted. Torsion of either appendage produces pain similar to that experienced with testicular torsion, but the onset is more gradual. The cremasteric reflex is not lost with torsion of an appendage. Color Doppler ultrasonography often demonstrates increased blood flow that may be indistinguishable from epididymitis. Occasionally a hypoechoic mass near the upper pole of the testis, the torsed appendage, may be visualized.

Torsion of a testicular appendage may be misinterpreted as epididymitis. However, if the urinalysis is normal, no antibiotic therapy is required. Management entails symptomatic treatment to minimize inflammation and edema. Normal activity may both worsen and prolong the symptoms. Non-steroidal anti-inflammatory drugs (NSAIDs) may offer symptomatic relief to some patients. The inflammation usually resolves within 1 week, although the testicular examination may not be completely normal for several weeks, with induration in the region of the head of the epididymis persisting for that interval.

Epididymitis or orchitis

Epididymitis in adolescents and young adults is often unrelated to sexual activity and does not present with a UTI. In prepubertal boys, however, bacterial epididymitis is often associated with a urinary tract anomaly.[201] Any episode of epididymitis and UTI should be investigated with a renal/bladder sonogram and a voiding cystourethrogram (VCUG) to rule out structural problems. The cause of epididymitis in the majority of young men can often not be determined, however.

Treatment includes empiric antibiotic therapy until the results of a urine culture are known. If the culture is negative, the symptoms are most likely to be due to abacterial chemical epididymitis caused by the retrograde reflux of urine into the vas deferens. Bedrest and scrotal elevation are often helpful. Symptoms may be alleviated with NSAIDs and analgesics. As with appendiceal torsion, the pain and swelling generally resolve within 1 week. Resolution of epididymal induration may require several weeks.

Scrotal trauma

Severe testicular injury is uncommon and usually results from either a direct blow to the scrotum or a straddle injury. Damage generally occurs when the testis is forcefully compressed against the pubic bones. A spectrum of injuries may occur. Traumatic epididymitis is a non-infectious inflammatory condition that usually occurs within a few days after a blow to the testis.[202] Treatment is similar to that of non-traumatic abacterial epididymitis. Scrotal trauma can also result in intratesticular hematoma, hematocele, or laceration of the tunica albuginea (testicular rupture). Color Doppler ultrasonography is the imaging technique of choice (see Figure 72.16). Testicular rupture is a surgical emergency requiring debridement of devascularized tissue and closure of the tunica albuginea. Isolated hematomas and hematoceles are managed on an individual basis.

Lacerations of the scrotum itself are a fairly common occurrence in active boys, usually the consequence of bicycle accidents or getting caught on a fence. Most are superficial and do not involve the tunica vaginalis, requiring only minor suturing with sedation and local anesthesia. Deeper injuries may require a trip to the operating room.

Other acute scrotal disease

Acute idiopathic scrotal edema is another cause of an acute scrotum (Figure 72.20). This condition is characterized by the rapid onset of significant edema without tenderness. Erythema may be present. The patient is usually afebrile and all diagnostic tests are negative. The etiology of this condition remains unclear. Treatment consists of bedrest and scrotal elevation. Analgesics are rarely needed.

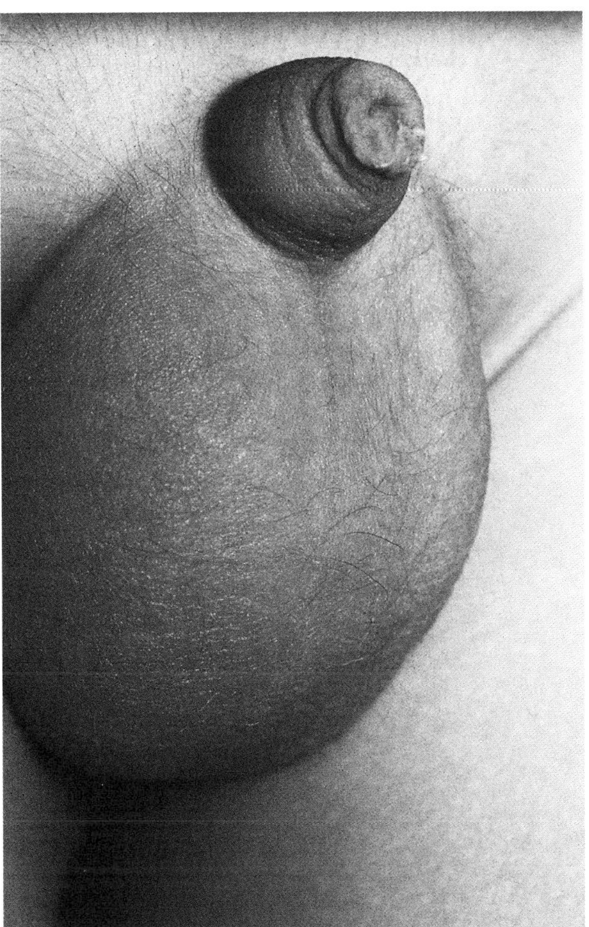

Figure 72.20 Idiopathic scrotal edema.

Schönlein–Henoch purpura, a systemic vasculitic syndrome of uncertain etiology, is characterized by non-thrombocytopenic purpura, arthralgia, renal disease, abdominal pain, gastrointestinal bleeding and, occasionally, scrotal pain and swelling.[203] The onset can be acute or insidious. Hematuria may be present. The syndrome has no specific treatment.

The overriding need in the child with scrotal edema is to rule out testicular pathology. Color Doppler sonography may be helpful, but it may also be possible to make this determination clinically. If the testes can be manipulated gently into the superficial inguinal pouches and palpated, their non-involvement in the inflammatory process may be proven and no further diagnostic studies need be carried out.

Hernia and hydrocele

Inguinal hernia and hydrocele in childhood is most commonly due to patency of the processus vaginalis, an extension of peritoneum that forms in the first trimester in proximity to the gubernaculum of both sexes.[204] In males, the processus vaginalis migrates distally through the inguinal canal with the masculinized gubernaculum, facilitates descent of the testis, persists distally as the tunica vaginalis, and normally becomes obliterated proximally. In females, the processus vaginalis develops but does not enlarge substantially. In both sexes, failure of closure of the processus creates a potential site for clinical hernia formation, characterized by passage of fluid or intra-abdominal viscera into the persisting sac.

The timing of closure of the processus vaginalis and its relationship to clinical hernia formation can be inferred from data obtained at autopsy, inguinal exploration, intraoperative laparoscopy, and studies of patients requiring ventriculoperitoneal shunts. These studies suggest that the processus is open in more than 80% of individuals at birth, and closure is most common in the first year of life but may occur much later. Patency persists in 15–30% of adults.[205,206] However, clinical hernias develop in fewer than 30% of newborns and 10% of 1 year olds after placement of a ventriculoperitoneal shunt.[207] Similarly, contralateral patency of the processus vaginalis has been reported to be as high as 40–50% of children with unilateral inguinal hernias.[208] However,

context of hernia repair if they suggest an additional diagnosis that requires treatment, are confused with normal tissue or are removed inadvertently, producing morbidity. Additional diagnoses of significance include persistent müllerian duct syndrome (usually associated with cryptorchidism), intersex abnormalities in phenotypic females, and testicular, vasal, or epididymal anomalies (see below). Since androgen insensitivity syndrome is present in about 1% of girls undergoing hernia repair,[213] routine exposure of the ovary and/or vaginal examination under anesthesia is warranted in these cases.

Incompletely developed portions of vas or epididymis have been identified by microscopic analysis of excised hernia sac tissue in 1.5–4% of cases and may cause concern of vasal injury. These can be differentiated from normal vas and epididymis by their small mean diameter of 0.17–0.26 mm vs >0.7 mm for normal ducts.[214,215] Serious injury to the normal vas, bladder, ureter, or testis during hernia/hydrocele repair is uncommon (2%).[206,216,217] Even in the subset of boys requiring hernia repair in infancy for incarceration, the rate of testicular atrophy is low (2%).[218] Hernia recurrence is also rare (<0.5%). Postoperative (new or persistent) hydrocele may be found in 1.5–3.5% of cases but the majority resolve spontaneously within 1 year.

A more severe and unusual form of hydrocele is the abdominoscrotal hydrocele (ASH), which extends from scrotum to retroperitoneum but has no demonstrable communication with the peritoneal cavity.[219–221] Presentation is usually unilateral but may be bilateral. Bimanual examination confirms an abdominoscrotal mass which transmits a fluid wave; ultrasound may be useful to confirm the diagnosis in some cases. Often present at birth, the ASH may become quite large, extending laterally to the level of the umbilicus or higher. They often do not regress and may enlarge with time. They may rarely cause pain, lower extremity edema, hydronephrosis, and testicular atrophy.[221,222]

Proposed etiologies include isolated closure of the processus vaginalis at the internal ring with gradual upward extension of the hydrocele retroperitoneally, or incomplete proximal obliteration of the processus producing a one-way valve mechanism with continued accumulation of fluid.[219,220] Associated undescended testis may be present. ASH repair is generally performed through a standard inguinal incision, although inbrication of the wall transcrotally may be safer.[222] The sac is transected, the distal portion opened widely, and the retroperitoneal portion excised completely to prevent recurrence. Extreme care must be taken to avoid injury to local retroperitoneal structures, such as the vas or ureter, which may be difficult to identify in the folds of the large hydrocele wall.[219] For this reason the scrotal approach may be preferable. Concomitant orchidopexy is performed, if indicated.

Testicular abnormalities

Congenital testicular anomalies other than cryptorchidism are rare but are often found in association with abnormal testicular descent. Those associated with intersex disorders are reviewed elsewhere (see Chapter 68).

Defects of number and position

Anorchism and monorchism

Absence of one or both testes in otherwise normal phenotypic males is identified in as many as 35% of patients evaluated for non-palpable testes.[224–226] In the majority, the vas and spermatic vessels are present but end blindly distal to the internal inguinal ring, a condition called vanishing testis. Several observations indicate that the likely cause of vanishing testis is antenatal torsion. These include presence of hemosiderin or calcification in 15–85% of specimens examined histologically,[224–226] absence of developmental abnormalities in the contralateral testis,[227] and sonographic confirmation of prenatal testicular disappearance in a patient with extravaginal torsion.[228] The diagnosis of anorchism can be made after the first 3 months of age if both elevation of plasma gonadotropins and lack of testosterone response to hCG stimulation are present.[229] However, testosterone levels are elevated until about 2 months of age in the normal male. Therefore, absence of measurable levels in this age group suggests anorchia. During mid-childhood, gonadotropin levels may be normal in anorchid boys, but a GnRH stimulation test will reveal an exaggerated gonadotropin response. Contralateral testicular enlargement and elevated FSH levels are present in some, but not all, patients with monorchism.[230] Therefore, diagnosis must be based on laparoscopic and/or surgical findings of blind-ending spermatic vessels. Reduced levels of serum müllerian inhibiting substance may also prove useful in the diagnosis of anorchism.[232]

Polyorchidism

Supernumerary testis is a rare entity, with fewer than 100 case reports in the literature.[233–235] The proposed

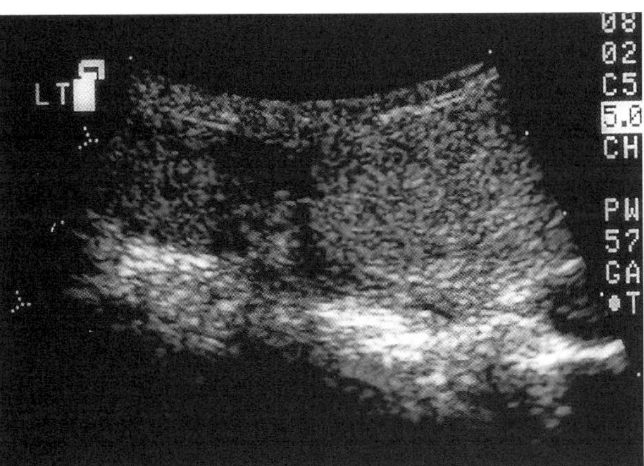

Figure 72.22 Polyorchidism: ultrasound image showing two normal testes on the left side.

etiology is complete duplication of the genital ridge or separation of the ridge into two or more parts. The extra testis is most commonly located in the scrotum (75%), but may be inguinal (20%) or retroperitoneal (5%). The condition is rarely bilateral (5%). Associated ductal structures on the affected side may be single or duplicated. The anatomic variants described in the literature include shared epididymis and vas (47%), duplicated epididymis and common vas (33%), duplicated epididymis and vas (11%), and absence of both adjacent to the accessory testis (5%). Associated genital anomalies are common and in decreasing order of frequency include inguinal hernia, undescended orthotopic testis, spermatic cord torsion, hydrocele, testicular tumor, and varicocele. The diagnosis is suspected by physical findings and can often be confirmed sonographically (Figure 72.22). Surgical intervention is indicated for torsion, hernia/hydrocele, suspected tumor, or cryptorchidism.

Testicular exstrophy

Congenital extrusion of one or both testes outside the scrotum is one of the rarest testicular anomalies.[236,237] There are inadequate data to support any specific etiology, but theories include gubernacular malfunction, scrotal ischemia, or local mesodermal abnormality. No associated anomalies are reported. Treatment is simple scrotal orchidopexy and closure.

Transverse testicular ectopia

The presence of both testes on the same side, each with an intact ipsilateral blood supply, epididymis, and vas, is an uncommon malformation.[238,239] The most frequent associated anomalies include inguinal hernia (98%) and persistent müllerian duct syndrome (30%). The absence of a normal attachment of the gubernacular remnant suggests that anomalous development of this structure may predispose to transverse ectopy. Laparoscopy may be useful for both diagnosis and management.[240–243] Depending on presentation, orchiectomy or orchidopexy is performed with partial excision of müllerian remnants as required to facilitate scrotal placement of the testis.

Other testicular anomalies

Gonadal fusion anomalies

Splenogonadal fusion is a rare anomaly characterized by an abnormal attachment between the left gonad or its internal ductal system and the spleen or accessory splenic tissue.[244–247] Almost 150 cases have been reported, with the majority occurring in males. Patients most commonly present with a scrotal mass, inguinal hernia, or undescended testis. Rare presentations include bowel obstruction, ambiguous genitalia, and acute enlargement or traumatic rupture of the scrotal spleen. Two variants are described: a continuous form characterized by a fibrous connection between gonad and spleen which may contain accessory 'spleenlets', and a discontinuous form, with no connection between the gonad and the orthotopic spleen. These subtypes occur with similar frequency. Other congenital anomalies are present in about one-third of cases, including limb, skull or cardiac defects, micrognathia, diaphragmatic hernia, imperforate anus, spina bifida, and hypospadias. Proposed etiologies include adhesion between splenic and gonadal tissue at 5–9 weeks' gestation due to simple fusion or inflammation[244] and migration of splenic cells into a persistent diaphragmatic gonadal ligament.[246] Treatment is based on associated findings, but care should be taken to avoid injury to the associated normal testis.[244]

A single case of hepatogonadal fusion has appeared in the relatively recent literature.[248] This patient presented with a right inguinal hernia, and had a histologically proven liver nodule attached to the upper testicular pole and a fibrous attachment to the porta hepatis. No other anomalies were present.

Testicular hypertrophy and macroorchidism

Testicular volume is usually less than 2 ml prior to puberty.[249,250] After the age of 9–10 years, testicular size is markedly variable but correlates with Tanner stage.[249] Unilateral or bilateral enlargement of the testis has many etiologies. Malignant lesions, including primary testicular tumors and leukemia, are rare but should be ruled out initially. Benign causes of increased testicular size include asymmetric pubertal enlargement,[251,252] compensatory hypertrophy in some cases of monorchism or cryptorchidism,[253] macroorchidism associated with fragile X and other mental retardation syndromes,[254,255] nodular enlargement in patients with congenital adrenal hyperplasia[256] and isosexual precocity due to central nervous system (CNS) lesions, excess gonadotropins, testotoxicosis, hypothyroidism, and other syndromes.[257]

Testicular size discrepancy at puberty in otherwise normal boys is an uncommon finding. If a history of previous inguinal surgery or testicular injury is absent, the proposed cause is asymmetric response of the testis to normal maturational stimulation.[252] Exaggerated bilateral, benign testicular enlargement is also reported.[251] These patients should be evaluated with testicular sonography and, if a tumor is not identified, no further steps are indicated. Over time, the size discrepancy in unilateral cases may persist or resolve.[252]

Microlithiasis

Microlithiasis is a condition usually reported in adult men, but also found in children.[258] It is characterized by ultrasonic and/or histologic evidence of multiple calcifications within the testicular parenchyma (Figure 72.23).[259] Adult men with microlithiasis often present with other testicular disease, and associated germ cell tumors have been reported in as many as 40%.[260] By contrast, the prevalence of microlithiasis in men who have had testicular sonography for other reasons is 0.6%.[261] The exact incidence in the general population is unknown, but a study of 1504 young asymptomatic men 10–35 years old found a 5.6% prevalence of testicular microlithiasis.[262] A recent study by Wasniewska et al[263] revealed a high prevalence of testicular microlithiasis in males with McCune–Albright syndrome. Microlithiasis identified by pathologic examination is not always evident by sonography. However, the histologic type may be helpful in determining the significance of the lesion.[259] Hematoxylin bodies are associated with germ cell tumors, whereas laminated calcifications may be present in association with testis tumors, but also occur in normal boys and in other diseases affecting the testis including cryptorchidism, epididymitis, inguinal hernia, and Klinefelter's syndrome.

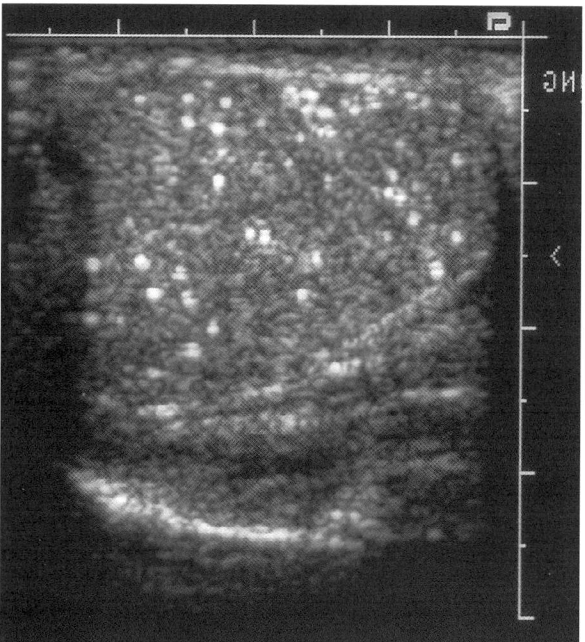

Figure 72.23 Testicular microlithiasis: typical appearance on ultrasound image.

Histologic microlithiasis is even rarer in the pediatric population, identified in only 1 of 2100 autopsies and 1 of 600 testicular biopsies.[264] In a multi-institutional series, Furness et al[258] studied 26 patients aged 6 months to 21 years (mean 12 years) in whom microlithiasis was diagnosed incidentally by sonogram. Reasons for evaluation included hydrocele, epididymitis, varicocele, trauma, testicular or appendix torsion, testicular mass, and unilateral testicular enlargement. There were no cases of clinically evident tumor during a mean follow-up period of slightly more than 2 years. Additionally, long-term data are required to identify the clinical significance, if any, of testicular microlithiasis in children. For the present, self-examination, yearly ultrasound imaging, and selected biopsy should be used in the surveillance of these patients.

Abnormalities of accessory organs

Cystic dysplasia of rete testis

Cystic dysplasia of the rete testes (also called cystic dysplasia of the testis) has been reported 32 times in the literature.[265–267] This lesion is believed to be due to a defect in fusion between the rete testis and efferent ducts. Cystic dysplasia is usually unilateral but may be bilateral, and patients often present in childhood with a testicular or scrotal mass. The diagnosis may be made by identifying multiple small cysts on the medical aspect of the testis, although most of the testicular parenchyma may be compressed by the mass. Associated genitourinary anomalies are common, suggesting that an associated wolffian duct anomaly may be present. Almost all cases are associated with renal anomalies. The most common are agenesis, dysplasia or hypoplasia, or hydronephrosis. Abdominal cryptorchidism is seen in one-third of patients. Preferred treatment is local excision, but an inguinal approach with control of the cord vessels is recommended to rule out tumor. Orchiectomy is performed if testis sparing is not possible. Cimador et al[268] suggests a more conservative approach with serial ultrasonography.

Wolffian duct system

Since the mesonephric or wolffian duct is the precursor of both ureteral bud and the internal genital ducts, including vas, epididymis, and seminal vesicles, anomalous development frequently affects both the kidney and reproductive tract.[269] The caudal segment of the wolffian duct, or common mesonephric duct, is the site of the origin of the ureteral bud. The middle segment, or common vas precursor, becomes the vas and seminal vesicles, and the upper mesonephric duct becomes the distal vas and epididymis.[270] It is proposed that defects that appear before the 7th week of gestation (onset of ureteral bud differentiation) may interfere with normal renal and reproductive tract development and after that time the reproductive tract alone is affected.[269] The timing and extent of the development defect probably influence the eventual phenotype.

Agenesis

Absence of the vas deferens is the most common finding in patients with agenesis of wolffian duct derivatives.[269,271–273] The lesion may be bilateral or unilateral and in either form occurs in less than 1% of males. Vasal agenesis is usually discovered in adult patients with infertility or at the time of planned vasectomy, but may also present during inguinal exploration at any age. Both the unilateral and bilateral forms are associated with agenesis of the epididymis, seminal vesicle and/or kidney, but the association is more frequent in unilateral cases. The caput epididymis almost always persists. This observation supports other clinical data indicating similarities between the caput epididymis and the efferent ducts, with the implication that the caput arises from the gonadal ridge rather than the wolffian duct. Mutation of the transmembrane conductance regulator (*CFTR*) gene is the only known genetic etiology of vasal agenesis. *CFTR* gene mutations are more common in bilateral (64%) than unilateral (25%) disease and have not been found in patients with bilateral vasal agenesis in association with renal anomalies.[269] When vasal agenesis is diagnosed in childhood, renal and pelvic sonography and, if abnormal, VCUG should be performed. Vasal agenesis may be found in patients with cystic fibrosis, even when clinical evidence of the disease is absent.

Anomalies of epididymal attachment

Abnormalities of fusion or suspension of the epididymis are known to be common in patients with cryptorchidism. Turek et al[274] studied epididymal anatomy in a group of boys undergoing inguinal or scrotal exploration primarily for hydrocele and reported normal anatomy in 96%. However, two other studies have shown a higher incidence (31–39%) of mild suspension or fusion anomalies of the epididymis in boys with hernia/hydrocele, with a greater frequency in those patients with a patent processus vaginalis.[275,276] The clinical significance of partial epididymal detachment or a long looping epididymis in patients with a normally positioned testis is unclear.

Epididymal cysts

Cysts of the epididymis (spermatocele) (Figure 72.24) usually appear during puberty or adulthood and are asymptomatic. The etiology is unknown but

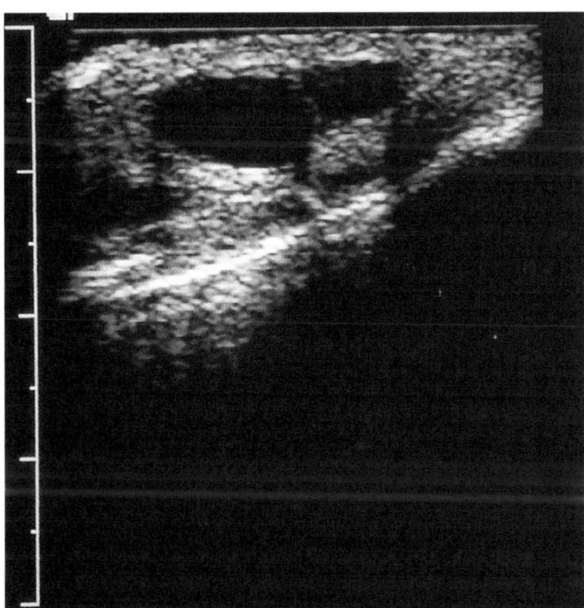

Figure 72.24 Epididymal cysts in a patient with polyorchidism.

proposed theories include dilated efferent ducts that have failed to fuse with the epididymis[269,277] and/or part of a testicular dysgenesis syndrome caused by an endocrine abnormality.[278,279] Conditions associated with a higher incidence of epididymal cysts include cryptorchidism, Von Hippel–Lindau disease and fetal exposure to diethylstilbestrol. Intervention is not usually required, but both excision[280] and sclerotherapy[281,282] have been used successfully in symptomatic patients. Two cases of torsion of an epididymal cyst have been reported.[283]

Other vasal anomalies

Ectopy of the vas deferens,[270,284,285] also called persisting mesonephric duct,[286] is characterized by ectopic insertion of the vas into the urinary tract. Most commonly, fusion of the vas and ureter occurs proximal to the bladder[287] (vasoureteric insertion), but direct entry of the vas into the bladder (vasovesical insertion) may occur. Approximately 30 cases are reported in the English literature. Proposed mechanisms include ectopic insertion of the ureteral bud and/or aberrant development of the proximal vas precursor.[270,286] Patients are asymptomatic or present with UTIs and/or epididymitis. Other congenital anomalies are common, including agenesis of the seminal vesicles, imperforate anus, hypospadias, ureteral reflux and/or ectopy, and renal anomalies. The triad of imperforate anus, hypospadias, and ectopic vas was reported in 21% of cases.[288] The diagnosis may be made by cystourethrography, retrograde ureterography, or at the time of ureteroneocystostomy. Treatment is based on anatomic findings and clinical indications.

True duplication of the vas deferens is extremely rare. Binderow et al[289] reported a single case found at the time of inguinal hernia repair in a boy with a normal urinary tract. The authors proposed wolffian duct duplication or ductal bifurcation in the region of the proximal vas precursor as the etiology.

Seminal vesicle cysts

Seminal vesicle cysts are another rare manifestation of anomalous wolffian duct development.[290–292] They may be congenital or acquired.[293] Most are associated with renal agenesis with or without ureteral ectopy. Presentation is predominantly in adulthood with pain during micturition, defecation or ejaculation, UTI, or infertility. A palpable mass is appreciated on rectal examination. The diagnosis may be confirmed by abdominal or transrectal sonogram. A computed topographic scan may be useful to visualize the semi-

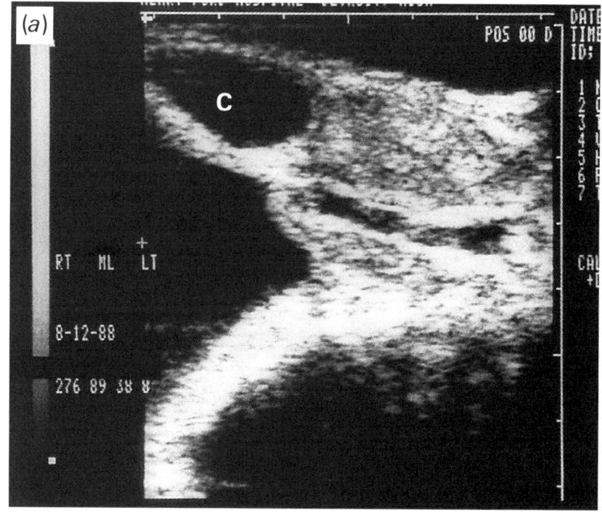

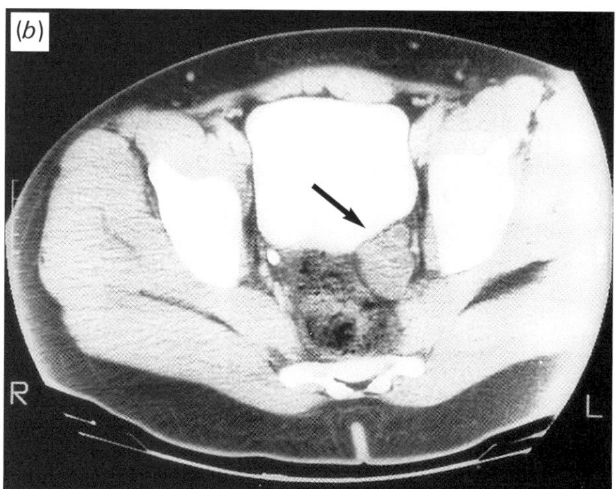

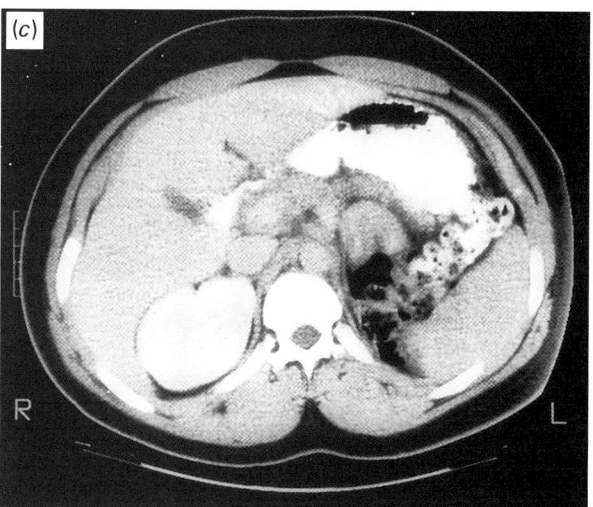

Figure 72.25 Seminal vesical cyst in an adolescent presenting with voiding symptoms and urinary tract infection: (*a*) sonogram showing a cystic structure posterior to the bladder in the left sagittal view (C); (*b*) computed tomographic (CT) scan confirming a fluid-filled structure (arrow) in the region of the left seminal vesicle; (*c*) absence of the left kidney on CT scan.

nal vesicle and confirm renal agenesis (Figure 72.25). Excision is indicated in symptomatic patients, either using an open technique, such as a transtrigonal approach,[292] or laparoscopically.[294–296]

References

1. Shapiro E. The sonographic appearance of normal and abnormal fetal genitalia. J Urol 1999; 162:530.
2. Ammini AC, Sabherwal U, Mukhopadhyay C et al. Morphogenesis of the human external male genitalia. Pediatr Surg Int 1997; 12:401–6.
3. Glenister TW. The origin and fate of the urethral plate in man. J Anat (London) 1921; 88:413–23.
4. Kurzrock EA, Baskin LS, Cunha GR. Ontogeny of the male urethra: theory of endodermal differentiation. Differentiation 1999; 64:115–22.
5. Kurzrock EA, Baskin LS, Li Y, Cunha GR. Epithelial–mesenchymal interactions in development of the mouse fetal genital tubercle. Cells Tissues Organs 1999; 164:125–30.
6. Oster J. Further fate of the foreskin: incidence of preputial adhesions, phimosis, and smegma among Danish schoolboys. Arch Dis Child 1968; 43:200–3.
7. Herzog LW, Alvarez SR. The frequency of foreskin problems in uncircumcised children. Am J Dis Child 1986; 140:254–6.
8. Kayaba H, Tamura H, Kitajima S et al. Analysis of shape and retractability of the prepuce in 603 Japanese boys. J Urol 1996; 156:1813–15.
9. Rickwood AMK. Medical indications for circumcision. BJU Int 1999; 83(Suppl 1):45–51.
10. Laumann EO, Mai CM, Zuckerman EW. Circumcision in the United States: prevalence, prophylactic effects, and sexual practice. JAMA 1997; 277:1052–7.
11. American Academy of Pediatrics: Task Force on Circumcision. Circumcision policy statement. Pediatrics 1999; 103:686–93.
12. Van Howe RS. Does circumcision influence sexually transmitted diseases? A literature review. BJU Int 1999; 83(Suppl 1):52–62.
13. Ashfield JE, Nickel KR, Siemens DR, MacNeily AE, Nickel JC. Treatment of phimosis with topical steroids in 194 children. J Urol 2003; 169:1106–8.
14. Griffiths DM, Atwell JD, Freeman NV. A prospective survey of the indications and morbidity of circumcision in children. Eur Urol 1985; 11:184–7.
15. Baskin LS, Canning DA, Snyder HM, Duckett J. Treating complications of circumcision. Pediatr Emerg Care 1996; 12:62–8.
16. Lander J, Brady-Fryer B, Metcalfe JB et al. Comparison of ring block, dorsal penile nerve block, and topical anesthesia for neonatal circumcision. A randomized clinical trial. JAMA 1997; 278:2157–62.
17. Baskin LS, Canning DA, Snyder HM, Duckett JW. Surgical repair of urethral circumcision injuries. J Urol 1997; 158:2269–71.
18. Peters K, Kass EJ. The use of electrosurgery for routine penile procedures. J Urol 1997; 157:1453–55.
19. Gearhart JP, Rock JA. Total ablation of the penis after circumcision with electrocautery: a method of management and long-term follow-up. J Urol 1989; 142:799–801.
20. Diamond M. Prenatal predisposition and the clinical management of some pediatric conditions. J Sex Marital Ther 1996; 22:139–74.
21. Persad R, Sharma S, McTavish J et al. Clinical presentation and pathophysiology of meatal stenosis following circumcision. Br J Urol 1995; 75:91–3.
22. Hensle TW. Editorial comment. J Urol 1996; 156:858–9.
23. Stenham A, Malrnfors G, Okmian L. Circumcision for phimosis: a follow-up study. Scand J Urol Nephrol 1986; 20:89–92.
24. American Academy of Pediatrics Urology Section. Urethral meatal stenosis in males. Pediatrics 1978; 61:778–80.
25. Cartwright PC, Snow BW, McNees DC. Urethral meatotomy in the office using topical EMLA cream for anesthesia. J Urol 1996; 156:857–9.
26. Oesch IL, Pinter A, Ransley PG. Penile agenesis: a report of six cases. J Pediatr Surg 1987; 22:172–4.
27. Skoog SJ, Belman AB. Aphallia: its classification and management. J Urol 1989; 141:589–92.
28. Stolar CJH, Wiener ES, Hensle TW et al. Reconstruction of penile agenesis by a posterior sagittal approach. J Pediatr 1987; 22:1076–80.
29. Hendren WH. The genetic male with absent penis and urethrorectal communication: experience with 5 patients. J Urol 1997; 157:1469–74.
30. Johnston WG Jr, Yeatman GW, Weigel JW. Congenital absence of the penis. J Urol 1977; 117:508–12.
31. Cifti AO, Senocak ME, Buyukpamukcu N. Male gender assignment in penile agenesis: a case report and review of the literature. J Pediatr Surg 1995; 30:1358–60.
32. Diamond M, Sigmundson HK. Sex reassignment at birth. Long-term review and clinical implications. Arch Pediatr Adolesc Med 1997; 151:298–304.
33. Schober JM, Carmichael PA, Hines M, Ransky PG. The ultimate challenge of cloacal exstrophy. J Urol 2002; 167:300–4.
34. Reiner WG, Kropp BP. A 7-year experience of genetic males with severe phallic inadequacy assigned female. J Urol 2004; 172:2395–8.
35. Reiner WG, Gearhart JP. Discordant sexual identity in some genetic males with cloacal exstrophy assigned to female sex at birth. N Engl J Med 2004; 350(4):333–41.
36. Gilbert DA, Jordan GH, Devine CG Jr et al. Phallic construction in prepubertal and adolescent boys. J Urol 1993; 149:1521–6.
37. Marti-Bonmati L, Menor F, Gonez J et al. Value of sonography in true complete diphallia. J Urol 1989; 142:356–7.
38. Zolfaghari A, Pourissa M, Hajialilou SH, Amjadi M. True complete diphallia. A case report. Scand J Urol Nephrol 1995; 29:233–5.
39. Hollowell JG Jr, Witherington R, Balagas AJ, Burr IN. Embryologic considerations of diphallus and associated anomalies. J Urol 1997; 117:728–32.
40. Karna P, Kapur S. Diphallus and associated anomalies with balanced autosomal chromosomal translocation. Clin Genet 1994; 46:209–11.

41. Maruyama K, Takahashi A, Kobayashi T, Hatakeyama S, Matsuo Y. Diphallia and the VATER association. J Urol 1999; 162:2144.
42. Pomerantz P, Hanna M, Levitt S, Kogan S. Isolated torsion of penis. Urology 1978; 11:37–9.
43. Ben-Ari J, Merlob P, Mimouni F, Reisner SH. Characteristics of the male genitalia in the newborn: penis. J Urol 1985; 134:521–2.
44. Fisher PC, Park JM. Penile torsion repair using dorsal dartos flap rotation. J Urol 2004; 171:1903–4.
45. Perlmutter AD, Chamberlain JW. Webbed penis without chordee. J Urol 1972; 107:320–1.
46. Redman JF. A technique for the correction of penoscrotal fusion. J Urol 1985; 133:432–3.
47. Cromie WJ, Ritchey ML, Smith RC, Zagaja GP. Anatomical alignment for the correction of buried penis. J Urol 1998; 160:1482–4.
48. Bergeson PS, Hopkin RJ, Bailey RB et al. The inconspicuous penis. Pediatrics 1993; 92:794–9.
49. Little JR. The inconspicuous or 'disappearing' penis. Pediatrics 1994; 94:240–2.
50. Herndon CDA, Casale AJ, Cain MP, Rink RC. Long-term outcome analysis of the surgical treatment of concealed penis. J Urol 2003; 170:1695–97.
51. Maizels M, Zaontz M, Donovan J et al. Surgical correction of the buried penis: description of a classification system and a technique to correct the disorder. J Urol 1986; 136:268–71.
52. Chuang J-H. Penoplasty for buried penis. J Pediatr Surg 1995; 30:1256–7.
53. Lee PA, Mzur T, Danish R et al. Micropenis. 1. Criteria, etiologies and classification. Johns Hopkins Med J 1980; 146:156–63.
54. Aaronson IA. Micropenis: medical and surgical implications. J Urol 1994; 152:4–14.
55. Sinnecker GH, Hiort O, Dibbelt L et al. Phenotypic classification of male pseudohermaphroditism due to steroid 5α-reductase deficiency. Am J Med Genet 1996; 63:223–30.
56. Quigley CA, DeBellis A, Marschke KB et al. Androgen receptor defects: historical, clinical, and molecular perspectives. Endroer Rev 1995; 16:271–321.
57. Lee PA, Danish RK, Mazur T, Migeon CJ. Micropenis. II. Primary hypogonadism, partial androgen insensitivity syndrome, and idiopathic disorders. Johns Hopkins Med J 1980; 147:175–81.
58. Money J, Lehne GK, Pierre-Jerome F. Micropenis: gender, erotosexual coping strategy, and behavioral health in nine pediatric cases followed to adulthood. Compr Psychiatry 1985; 26:29–42.
59. Kogan SJ, Williams DI. The micropenis syndrome: clinical observations and expectations for growth. J Urol 1977; 118:311–13.
60. Okuyama A, Itatani H, Aono T et al. Prognosis of sexual maturation in prepubertal boys with micropenis. Arch Androl 1980; 5:265–9.
61. Choi SK, Han SW, Kim DH, de Lignieres B. Transdermal dihydrotestosterone therapy and its effects on patients with microphallus. J Urol 1993; 150:657–60.
62. Levy JB, Husmann DA. Micropenis secondary to growth hormone deficiency: does treatment with growth hormone alone result in adequate penile growth? J Urol 1996; 156:214–16.
63. Sutherland RS, Kogan BA, Baskin LS et al. The effect of prepubertal androgen exposure on adult penile length. J Urol 1996; 156:783–7.
64. Reilly JM, Woodhouse CRJ. Small penis and the male sexual role. J Urol 1989; 142:569–71.
65. Dewan PA, Tan HL, Auldist AW, Moss DI. Priapism in childhood. Br J Urol 1989; 64:541–5.
66. Friedman J. Priapism: an unusual presentation of appendicitis. Pediatr Emerg Care 1998; 14:143–4.
67. Ramos CE, Park JS, Ritchey ML, Benson GS. High flow priapism associated with sickle cell disease. J Urol 1995; 153:1619–21.
68. Callewaert P, Stockx L, Bogaert G, Baert L. Posttraumatic high-flow priapism in a 6-year-old boy: management by percutaneous placement of bilateral vascular coils. Urology 1998; 52:134–7.
69. Tarry WF, Duckett JW Jr, Snyder HM. 3rd. Urological complications of sickle cell disease in a pediatric population. J Urol 1987; 138:592–4.
70. Hamre MR, Harmon EP, Kirkpatrick DV et al. Priapism as a complication of sickle cell disease. J Urol 1991; 145:1–5.
71. Fowler JE Jr, Koshy M, Strub M, Chinn SK. Priapism associated with the sickle cell hemoglobinopathies: prevalence, natural history and sequelae. J Urol 1991; 145:65–8.
72. Sharpsteen JR Jr, Powars D, Johnson C et al. Multisystem damage associated with tricorporal priapism in sickle cell disease. Am J Med 1993; 94:289–95.
73. Miller ST, Rao SP, Dunn EK, Glassberg KI. Priapism in children with sickle cell disease. J Urol 1995; 154:844–7.
74. Adeyoju AB, Olujohunabe AG, Morris J et al. Priapism in sickle-cell disease; incidence, risk factors and complications – an international multicentre study. BJU Int 2002; 90:898–902.
75. Maples BL, Hagemann TM. Treatment of priapism in pediatric patients with sickle cell disease. Am J Health Syst Pharm 2004; 61:355–63.
76. Seeler RA. Intensive transfusion therapy for priapism in boys with sickle cell anemia. J Urol 1978; 110:360–1.
77. Montague DK, Jarow J, Broderick GA et al. American Urological Association guideline on the management of priapism. J Urol 2003; 170:1318–24.
78. Siegel JF, Rich MA, Brack WA. Association of sickle cell disease, priapism, exchange transfusion and neurological events: ASPEN syndrome, J Urol 1993; 150:1480–2.
79. Chakrabarty A, Upadhyay J, Dhabuwala CB et al. Priapism associated with sickle cell hemoglobinopathy in children: long-term effects on potency. J Urol 1996; 155:1419–23.
80. Bochinski DJ, Deng DY, Lue TF. Management of priapism. AUA Update Ser 2004; 23:17–23
81. Mykulak DJ, Glassberg KI. Impotence following childhood priapism. J Urol 1990; 144:134–5.
82. Emond AM, Holman R, Hayes RJ, Serjeant GR. Priapism and impotence in homozygous sickle cell disease. Arch Intern Med 1980; 140:1434–7.
83. Noe HN, Wilimas J, Jerkins GR. Surgical management of priapism in children with sickle cell anemia. J Urol 1981; 126:770–1.

84. Virag R, Bachir D, Lee K, Galacteros F. Preventive treatment of priapism in sickle cell disease with oral and self-administered intracavernous injection of etilefrine. Urology 1996; 47:777–81.
85. Okpala I, Westerdale N, Jegede T et al. Etilefrine for the prevention of priapism in adult sickle cell disease. Br J Haematol 2002; 118:918–21.
86. Al Jam'a AH, Al Dabbous IA. Hydroxyurea in the treatment of sickle cell associated priapism. J Urol 1998; 159:1642.
87. Bialecki ES, Bridges KR. Sildenafil relieves priapism in patients with sickle cell disease. Am J Med 2002; 113:252.
88. Levine LA, Guss SP. Gonadotropin-releasing hormone analogues in the treatment of sickle cell anemia-associated priapism. J Urol 1993; 150:475–7.
89. Dahm P, Rao DS, Donatucci CF. Antiandrogens in the treatment of priapism. Urology 2002; 59:138.
90. Walker JR, Casale AJ. Prolonged penile erection in the newborn. Urology 1997; 50:796–9.
91. Wright JE. Congenital absence of the scrotum: case report and description of an original technique of construction of a scrotum. J Pediatr Surg 1993; 28:264–6.
92. Verga G, Avolio L. Agenesis of the scrotum: an extremely rare anomaly. J Urol 1996; 156:1467.
93. Montero M, Mendez R, Tellado M et al. Agenesis of the scrotum. Pediatr Dermatol 2001; 18:141–2.
94. Sule JD, Skoog SJ, Tank ES. Perineal lipoma and the accessory labioscrotal fold: an etiological relationship. J Urol 1994; 151:475–7.
95. Ratan SK, Rattan KN, Schgal T, Ratan J. Perineal accessory scrotum. Ind J Pediatr 2003; 70:679–80.
96. Coplen DE, Mikkelsen D, Manley CB. Accessory scrotum located on the distal penile shaft. J Urol 1995; 154:1908.
97. Spears T, Franco I, Reda EF et al. Accessory and ectopic scrotum with VATER association. Urology 1992; 40:343–5.
98. Lamm DL, Kaplan GW. Accessory and ectopic scrota. Urology 1977; 9:149–53.
99. Elder JS, Jeffs RD. Suprainguinal ectopic scrotum and associated anomalies. J Urol 1982; 127:336–8.
100. Hoar RM, Calvano CJ, Reddy PP et al. Unilateral suprainguinal ectopic scrotum: the role of the gubernaculum in the formation of an ectopic scrotum. Teratology 1998; 57:64–9.
101. Chowdhary SK, Suri S, Narasimhan KL, Rao KL. Ectopic scrotum and patent urachus. Pediatr Surg Int 2001; 17:75–6.
102. Parida SK, Hall BD, Barton L, Fujimoto A. Penoscrotal transposition and associated anomalies: report of five new cases and review of the literature. Am J Med Genet 1995; 59:68–75.
103. Bartsch O, Kuhnle U, Wu LL et al. Evidence for a critical region for penoscrotal inversion, hypospadias, and imperforate anus within chromosomal region 13q32.2q34. Am J Med Genet 1996; 65:218–21.
104. Glenn JF, Anderson EE. Surgical correction of incomplete penoscrotal transposition. J Urol 1973; 110:603–5.
105. Levy JB, Darson MF, Bite U, Kramer SA. Modified pudendal–thigh flap for correction of penoscrotal transposition. Urology 1997; 50:597–600.
106. Sadler BT, Greenfield SP, Wan J, Glick PL. Intrascrotal epidermoid cyst with extension into the pelvis. J Urol 1995; 153:1265–6.
107. LeVasseur JG, Perry VE. Perineal median raphe cyst. Pediatr Dermatol 1997; 14:391–2.
108. Rattan J, Rattan S, Gupta DK. Epidermoid cyst of the penis with extension into the pelvis. J Urol 1997; 158:593.
109. Steeno O, Knops J, Declerk L et al. Prevention of fertility disorders by detection and treatment of varicocele at school and college age. Andrologia 1976; 8:47–53.
110. Oster J. Varicocele in children and adolescents. An investigation of the incidence among Danish school children. Scand J Urol Nephrol 1971; 5:27–32.
111. Dubin L, Amelar RD. Varicocelectomy as therapy in male infertility: a study of 504 cases. J Urol 1975; 113:640–1.
112. Dubin L, Amelar RD. Varicocele size and results of varicocelectomy in selected subfertile men with varicocele. Fertil Steril 1970; 21:606–9.
113. Fariss BL, Fenner DK, Plymate SR et al. Seminal characteristics in the presence of a varicocele as compared with those of expectant fathers and prevasectomy men. Fertil Steril 1981; 35:325–7.
114. Szabo R, Kessler R. Hydrocele following internal spermatic vein ligation: a retroperitoneal study and review of the literature. J Urol 1984; 132:924–5.
115. Tinga DJ, Jager S, Bruijnen CL, Kremer J, Mensink HJ. Factors related to semen improvement and fertility after varicocele operation. Fertil Steril 1984; 41:404–10.
116. Steckel J, Dicker AP, Goldstein M. Relationship between varicocele size and response to varicocelectomy. J Urol 1993; 149:769–71.
117. Sigman M, Jarow JP. Ipsilateral testicular hypertrophy is associated with decreased sperm counts in infertile men with varicoceles. J Urol 1997; 158:605–7.
118. Johnson L, Petty CS, Neaves WE. A comparative study of daily sperm production and testicular composition in humans and rats. Biol Reprod 1980; 22:1233–43.
119. Rey RA, Campo SM, Bedecarras P et al. Is infancy a quiescent period of testicular development? Histological, morphometric, and functional study of the seminiferous tabules of the cebus monkey from birth to end of puberty. J Clin Endocrinol Metab 1993; 76:1325–31.
120. Haans LC, Laven JS, Mali WP et al. Testis volumes, semen quality and hormonal patterns in adolescents with and without a varicocele. Fertil Steril 1991; 56:731–6.
121. Zorgniotti AW, MacLeod J. Studies in temperature, human semen quality and varicocele. Fertil Steril 1973; 24:854–63.
122. Robinson P, Rock J, Menkin MF. Control of human spermatogenesis by induced changes of intrascrotal temperature. JAMA 1968; 204:290–7.
123. Amelar RD, Dubin L. Right varicocelectomy in selected infertile patients who have failed to improve after previous left varicocelectomy. Fertil Steril 1987; 47:833–7.
124. Levine RJ, Mathew RM, Chenault CB et al. Differences in the quality of semen in outdoor workers during summer and winter. N Engl J Med 1990; 323:12–16.
125. Agger P. Scrotal and testicular temperature: its relation to sperm count before and after operation for varicocele. Fertil Steril 1971; 22:286–97.

126. Kass EJ, Salisz JA. The significance of scrotal temperature elevation in an adolescent with a varicocele. In: Zorgniotti AW, ed. Temperature and Environmental Effects on the Testis. New York: Plenum Press, 1991: 245–51.
127. Charney CW. Effect of varicocele on fertility. Fertil Steril 1962; 13:47.
128. Ibrahim AA, Awad HA, El-Haggar S, Mitawi BA. Bilateral testicular biopsy in men with varicocele. Fertil Steril 1977; 28:663–7.
129. Wang Y-X, Lei C, Dong S-G et al. Study of bilateral histology and meiotic analysis in men undergoing varicocele ligation. Fertil Steril 1991; 55:152–5.
130. Hienz HA, Voggenthaler J, Weissbach L. Histological findings in testes with varicocele during childhood and their therapeutic consequences. Eur J Pediatr 1980; 133: 139–46.
131. Kass EJ, Chandra RS, Belman AB. Testicular histology in the adolescent with a varicocele. Pediatrics 1987; 79:996–8.
132. Hadziselimovic F, Leibundgut B, Da Rugna D, Buser MW. The value of testicular biopsy in patients with varicocele. J Urol 1986; 135:707–10.
133. Hadziselimovic F, Herzog B, Jenny P. The chance for fertility in adolescent boys after corrective surgery for varicocele. J Urol 1995; 154:731–3.
134. Hadziselimovic F, Herzog B, Liebundgut B, Jenny P, Buser M. Testicular and vascular changes in children and adults with varicocele. J Urol 1989; 142:583–5.
135. Weiss DB, Rodriguez-Rigau LJ, Smith KD, Steinberger E. Leydig cell function in oligospermatic men with varicocele. J Urol 1978; 120:427–30.
136. Ando S, Giacchetto C, Bealdi E et al. The influence of age on Leydig cell function in patients with varicocele. Int J Androl 1982; 7:104–18.
137. Spera G, Medolago-Albani L, Coia L et al. Histological, histochemical, and ultrastructural aspects of interstitial tissue from the contralateral testis in infertile men with monolateral varicocele. Arch Androl 1983; 10:73–8.
138. Su L, Goldstein M, Schlegel PN. The effect of varicocelectomy on serum testosterone levels in infertile men with varicoceles. J Urol 1995; 154:1752–5.
139. Nagao RR, Plymate SR, Berger RE et al. Comparison of gonadal function between fertile and infertile men with varicoceles. Fertil Steril 1986; 46:930–3.
140. Hudson RW, Perez-Marrero RA, Crawford VA, McKay DE. Hormonal parameters of men with varicoceles before and after varicocelectomy. Fertil Steril 1985; 43:905–10.
141. Bickel A, Dickstein G. Factors predicting the outcome of varicocele repair for subfertility: the value of the luteinizing hormone-releasing hormone test. J Urol 1989; 142:1230–4.
142. Fujisawa M, Hayashi A, Imanishi O et al. The significance of gonadotropin-releasing hormone test for predicting fertility after varicocelectomy. Fertil Steril 1994; 61:779–82.
143. Atikeler K, Yeni E, Semercioz A et al. The value of the gonadotropin-releasing hormone test as a prognostic factor in infertile patients with varicocele. Br J Urol 1996; 78:632–4.
144. Bablok L, Czaplicki M, Fracki S et al. Relationship between semen quality improvements after varicocelectomy and preoperative levels of hypophyseal and gonadal hormones. Int Urol Nephrol 1997; 29:345–9.
145. Lipshultz LI, Caminos-Torres R, Greenspan CS, Snyder PJ. Testicular function after orchiopexy for unilaterally undescended testis. N Engl J Med 1976; 295:15–18.
146. Dickerman Z, Landman J, Prager-Lewin R, Laron Z. Evaluation of testicular function in prepubertal boys by means of the luteinizing hormone-releasing hormone test. Fertil Steril 1978; 29:655.
147. Kass EJ, Freitas JE, Salisz JA, Steinert BW. Pituitary gonadal dysfunction in adolescents with varicocele. Urology 1993; 42:179–81.
148. Barwell R. One hundred cases of varicocele treated by the subcutaneous wire loop. Lancet 1978.
149. Kass EJ, Belman AB. Reversal of testicular growth failure by varicocele ligation. J Urol 1987; 137:475–6.
150. Laven JD, Haans LCF, Mali WPTh et al. Effects of varicocele treatment in adolescents: a randomised study. Fertil Steril 1992; 58:756–62.
151. Yamamoto M, Katsuno S, Yokoi K et al. The effect of varicocelectomy on testicular volume in infertile patients with varicoceles. Nagoya J Med Sci 1995; 58:47–50.
152. Vasavada S, Ross J, Nasrallah P, Kay R. Prepubertal varicoceles. Urology 1997; 50:774–7.
153. Salzhauer EW, Sokol A, Glassberg KI. Paternity after adolescent varicocele repair. Pediatrics 2004; 114:1631–3.
154. Zachmann M, Prader A, Kind HP et al. Testicular volume during adolescence: cross-sectional and longitudinal studies. Helv Paediatr Acta 1974; 29:61–72.
155. Daniel WA, Feinstein RA, Howard-Peebles P, Baxley WD. Testicular volumes of adolescents. J Pediatr 1982; 101:1009–12.
156. Behre HM, Nashan D, Nieschlag E. Objective measurement of testicular volume by ultrasonography: evaluation of the technique and comparison with orchidometer estimates. Int J Androl 1989; 12:395–403.
157. Janczewski Z, Bablok L. Semen characteristics in pubertal boys. Semen quality after first ejaculation. Arch Androl 1985; 15:199–205.
158. Cayan S, Akbay E, Bozlu M et al. The effect of varicocele repair on testicular volume in children and adolescents with varicocele. J Urol 2002; 168:731–4.
159. Okuyama A, Nakamura M, Namiki M et al. Surgical repair of varicocele at puberty: preventive treatment for fertility improvement. J Urol 1988; 139:562–4.
160. Paduch DA, Niedzielski J. Repair versus observation in adolescent varicocele: a prospective study. J Urol 1997; 158:1128–32.
161. Lenzi A, Gandini L, Bagolan P et al. Sperm parameters after early left varicocele treatment. Fertil Steril 1998; 69:347–9.
162. Hosli PO. Varicocele – results after early treatment in children and adolescents. Z Kinderchir 1988; 43:213–15.
163. Belloli G, D'Agostino S, Zen F, Ioverno E. Fertility rates after successful correction of varicocele in adolescence and adulthood. Eur J Pediatr Surg 1995; 5:216–18.
164. Sayfan J, Siplovich L, Koltun L, Benyamin N. Varicocele treatment in pubertal boys prevents testicular growth arrest. J Urol 1997; 157:1456–7.

165. Kass EJ, Freitas JE, Bour JB. Adolescent varicocele: objective indications for treatment. J Urol 1989; 142:579–82.
166. Mandressi A, Buizza C, Antonelli D, Chisnea S. Is laparoscopy a worthy method to treat varicocele? Comparison between 160 cases of two-port laparoscopic and 120 cases of open inguinal spermatic vein ligation. J Endourol 1996; 10:435–41.
167. Abdulmaaboud MR, Shokeir AA, Forage Y et al. Treatment of varicocele: a comparative study of conventional open surgery, percutaneous retrograde sclerotherapy, and laparoscopy. Urology 1998; 52:294–300.
168. Lenz M, Hof N, Kersting-Sommerhoff B, Bauer W. Anatomic variants of the spermatic vein: importance for percutaneous sclerotherapy of idiopathic varicocele. Radiology 1996; 198:425–31.
169. Punekar SV, Prem AR, Ridhorkar VR et al. Post-surgical recurrent varicocele: efficacy of internal spermatic venography and steel-coil embolization. Br J Urol 1996; 77:124–8.
170. Perala JM, Leinonen SAS, Suramo IJI, Hellstrom PA, Seppanen EJ. Comparison of early deflation rate of detachable latex and silicone balloons and observations on persistent varicocele. J Vasc Interv Radiol 1998; 9:761–5.
171. Lord DJ, Burrows PE. Pediatric varicocele embolization. Tech Vasc Interv Radiol 2003; 6:169–75.
172. Miersch WDE, Schoeneich G, Winter P, Buszello H. Laparoscopic varicocelectomy: indication, technique and surgical results. Br J Urol 1995; 76:636–8.
173. Belloli G, Musi L, D'Agostino S. Laparoscopic surgery for adolescent varicocele: preliminary report on 80 patients. J Pediatr Surg 1996; 31:1488–90.
174. Humphrey GME, Najmaldin AS. Laparoscopy in the management of pediatric varicoceles. J Pediatr Surg 1997; 32:1470–2.
175. Kattan S. Incidence and pattern of varicocele recurrence after laparoscopic ligation of the internal spermatic vein with preservation of the testicular artery. Scand J Urol Nephrol 1998; 32:335–40.
176. Koyle MA, Oottamasathien S, Barqawi A, Rajimwale A, Furness PD 3rd. Laparoscopic Palomo varicocele ligation in children and adolescents: results of 103 cases. J Urol 2004; 172:1749–52.
177. Ivanissevich O. Left varicocele due to reflux; experience with 4,470 operative cases in forty-two years. J Int Coll Surg 1918; 34:742.
178. Atassi O, Kass EJ, Steinert BW. Testicular growth after successful varicocele correction in adolescents: comparison of artery-sparing techniques with the Palomo procedure. J Urol 1995; 153:482–3.
179. Palomo A. Radical cure of varicocele by a new technique: preliminary report. J Urol 1949; 61:604.
180. Hsu TH, Huang JK, Ho DM et al. Role of the spermatic artery in spermatogenesis and sex hormone synthesis. Arch Androl 1993; 31:191–7.
181. Parrott TS, Hewatt L. Ligation of the testicular artery and vein in adolescent varicocele. J Urol 1994; 152:791–3.
182. Stern R, Kistler W, Scharli AF. The Palomo procedure in the treatment of boys with varicocele: a retrospective study of testicular growth and fertility. Pediatr Surg Int 1998; 14:74–8.
183. Kass EJ, Marcol B. Results of varicocele surgery in adolescents: a comparison of techniques. J Urol 1992; 148:694–6.
184. Minevich E, Wacksman J, Lewis AG, Sheldon CA. Inguinal microsurgical varicocelectomy in the adolescent: technique and preliminary results. J Urol 1998; 159:1022–4.
185. Marmar JL, Kim Y. Subinguinal microsurgical varicocelectomy: a technical critique and statistical analysis of semen and pregnancy data. J Urol 1994; 152:1127–32.
186. Goldstein M, Gilbert BR, Dicker AP et al. Microsurgical inguinal varicocelectomy with delivery of the testis: an artery and lymphatic sparing technique. J Urol 1992; 148:1808–11.
187. Lima M, Domini M, Libri M. The varicocele in pediatric age: 207 cases treated with microsurgical technique. Eur J Pediatr Surg 1997; 7:30–3.
188. Lemack GE, Uzzo RG, Schlegel PN, Goldstein M. Microsurgical repair of the adolescent varicocele. J Urol 1998; 160:179–81.
189. Caesar RE, Kaplan GW. The incidence of the cremasteric reflex in normal boys. J Urol 1994; 152:779–80.
190. Rabinowitz R. The importance of the cremasteric reflex in acute scrotal swelling in children. J Urol 1984; 132:89–90.
191. Kass EJ, Stone KT, Cacciarelli AA, Mitchell B. Do all children with an acute scrotum require exploration? J Urol 1993; 150:667–9.
192. al Mufti RA, Ogedegbe AK, Lafferty K. The use of Doppler ultrasound in the clinical management of acute testicular pain. Br J Urol 1995; 76:625–7.
193. Lewis AG, Bukowski TP, Jarvis PD et al. Evaluation of acute scrotum in the emergency department. J Pediatr Surg 1995; 30:277–82.
194. Watkin NA, Reiger NA, Moisey CU. Is the conservative management of the acute scrotum justified on clinical grounds? Br J Urol 1996; 78:623–7.
195. Deeg KH, Wild F. Colour Doppler imaging – a new method to differentiate torsion of the spermatic cord and epididymo-orchitis. Eur J Pediatr 1990; 149:253–5.
196. Dewire DM, Begun FP, Lawson RK et al. Color Doppler ultrasonography in the evaluation of the acute scrotum. J Urol 1992; 147:89–91.
197. Wilbert DM, Schaerfe CW, Stren WD et al. Evaluation of the acute scrotum by color-coded Doppler ultrasonography. J Urol 1993; 149:1475–7.
198. Brown JM, Hammers LW, Barton JW et al. Quantitative Doppler assessment of acute scrotal inflammation. Radiology 1995; 197:427–31.
199. Kass EJ, Lundak B. The acute scrotum. Pediatr Clin North Am 1997; 44(5):1251–66.
200. Stone KT, Kass EJ, Cacciarelli AA, Gibson DP. Management of suspected antenatal torsion: what is the best strategy? J Urol 1995; 153:782–4.
201. Siegel A, Snyder H, Duckett JW. Epididymitis in infants and boys: underlying urogenital anomalies and efficacy of imaging modalities. J Urol 1987; 138:1100–3.
202. Gordon LM, Stein SM, Ralls PW. Traumatic epididymitis: evaluation with color Doppler sonography. AJR Am J Roentgenol 1996; 116:1323–5.

203. Wara DW, Emery HM. Collagen vascular diseases. In: Rudolph AM, ed. Rudolph's Pediatrics, 19th edn. Norwalk, CT: Appleton & Lange, 1991:490–1.
204. Heyns CF. The gubernaculum during testicular descent in the human fetus. J Anat 1987; 153:93–112.
205. Rowe MI, Copelson LW, Clatworthy HW. The patent processes vaginalis and the inguinal hernia. J Pediatr Surg 1969; 4:102–7.
206. Bronsther B, Abrams MW, Elboim C. Inguinal hernias in children – a study of 1000 cases and a review of the literature. J Am Med Women's Assoc 1972; 27:522–35.
207. Clarnette TD, Lam SKL, Hutson JM. Ventriculo-peritoneal shunts in children reveal the natural history of closure of the processus vaginalis. J Pediatr Surg 1998; 33:413–16.
208. Miltenburg DM, Nuchtern JG, Jaksic T et al. Laparoscopic evaluation of the pediatric inguinal hernia – a meta-analysis. J Pediatr Surg 1998; 33:874–9.
209. Miltenburg DM, Nuchtern JG, Jaksic T et al. Meta-analysis of the risk of metachronous hernia in infants and children. Am J Surg 1997; 174:741–4.
210. Skoog SJ, Conlin MJ. Pediatric hernias and hydroceles. Urol Clin North Am 1995; 22:119–30.
211. Lord PH. A bloodless operation for the radical cure of idiopathic hydrocele. Br J Surg 1964; 51:914.
212. Bloom DA, Wan J, Key D. Disorders of the male external genitalia and inguinal canal. In: Kelalis PP, King LR, Belman AB, eds. Clinical Pediatric Urology, 3rd edn. Philadelphia: WB Saunders, 1992:1015–49.
213. Atwell JD. Inguinal hernia in female infants and children. Br J Surg 1962; 50:294–7.
214. Popek EJ. Embryonal remants in inguinal hernia sacs. Hum Pathol 1990; 21:339–49.
215. Gill B, Favale D, Kogan SJ et al. Significance of accessory ductal structures in hernia sacs. J Urol 1992; 148:697–8.
216. Rodman JF. Cystectomy: a catastrophic complication of herniorrhaphy. J Urol 1985; 133:97–8.
217. Morecroft JA, Stringer MD, Higgins M et al. Follow-up after inguinal herniotomy or surgery for hydrocele in boys. Br J Surg 1993; 80:1613–14.
218. Puri P, Guiney EJ, O'Donell B. Inguinal hernia in infants: the fate of the testis following incarceration. J Petiatr Surg 1984; 19:44–6.
219. Serels S, Kogan S, Bilateral giant abdominoscrotal hydroceles in childhood. Urology 1996; 47:763–5.
220. Gentile DP, Rabinowitz R, Hulbert WC. Abdominoscrotal hydrocele in infancy. Urology 1998; 51(Suppl 5A):20–2.
221. Mohamed AA, Stockdale EJ, Varghese J, Youngson GG. Abdominoscrotal hydrocoeles: little place for conservatism. Pediatr Surg Int 1998; 13:186–8.
222. Chamberlain SA, Kirsch AJ, Thall EH et al. Testicular dysmorphism associated with abdominoscrotal hydroceles during infancy. Urology 1995; 46:881–2.
223. Belman AB. Abdomenoscrotal hydrocele in infancy. Review and presentation of scrotal approach for correction. J Urol 2001; 165:225.
224. Turek PJ, Ewalt DH, Snyder HM et al. The absent cryptorchid testis: surgical findings and their implications for diagnosis and etiology. J Urol 1994; 151:718–21.
225. Merry C, Sweeney B, Puri P. The vanishing testis: anatomical and histological findings. Eur Urol 1997; 31:65–7.
226. Cendron M, Schned AR, Ellsworth PI. Histological evaluation of the testicular nubbin in the vanishing testis syndrome. J Urol 1998; 160:1161–2, discussion 1163.
227. Huff DS, Wu H-Y, Snyder HM et al. Evidence in favor of the mechanical (intrauterine torsion) theory over the endocrinopathy (cryptorchidism) theory in the pathogenesis of testicular agenesis. J Urol 1991; 146:630–1.
228. Gong M, Geary ES, Shortliffe LMD. Testicular torsion with contralateral vanishing testis. Urology 1996; 48:306–7.
229. Lustig RH, Conte FA, Kogan BA, Grumbach MM. Ontogeny of gonadotropin secretion in congenital anorchism: sexual dimorphism versus syndrome of gonadal dysgenesis and diagnostic considerations. J Urol 1987; 138:587–91.
230. Huff DS, Snyder HM, Hadziselimovic F et al. An absent testis is associated with contralateral testicular hypertrophy. J Urol 1992; 148:627–8.
231. Palmer LS, Gill B, Kogan SJ. Endocrine analysis of childhood monorchism. J Urol 1997; 158:594–6.
232. Lee MM, Donahoe PK, Silverman BL et al. Measurements of serum müllerian inhibiting substance in the evaluation of children with nonpalpable gonads. N Engl J Med 1997; 336:1480–6.
233. Thum G. Polyorchidism: case report and review of the literature. J Urol 1991; 145:370–2.
234. Merida MG, Miguelez C, Galiano E, Lopez Perez GA. Polyorchidism: an exceptional case of three homolateral testes. Eur Urol 1992; 21:338–9.
235. Lawrentschuk N, MacGregor RJ. Polyorchidism: a case report and review of the literature. Aust N Z J Surg 2004; 74:1130–2.
236. Heyns CF. Exstrophy of the testis. J Urol 1990; 144:724–5.
237. Gupta DK, Bajpai M, Rattan S. Testicular exstrophy: bilateral presentation in a newborn. J Urol 1997; 158:599.
238. Golladay ES, Redman JF. Transverse testicular ectopia. Urology 1982; 14:181–6.
239. Gauderer MWL, Grisoni ER, Stellato TA et al. Transverse testicular ectopia. J Pediatr Surg 1982; 17:43–7.
240. Gornall PG, Pender DJ. Crossed testicular ectopia detected by laparoscopy. Br J Urol 1987; 59:283.
241. Balaji KC, Diamond DA. Laparoscopic diagnosis and management of transverse testicular ectopia. Urology 1995; 46:879–80.
242. Hafez AT, Khoury AE. Crossed ectopic testis: another factor favouring laparoscopy for the impalpable testis. BJU Int 2001; 87:414.
243. Dean GE, Shah SK. Laparoscopically assisted correction of transverse testicular ectopia. J Urol 2002; 167:1817.
244. Karaman MI, Gonzales ET. Splenogonadal fusion: report of 2 cases and review of the literature. J Urol 1996; 155:309–11.
245. Balaji KC, Caldamone AA, Rabinowitz R et al. Splenogonadal fusion. J Urol 1996; 156:854–6.
246. Cortes D, Thorup JM, Visfeldt J. The pathogenesis of cryptorchidism and splenogonadal fusion: a new hypothesis. Br J Urol 1996; 77:285–90.
247. McPherson F, Frias JL, Spicer D, Opitz JM, Gilbert-Barness EF. Splenogonadal fusion-limb defect 'syndrome'

and associated malformations. Am J Med Genet A 2003; 120:518–22.
248. Ferro F, Lais A, Boldrini R et al. Hepatogonadal fusion. J Pediatr Surg 1996; 31:435–6.
249. Schonfeld WA. Primary and Secondary sexual characteristics. Study of their development in males from birth through maturity, with biometric study of penis and testes. Am J Dis Child 1943; 539–49.
250. Fujieda K, Matsuura N. Growth and maturation in the male genitalia from birth to adolescence. 1. Change of testicular volume. Acta Paediatr Jpn 1987; 29:214–19.
251. Nisula BC, Loriaux DL, Sherins RJ, Kulin HE. Benign bilateral testicular enlargement. J Clin Endocrinol Metab 1974; 38:440–5.
252. Lee PE, Marshall FF, Greco JM, Jeffs RD. Unilateral testicular hypertrophy: an apparently benign occurrence without cryptorchidism. J Urol 1982; 127:329–31.
253. Laron Z, Dickerman Z, Ritterman I, Kaufman H. Follow-up of boys with unilateral compensatory testicular hypertrophy. Fertil Steril 1980; 33:297–301.
254. Simko A, Hornstein L, Sonkop S, Bagumery N. Fragile X syndrome: recognition in young children. Pediatrics 1989; 83:547–52.
255. Lindsay S, Splitt M, Edney S et al. PPM-X: a new X-linked mental retardation syndrome with psychosis, pyramidal signs, and macroorchidism maps to Xq28. Am J Hum Genet 1996; 58:1120–6.
256. Rutgers JL, Young RH, Scully RE. The testicular 'tumor' of the adrenogenital syndrome: a report of six cases and review of the literature on testicular masses in patients with adrenocortical disorders. Am J Surg Pathol 1988; 12:503–13.
257. Kletter GB, Kelch RP. Disorders of puberty in boys. Endocrinol Metab Clin North Am 1993; 22:455–77.
258. Furness PD, Husmann DA, Brock JW. Multi-institutional study of testicular microlithiasis in childhood: a benign or premalignant condition? J Urol 1998; 160:1151–4.
259. Renshaw AA. Testicular calcifications: incidence, histology and proposed pathological criteria for testicular microlithiosis. J Urol 1998; 160:1625–8.
260. Backus ML, Mack LA, Middleton WD et al. Testicular microlithiasis: imaging appearances and pathologic correlation. Radiology 1994; 192:781–5.
261. Hobarth K, Susani M, Szabo N, Kratzik C. Incidence of testicular microlithiasis. Urology 1992; 40:464–7.
262. Peterson AC, Bauman JM, Light DE, McMann LP, Costabile RA. The prevalence of testicular microlithiasis in an asymptomatic population of men 10 to 35 years old. J Urol 2001; 166:2061–4.
263. Wasniewska M, De Luca F, Bertelloni S et al. Testicular microlithiasis: an unreported feature of McCune–Albright syndrome in males. J Pediatr 2004; 145:670–2.
264. Nistal M, Paniagua R, Dfez-Pardo JA. Testicular microlithiasis in 2 children with bilateral cryptorchidism. J Urol 1979; 121:535–7.
265. Bonnet JP, Aigrain Y, Ferkadji L. Cystic dysplasia of the testis with ipsilateral renal agenesis. A case report and review of the literature. Eur J Pediatr Surg 1997; 7:57–9.
266. Wojcik LJ, Hansen K, Diamond DA et al. Cystic dysplasia of the rete testis: a benign congenital lesion associated with ipsilateral urological abnormalities. J Urol 1997; 158:600–4.
267. Camassei FD, Francalanci P, Ferro F, Capozza N, Boldrini R. Cystic dysplasia of the rete testis: report of two cases and review of the literature. Pediatr Dev Pathol 2002; 5:206–10.
268. Cimador M, Rosone G, Castagnetti M et al. [Cystic dysplasia of rete testis associated with ipsilateral renal agenesis. Case report] Minerva Pediatr 2003; 55:175–9. [Italian]
269. Vohra S, Morgentaler A. Congenital anomalies of the vas deferens, epididymis and seminal vesicles. Urology 1997; 49:313–21.
270. Gibbons MD, Cromie WJ, Duckett JW. Ectopic vas deferens. J Urol 1978; 120:597–604.
271. Charney CW, Gillenwater JY. Congenital absence of the vas deferens. J Urol 1965; 93:399–401.
272. Donahue RE, Fauver HE. Unilateral absence of the vas deferens. A useful clinical sign. JAMA 1989; 261:1180–2.
273. Anguiano A, Oates RD, Amos JA et al. Congenital bilateral absence of the vas deferens: a primarily genital form of cystic fibrosis. JAMA 1992; 267:1794–7.
274. Turek PJ, Ewalt DH, Snyder HM, Duckett JW. Normal epididymal anatomy in boys. J Urol 1994; 151:726–7.
275. Elder J. Epididymal anomalies associated with hydrocele/hernia and cryptorchidism: implications regarding testicular descent. J Urol 1992; 148:624–6.
276. Barthold JS, Redman JF. Association of epididymal anomalies with patent processus vaginalis in hernia, hydrocele and cryptorchidism. J Urol 1996; 156:2054–6.
277. Comiter CV, Bruning CO III, Morgentaler A. Detached ciliary tufts in the epididymis: a lesson in applied anatomy. Urology 1995; 46:740–2.
278. Skakkebaek NE, Rajpert-DeMeyts E, Main KM. Testicular dysgenesis syndrome: an increasingly common developmental disorder with environmental aspects. Hum Reprod 2001; 16:972.
279. Homayoon K, Suhre CD, Steinhardt GF. Epididymal cysts in children: natural history. J Urol 2004; 171:1274–6.
280. Padmore DE, Norman RW, Millard OH. Analyses of indications for and outcomes of epididymectomy. J Urol 1996; 156:95–6.
281. Daehlin L, Tonder B, Kapstad L. Comparison of polidocanol and tetracycline in the sclerotherapy of testicular hydrocele and epididymal cyst. Br J Urol 1997; 80:468–71.
282. Pieri S, Agresti P, Morucci M, Carnabuci A, De Medici L. A therapeutic alternative in the treatment of epididymal cysts: percutaneous sclerotherapy. Radiol Med (Torino) 2003; 105:462–70.
283. Yilmaz E, Batislam E, Bozdogan O, Basar H, Basar MM. Torsion of an epididymal cyst. Int J Urol 2004; 11:182–3.
284. Nesbitt JA, King LR. Ectopia of the vas deferens. J Pediatr Surg 1990; 25:335–8.
285. Kriss VM, Miller SD, McRoberts WJ. Ectopia of the vas deferens. Pediatr Radiol 1995; 25:381–2.
286. Schwartz R, Stephens FD. The persisting mesonephric duct: high junction of vas deferens and ureter. J Urol 1978; 120:592–6.

287. Borger JA, Belman AB. Uretero-vas deferens anastomosis associated with imperforate anus: an embryologically predictable occurrence. J Pediatr Surg 1975; 10:255–7.
288. Hicks CM, Skoog SJ, Done S. Ectopic vas deferens, imperforate anus and hypospadias: a new triad. J Urol 1989; 141:586–8.
289. Binderow SR, Shah KD, Dolgin SE. True duplication of the vas deferens. J Pediatr Surg 1993; 28:269–70.
290. Fuselier HA, Peters DH. Cyst of seminal vesicle with ipsilateral renal agenesis and ectopic ureter: case report. J Urol 1976; 116:833–5.
291. Roehrborn CG, Schneider H-J, Rugerdorff EW, Hamann W. Embryological and diagnostic aspects of seminal vesicle cysts associated with upper urinary tract malformation. J Urol 1986; 135:1029–32.
292. Zaontz MR, Kass EJ. Ectopic ureter opening into seminal vesicle cyst associated with ipsilateral renal agenesis. Urology 1987; 24:523–5.
293. Patel B, Gujral S, Jefferson K, Evans S, Persad R. Seminal vesicle cysts and associated anomalies. BJU Int 2002; 90:265–71.
294. Carmignani G, Gallucci M, Puppo P et al. Video laparoscopic excision of a seminal vesicle cyst associated with ipsilateral renal agenesis. J Urol 1995; 153:437–9.
295. Valla JS, Carfagna L, Tursini S et al. Congenital seminal vesicle cyst: prenatal diagnosis and postnatal laparoscopic excision with an attempt to preserve fertility. BJU Int 2003; 91:891–2.
296. Basillote JB, Shanberg AM, Woo D et al. Laparoscopic excision of a seminal vesicle cyst in a child. J Urol 2004; 171:369–71.

Hernia, hydroceles, testicular torsion, and varicocele

73

Hiep T Nguyen

Problems associated with the testis such as hernia/hydrocele, testicular torsion, and varicocele are common in infants and children. Although these diagnoses can be difficult to make at times, problems associated with the testes mandate accurate and prompt recognition in order to prevent potential testicular damage or loss. Management options are often diverse and controversial, requiring the clinician to be aware of these issues in counseling the patients or their parents. These conditions can be corrected surgically, but there may be long-term consequences such as testicular atrophy and infertility that require further follow-up care after surgical management.

Hernia and hydrocele

Definition and incidence

A hernia is defined as a protrusion of organ or tissue through an abnormal opening in the abdominal wall muscle or fascia. A direct inguinal hernia results from a weakness in the floor of the inguinal canal, allowing abdominal content and fluid to herniate through the external ring, medial to the epigastric vessels. In contrast, an indirect inguinal hernia results from a patent processus vaginalis (PV), allowing abdominal content and fluid to herniate through the internal ring. A direct inguinal hernia is uncommon in children. A hydrocele is defined as an accumulation of fluid around the testis. A communicating hydrocele results from a patent PV in which the opening through the internal ring is small, allowing fluid but not bowel to enter the scrotum. A non-communicating hydrocele results from a patent PV in which the opening through the internal ring is closed but the rest of the PV is not completely obliterated. Since there is no communication with the peritoneum, the fluid in the non-communicating hydrocele originates from the mesothelial lining of tunica vaginalis as a result of inflammation of the testis or epididymitis. A communicating hydrocele is common in young children, whereas a non-communicating hydrocele is more common in adolescents.

Hernia and hydrocele occur in approximately 1–3% of full-term infants but are three times more common in premature infants.[1,2] With regards to hernia, the male to female ratio is 8 to 1. A hernia/hydrocele occurs more often on the right than left (2:1) and is present bilaterally in 16% of affected patients.[1] Ten percent of children with a hernia/hydrocele will have a positive family history. Approximately one-third of the children with a hernia/hydrocele will be diagnosed before 6 months of age. An increased incidence of hernia/hydrocele is seen in patients with cystic fibrosis (15%),[3] connective tissue disease such as Ehlers–Danlos syndrome and Hunter–Hurler syndrome,[4,5] and congenital hip dislocation.[6] Children with a ventriculoperitoneal (VP) shunt or on continuous ambulatory peritoneal dialysis (CAPD) are also at higher risk of developing a hernia/hydrocele.[7]

Etiology and pathophysiology

In the male fetus, the testes develop from the cranial end of the mesonephros. The gubernaculum forms from a band of condescended mesenchyme, connecting to the lower pole of each testis. Around the 8th week of gestation, an outpouching of mesothelial cells from the coelomic cavity grows into the substance of gubernacular mesenchyme, forming the processus vaginalis. The PV is composed of a lining of simple mesothelium, surrounded by a fibrous layer of variable thickness and fatty connective tissue containing blood vessels, nerve trunks, lymph nodes, and variable amount of muscle.[8] The skeletal muscles of the PV are derived from the transverse abdominis muscle and the smooth muscle component is derived from the dartos muscles. Occasionally, the lining of PV undergoes proliferation due to chronic irritation. It may contain papillary structures or nodules. On histologic examination, fibrin deposition, extensive scarring, and psammoma bodies may be evident. In addition, mesothelial hyperplasia may be present with multinucleated cells, forming tubule-like structures within the fibrous tissue. These structures may appear to invade into the fibrous subserosa of the irritated PV. These features are often confused with those of rhabdomyosarcoma, mesothelioma, and metastatic carcinoma.[9]

By the 28th week of gestation, the testes begin to move from the posterior abdominal wall to the internal ring, as a result of growth of the fetal trunk and pelvis. The PV forms a channel through which the testes descend into the scrotum. It is believed that testicular descent is directed by the gubernacula[10] and assisted by the PV, which allows transmission of the abdominal pressure to the fetal testes, causing their descent through the inguinal canal.[11] The passage through the inguinal canal takes approximately 3 days and appears to be regulated by the genitofemoral nerve and the release of the calcitonin gene-related peptide (CGRP).[12,13] The testes enter the scrotum between the 32nd and 38th weeks of gestation; in some patients this process may be delayed up to the 40th week of gestation.

After the descent of the testes, the entrance to the inguinal canal, the internal ring, closes and the lumen of the PV is obliterated. Progressive fibrous obliteration of the PV occurs in a cephalad direction, beginning above the epididymis.[14] Organ culture of the PV from human infants demonstrates the presence of CGRP receptor on the mesechymal fibroblasts but not the epithelial cells. Addition of CGRP induces fusion of the PV through its effects on the fibroblasts.[13] In addition, it is observed that patency of the PV is often seen in association with epididymal abnormalities.[15] Since epididymal development is dependent on androgen stimulation, it is speculated that closure of the PV is also regulated by androgen. Another suggested mechanism to account for the persistently patent PV is the failure of the smooth muscle in PV to regress. Normally, these muscles disappear after taking part in the descent of the testis, a process that appears to be regulated by the autonomic system. In patients with a hernia, the muscles fail to undergo apoptosis and therefore maintain the patency of the PV.[16–19]

In the female fetus, the ovaries descend in a similar manner except that the process is halted in the pelvis. The cranial portion of the gubernaculum forms the ovarian ligament, and the caudal portion forms the round ligament, which runs from the uterus to the labia majora. It appears that the gubernaculum also plays a role in guiding ovarian descent.[20] Only rudimentary development of the PV occurs, forming the canal of Nuck.

Presentation and diagnosis

Children with a hernia/hydrocele often present with a history of a painless lump or bulge in the groin, scrotum, or labium (Figure 73.1). In younger children,

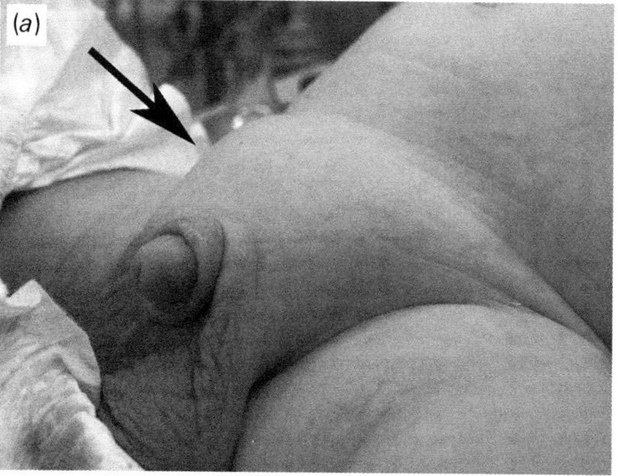

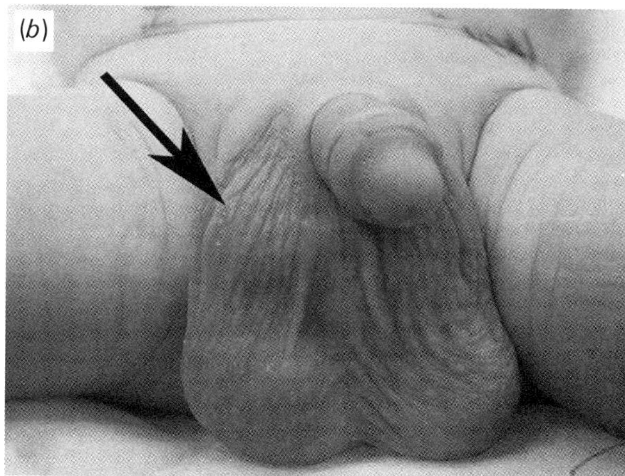

Figure 73.1 On physical examination, a bulge (arrows) can be seen in the groin (*a*) or in the scrotum (*b*), distinct from the testis in infants with an inguinal hernia.

this bulge may be more obvious while the child is crying, straining, or doing maneuvers that increase abdominal pressure. In older children, the hernia/hydrocele often gets larger during the day and smaller at night or during time of recumbency. Occasionally, a child may present with symptoms similar to that of acute testicular torsion, resulting from torsion of the hernia sac.[21,22] Approximately 10% of patients with an inguinal hernia present to medical attention with symptoms of bowel obstruction such as nausea, vomiting, abdominal distention, or localized or generalized abdominal tenderness.

On physical examination, bowel can be palpated or heard during manipulation of the inguinal or scrotal bulge in patients with a hernia. Occasionally, a silk glove sign can be detected on examination, as the layers of PV can be felt around the spermatic cord, feeling like silk rubbing on silk. It has been suggested that the silk glove sign is not from an empty hernia sac but from the hypertrophied cremasteric muscle fibers.[23] Unfortunately, this physical finding is very inaccurate in the absence of finding an obvious hernia/hydrocele.[24] It should be noted that in many patients with a hernia, there are no findings on physical examination, and the diagnosis is dependent upon the clinical history alone.

Typically, a non-tender bluish discoloration to scrotum and a soft mass around the testis is noted in patients with a hydrocele. In others, a painless mobile cystic swelling may be found anywhere along the spermatic cord. Termed a cord or encysted hydrocele, it is not reducible and can often be confused with a hernia.[25] Rarely, a child may present with an abdominoscrotal hydrocele in which a scrotal hydrocele has a dumbbell-shaped extension through the internal ring into the abdomen that forms an intra-abdominal cystic mass. In most patients, the hydrocele contains an exudative fluid. However, other fluid types have also been found in association with a hydrocele. A meconium hydrocele results from an in-utero perforation of bowel and subsequent inflammation and calcification of the meconium.[26] A pyocele can develop in association with acute appendicitis,[27,28] infection of the epididymis or testis, tuberculosis peritonitis,[29,30] or primary bacterial infection.[31] A pneumocele may develop as a consequence of necrotizing enterocolitis or other causes of bowel perforation.[32] A hematocele can form as a result of blunt abdominal trauma with associated splenic injury or scrotal injury.[33] A hydrocele may also contain ascites fluid such as bile, chyle, urine, cerebrospinal fluid in patients with a VP shunt, or dialysate fluid in patients on peritoneal dialysis. Hydrocele may also occur in girls, arising from the canal of Nuck.[34]

Being able to distinguish a hernia from a hydrocele on physical examination is often difficult. It has been suggested that transillumination may be used to identify a hydrocele (Figure 73.2). However, it

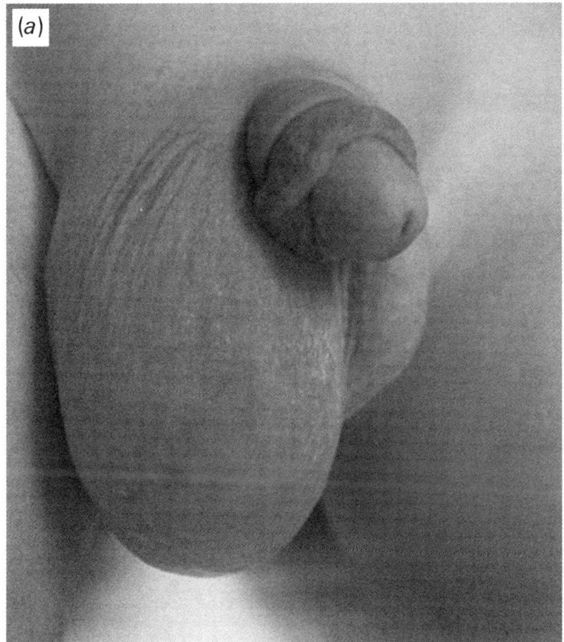

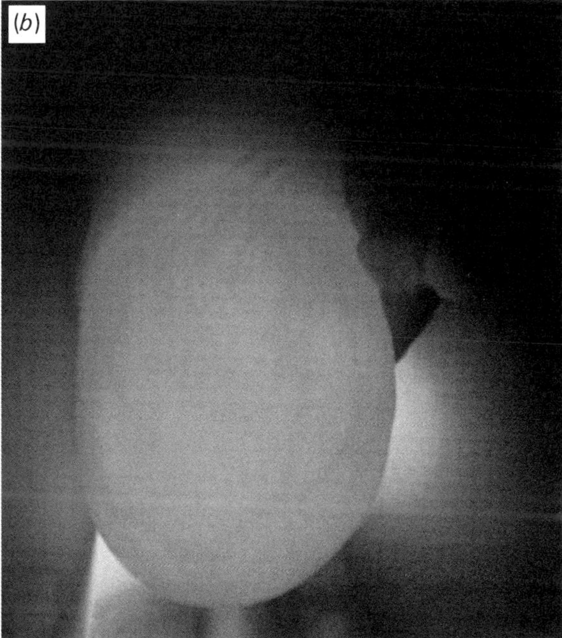

Figure 73.2 On physical examination of a boy with a hydrocele, scrotal swelling can be seen involving the testis (*a*) and this does transilluminate (*b*).

should be noted that since bowel fluid and air will transmit light in a similar manner as hydrocele fluid, this finding is not reliable. A scrotal mass that is easily reducible suggests a large patent PV representing either a hernia or a large communicating hydrocele. In contrast, a mass that is not reducible is likely to represent either a non-communicating hydrocele, one with a small patent internal ring, or an incarnated hernia.

In most patients with a hernia/hydrocele, the diagnosis can be made by clinical history and physical examination. In those few patients in whom the diagnosis cannot be well established, further radiologic examination may be helpful. In addition, when the testis cannot be palpated on physical examination, further radiologic imaging is required to rule out potentially serious pathologies such as undescended testis, infection, or testicular cancer. Ultrasonography (US) is widely used in evaluating inguinal and scrotal pathology. In patients with a hernia, fluid- or air-filled loops of bowel may be identified in the inguinal canal or scrotum. When there is omental herniation, a hyperechoic mass can be seen. However, it should be noted that US often fails to detect herniated bowel loops since the herniation is often periodic. In the absence of finding bowel or fluid in the inguinal canal, an increased cord width, as measured by US (7.2 ± 2.0 mm compared with 3.6 ± 0.8 mm in a normal inguinal canal), has been used to diagnose hernia.[35] In contrast, a hydrocele on US can be identified by identifying fluid in between tunical layers and the normal testis/epididymis. The hydrocele may contain loculations. Fine particulate matter seen on US may represent pus or blood, whereas calcification (seen as hyperechoic shadowing masses) suggests the presence of meconium.

Aside from US, other imaging techniques are seldom helpful in the diagnosis of a hernia/hydrocele. A KUB (kidney, ureter, and bladder X-ray) may demonstrate air or calcification in the scrotum, suggesting the presence of a pneumocele or meconium hydrocele, respectively. Herniography has been utilized in the diagnosis of a hernia.[36] Iothalamate solution (60%) is injected into the peritoneum. The patient is placed in an upright position for 10 minutes; a KUB or a computed tomography (CT) scan is obtained to identify contrast lining the patent PV/hernia sac.[37,38] Because of potentially serious complications such as bowel injury, contrast reaction, and peritoneal irritation, its use is limited to special circumstances such as in evaluating chronic groin pain.[39,40]

Management and techniques

Hernia repair

Currently, there is no effective medical management of a hernia; the use of a truss is primarily of historical interest. Since inguinal hernia is likely to persist indefinitely, it is recommend that children who are diagnosed with an inguinal hernia undergo surgical repair to prevent bowel incarceration and potential testicular atrophy. This is of particular importance in premature infants and neonates, who are higher risk of developing bowel incarceration while waiting for surgery.[41] In extremely premature infants, hernia repair can be safely deferred until the child is ready to be discharged from the neonatal unit.[42] It is reported that the success rate for hernia repair approaches 99%.

The type of surgical repair is dependent on the type of inguinal hernia. The direct inguinal hernia requires reconstruction of the floor of the inguinal canal with or without the use of prosthetic materials such as polypropylene, Dacron (polyethylene terephthalate), or PTFE (polytetrafluoroethylene). Since it is an uncommon type of hernia in children, a review of all types of direct inguinal hernia repair is beyond the scope of this chapter but is provided by Read.[43] Repair of the indirect hernia can be approached with either an open or a laparoscopic technique. Czerny and Banks first introduced the concept of high ligation of the hernia sac in 1877. In brief, an inguinal incision, which is preferably hidden in a skin crease, is made approximately one-third the distance from the pubic tubercle to the anterior iliac spine. Scarpa's fascia is next incised and the external oblique fascia is exposed. The shelving edge of the fascia is then defined with blunt dissection; this will allow for easier closure of the external oblique fascia later. To expose the inguinal canal, the fascia is incised along the direction of the fibers, parallel to the shelving edge over the external ring. After identifying the spermatic cord, the cremasteric muscles are separated to expose the hernia sac, which is located anterior and medial to the vas and testicular vessels. The hernia sac is carefully dissected from adjacent structures and divided between hemostats (Figure 73.3). The hernia sac is next freed proximally to the internal ring, where it is ligated with absorbable sutures. The distal portion of the hernia sac may be opened down to the testis to prevent hydrocele formation, although the necessity of this step is debated. A similar technique is done for the repair of inguinal hernia in girls (Figure 73.4). It is important in these patients to open the hernia sac to ensure that there are no herniated structures such as gonads or fal-

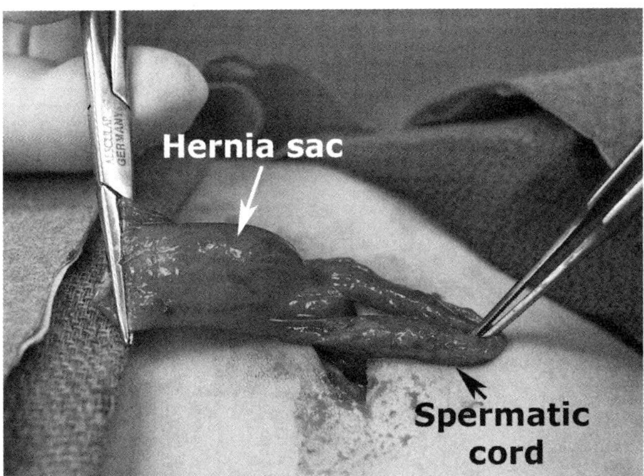

Figure 73.3 During the repair of an inguinal hernia, the hernia sac, which is located anterior medial to the spermatic cord, is carefully dissected away from the cord, ligated, and divided.

lopian tubes. Variations of this technique include approaching the hernia sac through a scrotal[44] or a low inguinal groove incision.[45] However, it should be noted that these approaches might limit the ability to ligate the hernia sac near the internal ring.

The repair of the indirect hernia may also be performed by laparoscopy. The internal ring can be approached either transperitoneally or preperitoneally[46] and the opening closed with a metal clip or sutures.[47] The surgical success rate using this technique is approximately 97%.[48,49] The laparoscopic approach is especially useful in patients with recurrent hernia. It allows for identification of the etiology of the recurrence such as incomplete ligation of the hernia sac, the de-novo development of a direct hernia, and the presence of other types of hernias such a femoral hernia.[50,51] More recently, the use of needlescopic hernia repair has been advocated. In brief, a 1.7 mm needle laparoscope is introduced through the umbilicus to visualize the opened internal ring. Through a second port positioned laterally, a grasper may be placed in the abdomen to help in the traction of the spermatic cord. A 2–3 mm incision is then made in skin directly over the internal ring and a suture is passed percutaneously anterolateral to the internal ring to perform an extraperitoneal high ligation of the hernia sac.[52] Long-term results and complication rates using this technique are not yet known.

Hydrocele repair

Unlike hernias, hydroceles may resolve spontaneously during the first year of life. Thus, in the absence of a hernia, surgical treatment for hydroceles can be deferred and observation is warranted. In older children who acutely present with a hydrocele, the underlying etiology such as epididymitis or orchitis should be treated. If the hydrocele persists several months after treatment, surgical repair may be considered. In young children, the hydrocele repair is performed in a similar manner to those described for repair of the indirect hernia, since these patients are likely to have a patent PV. In older children, the hydrocele repair can be performed through a midline or transverse scrotal incision since there is a low likelihood of a patent PV. The tunica vaginalis can be excised, everted (the bottle procedure), or imbricated (Lord's procedure). Sclerotherapy has been used in the treatment of hydroceles. The hydrocele is injected with a sclerosant such as tetracycline or polidocanol.[53] Complications include pain, long-term hazards of the sclerosant, and leakage

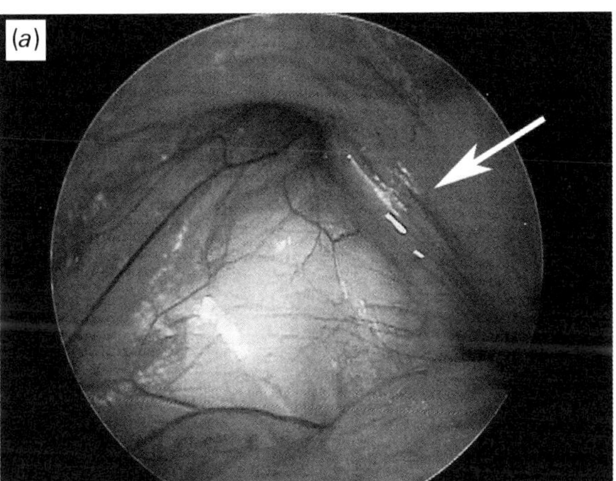

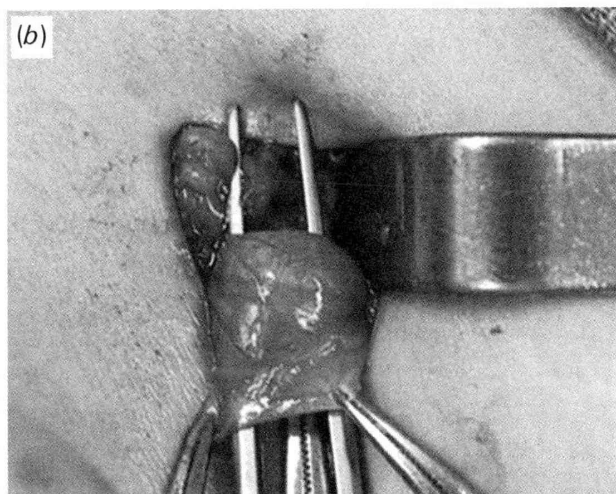

Figure 73.4 Inguinal hernia can also develop in girls. (*a*) On laparoscopy, an opened internal ring can be seen with the ovarian ligament (arrow) entering it. (*b*) On inguinal exploration, a hernia sac is identified. The hernia sac should be carefully examined to make sure that there are no structures herniating through the sac.

of the sclerosant through a patent PV. In addition, recurrence following treatment is common. Consequently, sclerotherapy is not recommended for children.

Potential structures encountered in the hernia sac during surgery

Numerous structures can be potentially encountered in the hernia sac; therefore, great care should be taken when dividing the sac. Typically, the hernia sac may contain intestine (small bowel, large bowel, appendix, and Meckel's diverticulum) or omentum. Occasionally, the bladder or intra-abdominal catheters such as a CAPD catheter or a VP shunt may herniate through the sac.[54] Less frequently, ectopic tissue such as that from the adrenal cortex,[55] spleen,[56] liver,[57] kidney,[58] and brain[59] can be found in the hernia sac. In a few rare cases (<0.1% of hernia repairs on adults and even less in children[60]), an unexpected discovery of a neoplasm is made during a hernia repair. Types of neoplasm found in the hernia sac include primary mesothelioma and liposarcomas,[55] extrarenal Wilms' tumor,[61] and metastatic cancer from the gastrointestinal tract, the ovaries, and the prostate.[8]

More frequently, the gonads and their associated structures may be encountered in the hernia sac. Despite having a palpable testis in the ipsilateral hemiscrotum, an additional testicle may be found at the time of hernia repair in boys with supernumerary testis[62] or cross-testicular ectopia. In approximately 2–3% of phenotypic girls undergoing hernia repair, a testis may be found in the sac, suggesting the diagnosis of complete androgen insensitivity syndrome (CAIS).[63,64] In these patients, the testis can either be removed after puberty to reduce the risk of germ cell malignancy (such as gonadoblastoma) or at the time of hernia repair to reduce the risk of virilization when the androgen insensitivity is not complete. An ovary can also be found in the hernia sac in 4% of girls undergoing surgery. Approximately 25% of these patients will have evidence of torsion effects or infarction in the herniated ovary.[65] Less often, genital duct structures are identified at the time of surgery or during pathologic evaluation. Functional wolffian duct derivatives such an accessory vas or epididymis may be seen separate from the spermatic cord, and should not be confused with true vasal injury. In patients with hernia uterine inguinale who have an anti-müllerian inhibiting factor or its receptor defect, persistent müllerian structures such as a uterus may be found in the hernia sac.[66,67] Owing to the close relationship with wolffian duct structures, great care has to be taken in excising the persistent müllerian structures. In 2–6% of the cases, non-functional müllerian or wolffian remnants structures can be identified in the hernia sac.[68,69] These structures are characterized by ciliated low columnar cells with occasional interspersed pale round cells, occurring singly, in small groups, or in large clusters.[70] They are smaller than functional duct derivatives and lack significant muscular coats. Given the potential for finding various structures in the sac, some clinicians have recommended sending the hernia sac routinely for pathologic examination. However, Miller et al[71] observed that in their series of 456 patients, only four cases (0.88%) had unexpected findings on pathologic evaluation of the hernia sac. None of these cases were of clinical significance (i.e. changed the patient management). The authors concluded that the routine histologic evaluation of inguinal hernia sacs in children is an unnecessary expense and should be reserved for select cases at the discretion of the surgeon.

Management of the contralateral patent processus vaginalis

In children who present with a unilateral hernia, much controversy exists as to the management of the contralateral side. Some surgeons recommend routinely exploring the opposite side for a patent PV, whereas others are more selective based upon clinical criteria such as age or sex.[72,73] Some utilize further radiologic imaging such as US[74] or perform diagnostic pneumoperitoneum[75] or laparoscopy through the umbilicus[76,77] or hernia sac[78,79] to diagnose a patent PV. Others just recommend observation for the development of a contralateral hernia. From autopsy studies, it is observed that the incidence of a patent PV is 90% in preterm infants, 80% in newborns, 60% in children less than 1 year of age, and 15–30% in adults.[80,81] From studies in which the patency of the contralateral PV was assessed in children with a unilateral hernia, it was observed that the incidence of a patent PV was also age dependent: approximately 60% of children <2 months of age who had a unilateral hernia had a patent contralateral PV; this incidence declined during the first 2 years of life and stabilized at 40% in children from 2 to 16 years of age.[73,82]

Several studies have also observed that the incidence of a contralateral hernia developing following unilateral hernia repair ranged from 3.6 to 10% (an average of approximately 7%),[83–87] far exceeding the rate of a patent PV. Chertin et al similarly found that the incidence of developing a contralateral hernia in 300 girls who presented with a unilateral hernia and underwent a unilateral repair was 8%.[88] Using a univariate analysis with the Cox regression models, Ikeda et al observed that a left-sided hernia and a positive family history were significantly associated with the metachronous development of a contralateral hernia.[89] However, the incidence was at most 10%. Miltenburg et al performed a meta-analysis of the risk of metachronous hernia in infants and children and found that there was a 7% risk of developing a contralateral hernia following unilateral repair.[90] Gender and age were not risk factors. Similar to the findings by Ikeda et al,[89] there was an 11% risk of metachronous hernia if the original hernia was on the left side, a risk that was 50% greater than if the original hernia was on the right. Of patients who developed a metachronous hernia, 90% did so within 5 years, with a complication rate of 0.5%.[76] Based upon these findings, it can be concluded that patients with a patent PV do not necessarily progress to develop a clinically apparent inguinal hernia. Concurrent management of a contralateral PV is of probable benefit in premature and young infants where the risk of a second anesthesia is high and in children with risk factors for hernia recurrence such as cystic fibrosis or connective tissue disease. Interestingly, it was observed that in a study in which the parents were presented with the above issues and asked to choose between unilateral hernia repair only or with concomitant evaluation and repair of a contralateral patent PV for their child, 85% of the parents chose the latter.[91] Approximately 80% of those who chose contralateral exploration indicated that convenience was the primary motive in their choice and only 19% had concerns about their child undergoing a second anesthesia if a contralateral hernia develops later.

Complications of hernia/hydrocele repair

In general, the complication rate is higher in patients undergoing hernia repairs compared with those undergoing hydrocele repairs and in emergent compared with elective repair. The primary concern is associated with the anesthetic risk;[92] this is of particular significance in premature infants and in those <3 months of age. Improvements in pediatric anesthesia techniques such as the use of a laryngeal mask[93] with caudal[94] or local anesthesia and the use of regional anesthesia in premature infants[95] have greatly decreased the risk of potential anesthetic complications. Early complications associated with a hernia/hydrocele repair include local edema, hematoma, and wound infection. Early recurrence of inguinal/scrotal swelling result from a missed hernia or refilling of the potential space with fluid. Late complications include iatrogenic, upward displacement of the testis (incidence of 1% in children undergoing hernia repair),[96] paravesical abscess,[97] damage to spermatic cord, and recurrence. The incidence of spermatic cord injury during uncomplicated inguinal hernia surgery is approximately ≤1% during hydrocele repair.[98] However, if the hernia is incarcerated, the risk of spermatic cord injury increases significantly to 6–10%, with a subsequent testicular atrophy rate of 4%.[99] It is suggested that the bowel incarceration induces ischemia on the spermatic cord as a result of pressure. The rate of recurrence following open hernia/hydrocele repair is approximately 1–3%; however, it may be as high as 20% in premature infants undergoing repair.[43] Recurrence may be caused by failure to dissect a complete sac, tearing of the sac, or slipped sutures in ligating the sac. Moreover, in patients with recurrent hernia, other pathologies such as connective tissue diseases should be considered. Hydrocele formation following hernia repair either with an open or laparoscopic approach occurs in less than 1% of the patients.[48,49]

Testicular and appendiceal torsion

Definition and incidence

Normally, the tunica vaginalis covers the anterior surface of the testis, epididymis, and various distances over the spermatic cord. Attachment with the gubernaculum and scrotal wall posteriorly allows the testis to be fixed, preventing it from twisting around the vascular mesentery. However, when these attachments are not secure, torsion of the testis may occur, leading to vascular compromise. Although, testicular torsion can occur at any age, there is a bimodal distribution in the age of presentation, during puberty and during the neonatal period. More commonly in adolescents, testicular torsion involves torsion of the spermatic cord within the tunica vaginalis (intravaginal torsion). Owing to abnormal fixation of the testis and epididymis, the testis is freely suspended within the tunical cavity. This bell clapper deformity allows the testis to adopt a horizontal position in the scrotum (Figure 73.5a). It is found in 12% of testes at postmortem, and frequently occurs bilaterally.[100] It is the

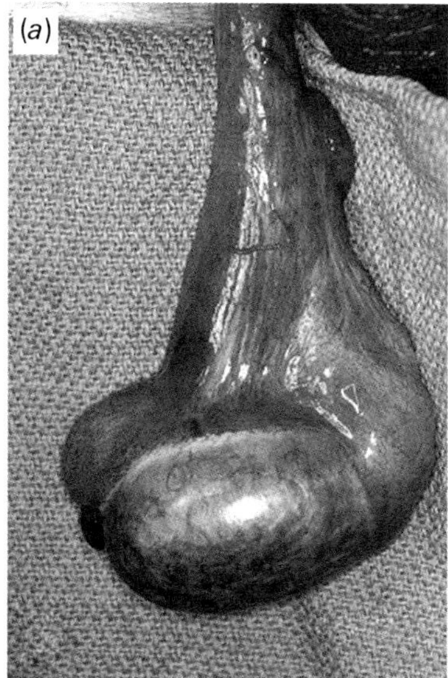

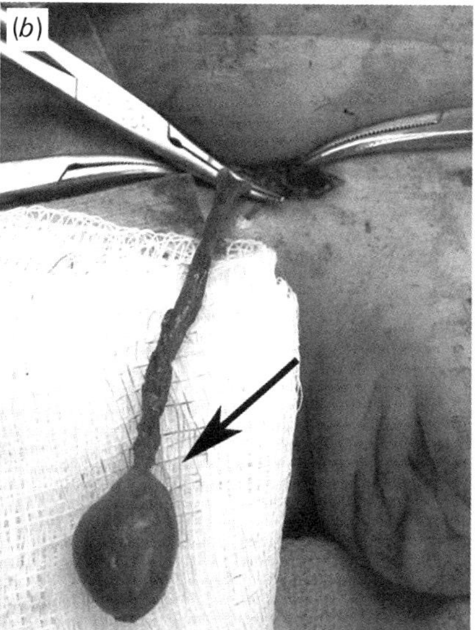

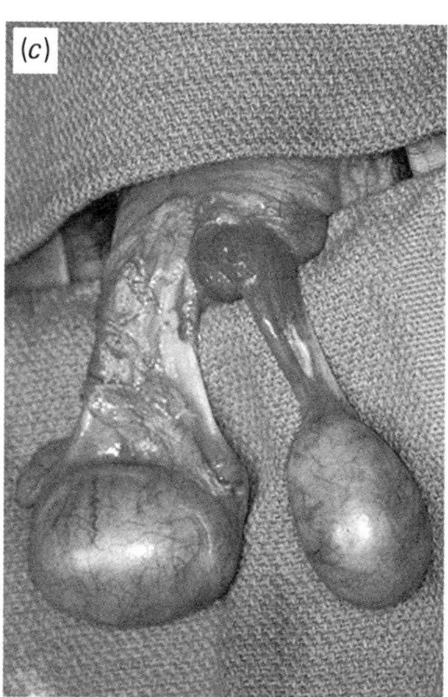

Figure 73.5 (*a*) In adolescents, testicular torsion occurs intravaginally, commonly due to the bell clapper deformity. (*b*) In neonates, testicular torsion occurs extravaginally, in which the entire cord is twisted about its axis (arrow). (*c*) In children with intermittent torsion, such as the one shown here who presented with intermittent left testicular pain, a bell clapper deformity (left testis) is often seen on the affected side.

most common etiology of torsion in adolescents, in whom rapidly increasing testicular mass associated with puberty increases the chance of the testis rotating. Intravaginal testicular torsion can also occur intermittently, spontaneously twisting and untwisting (Figure 73.5b).

Approximately 10% of all testicular torsion occurs in newborns. In 70% of these patients, torsion occurs prenatally and is diagnosed at the time of birth. In the other 30% of patients, torsion occurs in previously normal testes.[101] Testicular torsion in newborns occurs primarily extravaginally. In the neonatal period, the descending or recently descended testis and its coverings are very mobile within the scrotum, creating a risk for the spermatic cord to twist en masse (Figure 73.5c). Multiparity, excessive uterine pressure, and a strong cremasteric contraction have been suggested as etiologic factors for extravaginal torsion.[102]

Torsion of the testicular appendages may also occur. The appendix testis is a vestigial remnant of the müllerian system located on the upper pole of the testis. It is found in 90% of males and bilaterally in 60% (Figure 73.6a). Appendages may also be found on the epididymis (Figure 73.6b), epididymotesticular groove, or the cord itself. These appendages are remnants of the wolffian system. Approximately 95% of the appendiceal torsions involve the appendix testis. The peak age of presentation is around 10 years.[103] It has been suggested that hormonal stimulation during pubertal development increases the size of the testicular appendages, making them more susceptible to twisting around their small blood supply. In a review of 100 boys

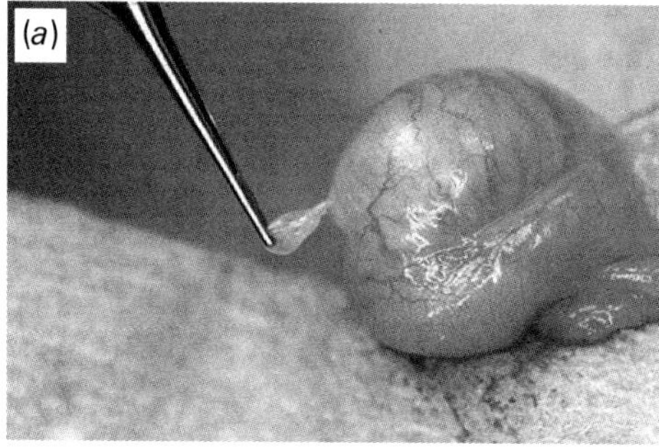

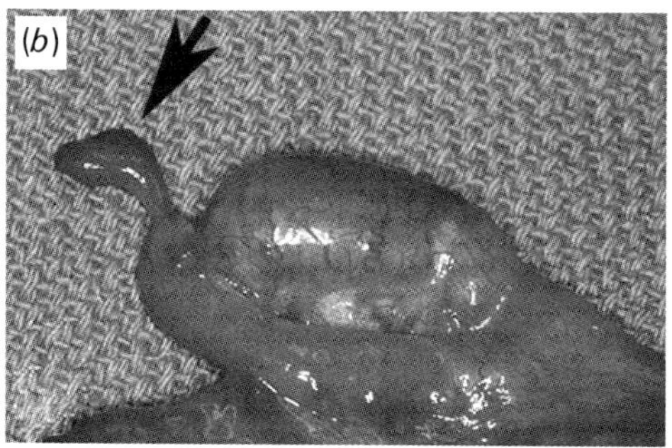

Figure 73.6 Acute testicular pain can also be due to torsion of the testicular appendages such as the appendix testis (*a*) and appendix epididymis (*b*) (arrow).

<15 years of age who presented with acute scrotal pain, Melekos et al[103] observed that 42% had testicular torsion and 32% had appendiceal torsion.

Presentation and diagnosis

Children and adolescents who present with an acute painful scrotum require prompt evaluation. Timely and accurate diagnosis is required to prevent testicular loss. Whereas the differential diagnosis is extensive (Table 73.1), the diagnosis can be determined based upon history, physical examination, and limited laboratory and radiologic evaluation. Typically, adolescents with intravaginal testicular torsion will present with acute onset of severe scrotal pain. In a series of 670 patients with acute testicular torsion, 89% of the patients presented with a complaint of acute-onset ipsilateral testicular pain.[104] The remaining patients presented only with pain referred to the ipsilateral lower abdomen, groin, or thigh. The majority of these patients were later found to have torsion in the undescended testis. Associated trauma and recent exercise was seen in 4% and 10% of the patients, respectively. About 11% of the patients were awakened from sleep with pain. Nausea and vomiting were associated with testicular torsion in 39% of the patients, whereas urinary symptoms such as dysuria and urgency were usually absent (<5%). Interestingly, 36% of the patients had a previous history of testicular pain or swelling. A prior history of ipsilateral orchidopexy does not exclude the diagnosis of testicular torsion. Inadequate fixation or the development of single adhesions forming an axis for the testis to twist has been observed in patients with a prior history of orchidopexy who presented with a recurrent testicular torsion.[105] Physical examination of the torsed testis is often very difficult due to the severity of the pain. Important signs of testicular torsion include a firm testicle high-riding in the scrotum, an abnormal transverse orientation of the testis, and the absence of a cremasteric reflex.[106] None of these physical findings is foolproof, and the clinician must maintain a high degree of suspicion. In many cases, acute hydrocele or marked scrotal edema develops when several hours have passed since the onset of the scrotal pain. Fever and an elevated white blood cell count are seldom associated with testicular torsion. Intermittent testicular torsion has a similar presentation to that of intravaginal torsion, except that the episode is self-limited with resolution of symptoms after the cord spontaneously untwists. Many patients who present with acute testicular torsion have a history of prior episodes consistent with intermittent testicular torsion. Those patients with intermittent torsion are likely to have normal physical examination at the time of evaluation, when the pain has resolved. In contrast to those patients with intravaginal torsion, patients with extravaginal neonatal torsion typically present with painless swelling and scrotal discoloration. A firm testis with an associated hydrocele is often noted incidentally on newborn examination or during diaper change. Interestingly, associated scrotal erythema is not often present, but the overlying skin is discolored by the underlying hemorrhagic necrosis.

Table 73.1 Differential diagnosis for acute/subacute scrotum

Testicular torsion
Appendiceal torsion (testis or epididymis)
Epididymitis/epididymo-orchitis
Inguinal hernia (reducible or incarcerated)
Hydrocele
Trauma (mechanical, burns, or animal/insect bite)
Testicular neoplasms
Spermatocele
Varicocele
Dermatologic lesions
Inflammatory vasculitis (Henoch–Schönlein purpura)
Idiopathic scrotal edema
Referred pain

Patients with appendiceal torsion can also present with pain similar to those with intravaginal testicular torsion. However, the presentation for appendiceal torsion can be quite variable, from an insidious onset of scrotal discomfort to acute severe scrotal pain. Consequently, it is often difficult to differentiate appendiceal torsion from other causes of acute scrotum. At the earlier stages, the pain may be localized to the upper pole of the testis or epididymis, and a firm nodule can sometimes be palpated in this region of the scrotum. The pain is more often of a gradual onset rather than developing acutely, and associated symptoms such as nausea, vomiting, and abdominal pain are unusual. On physical examination, the infarcted appendage can be seen through the scrotal skin as a blue dot; this is considered pathognomonic for appendiceal torsion. However, the blue dot sign is only seen in approximately 20% of patients with an appendiceal torsion.[103] In the latter stages, scrotal wall edema and erythema can develop, distorting the physical examination. The cremasteric reflex is usually preserved and the testis remains mobile.

In those patients who are suspected of having testicular torsion on a clinical basis, prompt surgical exploration is mandatory. Adjunctive radiologic tests should only be obtained when their purpose is to confirm the absence of testicular torsion so that surgical exploration can be avoided. These tests are also of use in patients in whom the duration of symptoms suggests a non-salvageable testis if torsion is the cause. In these limited cases, color or power Doppler US or ^{99m}Tc-radioisotope scintigraphy may be obtained to evaluate testicular blood flow. Both of these tests depend on the availability of equipment and personnel. False-negative results can occur with any of the above modalities. The choice of which study to obtain varies from institution to institution, depending on local experience and the availability and reliability of the tests. Color Doppler US studies can assess the anatomy of the scrotum and its content, while determining the presence or absence of testicular blood flow (as measured by velocity). The sensitivity of color Doppler US is reported to be as high as 90%, with a specificity of 99%.[107] However, caution must be used in the interpretation of these studies; almost 40% of patients, especially those younger than 8 years of age, may fail to demonstrate flow on the asymptomatic side.[108,109] Power Doppler US measures blood flow by detecting the number of red blood cells as opposed to the velocity of flow. Although blood flow is more consistently detected in younger children with power Doppler,[108] evidence from animal studies suggests that power Doppler and color Doppler are equally effective in the detection of torsion.[110] Radionuclide imaging was originally the study of choice for ruling out testicular torsion. However, it only allows for the assessment of blood flow. Its positive predictive value has been reported to be around 75%, with a sensitivity of 90% and a specificity of 89%.[111] Hyperemia of the scrotal wall can give false impressions of testicular blood flow. In addition, it is difficult to image children with small scrotal sacs or testes using this study.

Effects of unilateral torsion on testicular function

Ischemic damage from torsion is related to the duration of the torsion and the number of revolutions of the spermatic cord. Studies in dogs have demonstrated that no spermatogenic or Sertoli cells are viable after 6 hours of testicular ischemia, and all Leydig cells are lost after 10 hours of ischemia.[112] However, in humans, severe testicular atrophy can be seen as early as 4 hours when the degree of torsion is greater than 360°.[113] It is likely that when the cord is torsed >360°, the artery becomes completely occluded. In contrast, when the torsion is <360°, arteriolar stasis develops secondary to venous occlusion and edema. In general, testicular atrophy is rare before 8 hours of torsion but is common after this time period.[114] The mechanism of testicular damage appears to be related to a combination of ischemia and reperfusion injury, resulting from activation of the xanthine oxidase system in parenchymal cells or from leukocytes adherent to the reperfused venule walls.

The effects of ischemia do not seem to be limited to the torsed testis. In patients who had treatment of testicular torsion within 4 hours of the onset of symptoms, half of the patients had abnormal semen analysis in follow-up, suggesting injury to both testes.[114] Studies in rats have confirmed that unilateral torsion can induce bilateral testicular damage and reduced fertility.[115,116] Several mechanisms have been suggested to explain these observations, including an immunologic cause, congenital dysplasia, and damage of the normal testis by reflex vasoconstriction. It is suggested that torsion disrupts the normal blood–testis barrier, allowing the release of sperm antigens from the damaged testis. The antigens induce formation of autoantibodies, which can then attack the unaffected testis. In rats, it has been demonstrated that orchidectomy of the torsed testis, treatment with perioperative antilymphocyte globulin, and splenectomy,[117] or administration of immunosuppressants such as steroids and cyclosporine,[118] can prevent contralateral testicular damage. Similarly, in humans, patients with torsion for >24 hours who had undergone an orchidectomy are more likely to have a normal semen analysis than those in whom the torsed testis was left in place.[114] Although there is ample evidence in animal studies that damage of the contralateral testis is mediated by an immune response, direct evidence in human studies is lacking. Antitestis antibodies have been found in only approximately 10–20% of patients who had a testicular torsion.[119,120] In addition, their presence does not correlate with infertility or with any testicular exocrine or endocrine dysfunction. An alternative explanation for the observed abnormal semen parameters in patients with unilateral torsion is the presence of underlying congenital dysplasia in the unaffected testis. Biopsies from the contralateral testis at the time of treatment for unilateral torsion demonstrate abnormalities such as desquamation of the germinative epithelium, atrophy of the Leydig cells, and malformation of spermatoblasts in 88% of the cases.[121] The presence of these abnormalities so soon after the onset of torsion suggests that there may be pre-existing underlying pathology in contralateral testis. However, this explanation does not explain the consistent correlation between the duration of torsion and total sperm count, unless the damage is compounded by another mechanism.[122] The most recent explanation of the observed damage in the non-torsed testis is that it is caused by ischemia induced by reflex vasoconstriction. In animal studies,[123–125] unilateral testicular torsion induces an immediate and progressive decrease in blood flow to the contralateral testis followed by a gradual increase after detorsion. Like the affected side, the contralateral testis can be damaged by a combination of ischemia and reperfusion injury. The effect of torsion on contralateral testicular blood flow appears to be mediated by sympathetic nerve discharges from the genitofemoral nerve.[126]

Several studies have suggested that testicular damage after torsion can be limited by cooling of the testes, suppressing immune-mediated damage, and chemical sympathectomy to prevent reflex vasoconstriction. In animal studies, external cooling of the testis can delay the effects of ischemia for a few hours.[127] In addition, verapamil, surfactant, allopurinol, platelet-activating factor inhibitors, and hyperbaric oxygen have been used in attempt to decrease reperfusion injury.[118,128,129] Similarly, immunosuppression with steroids, cyclosporine, and azathioprine has also been used to reduce testicular damage induced by an immune response.[130] Drugs such as capsaicin, 6-hydroxydopamine hydrobromide, guanethidine monosulfate, and nitric oxide have been shown in animal studies to reduce testicular damage by preventing vasospasm and hypoxia in the contralateral testis.[131,132] Apart from hypothermia, the other methods of limiting testicular damage following unilateral torsion have been used in humans.[133]

Treatment

When suspected of having testicular torsion, the patient should be taken to surgery without delay. Manual detorsion may be tried if surgical intervention cannot be done for a period of time. The testis should be turned caudal to cranial, and medial to lateral.[134] If the first attempt is unsuccessful, the testis should be turned in the opposite direction. If the detorsion is successful, the pain should resolve immediately. However, this process is often very painful, and manual detorsion may not completely correct the obstructed blood flow. Consequently, surgical intervention is still required following manual detorsion.

Fixation can be accomplished by securing the testis to the septum or placement into a dartos pouch. For trans-septal fixation, the scrotum is opened through an incision in the median raphe. For the pouch fixation, the incision is made transversely following the skin creases of the scrotum. When using the latter method, the dartos pouch is made after the skin is incised. The tunica vaginalis is then entered, and the testis is examined. The spermatic cord should be detorsed to restore blood flow. The affected testis should be placed in a warm sponge and observed for several minutes to determine viability. If it is nonviable, the necrotic testis should be removed. Exploration of the contralateral testis should also be performed and, in all cases, the contralateral testis must be fixed. The testicles can be fixed to the median septum with three or four fine, non-reactive and nonabsorbable sutures. These sutures can be brought through the septum, enabling the contralateral side to be fixed concurrently. Alternatively, a dartos pouch is created and fixation relies on scarification of the testis. The tunica vaginalis is everted and the testicle placed into the dartos pouch. A non-absorbable suture is then used to secure the dartos tissue around the cord. This technique is advantageous in that complications such as abscess formation and tubular atrophy are uncommon. In addition, there have been no reported cases of recurrent torsion with this technique. Intermittent torsion is corrected using either of the above techniques on a semiemergent basis. As a result of the effects of torsion on the function of the affected and unaffected testis, these patients will require further follow-up care to evaluate for infertility.

The treatment of neonatal torsion is controversial. Some clinicians suggest that surgical exploration is unnecessary, whereas others advocate immediate surgical exploration and fixation of the contralateral side. It is rare to salvage the affected testis in a patient with unilateral neonatal torsion; out of more than 30 cases of bilateral neonatal torsion reported in the literature, only two testicles have been successfully salvaged.[135] Important reasons for exploration are to exclude tumor and to prevent possible unilateral torsion from becoming bilateral anorchia.[101] In the rare case of bilateral neonatal torsion, a more conservative approach can be taken. The newborn's general condition and anesthetic considerations should be evaluated to determine whether or not to proceed with surgical intervention.

The treatment of twisted testicular appendages is non-surgical if the diagnosis is certain. Conservative therapy with limitation of activity, scrotal elevation, and administration of non-steroidal analgesics is highly effective. Most of the symptoms will dissipate once the acute changes of acute necrosis resolve. In rare instances, surgical exploration may be undertaken if conservative management fails. Simple excision of the torsed appendage is curative. Although an asymptomatic appendage is likely to be present on the contralateral side, exploration of the unaffected testis is not indicated. Some clinicians have advocated surgical treatment for the management of appendiceal torsion because these patients seem to recover more rapidly and return to normal activity quicker than those treated conservatively.[136]

Varicocele

Definition and incidence

A varicocele is caused by abnormal dilation of the internal spermatic vein and the pampiniform plexus of the testis. There are three primary vascular suppliers to the testis: the internal spermatic, the vassal, and cremasteric artery and vein. At testicular levels, there is free communication between the arteries. The pampiniform plexus is formed from veins providing the drainage from the testis and epididymis. As this plexus courses toward its drainage into the renal vein on the left and the inferior vena cava on the right, it becomes the internal spermatic vein. Like the arteries, there is free communication between the pampiniform plexus and the vasal vein, which drains via the inferior vesical vein into the hypogastric vein, and the cremasteric vein, which drains via the inferior epigastric vein into the external iliac vein. In addition, the distal portion of the pampiniform plexus is also drained via the anterior scrotal vein into the femoral vein.

A varicocele is rarely seen in boys less than 10 years of age.[137] Its incidence rapidly increases between 10 and 15 years of age, and it is seen in approximately 15% of male adults.[138] There appears to be a causal relationship between pubertal development and varicocele formation. Varicocele may be classified by size during examination with the patient standing: grade I varicocele is not visible but becomes palpable during the Valsava maneuver; grade II varicocele is easily palpable on examination without the need for the Valsava maneuver; and grade III varicocele is clearly visible on examination. Grade I varicocele is seen in approximately 9% of adolescent males, whereas grade II is seen in 4% and grade III in 2%.[139] The true incidence of varicocele may be underestimated, since many adolescent males do not routinely undergo proper testicular examination in the upright position. Approximately 90% of varicoceles detected are found on the left side, whereas bilateral varicoceles occur in 2–10% of the cases. An isolated, right-sided varicocele is uncommon, and its presence should raise the suspicion of a pelvic mass compressing venous return.

Etiology and pathophysiology

There are many theories as to the etiology of a varicocele. It is speculated that there are incompetent or absent valves in the left spermatic vein, which allows retrograde blood flow into the pampiniform plexus.[140] It has also been hypothesized that the anatomic differences between the left and right spermatic veins (with the left being longer and having a right angle insertion into the left renal vein) allow for preferential transmission of higher hydrostatic pressures to the left pampiniform plexus. Alternatively, it has been suggested that a varicocele develops as a consequence of the left renal vein being compressed as it passes between the aorta and the superior mesenteric artery. However, this 'nutcracker effect' has not been seen clinically.[141] Finally, it is hypothesized that a varicocele develops from abnormal embryonic transformation of the primary venous system into the secondary system. The inferior vena cava is formed as the subcardinal, the posterior cardinal, and the supracardinal veins involute. Disordered involution may cause a persistence of intercardinal anastomoses that could lead to the formation of the varicocele.[141]

Although the etiology of a varicocele remains unclear, its effect on the testis is well documented. Biopsies from the testes of men with unilateral varicocele and fertility problems demonstrate incomplete maturational arrest at the spermatid and spermatocyte levels.[142,143] In addition, there is decreased spermatogenesis and seminiferous tubular thickening with decreased tubular diameter. Interestingly, these changes are seen in both testes but are more severe on the varicocele side.[142] It has also been observed that there are changes in the other components of the testis. Leydig cell hyperplasia is seen in association with varicocele. Its presence can be used for prognosis, since the pregnancy rate was observed to be decreased from 40% to 5% in partners of men with a varicocele who have Leydig cell hyperplasia on testicular biopsy.[144] Sertoli cell abnormalities have also been reported in men with varicocele. On light and electron microscopy, spermatids are seen to be maloriented relative to Sertoli cells, and Sertoli–germ cell junctional complexes appear to be structurally abnormal.[145] Finally, the testicular microvasculature is also affected in adolescents and men with varicocele, in which proliferative endothelial lesions in the capillaries are seen. These vascular lesions precede the testicular changes and are reversible with surgical correction.[146] All of these findings must be interpreted with caution, as they come from men with fertility problems. Most men with varicocele are fertile.

Varicocele is also associated with specific biochemical changes. It has been observed that there is decreased intratesticular testosterone concentration in some adult men with varicocele.[147] It is not surprising that this decrease correlates with impaired spermatogenesis and Leydig cell changes in men with varicocele.[147,148] Similarly, a decrease in serum testosterone has been noted in some men with bilateral grade III varicoceles.[149] However, this observation is not seen in patients with other grades of varicocele.[150] Inhibin B is a glycoprotein produced by Sertoli cells that can potentially serve as a maker of Sertoli cell function in patients with varicocele. It is observed that serum inhibin B levels tend to be positively correlated with sperm concentration in some patients.[150,151] In comparison, it is more consistently observed that men[152,153] and adolescents[154] with varicocele have elevated gonadotropic hormones such as follicle-stimulating hormone (FSH). In addition, excessive gonadotropin (in particular FSH) response to gonadotropin-releasing hormone (GnRH) is seen in some adolescents with varicocele. In one study,[155] it was observed that 31% of adolescents with a unilateral varicocele had an abnormal response to GnRH stimulation, and 75% of those with testicular hypotrophy of >3 ml differential had an abnormal response. However, it should be noted that 54% of those who did not have elevated FSH and luteinizing hormone (LH) in response to GnRH stimulation also had hypotrophy. Aragona et al[156] observed a correlation between abnormal testis histology and an exaggerated response to GnRH. This abnormal GnRH response appears to be limited to those patients at Tanner stage V. Approximately 40% of the Tanner stage V patients had an exaggerated response to GnRH, whereas those patients with Tanner stages III and IV had no difference in LH or FSH response to GnRH.[157] Unfortunately, the use of GnRH as a predictor for the need for surgery is limited, since it does not correlate with the grade of the varicocele, testicular hypotrophy, or fertility.[157,158]

Since 98% of the testicular mass is composed of seminiferous tubules and germinal cells, it is not surprising that the histologic, deleterious effects of varicocele may be seen grossly by changes in testicular volume. The average size of the testis in an adult male is 24 ± 3 ml. Normally, there is no more than 2 ml difference. It has long been noted that the ipsilateral testis of patients with a unilateral varicocele can be significantly smaller than the contralateral side.[159] It should be noted, however, that in adult men, although a varicocele can cause significant ipsilateral testicular atrophy/hypotrophy, there does not seem to be a correlation between loss of testicular volume and fertility status in men with a left varicocele.[160] In adolescents, absolute changes in testicular volume cannot be used, since the testis is growing during puberty. Consequently, the percent volume loss compared with the right side is utilized. Like adult men, adolescents with a unilateral varicocele may have a significant amount of testicular volume loss. It remains a topic of debate as to what percentage of volume loss is considered significant (10% vs 25%).[161,162] Nevertheless, it has been observed that volume loss is seen in 34% of adolescents with grade II varicocele and 81% with grade III varicocele.[138] Several prospective studies[156,161,163] have demonstrated that in adolescents the testicular volume either fails to increase or even decreases in the presence of the varicocele.

The effects of the varicocele can also be seen in the semen quality. A 'stress pattern' can be observed in the semen of adults with a varicocele in approximately 90% of cases.[164] These characteristic changes consist of subnormal motility, an increase in immature forms, a shift from oval to tapered, and amorphous sperm forms.[165] These changes may worsen over time.[166] In adolescents, varicocele is associated with impairment in sperm motility and morphology, with no significant difference in sperm counts.[167] Surgical correction of the varicocele in adulthood[168–170] or in adolescence[161,171–173] results in improved semen parameters. In the only prospective study,[174] only improvement in sperm concentration was noted in adolescents with a unilateral varicocele who underwent surgical correction.

Several theories have been suggested for the etiology of how a varicocele induces these changes to the testis. It is speculated that these changes may be mediated by increased venous pressure or retrograde flow of toxic metabolites from the adrenal gland. Currently, the most plausible theory is that a varicocele induces thermal damage to the testis. Intratesticular temperature is normally maintained at approximately 33–34°C. A countercurrent heat exchange between the blood coming down and the blood leaving the testis allows the testis to be maintained at a lower temperature. It is suggested that a varicocele disrupts this countercurrent heat exchange and induces testicular hyperthermia, which interferes with normal spermatogenesis.[175] This theory has been demonstrated in animal models of varicocele (reviewed by Turner[176]). In primates,[177] dogs,[178] and rats,[179] partial ligation of the left renal vein results in varicosity of the left spermatic vein and the pampiniform plexus. The surgically created varicocele induces bilateral increases in testicular blood flow and temperature, resulting in decreases in intratesticular testosterone and sperm output.[176] These effects do not appear to be immunologically or neurologically mediated[180] and are reversed with varicocelectomy.[181,182]

Presentation and diagnosis

The majority of adolescents who present with a unilateral varicocele are asymptomatic; pain or a dull nagging ache is the presenting symptom only in approximately 3% of the patients.[183] The varicocele is usually detected on a physical examination as a scrotal swelling/mass. To evaluate for the presence of a varicocele, it is essential to examine the patient standing up and then performing the Valsava maneuver. In addition, the testes should be carefully evaluated for their size and consistency. Several methods of testicular measurements, including rulers and calipers, orchidometers, and US, have been employed. Measurement using orchidometers such as the Prader or Rochester (Takihara) is readily available and inexpensive; however, the accuracy of the measurement is highly dependent upon the experience of the examiner. In comparison, measurement using testicular US is better correlated with actual testicular volume[184,185] but is more costly. Another advantage of using US in evaluating varicocele is its ability to pick up unexpected pathology such as a retroperitoneal mass, intratesticular varicocele, or testicular mass. An intratesticular varicocele is seen on scrotal Doppler US as an intratesticular anechoic lesion with active Doppler flow. It is found in association with traditionally large extratesticular varicoceles and has been shown to resolve following spermatic vein ligation.[186]

When possible, a semen analysis should be obtained. Semen quality is a good indicator of testicular function in adults with varicocele. However, it should be noted that its use in adolescents with a varicocele has some potential limitations: often it is very difficult to obtain semen analysis in adolescents due to ethical concerns. In addition, normal semen parameters have not been well defined prior to sexual maturity; between 12 and 19 years of age, spermatozoa are absent and semen parameters reach adult values 29–33 months after the onset of puberty.[187] Consequently, the interpretation of semen parameters is problematic in adolescents who are undergoing pubertal changes, and most practitioners do not routinely obtain semen specimens.

Serum measurement of FSH with or without GnRH stimulation may be potentially helpful in identifying those patients with testicular dysfunction induced by a varicocele. However, as indicated previously, elevation in FSH levels and abnormal GnRH responses do not always correlate with abnormal semen parameters or fertility. In addition, not all patients with testicular dysfunction have elevated FSH or abnormal response to GnRH. Consequently, their routine use in evaluating adolescents with varicocele is limited.

In a very selected group of patients, further radiologic imaging may be utilized in the evaluation of a varicocele. Internal spermatic vein venography can delineate the anatomy of the varicocele; however, it is costly and invasive. Its use tends to be limited to selected patients with recurrent varicocele[188] or during intraoperative evaluation.[189] Another method in the evaluation of a varicocele is the use of scrotal thermography to measure the scrotal temperature.[190,191] It is suggested that the observed increase in testicular temperature might identify those patients at risk for varicocele-induced testicular damage. Owing to a lack of correlation with outcome, this method is not in common use in the USA today. Color Doppler US may also be used to evaluate for the presence of a varicocele (Figure 73.7). It is able to define the number of dilated veins as well as the severity of dilation. However, with these various radiologic methods, many subclinical varicoceles can be identified (i.e. those that are not palpable on physical examination but are visualized with radiologic imaging.). Using contact thermography and venography, approximately 7% of those with a left-sided and 86% of those with right-sided varicocele are identified in the absence of findings on physical examination in adolescents who present for evaluation of a varicocele.[192] Because subclinical varicoceles are seen in approximately 60% of men attending fertility clinics but also in 40% of fertile men,[193,194] the clinical rele-

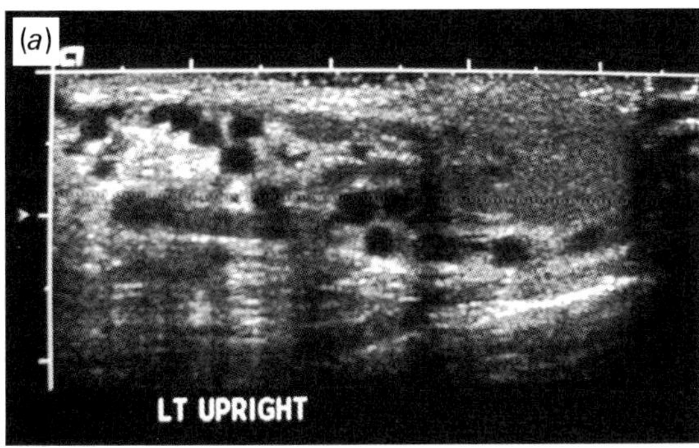

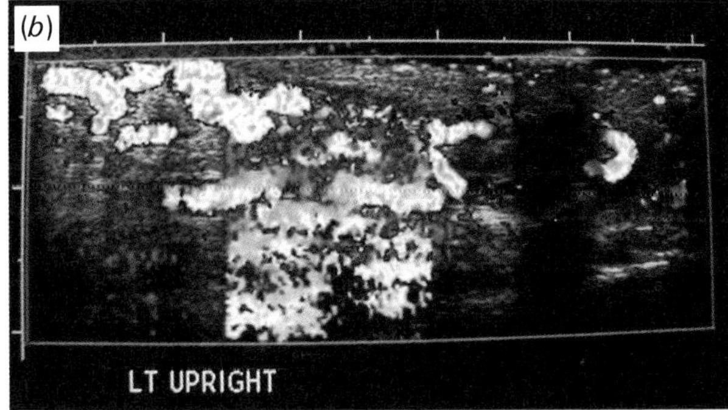

Figure 73.7 On ultrasonography (US), a varicocele can be identified by its 'Swiss-cheese' appearance (*a*). Doppler US can demonstrate retrograde flow in the varicocele (*b*).

vance and therefore the importance of diagnosing subclinical varicoceles are highly debated.

Treatment

Since 15% of adult men have a varicocele but only 20% of them have infertility, observation is a valid option in the management of patients with a varicocele. The risk in observing these patients is that some of them may demonstrate deterioration in the semen parameters and may progress to infertility. Although surgical correction reverses these changes in at least 50% of adult men, in others it does not, suggesting a potential for developing irreversible damage. Consequently, early surgical correction of adolescent varicocele has been advocated. This recommendation is based upon the assumption that adolescent varicocele is a progressive disease. In the only prospective longitudinal study in adults,[195] semen quality in men with untreated varicocele did not decline with time. However, most of the men had a semen quality at baseline that was worse than that of the controls. In the two studies of adolescent varicocele,[173,174] the authors observed lower semen quality in those who underwent varicocele repair compared with those who were not treated. However, it should be noted that in the first study there was no sequential semen analysis and in the second, the untreated group had similar semen parameters compared with controls. In another study,[196] a group of adolescents with a unilateral varicocele was followed with serial examinations, with a mean follow-up between the first and second examinations of 16 months. There was neither an increase in varicocele grade nor a change in testicular volume differentials over time, suggesting that perhaps adolescent varicocele is not a progressive disease. However, the limitations of this study are length of follow-up time and correlation with other parameters such as semen analysis. Currently, there are no convincing data supporting or refuting the premise that adolescent varicocele is a progressive disease.

Consequently, with the goal of preserving fertility, it is important to identify those adolescents with varicocele who would benefit from early intervention. It is generally agreed upon that an indication for surgical intervention is for symptoms such as pain. Although an uncommon complaint, 80–90% of those patients who undergo varicocele repair will have resolution of their symptoms.[183] In addition, those adolescents with bilateral varicoceles may benefit from surgery, since it is difficult to follow their testicular growth as both sides are affected. Similarly, in older patients with abnormal semen parameters on serial evaluation, surgical intervention would be indicated, allowing for potential improvement in semen parameters[172,173] and fertility.[197]

Other indications for varicocele repair in adolescents are more controversial. When semen analysis is not available, marked testicular volume differential is used as an indication for surgery. In adult men with a unilateral varicocele, testicular hypotrophy is associated with decreased total motile sperm counts.[198] However, there does not appear to be a correlation between the loss of testis volume and fertility status.[160] Nevertheless, surgical intervention does reverse the growth loss in adolescents with a unilateral varicocele.[167,172–174] Although it remains unclear whether varicocele repair solely for the purpose of reversing testicular hypotrophy improves future fertility potential, most would agree on this as an indication for intervention, in the absence of semen analysis. Size (i.e. grade) of the varicocele has also been suggested as a potential indicator for surgical intervention. It was observed that in infertile patients with grade III varicocele, there was a greater improvement in sperm concentration and motility than in those patients with grade I or II varicocele.[199] However, there was no difference in fertility rates in those with large or small varicocele who underwent repair.[199,200] Consequently, the grade of the varicocele in itself is not predictive of the need for surgical intervention. Similarly, the finding of a 'soft' testis in association with the varicocele is not a strong indication for surgery. This finding is quite subjective and difficult to quantify; consequently, there is a lack of data of proven value for predicting the need for early intervention. Finally, parental and adolescent preferences often play a role in determining the treatment of varicocele: they may feel that surgery may be of some psychological benefits, restoring normal scrotal appearance and allowing them not to worry about potential future complications.

Techniques of varicocele repair

There are several techniques that can be employed in the treatment of a varicocele, including percutaneous, open, and laparoscopic approaches. With percutaneous techniques, the dilated veins can be sclerosed with a chemical agent or occluded with coils or a balloon. Access can be obtained percutaneously in a retrograde manner via the femoral or jugular vein or in an antegrade manner via the varicocele itself.[201,202] The advantages of the percutaneous techniques include being less costly and having a shorter recovery time compared with open surgery. In older patients, these techniques can be performed under local anesthesia, alleviating the need and risk of general anesthesia. However, it should be noted that in 15–27% of the patients undergoing transvenous occlusion, the procedure could not be performed as a result of difficulties in reaching the varicocele.[203] Potential complications include extravasation of contrast material, coil migration, postprocedure hydrocele formation (11%), and recurrence (5%).

Open surgical correction of varicocele has conventionally been the standard treatment of varicocele for many years. This treatment can be performed inguinally, retroperitoneally, or subinguinally. The Ivanissevich repair utilizes an incision in the inguinal region with the patient in reverse Trendelenburg position. The spermatic cord is exposed and mobilized in the inguinal canal. Under loupe magnification, all veins are ligated. The testicular artery, which may be dilated with warm saline or papaverine and identified visually or with Doppler US, can be spared or mass ligated with the veins. The advantage of this procedure is that it is easy to perform because of its anatomic familiarity and easy access to the cord. With this technique, there is a 3–8.6% incidence of hydrocele postoperatively and a 16% recurrence rate in the treatment of adolescent varicocele. Both the hydrocele rate and the recurrence rate can be reduced using microscopic dissection. Sparing the artery decreases the risk of hydrocele formation by sparing the lymphatic vessels surrounding the artery but increases the risk of recurrence from missed venous connections.

The Palomo technique utilizes a muscle-splitting incision one–two fingerbreaths medial and anterior to the superior iliac crest and the same distance above the estimated position of the internal ring, providing access to the retroperitoneum. The vessels are identified on the posterior aspect of the peritoneum; they may be better visualized by providing traction on the testis. As with the inguinal approach, the testicular artery can be ligated with the vein. The advantages of this technique are that above the inguinal canal there are fewer venous branches requiring ligation and that the vas and its associated vessels have separated from the rest of the cord, minimizing the risk of their injury. However, this approach is often more anatomically difficult and could miss scrotal or pelvic collaterals feeding into the varicocele. The incidence of hydrocele postoperatively is approximately 7%. Similar to that of the Ivanissevich repair, the rate of recurrence is around 11–14% with sparing of the artery or 2% by not sparing of the artery. Several studies[204] have demonstrated that ligation of the artery during Palomo repair can be safely performed and does not result in testicular atrophy.

The subinguinal technique utilizes a low transverse inguinal incision to expose the cord below the external ring. The external oblique aponeurosis is opened and the testis is delivered out of the scrotum. Using an operating microscope, the artery and lymphatic vessels are identified and spared, while all the external spermatic veins and scrotal veins are ligated. By being able to identify and preserve the artery and lymphatic vessels, the incidence of postoperative hydrocele is very low (approximately 0.8%) with a 2.1% recurrence rate.[205]

Over the past decade, the laparoscopic approach to varicocele repair has gained in popularity. It can be performed with a transperitoneal or a preperitoneal approach. For the transperitoneal approach, an incision is made in the umbilicus and is extended down to the midline fascia. A pneumoperitoneum is created with a Veress needle or by the open Hassan technique. The abdomen is insufflated to 12–14 cmH_2O. Two additional ports are placed: one in the midline near the

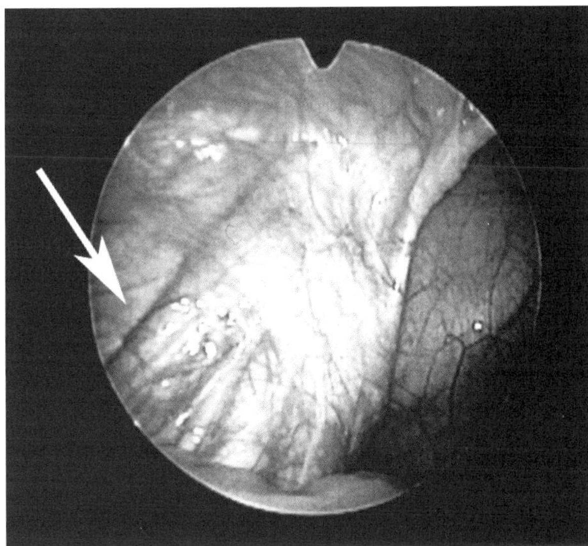

Figure 73.8 On laparoscopy, the spermatic veins (arrow) can be easily identified in the retroperitoneum. Above the level of the internal ring, the vas and its vessels have separated away from the cord, minimizing its injury during the dissection.

pubis and the second in between the other two. The position of the ports should allow the instruments to triangulate the work area. The patient is placed in steep Trendelenburg position to allow the bowel to move out of the pelvis. Collaterals can be accessed by compressing on the main vein and squeezing the testis[206] (Figure 73.8). The vessels are mobilized from the peritoneum and ligated. The artery may be identified with a Doppler US and spared.[207] After the completion of the procedure, the abdominal pressure should be reduced and the area carefully inspected for bleeding. The advantages of this technique include a shorter postoperative convalescence due to avoidance of a larger inguinal or abdominal incisions, better visualization,[208] and the capacity to treat other associated problems such as bilateral varicoceles or concurrent inguinal hernia.[209] The laparoscopic Palomo can be safely performed in patients who have undergone prior inguinal surgery without a risk of testicular atrophy.[210] The disadvantages include the requirement for general anesthesia, the cost, and the potential for bowel injury, bleeding, and peritonitis. Using this technique, the incidence of postoperative hydrocele is approximately 7% and the recurrence rate is 15%.[211–213]

Treatment of postoperative hydrocele and recurrence

Esposito et al[214] observed that the median incidence of postoperative hydrocele after varicocele surgery was about 12%. The incidence is higher after an artery non-sparing vs a sparing procedure (17.6% compared with 4.3%). Interestingly, no difference in postoperative hydrocele rate was observed between those surgeries performed by laparoscopic or by open techniques. Hydroceles are infrequently detected within 6 months of varicocele repair, generally occurring after 6 months up to 3 years following surgery.[215] Total hydrocele regression occurs in approximately 80% of the patients following clinical observation or being treated with simple scrotal puncture.[214] However, some patients may require open hydrocele repair.

Recurrence following varicocele repair is usually noted several months after surgery.[216] A lower recurrence rate is seen when performing mass ligation compared with artery sparing surgery.[204,217] It is uncommon that recurrence is a result of delayed recanalization.[216] Reoperation is indicated when the indications for the original surgery persist. Intraoperative venography may be helpful in defining collaterals that were missed during the initial surgery. This can be accomplished by placing the patient in a reverse Trendelenburg position and making a small scrotal incision to expose the dilated veins. The vein is cannulated with an angiocatheter directed away from the testis. The catheter is then injected with 30% contrast at a volume of 1 ml/kg body weight. After an X-ray is obtained, the vein is flushed with normal saline solution. It is generally recommended that the cord be approached at a higher level in order to ligate the missed collaterals.

References

1. Rowe MI, Marchildon MB. Inguinal hernia and hydrocele in infants and children. Surg Clin North Am 1981; 61(5):1137–45.
2. Boocock GR, Todd PJ. Inguinal hernias are common in preterm infants. Arch Dis Child 1985; 60(7):669–70.
3. Holsclaw DS, Shwachman H. Increased incidence of inguinal hernia, hydrocele, and undescended testicle in males with cystic fibrosis. Pediatrics 1971; 48(3):442–5.
4. McEntyre RL, Raffensperger JG. Surgical complications of Ehlers–Danlos syndrome in children. J Pediatr Surg 1977; 12(4):531–5.
5. Reed WB, Horowitz RE, Beighton P. Acquired cutis laxa. Primary generalized elastolysis. Arch Dermatol 1971; 103(6):661–9.
6. Uden A, Lindhagen T. Inguinal hernia in patients with congenital dislocation of the hip. A sign of general connective tissue disorder. Acta Orthop Scand 1988; 59(6):667–8.
7. Grosfeld JL, Minnick K, Shedd F et al. Inguinal hernia in

children: factors affecting recurrence in 62 cases. J Pediatr Surg 1991; 26(3):283–7.
8. Taylor GP. Pathology of the pediatric regio inguinalis: mysteries of the hernia sac exposed. Pediatr Dev Pathol 2000; 3(6):513–24.
9. Rosai J, Dehner LP. Nodular mesothelial hyperplasia in hernia sacs: a benign reactive condition simulating a neoplastic process. Cancer 1975; 35(1):165–75.
10. Heyns CF. The gubernaculum during testicular descent in the human fetus. J Anat 1987; 153:93–112.
11. Tanyel FC, Dagdeviren A, Muftuoglu S et al. Inguinal hernia revisited through comparative evaluation of peritoneum, processus vaginalis, and sacs obtained from children with hernia, hydrocele, and undescended testis. J Pediatr Surg 1999; 34(4):552–5.
12. Clarnette TD, Hutson JM. Exogenous calcitonin gene-related peptide can change the direction of gubernacular migration in the mutant trans-scrotal rat. J Pediatr Surg 1999; 34(8):1208–12.
13. Cook BJ, Hasthorpe S, Hutson JM. Fusion of childhood inguinal hernia induced by HGF and CGRP via an epithelial transition. J Pediatr Surg 2000; 35(1):77–81.
14. Momoh JT. Obliteration of processus vaginalis and inguinal hernial sacs in children. Can J Surg 1982; 25(5):483–5.
15. Barthold JS, Redman JF. Association of epididymal anomalies with patent processus vaginalis in hernia, hydrocele and cryptorchidism. J Urol 1996; 156(6):2054–6.
16. Tanyel FC, Muftuoglu S, Dagdeviren A, Kaymaz FF, Buyukpamukcu N. Myofibroblasts defined by electron microscopy suggest the dedifferentiation of smooth muscle within the sac walls associated with congenital inguinal hernia. BJU Int 2001; 87(3):251–5.
17. Tanyel FC, Erdem S, Buyukpamukcu N, Tan E. Smooth muscle within incomplete obliterations of processus vaginalis lacks apoptotic nuclei. Urol Int 2002; 69(1):42–5.
18. Tanyel FC, Ulusu NN, Tezcan EF, Buyukpamukcu N. Total calcium content of sacs associated with inguinal hernia, hydrocele or undescended testis reflects differences dictated by programmed cell death. Urol Int 2003; 70(3):211–15.
19. Tanyel FC, Okur HD. Autonomic nervous system appears to play a role in obliteration of processus vaginalis. Hernia 2004; 8(2):149–54.
20. Clarnette TD, Lam SK, Hutson JM. Ventriculo-peritoneal shunts in children reveal the natural history of closure of the processus vaginalis. J Pediatr Surg 1998; 33(3):413–16.
21. Matsumoto A, Nagatomi Y, Sakai M, Oshi M. Torsion of the hernia sac within a hydrocele of the scrotum in a child. Int J Urol 2004; 11(9):789–91.
22. Myers JB, Lovell MA, Lee RS, Furness PD 3rd, Koyle M. Torsion of an indirect hernia sac causing acute scrotum. J Pediatr Surg 2004; 39(1):122–3.
23. Brisson P, Patel H, Feins N. Cremasteric muscle hypertrophy accompanies inguinal hernias in children. J Pediatr Surg 1999; 34(9):1320–1.
24. Gilbert M, Clatworthy HW Jr. Bilateral operations for inguinal hernia and hydrocele in infancy and childhood. Am J Surg 1959; 97(3):255–9.
25. Rathaus V, Konen O, Shapiro M et al. Ultrasound features of spermatic cord hydrocele in children. Br J Radiol 2001; 74(885):818–20.
26. Ring KS, Axelrod SL, Burbige KA, Hensle TW. Meconium hydrocele: an unusual etiology of a scrotal mass in the newborn. J Urol 1989; 141(5):1172–3.
27. Mendez R, Tellado M, Montero M et al. Acute scrotum: an exceptional presentation of acute nonperforated appendicitis in childhood. J Pediatr Surg 1998; 33(9):1435–6.
28. Nagel P. Scrotal swelling as the presenting symptom of acute perforated appendicitis in an infant. J Pediatr Surg 1984; 19(2):177–8.
29. Reeve HR, Weinerth JL, Peterson LJ. Tuberculosis of epididymis and testicle presenting as hydrocele. Urology 1974; 4(3):329–31.
30. Guy RJ. Tuberculous epididymitis presenting as acute hydrocele. J R Nav Med Serv 1995; 81(1):33–6.
31. Pachter EM, Horowitz M, Glassberg KI. Infected hydrocele in a neonate. J Urol 1997; 157(4):1464–5.
32. Linn RH, Sage WH 3rd, Walsh JJ. Scrotal pneumocele complicating pneumoperitoneum. Am Rev Tuberc 1956; 74(4):622–3.
33. Skoog SJ, Belman AB. The communicating hematocele: an unusual presentation for blunt splenic trauma. J Urol 1986; 136(5):1092–3.
34. Park SJ, Lee HK, Hong HS et al. Hydrocele of the canal of Nuck in a girl: ultrasound and MR appearance. Br J Radiol 2004; 77(915):243–4.
35. Erez I, Rathause V, Vacian I et al. Preoperative ultrasound and intraoperative findings of inguinal hernias in children: a prospective study of 642 children. J Pediatr Surg 2002; 37(6):865–8.
36. Swischuk LE, Stacy TM. Herniography: radiologic investigation of inguinal hernia. Radiology 1971; 101(1):139–46.
37. Nadkarni S, Brown PW, van Beek EJ, Collins MC. Herniography: a prospective, randomized study between midline and left iliac fossa puncture techniques. Clin Radiol 2001; 56(5):389–92.
38. Markos V, Brown EF. CT herniography in the diagnosis of occult groin hernias. Clin Radiol 2005; 60(2):251–6.
39. Calder F, Evans R, Neilson D, Hurley P. Value of herniography in the management of occult hernia and chronic groin pain in adults. Br J Surg 2000; 87(6):824–5.
40. Heise CP, Sproat IA, Starling JR. Peritoneography (herniography) for detecting occult inguinal hernia in patients with inguinodynia. Ann Surg 2002; 235(1):140–4.
41. Leung WY, Poon M, Chung KW, Kwok WK. Should we perform early operations in children who have reducible inguinal hernia? Hong Kong Med J 1998; 4(3):337.
42. Gonzalez Santacruz M, Mira Navarro J, Encinas Goenechea A et al. Low prevalence of complications of delayed herniotomy in the extremely premature infant. Acta Paediatr 2004; 93(1):94–8.
43. Read RC. Recent advances in the repair of groin herniation. Curr Probl Surg 2003; 40(1):13–79.
44. Fearne C, Abela M, Aquilina D. Scrotal approach for inguinal hernia and hydrocele repair in boys. Eur J Pediatr Surg 2002; 12(2):116–17.

45. Gokcora IH, Yagmurlu A. A novel incision for groin pathologies in children: the low inguinal groove approach. Hernia 2003; 7(3):146–9.
46. Ger R. Historical aspects of laparoscopic hernia repair. Semin Laparosc Surg 1998; 5(4):212–16.
47. Gorsler CM, Schier F. Laparoscopic herniorrhaphy in children. Surg Endosc 2003; 17(4):571–3.
48. Schier F, Montupet P, Esposito C. Laparoscopic inguinal herniorrhaphy in children: a three-center experience with 933 repairs. J Pediatr Surg 2002; 37(3):395–7.
49. Shalaby R, Desoky A. Needlescopic inguinal hernia repair in children. Pediatr Surg Int 2002; 18(2–3):153–6.
50. Perlstein J, Du Bois JJ. The role of laparoscopy in the management of suspected recurrent pediatric hernias. J Pediatr Surg 2000; 35(8):1205–8.
51. Schier F. Direct inguinal hernias in children: laparoscopic aspects. Pediatr Surg Int 2000; 16(8):562–4.
52. Prasad R, Lovvorn HN 3rd, Wadie GM, Lobe TE. Early experience with needleoscopic inguinal herniorrhaphy in children. J Pediatr Surg 2003; 38(7):1055–8.
53. Daehlin L, Tonder B, Kapstad L. Comparison of polidocanol and tetracycline in the sclerotherapy of testicular hydrocele and epididymal cyst. Br J Urol 1997; 80(3):468–71.
54. Crofford MJ, Balsam D. Scrotal migration of ventriculoperitoneal shunts. AJR Am J Roentgenol 1983; 141(2):369–71.
55. Mares AJ, Shkolnik A, Sacks M, Feuchtwanger MM. Aberrant (ectopic) adrenocortical tissue along the spermatic cord. J Pediatr Surg 1980; 15(3):289–92.
56. Carragher AM. One hundred years of splenogonadal fusion. Urology 1990; 35(6):471–5.
57. Ferro F, Lais A, Boldrini R et al. Hepatogonadal fusion. J Pediatr Surg 1996; 31(3):435–6.
58. Orlowski JP, Levin HS, Dyment PG. Intrascrotal Wilms' tumor developing in a heterotopic renal anlage of probable mesonephric origin. J Pediatr Surg 1980; 15(5):679–82.
59. Magee JF, Barker NE, Blair GK, Steinbok P. Inguinal herniation with glial implants: possible complication of ventriculoperitoneal shunting. Pediatr Pathol Lab Med 1996; 16(4):591–6.
60. Nicholson CP, Donohue JH, Thompson GB, Lewis JE. A study of metastatic cancer found during inguinal hernia repair. Cancer 1992; 69(12):3008–11.
61. Fernandes ET, Kumar M, Douglass EC et al. Extrarenal Wilms' tumor. J Pediatr Surg 1989; 24(5):483–5.
62. Hancock RA, Hodgins TE. Polyorchidism. Urology 1984; 24(4):303–7.
63. Barthold JS, Kumasi-Rivers K, Upadhyay J, Shekarriz B, Imperato-Mcginley J. Testicular position in the androgen insensitivity syndrome: implications for the role of androgens in testicular descent. J Urol 2000; 164(2):497–501.
64. Sultan C, Lumbroso S, Paris F et al. Disorders of androgen action. Semin Reprod Med 2002; 20(3):217–28.
65. Boley SJ, Cahn D, Lauer T, Weinberg G, Kleinhaus S. The irreducible ovary: a true emergency. J Pediatr Surg 1991; 26(9):1035–8.
66. El-Gohary MA. Laparoscopic management of persistent müllerian duct syndrome. Pediatr Surg Int 2003; 19(7):533–6.
67. Loeff DS, Imbeaud S, Reyes HM, Meller JL, Rosenthal IM. Surgical and genetic aspects of persistent müllerian duct syndrome. J Pediatr Surg 1994; 29(1):61–5.
68. Gill B, Favale D, Kogan SJ et al. Significance of accessory ductal structures in hernia sacs. J Urol 1992; 148(2 Pt 2):697–8.
69. Popek EJ. Embryonal remnants in inguinal hernia sacs. Hum Pathol 1990; 21(3):339–49.
70. Walker AN, Mills SE. Glandular inclusions in inguinal hernial sacs and spermatic cords. Müllerian-like remnants confused with functional reproductive structures. Am J Clin Pathol 1984; 82(1):85–9.
71. Miller GG, McDonald SE, Milbrandt K, Chibbar R. Routine pathological evaluation of tissue from inguinal hernias in children is unnecessary. Can J Surg 2003; 46(2):117–19.
72. Clausen EG, Jake RJ, Binkley FM. Contralateral inguinal exploration of unilateral hernia in infants and children. Surgery 1958; 44(4):735–40.
73. Rowe MI, Copelson LW, Clatworthy HW. The patent processus vaginalis and the inguinal hernia. J Pediatr Surg 1969; 4(1):102–7.
74. Hata S, Takahashi Y, Nakamura T et al. Preoperative sonographic evaluation is a useful method of detecting contralateral patent processus vaginalis in pediatric patients with unilateral inguinal hernia. J Pediatr Surg 2004; 39(9):1396–9.
75. Downey EC, Maher DP, Thompson WR. Diagnostic pneumoperitoneum accurately predicts the presence of patent processus vaginalis. J Pediatr Surg 1995; 30(9):1271–2.
76. Miltenburg DM, Nuchtern JG, Jaksic T, Kozinetiz C, Brandt ML. Laparoscopic evaluation of the pediatric inguinal hernia – a meta-analysis. J Pediatr Surg 1998; 33(6):874–9.
77. Bhatia AM, Gow KW, Heiss KF, Barr G, Wulkan ML. Is the use of laparoscopy to determine presence of contralateral patent processus vaginalis justified in children greater than 2 years of age? J Pediatr Surg 2004; 39(5):778–81.
78. Eller Miranda M, Duarte Lanna JC. Videolaparoscopy of the contralateral internal inguinal ring via the hernia sac in children with unilateral inguinal hernia – initial experience in Brazil, with a meta-analysis. Pediatr Surg Int 2002; 18(5–6):463–9.
79. Lotan G, Efrati Y, Stolero S, Klin B. Transinguinal laparoscopic examination: an end to the controversy on repair of inguinal hernia in children. Isr Med Assoc J 2004; 6(6):339–41.
80. Hessert W. The frequency of congenital sacs in oblique inguinal hernia. Surg Gynecol Obstet 1910; 10:252.
81. Mitchell GAG. The condition of the peritoneal vaginal process at birth. J Anat 1939; 75:658–61.
82. Geisler DP, Jegathesan S, Parmley MC et al. Laparoscopic exploration for the clinically undetected hernia in infancy and childhood. Am J Surg 2001; 182(6):693–6.
83. Ballantyne A, Jawaheer G, Munro FD. Contralateral groin exploration is not justified in infants with a unilateral inguinal hernia. Br J Surg 2001; 88(5):720–3.
84. Lym L, Ross JH, Alexander F, Kay R. Risk of contralateral hydrocele or hernia after unilateral hydrocele repair in

children. J Urol 1999; 162(3 Pt 2):1169–70, discussion 1171.

85. Nassiri SJ. Contralateral exploration is not mandatory in unilateral inguinal hernia in children: a prospective 6-year study. Pediatr Surg Int 2002; 18(5–6):470–1.
86. Shabbir J, Moore A, O'Sullivan JB et al. Contralateral groin exploration is not justified in infants with a unilateral inguinal hernia. Ir J Med Sci 2003; 172(1):18–19.
87. Tackett LD, Breuer CK, Luks FI et al. Incidence of contralateral inguinal hernia: a prospective analysis. J Pediatr Surg 1999; 34(5):684–7, discussion 687–8.
88. Chertin B, De Caluwe D, Gajaharan M, Piaseczna-Piotrowska A, Puri P. Is contralateral exploration necessary in girls with unilateral inguinal hernia? J Pediatr Surg 2003; 38(5):756–7.
89. Ikeda H, Suzuki N, Takahashi A et al. Risk of contralateral manifestation in children with unilateral inguinal hernia: should hernia in children be treated contralaterally? J Pediatr Surg 2000; 35(12):1746–8.
90. Miltenburg DM, Nuchtern JG, Jaksic T, Kozinetz CA, Brandt ML. Meta-analysis of the risk of metachronous hernia in infants and children. Am J Surg 1997; 174(6):741–4.
91. Holcomb GW 3rd, Miller KA, Chaignaud BE, Shew SB, Ostlie DJ. The parental perspective regarding the contralateral inguinal region in a child with a known unilateral inguinal hernia. J Pediatr Surg 2004; 39(3):480–2, discussion 480–2.
92. Burd RS, Heffington SH, Teague JL. The optimal approach for management of metachronous hernias in children: a decision analysis. J Pediatr Surg 2001; 36(8):1190–5.
93. Shimbori H, Ono K, Miwa T et al. Comparison of the LMA-ProSeal and LMA-Classic in children. Br J Anaesth 2004; 93(4):528–31.
94. Passariello M, Almenrader N, Canneti A et al. Caudal analgesia in children: S(+)-ketamine vs S(+)-ketamine plus clonidine. Paediatr Anaesth 2004; 14(10):851–5.
95. Broadman LM. Use of spinal or continuous caudal anesthesia for inguinal hernia repair in premature infants: are there advantages? Reg Anesth 1996; 21(6 Suppl):108–13.
96. Surana R, Puri P. Iatrogenic ascent of the testis: an under-recognized complication of inguinal hernia operation in children. Br J Urol 1994; 73(5):580–1.
97. Imamoglu M, Cay A, Sarihan H, Ahmetoglu A, Ozdemir O. Paravesical abscess as an unusual late complication of inguinal hernia repair in children. J Urol 2004; 171(3):1268–70.
98. Johnstone MS. Inguinal hernia repair. In: Stringer MD, Oldham KT, Mouriquand PDE, Howard ER, eds. Pediatric Surgery and Urology: Long Term Outcomes. Philadelphia: WB Saunders, 1998: 257–63.
99. Kurkchubasche AG, Tracy TFJ. Unique features of groin hernia repair in infants and children. In: Fitzgibbons RJJ, Greenburg AG, eds. Nyhus and Condon's Hernia, 5th edn. Philadelphia: Lippincott, 2002: 435–51.
100. Caesar RE, Kaplan GW. Incidence of the bell-clapper deformity in an autopsy series. Urology 1994; 44(1):114–16.
101. Das S, Singer A. Controversies of perinatal torsion of the spermatic cord: a review, survey and recommendations. J Urol 1990; 143(2):231–3.
102. Barca PR, Dargallo T, Jardon JA et al. Bilateral testicular torsion in the neonatal period. J Urol 1997; 158:1957–9.
103. Melekos MD, Asbach HW, Markou SA. Etiology of acute scrotum in 100 boys with regard to age distribution. J Urol 1988; 139(5):1023–5.
104. Anderson JB, Williamson RC. Testicular torsion in Bristol: a 25-year review. Br J Surg 1988; 75(10):988–92.
105. Thurston A, Whitaker R. Torsion of testis after previous testicular surgery. Br J Surg 1983; 70(4):217.
106. Rabinowitz R. The importance of the cremasteric reflex in acute scrotal swelling in children. J Urol 1984; 132:89–90.
107. Baker LA, Sigman D, Mathews RI, Benson J, Docimo SG. An analysis of clinical outcomes using color Doppler testicular ultrasound for testicular torsion. Pediatrics 2000; 105(3):604–7.
108. Bader TR, Kammerhuber F, Herneth AM. Testicular blood flow in boys as assessed at color Doppler and power Doppler sonography. Radiology 1997; 202:559–64.
109. Ingram S, Hollman A. Colour Doppler sonography of the normal paediatric testis. Clin Radiol 1994; 49:266–7.
110. Lee FT Jr, Winter DB, Madsen FA et al. Conventional color Doppler velocity sonography versus color Doppler energy sonography for the diagnosis of acute experimental torsion of the spermatic cord. AJR Am J Roentgenol 1996; 167:785–90.
111. Levy OM, Gittelman MC, Strashun AM, Cohen EL, Fine EJ. Diagnosis of acute testicular torsion using radionuclide scanning. J Urol 1983; 129(5):975–7.
112. Smith G. Cellular changes from graded testicular ischemia. J Urol 1955; 73:355–62.
113. Tryfonas G, Violaki A, Tsikopoulos G et al. Late postoperative results in males treated for testicular torsion during childhood. J Pediatr Surg 1994; 29(4):553–6.
114. Bartsch G, Frank S, Marberger H, Mikuz G. Testicular torsion: late results with special regard to fertility and endocrine function. J Urol 1980; 124(3):375–8.
115. Cosentino MJ, Nishida M, Rabinowitz R, Cockett AT. Histological changes occurring in the contralateral testes of prepubertal rats subjected to various durations of unilateral spermatic cord torsion. J Urol 1985; 133(5):906–11.
116. Cosentino MJ, Rabinowitz R, Valvo JR, Cockett AT. The effect of prepubertal spermatic cord torsion on subsequent fertility in rats. J Androl 1984; 5(2):93–8.
117. Nagler HM, White RD. The effect of testicular torsion on the contralateral testis. J Urol 1982; 128(6):1343–8.
118. Madarikan BA. Testicular salvage following spermatic cord torsion. J Pediatr Surg 1987; 22(3):231–4.
119. Zanchetta R, Mastrogiacomo I, Graziotti P, Foresta C, Betterle C. Autoantibodies against Leydig cells in patients after spermatic cord torsion. Clin Exp Immunol 1984; 55(1):49–57.
120. Mastrogiacomo I, Zanchetta R, Graziotti P et al. Immunological and clinical study of patients after spermatic cord torsion. Andrologia 1982; 14(1):25–30.
121. Hagen P, Buchholz MM, Eigenmann J, Bandhauer K. Testicular dysplasia causing disturbance of spermiogene-

sis in patients with unilateral torsion of the testis. Urol Int 1992; 49(3):154–7.

122. Thomas WE, Cooper MJ, Crane GA, Lee G, Williamson RC. Testicular exocrine malfunction after torsion. Lancet 1984; 2(8416):1357–60.
123. Salman AB, Mutlu S, Iskit AB et al. Hemodynamic monitoring of the contralateral testis during unilateral testicular torsion describes the mechanism of damage. Eur Urol 1998; 33(6):576–80.
124. Tanyel FC, Buyukpamukcu N, Hicsonmez A. Contralateral testicular blood flow during unilateral testicular torsion. Br J Urol 1989; 63(5):522–4.
125. Kolettis PN, Stowe NT, Inman SR, Thomas AJ Jr. Acute spermatic cord torsion alters the microcirculation of the contralateral testis. J Urol 1996; 155(1):350–4.
126. Otcu S, Durakogugil M, Orer HS, Tanyel FC. Contralateral genitofemoral sympathetic nerve discharge increases following ipsilateral testicular torsion. Urol Res 2002; 30(5):324–8.
127. Power RE, Scanlon R, Kay EW, Creagh TA, Bouchier-Hayes DJ. Long-term protective effects of hypothermia on reperfusion injury post-testicular torsion. Scand J Urol Nephrol 2003; 37(6):456–60.
128. Akgur FM, Kilinc K, Aktug T, Olguner M. The effect of allopurinol pretreatment before detorting testicular torsion. J Urol 1994; 151(6):1715–17.
129. Palmer JS, Cromie WJ, Lee RC. Surfactant administration reduces testicular ischemia-reperfusion injury. J Urol 1998; 159(6):2136–9.
130. Pakyz RE, Heindel RM, Kallish M, Cosentino MJ. Spermatic cord torsion: effects of cyclosporine and prednisone on fertility and the contralateral testis in the rat. J Androl 1990; 11(5):401–8.
131. Dokucu AI, Ozturk H, Ozdemir E et al. The protective effects of nitric oxide on the contralateral testis in prepubertal rats with unilateral testicular torsion. BJU Int 2000; 85(6):767–71.
132. Oguzkurt P, Okur DH, Tanyel FC, Buyukpamukcu N, Hicsonmez A. The effects of vasodilatation and chemical sympathectomy on spermatogenesis after unilateral testicular torsion: a flow cytometric DNA analysis. Br J Urol 1998; 82(1):104–8.
133. Visser AJ, Heyns CF. Testicular function after torsion of the spermatic cord. BJU Int 2003; 92(3):200–3.
134. Kiesling VJ Jr, Schroeder DE, Pauljev P, Hull J. Spermatic cord block and manual reduction: primary treatment for spermatic cord torsion. J Urol 1984; 132(5):921–3.
135. Cooper CS, Snyder OB, Hawtrey CE. Bilateral neonatal testicular torsion. Clin Pediatr 1997; 36:653–6.
136. Cuckow PM, Frank JD. Torsion of the testis. BJU Int 2000; 86(3):349–53.
137. Akbay E, Cayan S, Doruk E, Duce MN, Bozlu M. The prevalence of varicocele and varicocele-related testicular atrophy in Turkish children and adolescents. BJU Int 2000; 86(4):490–3.
138. Steeno O, Knops J, Declerck L, Adimoelja A, van de Voorde H. Prevention of fertility disorders by detection and treatment of varicocele at school and college age. Andrologia 1976; 8(1):47–53.
139. Niedzielski J, Paduch D, Raczynski P. Assessment of adolescent varicocele. Pediatr Surg Int 1997; 12(5–6):410–13.
140. Sigmund G, Gall H, Bahren W. Stop-type and shunt-type varicoceles: venographic findings. Radiology 1987; 163(1):105–10.
141. Braedel HU, Steffens J, Ziegler M, Polsky MS, Platt ML. A possible ontogenic etiology for idiopathic left varicocele. J Urol 1994; 151(1):62–6.
142. Ibrahim AA, Awad HA, El-Haggar S, Mitawi BA. Bilateral testicular biopsy in men with varicocele. Fertil Steril 1977; 28(6):663–7.
143. Agger P, Johnsen SG. Quantitative evaluation of testicular biopsies in varicocele. Fertil Steril 1978; 29(1):52–7.
144. McFadden MR, Mehan DJ. Testicular biopsies in 101 cases of varicocele. J Urol 1978; 119(3):372–4.
145. Cameron DF, Snydle FE, Ross MH, Drylie DM. Ultrastructural alterations in the adluminal testicular compartment in men with varicocele. Fertil Steril 1980; 33(5):526–33.
146. Hadziselimovic F, Herzog B, Liebundgut B, Jenny P, Buser M. Testicular and vascular changes in children and adults with varicocele. J Urol 1989; 142(2 Pt 2):583–5, discussion 603–5.
147. Weiss DB, Rodriguez-Rigau LJ, Smith KD, Steinberger E. Leydig cell function in oligospermic men with varicocele. J Urol 1978; 120(4):427–30.
148. Hadziselimovic F, Leibundgut B, Da Rugna D, Buser MW. The value of testicular biopsy in patients with varicocele. J Urol 1986; 135(4):707–10.
149. Younes AK. Low plasma testosterone in varicocele patients with impotence and male infertility. Arch Androl 2000; 45(3):187–95.
150. Bohring C, Krause W. Serum levels of inhibin B in men with different causes of spermatogenic failure. Andrologia 1999; 31(3):137–41.
151. Hipler UC, Hochheim B, Knoll B, Tittelbach J, Schreiber G. Serum inhibin B as a marker for spermatogenesis. Arch Androl 2001; 46(3):217–22.
152. Ibrahim II, Abdalla MI, Girgis SM et al. FSH, LH, E2, progesterone, and testosterone in peripheral blood, spermatic vein, and semen of subfertile men with varicocele. Arch Androl 1983; 10(2):173–7.
153. Bruno B, Francavilla S, Properzi G, Martini M, Fabbrini A. Hormonal and seminal parameters in infertile men. Andrologia 1986; 18(6):595–600.
154. Guarino N, Tadini B, Bianchi M. The adolescent varicocele: the crucial role of hormonal tests in selecting patients with testicular dysfunction. J Pediatr Surg 2003; 38(1):120–3, discussion 120–3.
155. Kass EJ, Freitas JE, Bour JB. Adolescent varicocele: objective indications for treatment. J Urol 1989; 142(2 Pt 2):579–82, discussion 603–5.
156. Aragona F, Ragazzi R, Pozzan GB et al. Correlation of testicular volume, histology and LHRH test in adolescents with idiopathic varicocele. Eur Urol 1994; 26(1):61–6.
157. Osuna JA, Lozano JR, Cruz I, Tortolero I. Pituitary and testicular function in adolescents with varicocele. Arch Androl 1999; 43(3):183–8.
158. Fideleff HL, Boquete H, Ruibal G et al. Varicocele in prepubertal boys. Evaluation of clinical Doppler and hormonal findings. Medicina (B Aires) 1996; 56(6):679–82.

159. Lipshultz LI, Corriere JN Jr. Progressive testicular atrophy in the varicocele patient. J Urol 1977; 117(2):175–6.
160. Pinto KJ, Kroovand RL, Jarow JP. Varicocele related testicular atrophy and its predictive effect upon fertility. J Urol 1994; 152(2 Pt 2):788–90.
161. Sayfan J, Siplovich L, Koltun L, Benyamin N. Varicocele treatment in pubertal boys prevents testicular growth arrest. J Urol 1997; 157(4):1456–7.
162. Parrott TS, Hewatt L. Ligation of the testicular artery and vein in adolescent varicocele. J Urol 1994; 152(2 Pt 2):791–3; discussion 793.
163. Haans LC, Laven JS, Mali WP, te Velde ER, Wensing CJ. Testis volumes, semen quality, and hormonal patterns in adolescents with and without a varicocele. Fertil Steril 1991; 56(4):731–6.
164. Baker HW, Burger HG, de Kretser DM et al. Testicular vein ligation and fertility in men with varicoceles. Br Med J (Clin Res Ed) 1985; 291(6510):1678–80.
165. MacLeod J. Seminal cytology in the presence of varicocele. Fertil Steril 1965; 16(6):735–57.
166. Chehval MJ, Purcell MH. Deterioration of semen parameters over time in men with untreated varicocele: evidence of progressive testicular damage. Fertil Steril 1992; 57(1):174–7.
167. Paduch DA, Niedzielski J. Semen analysis in young men with varicocele: preliminary study. J Urol 1996; 156(2 Pt 2):788–90.
168. Parsch EM, Schill WB, Erlinger C, Tauber R, Pfeifer KJ. Semen parameters and conception rates after surgical treatment and sclerotherapy of varicocele. Andrologia 1990; 22(3):275–8.
169. Rodriguez-Rigau LJ, Smith KD, Steinberger E. Relationship of varicocele to sperm output and fertility of male partners in infertile couples. J Urol 1978; 120(6):691–4.
170. Dubin L, Amelar RD. Varicocelectomy: 986 cases in a twelve-year study. Urology 1977; 10(5):446–9.
171. Lenzi A, Gandini L, Bagolan P, Nahum A, Dondero F. Sperm parameters after early left varicocele treatment. Fertil Steril 1998; 69(2):347–9.
172. Laven JS, Haans LC, Mali WP et al. Effects of varicocele treatment in adolescents: a randomized study. Fertil Steril 1992; 58(4):756–62.
173. Okuyama A, Nakamura M, Namiki M et al. Surgical repair of varicocele at puberty: preventive treatment for fertility improvement. J Urol 1988; 139(3):562–4.
174. Yamamoto M, Hibi H, Katsuno S, Miyake K. Effects of varicocelectomy on testis volume and semen parameters in adolescents: a randomized prospective study. Nagoya J Med Sci 1995; 58(3–4):127–32.
175. Salisz JA, Kass EJ, Steinert BW. The significance of elevated scrotal temperature in an adolescent with a varicocele. Adv Exp Med Biol 1991; 286:245–51.
176. Turner TT. The study of varicocele through the use of animal models. Hum Reprod Update 2001; 7(1):78–84.
177. Harrison RM, Lewis RW, Roberts JA. Pathophysiology of varicocele in nonhuman primates: long-term seminal and testicular changes. Fertil Steril 1986; 46(3):500–10.
178. Al-Juburi A, Pranikoff K, Dougherty KA, Urry RL, Cockett AT. Alteration of semen quality in dogs after creation of varicocele. Urology 1979; 13(5):535–9.
179. Saypol DC, Howards SS, Turner TT, Miller ED Jr. Influence of surgically induced varicocele on testicular blood flow, temperature, and histology in adult rats and dogs. J Clin Invest 1981; 68(1):39–45.
180. Green KF, Turner TT, Howards SS. Effects of varicocele after unilateral orchiectomy and sympathectomy. J Urol 1985; 134(2):378–83.
181. Hurt GS, Howards SS, Turner TT. Repair of experimental varicoceles in the rat. Long-term effects on testicular blood flow and temperature and cauda epididymidal sperm concentration and motility. J Androl 1986; 7(5):271–6.
182. Green KF, Turner TT, Howards SS. Varicocele: reversal of the testicular blood flow and temperature effects by varicocele repair. J Urol 1984; 131(6):1208–11.
183. Diamond DA. Adolescent varicocele: emerging understanding. BJU Int 2003; 92(Suppl 1):48–51.
184. Paltiel HJ, Diamond DA, Di Canzio J et al. Testicular volume: comparison of orchidometer and US measurements in dogs. Radiology 2002; 222(1):114–19.
185. Diamond DA, Paltiel HJ, DiCanzio J et al. Comparative assessment of pediatric testicular volume: orchidometer versus ultrasound. J Urol 2000; 164(3 Pt 2):1111–14.
186. Diamond DA, Roth JA, Cilento BG, Barnewolt CE. Intratesticular varicocele in adolescents: a reversible anechoic lesion of the testis. J Urol 2004; 171(1):381–3.
187. Janczewski Z, Bablok L. Semen characteristics in pubertal boys. I. Semen quality after first ejaculation. Arch Androl 1985; 15(2–3):199–205.
188. Punekar SV, Prem AR, Ridhorkar VR, Deshmukh HL, Kelkar AR. Post-surgical recurrent varicocele: efficacy of internal spermatic venography and steel-coil embolization. Br J Urol 1996; 77(1):124–8.
189. Tauber R, Pfeiffer D, Bruns T. Phlebography: why it is important to study radiological imaging of spermatic veins. Arch Ital Urol Androl 2003; 75(1):62–7.
190. Lewis RW, Harrison RM. Contact scrotal thermography: application to problems of infertility. J Urol 1979; 122(1):40–2.
191. Tucker AT. Infrared thermographic assessment of the human scrotum. Fertil Steril 2000; 74(4):802–3.
192. Gat Y, Zukerman ZV, Bachar GN, Feldberg DO, Gornish M. Adolescent varicocele: is it a unilateral disease? Urology 2003; 62(4):742–6, discussion 746–7.
193. Meacham RB, Townsend RR, Rademacher D, Drose JA. The incidence of varicoceles in the general population when evaluated by physical examination, gray scale sonography and color Doppler sonography. J Urol 1994; 151(6):1535–8.
194. Kursh ED. What is the incidence of varicocele in a fertile population? Fertil Steril 1987; 48(3):510–11.
195. Lund L, Larsen SB. A follow-up study of semen quality and fertility in men with varicocele testis and in control subjects. Br J Urol 1998; 82(5):682–6.
196. Diamond DA, Zurakowski D, Atala A et al. Is adolescent varicocele a progressive disease process? J Urol 2004; 172(4 Pt 2):1746–8, discussion 1748.
197. Madgar I, Weissenberg R, Lunenfeld B, Karasik A, Goldwasser B. Controlled trial of high spermatic vein ligation for varicocele in infertile men. Fertil Steril 1995; 63(1):120–4.

198. Sigman M, Jarow JP. Ipsilateral testicular hypotrophy is associated with decreased sperm counts in infertile men with varicoceles. J Urol 1997; 158(2):605–7.
199. Steckel J, Dicker AP, Goldstein M. Relationship between varicocele size and response to varicocelectomy. J Urol 1993; 149(4):769–71.
200. Dubin L, Amelar RD. Varicocele size and results of varicocelectomy in selected subfertile men with varicocele. Fertil Steril 1970; 21(8):606–9.
201. Fette A, Mayr J. Treatment of varicoceles in childhood and adolescence with Tauber's antegrade scrotal sclerotherapy. J Pediatr Surg 2000; 35(8):1222–5.
202. Mazzoni G, Spagnoli A, Lucchetti MC et al. Adolescent varicocele: Tauber antegrade sclerotherapy versus Palomo repair. J Urol 2001; 166(4):1462–4.
203. Porst H, Bahren W, Lenz M, Altwein JE. Percutaneous sclerotherapy of varicoceles – an alternative to conventional surgical methods. Br J Urol 1984; 56(1):73–8.
204. Atassi O, Kass EJ, Steinert BW. Testicular growth after successful varicocele correction in adolescents: comparison of artery sparing techniques with the Palomo procedure. J Urol 1995; 153(2):482–3.
205. Cimador M, Castagnetti M, Ajovalasit V et al. Subinguinal interruption of dilated veins in adolescent varicocele: should it be considered a gold standard technique? Minerva Pediatr 2003; 55(6):599–605.
206. Nyirady P, Kiss A, Pirot L et al. Evaluation of 100 laparoscopic varicocele operations with preservation of testicular artery and ligation of collateral vein in children and adolescents. Eur Urol 2002; 42(6):594–7.
207. Cohen RC. Laparoscopic varicocelectomy with preservation of the testicular artery in adolescents. J Pediatr Surg 2001; 36(2):394–6.
208. Bebars GA, Zaki A, Dawood AR, El-Gohary MA. Laparoscopic versus open high ligation of the testicular veins for the treatment of varicocele. JSlS 2000; 4(3):209–13.
209. Esposito C, Monguzzi GL, Gonzalez-Sabin MA et al. Laparoscopic treatment of pediatric varicocele: a multicenter study of the Italian Society of Video Surgery in Infancy. J Urol 2000; 163(6):1944–6.
210. Barqawi A, Furness P 3rd, Koyle M. Laparoscopic Palomo varicocelectomy in the adolescent is safe after previous ipsilateral inguinal surgery. BJU Int 2002; 89(3):269–72.
211. Esposito C, Monguzzi G, Gonzalez-Sabin MA et al. Results and complications of laparoscopic surgery for pediatric varicocele. J Pediatr Surg 2001; 36(5):767–9.
212. Itoh K, Suzuki Y, Yazawa H et al. Results and complications of laparoscopic Palomo varicocelecctomy. Arch Androl 2003; 49(2):107–10.
213. Koyle MA, Oottamasathien S, Barqawi A, Rajimwale A, Furness PD 3rd. Laparoscopic Palomo varicocele ligation in children and adolescents: results of 103 cases. J Urol 2004; 172(4 Pt 2):1749–52, discussion 1752.
214. Esposito C, Valla JS, Najmaldin A et al. Incidence and management of hydrocele following varicocele surgery in children. J Urol 2004; 171(3):1271–3.
215. Misseri R, Gershbein AB, Horowitz M, Glassberg KI. The adolescent varicocele. II: the incidence of hydrocele and delayed recurrent varicocele after varicocelectomy in a long-term follow-up. BJU Int 2001; 87(6):494–8.
216. Levitt S, Gill B, Katlowitz N, Kogan SJ, Reda E. Routine intraoperative post-ligation venography in the treatment of the pediatric varicocele. J Urol 1987; 137(4):716–18.
217. Kass EJ, Marcol B. Results of varicocele surgery in adolescents: a comparison of techniques. J Urol 1992; 148 (2 Pt 2):694–6.

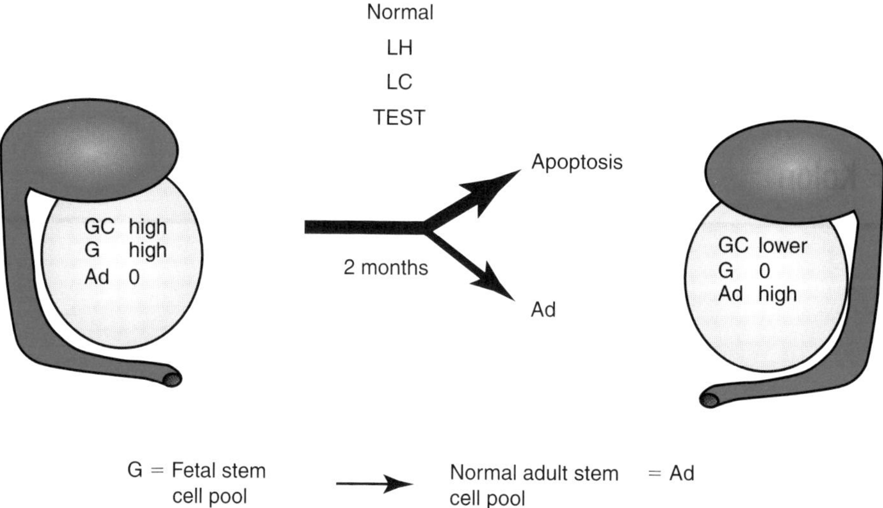

Figure 74.1 Third step in maturation: differentiation of fetal gonocytes into adult dark (Ad) spermatogonia. GC = germ cell, G = gonocyte, LH = luteinizing hormone, LC = Leydig cell, TEST = testosterone.

(two prenatal and two postnatal) prior to the final maturational changes at puberty.

Differentiation of the bipotential gonad into the testis occurs under control of the *SRY* (sex-related gene on the Y chromosome) gene. In the first step in maturation, primordial germ cells enter the emerging testicular cords and differentiate into gonocytes. These gonocytes constitute the fetal stem cell pool of the germ cell line and lie in the center of the testicular cords. Human chorionic gonadotropin (hCG) stimulates fetal Leydig cell development, proliferation, and testosterone secretion. Gonocyte proliferation expands the fetal stem cell pool, whereas fetal Sertoli cells simultaneously differentiate and begin to secrete müllerian inhibiting substance (MIS). Masculinization of the mesonephric (wolffian) duct, paramesonephric (müllerian) duct, and external genitalia begin. MIS causes regression of müllerian structures and testosterone causes development of the wolffian duct to form the epididymis and vas deferens.[14,15]

In the second step in maturation, the level of hCG, number of fetal Leydig cells, and the level of testosterone reach their peaks during the 13th week of gestation. Gonocytes begin to migrate to the basement membranes of the seminiferous tubules and differentiate into fetal spermatogonia. Since they are stem cells, gonocytes can replenish their own numbers. Masculinization of the external genitalia and resorption of the paramesonephric ducts is completed. Maculinization of the mesonephric duct into the epididymis continues and the swelling of the gubernacula begins. Differentiation of fetal spermatogonia continues throughout fetal life. Canalization of the rete testis and mesonephric tubules begins in week 12 and is completed by puberty. Testicular descent occurs in the 7th month of gestation and depends on multiple factors discussed earlier.

The third step occurs postnatally during the 2nd month after birth (Figure 74.1). By now the seminiferous tubules contain numerous germ cells. Approximately half are gonocytes and the rest are fetal spermatogonia. A surge in luteinizing hormone (LH) and follicle-stimulating hormone (FSH) levels stimulates proliferation of fetal Leydig cells, in turn causing a surge in testosterone. Some gonocytes attach to the tubule basement membrane and are transformed. A minority of gonocytes differentiate into adult dark (Ad) spermatogonia, whereas the majority undergo apoptosis and disappear, lowering the total germ cell number. Thus, the gonocyte fetal stem cell pool is replaced by Ad spermatogonia, making up the adult stem cell pool. The transformation and disappearance of gonocytes is normally completed by 6 months of age. The levels of gonadotropins and testosterone fall as fetal Leydig cells regress into inactive juvenile Leydig cells. Some Ad spermatogonia mature into adult pale (Ap) spermatogonia. Fetal Sertoli cells mature into Sa Sertoli cells. This third step is extremely important since the transformation of the fetal stem cell pool into the adult stem cell pool (Ad spermatogonia) is a prerequisite for future maturation of the testis.

At approximately 5 years of age, the fourth important maturational step commences with the onset of meiosis. Simultaneous transient peaks of LH, number and size of juvenile Leydig cells, and testosterone

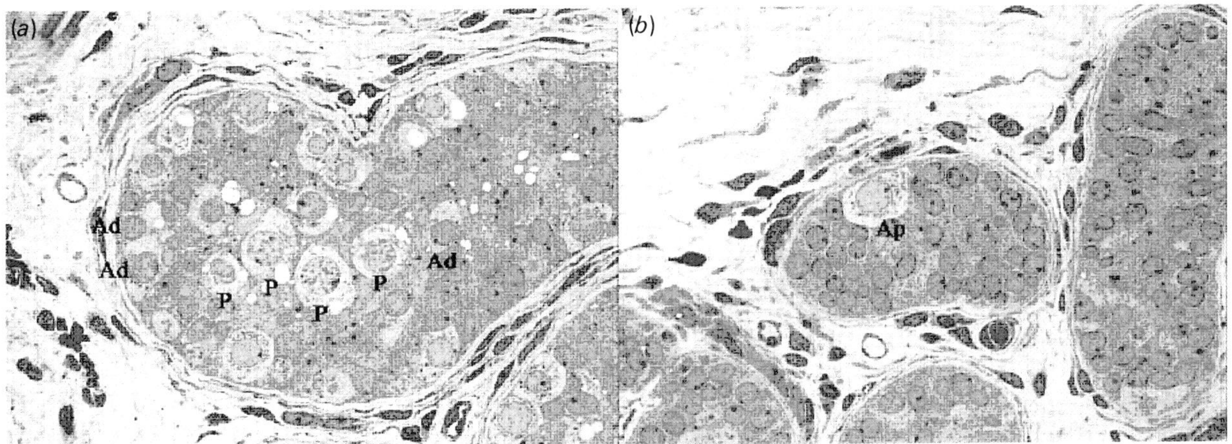

Figure 74.2 (*a*) Descended testis biopsy showing adult dark (Ad) spermatogonia and primary spermatocytes (P). (*b*) Cryptorchid testis biopsy showing paucity of Ad spermatogonia and persistence of fetal gonocytes with an adult pale (Ap) spermatogonium.

occur. The increased testosterone stimulates an increase in Ad spermatogonia and the total germ cells. It also triggers the maturation of the mitotic Ad spermatogonia into primary spermatocytes that are germ cells in prophase of the first meiotic division. Sa Sertoli cells mature into Sb Sertoli cells.

Final germ cell maturation at puberty depends on adequate completion of the two prepubertal developmental milestones. The pubertal surge in LH and FSH stimulates the inactive juvenile Leydig cells to multiply and mature into adult Leydig cells. They produce the high pubertal surge in testosterone that triggers the final maturation to secondary spermatocytes, early and late spermatids, and sperm. Sertoli cells undergo their final maturation into Sc Sertoli cells. Complete spermatogenesis is usually accomplished by 13–15 years of age.

In the cryptorchid testis, the number of Leydig cells is decreased and they appear atrophic (Figure 74.2). In the first 6 months of life, the total number of germ cells is within the normal range in cryptorchid testes; however, the number of spermatogonia remains low and does not increase with age. This gives evidence for the lack of transformation of gonocytes into Ad spermatogonia in the cryptorchid testis. The normal postnatal development of Leydig cells and germ cell transformation parallels the normal gonadotropin and resultant testosterone surge around 60–90 days of life.[16]

Etiology

Despite the relatively frequent incidence of cryptorchidism, the etiology and molecular markers of future fertility or malignancy remain obscure.[13] Cryptorchidism is a well-known manifestation of chromosomal abnormalities and a common component of over 50 syndromes of multiple congenital anomalies.[17] Cryptorchidism, when associated with other congenital anomalies like hypospadias, has a higher incidence of chromosomal anomalies (12–25%) than when it occurs as an isolated defect (3–4%).[18–21] However, at present, there is no consistent chromosomal disorder associated with isolated cryptorchidism.

Cryptorchidism accompanies defects in every intrinsic step of the hypothalamic–pituitary–testicular–end organ axis as well as defects in extrinsic pathways that affect the axis such as extratesticular cholesterol synthesis, adrenal steroidogenesis, placental 'insufficiency', and maternal or environmental endocrine disruptors. Hypogonadism results from defects in the hypothalamic–pituitary–testicular axis and is characterized by cryptorchidism, hypospadias, small penis, chordee, minor scrotal anomalies, inguinal hernia, hydrocele, and epididymal anomalies. Huff et al proposed a cryptorchidism sequence, since over 70% of examined cryptorchid boys had one or more of these late defects of masculinization associated with the endocrinopathy of hypogonadism. He classifies the multiple conditions upstream from cryptorchidism into errors of blastogenesis, organogenesis, sexual differentiation, and late masculinization; the cascade of events downstream from cryptorchidism are testicular atrophy, microlithiasis, intrauterine torsion, Sertoli cell nodules, and, most importantly, germ cell maldevelopment. The abnormal proliferation and maturation of germ cells in and controls. Further evaluation should be carried out to fully characterize the role of these posterior *HOX* genes in abnormal testicular descent. Many other gene products have been targeted as being expressed in testicular differentiation (i.e. *PAX5*, *SRY*, *SOX9*, *DAX1*, *MIS*) but not specifically in cryptorchidism.[67,68]

Hormonal factors

It has been theorized that this spontaneous descent in infancy may occur as a result of the normal gonadotropin surge that occurs around 60–90 days of life.[69–72] Gendrel et al and Job et al reported blunting of this surge in boys with UDT that remain undescended in the first year of life.[69,70] They demonstrated a significant difference in the polynomial regression curves comparing the testosterone levels of persistently cryptorchid testes with those having delayed spontaneous descent. However, the positive predictive value that bilateral UDT will have abnormally low testosterone levels is only about 23%.[69] In contrast, Barthold et al examined gonadotropin and testosterone, estradiol, inhibin B, leptin, and sex hormone-binding globulin in a cohort of cryptorchid boys. They failed to identify any significant differences in hormonal levels in their cohort compared with controls.[73]

An endocrine disruptor is an environmental chemical that interferes with the production, transport, and metabolism of hormones in the body.[74] Some of these agents have estrogenic activity, whereas others act as agonists and antagonists of androgens.[74,75] Endocrine disruptors have been hypothesized to play a role in cryptorchidism, as androgens contribute significantly in the physiology of germ cell development and testicular descent. Several environmental chemicals have antiandrogenic effects in rodent models. Although these agents act by many different mechanisms, they all produce similar effects on the developing male reproductive tract. At high in-utero doses, antiandrogens are associated with UDT and agenesis of the epididymis, whereas at lower doses hypospadias and decreased anogenital distances are seen. Boys exposed to the antiandrogenic effects of diethylstilbesterol in utero have an increased number of genital abnormalities, including cryptorchidism.[76] Phthalate esters inhibit testosterone synthesis during fetal life and produce dose-related abnormalities of the male reproductive tract such as focal hyperplasia of fetal Leydig cells that persists postnatally, as well as agenesis of the gubernaculum.[77–80] In animal models, phthalates reduce cholesterol transport across the mitochondrial membrane, decrease testosterone biosynthesis, and reduce expression of the *insl3* gene.[81,82] Animal research findings demonstrate a coordinated, dose-dependent reduction in expression of key genes involved in cholesterol transport and steroidogenesis, and a corresponding reduction in testosterone in fetal testes at low dibutyl phthalate (DBP) doses which do not produce male reproductive tract anomalies.[77] Similar studies have been carried out in adult rats to determine the pattern of gene expression in the proximal wolffian duct, which gives rise to the epididymis, following prenatal exposure to DBP. Changes in mRNA expression were observed in genes involved in testosterone biosynthesis and testicular descent, including the insulin-like growth factor pathway and the androgen receptor.[83] These alterations in expression of genes at phthalate doses that do not produce isolated UDT suggest that gene–environment interactions could occur in human populations. It has been hypothesized that fetuses with susceptible genotypes exposed in utero to environmentally relevant doses of phthalates may be at the greatest risk for developing UDT. Findings with the phthalates are of particular concern because exposure is ubiquitous and phthalates are widely used in many consumer products. The phthalate monoester metabolites have been found in the urine samples of >75% of approximately 2550 participants in the 1999–2000 National Health and Nutrition Examination Survey (NHANES).[84,85] Familial clustering of hypospadias and UDT among first-degree relatives has been suggested as evidence for a genetic component for these anomalies. However, another etiologic possibility is the role of exposure to environmental contaminants in familial clusters because of the high probability of shared exposures among first-degree relatives.[86]

These animal findings further advocate a multifactorial and complex etiology of cryptorchidism. UDT is a variable and multifactorial phenotypic trait that probably involves several candidate genes as well as clinical (hormonal) and environmental risk factors rather than a causative single gene mutation. It is likely that a shift in the dynamic equilibrium of these factors is involved.

Other factors

Secondary cryptorchidism can occur after inguinal surgery, either as a result of scar tissue or the difficulty in diagnosing UDT in a young boy with a hernia. An ascending testis is one that appeared descended at birth and later ascended. Reports suggest that an ascending testis has similar testis biopsy histology to a UDT.[87] Yearly examination should occur in questionable cases to identify a true UDT.

Diagnosis

History and physical examination

A thorough history should include prematurity (incidence of UDT in premature boys is as high as 30%), maternal use/exposure to exogenous hormones (estrogens), lesions of the central nervous system (myelomeningocele), and previous inguinal surgery. Document a family history of cryptorchidism and other congenital anomalies, neonatal deaths, precocious puberty, infertility, and consanguinity. It is also important to know if the testes were ever palpable in the scrotum at the time of birth or within the first year of life. Testicular retraction, due to a strong cremasteric reflex, is most apparent between 4 and 6 years of age and may lead to an inaccurate diagnosis of UDT.[16]

An undescended testis can be classified by its location. It may be located in the abdomen, the inguinal canal, the superficial inguinal pouch, the upper scrotum, or rarely ectopic (perineum, contralateral scrotum, or femoral). However, for treatment purposes, the main distinction that needs to be made is whether or not the testis is palpable.

The patient should be examined supine in the frog-leg position with both legs free. With warmed hands, check the size, location, and texture of the contralateral descended testis (CDT). Begin examination of the UDT at the anterior superior iliac spine and sweep the groin from lateral to medial with the non-dominant hand. Once the testis is palpated, grasp it with the dominant hand and continue to sweep the testis toward the scrotum with the other hand. With a combination of sweeping and pulling, it is sometimes possible to bring the testis to the scrotum. Maintain the position of the testis in the scrotum for a minute, so that the cremaster muscle is fatigued. Release the testis and, if it remains in place, it is a retractile testis. If it immediately pops back to a prescrotal position, it is a UDT.

For the difficult-to-examine patient (chubby 6 month-olds or obese youths), the sitting cross-legged position or the baseball 'catcher's position' can also help relax the cremaster muscle. Wetting the fingers of the non-dominant hand with lubricating jelly or soap can increase the sensitivity of the fingers in palpating the small, mobile testis.

A retractile testis is often confused with a UDT. The key to distinguishing a retractile testis from a UDT is demonstrating that the testis can be delivered into the scrotum. The retractile testis will stay in the scrotum after the cremaster muscle has been overstretched, whereas the low UDT will immediately pop back to its undescended position after being released. If there is any question, the child should be seen in follow-up for a repeat examination. Miller et al have also recommended the use of hCG stimulation to help distinguish between a retractile and an undescended testis in the hard-to-examine child.[88]

An atrophic or vanishing testis can be found anywhere along the normal path to the scrotum. The etiology is thought to be due to neonatal vascular ischemia, possibly due to torsion.[89] The CDT may be hypertrophied in these boys, but this is not a reliable diagnostic sign.

Upon surgical exploration, 60–80% of non-palpable testes are present in the inguinal canal or in the intra-abdominal location, whereas up to 40% are absent or an inguinoscrotal nubbin of fibrous tissue and hemosiderin. Presence of bilateral UDT should raise suspicion of an endocrine disorder or an intersex state that should be evaluated. Cryptorchidism associated with hypospadias, especially proximal, should also raise the possibility of the intersex state and occurs in 30–40% of the patients, mainly consisting of defects in the testosterone synthesis pathway.[90]

Laboratory tests

In boys with unilateral or bilateral UDT where one testis is palpable, no further laboratory evaluation is necessary to aid the diagnosis. In boys with bilateral UDT where neither testis is palpable and also in boys with associated hypospadias, chromosomal and endocrinologic evaluation may be carried out but is not always necessary.[19] These levels should be drawn during the maternal newborn gonadotropin surge or at 60–90 days of life. In patients ≤ 3 months with bilateral non-palpable UDT, LH, FSH, and testosterone levels will help determine whether the testes are present; >3 months of age, an hCG stimulation test will aid in the diagnosis of the absent testes. A weight-based single injection of hCG (100 IU/kg) is usually sufficient to detect a rise in serum testosterone 4–5 days later.[91] A failure to see a measurable increase in testosterone in combination with elevated LH and

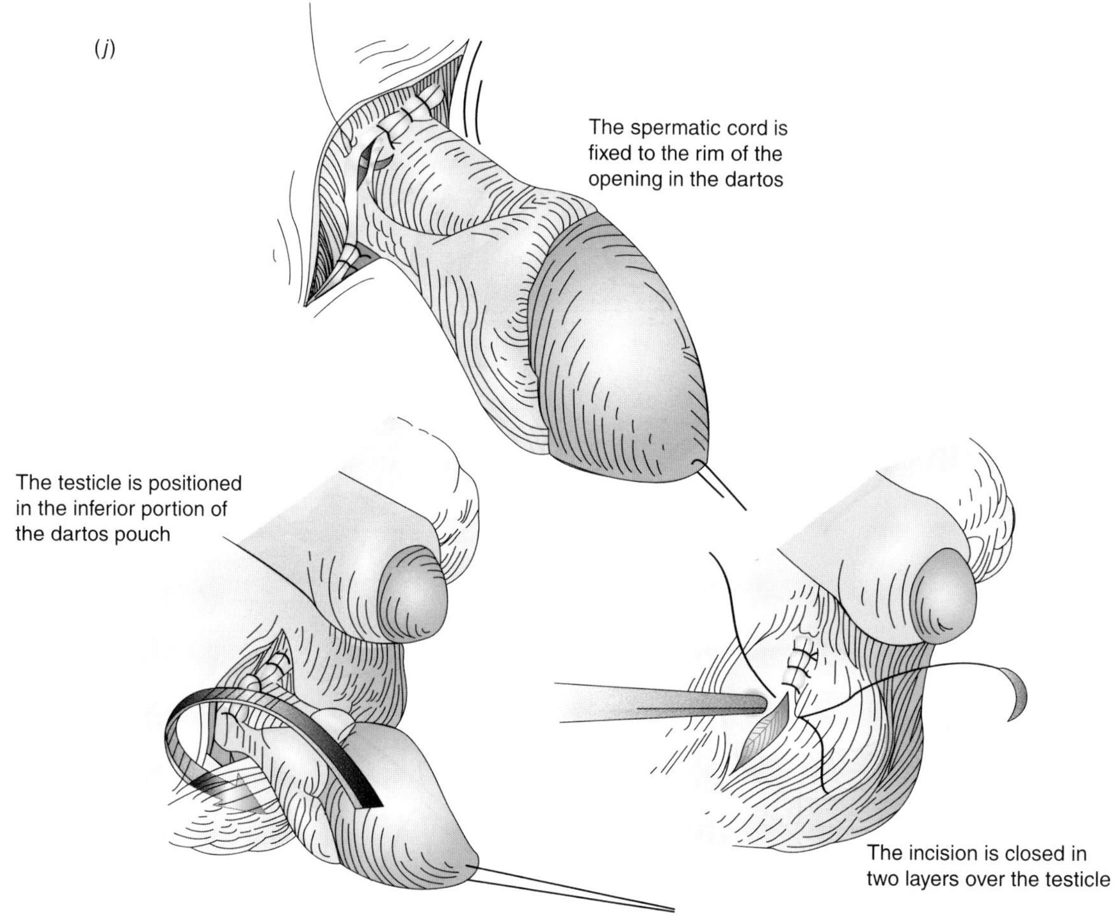

scrotum. This vessel can be transected without repercussions. If necessary, the internal oblique muscle can be incised for 1–2 cm and dissection of the lateral investing fascia can be carried further into the retroperitoneum (Figure 75.2c).

If after completing the dissection of the cord the testis still does not reach the scrotum, the floor of the canal can be incised and the testis brought on the lateral side of the epigastric vessels, or the epigastric vessels can be divided (Prentis maneuver) (Figure 75.2g). Some feel that this maneuver may add 5–10 mm of additional length to the cord. Care should be taken during the division of the floor of the canal, especially if the bladder is distended, as it is possible to inadvertently injure the bladder.

Once adequate length has been achieved, fixation of the testis in the scrotum is accomplished within a subdartos pouch (Figure 75.2h). Avoid a pouch that is laterally placed, as this will yield an unsatisfactory result. A natural tendency but one which is incorrect is to follow the path of the ectopically located testis and use this to enter the scrotum to create the subdartos pouch. Instead, creating the neocanal along the base of the penis will avoid the tendency to drift laterally and result in a poorly placed testis. With a finger in the scrotum, the location for the pouch is selected and an incision is made. The pouch is created using a tenotomy scissor, with the larger portion of the dissection directed inferiorly. The pouch should be generous in size so that the testis can fit without excessive tension. A clamp is passed on the fingertip into the inguinal region and a portion of the cauda gubernaculum or a fixation stitch is pulled into the scrotum (Figure 75.2i). The testis is fixed in the scrotum using absorbable stay sutures at three points or, if a fixation stitch is used, this suture is loaded on a free Keith needle and brought out the inferior wall of the scrotum (Figure 75.2j). The scrotum is closed and the fixation stitch is tied loosely at the skin level, either to itself or over a pledget, depending on the amount of tension.

The staged orchidopexy

In cases where inguinal exploration is performed and where it is not feasible to perform a vessel ligation to bring the testis down in either one or two stages, the staged orchidopexy may be necessary. The testis can be fixed to the pubic tubercle to prevent it from pulling up higher into the groin. Historically, silastic sheeting was used to wrap the cord to facilitate subsequent dissection. The second-stage procedure is carried out 6 months to 1 year later in the hopes of achieving greater length on the cord. With modern techniques of orchidopexy, the staged procedure is rarely necessary.

Orchidopexy by spermatic vessel transection

Orchidopexy by spermatic vessel transection was first described by Bevin in 1903.[31] It was not popularized until Fowler and Stephens better characterized the blood supply of the testis in 1959.[51] The Fowler–Stephens analysis revealed that the testicular artery receives constant collateral communication from the vasal and cremasteric arteries before it reaches the testis. They believed that transection of the main artery too close to the testis would cut off collateral blood supply and lead to atrophy. They advocated temporarily occluding the internal spermatic vessels to test the capacity of the testicle's collateral blood supply, as well as high ligation of the vessels above the collaterals. Johnston[52] advocated leaving a medial broad strip of peritoneum along with the vas to further preserve collateral blood supply (Figure 75.3). Success rates as high as 89% have been reported utilizing their technique.[53]

Recent studies of the vascular anatomy by Jarow[54] indicate that large-caliber anastomotic channels exist between the testicular and vasal arteries. These channels typically run beneath the tunica albuginea and communicate with the inferior pole of the testes. Koff feels that high ligation may in fact contribute to testicular ischemia by limiting dissection between the ascending and descending vasal loops to unfold the testis. He also proposes that additional collateral blood flow can be derived from the distal spermatic vessels that are left intact. Koff modified the Fowler–Stephens procedure by[55] dividing the vessels as close to the testis as possible (Figure 75.4). He achieved a success rate of 93% in a series of 39 low-spermatic transactions, excluding those with prior inguinal surgery. From our own series of laparoscopic Fowler–Stephens orchidopexies[56] we have had an overall success rate of 85%, but when patients who also had prior inguinal surgery or manipulations of the cord are eliminated the success rate is 96%. The principles of both high and low ligation are similar in that avoidance of manipulation of the vas and cord should be of the highest priority to prevent damaging the delicate blood supply. Preservation of the peritoneum between the vessels and vas is essential to the success of the procedure.

Wang and Shaul[57] have emphasized preservation of the gubernacula in Fowler–Stephens procedures, and have had success rates comparable with those reported by Chang et al[58] and Samadi et al[59] when virgin cases only were included.

Jones incision for the non-palpable testis

When the testis is non-palpable on examination in the office and is subsequently found to be a high canalicular or peeping testis at the time of surgery, the Jones approach[60] is potentially useful. The technique was combined with diagnostic laparoscopy by Gheiler et al,[61] with 18 out of 19 testes achieving satisfactory

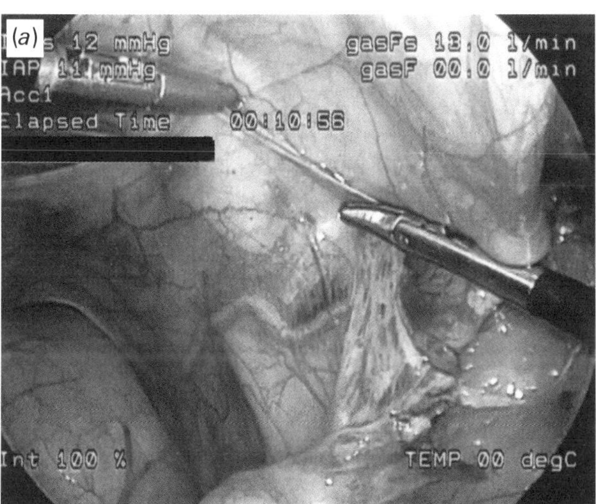

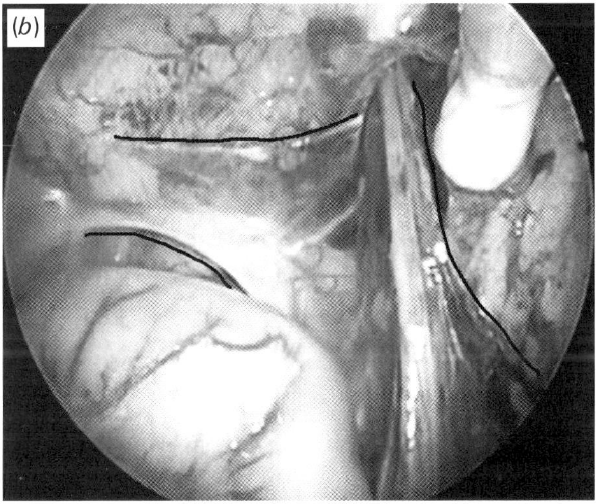

Figure 75.3 (*a*) Peritoneal tongue in a Fowler–Stephens orchidopexy. (*b*) Peritoneal triangle with vas in the center.

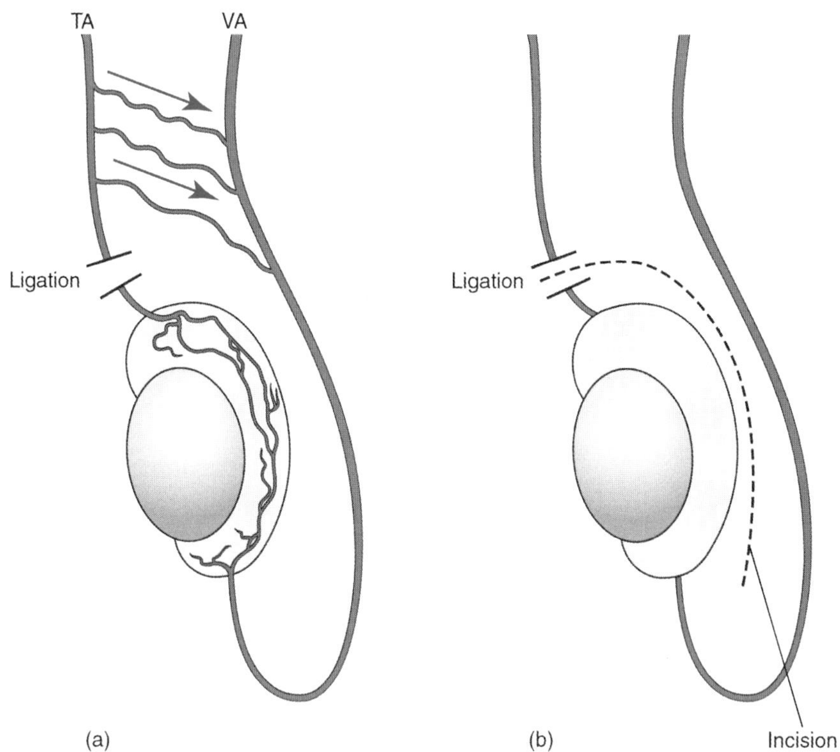

Figure 75.4 Low spermatic vessel ligation as advocated by Koff. (Reproduced from Koff and Seth,[55] with permission.)

scrotal positioning. The one failure was in a patient who underwent simultaneous Fowler–Stephens orchidopexy. The technique involves making an incision medial to the anterior superior iliac spine (ASIS) (Figure 75.5a). The muscle is split and the retroperitoneum is entered (Figure 75.5b). The peritoneum is mobilized medially and the internal inguinal ring is identified (Figure 75.5c). The sac is identified and opened and the testis is brought into the field (Figure 75.5d). The hernia sac is ligated and the spermatic vessels are mobilized by incising the lateral spermatic fascia superiorly (Figure 75.5e). The subcutaneous tissue is mobilized off the external oblique fascia to the level of the pubic tubercle (Figure 75.5f). An opening large enough to allow the testis to pass through the abdominal wall at the pubic tubercle is made and the testis is delivered (Figure 75.5h). The testis is then fixed in the scrotum in a subdartos pouch.

Microvascular autotransplantation of the testis

With the advent of microvascular surgery in the 1970s the first reported cases of microvascular autotransplantation of the testis were reported by Silber and Kelly[62] in 1976. A large series of 27 autotransplantations reported a success rate of 96%.[63] Docimo[64] reported a combined success rate in the literature of 83.7% in a total of 86 cases reported up to 1995 (Table 75.3). The procedure, as described by Bukowski et al,[63] is as follows: a high inguinal incision is used to avoid injuring the inferior epigastric vessels. The dissection is then carried down to the level of the inferior epigastric vessels. The retroperitoneum is entered and the colon is mobilized. The testicle is identified and the testicular vessels are isolated and divided as proximally as possible. The testis is mobilized in a fashion similar to the Fowler–Stephens mobilization, maintaining a wide strip of peritoneum which is taken with the vas deferens. The testis is brought through an anterior abdominal incision and placed in the scrotum in a subdartos pouch. Care is taken to make sure that there is no tension on the vas deferens, which can be mobilized back to the bladder if needed. The inferior epigastric vessels are isolated. Small branches are ligated until 8–9 cm has been freed beneath the rectus muscle towards the umbilicus. The inferior epigastric vessels are ligated distally and clips are placed proximally. The proximal vessels are opened and flushed with heparinized saline. The testicular artery is then anastomosed to the inferior

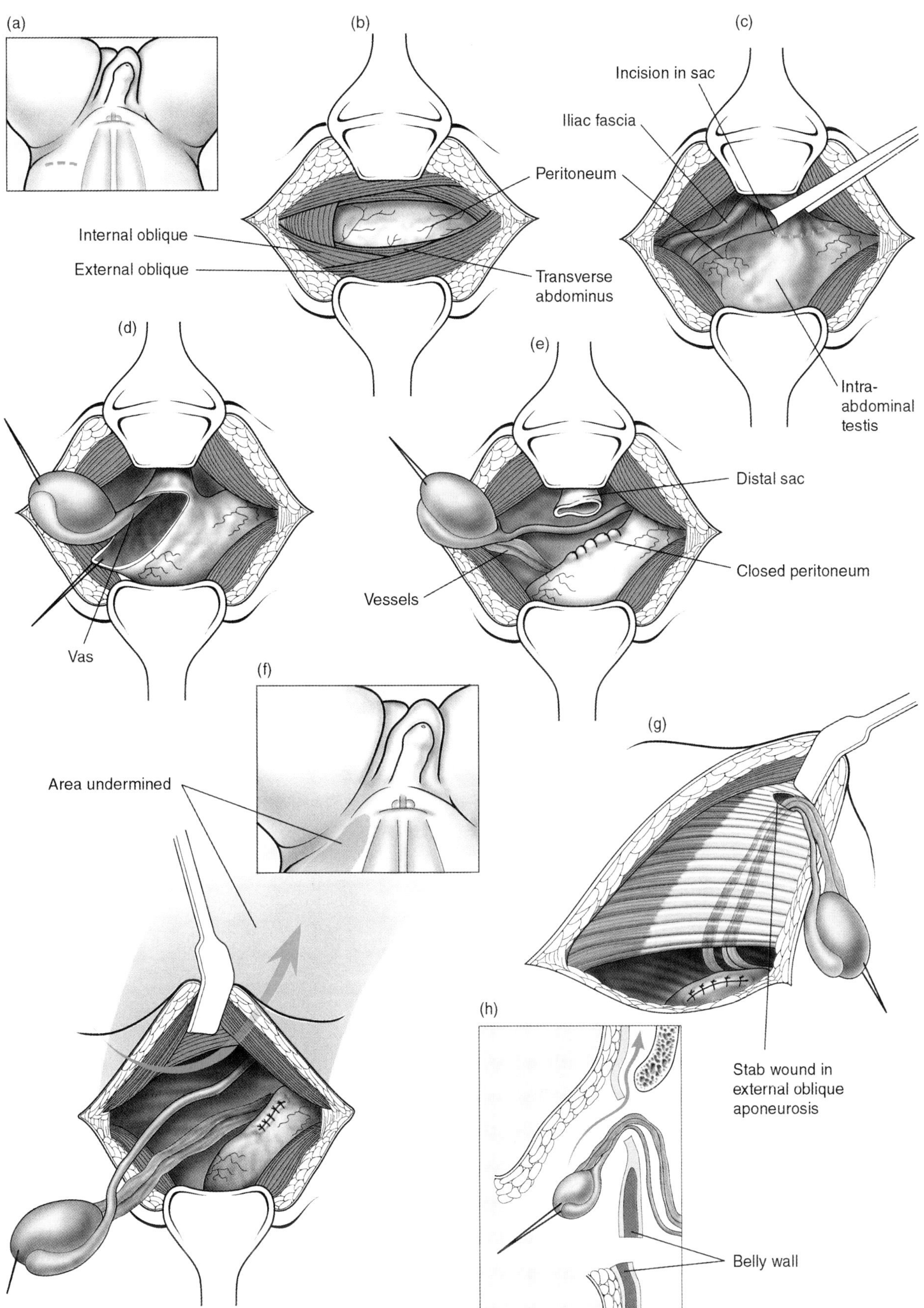

Figure 75.5 The Jones technique for orchidopexy. For details, see text.

Table 75.3 Success of orchiopexy by anatomic position of testis and procedure

	Preoperative position of tests No. successes/total no. (%)				Type of orchiopexy No. successes/total no. (%)					
	Abdominal	Peeping	Canalicular	Distal	Inguinal	Fowler–Stephens	Staged Fowler–Stephens	Trans-abdominal	Two-stage	Microvascular
Overall	623/842 (74.0)	242/294 (82.3)	593/681 (87.1)	624/674 (92.6)	1388/1566 (88.6)	214/321 (66.7)		65/80(81.3)	180/248 (72.6)	72/86(83.7)
After 6 months	420/564 (74.5)	229/279 (82.1)	397/473 (83.9)	603/653 (92.3)	1110/1285 (86.4)	109/174 (62.6)	43/56 (76.8)	44/57(77.2)	106/149 (71.1)	71/85(83.5)
To age 6 years	148/211 (70.1)	7/7(100)	245/257 (95.3) $p<0.05$	Not available	535/588 (91.0) $p<0.05$	9/19(47.4)	43/56(76.8) 32/43(74.4)	11/15(73.3)	67/84 (79.8) $p<0.05$	35/43(81.4)
Older than 6 years	107/166 (64.5)	229/279 (82.1)	143/199 (71.9)	159/197(80.7)	364/428 (85.0)	31/58(53.4)	9/11(81.8)	33/42(78.6)	43/69 (62.3)	37/43(86.0)
Through 1985	239/345 (69.4) $p<0.05$	235/287 (81.9)	263/336 (78.3) $p<0.05$	605/655(92.4)	811/889 (91.2)	138/210 (65.7)	Not available	44/57(77.2)	138/183 (75.4)	23/25(91.7) $p<0.05$
After 1985	384/497 (77.3)	7/7(100)	330/345 (96.7)	19/19(100)	577/677 (85.3)	76/111 (68.5)	43/56(76.8)	21/23(91.3)	42/65 (64.6)	49/61(80.3)

Data from Docimo[64]

epigastric artery. The testicular artery typically measures 0.5–1 mm in diameter, whereas the epigastric artery is 1–1.5 mm in diameter. The veins are usually similar in size, measuring 1 mm in diameter. An end-to-end or end-to-side anastomosis is used. Patients are typically kept immobilized for 24 hours. Tackett et al[65] reported on 17 cases of microvascular anastomosis and laparoscopic testicular mobilization, thereby minimizing the intra-abdominal dissection. The overall success rate was 88% (15/17). Although the success rates with this procedure are quite impressive, they are probably not better than the success rates obtained by meticulous vessel transections solely. In our series and those of Kogan[53] and Koff[55] similar results were obtained without utilizing the microvascular anastomosis. The indications for microvascular autotransplantation are therefore unclear.

Therapeutic laparoscopy for the undescended testis

Laparoscopic vessel ligation

Bloom[66] was the first to combine diagnostic laparoscopy and operative intervention when he fulgurated the vessels of intra-abdominal testes and performed a second-stage open Fowler–Stephens orchidopexy at a later date.

Laparoscopic orchidopexy

Laparoscopic orchidopexy seemed to be the logical extension to early attempts at vessel ligation by Bloom[66] and routine diagnostic laparoscopy. The procedure allows the surgeon to transition from a diagnostic mode to an operative procedure. Laparoscopic orchidopexy was first described by Jordan et al in 1992.[67] Subsequently, there have been numerous reports describing this technique.[68–72] Our original series was the largest series of laparoscopic orchidopexies, and now consists of 203 procedures.[72] Our success rate in getting the testis in a scrotal position without atrophy is 95% in the cases not involving vessel transections.[59]

The original description by Jordan et al[67] remains relatively unchanged, except for some minor variations in how to bring the testis out of the abdomen. Routine laparoscopy is performed via an infra- or supraumbilical incision. Open trocar placement is preferred in our series (Figure 75.6). The bladder should be emptied by catheterization and the catheter should remain throughout the procedure to prevent

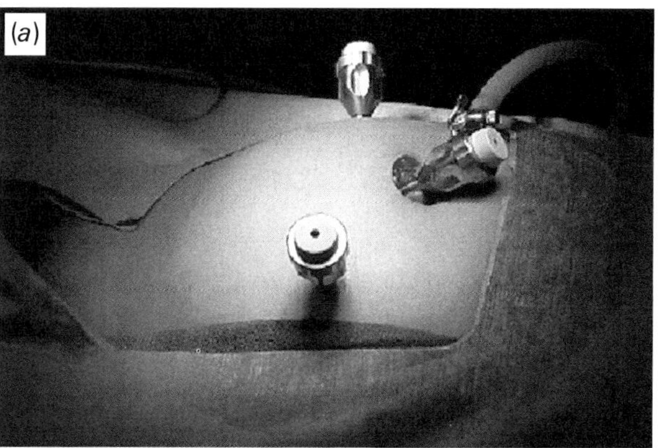

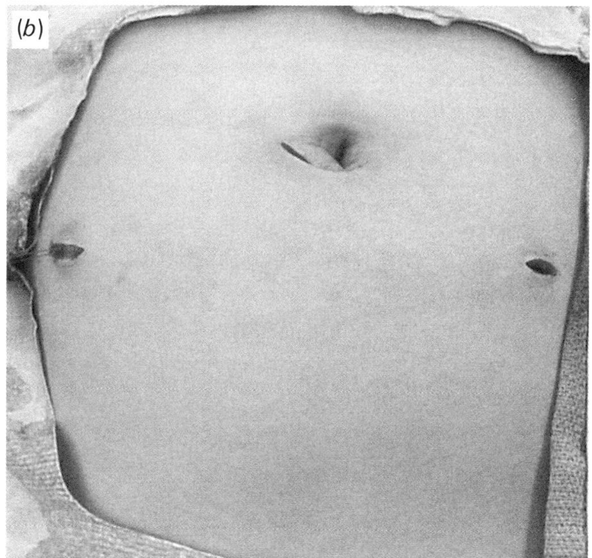

Figure 75.6 (*a* and *b*) Trocar placement.

injury to the bladder. This is especially critical at the time that the neoring is created. In the prune belly patient, extra caution is necessary when placing the initial trocar, since the urachal diverticulum may extend all the way to the umbilicus. In these cases a supraumbilical incision should be used.

Once in the abdomen, inspection of the internal ring should be performed. The vas and vessels should be seen approaching the ring. The vessels are generally thinner and the vas will tend to have prominent vessels traveling with it in cases of atrophy (see Figure 75.1). A closed ring does not always signify an absent testis. Very high abdominal testes may not have any attachments to the internal ring and may be situated behind the bowel (Figure 75.7). If no vessels or vas are seen approaching the ring, additional trocars should be inserted to reflect the colon. The contralateral side can be used as reference in cases of unilateral undescended testis. The testis will be found within 1 cm of the ring in the majority of cases. Peeping

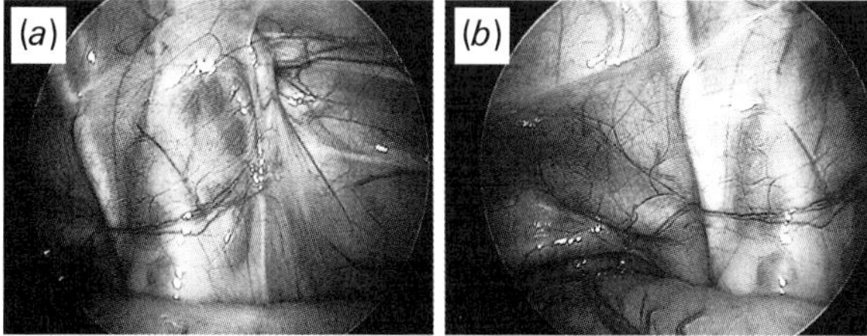

Figure 75.7 (*a, b*) Closed internal rings with absence of vas. In both the testis was out of sight. (*c*) Note the absent vas in the peritoneal triangle. (*d*) Note the testis with absence of epididymal structures.

testes can be pushed into the abdomen by pressing on the canal (Figure 75.8).

Once the decision to perform a laparoscopic orchidopexy has been made, the working trocars are placed under direct vision. The size of the working trocars depends on the need for vascular clips. The smallest clip applicator currently available is 5 mm. Trocars are placed at the level of the umbilicus and along the mid clavicular line. Inspection of the placement site will help avoid injury to the epigastric vessels. In very young children placement of the trocars above the level of the umbilicus is helpful to avoid crossing instruments. Once the trocars are in place, two grasping forceps can be used to pull on the gubernaculum and bring as much of it into the abdomen as possible (Figure 75.9). Sometimes, the vas is looping into the gubernacular tissue, and can be injured during this maneuver or gubernacular division. The gubernaculum is transected using an electrified scissor with a minimal amount of cautery to prevent dissipation of heat to the vas. The dissection is carried medially over the bladder, incising the peritoneum distal to the vas and moving towards the contralateral median umbilical ligament. A generous segment of peritoneum should be maintained between the cut edge and the vas. The dissection is then carried lateral to the spermatic vessels to the colon (Figure 75.10). The peritoneum is then incised medially over the proximal spermatic vessels. This is critical in providing additional length for proper mobilization of the testis into

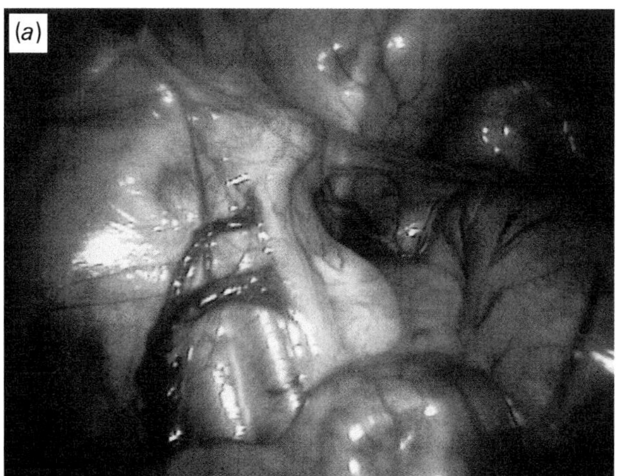

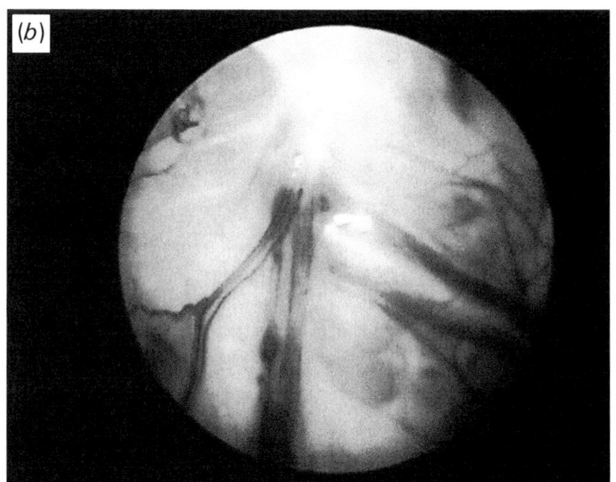

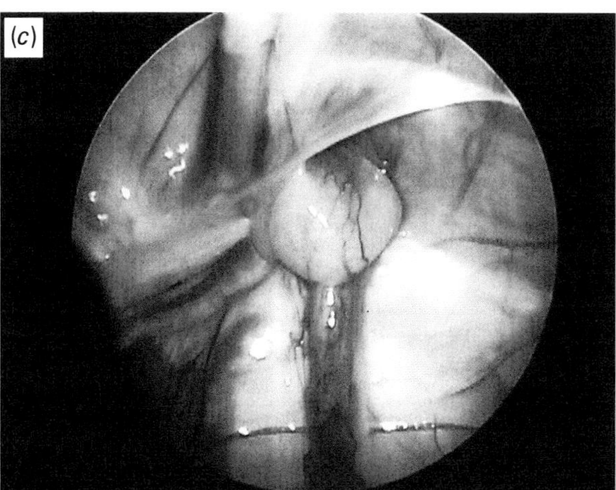

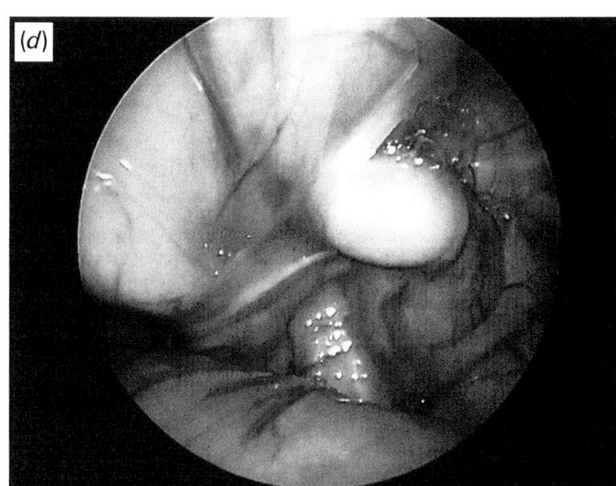

Figure 75.8 (*a*) Intra-abdominal testis. (*b*) Normal contralateral internal ring. (*c* and *d*) Peeping testis.

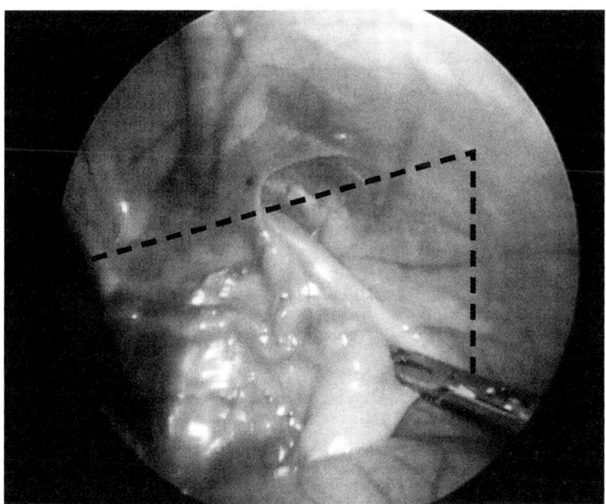

Figure 75.9 Gubernacular fibers. Dashed lines are incision lines of the peritoneum.

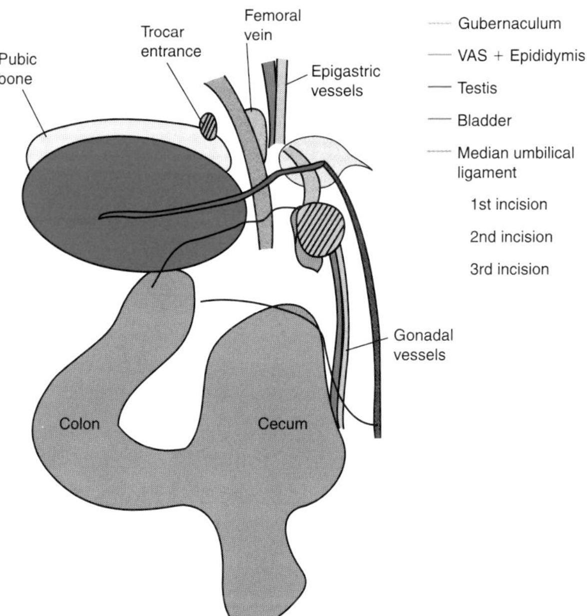

Figure 75.10 Representive view of the pelvis with incision lines.

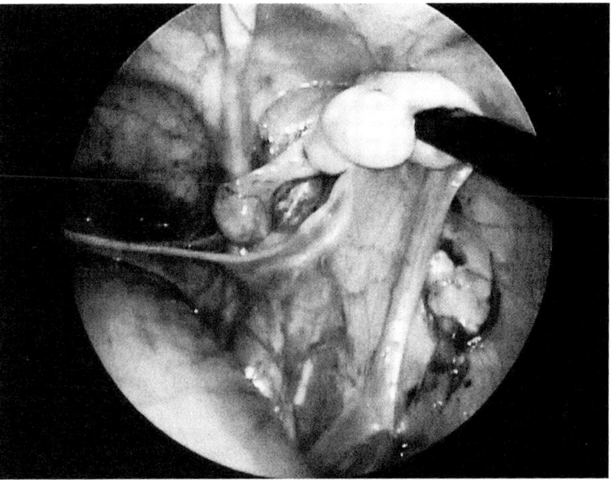

Figure 75.11 Testis freed up after incising over the bladder and lateral pelvic wall.

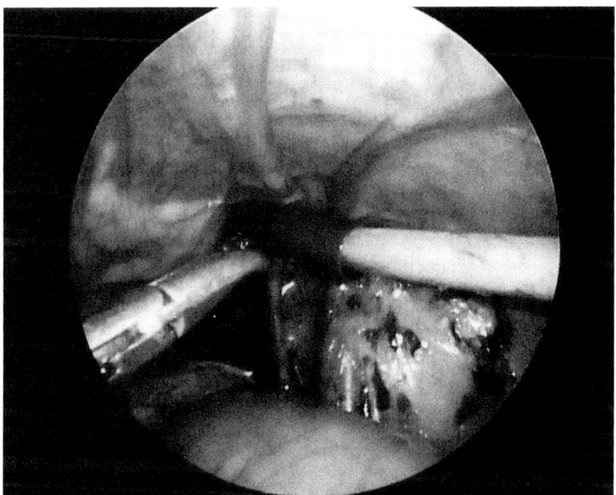

Figure 75.12 Neoinguinal ring between bladder and medium umbilical ligament.

the scrotum (Figure 75.11). This also leaves a generous triangle of peritoneum between the vessels and vas in case vessel transection is necessary.

Laparoscopic Fowler–Stephens orchidopexy as performed in our series consists of the high ligation technique. A large wide wedge-shaped strip of peritoneum has been preserved (see Figure 75.3). We have encountered only two failed Fowler–Stephens orchidopexies to date using the laparoscopic one-stage Fowler–Stephens orchidopexy in a virgin case.

The testis is brought out of the abdomen via a neoinguinal canal created in the anterior abdominal wall near the pubic tubercle (Figure 75.12). We prefer to bring the testis out medial to the median umbilical ligament and lateral to the bladder. This is done by dissecting in the space between the aforementioned structures and getting down to the pubis. The scrotum is invaginated by the index finger, and the endodissector is placed over the pubic bone and the external inguinal ring is palpated with the dissector and the finger invaginating the scrotum. Once the ring is identified, the dissector is driven into the scrotum guided by the index finger (Figure 75.13). A small scrotal incision is made and the dissector is brought out into the field. A subdartos pouch is created and a 5 mm trocar is placed over the dissector and guided into the abdomen (Figure 75.14). This trocar can be used to apply clips if a vessel transection

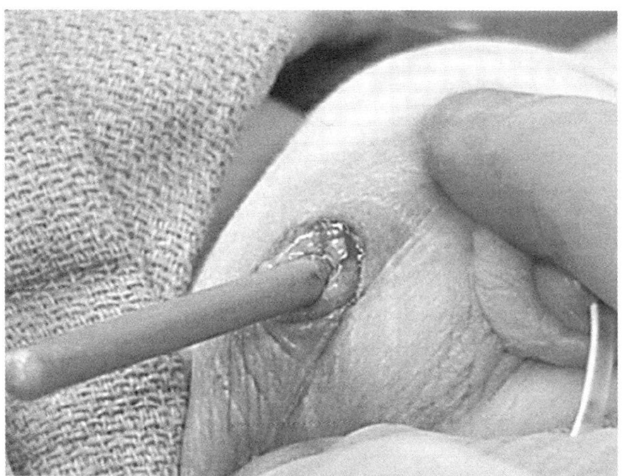

Figure 75.13 A subdartos pouch has been created.

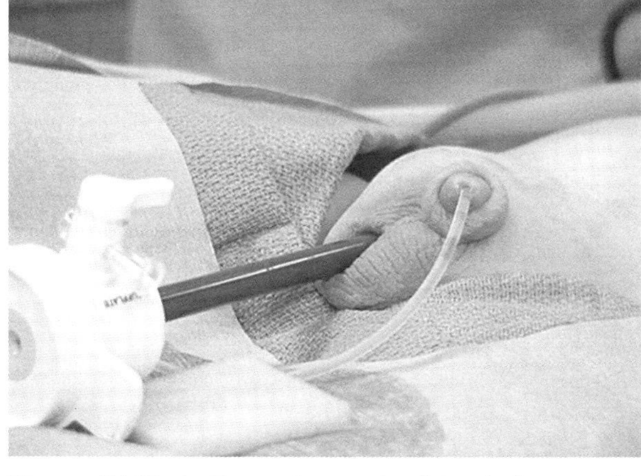

Figure 75.14 A 5 mm trocar back-loaded over the instrument.

is necessary while using microinstrumentation. The gubernacular attachments of the testis are grasped with an endoallis clamp and the testis is delivered into the field. The testis is fixed in the scrotum in the usual fashion.

If testicular positioning is inadequate, further dissection can be done while holding the testis in the scrotum. If the length is inadequate, vessel transection can be done at this point with a clip applier. Since the vas and its vessels have never been touched, this allows a successful Fowler–Stephens orchidopexy. Concerns regarding the possible development of hernias at the internal ring and along the inguinal canal have been largely unfounded; thus we do not attempt to close the ring. There is one reported hernia after laparoscopic orchidopexy,[73] but this seems to be a rare exception.

Risks and complications

Risks of orchidopexy include bleeding, infection, testicular atrophy, testicular malposition, and recurrence of inguinal hernia. Complications associated with laparoscopic orchidopexy are the same, with the addition of possible injuries from cautery or trocar placement. Injury to the iliac vessels during dissection is possible during open or laparoscopic orchidopexy. Avulsion of the gonadal vessels or inadvertent Fowler–Stephens orchidopexy is another complication, more commonly reported with the laparoscopic approach. This usually occurs during delivery of the testis into the scrotum. This can also occur when the surgeon pulls vigorously on the testis during dissection. We have encountered this complication without the loss of the testis. The proximal vessels may retract and go into spasm, making identification difficult. These vessels need to be found and clipped. The vessels from the testis can generally be pulled into the scrotum and ligated. Another potential catastrophic complication is injury to the femoral vessels. This can be avoided by making sure that the endodissector is passed from the ipsilateral port and aimed medially at all times during development of the neocanal. Also dissecting down to the pubic bone in the window between the bladder and the medial umbilical ligament will prevent injuries to the femoral vessels as well as injuries to the bladder. Bladder injuries may occur when the bladder is not decompressed throughout the procedure. Obstruction of the ureter due to tension on the vas has been reported rarely, and has been associated with the Fowler–Stephens procedure.

Much controversy exists in the literature and has been publicly expressed about the risks of adhesions postlaparoscopy. We have not encountered adhesions in our patients that have had multiple laparoscopic procedures nor have we encountered any episodes of bowel obstruction postlaparoscopy secondary to adhesions. Bowel obstruction is a potential complication of laparoscopy in the immediate postoperative period. This is due to herniation of bowel into a trocar site that was inadequately closed. Closure of all trocars sites 5 mm or greater is recommended for children. The advent of microendoscopic equipment and non-cutting trocar technology reduces the risk of herniation and bowel obstruction.

Outcomes of orchidopexy

Conventional orchidopexy for the peeping testis has a satisfactory scrotal placement rate of 82% and for the intra-abdominal testis a rate of 74%.[64] Hazebroek et al[38] had an atrophy rate of 16% for open orchidopexies for peeping or intra-abdominal testis on long-term follow-up. They had a 33% atrophy rate for their vessel transection orchidopexies that included one-stage, two-stage, and revascularization procedures. Laparoscopic orchidopexy achieved a 97% combined satisfactory scrotal placement in our series[59] of patients and there were similar results in other large series. Results with Fowler–Stephens orchidopexy are also superior to those reported in the cumulative literature. The staged Fowler–Stephens procedure was thought to be a better alternative to one-stage vessel transection, allowing collateral blood supply to mature and support transplantation of the testis more readily. This concept was supported by work done by Pascual et al[74] in rats utilizing a xenon washout technique to measure blood flow at 1 hour and 30 days after ligation. Results demonstrated an 80% reduction in blood flow at 1 hour after ligation. However, 30 days later, blood flow returned to normal pretreatment values. Some authors have reported very high success rate with this technique.[68,75] However a review of the literature by Docimo[64] in 1995 revealed no significant difference statistically between one-stage and two-stage vessel transactions prior to the era of laparoscopic orchidopexy. He found that staged Fowler–Stephens orchidopexy had an overall success rate of 76.8% (43/56 testis). When compared with one-stage Fowler–Stephens orchidopexy during the same time period (post 1985), the success rate was 68.5% (76 of 111). These results again tend to prove that meticulous preservation of the vasal blood supply is the most important factor in cases of spermatic vessel transection. Despite this, the majority of laparoscopic practitioners still adhere to the superiority of the staged procedure.

The expense of laparoscopic procedures has been a concern in the past. Lorenzo et al[76] reported on a computer-based analysis of costs for surgery for non-palpable testis and found that there was no difference between open and laparoscopic approaches. The costs of laparoscopy continue to decrease as reusable instruments improve and operative times decrease with experience.

References

1. Levitt SB, Kogan SJ, Engel RM et al. The impalpable testis: a rational approach to management. J Urol 1978; 120:515–20.
2. Wenzler DL, Bloom DA, Park JM. What is the rate of spontaneous testicular descent in infants with cryptorchidism? J Urol 2004; 171(2):849–51.
3. Franco I, Palmer LS, Kolligian M et al. Is laparoscopy the ideal means of evaluating the child with an impalpable testis. J Soc Laparoendosc Surg 2000; 4(4):338.
4. Borrow M, Gough MH. Bilateral absence of testes. Lancet 1970; 1:366.
5. Belman B, Rushton HG. Is the vanishing testis always a scrotal event? BJU Int 2001; 87:480.
6. Van Savage JG. Avoidance of inguinal incision in laparoscopically confirmed vanishing testis syndrome. J Urol 2001; 166:1421–4.
7. Snodgrass W, Chen K, Harrison C. Initial scrotal incision for unilateral nonpalpable testis. J Urol 2004; 172:1742–5.
8. Koff SA. Does compensatory testicular enlargement predict monorchidism. J Urol 1991; 146:632–4.
9. Huff DS, Snyder HM 3rd, Hadziselimovic F, Blyth B, Duckett JW et al. An absent testis is associated with contralateral testicular hypertrophy. J Urol 1992; 148:627–9.
10. Hurwitz RS, Kaptein JS. How well does contralateral testis hypertrophy predict the absence of the nonpalpable testis? J Urol 2001; 165:588–92.
11. Lunderquist A, Rafstedt S. Roentgenologic diagnosis of cryptorchidism. J Urol 1967; 98:219–23.
12. White JJ, Haller JA Jr, Dorst JP. Congenital inguinal hernia and inguinal herniography. Surg Clin N Am 1970; 50:823–37.
13. Notkovich H. Variations of the testicular and ovarian arteries in relation to the renal pedicle. Surg Gynecol Obstet 1956; 103:487–95.
14. Weiss RM, Glickman MG, Lytton B. Preoperative. Localization of non-palpable undescended testis. In: Birth Defects, Original Article Series XIII, Vol. 5. New York: Alan R Liss, 1977: 273.
15. Khademi M, Seebode JJ, Falla AA. Selective spermatic arteriography for localization for an impalpable undescended testis. Radiology 1980; 136:627–34.
16. Rubin SZ, Gershater R. Testicular venography as an accurate indicator of true cryptorchidism. Can J Surg 1981; 33:360–2.
17. Rubin SZ, Mueller DL, Amundson GM, Wesenberg RL. Ultrasonography and the impalpable testis journal. Aust N Z J Surg 1986; 56:609–11.
18. Graif M, Czerniak A, Avigad I et al. High-resolution sonography of the undescended testis in childhood: in analysis of 45 cases. Isr J Med Sci 1990; 33:382–5.
19. Cain MP, Garra B, Gibbons MD. Scrotal-inguinal ultrasonography: a technique for identifying the nonpalpable inguinal testis without laparoscopy. J Urol 1996; 33:791–4.
20. Weiss RM, Carter AR, Rosenfield AT. High resolution real-time ultrasonography in the localization of the undescended testis. J Urol 1986; 135:936–8.
21. Malone PS, Quiney EJ. A comparison between ultrasonography and laparoscopy in localizing the impalpable undescended testis. Br J Urol 1985; 57:185–6.
22. Wolverson MK, Houttuin E, Heiberg E, Sundaram M, Shields JB. Comparison of computed tomography with

high-resolution real-time ultrasound in the localization of the impalpable undescended testis. Radiology 1983; 146:133–6.
23. Tripathi RP, Jena AN, Gulati P et al. Undescended testis: evaluation by magnetic resonance imaging. Indian Pediatr 1992; 29:433–8.
24. Sarihan H, Sari A, Abes M, Dinc H. The nonpalpable undescended testis. Value of magnetic resonance imaging. Minerva Urol Nefrol 1998; 29:233–6.
25. Landa HM, Gylys-Morin V, Mattrey RF et al. The magnetic resonance imaging of the cryptorchid testis. Eur J Pediatr 1987; 29:S16–17.
26. Fritzsch PJ, Hricak H, Kogan BA, Winkler ML, Tanagho EA. Undescended testis: value of MR imaging. Radiology 1987; 164:169–73.
27. Lam WW, Tam PK, Ai VH et al. Gadolinium-infusion magnetic resonance angiogram: a new, noninvasive, and accurate method of preoperative localization of impalpable undescended testis. J Pediatr Surg 1998; 33:123–6.
28. Yeung CK, Tam YH, Chan YL, Lee KH, Metreweli C. A new management algorithm for impalpable undescended testis with gadolinium enhanced magnetic resonance angiography. J Urol 1999; 162:998–1002.
29. Polascik TJ, Chan-Tack KM, Jeffs RD, Gearhart JP. Reappraisal of the role of human chorionic gonadotropin in the diagnosis and treatment of the nonpalpable testis: a 10-year experience. J Urol 1996; 156:804–6.
30. Hjertkvist M, Lackgren G, Ploen L, Bergh A. Does HCG treatment induce inflammation-like changes in undescended testes in boys? J Pediatr Surg 1993; 28:254–8.
31. Bevin AD. The surgical treatment of undescended testicle: a further contribution. JAMA 1903; 41:718.
32. Plotzker ED, Rushton HG, Belman AB, Skoog SJ. Laparoscopy for nonpalpable testis in childhood: is inguinal exploration also necessary when vas and vessels exit the internal ring? J Urol 1992; 148:635–7, discussion 638.
33. Cendron M, Schened AR, Ellsworth PI. Histological evaluation of the testicular nubbin in the vanishing testis syndrome. J Urol 1998; 160:1161–3.
34. El-Gohary MA. The role of laparoscopy in the management of impalpable testis. Pediatr Surg Int 1979; 33:463–5.
35. Rappe BJ, Zandberg AR, De Vries JD, Froeling FM, Debruyne FM. The value of laparoscopy in the management of impalpable cryptorchid testis. Eur Urol 1992; 21:164–7.
36. Humphrey GM, Najmaldin AS, Thomas DF. Laparoscopy in the management of the impalpable undescended testis. Br J Surg 1998; 60:983–5.
37. Mark SD, Davidson PJ. The role of laparoscopy in evaluation of the impalpable undescended testis. Aust N Z J Surg 1997; 67:332–4.
38. Hazebroek FW, Molenaar JC. The management of the impalpable testis by surgery alone. J Urol 1992; 148 (2 Pt):620–31.
39. Boddy SA, Corkery JJ, Gornall P. The place of laparoscopy in the management of the impalpable testis. Br J Surg 1985; 72:918–19.
40. Gulanikar AC, Anderson PA, Schwarz R, Giacomantonio M. Impact of diagnostic laparoscopy in the management of unilateral impalpable testis. Br J Urol 1996; 77:455–7.
41. Lawson A, Gornall P, Buick RG, Corkery JJ. Impalpable testis: testicular vessel division in treatment. Br J Urol 1991; 78:1011–12.
42. Oesch I, Ransley PG. Unilaterally impalpable testis. Eur Urol 1987; 13:324–6.
43. Barqawi AZ, Blyth B, Jordan G, Ehrlich RM, Koyle MA. Role of laparoscopy in patients with previous negative exploration for impalpable testis. Urology 2003; 61:1234–7, discussion 1237.
44. Lakhoo K, Thomas DF, Najmaldin AS. Is inguinal exploration for impalpable testis an outdated operation? Br J Urol 1996; 77:452–4.
45. Perovic S, Janic N. Laparoscopy in the diagnosis of nonpalpable testis. Br J Urol 1994; 73:310–13.
46. Kanemoto K, Hayashi Y, Kojima Y et al. The management of nonpalpable testis with combined groin exploration and subsequent transinguinal laparoscopy. J Urol 2002; 167:674–6.
47. Tennenbaum SY, Lerner SE, McAleer IM et al. Preoperative laparoscopic localization of the nonpalpable testis: a critical analysis of a 10-year experience J Urol 1994; 151:732–4.
48. Zaccara A, Spagnoli A, Copitanucci ML et al. Impalpable testis and laparoscopy: when the gonad is not visualized. JSLS 2004; 8:39–42.
49. Cisek LJ, Peters CA, Atala A et al. Current findings in diagnostic laparoscopic evaluation of the nonpalpable testis. J Urol 1998; 160:1145–9, discussion 1150.
50. O'Hali W, Anderson P, Giacomantonio M. Management of impalpable testis. Indications for abdominal exploration. J Pediatr Surg 1997; 148:918–20.
51. Fowler R, Stephens FO. The role of testicular vascular anatomy in the high undescended testes. Aust N Z J Surg 1959; 29:92.
52. Johnston JH. Prune belly syndrome. In: Eckstein HB, Henfellner R, Williams DJ, eds. Surgical Pediatric Urology. Philadelphia: WB Saunders, 1977: 240.
53. Kogan SJ, Houman BZ, Reda EF, Levitt SB. Orchidopexy of the high undescended testis by division of the spermatic vessels: a critical review of 38 selected transections. J Urol 1989; 141:1416–19.
54. Jarow JP. Intratesticular arterial anatomy. J Androl 1990; 11:255–9.
55. Koff FA, Seth PS. Treatment of high undescended testes by lower spermatic vessel ligation: an alternative to the Fowler–Stephens technique. J Urol 1996; 156:799–803.
56. Lindgren BW, Franco I, Brick S et al. Laparoscopic Fowler–Stephens orchidopexy for the high abdominal testis. J Urol 1999; 162:990–4.
57. Wang KS, Shaul DB. Two-stage laparoscopic orchidopexy with gubernacular preservation: preliminary report of a new approach to the intra-abdominal testis. Pediatr Endosurg Innov Techn 2004; 8(3):250–53.
58. Chang B, Palmer LS, Franco I. Laparoscopic orchidopexy: a review of a large clinical series. BJU Int 2001; 87:490–3.
59. Samadi AA, Palmer LS, Franco I. Laparoscopic orchiopexy: report of 203 cases with review of diagnosis, operative technique, and lessons learned. J Endourol 2003; 17:365–8.
60. Jones PF, Bagley FH. An abdominal extraperitoneal

approach for the difficult orchidopexy. Br J Surg 1979; 56:14–18.
61. Gheiler EL, Spencer-Barthold J, Gonzalez R. Benefits of laparoscopy and the Jones technique for the nonpalpable testis. J Urol 1997; 158:1948–51.
62. Silber SJ, Kelly J. Successful autotransplantation of an intraabdominal testis to the scrotum by microvascular technique. J Urol 1976; 115:452–4.
63. Bukowski TP, Wacksman FJ, Billmire DA et al. Testicular autotransplantation: a seventeen year review of an effective approach to the management of the intraabdominal testes. J Urol 1995; 154:558–61.
64. Docimo SG. The results of surgical therapy for cryptorchidism; a literature review and analysis. J Urol 1995; 154:1148–52.
65. Tackett LD, Wacksman J, Billmire D, Sheldon CA, Minevich E. The high intra-abdominal testis: technique and long-term success of laparoscopic testicular autotransplantation. J Endourol 2002; 16:359–61.
66. Bloom DA. Two-step orchidopexy with pelviscopic clip ligation of the spermatic vessels. J Urol 1991; 145:1030–1.
67. Jordan GH, Robey EL, Winslow BH. Laparoendoscopic surgical management of the abdominal/transinguinal undescended testicle. J Endourol 1992; 6:159.
68. Caldamone AA, Maral JF. Laparoscopic stage II Fowler–Stephens orchidopexy. J Urol 1994; 152:1253–6.
69. Jordan GH, Winslow BH. Laparoscopic single and staged orchidopexy. J Urol 1994; 152:1249–52.
70. Poppas DP, Lemack GE, Mininberg DT. Laparoscopic orchidopexy: clinical experience and description of technique. J Urol 1996; 155:708–11.
71. Docimo SG, Moore RG, Adams J et al. Laparoscopic orchidopexy for the high palpable undescended testis: preliminary experience. J Urol 1995; 154:1513–15.
72. Lindgren BW, Darby EC, Faiella L et al. Laparoscopic orchidopexy: procedure of choice for the nonpalpable testis? J Urol 1998; 159:2132–5.
73. Metwalli AR, Cheng EY. Inguinal hernia after laparoscopic orchiopexy. J Urol 2002; 168:2163.
74. Pascual JA, Villanueva-Meyer JS, Salido E et al. Recovery of testicular blood flow following ligation of testicular vessels. J Urol 1989; 142:549–52.
75. Elder JS. Two stage Fowler–Stephens orchidopexy in the management of intraabdominal testes. J Urol 1992; 148:1239–41.
76. Lorenzo AJ, Samuelson ML, Docimo SG, Baker LA, Lotan Y. Cost analysis of laparoscopic versus open orchiopexy in the management of unilateral nonpalpable testicles. J Urol 2004; 172:712–16.

Testicular tumors

76

Jonathan H Ross

Introduction

Prepubertal testicular tumors are less common than other pediatric urologic tumors such as neuroblastoma and Wilms' tumor, and testicular tumors are far more common in adults than in children. Historically, the management of pediatric testicular tumors has been based on experience in adults. Indeed, testicular tumors in adults and children have many similarities. Both usually present with a testicular mass and are treated initially with excision of the primary tumor. In both children and adults, testicular tumors are particularly sensitive to platinum-based chemotherapy, which has revolutionized the management of testicular cancer throughout the age spectrum.[1,2] However, there are important differences between testis tumors occurring in children and adults. These differences occur in the tumor histopathology, malignant potential, and pattern of metastatic spread. The patients themselves are also dissimilar, with different concerns regarding surgical morbidity and preservation of testicular function. The introduction of a Prepubertal Testicular Tumor Registry by the Section on Urology of the American Academy of Pediatrics (AAP) in 1980 allowed for the accrual of valuable epidemiologic information.[3] Recent multicenter and prospective clinical trials have further advanced our understanding of these tumors and their management.[4–6]

Epidemiology

There is a bimodal age distribution for testis tumors, with one peak occurring in the first 2 years of life, and a second larger peak occurring in young adulthood. The incidence of pediatric testis tumors is 0.5–2.0 per 100 000 children, accounting for 1–2% of all pediatric tumors.[7] Testis tumors are categorized, based on the presumed cell of origin, into stromal tumors and germ cell tumors. In the Prepubertal Testicular Tumor Registry of the Section on Urology of the AAP, the majority of primary testis tumors were yolk sac tumors followed by teratomas and stromal tumors.[3] However, selection bias can lead to an overrepresentation of malignant tumors in registries. Indeed several recent studies have found teratoma to be more common than yolk sac tumor.[8–12] Table 76.1 summarizes the distribution of testis tumors in the Prepubertal Testicular Tumor Registry and a multicenter review of prepubertal testicular tumor pathology specimens. Because teratomas and most stromal tumors are benign in children, the percentage of prepubertal testis tumors that have malignant potential is much lower than the 90% of tumors in adults.

Evaluation

The majority of patients with a testicular tumor will present with a testicular mass noted by the patient, a parent, or a healthcare provider. These masses are usually hard and painless. Occasionally, patients may present with a hydrocele or pain due to torsion or bleeding into the tumor. Physical examination can usually distinguish testicular tumors from other scrotal masses such as hydroceles, hernias, or epididymal cysts. When the physical examination is equivocal, an ultrasound of the testicles can resolve the issue. Ultrasound can also assist in characterizing the lesion. Although ultrasound cannot reliably distinguish malignant from benign testicular tumors, cystic tumors are more likely to be benign in children.

Tumor markers typically utilized in the evaluation and management of adult testis tumors include human

Table 76.1 Distribution of tumor types in the 395 primary testis tumors registered in the Prepubertal Testicular Tumor Registry of the Section on Urology of the American Academy of Pediatrics[3] and 98 tumors in a multicenter consecutive series of patients[12]

Tumor type	Percent of tumors in Registry	Percent of tumors in multicenter study
Germ cell:		
Yolk sac	62	15
Teratoma and epidermoid cyst	26	62
Stromal:		
Leydig cell	1	4
Sertoli cell	3	3
Juvenile granulosa cell	3	5
Unspecified stromal	4	1
Gonadoblastoma	1	2

chorionic gonadotropin (hCG) and alpha-fetoprotein (AFP). Whereas hCG is elaborated in a significant number of mixed germ cell tumors, this tumor type is vanishingly rare in prepubertal patients. It is therefore not a helpful marker for this population. On the other hand, the AFP level is elevated in 90% of patients with yolk sac tumor and can be very helpful in the preoperative distinction between yolk sac and other tumors (almost all of which are benign). One caveat is that the AFP level is quite high in normal infants. The AFP levels are highly variable in infants; typical levels range from approximately 50 000 ng/ml in newborns, to 10 000 ng/ml by 2 weeks of age, 300 ng/ml by 2 months, and 12 ng/ml by 6 months of age.[13] Therefore, AFP levels among patients with yolk sac tumor and benign tumors overlap in the first 6 months of life, making it a less helpful indicator for distinguishing tumor types in young infants (Figure 76.1).[14]

Since many, if not most, prepubertal patients will have a benign tumor, the metastatic evaluation may be deferred until a histologic diagnosis of the primary tumor is obtained. A preoperative metastatic evaluation may be undertaken in patients over 6 months of age with an elevated AFP level, who probably harbor a yolk sac tumor. Metastases from yolk sac tumor typically occur in the lungs and the retroperitoneal lymph nodes. A chest X-ray or chest computed tomography (CT) scan and abdominal CT are obtained. Postoperative AFP levels are also followed. The half-life of AFP is approximately 5 days. Failure of an elevated AFP to decline as expected after removal of the primary tumor is evidence of persistent metastatic disease.

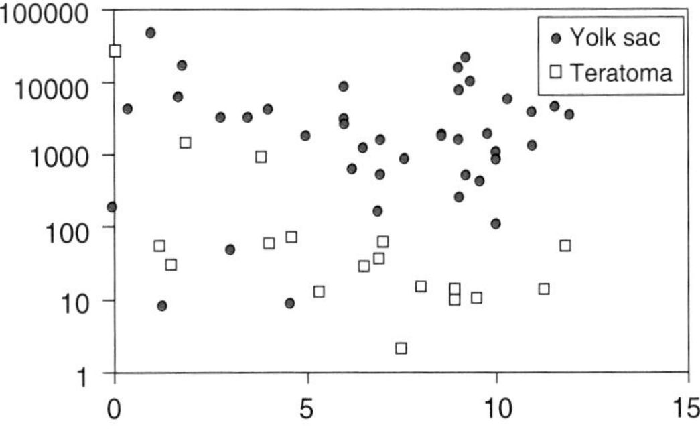

Figure 76.1 Alpha-fetoprotein (AFP) level (ng/ml) as function of age for infants with yolk sac tumor in the Prepubertal Testicular Tumor Registry of the Section on Urology of the American Academy of Pediatrics. (Reprinted from Ross et al,[3] with permission.)

Surgical management

The standard initial treatment for a malignant testicular tumor is an inguinal orchiectomy with early control of the vessels. In prepubertal patients, this approach should be applied only to patients >6 months of age with an elevated AFP.[3] In all other patients, a benign tumor is likely to be present, and the initial surgical management should be an excisional biopsy with frozen section analysis. The exploration is accomplished through an inguinal incision, with occlusion of the testicular vessels (Figure 76.2). Failure to follow these guidelines, particularly scrotal violations, may increase the recurrence rate if the tumor proves to be a yolk sac tumor.[15] If the frozen section reveals a likely malignancy, then the entire testis is removed. If a benign histology is confirmed (usually teratoma), the remaining testis is closed with chromic suture and returned to the scrotum. Even large tumors can be enucleated with preservation of significant testicular tissue (Figure 76.3).

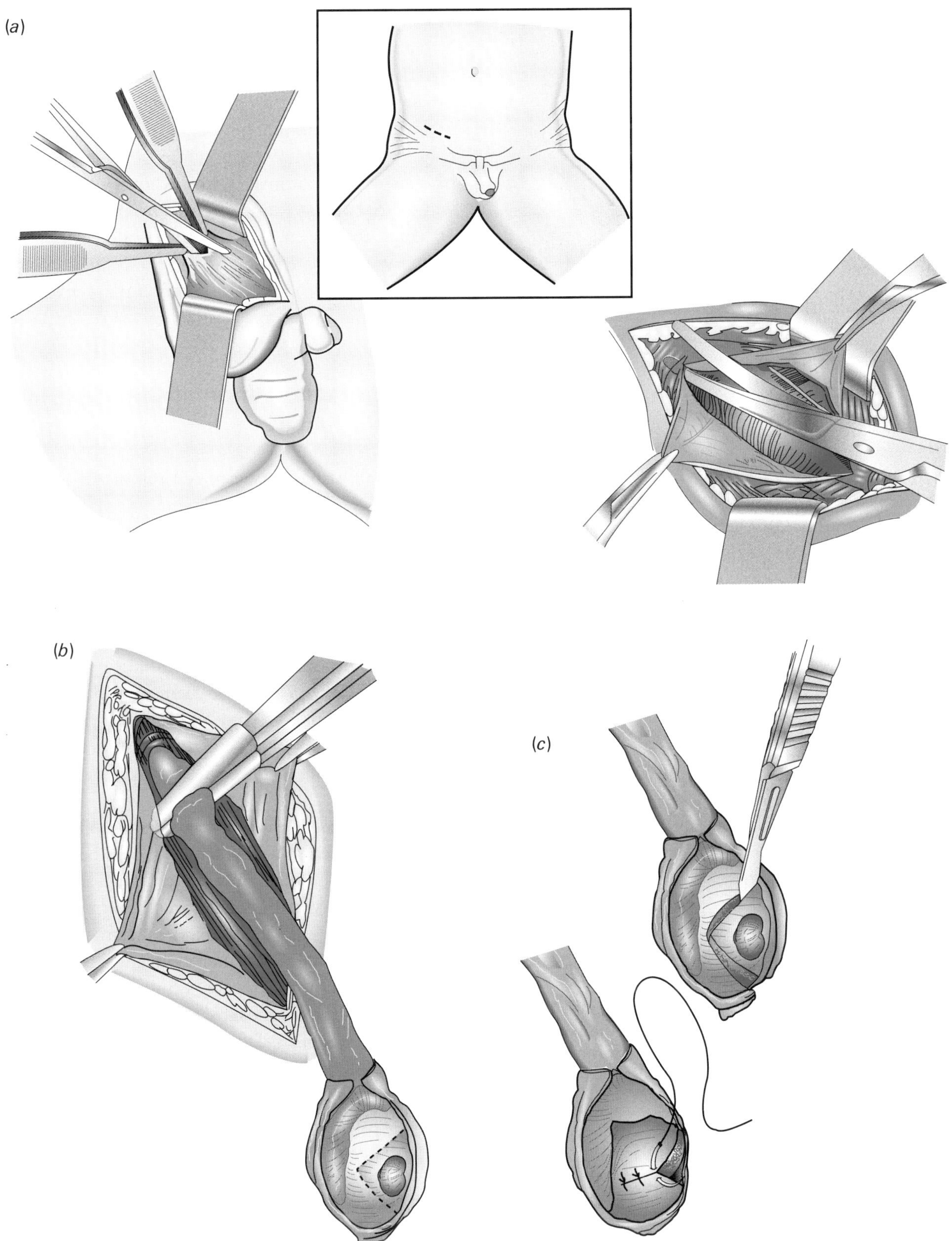

Figure 76.2 Inguinal exploration with testis-sparing tumor excision. (*a*) An inguinal incision is made and Scarpa's fascia is opened, exposing the external oblique aponeurosis. This is opened along the length of its fibers through the external ring, exposing the spermatic cord structures. (*b*) The vessels are temporarily occluded and the testis delivered into the operative field. The hydrocele sac is opened and the tumor sharply excised. If a benign tumor is confirmed on frozen section, then the remnant testis is closed and returned to the scrotum.

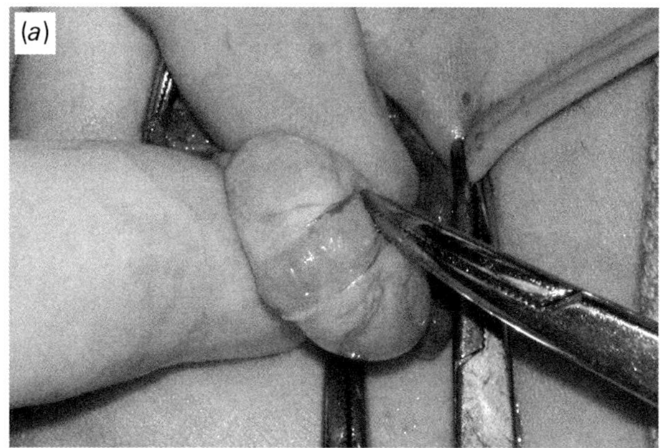

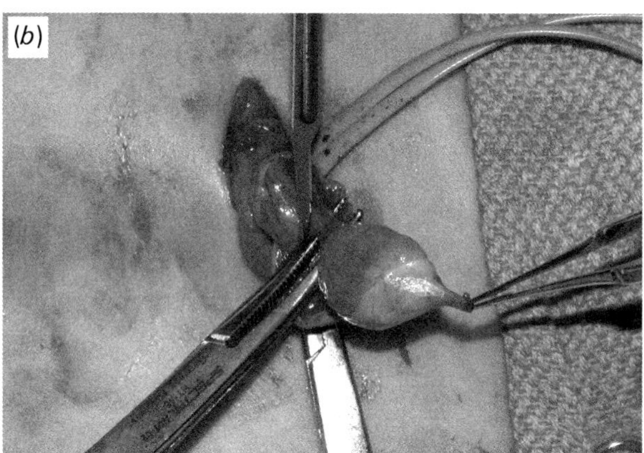

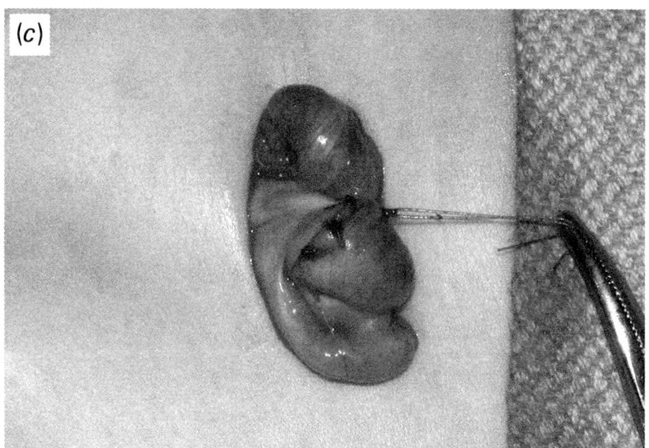

Figure 76.3 Enucleation of a benign tumor. (*a*) With the vessels occluded, an incision is made in the testicular tunic, exposing the cystic tumor. (*b*) The tumor is enucleated and detached from the testis. (*c*) The testis is closed with interrupted suture.

One concern with this approach is the malignant potential of the remnant testicular tissue. In adults, 88% of testicles with teratoma harbor carcinoma in situ (CIS) elsewhere in the testis, and so orchiectomy is still an appropriate management in postpubertal patients.[16] However, in studies of prepubertal teratoma, with the exception of one case, no such finding has been evident.[17–19] Rushton et al reviewed the histopathology of 17 testes removed for teratoma.[18] No multifocal tumor or CIS was found in any specimen. In initial small series of testis-sparing surgery for prepubertal benign tumors, there have been no cases of recurrent tumor in the preserved testicular remnant.[10,11,17,18,20] In 1999, Sugita et al reported on 27 patients with teratoma, 17 of whom were treated with partial orchiectomy.[11] With a mean follow-up of 10 years, there were no recurrences and no cases of testicular atrophy. In these studies, testes undergoing testis-sparing tumor excision appear to maintain normal testicular volume postoperatively.

Adjuvant therapy for malignant testicular tumors

Virtually all malignant germ cell tumors in children are yolk sac tumors. The typical mixed germ cell tumors seen in adults occur only after puberty. There is little data regarding the behavior of mixed germ cell tumors in adolescents, although they appear to exhibit behavior similar to that seen in adults.[21] It is therefore assumed that they should be managed as in adults with observation, retroperitoneal lymph node dissection (RPLND), and/or chemotherapy, depending on the specific histology and stage of the disease. This seems a reasonable approach until further studies in adolescents with testicular malignancies are undertaken.

Yolk sac tumor is a yellow to pale gray solid tumor. It has been referred to by a variety of other names, including endodermal sinus tumor, orchioblastoma, juvenile embryonal carcinoma, mesoblastoma vitellinum, clear cell adenocarcinoma, extraembryonal mesoblastoma, and archenteronoma.[7] A variety of histologic patterns may occur. Positive staining with AFP supports the diagnosis of yolk sac tumor. Classic glomeruloid (Schiller–Duval) bodies and embryoid bodies may be present. These structures are clusters of cells resembling the structures for which they are named (Figure 76.4).

As with most malignancies, adjuvant therapy for yolk sac tumor is based on tumor stage. Different cancer study groups employ different staging systems. However, detailed staging is unnecessary, since the number of patients with metastatic testis tumors in all series is very small, and stratifying response rates and tumor behavior based on the extent of metastatic disease is impossible. Indeed, in large studies, all metastatic yolk sac tumors are treated the same, regardless of the extent or location of metastatic dis-

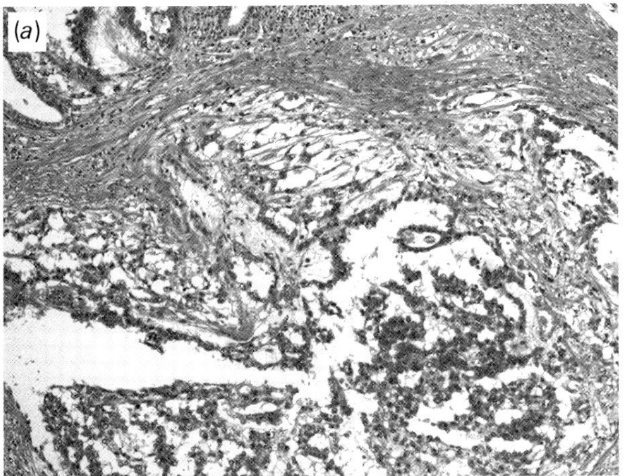

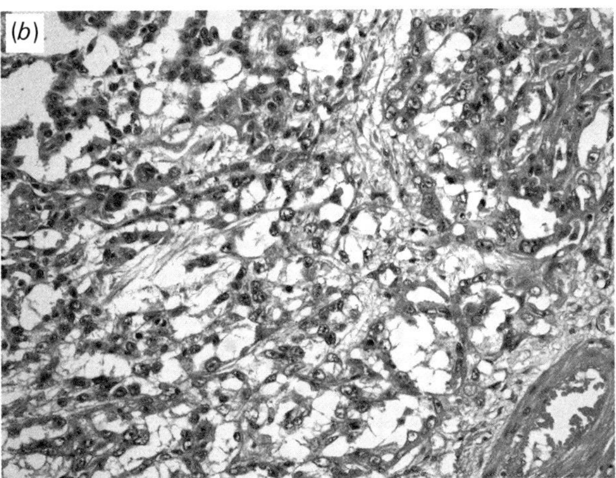

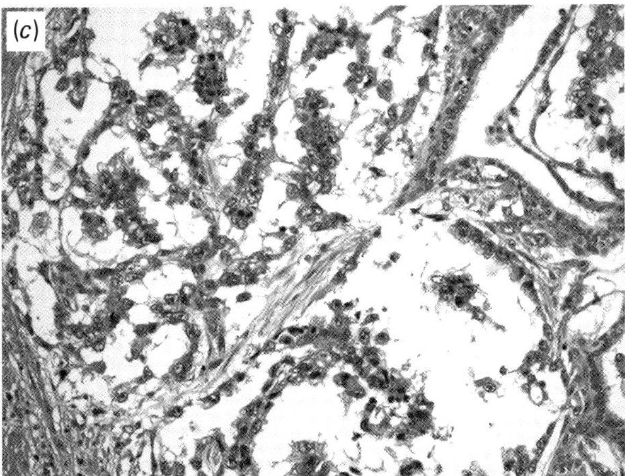

Figure 76.4 Histopathology of a yolk sac tumor; (*a*) ×100 magnification; (*b* and *c*) ×200 magnification.

ease. Therefore, the important distinction for yolk sac tumors is between stage 1 disease (disease limited to the testis and completely excised) and those tumors with any degree of residual or metastatic disease.

The majority of prepubertal testis tumors present with stage 1 disease.[3] Recent studies suggest that these patients can be safely managed with observation followed by chemotherapy for patients who recur.[4–6,22–24] The United Kingdom Children's Cancer Study Group, the German Society of Pediatric Oncology, and the United States Pediatric Intergroup Study (now the Children's Oncology Group) have recently reported their results employing observation for stage 1 yolk sac tumor of the testis and platinum-based chemotherapy for patients with recurrent or metastatic disease.[4–6] Most patients with recurrent or metastatic disease received four cycles of chemotherapy. The potential toxicities of the chemotherapy regimens employed include myelosuppression, ototoxicity and renal toxicity from platinum-based agents, and pulmonary toxicity from bleomycin. High-grade ototoxicity was rare in the United Kingdom study, which utilized carboplatin rather than cisplatin; however, carboplatin is more myelotoxic.

A summary of the three large multicenter studies is presented in Table 76.2. Eighty-four percent of all patients presented with stage 1 disease. Overall, the recurrence rate for patients with stage 1 tumors managed with observation was 17%, and all were cured with chemotherapy. The overall survival of all patients receiving chemotherapy for recurrent or metastatic disease was 98%. Clearly, the outlook for prepubertal testis tumors is excellent. Stage 1 tumors are best managed with orchiectomy and observation. Observation should include frequent chest and abdominal imaging and measurement of AFP levels. Patients with recurrent disease or metastatic disease can expect excellent results with platinum-based multiagent chemotherapy. Future studies will focus on reducing the morbidity for those patients requiring chemotherapy by reducing the number of agents and/or cycles of therapy administered.

Another shift in the management of prepubertal testis tumors has been away from performance of RPLND, once a standard component of management.[25–27] The rationale for this dissection in select adult patients is the likelihood of retroperitoneal disease and the ability to avoid the morbidity of chemotherapy in some patients. Several characteristics of prepubertal tumors argue against its use in children. Most prepubertal patients have clinical stage 1 disease and the recurrence rate for these patients with observation alone is only 17%. Nearly all the recurrences can be salvaged with chemotherapy. For those with metastatic disease, it appears that only a minority of prepubertal patients have disease limited to the retroperitoneum.[28] The majority have disease in the chest (with or without retroperitoneal disease). Finally, the morbidity of abdominal surgery is greater

Table 76.2 Results of three large multicenter studies of pediatric testicular yolk sac tumors

	Number of patients	Percent with stage 1 tumors	Recurrence rate of stage 1 tumors on observation	Chemotherapy for recurrent or metastatic disease	Survival for stage 1 tumors	Survival for those patients with residual disease/ metastases
United Kingdom Children's Cancer Study Group[4]	73	70%	22%	Bleomycin, etoposide, carboplatin	100%	100%
German Cooperative Studies[5]	110	95%	15%	Bleomycin, vinblastine, cisplatin	100%	80%
US Pediatric Intergroup Study[6]	79	82%	18%	Bleomycin, etoposide, cisplatin	100%	100%
Total	262	84%	17%		100%	98%

for children than for adults. Children have a particularly high rate of postoperative bowel obstruction. It is also unclear that a nerve-sparing approach is technically feasible in small children. For prepubertal testis tumors, RPLND is limited to patients with persistent retroperitoneal masses following chemotherapy, an extremely rare occurrence.

Teratoma and epidermoid cyst

Teratoma is the most common benign tumor in prepubertal patients. The median age of presentation is 13 months, with several patients presenting in the neonatal period.[14,29] Histologically, teratomas consist of tissues representing the three germinal layers: endoderm, mesoderm, and ectoderm. Epidermoid cysts are benign tumors composed entirely of keratin-producing epithelium. They are distinguished from dermoid cysts, which contain skin and skin appendages, and from teratomas, which contain derivatives of other germ cell layers. Teratomas and epidermoid cysts are universally benign in prepubertal children. On ultrasonography, most epidermoid cysts appear as discrete intratesticular masses, with areas of increased echogenicity corresponding to the keratin debris or peripheral calcification.[30,31]

At the time of inguinal exploration, an excisional biopsy with frozen section should be performed to confirm the diagnosis.[17,18] In older children with teratoma, surrounding testicular parenchyma must be carefully evaluated. If there is histologic evidence of pubertal changes, then an orchiectomy should be performed since teratomas are potentially malignant in postpubertal males. Biopsies of surrounding testicular parenchyma are probably unnecessary in prepubertal patients.[18,19,30] Whereas 88% of testes removed for adult teratoma contain areas of intratubular germ cell neoplasia, this has generally not been the case for epidermoid cysts or for pediatric teratoma.[16–19]

For patients with epidermoid cyst and prepubertal patients with teratoma, no radiographic studies or follow-up for the development of metastatic disease are required. Because of the potential for malignancy, postpubertal patients with teratoma should be evaluated and followed on the same protocol as adults with potentially malignant germ cell tumors.

Gonadal stromal tumors

Stromal tumors comprise Leydig cell, Sertoli cell, juvenile granulosa, and mixed or undifferentiated tumors. Stromal testis tumors are rare in children, and there are no large series to guide their management. However, anecdotal reports and small series in the literature offer some experience on which to base therapy.[32]

Leydig cell tumors are universally benign in children.[7,32] They usually present between 5 and 10 years of age with precocious puberty. Congenital adrenal hyperplasia (CAH) can also lead to precocious puberty and testicular masses. Patients with Leydig cell tumors typically have elevated testosterone levels with low or normal gonadotropin levels, whereas patients with CAH will usually have elevated levels of 17-hydroxyprogesterone. Leydig cell tumors may be treated by testis-sparing excision.[33] Persistence of androgenic effects may be due to a contralateral tumor, but this is rare in children. Because Leydig cell tumors are sometimes difficult to detect on physical examination, an ultrasound may be necessary to rule out a contralateral tumor. However, even after successful removal of a solitary tumor, androgenic changes are not completely reversible, and some children may proceed through premature puberty as a result of the activation of the hypothalamic–pituitary–gonadal axis.

Sertoli cell tumors are rare in children. The median age of patients in the Prepubertal Testicular Tumor Registry was 6 months, with a range of 4 months to 10 years.[32] Sertoli cell tumors are usually well circumscribed and often lobulated. Cysts are common. Approximately 10% of adult Sertoli cell tumors are malignant. Sertoli cell tumors are usually hormonally inactive in children, although they may occasionally cause gynecomastia or isosexual precocious puberty. Although all reported cases to date have been benign in children <5 years of age, there have been a few cases of malignant Sertoli cell tumors in older children.[34,35] Orchiectomy is usually sufficient treatment in infants and young children. A metastatic evaluation could be considered in older children and in patients with worrisome histologic findings. When metastatic disease is present, aggressive combination treatment, including RPLND, chemotherapy, and radiation therapy, should be considered.

The large cell calcifying Sertoli cell tumor is a clinically and histologically distinct entity, with a higher incidence of multifocality and hormonal activity.[7,36–39] These tumors are composed of large cells with abundant cytoplasm and varying degrees of calcification, ranging from minimal amounts to massive deposits. Whereas standard Sertoli cell tumors are more common in adults, large cell calcifying Sertoli cell tumors are found predominantly in children and adolescents. Most present with a testicular mass. Approximately one-quarter of patients have bilateral and multifocal tumors. The presence of calcifications results in a characteristic ultrasound appearance including multiple hyperechoic areas.

Approximately one-third of patients with large cell calcifying Sertoli cell tumor have an associated genetic syndrome and/or endocrine abnormality. The two most common associated syndromes are Peutz–Jeghers syndrome, which is characterized by mucocutaneous pigmentation and hamartomatous intestinal polyposis, and Carney's syndrome, which is characterized by myxomas of the skin, soft tissues and heart, myxoid changes of the breast, lentigines of the face and lips, cutaneous blue nevi, Cushing's syndrome, pituitary adenoma, and schwannoma. Screening for these syndromes in patients with large cell calcifying Sertoli cell tumors is important since the patients and their first-degree relatives are at risk for the potentially lethal associated anomalies. Whereas occasionally malignant in adults, large cell calcifying Sertoli cell tumors have been universally benign in patients under 25 years of age, and inguinal orchiectomy is sufficient treatment for children.

Testicular juvenile granulosa cell tumor is a stromal tumor bearing a light-microscopic resemblance to ovarian juvenile granulosa cell tumor. However, the histologic origin of this tumor in testicles is unclear. Granulosa cell tumors occur almost exclusively in the first year of life, most in the first 6 months. Of 22 tumors diagnosed in newborns in the Prepubertal Testicular Tumor Registry, six were juvenile granulosa cell tumors, six were yolk sac tumors, and six were unspecified stromal tumors.[29] Structural abnormalities of the Y chromosome and mosaicism are common in boys with juvenile granulosa cell tumor.[34] Several cases have been described in association with ambiguous genitalia.[40] These tumors are hormonally inactive and benign. Although these children should undergo chromosomal analysis, no treatment or metastatic evaluation is required beyond testis-sparing excision.[32,41]

Undifferentiated stromal tumors consist of areas of gonadal stromal neoplasia and undifferentiated regions of spindle cells that may exhibit a high mitotic rate. These stromal tumors have an epidemiology similar to that of granulosa cell tumors.[32] Although some of these tumors have histologic characteristics commonly associated with malignancy, most behave in a benign fashion. There are inadequate data in the literature to formulate rigid guidelines for managing these tumors. Whereas aggressive behavior has not occurred in young infants, there are reports of such behavior in older children. Unfortunately, histologic features do not appear to correlate with invasive or metastatic potential. Since orchiectomy cures most of these patients, aggressive treatment is probably not appropriate in the absence of radiographic evidence of metastatic disease. However, given the uncertainty, postoperative evaluation and follow-up for the development of metastatic disease seem prudent for patients with this rare tumor.

Gonadoblastoma

Gonadoblastomas are benign tumors that typically arise in dysgenetic gonads. They contain both germ cell and stromal elements.[42] Dysgenetic or 'streak' gonads are gonads that have failed to develop normally and contain fibrous tissue and primitive ovarian structures. If the gonad has features of primitive testicular development, it is usually referred to as a dysgenetic testis rather than a streak gonad. Gonadoblastoma arises almost exclusively in the dysgenetic gonads of patients with a Y chromosome or evidence of some Y chromatin in their karyotype. Dysgenetic gonads in patients without Y chromatin, such as patients with Turner's syndrome or XX gonadal dysgenesis, seem to be at little risk. Gonadoblastomas have been reported in 3% of true hermaphrodites and in 10–30% of patients with mixed gonadal dysgenesis or pure gonadal dysgenesis in the presence of Y chromatin.[43,44] They also occur commonly in dysgenetic testes.[45]

Although gonadoblastomas are benign, they are prone to the development of malignant degeneration, and overt malignant behavior is seen in 10% of cases.[44] Most cases of malignancy occur after puberty, but there have also been cases reported in children.[44] Therefore, early prophylactic removal of dysgenetic gonads should be performed. If malignant elements are present, a metastatic evaluation should be undertaken. Dysgerminoma (or seminoma) is the most common malignancy to occur in association with gonadoblastoma. Like their counterpart in normal testicles, these tumors are very radiosensitive, and the outlook for these patients is generally favorable.

Testis tumors in congenital adrenal hyperplasia

Congenital adrenal hyperplasia in boys often presents with precocious puberty. Adrenal rests, commonly present along the spermatic cord and in the testicular hilum, may hypertrophy in patients with CAH, leading to testicular nodules that are clinically indistinguishable from testicular tumors. Indeed, the presentation of a testicular mass and precocious puberty is typical of patients with Leydig cell tumors as well. In patients with CAH these nodules are often multifocal and bilateral.[46–48] The diagnosis of CAH can generally be made by demonstrating an elevated serum 17-hydroxyprogesterone level. In this setting, the nodules will usually resolve or significantly reduce in size with steroid replacement. If this occurs, the patient may be followed with serial examinations.[49] Any nodule that fails to respond should be biopsied. Large nodules that fail to regress may be safely enucleated.[49,50]

Leukemia

Historically, the urologist has played an important role in the evaluation of patients with acute lymphoblastic leukemia (ALL) because of the concept that the testis was a site protected from therapy by the 'blood–testis barrier'. Approximately 20% of ALL patients have microscopic involvement at diagnosis, and pretreatment biopsy was common.[51] Following treatment, biopsy was undertaken to detect the 10% of patients with persistent testicular disease. However, with current chemotherapy, most patients with microscopic testicular involvement achieve a complete remission. Conversely, some patients without histologic evidence of testicular involvement at diagnosis will ultimately relapse in the testicles. Therefore, pretreatment testicular biopsy is no longer recommended since it does not predict those at risk for persistent or relapsing disease. Modern treatment has reduced the post-treatment relapse rate to <1%. Therefore, post-treatment biopsy in the absence of clinical evidence of persistent disease is also unnecessary.[52] Rare patients with persistent or recurrent testicular enlargement following chemotherapy should undergo testicular biopsy to confirm the presence of ALL. In most cases the patient will have relapsed at other sites and further systemic treatment will be required. Typically, the testicles are also treated with radiation.

References

1. Einhorn LH, Williams SD. Chemotherapy of disseminated testicular cancer. Cancer 1980; 46:1339–44.
2. Flamant F, Baranzelli MD, Kalifa C, Lemerle J. Treatment of malignant germ cell tumors in children: experience of the Institut Gustave Roussy and the French Society of Pediatric Oncology. Crit Rev Oncol Hematol 1990; 10:99–110.
3. Ross JH, Rybicki L, Kay R. Clinical behavior and a contemporary management algorithm for prepubertal testis tumors: a summary of the Prepubertal Testis Tumor Registry. J Urol 2002; 168:1675–9.
4. Mann JR, Raafat F, Robinson K et al. The United Kingdom Children's Cancer Study Group's second germ cell tumor study: carboplatin, etoposide, and bleomycin are effective treatment for children with malignant extracranial germ cell tumors, with acceptable toxicity. J Clin Oncol 2000; 18:3809–18.
5. Haas RJ, Schmidt P, Gobel U, Harms D. Testicular germ cell tumors, an update. Results of the German cooperative studies 1982–1997. Klin Padiatr 1999; 211:300–4.
6. Giller R, Cushing B, Marina N et al. Outcome of surgery alone or surgery plus cisplatin/etoposide/bleomycin (PEB) for localized gonadal malignant germ cell tumors

(MGCT) in children: a pediatric intergroup report (CCG8891/POG9048). Med Ped Oncol 1997; 29:413.
7. Coppes MJ, Rackley R, Kay R. Primary testicular and paratesticular tumors of childhood. Med Pediatr Oncol 1994; 22:329–40.
8. Rushton HG, Belman AB. Testis-sparing surgery for benign lesions of the prepubertal testis. Urol Clin North Am 1993; 20:27–37.
9. Farivar-Mohseni H, Bagli DJ, McLorie G, Pippi Salle J, Khoury A. Prepubertal testicular and paratesticular tumours. J Urol 1996; 155(Suppl):392A.
10. Shukla AR, Woodard C, Carr MC et al. Testicular teratoma at the Children's Hospital of Philadelphia: the role of testis preserving surgery. J Urol 2002; 167(Suppl):109.
11. Sugita Y, Clarnette TD, Cooke-Yarborough CC et al. Testicular and paratesticular tumours in children: 30 years' experience. Aust N Z J Surg 1999; 69:505–8.
12. Pohl HG, Shukla AR, Metcalf PD et al. Prepubertal testis tumors: actual prevalence rate of histological types. J Urol 2004; 172:2370–2.
13. Wu JT, Book IL, Sudar K. Serum alpha-fetoprotein (AFP) levels in normal infants. Pediatr Res 1981; 15:50–2.
14. Grady R, Ross JH, Kay R. Epidemiologic features of teratomas of the testis in a prepubertal population. J Urol 1997; 158:1191–2.
15. Schlatter M, Rescorla F, Giller R et al. Excellent outcome in patients with stage I germ cell tumors of the testes: a study of the Children's Cancer Group/Pediatric Oncology Group. J Pediatr Surg 2003; 38:319–24.
16. Manivel JC, Reinberg Y, Nehans GA, Fraley EE. Intratubular germ cell neoplasia in testicular teratoma and epidermoid cysts – correlation with prognosis and possible biologic significance. J Urol 1989; 64:715.
17. Ross JH, Kay R, Elder J. Testis sparing surgery for pediatric epidermoid cysts of the testis. J Urol 1993; 149:353–6.
18. Rushton HG, Belman AB, Sesterhenn I, Patterson K, Mostofi FK. Testicular sparing surgery for prepubertal teratoma of the testis: a clinical and pathological study. J Urol 1990; 144:726–30.
19. Renedo DE, Trainer TD. Intratubular germ cell neoplasia (ITGCN) with p53 and PCNA expression and adjacent mature teratoma in an infant testis. Am J Surg Pathol 1994; 18:947–52.
20. Pearse BI, Glick RD, Abramson SJ et al. Testicular-sparing surgery for benign testicular tumors. J Pediatr Surg 1999; 34:1000–3.
21. Terenziani M, Piva L, Spreafico F et al. Clinical stage I nonseminomatous germ cell tumors of the testis in childhood and adolescence: an analysis of 31 cases. J Pediatr Hematol Oncol 2002; 24:454–8.
22. Lo Curto M, D'Angelo P, Arrighini A et al. Malignant germ cell tumours in childhood: the Italian experience. In: Jones WG, Appleyard I, Harnden P, Joffe JK, eds. Germ Cell Tumours IV. London: John Libbey & Co, 1998: 227–31.
23. Baranzelli MC, Patte C. The French experience in paediatric malignant germ cell tumours. In: Jones WG, Appleyard I, Harnden P, Joffe JK, eds. Germ Cell Tumours IV, London: John Libbey & Co, 1998: 227–31.
24. Lin JN, Wang KL, Hung IJ, Yang CP. Management of yolk sac tumor of the testis in children. J Formos Med Assoc 1994; 93:393–6.
25. Fernandes ET, Etcubanas E, Rao BN et al. Two decades of experience with testicular tumors in children at St Jude Children's Research Hospital. J Pediatr Surg 1989; 24:677–82.
26. Hopkins TB, Jaffe N, Colodny A, Cassady JR, Filler RM. The management of testicular tumors in children. J Urol 1978; 120:96–102.
27. Kaplan WE, Firlit CF. Treatment of testicular yolk sac carcinoma in the young child. J Urol 1981; 126:663–4.
28. Grady RW, Ross JH, Kay R. Patterns of metastatic spread in prepubertal yolk sac tumor of the testis. J Urol 1995; 153:1259–61.
29. Levy DA, Kay R, Elder JS. Neonatal testis tumors: a review of the Prepubertal Testis Tumor Registry. J Urol 1994; 151:715–17.
30. Reinberg Y, Manivel JC, Llerena J, Niehans G, Fraley EE. Epidermoid cyst (monodermal teratoma) of the testis. Br J Urol 1990; 66:648–51.
31. Maxwell AJ, Mamtora H. Sonographic appearance of epidermoid cyst of the testis. J Clin Ultrasound 1990; 18:188–90.
32. Thomas JC, Ross JH, Kay R. Stromal testis tumors in children: a report from the prepubertal testis tumor registry. J Urol 2001; 166:2338–40.
33. Konrad D, Schoenle EJ. Ten-year follow-up in a boy with Leydig cell tumor after selective surgery. Horm Res 1999; 51:96–100.
34. Cortez JC, Kaplan GW. Gonadal stromal tumors, gonadoblastomas, epidermoid cysts, and secondary tumors of the testis in children. Urol Clin North Am 1993; 20:15–26.
35. Kolon TF, Hochman HI. Malignant Sertoli cell tumor in a prepubescent boy. J Urol 1997; 158:608–9.
36. Niewenhuis JC, Wolf MC, Kass EJ. Bilateral asynchronous Sertoli cell tumor in a boy with the Peutz–Jeghers syndrome. J Urol 1994; 152:1246–8.
37. Proppe KH, Scully RE. Large-cell calcifying Sertoli cell tumor of the testis. Am J Clin Pathol 1980; 74:607–19.
38. Kratzer SS, Ulbright TM, Talerman A et al., Large cell calcifying Sertoli cell tumor of the testis: contrasting features of six malignant and six benign tumors and a review of the literature. Am J Surg Pathol 1997; 21:1271–80.
39. Chang B, Borer JG, Tan PE, Diamond DA, Large-cell calcifying Sertoli cell tumor of the testis: case report and review of the literature. Urology 1998; 52:520–2.
40. Young RH, Lawrence WD, Scully RE. Juvenile granulosa cell tumor – another neoplasm associated with abnormal chromosomes and ambiguous genitalia, a report of 3 cases. Am J Surg Pathol 1985; 9:737.
41. Shukla AR, Huff DS, Canning DA, Filmer RB, Snyder HM 3rd. Juvenile granulosa cell tumor of the testis: contemporary clinical management and pathological diagnosis. J Urol 2004; 171:1900–2.
42. Rutgers JL, Scully RE. Pathology of the testis in intersex syndromes. Semin Diagn Pathol 1987; 4:275.
43. Savage MO, Lowe DG. Gonadal neoplasia and abnormal sexual differentiation. Clin Endocrinol 1990; 32:519.
44. Ramani P, Yeung CK, Habeebu SS. Testicular intratubu-

Clinical and biologic features

Neuroblastoma ranks as the most common extracranial solid malignancy of childhood[5] and early infancy. The incidence may be increasing slightly.[5,6] In children presenting with neuroblastoma, 65% will occur in the retroperitoneum, of which 40% will originate in the adrenal gland.[7]

Few, if any, environmental risk factors have been identified for neuroblastoma. Recently, maternal vaginal infections, their treatment, and prenatal maternal hormone use have been weakly suggested to increase the risk of neuroblastoma in offspring.[8] Pesticide exposure has been suggested as being associated with an increased risk of carcinogenesis in children compared with adults; the risk included, but was not specific for, neuroblastoma.[9]

While newer molecular modalities are helping to refine prognostic groupings and treatment assignment, the overwhelming variables distinguishing high from low-risk groups continue to be age at diagnosis, tumor stage, and histologic grade.[10] Diagnosis before 12 months of age is more clinically favorable than later diagnosis.

Any predisposition for neuroblastoma appears to follow an autosomal dominant pattern, as elucidated by the two-hit hypothesis of Knudson and Strong.[11] Also described for Wilms' tumor and pheochromocytoma, inherited forms of neuroblastoma may occur in patients who harbor a mutation in a gene that preexisted in a parental germ line (preconception or germinal mutation). A subsequent spontaneous mutation of the other copy of the same gene (a somatic mutation) in a cell of the appropriate background (neural crest cell) leads to malignant transformation of that cell. This has led to estimates that over one-fifth of all neuroblastoma may be of the inherited variety.[11] The occurrence of non-familial neuroblastoma must therefore await these two critical mutations or 'hits' as two independent spontaneous events. This explains the reduced likelihood (incidence) of non-familial or sporadic disease. With one of two mutations possibly present in all cells of a given child with a strong family history of neuroblastoma, it is easy to see why earlier incidence, bilaterality and multifocality, and higher recurrence rates are the norm in those with familial disease. Exceptions to the two-hit hypothesis have been reported (familial neuroblastoma in older children), suggesting that other genetic mechanisms may also underlie familial disease.[12] While several reports exist of neuroblastoma being found in children with a chromosomal abnormality, few chromosomal predispositions have been definitively associated with neuroblastoma. Abnormal rearrangements have been described involving chromosomes 1 and 17 (see below). Deletions involving 1p36 have implicated this region as containing a neuroblastoma tumor suppressor gene, and gains in the 17q region have been associated with poor prognosis.[12–17] In addition, FISH analysis for chromosome alteration in 3p and 11q may define patients with a poorer prognosis.[18] Finally, loss of heterozygosity (LOH), a molecular phenotype characterized by the loss of the subtle differences that normally exist between the two allelic (parental) copies of any gene signifying that one of the copies is missing, has been identified as a more general phenomenon in neuroblastoma. Subjects with LOH are, therefore, homozygous instead of heterozygous for that particular chromosomal region. When a disease becomes evident in association with LOH in particular regions of a chromosome, this implies that the missing region of that chromosome encodes a gene or genes responsible for suppressing that disease, i.e. tumor suppressor genes. Although LOH does not identify the missing gene itself, LOH in neuroblastoma has been reported in a number of chromosomes, including 1p, 11q and 14q, 2q, 9p, and 18q.[19]

Clinical manifestations: primary, metastatic, and paraneoplastic features

The presenting signs and symptoms are variable and may reflect the effects of the tumor, the presence of metastatic disease, or the results of tumor hormone production. As mentioned earlier, prenatal screening may also identify neuroblastoma. Infants may present with an abdominal mass that is often huge. In spite of the size, which makes the tumors detectable at birth, their prognosis is often excellent with respect to cure, although some neurological defects may persist.[20] A unique feature of neuroblastoma in children is the potential for widespread liver metastatic disease that may signify stage 4S disease (Figure 77.1).

Children with stage 4S have a potential survival rate of up to 90%, in spite of metastases to either liver, skin, or bone marrow, but not to cortical bone. Subcutaneous nodules are another manifestation of this early presentation.[22] In some patients, tumors regress spontaneously. Alternatively, metastases may regress following excision of the primary tumor.[23–25] In children >1 year of age the size of the abdominal mass is variable and may not be the presenting symptom. Malaise and/or pain reflecting the presence of

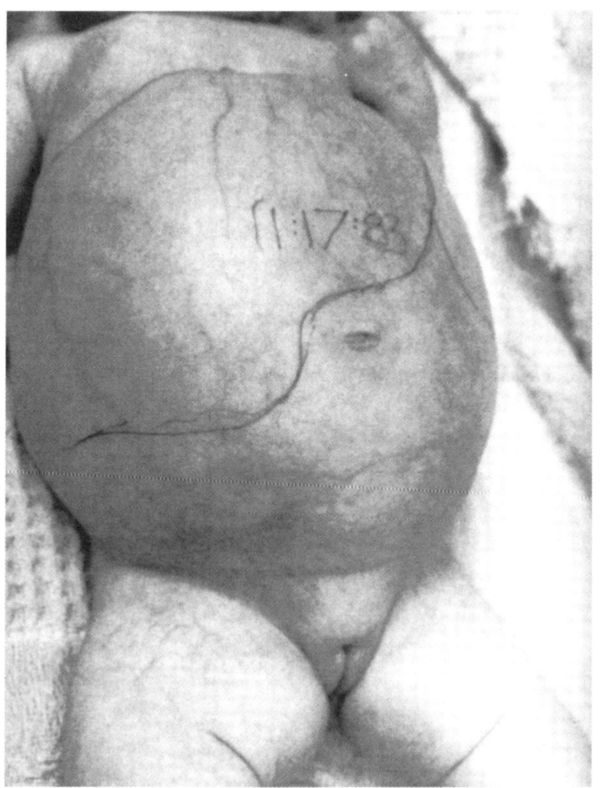

Figure 77.1 Neuroblastoma metastatic to liver. Stage 4S neuroblastoma underwent spontaneous regression. (Reproduced from Snyder et al,[21] with permission.)

metastatic disease is the presenting complaint in up to 60%. Anemia (from bone marrow involvement in 50% of patients) is also a common presenting sign. The new or sudden onset of constipation or urinary retention may herald the well-known propensity of neuroblastoma to invade the spinal cord. In addition, transient pain attributable to bony metastases may mimic rheumatoid arthritis. Lung or brain metastases are common sites of relapse and late-stage disease.

Paraneoplastic syndromes occur in fewer than 5% of neuroblastoma patients. Intractable diarrhea may result from the secretion of vasoactive intestinal peptide (VIP).[26] However, this symptom, mimicking malabsorption syndrome, is more often associated with the better-differentiated ganglioneuroma or intermediately differentiated ganglioneuroblastoma. Resolution follows removal of the tumor. Another unusual symptom is cerebellar ataxia and opsomyoclonus (dancing feet, dancing eyes; myoclonic encephalopathy of infants). This syndrome is of unknown pathogenesis and is more often associated with thoracic tumors.[7] Whereas symptoms of catecholamine excess (palpitations, tachycardia, and hypertension) are rare in neuroblastoma, they can occur from excess circulating tumor-derived norepinephrine. However, norepinephrine is less potent than its metabolite, epinephrine, in inducing these symptoms. These symptoms are more commonly found in patients with pheochromocytoma where the enzyme responsible is phenylethanolamine *N*-methyltransferase (PNMT), which catalyzes the conversion of norepinephrine to epinephrine.

Gross, histologic, molecular pathology, and markers

Neuroblastomas arise from cells of neural crest origin, which ultimately form the sympathetic nervous systems (sympathogonia). The sites of origin may be found at any location in the sympathetic nervous system with over one-half occurring in the neonatal abdominal cavity, and up to two-thirds from the adrenal gland. The remainder occurs in the sympathetic ganglia and, more rarely, in the organ of Zuckerhandl. The spectrum of biologic behavior or potential of these tumors is broad. Malignant neuroblastomas constitute the majority. Ganglioneuroblastoma and ganglioneuroma represent progressively more benign forms of the tumor, reflecting more indolent clinical manifestations, better prognoses, as well as distinct morphology and biochemical profiles.

The histopathologic features that define the malignant potential are unique. Homer Wright pseudorosettes, the diagnostic histologic presence of eosinophilic neutrophils surrounded by neuroblasts, occur in only one-half of cases.[27] The presence of associated neuropils (pigmented neuritic processes) is pathognomonic for neuroblastoma. The other type of cell is the Schwann cell, which may be recruited into the tumor and constitutes the schwannian stroma, which makes up the mesenchymal component of the tumor. The degree of histologic differentiation is classified according to a variety of schemes but the most popular is that developed by Shimada, which has recently been revised by Joshi (Table 77.2), and a combination of the two is the basis of planned prospective trials.[29]

Molecular pathology

Molecular understanding of neuroblastoma has identified several newer features of the disease that may aid in all aspects of its management, including diagnosis, natural history, prognostic stratification, and treatment selection. These include analyses of nuclear and chromosomal material, and neuronal phenotyping through assessment of various neuron-associated

Table 77.2 Histopathologic classifications of Shimada and Joshi

Prognosis	Histopathologic features/age
Favorable	
Shimada	Stroma rich, all ages, no nodular pattern
	Stroma poor, age 1.5–5 years, differentiated, MKI <100
	Stroma poor, age <1.5 years, MKI <200
Joshi	Grade 1, all ages; grade 2, <1 year
Unfavorable	
Shimada	Stroma rich, all ages, nodular pattern
	Stroma poor, age >5 years
	Stroma poor, age 1.5–5 years, undifferentiated
	Stroma poor, age 1.5–5 years, differentiated, MKI >100
	Stroma poor, age <1.5 years, MKI >200
Joshi	Grade 2, age >1 year; grade 3, all ages

Grade 1 = low mitotic rate (<10 mitotic figures per 10 high power fields) and calcification present; grade 2 = either low mitotic rate or calcification present; grade 3 = neither low mitotic rate nor calcification present.
MKI = mitosis–karyorrhexis index (number of mitoses and karyorrhexis per 5000 cells).
Adapted from Brodeur and Castleberry,[28] with permission.

growth factors. Whereas karyotyping has identified specific chromosomal abnormalities (see below), analysis of DNA ploidy has also revealed significant information. Paradoxically, neuroblastomas of the hyperdiploid variety are more likely to respond favorably to chemotherapy. Diploid or near-diploid tumors are associated with higher-stage disease (including unresectable tumors), poorer prognosis, a lower response to chemotherapy, and recurrence or progression.[30–33]

The most widely reported genetic marker for neuroblastoma has been amplification of the *MYCN* (or N-myc) proto-oncogene.[24,34] The association between *MYCN* amplification and high-grade,[35] advanced stage disease at presentation, rapid progression, and overall poor prognosis is well established. Recently, an etiologic relationship between *MYCN* and neuroblastoma has been demonstrated by two complementary studies. Chan and co-workers from the Hospital for Sick Children in Toronto reported that elevations in MYCN protein expression in neuroblastoma tissues is independently associated with poor prognosis in high-stage disease (III, IV, IVS) even in the absence of *MYCN* gene amplification.[36] Furthermore, MYCN protein levels were prognostic, independent of the most significant clinical variables of age or stage,[36] thus strongly supporting the concept that *MYCN* expression is directly involved in the cellular events of neuroblastoma progression. Conversely, in the subgroup of patients who did well with normal *MYCN* gene expression, MYCN protein levels were undetectable.[36] In a related animal study, the targeted overexpression of the *MYCN* gene in neuroectodermal cells led to the development of neuroblastoma in *MYCN* transgenic mice.[37] MYCN tumorigenesis is further augmented in the absence of the recognized tumor suppressor genes *NF1* or *RB1*.[37] This demonstrates that *MYCN*'s transforming effect can be influenced by other genes, which is consistent with the emerging concept of multistep processes in malignant transformation. MYCN gene amplification is present in approximately 40% of patients with advanced stage III or IV disease (compared with <10% in low-stage patients) and its absence augurs a slower disease progression in these patients.

A recent report by Wei et al[38] at the National Cancer Institute has proposed an artificial neural network to define 19 predictable genes which would substratify prognosis groupings beyond *MYCN* amplification. Also, Weber et al[39] has shown that coexpression of insulin receptor-related activity and insulin-like growth factor correlated with enhanced apoptosis and differentiation in neuroblastomas.

As mentioned above, deletions of chromosome 1 and gains in chromosome 17 have been shown to carry strong prognostic information in advanced neuroblastoma. A landmark report from a collaborative group in Europe has shown a very powerful association between gains in chromosome 17q and adverse neuroblastoma outcome. The study is important because of its large numbers, the availability of all clinical and genetic data variables for 85% of the patients in the cohort, and the close coordination between a team of basic and clinical researchers. In total, 313 children from six European centers were studied. Often, but not exclusively, the gain of 17q was linked to the loss of 1p. Most significantly, in univariate and multivariate analyses, 17q gain was independently predictive of poor outcome (30.6% 5-year survival with 17q gain vs 86% 5-year survival without

Table 77.3 Genetic neuroblastoma profiles

Feature	Type 1	Type 2	Type 3
MYCN amplification	None	None	Present
DNA ploidy	Hyperdiploid	Near-diploid	Near-tetraploid
LOH	Rare	25–50%	Present
Neurotropin gene expression	High	Low/absent (except TRK-B, high)	
Age	1 year	>1 year	
Stage	1, 2, 4S	3, 4	
3-year survival	95%	25–50%	<5%

LOH = loss of heterozygosity; TRK = tyrosine kinase receptor.
Adapted from Brodeur,[44] with permission.

17q gain).[40] Prognosis may be further predicted by more chromosome changes on 3p and 11q.[18]

A long-standing notion in tumorigenesis states that transformation (neoplasia) is the result of aberrant differentiation pathways leading away from the normal cell phenotype. As a result, neuroblastoma may represent an aberration of normal neuronal development. As such, several neuronal differentiation markers have been investigated in this disease, including chromogranin A, neuropeptide Y, and receptors for neurotropins such as nerve growth factor. Neuropeptide Y is detectable in abundance in the serum of neuroblastoma patients and may be useful in following tumor burden both before and after therapy.[41] In tumor tissue, it reaches its highest levels in poorly differentiated neuroblastoma, compared with ganglioneuroblastoma or ganglioneuroma.[41] Conversely, chomogranin A derivatives may become useful markers of more favorably differentiated tumors.[41]

Acting through various receptors, neurotropic factors are, by definition, involved in the differentiation of neural tissues. One family of neurotropin receptors, the tyrosine kinase receptors TRK-A, TRK-B, and TRK-C, is showing promise in understanding neuroblastoma biology. It appears that *TRK-A* gene expression is associated with favorable outcome, yielding its highest expression in more well-differentiated tumors.[42,43] Furthermore, TRK-A levels are inversely correlated with *MYCN* gene expression.[42] Expression of TRK-C and shortened forms of TRK-B also portend better outcome.[42] Together, these observations have also led to speculation that functioning, intact neurotropin/TRK receptor pathways in these tumors may be further linked to their propensity to mature (differentiate) into ganglioneuromas, or regress through a cell-death pathway (from a presumed eventual unavailability of factor for the receptor, or receptor malfunction). However, as our knowledge of the role of these pathways evolves, it is becoming clear that they carry potential as powerful markers of disease, or even as molecular therapeutic targets to manipulate neuroblastomas to assume differentiation or regression pathways.

Drawing on the foregoing discussion, neuroblastomas may be stratified into specific prognostic subgroups based on the genetic interplay represented by *MYCN* expression, LOH, DNA ploidy, and neurotropin receptor expression. Combined with age and stage, three genetic neuroblastoma profiles can be determined with differing survival rates (Table 77.3).

Diagnosis, staging, and treatment

The diagnosis of neuroblastoma is confirmed by histologic sampling of tumor tissue or bone marrow. Standard light and electron microscopic evaluation may be followed by immunohistochemical identification of tissue of neuronal origin. The vast majority of the tumors secrete catecholamines synthesized from the amino acid tyrosine in the sequence: dopa, dopamine [both excreted as homovanillic acid (HVA)], and finally norepinephrine. In contrast to pheochromocytomas, neuroblastomas lack the ability to convert norepinephrine to epinephrine. Norepinephrine and epinephrine are both excreted as VMA.

Imaging techniques

Traditionally, the presentation of an abdominal neuroblastoma has been either by the discovery of an abdominal mass on physical examination, or the result of investigations to explain symptoms related to either metastatic disease or the neurendocrine manifestations of the tumor. Abdominal ultrasonography will detect a great percentage of those tumors that occur in the abdominal cavity. Occasionally they are

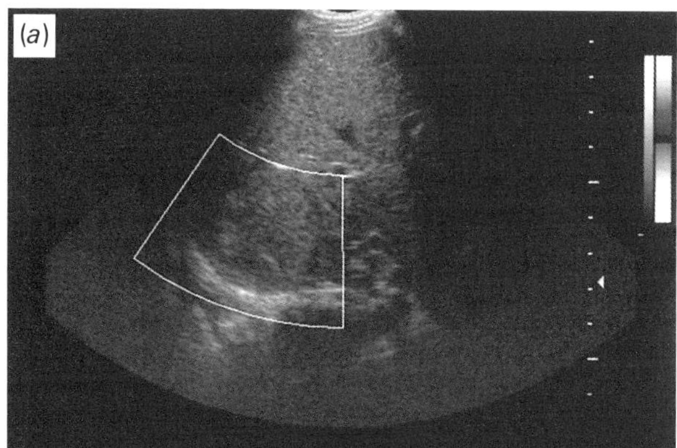

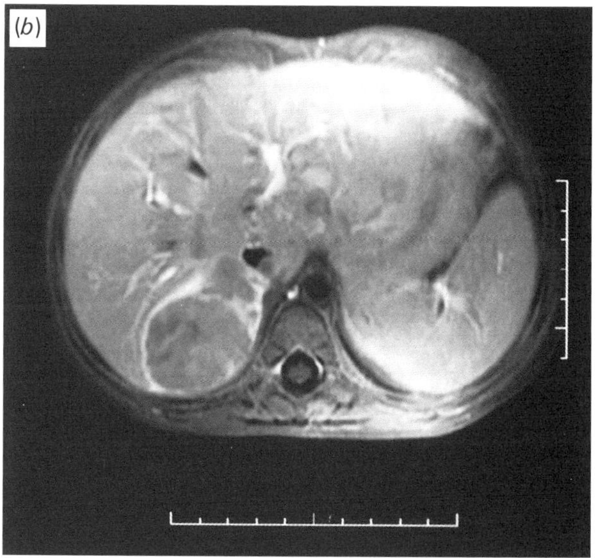

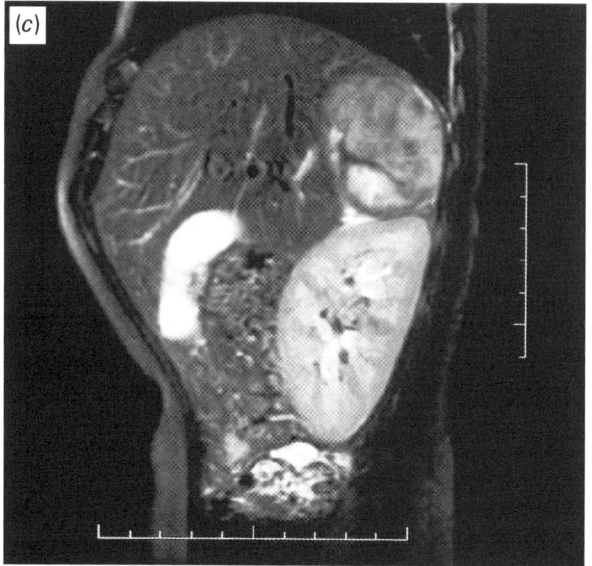

Figure 77.2 (*a*) Ultrasound image of a neuroblastoma discovered in a 1-year-old child as 'incidentaloma' in the course of investigating contralateral antenatally diagnosed hydronephrosis. A prior sonogram 6 months earlier with good views of the same area showed no evidence of mass lesion. (*b* and *c*) Transverse and sagittal magnetic resonance images of the same lesion, showing relationships in the retroperitoneum.

found as an incidental finding in the course of pursuing an otherwise unrelated symptom. With increased sonographic screening this has now become a more common cause for presentation of these tumors.[45] In the authors' recent experience at a large children's hospital there have been two instances in the past year when children who were being followed in the course of an investigation for antenatal hydronephrosis had neuroblastomas that became apparent and had not been present on prior examinations (Figure 77.2).

Diagnostic imaging techniques are evolving and improving with great rapidity, and there is no consensus as to which method is best. The choices include ultrasonography, computed tomography (CT), and magnetic resonance imaging (MRI). The availability and the non-invasive nature of ultrasonography endorse this technology as the choice for the initial screening test. The time required for both CT and MRI makes their selection for young children more critical. Either of these techniques may be used to delineate and define the extent of the disease. Availability may be the most critical determinant of which technique should be used (Figures 77.2 and 77.3).

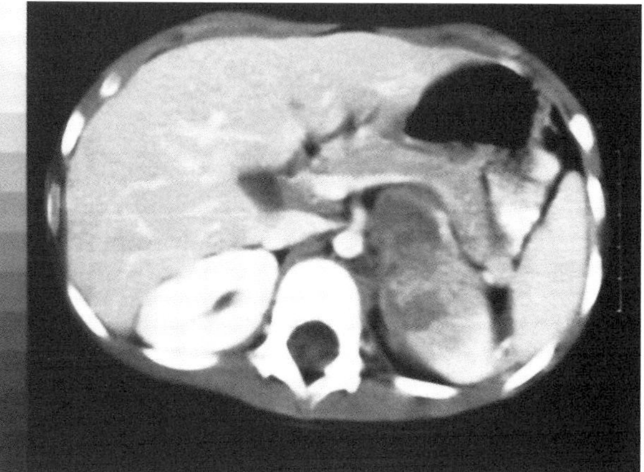

Figure 77.3 Transverse computed tomographic scan of retroperitoneal recurrence of a previously excised stage 3 neuroblastoma.

In seeking metastatic disease a chest radiograph is a useful initial step. Radioisotope bone scanning using

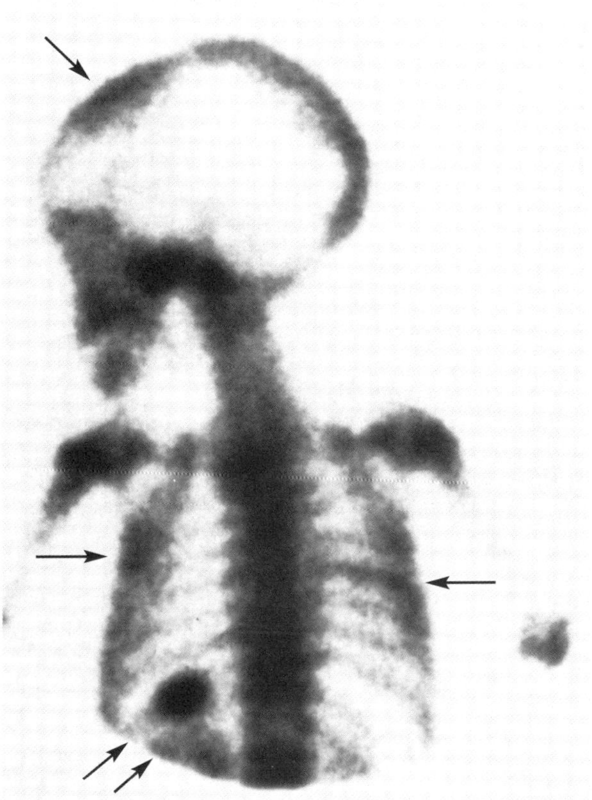

Figure 77.4 Posterior view of thorax and skull. Increased uptake is seen in skull, upper thoracic spine and left and right ribs (arrows) as a result of metastatic neuroblastoma. The decreased uptake at T12 is an unusual manifestation of metastatic tumor. The right suprarenal uptake of tracer is within the primary tumor (double arrow).

technetium 99m (^{99m}TC)-methylene diphosphonate is more accurate than a standard X-ray skeletal survey for the detection of bony metastases (Figure 77.4).

Prognostic markers

Both clinical and biochemical markers have evolved that are helpful in the management of neuroblastoma. The best recognized are the traditional clinical parameters of age at diagnosis and tumor stage. Patients diagnosed at 1 year of age appear to show consistently better survival outcomes than older children, even in the presence of advanced disease at presentation. Survival also stratifies dramatically with respect to disease stage, with 75–90% 5-year survival for stage 1, 2, and 4S patients, compared with 10–30% 2-year survival for stage 3–4 disease.

Various biochemical and cell-associated parameters have also been assessed for their prognostic ability in the management of neuroblastoma. Serum ferritin is elevated during periods of rapid tumor growth and/or large tumor burden. Whether this reflects a growth requirement for ferritin by the tumor or is a product of neuroblastoma cell metabolism is unknown. Ferritin levels appear to discriminate between stage 4 and stage 4S disease.[46] Lactate dehydrogenase (LDH) is elaborated non-specifically in several tumor types, including neuroblastoma, where it may reflect rapid tumor cell turnover and tumor burden.[47] Neuron-specific enolase is a cytoplasmic enzyme found in cells of neural origin.[48] Neuroblastoma prognosis appears worse if elevated levels are detected in serum, although this marker is not specific to neuroblastoma.[48] Serum and tissue ganglioside GD2 is a glycosphingolipid shed by neuroblastoma tumor cells. It may reflect tumor burden, and decreasing levels may be seen as a positive response to successful reduction of tumor load. The presence of GD2 on the cell surface has attracted interest in targeting this molecule using immunotherapy strategies.[49–51] Finally, matrix metalloproteinases (MMPs) are cellular enzymes required to break down the extracellular matrix and facilitate cell movement through the matrix during the metastatic process. Very recently, tumor cell expression of a membrane-associated MMP was found to correlate with advanced stage and poor outcome in neuroblastoma.[47]

Staging

A disease with such diverse manifestations as neuroblastoma in childhood needs a comprehensive staging system to allow precise diagnostic criteria and a method for categorizing and quantifying disease. Such a staging system then acts as a template upon which diagnostic criteria can be applied to various subgroups of disease, and permits definition of outcome measures that will allow collaboration between centers in implementing and assessing clinical trials. An international working group published the outcome of its deliberations in 1988.[52] The staging system recommended is known as the International Neuroblastoma Staging System (INSS) and the response criteria are referred to as the International Neuroblastoma Response Criteria (INRC). This staging system has now replaced previous systems by Evans, originally established by the Pediatric Oncology Group (POG). Table 77.4 outlines the three staging systems, thus facilitating some comparison of previously published data.

Treatment

Therapy of neuroblastoma requires close coordination of medical, surgical, and radiation oncologists

Table 77.4 Neuroblastoma staging systems

Evans and D'Angio	POG	INSS
Stage I Tumor confined to the organ or structure of origin	*Stage A* Complete gross resection of structure of origin/primary tumor, with or without microscopic residual. Intracavitary lymph nodes, not adhered to and removed with primary (nodes adhered to or with tumor resection may be positive for tumor without upstaging patient to stage C), histologically free of tumor. If primary in the abdomen or pelvis, liver histologically free of tumor	*Stage I* Localized tumor with complete gross excision without microscopic residual disease; representative ipsilateral lymph nodes negative for tumor microscopically (nodes attached to and removed with the primary tumor may be positive)
Stage II Tumor extending in continuity beyond the organ or structure of origin but not crossing the midline. Regional lymph nodes on the ipsilateral side may be involved	*Stage B* Grossly unresected primary tumor. Nodes and liver same as stage A	*Stage 2A* Localized tumor with incomplete gross excision; representative ipsilateral non-adherent lymph nodes negative for tumor microscopically
Stage III Tumor extending in continuity beyond the midline. Regional lymph nodes may be involved bilaterally	*Stage C* Complete or incomplete resection of primary. Intracavitary nodes not adhered to primary histologically positive for tumor. Liver as in stage A	*Stage 2B* Localized tumor with or without complete gross excision, with ipsilateral non-adherent lymph nodes positive for tumor. Enlarged contralateral lymph nodes must be negative microscopically.
Stage IV Remote disease involving the skeleton, bone marrow, soft tissue, distant lymph node groups, etc. (see stage IV–S)	*Stage D* Any dissemination of disease beyond intracavitary nodes (i.e. extracavitary nodes, liver, skin, bone marrow, bone)	*Stage 3* Unresectable unilateral tumor infiltrating across the midline, with or without regional lymph node involvement; or localized unilateral tumor with contralateral regional lymph node involvement; or midline tumor with bilateral extension by infiltration (unresectable) or by lymph node involvement
State IV–S Patients who would otherwise be stage I or II, but who have remote disease confined to liver, skin, or bone marrow (without radiographic evidence of bone metastases on complete skeletal survey)	*Stage DS* Infants <1 year of age with stage IV–S disease (see Evans and D'Angio)	*Stage 4* Any primary tumor with dissemination to distant lymph nodes, bone, bone marrow, liver, skin, and/or other organs (except as defined for stage 4S)
		Stage 4S Localized primary tumor as defined for stage 1, 2A, or 2B with dissemination limited to skin, liver, and/or bone marrow (limited to infants <1 year of age)

POG = Pediatric Oncology Group; INSS = International Neuroblastoma Staging System.
From Halperin et al.[53]

and clearly represents a prime example of multimodal cancer therapy. Surgical intervention plays a dual role. At the time of diagnosis, open or laparoscopic approaches may be necessary to obtain adequate and thorough samples for histologic and molecular diagnosis and marker analysis. Needle biopsy materials are most often inadequate for these purposes. For selected tumors, primary surgical excision may be possible, particularly for small, locally confined cases. In this regard, laparoscopic surgery may be considered and has been used successfully for small tumors identified by screening.[54] Laparoscopy is safe and feasible for adrenal tumors.[55] Given that infant screening detects tumors that are generally biologically favorable, laparoscopic surgery may be a safe modality on oncologic grounds. Open surgical dissection is also employed to both assess response to therapy and excise residual disease after initial courses of chemotherapy have been completed. Recent reports have suggested a higher incidence of nephrectomy in children with neuroblastoma who were treated with primary surgical intervention.[56]

Chemotherapy is a major component of the treatment of neuroblastoma. Both single-agent and synergistic multiagent drug regimens are used, combining cell-cycle-specific and cell-cycle-independent drugs to achieve the maximum ratio of therapeutic benefit to toxicity. Ionizing radiation has a role in neuroblastoma treatment as the tumor is radiosensitive. It is most useful in achieving local control on the one hand, and palliation of disease uncontrollable by other modalities on the other. As a primary modality, however, radiotherapy is limited by the extensive metastatic proclivity of many neuroblastomas. The agent metaiodobenzylguanidine (MIBG), used in the localization of neuroblastomas and pheochromocytomas, has been studied for its ability to bind to neuroblastoma tumors systemically and carry with it radioligands such as iodine-131 that are toxic to the tumor cells.[51,57,58] This approach has also been used as a surgical adjunct to guide tumor tissue resection using the gamma camera intraoperatively once the tumor is radiolabeled by preoperative injection of [I^{131}]MIBG.[59]

Given the aggressive nature of advanced and higher staged disease, efforts continue to attempt improved disease control in this subset of patients while refining therapy to limit toxicity in lower stage and more favorable disease.

Treatment strategy

The ability to stratify patients into distinctly risk-related groups, by application of the varied but highly accurate histologic and molecular diagnostic and staging methodologies, has permitted the much more judicious and specific use of the therapeutic regimens.

Stage 1 and 2 tumors (low risk) are treatable by primary surgical resection alone, with no need for initial chemotherapy or radiotherapy. A prognosis of up to 89% survival has been reported in this group of patients.[2,58,60] Kushner et al[61] have shown that excellent results (80 to survival) can be achieved even with reduction in the number of chemotherapy cycles from 7 to 5. In another report, the same authors[62] have shown that surgery alone is a potentially curable treatment for recurrent disease. Stage 4S tumors will undergo spontaneous remission and are thus considered low risk. However, if symptoms are present related to severe hepatic metastatic disease or respiratory compromise, patients may benefit from chemotherapy or radiation therapy in small doses.

Stage 3 tumors (intermediate risk) still have an excellent overall survival rate of up to 89%[60] but chemotherapy is advised following primary surgical excision. Second-look surgery may also be appropriate after chemotherapy. The goal of therapy in this group is to reserve more intense therapy for those children with biologically unfavorable tumors.

Patients with stage 4 disease (high risk) have derived minimal benefits from even the most intensive regimens. Multiagent chemotherapy remains the standard primary treatment strategy for these patients. Only a number of adolescents have developed stage 4 neuroblastomas and their prognosis remains poor.[63] There have been isolated applications of ablative chemotherapy and bone marrow transplantation and these intensive therapeutic approaches are currently being explored in multicenter trials. The overall prognosis in this group of children remains very low (15–35% survival).[64] An additional risk of bone marrow transplant is Epstein–Barr virus-related lymphoproliferative disease (EBV-LPD). Powell et al[65] from the Children's Hospital of Philadelphia outlined an incidence of 4% of neuroblastoma patients who received a bone marrow transplant and developed EBV-LPD. Treatment of the lymphoprofilerative disease was successful in four of the five patients.

Ganglioneuroma

A more histologically benign counterpart of neuroblastoma is the ganglioneuroma. Ganglioneuroblastoma is an intermediate malignant classification between ganglioneuroma and neuroblastoma, and for treatment purposes is regarded with neuroblastoma. Ganglioneuromas are most often seen in older children and present as abdominal masses. It is intriguing to hypothesize that late development of a more benign variant may represent a 'second hit', but these tumors do not exhibit an 'explosive' form of metastatic behavior.[66] Nonetheless, by virtue of their inexorable growth and distortion

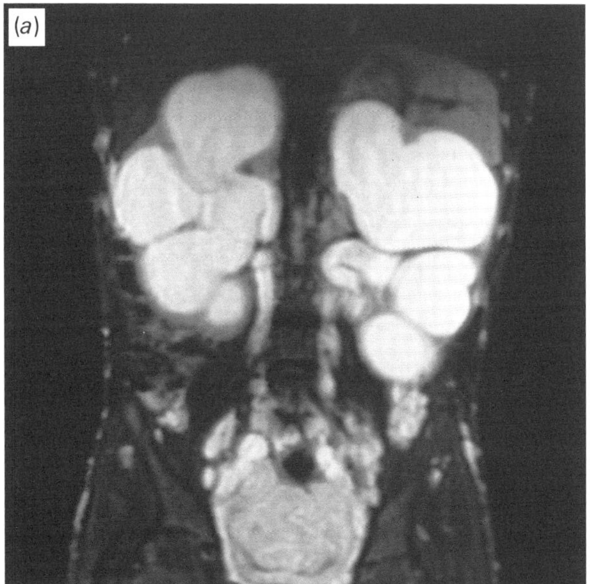

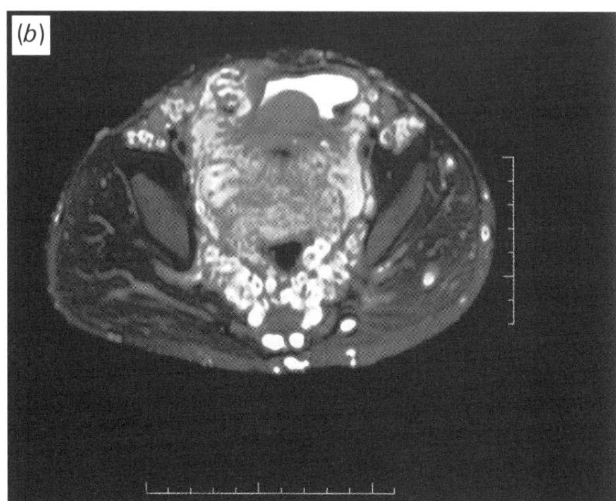

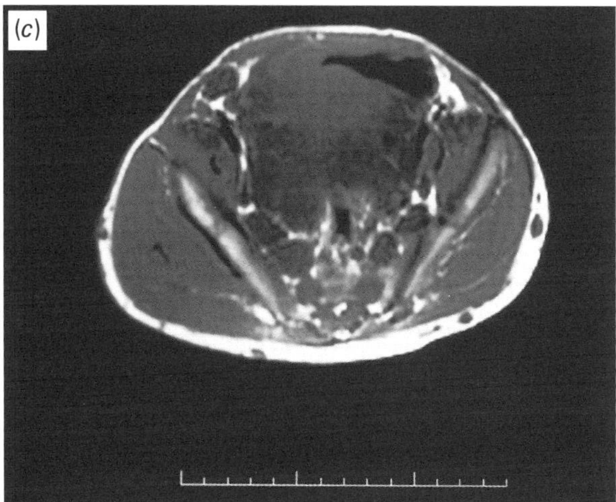

Figure 77.5 (*a*) Magnetic resonance scan of patient with a ganglioneuroma, showing obstruction of the ureters. (*b*) Primary neuronal masses displacing the bladder anteriorly and the rectum posteriorly. (*c*) T2-weighted image of the same pelvic area as in (*b*), showing the different appearance of neural tissues.

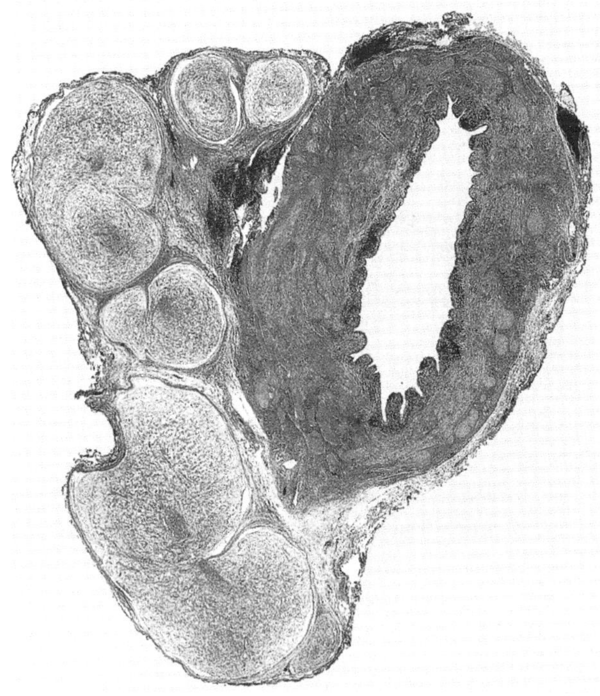

Figure 77.6 Pathologic section of area of excised ureter, with ureter encased in, but not invaded by tumor tissue.

of adjacent tissues they can have a very morbid clinical course. Such a case is illustrated in Figure 77.5, in which both gastrointestinal and genitourinary tissues are grossly displaced. The urologic system, in particular, may exhibit such profound destruction that urinary diversion may be deemed necessary. The figures illustrate the results of MRI, which can provide eloquent detail of the soft-tissue involvement by these tumors, while there is no evidence of direct histologic invasion of the compressed tissues (Figure 77.6).

The correlation of the MRI features with latent malignant potential in these tumors has been documented by Ichikawa et al.[67] They were able to show that punctate calcification on the CT scan and low or intermediate attenuation are common in ganglioneuromas. The MR images are mainly of low intensity on T1-weighted images (T_1WI) and of high intensity on T2-weighted images (T_2WI). Dynamic MR studies show a lack of early involvement but gradually increasing enhancement. The authors concluded that the absence of these features, judged 'typical' for ganglioneuroma, should suggest a potential for a more malignant course. The slow-growing nature of ganglioneuromas may also have a devastating effect on vascular and neurologic function by virtue of its compressive effects on adjacent structures. Figure 77.7 demonstrates extension along the sacral nerve prior to

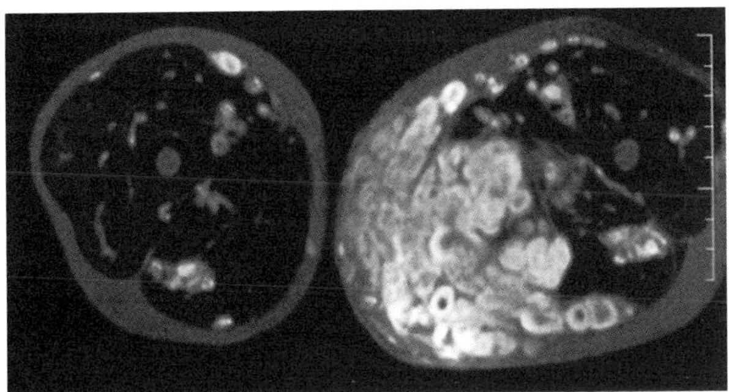

Figure 77.7 Extension of ganglioneuroma down the sheath of the sacral nerve.

the appearance of clinical degeneration. This and other cases have demonstrated the potential for clinical morbidity that may be associated with ganglioneuroma despite its non-metastatic nature. To prevent these localized effects, incomplete surgical resection may be justified in the absence of effective chemotherapy or radiotherapy.

Pheochromocytoma

Clinical features and presentation

Pediatric pheochromocytoma is an extremely uncommon primary tumor of the adrenal medulla, although it is the most common hyperfunctioning form of this tissue in children. Over a period of 5 years at the Hospital for Sick Children in Toronto, of 30 patients presenting with a primary adrenal tumor, only one, a 16-year-old girl, had a pheochromocytoma (pers comm). The tumors arise in the autonomic system, with 90% originating in the adrenal gland. Catecholamine production is the norm and is the basis for both the clinical manifestations and laboratory diagnosis. Pediatric pheochromocytomas can be seen in association with a variety of diseases including neurofibromatosis, von Hippel–Lindau disease, Sturge–Weber syndrome, and multiple endocrine neoplasias (MEN-2). Those associated with MEN-2 are more likely to occur later in life and are more likely to be bilateral. Almost 25% of patients with apparently sporadic pheochromocytoma may be carriers of the mutations, thus justifying an in-depth analysis.[68]

Imaging, biochemical features, and new prognostic markers

The diagnosis of pheochromocytoma in childhood is suggested by the rare coexistence of hypertension and abdominal mass detectable on sonographic evaluation. Non-palpable pheochromocytoma causing secondary hypertension in children is exceedingly rare. The diagnosis is confirmed by means of either serum or urine confirmation of hypersecretion of catecholamines.

As stated previously, the principal catecholamine that produces the classic characteristic symptoms of flushing, palpitations, hypertension (vasoconstriction), and anxiety in patients with pheochromocytoma is epinephrine. Epinephrine is a metabolite of its precursor, norepinephrine. The latter is a less potent mediator of the clinical constellation seen in pheochromocytoma. However, compared with neuroblastoma, both catecholamines are more commonly produced by pheochromocytomas. Pheochromocytomas, particularly those of adrenal origin, produce the enzyme PNMT, which catalyzes the conversion of norepinephrine to epinephrine. As such, the norepinephrine to epinephrine ratio has been used to distinguish pheochromocytomas of adrenal from those of extraadrenal origin. Weise et al[69] have recently endorsed the sensitivity of the ratio of free metanephrines, and this has been confirmed by others.[70]

With respect to diagnostic imaging, the initial methodology in suspected cases is ultrasonography (Figure 77.8). Thereafter, either CT or MRI can be employed to confirm the diagnosis of an adrenal or a

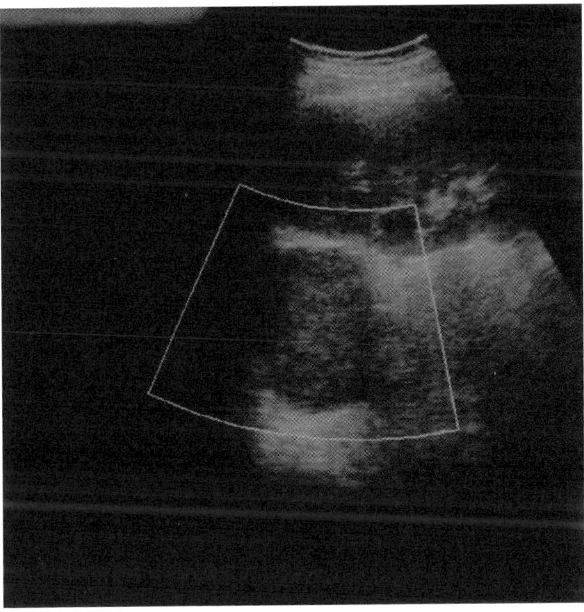

Figure 77.8 Ultrasound image of a left suprarenal tumor in a 16-year-old child presenting with hypertension.

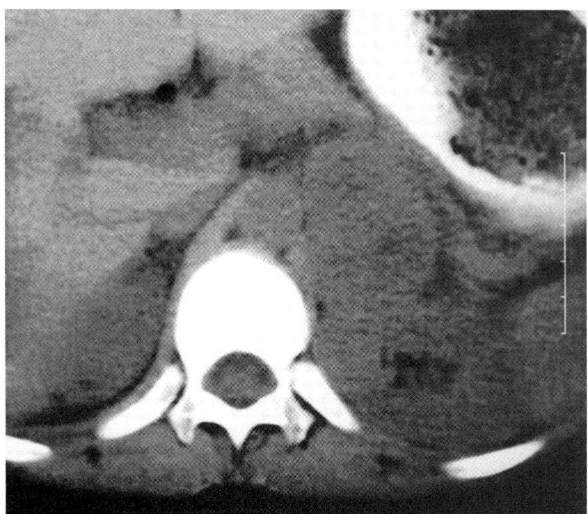

Figure 77.9 Computed tomographic image of left suprarenal pheochromocytoma, as seen in ultrasound in Figure 77.8.

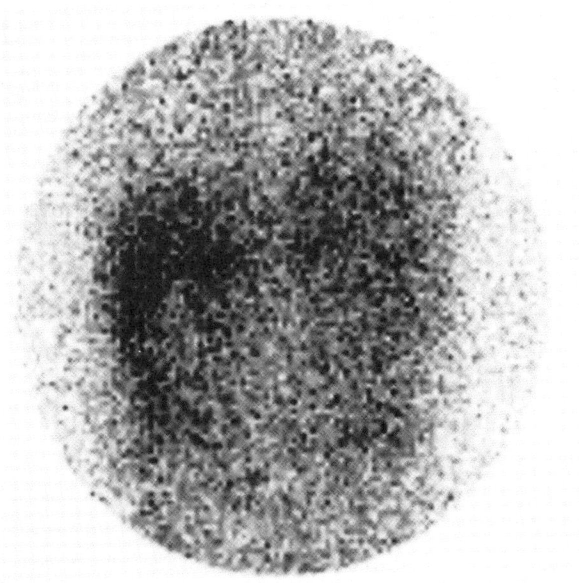

Figure 77.10 MIBG abdominal scan, with uptake of radionuclide in the left suprarenal area, in a 16-year-old patient with pheochromocytoma.

para-adrenal mass (Figure 77.9). Serologic or creatinine-specific measures of catecholamine excretion in the urine are then undertaken. The most specific diagnostic imaging methodology is radionuclide scanning using [I^{131}]MIBG scintigraphy (Figure 77.10). With this approach, the sensitivity is greater than 90%.[71] [I^{131}]MIBG scanning is particularly valuable in the localization of tumors that are outside the adrenal gland.[72,73]

One of the persisting challenges in pheochromocytoma management remains the inability to define precisely whether a given tumor is benign or malignant. The current gold standard criterion for malignancy remains the appearance of metastases. As a predictor of malignancy, this is analogous to predicting that automobile brakes are defective based on the occurrence of a collision. Clearly, more accurate markers for determining malignancy of pheochromocytoma are needed. Recent studies have identified biologic features of pheochromocytomas that may hold promise in determining the metastatic proclivity of the tumor. For example, telomeres comprise repeated nucleotide sequences on the ends of chromosomes. During normal cell aging, they progressively shorten with successive normal cell replications. In normal cells, this shortening is thought to be associated with waning activity of the enzyme that produces the telomeres. Recent retrospective molecular analysis of pheochromocytoma tumors known to be benign or malignant reveals that telomerase, the RNA polymerase enzyme responsible for the production of telomeres, shows increased activity exclusively in tumors known to be malignant.[74,75] Similarly, antibody-based approaches that detect proliferating cells are being used increasingly to describe the malignant phenotype in tumors. One such antibody, MIP-1, selectively recognizes cells engaged in the cell cycle (i.e. scheduled to undergo mitosis, but not necessarily in the process of mitosis). Its predictability was explored in a survey of pheochromocytomas in which malignancy was confirmed by the existence of metastases. A positive MIB-1 labeling index (defined as >3% of tumor cells staining positive for MIB-1 vs the total number of cells counted) showed a specificity of 100% (benign tumors stained negative) and sensitivity of 50% (half of the malignant tumors stained positive).[76] Although sensitivity was poor, the ability to define benign disease accurately in this manner would be clinically reassuring.

Therapy

The historic importance of pheochromocytomas with respect to surgery is not the technical nature of their excision but the associated anesthetic risks. These relate to the potential for drastic changes in the excretion of catecholamines upon manipulation and subsequent removal of the tumor. The challenges revolve around stabilization of blood pressure intraoperatively and the prevention of potential cardiovascular collapse at the time of tumor removal or ligation of the veins delivering catecholamines to the systemic circulation. In infants, particularly in the preoperative state, these risks are a great concern. In view of the high specificity and reduced invasiveness of modern serologic and radionuclide diagnostic methodologies, risk factors are reduced. Prevention of problems in the treatment of pheochromocytoma is considered one of the primary goals. As in adults, the mainstay of preoperative therapy includes blockade of α-adrenergic receptors (phenoxybenzamine) accompanied by adequate systemic volume repletion once the vasoconstrictive and volume-contracted state has been overcome. Cardiac β-blockade (propranolol) in every case to prevent reflex tachyarrhythmias remains controversial but should at least be considered in selected cases. Clearly, preoperative pharmacologic management of affected children should be undertaken in collaboration with the pediatric endocrinologist and anesthesiologist. If adequate blockade and volume replacement are achieved preoperatively, manipulation of the tumor is usually not accompanied by large variations in blood pressure and large additional volume requirements are usually not found necessary upon tumor removal.

Perianesthetic risks and outcomes of surgical resection have been recently outlined and still rely mainly on premedication and β-adrenergic blockade.[77] In this paper, the authors outline the methodologies of perioperative adrenal modulation, and confirm the absence of mortality, myocardial infarctions, or cerebrovascular events in a large series of patients (n = 41). They do confirm, however, a substantial morbidity, with 41 patients noting substantial intraoperative events, most commonly hypertension, or other intraoperative hemodynamic lability.

Open surgical excision by the flank or posterior lumbotomy approach has been the classic means of treatment. However, Rutherford et al[78] have published an excellent review of the laparoscopic experience of excision of these tumors. Laparoscopic removal is now the standard of care, although the limited operating space may be challenging in smaller children. Hwang et al[79] at the National Cancer Institute have confirmed the safety of this approach in children. They noted that patients treated laparoscopically have a significant reduction in recovery time as well as a low complication rate. It may well be that this will become the most widely accepted method of surgical excision.

Sacrococcygeal teratoma

Sacrococcygeal teratoma (SCT) is the most common neoplasm in the newborn, and one of the first tumors successfully excised surgically.[80] Virchow coined the term 'teratoma', referring to a coccygeal growth with diverse anatomic characteristics. The tumors originate from all three embryologic tissues: ectoderm, mesoderm, and endoderm. Although they have provoked great interest because of their occurrence early in life and their dramatic appearance at birth, they have achieved even more current interest because of the facility and frequency with which they can be diagnosed by antenatal ultrasonography.[81,82] Antenatal diagnosis is now the rule, with diagnosis, definition of intrauterine risk factors and, in some limited cases, intrauterine treatment being feasible.[83–85] The appearance and character of the tumors are highly variable since they may be internal or external. SCTs have no known etiology. They are usually benign, but may undergo malignant degeneration.

Pathology

A teratoma is a neoplasm composed of multiple tissues that are foreign to the area in which it arises. Teratomas are grouped into those benign lesions with mature tissue (70%), those having malignant anaplastic elements (20%), and a third, embryonic group (10%) that may contain histologically immature-appearing benign tissue that does not progress to mature organ formation.[86] This latter group carries a generally favorable prognosis following total excision. In the benign varieties, elements such as skin, teeth, central nervous system (CNS) tissue, cartilage, bone, and respiratory and alimentary mucosa may be seen.

Infants diagnosed with SCT at >1 year of age as well as older children are more likely to have malignant elements. To detect these elements, the pathologist must undertake an extensive search through all of the varied elements within the tumor. The term 'yolk sac' or endodermal sinus tumor is the name appropriately used for the malignant elements in such tumors. These tissues represent a separate element of the teratomatous cell line. Elevated serum levels of α-fetoprotein may be seen in these cases.

Clinical features and presentation

The traditional mode of presentation of these tumors has been discovery at birth. In most developed countries where antenatal sonography is now either mandatory or prevalent, they are discovered by antenatal sonography. A review[87] of antenatally diagnosed SCTs demonstrated a high incidence of in-utero mortality (19%) coupled with a perinatal mortality of 14%. The hydrops causing this in-utero mortality may now be predicted by ultrasound[85] and MRI.[83] They may also be treated.[84] The incidence of premature labor in this series was 50%. Thus, although the pathology of SCT is often benign, the overall outcome is associated with considerable morbidity and mortality. Those clinical features in the antenatal state that correlated with a poorer prognosis included polyhydramnios (an early sign of fetal distress and predictor of placental megaly-hydrops fetalis), tumor hypervascularity, or the presence of a solid tumor (a risk factor for both malignancy and vascular steal syndrome), large tumor size at delivery (>10 cm in its greatest dimension), and a fast rate of tumor growth relative to cranial growth.

A solid tumor is the most ominous predictor of poor outcome. A fetus with a solid tumor has a mortality rate of 66% compared with a mortality of 11% for cystic or mixed tumors. Thus, mothers carrying a fetal diagnosis of SCT at the time of clinical obstetric presentation are definitely at risk for prenatal and perinatal complications. The presence of polyhydramnios appears to be a relative predictor or warning sign of premature labor.

There is a 5–25% association with other congenital anomalies in infants with benign SCT. Seventy-five percent of the infants are female, harboring primarily benign tumors.[71] The sex distribution is more evenly distributed between males and females in those whose tumors develop malignant degeneration.

Classification

The classification of SCT was proposed in 1974 by Altman and comprises: type 1, totally external; type 2, primarily external with internal component; type 3, almost completely internal; and type 4, totally internal[81] (Figure 77.11).

Today, since most SCTs may well be diagnosed in the antenatal state following obstetric ultrasonography, an improved prognosis may be anticipated following delivery by cesarean section. The latter is advised as an initial attempt to decrease perinatal mortality and morbidity. The major early cause for morbidity relates to tumor rupture, for which cesarean section is the best prophylaxis. In Altman's classification, large tumors were defined as being >10 cm, and these appear to be associated with greater morbidity.

When not diagnosed prior to birth, external tumors are found at delivery. Internal tumors may present as an abdominal mass, with the diagnosis of SCT noted by neonatal ultrasonography. Prior to the widespread use of prenatal ultrasound, some authors[88] had proposed that all newborns should have a rectal examination to exclude internal SCT, but acknowledged that the rarity of the tumor would result in positive identification in only 1 out of 400 000 babies.

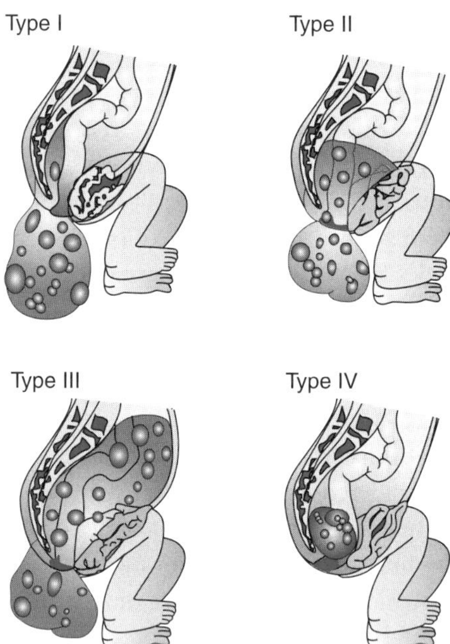

Figure 77.11 Classification of sacrococcygeal teratomas. Type 1: tumors are predominantly external (sacrococcygeal) with only a minimal presacral component. Type 2: tumors present externally but with a significant intrapelvic extension. Type 3: tumors are apparent externally but the predominant mass is pelvic and extends into the abdomen. Type 4: tumors are presacral with no external presentation. (Adapted from (Altman et al,[81] with permission.)

Laboratory

Tumors that undergo malignant degeneration may produce α-fetoprotein and/or β-human chorionic gonadotropin (β-hCG). These proteins are indicators of malignant degeneration in the dermal sinus or choriocarcinomatous components of the tumor.[80,89]

Imaging

Imaging studies for complete assessment include CT and MRI. Radiographic detection of calcification does not distinguish between benign and malignant tumors (Figures 77.12 and 77.13).

Treatment

With the increasing availability of antenatal diagnosis, the question of antenatal intervention has had a logical appeal. Other forms of intrauterine therapy, such

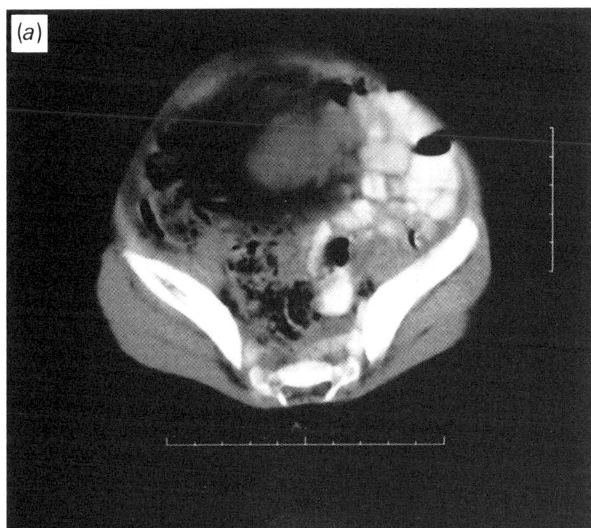

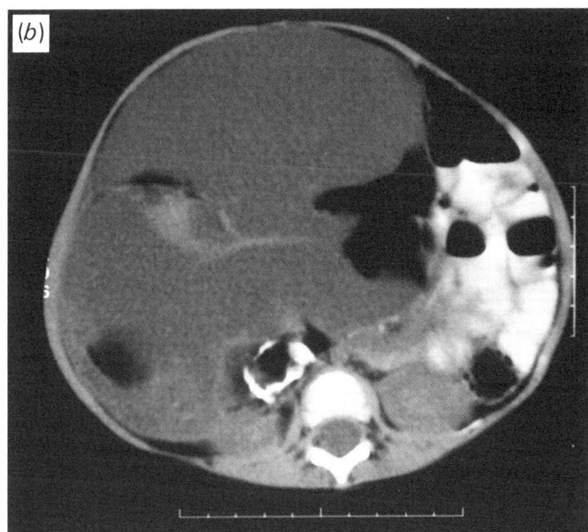

Figure 77.12 Computed tomographic images of cystic teratoma in a 6-month-old child, arising from the pelvis (*a*) and filling the abdomen (*b*).

as intrauterine transfusion and decompression of a dilated urinary tract, have been successful as early as 16 weeks' gestational age. It has been speculated that ligating the blood supply to the tumor prenatally may be effective in decreasing its size and/or controlling the hyperdynamic state in the perinatal period.[90,91] The Children's Hospital of Philadelphia has reported success in antenatal debulking in four fetuses out of 30 presenting in the period 1995–2003. Although one fetus died and the other three experienced significant morbidity, the authors consider the intervention potentially lifesaving in view of the higher mortality (16/30) of the overall group.[84]

Postnatal therapy of SCT is primarily surgical. Devascularization of the tumor may be of benefit; however, this is best applied as the first intraoperative component of surgical removal.[90,91] Complete surgical excision should be the rule, with en bloc removal of the involved portion of the coccyx. A laparoscopic approach may help with both control of the blood supply in infants or in dissection of the internal extensions of the tumor.[92] Burdis and coworkers at the Children's Hospital of Philadelphia have used cardiopulmonary bypass to facilitate removal of large tumors.[93]

The three clinical groups of presentations comprise:

- antenatal detection
- those that appear at birth or in the neonatal period with large, benign tumors
- those that appear later (>1 year of age), which are often smaller, fixed, and malignant.

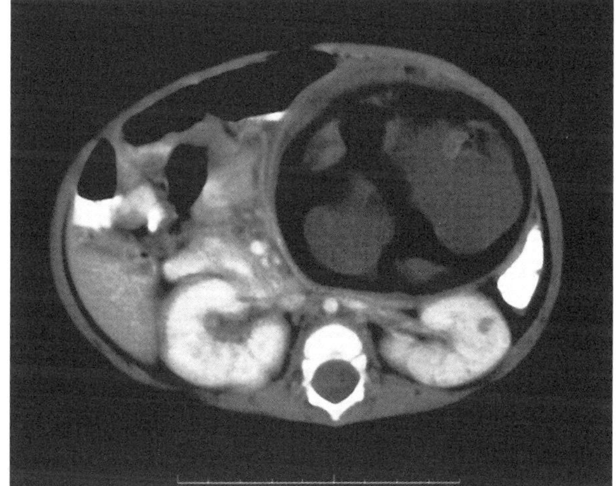

Figure 77.13 Computed tomographic image of a more solid teratoma filling the central abdomen in a 6-month-old child.

In the first two groups, total removal is the rule and is best achieved by a midline sacral or chevron incision. The coccyx should be removed in the process of excising the tumor. With the retroperitoneal extension of the teratoma, urinary, internal genital, and gastrointestinal organs may be displaced. They can usually be dissected free, with minimal injury to the viscera, and good access to the vascular supply of the tumor is usually afforded by this retroperitoneal approach. However, in more extensive cases, anterior abdominal exploration may be warranted. A generous surgical exposure to obtain control of the presacral vessels is recommended. Avulsion of the vessels is a hazard to be avoided. In these instances, laparoscopic approaches prelaparotomy may be of benefit. In some rare instances, SCT may involve the dura or extend to the spine. This potential extension can be defined by meticulous preoperative imaging.[94–96] An inadvertent entry into the dura may result in a cerebrospinal fluid leak, which is associated with a higher morbidity. Modern imaging techniques, particularly MRI, will allow a clearer definition of these potential extensions to the CNS.

The third group represents those children in whom tumors present at an age >1 year. These tumors are generally symptomatic, fixed, and firm. Diagnosis is established by ultrasound and/or physical examination and confirmed by CT or MRI. These tumors are often of a malignant variety and serum α-fetoprotein is a sensitive marker. The appropriate surgical approach is initially directed at biopsy, followed by either multiagent chemotherapy or radiotherapy, in an attempt to decrease the size of the tumor, followed by surgical removal.

Results of therapy

Antenatal therapy may be advisable in a limited number of select fetuses, especially those at risk from high-output heart failure.[83–85] In postnatal excisions, those undertaken in infancy for both external and internal SCT are remarkably successful in achieving complete removal of tumors with relatively little long-term morbidity.[97] Incontinence is rare.[71] However, in those cases where high sacrococcygeal extension is present necessitating transabdominopelvic excision, long-term fecal soiling and incontinence may be more prevalent. These sequelae may be related to more direct injury of skeletal muscular components or to some more occult neurogenic impairment of the viscera.[98] These sequelae may also be seen in the newborns after the excision of large, benign tumors.

Malignant SCT is rare in children under 6 months of age but, beyond that, the incidence rises sharply.[99] Malignant tumors may invade adjacent tissues or may recur in up to 40% of cases. Chemotherapeutic regimes, established in the 1990s, have added considerably to the improved outcomes.[100,101]

Long-term follow-up

An evaluation of long-term follow-up in children with SCT showed that mature teratomas may have a recurrence rate of up to 11%. Further treatment with surgical excision and combined chemotherapy resulted in an 85% cure rate.[102] On long-term follow-up, a 3% recurrence rate was noted for immature teratomas. They were detected by a rising α-fetoprotein level 6 months after the initial procedure. These responded well to local excision. Endodermal sinus tumors detected and treated initially with surgical excisions represented only 9% of the tumors presenting at birth, whereas they represented 27% of the patients presenting at an older age. With long-term follow-up, 89% are still alive in spite of the higher recurrence rate.

Adrenal carcinoma

Adrenal carcinoma represents fewer than 0.0001% of neoplastic tumors in children. The most common presentation is abnormal virilization, occurring in two-thirds.[103] Symptoms consistent with Cushing's syndrome account for most of the remainder. Individual case reports have reported occasional aldosterone-secreting tumors. Given the widespread availability of ultrasound imaging technology, the most common presentation currently is that of an incidental finding on an abdominal ultrasound.

Adrenocortical tumors may also be a component of more global genetic malformations. These include children with congenital adrenal hyperplasia, multiple endocrine syndromes (MEN 1), and Beckwith–Wiedemann syndrome.

Clinical presentation

Virilizing adrenal tumors

Of the functioning adrenal cortical tumors, virilizing forms account for two-thirds, usually occurring in children >2 years. The tumors produce dehydroepiandrosterone (DHEA), a weak androgen but one that is converted to Δ^4-androstenedione and testosterone, which are more potent virilizing hormones. Boys with such tumors present with signs of precocious puberty. Girls respond with an increase in clitoral size, similar to that seen with congenital adrenal hyperplasia (Figure 77.14). Pubic and axillary hair may be seen in children of either gender.

Other causes of premature virilization in boys include interstitial cell tumors of the testis or as a delayed manifestation of congenital adrenal hyperplasia. Clinical evaluation may give some clues towards distinguishing the underlying etiology. Unilateral or asymmetric testicular enlargement suggests a Leydig cell tumor. In patients with centrally stimulated precocious puberty, testicular enlargement is bilateral.

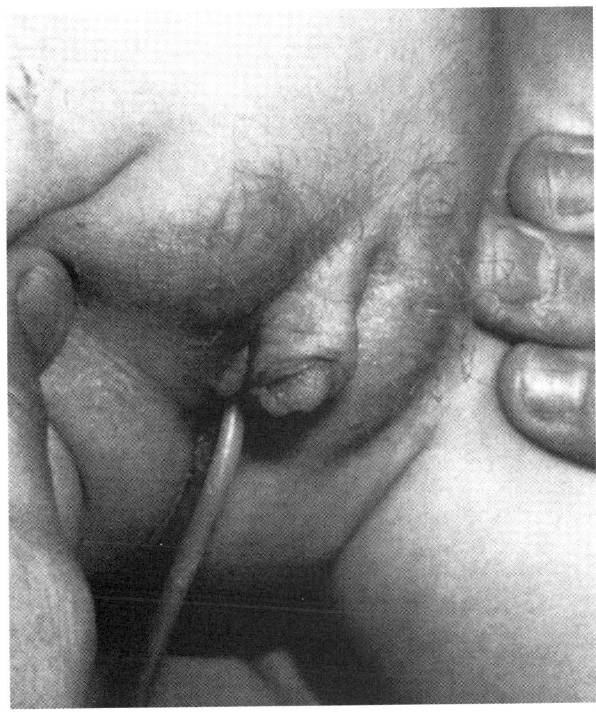

Figure 77.14 Virilizing adrenal carcinoma in a 5-year-old girl. Note clitoral hypertrophy and pubic hair. There is no posterior labial fusion, as would be seen in congenital adrenal hyperplasia.

With virilizing adrenal tumors, the testes are usually small.

The differential diagnosis in female children includes ovarian arrhenoblastoma and other rare tumors of the adrenal cortex.

Cushing's syndrome

Approximately one-third of children with adrenocortical tumors have the stigmata of Cushing's syndrome. Carcinoma may be responsible in up to one-half, with the others having bilateral adrenal hyperplasia. A benign adenoma may rarely be seen. The clinical appearance is in response to the excessive production of cortisol. This leads to protein catabolism, increased gluconeogenesis, and the typical obesity associated with cortisol excess. The moon facies and truncal obesity (Figure 77.15) of Cushing's disease are generally obvious when they are present in infants.

The differential diagnosis in patients exhibiting excess adrenocortical activity includes adrenal adenomas and iatrogenic administration of steroids. This latter iatrogenic excess is commonly seen in children receiving transplanted organs.

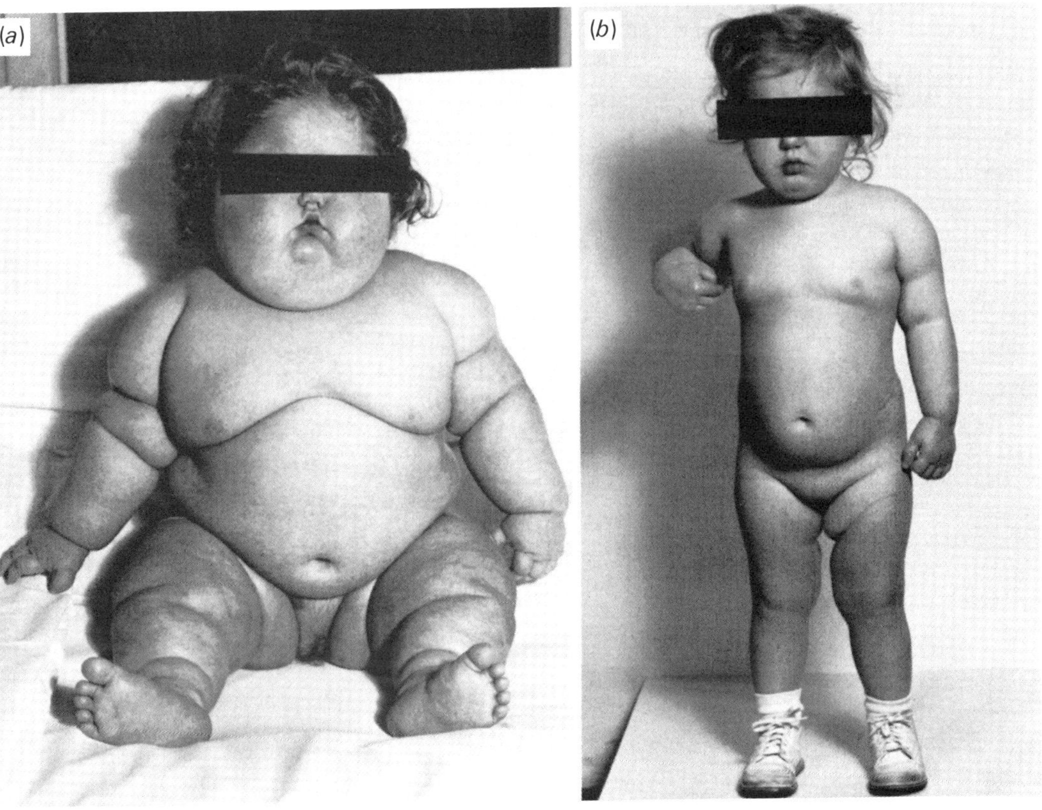

Figure 77.15 (*a*) Striking features of cortisol excess in a 17-month-old girl with adrenocortical carcinoma. In addition, pubic hair and mild enlargement of the clitoris were present. (*b*) At 10 months after removal of the adrenocortical carcinoma, there was complete regression of the signs of Cushing's syndrome.

Feminizing adrenal tumors

Feminizing adrenal tumors are rare. They occur more frequently in males, and in these cases the more commonly seen primary gynecomastia must be excluded.

Diagnostic evaluation

The critical diagnostic feature is the biochemical demonstration of adrenal hyperfunction. Urinary steroids typically show a markedly elevated 17-ketosteroid level. The free cortisol, DHA, and 17-hydroxysteroid levels may also be elevated.[104] Radioimmune assays of serum hormonal levels usually show elevation of DHEA, Δ^4-androstenedione, testosterone, and cortisol.[105] Serum estrogen levels are elevated in the rare feminizing cases.[106] Occasionally, an elevated serum aldosterone level can be demonstrated in cases of adrenocortical carcinoma.[107]

In Cushing's syndrome caused by adrenocortical carcinoma, the plasma cortisol level and urinary corticosteroids are markedly elevated above the levels typically seen with adrenal hyperplasia or an adrenal adenoma. A significant elevation in 17-ketosteroids, pregnanetriol, and estrogens may suggest carcinoma. The adrenocorticotropic hormone (ACTH) stimulation test produces no change in adrenocortical carcinomas, whereas those patients with adrenal hyperplasia show an exaggerated normal response. In exogenous obesity, which occasionally may enter the differential diagnosis, the ACTH test result is normal. When benign adenomas are present, the ACTH test exhibits a subnormal response. Metyrapone blocks 17β-hydroxylation in the adrenal cortex and leads to a fall in cortisol level with an increase in endogenous ACTH. Thus, a test with metyrapone produces results similar to those produced by the ACTH test. The diurnal variation usually seen in normal cortisol levels is absent with both tumors and adrenal hyperplasia. Dexamethasone blocks ACTH release in normal patients. The dexamethasone suppression test is useful to separate adrenal hyperplasia from tumors in that a large dose (8 mg) typically suppresses hyperplasia but not a tumor[108] (Table 77.5).

Modern diagnostic imaging has led to the greatest advances over the past decade (see section on imaging techniques under Neuroblastoma.) In addition to the ultrasound findings, MRI scanning has led to tremendous advances in the ability to distinguish adrenal carcinoma from benign adenomas.[109,110]

Treatment

Treatment of adrenal cortical carcinoma is surgical. In children, open surgical removal may be accomplished by large, transverse abdominal incisions or, in some instances, by extended flank incisions. Laparoscopic removal is now widely used in adults and is improving in children.[79] The advances in imaging allow more limited surgical approaches than may have been previously encountered. Tumor diameter of >5 cm is a reasonable predictor of malignancy, whereas small adenomas may be approached in a more limited manner. Preoperative care must recognize the need for corticosteroid replacement in cases where corticoid excess is anticipated.

The prognosis for adrenal carcinoma is poor. Surgery is the primary mode of therapy and chemotherapy has not been effective in controlling widespread disease.

Table 77.5 Test results with various adrenocortical lesions

Condition	Plasma cortisols		Dexamethasone test[a]		Metyrapone test response	Plasma ACTH
	Concentration	Diurnal rhythm	Low-dose suppression	High-dose suppression		
Normal	Normal	Yes	Yes	Yes	Yes	Normal
Cushing's disease	High	No	No	Yes	Yes	Increases
Tumor	High	No	No	No	No	Decrease
Non-ACTH-dependent hyperplasia	High	No	No	No	No	Decrease
Ectopic ACTH syndrome	High	No	No	No	No	Increase

[a]Low dose = 0.22 mg/10 kg for 2 days; high dose = 0.84 mg/10 kg for 3 days.
ACTH = adrenocorticotropic hormone.

Lymphangiomas

Lymphangiomas are benign tumors comprising a mass of anastomosing lymphatic channels. These are rare and most commonly affect the extremities. Most are congenital and may not become evident until a few years of age. When in the retroperitoneum, they are found by the evaluation of abdominal pain, which may be caused by the onset of spontaneous hemorrhage into the mass. However, they may extend through the inguinal canal and present with the misdiagnosis of hernia. Diagnosis is made on CT, at which time the low-density characteristic of lymphatic tissue is noted.

Surgical excision of the majority of the wall of the tumor is ideal, but may not be technically possible without causing significant damage to adjacent organs. Large cysts may be drained into the peritoneal cavity.

Neurofibroma

Patients with neurofibromatosis (von Recklinghausen's disease) may present with abdominal neurofibromas similar to but as a more benign variant of ganglioneuromas. As outlined in the previous section on benign ganglioneuromas, partial excision may be an appropriate surgical treatment.

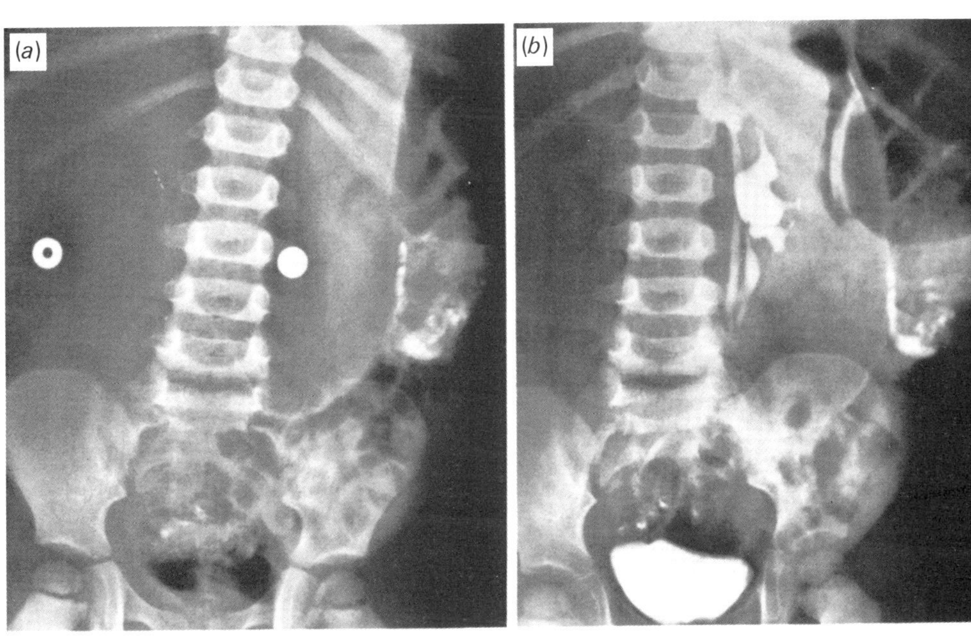

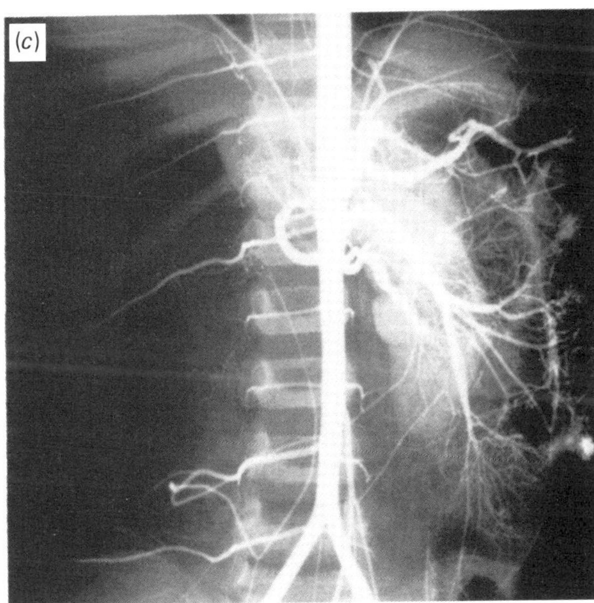

Figure 77.16 Retroperitoneal lipoma. (*a*) Abdominal film (KUB) demonstrating a retroperitoneal mass obliterating the right psoas shadow and displacing the bowel to the left. (*b*) Excretory urogram showing the right kidney and ureter displaced across the midline to the left. Note the absence of hydronephrosis. (*c*) Aortogram shows displacement of the right renal artery. The right kidney is now superior to the left kidney. The absence of neovascularity suggests the benign nature of the tumor.

Lipoma

Retroperitoneal lipomas are usually benign, presenting as an abdominal mass in infants and young children (Figure 77.16). CT defines the characteristically low-density lesions. These are generally benign and well encapsulated. Local excision is the treatment of choice.

Other malignant retroperitoneal tumors

Hodgkin's and non-Hodgkin's lymphomas may involve intra-abdominal viscera including the urinary and gastrointestinal tracts. Lateral deviation of the ureters is the most common genitourinary feature; however, ureteral obstruction may be the primary presenting symptom. Ureteral catheterization may become necessary in advance of chemotherapy.

Liposarcoma

Liposarcoma is rare in children, being seen more often in the teenage years leading into young adulthood. If it is identified early, surgical excision may result in complete cure.

Fibrosarcoma

Fibrosarcoma may be difficult to distinguish from neurofibroma. These lesions also occur primarily in the extremities, although retroperitoneal sites may be seen.

References

1. Beckwith JB, Perrin EV. In situ neuroblastoma: a contribution to the natural history of neural crest tumors. Am J Pathol 1963; 43:1089–94.
2. Castleberry RP. Neuroblastoma. Eur J Cancer 1997; 33:1430–7, discussion 1437–8.
3. Woods WG, Tuchman M, Robison LL et al. A population-based study of the usefulness of screening for neuroblastoma. Lancet 1996; 348:1682–7.
4. Woods WG, Tuchman M, Robison LL et al. Screening for neuroblastoma is ineffective in reducing the incidence of unfavourable advanced stage disease in older children. Eur J Cancer 1997; 33:2106–12.
5. Gurney JG, Ross JA, Wall DA et al. Infant cancer in the U.S.: histology-specific incidence and trends, 1973 to 1992. J Pediatr Hematol Oncol 1997; 19:428–32.
6. Kenney LB, Miller BA, Ries LA et al. Increased incidence of cancer in infants in the U.S.: 1980–1990. Cancer 1998; 82:1396–400.
7. Bonovarus A, Kirks DR, Grossman H. Imaging of neuroblastoma: an overview. Pediatr Radiol 1986; 16: 89–106.
8. Michalek AM, Buck GM, Nasca PC et al. Gravid health status, medication use, and risk of neuroblastoma. Am J Epidemiol 1996; 143:996–1001.
9. Zahm SH, Ward MH. Pesticides and childhood cancer. Environ Health Perspect 1998; 106(Suppl 3):893–908.
10. Saito T, Tsunematsu, Y, Saeki M. Trends of survival in neuroblastoma and independent risk factors for survival at a single institution. Med Pediatr Oncol 1997; 29:197–205.
11. Knudson AG Jr, Strong LC. Neuroblastoma and pheochromocytoma. Am J Hum Genet 1972; 24:512–32.
12. Ichimiya S, Nimura Y, Kageyama H et al. p73 at chromosome 1p36.3 is lost in advanced stage neuroblastoma but its mutation is infrequent. Oncogene 1999; 18:1061–6.
13. Caron H. Allelic loss of chromosome 1 and additional chromosome 17 material are both unfavourable prognostic markers in neuroblastoma. Med Pediatr Oncol 1995; 24:215–21.
14. Caton H, van Sluis P, de Kraker J. Allelic loss of chromosome 1p as a predictor of unfavourable outcome in patients with neuroblastoma. N Engl J Med 1996; 334:225–30.
15. Lastowski M, Cotterill S, Pearson AD. Gain of chromosome arm 17q predicts unfavourable outcome in neuroblastoma patients. U.K. Children's Cancer Study and the U.K. Cancer Cytogenetics Group. Eur J Cancer 1997; 33:1627–33.
16. Lastowski M, Roberts P, Pearson AD. Promiscuous translocations of chromosome arm 17q in human neuroblastomas. Genes Chromosomes Cancer 1997; 19:143–9.
17. Plantaz D, Mohapatra G, Matthay KK et al. Gain of chromosome 17 is the most frequent abnormality detected in neuroblastoma by comparative genomic hybridization. Am J Pathol 1997; 150:81–9.
18. Spitz P, Hero B, Ernestus K, Berthold F. FISH analyses for alterations in chromosomes 1, 2, 3, and 11 define high-risk groups in neuroblastoma. Med Pediatr Oncol 2003; 41:30–5.
19. Takita J, Hayashi Y, Yokata J. Loss of heterozygosity in neuroblastomas – an overview. Eur J Cancer 1997; 33:1971–3.
20. Luis AL, Martinez L, Hernandez F et al. [Congenital neuroblastomas]. Cir Pediatr 2004; 17:89–92. [Spanish]
21. Snyder HM, D'Angio GJ, Evans AE et al. Pediatric oncology. In: Walsh PC, Girres RF, Permutter AD, Raney RB, eds. Campbell's Urology, 5th edn. Philadelphia: WB Saunders, 1986: 2269.
22. Peled N, Baby NP, deNanosssy Q. The computed tomographic appearance of subcutaneous nodules occurring in metastatic neuroblastoma. Can Assoc Radiol J 1992; 43:441–2.
23. Evans AE, Albo V, D'Angio GJ et al. Factors influencing

survival of children with non-metastatic neuroblastoma. Cancer 1976; 38:661–2.

24. Brodeur GM, Seeger RC, Schwab M et al. Amplification of n-myc in untreated human neuroblastomas correlates with advanced stage of disease. Science 1984; 224:1121–4.
25. Levitt GA, Platt KA, De Byrne R, Sebire N, Owens CM. 4s neuroblastoma: the long-term outcome. Pediatr Blood Cancer 2004; 43:120–5.
26. Mendelsohn G, Eggleston JC, Olson JL. Vasoactive intestinal peptide and its relationship to ganglion cell differentiation in neuroblastic tumors. Lab Invest 1979; 41:144–9.
27. Black CT, Atkinson JB. Neuroblastoma. Semin Pediatr Surg 1997; 6:2–10
28. Brodeur GM, Castleberry RP. Neuroblastoma. In: Pizzo PA, Poplack DG, eds. Principles and Practice of Pediatric Oncology. Philadelphia: JB Lippincott, 1997: 7712.
29. Shimada H, Chatten J, Newton WA. Jr. Histopathologic prognostic factors in neuroblastic tumors: definition of subtypes of ganglioneuroblastoma and an age-linked classification of neuroblastomas. J Natl Cancer Inst 1984; 73: 405–16.
30. Morris JA, Schochat SJ, Smith EI et al. Biological variables in thoracic neuroblastoma: a Pediatric Oncology Group study. J Pediatr Surg 1995; 30:296–302; discussion 302–3.
31. Bowman LC, Castleberry RP, Cantor A et al. Genetic staging of unresectable or metastatic neuroblastoma in infants: a Pediatric Oncology Group study. J Natl Cancer Inst 1997; 89:373–80.
32. Cheung NK, Kushner BH, LaQuaglia MP et al. Survival from non-stage 4 neuroblastoma without cytotoxic therapy: an analysis of clinical and biological markers. Eur J Cancer 1997; 33:2117–20.
33. Katzenstein HM, Bowman LC, Vrondeur GM et al. Prognostic significance of age, MYCN oncogene amplification, tumor cell ploidy, and histology in 110 infants with stage D(S) neuroblastoma: the pediatric oncology group experience – a pediatric oncology group study. J Clin Oncol 1998; 16:2007–17.
34. Seeger RC, Brodeur GM, Sather H et al. Association of multiple copies of the N-myc oncogene with rapid progression of neuroblastomas. N Engl J Med 1985; 313:1111–16.
35. Shimada H, Stram DO, Chatten J. Identification of subsets of neuroblastomas by combined histopathologic and N-myc analysis. J Natl Cancer Inst 1995; 87:1470–6.
36. Chan HS, Gallie BL, DeBoer G et al. MYCN protein expression as a predictor of neuroblastoma prognosis. Clin Cancer Res 1997; 3:1699–706.
37. Weiss WA, Aldape K, Mohapatra G et al. Targeted expression of MYCN causes neuroblastoma in transgenic mice. EMBO J 1997; 16:2985–95.
38. Wei JS, Greer BT, Westermann F et al. Prediction of clinical outcome using gene expression profiling and artificial neural networks for patients with neuroblastoma. Cancer Res 2004; 64:6883–91.
39. Weber A, Huesken C, Bergmann E et al. Coexpression of insulin receptor-related receptor and insulin-like growth factor 1 receptor correlates with enhanced apoptosis and dedifferentiation in human neuroblastomas. Clin Cancer Res 2003; 9:5683–92.
40. Bown N, Cotterill BA, Lastowska M et al. Gain of chromosome arm 17q and adverse outcome in patients with neuroblastoma. N Engl J Med 1999; 340:1954–61.
41. Kogner P, Björk O, Theodorsson E. Neuropeptide Y in neuroblastoma: increased concentration in metastasis, release during surgery, and characterization of plasma and tumor extracts. Med Pediatr Oncol 1993; 21(5):317–22.
42. Brodeur GM, Nakagawara A, Yamashiro DJ et al. Expression of TrkA, TrkB and TrkC in human neuroblastomas. J Neurooncol 1997; 31:49–55.
43. Combaret V, Gross N, Lasset C et al. Clinical relevance of TRKA expression on neuroblastoma: comparison with N-MYC amplification and CD44 expression. Br J Cancer 1997; 75:1151–5.
44. Broeder GM. Clinical and biological aspects of neuroblastoma. In: Vogelstein B, Kinzler KW, eds. The Genetic Basis of Human Cancer. New York: McGraw-Hill, 1998.
45. Graham DJ, McHenry CR. The adrenal incidentaloma: guidelines for evaluation and recommendations for management. Surg Oncol Clin North Am 1998; 7:749–64.
46. Hann HW, Evans AE, Cohen IJ, Leitmeyer JE. Biologic differences between neuroblastoma stages IV-S and IV. Measurement of serum ferritin and E-rosette inhibition in 30 children. N Engl J Med 1981; 305:425–9.
47. Sakakibara M, Koizumi S, Saikawa Y et al. Membrane-type matrix metalloproteinase-1 expression and activation of gelatinase A as prognostic markers in advanced pediatric neuroblastoma. Cancer 1999; 85:231–9.
48. Massaron S, Seregni E, Luksch R et al. Neuron-specific enolase evaluation in patients with neuroblastoma. Tumour Biol 1998; 19:261–8.
49. Cheung IY, Barber D, Cheung NK. Detection of microscopic neuroblastoma in marrow by histology, immunocytology, and reverse transcription-PCR of multiple molecular markers. Clin Cancer Res 1998; 4:2801–5.
50. Cheung NK, Kushner BH, Cheung IY. Anti-G(D2) antibody treatment of minimal residual stage 4 neuroblastoma diagnosed at more than 1 year of age. J Clin Oncol 1998; 16:3053–60.
51. Klingebiel T, Bader P, Bares R et al. Treatment of neuroblastoma stage 4 with 131I-meta-iodo-benzylguanidine, high-dose chemotherapy and immunotherapy. A pilot study. Eur J Cancer 1998; 34:1398–402.
52. Brodeur GM, Seeger RC, Barrett A et al. International criteria for diagnosis, staging, and response to treatment in patients with neuroblastoma. J Clin Oncol 1988; 6:1874–81.
53. Halperin EC, Constine LC, Tarbell NJ et al. Neuroblastoma. In: Halperin EC, ed. Pediatric Radiation Oncology, 2nd edn. New York: Raven Press, 1994: 182–3.
54. Nakajima K, Fuzukawa M, Fukui Y et al. Laparoscopic resection of mass-screened adrenal neuroblastoma in an 8-month-old infant. Surg Laparosc Endosc 1997; 7:498–500.
55. De Lagausie P, Berrebi D, Michon J et al. Laparoscopic adrenal surgery for neuroblastomas in children. J Urol 2003; 170:932–5.
56. Cañete A, Jovani C, Lopez A et al. Surgical treatment for neuroblastoma: complications during 15 years' experience. J Pediatr Surg 1998; 33:1526–30.

57. Mastrangelo R, Tornesello A, Mastrangelo S. Role of 131I-metaiodobenzylguanidine in the treatment of neuroblastoma. Med Pediatr Oncol 1998; 31:22–6.
58. Matthay KK, DeSantes K, Hasegawa B et al. Phase I dose escalation of 131I-metaiodobenzylguanidine with autologous bone marrow support in refractory neuroblastoma. J Clin Oncol 1998; 16:229–36.
59. Heij HA, Rutgers EJ, de Kraker J, Vos A. Intraoperative search for neuroblastoma by MIBG and radioguided surgery with the gamma detector. Med Pediatr Oncol 1997; 28:171–4.
60. Nitschke R, Smith EI, Altshuler G et al. Postoperative treatment of nonmetastatic visible residual neuroblastoma: a Pediatric Oncology Group study. J Clin Oncol. 1991; 9:1181–8.
61. Kushner BH, LaQuaglia MP, Kramer K, Cheung NK. Radically different treatment recommendations for newly diagnosed neuroblastoma: pitfalls in assessment of risk. J Pediatr Hematol Oncol 2004; 26(l):35–9.
62. Kushner BH, Kramer K, LaQuaglia MP, Cheung NK. Curability of recurrent disseminated disease after surgery alone for local-regional neuroblastoma using intensive chemotherapy and anti-G(D2) immunotherapy. J Pediatr Hematol Oncol 2003; 25:515–19.
63. Gaspar N, Hartmann O, Munzer C. Neuroblastoma in adolescents. Cancer 2003; 98:349–55.
64. Stram DO, Matthay KK, O'Leary M. Consolidation chemoradiotherapy and autologous bone marrow transplantation versus continued chemotherapy for metastatic neuroblastoma: a report of two concurrent Children's Cancer Group studies. J Clin Oncol 1996; 14:2417–26.
65. Powell JL, Bunin NJ, Callahan C. An unexpectedly high incidence of Epstein-Barr virus lymphoproliferative disease after CD34+ selected autologous peripheral blood stem cell transplant in neuroblastoma. Bone Marrow Transplant 2004; 33:651–7.
66. Moschovi M, Arvanitis D, Hadjigeorgi C et al. Late malignant transformation of dormant ganglioneuroma? Med Pediatr Oncol 1997; 28:377–81.
67. Ichikawa T, Ohtomo K, Araki T et al. Ganglioneuroma: computed tomography and magnetic resonance features. Br J Radiol 1996; 69(818):114–21.
68. Neumann HP, Bausch B, McWhinney SR et al; Freiburg-Warsaw-Colombus Pheochromocytoma Study Group. Germ-line mutations in nonsyndromic pheochromocytoma. N Engl J Med 2002; 346:1459–66.
69. Weise M, Merke DP, Pacak K, Walther MM, Eisenhofer G. Utility of plasma free metanephrines for detecting childhood pheochromocytoma. J Clin Endocrinol Metab 2002; 87:1955–60.
70. Lenders JW, Pacak K, Walther MM et al. Biochemical diagnosis of pheochromocytoma: which test is best? JAMA 2002; 287:1427–34.
71. Ein LH, Adeyemi SD, Mancer K. Benign sacrococcygeal teratomas in infants and children: a 25 year review. Ann Surg 1980; 191:382–4.
72. Francis IR, Korobkin M. Pheochromocytoma. Radiol Clin North Am 1996; 34:1101–12.
73. Nielsen JT, Nielsen BV, Rehling M. Location of adrenal medullary pheochromocytoma by I-123 metaiodobenzylguanidine SPECT. Clin Nucl Med 1996; 21:695–9.
74. Kinoshita H, Ogawa O, Mishina M et al. Telomerase activity in adrenal cortical tumors and pheochromocytomas with reference to clinicopathologic features. Urol Res 1998; 26:29–32.
75. Kubota Y, Nakada T, Sasagawa I, Yanai H, Itoh K. Elevated levels of telomerase activity in malignant pheochromocytoma. Cancer 1998; 82:176–9.
76. Clarke MR, Weyant RJ, Watson CG, Carty SE. Prognostic markers in pheochromocytoma. Hum Pathol 1998; 29:522–6.
77. Kinney MA, Warner ME, van Heerden JA et al. Perianesthetic risks and outcomes of pheochromocytoma and paraganglioma resection. Anesth Analg 2000; 91:1118–23.
78. Rutherford JC, Gordon RD, Stowasser M, Tunny TJ, Klemm SA. Laparoscopic adrenalectomy for adrenal tumours causing hypertension and for 'incidentalomas' of the adrenal on computerized tomography scanning. Clin Exp Pharmacol Physiol 1995; 22:490–2.
79. Hwang J, Shoaf G, Uchio EM et al. Laparoscopic management of extra-adrenal pheochromocytoma. J Urol 2004; 171:72–6.
80. Wolley MM. Teratoma. In: Welch KJ, Bandolph JG, Revich MM et al, eds. Pediatric Surgery, 14th edn. Chicago: Year Book, 1986: 265–76.
81. Altman RP, Randolph JG, Lilly JR. Sacrococcygeal teratoma: American Academy of Pediatrics Surgical Section Survey – 1973. J Pediatr Surg 1974; 9(3):389–98.
82. Ein SH, Mancer K, Adeyemi SD. Malignant sacrococcygeal teratoma – endodermal sinus, yolk sac tumor – in infants and children: a 32-year review. J Pediatr Surg 1985; 20:473–7.
83. Avni FE, Guiband L, Robert Y. MR imaging of fetal sacrococcygeal teratoma: diagnosis and assessment. AJR Am J Roentgenol 2002; 178:179–83.
84. Hedrick HL, Flake AW, Crombleholme TM et al. Sacrococcygeal teratoma: prenatal assessment, fetal intervention, and outcome. J Pediatr Surg 2004; 39:430–8, discussion 430–8.
85. Neubert S, Trautmann K, Tanner B et al. Sonographic prognostic factors in prenatal diagnosis of SCT. Fetal Diagn Ther 2004; 19:319–26.
86. Mahour HG, Wooley MM, Trivedi SN, Landing BH. Sacrococcygeal teratoma. J Pediatr Surg 1975; 10:183–8.
87. Holterman AX, Filiatrault D, Lallier M, Youssef S. The natural history of sacrococcygeal teratomas diagnosed through routine obstetric sonogram: a single institution experience. J Pediatr Surg 1998; 33:899–903.
88. Rauch F, Schonau E, Woitge H, Remer T, Seibal M. Urinary excretion of hydroxy-pyridinium cross-links of collagen reflects skeletal growth velocity in normal children. Exp Clin Endocrinol 1994; 102:94–7.
89. Tsuchida K, Kaneko M, Fukui M, Sakaguchi H, Ishiguro T. Three different types of alpha-fetoprotein in the diagnosis of malignant solid tumors: use of a sensitive lectin-affinity immunoelectrophoresis. J Pediatr Surg 1989; 24:350–5.
90. Robertson FM, Crombleholme TM, Frantz ID 3rd et al. Devascularization and staged resection of giant sacrococcygeal teratoma in the premature infant. J Pediatr Surg 1995; 30:309–11.

91. Angel CA, Murillo C, Mayhew J. Experience with vascular control before excision of giant, highly vascular sacrococcygeal teratomas in neonates. J Pediatr Surg 1998; 33:1840–2.
92. Bax NM, van der Zee DC. The laparoscopic approach to sacrococcygeal teratomas. Surg Endosc 2004; 18:128–30.
93. Burdis L, Koch DD. The use of cardiopulmonary bypass and extracorporeal membrane oxygenation for support during removal of two teratomas and hydrops fetalis. J Extra Corpor Technol 2004; 36:182–4.
94. Gross RE, Clatworthy HW, Mecker IA. Sacrococcygeal teratomas in infants and children: a report of 40 cases. Surg Gynecol Obstet 1951; 92:341–54.
95. Donnellan WA, Swenson O. Benign and malignant sacrococcygeal teratomas. Surgery 1968; 64:834–46.
96. Ashcraft KW, Holder TN. Hereditary presacral teratoma. J Pediatr Surg 1974; 9:691–7.
97. Shanbhogue LK, Bianchi A, Doig CM, Gough DC. Management of benign sacrococcygeal teratoma: reducing mortality and morbidity. Pediatr Surg 1990; 5:41–4.
98. Bass J, Luks F, Yazbeck S. Long-term follow-up of sacrococcygeal teratomas with emphasis on anorectal function. Pediatr Surg Int 1991; 6:119–21.
99. Hickey RC, Layton JM. Sacrococcygeal teratoma: emphasis on the biological history and early therapy. Cancer 1954; 7:1031–43.
100. Shanbhogue LK, Gough DC, Jones PM. Malignant sacrococcygeal teratoma: improved survival with chemotherapy. J Pediatr Surg 1989; 4:202–4.
101. Bilik R, Shandling B, Pope M et al. Malignant benign neonatal sacrococcygeal teratoma. J Pediatr Surg 1993; 28:1158–60.
102. Göbel U, Calaminus G, Engert J et al. Teratomas in infancy and childhood. Med Pediatr Oncol 1998; 31:8–15.
103. Hayles AB, Hahn HB, Sprague RG et al. Hormone-secreting tumors of the adrenal cortex in children. Am J Med 1996; 41:581.
104. Lipsett MB, Wilson H. Adrenocortical cancer: steroid biosynthesis and metabolism evaluated by urinary metabolites. J Clin Endocrinol Med 1962; 22:906–15.
105. Saez J, Lorans B, Morera AM, Bertrand J. Studies of androgens and their precursors in adrenocortical virilizing carcinoma. J Clin Endocrinol Metab 1971; 32:462–9.
106. Axelrod J, Black IB. The clinician and the biologic clock. N Eng J Med 1968; 279:216–17.
107. Jackson WP, Zilberg B, Lewis B, McKenzie D. Cushing's syndrome in childhood; report of case of adrenocortical carcinoma with excessive aldosterone production. Br Med J 1958; 34:130–3.
108. Liddle GW, Tests of pituitary-adrenal suppressibility in the diagnosis of Cushing's syndrome. J Clin Endocrinol Metab 1960; 20:1539–60.
109. Schwartz LH, Panicek DM, Doyle MV et al. Comparison of two algorithms and their associated charges when evaluating adrenal masses in patients with malignancies. AJR Am J Roentgenol 1997; 168:1575–8.
110. McGrath PC, Sloan DA, Schwartz RW, Kenady DE. Advances in the diagnosis and therapy of adrenal tumors. Curr Opin Oncol 1998; 10:52–7.